PEDIATRIC NEPHROLOGY

SECOND EDITION

MALCOLM A. HOLLIDAY, M.D.

Professor of Pediatrics
Children's Renal Center
University of California, San Francisco
San Francisco, California

T. MARTIN BARRATT, M.B., F.R.C.P.

Professor of Paediatric Nephrology
Department of Nephrology
Institute of Child Health
London, England

ROBERT L. VERNIER, M.D.

Professor of Pediatrics
Department of Pediatrics
University of Minnesota
Minneapolis, Minnesota

WILLIAMS & WILKINS
Baltimore • Hong Kong • London • Sydney

Editor: Nancy Collins
Associate Editor: Vicki Vaughn
Copy Editor: CRACOM Corporation
Design: Joanne Janowiak
Illustration Planning: Reginald Stanley
Production: Anne G Seitz

Accurate indications, adverse reactions, and dosage schedules for drugs are provided in this book, but it is possible that they may change. The reader is urged to review the package information data of the manufacturers of the medications mentioned.

Printed in the United States of America

Library of Congress Cataloging-in-Publication Data

Main entry under title:

Pediatric nephrology.

Edition of 1975: Editor, Mitchell I. Rubin and associate editor, T. Martin Barratt.
Includes bibliographies and index.
1. Pediatric nephrology. I. Maldolm A. (Malcolm Alexander), 1924–II. Vernier, Robert L., 1924– III. Barratt, T. Martin. IV. Rubin, Mitchell I. [DNLM: 1. Kidney Diseases—in infancy & childhood. 2. Urinary Tract Infections—in infancy & childhood. WS 320 P371] RJ466.P366 1986 618.92'61 85-16933
ISBN 0-683-04101-0

88 89 90 91 10 9 8 7 6 5 4 3 2

PEDIATRIC NEPHROLOGY

SECOND EDITION

Preface

In the foreword to the first edition of *Pediatric Nephrology*, Mitchell Rubin, senior editor, stated the case for specialized care by pediatricians for children. While that viewpoint is now widely accepted, other specialists often provide care to children with kidney disease so that a modern text must address a broad audience of physicians.

The first goal of the editors is to produce a book that is both text and reference for pediatric nephrologists, pediatricians, and general nephrologists while providing useful information to urologists, neonatologists, and family physicians.

The editors of this edition have a 12 year gap to close since the first edition appeared. There is much new information to present and new perspectives to review. This has required extensive reorganization of the text.

A feature of the book is the integration of body composition, metabolism, and renal and electrolyte physiology with nutrition and fluid therapy in patients from 700 gm to 70 kg. How to measure and evaluate growth and change in function with growth is given detailed treatment.

The section on basic mechanism gives the reader a comprehensive review of processes that have important bearing on kidney disease. The use of new imaging procedures and interpretation of clinical and laboratory data precede the sections on clinical topics. An essay on "Medicine in an Unjust World" is followed by a brief look at nephrology from various parts of the world. These remind us that problems and diseases in other societies differ from those in the Western World.

Specific glomerular diseases occurring alone or with systemic disease are covered individually and followed by a chapter on therapy. The section on metabolic and tubular disorders describes inherited and acquired disorders in which functional disturbances predominate. The chapter on syndromes that was so well received in the first edition is updated as is the chapter on cystic diseases.

The section on genitourinary disorders is introduced with a detailed review of the natural course and treatment of urinary tract infection; differences between children and adults are described. The remainder of the section describes the major genitourinary diseases in children and common problems such as eneuresis and circumcision. Hypertension—how it arises, how it is defined, diagnosed, and treated should be helpful to many physicians.

A large section describes the problem of children with reduced renal function and the consequences of different degrees of loss of function at different ages. Principles and clinical management of the metabolic abnormalities of renal failure are discussed along with newer methods for measuring renal injury and arresting its progression. The various forms of dialysis and hemofiltration are reviewed; transplantation immunology and results of renal transplantation in children are given detailed treatment as are common complications of renal failure.

A final section addresses topics in perinatal nephrology: the development of renal function in utero, and the adaptive capacities of the low birth weight and term infant to electrolyte and nutrition disorders. Nephrological and urological conditions in the newborn are described.

The editors' other goals are to produce a text that keeps a balance between mechanisms and clinical practice, and a perspective between how the kidney is affected by disease and how the body responds to disease of the kidney.

We sought a compromise between the encyclopedic bibliography and one that listed only "key" references. Where the material is new or controversial, primary sources were cited; where the material is well established, comprehensive review articles were cited to lead to primary sources for those needing them. We set out to accomplish these goals with a one volume text.

We owe a large debt to the contributors, most of whom are active in pediatric nephrology. Many of these people suffered through revisions in order to meet the goals we set. We also express gratitude to managing editor Anne Schmid, those who indexed, the staff of Willliams & Wilkins, Kathleen Gallagher, and all the others who redrafted manuscripts, met deadlines, and contributed to the final product.

Contributors

Raymond D. Adelman, M.D.
Associate Professor of Pediatrics
Director of Pediatric Nephrology
University of California School of Medicine, Davis
Sacramento, CA

George A. O. Alleyne, M.D.
Director, Area Health Programs Development
Pan American Health Organization
Washington, DC

Anita Aperia, M.D.
Professor of Pediatrics and Developmental Physiology
Department of Developmental Physiology
Huddinge University Hospital & St. Gorans
Children's Hospital
Stockholm, Sweden

J. Williamson Balfe, M.D.
Associate Professor of Pediatrics
University of Toronto
Division of Nephrology
Department of Pediatrics
The Hospital for Sick Children
Toronto, Ontario, Canada

T. Martin Barratt, M.B., F.R.C.P.
Professor of Paediatric Nephrology
Department of Nephrology
Institute of Child Health
Consultant Pediatric Nephrologist Hospital for Sick Children
London, England

Michel Bergeron, M.D.
Professor of Physiology
Départment de Physiologie
Université de Montréal
Montréal, Québec, Canada H3C 3T8

A. Caroline Berry, M.B., Ph.D.
Paediatric Research Unit
Guy's Hospital
London, England

Norma N. Bibiloni, M.D.
Department of Nephrology
Hospital de Ninos de la Plata
La Plata, Argentina

Glen H. Bock, M.D.
Attending Pediatric Nephrologist
Children's Hospital National Medical Center
Assistant Professor
Department of Child Health and Development
George Washington University School of Medicine
Washington, DC

Beverley E. Booth, M.D.
CMC and Brown Memorial Hospital
Ludhiana 141008
Punjab, India

David M. Brown, M.D.
Dean
Professor, Laboratory Medicine and Pathology and Pediatrics
University of Minnesota Medical School
Mayo Memorial Building
Minneapolis, MN

Barbara A. Burke, M.D.
Professor, Department of Laboratory Medicine and Pathology
University of Minnesota
Minneapolis, MN

J. Stewart Cameron, M.D., F.R.C.P.
Professor of Renal Medicine
Guy's Hospital and Medical School London, England.
London, England

Alfonso Campos, M.D.
Assistant Professor
Department of Pediatrics
University of South Florida
Tampa, FL

Cyril Chantler, M.D., F.R.C.P.
Professor of Paediatrics
Guy's Hospital and Medical School
London, England

Russell W. Chesney, M.D.
Professor and Vice Chairman
Department of Pediatrics
University of California, Davis
Sacramento, CA

H. M. Coovadia M.Sc., M.D.
Associate Professor
Department of Pediatrics and Child Health
University of Natal
Faculty of Medicine
Congella, Durban, Republic of South Africa

Shermine Dabbagh, M.D.
Children's Hospital of Pittsburgh
Pittsburgh, PA

Ralph B. Dell, M.D.
Professor of Pediatrics
Director, Division of Nutrition and Metabolism
Department of Pediatrics
The College of Physicians & Surgeons of Columbia University
New York, NY

Michael J. Dillon, M.B., F.R.C.P., D.C.H.
Consultant Physician and Pediatric Nephrologist
The Hospital for Sick Children
Great Ormond Street
London, England

Raymond Donckerwolcke, M.D.
Pediatric Nephrologist
University of Utrecht
Director, Dialysis and Transplant Program, Children's Hospital
Utrecht, The Netherlands

Demetrius Ellis, M.D.
Associate Professor of Pediatrics and Nephrology
Director of Pediatric Nephrology
Children's Hospital of Pittsburgh
University of Pittsburgh School of Medicine
Pittsburgh, PA

Robert B. Ettenger, M.D.
Associate Professor of Pediatrics
UCLA School of Medicine
Director, Renal Transplant Program
Division of Pediatric Nephrology
UCLA Center for the Health Sciences
Los Angeles, CA

Leonard G. Feld, M.D., Ph.D.
Assistant Professor of Pediatrics
State University of New York at Buffalo
School of Medicine
Chief of Nephrology
Children's Hospital of Buffalo
Buffalo, NY

Richard N. Fine, M.D.
Professor of Pediatrics
UCLA School of Medicine
Head, Division of Pediatric Nephrology
UCLA Center for the Health Sciences
Los Angeles, CA

Alfred J. Fish, M.D.
Professor, Department of Pediatrics
University of Minnesota
Minneapolis, MN

John W. Foreman, M.D.
Associate Professor of Pediatrics
Medical College of Virginia
Virginia Commonwealth University
Richmond, VA

Aaron L. Friedman, M.D.
Associate Professor
Department of Pediatrics
University of Wisconsin Center for Health Sciences
Madison, WI

Prasit Futrakul, M.D.
Pediatric Nephrology Division
Chulalongjorn Medical School Hospital
Bangkok, Thailand

Rafael Garcia, M.D.
Associate Professor of Medicine
Renal Services and Laboratory
Hospital Universitario and Universidad del Zulia
Maracaibo, Zulia Venezuela

Dennis F. Geary, M.B., M.R.C.P.
Department of Nephrology
The Hospital for Sick Children
Toronto, Canada

Frederick G. Germuth, M.D.
Director of Experimental Immunopathology
St. Johns Mercy Medical Center
St. Louis, MO

Enid F. Gilbert, M.D.
Department of Pathology
University of Wisconsin
Center for Health Sciences
Madison, WI

Giulio Gilli, M.D.
Kinderklinik "Florence Nightingale" Hospital
Krenzbergstrasse 79
Federal Republic of Germany

Noemia Perli Goldraich, M.D., M.Sc., Ph.D.
Professor of Pediatric Nephrology
Associate Professor, Department of Internal Medicine
Universidade Federal do Rio Grande do Sul
Porto Alegre, RS, Brazil

Isky Gordon, M.B., F.R.C.R.
Honorary Senior Lecturer
Department of Radiology
Hospital for Sick Children
London, England

Gustavo Gordillo-Paniagua, M.D.
Chief of the Department of Nephrology
Hospital Infantil de Mexico
Calle ds Marquez Mexico

Marie-Claire Gubler, M.D.
Hôpital des Enfants-Malades
Paris, Cedex, France

Jean-Pierre Guignard, M.D.
Associate Professor of Pediatrics
Department of Pediatrics
Centre Hospitalier Universitaire Vaudois
Lausanne, Switzerland

Arthur C. Guyton, M.D.
Professor and Chairman, School of Medicine
Department of Physiology and Biophysics
University of Mississippi Medical Center
Jackson, MS

Renee Habib, M.D.
Directeur de Recherches á l'INSERM
I.N.S.E.R.M.U. 192
Hôpital des Enfants-Malades
Paris, Cedex, France

George Haycock, M.B., F.R.C.P.
Consultant Paediatric Nephrologist
Department of Pediatrics
Guy's Hospital
London, England

William C. Heird, M.D.
Associate Professor of Pediatrics
Department of Pediatrics
The Columbia University College of Physicians & Surgeons
New York, NY

Ronald J. Hogg, M.D.
Chief, Division of Pediatric Nephrology
Associate Professor of Pediatrics
Department of Pediatrics
University of Texas
Dallas, TX

P. C. Holland, M.B., M.R.C.P.
Research Fellow
Department of Immunology
Institute of Child Health
London, England

Malcolm A. Holliday, M.D.
Professor of Pediatrics
Children's Renal Center University of California, San Francisco
San Francisco, CA

Iekuni Ichikawa, M.D.
Professor of Pediatrics
Division of Nephrology
Vanderbilt Medical School
Nashville, TN

Gunilla Kallenius, M.D.
Department of Pediatrics
Karolinska Hospital
Karolinska Institute and National Bacteriological Laboratory
Stockholm, Sweden

Solomon A. Kaplan, M.D.
Professor of Pediatrics
Chief, Division of Endocrinology
Department of Pediatrics
UCLA Center for Health Sciences
Los Angeles, CA

R. H. Kauffmann, M.D.
Department of Nephrology
University Hospital
The Netherlands

Youngki Kim, M.D.
Associate Professor
Department of Pediatrics and Laboratory Medicine
University of Minnesota Medical School
Minneapolis, MN

Claire Kleinknecht, M.D.
Maitre de Recherches Institut National de la Sante et de la Recherche Medicale
Hôpital des Enfants-Malades
Paris, Cedex, France

Barry A. Kogan, M.D.
Chief of Pediatric Urology
Assistant Professor of Urology
Department of Urology and Pediatrics
University of California, San Francisco
San Francisco, CA

Benjamin H. Landing, M.D.
Anatomic Pathology Division
Children's Hospital of Los Angeles
Los Angeles, CA

Eunice J. Larson, M.D.
Department of Pathology
Miller Children's Hospital
Longbeach, CA

M. Levin, M.B., M.R.C.P.
Lecturer, Department of Nephrology
Institute of Child Health
London, England

Robert L. Lynch, Ph.D., M.D.
Associate Professor of Pediatrics and Internal Medicine
Director, Division of Pediatric Nephrology
St. Louis University School of Medicine
St. Louis, MO

John D. Mahan, Jr., M.D.
University of Minnesota Medical School
Mayo Memorial Building
Minneapolis, MN

G. A. Manzoni, M.D.
Research Fellow Department of Urology
Hospital for Sick Children
London, England

S. Michael Mauer, M.D.
Professor of Pediatrics
University of Minnesota Medical School
Mayo Memorial Building
Minneapolis, MN

A. James McAdams, M.D.
Professor of Pediatrics and Pathology
University of Cincinnati College of Medicine
Children's Hospital Medical Center
Cincinnati, OH

Wallace W. McCrory, M.D.
Professor of Pediatrics
Division of Pediatric Nephrology
New York Hospital-Cornell Medical Center
New York, NY

S. R. Meadow, M.B., F.R.C.P.
Professor of Pediatrics
Department of Pediatrics and Child Health
St. James University Hospital
Leeds, England

Otto Mehls, M.D.
Professor of Pediatrics
Klinikum der Universitat Heidelberg
Kinderklinik
Federal Republic of Germany

Tyrone Melvin, M.D.
Medical Fellow
University of Minnesota
Mayo Memorial Building
Minneapolis, MN

Laurie C. Miller, M.D.
Postdoctoral Research Fellow
Department of Pediatrics
University of Minnesota
Minneapolis, MN

Kenneth Miller, M.D.
Assistant Professor of Pediatrics
Department of Pediatrics
University of Illinois
Lutheran General Hospital
Park Ridge, IL

R. Mollby, M.D.
Karolinska Institute and National Bacteriological Laboratory
Stockholm, Sweden

R. Curtis Morris, Jr., M.D.
Professor of Medicine and Pediatrics
University of California, San Francisco
San Francisco, CA

Dirk E. Müller-Wiefel, Ph.D., M.D.
Klinikum der Universitat Heidelberg
Kinderklinik
Federal Republic of Germany

Ricardo Munoz-Arizpe, M.D.
Investigator
Department of Nephrology
Hospital Infantil de Mexico
Mexico, D.F.

Rosario Nadorra, M.D.
Department of Pathology
Children's Hospital of Los Angeles
Los Angeles, CA

Jacob L. Ngu, M.D.
Professor of Internal Medicine
Nlongkak, Taounde
United Republic of Cameron

John M. Opitz, M.D.
Genetics and Birth Defects Unit
Shodair Children's Hospital
Helena, MT

Thomas S. Parrott, M.D.
Clinical Assistant Professor of Surgery (Urology)
Chief of Urology
Emory University School of Medicine
Scottish Rite Hospital
Atlanta, GA

Jeffrey L. Platt, M.D.
Instructor, Department of Pediatrics
University of Minnesota
Minneapolis, MN

Milana Popović-Rolović, M.D., D.Sci.
Professor of Pediatrics
Chief, Department of Pediatrics
Children's University Hospital
Beograd, Yugoslavia

Anthony A. Portale, M.D.
Assistant Professor of Pediatrics and Medicine
University of California, San Francisco
San Francisco, CA

Michael A. Preece, M.D.
Professor of Paediatrics
Department of Growth and Development
Institute of Child Health
London, England

Wolfgang Rascher, M.D.
Department of Pharmacology
Klinikum der Universitat Heidelberg, Kinderklinik
Federal Republic of Germany

Wolfgang Rauh, M.D.
Head of Department of Pediatrics
Federal Republic of Germany

Jack Resnick, M.D.
Captain, U.S.N.R.
Department of Radiology
Naval Hospital
San Diego, CA

Eberhard Ritz, M.D.
Klinikum der Universitat Heidelberg
Kinderklinik
Federal Republic of Germany

Jean E. Robillard, M.D.
Department of Pediatrics
University of Iowa
College of Medicine
Iowa City, IA

Eugene Rodriguez, Sc.D.
Immunochemist
Division of Experimental Immunopathology
St. Johns Mercy Medical Center
St. Louis, MO

Bernardo Rodríguez-Iturbe, M.D.
Professor of Medicine
Renal Service and Laboratory
Hospital Universitario & Universidad del Zulia
Maracaibo, Zulia, Venezuela

Edward J. Ruley, M.D.
Chairman, Department of Nephrology
Children's Hospital National Medical Center
Associate Professor
Department of Child Health and Development
George Washington University School of Medicine
Washington, DC

Tadasu Sakai, M.D.
Department of Pediatric Nephrology
Kitasato University Hospital
Kitasato, Sagamihra-Shi
Kanagawa, Japan

Karl Schärer, M.D.
Pediatrics, Head,
Division of Pediatric Nephrology,
University Children's Hospital
Federal Republic of Germany

George J. Schwartz, M.D.
Associate Professor of Pediatrics and Physiology/Biophysics
Albert Einstein College of Medicine
Bronx, NY

Charles R. Scriver, M.D., F.R.C.S.
Professor of Biology, Genetics and Pediatrics
Department of Biochemical Genetics
McGill University
Montreal Children's Hospital Research Institute
Montreal, Quebec, Canada

Stanton Segal, M.D.
Professor of Pediatrics and Medicine
Director, Division of Biochemical Development
University of Pennsylvania School of Medicine
The Children's Hospital of Philadelphia
Philadelphia, PA

Hannsjorg W. Seyberth, M.D.
Professor of Pediatric Nephrology
Klinikum der Universitat Heidelberg, Kinderklinik
Federal Republic of Germany

Alan R. Sinaiko, M.D.
Associate Professor of Pediatrics and Pharmacology
University of Minnesota Medical School
Minneapolis, MN

Howard McC. Snyder III, M.D.
Associate Director
Division of Urology
Children's Hospital of Philadelphia
Philadelphia, PA

R. N. Srivastava, M.D.
Associate Professor
Department of Pediatrics
All India Institute of Medical Sciences
Ansari Nagor
New Delhi, India

F. Bruder Stapleton, M.D.
Professor of Pediatrics Chief, Section of Nephrology
University of Tennessee
Center for Health Sciences
Memphis, TN

S. B. Svenson, M.D.
Karolinska Institute and National Bacteriological Laboratory
Stockholm, Sweden

M. deSwiet, M.D., F.R.C.P.
Consultant Physician
Department of Paediatrics
Cardiothoracic Institute
Brompton Hospital
Fulham Road
London, England

Richard S. Trompeter, M.B., M.R.C.P.
Senior Lecturer in Pediatrics
Consultant Pediatric Nephrologist
Department of Paediatrics
Royal Free Hospital
London, England

William R. Turner, Jr., M.D.
Professor of Urology and Pediatrics
Medical University of South Carolina
Charleston, SC

Herbert E. Ulmer, M.D.
Division of Pediatric Cardiology
University Children's Hospital
Federal Republic of Germany

R. M. Valentijn, M.D.
Department of Nephrology
University Hospital
The Netherlands

Leender A. Van Es, M.D.
Department of Nephrology
University Hospital
The Netherlands

Robert L. Vernier, M.D.
Professor of Pediatrics
Department of Pediatrics
University of Minnesota
Minneapolis, MN

Clark D. West, M.D.
Professor of Pediatrics
Associate Director
Department of Pediatrics
University of Cincinnati College of Medicine
Children's Hospital Medical Center
Cincinnati, OH

Jan Winberg, M.D.
Professor of Pediatrics
Department of Pediatrics
Karolinska Hospital
Stockholm, Sweden

John R. Woodard, M.D.
Professor of Surgery (Urology)
Associate Professor of Pediatrics
Director of Pediatric Urology
Chief of Urology
Division of Pediatric Urology
Emery University School of Medicine
Henrietta Egleston Hospital for Children
Atlanta, GA

Ji-Yun Yang, M.D.
Associate Professor of Pediatrics
Chief, Nephrology Division
Pediatric Department
The First Teaching Hospital of Beiging
Medical College Beiging
Peoples Republic of China

Aida Yared, M.D.
Research Fellow
Division of Nephrology
Vanderbilt University Medical School
Nashville, TN

Contents

5 Epidemiology

6 Congenital Disease

7 Glomerular Disease

8 Metabolic and Tubular Disease

9 Genitourinary Tract Disease

1

The Body, The Kidney, and Growth

CHAPTER **1**

Body Composition, Metabolism, and Growth

MALCOLM A. HOLLIDAY

INTRODUCTION

Nephrology is the study of renal function, of diseases that affect the kidney, and of the consequences of living with reduced renal function. Pediatric nephrology focuses on children from infancy through childhood and adolescence into maturity. Renal function operates to maintain a normal volume and composition of body fluids, particularly extracellular fluid (ECF), and has endocrine and metabolic functions as well. For this reason, the discipline of nephrology encompasses not only the physiology of regulating the volume and physicochemical state (ion concentration, pH and osmolality) of body fluids, but also factors that modify them. It also encompasses body composition, reflected by its metabolic and nutritional status, since the loss of renal function affects these as well as the body fluids.

The kidneys can accommodate a wide range of dietary intake, metabolic input, and nonrenal losses. In primitive settings the tolerance to a varied diet improves the chances of meeting nutrient requirements from the erratic food sources used to satisfy hunger. In modern cultures, this tolerance makes it possible for an individual to eat "what he wants when he wants it." In either case, normal body composition is sustained despite extraordinary changes in intake and metabolic input, because these are balanced by regulated losses (Table 1.1). It follows that a loss of renal function compromises this tolerance and potentially the ability to sustain normal body composition. For children, renal function is an essential factor that allows a varied intake to support growth and change in body composition. In children with reduced renal function, both growth and body composition are compromised. Because there is an important relationship between diet and renal function and there are dietary consequences of impaired renal function, this chapter describes the relation between body composition and energy metabolism as an appropriate beginning to the study of nephrology.

MODELS

The integration of kidney function into clinical well-being should include consideration of intake and body composition. From this perspective, a model of body composition is a good place to begin. (Fig. 1.1). This model divides the extracellular and the cellular phases of the body into several parts and each has structural and fluid components. The ECF phase is the environment for cells and has several parts each with fluid components. The cellular phase is divided into three parts, based on differences in their metabolism (1). The model describes exchanges of solutes between cells and ECF and exchange between the body and the outside.

The flow of solutes into and out of ECF is described more specifically by the model illustrated in Figure 1.2, *A*. In this model, ECF is the pool subject to change when intake from the environment (input) and excretion into the environment (output) occurs, and when there is release from cells into ECF (input) or uptake by cells from ECF (output). ECF composition is monitored when plasma is analyzed for electrolytes, minerals, and other constituents. The ECF-based model is useful for interpreting laboratory results. Stability is achieved when the input from intake and from cells equals output from excretion and cell uptake.

The intake of nutrients and excretion of products by the kidney, gastrointestinal tract, and skin in relation to total body mass, is the other model (Fig. 1.2 *B,*). This model describes body composition and the changes that occur when intake and excretion do not balance. The imbalance may affect cells, ECF, or both. There is a presumption of no change when intake and excretion balance. However, shifts between cells and ECF may have occurred; thus the value of the complementary model. Changes in ECF composition, intake, excretion, and metabolism have to be integrated, using both models to give an accurate description of a change in body composition. At a practical level, this is rarely possible, but the intellectual exercise of considering both models will improve the interpretation of laboratory results (chapter 19) and planning supportive therapy (chapter 11).

These models are also useful in describing growth. This chapter describes the changes in body composition represented by the model in Figure 1.1 while growth occurs as a basis for integrating the changes in metabolism, nutritional requirements, body composition, and renal function. Changes in metabolic rate and nutritional requirements during growth correlate with the development of renal function. The models of Figures 1.1 and 1.2 are useful in describing the metabolic differences between children and adults as a result of differences in both size and composition. Whereas input and renal function are proportional during growth, pool size in relation to turnover, as judged from ECF, body content of any specific nutrient, or total body mass, is smaller. Nutrient in this sense includes water, electrolytes, minerals, and glucose, as well as the conventional nutrients.

EXTRACELLULAR PHASE

General Characteristics

The extracellular phase in adult males is 30% to 40% of body weight and slightly less in females. Two thirds of this phase is ECF, and one third is bone solids and connective tissue protein (2). The fluid compartments are plasma and interstitial fluid (ISF), including connective tissue fluid (3). These have certain properties in common, e.g., Na and Cl concentrations are high and small molecular weight solutes are freely diffusible among the phases. Regulation of the physicochemical state of ECF is described in detail in Section II of this textbook. Chapter 6 provides a description of ECF, i.e., how its volume and composition are maintained. Guyton and his colleagues (4) have provided a model of ECF that integrates the components into an entity and describes the circulation of ECF (Fig. 1.3).

Table 1.1
Minimum and Maximum Values for Intake[a] of Several Nutrients whose Tolerance is Affected by Loss of Renal Function

	Minimum	Maximum	RDA	Average (US)
Sodium (mEq)	10	400	—	200
Water (ml)	1200	12,000	—	3000
Potassium (mEq)	20	400	—	200
Hydrogen ion (mEq)	−100	300	—	70
Calcium (mg)	400	>2000	800	1000
Phosphorus (mg)	500	4500	800	1500
Protein (gm)	30	300	56	110

[a] Values for 70 kg male 23 to 50 years of age.

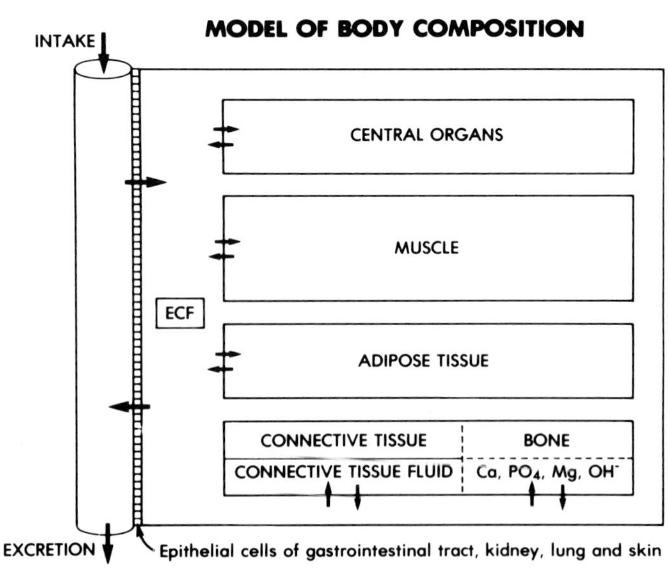

Figure 1.1. Diagram of body composition describing the extracellular and cellular phases.

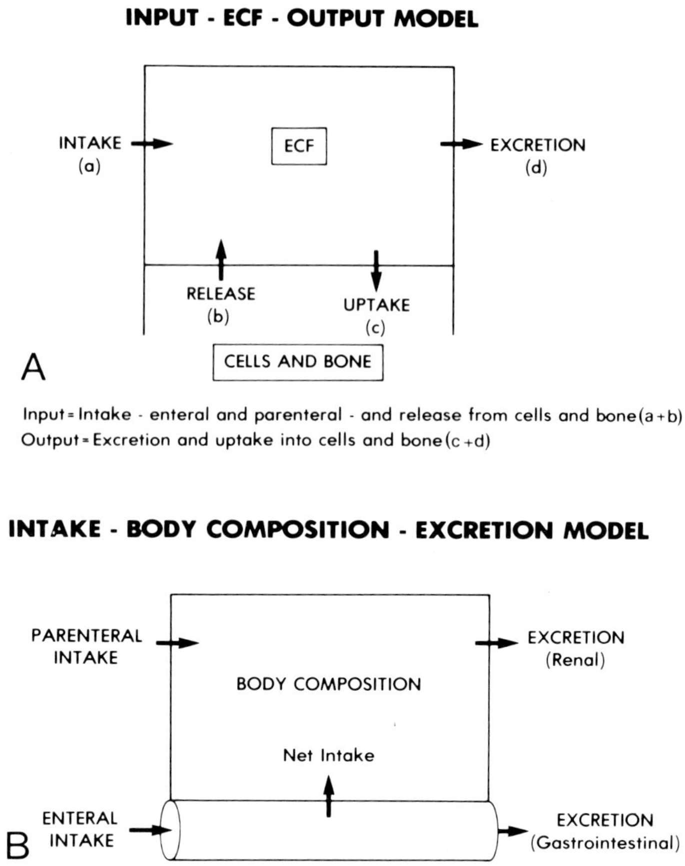

Figure 1.2. **A,** The input-ECF-output model in which input is intake (*a*) from environment and release (*b*) from cells and output is uptake by cells (*c*) and excretion (*d*). **B,** The intake-body composition-excretion model which is used in defining metabolic balance in which balance = Intake − (GI—other nonrenal/urinary) losses.

Components

Plasma

Plasma constitutes 4% to 5% of body weight and is the interface between the major organs and structures within the body and between these organs and structures and the epithelial cells that, in turn, interact with the outside environment.

Plasma contains proteins that among other functions provide a gradient across capillaries to return fluid ultrafiltered by hydrostatic pressure. Together hydrostatic and oncotic forces comprise the Starling forces (4) that regulate the exchange of fluid between capillaries and interstitial spaces. There is a net loss of fluid from capillaries to the interstitial space, because the hydrostatic pressure exceeds peripheral capillary oncotic pressure. The fluid lost from plasma in this manner is returned via lymph flow to the venous circulation (Fig. 1.4). The flow is abetted by a negative

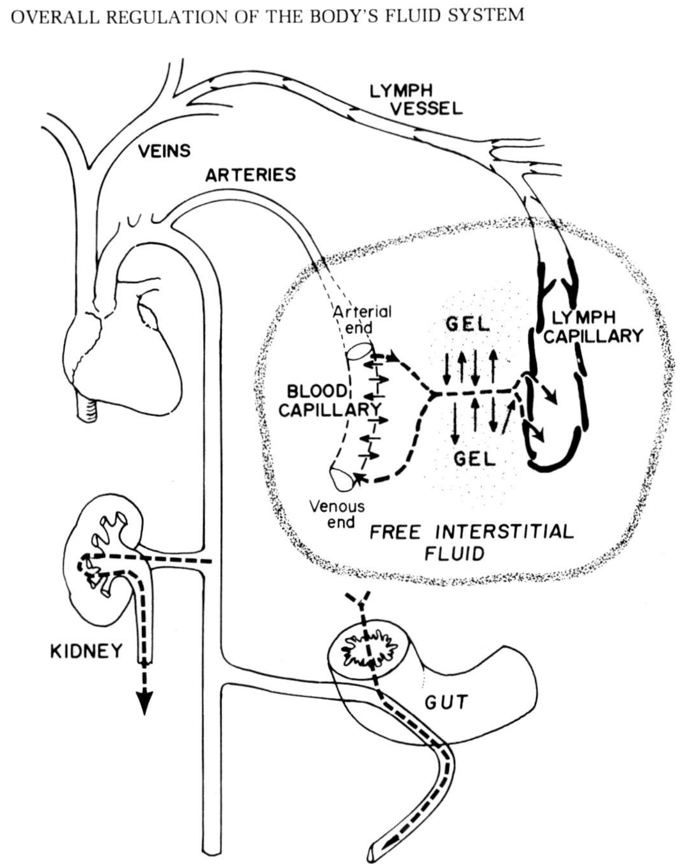

Figure 1.3. The circulation of ECF from blood to interstitial fluid to lymphatics and back to blood.

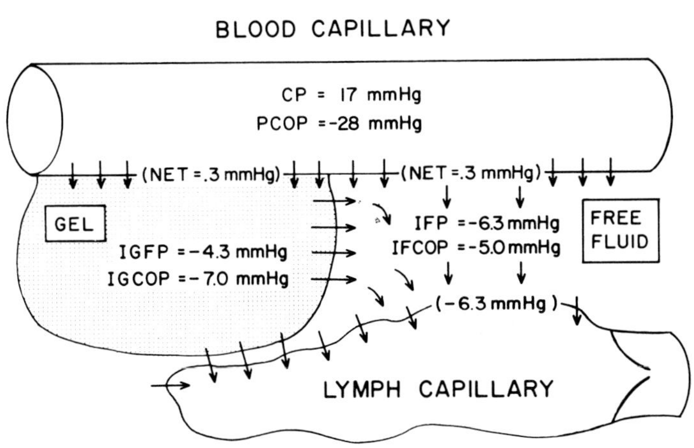

Figure 1.4. The forces moving fluid out in mm Hg are capillary pressure (CP = 17) plus negative interstitial fluid pressure (IFP = −6.3) plus interstitial fluid colloid oncotic pressure (IFCOP = −5) totaling 28.3. The forces moving fluid into capillaries is the plasma colloid oncotic pressure (PCOP = −28). The net difference = .3; there results a net gain of fluid by the interstitial space and this is moved back to the circulation via lymphatics.

pressure in interstitial spaces that moves fluid through lymph channels to the lymphatic duct.

Plasma albumin pool accounts for approximately half the total albumin pool; the balance is distributed in ISF, but at varied concentrations, usually below those in plasma. Albumin accounts for more than half the peripheral capillary oncotic pressure that recovers fluid from ISF back into plasma. ISF expands and plasma volume contracts when Starling forces are changed that favor redistribution of fluid from plasma to ISF. However, the gel structure of ISF resists expansion and lymph return continues, so that plasma volume is maintained until the pressure gradient between the capillaries and ISF is dissipated.

Interstitial Fluid

ISF volume is a composite of the fluid that is in the interstices of the cells and that which is an integral part of connective tissue (3). Formerly, these were treated as separate components, but, because they are a continuum that exists as a gel of varying fluidity, they are now considered as one (4). More of the fluid (approximately 10% to 12% of body weight) is within the interstices of cells, and 8% to 10% is in the fluid phase of connective tissue, most of which is in skin (4). Some is also in the dense connective tissue of ligaments (Fig. 1.1). The ISF gel resists expansion when Starling forces are imbalanced until the gradient is dissipated; only then does edema fluid form (Fig. 1.5).

Lymph is a part of ISF and its circulation is essential in maintaining the balance between plasma and ISF. Circulation of lymph depends on muscle tone and activity acting counter to gravity. Prolonged quiet standing can lead to dissipation of the capillary-ISF pressure gradient, pooling of fluid in interstitial spaces and reduction in plasma volume, as well as to venous pooling. This reduces venous return and cardiac output, leading to oliguria. Head-out immersion in water or weightlessness in

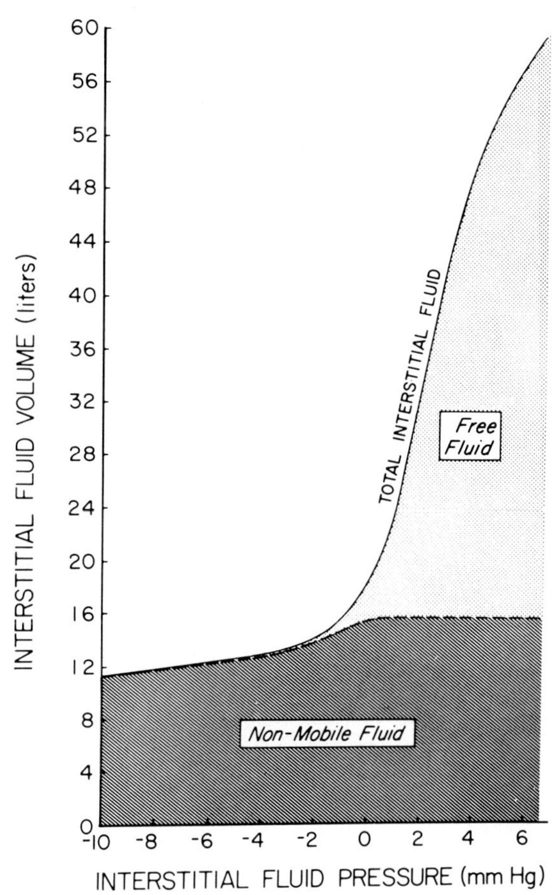

Figure 1.5. Diagram showing relation between capillary hydraulic pressure and volume. ISF pressure can decrease from −8 to near −0 before free fluid accumulates as edema.

space has the opposite effect, i.e., venous return increases and a diuresis is initiated.

Transcellular Fluids

These fluids are sometimes considered to be another phase of ECF. They are a composite of gastrointestinal, cerebrospinal, and respiratory epithelial cells whose total volume at any moment is small (2). Because they are secretions, their composition varies at different sites. Na and Cl are the principal electrolytes. Secretory and, hence, turnover rates are high. The formation of transcellular fluids from ECF represents a potential for loss of ECF if reabsorption does not balance secretion, e.g., in cholera, secretion increases and reabsorption is reduced, so that net losses can exceed 1 l/hour. Losses of gastrointestinal or cerebrospinal (CSF) fluids without adequate replacement causes ECF volume contraction or dehydration. Because losses of transcellular fluids from different sites have different composition, the site of loss can alter the residual ECF concentrations as well, e.g., loss of gastric fluid causes alkalosis and loss of duodenal fluid causes hyperchloremic acidosis.

Edema

Edema is an expansion of ECF in which plasma volume may be contracted or expanded. The former occurs when changes in Starling forces lead to redistribution of fluid from plasma to ISF. This occurs with tissue injury, some types of the nephrotic syndrome, heart failure, and liver disease. Circulation and perfusion may be impaired. Plasma and ISF volume both expand when salt and water intake exceeds excretion because of a change in renal function that limits salt excretion, i.e., the circulatory system is overexpanded (chapter 6).

Solid Phase

The solid phase consists of bone apatite, its structural base (the organic matrix of cartilage), the collagen and elastin of connective tissue, and the glycoproteins that form the gel of ISF. Bone apatite gives bone its rigidity and it also serves as a pool for Ca and P to maintain the much smaller Ca and P pools in ECF and cells when intake does not match output. There are rapidly and slowly exchangeable pools of Ca and P. Although collagen is the largest pool of body protein, once it is cross-linked, it does not degrade. Consequently, this large pool is not a source of amino acids when acute starvation or chronic malnutrition develop. The glycoproteins of ISF provide the "framework" for the gel of ISF, maintaining a constant relation between capillaries and cells. The gel is an efficient medium of exchange between plasma and cells.

CELL MASS

General Characteristics

The cell phase in normal adult males is 60% to 70% of body weight, i.e., it is the balance of body mass that is not extracellular. Between 55% and 70% of the cell phase is water. The model of body composition described in Figure 1.1 divides the cell phase into 3 components: the central organs, muscle, and adipose tissue. The cells of small specialized tissues are quantitatively not significant.

Cells, like ECF, have certain properties in common. Each cell is bounded by a membrane that separates it from ECF. Cells have a characteristic electrolyte pattern, and the principal ions are potassium, phosphorus, and proteins. Cells usually are 75% water; the balance is mostly soluble protein or protein of organelles or contractile proteins. The latter is the major cell protein. Cells that are storage cells, e.g., adipocytes, have less water, but within the cells the nonstorage phase is 75% water.

Cells take up nutrients, electrolytes, and other solutes from the environment by exchange diffusion, active transport, and pinocytosis from ISF. Similarly, they release metabolic end-products into ISF. Cells usually do not change composition or size significantly, except to grow larger. The uptake of solutes and nutrients by cells is balanced in a thermodynamic sense by release of energy and other solutes. Once cells attain their full size the content of water, electrolyte, mineral, carbon, and N remains constant except for those that store fat or glycogen. Muscle cells gain and lose contractile protein in response to change in nutritional status and workload.

The high K concentration in cells is maintained by an outward-oriented Na pump that pumps Na from cells in exchange for K. This results in a transmembrane potential across cells that is negative on the cell interior. The pump is a Na/K-dependent adenosine triphosphatase (Na-K-ATPase) that hydrolyzes ATPase to adenosine 5′-diphosphate (ADP) (5). Pump activity may account for a significant fraction of tissue oxygen consumption and, by inference, basal metabolic rate (BMR). Like BMR, pump activity is regulated by thyroid hormone (6). Changes in permeability of cell membrane also affect the relation between pump activity and cell composition.

Components

The three components of cell mass (Fig. 1.1) have very different rates of oxygen consumption and substrate utilization (Table 1.2) (7).

Central organs

Central organs, i.e., brain, liver, heart, and kidney, account for 66% of basal metabolism, although they are only 5% of body weight. These four organs have comparable rates of oxygen consumption (see Table 1.2). The brain, except in extended starvation (8), uses glucose for substrate (9). Its high rate of metabolism changes little under physiologic conditions (10). Its dependence on glucose for substrate is the principal reason that glucose specifically is needed in the resting state (9, 10). The liver and the gastrointestinal tract, i.e., the splanchnic area, increase metabolic rate after a meal, which is diet-induced thermogenesis (11). Part of the decrease in metabolism associated with malnutrition is a result of a reduction in diet-induced thermogenesis. Renal oxygen consumption varies with the rate of renal Na reabsorption or glomerular filtration rate (GFR), which changes very little except when GFR is reduced (12).

Muscle

In contrast to the central organs, muscle has a low metabolic rate. When an individual is in the basal state (1600 kcal/day in adult males),

Table 1.2
Organ Metabolic Rate (OMR) and Organ size in Adults: Relation to BMR[a]

	Weight (kg)	VO_2 (ml/100 gm/m)	OMR (kcal/ da)	OMR/BMR × 100 %
Brain	1.40	4.2	414	23.3 (18.3)[b]
Liver	1.60	4.1	464	26.1 (26.4)
Heart	0.30	8.6	182	10.2 (9.2)
Kidney	0.30	5.5	116	7.1 (7.2)
SUBTOTAL	3.6	—	1177	66.7 (61.1)
Skeletal muscle	28.3	0.26	500	28.1 (25.6)
TOTAL	31.9		1677	94.8 (86.7)

[a] Adapted from Holliday MA: Pediatrics 47:169, 1971.
[b] Adapted from Brozek J, Grande F: Human Biol 27:22, 1955.

resting muscle metabolism accounts for only 28% of oxygen consumption, although muscle mass is 40% of body weight and more than 85% of cell mass (7). With maximal physical activity, muscle oxygen consumption can increase ten- to twenty-fold for brief periods. When daily energy expenditure is 2700 kcal/day (the average for adult males in sedentary occupations), muscle accounts for 40% of total expenditure. With strenuous activity, muscle oxygen consumption is 60% to 80% of the total.

Muscle contractile protein is a large pool of protein (80 g/kg) that contributes significantly to the total turnover of protein of 3 to 5 g/kg/day (13). Synthesis and breakdown can vary independently. In an anabolic phase, as occurs postfeeding, synthesis increases, breakdown decreases, and muscle protein mass increases. The converse is true in a catabolic phase. Muscle protein mass of specific muscles increases when workload of those muscles increase and decreases when workload declines. When an individual becomes inactive or when dietary energy or protein intake is deficient, total muscle mass decreases. It decreases rapidly in response to acute starvation or catabolic stress as catabolism of protein and/or gluconeogenesis increase (14). By giving carbohydrate when food is withheld, the loss of N is reduced because the stimulus for gluconeogenesis is removed (15).

The pool of contractile protein in muscle is not labile in the sense that it is "storage" protein analogous to body fat. Rather, muscle and plasma proteins and protein from the gastrointestinal tract are labile in that the pools will decrease in response to catabolism and thereby provide amino acids, which can be used elsewhere as substrate for protein synthesis or as carbon sources for gluconeogenesis (16). These adaptations, made possible by the turnover of most body proteins, contrast with the very low rate of turnover of connective tissue protein. Collagen, once cross-linked, does not turnover.

Loss of muscle mass in malnutrition is an adaptive response for survival, but with this response is the disadvantage of the loss of muscle strength. Fasting individuals adapt in time by reducing body protein N losses (9). The time required to adapt to starvation is less in infants and even less still in infants who are malnourished (17). Thus, there is a built-in feedback system that stabilizes loss of body N or muscle mass as malnutrition develops. It is possible to reach a state of equilibrium when intakes of energy and protein are 50% to 70% of normal. Both body protein and energy reserves are depleted initially before this adaptive response develops.

Adipose Tissue

Adipose tissue, except for brown adipose tissue, has a low rate of metabolism. It is 60% to 85% storage fat. Fat, upon hydrolysis, yields glycerol and fatty acids in which the ratio of carbons is 1:20. Glycerol, like lactic acid and most amino acids, is potential substrate for synthesis of glucose (gluconeogenesis) when glucose is not available from intake. Fatty acids enter the Krebs cycle directly as acetate or are first synthesized into ketones. They cannot be used for net synthesis of glucose. Fatty acids and ketones are potential substrates for metabolism of muscle, heart, liver, and other organs. Brain can use ketones when it is adapted to fasting (8).

Adipose tissue is distinct among the components of body composition because it varies so widely as a percentage of body weight in the normal population. The range of body fat as a percentage of body weight is 10% to 20% in normal males and 15% to 30% in females (18).

Adipose tissue is reduced in well-trained runners. They have free access to food and control intake to maintain body fat (calorie storage) at low levels. Their calorie reserve is less, but they have a normal muscle mass. Body fat is also reduced in patients with malnutrition (19). Not having free access to food, they have reduced substrate reserves in both adipose tissue and muscle protein but not collagen protein. They balance their enforced low-calorie intake by expending fewer calories, i.e., they are less active (20).

Obese patients have 30% or more of body weight as fat. They may have larger than normal muscle mass or they may be inactive and have a decreased muscle mass (21). Brown adipose tissue has a high mitochondrial content that, when stimulated, releases much heat usually in response to cold stress. Its role, if any, in energy balance in adults is disputed (22).

BODY COMPOSITION DURING GROWTH

General Changes

Physical growth from a clinical perspective begins with birth and ends in late adolescence as the individual becomes an adult. Growth rate expressed as g/kg/day is greatest in the first 3 months (Table 1.3); growth in stature is greatest in the first 2 years (chapter 2). Changes in body composition, metabolism, and renal function are dramatic in the neonatal period. Change continues at a rapid rate in the first year of life (infancy) and is slower in childhood. Puberty is a period of relatively rapid change when compared with childhood. The pubertal growth spurt appears to be superimposed on the normal growth pattern of childhood. In the case of the low birth weight (LBW) infant, growth from 1 kg to 3.5 kg, which normally occurs in the third trimester of gestation, must occur in the less friendly environment of an intensive care nursery. Of particular concern to pediatric nephrologists are the special problems relating to metabolism and renal function in this group (chapters 54 and 55). The maximum rate of weight gain is greater (Table 1.3).

Differences in body composition at selected points in growth (Table 1.4) describe several trends. ECF volume as a fraction of body mass tends to decrease (23); central organ mass as a fraction of body weight decreases after the first year (1). By contrast, muscle mass increases (24). Body fat, low at birth, increases throughout the first year of life, and then decreases during childhood. Its course after that varies (25).

Changes in Each Period

Although there are trends to the change in body composition throughout growth, each period of growth (the neonatal period, up to 1 month, infancy to 1 year, childhood to puberty, and adolescence) has distinctive features. (LBW infants, who may triple their weight in reaching term weight, are a special case.)

Neonatal Period

Changes in metabolism at birth are marked as the infant adapts to the extrauterine world in which the kidney, lung, and gastrointestinal tract act for the placenta. ECF volume contracts as a result of a natriuresis. This contraction is the largest factor in the weight loss that occurs in the

Table 1.3
Growth Rate (gm/kg/day) for Each Quarter of the First Year of Life and for Period of Maximum Weight Gain During Adolescence

Age (months)	Average growth rate (gm/kg/day)
0–1 (LBW—1500 gm)	14.0
0–3	5.7
3–6	3.1
6–9	2.0
9–12	1.2
Adolescence[a]	.4

[a] Average weight gain at peak period of growth.

Table 1.4
Body Composition at Different Stages of Growth

Age (years)	Height (cm)	Body weight (kg)	Organ weight[a]	Muscle mass[b]	Body Fat[c]	ECF volume
			Body weight (%)			
LBW[d]	40	1.1	21	<10	3	50
NB[e]	50	3.5	18	20	12	40
0.25	60	5.5	15	22	11	32
1.50	80	11.0	14	23	20	26
5	110	19.0	10	35	15	24
10	140	31.0	8.4	37	15	25
14 (m)	160	50	5.7	42	12	21
Adult (m)	180	70	5.2	40	11	19
13 (f)	160	45	4.8	39	18	19
Adult (f)	162	55	4.4	35	20	16

[a] Sum of brain, liver, heart, and kidney. (1)
[b] Derived from creatinine excretion. (1)
[c] Interpolated values from literature. (23, 26)

first 2 weeks of life (23, 26). Plasma composition changes; bicarbonate concentration initially is low relative to adult norms (chapter 8) and phosphorus concentration is elevated (chapter 9). Renal blood flow and GFR increase rapidly as nutrient intake increases (chapter 4).

Infancy

During the first year of life, growth is rapid; body weight increases three-fold. The energy cost of growth in the first 4 months is 20% to 30% of total energy intake (27). Body fat increases from 12% to 20%; weight gain in the first 4 months is 40% fat (24). Dietary energy requirement increases at the same rate as body weight (28). Nutrient requirements are met in large degree from human milk, so that variations in the composition of diet are not large. Renal function increases at a rate greater than kidney weight, metabolic rate, surface area, or body weight (29).

LBW infants begin life with a low muscle and adipose tissue mass; a large fraction of their weight is ECF (26). For them, growth in this period is rapid; the energy cost of growth is half of the total energy intake (chapter 55B).

Childhood

As the infant is weaned and diet composition becomes diverse, the period of rapid growth ends. Organ function has matured to accommodate the challenge of a widely varying diet. Growth is relatively slow in childhood; there is a change in body composition and nutrient requirement relative to body size. Brain growth is rapid through the first 3 years of life, slows thereafter, and is complete by 5 years of age. Splanchnic organs (gastrointestinal tract and liver) and kidney size increase at a slower rate than body weight, whereas muscle mass increases at a faster rate (29).

Adolescence

Adolescence encompasses puberty, which is a period of sexual maturation and of rapid growth in body weight and stature. Females begin their pubertal growth spurt earlier than males. A larger proportion of their weight gain is fat, which is useful as a reserve for child bearing and lactation. Puberty for males begins later. Much of their weight gain is muscle; body fat may decrease. The composition of weight gain is influenced by sex hormones, e.g., estrogen controls the increase in body fat in females, and androgen controls the increase in muscle mass of males (chapter 2). Adolescents usually are active and their food intake is correspondingly increased. The energy cost of weight gain in this period is low (<3% of total), so that the characteristic high food intake and energy expenditure are more a result of the high level of physical activity. Increases in BMR and renal function are proportional to those of food intake.

ENERGY METABOLISM

Basal Metabolic Rate and Body Composition

Variation in the basal energy expenditure or BMR of adults, both male and female, is a result of variations in lean body mass (LBM), i.e., body weight minus body fat. The differences in BMR related to weight between males and females are largely a result of the differences in body fat (22). Although BMR is more a result of the central organs (Table 1.2), LBM is determined more by muscle mass. Among adults, central organ mass and muscle mass are proportional. Normal variations in BMR are a result of differences in thyroid hormone activity and probably its effect on Na pump activity (6).

Physical Activity

Total energy expenditure is a composite of BMR, physical activity, cold stress, and diet-induced thermogenesis. Variations in total energy expenditure are considerable and are a result mostly of variations in physical activity. Body composition has little relation to physical activity. The secular trend in our society has seen a decrease in physical activity and a decline in total energy requirement. The current emphasis on physical fitness has not increased energy expenditure by more than a few percent in most individuals because the periods of exercise are relatively short.

Change With Growth

Energy requirements during childhood are higher in relation to body weight and decline with growth (Fig. 1.6). The components of energy requirements include the energy cost of growth, which is quantitatively significant as a fraction of energy requirement only in infancy and in the special case of the LBW infant. However, endocrine factors affecting growth are sensitive to food intake, since small reductions in food intake affect growth in stature and weight throughout childhood, even though the energy cost of growth is very small (30).

BMR/kg declines as growth proceeds, i.e., body weight increases more rapidly than does BMR. The high proportion of BMR that is a result of central organ metabolism in adults has been noted. When the change in weight of these organs and the change in BMR are both compared with the change in body weight throughout growth, a parallel is evident (Fig. 1.7), which suggests a relationship between BMR and the sum of central organ weights (ΣOW). When log BMR is plotted against log ΣOW (Fig. 1.8, *line A*), the relationship is not quite linear. When BMR is adjusted by subtracting muscle metabolism to describe organ metabolic rate (OMR), the relationship is a straight line passing through zero. The slope of that line defines a composite of BMR/ΣOW throughout growth that corresponds with the adult composite value (Fig. 1.8, (*line B*). The rates of increase in OMR and ΣOW are the same from term birth to maturity. The ΣOW is the principal determinant of the changing relationship between BMR and body size, during growth.

Total energy requirement throughout growth, the sum of BMR, and the energy cost of growth and average physical activity parallels BMR through infancy and childhood and is between 1.6 and 2 × BMR. In infancy, physical activity is a small fraction; physical activity and the energy cost of growth nearly equals BMR (31). Thereafter, the energy cost of physical activity, on average, equals BMR. However, the range of

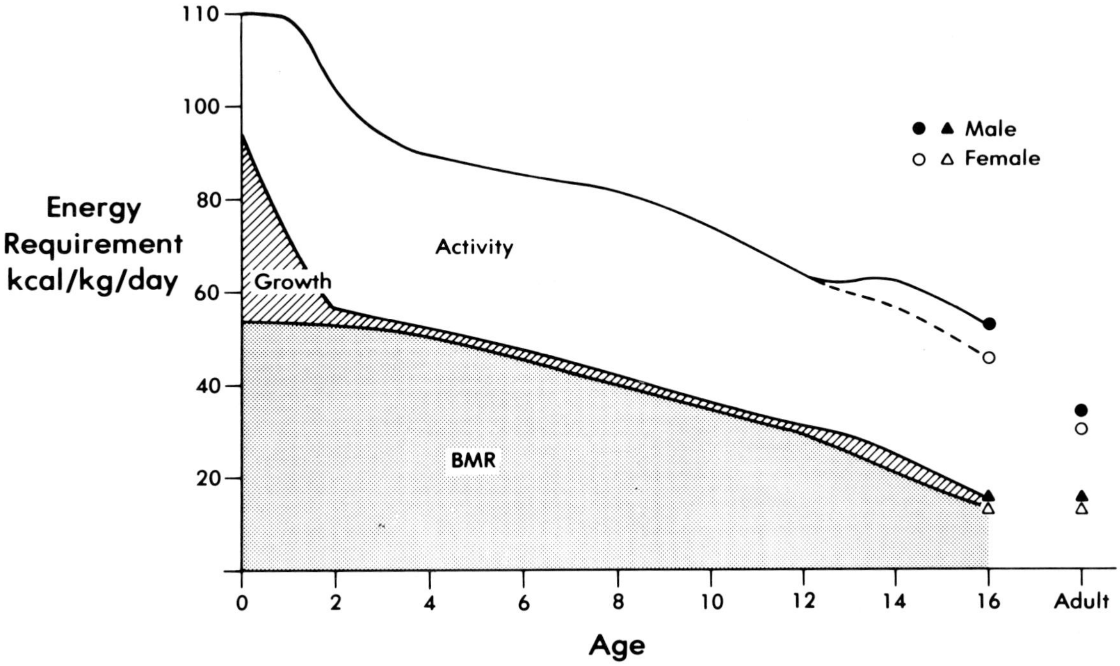

Figure 1.6. Changes in energy requirement/kg that occur during growth. While energy requirements for growth are quantitatively small after 2 years of age, growth rate is sensitive to inadequate intake.

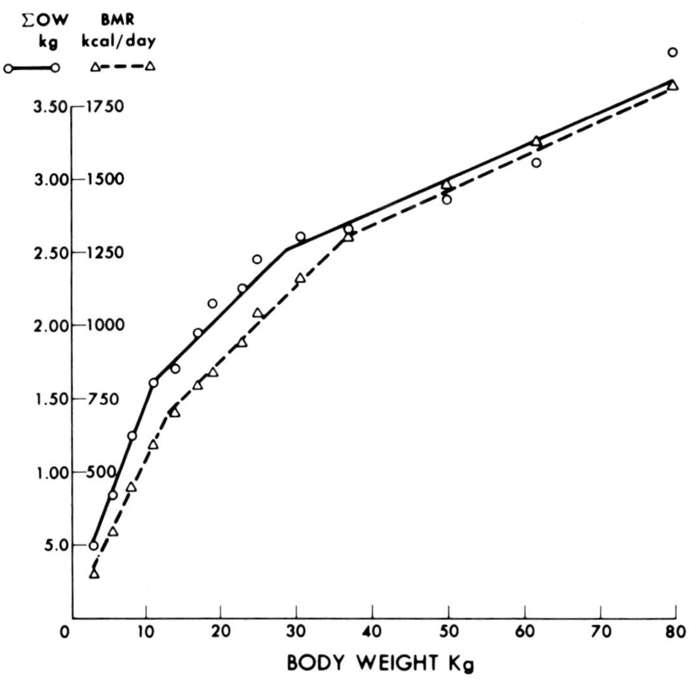

Figure 1.7. BMR and the weight of central organs (ΣOW) in relation to body weight during growth.

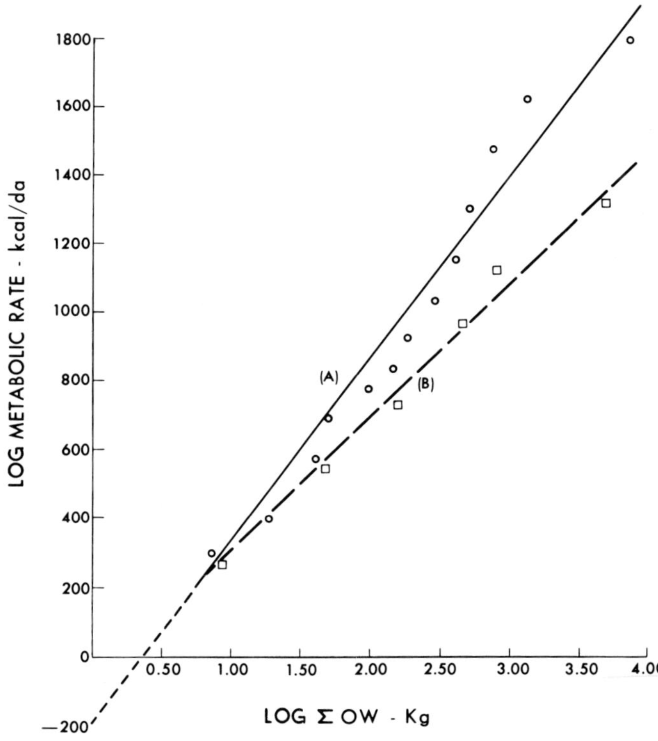

Figure 1.8. Relation of BMR with ΣOW (*line A*) and BMR adjusted by subtracting resting muscle metabolic rate to describe the central organ metabolic rates (OMR) with ΣOW (*line B*). The intercept of the latter is near-zero, and the slope defines an integrated metabolic rate for those organs, that is similar to the one derived from the values in adults in Table 1.1.

variability is great because activity levels vary so much among individuals (Fig. 1.9).

Brain

Comparison of the metabolism of specific organs at different ages to total BMR illustrates the dominant role that brain metabolism plays in setting the metabolic and nutritional needs of infants (Fig. 1.10). Glucose turnover increases with growth as brain size increases (32). Consequently, the glucose requirement relative to body weight is highest in infancy and declines with growth (Chap 11). The large brain size and its corresponding energy requirement are unique in humans and are responsible for an unusually high resting metabolism. This may be a factor in the slow

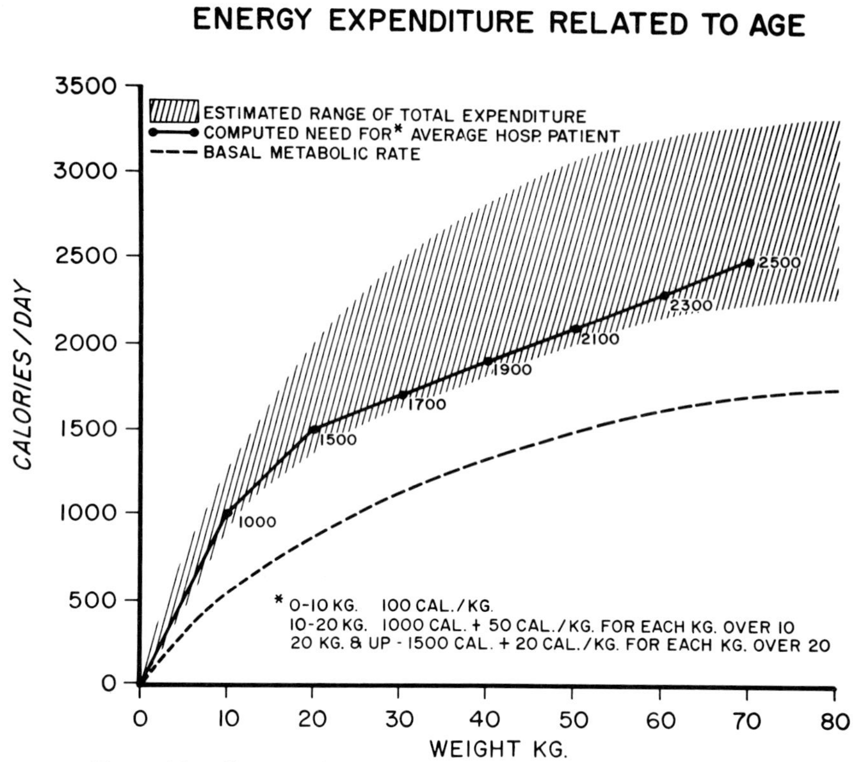

Figure 1.9. Change in BMR and total energy expenditure with growth.

growth of humans in relation to other species. Human milk differs from other mammalian milk in that it has a low protein and mineral content relative to its energy content, which is appropriate for the slower growth and the higher resting metabolism.

Renal Function

Renal function and renal size over the period of growth, by convention, is related to surface area. During the first year of life GFR/1.73 m^2 is low. The coefficients of variation of the normal values are high because maturation proceeds at different rates among normal infants. Thereafter, GFR/unit surface area is relatively constant (chapter 19). In the first year of life, when GFR is relatively low, the infant's principal nutrient source (milk) is balanced and provides little excretory load. During the first year of life, the child's diet becomes more varied and excretory load increases; GFR in the first year also increases more rapidly than surface area or BMR. Thereafter, GFR increases in proportion with BMR and with average energy or food intake increases (Table 1.5). The kidney in the first year of life is often described as immature. From a biologic perspective, the low kidney function during the first year of life is well adapted to the nature of the nutrient intake (human milk), since the excretory load from human milk is small. A low rate of kidney function is appropriate and entails a lower rate of energy expenditure.

The Low Birth Weight Infant

The relationship of energy metabolism to body composition is different during growth of the LBW infant. Metabolic rate, either as a derivative of body weight or ΣOW is low when the infant weighs 1 kg, but increases at a more rapid rate (1.3 times) than either body weight or ΣOW to attain the value characteristic of the term infant (1, 33). During this period of growth, resting energy requirement is less and energy needed for growth, particularly growth of adipose tissue, is high. Also, substrates that support growth, e.g., protein and minerals, are needed in relatively greater amounts (chapter 55B).

MEASUREMENT

The characteristics of body composition were originally derived postmortem from dissection and chemical analysis of animals and humans. Subsequently, body water and ECF, respectively, were estimated from the volume of distribution of compounds distributed into total body water (TBW) and a volume that approximates ECF. Today less invasive means are sought to estimate body fat, muscle mass, and skeletal mass for clinical purposes. However, the techniques of measuring the volume of distribution of compounds to identify ECF space and TBW are still used for clinical investigation.

Total Body Water and Lean Body Mass

The estimation of TBW in normal subjects defines the component LBM, which is the body mass minus its fat. LBM, after a certain point in infancy in humans and other species, is 70% water. LBM can be estimated in normal individuals from the measurement of TBW by the equation:

$$LBM = TBW/0.7$$

The difference between body weight and LBM (body weight − LBM) is fat. This method has been used to estimate fat in normal populations and as a reference measure of body fat in validating other less invasive measures (18). Estimating body fat by this indirect means incurs an error of ±10%, because body fat is the difference between two larger numbers—body weight and TBW—and the estimate of LBM from body water is a composite of different components of LBM. The method is unreliable for estimating either LBM or fat when wasting or edema are present.

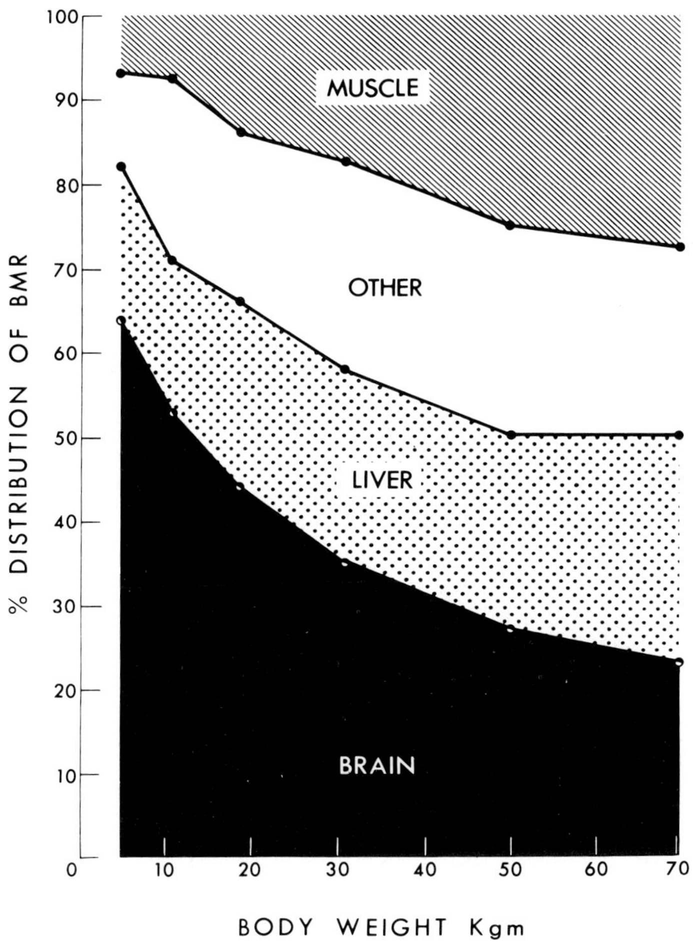

Figure 1.10. The relative contribution of brain metabolism to total BMR at various stages of growth.

Table 1.5
Relation of Energy Intake and BMR to GFR at Different Stages of Growth[a]

Age	Weight	Total energy intake (kcal/day)	BMR	GFR (ml/min)	GFR (ml/min/100kcal)	
					Total intake	BMR
0.25	5.5	600	300	(11)	1.8	3.7
1.5	11	1100	590	29	2.6	4.9
5.5	19	1790	830	60	3.4	7.2
9.5	31	2380	1160	83	3.5	7.1
14.0	50	3020	1480	112	3.7	7.6
Adult	70	3100	1600	130	4.2	8.1

[a] Adapted from Holliday MA: Body composition and energy needs during growth. In Falkner F, Tanner JM (eds): Human Growth. New York and London, Plenum Press, 1979.

Extracellular Fluid

ECF is estimated from the volume of distribution of compounds excluded from cells. No compound is ideal for this purpose (26). Three classes of compounds are used and each gives slightly different results. The first class includes inulin, sucrose, and sorbitol, which are totally excluded from cells and are cleared rapidly by the kidney. These compounds, when used in normal individuals define a volume of distribution that is smaller than plasma and ISF, including dense connective tissue fluid, because they distribute slowly into the latter (34).

Sulfate and ^{35}S-sulfate are also excluded from cells but reach equilibrium rapidly in all phases of ECF and appear to measure the true ECF space most accurately (35). Radiosulfate has been used in clinical research to measure ISF volume in patients with hemorrhagic shock (36). Both inulin and sulfate are cleared rapidly from body fluids by GFR, so that the accuracy of measurement is impaired.

Cl and Br are the third class of compounds used to measure ECF volume. They also distribute into cell fluid at low concentrations so that a correction should be made (26). Isotopes of either (^{36}Cl, ^{82}Br) or stable Br equilibrate in 2 to 3 hours into their volume of distribution; both are excreted slowly, so that losses during equilibration are minimal; stable Br can be used to measure ECF (37). Intracellular Cl and Br are reciprocally related to transmembrane potential difference (PD) across cell membranes. When the PD is low, as it is in severe uremia, alcoholic intoxication, and heart failure, intracellular Cl increases. In patients with severe uremia, dialysis restores PD to normal (38). Br has been used to define the ECF volume in adults and children with moderate uremia, where PD is in a normal range. In them, ECF volume estimated from the volume of distribution of Br is increased (chapter 49).

Na space, measured by isotope dilution, defines a volume of distribution that is slightly greater than that defined by Cl. It is subject to a variable error because intracellular Na increases under a variety of conditions (39).

An important characteristic of body fluids is derived from the simultaneous measure of ^{22}Na, ^{42}K, and TBW. The derived concentration of Na+K/TBW is proportional to Na concentration in serum (Na_s) over a wide range of values in a diverse population. The relationship indicates that most Na and K in body water is freely dissociated and osmotically active (39). In this same study, the relationship between Na_s and osmolality of body fluids is defined.

Cell Mass

Cell mass is estimated from the difference between TBW and ECF (40), the volume of distribution of isotopic potassium (^{42}K), or of the natural-occurring isotope (^{40}K) (41), and from creatinine production rate (42, 43).

Cell mass, estimated from the difference between TBW and ECF, can define differences from the norm, especially differences in muscle mass, as long as transmembrane potential and cell K concentrations are normal.

^{40}K is a measure of total body K used to define muscle mass. It is less reliable in patients who have muscle wasting, because the concentrations of K in intracellular water may be low. Its measurement is difficult and the required equipment is expensive and available in only a few places. It is primarily useful in clinical research (chapter 7). ^{42}K is not suitable for clinical use because it has a short half-life and it entails significant radiation exposure.

Creatinine production rate, estimated from excretion rates for 24 hours, is a measure of muscle mass in normal subjects. Muscle mass can be derived from the equations of Cheek (42), or it can be estimated by assuming 50 mg/day of creatinine is produced by 1 kg of muscle. It is, however, inaccurate when plasma levels of creatinine secondary to renal disease exceed 2 mg/dl or when creatinine production is increased as it is with catabolic stress.

It would be useful in clinical practice to be able to measure ECF volume, adipose tissue or body fat content, and muscle mass. There is no method for measuring ECF volume that is suitable for clinical use; sulfate (36) and bromide (37) can be used for clinical investigative studies.

Skin turgor and signs of tissue perfusion are the best clinical guides to reduction in ECF volume and effective blood flow, respectively. Body fat can be estimated accurately from measures of skinfold thickness. The estimate is reproducible in children (44) and adults (45) when it has been carefully standardized and norms developed (chapter 2).

The only method for measuring muscle mass that has been used successfully in clinical practice is the measurement of midarm circumference. It has been used in surveys of nutritional status where malnutrition is endemic (46). Its usefulness in clinical nephrology is not established. Creatinine production is also not useful in chronic renal failure (CRF), because a variable but increasing amount of creatinine is catabolized by bacteria in the gastrointestinal tract as pool size (serum concentration) increases. The difference between TBW and ECF has been used to derive a term for ICW and cell mass (40). A satisfactory measure of muscle mass or contractile protein would be helpful in assessing body composition and nutritional status. It would be useful for determining whether muscle protein mass has been reduced in patients with CRF and whether specific regimens had long-term effects to increase or decrease muscle mass.

Weight and Growth

Clinical Interpretation

Weight is the most commonly used index of body size and growth. The weight-for-height index is used to identify overweight or underweight patients. An independent measure of body fat (skinfold thickness) is the most commonly used method for defining obesity or malnutrition. Change in weight is the most common measure for assessing change in nutritional status. The difficulty in interpreting change in weight is the uncertainty in knowing whether change is a result of change in ECF, muscle, or adipose tissue.

Unexpected weight gain often is a result of retention of fluid (edema). Retention of fluid equal to 10% of body weight may occur without clinical signs of edema. Patients with CRF may gain in edema fluid and lose muscle and adipose tissue, so that weight stays the same but undetected changes in composition occur (muscle mass declines; ECF volume expands). This pattern has obscured the development of edema and wasting in children on hemodialysis (Table 1.6) and illustrates the need for a good method of measuring body composition in clinical practice.

Rate of weight gain (g/kg/day) is commonly used to define the rate of recovery from malnutrition; the energy cost of weight gain is 5 kcal/g weight gain (47). Infants recovering from malnutrition may gain 14 to 15 g/kg/day; adults may gain 7 g/kg/day under these conditions (48) (chapter 11).

Recording weight gain in relation to body weight (g/kg/day) is useful in correlating weight gain to diet and the disposition of calories and protein when expressed in relation to body weight, i.e., calories/kg/day or protein as g/kg/day. Weight expressed as centiles, while useful, is subject to a variety of interpretations. It is good practice in following growth to record change in weight in relation to change in height in centiles on growth charts that are now widely available.

Table 1.6
Changes in Body Composition in a 16-year-old Male on Hemodialysis and Immediately Posttransplant

Time on dialysis (month)	Body weight (kg)	ECF (Br) (L)	Body weight—ECF (kg)
13	55.9	14.9	41
15	57.3	18.7	38.6
18	58.3	14.6	42.7
32	54.5 (−3.8)	24.8 (+10.2)	29.7 (−13)
33[a]	47 (−7.5)	16 (−8.8)	31

References

1. Holliday MA: Metabolic rate and organ size during growth from infancy to maturity. Pediatrics 47:169, 1971.
2. Edelman IS, Leibman J: Anatomy of the body fluids. Am J Med 27:256, 1959.
3. Aukland K, Nicolaysen G: Interstitial fluid volume: local regulatory mechanisms. Physiol Rev 61:556, 1981.
4. Guyton AC, Taylor AE, Granger HJ: Circulatory Physiology. II. Dynamics and control of the body fluids. Philadelphia, W.B. Saunders Co., 1975.
5. Skou JC: Enzymatic basis for active transport of Na+ and K+ across cell membranes. Physiol Rev 45:596, 1965.
6. Smith TJ, Edelman IS: The role of sodium transport in thyroid thermogenesis. Fed Proc 38:2150, 1979.
7. Brozek J, Grande F: Body composition and basal metabolism in man. Correlation analysis versus physiological approach. Human Biol 27:22, 1955.
8. Owen OE, Morgan AP, Kemp HG, et al: Brain metabolism during fasting. J Clin Invest 46:1519, 1967.
9. Cahill GF, Herrera MG, Morgan AP, et al: Hormone-fuel interrelationships during fasting. J Clin Invest 45:1751, 1966.
10. Kennedy C, Sokoloff L: An adaptation of the nitrous oxide method to the study of cerebral circulation in children. J Clin Invest 36:1130, 1957.
11. Garrow JS: Energy Balance and Obesity in Man. New York, American Elsevier, 1974, p 5.
12. Thureau K: Renal Na reabsorption and O_2 uptake in dogs during hypoxia and hydrochlorthiazide infusion. Proc Soc Exp Biol Med 106:714, 1961.
13. Fern EB, Garlick PJ, McNurlan MA, et al: The excretion of isotope in urea and ammonia for estimating protein turnover in man with ^{15}N glycine. Clin Sci 61:217, 1981.
14. Cuthbertson DP: In Munro HN, Allison JB (eds): Mammalian Protein Metabolism. New York, Academic Press, 1964, vol 2, p 19.
15. Gamble JL: Physiological information gained from studies on the life raft ration. Harvey Lect Ser 42:247, 1946.
16. Young VW: Skeletal and cardiac muscle in regulation of protein turnover. In Munro HN (ed): Protein Metabolism. New York, Academic Press, 1970, vol 4, p 1641.
17. Kerr D, Ashworth A, Picou D, et al: Accelerated recovery from infant malnutrition with high calorie feeding. In Gardner LL, Amacher P (eds): Endocrine Aspects of Malnutrition. Santa Ynez, Calif., Kroc Foundation, 1973, p 467.
18. Keys A, Brozek J: Body fat in adult man. Physiol Rev 33:245, 1953.
19. Garrow JS, Fletcher K, Halliday D: Body composition in severe infantile malnutrition. J Clin Invest 44:417, 1965.
20. Ashworth A: An investigation of very low calorie intakes reported in Jamaica. Brit J Nutr 22:341, 1968.
21. Forbes GB: Lean body mass and fat in obese children. Pediatrics 34:308, 1964.
22. James WPT: Energy requirements and obesity. Lancet 2:386, 1983.
23. Friis-Hansen B: body composition during growth Pediatrics 47:264, 1971.
24. Foman SJ: Body composition of the male reference infant during the first year of life. Pediatrics 40:683, 1966.
25. Widdowson EM, Dickerson JWT: Chemical composition of the body. In Comer CL, Bronner L (eds): Mineral Metabolism. New York, Academic Press, 1964, vol 2, p 1.
26. Cheek DB: ECF volume: Its structure and measurement and the influence of age and disease. J Pediatr 58:103, 1961.
27. Foman SJ, Thomas LN, Filer LJ, et al: food composition and growth of normal infants fed milk-based formulas. Acta Paediat Scand (Suppl 223):1, 1971.
28. Joint FAO/WHO ad hoc Expert Committee: Energy and Protein Requirements. WHO Techn Rept Ser #522, 1973.
29. Holliday MA: Body composition and energy needs during growth. In Falkner F, Tanner JM (eds): Human Growth. New York and London, Plenum Press, 1979, p 126.
30. Malcolm L: Protein-energy malnutrition and growth. In Falker F, Tanner JM (eds): Human Growth, ed 1. New York and London, Plenum Press, 1979, vol 3, p 361.
31. Payne PR, Waterlow JC: Relative requirements for maintenance growth and physical activity. Lancet 2:210, 1971.
32. Bier DM, Leak RD, Haymond MW, et al: Measurement of "truc" glucose production rates in infancy and children with 6,6-didenteroglucose. Diabetes 26:1016, 1977.
33. Sinclair JC, Scopes JW, Silverman WA: Metabolic reference standards for the neonate. Pediatrics 39:724, 1967.

34. Nichols G, Nichols N, Weil W, et al: The direct measurement of the extracellular phase of tissues. J Clin Invest 32:1299, 1953.
35. Barratt M, Walser M: Extracellular fluid in individual tissues in whole animals: the distribution of radiosulfate and radiobromide. J Clin Invest 48:56,1969.
36. Middleton ES, Matthews R, Shires GR: Radiosulfate as a measure of the extracellular space in acute hemorrhagic shock. Ann Surg 170:174, 1969.
37. Kaufman L, Wilson CJ: Determination of extracellular fluid volume by fluorescent excitation analysis of bromide. J Nucl Med 14:812, 1972.
38. Knochel JP, Seldin DW: The pathophysiology of uremia. In Brenner BM, Rector FC (eds): The Kidney. W.B. Saunders Co., ed 2. Philadelphia, 1981, p 2150.
39. Edelman IS, Liebman J, O'Meara MP et al: Interrelations between serum sodium concentration, serum osmolality, and total exchangeable sodium, total exchangeable potassium and total body water. J Clin Invest 40:723, 1961.
40. Coles GA: Body composition in uremia. Quart J Med 41:25, 1971.
41. Patrick J: Assessment of body potassium stores. Kidney Intl 11:476, 1977.
42. Cheek DB: Human Growth: Body Composition, Cell Growth, Energy and Intelligence. Philadelphia, Lea & Febiger, 1968, p 189.
43. Forbes GB, Bruining GJ: Urinary creatinine excretion and lean body mass. Am J Clin Nutr 29:1359, 1976.
44. Brook CGD: Determination of body composition of children from skinfold measurements. Arch Dis Child 46:182, 1971.
45. Durnin JVGA, Rahaman MM: The assessment of the amount of fat in the human body from measurement of the skinfold thickness. Brit J Nutr 21:631, 1967.
46. Jelliffe DB, Jelliffe EFP: In Falkner F, Tanner JM (eds): Epidemiological Considerations in Human Growth. New York and London, Plenum Press, 1979, vol 3, p 395.
47. Spady DW, Payne PR, Picore D, et al: Energy balance during recovery from malnutrition. Am J Clin Nutr 29:1073, 1976.
48. Keys A, Brozek J, Henschel A, et al: The Biology of Human Starvation. Minneapolis, Minn., University of Minnesota Press, 1950.

CHAPTER 2

Statural Growth and Maturation

MICHAEL A. PREECE

INTRODUCTION

The growth of a child is generally assessed in terms of height and weight. However, growth is far too complex a phenomenon to be described by these simple measurements alone; changes in body composition and proportion also need to be considered. This wider view is particularly important when assessing growth in relation to chronic illness in which the growth pattern may be distorted, as well as globally retarded.

The study of growth encompasses not only the physical aspects of increase in size, but also the physiologic mechanisms that control it. This chapter will describe the biology of skeletal growth and emphasize the key role of the chondrocyte, review the endocrine control of normal growth, describe the normal pattern of growth, consider the methodology in its assessment, and present data on the normal variation of growth and standards by which it can be assessed.

BIOLOGY OF SKELETAL GROWTH

The Cartilage

The endocrine system influences skeletal growth mainly through its effect on the chondrocyte. Exceptions are parathyroid hormone (PTH) and vitamin D, which have major roles in influencing calcification and the maintenance of calcified tissues (chapter 9). This chapter will describe the general properties of the chondrocyte and its environment, its relevance to growth, and discuss its behavior in response to growth hormone (GH), thyroid, and the sex hormone axes. While such other hormones as the prostaglandins may interact with cartilage cells, their role in growth is unclear.

The Chondrocyte

For a description of cartilage and its functions see the comprehensive text of Stockwell (1). There are many important differences in chondrocytes and their matrix according to the cartilage source, e.g., articular or growth plate origin. Typical chondrocytes are ovoid cells with irregular surfaces and projecting cell processes. Size varies considerably with a greater diameter of 10 to 30 μm. The shape, size, and other characteristics of cell morphology are influenced by the type of cartilage, the position of the cell in the tissue, the cell density, age, and many other factors.

The Cell Membrane

The cell membrane has the usual structure of a bimolecular leaflet of phospholipids and cholesterol coated with protein, including glycoproteins. Immunologic studies suggest these are the receptor sites for hormones (2). Closely associated with the cell membrane are a number of small vesicles of at least two types: (1) spherical or flask-shaped, opening to the exterior, which enable several materials to enter the cell and (2) acanthosomes, which are fewer in number and probably are responsible as receptors for intake of specific proteins (3).

Cells generally have numerous processes, although those near tissue boundaries may be relatively smooth. These cell processes are continually changing shape and influence the pericellular matrix. The pericellular matrix is finely textured and different from the more remote fibrous matrix. In immature cartilage, especially fetal, a single specialized process, or cilium, may be present for which a specific role of chemoreceptor has been suggested (4).

Internally there is a single nucleus of about 0.004 μm in diameter with a deoxyribonucleic acid (DNA) content (about 7×10^{-12} g/chondrocyte) similar to other tissue cell types. In immature cells, and occasionally in more mature cells, microtubules are observed (5). They bind alkaloids, such as colchicine, vinblastine, and vincristine, which in turn inhibit cell function. The microtubules have important structural functions and are involved in collagen secretion (6). This provides a mechanism whereby drugs such as the vinca alkaloids may deleteriously affect growth. However, the intermittent or short-term use of these drugs would minimize their effect on growth.

The granular endoplasmic reticulum and the Golgi complex are the most prominent cytoplasmic organelles. The primary role of the Golgi complex is the packaging of secretory proteins, which are synthesized in the rough endoplasmic reticulum. A second major function of this complex in the chondrocyte is polysaccharide synthesis (7), which is essential to synthesis of proteoglycans secreted into the pericellular matrix.

In cartilage, lysosomes are involved in local control of the matrix. Exteriorization of lysosomal enzymes is important in normal degradation and turnover of the matrix (8), and thus relevant to the degenerative growth plate changes that occur before calcification (9).

Mitochondria in the chondrocyte also show some special features. They contain dense granules of calcium phosphate as a result of Ca^{++} uptake by transport systems in the inner membrane. In calcifying cartilage, this becomes exaggerated; it is far less prominent in noncalcifying tissue, suggesting a role in bone calcification (10).

Table 2.4.
Mean Height Velocities and Standard Deviations for Males and Females in the U.K. Centered on Peak-Height Velocity Age[a]

Age (years)	Males		Females	
	Mean (cm)	SD (cm)	Mean (cm)	SD (cm)
7.25			5.74	0.85
7.75			5.60	0.82
8.25			5.50	0.79
8.75			5.49	0.78
9.25	5.30	0.74	5.46	0.78
9.75	5.20	0.71	5.44	0.80
10.25	5.12	0.69	5.50	0.87
10.50			5.64	0.92
19.75	5.04	0.68	5.92	0.97
11.00			6.50	1.01
11.25	4.98	0.69	7.21	1.05
11.50			7.90	1.08
11.75	4.94	0.74	8.27	1.10
12.00			8.33	1.10
12.25	5.02	0.83	8.17	1.10
12.50			7.56	1.09
12.75	5.65	0.96	6.57	1.07
13.00			5.50	1.05
13.25	7.45	1.11	4.48	1.01
13.50	8.67	1.15		
13.75	9.35	1.19	2.86	0.91
14.00	9.46	1.20		0.77
14.25	9.22	1.19	1.86	
14.50	8.20	1.18		0.57
14.75	7.03	1.16	1.08	
15.25	4.70	1.09		
15.75	3.20	0.99		
16.25	2.08	0.84		
16.75	1.22	0.62		

From Tanner JM, Whitehouse RH, Takaishi M: Arch Dis Childh 41:454, 1966.

[a] Peak-Height Velocity Age: 12.0, Females and 14.0, Males.

tissue diameters, together with the standard deviations, are found in Tanner and coworkers (40), from which standards could be constructed readily.

Bone Diameters. In Figure 2.2, *A* the distance curves for the mean width of humerus and tibia from the age of 3-years onward are shown. These data, together with those in Fig. 2.2, *B* and *C*, are taken from (40) and give details of methods and further analysis of the growth of these tissue components. The humerus in males is, on average, slightly wider than the girls until the female adolescent spurt starts. The means are then equal for about 2 years, after which the greater growth spurt commences in males. In tibia width, there is no sex difference before the the onset of puberty but by maturity bones in both show a 13% greater width in the male than in the female.

Limb Muscle. In Fig. 2.2, *B*, where calf and arm muscle widths are illustrated, it can be seen that before puberty the curves are similar to those for bone, although the sex difference in the arm is somewhat greater for muscle. At puberty, there is a marked growth spurt in both limb muscles in males; in females, the arm muscle increases only slightly while the calf muscle comes to exceed that of boys between the ages of 11 and 15. By full maturity, the male preponderance is much greater in the arm (about 20%) than in the calf (10%).

Limb Fat. Figure 2.2, *C* shows the widths of the fat layer again for

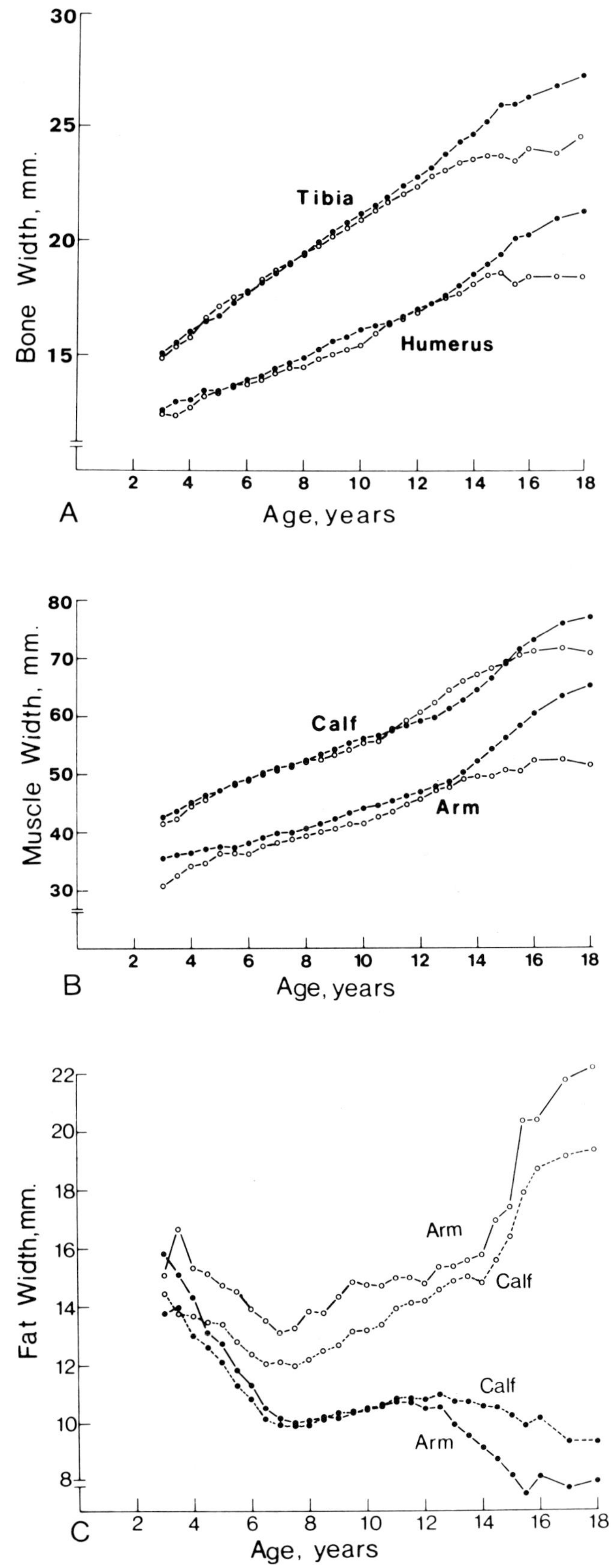

Figure 2.2. Distance curves of growth for limb bone (**A**), muscle (**B**), and fat (**C**) diameters for males (*filled circles*) and females (*open circles*). (From Tanner JM, Hughes PCR, Whitehouse RH: Ann Hum Biol 8:495, 1981.)

arm and calf. At both sites, males have less fat than females from age 4 years onward. The difference is increased during childhood, particularly at puberty. In both sexes, fat width falls from 3 to about 7 years, then starts to rise. In males, the rise is replaced from about 12 to 18 years by a further loss, which is greater in the arm than in the calf. In females, fat accumulates fairly continuously except for a period during puberty from 10 to 12 years of age, when arm fat remains fairly constant; note the marked increase in fat in postpubertal girls. Essentially, the same pattern is seen when triceps skinfold is used as a measure of limb fat. The changes tend to be less dramatic but clearly reflect the same events.

METHODOLOGY

Measurement of Skeletal Dimensions

For a more expanded discussion of these and other anthropometric techniques see Cameron (41). In all these measurements, it is important to assess the reliability of the results. There is a vast and confusing literature on this subject, but the simplest method of assessment is when the observer measures a number of subjects twice, long enough apart to have forgotten the first result. The standard error of measure (s_{meas}) can then be computed. Cameron (38) also provides examples of attainable s_{meas} values from major North American studies.

Height

This, in many ways, is the simplest and most frequent of anthropometric measurements, but it often the most abused. In many clinics, it is left to the most junior members of the staff so that the results thus obtained are often useless. It is only by attention to detail and by treating with respect what is often thought to be a rather simple measurement that useful information will result. For this reason, no apology is made for a rather didactic description of measurement technique.

The patient's shoes and socks should be removed, not only because they will affect the height but because they may conceal slight raising of the heels. The patient stands straight, so that the heels, buttocks, and shoulders are in contact with the vertical backboard of the stadiometer illustrated in Figure 2.3.

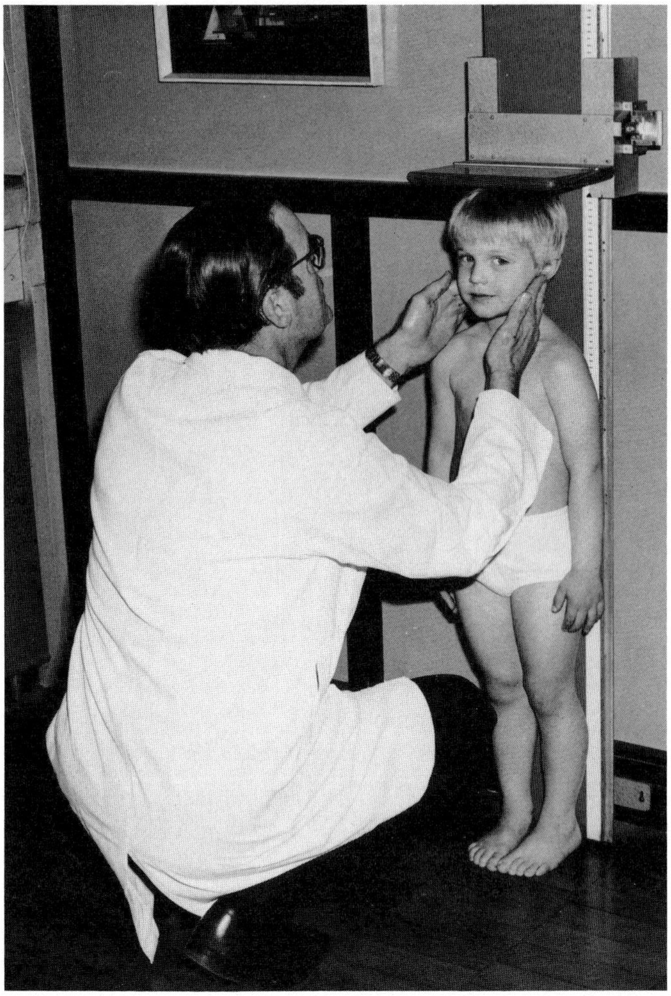

Figure 2.3. Measurement of height using a Harpenden stadiometer.

It may be necessary, particularly when young children are being measured, for an assistant to hold the heel down so that the undersides of the heels are in constant contact with the ground. The heels are placed together so that the medial malleoli are touching or occasionally, if the subject has genu valgum, so that the knees are together and feet slightly spread. The shoulders should be relaxed, sloping forward as naturally as possible to minimize lordosis. The head is positioned in the Frankfurt plane and the headboard of the stadiometer is slid down until it touches the patient's head. To ensure that the head stays in contact with the headboard and to minimize the effect of hair thickness, a weight of about 1 kg should be placed on the headboard.

The child is instructed to inhale, stand as tall as possible to aid the straightening of the spine, and then asked to exhale and relax. At this time, a little spinal traction may be exerted by gentle upward pressure on the mastoid processes. This stretching minimizes the diurnal variation, which may be as much as 2 cm without it. At this point, the measurement is read and preferably recorded by a second person.

Supine Length

The child is placed on the supine-length table or, if younger than 9 months, in the neonatometer (42), with the head held in the supinated Frankfurt plane (42). The head is held in this position by an assistant standing directly behind the headboard of the table or neonatometer. Especially when measuring young children and always when using the neonatometer, the assistant must apply downward pressure on the shoulders to prevent arching of the back. Having secured the head and shoulders of the child, the assistant applies gentle pressure to bring the head into contact with the headboard, while the observer having ensured that the legs are straight, the ankles are at right angles, and the toes are pointing directly upward, brings the footboard into firm contact against the child's heels. Only one heel is positioned when using the neonatometer. Such is the lack of cooperation from most infants that the observer will often find it necessary to apply downward pressure to the knee while maintaining a firm grip on the patient's foot.

Sitting Height

This is most easily measured using a sitting-height table, with the same instructions and encouragements used as for stature. Alternatively, an anthropometer may be used, but this technique is more difficult in relatively inexperienced hands (41). Subischial leg length is obtained by subtracting sitting height from stature. These measures are of particular value in assessing the growth of children with a disease process that particularly affects distinct areas of the body. For example, poor limb growth as a result of metaphyseal disease or poor vertebral growth secondary to abdominal radiation therapy will be seen clearly. In chronic renal disease, it is possible that subischial leg length may have extra importance related to the development of osteodystrophy.

The principal source of error in sitting height and, hence, subischial leg length is the influence of the thickness of gluteal muscle and fat. Marked changes, such as those due to the effects of diet, can lead to puzzling results in the trunk and limb dimensions.

Skinfold Measurements

These measurements are prone to many errors and, of the techniques described here, are the most difficult. However, they are by far the best assessment of subcutaneous fat; from them, extrapolations to total body fat and other measures of body composition are possible. The variation in the consistency of subcutaneous tissue and the individual way in which each measurer collects the fold of tissue seems to be the main source of error. The two most useful sites for measurement are the triceps and subscapular areas. The best instrument to use is the Harpenden skinfold caliper, which combines the requirements of a constant jaw pressure, easily read scale, and an ergonomic design to maximize accuracy.

Upper Arm Circumference

This measurement is one of the most straightforward to make and is used quite extensively. It reflects both subcutaneous fat and muscle bulk, so that it is a rather mixed measurement. However, in collaboration with tissue specific measurements, such as skinfold thickness, it may give additional valuable information. The child is positioned with the left arm completely relaxed and extended at the side. The measurement is taken midway between the acromium and the olecranon with an inextensible steel tape. It is important that the tape is in a plane perpendicular to the long axis of the limb and that the tissues are not compressed.

Maturity Indicators

Chronological age is a poor measure of maturity (43). The average maturing male completes his growth at 18 years of age, whereas an early developer may do so at 15 or 16 years; a late developer may still be growing at 20 years of age. The same is true of females, except that the whole process occurs about 2 years earlier. The growth of an early developer is advanced for the entire period of growth, including puberty, unless the advance is the result of a late-acquired factor. In precocious puberty, growth rate is accelerated but time of growth is shortened. The opposite applies in malnutrition, which leads to growth delay. In both cases, final height is reduced. Because these differences in the pattern of maturation are not accounted for by chronological age, other measures are needed to categorize a child as advanced or delayed in maturation (43). The variable pattern of an individual's maturation rate can be conveniently referred to as "tempo." Several measures of physiologic maturity have been advocated, all depending on defining a sequence of events that occur in an invariant order and which always occur in every individual that reaches maturity. Implicitly, each individual must reach the same final event at maturity.

Stages of Puberty

If the assessment of maturity is limited to the peripubertal stage of growth and development, the stages of puberty provide a convenient and reliable assessment of maturation. Almost universally, the systems in current use depend on the criteria formalized by Tanner (43). These depend on a rating of breast and pubic hair development on a 5-point scale and axillary hair on a 3-point scale for females and external genitalia, as well as pubic and axillary hair, on similar scales for males.

The breast stages for girls are illustrated in Figure 2.4 and are defined as follows:

Stage 1. Preadolescent: elevation of papilla only.

Stage 2. Breast-bud stage: elevation of breast and papilla as a small mound; enlargement of areolar diameter.

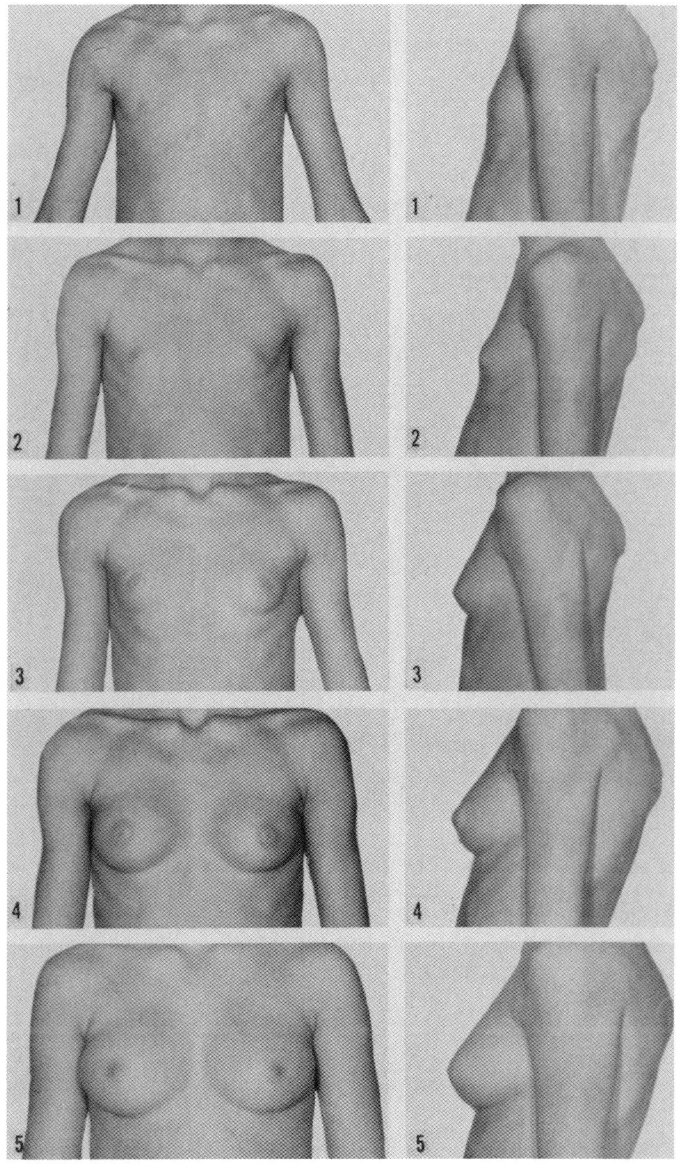

Figure 2.4. Standards for breast development ratings. (From Tanner JM: Growth at Adolescence, ed 2. Oxford, U.K., Blackwell Scientific Publication, 1962.)

Stage 3. Further enlargement and elevation of breast and areola with no separation of their contours.

Stage 4. Projection of areola and papilla to form a secondary mound above the level of the breast.

Stage 5. Mature stage: projection of papilla only, a result of recession of the areola to the general contour of the breast.

The Stage 4 development of the areolar mound does not occur in all girls, in 25% it is absent and in a further 25% it is relatively slight.

Genitalia stages for boys are shown in Figure 2.5 and are defined as follows:

Stage 1. Preadolescent: testes, scrotum, and penis are about the same size and proportion as in early childhood.

Stage 2. Enlargement of scrotum and testes. The skin of the scrotum reddens and changes in texture, with little or no enlargement of penis at this stage.

Stage 3. Enlargement of penis, which occurs at first mainly in length, and further growth of testes and scrotum.

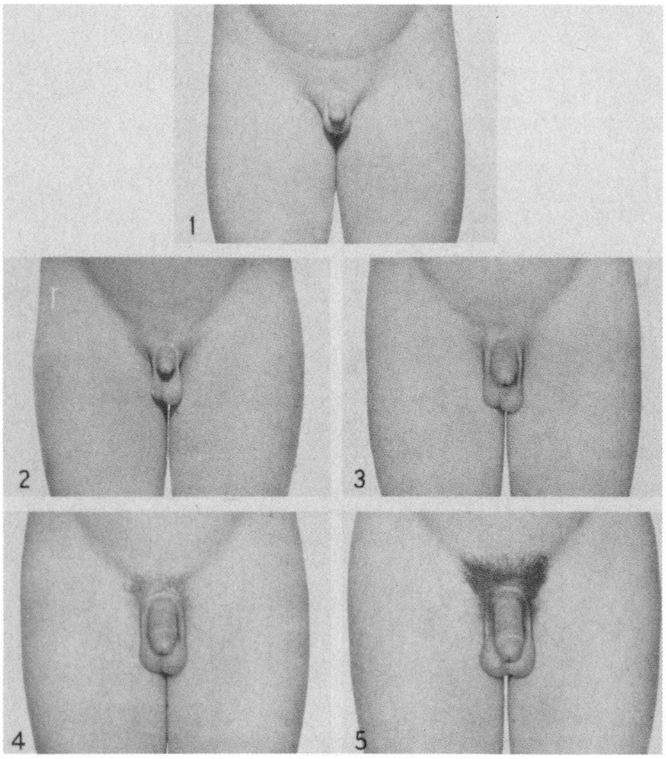

Figure 2.5. Standards for genitalia development ratings. (From Tanner JM: Growth at Adolescence, ed 2. Oxford, U.K., Blackwell Scientific Publications, 1962.)

Stage 4. Increased size of penis with growth in breadth, development of glans, further enlargement of testes and scrotum with increasing darkening of scrotal skin.

Stage 5. Genitalia are adult in size and shape.

Pubic hair stages for both sexes are illustrated in Figure 2.6 and are defined as follows:

Stage 1. Preadolescent: the vellus over the pubis is not further developed than over the abdominal wall.

Stage 2. Sparse growth of long, slightly pigmented downy hair, straight or only slightly curled, appearing chiefly at the base of the penis or along the labia.

Stage 3. Considerably darker, coarser, and more curled. The hair spreads sparsely over the junction of the pubis.

Stage 4. Hair now resembles adult type, but the area covered by it is still considerably smaller than in the adult with no spread to the medial surface of the thighs.

Stage 5. Adult in quantity and type, with distribution of the horizontal (or classically 'feminine') pattern. Spread to the medial surface of thighs but not up linea alba or elsewhere above the base of the inverse triangle.

Axillary in both sexes has only 3 stages: Stage 1, no hair; Stage 2, a small amount; and Stage 3, normal adult distribution. It is seldom, if ever, possible to see the actual transition from one stage to another. One can only be certain that a subject is in, say, Genitalia-2 (G2) but not yet G3. To underline this we usually talk of Stage G2+.

There are three major problems with pubertal stages. They are only relevant in the peripubertal child, they are relatively subjective, and the staging is unavoidably spread coarsely. Two maturity indicators that have been used in an endeavor to overcome these deficits have been skeletal and dental age.

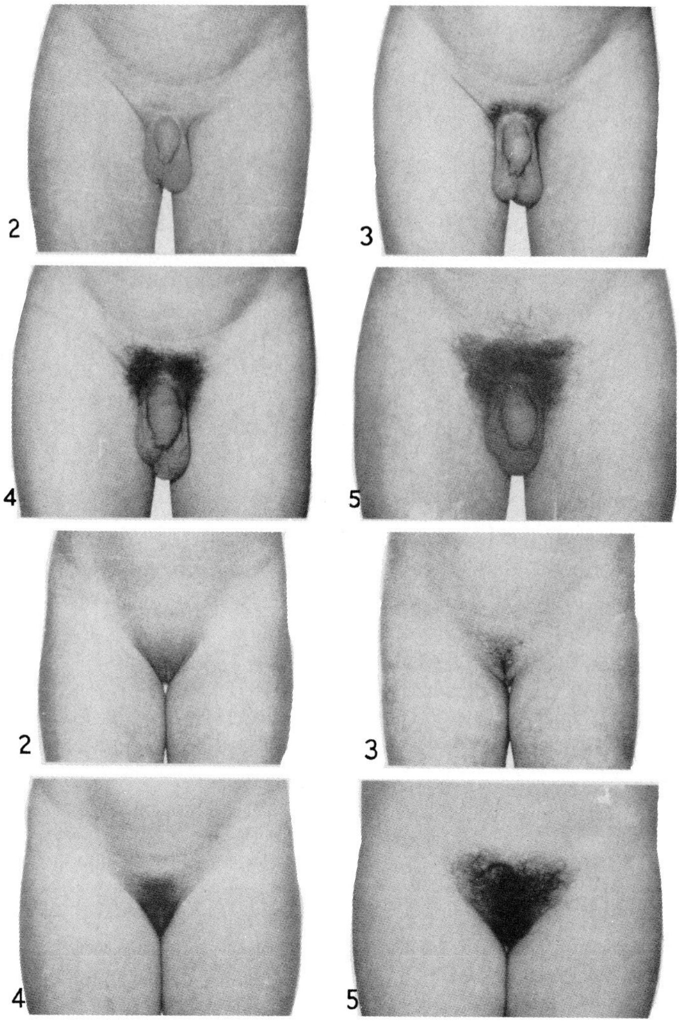

Figure 2.6. Standards for pubic hair development ratings for males and females. (From Tanner JM: Growth at Adolescence, ed 2. Oxford, U.K., Blackwell Scientific Publications, 1962.)

Skeletal Age

There are three current methods for assessing skeletal age, although there have been earlier methods that contributed to the evolution of newer techniques. The older method still in use is that first described in 1950 by Greulich and Pyle and subsequently revised in 1959 (44). In this method, a sequence of hand-wrist radiographs are displayed that are typical of children of specific chronologic age. While the authors intended the user to compare each bone of the patient's x-ray film carefully with the appropriate standard and then derive a median skeletal age, the tendency has been to find the example that most closely resembles the patient's and call that the skeletal "age." This is an unsatisfactory method, as the observer easily becomes focused on a few bones, especially the radius, ulna, and carpal bones, leading to a biased assessment. A further problem is that a Greulich and Pyle method was based mainly on the radiographs of the Brush Foundation Study (45), which consisted of socially advantaged children. They had relatively advanced skeletal maturation compared with other American children and even more when compared with European children. At present, the secular trend for earlier maturation has almost removed the social bias with respect to present-day Americans, but Europeans are still, on average, 9-months delayed. Thus, an average maturing European child, assessed by the

Greulich and Pyle method, will appear to have a skeletal age delay of 9 months.

Modifications of Greulich and Pyle have the same limitations and are based on the knee or foot and ankle (46, 47).

Preferred methods are those that use the bone-specific scoring systems for the hand-wrist (48) and the knee (49). In these, each bone is assessed according to a number of specific maturity indicators to which a score is attached. Only after scoring each indicator is it possible to derive a total maturity score, which may then be translated into a skeletal "age" by comparison with appropriate standards. Thus, it is impossible to use a short-cut as in the atlas method. The methods can be used for any population, although it is wise to develop specific standards for each country by first applying the methods to x-ray films of normal children of the appropriate background. The standards are derived from British (48), United States (49), and French (49a) children, respectively.

Dental Age

The concept of dental age has existed since the 1920s. Initially, it was based on a count of the number of erupted teeth, deciduous or permanent, but it has been refined in a number of ways. When purely dependent on visible teeth, it has the attraction of being immediate but is unfortunately very crude. In general, it offers little in the context of the present volume and will not be considered further. It was reviewed in more detail in Preece (50).

Summary

It is important to remember that some measures of maturity may be affected in the disease process. When this happens they may no longer represent a true maturity index, but a complex of maturational and pathological effects. In CRF, bone architecture is changed and the radiographic appearance of a hand-wrist or knee may no longer relate to the maturational processes. The appearances that would usually be interpreted as showing delayed maturation may be partly a result of bone disease. In this situation, caution in interpretation is required. Ideally, we should seek maturity indices that are not affected by the disease in question, but this is seldom possible; thus, established methods need to be used, but with caution.

It is important to consider how each maturity indicator correlates with others. Strikingly, there is poor correlation between any one system once chronological age (which measures the passage of time) has been taken into consideration (51). This is less surprising if we stop thinking of maturity indicators as direct measures of maturity but, rather, as measures of the inner biological clock, all using slightly different criteria. They show the same general pattern but the details and timing differ considerably.

Height Age

Since its use was suggested by Wilkins (52), the concept of height age has permeated much literature addressing growth disorders. This is unfortunate, since it incorporates a basic misunderstanding of the requirements for defining developmental age. An implicit assumption in developmental age is that all individuals reach the same mature endpoint. For stature, this is not so. A child may have a delayed height age for these reasons: delayed maturation, an absolute short final stature, or both. A child has a delayed skeletal age for only one reason: delayed maturation. Height age confounds these differences and may lead to a serious misclassification of diagnosis.

Height age is assigned by noting the age at which the average child of the same sex has the same height as the patient. It does not recognize that the child's family might be unusually short (or tall) and that, therefore, the population average is not relevant. Further, it takes no note of the normal variation of about 17 cm at adult size within a family, which is not dependent on maturity. The only valid way to use height as a measure of maturity is to compute an individual's height as a proportion of their own mature height, clearly a retrospective exercise and of little clinical value. Certainly height age has no place in modern auxological thinking.

Interpretation of Growth Data

Cross-sectional vs Longitudinal Methods

Cross-sectional standards are based on data obtained from a large number of children, each measured only on one occasion. In any one age group covering one year of chronological age, at least 100 children of each sex are required to produce even reasonable standards; for good estimates of the outer limits of normality, as many as 1000 children in each age band would be required (53). However, given that the numbers of children are available and that there are facilities for a large number of measuring teams, the logistics are not insuperable and standards can be developed fairly quickly.

In a longitudinal study, a much smaller number of children is needed, but they must be seen on multiple occasions at 3-, 6-, or 12-month intervals. The results develop a number of individual growth curves. By its very nature, the longitudinal study in its purest form has to be prolonged for as much as 20 years. This is clearly expensive in time, manpower, and the good will of the children. When the data collection is finished, the analysis is complex. For this reason, it is important to understand the arguments for and against the different types of standards (53).

Cross-sectional standards represent the status of a population in terms of the average size and its variance. This is fine if a child is assessed on one occasion or if one wishes to compare two populations of children as groups. This is not valid, however, if a single child, followed on many occasions as is usual in medical practice, is to be compared with a standard population. The problem would not arise if all children grew at the same tempo, i.e., if all children reached the same relative part of their growth curve at the same age, but this is not the case. This can be best illustrated by a particular example concentrating on the part of growth that is most affected by this, e.g., the adolescent growth spurt.

Figure 2.7, *A* depicts a series of individual velocity growth curves from 5 to 18 years of age, each growth spurt starting at a different time. These curves are quite typical of a small sample of children. If the mean velocity at each age is calculated and plotted, a curve such as the dotted line is generated, which bears no relationship to the true velocity curve of any single individual child. Translated into distance curve terms, the growth curve becomes flattened during adolescence and the spurt appears less prominent. Cross-sectional analysis introduces exactly this artifact.

Figure 2.7, *B* shows an alternative analysis, where each of the growth curves is aligned about its age of maximum velocity, then the averages are calculated. The mean velocity curve, again represented by the dotted line, now shows a good representation of an individual growth curve. Translated into distance curve terms, the mean height curve now closely represents the pattern of growth of an individual. Aligning the individual growth curves on a measure of developmental maturity, such as the age of peak velocity, are essential parts of longitudinal analysis and standards. In principle this effect could be seen at any age but it is most exaggerated in the first 3 years of life and in puberty. Between these age groups differences in means may be trivial but the variance differs and it is preferable to use one set of standards. In the case where children are followed through puberty and growth velocity scores are used, the scores can be recalculated once peak height velocity is determined and compared with norms developed in that manner (Table 2.4).

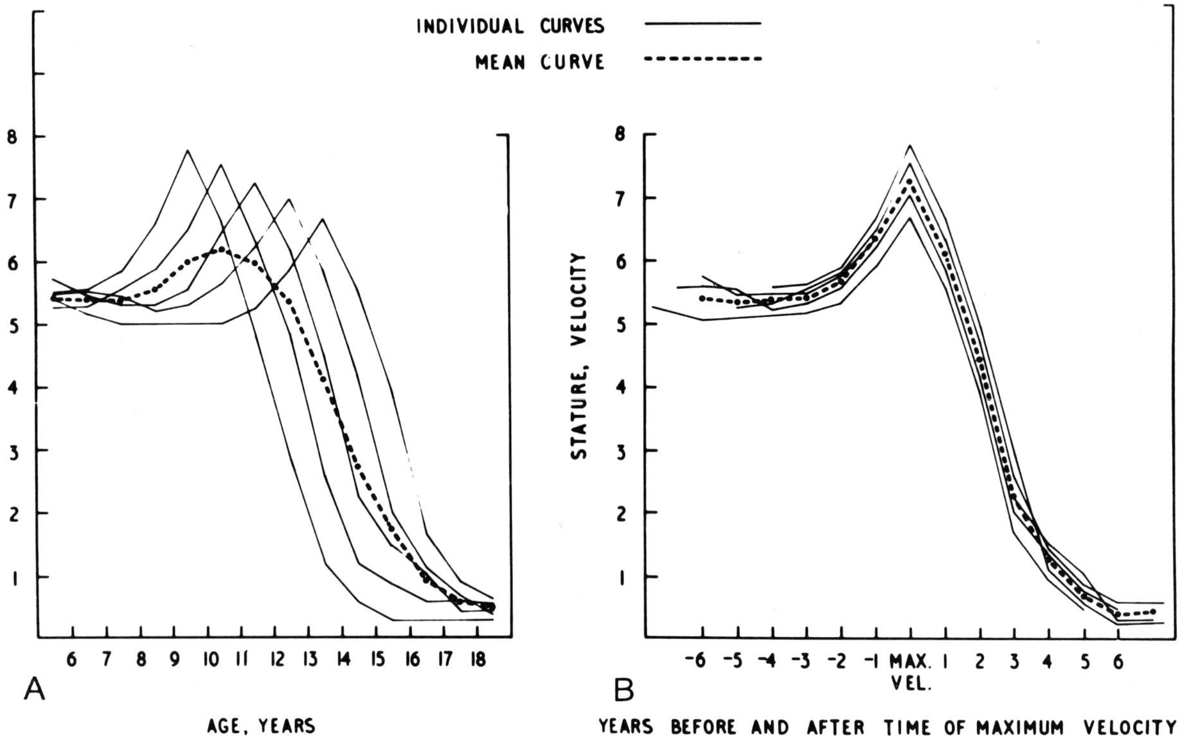

Figure 2.7. The relationship between individual and mean velocities during the adolescent growth spurt. **A**, The velocity curves are plotted against chronological age; **B**, They are plotted according to their time of maximum velocity. (From Tanner JM: Growth at Adolescence, ed 2. Oxford, U.K., Blackwell Scientific Publications, 1962.)

When children are to be observed on sequential occasions, their growth curves are best compared with longitudinal standards. Such longitudinal standards exist for many body dimensions in many countries and those data should be used. Further discussion of the mechanics and philosophy of growth standards may be found in Goldstein (53) or Healy (54).

Interpretation of Growth and its Changes

A frequent problem arises as to the best methods of expressing growth variables (height will be taken as a typical example) and of analyzing the changes. While children are within the normal range, transformation of the height to its centile is perfectly acceptable and is often the easiest way to explain the situation to the child and family. However, analysis in terms of centile values does not lend itself to statistical analysis and is clearly useless when the subjects are below the lowest published centile in height, which is the third or fifth centile.

In analyzing sets of growth data, especially in children outside the normal range, the use of Standard Deviation Scores (SDS) is more appropriate. In principle, any variable can be transformed provided the mean value and the standard deviation for each age and sex group are available. The width of the age band used for making the transformation should be quite narrow, ideally 6 months between 2 and 10 years of age and 3 months before 2 and between 10 and 16 years of age. The SDS is calculated from the relationship.

$$\mathrm{SDS} = \frac{x - x_i}{\mathrm{SD_i}} \qquad (1)$$

where x = actual measurement.

The mean value is x_i, and the standard deviation is $\mathrm{SD_i}$ for the i-th age band of the appropriate sex (55). In principle, there could be further subclassifications, such as ethnic or genetic origin or socioeconomic group, but numbers seldom allow for this. Fortunately, such differences are diminishing in western societies, as variations resulting from poor nutrition diminish. Comparing standards for height of UK and US children (Tables 2.1 and 2.2) show only slight differences. The SDS can be treated as a group independent of either age or sex. In a normal population the mean SDS will have a value of 0 and a standard deviation of 1; the 95% confidence limits will be between −2 and +2 SDS.

The use of SDS to assess the stature of a child or characterize a group of children is generally very powerful. However, there are major problems in using SDS of the distance curve to follow patients in a longitudinal study that covers several years. It is common practice to describe a stable SDS as "normal" growth when the SDS is below normal. This is misleading. For example, a group of children who maintain an average SDS of −3.0 for many years not only fails to catch up, as would be a reasonable expectation if health were restored, but incurs an increasing deficit in stature or "height deficit" (Table 2.5). Where SDS are used to describe progress in growth retarded children over more than 2 years, a statement describing change in height deficit with time provides additional useful information and is preferable to a statement that describes growth as percent of normal growth.

When SDS are applied to a population of subjects with delayed growth around the time of normal puberty, another problem can arise that becomes apparent from Fig. 2.8. As the normal population of adolescents enter their growth spurt (in this example, males at 12 years), the mean height normally increases rapidly. This is an inappropriate mean to use for calculating the patient's SDS as he is prepubertal. Some authorities advocate using the appropriate mean for skeletal age. In simple pubertal delay, this is probably acceptable. However, in many chronic illnesses, especially if corticosteroids have been used, skeletal age is poorly correlated with puberty and may not help. There is no generally accepted solution. However, an alternative we propose is to extend the prepubertal mean from age 10 in girls or age 12 in boys in a smooth curve, as shown in Figure 2.8, *A*, then using the appropriate values on this curve as the mean in the SDS calculation (Tables 2.1 and 2.2). The correct SD_i would be SD for age 10 years in females and 12 years in males. These extrapolated lines, while not exact, represent values observed over many years in patients with many different causes for severely delayed puberty. Similar figures, using local experience to supply the data, can be prepared when appropriate.

The male illustrated in Fig. 2.8, *A* at age 14 has a height of 136.2 cm that, using the population standards (Table 2.1), gives a SDS of (136.2 − 160.6)/6.6 = −3.70. One year later, having grown at a velocity of 3.8 cm/year, (Fig. 2.8, *B*) his height is 140 cm with a SDS of (140 − 168.7/6.6) = −4.35, apparently much worse. Using the modified calculations, in which the height is interpolated from the curve and the SD at 12 years is used to calculate the SDS, his initial SDS = (136.2 − 157)/6.5 = −3.20 and at 15 years is (140 − 160)/6.5 = −3.08. These latter figures give a more realistic expression of growth status for this prepubertal boy whose "normal" height at 14.0 years would be 157 cm (Fig. 2.8, *A*) and whose expected velocity is 3 cm/year. For comparative studies, it is advised to confine the study to ages between 3 and 10 years for females and 3 and 12 years for males, and to a period of 1 or 2 years. When it is important to include children past 10 years of age in females and 12 years of age in males who remain prepubertal, extending the growth curves without the normal growth spurt, (as illustrated above) appears to be the safest course.

The use of SDS can be extended to velocity measurements when these are available (Table 2.3). They do, however, suffer with the same problems as with stature in the child at adolescent age who has delayed puberty. This can be solved in a similar manner to that advised for distance (Fig. 2.8, *B*) expressed as cm/year and SDS.

There is further caution to be exercised with velocity measurements, whether expressed as cm/year or SDS. All the standards are based on velocities measured over a whole year; strictly, this should apply in the case of test subjects. In many situations, whole-year velocities are not practical, particularly in children with complex diseases where the course of the illness is unstable. In this case, shorter time intervals may be required but interpretation of results requires caution. Periods of less than 6 months are probably valueless.

The question now arises of what is the best way to compare growth in the same child in response to some change of management or differences in comparable groups given different treatment regimens. Two possibilities are evident: change in stature SDS before and after treatment or change in velocity SDS. At first it seems that there is little to choose between the two methods, but this is not so. A change in height SDS of 1 unit will appear to be equivalent at whatever the age of the child. However, such a change has quite different significance at different ages. Using velocities and their SDS automatically allows for this, as the increments in growth are standardized for age as opposed to the distance values when height SDS and their changes are studied. For this reason,

Table 2.5.
Relationship Between Standard Deviation Score (SDS) and Height Deficit of a Child at Different Ages Who Maintains a Score of −3.0 SDS Using UK Data[a]

Age (years)	Value of 1 SD (cm)	Height (cm)	Normal height (cm)	Height deficit (cm)
UK				
1	2.69	68.23	76.3	8.1
2	3.30	76.0	85.9	9.9
4	4.30	88.7	101.6	12.9
6	5.14	99.2	114.6	15.4
8	5.73	109.0	126.2	17.2
10	6.20	118.3	136.9	18.6
12	6.48	127.5	146.9	19.4
14	6.59	140.8	160.6	19.8
US				
10	6.20	118.9	137.5	18.6
12	7.51	127.2	149.7	22.5
14	8.48	137.7	163.1	25.4

[a] Data for 10 to 14 years using US data also given. SD for distance curves during puberty are greater in US.

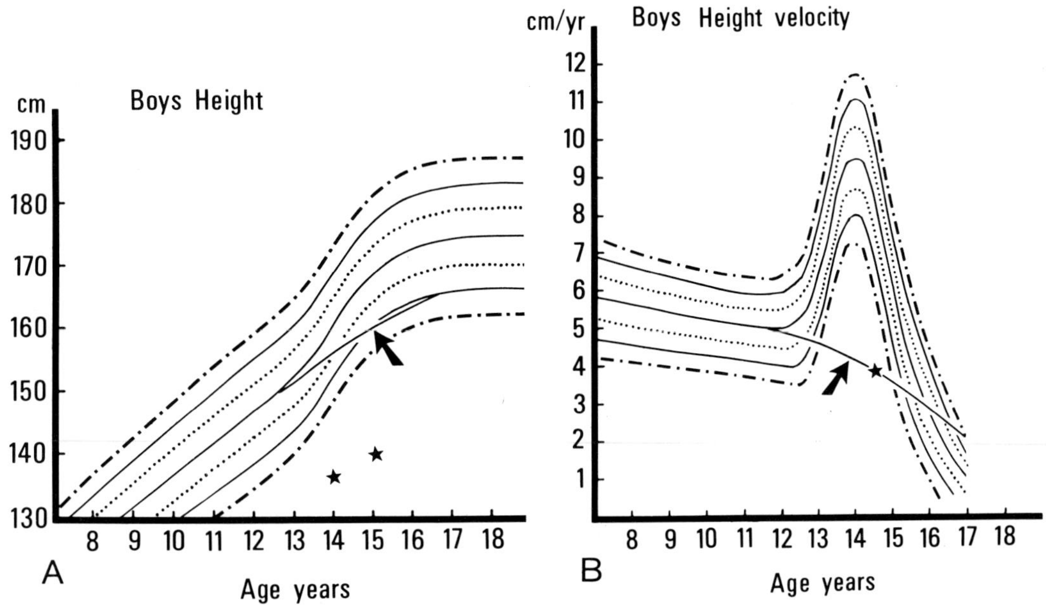

Figure 2.8. The normal distance (**A**) and velocity (**B**) standards from age 8 for males. In both figures the solid line marked with an arrow is a graphic extension of the 50th centile for males with delayed puberty. **A**, The two stars mark the height of such a male at 14 and 15 years of age and the single star marks his velocity.

it is preferable to use velocities when at all possible, as the principal means for comparing growth over time between two groups. Using distance SDS as supplemental data that describes each group relative to its norm may be useful.

The Fallacy of Ratio Standards

In many areas of medicine there is a tendency to quote certain biochemical and other results as a function of some measure of body size, most commonly weight or surface area and sometimes height. Pediatricians, because of the wide range in the size of patients, are especially prone to this; pediatric nephrology is no exception. There is, however, an important misconception in this practice that should be recognized by all who use such ratio standards, which is in effect what they are. The problems and assumptions of ratio standards have been extensively discussed by Tanner (56); a brief outline will be given here.

The use of a ratio, e.g., per surface area (SA) standard, implies that in a normal person the measure, say creatinine clearance (C_{Cr}), is proportional to SA; in fact, that the expression

$$C_{Cr} = k(\mathrm{SA}) \tag{2}$$

is valid over the range of SA for which the standard is used. The constant k would be the mean value of the C_{Cr}/m^2 values obtained in a study of normals. However, the formula implies that at zero SA, there is a zero C_{Cr}, i.e., the ratio line passes through the origin when extrapolated sufficiently. In fact, this is rarely the case and the relationship between variables, such as C_{Cr} and size, are more usually of the form of the regression equation:

$$C_{Cr} = a + b(\mathrm{SA}) \tag{3}$$

where a is significantly different from zero and usually positive. In this case the use of formula 2 when formula 3 is more correct will lead to identifying too many high values of C_{Cr} in small children and too many low ones in large children. If a in equation 3 is negative, the reverse would be true. C_{Cr} is used as an hypothetical example; but, before ratio standards such as equation 2 are used, the true relationship between the physiological measure and size must be checked. In certain situations, they may be correct but by no means in all.

There is a further problem, even when equation 2 is true. In serial measurement, it is more informative to provide the absolute measurement over time, as well as the ratio standard. In this way, changes in clearance with time can be envisioned, whereas changes in ratio incorporate both the changes in clearance and body size. When both are abnormal and changing at unpredictable rates, the ratio standard method above gives incomplete information.

NORMAL VARIATION IN GROWTH

Variation of Size by Age

Height Standards

Population Standards. In Figure 2.9 the curves use British standards for height for males (55), with the shape of the growth curve derived from analysis of normal longitudinal data. However, the range of normality, reflected by the centiles, was calculated from a much larger cross-sectional set of data so that the centiles conform to the shape of the individual's growth but with an overall spread to encompass the entire population. This is important, as longitudinal data are nearly always collected from a selected population of children, leading to an underestimate of population variance. The usual centiles, e.g., the 3rd, 10th, 25th, 50th, 75th, 90th, and 97th, are drawn to give guidance as to the normal variation in size. An alternative would be the use of +1, 2, or even 3 standard deviations. (Tables 2.1 and 2.2).

In Figure 2.9 there are two small shaded areas above the 97th and below the 3rd centile at the time of the adolescent growth spurt. These areas allow for the greater variance at this time in cross-sectional standards. Thus, a child who is seen for the first time, when we know nothing about his tempo and whose height lies in one of these areas, may be quite normal and just a little delayed or advanced in growth. A second visit will clarify the situation; if growth is normal, then the curve of growth will be closer to normal on subsequent visits.

It is conventional for children to be measured lying down until the age of 2 years and standing thereafter. For this reason, there is a small discontinuity in the standards at the age of 2 years as a child measured supine is about 1 cm taller than when measured standing. At the time of change-over from the supine to standing measurement, it is important that on at least two occasions both measurements are taken so that a correction can be made. Alternatively, it could be argued that children should be measured supine at all times, particularly when dealing with populations who are in the younger age groups. It would not be a major problem to adjust the standards accordingly, and in some countries this is routine.

Correction for Parental Height. The above standards are derived from population surveys; they can be made more accurate for a given child if the heights of the parents are taken into account. The easiest way of doing this is to plot the parents' centiles at the right-hand edge of the chart: age 19 for these standards. This is quickly done by plotting the actual height of the like-sexed parent and father's height, minus 12.5 cm, or the mother's height plus 12.5 cm, for the unlike-sexed parent. The 12.5 cm is the mean difference between adult men and women in the UK. (In the US, the difference is 13 cm.) When possible, this should be adjusted appropriately for other countries according to local data. The approximate position of the family 3rd and 97th centiles may be added by plotting the height of the parental mid-centile (the average between the parents' centile), and this height plus or minus 8 cm, which is obtained from the residual standard deviation for height after allowing for parents' heights (4.25 cm) multiplied by 1.88 (57).

The above technique also goes some way toward making allowances for large multiracial societies. An ideal would be race-specific standards (e.g. 58), but these are seldom available. Further, many differences that appear to be racial, are, in fact, environmental. Differences in standards because of race diminish considerably when measurements are made in the same country after environmental influences have asserted their effect (usually one or more generations).

Height Velocity Standards

Figure 2.10 shows the standards for height velocity for males. Once again the data are based on longitudinal observations and the extremes of normality are indicated by centiles. It is important to make two qualifications. In the first place, these normal values and the positions of the various centiles are based on velocity measurements taken over a whole year. If measurements were taken over a shorter time, then the spread between the 3rd and 97th centiles would be greater. This is because measurement errors assume greater importance as a percentage of the measured change and because there are substantial variations in growth velocity in any one year. This aspect has been explored more fully by Marshall (59), who has developed centiles for height velocity based on 3-month and 6-month velocity data. For this reason, it is important to interpret growth velocities cautiously when they are based upon periods of measurements of less than 1 year. In a perfect world no velocities should be compared to these standards unless they are calculated over a full year, but in practice this often is not possible.

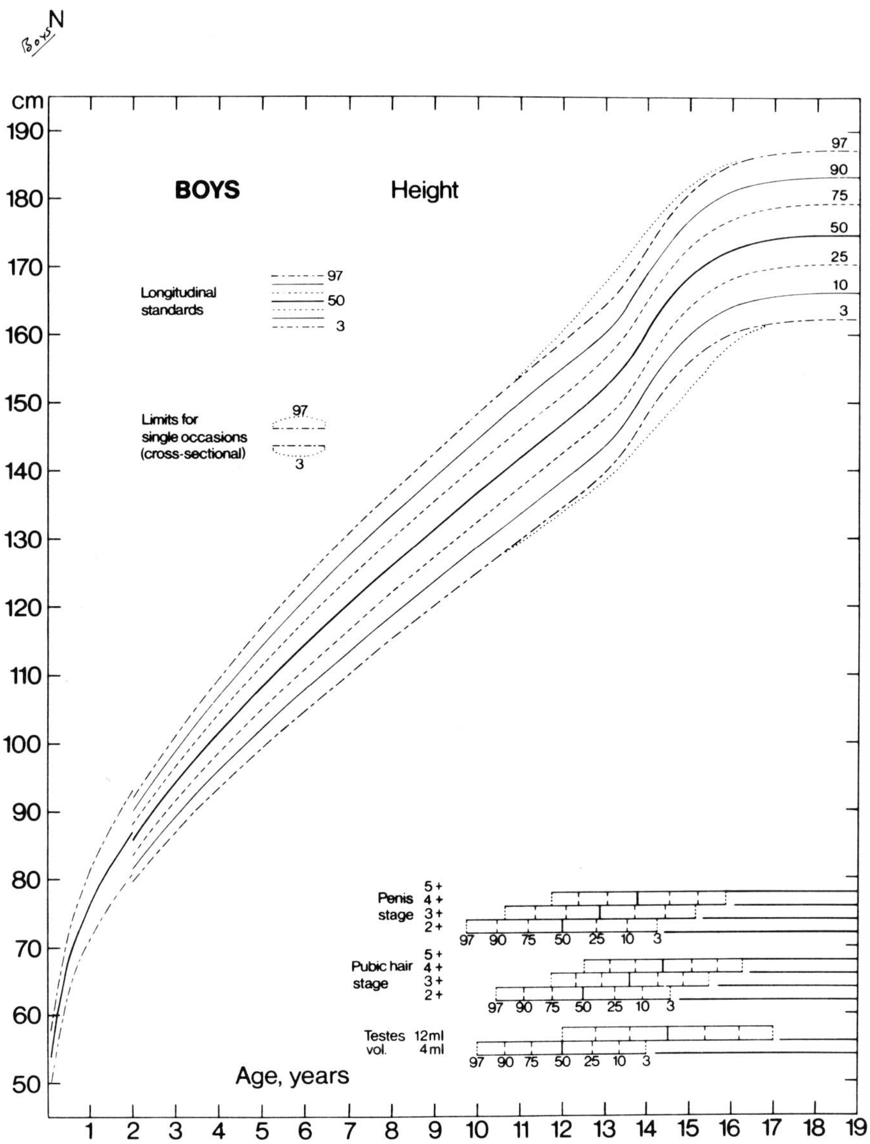

Figure 2.9. British standards for height for boys. (From Tanner JM, Whitehouse RH: Arch Dis Childh 51:170, 1976.)

The second comment that should be taken into account is that the various centiles for height velocity do have a different meaning to height centiles. On average over a year or more, any individual child who is growing normally should have a height velocity somewhere near the 50th centile for the population. If a child is to maintain the 10th centile for height, he should grow somewhere near the 40th centile for velocity. Similarly, a child who is maintaining his position on the 90th centile will have to grow at a slightly above average velocity but only at about the 60th centile. The child persistently growing at a 10th centile velocity will steadily fall further and further behind his peer group and soon become distinctly short and his SDS for height after 8 years of age will decline because SD is nearly constant.

In Fig. 2.10 there are two large grey areas flanking the adolescent growth spurt. The centiles are those for a child whose growth spurt occurs at an average age, i.e., 14 years. However, there is a normal variation in this age of attaining the peak growth spurt, i.e., approximately +2 years about the mean; the grey shaded areas in the Figure take this into account. In an individual case, the growth spurt should occur within the grey area with a shape similar to the centile centered at 14 years. Particularly in boys, earlier growth spurts tend to be more intense and later growth spurts less so; the same effect is seen in girls but to a less marked extent.

Other Standards. There are many other standards available for different measurements not illustrated here. Longitudinal standards exist for sitting height and subischial leg length (60) and cross-sectional standards for such measurements as biacromial and biiliac diameters and skinfold thickness.

A compendium of growth studies from all parts of the world has been prepared by Eveleth and Tanner (61) and is valuable source of reference data. There follows an abbreviated list of source references for the more important standards suitable for calculation of SDS and the comparison of patients from different countries: Belgium (62), Cuba (63), France (64), India (65), Italy (66), Japan (67), Sweden (68), United Kingdom (36.55), and the United States (69, 70).

For convenience, some tables of British and North American standards are included here. Table 2.1 gives the British height standards and

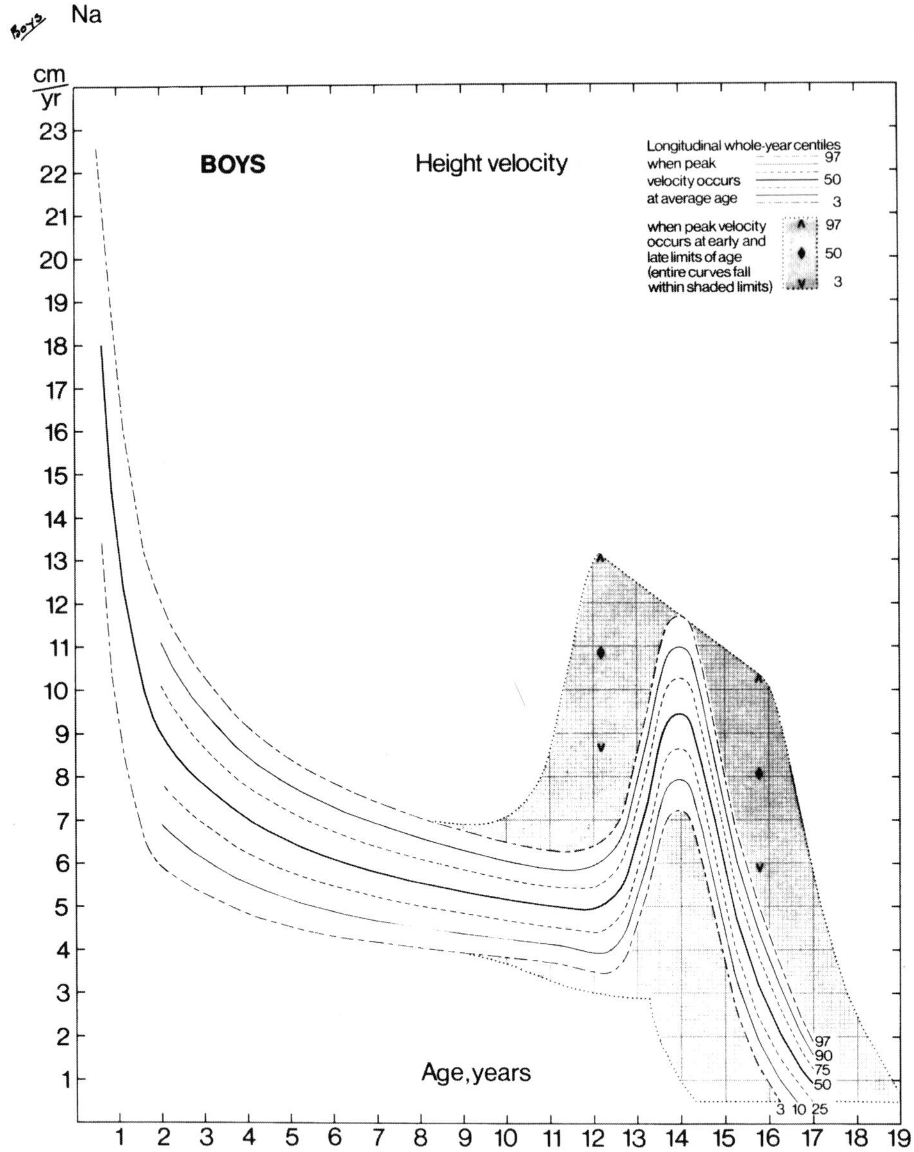

Figure 2.10. British standards for height velocity for boys. (From Tanner JM, Whitehouse RH: Arch Dis Childh 51:170, 1976.)

Table 2.3 the equivalent velocity standards (36). The latter are not centered on peak-height velocity age and are appropriate when the child has been seen only a few times and the age of peak velocity is unknown. The standard deviations beyond age 7.25 in females and 9.25 years in males have been recalculated from published data. Table 2.4 gives the centiles and standard deviations for older children after their growth curves have been centered at peak velocity age and are appropriate for retrospective analysis when this parameter is known. Table 2.2 gives North American height distance means and standard deviations (69); the latter have been calculated from the smoothed centiles tabulated in the original reference.

Variation of Tempo

As suggested, variation in growth exists not only in the size at a given stage of growth but also in the timing of reaching different stages of growth. This latter type of variation or tempo is seen with some children growing at a slow tempo, reaching each relative part of their growth curve at later and later chronological ages compared with the average. Other children grow at a fast tempo and attain the same points but earlier than average. A description of various maturity indicators that help in the assessment of this tempo have been described already, as well as the range of variation for the adolescent growth spurt.

Here the standards for puberty stages are described; they have been included on the stature standards illustrated in Figure 2.9. It is important to note the way in which these standards are constructed. The designation PH2, PH3, and so on represent the instant when these appearances first become visible. This is almost never observable; the physician can only see that a child has attained PH2 but not yet PH3. Therefore, we describe the child as being in PH2+, and the standards give the centiles for age of being in that stage. Thus, a male in PH2+ and aged 13 years is just above the 25th centile and a little older than average for that stage, although quite normal. In contrast, a similar male aged 15 years would be below the 3rd centile and suspiciously delayed.

Catch-up Growth

Apart from the normal patterns of growth observed in healthy children, there is the phenomenon of catch-up growth. This is the tendency of children, following a period of illness, malnutrition, or other insult that has led to poor growth to undergo a compensatory period at an above average velocity.

A general description of catch-up growth may be found in Prader (71), particularly related to the more commonly occurring pediatric illnesses. More mathematical descriptions are given in Forbes (72) and Tanner (73). The most striking feature is that after the disease is alleviated, growth in weight and height increase dramatically; however, as normal size approaches, the velocity falls gradually to normal. Overgrowth is not seen; the child simply returns to its previous growth channel.

This overall pattern, however, is not invariable. If the period of disease is more prolonged, the catch-up may be incomplete particularly if the child is near puberty. Particular disease processes, such as hypothyroidism, are more likely to allow complete recovery (74), whereas others do not. Corticosteroid excess is particularly likely to result in permanent short stature (75). The latter also has been seen in animal studies (76). This steroid effect may relate to their actions on proteoglycan synthesis in the chondrocyte.

There is some conflict as to the relative ease of catch up in height as opposed to weight. Using treated celiac disease as a model, Barr and coworkers (77) noted a more rapid weight gain, so that the children were overweight for height for a short period. The weight catch up was complete after 1 year of a gluten-free diet, whereas height (and skeletal maturity) took about 2 years to recover completely. It has been estimated that 5 to 6 calories above normal intake are required for every gram of catch-up weight gain following recovery from kwashiorkor (78) and that variations in calories are more important than variations in protein (79), as long as minimal protein requirements are met (chapter 11). In contrast, some animal studies suggest an easier catch up in length rather than weight (80). These may be differences between species and not of clinical importance.

The mechanism of catch up remains obscure. It seems unlikely that the classical hormones, especially GH, are causal. In all malnourished states, serum GH is elevated with poor growth and falls during the catch-up phase. It seems more likely that the mechanism involves the IGF's and probably chondrocyte metabolism itself (81, 82).

Other Factors Affecting Growth

Only a minority of children grow steadily throughout the year, with no variation in growth velocity. Earlier investigations (58) suggested increased growth between February and June in London children, with the maximum velocity being 2 to 3 times greater than the minimum. Further studies (83) in a different group of children in Orkney showed variability within the year in some 98% of children; however, this variation was strikingly seasonal in only 28% with peaks at the same time for 2 consecutive years.

The cause of this phenomenon remains unclear. Such factors as day length, sunlight, and ambient temperatures were specifically studied by Marshall (83) but, although statistically significant, they accounted for little of the variation. Some other cause or group of causes is clearly active. However, the presence of the effect is a major argument for whole year measurements of velocity whenever possible. In children under 2.0 years of age, measurements should be made quarterly. In a study using growth as a response measure, if whole year velocities are not possible, it is vital that the measurement periods be randomized with respect to season to minimize bias.

There remain a few other environmental factors that influence interpretation of growth data. The secular trend (84) and socioeconomic group differences (85) are potent factors in more long-term situations, but probably are not relevant here. Psychosocial factors, however, probably are important. There is no doubt that psychologic well being, or lack of it, may profoundly affect growth, which may be of great relevance in the chronically sick child.

Acknowledgment

I thank those colleagues, particularly Professors J. M. Tanner, C. Chantler, and Dr. C. M. Law, who helped to formulate this chapter, particularly some of the more personal views on methodology. I am grateful to Mrs. G. M. Sharp who took the manuscript through its many drafts.

References

1. Stockwell RA: Biology of cartilage cells. In Harrison RJ, McMinn RMH (eds): Biological Structure and Function. Cambridge, Cambridge University Press, vol 7, 1979.
2. Elves MW: A study of the transplantation antigens on chondrocytes from articular cartilage. J Bone Joint Surg 56B:178, 1974.
3. Roth TF, Porter KR: Yolk protein uptake in the oocyte of the mosquito *Aedes aegypti*. J Cell Biol 20:313, 1964.
4. Stockwell RA: The ultrastructure of cartilage canals and the surrounding cartilage in the sheep fetus. J Anat 109:397, 1971.
5. Weiss C, Rosenberg L, Helfet AJ: An ultrastructural study of normal young adult human articular cartilage. J Bone Joint Surg 50A:663, 1968.
6. Bornstein P: The biosynthesis of collagen. A Rev Biochem 43:567, 1974.
7. Horwitz AL, Dorfman A: Subcellular sites for synthesis of chondromucoprotein of cartilage. J Cell Biol 38:358, 1968.
8. Dingle JT: The secretion of enzymes into the pericellular environment. Phil Trans R Soc B 217:315, 1975.
9. Jibril AO: Proteolytic degradation of ossifying cartilage matrix and the removal of acid muco-polysaccharides prior to bone formation. Biochim Biophys Acta 136:162, 1967.
10. Martin JH, Matthews JL: Mitochondrial granules in chondrocytes. Calcif Tissue Res 3:184, 1969.
11. Mayne R, von der Mark K: Collagens of cartilage. In Hall BK (ed): Cartilage. New York and London, Academic Press, vol 2, 1983.
12. Jeffcoate SL: Hypophysiotrophic peptides. In Gray CH, James VHT (eds): Hormones in Blood. ed 3. London, Academic Press, vol 4, 1983.
13. Preece MA, Holder AT: The somatomedins: A family of serum growth factors. In O'Riordan JLH (ed): Recent Advances in Endocrinology and Metabolism. Edinburgh, Churchill Livingstone, vol 2, 1982.
14. Preece MA: The somatomedins. In Gray CH, James VHT (eds): Hormones in Blood. ed 3. London, Academic Press, vol 4, 1983a.
15. Rothstein H: Regulation of cell cycle by somatomedins. International Review of Cytology. New York, Academic Press, vol 78, 1982.
16. D'Ercole AJ, Decedue CJ, Furlanetto RW, et al: Evidence that somatomedin-C is degraded by the kidney and inhibits insulin degradation. Endocrinology 101:577, 1977.
16a. Goldberg AC, Tinvedi B, Delmiz JA, et al: Uremia reduces serum insulin-like growth factor I, increases serum insulin-like growth factor II and modifies their serum protein binding. J Clin Endo Metab 55:1040, 1982.
17. Schwalbe SL, Betts PR, Rayner PHW, et al: Somatomedin in growth disorders and chronic renal insufficiency in children. Brit Med J 1:697, 1977.
18. Lewey JE, Van Wyk JJ: Somatomedin and growth retardation in children with chronic renal insufficiency. Kidney Intl. 14:361, 1978.
19. Spencer EM, Uthne K, Arnold WC: Growth impairment with elevated somatomedin levels in children with chronic renal insufficiency. Acta Endocrinol. 91:36, 1979.
19a. Lynch RE, Furlanetto RW, Frans LB, et al: Serum RIA-Somatomedin-C (Sm-c) is depressed in children and adolescents with end stage renal disease. Kidney Intl 23:217(A), 1983.
20. Kilgore BS, McNatt ML, Meador S, et al: Alteraction of cartilage glycosaminoglycan protein acceptor by somatomedin and cortisol. Pediatr Res 13:96, 1979.
21. Preece MA: The effect of administered corticosteroids on the growth of children. Postgrad Med J 52:625, 1976.
22. Costin G, Kogut MD, Phillips LS, et al: Craniopharyngioma: The role of insulin in promoting postoperative growth. J Clin Endo Metab. 42:370, 1976.
23. Nagarajan L, Anderson WB: Insulin promotes the growth of F9 embryonal carcinoma cells apparently by acting through its own receptor. Biochem Biophys Res Commun. 106:974, 1982.
24. Holder AT, Wallis M, Biggs P, et al: Effects of growth hormone, prolactin and thyroxine on body weight, somatomedin-like activity and in vivo sulphation of cartilage in hypopituitary dwarf mice. J Endocrinol 85:35, 1980.

25. Holder AT, Wallis M: Actions of growth hormone, prolactin and thyroxine on serum somatomedin-like activity and growth in hypopituitary dwarf mice. J Endocrinol 77:223, 1977.
26. Preece MA, Cameron N, Donmall MC, et al: The endocrinology of male puberty. In Borms J (ed): Proceedings of the Third Congress of Auxology, Brussels, 1982, New York and London, Plenum Press, 1984.
27. Phillips LS, Herington AC, Daughaday WH: Steroid hormone effects on somatomedin. I. Somatomedin action in vitro. Endocrinology 97:780, 1975.
28. Silberberg M, Silberberg R: Steroid hormones and bone. In Bourne GH (ed): The Biochemistry and Physiology of Bone, ed 2. New York, Academic Press, vol 3, 1972.
29. Preece MA: Hormone treatment for very tall girls. J Obstet Gynaecol 3:S3 1982.
30. Fahmy A, Talley P, Frazier HM, et al: Ultra-structural effects of estrogen on epiphyseal cartilage. Calcif Tissue Res 7:139, 1971.
31. Strickland AL, Sprinz H: Studies of the influence of estradiol and growth hormone on the hypophysectomized immature rat epiphyseal cartilage growth plate. Am J Obstet Gynecol 115:471, 1973.
32. Wallace EZ, Rosman P, Toshav N, et al: Pituitary-adrenocortical function in chronic renal failure: studies of episodic secretion of cortisol and dexamethasone suppressibility. J Clin Endocrinol Metab 50:46, 1980.
33. Stewart-Bentley M, Gans D, Horton R: Regulation of gonadal function in uremia. Metabolism 23:1065, 1974.
34. Kretser DM, Atkins RC, Paulsen CA: Role of the kidney in the metabolism of luteinizing hormone. J Endocrinol 58:425, 1973.
35. Pimstone B, Epstein S, Hamilton SM, et al: Metabolic clearance and plasma half disappearance time of exogenous gonadotropin releasing hormone in normal subjects and in patients with liver disease and chronic renal failure. J Clin Endocrinol Metab 44:356, 1977.
36. Tanner JM, Whitehouse RH, Takaishi M: Standards from birth to maturity for height, weight, height velocity and weight velocity: British children, 1965. Arch Dis Child 41: 454, 613, 1966.
36a. Roche DP, Himes JH: Incremental growth charts. Am J Clin Nutr 33:2041, 1980.
36b. Tanner JM, Davies PW: Clinical longitudinal standards for height and height velocity for North American children. J Pediatr 107:317, 1985.
37. Smith DW, Truog W, McCann JJ, et al: Shifting linear growth during infancy and the genetics of growth in infancy. J Pediatr 89:225, 1976.
38. Cameron N: The Measurement of Human Growth. London, Croome Helm, 1984.
39. Preece MA: The development of skeletal sex differences at adolescence. In Russo P, Gass G (eds): Human Adaptation Department of Biological Sciences, Cumberland College of Health Sciences, Sydney, Australia, 1981.
39a. Tanner JM, Whitehouse RH: Revised standards for triceps and subscapular skinfolds in British children. Arch Dis Child. 50:142, 1975.
40. Tanner JM, Hughes PCR, Whitehouse RH: Radiographically determined widths of bone, muscle and fat in the upper arm and calf from age 3 to 18 years. Ann Hum Biol 8:495, 1981.
41. Cameron N: The methods of auxological anthropometry. In Falkner F, Tanner JM (eds): Human Growth. New York, Plenum Press, vol 2, 1978.
42. Davies DP, Holding RE: Neonatometer: a new infant length measure. Arch Dis Child 47:928, 1972.
43. Tanner JM: Growth at Adolescence, ed 2. Oxford, Blackwell Scientific Publications, 1962.
44. Greulich WW, Pyle SI: Radiographic Atlas of Skeletal Development of the Hand and Wrist, ed 2. Stanford Calif., Stanford University Press, 1959.
45. Todd TW: Atlas of Skeletal Maturation (hand). St. Louis, The C.V. Mosby Co., 1937.
46. Pyle SI, Hoerr NL: Radiographic Atlas of Skeletal Development of the Knee. Springfield, IL., Charles C Thomas, 1955.
47. Pyle SI, Hoerr NL: A Radiographic Standard of Reference for the Growing Knee. Springfield, IL., Charles C Thomas, 1969.
48. Tanner JM, Whitehouse RH, Marshall WA, et al: Assessment of skeletal maturity and prediction of adult height. London, Academic Press, 1975.
49. Roche AF, Wainer H, Thissen D: Skeletal Maturity, the Knee Joint as a Biological Indicator. London, Plenum Medical Book Company, New York 1975.
49a. Marti-Henneberg C, Patoris E, Nüranen A, et al: Bone maturation velocity in comptes Reudun sur la Croissauce et le développment de l'Enfant Normal, Paris, Paris Centre International de d'Enfance, 1974.
50. Preece MA: Are the number of teeth any help in assessing development? Arch Dis Childh 58:849, 1983.
51. Marshall WA: Inter-relationships of skeletal maturation, sexual development and somatic growth in man. Ann Hum Biol 1:29, 1974.
52. Wilkins L: The Diagnosis and Treatment of Endocrine Disorders in Childhood and Adolescence. Springfield, IL., Charles C Thomas, 1950.
53. Goldstein H: The design and analysis of longitudinal studies: their role in the measurement of change. London, Academic Press, 1979.
54. Healy MJR: Statistics of growth standards. In Falkner F, Tanner JM (eds): Human Growth. New York and London, Plenum Press, vol 1, 1978.
55. Tanner JM, Whitehouse RH: Clinical longitudinal standards for height, weight, height velocity and weight velocity and the stages of puberty. Arch Dis Childh 51:170, 1976.
56. Tanner JM: The fallacy of per-weight and per-surface area standards and their relation to spurious correlations. J Appl Physiol 2:1, 1949.
57. Tanner JM, Goldstein H, Whitehouse RH: Standards for children's height at ages 2–9 years, allowing for height of parents. Arch Dis Childh 45:755, 1970.
58. Hamill PVV, Johnston FE, Lemeshow S: Body Weight, Stature, and Sitting Height: White and Negro Youths 12–17 Years. DHEW Publication, series 11, No. 126, Rockville, Md., 1973.
59. Marshall WA: Evaluation of growth rate in height over periods of less than one year. Arch Dis Childh 46:414, 1971.
60. Tanner JM: Human growth standards: Construction and use. In Gedda L, Parisi P (eds): Auxology: Human Growth in Health and Disorder. London, Academic Press, 1978.
61. Eveleth PB, Tanner JM: Worldwide Variation in Human Growth. Cambridge, Cambridge University Press, 1976.
62. Ostyn M, Simons J, Beunen G, et al: Somatic and Motor Development of Belgian Secondary Schoolboys: Norms and Standards. Leuven, Leuven University Press, 1980.
63. Jordan JR: Desarollo humano en Cuba. La Habana, Editorial Cientifica-Tecnica, 1979.
64. Sempe P, Sempe M, Pedron G: Croissance et Maturation Osseuse. Paris, Theraplix, 1971.
65. Indian Council of Medical Research: Growth and Physical Development of Indian Infants and Children. Technical Report Series no. 18. New Delhi, ICMR, 1972.
66. Vizzoni L, Barghini G: Accrescimento staturo-ponderale nel commune di Carrara. Minerva Pediatr 21:1937, 1969.
67. Ministry of Education: Statistics of School Health Survey of 1977. Tokyo, MEJ 3-7816, 1978.
68. Karlberg P, Taranger J, Engstrom I, et al: The somatomedin development of children in a Swedish urban community. A prospective longitudinal study. I. Physical growth from birth to 16 years and longitudinal outcome of the study during the same age period. Courrier 30:special issue, 1980.
69. Hamill PVV, Johnston FE, Grams W, et al: NCHS Growth Curves 1:Height and Weight for Children Birth to 18 years. DHEW Publication, series 11, No. 165, Hyattsville, Md., 1977.
70. Roche AF, Malina RM: Manual of Physical Status and Performance in Childhood. New York and London, Plenum Press, 1983.
71. Prader A: Catch-up growth. In Barltrop D(ed): Paediatrics and Growth. London, Fellowship of Postgraduate Medicine, 1978.
72. Forbes GF: A note on the mathematics of 'catch-up' growth. Pediatr Res 8:929, 1974.
73. Tanner JM, editor: Control of Growth: Catch-up Growth in Man. In Brit Med Bull 37, 1981.
74. Prader A, Tanner JM, Harnack G-A Von: Catch-up growth following illness or starvation. J Pediatr 62:646, 1963.
75. Mosier HD, Smith FG, Schultz MA: Failure of catch-up growth after Cushing's syndrome in childhood. Am J Dis Child 124:251, 1972.
76. Mosier HD: Failure of compensatory (catch-up) growth in the rat. Pediatr Res 5:59, 1971.
77. Barr DGD, Shmerling DH, Prader A: Catch-up growth in malnutrition, studied in celiac disease after institution of gluten-free diet. Pediatr Res 6:521, 1972.
78. Kerr D, Ashworth A, Picou, D: et al: Accelerated recovery from infant malnutrition with high caloric feedings. Gardner LI, Amacher P (eds): Endocrine aspects of malnutrition. Santa Ynez, Calif., Kroc Foundation, 1973.
79. Waterlow JC: The rate of recovery of malnourished infants in relation to the protein and calorie levels of the diet. J Trop Pediatr 7:16, 1961.
80. Williams JPG, Tanner JM, Hughes PCR: Catch-up growth in male rats after growth retardation during the suckling period. Pediatr Res 8:149, 1974.
81. Pimstone BL, Wittmann W, Hansen JDL: Growth hormone and kwashiorkor. The Lancet 779, 1966.
82. Mosier HD, Dearden LC, Jansons RA: Cartilage sulfation during catch-up growth after fasting in rats. Endocrinology 102:386, 1978.
83. Marshall WA: The relationship of variations in children's growth rates to seasonal climatic variations. Ann Hum Biol 3:243, 1975.
84. van Wieringen JC: Secular growth changes. In Falkner F, Tanner JM (eds): Human Growth. New York and London, Plenum Press, vol 2, 1978.
85. Goldstein H: Factors influencing the height of seven-year-old children: results from the National Child Development Study. Hum Biol 43:92, 1971.

CHAPTER 3 Renal Structure and Development

WALLACE W. McCRORY

ANATOMY OF THE KIDNEY

The kidneys lie retroperitoneally in the lumbar region. The upper pole of each kidney lies opposite the twelfth thoracic vertebra, and the lower pole lies opposite the third lumbar vertebra. The right kidney is slightly lower than the left, and the size and length of each kidney increase with growth. When of normal size, both kidneys maintain length equal to four vertebral bodies. The hilus is the site through which pass the renal artery and vein, the lymphatics, a nerve plexus, and the renal pelvis. A tough fibrous capsule, the renal capsule, is loosely adherent to the surface of the renal parenchyma and surrounds the kidney. Two distinct regions can be identified on the cut surface of a bisected kidney: a pale inner region, the medulla, and a darker outer region, the cortex (Fig. 3.1).

The renal pelvis is the upper portion of the urinary tract that empties into the ureter. Viewed in a retrograde perspective, the pelvis is divided into three to five major calyces. Each major calyx is divided into 2 to 3 tubelike minor calyces, which attach to margins of the papillae and subtend them; their point of junction is called the fornix. The papillae expand into the renal pyramids, which are a mass of collecting tubules for urine formed in the attached nephrons. The medulla in the human kidney is made up of 8 to 18 striated triangular-shaped renal pyramids. The apex of each renal pyramid extends toward the renal pelvis forming a papilla. The base is positioned on the corticomedullary boundary. Ten to twenty-five small openings on the surface of each papilla, representing the distal ends of the collecting ducts (of Bellini), form the area cribosa.

The cortex in the human kidney forms a cap over the base of each renal pyramid; it extends downward between the individual pyramids to form the renal columns of Bertin. Along the base of the renal pyramids, i.e., at the corticomedullary junction, longitudinal elements termed the medullary rays of Ferrein extend vertically into the cortex. The medullary rays, despite the name, are considered a part of the cortex, formed by the collecting ducts and straight segments of the proximal and distal tubules (Fig. 3.2).

Blood Supply

The renal artery branches directly from the abdominal aorta and enters the kidney at the hilum, where it divides into three main branches. Two pass anteriorly and one posteriorly to the renal pelvis; each branch occasionally divides further. There is little or no anastomosis between these major arteries and each supplies three or four medullary pyramids and their corresponding cortical substance. Each major branch divides into interlobar arteries that ascend between adjacent medullary pyramids in a column of Bertin (Fig. 3.1). At the corticomedullary junction, the interlobar arteries break up into several branches, the arcuate arteries that run parallel to the surface of the kidney (Fig. 3.1). From these, branches pass peripherally into the cortex in a radial fashion, termed the interlobar arteries; from these, numerous side branches divide to become afferent glomerular arterioles. These break up almost at once into the capillary bed of the glomeruli. The afferent arteriole has a thick muscular coat; blood is thus supplied to the glomeruli at a high but controlled hydrostatic pressure. The capillaries reform into the efferent arteriole. The efferent arteriole of the cortical nephrons is slightly smaller than the afferent arteriole. They break up immediately beyond the glomerulus to form a freely anastomosing network of capillaries with low hydrostatic pressure that envelops the proximal and distal convolutions, portions of the ascending and descending limbs of the Henle loop, and the collecting ducts in the cortical zone. These capillary networks recombine into venules that coalesce to form interlobular veins.

The efferent arterioles of the juxtamedullary nephrons are of equal or greater diameter than the afferent. They give off branches that form an anastomosing peritubular network of capillaries around the cortical proximal and distal tubules in a pattern similar to that in the cortex. In addition, they send arteriolar branches directly into the medulla, following the descending limbs of Henle's loop to the tip of the medulla. These vessels turn with the bend of Henle's loop and return to the corticomedullary junction as venules, and then enter interlobular veins close to their junction with arcuate veins. These straight and vertically aligned vessels form the vasa recta and provide the blood supply to the medulla (1). Blood flowing through the vasa recta bypasses the proximal tubules. Most of the renal blood flow perfuses the cortical nephrons, the juxtamedullary nephrons and medulla receive about one fifth of the total renal blood flow in the adult.

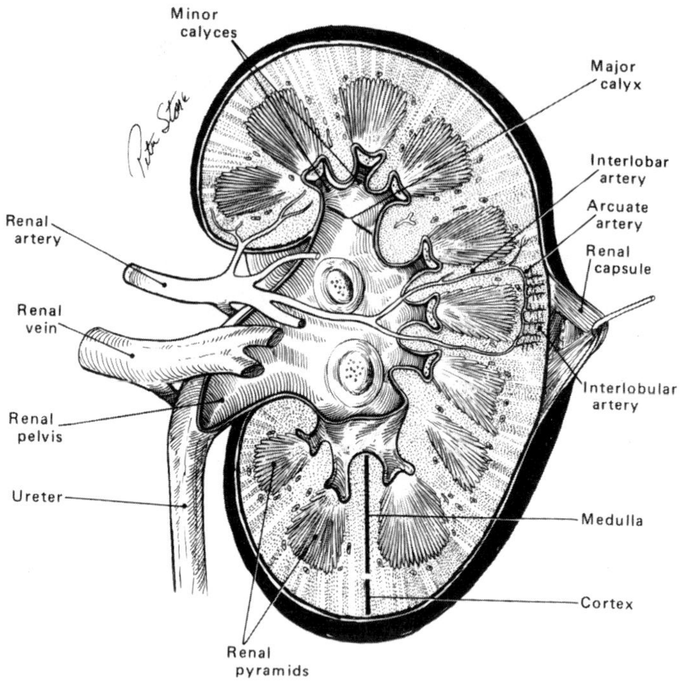

Figure 3.1. A kidney in longitudinal section. At the center are the papillae of renal pyramids lying perpendicular to the cut section. (With permission of Langley LL, Telford IR and Christensen JB: Dynamic Anatomy and Physiology, ed4, p. 637. McGraw-Hill, New York, 1980)

Nephron Structure

There are approximately a million nephrons in each kidney. Each nephron consists of several segments of different structure and function, and each segment is located in a definite position in the cortex or medulla (Fig. 3.2). The first part is the renal corpuscle or the glomerulus, and it consists of a tuft of capillaries situated within Bowman's capsule. Glomeruli vary in size; those situated in the deeper layers of the cortex—the juxtamedullary nephrons—are larger.

Glomerulus

Bowman's capsule, the epithelium-lined dilatation of the nephron, is invaginated by the tuft of capillaries, the glomerulus, thus acquiring a cap shape that is double-walled. There is a narrow slit-like space, the capsular space, between the outer or parietal layer (capsular epithelium) and the inner or visceral layer (glomerular epithelium), which closely invests the capillary tuft. The glomerulus has a vascular pole where afferent and efferent arterioles enter and leave and a urinary pole at the opposite side of the corpuscle. The capsular space is continuous with the lumen of the proximal convoluted tubules and the parietal (squamous) epithelium is continuous with the cuboidal or low columnar epithelium of the proximal convoluted tubule. The parietal layer of the Bowman capsule is composed of a simple squamous epithelium with nuclei that protrude slightly into the capsular space. The visceral layer of epithelium, made up of the podocytes, closely invests glomerular capillaries but does not form a simple and complete covering sheet.

These podocytes are stellate in form; their cell bodies are rarely in close contact with the basal laminae of glomerular capillaries (Fig. 3.3). From the cell body (*P* on Fig. 3.3), large arm-like "major processes" emerge and wrap around underlying glomerular capillary loops. Arising at nearly right angles from these major processes are numerous smaller processes: foot processes or pedicels (*F* on Fig. 3.3), which rest on the lamina rara externa of the glomerular basement membrane (GBM) and always interdigitate with foot processes from other podocytes. The portion of a foot process adjacent to the GBM is broader than the rest of the foot process, resulting in a characteristic bell-shaped appearance when viewed in cross section (Fig. 3.4). Adjacent foot processes are separated by a space (40 nm), the filtration slit (Fig. 3.4), which is spanned by a thin (60A) diaphragm that exhibits an orderly zipper-like substructure when viewed in sections tangential to the GBM. Glomerular podocytes and the filtration slits are coated with a thick, free surface coat that is rich in sialic acid.

Beneath the pedicels, the basal lamina is about 0.3 μm thick and composed of an amorphous material in which a network of fine filaments is embedded. The basal lamina shows a central electron-dense lamina, the lamina densa, about 0.1 μm thick, with an electron-lucent layer on the external and internal aspects. Internally, the endothelium of glomerular capillaries is greatly attenuated with numerous pores or fenestrae of about 80 nm in diameter.

The Tubule

The urinary tubule of each renal corpuscle begins with the convoluted portion of the proximal convoluted tubule (Fig. 3.2). The straight portion of the proximal tubule, the thin and thick limb segments, and the straight portion of the distal tubule form the loop of Henle. This enters the medullary ray and extends into the medulla, where it forms a loop and returns to the cortex via the same medullary ray. As the distal tubule returns to the cortex, it passes by the renal corpuscle from which the nephron originated (Fig. 3.2), forming the macula densa and then continues as the distal convoluted tubule within the cortex. The lengths of the loops of Henle vary with the position of the renal corpuscle in the cortex. Nephrons in the outer region of the cortex, the cortical nephrons, have short loops of Henle and no thin limbs, while nephrons that have renal corpuscles near the corticomedullary junction, juxtamedullary nephrons (15% to 20% of total), have long loops of Henle with long descending and ascending thin limb segments (Fig. 3.2). These thin limbs run parallel with the collecting ducts in the outer and inner zones of the medulla. In the human kidney, cortical nephrons extend into a terminal collecting duct, whereas several juxtamedullary nephrons empty into an arched connecting duct that courses peripherally in the cortex before it turns to enter a medullary ray as a collecting duct. All of the distal nephrons empty into their collecting ducts in the cortex (Fig. 3.2). These anatomic arrangements have functional significance in the processes of urinary dilution and concentration. The details of the structural characteristics of the various portions of the urinary tubule and their functional relationship are described in chapter 5.

Vascular Pole and Juxtaglomerular Apparatus

The juxtaglomerular apparatus is a triangular structure: the apex is the vascular pole of the glomerulus, the base is formed by the macula densa of the distal convoluted tubule, and the sides are the walls of the afferent and efferent arterioles. The cells within these limits are called the juxtaglomerular apparatus (1). Adjacent to the glomerulus, smooth muscle cells in the media of the afferent arteriole are replaced by large epithelioid cells whose cytoplasm contains big granules thought to be renin. These are the juxtaglomerular (JG) cells. In the afferent arteriole, the internal elastic lamina is absent, so that the JG cells lie adjacent to the endothelium and thus to blood in the lumen. The JG cells are also closely related to the macula densa, a specialized region of the distal convoluted tubule at its commencement. The macula densa lies between the afferent and efferent arterioles; it is part of the distal convoluted tubule but is formed of epithelial cells that differ from those that form the rest of this segment of the tubule. The macula densa lacks a basal

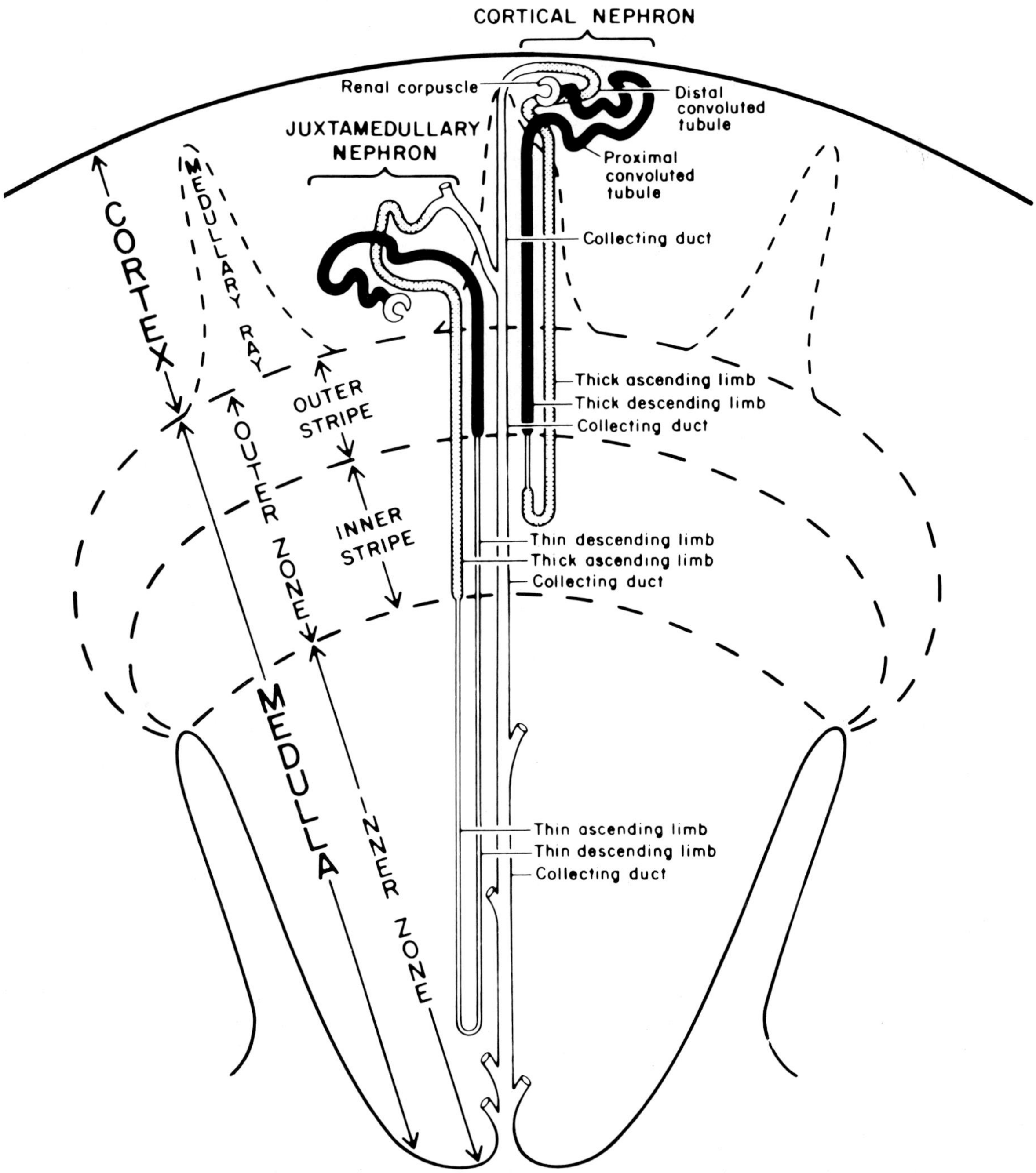

Figure 3.2. Schematic diagram of a cortical and juxtamedullary nephron showing the relationship of nephron segments to zones of the kidney. (With permission of Strauss MJ and Welt LG: Diseases of the Kidneys, ed3, p. 5. Little Brown and Co., Boston, 1979)

lamina and is in close contact with the JG mass and is not separated from it by any interposing peritubular capillary.

Renal Innervation

Relative to its size, the kidney has a rich, predominantly adrenergic innervation of the afferent and efferent arterioles, the JG apparatus, the proximal and distal convoluted tubules, and the thick ascending limb of the loop of Henle (2). Both histochemical and functional observations exclude a role for cholinergic innervation of the kidney. Dopamine-containing elements are found at the glomerular vascular pole. Efferent unmyelinated fibers predominate over afferent myelinated fibers. Direct or reflex-induced increases in efferent renal sympathetic nerve activity release norepinephrine and dopamine, but not epinephrine, into renal venous blood and urine. Both glomeruli and tubules possess alpha and beta adrenergic and dopamine receptors.

KIDNEY OF THE NEWBORN

The kidney of the normal newborn is anatomically distinguishable from the mature organ by both morphological and histological criteria (3). The external surface of the newborn kidney is lobulated, revealing the underlying structural organization. Cortical growth obliterates these lobulations so that the surface of the kidney becomes smooth.

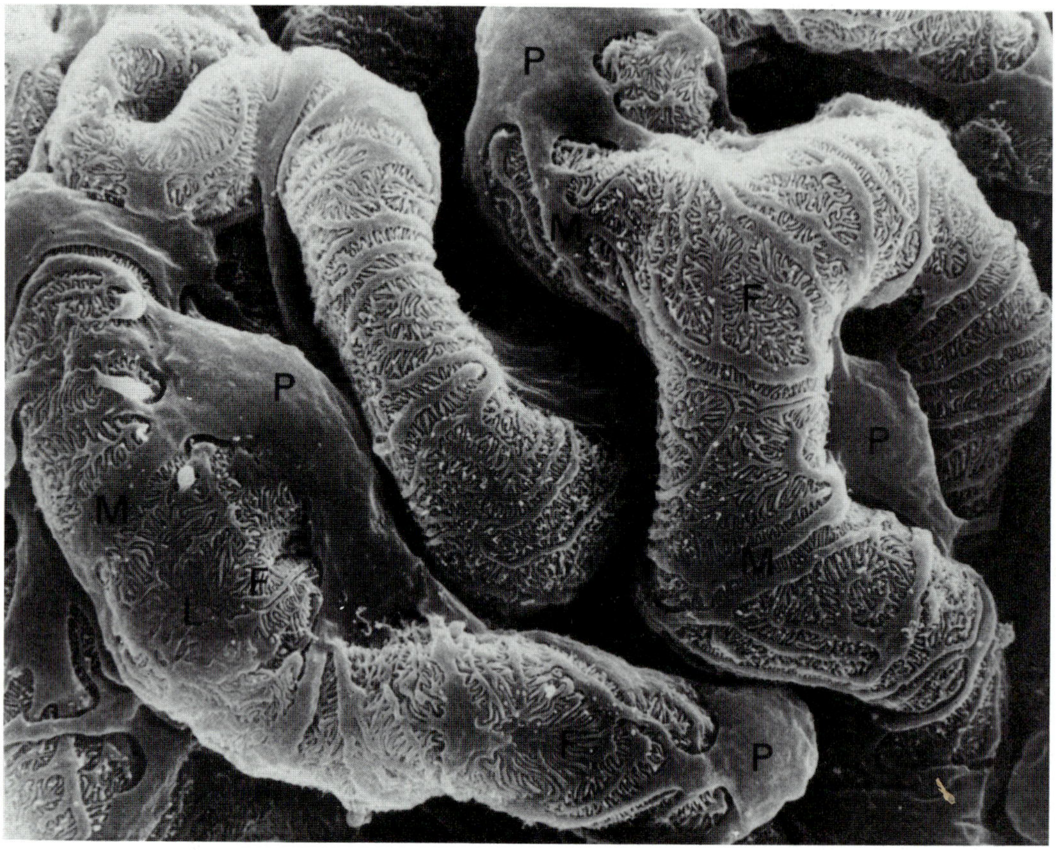

Figure 3.3. Glomerular epithelial podocytes (*P*) send their large major processes (*M*) and small foot processes (*F*) over winding glomerular capillary loops. Even in normal glomeruli, there are regions of focal foot process loss (*L*). (With permission of Allen DJ, Motta PM and Didio LJA: Three Dimensional Microanatomy of Cells and Surface Tissues, p. 105, Elsevier North Holland, Inc., 1981)

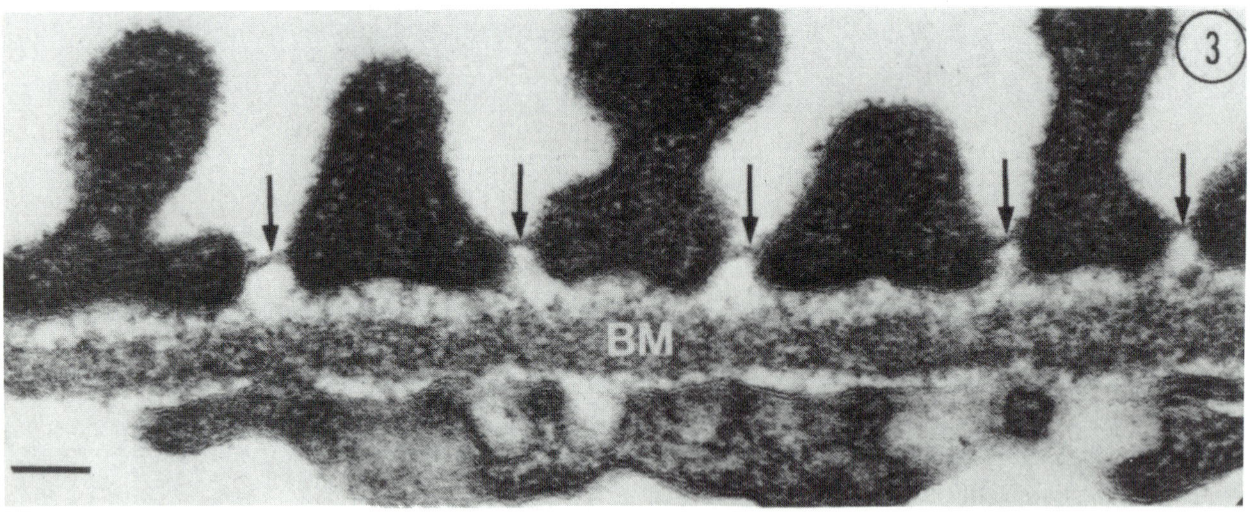

Figure 3.4. Higher magnification thin section through 5 podocyte foot processes. Filtration slits of varying width are bridged by slit diaphragms (*arrows*). Note that the bases of foot processes are spread out to varying extents over the basement membrane (*BM*). Vertically oriented strands of the lamina rara externa appear to insert onto these bases. A fuzzy surface coat is also evident. (With permission of Allen DJ, Motta PM and Didio LJA: Three Dimensional Microanatomy of Cells and Surface Tissues, p. 107, Elsevier North Holland, Inc., 1981)

Nephron induction ceases about the twenty-sixth week of gestation. The last generations of nephrons induced are located in the subcapsular region of the cortex in the normal full-term infant and are recognizable by their immaturity. The timing of the cessation of nephron induction is sufficiently precise so that the amount of nephrogenic activity present in the renal cortex at birth can serve as an anatomic index of gestational age (4). The kidney of the premature infant has nephrons characterized by their heavily cellular, primitive S-shaped or rudimentary tufts that lack a true vascular pole.

The size and configuration of nephrons in the different regions of the

Table 3.1.
Glomerular Diameter and Proximal Length for Three Cortical Levels of Nephrons in 23 Patients

Age	Mean glomerular diameter (cm)			Mean Proximal Length (m)		
	Outer	Middle	Inner	Outer	Middle	Inner
Months						
Newborn (full term)	0.106	0.115	0.129	1.26	1.73	2.46
1	0.105	0.109	0.123	2.29	2.94	3.37
3½	0.101	0.125	0.142	2.83	3.19	4.12
5	0.155	0.151	0.163	6.54	6.78	7.17
6	0.150	0.165	0.184	4.84	6.05	6.74
11	0.122	0.122	0.131	4.87	4.70	4.86
12	0.124	0.177	0.132	6.38	6.01	6.37
14	0.168	0.168	0.173	7.16	7.98	7.86
20	0.152	0.157	0.158	5.52	5.74	5.39
22	0.175	0.175	0.174	7.53	8.52	8.36
27	0.175	0.162	0.186	7.99	8.24	8.51
Years						
3	0.170	0.164	0.176	8.03	8.24	6.99
3	1.169	0.166	0.181	7.37	7.28	7.82
3½	0.178	0.178	0.188	6.29	7.14	7.50
3½	0.201	0.201	0.200	8.61	9.15	8.17
5	0.146	0.155	0.154	7.05	6.93	6.91
6	0.190	0.204	0.212	8.34	9.92	9.51
7½	0.215	0.221	0.230	10.72	10.94	12.91
8½	0.192	0.196	0.204	12.29	13.73	13.82
12	0.241	0.249	0.249	11.74	11.95	12.70
13	0.243	0.235	0.237	12.72	13.06	12.84
15	0.222	0.212	0.229	15.21	12.99	13.47
18	0.196	0.207	0.197	11.68	12.78	11.53
35[a]	0.287	0.280	0.283	21.5	19.4	17.8

[a] Data are for composite kidney at age 35. (From Fetterman GH, Shuploch NA, Phillip NS, et al: Pediatrics 35:601, 1965.)

cortex at birth and the changes that occur during postnatal development have been described by Fetterman and coworkers (5). The anatomic dimensions and characteristics of the nephrons in the kidney at birth differ from those in the adult (Table 3.1); the most striking finding is the physical underdevelopment of the proximal tubule relative to its corresponding glomerulus. The mean glomerular diameter in the newborn kidney is about 0.11 mm, about one-third that of the adult (0.28 mm). The mean length of proximal tubules, about 2 mm, is one-tenth that of the adult (20 mm). Nephron heterogeneity (variation in size between individual nephrons from the same level of the cortex) is another characteristic of the newborn kidney. Variation between lengths of the shortest and longest proximal tubules in infants (elevenfold) is greater than it is in adults (twofold).

Glomeruli vary in size but less so. The variations are related to the location in the cortex, reflecting differences in nephron age. The mean glomerular diameters in the 3 levels of the cortex of the newborn kidney are: outer 1.26 mm, middle 1.73 mm, and inner 2.46 mm. The differences in size contrast with the mature kidney, in which mean glomerular diameter is about the same at all levels (Table 3.1). These dimensional differences between nephrons in different levels of the cortex disappear by 12 to 14 months of age.

The differences in mean glomerular diameter in outer and inner levels of the kidney of the newborn are sufficient that one might anticipate differences in single nephron GFR. The higher GFR would be in the deeper-most mature nephrons. Although nephron heterogeneity is evident, individual glomeruli and their respective tubules are well-matched for size. The smallest (and least mature) glomeruli in the outer cortex have the shortest and least coiled proximal tubules; the largest (and most mature) glomeruli in the inner cortex have the longest and most coiled proximal tubules.

The postnatal increase in values for GFR and renal plasma flow are associated with the increases in physical dimensions of the individual nephrons (3). The heterogeneity of size, characteristic of the nephrons of the newborn kidney, disappears by the end of the first year of life. The low values for GFR and renal plasma flow characteristic of the neonatal period have increased more rapidly than kidney size during the first year, by which time GFR/g kidney is close to the value that pertains throughout the remainder of growth (3).

Individual nephron growth during organogenesis appears to be allometric; balance is preserved with respect to physical dimensions of individual glomeruli and their attached urinary tubules. Growth of nephrons in the early postnatal period decreases heterogeneity among nephrons. Tubular mass increases more than glomerular size, as nephrons assume the physical dimensions characteristic of maturity.

The heterogeneity of glomeruli and nephrons at birth develops as a consequence of the centripetal pattern of nephron formation during fetal life. The most mature units with respect to glomerular size, maturation, length of proximal and distal convolutions, and loops of Henle are located in the inner cortex. The least mature nephrons, with the shortest loops of Henle, occupy the outer cortex. All parts of the nephron increase in size as they mature (Table 3.1), but the most striking changes consist in elongation of the loops of Henle and increased tortuosity of the proximal convoluted tubules. By microdissection, the loops of Henle are invariably shortest in the most recently formed nephrons, growing progressively longer in older nephrons.

Fetterman and coworkers (5) found 20% of the loops of Henle still within the cortex in mature infants at birth. As the kidney increases in size after birth, all loops of Henle elongate so that the tips of all loops of Henle in the mature kidney are in the inner two thirds of the medulla. The thin portion of the loop of Henle of the youngest nephrons cannot be seen until some time after birth and remain limited to the descending limbs. In the mature kidney, only the loops of Henle that reach almost to the renal pelvis have thin portions that extend into the ascending limb.

EMBRYOGENESIS AND GROWTH

Embryogenesis

It is useful to distinguish between two processes responsible for developmental growth: *organogenesis*, the process of specific induction and differentiation of cells, and *maturation*, the process by which the organ acquires its full functional capacity. Renal function increases during growth and maturation in parallel with growth in renal size. This growth maintains an equilibrium between the renal work load (GFR) and nephron size.

Organogenesis of Nephrons

Renal organogenesis occurs sequentially from three anlage: pronephros, mesonephros, and metanephros. Nephron formation follows from the interaction of elements from the mesonephros (the ureteric bud) and the metanephros (6).

Pronephros

The pronephros begins with the development of individual paired tubules, pronephric tubules. The first tubules appear about the middle of the third week (8 to 9 somite embryo) and arise from a solid mass of mesenchymal cells, the nephrogenic cords, located between the lateral surface of the somite and the coelom. These pronephric tubules, about seven in all, persist for only a short time and undergo regression by the fifth week. Each proliferating tubular bud grows caudally until it fuses with the tubular bud of the next pronephric tubule, giving rise to the pronephric duct. The pronephric duct persists after the pronephric tubules regress (Fig. 3.5, *A*). This duct is important because it gives rise to the mesonephric duct. This, in turn, evolves into the ureteric bud.

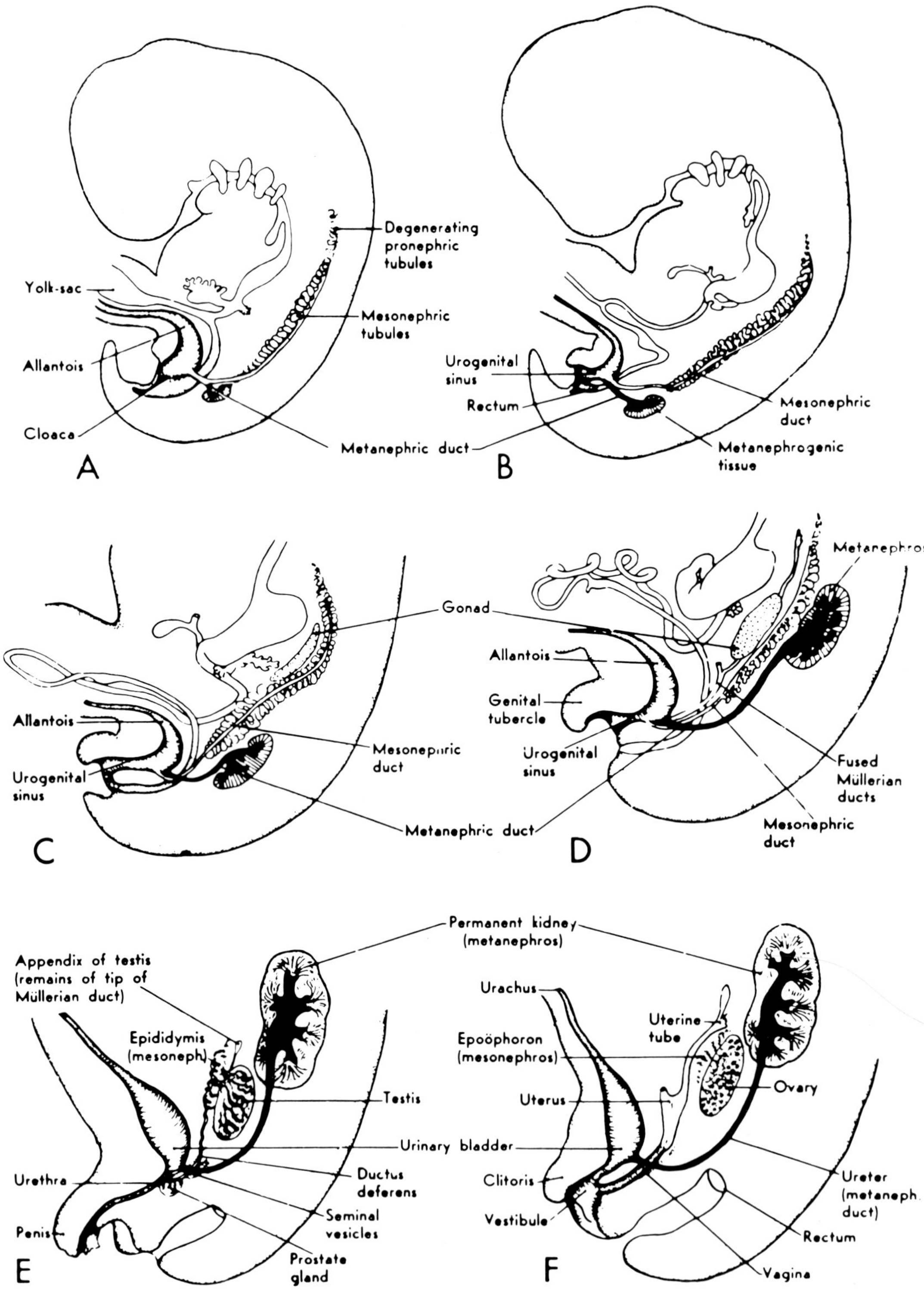

Figure 3.5. Relative size and positions of nephric organs of the human embryo at various stages of development. **A**, Early in fifth week (adapted from several sources covering 5 to 6 mm embryos). **B**, Early in sixth week (modified from Shikinami's 8 mm embryo). **C**, Seventh week (modified from Shikinami's 14.6 mm embryo). **D**, Eighth week (adapted from Shikinami's 23 mm embryo and the Kelly and Burnam 25 mm stage). **E**, Male at about 3 months, schematized. **F**, Female at about 3 months schematized. (With permission of Patton BM: Human Embryology, ed3, McGraw Hill, New York, 1968)

Mesonephros

The mesonephros appears in the third to fourth week as a more complex structure immediately caudal to the last of the pronephric tubules (Fig. 3.5, *A* and *B*). Vesicles induced by the mesonephros arise within the nephrogenic cords. The first vesicles differentiate at about the fourth week. As with the pronephros, the earliest nephrons are formed cephalad and begin to degenerate by the fifth week, while the more caudal nephrons are still differentiating, causing the mesonephros to shift caudally. The mesonephric nephrons degenerate by the eleventh to twelfth week.

The individual vesicles differentiate into primitive S-shaped tubules whose distal projections establish continuity with the mesonephric duct from which they are induced. The proximal ends broaden to form a two-layered cup, Bowman's capsule. The outer layer forms the parietal epithelium and the inner layer the visceral epithelium. The glomerulus is complete when capillaries vascularize this primitive Bowman's capsule. The tubules differentiate, forming convolutions, but no loop of Henle or distal portion. The tubule cells develop brush borders and organelles that are characteristic of transporting cells.

There is variation among species in the degree to which the mesonephros contributes to final renal architecture. In humans and rats, the mesonephros regresses completely by the eleventh to twelfth week as the metanephros begins to function. In sheep, pigs, and rabbits the mesonephros becomes a prominent organ and contributes to the formation of fetal urine for a variable time after the metanephros appears. The mesonephros and allantois are large in species that have a simple appositional type of placenta. They are small and short-lived in species, i.e., primates, in which the placenta is highly permeable hemochorial variety, and the allantois is rudimentary (7). The size and function of the mesonephros correlates with the size and function of the allantois.

Mesonephros of rabbits, cats, pigs, and other mammals excrete ferrocyanide and tubules excrete phenol red from the time these structures first appear until they degenerate (8). Mesonephric urine in fetal pigs and sheep is a glucose-free and protein-free fluid similar to an ultrafiltrate of fetal serum (9, 10). It is isoosmolar with body fluids and has the same concentrations of electrolyte and urea as fetal plasma.

Metanephros

The final phase of renal ontogeny is differentiation of the metanephros. This arises from the interaction of the ureteric bud with mesenchymal tissue. Normal differentiation of the ureteric bud from the mesonephric duct is essential to initiate the induction of duct-branching that finally produces the urinary collecting system and the induction of nephric vesicles that are responsible for individual nephron formation.

The ureteral bud arises during the fourth to fifth week of gestation as a small diverticulum at the caudal end of the mesonephric duct just proximal to the cloaca (Fig. 3.5, *A*). Growth of the ureteral bud proceeds dorsally, encountering the most caudal portion of the nephrogenic cord blastema. This then surrounds the growing and dividing ureteral bud as a condensed mass of cells that will form the metanephros. The metanephros migrates caudally (Fig. 3.5, *C* and *D*), coincident with rapid growth of the caudal somites and straightening out of the embryo from its curled configuration.

The ureteral bud begins dividing about the sixth week. The first few bud divisions are not associated with induction of nephrons. These appear on the third to fifth generation of ureteral bud branches (Fig. 3.6) at about 8 weeks. The nephron vesicles (first evidence of nephron differentiation) are attached to the ampullae of the terminal branches of the dividing bud.

Davies (11) has hypothesized that the ontogenesis of the metanephric kidney, with its capacity to dilute or concentrate urine and requiring a loop of Henle, emerged as the organism faced increased environmental pressures to conserve water by moving out of the sea and onto dry land.

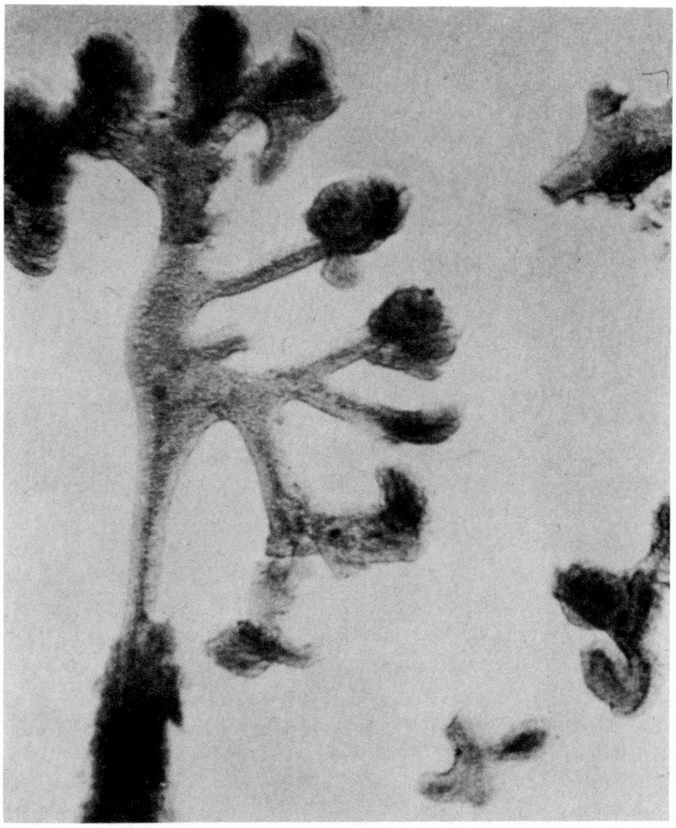

Figure 3.6. Microdissection of left kidney and ureter from 18 mm, 8-week embryo. Ureteral bud has divided 4 to 6 times in polar area and 3 to 4 times in interpolar area. All branches present at this stage will be expanded into renal pelvis and calyces during subsequent development. Renal vesicles derived from nephrogenic blastema are first present in relation to ampullary ends of third to fifth generation of ureteral bud branches. (With permission of Potter EL: Normal and Abnormal Development of the Kidney, Year Book Medical Publishers, Chicago, 1972)

Organogenesis of Nephronic Tubules

The mechanism responsible for differentiation of the pronephros is unknown. Its progeny, the wolffian duct and ureteral bud, induce nephron formation in the mesenchyme, possessing a nephrogenic potential, the mesonephros. The kidney is a classic example of inductive organogenesis in which epithelial and mesenchymal tissues interact (12). Tubules form from the nephrogenic mesenchyme as a result of inductive processes brought about by changes in the extracellular matrix (12). The undifferentiated mesenchyme releases fibronectin, but at this point no detectable laminin, type IV collagen, or basement membrane proteoglycan. During the inductive interaction, these specific components of the basement membrane: laminin, type IV collagen, basement membrane proteoglycan, appear and fibronectin is lost (13). Tubulogenesis follows from direct contact between interacting cells rather than from long-range diffusion of signal substances (14).

Differentiation of metanephric cells in culture produces glomeruli and tubules without the presence of blood vessels (15). As with in vivo nephrogenesis, mesenchymal cells aggregate and form a vesicle that elongates into an S-shaped loop; a biluminar cup at the end of the S-shaped loop forms the glomerulus.

The glomerular tuft in culture is a branching structure of basement membrane that is covered with epithelium. The epithelial cells develop foot processes separated by slit pores and bridged by slit diaphragms. The basement membrane of the tuft continues at the hilum with the basement membrane of the Bowman's capsule.

The lamina of basement membrane, lying between apposed layers of epithelium, enclose spaces for the ingrowth of glomerular capillaries *in vivo*. While the glomerulus can differentiate as an epithelial structure without vascular ingrowth, such glomeruli lack mesangial cells, endothelial cells, and JG complexes (15).

Continuity with vasculature is required for the endothelial cells of the glomerulus to differentiate (13). While differentiation of epithelial structures of the glomerulus requires inductive interaction, the development of the vasculature seems to involve an ingrowth of cells which deposit fibronectin and their basement-membrane-specific components (see previous section). These cells form the endothelium and probably the mesangium of the glomerulus. They contribute to the formation of the mature glomerular basement membrane made up of two layers (Fig. 3.4).

Nephron Formation

The nephrogenic elements or secretory units of the kidney arise separately from the collecting ductules, but require close physical association with duct tissue for successful differentiation (16). The first signs of nephron formation are condensation of circular masses of mesenchymal cells, which have close contact with the proliferating tissue of an ampulla that forms the tip of a branch of a collecting duct tubule (Fig. 3.7). The cell mass becomes spheroid, develops a central cavity (vesicle), elongates, and assumes a tubular form. Differential proliferation results in the formation of an S-shaped body. The example in Figure 3.8 shows the open communication between the nephron's lumen and the ampulla. Three portions of this S-shaped body are recognizable: (1) the upper limb continuous with the collecting tubule, which forms the connecting piece of the distal tubule; (2) the middle limb, the Stoerk complex, which subsequently forms the loop of Henle and proximal tubule; and (3) the lower limb, which has already formed the visceral and parietal epithelial layers that enclose Bowman's capsule.

As the glomerular anlage develops, a cleft appears between it and the lower limb. The cleft is penetrated by small vascular branches that arise from arteries within adjacent interstitial tissues, vascularizing the glomerulus. The cleft becomes deep and widened, as the Bowman capsule forms a hemisphere with a double layer of epithelial cells.

The outer layer consists of flat cells; the inner layer has thicker cuboidal cells, which give the primitive glomerulus the prominent visceral epithelial layer characteristic of fetal glomeruli (Fig. 3.8). The arterial branches that penetrate the cleft develop into a capillary network that fills the cavity of the hemisphere. Mesenchymal cells surrounding the

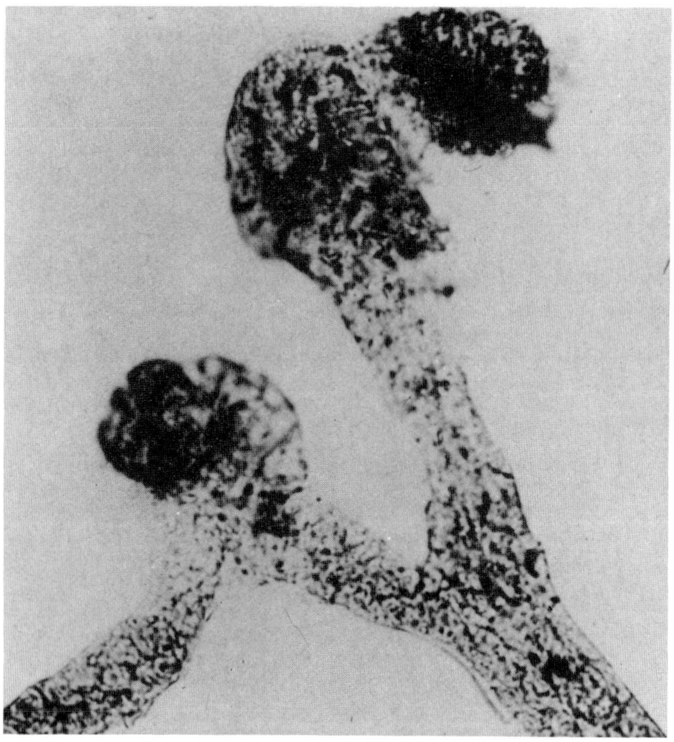

Figure 3.7. Earliest evidence of vesicle induction. A divided collecting tubule ends in two ampullae. At the lower left, a vesicle is seen as a disklike mass of deeply stained nephrogenic mesenchyme. Attached below is the connecting tubule of a previously induced nephron. Above and to the right is an ampulla with a fully developed spherical vesicle in which a central cavity can be seen dimly. (With permission of Oliver J: Nephrons and Kidneys: A Quantitative Study of the Developmental and Evolutionary Mammalian Renal Architectonics. Hoeber Medical Division, Harper and Row, New York, 1968)

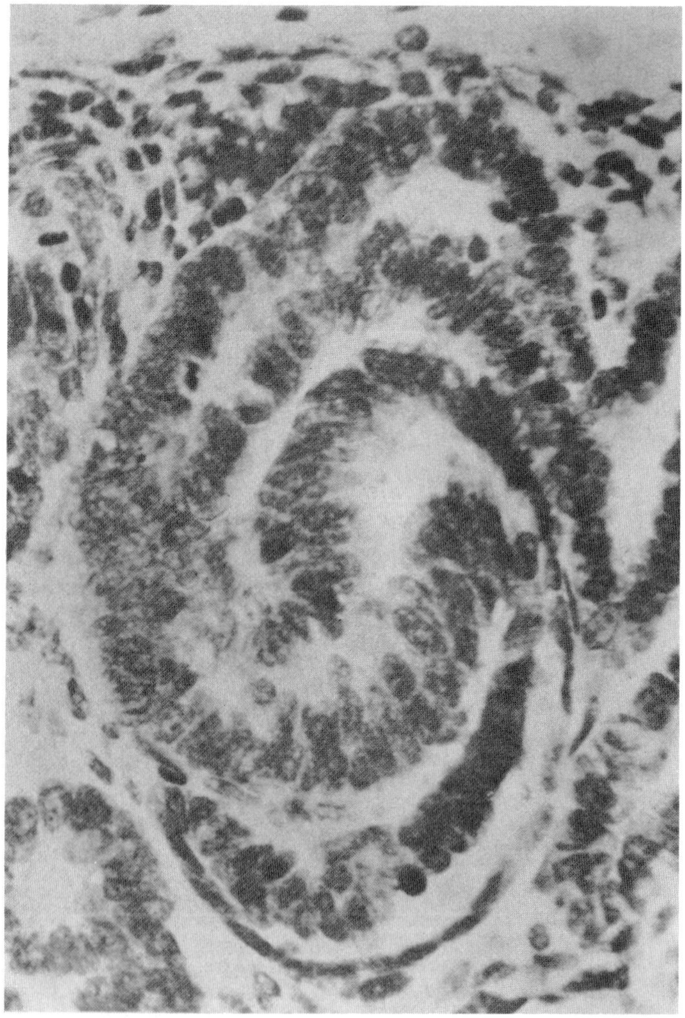

Figure 3.8. Nephron in S stage attached to ampulla before there is appreciable lengthening of the collecting tubule. Open communication between ampulla and nephron are shown in adjacent sections. (With permission of Oliver J: Nephrons and Kidneys: A Quantitative Study of the Developmental and Evolutionary Mammalian Renal Architectonics. Hoeber Medical Division, Harper and Row, New York, 1968)

capillary channels proliferate and locate within the glomerular stalk as mesangial cells. The rapid growth of the glomerulus and its capillary network pushes away the adjacent middle limb of the S-shaped body (Stoerk complex). This results in early positioning of the future macula densa of the distal tubule of the JG apparatus in close proximity to the vascular pole of the glomerulus (Fig. 3.9) (16). This position is retained throughout future nephronic development.

The upper edge of the Bowman capsule constricts and brings the efferent and afferent arteries together at the vascular pole of the glomerulus, opposite the exit of the proximal tubule.

Pelvicalyceal System

The ureteral bud branches that are proximal to the attachment of the earliest formed nephrons dilate to form the primitive renal pelvis and major calyces. This dilation occurs after formation of functioning glomeruli (Fig. 3.10) and is related to the excretion of urine (17). Additional divisions of the terminal bud branches occur in rapid succession; each division is associated with active nephron formation and results in new generations of tubules (Fig. 3.11, *A* & *B*).

The generations of ureteral bud branches that form the lobular collecting systems can be made out in the kidney of the thirteenth to fourteenth week fetus, because they open into the calyceal chambers. The calyces are evident as the broad chambers subtending a confluence of later generations of nephron-bearing tubular branches (Fig. 3.12, *A* & *B*). Each of the primitive tubular branches that empty into the minor calyces will ultimately form the papillary ducts. By 13 to 14 weeks, the minor calyces and their papillary ducts are well delineated and resemble those of the mature kidney.

The Renal Pyramids

In the early stages of development, 10 to 11 weeks, the first generations of ureteral bud branchings dilate to form the major and minor calyces; ducts of nephron-bearing collecting tubules open into this primitive minor calyceal system (Fig. 3.11, *B*). Each of these collecting ducts ultimately represent the final conduit for a fully organized collecting tree with branches forming the medullary collecting ducts. All generations of nephrons will have been moved to the periphery.

By 13 to 14 weeks, the minor calyces have developed their distinct cup shape, and the villiform plate of the papilla is being formed (Fig. 3.12, *A* & *B*), though how the plate is formed is unclear. Potter (17) ascribes it to a process of rapid growth of nephrons and ducts, which result in compression that restricts expansion of generations of duct tubules produced distal to the last generation involved in calyceal formation. By the end of 16 weeks, the papillae are sharply elevated and are similar to those of adult papillae. Developments responsible for the final shape of papillae and calyces take place during the fourth month, at which time the number of lobes in the mature kidney (average 14 to 16) are established.

The Collecting System

The collecting systems of the renal lobes in the mature kidney are highly systematized. The medullary portion is comprised of branches that collect urine formed by aggregates or clusters of cortical nephrons. The tubules of these cortical nephrons are within a renal lobe and connect with individual branches of collecting ducts. These converge into a single papillary duct that terminates in a single renal papilla. The centrifugal arborization of each of the collecting ducts forms a tree that starts with a single papillary duct that occurs during the early stages of nephrogenesis (Fig. 3.13).

Branching of the collecting system and nephron formation continues into 15 to 20 weeks. The last (fourteenth to fifteenth) generation of

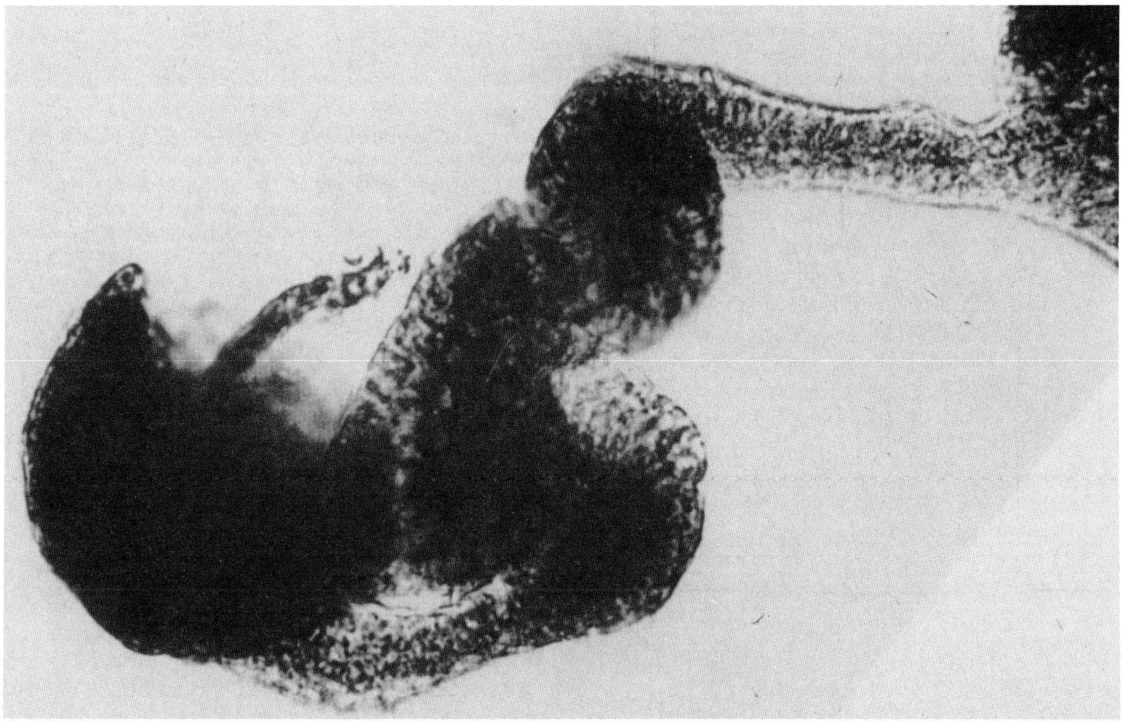

Figure 3.9. Vascularization of the rudimentary glomerulus. The dislocation of the two coils of the Stoerk complex from the glomerular cup occurs spontaneously. The edges of the cup have extended to form an ovoid hemisphere into the cavity of which a thick afferent vessel extends. The proximity that the arterial vessels would have to the first portion of the distal tubule before dissection is evident. (With permission of Oliver J: Nephrons and Kidneys: A Quantitative Study of the Developmental and Evolutionary Mammalian Renal Architectonics. Hoeber Medical Division, Harper and Row, New York, 1968)

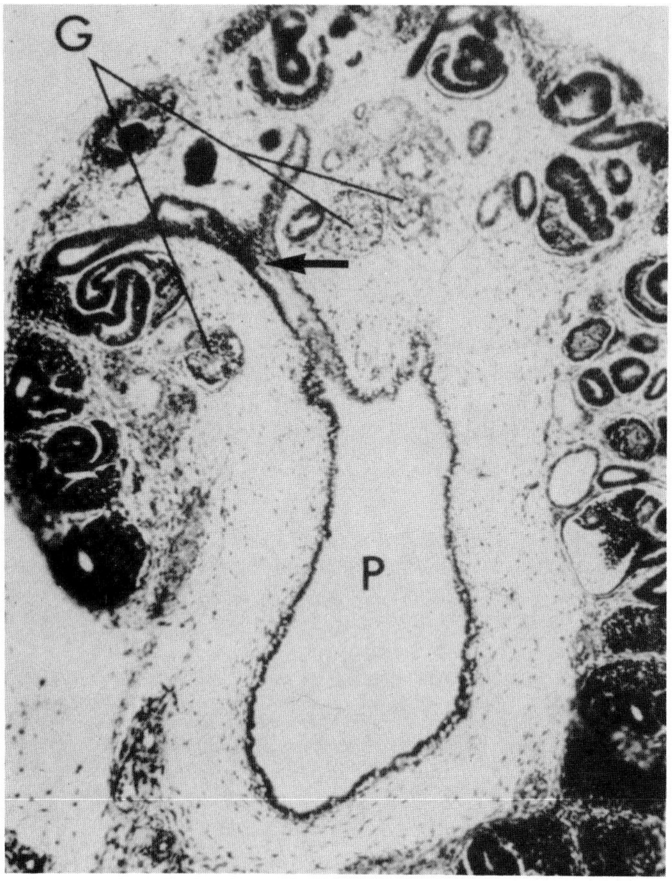

Figure 3.10. Kidney from 24 mm, 9-week embryo in cross section. Early branches of ureteral bud are dilated to form primitive renal pelvis (*P*). Dilation of proximal portions of next generation will leave terminal portions constricted (*arrow*), through which calyces will communicate with pelvis. Of eighteen well-formed glomeruli (*G*), three are visible in this section. (With permission of Potter EL: Normal and Abnormal Development of the Kidney, Year Book Medical Publishers, Chicago, 1972)

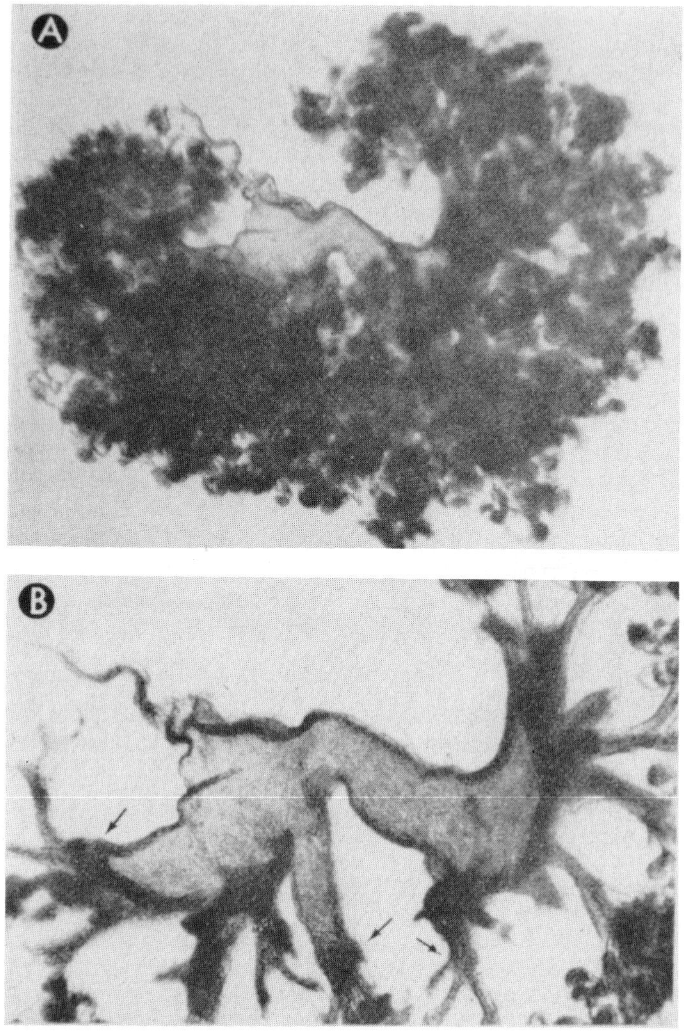

Figure 3.11. Kidney from 50 mm, 11-week human fetus. **A**, Entire kidney after preliminary microdissection. **B**, Most of the nephrons and collecting tubules have been removed to show ureter, renal pelvis, and earliest stages in formation of calyces. Tubules formed by third to fifth generation of ureteral bud branches have dilated to become the primitive renal pelvis, and many large tubules empty directly into it. Initial evidence of calyceal formation is indicated by arrows. Note small diameter of ureter. (With permission of Potter EL: Normal and Abnormal Development of the Kidney, Year Book Medical Publishers, Chicago, 1972)

collecting ducts formed continues to grow centrifugally and to induce nephrons for from three to five additional generations until 32 weeks. Extensions of the terminal generation of collecting ducts grow toward the outer cortex in spearlike tips. They form nephrons that are found in the middle and outer cortex in the mature kidney, about 80% of all nephrons. The nephrons located in the inner cortical region in the mature kidney (juxtamedullary) are formed during the period of collecting duct division. The last period of renal development begins at 32 to 36 weeks, when ampullae disappear and signal the end of nephron formation. Increases in renal mass that occur in this period (threefold increase in size) result from glomerular, interstitial, and tubular growth, particularly growth of the proximal tubule. Loops of Henle, distal tubules, and collecting ducts mature to complete the development of the kidney.

There have been a number of explanations for the segregation of nephron attachments to cortical collecting ducts. These have included proposals that nephron attachments migrate or change during development, or that the earliest nephrons left behind on the closed divided portion of the collecting system degenerate.

The view most widely accepted holds that the segregation of all nephron attachments to the terminal collecting duct arises as a consequence of the specialized growth processes. All nephrons are induced and form initial attachments only to ampullae. As the tip of an individual collecting duct divides to form new branches, an attached nephron can be carried forward with the advancing tip of one of the ampullae. This occurs with differential growth, allowing the attached nephron to move on one arm of the growing tip. In this manner, it allows accumulation of nephrons of different ages and at different stages of development on one arm of a dividing and extending duct branch. This process is known as the Peter transport process (18).

Oliver (16) observed movement by microdissection of attachments of nephrons to the periphery. They accumulate on later generations of bud branches and the early branches on which nephrons first appear later become nephron-free. The attached nephrons vary in stage of development, and the number on the different arms of the dividing terminal branches vary in accord with the branching process by dichotomous division of each bud (each ampulla induces one nephron) and the Peter transport process (18). This latter is operative during the formation of new branches of the collecting ducts. The nephrons that are produced during duct division and "carried forward" account for less than one

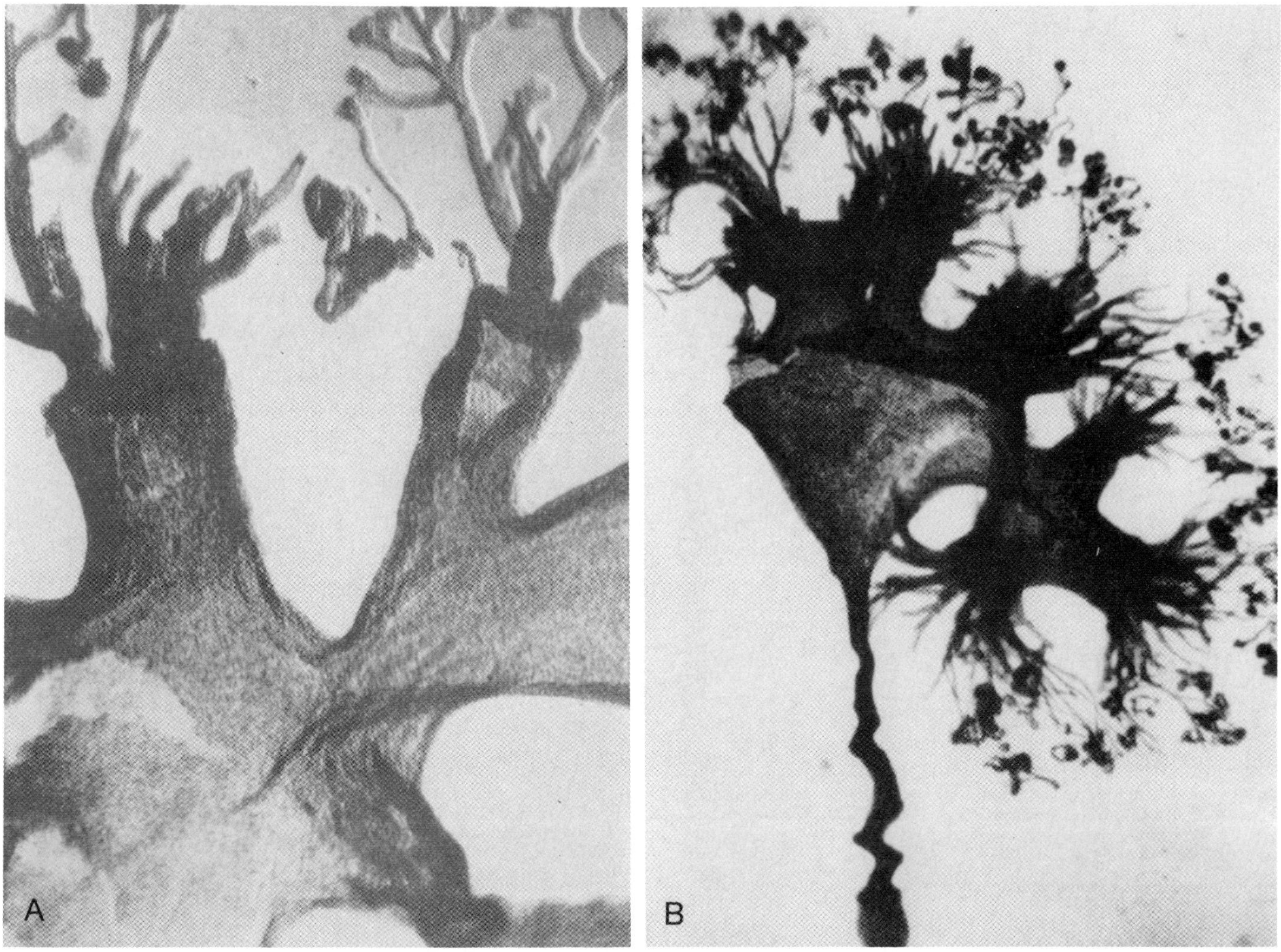

Figure 3.12. **A**, Kidney from a 74 mm, 13-week human fetus. Part of the ureter (*lower right*), interpolar portion of the renal pelvis, and 2 minor calyces are shown, as well as the total length of a few collecting tubules and 2 nephrons. The calyces are more distinctively cup-shaped than in earlier stages and begin to assume a definitive form. Five to six generations of collecting tubules are present distal to those that dilate to form the renal pelvis. **B**, Kidney from 90 mm, 14-week fetus. The upper third of the renal pelvis and most of last few generations of collecting tubules and nephrons have been removed to show calyces and proximal portions of tubules (papillary ducts) communicating with calyces. (With permission of Potter EL: Normal and Abnormal Development of the Kidney, Year Book Medical Publishers, Chicago, 1972)

third of the total nephrons formed. They ultimately constitute those found in the mature kidney in the inner juxtamedullary cortex. Those nephrons, whose attachments fail to move with the advancing ampullae, eventually disappear. They can be found in various stages of degeneration close to the renal pelvis during fetal life and sometimes even after birth.

Vascular Supply

Arteries from the aorta and veins from the vena cava adjacent to the primitive ureter are visible soon after the ureteral bud first divides. They give rise to branches that traverse the metanephric blastema surrounding the actively growing ampullae. The terminal branches of the arteries and veins extend to the periphery, where anastomosing small branches merge into the subcapsular network. By 14 to 15 weeks the vascular pattern of the fetal kidney already resembles that of the mature kidney (16, 17). At about 14 weeks, the branches of arteries near the junction of what will become the cortex and medulla elongate in a direction parallel to this zone, instead of remaining perpendicular as they were earlier. These represent the arcuate arteries. At maturity, the glomeruli in the outer two-thirds to three-quarters of the cortex usually are supplied by branches of the interlobular arteries. Those in the innermost part (juxtamedullary) are supplied by direct branches of arcuate, oblique, or even interlobular arteries. The differences between the vascular supply of the middle and outer cortical nephrons and the inner cortical nephrons are evident at 14 to 15 weeks.

THE URINARY TRACT AND GROWTH

Differentiation of the urinary tract occurs in synchrony with the early stages of metanephric development (3). The mesonephric duct communicates with the allantois and the cloaca at the fifth week of fetal life, when the ureteral bud appears. The urinary system separates from the rectum at about the sixth week, when the urorectal fold forms a septum isolating the urogenital sinus from the rectum (Fig. 3.5, *B*). The formation of a separate opening of the metanephric duct into the bladder occurs by the seventh week and becomes the vesicoureteral opening. This occurs via a complex process that absorbs the mesonephric duct distal to the ureteric bladder. The opening of the ureteral bud, which will become the ureteral orifice, migrates upward and laterally. That portion of the

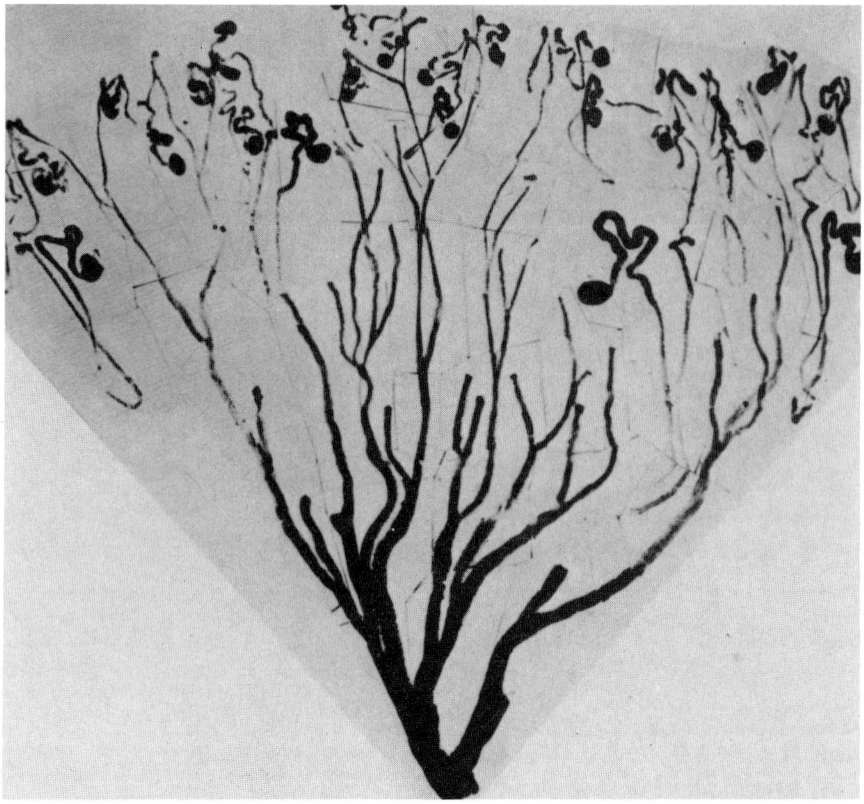

Figure 3.13. Collecting tree at 5 months. The tubules have divided 9 times in most instances, thus forming the fifteenth and final generation of the ductal systems, i.e., its closed divided portion has been established and now are all bifid. All the nephrons have been transported (Peter's transport process) to the periphery, and a separation into cortex and medulla is apparent. The nephrons appear in all configurations, from vesicles in those with well-developed loops of Henle; the former occur only at the periphery on the terminal budding ampullae. Note that every nephron is attached to an ampulla either directly by its connecting tubule or by an arcade; none has lagged behind. The kidney contains about one third the ultimate number of nephrons. The cortical region as it exists at this time will form only the juxtamedullary zone of the definitive cortex. (With permission of Oliver J: Nephrons and Kidneys: A Quantitative Study of the Developmental and Evolutionary Mammalian Renal Architectonics. Hoeber Medical Division, Harper and Row, New York, 1968)

ureteral bud that is above the bladder contracts to form a fibrous cord (urachus) (Fig. 3.5, *F*). When obstruction of the lower urinary tract is present, this fails to occur and urine is discharged via a patent urachus at the umbilicus.

The fetal ureter does not open into the bladder until about the ninth week, which concides with Gersh's (8) estimate of the time of onset of fetal renal function. Before this, a definite membrane is present at the anatomic junction of the ureter and urogenital sinus.

The Genital and Urinary Systems

The process responsible for the separation of the urinary from the genital system differs in the male and female (19, 20). The Y chromosome carries an inducer that transforms the primordial gonadal anlage into the masculine gonad. In the absence of the Y chromosome the bisexual gonad becomes the ovary. The primitive gonad of the male and female embryo goes through the undifferentiated period that lasts until the seventh week. Then, "obeying" the genetic impulse, it transforms into a testis or ovary.

The transformation of the potentially bisexual ductal system into male internal genitalia entails regression of the mullerian ducts. The regression of the mullerian ducts is induced by the mullerian regression factor produced by the fetal testis and differentiation of the mesonephric duct into wolffian ducts. In the male, the most cephalad portion of the wolffian ducts form the convoluted duct of the epidydimis; the caudal portion forms the ductus deferens, ejaculatory ducts, and seminal vesicles (Fig. 3.5, *E*). This process begins during the seventh to eighth week (19).

In the female the two mullerian ducts are maintained; by the end of the eighth week, the distal segments of these ducts join in the midline to form a single cord, the uterovaginal cord which opens into the urogenital sinus. The part of the urogenital sinus caudal to the opening of the mullerian duct forms the vaginal vestibule and contributes to the lower fifth of the vagina in the female. In the male, this part forms the intramontal part of the prostatic and membranous urethra. By the twelfth to thirteenth week, the median septum of the fused urogenital sinus is resorbed and the uterus, cervix, and part of the vagina (Fig. 3.5, *F*) evolve. At the same time, the mesenchymal wall that separates the urogenital sinus from the uterovaginal canal migrates downward, displaces the vagina posteriorly and inferiorly, and brings its opening to the perineum. The wolffian ducts regress completely, though a few remnants persist as epoophorons and Gartner ducts (20).

MALFORMATIONS

One approach to the classification of renal malformations would be to attempt to correlate the type of structural malformation observed with what might be predicted if one of the stages of renal development were adversely affected. This could facilitate the identification of the timing of teratogenic exposure in human renal malformations. This is, however,

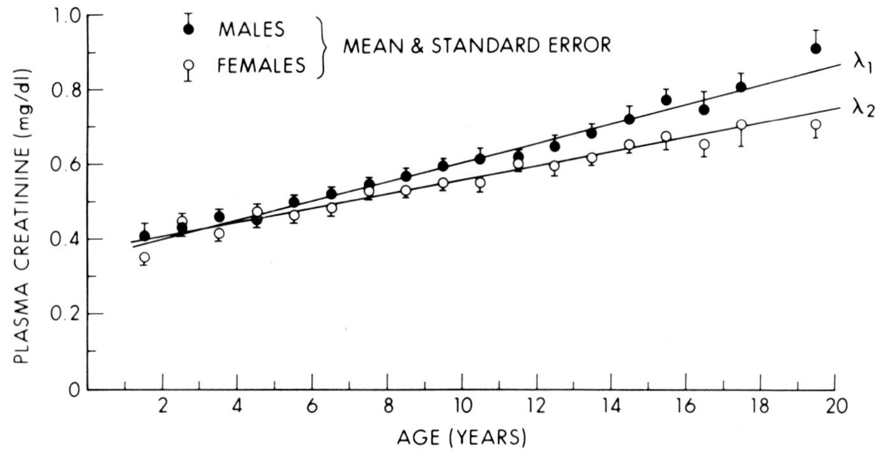

Figure 4.12. Mean plasma creatinine concentration (mg/dl) plotted against age for both sexes. The regression equations are: for males $y = 0.35 + 0.025 \times$ age and for females $y = 0.37 + 0.018 \times$ age. Reproduced with permission from Schwartz GJ, et al: J Pediat 88: 828, 1976.

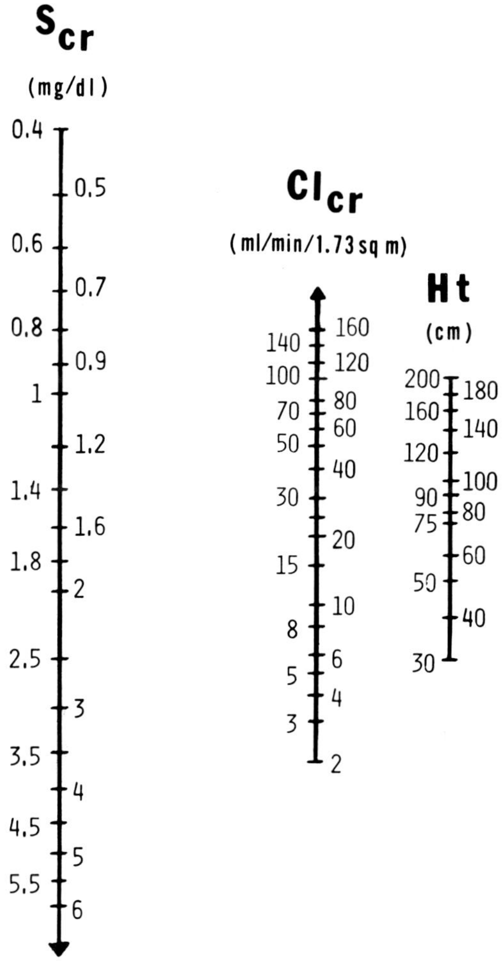

Figure 4.13. Normogram for rapid estimation of creatinine clearance in patients 1 to 18 years of age. A ruler used to connect the child's serum creatinine value (Cr_s) and height (Ht) will intersect the center line at a value approximating creatinine clearance (C_{Cr}). Reproduced with permission from Traub SL, Johnson CE: Am J Hosp Pharm 37: 195, 1980.

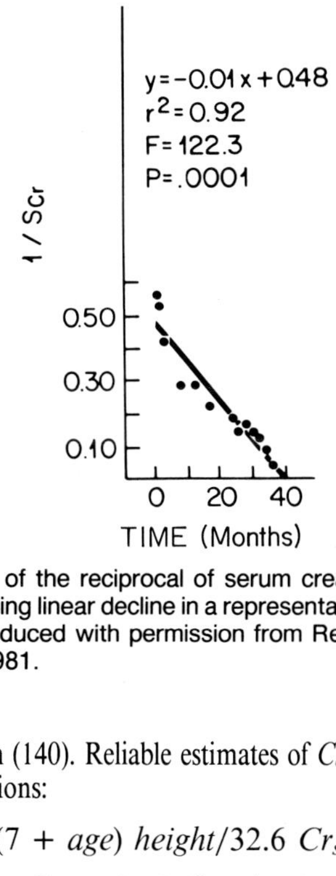

Figure 4.14. Plot of the reciprocal of serum creatinine ($1/Cr_s$) versus time (months) showing linear decline in a representative child with chronic renal failure. Reproduced with permission from Reimold EW: Am J Dis Child 135: 1039, 1981.

derive C_{Cr} from Cr_s as a per cent of normal by the equation: $C_{Cr}\% = Cr_s$ of normal individual for that age and size in relation to height, weight, and body surface (BSA). The formulae have been compiled recently by Traub and Johnson (140). Reliable estimates of C_{Cr} were derived from the following equations:

$$C_{Cr} = (7 + age)\ height/32.6\ Cr_s \times BSA$$

$$C_{Cr} = 0.48\ (height)Cr_s$$

where C_{Cr} is expressed in ml/min/1.73m^2, height in cm, age in year, Cr_s in mg/dl, and BSA in m^2. A normogram describing these relations is provided (Fig. 4.13).

Serum creatinine values are used to monitor the rate of deterioration of renal function in chronic renal failure. Since GFR $= U_x \times V/P_x$ in steady-state conditions, GFR is inversely proportional to plasma creatinine concentration. Hence, a doubling of serum creatinine level will reflect a decrease in GFR to half. An increase in Cr_s level from 1 to 2 mg% and from 4 to 8 mg% implies a fractional loss of half of the C_{Cr} between measures, but the fractional residual function is less in the second instance and the absolute decline is less. The rate of deterioration of GFR in most adults (141) and children (142, 143) with chronic renal failure, plotted as serial values of $1/Cr_s$ over time, describes a linear regression (Fig. 4.14), indicating that reduction in GFR in chronic renal failure in somewhat linear, while Cr_s increases exponentially. Plots using sufficient number of $1/Cr_s$ values over time are useful in predicting the time end-stage renal disease will develop.

References

1. Forster RP, Maes JP: Effect of experimental neurogenic hypertension on renal blood flow and glomerular filtration rate in intact denervated kidneys of unanesthetized rabbits with adrenal glands demedullated. Am J Physiol 150:534, 1947.
2. Schor N, Ichikawa I, Brenner BM: Glomerular adaptation to chronic dietary salt restriction or excess. Am J Physiol 238:F428, 1980.
3. Ichikawa I, Pfeffer JM, Pfeffer MA, et al: Role of Angiotensin II in the altered renal function of congestive heart failure. Circulation Res 55:669, 1984.
4. Jose PA, Slotkoff LM, Montgomery S, et al: Autoregulation of renal blood flow in the puppy. Am J Physiol 229:983, 1975.
5. Chevalier RL, Kaiser DL: Autoregulation of renal blood flow in the rat: effects of growth and uninephrectomy. Am J Physiol 244:F483, 1983.
6. Gilmore JP, Cornish KG, Rogers SD, et al: Direct evidence for myogenic autoregulation of the renal microcirculation in the hamster. Circulation Res 47:226, 1980.
7. Schnermann J, Briggs J: Concentration-dependent sodium chloride transport as the signal in feedback control of glomerular filtration rate. Kidney Intl 22:S82, 1982.
8. Wright FS, Schnermann J: Interference with feedback control of glomerular filtration rate by furosemide, triflocin and cyanide. J Clin Invest 53:1695, 1974.
9. McNay JL: Pharmacology of the renal circulation. Am J Med 62:507, 1977.
10. Gill JR, Melmon KL, Gillespie L, et al: Bradykinin and renal function in normal man: effects of adrenergic blockade. Am J Physiol 209:844, 1965.
11. Duchin KL, Peterson LN, Burke TJ: Effect of furosemide on renal autoregulation. Kidney Intl 12:379, 1977.
12. Adams PL, Adams FF, Bell PD, et al: Impaired renal blood flow autoregulation in ischemic acute renal failure. Kidney Intl 18:68, 1980.
13. Kopp U, Bradley T, Hjemdahl P: Renal venous outflow and urinary excretion of norepinephrine, epinephrine and dopamine during graded renal nerve stimulation. Am J Physiol 244:E52, 1983.
14. Kon V, Ichikawa I: Effector loci for renal nerve control of cortical microcirculation. Am J Physiol 245:F545, 1983.
15. Ammons WS, Koyama S, Manning JW: Neural and vascular interaction in renin response to graded renal nerve stimulation. Am J Physiol 242:R552, 1982.
16. Blair ML: Stimulation of renin secretion by α-receptor agonists. Am J Physiol 244:E37, 1983.
17. Hollenberg NK, Solomon HS, Adams DF, et al: Renal vascular response to angiotensin and norepinephrine in normal man. Circulation Res 31:750, 1972.
18. Rector JB, Stein JH, Bay WH, et al: Effect of hemorrhage and vasopressor agents on renal blood flow. Am J Physiol 222:1125, 1972.
19. Davalos M, Frega NS, Saker B, et al: Effect of exogenous angiotensin II on the isolated perfused rat kidney. Am J Physiol 235:F605, 1978.
20. Sakr HM, Dunham EW: Mechanism of arachidonic acid-induced vasoconstriction in the intact rat: possible involvement of thromboxane A_2. J Pharmacol Exptl Therap 221:614, 1982.
21. Stein JH, Ferris TF, Huprich JE, et al: Effect of renal vasodilatation on the distribution of cortical blood flow in the kidney of the dog. J Clin Invest 50:1429, 1971.
22. Vander AJ: Effects of acetylcholine, atropine, and physostigmine on renal function in the dog. Am J Physiol 206:492, 1964.
23. Mark AL, Eckstein JW, Abboud FM, et al: Renal vascular responses to isoproterenol. Am J Physiol 217:764, 1969.
24. Mizoguchi H, Dzau VJ, Siwek LG, et al: Effect of intrarenal administration of dopamine on renin release in conscious dogs. Am J Physiol 244:H39, 1983.
25. Spitalewitz S, Chou S-Y, Faubert PF, et al: Effect of diuretics on inner medullary hemodynamics in the dog. Circulation Res 51:703, 1982.
26. Vander AJ: Direct effects of prostaglandins on renal function and renin release in anesthetized dogs. Am J Physiol 214:218, 1968.
27. Adrendshorst WJ, Johnston PA, Selkurt EE: Effect of prostaglandin E1 on renal hemodynamics in nondiuretic and volume-expanded dogs. Am J Physiol 226:218, 1974.
28. Wong PC, Zimmerman BG, Kraft E, et al: Pharmacological evaluation in conscious dogs of factors involved in the renal vasodilator effect of captopril. J Pharmacol Exptl Therap 219:646, 1981.
29. Heinrich WL, Anderson RJ, Berns AS, et al: The role of renal nerves and prostaglandins in control of renal hemodynamics and plasma renin activity during hypotensive hemorrhage in the dog. J Clin Invest 61:744, 1978.
30. Cifuentes RF, Olley PM, Baefe JW, et al: Indomethacin and renal function in premature infants with persistent ductus arteriosus. J Pediatr 95:583, 1979.
31. Kawasaki A, Needleman P: Contribution of thromboxane to renal resistance in the isolated perfused hydronephrotic rabbit kidney. Circulation Res 50:486, 1982.
32. Iwamoto HS, Rudolph AM: Role of renin-angiotensin system in response to hemorrhage in fetal sheep. Am J Physiol 240:H848, 1981.
33. Rudolph AM, Heymann MA, Teramo AW, et al: Studies on the circulation of the previable human fetus. Pediatr Res 5:452, 1971.
34. Moore ES, Galvez MB, Pator JB, et al: Intrarenal blood flow in the baboon fetus. Pediatr Res 9:377, 1975.
35. Aperia A, Broberger O, Herin P, et al: Renal hemodynamics in the perinatal period. A study in lambs. Acta Physiol Scand 99:261, 1977.
36. Potter EL, Craig JM: Kidneys, ureters, urinary bladder and urethra. Pathology of the Fetus and the Infant. Chicago, Yearbook Medical Publishers, Inc., 1975, p 436.
37. Gruskin AB, Edelmann CM, Yuan S: Maturational changes in renal blood flow in piglets. Pediatr Res 4:7, 1970.
38. Aperia A, Herin P: Development of glomerular perfusion rate and nephron filtration rate in rats 17–60 days old. Am J Physiol 228:1319, 1975.
39. Strauss J, Daniel SS, Janis LS: Postnatal adjustment in renal function. Pediatrics 68:802, 1981.
40. Fawer C-L, Torrado A, Guignard, J-P: Maturation of renal function in full-term and premature neonates. Helvet Paediat Acta 34:11, 1979.
41 Rubin MI, Bruck E, Rapaport M: Maturation of renal function in childhood: clearance studies. J Clin Invest 28:1144, 1949.
42. Calcagno PL, Rubin MI: Renal extraction in para aminohippurate in infants and children. J Clin Invest 42:1632, 1963.
43. Guignard J-P, Torrado A, Mazouni SM, et al: Renal function in respiratory distress syndrome. J Pediatr 88:845, 1976.
44. Ichikawa I, Maddox DA, Brenner BM: Maturational development of glomerular ultrafiltration in the rat. Am J Physiol 236:F465, 1979.
45. Sulyok E, Nêmeth M, Tényi I, et al: Postnatal development of renin-angiotensin-aldosterone system, RAAS, in relation to electrolyte balance in premature infants. Pediatr Res 13:817, 1979.
46. Kotchen TA, Strickland AL, Rice TW, et al: A study of the renin-angiotensin system in newborn infants. J Pediatr 80:938, 1972.
47. Matson JR, Stokes JB, Robillard JE: Effect of inhibition of prostaglandin synthesis on fetal renal function. Kidney Intl 20:621, 1981.
48. Olbing J, Blaufox MD, Aschinberg LC, et al: Postnatal changes in glomerular blood flow distribution in puppies. J Clin Invest 52:2885, 1973.
49. Aperia A, Broberger O, Herin P: Maturational changes in glomerular perfusion rate and glomerular filtration rate in lambs. Pediatr Res 8:758, 1974.
50. Sraer JD, Sraer J, Ardaillou R, et al: Evidence for glomerular receptors for angiotensin II. Kidney Intl 6:241, 1974.
51. Ausiello DA, Kreisberg JI, Roy C, et al: Contraction of cultured rat glomerular cells of apparent mesangial origin after stimulation with angiotensin II and arginine vasopressin. J Clin Invest 65:754, 1980.
52. Sraer J, Sraer JD, Chansel D, et al: Evidence for glomerular receptors for parathyroid hormone. Am J Physiol 235:F96, 1978.
53. Schlondorff D, Yoo P, Alpert BE: Stimulation of adenylate cyclase in isolated rat glomeruli by prostaglandins. Am J Physiol 235:F458, 1978.
54. Folkert V, Schlondorff D: Inhibition and stimulation of prostaglandin synthesis in isolated rat glomeruli. Clin Res 27:414A, 1979.
55. Blantz RC, Konnen KS, Tucker BJ: Angiotensin II effects on the glomerular microcirculation and ultrafiltration coefficient of the rat. J Clin Invest 57:419, 1976.
56. Ichikawa I, Brenner BM: Evidence for glomerular actions of ADH and dibutyryl cyclic AMP in the rat. Am J Physiol 233:F102, 1977.
57. Ichikawa I, Humes HD, Dousa TP, et al: Influence of parathyroid hormone on glomerular ultrafiltration in the rat. Am J Physiol 234:F393, 1978.
58. Deen WM, Robertson CR, Brenner BM: A model of glomerular ultrafiltration in the rat. Am J Physiol 223:1178, 1972.
59. Robertson CR, Deen WM, Troy JL, et al: Dynamics of glomerular ultrafiltration in the rat. III. Hemodynamics and autoregulation. Am J Physiol 223:1191, 1972.
60. London GM, Safar ME, Levenson JA, et al: Renal filtration fraction, effective vascular compliance and partition of fluid volumes in sustained essential hypertension. Kidney Intl 20:99, 1981.
61. Arendshorst WJ: Autoregulation of renal blood flow in spontaneously hypertensive rats. Circulation Res 44:344, 1979.
62. Ichikawa I, Ferrone RA, Duchin KL, et al: Relative contribution of vasopressin and Angiotensin II to the altered renal microcirculatory dynamics in two-kidney Goldblatt hypertension. Circulation Res 53:592, 1983.
63. Blantz RC, Konnen KS, Tucker BJ: Glomerular filtration response to elevated ureteral pressure in both the hydropenic and the plasma-expanded rat. Circulation Res 37:819, 1975.
64. Dal Canton A, Stanziale R, Corradi A, et al: Effects of acute ureteral obstruction on glomerular hemodynamics in rat kidney. Kidney Intl 12:403, 1977.
65. Gaudio KM, Siegel NJ, Hayslett JP, et al: Renal perfusion and intratubular pressure during ureteral occlusion in the rat. Am J Physiol 238:F205, 1980.
66. Ichikawa I, Brenner BM: Local intrarenal vasoconstrictor-vasodilator interactions in mild partial ureteral obstruction. Am J Physiol 236:F131, 1979.
67. Dal Canton A, Corradi A, Stanziale R, et al: Glomerular hemodynamics before and after release of 24-hour bilateral ureteral obstruction. Kidney Intl 17:491, 1980.

68. Wilson DR: Nephron functional heterogeneity in the postobstructive kidney. Kidney Intl 7:19, 1975.
69. Venkatachalam MA, Bernard DB, Donohoe JF, et al: Ischemic damage and repair in the rat proximal tubule. Differences among the S1, S2 and S3 segments. Kidney Intl 14:31, 1978.
69a. Oliver J, MacDowell M: The renal lesion in epidemic hemorrhagic fever. J Clin Invest 36:99, 1957.
70. Baylis C, Ichikawa I, Willis WT, et al: Dynamics of glomerular ultrafiltration. IX. Effects of plasma protein concentration. Am J Physiol 232:F58, 1977.
71. Blantz RC, Rector FC, Seldin DW: Effects of hyperoncotic albumin expansion upon glomerular ultrafiltration in the rat. Kidney Intl 6:209, 1974.
72. Hoyer JR, Mauer SM, Michael AF: Unilateral renal disease in the rat. I. Clinical, morphologic and glomerular mesangial functional features of the experimental model produced by renal perfusion with aminonucleoside. J Lab Clin Med 85:756, 1975.
73. Ichikawa I, Rennke HG, Hoyer JR, et al: Role for intrarenal mechanisms in the impaired salt excretion of experimental nephrotic syndrome. J Clin Invest 71:91, 1983.
74. White RHR, Glasgow EF, Mills RJ: Clinicopathological study of nephrotic syndrome in childhood. Lancet i:1353, 1970.
75. Klahr S, Alleyne GAO: Effects of chronic protein-calorie malnutrition on the kidney. Kidney Intl 3:129, 1973.
76. Ichikawa I, Purkerson ML, Klahr S, et al: Mechanism of reduced glomerular filtration rate in chronic malnutrition. J Clin Invest 65:982, 1980.
77. Baylis C, Deen WM, Myers BD, et al: Effects of some vasodilator drugs on transcapillary fluid exchange in renal cortex. Am J Physiol 230:1148, 1976.
78. Ichikawa I, Brenner BM: Mechanism of action of histamine and histamine antagonists on the glomerular microcirculation in the rat. Circulation Res 45:737, 1979.
79. Myers BD, Deen WM, Brenner BM: Effects of norepinephrine and angiotensin II on the determinants of glomerular ultrafiltration and poximal tubule fluid reabsorption in the rat. Circulation Res 37:101, 1975.
80. Briggs AP, Fowell DM, Hamilton WF, et al: Renal and circulatory factors in the edema formation of congestive heart failure. J Clin Invest 27:810, 1948.
81. Heller BI, Jacobson WE: Renal hemodynamics in heart disease. Am Heart J 39:188, 1950.
82. Yared A, Kon V, Ichikawa I: Mechanism of preservation of glomerular perfusion and filtration during acute extracellular fluid volume depletion. Importance of intrarenal vasopressin-prostaglandin interaction for protecting kidneys from constrictor action of vasopressin. J Clin Ivest 75:1477, 1985.
83. Mogensen CE: Glomerular filtration rate and renal plasma flow in short-term and long-term juvenile diabetes mellitus. Scand J Clin Lab Invest 28:91, 1971.
84. Hostetter TH, Troy JL, Brenner BM: Glomerular hemodynamics in experimental diabetes. Kidney Intl 19:410, 1981.
85. Blantz C: The mechanism of acute renal failure after uranyl nitrate. J Clin Invest 55:621, 1975.
86. Baylis C, Rennke HR, Brenner BM: Mechanisms of the defect in glomerular ultrafiltration associated with gentamicin administration. Kidney Intl 12:344, 1977.
87. Maddox DA, Bennett CM, Deen WM, et al: Determinants of glomerular filtration in experimental glomerulonephritis in the rat. J Clin Invest 55:305, 1975.
88. Blantz RC, Wilson CB: Acute effects of antiglomerular basement membrane antibody on the process of glomerular filtration in the rat. J Clin Invest 58:899, 1976.
89. Ichikawa I, Hoyer JR, Seiler MW, et al: Mechanism of glomerulotubular balance in the setting of heterogeneous glomerular injury. Preservation of a close functional linkage between individual nephrons and surrounding microvasculature. J Clin Invest 69:185, 1982.
90. Steiner RW, Tucker BJ, Blantz RC: Glomerular hemodynamics in rats with chronic sodium depletion. Effect of saralasin. J Clin Invest 64:503, 1979.
91. Tucker BJ, Blantz RC: Mechanism of altered glomerular hemodynamics during chronic sodium depletion. Am J Physiol 244:F11, 1983.
92. Dilley JR, Corradi A, Arendshorst WJ: Effect of increased renal venous pressure on glomerular hemodynamics in the rat. Clin Res 30:446A, 1982.
93. Ichikawa I, Brenner BM: Importance of efferent arteriolar vascular tone in regulation of proximal tubule fluid reabsorption and glomerulotubular balance in the rat. J Clin Invest 65:1192, 1980.
94. Schor N, Ichikawa I, Rennke HG, et al: Pathophysiology of altered glomerular function in aminoglycoside-treated rats. Kidney Intl 19:288, 1980.
94a. Humes HD, Ichikawa I, Troy JL, et al: Evidence for a parathyroid hormone-dependent influence of calcium on the glomerular ultrafiltration coefficient. J Clin Invest 61:32, 1978.
95. Tucker BJ, Blantz RC: Factors determining superficial nephron filtration in the mature, growing rat. Am J Physiol 232:F97, 1977.
96. Deen WM, Robertson CR, Brenner BM: Glomerular ultrafiltration. Fed Proc 33:14, 1974.
97. Schor N, Ichikawa I, Brenner BM: Mechanisms of action of various hormones and vasoactive substances on glomerular ultrafiltration in the rat. Kidney Intl 20:442, 1981.
98. Baylis C, Brenner BM: Mechanism of the glucocorticoid-induced increase in glomerular filtration rate. Am J Physiol 234:F166, 1978.
99. Dworkin LD, Ichikawa I, Brenner BM: Hormonal modulation of renal function. Am J Physiol 244:F95, 1983.
100. Becker CG: Demonstration of actomyosin in mesangial cells of the renal glomerulus. Am J Path 66:97, 1972.
100a. Mahieu PR, Foidart JB, Dubois CH, et al: Tissue culture of normal rat glomeruli: contractile activity of the cultured mesangial cells. Invest Cell Pathol 3:121, 1980.
101. Larsson L, Aperia A, Wilton P: Effect of normal development on compensatory renal growth. Kidney Intl 18:29, 1980.
102. Horster M, Valtin H: Postnatal development of renal function: Micropuncture and clearance studies in the dog. J Clin Invest 50:779, 1971.
103. Merlet-Benichou C, Pegorier M, Muffat-Joly M, et al: Functional and morphologic patterns of renal maturation in the developing guinea pig. Am J Physiol 241:F618, 1981.
104. Odgen DA: Donor and recipient function 2 to 4 years after renal homotransplantation. Ann Intern Med 67:998, 1967.
105. Claësson I, Jacobsson B, Jodal U, et al: Compensatory kidney growth in children with urinary tract infection and renal scarring. An epidemiologic study. Kidney Intl 20:759, 1981.
106. Kaufman JM, Siegel NJ, Hayslett JP: Functional and hemodynamic adaptation to progressive renal ablation. Circulation Res 36:266, 1975.
107. Deen WM, Maddox DA, Robertson CR, et al: Dynamics of glomerular ultrafiltration in the rat. VII. Response to reduced renal mass. Am J Physiol 227:556, 1974.
108. Hayslett JP: Effect of age on compensatory renal growth. Kidney Intl 23:599, 1983.
109. Northrup TE, Malvin RL: Cellular hypertrophy and renal function during compensatory renal growth. Am J Physiol 231:1191, 1976.
110. Chevalier RL: Functional adaptation to reduced renal mass in early development. Am J Physiol 242:F190, 1982.
111. Carriere S, Gagnan-Brunette M: Compensatory renal hypertrophy in dogs: Single nephron glomerular filtration rate. Canad J Physiol Pharmacol 55:105, 1976.
112. Knutson DW, Chieu F, Bennett CM, et al: Estimation of relative glomerular capillary surface area in normal and hypertropic rat kidneys. Kidney Intl 14:437, 1978.
113. Preuss HG: Compensatory renal growth symposium: An introduction. Kidney Intl 23:571, 1983.
114. Allisson MEM, Wilson CB, Gottschalk CW: Pathophysiology of experimental glomerulonephritis in rats. J Clin Invest 53:1402, 1974.
115. Kramp RA, MacDowell M, Gottschalk CW, et al: A study by microdissection and micropuncture of the structure and the function of the kidneys and the nephrons of rats with chronic renal damage. Kidney Intl 5:147, 1974.
116. Gresham EL, Rankin JHG, Makowski EL, et al: An evaluation of fetal renal function in a chronic sheep preparation. J Clin Invest 51:149, 1972.
117. Robillard JE, Kulvinskas C, Sessions C, et al: Maturational changes in the fetal glomerular filtration rate. Am J Obstet Gynecol 122:601, 1975.
118. Horster M, Lewy JE: Filtration fraction and extraction of PAH during neonatal period in the rat. Am J Physiol 219:1061, 1970.
119. Kleinman LI, Lubbe RJ: Factors affecting the maturation of glomerular filtration rate and glomerular plasma flow in the newborn dog. J Physiol 223:395, 1972.
120. Guignard JP, Torrado A, Da Cunha O, et al: Glomerular filtration rate in the first three weeks of life. J Pediat 87:268, 1975.
121. Aperia A, Broberger O, Thodenius K, et al: Development of renal control of salt and fluid homeostasis during the first year of life. Acta Paediat Scand 64:393, 1975.
122. Lay KS, Barcalari E, Malkus H, et al: Acute effects of albumin infusion on blood volume and renal function in premature infants with respiratory distress syndrome. J Ped 97:619, 1980.
123. Spitzer A, Edelmann CM: Maturational changes in pressure gradients for glomerular filtration. Am J Physiol 221:1431, 1971.
124. Overman RR, Etteldorf JN, Bass AC, et al: Plasma and erythrocyte chemistry of the normal infant from birth to two years of age. Pediatrics 7:565, 1951.
125. Leake RD, Zakauddin S, Trygstad CW, et al: The effects of large volume intravenous fluid infusion on neonatal renal function. J Pediat 89:968, 1976.
126. Oh W, Oh MA, Lind J: Renal function and blood volume in newborn infant related to placental transfusion. Acta Paediat Scand 55:197, 1966.
126a. John E, Goldsmith DI, Spitzer A: Quantitative changes in the canine glomerular vasculature during development: Physiologic implications. Kidney Intl 20:223, 1981.
127. Fetterman GH, Shuplock NA, Philipp FJ, et al: The growth and maturation of human glomeruli from term to adulthood. Studies by microdissection. Pediatrics 35:601, 1965.
128. Spitzer A: Factors underlying the increase in glomerular filtration rate during postnatal development. In Spitzer A (ed): The Kidney During Development, Morphology and Function. New York, Masson Publishing U.S.A., Inc., 1982, p 127.
129. Hook JB, Hewitt WR: Development of mechanisms for drug excretion. Am J Med 62:497, 1977.

130. Graystone JE: Creatinine excretion during growth. In Cheek DB (ed): Human Growth. Philadelphia, Lea and Febiger, 1968, p 182.
131. Arant BS, Edelmann CM, Spitzer A: The congruence of creatinine and inulin clearances in children. Use of the Technicon Autoanalyzer. J Pediat 81:559, 1972.
132. Carrie BJ, Golbetz HV, Michaels AS, et al: Creatinine: An inadequate filtration marker in glomerular diseases. Am J Med 69:177, 1980.
133. Myers BM, Chui F, Hilberman M, et al: Transtubular leakage of glomerular filtrate in human acute renal failure. Am J Physiol 237:F319, 1979.
134. Eisenbach GM, Steinhausen M: Micropuncture studies after temporary ischemia of rat kidneys. Pflugers Archiv 343:11, 1973.
135. Mak RHK, Al Dahhan J, Azzopardi D, et al: Measurement of glomerular filtration rate in children after renal transplantation. Kidney Intl 23:410, 1983.
136. Stonestreet BS, Oh W: Plasma creatinine levels in low birth weight infants during the first three months of life. Pediatrics 61:788, 1978.
137. Sutphen JL: Anthropometric determinants of creatinine excretion in preterm infants. Pediatrics 69:719, 1982.
138. Schwartz GJ, Haycock GB, Chir B, et al: Plasma creatinine and urea concentration in children: Normal values for age and sex. J Pediat 88:828, 1976.
139. Lewis JS, Bunker ML, Getts SS, et al: Variability of creatinine excretion of normal, phenylketouric and galactosemic children, and children treated with anticonvulsant drugs. Am J Clin Nutr 28:310, 1975.
140. Traub SL, Johnson CE: Comparison of methods of estimating creatinine clearance in children. Am J Hosp Pharm 37:195, 1980.
141. Mitch WE, Walser M, Buffington GA, et al: A simple method of estimating progression of chronic renal failure. Lancet ii:1326, 1976.
142. Reimold EW: Chronic progressive renal failure. Rate of progression monitored by change of serum creatinine concentration. Am J Dis Child 135:1039, 1981.
143. Arbus GS, Bacheyie GS: Method for predicting when children with progressive renal disease may reach high serum creatinine levels. Pediatrics 67:871, 1981.

CHAPTER 5

RENAL TUBULAR FUNCTION

Ronald J. Hogg
F. Bruder Stapleton

INTRODUCTION

Our current level of knowledge regarding renal tubular function has evolved largely through a series of theoretical and technical advances in renal physiology over the past 35 years. During that time, renal physiologists have studied tubular handling of the glomerular filtrate in a variety of mammalian and nonmammalian species, using techniques ranging from clearance, micropuncture, and microcatheterization studies in vivo to isolated kidney, perfused tubule, and microvesicle studies in vitro. The integration of results from these diverse technologies has been painful at times but, in most cases, has produced a more comprehensive understanding of individual renal tubular transport processes. The extrapolation of results from studies on nonhuman species to normal human renal physiology must be carried out with caution, but this caveat should not undermine the tremendous impact that data obtained from animal studies have had on current concepts of normal and abnormal renal physiology.

This chapter will attempt to detail the major sites and processes involved with tubular modification of glomerular filtrate as it traverses the length of the nephron. Much of the information has been derived from animal studies but, where possible, the results have been derived from human studies. Most studies of renal tubular function have been performed on tubules from adult kidneys; however, more attention has been directed recently toward renal tubular function in human infants and experimental work evaluating tubular transport mechanisms in immature nephrons from other species has increased.

The terminology in Figure 5.1 (1) for individual nephron segments will be used throughout this chapter. In addition, the proximal tubule will be considered in terms of its further segmentation into S_1, S_2, and S_3 (2, 3) (Fig. 5.2). The S_1 segment represents the initial proximal convoluted tubule with a thick brush border and complex basolateral membrane; S_2 is the junction of the convoluted and straight portions of the proximal tubule with a short brush border; and S_3 is the terminal proximal straight tubule located in the innermost cortex and outermost medullary stripe (2).

SODIUM AND CHLORIDE TRANSPORT

Maturity

Because sodium (Na) and chloride (Cl) constitute the most important osmolar components of extracellular fluid (ECF), changes in their rate of excretion have a major effect on the maintenance of normal body homeostasis. Whereas the active reabsorption of the two ions varies between different nephron segments, the active reabsorption of one greatly influences the reabsorption of the other; thus, it is relevant to consider their renal tubular transport mechanisms in concert (chapter 6).

Proximal Tubules

NaCl reabsorption in the proximal convoluted and straight tubules has been investigated by all currently known techniques. The availability of accessible superficial convoluted segments in a number of species enables segmental analysis of NaCl transport to be evaluated in this nephron segment in vivo during variations of the physiologic state of the animal. Micropuncture studies show that approximately 60% to 70% of filtered NaCl is absorbed in the proximal tubule. Much of the NaCl transport in this segment is the result of active cotransport of Na with amino acids and glucose (4). In addition, some of the NaCl that is reabsorbed occurs as a result of Na-hydrogen exchange via a brush border membrane-bound antiporter with subsequent passive Cl diffusion (see Fluid Reabsorption). Some sodium reabsorption in the proximal straight tubule may be the result of an active transport mechanism involving this cation only (5).

Thin Descending Limb and Ascending Limb of Henle

NaCl transport in the thin descending limb has been evaluated using the isolated perfused tubule technique. An evaluation of intraspecies and interspecies heterogeneity involving NaCl transport in the thin limbs of Henle's loop was the subject of a series of studies by Imai (6). By comparing thin descending limbs of superficial and juxtamedullary nephrons in the hamster, he concluded that the initial segment of the juxta-

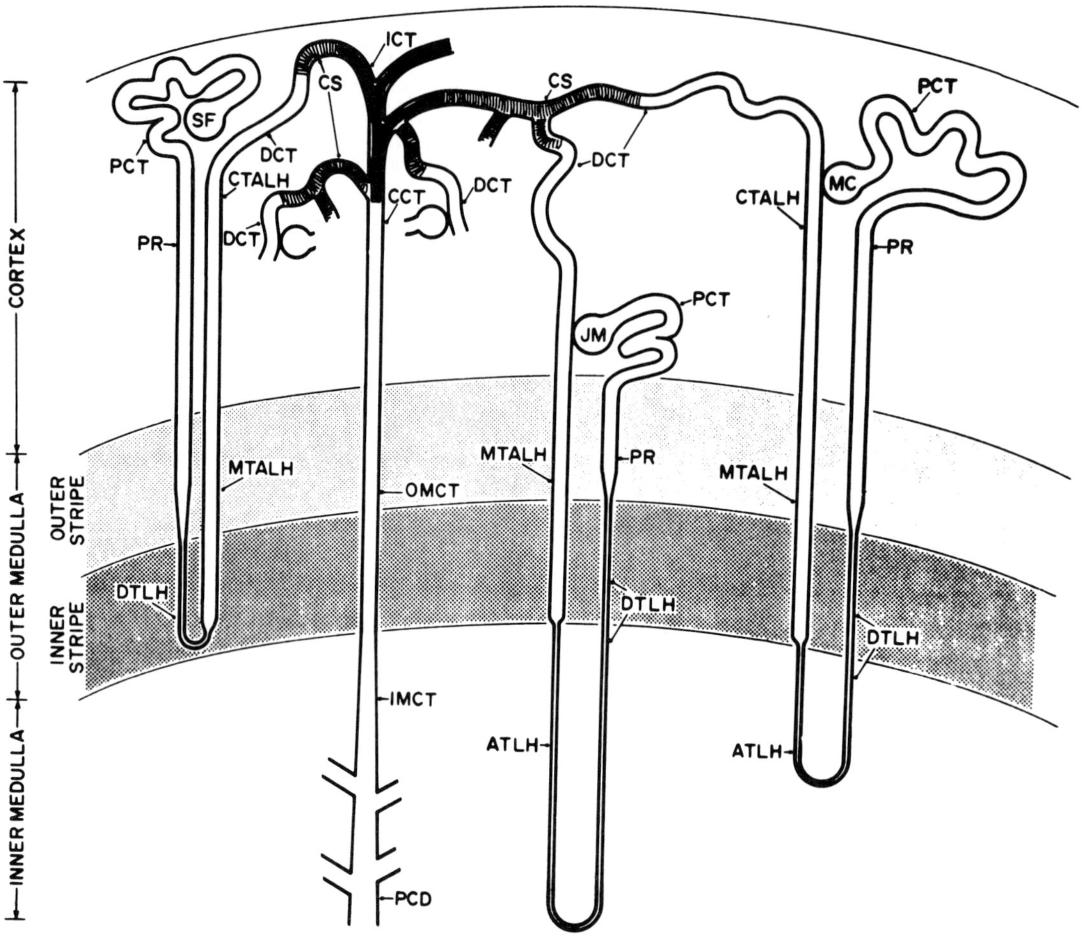

Figure 5.1. Anatomic configuration and terminology for renal tubule segments. Three populations of nephrons based on the location of their glomeruli: superficial (*SF*), midcortical (*MC*), and juxtamedullary (*JM*). The extent to which functional differences exist between these—and possibly other intermediate nephron populations—in mature and immature kidneys is unclear. *PCT*, proximal convoluted tubule; *PR*, pars recta; *DTLH*, descending thin limb of Henle; *ATLH*, ascending thin limb of Henle; *MTALH*, medullary thick ascending limb of Henle; *CTALH*, cortical thick ascending limb of Henle; *DCT*, distal convoluted tubule; *CS*, connecting segment; *ICT*, initial collecting tubule; *CCT*, cortical collecting tubule; *OMCT*, outer medullary collecting; *IMCT* inner medullary collecting tubule; and *PCD*, papillary collecting duct. (From Jacobson HR: Am J Physiol 241:F203, 1981.)

medullary descending limb of Henle is more permeable to Na than Cl in this species, whereas the opposite is true for superficial nephron segments (6). Similar results were found in the descending limb of the rat but smaller changes were found in the rabbit, confirming previous studies in this species (7). Isotopic permeability coefficients correlated well with the relative permeabilities (6). The physiologic relevance of variable Na and Cl permeability in the thin descending limbs is unclear at the present time.

In contrast to the species differences noted in descending limbs, the thin ascending limbs of juxtamedullary nephrons in various species have similar specific ion permeabilities. There are, of course, no thin ascending limb segments in superficial nephrons (Fig. 5.1). Chloride is the most permeable ion in this segment. This finding has been obtained in both in vitro studies of rabbit tubules (8) and in vivo studies in the rat papillae (9) and is consistent with the presence of significant passive reabsorption of NaCl in this segment.

Thick Ascending Limb of Henle

NaCl absorption in the thick ascending limb may account for 20% to 30% of the filtered NaCl. Net transport of NaCl in the rabbit medullary thick ascending limb is twofold to threefold higher than in the cortical thick ascending limb. NaCl transport also differs in these two segments in that the medullary thick ascending limbs have a higher transport capacity for NaCl, but the cortical segment is able to generate a steeper transepithelial concentration gradient. The mechanism of NaCl transport in the thick ascending limb has been subjected to a rigorous reevaluation in the last 4 years (10). Previous studies of NaCl transport in this segment (11, 12) had suggested the presence of a primary active Cl transport mechanism. This was apparently preserved when luminal Na was removed. However, with more stringent removal of Na from the lumen and bath solutions, NaCl transport was ablated, demonstrating that Cl transport in this segment is closely coupled to Na transport (Fig. 5.3) (10).

Modulations of NaCl Transport in the Thick Ascending Limb. In some species, active transport of NaCl across the medullary thick ascending limb is stimulated by antidiuretic hormone (ADH) (13, 14). The basolateral membrane potential of cells in this segment is decreased by ADH, which has led to the conclusion that Cl conductance channels in the basolateral membrane are opened up. This increase in NaCl transport appears to be induced by cyclic adenosine monophosphate (AMP) (17). However, the human medullary thick ascending limb lacks ADH-stimulated adenylate cyclase (15) and thus may not be sensitive to ADH as are those species which do demonstrate the ADH effect in this segment.

Prostaglandin inhibition of active NaCl transport in the thick ascend-

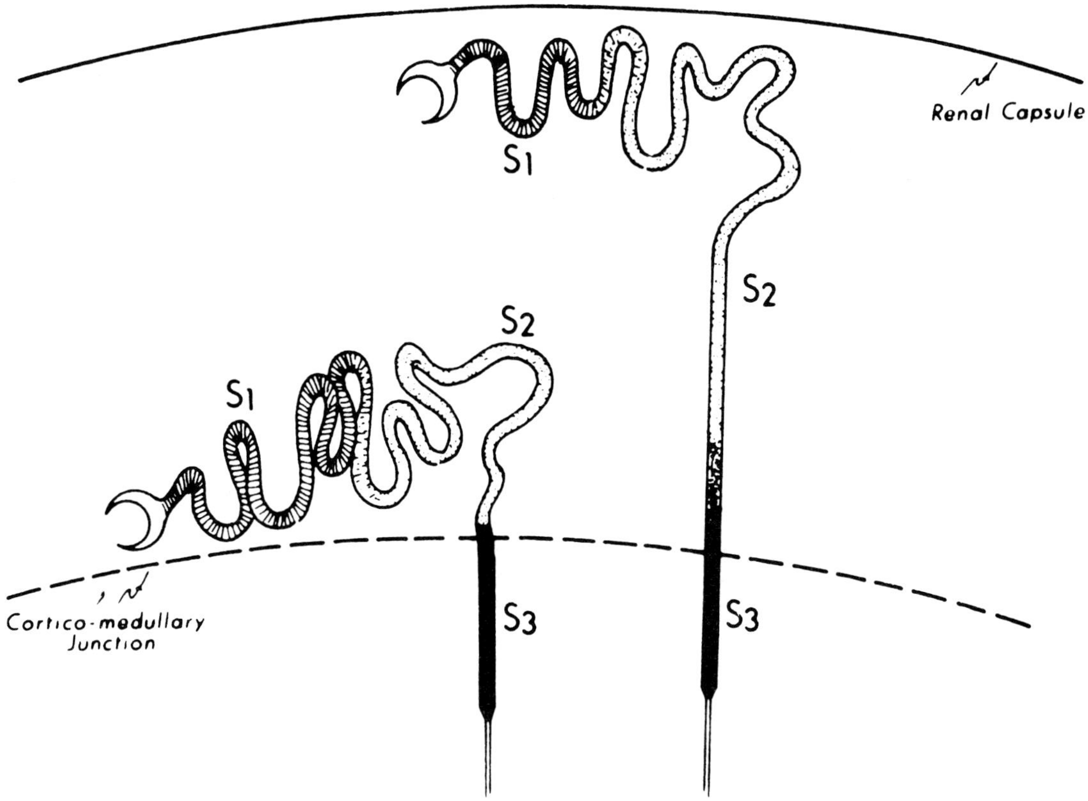

Figure 5.2. Schematic representation of the distribution of S_1, S_2, and S_3 segments in superficial and juxtamedullary proximal tubules. (From Woodhall PB, et al: J Clin Invest 61:1320, 1978, by copyright permission of The American Society for Clinical Investigation.)

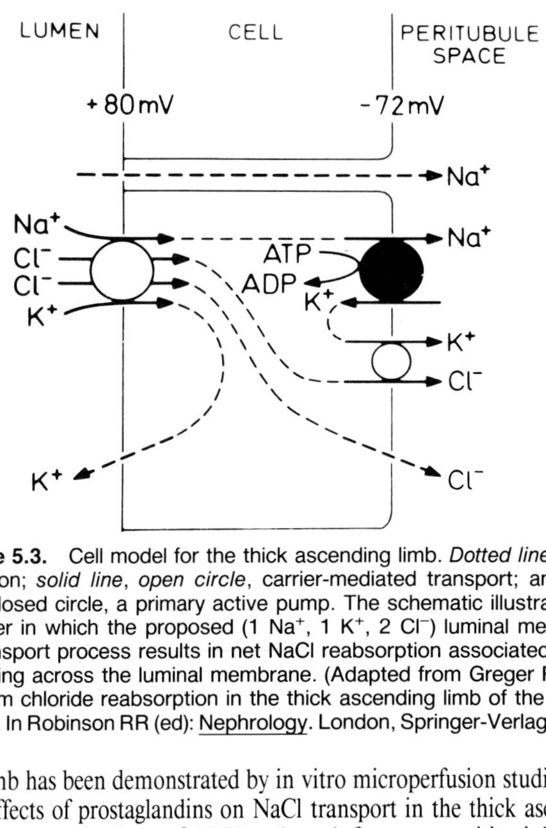

Figure 5.3. Cell model for the thick ascending limb. *Dotted line arrow*, diffusion; *solid line, open circle*, carrier-mediated transport; and solid line, closed circle, a primary active pump. The schematic illustrates the manner in which the proposed (1 Na^+, 1 K^+, 2 Cl^-) luminal membrane cotransport process results in net NaCl reabsorption associated with K recycling across the luminal membrane. (Adapted from Greger R, et al: Sodium chloride reabsorption in the thick ascending limb of the loop of Henle. In Robinson RR (ed): Nephrology. London, Springer-Verlag, 1984.)

ing limb has been demonstrated by in vitro microperfusion studies (16). The effects of prostaglandins on NaCl transport in the thick ascending limb are opposite those of ADH and result from competitive inhibition (17). Other studies have demonstrated an inhibitory effect of hypertonic peritubular media on NaCl transport by the thick ascending limb; hypertonicity modulates the extent to which ADH stimulates the reabsorption of NaCl (18). Increase in ambient potassium (K) concentration also reduces NaCl transport in the medullary thick ascending limb (19); details of the interrelationships of these different modulators of NaCl have been reviewed elsewhere (20).

Distal Tubule

Although NaCl transport in the distal nephron and collecting tubules has been studied by in vivo micropuncture and in vitro microperfusion techniques, the recent appreciation of heterogeneity of structure and function along the distal accessible segments of the nephron has made it difficult to ascribe data from micropuncture experiments to specific tubule segments. This heterogeneity also extends to different segments of the collecting tubule and pertains to the transport of Na and K ions (21). Whereas the cortical collecting tubule exhibits mineralocorticoid-dependent NaCl reabsorption and K secretion, the medullary collecting tubule does not show any significant active transport of these ions, either under normal conditions or following mineralocorticoid stimulation. Aldosterone increases Na reabsorption and K exchange in the cortical collecting duct as a result of an increase in Na,K-adenosine triphosphatase (ATPase) activity that is blocked if luminal Na uptake is inhibited by amiloride (22).

The stimulatory effect of mineralocorticoids on Na reabsorption in the collecting tubule may be contrasted with the effect of prostaglandin E_2, which inhibits both lumen-negative voltage and Na reabsorption when added to the peritubular fluid (23). Although we have known for sometime that Na is reabsorbed in the cortical collecting tubule, only recently have we known that Cl also is reabsorbed there (24). With the demonstration that NaCl is reabsorbed in the cortical collecting tubule, this segment is acting as the final diluting segment.

Developmental Aspects

Developmental aspects of sodium chloride reabsorption have been evaluated in a variety of species at different stages of maturation. The failure of newborn dogs to develop an appropriate natriuretic response following saline loading was studied by Kleinman (25) using the technique of distal blockade of sodium chloride reabsorption (using ethacrynic acid and chlorothiazide). He showed that proximal reabsorption of Na was depressed significantly in these animals following volume expansion and concluded that the failure to excrete a sodium load under normal conditions resulted from persistent augmentation of distal sodium reabsorption.

Micropuncture studies of NaCl reabsorption in the superficial loop of Henle (26) showed a depression of NaCl reabsorption, which increased in the diluting segment with maturation. The likely explanation for this involves an increase in NaCl reabsorption in the thick ascending limb (26).

Premature infants sometimes exhibit NaCl wasting. Sulyok & coworkers (27) who examined this disturbance in serial clearance studies of human infants, demonstrated that in the first week of life distal fractional Na reabsorption was depressed to 70%; over the next week this improved to approximately 84%. They postulated that the rapid improvement during the first postnatal week may have resulted from activation of the renin-angiotensin-aldosterone system.

The newborn human kidney is limited in its ability to excrete a Na load given acutely, although characteristically there is a normal natriuresis in the first week of life that leads to a contraction of ECF volume. Salt wasting in the low birth weight infant may reflect the maturational status of the fetal distal nephron at that point in gestation.

POTASSIUM

Maturity

The kidneys play a major role in the maintenance of normal K balance (chapter 7). The renal tubules are of primary importance in the excretion of K, since most filtered K is reabsorbed in the proximal segments of the nephron, leaving net K excretion to be determined predominantly by secretory mechanisms in the distal nephron (28). Most of the information regarding renal tubular handling of K has been obtained from in vivo studies of superficial nephrons and, to a lesser extent, juxtamedullary nephrons. Although some recent studies have been directed toward recycling of K between ascending and descending limbs of Henle's loop in deep nephrons, the bulk of K transport in the renal tubule appears to involve the superficial nephron.

Proximal Tubule

In vivo micropuncture studies in the rat indicate that approximately 50% of filtered K is reabsorbed in accessible superficial proximal convoluted tubules (29). The mechanisms involved in the reabsorption of K in the proximal tubule appear to be passive in nature, with early studies of this segment showing the tubular fluid to plasma concentration ratio (TF/P) of K to be near unity (30, 31). A more recent study (32) suggests that K reabsorption in the rat proximal tubule is less than that of Na or water; a subsequent review pointed out that those findings are consistent with the concept that K reabsorption in the proximal convoluted tubule is passive in nature, occurring down a concentration gradient that develops as a consequence of fluid reabsorption (33).

Studies of K transport in the proximal straight tubule, using only in vitro perfusion methods, have demonstrated net secretion of K into this segment (34). This finding has been corroborated and extended for the pars rectae of both superficial and juxtamedullary nephrons (35); it was reported that the rate of K secretion in late proximal straight tubules, i.e., S_3 segments, obtained from juxtamedullary nephrons is higher than it is in those from superficial nephrons (35). The physiological importance of this difference is likely to be small, however, since the pars recta of juxtamedullary nephrons is short. The permeability of juxtamedullary proximal straight tubules to K is much higher than it is in superficial proximal straight tubules (35). Hence, it is possible that K entry may occur by diffusion in the juxtamedullary S_3 segment to a greater extent, particularly if the K concentration in the outer medullary interstitium is elevated, as it appears to be. The inaccessibility of this segment of the nephron unfortunately precludes in vivo testing of this proposal.

Loop of Henle

The isolated thin descending limb of the rabbit has a high K permeability coefficient (0.4 μm/sec) (36). This information, combined with that obtained from in vivo studies on the exposed rat papilla (37), suggests that sufficient K could diffuse from the inner medullary interstitium into the descending thin limb to account for a high fractional delivery of K to the bend of Henle's loop; this has been found in rats under normal conditions (37) and with K loading (38). K transport in the thin ascending limb has not been well defined. However, this segment generally has a high solute permeability (8), a situation that should lead to net K reabsorption along the length of this segment (33).

The extent to which K transport occurs in the medullary thick ascending limb is uncertain, but may be important in view of the current interest in medullary recycling of K. Active K transport occurs in the rabbit thick ascending limb, although the rate is much less than that for Cl (19). The recycling of K across the luminal membrane may be more important (Fig. 5.3) (10). The electroneutral cotransport of ($1Na^+$, $1K^+$, $2Cl^-$) from lumen to cell across the luminal membrane is associated with K recycling from cell to lumen along K conductance pathways in the apical plasma membrane (10, 20). The apical membrane K conductance results in net K transepithelial flux being minimal, although there is considerable lumen to cell active K transport. Despite recent advances in knowledge regarding mechanisms of solute transport across the medullary segment of the thick ascending limb, there is still uncertainty regarding the potential K reabsorptive capacity of this segment. Studies of the cortical thick ascending limb have shown K transport to be voltage-dependent (39); net secretion is evident when the lumen-positive potential is <10 mV but K reabsorption is present when the potential difference is higher. The fractional delivery of K to the distal tubule of superficial nephrons is $<10\%$ of the filtered load; no comparable data are available for juxtamedullary nephrons.

Distal Convoluted and Cortical Collecting Tubule

K secretion is the net effect of transport processes that occur in the heterogeneous nephron segments that make up the distal nephron. Micropuncture experiments carried out on accessible superficial distal nephron segments in the rat have shown that the fractional delivery of K increases from the most proximal puncture site to more distal sites (40). These results almost certainly involve effects by more than one nephron segment. Studies of more specific nephron segments, using rabbit isolated tubules show active K transport into the cortical collecting tubule fluid (41). This effect is augmented by acute or chronic K loading or by administering mineralocorticoids. Despite this demonstration of active K transport in special circumstances, there is general agreement that K secretion in the distal nephron involves active cellular uptake of K across the basolateral membrane followed by passive diffusion into the lumen along K selective conductance pathways, i.e., active cellular uptake of K from interstitial fluid and diffusion into luminal fluid down a favorable electrochemical gradient. The rate of secretion varies with many physiological conditions (chapter 7) but appears to be most dependent on the electrochemical gradient between cell and lumen. This, in turn, may be enhanced significantly by increasing Na intake and its excretion rate (42). This process may be independent, to some extent, of the mineralocorticoid status of the animal (42, 43).

Medullary Collecting Tubule

Studies of K transport in rabbit collecting tubules taken from the inner strip of the outer medulla (21) have shown a striking difference from the situation observed in cortical collecting tubules. Both K and Na transport in the medullary segment are passive in nature and are not influenced by mineralocorticoids. This has led to the conclusion that passive K reabsorption may play a significant role in medullary K recycling when high concentrations of K are presented to the medullary collecting tubule (19, 21) (Fig. 5.4).

In summary, it appears that net K excretion is dependent on many factors, including secretion into superficial and probably juxtamedullary distal nephron segments, with most of this secretion occurring passively down an electrochemical gradient. The effect of medullary recycling of K on overall K homeostasis remains speculative (Fig. 5.4), but the finding that high peritubular K concentrations inhibit NaCl reabsorption in the thick ascending limb may provide some insight. The increased distal Na delivery, which results from this effect, may augment K secretion and net K excretion in such circumstances (19).

Developmental Aspects

The excretory capacity for K, a function of the activity of Na,K-ATPase, is low at birth and increases in early postnatal life (see p. 73) as K intake and excretion increase. Na in tubular fluid directly stimulates Na,K-ATPase activity; adrenal steroids, also influenced by Na and K intake, also stimulate Na,K-ATPase activity early in life (22) (chapter 7).

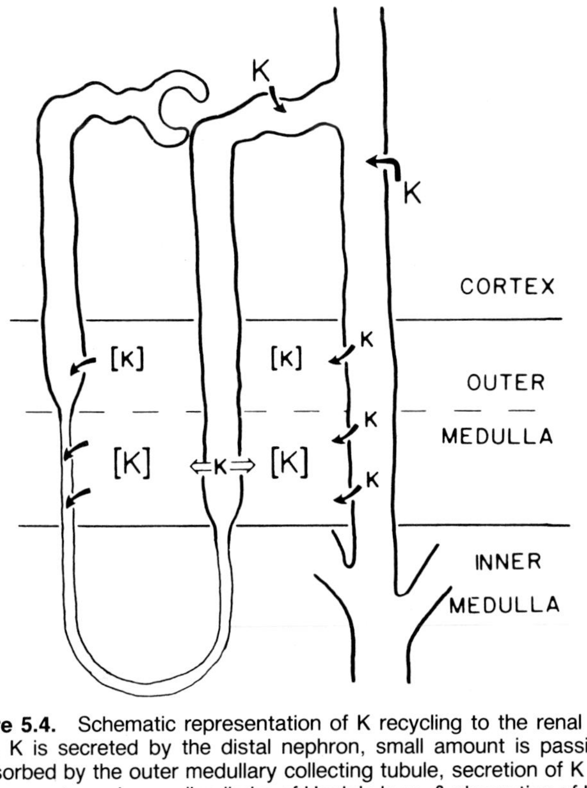

Figure 5.4. Schematic representation of K recycling to the renal medulla. K is secreted by the distal nephron, small amount is passively reabsorbed by the outer medullary collecting tubule, secretion of K into the pars recta or descending limbs of Henle's loop, & absorption of K by the medullary segment of the TAL. (From Stokes JB: J Clin Invest 70: 219, 1982, by copyright permission of The American Society for Clinical Investigation.)

HYDROGEN ION SECRETION

Maturity

The major tubular contribution to renal net acid excretion involves hydrogen ion (H^+) secretion, a process which appears to be shared by a number of nephron segments. The reaction of H^+ with tubular fluid bicarbonate, phosphate, and ammonia permits the kidney to excrete large acid loads (H^+) without the development of steep (>3.0) pH gradients between blood and tubular fluid. The renal tubule is able to vary its H^+ secretory rate in response to a large number of physiological perturbations (44) (chapters 8, 34). Although primary bicarbonate reabsorption has never been established, some recent studies have demonstrated the existence of both bicarbonate secretion and reabsorption by the cortical collecting tubule (Fig. 5.5) (45). Hence, different segments of the nephron may be able to acidify or alkalinize the glomerular filtrate and thus respond to a host of different physiological states.

Proximal Tubule

Specific details regarding the process of H^+ transfer from tubular cells to luminal fluid have been the subject of extensive research (46–48). The principal method (80% to 90%) of proton secretion into the proximal convoluted tubule involves a neutral Na^+-H^+ antiporter in the luminal membrane (47, 48). This mechanism also appears to be operative in the proximal straight tubule. When H^+ is secreted into the proximal tubule it reacts with bicarbonate to form carbonic acid, which then undergoes rapid dehydration in the presence of carbonic anhydrase to form carbon dioxide and water. Carbon dioxide, the partial pressure (pCO_2) of which is high throughout the renal cortex (49–51) of both rat and rabbit, enters the cell, where carbonic anhydrase catalyzes the formation of carbonic acid and subsequently bicarbonate from CO_2 and H_2O. The regenerated bicarbonate ions then exit the cell across the basolateral membrane into

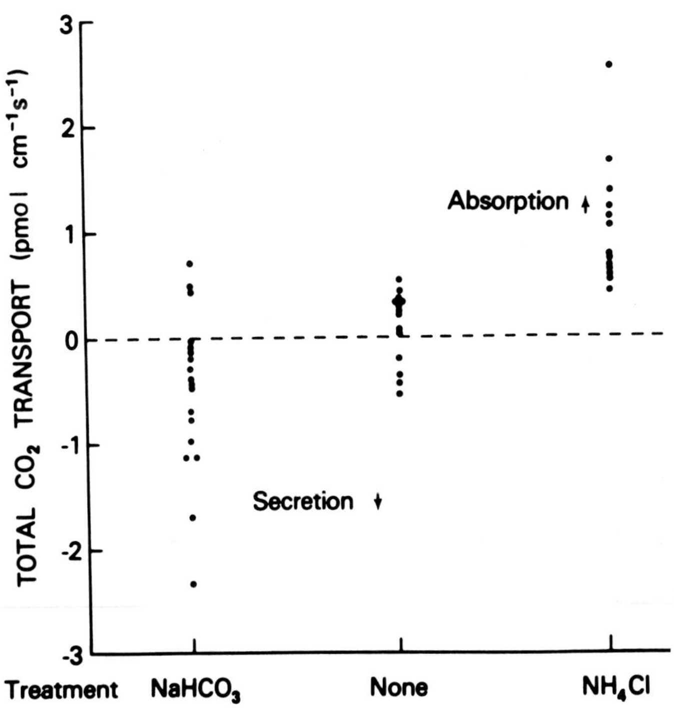

Figure 5.5. Effect of pretreatment of rabbits with NH_4Cl or $NaHCO_3$ on bicarbonate transport by their cortical collecting tubules in vitro. Treated animals received 15 mEq/kg NH_4Cl or 20 mEq/kg $NaHCO_3$ by gavage on the day preceding the experiment. (From McKinney TD, Burg MG: J Clin Invest 60:76, 1977, by copyright permission of The American Society for Clinical Investigation.)

peritubular capillaries, while H^+ is secreted into the tubular lumen via the $Na^+ - H^+$ antiporter. When luminal carbonic anhydrase is inhibited, the disequilibrium pH in the tubular fluid that follows has established H^+ secretion as a major factor in proximal tubule fluid acidification (52).

Bicarbonate ions exit the proximal tubule cell and return to the peritubular capillaries by a passive mechanism down an electrochemical gradient (Fig. 5.6) (53); this mechanism was recently demonstrated by showing inhibition of net bicarbonate reabsorption when the basolateral membrane potential difference was depolarized using barium ions (53). Thus, it would appear that the two major cell events associated with the bulk of bicarbonate reabsorption in the kidney are (1) cell-to-lumen hydrogen secretion via a brush border membrane $Na^+ - H^+$ antiporter and (2) subsequent cell-to-blood rheogenic bicarbonate exit across the basolateral membrane.

The relative roles of juxtamedullary and superficial nephrons in the acidification process have not been fully elucidated. In vivo micropuncture studies that compare acidification parameters in superficial and juxtamedullary nephrons reveal some interesting differences in pH and bicarbonate concentration between the two nephron populations (Fig. 5.7). The net effect on acidification does not differ, however, because the fractional delivery of bicarbonate to the last accessible convolution of the superficial proximal convoluted tubule is similar to that observed in the descending limb of juxtamedullary nephrons. This suggests that the proximal tubules of both nephron populations are able to reabsorb approximately 90% of filtered bicarbonate (54), which exceeds the fractional reabsorption of Na and water.

Loop of Henle

The nephron segments in the loop of Henle do not have a major role in the acidification process, although they may contribute to net acid excretion via recycling of ammonia. When the cortical thick ascending limb was studied directly by the isolated perfused tubule technique, no evidence for net bicarbonate transport was found (55).

Collecting Tubule

The role of collecting tubule segments (cortical, medullary, & papillary) in the acidification of the urine has been evaluated by in vivo and in vitro studies. In vivo micropuncture studies in the rat suggest that the collecting duct system may reabsorb as much as 2.5% of filtered bicarbonate (56). More recent studies have demonstrated that mineralocorticoids have a net effect on this distal acidification process (57). In vitro perfusion studies show that the rabbit cortical collecting segment is not involved in the process to as great an extent as the medullary segment (58). The disparity is consistent with recent studies of the morphology of the epithelium lining the two segments. Mitochondrial-rich cells, which are thought to be rich in carbonic anhydrase and represent the proton secreting cells, are much more abundant in the medullary segment. Although both cortical and medullary segments are responsive to mineralocorticoids, the effect of aldosterone differs in the two segments, Na/K exchange is greater in the cortical segment and H^+ secretion is greater in the medullary segments (21). Recent studies confirm the role of the medullary collecting duct in urine acidification (59) and demonstrate that Cl ions modify H^+ secretion and subsequent HCO_3 reabsorption in this segment. It has been suggested that H^+ secretion in this segment occurs via an apical membrane translocating ATPase and that the H^+ secretion occurs in parallel with Cl secretion (Fig. 5.8) (59).

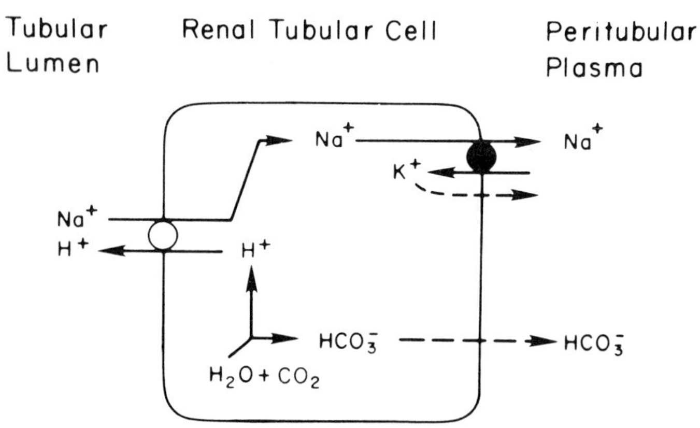

Figure 5.6. Proposed model for $NaHCO_3$ reabsorption in rabbit proximal convoluted tubule. *Solid line arrow with open circle*, ion exchange mechanism; *solid line arrow with closed circle*, ion pump; and *dotted line arrow*, rheogenic transport. (From Sasaki S, Berry CA: Am J Physiol 246:F889, 1984.)

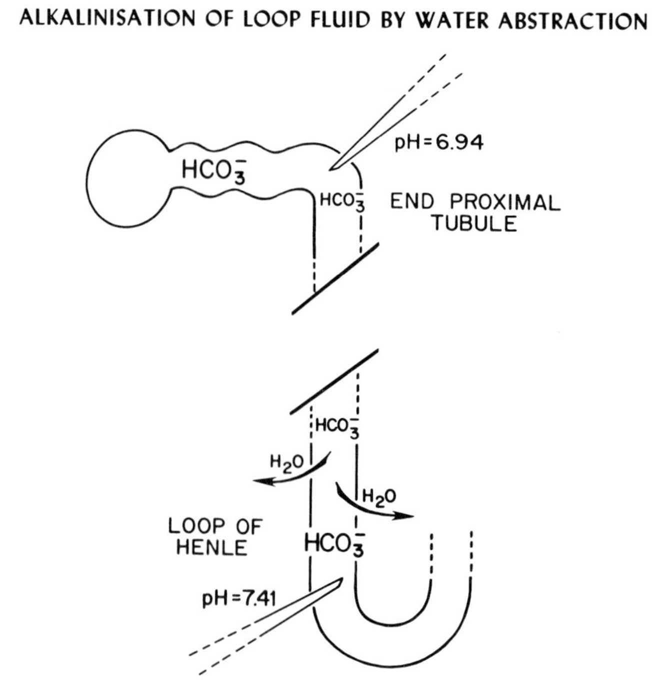

Figure 5.7. Schematic to show apparent alkalinization of tubular fluid that occurs between the proximal convoluted tubule and the bend of Henle's loop. The data are from in vivo rat micropuncture studies comparing superficial and juxtamedullary nephrons. This demonstrates the probable mechanism for alkalinization of the fluid in the descending limb, i.e., solute-free water abstraction in the descending thin limb.

Acidification in the inner medullary and papillary collecting duct has been examined by micropuncture and microcatheterization techniques (60, 61). HCO_3 reabsorption in this segment occurs in the absence or presence of a favorable concentration gradient. The process appears to be aldosterone sensitive (60) and produces a progressive decline in pH along the inner medullary collection duct (61). Hence, it appears that the entire length of the collecting duct participates in the acidification process.

Developmental Aspects

Developmental aspects of urinary acidification have been studied mainly using clearance techniques. Infants appear to have a relatively low renal tubular threshold for HCO_3 reabsorption under normal conditions (62). However, this decreased threshold can be increased mark-

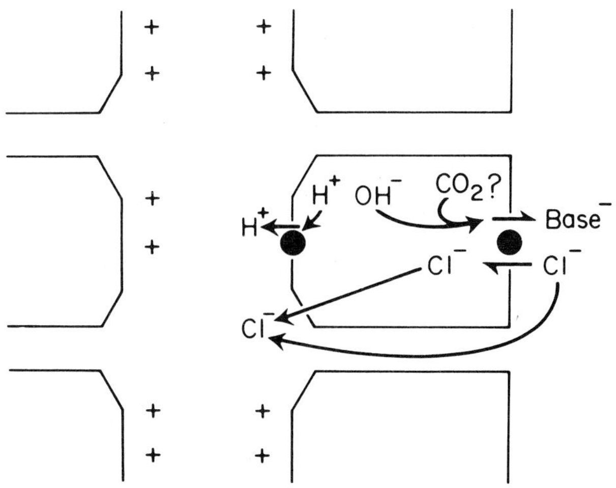

Figure 5.8. Proposed role of chloride (Cl^-) in the process of acidification in the medullary collecting duct. At the basolateral membrane (*right*), intracellular base exits via a chloride-base exchange mechanism; at the apical membrane chloride secretion, across chloride conductance channels, balances electrogenic proton secretion. (From Stone DK, et al: J Clin Invest 71: 1505, 1983, by copyright permission of The American Society for Clinical Investigation.)

edly when extracellular volume is reduced in both puppies (63) and fetal lambs (64). Normal net acid excretion in infants is comparable to that in adults, but the ability to respond to an increased acid load is less, suggesting that the rates of titratable acid and ammonium excretion in infants are close to their maximum capacity (62).

More direct studies of renal tubular HCO_3 transport have been carried out using the isolated perfused tubule of rabbits. The rate of HCO_3 reabsorption in juxtamedullary proximal convoluted tubules of newborn rabbits is one-third of that observed in comparable tubule segments from adult rabbits (65, 66). It was postulated that this decreased rate of HCO_3 flux may be responsible for the lower concentration of plasma HCO_3 in the human neonate. As development progresses, the maturation of the process of HCO_3 reabsorption in rabbits occurs in a nonlinear fashion. There is little change for the first 3 weeks of postnatal life and then a rapid surge that enables adult HCO_3 transport rates to be achieved by the sixth postnatal week. This sudden acceleration in the maturation of the transport rate suggests that an external triggering factor initiates the change. The increase at this age precedes the changes in Na,K-ATPase activity (66).

AMMONIA PRODUCTION AND SECRETION

Maturity

Proximal Tubule

Ammonia is produced from glutamine in all nephron segments, but the proximal tubule is thought to be the principal site of ammonia production (67). The ammonia is subsequently absorbed in the loop of Henle where tubular fluid is relatively alkaline (54, 68), then secreted into the acidic fluid of the collecting duct where it reacts with H^+ ions and is entrapped as amonium ions (67, 68).

Developmental Aspects

As stated above, the rate of ammonium excretion in infants appears to be close to maximum capacity (62). However, specific studies of segmental nephron ammonia production and secretion have not been performed during development.

FLUID TRANSPORT

Maturity

Reabsorption of filtered water by the renal tubules represents the most important aspect of adaptation to terrestrial existence. In most circumstances, more than 99% of filtered water is reabsorbed across the various nephron segments. The mechanisms underlying generation of the necessary osmotic gradients for reabsorption vary widely among nephron segments.

Proximal Tubules

The proximal tubule is responsible for the bulk of water reabsorption (70% to 80%) in the form of isosmotic volume absorption. The mechanisms that permit this apparently paradoxical combination of osmotically driven water transfer and isosmotic reabsorption have been reviewed (69). The most likely explanation for the osmotic water flux is the existence of a transepithelial osmolality difference generated by active reabsorption of various solutes in the proximal tubule, including Na, glucose, and amino acids. Schafer (69) proposed that the bulk of the evidence does not concur with the concept of a hyperosmolar third compartment in the intercellular spaces of the proximal tubule. A series of studies has demonstrated the existence of an hyperosmolar reabsorbate in proximal convoluted and straight tubules (70). There a small osmotic gradient between the reabsorption droplets and perfusate fluid. Although the osmotic gradient generated is small, it is sufficient when coupled with the high water permeability—hydraulic conductivity—to explain the significant water flux (71, 72). As a corollary to these experiments, it was postulated that solute reabsorption in the proximal tubule in vivo generates luminal fluid hypotonicity and subsequent osmotic water flow (69).

In addition to water flow secondary to active solute transport in the initial segment of the proximal tubule, some water flux in later sites may occur as the result of *passive volume absorption* wherein not only the water flux but also the events preceding this flux are passive in nature. There are two mechanisms that have been proposed to explain this passive component.

The first, termed *effective osmolality difference*, depends on the existence of differential permeabilities between the dominant luminal and peritubular anions, Cl and HCO_3. Since Cl appears to be more permeable than HCO_3 in superficial proximal tubules (73), the presence of higher HCO_3 concentrations on the peritubular side and higher Cl concentrations in luminal fluid (74) would produce an effective osmolality difference, favoring outward movement of water. However, studies of juxtamedullary nephrons (73) do not demonstrate any difference between Cl and HCO_3 permeability, suggesting that significant fluid reabsorption by this mechanism can be operative only in the superficial nephrons.

The second passive component involves *preferential passive reabsorption* of Cl down a favorable electrochemical gradient in the distal part of the proximal convoluted tubule. The contribution of this "truly" passive component of fluid reabsorption is estimated to make a small contribution to overall fluid reabsorption in this segment (69).

Finally, the role of *physical forces* on fluid reabsorption in the proximal tubule should be considered. Lowering the proximal tubule peritubular protein oncotic pressure reduces net volume reabsorption in this segment (3, 75–77). The most widely accepted mechanism for this phenomenon has been thought to involve back-leak of solutes and water across the paracellular spaces. However, there is recent evidence (78) in favor of a direct effect of peritubular oncotic pressure—more specifically protein—on transcellular or paracellular NaCl reabsorption (Fig. 5.9).

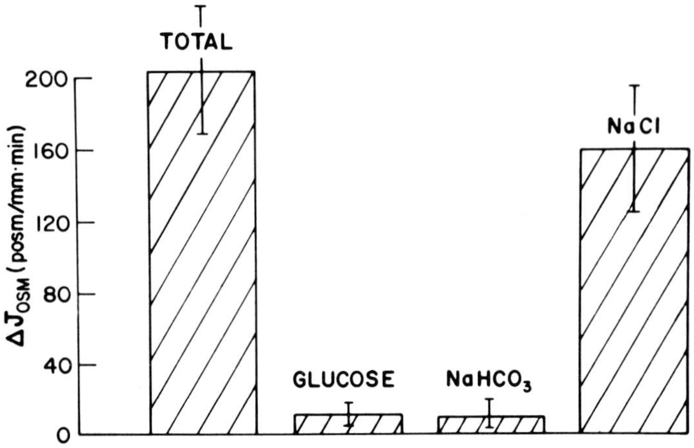

Figure 5.9. Evaluation of the effect of removal of bath protein on solute fluxes across the isolated perfused rabbit proximal convoluted tubule. The change in the solute fluxes (ΔJ_{osm}) of glucose, $NaHCO_3$, and NaCl are compared with the total. At least 80% of the change in the total flux can be account for by the change in NaCl. (From Berry CA, Cogan MG: J Clin Invest 68:506, 1981, by copyright permission of The American Society for Clinical Investigation.)

Loop of Henle

Abstraction of water occurs subsequently in the thin descending limb of Henle's loop, leading to progressive concentration of the tubular field (7). This process is quantitatively much more important in the juxtamedullary nephrons where, in some species, up to 80% of water delivered out of the proximal tubule may be reabsorbed in this segment. Less than 10% of filtered water reaches the hairpin bend of the loop of Henle. This water abstraction in most species occurs in the absence of any solute flux and results in the delivery of highly concentrated tubular fluid to the inner medulla, an integral component of the concentrating mechanism. Outward movement of water in this segment appears to be the result of osmotic forces and does not depend on any interaction between epithelium and endogenous hormones.

Although the thin ascending limb is highly permeable to a variety of solutes, it appears from in vitro microperfusion studies of the rabbit tubule that it is impermeable to water. Reabsorption of solute from this segment in the absence of water reabsorption leads to progressive dilution of the luminal contents (8). In both the medullary and cortical portions of the thick ascending limb the hydraulic conductance also is low. Thus, in these segments, as in the thin limbs, solute but not water reabsorption occurs; further dilution of tubular fluid results.

Distal Tubule and Collecting Tubules

Studies of water reabsorption in the distal nephron have been complicated by the heterogeneity of the accessible *distal nephron* from in vivo micropuncture studies. Micropuncture studies performed in this area have included more than one specific nephron segment. It would appear from studies of the rabbit distal convoluted tubule and cortical collecting tubule by in vitro perfusion studies that a considerable difference exists between the two segments in terms of the transport of water.

In both cases, the osmotic water permeability is low in the absence of ADH. However, when vasopressin is added to the bath during perfusion of cortical collecting tubules, a considerable increase in the osmotic water permeability ensues (79); this also occurs in the medullary and papillary segments of the collecting duct (80). The reabsorption of water from the collecting duct system is a transcellular process that is stimulated by the production of intracellular cyclic AMP. It should be noted that the absolute rate of papillary collecting duct water reabsorption may be greater in the absence of ADH (81). However, the ability of the collecting duct to produce a concentrated urine is dependent on the presence of circulating vasopressin (see Chapter 6).

Developmental Aspects

Developmental aspects of fluid reabsorption in individual nephron segments have been studied by a number of methods. The in vitro microperfusion technique was used to evaluate the rabbit proximal convoluted tubule (82) by measuring the hydraulic and osmotic water conductance of mid- to late-proximal tubule segments taken from the superficial cortex at three stages of development: immature (2 to 6-days postnatal), maturing (10 to 14 days), and mature (30 to 38 days). An age-dependent postnatal decrease of hydrostatic and osmotic water permeability of these tubules was demonstrated; it was concluded that in the neonatal rabbit, proximal tubule fluid reabsorption may depend more on transepithelial pressure gradients than in mature animals.

A recently described maturation phenomenon may have important implications regarding fluid reabsorption in immature proximal convoluted tubules (83). The most superficial proximal tubules with open lumens from rabbits <36 hours old (situated in the mid-cortex) had a higher Cl to Na permeability ratio than similarly placed nephrons in mature animals or juxtamedullary nephrons in the same neonatal animals. It was concluded that the higher Cl to Na permeability ratios observed in these deep nephrons also may indicate more significant passive volume reabsorption in immature proximal tubules via the effective osmolality difference (83).

These findings are compatible with clearance studies carried out in the newborn of different species, particularly puppies (84), using the technique of distal blockade of NaCl reabsorption (achieved by amiloride and ethacrynic acid). The conclusion of this study was that the proximal tubules of newborn dogs can generate a transtubular Cl gradient, as evidenced by the presence of a urine to plasma chloride gradient of 1.34 during distal blockade. The inhibition of proximal HCO_3 reabsorption with acetazolamide resulted in a decrease in the Cl gradient associated with a dramatic increase in excretion of water (as well as Na, Cl, and HCO_3). Thus, the newborn dog possesses Cl selective proximal tubules that, in the presence of intact HCO_3 reabsorption, generate a transtubular Cl gradient that may, in turn, contribute significantly to passive volume reabsorption.

PHOSPHORUS, CALCIUM, AND MAGNESIUM

The renal handling of phosphorus (P), calcium (Ca), and magnesium (Mg) is a complex interdependent process. These minerals are subject to regulation by hormones, acid base homeostasis, ECF volume, and other modulators. This discussion will focus on tubular transport under physiological conditions, with less attention to physiological preparation, e.g., micropuncture and perfusion (chapters 10, 32).

Phosphorus

Maturity

Regulation of urinary P excretion plays an essential role in body phosphorus homeostasis. Plasma P exists primarily as inorganic phosphate, which is measured in the clinical laboratory and expressed as mg of phosphorus. Approximately 90% of plasma inorganic P is filtered at the glomerulus. Net tubular reabsorption of phosphate occurs; fractional excretion of P is <20%. The tubular maximum (TmP) for P has been used as a clinical measure of tubular phosphate transport and was once considered to be independent of glomerular filtration (GFR) (85). More recent data indicate that TmP varies with changes in GFR and that TmP/GFR is a more reliable measure of tubule function (86). Normal values for TmP/GFR range from 2.5 to 4.2 mg/dl/100 ml GFR in adults. The mean and SD in newborns and for children 1 to 12 years of age are 4.4 ± 0.6 mg/dl GFR (87).

Proximal Tubule. Approximately 70% to 75% of filtered P is reabsorbed in the proximal tubule. There is a marked axial heterogeneity in P transport capacity (88), e.g., the permeability or transport capacity for P of the S_1 segment is four times that of the S_2 segment; approximately 60% of the total proximal tubular P reabsorption occurs in the first 10% of proximal tubule length. In the remainder of the proximal tubule, there is no change in the TF/P phosphate:inulin ratio. Whether heterogeneity between P transport in superficial and deep nephrons exists is unclear (89, 90). Throughout the proximal tubule, P transport is unidirectional, i.e., backflux is insignificant (91). P transport across the brush border membrane in S_1 is dependent on the electrochemical forces that effect Na transport (92). This cotransport system is saturable and is inhibited by arsenic or ouabain (92, 93). Transport of P across the basolateral membrane also is dependent on Na transport and may be passive down an electrochemical gradient (94). Reabsorption of P in the S_2 segment occurs at a slower rate but, unlike reabsorption in the S_1 segment, it is quite sensitive to parathyroid hormone (PTH) (95) (chapters 10 and 30).

Loop of Henle and the Distal Tubule. Whether tubular reabsorption of P occurs distal to the pars recta is controversial; it is, in any case, small and of limited significance under normal physiological conditions. Net transport of P does not occur in isolated segments from descending and ascending limbs of Henle's loop studied by microperfusion (96). P reabsorption that may occur in Henle's loop is sensitive to PTH, e.g., 86% of isotopic P injected into the late proximal tubule is recovered in the final urine when PTH is present and only 50% is recovered in its absence (97). Furthermore, the P content of the final urine is regularly less than the P delivered to the accessible, distal tubule suggesting further reabsorption beyond this site (88, 98). Both PTH-sensitive and PTH-insensitive transport occurs in the distal nephron (99). Distal P reabsorption is very sensitive to PTH inhibition.

Developmental Aspects

Renal P clearance is low in utero and during the early postnatal period, despite a high serum P concentration (100, 101). Both exogenous PTH and ECF volume expansion increase renal P clearance in fetal lambs (102). Tubular reabsorption of P is higher in newborns (88%) than it is in adult guinea pigs (79%) (103). In accessible proximal tubules, fractional reabsorption of P is 77% in newborns and 64% in adults; distal fractional reabsorption is 17.5% and 8.5% in newborn and adult guinea pigs, respectively. Tubular P reabsorption, therefore, occurs in both the proximal and distal tubule during the neonatal period. When P kinetics were examined in guinea pig brush-border vesicles, there was no difference in either Km or Vmax to explain P retention during development (104). Measurements of intracellular P concentration are consistent with the hypothesis that low intracellular P concentrations create a steep concentration gradient for passive diffusion across the luminal membrane into cells.

Calcium

Maturity

Ca is excreted by the kidney through the processes of glomerular filtration and tubular reabsorption. Ultrafilterable Ca consists of ionized and complexed Ca that represents approximately 60% of the total plasma Ca. Tubular reabsorption of Ca occurs throughout the nephron, with reabsorption of 60% of filtered Ca in the proximal tubule, 20% between the late proximal and early distal tubule, 10% in the distal convoluted tubule, and the remainder in the collecting system. The fractional excretion of Ca is <2% in normal humans (105).

Proximal Tubule. Throughout the proximal tubule, the Ca TF/UF ratio is between 1.0 and 1.2, suggesting isosmotic passive reabsorption. Microperfusion experiments have demonstrated that the proximal tubule is highly permeable to Ca with the back-leak flux equal to three times the net unidirectional flux (106). Ca reabsorption is dependent on the presence of luminal Na (107, 108).

Experiments assessing proximal tubule Ca transport by luminal and peritubular capillary perfusion suggest that passive diffusion accounts for 80% of net transport, active transport for 20% (107). While the bulk of luminal membrane transport is passive, the presumably low intracellular Ca and the negative intracellular potential difference require active transport at the basolateral membrane. Active basolateral transport can occur through Ca-Na countertransport or by the action of Ca-activated ATPase, which is present in basolateral but not brush-border membranes (109). A current hypothesis is that bulk transcellular Ca transport occurs through Na-Ca countertransport while Ca-activated ATPase provides the fine regulation of Ca extrusion (105). The role of the proximal straight or S_2 segment in Ca reabsorption is uncertain; however, it appears that active Ca transport occurs in excess of Na reabsorption.

Loop of Henle. Studies of Ca transport in the thin descending limb of the loop of Henle suggest a low permeability to Ca (110, 111); no measurements of Ca transport have been made in the thin ascending limb. In the thick ascending limb, Ca is reabsorbed in association with NaCl in both cortical and medullary segments. Secondary active Cl transport in these segments generates a lumen-positive PD, which creates a favorable electrochemical gradient for passive Ca absorption (111, 112). On the other hand, an active component of Ca transport is suggested by the fact that PTH increases Ca reabsorption in cortical thick ascending limbs independent of any change in PD (113). Heterogeneity in Ca transport between cortical and medullary thick ascending limbs has been found (113), in which PTH stimulates Ca reabsorption in cortical but not medullary segments. In contrast, furosemide inhibits Ca reabsorption only in medullary segments (113). This suggests that Ca transport is passive in the medullary segment of the thick ascending limb of Henle and active in the cortical segment.

Distal Tubule. In the distal convoluted tubule, active reabsorption of Ca is independent of Na and PD (114). Ca reabsorption in this segment is increased by increasing PTH levels and by increased HCO_3 delivery (115, 116). Ca reabsorption is also increased by thiazide diuretics by a mechanism independent of PTH (115). Relatively little is known about Ca transport in the collecting tubule. It has been found that Ca reabsorption occurs in granular (but not light) cortical collecting tubule segments (117).

Developmental Aspects

Ca transport during early development has not been examined extensively; in general, urinary Ca excretion is minimal during the neonatal period (118, 119). Clearance studies demonstrate a close relationship between urinary Ca excretion and both Na intake and excretion in premature neonates ranging in gestational age from 28 to 36 weeks (120). Term and premature neonates demonstrate a calciuric response to furosemide and anticalciuric response to thiazide diuretics, which is similar to responses adults demonstrate (121).

Magnesium

Maturity

Mg transport by the renal tubules differs from Ca and P in both magnitude and location of maximal nephron transport. Approximately 70% ot 80% of plasma Mg is filtered at the glomerulus (122). Of the ultrafilterable Mg, 25% to 30% is complexed to oxalate, citrate, and P. In man, 5% to 20% of filtered Mg is excreted in the final urine.

Unlike Ca and P, the primary nephron site for regulation of renal Mg excretion is the loop of Henle. Whether a tubular maximum (Tmax) for Mg transport exists is unclear. Massry (123) defined a Tmax Mg in dogs of 280 μg/min/kg. These studies were performed with an increased serum Mg concentration and demonstrated a marked splay. More recently, Tmax for Mg was not found in microperfusion studies in rats, even with high Mg perfusate concentration (124).

Proximal Tubule. The proximal tubule is relatively impermeable to Mg; only 20% to 30% of the filtered load is reabsorbed in this segment (125). In micropuncture studies in rats there was a rise in TF/UF Mg of 1.5 to 2.0 in the late proximal tubule, in contrast to the isotonic reabsorption of Na and Ca in this segment (126). In microperfusion studies, absolute Mg reabsorption in the proximal tubule rises when Mg delivery is increased; however, regardless of the perfusate Mg concentration, TF/UF Mg rises along this segment (127). Neither backflux nor tubular secretion of Mg occurs in the early proximal tubule, since isotopic Mg injected into peritubular capillaries does not enter the tubular lumen (128).

Loop of Henle. Whether Mg secretion occurs into the S_2 or S_3 segments of the proximal tubule or into the thin descending limb of Henle's loop is controversial. In tubular fluid collections from the bend of Henle's loop of juxtamedullary nephrons, a greater fractional delivery of Mg was found than at the end of the accessible proximal tubule of superficial nephrons (110). However, recent studies of perfused superficial loops of Henle with magnesium-free solutions found no Mg in distal collections (127). If tubular secretion of Mg exists, its role in Mg homeostasis under physiological conditions is unclear.

The principal site of Mg reabsorption is the thick ascending limb of the loop of Henle; 50% to 60% of filtered Mg is reabsorbed between the late proximal and early distal tubule (126). Since Mg secretion may occur in the descending limb, the site of maximal reabsorption is deduced to be the thick ascending limb. In perfusion studies of superficial nephrons, absolute tubular Mg reabsorption in the loop of Henle increases as the Mg concentration in the perfusate increases from 0 to 10 mEq/L, with approximately 80% of the delivered Mg being reabsorbed at any luminal Mg concentration (127). Hypermagnesemia and hypercalcemia both reduce Mg reabsorption in this segment (125, 127). Recent evidence suggests that Mg reabsorption in the thick ascending limb is voltage-dependent (129). As secondary active Cl transport generates increased luminal electropositivity, a favorable gradient for passive Mg entry into the cells is created. This concept of active Cl transport with passive Mg uptake is supported by the finding that Mg reabsorption is inhibited by furosemide (129). The membrane transport system for cellular Mg efflux is currently unknown.

Distal and Collecting Tubules. Even less is known concerning Mg transport in more distal nephron segments. In the distal convoluted tubule, 2% to 5% of filtered Mg is reabsorbed. Mg reabsorption in this segment increases when Mg delivery is elevated. In the cortical collecting tubule, 1% to 3% of filtered Mg is reabsorbed (125). However, Shareghi and Agus (130) found no net Mg transport in the "light" segment of rabbit cortical collecting tubules.

ORGANIC COMPOUNDS: GLUCOSE, AMINO ACIDS, AND ORGANIC ACIDS

Glucose

Maturity

Despite nearly complete glomerular filtration, glucose (d-glucose) has an exceedingly low renal clearance. Increasing the quantities of filtered glucose results in increasing reabsorption of glucose until a maximal reabsorptive rate is attained. This tubular maximum for glucose (TmG) is calculated as:

$$\text{TmG} = (\text{PG} \times \text{GFR}) - (\text{UG} \times \text{V})$$

where PG is plasma glucose, UG is urinary glucose concentration, and V is urine volume.

TmG has been used extensively as a measure of proximal tubular reabsorptive capacity and as a means of assessing the balance between glomerular filtration and tubular function, as measured by TmG (130). In early studies, Shannon and Fischer (131) believed that TmG was independent of acute changes in GFR; this hypothesis is supported by studies in isolated microperfused rabbit tubules (132). TmG in adults is constant (TmG/C_{In} 2.5 mg/ml). Whereas absolute TmG is lower in infants and children, TmG adjusted to GFR (TmG/C_{In}) in children (2.8 mg/ml), infants (2.9 mg/ml), and premature infants (2.5 mg/ml) is comparable to that in adults (2.21–2.84 mg/ml) (133–135). TmG/C_{In} in fetal sheep is, if anything, greater than it is in adults (136). Reexamination of TmG/C_{In} in carefully controlled experiments suggests that TmG is related to GFR and expansion of ECF depressant Mg/C_{In} in both mature and immature animals (137–139).

Proximal Tubule. The primary site of glucose reabsorption is the early proximal tubule or S_1 segment (140, 141). Micropuncture studies have demonstrated that >98% of filtered glucose is reabsorbed in the proximal tubule. Glucose is reabsorbed avidly in the first 3 mm of the proximal tubule (141), being cotransported with Na across the luminal cell membrane (141–144). While Na-independent transport of glucose also may be present at physiological plasma glucose concentrations, luminal transport is primarily Na-dependent (142). Active glucose reabsorption is inhibited by phlorizin (145). Na-dependent glucose transport is nearly 100 times more sensitive to phlorizin than is the Na-independent flux. Na transport is driven by Na,K-ATPase; for this reason, Na-glucose cotransport is inhibited by ouabain (140). The glucose transport carrier in the luminal brush border appears to be specific for D-glucose. As intracellular glucose concentration increases, passive efflux occurs across the basolateral proximal tubule cell membrane. The passive (facilitated) glucose permeability of the basolateral cell membrane is 4 times greater than the luminal cell membrane (146). Net glucose reabsorption in the proximal tubule is increased by large doses of thyroid and inhibited by insulin (130). The only additional site of glucose reabsorption is located between the late distal tubule and final urine (141). The specific transport site and mechanism are unknown.

Developmental Aspects

Development of cellular glucose transport in rabbit proximal tubules has been examined in perfused S_1 segments of juxtamedullary nephrons from 1 to 6 weeks postnatal age and compared with transport in adult S_1 segments (165). Glucose reabsorption is low in rabbits 1 to 4 weeks of age and rises to adult levels thereafter. Passive glucose diffusion does not vary with postnatal age. In these young rabbits, basolateral membrane surface area increased before maturation of glucose reabsorption. It was speculated that maturational increases in glucose reabsorption might occur from increasing activity of Na-K-ATPase, delayed insertion of Na "pumps" into new cell membranes or inherent limitations of the immature proximal tubule cell to produce ATP.

Amino Acids

Maturity

Renal tubular amino acid (AA) transport interests pediatric nephrologists who encounter patients with hereditary forms of specific aminoaciduria (Chapter 31). Following ultrafiltration, AA are reabsorbed so that only 1% of those filtered are excreted by the kidneys (147).

Proximal Tubule. Stop-flow experiments place the site of reabsorption primarily in the proximal tubule (148), a finding confirmed by Bergeron and Morel (149) who found no significant reabsorption of microinjected AA beyond the proximal tubule in rats. Based on clearance studies that determined the tubular maximum (Tm) for reabsorption of AA, it was postulated that multiple transport processes were available for AA reabsorption (147). Similar conclusions were drawn from the demonstration of high renal clearance of AA during infancy, with a maturational decline in AA clearance that was not synchronous for all AA (150). Currently, net reabsorptive transport systems in the proximal tubule are proposed to exist for 5 groups of AA: (1) neutral, (2) acidic, (3) basic, (4) alanine and glycine, and (5) B-amino acids (151).

The major site of AA reabsorption is the S_1 segment of the proximal tubule (152). For all AA, there is active transport from the tubular lumen across the brush border membrane, which is dependent on Na cotransport (151). Individual AA demonstrate considerable differences in apical membrane transport rates. Carriers are located within the brush border membrane that are specific for a class of AA (153). Much has been learned of the specificity of membrane carriers by studies of patients with aminoacidurias. Both high and low affinity transport systems for proline, glycine, and α-aminoisobutyric acid have been shown in cortical kidney slices (154). Active transport of the D-isomers of AA is insignificant compared with most of the L-isomers. It appears that D-forms use the same transport systems but are transported at a much lower rate (151).

In general, net transepithelial AA reabsorption results from active luminal membrane transport, leading to a high intracellular AA concentration (153) and subsequent passive efflux across the basolateral membrane. In addition, glycine is actively transported across the basolateral membrane into the cell (155). Net transepithelial secretion of cysteine has been observed in a few patients with cystinuria, which suggests active cell uptake from the peritubular fluid under some conditions. The physiological importance of active basolateral transport of AAs into cells

Table 5.1.
Organic Acids Secreted by the Proximal Tubule

Endogenous Acids	Exogenous Acids
Uric acid	Diuretics
Hippurates	Furosemide
Oxalate	Thiazides
Prostaglandins	Acetazolamide
Bile Salts	Antibiotics
Benzoates	Penicillins
Cyclic AMP	Cephalosporins
	Salicylates
	Probenecid
	Iodinated Contrast Media
	Morphine Sulfate

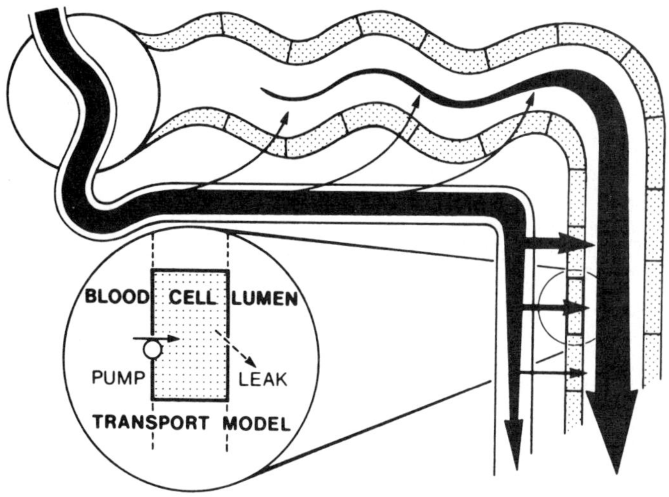

Figure 5.10. Mechanism of renal excretion of iodohippurate sodium 131; width of solid black arrows indicates relative concentration. Inset, mechanism of transcellular hippurate transport. (From Tune BM, Burg MB, Patlak CS: Am J Physiol 217:1057, 1969. Copyright 1976, American Medical Association.)

is uncertain; it may meet cellular nutrient requirements rather than be a part of transepithelial transport (156). Finally, there is a small passive paracellular backleak for most AA (153).

Developmental Aspects

The mechanisms underlying maturation of tubular AA transport have been reviewed (157). Aminoaciduria during infancy may be explained by decreased cellular uptake or efflux or increased tubular backleak. Some controversy exists concerning whether cellular AA uptake is lower in immature nephrons. Decreased AA uptake has been reported in neonatal kidney slices and isolated tubule segments (158–160); however, no developmental differences in cellular uptake of glycine, cystine, and proline in either cortical kidney slices or isolated rat tubules was found by Segal and coworkers (161, 162). Maturational increase in uptake of AAs during development may reflect either increased numbers of membrane carriers or increasing transport capacity of available carriers.

Organic Acids

Maturity

A large number of endogenous and exogenous organic acids are secreted into the proximal renal tubule fluid (Table 5.1) (163). Epithelial transport of organic acids, such as *p*-aminohippurate (PAH), is unidirectional (peritubular capillaries to tubular lumen) whereas transport of others, e.g., uric acid, show bidirectional epithelial transport. Much of our current understanding of tubular secretory processes has been the result of studies of renal transport of PAH. Since PAH is almost completely extracted from renal blood perfusing mature mammalian kidneys, its clearance has been utilized to estimate RBF (164) except in infants where its renal extraction is incomplete (165, 166).

PAH is actively transported into proximal renal tubule cells across the basolateral membrane and subsequently diffuses passively into the tubular lumen (167) (Fig. 5.10). PAH secretion demonstrates considerable intranephron variability in some species. It is secreted to the greatest extent in the S_2 segment in rabbits and presumably in man; however, a more homogeneous pattern of PAH secretion has been demonstrated in other mammalian species (168). Most, but not all, organic acids are secreted in the S_2 segment to the greatest extent. Oxalate, however, is secreted primarily in the S_1 segment (169).

Active transport of PAH across the basolateral membrane is dependent on K and Na and may be inhibited by ouabain (170–172) pointing to a relationship between PAH transport and Na, K-ATPase activity. While characterization of the binding sites, membrane carriers, and carrier affinities for PAH is incomplete, nephron heterogeneity of PAH secretion, in part, appears to be the result of varying density of PAH transporters in the basolateral membranes of the S_2 segment (173). Within the cell, PAH is bound to reduced glutathione (GSH) S transferase (ligandin) (174), which is not rate-limiting (175). PAH may "leak" across the apical membrane by diffusion, facilitated diffusion, or perhaps by a carrier-mediated process (167, 176, 177). Permeability characteristics of the apical membrane greatly influence transepithelial secretion.

In the case of other organic acids, e.g., the several cephalosporin antibiotics (chapter 14), the proximal tubule's apical membrane conductance varies (178). Cephalothin, for instance, simulates PAH transport with diffusion down a concentration gradient from the cell into the tubular lumen. Cephaloridine, on the other hand, is transported into the cell, where it accumulates with little diffusion out of the cell, trapping within the cell, which accounts for its greater nephrotoxicity (178).

Secretion of most organic acids by the proximal tubule is inhibited by probenicid and stimulated by acetate (179). An interesting phenomenon associated with PAH secretion in nonperfused rabbit tubules is that the high concentration of PAH in the tubule lumen results in transepithelial fluid secretion (180). The effect of PAH as a secretogogue has been shown in a nonperfused human proximal S_2 segment dissected from a nephrectomy specimen of a 9-year-old girl (181) (Fig. 5.11).

Developmental Aspects

The mechanism for organic acid transport in neonates is less developed, e.g., in vivo renal extraction of PAH, uptake of PAH by cortical kidney slices, and intrinsic capacity for PAH transport by microperfused proximal tubules are decreased in fetal or neonatal tissues (165, 166). Both cellular uptake and release of PAH in renal cortical slices from young rabbits are impaired. Kinetics of accumulation of PAH by cortical slices were related to diminished numbers of PAH transport sites and to an altered relationship between uptake and efflux (182). On the other hand, ligand plays no role in the developmental maturation of PAH uptake (166, 182).

PAH uptake in renal cortical slices from newborn animals can be stimulated by prior administration of procaine penicillin or acetate (166). The intrinsic PAH transport capacity increased by 90%/unit length of tubule over the period of 1 to 10 weeks (183). However, the mechanism of substrate stimulated and age-related maturation of PAH transport remains imprecise.

Uric Acid

Maturity

Uric acid, an endogenous organic acid, is filtered and undergoes both reabsorption and secretion in man, such that there is net reabsorption; excretion is 6% to 12% of the filtered load (184). Studies of renal urate transport mechanisms in humans have, by necessity, relied on clearance studies and the use of inhibitors of tubular urate transport. Studies that evaluate uric transport in nephron segments in experimental animals must be viewed with caution because renal urate-handling varies among species. However, rats, dogs—except Dalmations—and chimpanzees have urate transport systems, at least qualitatively, similar to that in humans (185).

A large percent of tubular reabsorption of urate in rats occurs in the S_1 segment of the proximal tubule, prior to tubular secretion (186). Reabsorption results from both active transport and passive diffusion. Urate reabsorption in man is active since probenecid inhibits reabsorp-

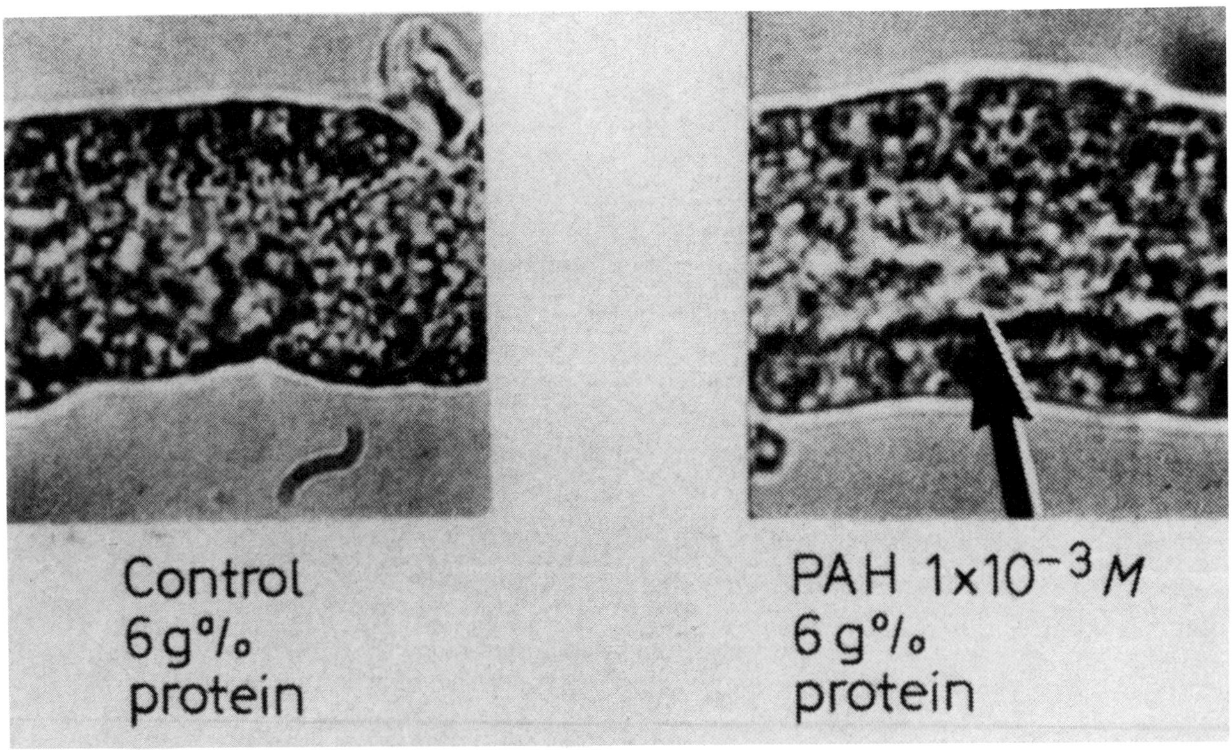

Figure 5.11. Human proximal straight tubule incubated in 1 mM PAH at 37° C. Note lumen in the center of the tubule (*arrow*). (X400.) (From Stapleton FB, Linshaw MA: Renal Physiol 1:334, 1978, by permission of S. Karger AG, Basel.)

tion and, with administration of pyrazinamide, an inhibitor of urate secretion, reabsorption occurs against a chemical gradient (185, 187). Reabsorption also is influenced by ECF volume (188, 189), i.e., uric acid excretion increases during saline infusion; however, this effect is blocked by pyrazinamide, suggesting that some reabsorption occurs distal to secretory sites. Uric acid reabsorption appears to be independent of Na reabsorption (190).

Tubular Secretion. Because excretion may exceed filtered load in man, tubular secretion of uric acid is certain (191). As much as 80% of urate excretion appears to be by tubular secretion. Active secretion appears to follow the PAH model, but urate and PAH appear to be secreted separately (192, 193) since pyrazinamide inhibits urate but not PAH excretion. Furthermore, plasma PAH levels adequate to saturate PAH secretion do not inhibit urate secretion (192). Secretion increases as uric acid levels increase (194).

Reabsorption of uric acid in rat nephrons also occurs distal to secretory sites in the S_2 or S_3 segment of the proximal tubule. "Postsecretory" reabsorption in humans is inferred from studies in which pyrazinamide administration inhibited the uricosuric effect of probenecid without altering probenecid excretion (195, 196). Whether extensive bidirectional transport of uric acid occurs within the same segment in man is unknown. Tubular transport of uric acid beyond the proximal tubule seems unlikely.

In micropuncture and microperfusion experiments, urate reabsorption is influenced by urinary flow rate (197), luminal hexose sugars (198), and anion exchange inhibitors (199, 200). Urate transport across renal brush border vesicles is stimulated by increasing the intravesical pH relative to that of the bathing fluid (176) and by increasing an outwardly directed chloride gradient (177).

Developmental Aspects

Renal urate handling in children differs from that in adults. Fractional excretion of urate declines from 61% in premature infants with a gestational age of 29 to 33 weeks to 38% in term neonates (201); this occurs as the filtered load of urate increases and is correlated with fractional excretion of Na and urine flow. The maturational pattern in dogs is similar (202). The postnatal decline in urate clearance results from increasing net tubule reabsorption of urate, possibly related to a contracting ECF volume.

Tubular Transport. Net tubular transport in children aged 3 to 14 years is less than it is in adults, but approaches adult values early in adolescence (203). Tubular secretory capacity, however, may be relatively greater in children than it is in adults (204).

Studies of renal tubular urate transport in early life have been limited to neonatal rabbit and fetal mouse kidney slices. Urate uptake is less in fetal and postnatal renal cortical slices than it is from mature rabbits or mice (166, 178). Urate uptake in neonatal rabbit kidney slices is not stimulated by procaine penicillin administration as it is in slices from adults (166).

Urea

Although urea excretion is a means to remove excess nitrogen from the body, it also plays a major role in facilitating a number of renal tubular functions, including water abstraction from the thin descending limb (7), passive NaCl reabsorption from the thin ascending limb (8), and active secondary Cl reabsorption from the thick ascending limb through its contribution to medullary hypertonicity (18). Urea also has a pivotal role in the operation of the medullary countercurrent multiplication system (Chapter 6). It is, therefore, appropriate to consider how urea is transported across various nephron segments. In general terms, urea is handled differently in the loops of Henle by superficial and juxtamedullary nephrons resulting from, in part, the different permeability characteristics of the thin limbs.

Proximal Tubules

Urea is passively reabsorbed in the proximal convoluted tubule (205). Studies of urea transport in the perfused pars recta of the rabbit have resulted in conflicting evidence. In one study, active secretion was demonstrated (206); in another, passive urea secretion was suggested on the basis of a high urea permeability (207). The latter study may have overlooked a small secretory component. It therefore appears that both active and passive urea secretion may occur in the pars recta (207).

Loop of Henle. Urea transport in the thin descending limb varies among species as well as between superficial and juxtamedullary nephrons. Net urea secretion (208), defined as a fractional delivery rate of urea to the end of the descending limb that is greater than the filtered load occurs in the thin, limb of the exposed rat papillae. Urea also enters into the prebend portion of the descending limb of hamsters (209). However, urea is relatively impermeant in the descending limb of the in vitro perfused nephron of the rabbit (205). The discrepancies among these studies are probably the result of species differences, since epithelial structure and histopathology of the initial descending limb segments among them varies (210).

The thin ascending limb has a moderately high urea permeability coefficient (8, 211) that allows urea entry to occur down its concentration gradient into the postbend segment (209). However, since most of the thin ascending limb is inaccessible to in vivo studies, it is not possible to determine whether reabsorption of urea occurs along the remainder of this segment, after the tubular fluid urea concentration has reached equilibration with the interstitial concentration.

Medullary and cortical segments of the thick ascending limbs have differing urea permeabilities. Whereas the medullary segment has a low urea permeability (212, 213), the cortical segment has a higher urea permeability (207, 213), so that passive urea reabsorption from the cortical thick ascending limb may be substantial. The importance of this is in the possibility that reabsorbed urea may enter the pars recta by active and passive means, providing a mechanism for urea recycling into both short- and long-looped nephrons.

Collecting Tubules. Considerable heterogeneity of urea transport processes exists along the length of the collecting tubules. The cortical collecting tubules of rats (213) and outer medullary collecting ducts of rabbits (212) have a very low urea permeability coefficient unaffected by vasopressin (214). The papillary collecting duct segments of both species have a much higher one that is sensitive to vasopressin (80, 215). Taken together, these studies are consistent with the concept that urea remains within the collecting duct system proximal to the papillary region, whereas beyond that it is reabsorbed into the inner medulla. This process may be modulated by prostaglandins (216), and it is suggested that prostaglandins inhibit papillary collecting duct urea reabsorption.

INDIVIDUAL RENAL TUBULAR FUNCTIONS IN THE COUNTERCURRENT MULTIPLICATION SYSTEM

Tubular Transport

The segmental analysis of renal tubular transport mechanisms that has formed the basis for this chapter may lead to the conclusion that the nephron is unnecessarily complicated and inefficient in its diverse functions. However, the various modifications of tubular fluid that occur along the length of the nephron allow for fine adjustments of urinary volume and solute concentrations subsequent to a wide range of physiological conditions. This concept of renal tubular function (217) may be exemplified most clearly by the processes of urinary concentration and dilution.

The production of urine, ranging in osmolality from 50 to 1000 to 5000 mOsm/kg H_{20} (Umax varies between species), depends on the functional integrity of many of the discrete tubular transport mechanisms that have been described. The 3 basic requirements involve (1) generation and maintenance of an hypertonic renal medulla, (2) formation of dilute distal tubular fluid, and (3) a mechanism whereby this tubular fluid subsequently loses water to the hypertonic renal medulla. The final urine osmolality varies according to the physiological state of the animal.

Some of the individual tubular transport processes involved in the elaboration of hypertonic and hypotonic urine are depicted in Fig. 5.12 (218). This schema depicts a long-looped nephron and assumes that fluid reabsorbed from the proximal tubule is isotonic. The sequence of events shown in Fig. 5.12 summarizes our current understanding of the passive model of the countercurrent multiplication system.

When the tubular fluid passes along the thin descending limb of Henle's loop, the contents become progressively more concentrated as the result of water abstraction, an event that, in some species, is accompanied by addition of solute. The tubular fluid that reaches the hairpin bend of Henle's loop has a high osmolality with higher concentrations of Na and Cl and lower concentrations of urea as compared with adjacent vasa recta and, presumably therefore, the surrounding interstitium. The specific membrane characteristics of the thin ascending limb then allow NaCl reabsorption from this segment to occur pari passu with a lesser degree of urea entry, leading to progressive dilution of luminal contents associated with accumulation of urea (8).

As tubular fluid passes into the medullary and cortical segments of the thick ascending limb, further dilution results from active NaCl transport out of the lumen. This separation of solute from water constitutes the primary event in the generation of the hypertonic renal medulla, the first requirement for varying the urine osmolality. The low urea permeability of the initial portion of the collecting tubule prevents urea reabsorption, but urea may diffuse passively out of the distal medullary and papillary segments to be recycled into the inner medulla and contribute to the maintenance of the hypertonic inner medulla (213). Despite the possibility of some urea reabsorption, the tubular fluid that enters the distal tubule of the juxtamedullary nephron is thought to be hypotonic, with urea being its major osmotic component. This fulfills the second of the requirements listed.

The tubular fluid is further modified in the various segments of the collecting duct system. The hydraulic conductance of all 3 major segments of this system is varied tremendously, in response to ADH. When physiological conditions require the excretion of free water, ADH is not secreted and fractional water reabsorption is low, although the absolute rate is paradoxically higher than it is in the presence of ADH (81). When water conservation is required, ADH is secreted, inducing high fractional water reabsorption, resulting in a highly concentrated urine. The third

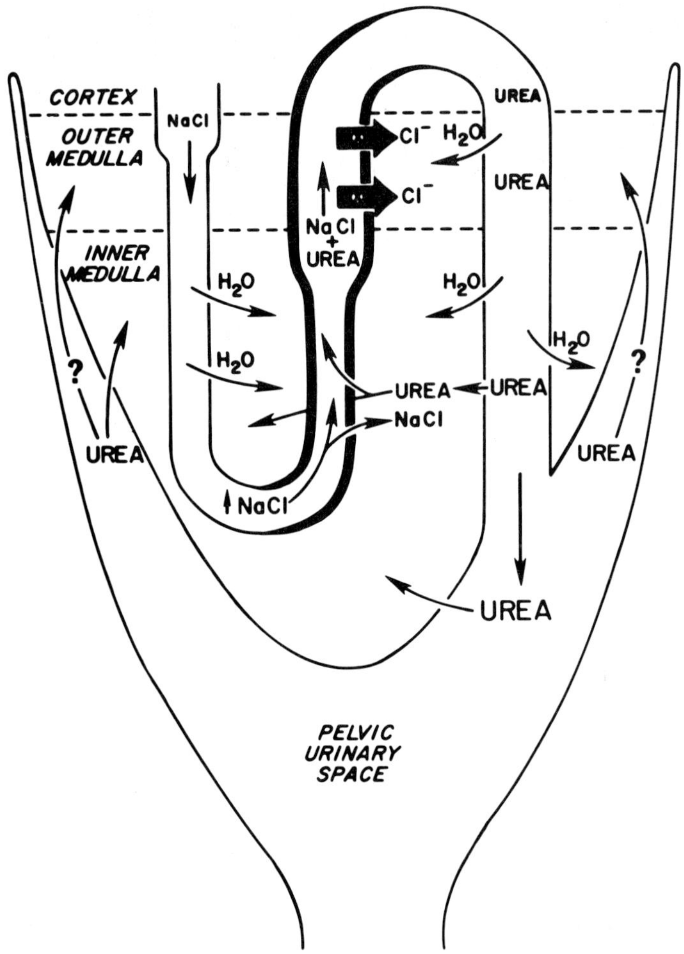

Figure 5.12. General features of the countercurrent multiplication system. (From Hogg RJ, Kokko JP: Rev Physiol Biochem Pharmacol 86: 95, 1979.)

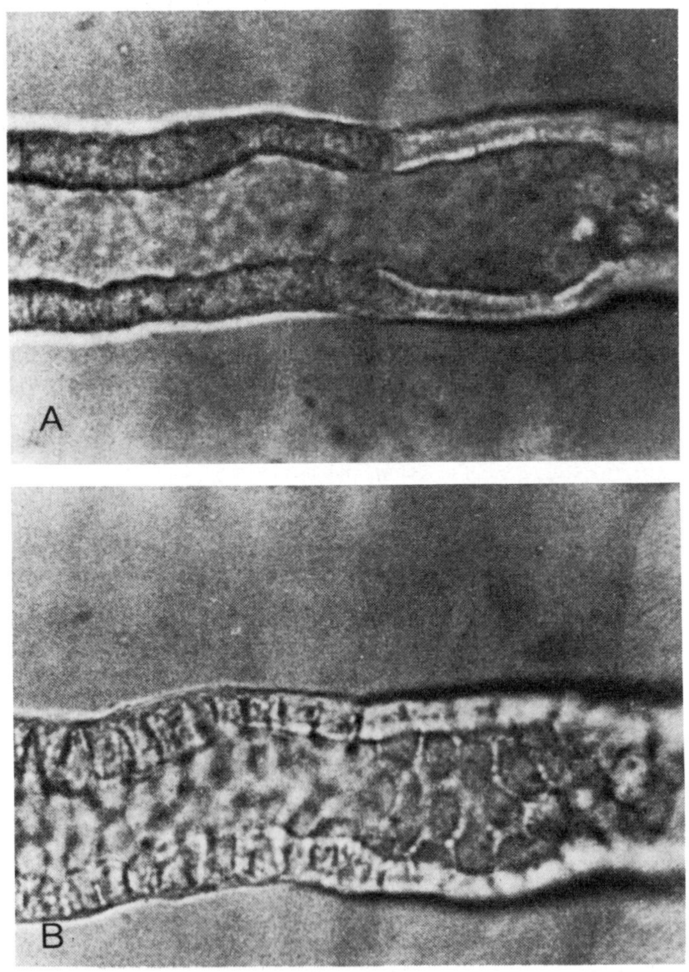

Figure 5.13. Micrograph of isolated perfused human fetus collecting duct. Focal plane at the central axis on the right and at apical surface of the cells on the left. **A**, before vasopressin; **B**, after vasopressin. (X520.) (From Abramow M, Dratwa M: Nature 250:492, 1974. Reprinted by permission. Copyright Macmillan Journals Limited.)

requirement for the generation of maximally dilute or concentrated urine is thus satisfied. The reabsorption of urea across the papillary collecting ducts increases the medullary tonicity and enhances the subsequent abstraction of water from the thin descending limb, thus completing the cycle (Fig. 5.12).

The many discrete and specific tubular transport systems described in this overview of the countercurrent multiplication system are thus integrated into a highly efficient and flexible system for varying the extent to which water is excreted. There are, of course, many other aspects of the concentrating mechanism that are beyond the scope of this chapter but are reviewed elsewhere (219).

Developmental Aspects

The newborn kidney is unable to concentrate urine to the same extent as the mature organ. Neonatal kidneys normally excrete urine with a low concentration of urea, a feature that may be attributed to the fact that most of the N that is ingested is utilized for net protein gain at this age (220). Since urea has a pivotal role in the concentrating mechanism it is not surprising that the newborn's ability to concentrate is less. Administration of a high protein diet to the newborn infant results in increased urea excretion and enhancement of the concentrating capacity (220).

Other studies have evaluated the concentrating mechanism in the fetus and neonate. Plasma arginine vasopressin levels, measured in chronically catheterized, unstressed fetal sheep, rise with infusion of hypertonic saline (221), i.e., the osmoreceptor control of vasopressin secretion is responsive by the third trimester of pregnancy in sheep. No age-related differences in ADH initiated cyclic AMP accumulation are noted in fetal life; however, the medulla from the newborn dog is slightly less responsive when tissue cyclic AMP was related to tissue protein.

Finally, the direct effect of vasopressin on water transport across a human fetus medullary collecting tubule, using the isolated perfused tubule technique (Fig. 5.13), confirmed the end-organ responsiveness to ADH in the human collecting duct during early development (223). From these studies, it could be concluded that, in infants, delay in ability to concentrate urine maximally results from inadequate generation and maintenance of an hypertonic medulla rather than failure of the collecting tubules to permit water reabsorption and subsequent concentration of tubular fluid.

SODIUM, POTASSIUM-ADENOSINE TRIPHOSPHATASE AND RENAL TUBULAR TRANSPORT

Many renal tubular transport mechanisms depend on cyclic AMP or Na, K-ATPase for the transcellular movement of water or solutes. Detailed descriptions of the segmental activity of these transport mediators are reviewed elsewhere (1, 224–226). It is relevant, however, to add a short discussion here of the development of Na, K-ATPase in the immature nephron.

The distribution pattern of Na, K-ATPase in individual nephron segments is qualitatively similar in neonatal and mature animals, but activity is lower in the neonate. The enzyme activity is greatest in the distal nephron; the juxtamedullary proximal convoluted tubules possess Na, K-ATPase activity levels twice as high as the superficial segments (227). The enzyme activity (Fig. 5.14) is particularly low in the immature superficial (subcapsular) proximal convoluted tubule. The age-related increase in proximal convoluted tubule Na, K-ATPase activity is of the same order (227) as the maturational development of the increase in membrane area—approximately 260%—progressing from neonatal to mature rabbits (82).

There is a gradual increase of Na, K-ATPase activity in the S_1 segment from rabbit juxtamedullary proximal convolutions from 1 to 6 weeks of age followed by a rapid surge in enzyme activity in the 7th week (66,

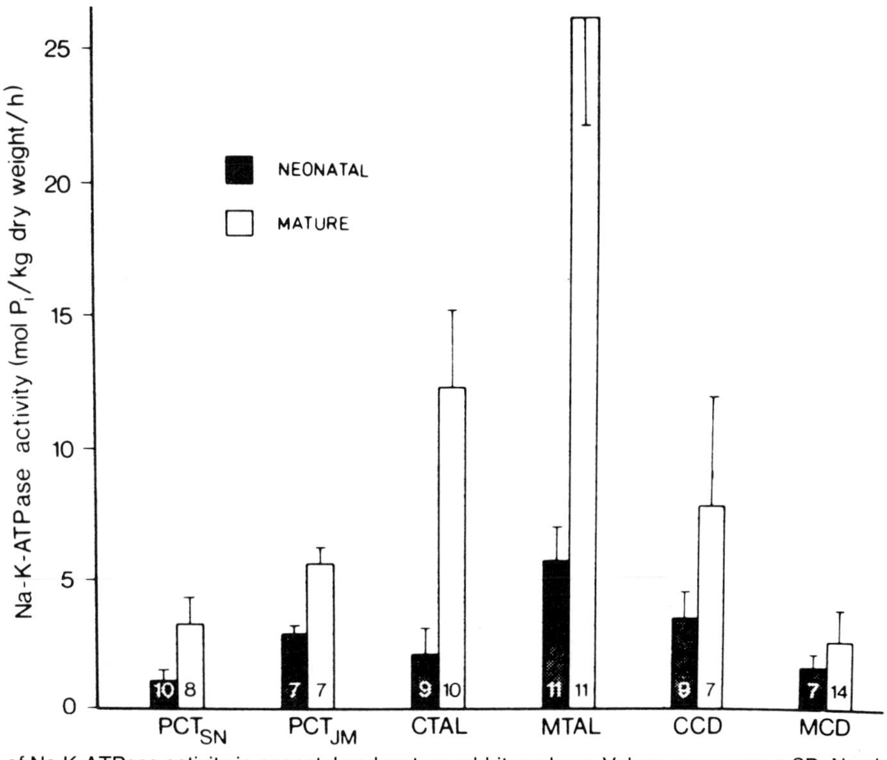

Figure 5.14. Distribution of Na,K-ATPase activity in neonatal and mature rabbit nephron. Values are means ± SD. Numbers in bars indicated number of analyzed tubular segments. *PCT_{SN}*, proximal convoluted tubule (early segment) from subcapsular nephron; *PCT_{JM}*, proximal convoluted tubule (early segment) from juxtamedullary nephron; *CTAL*, cortical thick ascending loop of Henle; *MTAL*, medullary thick ascending loop of Henle; *CCD*, cortical collecting duct; *MCD*, medullary collecting duct. (From Schmidt U, Horster M: Am J Physiol 233:F55, 1977.)

82). Since the surge in Na, K-ATPase followed the big increase in transport rates of Na, HCO_3, and glucose in this segment, it was concluded that the change in enzyme activity is secondary to the change in transport. The findings are compatible with studies of the effect of amiloride, an agent that blocks Na reabsorption, on aldosterone stimulation of Na, K-ATPase. Giving amiloride, the aldosterone-stimulated increase in Na, K-ATPase activity was blocked. Since amiloride is a diuretic agent that inhibits the entry of Na ions, the conclusion reached by these investigators is that Na, K-ATPase is activated by the availability of Na at the pump site. The mechanisms by which increased Na is delivered to this site is a matter of speculation at the present time.

CONCLUSION

Individual renal tubular segments are characterized by specific transport properties that enable tremendous variation in urinary solute content. The integration of the many separate processes may vary but appears to provide functional integrity in assuring glomerulotubular balance and maintenance of body composition at all stages of growth. Further study will extend our understanding of individual tubular functions, as they contribute to overall renal function in the mature and the developing human kidney.

References

1. Jacobson HR: Functional segmentation of the mammalian nephron. Am J Physiol 241:F203, 1981.
2. Woodhall PB, Tisher CC, Simonton CA, et al: Relationship between Para-aminohippurate secretion and cellular morphology in rabbit proximal tubules. J Clin Invest 61:1320, 1978.
3. Tisher CC: Anatomy of the kidney. In Brenner BM, Rector FC Jr (eds): The Kidney. Philadelphia, W.B. Saunders Co., 1976, p 23.
4. Burg MB, Patlak C, Green N, et al: Organic solutes in fluid absorption by renal proximal convoluted tubules. Am J Physiol 231:627, 1976.
5. Kawamura S, Imai M, Seldin DW, et al: Characteristics of salt and water transport in superficial and juxtamedullary straight segments of proximal tubules. J Clin Invest 55:1269, 1975.
6. Imai M: Ninth International Congress of Nephrology, 1984.
7. Kokko JP: Sodium chloride and water transport in the descending limb of Henle. J Clin Invest 49:1838, 1970.
8. Imai M, Kokko JP: Sodium chloride, urea, and water transport in the thin ascending limb of Henle. Generation of osmotic gradients by passive diffusion of solutes. J Clin Invest 53:393, 1974.
9. Hogg RJ, Kokko JP: Comparison between the electrical potential profile and the chloride gradients in the thin limbs of Henle's loop in rats. Kidney Intl 14:428, 1978.
10. Greger R, Wittner M, Schlatter E, et al: Sodium chloride reabsorption in the thick ascending limb of the loop of Henle. In Robinson RR (ed): Nephrology. London, Springer-Verlag, 1984, p 224.
11. Rocha AS, Kokko JP: Sodium chloride and water transport in the medullary thick ascending limb of Henle. J Clin Invest 52:612, 1973.
12. Burg MB, Green N: Function of the thick ascending limb of Henle's loop. Am J Physiol 224:659, 1973.
13. Hall DA, Varney DM: Effect of vasopressin on electrical potential difference and chloride transport in mouse medullary thick ascending limb of Henle. J Clin Invest 66:792, 1980.
14. Sasaki S, Imai M: Effects of vasopressin on water and NaCl transport across the in vitro perfused medullary thick ascending limb of Henle's loop of mouse, rat, and rabbit kidney. Pfluegers Arch 383:215, 1980.
15. Chabardes D, Gagnan-Brunette M, Imbert-Teboul M, et al: Adenylate cyclase responsiveness to hormones in various portions of the human nephron. J Clin Invest 65:439, 1980.
16. Stokes JB: Effect of prostaglandin E_2 on chloride transport across the rabbit thick ascending limb. J Clin Invest 64:495, 1979.
17. Culpepper RM, Andreoli TE: Interactions among prostaglandin E_2, antidiuretic hormone, and cyclic adenosine monophosphate in modulating Cl^- absorption in single mouse medullary thick ascending limbs of Henle. J Clin Invest 71:1588, 1983.
18. Hebert SC, Culpepper RM, Andreoli TE: NaCl transport in mouse medullary thick ascending limbs. III. Modulation of the ADH effect by peritubular osmolality. Am J Physiol 241:F443, 1981.
19. Stokes JB: Consequences of potassium recycling in the renal medulla. Effects on ion transport by the medullary thick ascending limb of Henle's loop. J Clin Invest 70:219, 1982.
20. Hebert SC, Andreoli TE: Control of NaCl transport in the thick ascending limb. Am J Physiol 246:F745, 1984.
21. Stokes JB: Na and K transport across the cortical and outer medullary collecting duct of the rabbit: evidence for diffusion across the outer medullary portion. Am J Physiol 242:F514, 1982.
22. Petty KJ, Kokko JP, Marver D: Secondary effect of aldosterone on Na-K-ATPase activity in the rabbit cortical collecting tubules. J Clin Invest 68:1514, 1982.
23. Stokes JB, Kokko JP: Inhibition of sodium transport by prostaglandin E_2 across the isolated, perfused rabbit collecting tubule. J Clin Invest 59:1099,1977.
24. Hanley MJ, Kokko JP: Study of chloride transport across the rabbit cortical collecting tubule. J Clin Invest 62:39, 1978.
25. Kleinman LI: Renal sodium reabsorption during saline loading and distal blockade in newborn dogs. Am J Physiol 228:1403, 1975.
26. Zink H, Horster M: Maturation of diluting capacity in loop of Henle of rat superficial nephrons. Am J Physiol 233:F519, 1977.
27. Sulyok E, Varga F, Gyory E, et al: Postnatal development of renal sodium handling in premature infants. J Pediatr 95:787, 1979.
28. Wright FS: Potassium transport by successive segments of the mammalian nephron. Fed Proc 40:2398, 1981.
29. Malnic G, Klose RM, Giebisch G: Micropuncture study of renal potassium excretion in the rat. Am J Physiol 206:674, 1964.
30. Litchfield JB, Bolt PA: Micropuncture study of renal excretion of water, K, Na and Cl in the rat. Am J Physiol 203:667, 1962.
31. Blommer HA, Rector FC Jr, Seldin DW: The mechanism of potassium reabsorption in the proximal tubule of the rat. J Clin Invest 42:277, 1963.
32. LeGrimellec C: Micropuncture study along the proximal convoluted tubule. Electrolyte reabsorption in first convolutions. Pfluegers Arch 354:133, 1975.
33. Jamison RL, Work J, Schafer JA: New pathways for potassium transport in the kidney. Am J Physiol 242:F297, 1982.
34. Grantham JJ, Qualizza PB, Irwin RL: Net fluid secretion in proximal straight renal tubules in vitro: role of PAH. Am J Physiol 226:191, 1974.
35. Work J, Troutman SL, Schafer JA: Transport of potassium in the rabbit pars recta. Am J Physiol 242:F226, 1982.
36. Rocha AS, Kokko JP: Membrane characteristics regulating potassium transport out of the isolated perfused descending limb of Henle. Kidney Intl 4:326, 1973.
37. Jamison RL, Lacy FB, Pennell JP, et al: Potassium excretion by the descending limb or pars recta of juxtamedullary nephron in vivo. Kidney Intl 9:323, 1976.
38. Battilana CA, Dobyan DC, Lacy FB, et al: The effect of chronic potassium loading on potassium secretion by the pars recta or descending limb of the juxtamedullary nephron in the rat. J Clin Invest 62:1093, 1978.
39. Burg MB, Bourdeau JE: Function of the thick ascending limb of Henle's loop. In Vogel HG, Ullrich KJ (eds): New Aspects of Renal Function. Excerpta Medica, 1978, p 91, Amsterdam-Oxford.
40. Peterson LN, Wright FS: Effect of sodium intake on renal potassium excretion. Am J Physiol 233:F225, 1977.
41. Grantham JJ, Burg MB, Orloff J: The nature of transtubular Na and K transport in isolated rabbit renal collecting tubules. J Clin Invest 49:1815, 1970.
42. Young DB, Jackson TE, Tipayamoutri U, et al: Effects of sodium intake on steady-state potassium secretion. Am J Physiol 246:F772, 1984.
43. Wingo CS, Seldin DW, Kokko JP, et al: Dietary modulation of active potassium secretion in the cortical collecting tubule of adrenalectomized rabbits. J Clin Invest 70:579, 1982.
44. Bichara M, Paillard M, Corman G, et al: Volume expansion modulates $NaHCO_3$ and NaCl in the proximal tubule and Henle's loop. Am J Physiol 247:F140, 1984.
45. McKinney TD, Burg MB: Bicarbonate transport by rabbit cortical collecting tubules. Effect of acid and alkali loads in vivo on transport in vitro. J Clin Invest 60:76, 1977.
46. Burg M, Green N: Bicarbonate transport by isolated perfused rabbit proximal convoluted tubules. Am J Physiol 233:F307, 1977.
47. Murer H, Hopfer U, Kinne R: Sodium/proton antiport in brush-border membrane vesicles isolated from rat small intestine and kidney. Biochem J 154:597, 1976.
48. Mircheff AK, Ives HE, Yee VJ, et al: Na^+/H^+ antiporter in membrane populations resolved from a renal brush border vesicle preparation. Am J Physiol 246:F853, 1984.
49. DuBose TD Jr, Pucacco LR, Seldin DW, et al: Direct determination of PCO_2 in the rat renal cortex. J Clin Invest 62:338, 1978.
50. Hogg RJ, Pucacco LR, Carter NW, et al: In situ Pco_2 in the renal cortex, liver, muscle, and brain of the New Zealand white rabbit. Am J Physiol 247, F491–498, 1984.
51. Maddox DA, Atherton LJ, Deen WM, et al: Proximal HCO_3^- reabsorption and the determinants of tubular and capillary Pco_2 in the rat. Am J Physiol 247:F73, 1984.
52. DuBose TD Jr, Pucacco LR, Carter NW: Determination of disequilibrium pH in the rat kidney in vivo: evidence for hydrogen secretion. Am J Physiol 240:F138, 1981.

53. Sasaki S, Berry CA: Mechanism of bicarbonate exit across basolateral membrane of the rabbit proximal convoluted tubule. Am J Physiol 246:F889, 1984.
54. DuBose TD Jr, Lucci MS, Hogg RJ, et al: Comparison of acidification parameters in superficial and deep nephrons of the rat. Am J Physiol 244:F497, 1983.
55. Freidman PA, Andreoli TE: CO_2 stimulated NaCl absorption in the mouse renal cortical thick ascending limb of Henle. J Gen Physiol. 80:683, 1982.
56. Malnic G, de Mello-Aires M, Giebisch G: Micropuncture study of renal tubular hydrogen ion transport in the rat. Am J Physiol 222:147, 1972.
57. Kornandakieti C, Tannen RL: H^+ transport by the aldosterone-deficient rat distal nephron. Kidney Intl 25:629, 1984.
58. Lombard WE, Kokko JP, Jacobson HR: Bicarbonate transport in cortical and outer medullary collecting tubules. Am J Physiol 244:F289, 1983.
59. Stone DK, Seldin DW, Kokko JP et al: Anion dependence of rabbit medullary collecting duct acidification. J Clin Invest 71:1505, 1983.
60. Graber ML, Bengele HH, Schwartz JH, et al: pH and P_{CO_2} profiles of the rat inner medullary collecting duct. Am J Physiol 241:F659, 1981.
61. Higashihara E, Carter NW, Pucacco L, et al: Aldosterone effects on papillary collecting duct pH profile of the rat. Am J Physiol 246:F725, 1984.
62. Edelmann CM Jr, Rodriguez-Soriano J, Boichis H, et al: Bicarbonate reabsorption and hydrogen ion excretion in normal infants. J Clin Invest 46:1309, 1967.
63. Moore ES, Fine BP, Satrasook SS, et al: Renal reabsorption of bicarbonate in puppies: effect of extracellular volume contraction on the renal threshold for bicarbonate. Pediatr Res 6:859, 1972.
64. Robillard JE, Sessions C, Burmeister L, et al: Influence of fetal extracellular volume contraction on renal reabsorption of bicarbonate in fetal lambs. Pediatr Res 11:649, 1977.
65. Schwartz GJ, Evan AP: Development of solute transport in rabbit proximal tubule. I. HCO_3^- and glucose absorption. Am J Physiol 245:F382, 1983.
66. Schwartz GJ, Evan AP: Development of solute transport in rabbit proximal tubule. III. Na-K-ATPase activity. Am J Physiol 246:F845, 1984.
67. Buerkert J, Martin D, Trigg D: Ammonium handling by superficial and juxtamedullary nephrons in the rat; evidence for an ammonia shunt between the loop of Henle and the collecting duct. J Clin Invest 70:1, 1982.
68. Buerkert J, Martin D, Trigg D: Segmental analysis of the renal tubule in buffer production and net acid formation. Am J Physiol 244:F442, 1983.
69. Schafer JA: Mechanisms coupling the absorption of solutes and water in the proximal nephron. Kidney Intl 25:708, 1984.
70. Barfuss DW, Schafer JA: Hyperosmolality of absorbate from isolated proximal straight tubules. Am J Physiol 247:F130, 1984.
71. Andreoli TE, Schafer JA, Troutman SL: Perfusion rate dependence of transepithelial osmosis in isolated proximal convoluted tubules: estimation of the hydraulic conductance. Kidney Intl 14:263, 1978.
72. Jacobson HR, Kokko JP: Intrinsic differences in various segments of proximal convoluted tubules. J Clin Invest 57:818, 1976.
73. Holmberg C, Kokko JP, Jacobson HR: Determination of chloride and bicarbonate permeabilities in proximal convoluted tubules. Am J Physiol 241:F386, 1981.
74. Vari RC, Ott CE: In vivo proximal tubular fluid-to-plasma chloride concentration gradient in the rabbit. Am J Physiol 242:F575, 1982.
75. Lewy JE, Windhager EE: Peritubular control of proximal tubular fluid reabsorption in the rat kidney. Am J Physiol 214:943, 1960.
76. Brenner BM, Falchuk KH, Keinowitz RI, et al: The relationship between peritubular capillary protein concentration and fluid reabsorption by the renal proximal tubule. J Clin Invest 48:1519, 1969.
77. Imai M, Kokko JP: Transtubular oncotic pressure gradients and net fluid transport in isolated proximal tubules. Kidney Intl 6:138, 1974.
78. Berry CA, Cogan MG: Influence of peritubular protein on solute reabsorption in the rabbit proximal tubule. J Clin Invest 68:506, 1981.
79. Grantham JJ, Burg MB: Effect of vasopressin and cyclic AMP on permeability of isolated collecting tubules. Am J Physiol 211:255, 1966.
80. Rocha AS, Kudo LH: Water, urea, sodium, chloride and potassium transport in the in vitro isolated perfused papillary collecting duct. Kidney Intl 22:485, 1982.
81. Jamison RL, Buerkert J, Lacy F: Micropuncture study of collecting tubule function in rats with hereditary diabetes insipidus. J Clin Invest 50:2444, 1971.
82. Horster M, Larsson L: Mechanisms of fluid absorption during proximal tubule development. Kidney Intl 10:348, 1976.
83. Holmberg C, Tisher CC, Jacobson HR, et al: Na to Cl permeability in newborn rabbit superficial and juxtamedullary proximal convoluted tubules. Mineral Electrolyte Metab Vol 2, p 215–222, 1985.
84. Haramati A, Kleinman LI: Chloride concentration gradient in newborn dogs in the presence of distal nephron blockade. Am J Physiol 239:F328, 1980.
85. Pitts RF, Alexander RS: The renal absorptive mechanism for inorganic phosphate in normal and acidotic dogs. Am J Physiol 147:648, 1944.
86. Bijvoet OLM, Walton RJ: Nomogram for derivation of renal threshold phosphate concentration. Lancet 2:309, 1979.
87. Stark H, Eisenstein B, Tieder M: Tp/GFR as a measure of renal Po_4 handling in children. Eur J Pediatr 140:181, 1983.
88. Strickler JC, Thompson DD, Klose RM, et al: Micropuncture study of inorganic phosphate excretion in the rat. J Clin Invest 43:1596, 1964.
89. Knox FG, Haas JA, Berndt T, et al: Phosphate transport in superficial and deep nephrons in phosphate-loaded rats. Am J Physiol 233:F150, 1977.
90. Haramati A, Haas JA, Knox FG: Adaptation of deep and superficial nephrons to changes in dietary phosphate intake. Am J Physiol 244:F265, 1983.
91. Dennis VW, Woodhall PB, Robinson RR: Characteristics of phosphate transport in isolated proximal tubule. Am J Physiol 231:979, 1976.
92. Dennis VW, Brazy PC: Sodium, phosphate, glucose, bicarbonate and alanine interactions in the isolated proximal convoluted tubule of rabbit kidney. J Clin Invest 62:387, 1978.
93. Hoffman N, Thees M, Kinne R: Phosphate transport by isolated renal brush border vesicles. Pfluegers Arch 367:147, 1976.
94. Kinne R, Berner W, Hoffman N, et al: Phosphate transport by isolated renal and intestinal plasma membranes. Clin Res 429A, 1977.
95. Ullrich KJ, Rumrich G, Klose S: Phosphate transport in the proximal convolution of rat kidney. Pfluegers Arch 372:269, 1977.
96. Rocha AS, Magaldi JB, Kokko JP: Calcium and phosphate transport in isolated segments of rabbit Henle's loop. J Clin Invest 59:975, 1977.
97. Brunette MG, Taleb L, Carrere S: Effect of parathyroid hormone on phosphate reabsorption along the nephron of the rat. Am J Physiol 225:1076, 1973.
98. Amiel C, Kuntziger H, Richet G: Micropuncture study of handling of phosphate by proximal and distal nephrons in normal and parathyroidectomized rat. Evidence for distal reabsorption. Pfluegers Arch 347:93, 1970.
99. Pastoriza-Munoz E, Colendres RE, Lassiter WE, et al: Effect of parathyroid hormone on phosphate reabsorption in rat distal convolution. Am J Physiol 235:F321, 1978.
100. Moore ES, Ocampo M, Langmas CB, et al: Renal phosphate clearance in the fetus. Sem Nephrol 3:81, 1983.
101. Spitzer A, Kaskel FJ, Feld LG, et al: Renal regulation of phosphate homeostasis during growth. Sem Nephrol 3:87, 1983.
102. Moore ES, Chung EE, Cevallos EE, et al: Renal phosphate clearance in fetal lambs. Pediatr Res 12:1066, 1978.
103. Kaskel FJ, Kumar AM, Feld L, et al: Renal tubular reabsorption of phosphate during development. Pediatr Res 18:370A, 1984.
104. Cloi Y, Kinne R, Spitzer A: Cellular mechanism of renal phosphate transport by the newborn. Pediatr Res 18:370A, 1984.
105. Suki WN: Calcium transport in the nephron. Am J Physiol 237:F1, 1979.
106. Murayama Y, Morel F, LeGrimellac C: Phosphate, calcium and magnesium transfers in proximal tubules and loops of Henle as measured by single nephron microperfusion experiments in the rat. Pfluegers Arch 333:1, 1972.
107. Ullrich KJ, Rumrich G, Klos S: Active Ca^{++} reabsorption in the proximal tubule of the rat kidney. Pfluegers Arch 364:223, 1976.
108. Friedman PA, Figueredo JR, Maack T, et al: Sodium-calcium interactions in the renal proximal convoluted tubule of the rabbit. Am J Physiol 240:F558, 1981.
109. Kinne-Saffian E, Kinne R: Localization of a calcium-stimulated ATPase in the basal-lateral plasma membranes of the proximal tubule of rat kidney cortex. J Membr Biol 17:263, 1974.
110. Jamison RL, Frey NR, Lacy FB: Calcium reabsorption in the thin loop of Henle. Am J Physiol 227:745, 1974.
111. DeRouffignac CF, Morel F, Moss N, et al: Micropuncture study of water and electrolyte movements along the loop of Henle in Psammomys with special reference to magnesium, calcium and phosphorus. Pfluegers Arch 344:309, 1973.
112. Eknoyan G, Suki WN, Martinez-Maldonado M: Effect of diuretics on urinary excretion of phosphate, calcium and magnesium in thyroparathyroidectomized dogs. J Lab Clin Med 76:257, 1970.
113. Suki WN, Rouse D, Ng RCK, et al: Calcium transport in the thick ascending limb of Henle. Heterogeneity of function in the medullary and cortical segments. J Clin Invest 66:1004, 1980.
114. Costanzo LS, Windhager EE: Calcium and sodium transport by the distal convoluted tubule of the rat. Am J Physiol 235:F492, 1978.
115. Costanzo LS, Weiner IM: Relationship between clearance of Ca and Na; effect of distal diuretics and PAH. Am J Physiol 230:67, 1976.
116. Peraino RA, Suki WN: Urine HCO_3^- augments Ca^{2+} reabsorption independent of systemic acid base changes. Am J Physiol 238:F394, 1980.
117. Shareghi GR, Stoner LC: Calcium transport across segments of the rabbit distal nephron in vitro. Am J Physiol 235:F367, 1978.
118. Arant BS, Jr, Stapleton FB, Engle WD, et al: Urinary excretion of calcium in human neonates. Eur J Pediatr 140:184A, 1983.
119. Greer FR, Chesney RW: Disorders of calcium metabolism in the neonate. Sem Nephrol 3:100, 1983.
120. Brown DR, Steranka BH: Renal calcium excretion in the hypocalcemic premature human neonate. Pediatr Res 15:1100, 1981.
121. Hofnagle KG, Khan SN, Penn D, et al: Renal calcifications. A complication of long-term furosemide therapy in preterm infants. Pediatrics 70:367, 1982.
122. Walser M: Divalent cations: physicochemical state in glomerular filtrate and urine

acid renal extraction. In Orloff J, Berliner RW, (ed): Handbook of Physiology. Washington, American Physiological Society, 1978, p 555.
123. Massry SG, Coburn JW, Ullman CR: Renal handling of magnesium in the dog. Am J Physiol 216:1460, 1969.
124. Wong NLM, Quamme GA, Dirks JH; Tubular maximum reabsorption capacity for magnesium in the dog. Kidney Intl 16:658, 1979.
125. Quamme GA, Dirks JH: Magnesium transport in the nephron. Am J Physiol 239:F393, 1980.
126. Morel F, Roinel N, LeGrimellac C: Electroprobe analysis of tubular fluid composition. Nephron 6:350, 1969.
127. Quamme GA, Dirks JH: Intraluminal and contraluminal magnesium on magnesium and calcium transfer in the rat nephron. Am J Physiol 238:F187, 1980.
128. Brunette M, Aras M: A micropuncture study of nephron permeability to calcium and magnesium. Am J Physiol 221:1442, 1971.
129. Shareghi GR, Agus ZS: Magnesium transport in the cortical thick ascending limb of Henle's loop of the rabbit. J Clin Invest 69:759, 1982.
130. Mudge GH, Berndt WO, Vatlin H: Tubular transport of urea, glucose, phosphate, uric acid, sulfate and thiosulfate. In Orloffo J, Berliner RW (eds): Handbook of Physiology. Washington, American Physiological Society, 1973, p 594.
131. Shannon JA, Fischer S: The renal reabsorption of glucose in the normal dog. Am J Physiol 122:765, 1938.
132. Tune BN, Burg MB: Glucose transport by proximal renal tubules. Am J Physiol 221:580, 1971.
133. Brodehl J, Franken A, Gellisen K: Maximal tubular reabsorption of glucose in infants and children. Acta Paediatr Scand 61:413, 1972.
134. Arant BS Jr: Developmental patterns of renal functional maturation compared in the human neonate. J Pediatr 92:705, 1978.
135. Tudvad F: Sugar reabsorption in prematures and fullterm babies. Scand J Clin Lab Invest 1:281, 1949.
136. Robillard JE, Sessions C, Kennedy RL, et al: Maturation of the glucose transport process by the fetal kidney. Pediatr Res 12:680, 1978.
137. Arant BS Jr: Glomerulotubular balance following saline loading in the developing canine kidney. Am J Physiol 35:F417, 1978.
138. Kwong T-F, Bennett CM: Relationship between glomerular filtration rate and maximum tubular reabsorption rate of glucose. Kidney Intl 5:23, 1974.
139. Robson AM, Srivastava PL, Bricker NS: The influence of saline loading on renal glucose reabsorption in the rat. J Clin Invest 47:329, 1965.
140. Burg MB: Renal handling of sodium, chloride, water amino acids and glucose. In Brenner BM, Rector FC Jr (eds): The Kidney. Philadelphia, W.B. Saunders Co., 1981, p 328.
141. Frohnert PP, Holimann B, Zweikel R, et al: Free flow micropuncture studies of glucose transport in the rat nephron. Pfluegers Arch 315:66, 1970.
142. Busse D, John A, Steinmarer G: Carrier mediated transfer of d-glucose in brush border vesicles derived from rabbit renal tubules: Na^+-dependent versus Na^+-independent transfer. Biochim Biophys Acta 401:231, 1975.
143. Aronson PS, Sacktor B: Transport of d-glucose by brush border membranes isolated from the renal cortex. Biochim Biophys Acta 356:231, 1974.
144. Kippen I, Herayama B, Klinenberg JR, et al: Transport of p-aminohippuric acid, uric acid and glucose in highly purified rabbit renal brush border membranes. Biochim Biophys Acta 556:161, 1979.
145. Silverman M: Glucose transport in the kidney. Biochim Biophys Acta 457:303, 1976.
146. Kleinzeller A, Kolunska K, Benes I: Transport of glucose and galactose in kidney cortex cells. Biochem J 104:843, 1967.
147. Segal S, Thier SO: Renal handling of amino acids. In Orloff J, Berliner RW (eds): Handbook of Physiology. Washington, American Physiological Society, 1973, p 653.
148. Brown JL, Samiy AH, Pitts RF: Localization of amino nitrogen reabsorption in the nephron of the dog. Am J Physiol 200:370, 1961.
149. Bergeron M, Morel F: Amino acid transport in rat renal tubules. Am J Physiol 216:1139, 1969.
150. Brodehl J, Gillissen K: Endogenous renal transport of free amino acids in infancy and childhood. Pediatrics 42:395, 1968.
151. Ullrich KJ: Sugar, amino acid and sodium co-transport in the proximal tubule. Ann Rev Physiol 41:181, 1979.
152. Eisenbach GM, Weise M, Stolte H: Amino acid reabsorption in the rat nephron. Pfluegers Arch 357:63, 1975.
153. Schafer JA, Barfuss DW: Membrane mechanisms for transepithelial amino acid absorption and secretion. Am J Physiol 238:F335, 1980.
154. Scriver CR, Mohyuddin F: Amino acid transport in kidney heterogeneity of α-aminobutyric uptake. J Biol Chem 243:3207, 1968.
155. Barfuss DW, Mays JM, Schafer JA: Peritubular uptake and transepithelial transport of glycine in isolated proximal tubules. Am J Physiol 238:F324, 1980.
156. Silbernagl S, Pfaller W, Deeten P: Molecular specificity of tubular amino acid reabsorption. Rev Physiol Biochem Pharma 74:105, 1978.
157. Segal S: Regulatory aspects of transport during development. In Spitzer A (ed): The Kidney during Development: Morphology and Function. New York, Masson Publishing, 1980, p 363.
158. Solomon S, Bengele HH, Evan AP: Amino acid uptake by fetal kidney slices. Biol Neonate 29:257, 1976.
159. Chesney RW, Jax DA: Developmental aspects of renal B amino acid transport. II. Ontogeny of uptake and efflux process and effect of anoxia. Pediatr Res 13:861, 1979.
160. Friedman AL, Jax DK, Chesney RW: Developmental aspects of renal B amino acid transport. III. Ontogeny of transport in isolated renal tubule segments. Pediatr Res 15:10, 1981.
161. Segal S, Rea C, Smith I: Separate transport systems for sugars and amino acids in developing rat kidney cortex. Proc Natl Acad Sci USA 68: 372, 1971.
162. Roth KS, Hwang S-M, London JW, et al: Ontogeny of glycine transport in isolated rat renal tubules. Am J Physiol 233:F241, 1977.
163. Irish JM III, Grantham JJ: Renal handling of organic acids and cations. In Brenner BM, Rector FC Jr (eds): The Kidney, ed. 2. Philadelphia, W.B. Saunders Co., 1981, p 619.
164. Smith HW, Goldring W, Chasis H: The measurement of the tubular excretory mass, effective blood flow and filtration rate in the normal kidney. J Clin Invest 17:263, 1938.
165. Calcagno PL, Rubin MI: Renal extraction of para aminohippurate in infants and children. J Clin Invest 42:1632, 1963.
166. Hook JB, Hewitt WR: Development of mechanisms for drug excretion. Am J Med 62:197, 1977.
167. Tune BM, Burg MB, Patlak CS: Characteristics of *p*-amminohippurate transport in proximal tubules. Am J Physiol 217:1057, 1969.
168. Schali C, Roch-Ramel F: Uptake of [^{3}H] PAH and [^{14}C] urate into isolated proximal tubular segments of the pig kidney. Am J Physiol 241:F591, 1981.
169. Weinman EJ, Frankfurt SJ, Ince A, et al: Renal tubular transport of organic acids. Studies with oxalate and para-aminohippurate in the rat. J Clin Invest 61:801, 1978.
170. Maxild J, Moeller JV, Sheikh MI: Kinetics of p-aminohippurate transport in rabbit kidney slices: Role of Na^+. Biochem Biophys Acta 601:490, 1980.
171. Maxild J, Moeller JV, Sheikh MI: Involvement of Na-K-ATPase in *p*-aminohippurate transport by rabbit kidney tissue. J Physiol 315:189, 1981.
172. Spencer AM, Sack J, Hong SK: Relationship between PAH transport and Na-K-ATPase activity in the rabbit kidney. Am J Physiol 236:F126, 1979.
173. Shimomura A, Chunko AM, Grantham, JJ: The basis of heterogeneity of para-aminohippurate secretion. Am J Physiol 241:F565, 1981.
174. Habig WH, Pabst MJ, Fleischer G, et al: The identity of glutathione S-transferase with ligandin, a major binding protein of liver. Proc Natl Acad Sci USA 71:3879, 1974.
175. Hook JB, Hewitt WR, Pegg DG, et al: Studies on the mechanism of substrate stimulation of renal organic acids transport in newborn rabbits. In Spitzer A (ed): The Kidney during Development. New York, Masson Publishing, 1982, p 345.
176. Blomstedt JW, Aronson PS: pH gradient-stimulated transport of urate and p-Aminohippurate in dog renal microvillus membrane vesicles. J Clin Invest 65:931, 1980.
177. Kahn AM, Aronson PS: Urate transport via anion exchange in dog renal microvillus membrane vesicles. Am J Physiol 244:F56, 1983.
178. Tune BM: Relationship between the transport and toxicity of cephalosporins in the kidney. J Infect Dis 132:189, 1975.
179. Weiner IM: Transport of weak acids and bases. In Orloff J, Berliner RW (eds): Handbook of Physiology. Washington, American Physiological Society, 1973, p 521.
180. Irish JM III, Grantham JJ: Role of luminal PAH in fluid secretion in proximal straight tubules. Fed Proc 36:592, 1975.
181. Stapleton FB, Linshaw MA: Regulation of cell volume in a human proximal straight tubule. Renal Physiol 1:334, 1978.
182. Cole BR, Brocklebank JT, Capps RG, et al: Maturation of *p*-aminohippuric acid transport in the developing rabbit kidney: interrelationships of the individual components. Pediatr Res 12:992, 1978.
183. Schwartz GJ, Goldsmith DI, Fine LG: *p*-Amino-hippurate transport in the proximal straight tubule: Development and substrate stimulation. Pediatr Res 12:793, 1978.
184. Reiselbach RE, Steele TH: Influence of the kidney upon urate homeostasis in health and disease. Am J Med 56:665, 1974.
185. Weiner IM: Urate transport in the nephron. Am J Physiol 237:F85, 1979.
186. Weiner IM, Tinker JP: Pharmacology of pyrazinamide: metabolic and renal function studies related to the mechanism of drug induced urate retention. J Pharmacol Exp Ther 180:411, 1972.
187. Diamond HS, Meisel AD: Post-secretory reabsorption of urate in man. Arth Rheum 18:805, 1978.
188. Weinman EJ, Eknoyan E, Suki WN: The influence of the extracellular fluid volume on the tubular reabsorption of uric acid. J Clin Invest 55:283, 1975.
189. Manual MA, Steele TH: Pyrazinamide suppression of the uricosuric response to sodium chloride infusion. J Lab Clin Med 83:417, 1974.

190. Weinman EJ, Knight TF, McKenzie R, et al: Dissociation of urate from sodium transport in the rat proximal tubule. Kidney Intl 10:295, 1976.
191. Praetorius E, Kirk JE: Hypouricemia: with evidence for tubular elimination of uric acid. J Lab Clin Med 35:856, 1950.
192. Boner G, Steele TH: Relationship of urate and PAH secretion in man. Am J Physiol 225:100, 1973.
193. Shimomura A, Chonko A, Tanner R, et al: Nature of urate transport in isolated rabbit tubules. Am J Physiol 241:F565, 1981.
194. Steele TH, Rieselbach R: The renal mechanism for urate homeostasis in normal man. Am J Med 43:868, 1967.
195. Diamond HS, Paolino JS: Evidence for a post-secretory reabsorptive site for uric acid in man. J Clin Invest 52:1481, 1973.
196. Meisel AD, Diamond HS: Inhibition of probenecid uricosuric by pyrazinamide and paraaminohippurate. Am J Physiol 32:F222, 1976.
197. Senekjian HO, Knight TF, Sansom SG, et al: Effect of flow rate and extracellular fluid volume on proximal tubule rate and water reabsorption. Kidney Intl 17:155, 1980.
198. Knight TF, Senekjian HO, Sansom S, et al: Effects of intraluminal D-glucose and probenecid on urate reabsorption in the rat proximal tubule. Am J Physiol 236:F526, 1979.
199. Dantzler WH, Bentley SK: Effect of inhibitors in lumen on PAH and urate transport by isolated renal tubules. Am J Physiol 236:F379, 1979.
200. Weinman EJ, Sansom SC, Bennett S, et al: Effect of anion exchange inhibitors and para-aminohippurate on the transport of urate in the rat proximal tubule. Kidney Intl 23:832, 1983.
201. Stapleton FB: Renal uric acid clearance in human neonates. J Pediatr 103:290, 1983.
202. Stapleton FB, Arant BS Jr: Ontogeny of renal uric acid excretion in the mongrel puppy. Pediatr Res 15:1513, 1981.
203. Stapleton FB, Linshaw MA, Hassanein K, et al: Uric acid excretion in normal children. J Pediatr 92:911, 1978.
204. Stapleton FB: Developmental aspects of renal excretion of uric acid. In Sptizer A (ed): The Kidney during Development. New York, Masson Publishing, 1982, p 355.
205. Kokko JP: Urea transport in the proximal tubule and the descending limb of Henle. J Clin Invest 51:1199, 1972.
206. Kawamura S, Kokko JP: Urea secretion by the straight segment of the proximal tubule. J Clin Invest 58:604, 1976.
207. Knepper MA: Urea transport in nephron segments from medullary rays of rabbits. Am J Physiol 245:F622, 1983.
208. Pennell JP, Sanjana V, Frey NR, et al: The effect of urea infusion on the urinary concentrating mechanism in protein depleted rats. J Clin Invest 55:399, 1975.
209. Marsh DJ: Solute and water flows in thin limbs of Henle's loop in the hamster kidney. Kidney Intl 14:428, 1978.
210. Kriz W: Structural organization of the renal medullary counterflow system. Fed Proc 42:2379, 1983.
211. Imai M: Function of the thin ascending limb of rats and hamsters perfused in vitro. Am J Physiol 232:F201, 1977.
212. Rocha AS, Kokko JP: Permeability of medullary nephron segments to urea and water: effect of vasopressin. Kidney Intl 6:379, 1974.
213. Knepper MA: Urea transport in isolated thick ascending limbs and collecting ducts from rats. Am J Physiol 245:F634, 1983.
214. Schafer JA, Andreoli TE: The effect of antidiuretic hormone on solute flows in mammalian collecting tubules. J Clin Invest 51:1279, 1972.
215. Morgan T, Sakai F, Berliner RW: In vitro permeability of medullary collecting ducts to water and urea. Am J Physiol 214:574, 1968.
216. Roman RJ, Lechene C: Prostaglandin E_2 and $F2\alpha$ reduces urea reabsorption from the rat collecting duct. Am J Physiol 241:F53, 1981.
217. Knepper M, Burg M: Organization of nephron function. Am J Physiol 244:F579, 1983.
218. Hogg RJ, Kokko JP: Renal countercurrent multiplication system. Rev Physiol Biochem Pharmacol 86:95, 1979.
219. Hogg RJ, Kokko JP: Urine concentrating and diluting mechanisms in mammalian kidneys. In Brenner BM, Rector FC Jr (eds): The Kidney. Philadelphia, W.B. Saunders Co. 1986. 3rd edition. Chapter 8, pp 251–279.
220. Edelmann CM, Barnett HL, Troupkou V: Renal concentrating mechanisms in newborn infants. Effect of dietary protein and water content, role of urea, and responsiveness to antidiuretic hormone. J Clin Invest 39:1062, 1960.
221. Weitzman RE, Fisher DA, Robillard J, et al: Arginine vasopressin response to an osmotic stimulus in the fetal sheep. Pediatr Res 12:35, 1978.
222. Lu L-T, Bailie MD, Hook JB: Effect of antidiuretic hormone and theophylline on cyclic AMP in renal medulla of newborn and adult rabbits and dogs. Gen Pharmac 6:181, 1975.
223. Abramow M, Dratwa M: Effect of vasopressin on the isolated human collecting duct. Nature 250:492, 1974.
224. Morel F: Sites of hormone action in the mammalian nephron. Am J Physiol 240:F159, 1981.
225. Morel F, Imbert-Teboul M, Chabardes D: Distribution of hormone-dependent adenylate cyclase in the nephron and its physiologic significance. Ann Rev Physiol 43:569, 1981.
226. Marver D, Kokko JP: Renal target sites and the mechanism of action of aldosterone. Mineral Electrolyte Metab 9:1, 1983.
227. Schmidt U, Horster M: Na-K activated ATPase: Activity maturation in rabbit nephron segments dissected in vitro. Am J Physiol 233:F55, 1977.

2

Body Fluids and Nutrition

CHAPTER 6 Sodium and Water

6A Physiology of Sodium, Chloride, and Water

GEORGE HAYCOCK

Sodium (Na) and its anion chloride (Cl) are the principal solutes of extracellular fluid (ECF) and are, therefore, the main determinants of ECF volume. A description of the regulation of body Na is, in effect, a description of how ECF volume is controlled. The concentration of Na in ECF virtually defines the osmolality of body fluids, which in turn is set largely by factors controlling water intake and excretion.

The regulation of body Na is largely effected by its renal excretion. Intake generally exceeds extrarenal losses and is, therefore, in excess of the sum of requirement and non-renal losses. Renal excretion can vary from near zero, when intake is marginal, to more than 1000 mEq daily. Redistribution, nonrenal losses, or renal disease can cause changes in body Na or its distribution, with physical signs indicative of deficiency or excess. The effects of ECF volume depletion are mediated by contraction of the effective intravascular (plasma) or interstitial fluid (ISF) volume. However, plasma and ISF volume may be contracted when total ECF is increased but sequestered as edema. Retention of Na and Cl secondary to renal disease causes expansion of ECF volume, including both effective plasma and ISF volume i.e., edema may be present either with depletion or excess of plasma volume.

The regulation of body water involves the control of renal excretion of water in relation to intake, which usually is in excess of minimum requirement, and the excess is excreted. The tonicity (effective osmolality) of body fluids remains normal. The manner in which NaCl and water are distributed and the controls that affect their turnover are the subject of this chapter. Abnormalities of ECF volume and osmolality also are considered.

DISTRIBUTION OF BODY FLUIDS

Water accounts for about 45% to 65% of total body weight in adults and for a greater proportion in infants and young children. Between one-third and one-half of body water is ECF (chapter 1). The recognition that the cell, the basic unit of life, lives in the ECF was a major step toward developing the modern concepts of biology. The difference in composition between intracellular fluid (ICF) and ECF raises questions as to how the two fluids, so different in compositions interact and how the normal volume and composition of each is maintained. From an evolutionary perspective, the adaptation of life to dry land necessitated the development of intricate systems governing the exchange between cells and ECF and the maintenance of ECF as a suitable environment for cells.

The Semipermeable Membrane

The cell membrane that separates major compartments of body fluids is a lipid bilayer impermeable to water. Dispersed throughout the membrane are "pores" through which water passes freely by diffusion. The area occupied by these pores is small, about $\frac{1}{5000}$ of the total membrane area, but is sufficient to present no measurable hindrance to the free movement of water between the two fluid phases; the passage of solutes, however, is restricted, i.e., the membrane is semipermeable. The steady state that exists in health is a dynamic equilibrium in which entry and egress of water are matched by a balance of opposing osmotic and energy-dependent forces.

The membrane that separates cells from ECF shares characteristics with the capillary membranes that separate plasma from ISF. The properties of these membranes are the principal determinants of the fluid distribution between these various phases in the body. However, other factors affect how plasma and ISF are partitioned, including the Gibbs-Donnan effect, the Starling forces, and the function of the lymphatic system.

Properties

A semipermeable membrane is one that separates two solutions and is permeable to their common solvent but is impermeable to one or more solutes in them. This provides the physical basis of the forces governing fluid exchange between cells and ECF. If one solution has a higher solute concentration, it also has a lower concentration of solvent, i.e., the solvent is "diluted" by the solute in the solution. This favors net movement of solvent by diffusion from the less concentrated solution across the membrane to the more concentrated one, until osmotic equilibrium is reached or until it is opposed by the hydrostatic pressure of equal strength.

The osmotic pressure of a solution is measured by the hydrostatic pressure required to prevent movement from pure solvent to the solution. This pressure is a function of the number of dissolved particles per unit of solvent (water). The osmotically effective concentration of solute is expressed as osmolality; one osmol is the number of particles in a gram mole of a nondissociating solute (6.0225×10^{23}: Avogadro's number). The normal osmolality of mammalian body fluids is 290 mOsm/kg water.

Equilibrium between ECF and ICF is maintained by the movement of water in response to alteration in osmolality of either. This water movement is driven by the kinetic energy of the random thermal movement of water molecules themselves (diffusion). The greater the flux across the membrane, the greater the tendency for the concerted movement of these molecules to "sweep" other molecules along with them in a streaming effect known as bulk flow, which significantly increases the rate of net water movement above that which would be predicted from diffusion alone. The greater the underlying rate of diffusion, the greater the enhancing effect of bulk flow. Bulk flow occurs whenever there is net water movement by diffusion, as occurs across capillary membranes. Bulk flow also increases the net rate of movement of permeant solutes.

Partition of Water between ECF and ICF

The partition of water is determined by the distribution of solute on either side of the cell membrane. The principal osmotically active solutes in these solutions are Na, K, and their associated anions. The activity of the Na pump prevents net gain of Na by cells and loss of K from them and, therefore, is central to preserving the balance between the two compartments. ICF is rich in negatively-charged macromolecules and attracts permeant cations into cells. This attraction, unopposed, would lead to gain in cell cations and water; it is offset by the asymmetric action of the Na pump, which transports three Na ions out of the cell for each two K ions transported in, so that cation and solute influx and efflux are equal. Therefore, cell volume is regulated by active transport of Na out of the cell.

Characteristics of Extracellular Fluid

ECF is divided into intravascular (plasma), ISF including fluid in connective tissue and bone, and transcellular fluid. Plasma and ISF are separated by capillary membrane. Transcellular fluid is ECF that is secreted into and reabsorbed from the gastrointestinal tract and other spaces lined by epithelial cells. Its turnover depends on active transport; the rate of turnover is large, but residual fluid in these spaces is usually small. Transcellular fluid makes no contribution to changes in volume and composition of the ECF except when reabsorption is not complete and there are net losses, e.g., gastrointestinal secretions.

The Capillary Membrane

The semipermeable membrane separating the two principal components of the ECF—plasma and ISF—is different from the semipermeable membrane surrounding cells in important ways. Anatomically, the capillary wall consists of two layers, a thin monolayer of endothelial cells and an outer basement membrane. Although the relative contribution of the two layers to the restriction of large solute movement across the capillary is not fully determined, the two together may be considered as a membrane freely permeable to water and small solutes, but less permeable to larger molecules—the plasma proteins. The capillary membrane is part of the system that controls the flow of ECF between plasma and ISF. The permeability of capillary walls to various molecular species is summarized in Table 6.1 (1). The values for water and NaCl are very high and nearly identical, so that equilibrium of both salt and water across the capillary wall occurs rapidly; NaCl does not exert an osmotic force across capillaries. Even substances such as mannitol do so only transiently. Despite the low permeance of albumin relative to water, some filtration of albumin from plasma into ISF occurs. The return of albumin from ISF by the lymphatic system balances the transfer of albumin to ISF across the capillary membrane. The fluid that is transferred contains, on average, about 2 g/dl protein. Regional variations in this value are considerable, e.g., hepatic lymph contains protein at a concentration close to that in plasma.

The Gibbs-Donnan Effect

Plasma proteins are polyanionic—negatively charged at plasma pH—and their distribution across the capillary wall is asymmetric. This affects the distribution of permeant ions, such as Na and Cl. The excess of anionic protein in plasma compared with ISF displaces Cl into ISF. The distribution to establish electroneutrality is offset by the creation of a potential osmotic gradient. This results in diffusion of Cl from ISF into plasma, creating an electrical potential difference across the dividing membrane, plasma being negative with respect to ISF. The distribution is described by the Nernst equation (2):

$$E = \frac{RT}{F} \times \ln \frac{\mathrm{Cl}_i}{\mathrm{Cl}_e} \qquad (1)$$

At 37° C: $E = 61 \times \ln \frac{\mathrm{Cl}_i}{\mathrm{Cl}_e}$ where E = transmembrane potential difference in millivolts, R, T, and F are gas constant, the absolute temperature, and Faraday's constant, and Cl_i and Cl_e are the concentrations (more strictly, the activities) of Cl in ISF and plasma, respectively.

The resulting electrochemical gradient for Cl causes redistribution of Na until a new equilibrium is reached. This occurs when the Nernst potential calculated from Na distribution is identical to that calculated from Cl distribution but opposite in sign.

The resulting distribution of ions is known as a Gibbs-Donnan distribution (3), which applies to their concentration in the solvent phase—water. The ratio of ISF:plasma concentration for any ionic species is the Gibbs-Donnan Factor for that species. This corrects for a number of interfering factors, such as interactions between proteins and other ions in their immediate vicinity (4). The theoretically derived Gibbs-Donnan distribution between plasma and ISF applies to the aqueous phase of the

Table 6.1.
Permeability of Capillary Walls to Some Important Molecular Species.

Substance	Permeability
Water	1
NaCl	0.96
Urea	0.8
Glucose	0.6
Inulin	0.2
Hemoglobin	0.01
Albumin	<0.0001

(From Landis EM, Pappenheimer JR: Exchange of substances through the capillary walls. In Hamilton WF, Dow P (eds): Handbook of Physiology. Washington, D. C., American Physiological Society, 1963, vol 2, p 961.)

two solutions. Measured values for electrolytes in plasma are lower than would be predicted, since only 92% of the volume of plasma consists of solvent (water); a smaller correction is applied to ISF.

The Gibbs-Donnan effect has three important consequences. First, the ionic composition of the aqueous phase of plasma and ISF differ. Second, the total osmolal concentration in plasma is higher than it would be if the proteins were uncharged. Third, the oncotic pressure of plasma proteins is affected. The latter is a polynomial function of the concentration of protein expressed in the following equation (5):

$$\text{oncotic pressure} = ac + bc^2 + dc^3 \qquad (2)$$

where c represents protein concentration, and a, b, and d are empirically derived coefficients. For whole human plasma with a normal albumin:globulin ratio, the values are a, 2.1; b, 0.16; and d, 0.009; while for a solution of pure albumin a, 2.0; b, 0.18; and d, 0.012.

Figure 6.1 shows this relationship graphically and compares it with that derived for connective tissue proteoglycan. The oncotic pressure of normal arterial plasma with a protein concentration of 7 g/dl is approximately 28 torr, of which 80% is contributed by albumin. The oncotic pressure of ISF, with an average protein concentration of about 2 g/dl is 5 torr.

Starling Forces Between Plasma and ISF

The oncotic pressure gradient of 23 torr between plasma and interstitial space is opposed by the hydrostatic pressure within the capillaries as a function of blood pressure. The hydrostatic pressure in peripheral capillaries falls from about 25 torr at the arterial end to about 10 at the venous end. The interstitial space has a negative hydrostatic pressure (16) on the order of −7 torr relative to atmospheric pressure, owing to the pumping action of muscles on lymphatics (7). Summating the oncotic and hydrostatic pressure gradients gives a net outward (plasma to ISF) pressure of about 8 torr at the arterial end and a net reabsorptive force of about 7 torr at the venous end of the capillary bed. The result is that about 90% of the fluid filtered from plasma to interstitium is passed through the arterial segment of capillaries and is reabsorbed at the venous segment. The remaining 10% is returned to the circulation via the lymphatics. The forces controlling fluid exchange between plasma and lymph are termed Starling forces (8). There is a filtration of 15 to 20 ml/min from plasma to ISF; this contrasts with the more than 200 l/min which exchanges between the two compartments as a result of diffusion and bulk flow (1, 8, 9).

The Lymphatic System

Most of the fluid filtered from the arterial segment of the capillary bed is reabsorbed across its venous segments. A smaller fraction, usually 10%, is returned by the lymphatic system. The edges of the lymphatic endothelial cells overlap in such a way that they function as nonreturn valves, preventing backleak of fluid to the ISF. Afferent lymphatic channels contain valves similar to those found in systemic veins, so that compression of the lymphatics from muscle action cause centripetal movement of lymph into the lymphatic duct. Additional pumping is provided by intrinsic contractility of the lymphatic vessels themselves, although muscular action and changes in body posture are probably more important. Lymph flow increases up to 20-fold during muscular exertion and decreases during rest. Disturbances in lymphatic function can cause edema and contraction of plasma volume.

Properties of ISF

ISF is a complex network of solutions and gels in contact with one another and with plasma across capillary membranes (9). The relative proportions of the compartments are given in Figure 6.2 (10). Except for gastrointestinal fluid, the transcellular fluids seldom affect the dynamics of ECF significantly. The measurement of ECF is discussed in Chapter 1.

The ISF is located mostly in the interstices of the filamentous macromolecules composing the intercellular ground substance, with which it forms a gel. The major components of this ground substance are collagen and proteoglycans. The latter are chiefly responsible for the physical and chemical properties of the system.

Proteoglycans are complex polysaccharide chains consisting of repeating disaccharide subunits linked at one end to a protein core (11). Small quantities of ECF are present as free fluid in channels within and adjacent to the gel, but under normal circumstances most of the interstitial water is in the gel phase. The polyanionic nature of the proteoglycan molecules leads to the establishment of a Donnan equilibrium between the gel and

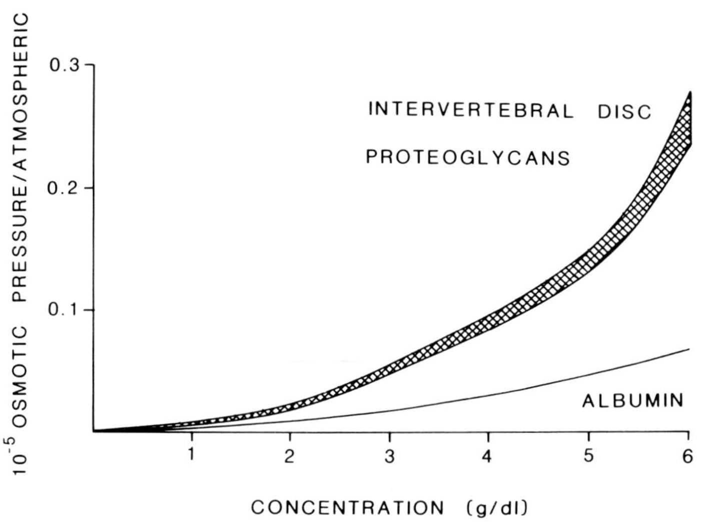

Figure 6.1. The relationship between concentration and osmotic pressure for serum albumin and a representative connective tissue proteoglycan. (Redrawn from Comper WD, Laurent TC: Physiol Rev 58:225, 1978.)

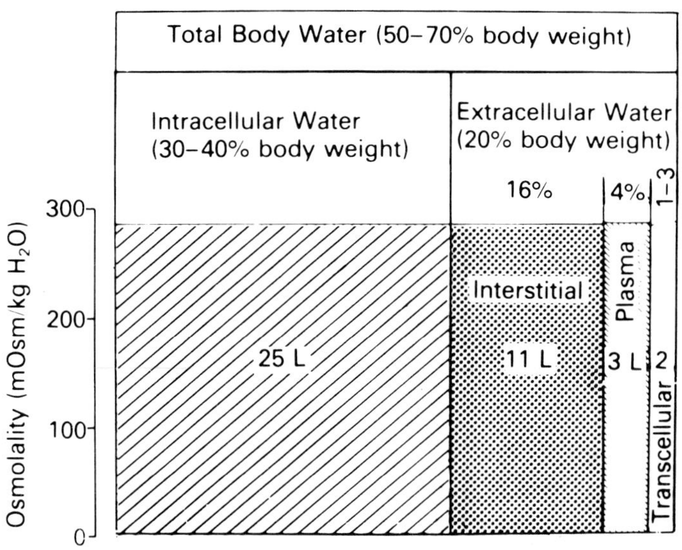

Figure 6.2. Approximate sizes of the major body fluid compartments. (Reproduced with permission from Valtin H: Renal Function: Mechanisms Involved in Fluid and Solute Balance, ed. 2. Boston, Little, Brown, 1982.)

free fluid components of the system and an osmotic gradient favoring water movement into the gel, so that the interstitium is not fluid. Resistance to water loss from the gel rises sharply with dehydration, i.e., oncotic pressure rises rapidly (Figure 6.1), which is an important homeostatic defense of the immediate environment of the cells. This property also contributes to the elasticity of tissues, such as articular cartilage and intervertebral disks, encouraging rapid restoration of normal hydration after expulsion of water under compression.

The molecular structure of the proteoglycan matrix is such that, while diffusional movement of water and solute occurs almost as freely as it does in solutions, bulk flow is almost nonexistent. Thus, exchange of water, electrolytes, nutrients, and excretory products takes place by diffusion between plasma and cells, while distortion of the intercellular matrix under the influence of gravitational and other physical forces is resisted. This contrasts with the situation in states of edema, where the free fluid component of the interstitium is greatly expanded and the structural stability of the system is compromised.

The net balance of Starling forces between plasma and ISF favors filtration from the circulation to ISF. Efficient removal of this filtrate by means of lymphatic pumping maintains the gel-like character of the interstitium. The hydrostatic pressure in the interstitial space is negative as lymph is pumped out (6). This negative hydrostatic pressure contributes to the balance of forces leading to filtration from capillaries to ISF. It is a critical determinant of the circulation of the ISF and in the maintenance of its normal volume and composition.

CONTROL OF SODIUM

The control of Na excretion is part of a larger control system that maintains the various components of ECF volume and the distribution of fluid among its phases, most particularly plasma and ISF.

Intake

Na intake as NaCl varies widely among cultures and individuals widely from levels of <10 mEq (250 mg Na) daily to >1000 (25 g Na). Within this range, renal and nonrenal control of output can vary to balance intake. Salt intake is largely a cultural and learned response, as opposed to an appetite, such as thirst and hunger. Nonetheless, there is an appetite for salt related to physiologic need. This can be elicited in extreme salt deficiency or suppressed by salt excess, but salt appetite is not important in regulating salt intake in daily experience. Water intake is regulated to maintain constant body osmolality and replace renal and nonrenal losses. The control of NaCl turnover entails an implied effect on water turnover. Water excretion is controlled separately from that of solute by a separate system.

Sodium Excretion

The control of Na and Cl excretion maintains ECF volume and body osmolality in the face of changes in input and output in a steady functioning state. This control is vested in factors affecting intake and, to a much greater extent, renal function, i.e., control over excretion of an intake that exceeds minimum.

Changes in Na excretion may be initiated by events of several different kinds. These include:

(1) Change in intake: increased or decreased intake of NaCl (intake of other Na salts is usually less consequential as their excretion is rapid and they have little influence on ECF volume).

(2) Increased losses from non-renal routes, leading to net loss of NaCl and water (ECF volume contraction).

(3) Changes in intravascular volume due to alteration in Starling forces: loss of oncotic pressure, resulting from hypoalbuminemia, as occurs from albuminuria in nephrosis or sequestration of fluid in local injury, i.e., "third space" losses; increased transcapillary hydrostatic pressure gradient, as occurs with quiet standing; decreased transcapillary hydrostatic pressure, as occurs with head-out water immersion; and special consequences of modern therapy, e.g., intravenous fluids, diuretics.

Feedback Loops

Interlocking of NaCl and Water Control

In general, disturbances in ECF volume modulate Na excretion (Fig. 6.3), while changes in tonicity, i.e., effective osmolality, modulate the excretion of water. The osmoregulatory system, discussed later in this chapter, maintains the tonicity of body fluids between narrow limits by the effects on thirst and water excretion. Maximal responses in either direction are elicited by deviations of 1.5% from the normal value of 290 mOsm/kg water. Since the major osmotically active solute in ECF

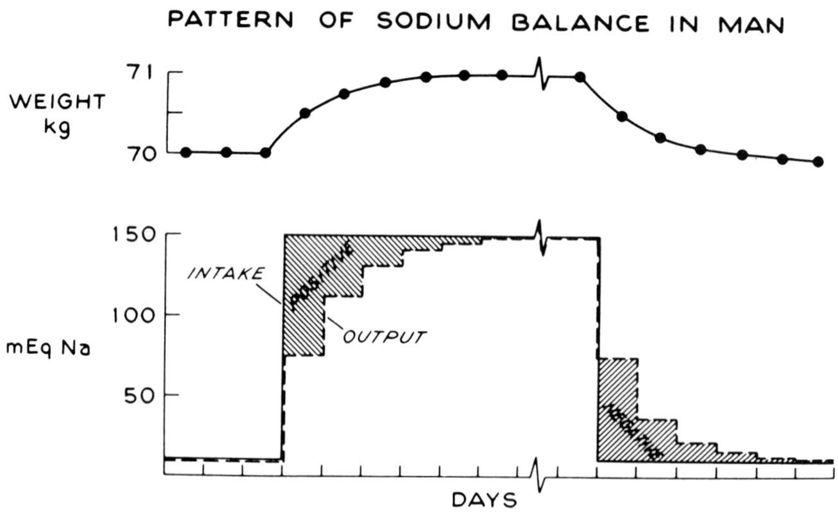

Figure 6.3. The renal response to alteration of sodium intake. Increasing intake leads to transiently positive sodium balance, ECF volume expansion and weight gain; reducing it leads to the opposite effects. Parallel changes in water balance prevent measurable changes in ECF sodium concentration. The observed changes in urinary sodium excretion evidently occur in response to changes in ECF volume rather than to changes in its composition.

is NaCl, the principal determinant of ECF volume is the NaCl content of the body. The sequence of events following a moderate reduction in ECF volume illustrates this principle. The primary response to volume depletion is a reduction in Na excretion rate that leads to a transient elevation of Na concentration, slight hypertonicity, thirst, and water intake. The retention of water is such that net losses of Na and water are proportional. With repletion of body Na, there is proportionate retention of water until normal volume is restored. Similarly, states of abnormal Na retention are usually accompanied by proportionate retention of water; the result is the expansion of ECF and the formation of edema.

The renal control of NaCl and salt excretion is affected by the interaction of two interlocking feedback loops: a volume responsive loop, which is the principal regulator of Na excretion but capable of directly influencing water excretion, and a tonicity-responsive loop, which is the principal regulator of renal water handling.

Nature of the Feedback System

The systems regulating renal NaCl and water excretion are based on the principle of negative feedback, in which deviations from normal status are sensed and elicit responses opposite in sign from the initiating stimulus. Its components are an afferent (sensory) component, an efferent (messenger) component, and an effector organ. The messenger is necessary if the stimulus is sensed at a site that is remote from the effector organ. When information is sensed in the effector itself, the messenger is not needed. Where the efferent system consists of several sensors, sometimes at different sites, messages might be integrated into an appropriate overall response.

The loops that regulate NaCl excretion have sensors in various parts of the body. The messengers are several, but the effector is the kidney. Some of these loops respond to signals sensed within the kidney; others are activated by signals sensed remotely. "Short" and "long" loops generally respond in the same direction, i.e., reinforce one another. The redundancy of these systems controlling NaCl excretion provides backup controls when one or more of these systems is impaired. Failure or imperfect operation of any one component is buffered by the capacity of the remainder to compensate. A further advantage is a high damping factor. If only one mechanism operated with a fixed response time, the amplitude of oscillation would be greater than with several operating at different response times.

The Afferent Component

Intrathoracic Receptors. An increase in intrathoracic blood volume, such as that produced by head-out immersion (12, 13), increases the effective arterial blood volume by increasing venous and lymphatic return to the heart. The natriuretic response is brisk even though total ECF volume is not increased. The sensors for the change are thought to be intracardiac. Section of the cardiac nerves abolishes the natriuretic response (14). Nerve stimulation caused by left atrial distension is a major factor in inducing the natriuresis (15); nerve input from the right ventricle may contribute (16). The effect of right atrial dilatation is less clear (17). Quiet standing produces opposite circulatory effects to those of water immersion and is antinatriuretic.

Arterial Receptors. Alterations in central arterial pressure also affect the Na excretion rate. Hypotension or underfilling of the high pressure compartment results in a decrease in Na excretion. If salt intake continues, NaCl is retained, ECF expands, and weight increases. This mechanism may be important in the NaCl retention characteristic of congestive cardiac failure. Stimuli capable of activating the arterial volume receptors include arteriovenous fistulae (18, 19), vasodilation as occurs with certain drugs, and depletion of ECF volume as occurs with loss of ECF or its sequestration as edema. Stimuli arising from reduction in effective arterial volume override any effect that venous filling might have and antinatriuresis results.

The effect of arterial pressure on NaCl excretion is mediated by afferent nervous impulses arising in the carotid sinus (20, 21). Although only a small proportion of the blood volume (15%) is normally in the high pressure or arterial compartment, this compartment is much more sensitive to volume changes than the venous compartment. The relationship between the holding capacity of the arterial circuit and its degree of fullness at any particular time is termed the effective arterial volume.

Hepatic and Portal Venous Receptors. Receptors in the liver and portal vein also affect NaCl excretion. Infusion of saline into the portal vein produces a greater natriuretic effect than equivalent infusions into systemic veins (22).

Central Nervous System Receptors. Altering the Na concentration of the cerebrospinal fluid (CSF) affects Na excretion (23). Observations of this effect were obtained as a result of grossly unphysiological manipulations, and it is not certain whether receptors in the CNS are involved in the day-to-day control of ECF volume.

Interstitial Baroreceptors. Interstitial fluid pressure may be sensed and act as a natriuretic stimulus. The oncotic pressure of infused fluid influences the Na excretion according to the pressure of the infused fluid (1, 24–26). The effect is further modified by the state of hydration of the subject (27). Infusing saline or Ringer's solution produces a much greater natriuresis than infusing plasma or whole blood. Hyperoncotic albumin infusions are antinatriuretic and may even inhibit an established diuresis (24). This is the reverse of what would be expected plasma or arterial volume alone were the perceived stimulus for Na excretion. It is the effect of these fluids on ISF volume, rather than intravascular volume, that correlates with Na excretion. Receptors have been identified in the pulmonary interstitium that might serve this function (28); this may be the 'effective' ISF volume. The different natriuretic effects of hyperoncotic and hypooncotic solutions may be mediated by the effect of changes in renal interstitial pressure on segmental tubular Na reabsorption (29, 30).

Intrarenal Receptors. Sensors are located in each kidney that initiate afferent impulses via the sympathetic system which result in efferent output to both kidneys. The efferent output may be either alpha-adrenergic or dopaminergic (31). Stimuli arising from changes in arterial perfusion, venous occlusion, or ureteral obstruction in one kidney mediate an effect on the contralateral kidney. For example, unilateral ureteral obstruction causes vasodilatation of both the affected and opposite kidney in rats (31a). Renal denervation abolishes this "reno-renal reflex." The significance of these experimental findings in the daily control of Na excretion or the role the reflex may play in disease is not clear (31b).

The Effector Component

The controls that regulate the urinary excretion of Na constitute the effector component. An adult with normal renal function filters about 25,000 mEq Na daily. On a normal western diet, only about 150 mEq will be excreted, i.e., 24,850 mEq are reabsorbed by the tubules:

$$Na_E = Na_F - Na_R$$

where subscripts denote excreted, filtered, and reabsorbed Na, respectively. A small percentage change in either Na_F or Na_R, not accompanied by a similar change in the other quantity, will lead to a large change in Na_E. In the above example, a 1% increase in glomerular filtration rate (GFR) and Na_F would produce an increase in Na_E of >160% in Na_E, equivalent to the loss of almost 2 L of ECF/day, unless Na_R were to increase in a compensatory fashion. Na_E is regulated by mechanisms maintaining proportionality or coupling between Na_F and Na_R. How these are coupled has proved unexpectedly difficult with the accuracy necessary to determine this when Na_E is in the physiological range.

Investigators have attempted to overcome this problem in a number of ways. One is to study the effects of acute changes in ECF volume on renal function. The magnitude of the "volume expansion" employed in these experiments is usually so massive as to bear little resemblance to any likely physiological state. Another strategy has been to constrain one variable, usually GFR, while observing the changes in the other (Na_R) produced by various natriuretic stimuli. A third approach is based on the study of the failing kidney, in which reduction of nephron numbers places increasing stress on the kidney's homeostatic reserve, "amplifying" the natriuretic demand per residual nephron and rendering it more transparent to investigation.

Glomerular Filtration Rate

GFR and, hence, Na_F change in the same direction as Na_E in response to a number of maneuvers (32, 33). This initially led many investigators to conclude that small changes in GFR would account for changes in Na_E. This was an inadequate explanation in that the absolute changes in Na_F greatly exceeded those in Na_E and a change in tubular reabsorption (Na_R) also must have occurred. On the other hand, changes in GFR and Na_F may occur with little or no change in Na_E (24, 30, 34, 35). When GFR was increased by protein feeding, dexamethasone administration, plasma protein dilution, dopamine infusion, or ECF volume expansion, GFR rose by 30%. Only in the case of volume expansion did Na_E increase; the natriuretic effect of expansion must have been a result of a smaller change in Na_R (35) than when other factors increased Na_F.

Changes in renal mass, whether made acutely by nephrectomy or gradually by progressive disease, do not affect Na balance until renal failure is severe. Since GFR and Na_F are reduced in these examples, changes in tubular function must occur in order that ($Na_F - Na_R$) remains sensitive to changes in Na intake. These and other findings focus the study of control of Na excretion on the tubule, which raises the question of which segments affect these changes and in response to what controls.

Proximal Tubular Reabsorption of Na

Normally, two thirds of Na_F is reabsorbed in the proximal tubule; small changes in this transport function could easily account for the observed changes in Na excretion. As in the case of GFR, Na_R is difficult to measure with the accuracy necessary to explain the relatively small changes in Na_E seen in normal conditions. Therefore, heroic manipulations of the system have been employed to obtain results capable of interpretation. Because the proximal tubule is not accessible to direct study in man and intact animals, most of the evidence bearing on the subject has been acquired by micropuncture studies and, more recently, by the study of isolated, perfused segments of rabbit tubules.

Saline volume expansion depresses fractional proximal reabsorption of Na, even when GFR is coincidentally reduced (36). Conversely, volume contraction results in an increase in proximal reabsorption (37). These and similar studies establish that changes in ECF volume usually stimulates an effect on proximal tubular reabsorption of Na sufficient to account for observed changes in Na_E without the need for an associated change in GFR.

Resorption of Na from the proximal tubule is achieved by active transport across the tubular epithelium and by Starling forces acting between the peritubular capillaries and the interstitium.

Active Sodium Transport. Several active transport systems are involved in Na transport in the proximal tubule. In the early (S_1) proximal tubule HCO_3 is reabsorbed in preference to Cl (38). The transport of Na and HCO_3 are interdependent. This is shown by the fact that both ouabain and acetazolamide are effective in inhibiting $NaHCO_3$ reabsorption (39). The reabsorption of HCO_3 involves the synthesis of new HCO_3 from CO_2 and H_2O by carbonic anhydrase. The reaction yields a proton ($H+$) that is secreted into the tubular lumen in exchange for Na via a Na-proton "antiport" demonstrated in rat kidney brush border membrane vesicles (40). The proton combines with filtered HCO_3 to form H_2CO_3, which is then dehydrated by luminal carbonic anhydrase to H_2O and CO_2. The latter diffuses down its concentration gradient into the tubular epithelial cells and into body fluids, completing the cycle (chapter 5).

Na is cotransported with other substances, including glucose (41) and amino acids (42) in the early proximal tubule. This is effected by carrier-coupled cotransport, not by utilization of the organic molecules as energy sources; thus, the nonmetabolized analogs alpha-methyl, D-glucoside, and cycloleucine are effective substitutes for glucose and leucine, respectively, in promoting Na transport (43).

The lumen-negative transepithelial potential difference measured in the early proximal tubule is the result of active Na transport (44). The preferential reabsorption of HCO_3 and organic solutes leads to Cl becoming progressively concentrated as fluid passes down the tubule (45), with the development of a concentration gradient for Cl between lumen and peritubular fluid. Cl, therefore is reabsorbed by passive diffusion down this gradient in the middle (S_2) portion of the proximal tubule. This leads to reversal of the potential difference, so that it becomes lumen-positive (46). This potential reversal augments the continuing active reabsorption of Na by creating an electrical gradient favoring it. Thus, although Na is actively transported all along the proximal tubule, the early preferential reabsorption of HCO_3 facilitates this transport at more distal sites.

An additional factor promoting the reabsorption of Na and other permeant solutes in the proximal tubule (as well as at more distal sites) is the movement of water through the intercellular channels of the epithelium. Adjacent cells are closely applied to one another at the luminal end of the intercellular space, at the "tight junction." This junction is thought to present some resistance to the passage of water and solute, although it is not impermeable. If Na is extruded from the tubular cells into the lateral intercellular space, this will make the fluid in that space slightly hypertonic to tubular fluid. This causes water to enter the intercellular space across the tight junction by osmosis, raising the pressure in the intercellular space and driving fluid across the basement membrane at the basal (antiluminal) end of the space, and into the peritubular interstitium. The resulting water flux across the epithelium carries Na and other solutes with it by "solvent drag," essentially another manifestation of bulk flow. The existence of this 'paracellular shunt pathway' is accepted widely and models have been constructed to account for fluid movement through it (47), but the relative importance of flow between and through the cells remains uncertain.

Peritubular Physical Forces. Physical factors, i.e., Starling forces, operate between the peritubular capillaries and the renal interstitium and affect Na_R (48–50). Altering hydrostatic and oncotic pressures in the capillaries and tubules affects proximal tubular reabsorption in the predicted direction (49, 50). Changing the protein concentration in the bath surrounding an isolated, perfused rabbit proximal tubule affects the rate of Na transport, presumably by adding an oncotic gradient to the forces favoring reabsorption (51, 52). Although both active transport and physical forces are necessary for proximal tubular Na reabsorption, many physiologists believe that the physical factors provide the rate-limiting step in the process. If this is so, it implies that control of Na reabsorption is accomplished by modulating these forces rather than by adjusting the rate of active transport. For these reasons, it is impossible to separate glomerular and tubular functions in attempting to understand Na reabsorption in this part of the nephron because glomerular hemodynamics profoundly affect the Starling forces in the peritubular capillaries.

Glomerulotubular Balance

The rate of delivery of fluid to the distal nephron is an important determinant of many regulatory functions, notably those concerned with K and H+ excretion. Since this rate is the difference between GFR and proximal tubular reabsorption, the coupling of the two processes is a basic prerequisite for the control of tubular function; it is known as glomerulotubular balance. The definition of the term has varied and is not always used in the same sense by different authors. It is used here as recommended by de Wardener (53) to mean that "sudden changes in filtration rate are accompanied by simultaneous and parallel compensatory changes in tubular reabsorption, so that the effect on Na excretion is clamped down." At least three mechanisms contribute to this balance: active transport, physical forces, and tubuloglomerular feedback.

Active Transport. Na transport in the early proximal tubule is dependent on the parallel reabsorption of HCO_3 (39, 40) and the cotransport of organic solutes (41–43). A rise in GFR will automatically increase the delivery of these solutes to the tubule, increasing Na reabsorption by these transport systems (54) and enhancing Na reabsorption downstream as a result of an increase in the Cl concentration gradient and, hence, Cl reabsorption.

Physical Forces. The operation of peritubular physical forces also preserves glomerulotubular balance. The peritubular capillary plexus in most nephrons in the mammalian cortex is in series with, and downstream from, the glomerulus. The physical forces operating in the peritubular environment, therefore, are determined largely by glomerular hemodynamics in a way that contributes importantly to maintaining glomerulotubular balance (55). When GFR and filtration fraction increase, as occurs with efferent arteriolar constriction, the protein concentration of postglomerular plasma rises and peritubular capillary hydrostatic pressures falls, favoring increased reabsorption from the tubule and countering the tendency to natriuresis. In contrast, when increases in GFR are associated with proportionate or greater increases in plasma flow, the filtration fraction is unchanged or reduced. Peritubular hydrostatic pressure is unchanged or may even increase and less "clamping" occurs, i.e., Na delivery to the distal nephron will increase. Glomerulotubular balance is reset. Intrarenal infusion of acetylcholine (56), prostaglandins, or bradykinin (57), systemic administration of dopamine (58), and renal denervation (59) are examples. All of these are natriuretic stimuli and mimic the effect of ECF volume expansion with saline.

Tubuloglomerular Feedback. Individual nephron filtration rate is regulated by negative feedback, which acts to sustain glomerulotubular balance (60). The ascending limb of the loop of Henle is intimately associated with the afferent and efferent arterioles of its own glomerulus, with which it forms the juxtaglomerular apparatus (JGA). The sensed stimulus probably is the rate of delivery of Cl to the macula densa and JGA (61). Increased Cl delivery causes release of renin and local production and conversion of angiotensin (62), which constricts afferent and efferent arterioles (63). This counters a potential loss of salt and water by a reflex fall in GFR.

Factors that change GFR and, therefore, Na_F, usually set processes in operation that increase proximal Na reabsorption or, in a negative feedback loop, reduce GFR. Glomerulotubular balance is preserved and distal delivery of Na is clamped or modulated. Exceptions are volume contraction or expansion, and other natriuretic or antinatriuretic stimuli.

Distal Nephron Na Reabsorption. Current evidence suggests that the distal nephron, which includes the collecting duct, is the predominant site for regulating or "fine-tuning" the rate of Na_E. There is a dissociation between natriuresis and fractional delivery of Na from the proximal tubule in volume expansion produced by different fluids (29). Differences in Na_E affected by infusions of hyperoncotic albumin and Ringer's solution are principally a result of the effect on Na_R in the collecting duct (30). Na_R reabsorption is inhibited by volume expansion in both the ascending limb of Henle and the collecting duct. Na_R in both sites is regulated to effect appropriate changes in Na_E (64–66). Massive volume expansion with isotonic saline appears to cause secretion by the medullary collecting duct, but this has been demonstrated only under highly unphysiological conditions (67).

Redundancy of Mechanisms. It might appear from the previous that the renal response to natriuretic and antinatriuretic stimuli is complex to the point of redundancy. Even if glomerular filtration and Na_R in substantial segments of the tubule are constrained by experimental conditions from responding "appropriately," whatever part of the nephron remains seems able to alter Na handling in a parallel and appropriate way. This probably reflects the extreme importance of Na homeostasis to survival. If one primary mechanism for regulating Na_E should fail, compensatory responses from other tubule segments compensate in each a way that any resulting disturbance of extracellular volume is minimized. It seems reasonable to assume, in the absence of evidence to the contrary, that the relatively small changes in Na_E required under normal conditions are mediated by small, parallel adjustments in several or all of these processes acting in harmony.

The Efferent Component

The efferent component regulating Na_E is the term used for the varied processes that respond to the afferent stimuli and initiate responses in the effector system to modulate Na_E. Both renal and extrarenal factors are capable of influencing this effector system—renal Na_E; some or all of these combine to form an appropriate efferent (messenger) component, usually resulting in an appropriate renal response to natriuretic and antinatriuretic stimuli detected elsewhere in the body.

Intrarenal Mechanisms

The maintenance of glomerulotubular balance is achieved mainly by intrarenal mechanisms, i.e., changes in the filtration rate of preferentially reabsorbed solutes (54), altered peritubular physical forces (55), and tubuloglomerular feedback (60). The isolated kidney is capable of responding to altered perfusion pressures with changes in Na_E (68), even though autoregulation of renal blood flow (RBF) is preserved (69). Intrarenal factors also modulate Na_E independently of extrarenal controlling influences, by affecting Na_R beyond the proximal tubule. Vasodilator drugs increase Na_E. Altered peritubular oncotic pressure and hydrostatic pressure may affect Na_R at several tubule sites (24, 36). There is a relationship between medullary tonicity and Na_R in the ascending limb of the loop of Henle. When tonicity is reduced by volume expansion with saline, reduction in Na_R follows washout of medullary solute that had resulted from increased vasa recta blood flow (57).

Natriuresis produced in the rat by saline volume expansion is prevented by renal artery constriction that reduces renal arterial pressure if it is applied before volume is expanded but not after the natriuresis is established (70–72). Natriuresis occurs in the contralateral kidney with the unconstricted artery, irrespective of the timing of the volume expansion, pointing to some intrarenal event that occurs in response to increased perfusion pressure at the onset of volume expansion. This event is necessary to "set" the kidney in the natriuretic mode.

Recent micropuncture experiments suggest that disturbances in intrarenal control mechanisms may be important in the abnormal Na handling associated with the nephrotic syndrome (73).

Intrarenal Redistribution of Blood Flow

The nephron population is heterogeneous both in structure and blood supply. Redistribution of function among different nephron subpopulations might be a factor that affects Na_E (74–76). Evidence that supports this view is the effect of increase in blood flow to the deep (juxtamedullary) nephrons and to the medullary vasa recta circulation in response to volume expansion with saline. In one study, intrarenal distribution of blood flow was accompanied by a change in nephron filtration rate in the opposite direction. An increase in medullary blood flow that followed volume expansion with saline was accompanied by an increase in superficial nephron GFR and a decrease in juxtamedullary nephron GFR (75). However, other studies have not elicited the same results (77–80). The role of intrarenal redistribution of blood flow and disparate change in GFR in different regions of the kidney in the physiological regulation of renal Na handling is not established.

Renal Nerves

The kidneys are richly innervated with afferent and efferent fibers. The latter are postganglionic sympathetic neurones derived mainly from the splanchnic nerves (81). Section of the renal nerves leads to a natriuresis (82), while low level electrical stimulation is antinatriuretic (83–85). These effects are probably mediated by the release of norepinephrine (noradrenaline) from nerve endings terminating at the afferent and efferent arterioles at the basement membrane of both proximal and distal tubules. The relative importance of hemodynamic alterations and of direct action on tubular Na transport is unknown. Although renal nerve stimulation causes both renin (83) and prostaglandins (86) to be released from the kidney, pharmacological blockade of the action of these substances does not abolish the effect on Na excretion (87, 88). This suggests a direct action on renal function independent of these hormones.

The clinical observation that the transplanted and, therefore, denervated human kidney is capable of efficient Na homeostasis is evidence that the action of the renal nerves is not central to regulating Na_E. This is not to say that it plays no role in the intact subject, given the redundancies already described. Renal nerves may contribute to the altered Na handling observed in cardiac failure and hypertension (89, 90).

The Renin-Angiotensin-Aldosterone System

Aldosterone increases renal tubular Na_R at a site distal to the proximal tubule; its action is principally on the cortical and medullary collecting duct (91, 92). At the cellular level, aldosterone stimulates the activity of Na^+, K^+-ATPase in the basolateral cell membrane, but it also enhances "leakage" of Na from the tubular lumen across the apical membrane into the cell (93). Electrochemical neutrality is preserved by the countermovement of K and H^+ not, as in other tubule segments, by the associated transport of Cl or HCO_3. Aldosterone promotes the excretion of K and H^+ as well as conserving Na (94).

Two important factors in controlling the rate of release of aldosterone are angiotensin-II and the ECF/K concentration (91). Angiotensin-II production is controlled to a large extent by plasma renin concentration. The relationship between plasma renin concentration (or activity) and ECF volume (95) closes a feedback loop in which volume depletion, via renin and angiotensin, stimulates aldosterone release and distal tubular Na_R. Conversely, volume expansion suppresses the renin-angiotensin-aldosterone system (RAAS) and is natriuretic.

The importance attributed to aldosterone in Na homeostasis has been somewhat obscured by other factors. This is because, within certain limits, adrenalectomy has not abolished regulation of Na balance either with hormone deficiency or fixed replacement at various hormone levels. For example, subjects placed on supramaximal doses of mineralocorticoid undergo a transient period of renal Na retention, after which Na_E again increases to match dietary input and external balance is reestablished (96). This "mineralocorticoid escape" phenomenon is accompanied by weight gain in a comparable manner to that observed in the renal adjustment to an increased NaCl intake.

However, a number of observations indicate that intact functioning of the RAAS is important to volume and electrolyte homeostasis in clinical experience. In the absence of aldosterone, severe restriction of Na intake is not tolerated. The clinical features of Addison's disease and the salt-losing forms of adrenal hyperplasia are those of NaCl depletion. With mineralocorticoid excess, external Na balance is less well maintained; in adrenal insufficiency treated with a fixed mineralocorticoid replacement regimen there is an exaggerated expansion of ECF volume in response to an increase in NaCl intake (97, 98). The RAAS exerts a clinically important control to modulate changes in ECF volume in response to given stresses.

The ability to regulate K excretion independently of Na_E is also dependent on the RAAS. At least three factors combine to determine the rate of distal tubular K secretion: the rate of Na delivery to the distal tubule, the ECF/K concentration, and the plasma aldosterone concentration. Normally, volume expansion increases distal Na delivery and decreases aldosterone activity, while volume contraction produces the opposite effects. The net effects on K excretion are, therefore, mutually opposed. On the other hand, volume expansion that occurs in primary (inappropriate) mineralocorticoid excess leads to increased distal Na delivery in the presence of high levels of mineralocorticoid activity and thus to renal K wasting. The same logic applies to H^+ excretion. Under these conditions the effect of hyperaldosteronism on Na balance is limited while that on K and H^+ balance is persistent (chapter 7).

In summary, in aldosterone excess, volume expansion, hypertension, and hypokalemic alkalosis occur, and will be exaggerated by a high Na intake. In case of aldosterone deficiency, volume contraction, hypotension, and hyperkalemic acidosis occur and will be exaggerated by low intake. (The role of aldosterone in disorders of acid-base and K homeostasis is also discussed in chapters 7, 8, 14.)

Prostaglandins

The most important prostaglandins produced by the kidney are PGE_2 and PGI_2 (prostacyclin); their importance in regulation of Na_E is not clear. PGE_2 given acutely initiates natriuresis. The infusion of arachidonic acid (a precursor of the prostaglandins) into the renal artery has the same effect (99). Inhibiting prostaglandin synthesis causes Na retention (100–103). These effects may be mediated by alterations in RBF and GFR, both of which are increased by prostaglandins and decreased by inhibitors of prostaglandin synthetase. Renal excretion of PGE_2 increases with ECF volume contraction and with hemorrhage (104). Prostaglandins may be important in maintaining renal perfusion in volume depletion states (104). Angiotensin-II is a powerful stimulus to the renal synthesis of PGE_2 (105).

Renal clearance studies (101) suggest that prostaglandins act on tubular transport independent of changes in GFR, a view supported by studies on the isolated perfused tubule. Its action appears to be on Cl reabsorption in the medullary thick ascending limb, where a significant fraction of Na_R takes place (106) (chapter 16).

Catecholamines

Norepinephrine infused in pharmacological amounts reduces renal plasma flow, GFR, and Na_E (107); dopamine has opposite effects (108, 109). Low doses of epinephrine may reduce Na_E and not affect GFR (110). These findings suggest either a direct effect on tubular Na transport or an indirect effect mediated by altered peritubular hemodynamics. Norepinephrine infusion redistributes RBF (111) and may thereby affect physical factors that modulate Na_E. The kidney of normal man contains specific dopaminergic receptors (112), blockade of which abolishes the natriuretic response produced by lower body positive pressure (113); conversely, adrenergic blockade prevents the reduction of Na_E associated with Na deprivation (114). Urinary dopamine excretion increases in response to an increase in dietary Na intake in normal man (115), but not in patients with chronic renal disease (116). The latter observation may be a factor in the NaCl retention and hypertension commonly observed in this condition.

Dopamine and norepinephrine probably act as intrarenal messengers rather than as true hormones. L-dopa, a precursor of dopamine, when infused into the renal artery increases GFR and Na excretion (117). A controlling step in the conversion of L-dopa to dopamine is the intra renal decarboxylation of L-dopa; this process may be regulated by some proximal "messenger" of Na or volume status (118).

The Kallikrein-Kinin System

Kallikrein is a peptidase produced in the kidney, probably in the distal convoluted tubule (119). Kinins are vasodilators and natriuretic substances; they increase GFR (120) and diminish tubular Na_R (121). Proximal tubular Na reabsorption in superficial nephrons is not influenced by bradykinin. Its effect is either on more distal segments or proximal Na_R of deeper nephrons (122). Bradykinin is degraded by the enzyme kininase-II, which is the same as the antiotensin-converting enzyme (ACE). Increased activity of ACE increases angiotensin-mediated vasoconstriction and reduces kinin-dependent vasodilatation. Inhibition of the enzyme, e.g., with Captopril, has the opposite effects. Kinins may act by stimulating prostaglandin release (123), and PGE_2 appears to stimulate kallikrein activity (124). In general, activity of the kallikrein-kinin system increases in conditions associated with natriuresis, e.g., a high Na intake is associated with high levels of activity, a low intake with low levels (125).

Other Natriuretic Factors

As the previous discussion reveals, numerous pharmacologically active substances are capable of influencing renal Na handling in a variety of pathological situations. Evidence in favor of the existence of a natriuretic hormone, active under physiological conditions, has been accumulating steady over the last 2 decades.

de Wardener and his coworkers (126) demonstrated that volume expansion with saline is natriuretic in experiments where GFR falls. This occurs even though maximal doses of mineralocorticoids and vasopressin have been given. The effect persists when the kidney is denervated. It is transmitted to an isolated kidney perfused with the blood of a volume-expanded dog and to a second animal cross-circulated with the dog's blood. The natriuresis appears to be a result of some change in the blood of the expanded dog. The same effect is observed when dogs are expanded with blood with which they were already in equilibrium (127–129). Natriuresis is observed when arterial and venous pressures are held constant in the isolated perfused kidney (128) and the autotransplanted kidney (130). Similar results have been obtained in rats (131).

These later results (127–129), unlike the original (126), cannot be explained by changes in the physical composition of the blood perfusing the experimental kidney, such as dilutional reduction in plasma protein concentration. They can best be explained by an increase in a specific natriuretic factor in the blood as a result of the volume expansion (131). Natriuretic activity is detectable in the urine of healthy males undergoing head-out water immersion (132). The alternative explanation, that a decrease in the concentration of an antinatriuretic factor might be responsible, is unlikely in view of the fact that the kidney of the salt-depleted rat is more responsive to acute volume expansion by prior cross-circulation with rats that have been salt-loaded (133).

Bricker and coworkers (134–137) studied the natriuretic properties of urine and serum from uremic patients and animals. Urine from nephrotic uremic patients lacks natriuretic activity, while that from nonedematous uremic patients was highly natriuretic (136).

The presence of natriuretic activity in uremic urine is inferred from its inhibition of Na transport in frog skin and toad bladder (138, 139), in isolated renal tubular fragments (140), and in leukocytes (141). Na^+, K^+-ATPase activity is also inhibited in various experimental systems (142–144). An extract of uremic urine abolishes Na transport in the isolated rabbit collecting duct, probably the principal renal site of activity of the natriuretic hormone. The kidney in uremia shows enhanced end-organ responsiveness to its effects (145).

Whether more than one substance is responsible for the natriuretic activity demonstrated in salt-loaded and uremic subjects has not yet been established. The recent identification of a natriuretic peptide in rat cardiac atria and its subsequent amino acid sequencing and synthesis (145a, 145b) represent a potentially important advance in this field. This substance may be involved in the pathogenesis of edema of heart failure; deficiency of the factor in a strain of hamsters prone to degenerative cardiomyopathy is associated with an edema-forming tendency (145c).

The existence of other natriuretic factors also seems likely. Two natriuretic fractions of urine have been described, one of molecular weight $>30{,}000$ and the other near 400 (146, 147). Immunological crossreactivity with digoxin has been described (148), a property unlikely to be possessed by a peptide. Thus, although the existence of natriuretic factors other than atrial natriuretic peptide seems highly probable, their importance relative to the other factors discussed in the day-to-day regulation of Na_E remains unknown.

The site or sites of manufacture and release have not been identified, although the brain (149), the hypothalamus (150), and the liver (151) have been proposed. The last because saline infused into the portal vein is more natriuretic than an equivalent quantity administered via a systemic vein (22). The abolition of this effect by vagotomy suggests that the liver is sensing volume changes but that the effector limb is initiated elsewhere (152).

Many other hormones, including antidiuretic hormone, thyroxine, calcitonin, glucagon, prolactin, estrogen, and progesterone have all been shown to be capable of influencing Na_E in pharmacological doses, but are probably not directly involved in its physiological control (153).

BODY WATER AND OSMOLALITY

Control of Intake

Water intake is continuously required to meet renal and nonrenal losses. The latter is reduced to a minimum when intake is insufficient or marginal but can be increased to 20 or more times that amount when intake exceeds requirement.

Factors Regulating Intake

The major factor that stimulates thirst is a rise in the effective osmolality or tonicity of ECF that causes a transfer of water from cells. Solutes that do not affect cell volume do not stimulate thirst, hence the relevance of tonicity rather than total osmolality. A decrease in effective plasma volume also stimulates thirst probably by activating carotid sinus baroreceptors but also by a direct effect of angiotensin-II on the thirst center. The drive for water, represented by thirst, is powerful and the consequences of failing to respond include hyperosmolar and hypernatremic states that may cause serious CNS damage and death. Only young infants, comatose individuals or, rarely, patients with adipsia secondary to a specific brain lesion fail to develop a compulsive desire for water in response to these stimuli.

The stimulus, a rise in plasma osmolality, is usually secondary to a rise in plasma Na concentration. Hyperglycemia is also effective while a raised plasma urea concentration is not, because urea permeates cells freely. An acute change in urea concentration can affect cell volume transiently because the reflection coefficient for urea is not zero and some lag in equilibration occurs when the concentration changes suddenly. The effective stimulus is a decrease in cell volume secondary to an osmotically induced shift of water to ECF from ICF. The other independent signal arises from ECF volume depletion acting through neural stimuli perceived by baroreceptors in the low capacitance vessels and from a release of angiotensin-II, usually in response to ECF volume depletion.

Whereas intake of water among most land-based mammals is thirst-driven, and, therefore, tends to be the minimum needed to meet requirement, intake in humans is influenced by cultural and personal factors, so that a generous or even exaggerated intake may occur purely on the basis of such preferences. Behavioral disorders may become manifest as compulsive water drinking and give full expression to this generous capacity. CNS lesions and abnormalities in the controls of body water also may stimulate or depress thirst and water intake inappropriately.

The nonrenal losses of water are insensible water losses (IWL) and losses of transcellular fluids; the latter are insignificant in health. The minimal renal loss of water is that needed to excrete solute at maximal osmolal concentration (1200 mOsm/1); the maximum is that which excretes ordinary solute loads at 40 mOsm/kg. In the adult, a low average rate of solute excretion (720 mOsm/day) sets the limits for unit volume between 0.6 and 18.0 l/day. Unfortunately, the factors that lead to compulsive water drinking often reduce this tolerance and lesser quantities may induce hypoosmolar states.

Body Water

Body water, being freely diffusible, is in equilibrium in relation to distribution of nondiffusible solutes (see semipermeable membranes, p. 81). Cell solutes enveloped by cell membranes constitute the effective osmolar content of cells and determine cell water content. Sudden change in cell solute content has been documented only following electric shock therapy. Slower change in solute content of certain cells, e.g., brain (153a), red cells (153b), and kidney (153c), occurs when cells are maintained in hypoosmolal or hyperosmolal states. Acute changes in ECF osmolality affect cell volume immediately: hypoosmolality leads to cell swelling, hyperosmolality to shrinking. Prolonged hypoosmolality leads to loss of solute from brain (153a), red cells (153b), and renal tubular cells (153c); the converse occurs with hyperosmolality. The osmolality of body fluids (Posm) is predicted from serum Na, glucose, and urea levels. Posm over a wide range of disorders in body fluid is a function of the net change in total body Na + K and total body water and not of body Na per se (153d).

The ECF solute content is determined by ECF Na and Cl content and, on occasion, glucose and other poorly permeant substances given intravenously, e.g., contrast media. The regulation of body water through the stimulus for thirst and control of water excretion usually assures a body water content that sustains normal osmolality in total body water distributed in accordance with the effective solute content of cells and ECF.

Control of Excretion

The minimum and maximum rates of urinary water excretion are set within limits by the rate of urinary solute excretion. This, in turn, is set by dietary and metabolic factors, not by the need to conserve or excrete water. An organism consuming a varied diet that leads to variations in solute excretion and subject to uncontrollable changes in nonrenal water losses, must regulate water intake over a wide range. The capacity for this is affected by the abilities to sense the need for replacing and conserving water (the effector limit). The latter is controlled by a feedback system analogous to that controlling Na_E. It has an afferent or sensing limb and an efferent limb—the renal concentrating and diluting mechanism. Renal mechanisms regulate water excretion in response not simply to requirement, but also to intake in excess of requirement. The latter is independent of the rate of solute excretion and is manifest by the ability to excrete concentrated or dilute urine.

The Effector Limb

The ability to excrete both concentrated and dilute urine depends on the following three properties of the kidney: (1) the capacity to reabsorb solute without water in one segment of the nephron, (2) the presence of a mechanism to amplify the resulting medullary hypertonicity in the medulla, and (3) variable water permeability in the distal nephron.

The second of these depends not only on the permeability and transport functions of different tubular segments but also on the anatomical arrangement of the various structures that make up the renal medulla and their relationships to one another. They comprise the renal countercurrent multiplier system, which is essential to the concentrating process and which elegantly employs the same energy source to power both dilution and concentration.

Countercurrent Multiplication. The principles of countercurrent exchange and multiplication have been known to engineers for many years, and natural examples are widespread in biological systems (154). A simple countercurrent exchanger is shown in Figure 6.4, *A*. Solvent flows from right to left in the upper channel, while a solution of solute x flows from left to right in the lower one. The two are separated by a membrane permeable to x but not to the solvent. At all points along the axis of flow a gradient exists for diffusion of x from the lower to the upper channel. If the two channels shown are replaced by two sets of pipes interdigitating with each other, so that each element is surrounded by pipes running in the opposite direction to itself, extremely efficient exchange can be achieved. A countercurrent multiplier, illustrated in Figure 6.4, *B*, differs from an exchanger in the following two respects: (1) instead of two pipes, or systems of pipes, counterflow occurs by the entire system of tubes bending back on itself; and (2) solute transfer takes place by active transport rather than by diffusion. Thus, in the illustration, x is pumped from the lower to the upper channel, leading to the establishment of an axial concentration gradient as a result of "trapping" of solute in the loop. The degree of concentration of solute achieved in this way depends on several factors, including the flow rate through the loop, the length of the loop, and the power of the pump.

The Medulla as a Countercurrent Multiplier. The arrangement of the loops of Henle in the medulla is consistent with their functioning as a countercurrent multiplier (155, 156). Two characteristics of the system (not shown in Figure 6.4, *B*) are that, irrespective of the state of diuresis or antidiuresis, the fluid entering the loop is isotonic while that leaving the ascending limb is always hypotonic, suggesting that the "single effect" driving the system is active solute reabsorption in the ascending limb of the loop. The different effects of osmotic diuresis produced by NaCl, urea, mannitol, and glucose on early distal tubular fluid:plasma osmolar ratio indicate that NaCl is the actively reabsorbed solute and also that urea is handled differently from other nonactively transported solutes (157). Another characteristic is that the fluids from all the tubular elements at the same level in the medulla (ascending and descending limbs of Henle's loop, ascending and descending vasa recta, and collecting duct) are near identical osmolality. In one study (158), the fluid in the collecting duct appeared to be slightly more dilute than that in the loop at the same level, supporting the view that the final concentration of urine is achieved by the osmotic extraction of water from the collecting duct fluid. Another important characteristic is that more water is removed from the fluid in the ascending limb than is added to the fluid in the descending limb, indicating that net water reabsorption occurs in the loop. The removal of water from the medulla by the vasa recta uses the principle of countercurrent exchange (159, 160).

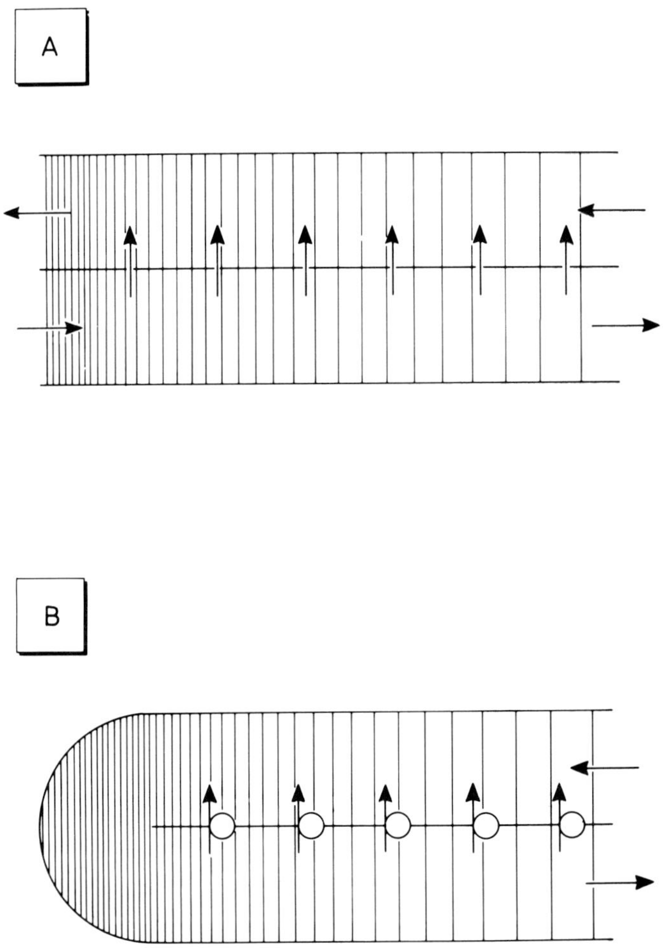

Figure 6.4.
A. Countercurrent exchange. Countercurrent flow takes place in the two channels illustrated, the density of the shading representing the concentration of a permeant solute, *x*. The fluid in the lower channel enters the system concentrated with respect to *x*, while that in the upper channel enters as pure solvent. At all points along the axis of flow, a concentration gradient favors diffusion of *x* from the lower to the upper channel (*vertical arrows*). With multiple, interdigitating channels running in each direction, highly efficient transfer of solute from one fluid to the other may be achieved.
B. Countercurrent multiplication. A countercurrent multiplier differs from an exchanger in two respects: (*a*) the two channels shown in *A* become a single tube reversed on itself, and (*b*) solute moves by active transport from the lower to the upper element. Solute is thus trapped in the loop with the establishment of a standing osmotic gradient.

The "Single Effect". Reabsorption of NaCl from the ascending limb of the loop of Henle is the "single effect" that powers the countercurrent system; Cl is the principal actively reabsorbed species (161, 162). The resulting interstitial hypertonicity concentrates the fluid in the descending limb of the loop either by osmotic removal of water or by the addition of NaCl by diffusion. In either case, the solute concentration at the bend of the loop is raised and Cl transport from the ascending limb is facilitated on the next pass. Whether concentration in the descending limb occurs by water removal or solute addition depends on the relative permeability of this tubule segment to water and solute. Both may occur; the net reabsorption of water known to occur in the loop (159, 160) indicates that water removal accounts for at least some of the effect. Water removed from the descending limb, as well as solute reabsorbed from the ascending limb, are removed from the medulla via the ascending vasa recta.

For the medullary concentrating system to operate strictly as a countercurrent multiplier, solute, i.e., NaCl, must be absorbed actively along the length of the exit limb. Active reabsorption along only the outer medullary portion of the exit loop, the thick ascending limb, will not suffice (163). However, the presence of active NaCl transport along the thin segment of the ascending or exit limb of Henle's loop in the inner medulla remains controversial. The ultrastructural features of the epithelium do not have components for electrogenic transport. Both in vitro studies in rats and in vivo perfusion studies of rabbit tubules have not demonstrated active NaCl transport (164–167), whereas micropuncture studies in golden hamsters appear to show Na and Cl movement out of the thin ascending limb (168–172), and electrophysiological findings in some cases strongly favor active transport (171, 172). The permeability characteristics of the thin ascending limb, particularly the low reflection coefficient for Cl (164–166), are not those to be expected of a Cl transporting epithelium. Some of the inconsistencies among these results may reflect species differences.

The Role of Urea. In the absence of convincing evidence of active NaCl reabsorption from the thin ascending limb, the question arises whether some additional factor might allow the generation of a medullary osmotic gradient increasing to the papillary tip, by multiplication of a single effect confined to the outer medulla. Theoretical considerations and experimental observations point to a possible role for urea. The contribution of renal handling of urea to the renal handling of water differs from that of other urinary solutes (157). For example, the addition of urea to the diet of rats on a low protein intake increased urinary concentration more than an osmotically equivalent amount of inorganic salts (173).

The increase in urinary osmolality induced by feeding urea was greater than could be accounted for by the rise in urinary urea concentration, i.e., the concentration of nonurea solute was also increased (174–177). Edelmann and coworkers (178) observed this effect in newborn human infants. These findings, together with the earlier observation that fractional urea excretion varies directly with urine flow (179, 180), suggest that passive back-diffusion of urea from the collecting duct recycles and concentrates urea within the countercurrent multiplier system. Supporting this view is the finding that as much as 35% to 40% of filtered urea is reabsorbed in the medullary collecting duct of the hamster under hydropenic conditions (181, 182).

Models of the Medullary Concentrating Mechanism. Understanding of the medullary concentrating mechanism has been enhanced by the use of computer simulations based on a variety of mathematical models of the countercurrent system. Two of these, the "central core" models developed by Stephenson (183) and by Kokko and Rector (184), purport to account for inner medullary solute concentration without inner medullary active solute transport, as a consequence of urea recycling and distinctive permeability characteristic of medullary segments to water, urea, Na, and Cl.

The central core is seen as a compartment that is closed at the papillary end and open at the corticomedullary junction and consists of the medullary interstitium and the ascending and descending vasa recta. The walls of these are postulated to be so permeable to water and solute that horizontal equilibration at any level within the medulla bay is instantaneous. Water and solute move between the core and the adjacent tubular structures, e.g., the ascending and descending limbs of the loop and the medullary collecting duct. Water and solute that accumulates in the core as a result of net reabsorption is returned to the systemic circulation by expansion through the "open" end of the core, i.e., via the ascending vasa recta.

Under antidiuretic conditions (184) water is osmotically removed from the fluid traversing the outer medullary collecting duct, leading to concentration of urea within the lumen and the establishment of a concentration gradient favoring diffusion of urea into the inner medullary interstitium. Osmotic removal of water from the relatively hypotonic fluid in the descending limb raises the concentration of Na and Cl progressively as the bend of the loop is approached, so that their concentration at the beginning of the ascending limb exceeds that in the surrounding interstitium. Na and Cl, therefore, diffuse out of the thin ascending limb down the resulting concentration gradient, to produce dilution of the luminal fluid as it ascends through the inner medulla. As a result, some of the urea in the interstitium diffuses into the ascending limb and is thereby recycled via the collecting duct back to the medulla. By these means, the "single effect" (active reabsorption of NaCl in the thick ascending limb) leads to "passive" NaCl reabsorption in the thin segment of the ascending limb and the development of a progressively more concentrated medullary interstitium toward the papillary tip.

This model works only if the fluid in the thin ascending limb is more dilute than that of the core structures at the same level; this in turn requires that the rate of entry of urea be less than the rate of outward diffusion of salt, i.e., it depends on distinctive permeabilities and reflection coefficients of the ascending and descending limbs of the loop to water, urea, and NaCl. In particular, the ascending limb of the loop must have high water permeability and low solute permeability, while the thin descending limb must be impermeable to water, moderately permeable to urea, and permeable to NaCl. Experimental data from the thin ascending limb support these predictions (164, 165, 167, 185, 186), but from the descending limb suggest it is permeable to solute, so that the rise in osmolality in this segment as it approaches the papillary tip must be a result of addition of solute, predominantly urea (159, 165, 170, 187–190) rather than to water removal, at least at physiological perfusion pressure (191). If this is so, the Kokko-Rector model cannot account for osmotic concentration in the inner medulla in the absence of active reabsorption of NaCl from the thin ascending limb.

These considerations led Bonventre and Lechene (192) to develop an alternative "passive" model, in which the fluid in the descending limb at the point of entry into the inner medulla is hypertonic to the surrounding interstitium, having been concentrated either by the addition of solute or by removal of water in the outer medulla. This leads to solute recycling in quite a different manner from that predicted by other models. Urea enters the interstitium from both the collecting duct and thin ascending limb, achieving a very high concentration at the bend of the loop, while NaCl is reabsorbed from all inner medullary tubule segments. This formulation satisfies the requirements for mass balance in the inner medulla, provides an explanation for papillary solute concentration in the absence of active salt transport in the thin ascending limb, and predicts segmental tubular permeability characteristics in good agreement with the results of experimental determinations. The inner medullary concentration profiles predicted by the Kokko-Rector and Bonventre-Lechene models are shown in Figure 6.5. A recent symposium reviews current concepts of the urinary concentrating mechanisms (192a).

The ureter may play a role in the process of concentrating urine in rodents, which have a single papilla projecting into the upper ureter (192b, 192c), but this process is unlikely to be significant in the human kidney with multiple papillae.

Excretion and Reabsorption of Free Water. The urinary solute excretion rate is determined by dietary and metabolic factors. The range of solute excretion of an adult is 500 to 1600 mOsm/day. Taking a representative value of 720 mOsm/day (0.5 mOsm/min)($U_{osm}V$) and assuming a plasma osmolality of 280 mOsm/kg or virtually 0.28 mOsm/ml (Posm) and urinary osmolality that is the same, volume of urine (V) at isosmolar concentration is 1.78 ml/min. The osmolar clearance

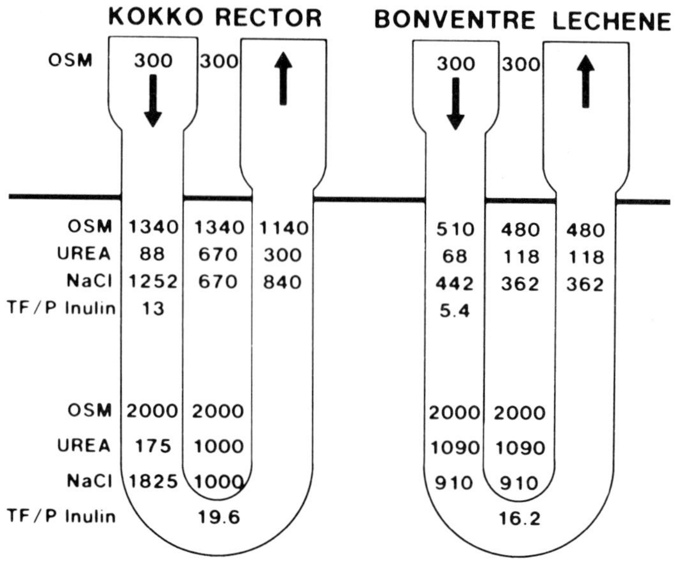

Figure 6.5. Concentration profiles in the ascending and descending limbs of the loop of Henle and the medullary interstitium, as predicted by the models of Kokko and Rector (184) and Bonventre and Lechene (192), respectively. All concentrations are expressed in milliosmoles per kilogram of H_2O. *TF/P inulin* = tubular fluid:plasma inulin concentration ratio at the point indicated. (Reproduced with permission from Stephenson JL, et al: Fed Proc 42:2377, 1983.)

(Cosm) is equal to the rate of urine flow (Equation 1b) because Uosm/Posm = 1.0.

$$\text{Cosm} = \text{V} \times \text{Uosm/Posm} \quad (1)$$

When water excretion is greater, urine will be hypotonic to plasma and $V > C_{osm}$. The difference between the two is free water clearance (C_{H_2O}):

$$\text{(a) } C_{H_2O} = V - C_{Osm} \qquad \text{(b) } C_{H_2O} = V(1 - U_{osm}/P_{osm}) \quad (2)$$

When water diuresis is maximal (U_{osm} = 40 mOsm/kg or 0.04 mOsm/ml, C_{H_2O} measures the capacity of the kidney to excrete free water. When $U_{osm}V$ is 0.5 mOsm/min, V = 12.46 ml/min (Equation 1a), the maximal rate of C_{H_2O} is 10.68 ml/min (Equation 2b). When the rate of water excretion is less than that used for the excretion of isotonic urine, urine will be hypertonic to plasma and $C_{osm} > V$ and C_{H_2O} is negative. Expressed as a positive value (Cosm − V), this becomes free water reabsorption (Tc_{H_2O}) and represents the free water reabsorbed (Equation 3):

$$Tc_{H_2O} = V(U_{osm}/P_{osm} - 1) \quad (3)$$

Maximal Tc_{H_2O} is the renal capacity to reabsorb free water. Like C_{H_2O} it is limited by solute excretion rate. Taking the same solute excretion rate, 0.5 mOsm/min, and maximal urinary osmolality of 1,200 mOsm/kg or 1.2 mOsm/ml (Uosm), V is 0.42 ml/min (Equation 1a) and Tc_{H_2O} is 1.36 ml/min (Equation 3). At normal solute excretion rates, the capacity to excrete free water greatly exceeds the capacity to reabsorb it, i.e., the protection against overhydration and dilution is greater than the protection against dehydration and concentration.

The Efferent Limb

The efferent limb regulating free water excretion or reabsorption is pituitary antidiuretic hormone (ADH). Fluid entering the distal convoluted tubule is hypotonic to plasma during both diuresis and antidiuresis (157). The osmolality of the final urine is determined by ADH acting on the distal nephron segments. It regulates the permeability of the distal tubule and collecting duct to water. In water diuresis and the absence of ADH, resistance to water reabsorption is high and tubular fluid is progressively diluted by reabsorption of NaCl until the limiting value of 40 mOsm/kg is approached. In antidiuresis, ADH causes the tubule to become more permeable, water is reabsorbed into the hypertonic medullary interstitium, and tubular fluid is concentrated. ADH in humans is arginine vasopressin, a nonapeptide having the following structure (193):

Cys-Tyr-Phe-Glm-Asn-Cys-Pro-Arg-Gly(NH_2)

The control of urine volume by the pituitary was first demonstrated when antidiuresis was induced in patients with diabetes insipidus and in normal volunteers by injecting extracts of the posterior pituitary (194, 195). This effect was demonstrated in the isolated kidney by 1924 (196). The release of ADH from the pituitary by the intravenous injection of hyperosmotic solutions was demonstrated in 1945 (197). These observations were confirmed by Verney (198) who, in 1947, noted that a hypertonic solution infused into the carotid artery was a more potent stimulus to ADH release than an equivalent quantity infused into a peripheral vein (199). He postulated the existence of an osmoreceptor within the distribution of the internal carotid artery, probably the anterior hypothalamus (200). Subsequent studies located the sensitive areas to the supraoptic and paraventricular nuclei (201); ablation of that area produces deficiency of both ADH and oxytocin. ADH is synthesized in cells in the hypothalamic nuclei and is released from the axonal endings of these cells in the posterior pituitary.

The Afferent Limb—Control of ADH Release

ADH release is governed predominantly by osmoreceptors and baroreceptors that constitute the afferent limb of the system.

Intracranial Osmoreceptors. Verney's contention (199) was that the signal to ADH release was osmolar because antidiuresis could be induced by the intracarotid injection of hypertonic solutions of sucrose, glucose, and Na sulphate as well as NaCl. He concluded that the osmoreceptor was located in specialized cells in the anterior hypothalamus. These sensed changes in the osmolality or tonicity because they caused changes in cell volume resulting from osmotically induced water movement. While this interpretation has been challenged from studies in which ADH release varied in response to cerebral ventricular perfusion (202–209), these results have been questioned because cerebral ventricular perfusion studies cause widespread, nonspecific disturbances of brain function and are likely to have little relevance to physiological events (210).

The hypothalamic osmoreceptor hypothesis has been supported by in vitro studies of "hypothalamo-neurohypophysial" explants. Raising the osmolality of the culture medium with NaCl or mannitol caused the rate of vasopressin release from the explant to increase, while doing so with glucose or urea did not. The difference can be explained most readily by the rapid penetrance of the two latter substances into the cells of the preparation, so that tonicity is not affected (211, 212).

Extrarenal Osmoreceptors. The thinking of Verney (210) has been so dominant that it may have inhibited the formulation of alternative hypotheses (210). A few attempts have been made to identify extracranial osmoreceptors. The infusion of limited volumes of hypotonic saline solutions into the portal vein of rats (213) and dogs (214) is followed by a rise in the rate of water excretion, which is not duplicated when similar quantities are infused into peripheral veins; conversely, intraportal infusion of limited quantities of hypertonic saline causes water excretion to increase, while equivalent infusion into peripheral veins does not (215).

The tonicity of the ECF is accepted as the principal physiological determinant of the rate of secretion of ADH under most circumstances. Because regional differences in tonicity of ECF must occur rarely outside the experimental laboratory, the location of the osmoreceptors has little clinical significance.

Threshold and Sensitivity of the Osmoreceptor. If it is accepted that the physiological role of the osmoreceptor mechanism is the regulation of the tonicity of the body fluids, by regulating the excretion or reabsorption of free water by ADH, it performs this function with remarkable efficiency. The development of a sensitive and reliable radioimmunoassay for ADH (216) enabled the relation of Posm to ADH to be stated in quantitative terms. In the absence of interfering nonosmotic influences, the plasma concentration of ADH is a linear function of Posm above a "threshold" value of 285 mOsm/kg in normal individuals and patients with primary polydipsia and nephrogenic diabetes insipidus; patients with pituitary diabetes insipidus respond subnormally or not at all (Figure 6.6) (216).

Furthermore, a close relationship is observed between plasma arginine vasopressin (AVP) and urinary osmolality within the limits of renal concentrating and diluting capacity in subjects with normal renal func-

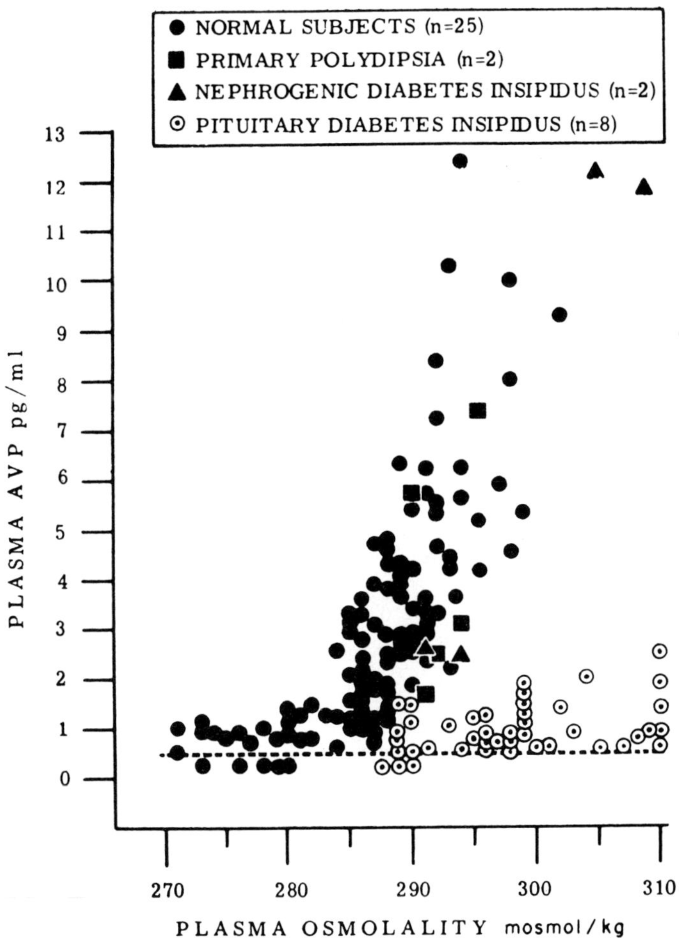

Figure 6.6. The relationship between plasma osmolality and plasma immunoreactive AVP in normal subjects and in patients with primary polydipsia, nephrogenic diabetes insipidus, and pituitary diabetes insipidus. The first three groups (*solid black symbols*) show essentially the same relationship between the two variables, indicating normal responsiveness of the neurohypophyseal secretory system to changes in ECG tonicity. (Reproduced with permission from Robertson GL, et al: J Clin Invest 52:2340, 1974.)

tion, with the exception of patients with nephrogenic diabetes insipidus (Figure 6.7) (217).

In normal individuals AVP is secreted when Posm exceeds 285 mOsm/kg. Maximally concentrated urine is produced at AVP concentrations of 5 pg/ml, which normally develops when Posm exceeds 293 mOsm/kg. Thus small changes in osmolality produce large changes in free water excretion, giving great power to the feedback loop responsible for osmoregulation. The continued rise of plasma AVP levels as plasma osmolalities exceed 294 mOsm/kg, despite the absence of any further effect in increasing free water conservation at such levels, may be related to the pressor rather than the antidiuretic effect of the hormone, since the most common situation in which such hypertonicity is encountered is severe dehydration. The relationship between plasma osmolality and plasma AVP is more accurately defined by an exponential rather than a linear function (218), in which case there cannot be a precise threshold for establishing maximal AVP stimulation. However, the threshold-linear concept is adequate for clinical purposes (218, 219).

The osmolar threshold for release in rats is altered by nonosmolar stimuli capable of influencing AVP release independently of osmotic pressure. For example, hypovolemia without hyperosmolality (220) and pharmacologically induced hypotension (221) both shift the threshold to the left, i.e., lower the minimum value of plasma osmolality at which AVP is released, but do not alter the slope or the sensitivity of the osmoreceptor. These observations emphasize the interaction of osmolar and nonosmolar factors to regulate AVP secretion. It is useful to separate them for investigative purposes, but such separation is essentially artificial and leads to a simplistic view of the control of water excretion in the intact subject.

Nonosmolar Control of ADH Release. The most clearly defined of these nonosmolar stimuli affecting AVP release is plasma volume contraction. The relation between the percentage reduction in blood volume and plasma AVP appears to be exponential; there is a detectable rise when volume is reduced by 8%, which increases steeply as volume is reduced by 20% to levels far above the maximal antidiuretic concentration of 5 pg/ml (220) (Figure 6.8). While volume contraction is well recognized as a potent stimulus to AVP release, the nature of the afferent signal(s) involved continues to be debated, as does the question of whether other nonosmolar stimulants and antagonists to ADH secretion share a common pathway with volume-mediated stimuli or act via other pathways.

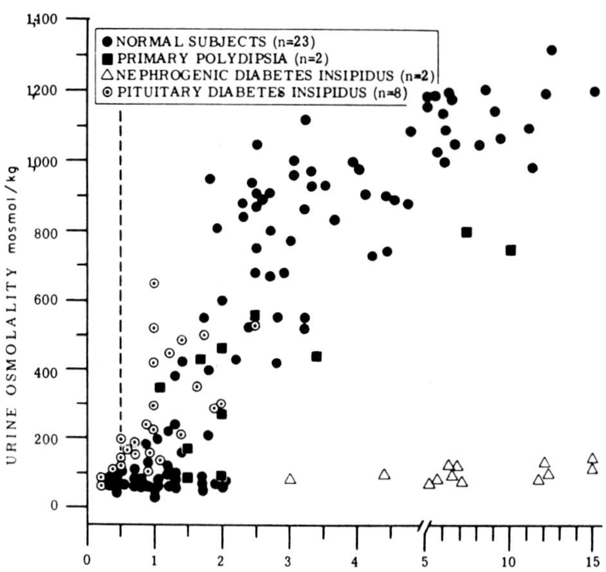

Figure 6.7. The relationship between plasma AVP concentration and urinary osmolality in normal subjects and in patients with primary polydipsia, nephrogenic diabetes insipidus, and pituitary diabetes insipidus. Patients with primary polydipsia show slightly reduced concentrating ability due to washout of medullary solute, whereas those with nephrogenic diabetes insipidus show no response at all. For other subjects, maximum urinary concentration is seen at a plasma AVP concentration of about 5 pg/ml. (Reproduced with permission from Robertson GL, et al: J Clin Invest 52:2340, 1974.)

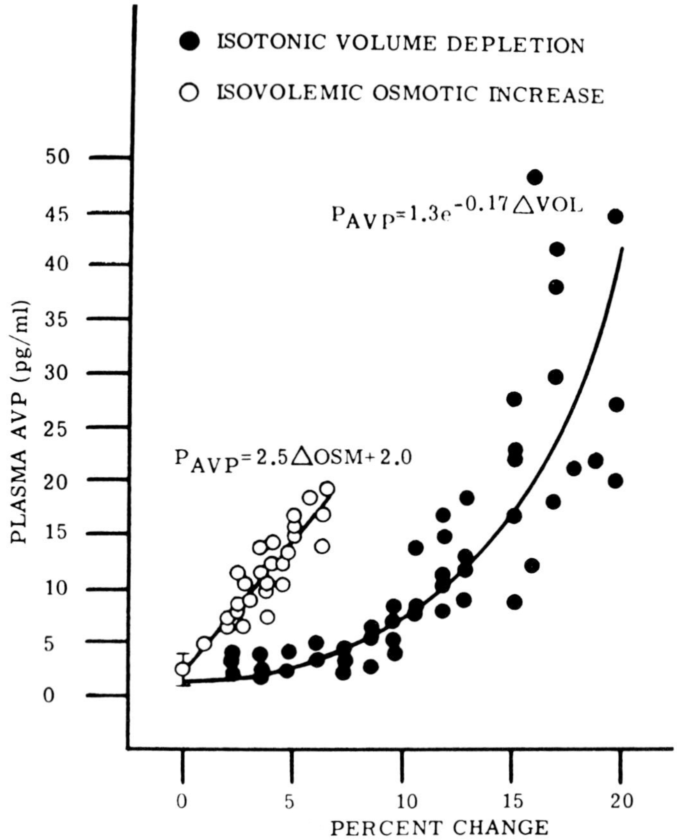

Figure 6.8. The relationship between changes in plasma osmolality (*open circles*) and volume depletion (*solid circles*) and plasma AVP concentration in conscious rats. The former relationship is linear over the range of values studied, while the latter approximates to an exponential function. (Reproduced with permission from Dunn FL, et al: J Clin Invest 52:3212, 1973.)

Norepinephrine and alpha-adrenergic drugs induce water diuresis (222–225). The effect is dependent on the presence of endogenous ADH, since no effect is elicited in ADH-deficiency (226–228). The diuretic effect of norepinephrine is abolished by alpha-adrenergic blockade (224) and by baroreceptor denervation (carotid sinus denervation and bilateral vagotomy) (229).

Conversely, beta-adrenergic stimulation is antidiuretic and is dependent on the presence of endogenous ADH (227, 228, 230) and intact baroreceptor innervation (231). It is likely, therefore, that the effects of volume contraction, alpha- and beta-adrenergic stimulation and blockade, and vasodilation on ADH secretion and water excretion are all mediated by baroreceptors. Although both high pressure (carotid sinus) and low pressure (left atrial) receptors appear to be involved, the former probably are more important (232). Direct effects of catecholamines on hypothalamic release of ADH and on the water permeability of distal tubule have not been excluded, but seem relatively unimportant in comparison with the baroreceptor-mediated response.

There remains the question of whether nonosmolar factors influence ADH release directly or indirectly by way of baroreceptor stimulation. Hypoxia (232), emesis (233), pain (232–234), and drugs such as nicotine (235), which stimulate ADH release also directly affect autonomic function and might directly stimulate baroreceptor responses. Responses to hypoxia (232) and nicotine (234, 235) are abolished by baroreceptor denervation. Because these stimuli increase arterial blood pressure their effect on ADH may be mediated by alterations in baroreceptor tone or sensitivity, as opposed to alterations in the magnitude of the pressure stimulus.

6B Clinical Disorders of Sodium, Chloride, and Water

GEORGE HAYCOCK

DEHYDRATION

Dehydration is the most common worldwide disorder of water and electrolyte homeostasis. It affects many millions of infants and children and causes much mortality and morbidity. The major cause of dehydration is gastroenteritis. This discussion concentrates on dehydration caused by diarrhea. However, the pathophysiology and management of diarrheal dehydration apply to dehydration as a result of other causes. Specific differences are mentioned where relevant.

Pathophysiology

Isotonic and Hypotonic Dehydration

The composition of the ECF as dehydration develops is determined by a number of factors: (1) the nature of the intake and gastrointestinal losses and the effect of, (2) volume contraction per se, (3) K depletion, (4) metabolic acidosis, and (5) redistribution of Na and K between ECF and ICF.

Intake and Gastrointestinal Losses. Diarrheal fluid contains the same electrolytes that are in ECF, but in different concentrations. The sum of the concentrations of electrolytes is less than their sum in ECF (236) so that losses might be anticipated to lead to hypertonicity or hypernatremia. In fact, dehydration usually is isotonic or hypotonic. While appetite is usually reduced, thirst is not, so that fluid intake continues. The fluids taken usually have Na + K concentrations less than those of the diarrheal fluid itself. Thus, the net loss of Na + K is usually proportional to or less than the net loss of water, resulting in isotonic or hypotonic dehydration. Even in infancy, when hypertonicity is most likely to occur, it is unusual for the Na + K composition of replacement fluid to be much higher than 50 mEq/l. However, carbohydrate in milk, either as disaccharide, monosaccharide, or smaller fragments that are not absorbed, leads to osmotic diarrhea and hypotonic gastrointestinal losses that may cause hypertonicity. In most cases, evaluation of the kind and quantity of intake and of gastrointestinal losses correctly predicts the type of dehydration.

Volume Contraction. Net fluid losses from the gastrointestinal tract initially deplete ECF. This sets in motion the responses to ECF volume contraction, a reduction in GFR and enhancement of proximal and distal tubular Na reabsorption. These are mediated both by alterations in the intrarenal controls and by release of volume-sensitive hormones, notably aldosterone and ADH. The high levels of aldosterone affect the subsequent development of dehydration particularly by contributing to K depletion. High levels of ADH cause maximal free water reabsorption. These responses result in the production of urine of low volume, high osmolality, and very low concentration of Na, irrespective of the plasma Na concentration. These responses override those that regulate the tonicity of body fluids, which then is determined by nonrenal events.

Potassium Depletion. Balance studies performed during the recovery phase of diarrheal dehydration (237, 238) have shown that the retention of K equals or exceeds that of Na. Although gastrointestinal fluid has 15 to 30 mEq/l of K, intestinal losses alone are insufficient to account for the estimated deficits (239, 240), so that other mechanisms must be involved. In the absence of vomiting, the urine is the only plausible vehicle for nonintestinal K loss, probably by the following sequence of events (241). Initial intestinal K loss causes a reduction in ECF K concentration and K moves down the resulting concentration gradient from ICF to ECF. However, the high circulating aldosterone concentration secondary to volume contraction causes most of this K to be excreted in the urine, maintaining the concentration gradient and perpetuating the loss of intracellular K. In support of this hypothesis is the observation that the severity of K depletion is proportional to the volume of stool lost rather than to the K content of the stool, which implicates volume contraction as the key factor. It follows that K repletion cannot be achieved until ECF volume has been restored (242).

Metabolic Acidosis. In the absence of other interfering factors, volume contraction alone causes metabolic alkalosis by mechanisms discussed in chapter 8. Diarrheal dehydration, especially when severe, is usually accompanied by metabolic acidosis. This acidosis is variable in severity and multifactorial in origin. Gastrointestinal fluid may have a high concentration of bicarbonate or organic anions, i.e., net acid intake is high. Starvation and volume contraction may increase production of keto acids or lactic acid. Volume contraction also interferes with correction of the acidosis, since the reduction in GFR limits the capacity of the kidney to excrete net acid (242). Carbohydrate malabsorption leads to production of organic acids by bacterial fermentation, increasing net acid intake and preventing reabsorption of HCO_3 (243). Hypernatremia also increases the degree of acidosis (259).

Redistribution Between ICF and ECF. Although Na and K losses often are equal (237, 238) and do not reflect ECF volume losses, change in body Cl (237–239), bromine (Br) (243a), or saccharide (244) spaces define the loss of ECF volume in isotonic dehydration. K loss from the cells is balanced by gain in Na, an effect facilitated by hyperaldosteronism (245). The K loss from cells is not accompanied by proportional loss of water but by a gain in Na; the brunt of volume contraction falls on ECF (243a). Replacement of K and correction of acidosis are necessary to reverse these ionic shifts. In hypotonic dehydration, where net Na + K loss exceeds net water loss, water enters cells and ICF volume expands; ECF volume contraction is greater than that accounted for by external losses (245a).

Hypertonic Dehydration

In 1947, Rapoport (246) first described dehydrated children in whom plasma Na concentration was elevated. Subsequently the condition of hypernatremic or hypertonic dehydration in infancy was widely recognized (247–251). Its pathophysiology is complex and still the subject of debate. Although the tonicity of body water is the net result of the external balance of Na + K and water (153d), in diarrheal dehydration, the cause of hypertonicity is a disproportionate loss of water to Na + K.

It has been suggested that the principal cause of hypernatremia in diarrheal dehydration is the administration of fluid with too high a concentration of Na (248, 252–254). This hypothesis alone fails to explain why only a minority of infants and children fed such fluids develop hypernatremia and why hypernatremic dehydration is rapidly and safely corrected with solutions containing as much as 90 mEq/l Na (255–257), which is a value considerably higher than that found in most of the formulas suspected of causing the condition. Further, the infant kidney can maintain water balance in the absence of severe dehydration on an intake of cow's milk made up to twice normal strength even in the presence of mild diarrhea (258).

A better explanation is found in the effect of relatively high carbohydrate content of many oral preparations. Glucose at a concentration of 5% is poorly absorbed by children with gastroenteritis. The nonabsorbed fraction retards intestinal absorption of water by its osmotic effect. Degradation by intestinal bacteria increases the osmotic effect further by producing organic acids of lower molecular weight (259). The result of malabsorption is fermentative diarrhea with copious losses of fluid having a low Na content (260, 261). These effects have been observed during feeding of infants with fluids high in glucose (262), glucose polymers, and lactose, e.g., boiled skimmed milk (252) and concentrated milk (251) or formulas (263), as well as with 5% glucose.

Once hypertonic dehydration is established, it tends to be self-perpetuating. Volume contraction leads to renal Na conservation. K depletion, usually present in this as in other forms of dehydration, further impairs Na excretion (264), in part by promoting renin release (265). Insulin resistance (266, 267) occurs in association with hypertonicity and may lead to hyperglycemia and additional renal water loss resulting from osmotic diuresis.

With hypertonicity, there is net movement of water out of cells and ICF volume decreases, which affects intracellular metabolism, particularly that of the nervous system (268). An additional phenomenon in the CNS, which complicates intracellular dehydration with a tendency to worsen hypertonicity, is the production of "idiogenic osmols" (269, 270). Development of significant idiogenic osmols is not consistent with the relations established between total body Na + K and total body water in patients having a wide range of disorders in body osmolality (153d), but there is evidence for idiogenic osmols contributing to the ICF of brain (270a). This has the benefit in this case of stabilizing brain volume (153a).

Clinical Features

Isotonic and Hypotonic Dehydration

The signs of isotonic and hypotonic dehydration are those of ECF volume contraction. For any given degree of dehydration in terms of total body water, these signs will be more prominent in hypotonic dehydration because of the shift in water from ECF to ICF. Volume contraction resulting from dehydration affects both intravascular and ISF compartments of ECF. In mild dehydration, the vascular compartment is protected to some extent because any reduction in plasma volume tends to draw fluid into the circulation, which is a result of alteration of Starling forces, although this is offset by the nature of the gel structure of ISF (p. 83). In clinical terms, the signs of mild to moderate dehydration are those of depletion of the ISF, whereas circulatory disturbances become apparent as severity increases.

Reduction of ISF volume produces loss of skin turgor, recognizable as a loss of elasticity when a fold of skin is pinched between finger and thumb in infants, and depression of the fontanelle. Loss of fluid from intraorbital connective tissue causes a hollow-eyed appearance; the effect is similar in some respects to that observed in severe malnutrition when the changes are a result of loss of orbital fat. The child is usually listless, miserable, and thirsty.

Reduction of circulating volume sufficient to produce definite clinical signs occurs only in moderately severe to severe dehydration. Tachycardia, out of proportion to any accompanying fever, is present. Vasoconstriction of arterioles to less vital structures occurs and offers protection to the circulation to vital organs. This peripheral vasoconstriction is reflected by a fall in skin temperature, particularly in the extremities. Capillary return is delayed, i.e., if an area of skin is blanched by pressure, color is slow to return. Measurement of the "gap" between central (rectal) and peripheral (toe) temperature is a simple, sensitive, and valuable method for assessing circulatory inadequacy (271, 272). Abdominal pain is common and probably indicates underperfusion of the splanchnic circulation.

As a late event, cerebral perfusion may be impaired. These signs presage imminent circulatory collapse and require treatment as an extreme emergency.

Oliguria of the "prerenal" type is present in all children if renal function is intact. The urine is of small volume, with high osmolar, urea, and creatinine concentrations and low Na concentrations; percent fractional Na excretion (Na clearance/GFR) is low, typically $<0.5\%$. Exocrine secretions are reduced in volume, leading to dry mouth and eyes.

It is customary and convenient to express the severity of dehydration in terms of percentage loss of body weight. In well nourished children, loss of <5% body weight is attended by little or no objective evidence of dehydration. This is commonly known as "mild" dehydration; between 5% and 10% weight loss is "moderate" dehydration with signs of interstitial volume loss predominating; at 10% or more weight loss dehydration is severe and signs of circulatory failure are common. These percentages apply to children with isotonic volume depletion. The losses of fluid attributable to ECF volume contraction in acute diarrhea are 60% of the total weight loss, i.e., 10% weight loss, the loss of ECF is 6% of body weight. The balance is the effect of acute starvation. Because of the internal redistribution of body water that accompanies hypotonic dehydration, these children show relatively more clinical signs of dehydration at any level of weight loss. Clinical features of ECF dehydration are summarized in Table 6.1.

Hypertonic Dehydration

To the extent that hypertonic dehydration involves some contraction of the ECF, clinical signs will be present but to a lesser degree in relation to absolute volume loss than in isotonic and hypotonic dehydration. However, the loss of cell volume characteristic of the condition imparts a distinctive "doughy" texture to the skin and subcutaneous tissues. More importantly, it gives rise to changes in neurological function, resulting from shrinkage of neurones and perhaps to alterations in ICF composition. Permanent brain damage is common; the incidence rises with the severity of the hypertonicity.

Management

Correction of Circulatory Insufficiency

Irrespective of the type of dehydration involved, restoration of adequate circulating volume takes priority over other considerations if shock or impending shock is present. This should be achieved by the intravenous infusion of a colloid-containing fluid. Plasma or plasma equivalent (Plasmanate or human plasma protein fraction) is ideal and should be administered rapidly until perfusion is restored. Closing of the central-peripheral temperature gap is the best guide for restoration of perfusion (271, 272). Plasma expanders, such as dextrans, dissolved in isotonic saline are a good second best. Typically, 20 ml/kg or more will be required. If colloidal solutions are not available, an isotonic electrolyte solution may be used, bearing in mind that larger volumes will be required as a result of the larger volume of distribution.

Repair of Dehydration and Electrolyte Imbalance

In the child who presents without circulatory insufficiency or in whom resuscitation has been achieved, attention must be directed to the reversal of the underlying disorder of fluid and electrolyte balance. There has been a substantial revision of "traditional" views as to how this may best be achieved, partly through better understanding of the pathophysiology of dehydration and partly as a result of the conspicuous success of oral rehydration programs in the management of dehydrated children in both tropical (256) and nontropical (257) settings.

Isotonic/Hypotonic Dehydration. The traditional approach to rehydration of children with isotonic or hypotonic dehydration divides the treatment program into 4 phases: (1) circulatory resuscitation, (2) restoration of ECF volume, (3) correction of ECF and ICF composition (K repletion), and (4) restoration of nutritional status. These phases are carried out sequentially. In this approach K is omitted until urine output is established. Alkali as such is not given unless acidosis is severe, but Ringer's solution or saline-bicarbonate solutions expand ECF and improve acid-base status at the same time. The fluid given in phase 2 is calculated on the basis of the estimated ECF deficit and is supplemented by an allowance for maintenance fluid therapy (chapter 11).

The rationale behind this approach rests on the avoidance of Na overload and of the risk of hyperkalemia. In addition, fasting to "rest the gastrointestinal tract" is practiced to prevent continuing diarrhea. All these arguments have been challenged by advocates of rapid oral rehydration using a single glucose-polyelectrolyte fluid, which is sometimes alternated with water and followed by early feeding.

Hypertonic Rehydration. Giving solute-free water to children with hypernatremic dehydration is ineffective and dangerous. It is ineffective because it fails to correct the complex disturbance of water and electrolyte balance present and dangerous because rapid lowering of hypertonicity leads to a shift of water into brain cells that may produce brain edema (269, 270). Solute-free water must be made available relatively slowly and, in the presence of K and alkali, to allow for the redistribution of Na + K to occur in brain (270a).

These considerations have led to the establishment of the following ground rules for the conventional management of hypernatremia: (1) the rehydrating fluid following circulatory resuscitation should be relatively hypotonic, (2) it should contain K and alkali, and (3) it should be given slowly with the intention of restoring normal hydration over a period of 1 to 2 days rather than hours.

Many different regimens have been reported within the above guidelines. Finberg and coworkers (273) have recommended from their extensive experience a solution with the following composition: Na—50 to 75 mEq/l; K—10 to 40 mEq/l; Cl to balance the Na + K; and glucose—5%. Using this fluid at appropriate intakes, only 2 of 67 children with severe hypernatremic dehydration died (273).

An alternative is to use a single oral rehydration solution. This approach is based on the following: Na is absorbed in the intestine by active cotransport with glucose and certain other organic molecules; its absorption is greatly enhanced by the presence of glucose in equimolar quantities (275, 276). More glucose causes osmotic diarrhea and no glucose inhibits Na, Cl, and water absorption. This has led to the use of solutions for oral rehydration with the following composition: Na—50 to 90 mEq/l; K—15 to 30 mEq/l; bicarbonate 20-30 mEq/l; Cl to balance; and glucose—2 to 2.5%. The principle was first employed in the 1960s for the treatment of cholera. With oral rehydration therapy, the mortality, morbidity, and complexity of treatment was reduced dramatically (277-280). The solution contained the following: Na—120 mEq/l with Cl and glucose, 111 mMol or 20 g/l; K and HCO_3 were added. The high Na concentration reflects the composition of cholera stools. A similar approach has been successful in treating infants and children with noncholera diarrhea using the World Health Organization (WHO) solution that has the following composition: Na—90 mEq/l; K—20 mEq/l; Cl—80 mEq/l; HCO_3—30 mEq/l; and glucose—111 mMol or 20 g/l (255, 256, 278). Despite some caveats concerning the high Na concentration of this fluid, particularly in the treatment of well-nourished western children (281), the anticipated hazards of hypernatremia, fluid overload and hyperkalemia, have not occurred. Controlled studies, comparing the WHO solution with one that has Na and Cl concentrations of 50 and 40 mEq/l, respectively, have shown both to be equally effective in treating children with acute diarrheal dehydration in the United States and Panama (257). A particularly interesting finding was that initial hypernatremia (Na >150 mEq/l) was rapidly and safely corrected by either solution.

These results are in accordance with current understanding of the pathophysiological mechanisms of hypernatremic dehydration. Oral rehydration fluid was deliberately administered rapidly to achieve ECF volume expansion and to correct acidosis and K depletion. Volume repletion suppresses aldosterone and other sodium-retaining mechanisms. Renal regulation of excess Na, Cl, K, and water completes the adjustment of ECF to normal. This factor accounts for the seemingly paradoxical finding that a single orally administered solution rapidly corrects hypotonic, isotonic, and hypertonic dehydration. The greater natriuretic effect of oral as opposed to intravenous saline (151, 282) also contributes to the more rapid correction of hypernatremia when the oral route is used.

Other Causes of Dehydration

Many disorders other than diarrhea may result in dehydration. They may differ with regard to whether K depletion is present and whether there is an associated acid-base disorder (Table 6.2). The physiological responses to renal handling of Na and water are generally similar to those described with diarrheal dehydration. Primary disorders of renal function or of aldosterone or ADH release are important exceptions.

HYPONATREMIC STATES

Causes

Hyponatremia (plasma Na <130 mMol/1) may be a result of abnormal water retention or to primary Na loss. Hyponatremia because of water retention may occur in the presence of increased, normal, or decreased body Na. Primary Na loss, on the other hand, is usually accompanied by some degree of water loss. Within these two broad categories, many disorders involving various organ systems may present with hyponatremia. The major causes are listed in the box on this page.

Pseudohyponatremia

Routine laboratory measurements are performed on whole plasma. Normal plasma is 94% water by volume, and other electrolytes are dissolved in this water. The remaining 6% is mostly protein. The Na concentration in plasma water (Na_{PW}) therefore is higher than that in whole plasma by a factor varying in proportion with the fraction of the plasma that is nonaqueous. Na_{PW} is calculated as follows:

$$Na_{PW} = Na_P \times [100/(100 - x)] \quad (1)$$

where Na_{PW} and Na_P are the Na concentrations in plasma water and whole plasma, respectively, and x is the nonaqueous phase of plasma.

Table 6.2.
Causes of Dehydration and ECF Volume Contraction

Physiological cause	Acid-base disorder	Potassium depletion
Gastrointestinal		
diarrhea	acidosis	+
pyloric stenosis	alkalosis	+
laxatives	alkalosis	+
Urinary losses		
diabetic ketoacidosis	acidosis	+
diuretics		
thiazides, loop diuretics	alkalosis	+
potassium-sparing	variable	−(retention)
mineralocorticoid deficiency	acidosis	−(retention)
renal tubular acidosis	acidosis	+
Bartter's syndrome	alkalosis	+
diabetes insipidus	variable	−
hypokalemic nephropathy	alkalosis	+
salt-losing renal disease	variable	−
Other		
heatstroke	acidosis	−
water deprivation	variable	−
starvation	acidosis	+

CAUSES OF HYPONATREMIA

- Pseudohyponatremia
  - Hyperlipidemia (>5 gm/dl)
  - Hyperproteinemia (>10 gm/dl)
- Osmotic redistribution of water
  - Hyperglycemia
  - Mannitol, contrast media
- Excess water intake
  - Compulsive water drinking
- Reduced renal water excretion
  - Acute renal failure
  - Chronic renal failure
  - Congestive cardiac failure
  - Nephrotic syndrome
  - Cirrhosis of the liver
  - Glucocorticoid deficiency
  - Hypothyroidism
  - Antidiuretic Drugs
  - Stress
  - Inappropriate ADH secretion
- Excessive sodium loss
  - Renal
    - Mineralocorticoid deficiency
    - Diuretics
    - Polyuric acute renal failure
    - Salt-wasting renal disease
    - Renal tubular acidosis
    - Metabolic alkalosis
    - Bartter's syndrome
  - Gastrointestinal
    - Diarrheal dehydration
    - Renewal of gastrointestinal fluid by suction
    - Intestinal fistula
    - Laxative abuse
  - Transcutaneous
    - Cystic fibrosis and heat stress
    - Heat losses with inadequate salt replacement
  - Sequestration or "third space" losses associated with inappropriate fluid therapy
    - Burns
    - Major trauma including surgical procedures

When x is 6% and Na_P is 141 mMol/l, Na_{PW} is 150. An increase in the nonaqueous phase to >10% occurs in hyperproteinemia (rarely, if ever, seen in childhood) and hyperlipemia. In the latter case, gross lipemia in plasma is visible in blood samples. Measurement of the Na concentration after removal of lipid by centrifugation will correct for this effect. Plasma osmolality, which measures the solute concentration in plasma water, is not reduced by hyperlipemia. In normal plasma, osmolality may be estimated from the formula (153d):

$$\text{Osmolality (mOsm/kg)} = (2 \times \text{Na}) + \text{glucose} + \text{urea} + 10 \quad (2)$$

The terms on the right hand side of the equation are in mMol/l (glucose in mMol/l = mg/dl ÷ 18; urea in mMol/l = BUN (mg/dl) ÷ 2.8). If the measured osmolality is >20 mOsm/kg higher than the value calculated in this way, either pseudohyponatremia is present or an unmeasured osmotically active substance, such as mannitol or alcohol, is present.

Hyperglycemia

Acutely induced hyperglycemia raises the tonicity of ECF and causes an osmotic shift of water out of cells and dilutional hyponatremia results. The Na_P falls by 1 mMol/l for every 2 to 3 mMol/l rise in plasma glucose (1.35 to 1.6 mMol/l/100 mg/dl glucose (283, 284). Unless the Na_P is lower than can be accounted for by this relationship, prompt correction of hyperglycemia will normalize plasma Na.

However, sustained hyperglycemia as occurs with diabetes mellitus will cause an osmotic diuresis, leading to ECF volume depletion. Hyponatremia will develop as the patient continues to drink water. In the patient with diabetic ketoacidosis or nonketotic hyperglycemia, the latter mechanism is more important and volume repletion must be undertaken along with insulin therapy to lower blood sugar.

Other Osmotically Active Substances

Mannitol (molecular weight—180 daltons) and x-ray contrast media act in an analogous way to glucose increase tonicity and lower Na_P. Mannitol in the treatment of cerebral edema removes cell and interstitial brain water. The osmotic diuresis induced by either may cause ECF volume contraction.

Urea, ethanol, methanol, and polyethylene glycol (antifreeze) raise the osmolality. For example, ethanol (molecular weight—46 daltons) contributes 22 mOsm/kg for every 100 mg/dl measured. Because these substances are permeant and enter cells rapidly they produce only transient shifts of water between ECF and ICF. Equilibration takes place by movement of solute (285). For this reason, hyperosmolality in the presence of normal Na_P is the usual finding.

Excess Water Intake (Water Intoxication)

In health, the capacity to excrete solute-free water is so large that it requires an extraordinary water overload to cause hyponatremia. However, water intoxication and encephalopathy has followed prodigious water drinking in adults (286, 287). Water intoxication because of compulsive drinking of this severity is rare in childhood (288), but water intoxication and seizures have been described in association with attempts at oral rehydration with water (289). Water overload also can be induced by pulmonary absorption of nebulized water during mechanical ventilation or by colonic absorption of water from tap-water enemas used in the management of Hirschsprung's disease.

A variant of compulsive water drinking occurs in the occasional psychotic patient who combines a disorder of thirst with abnormal ADH release (290). The close relationship believed to exist between the neurological mechanisms responsible for thirst and ADH release (291, 292) suggests that some alteration in brain function produced by psychosis is capable of activating thirst and water-retaining mechanisms in a synchronous fashion.

Reduced Renal Water Excretion

A number of factors limit the capacity of the kidney to excrete solute-free water. These include: (1) Reduced solute delivery to the distal nephron, i.e., the thick ascending limb of the loop of Henle, often secondary to a reduction in single nephron GFR and increased Na reabsorption in the proximal tubule; (2) Low solute excretion rate, in which the human kidney cannot dilute urine <40 mOSm/kg water.

Increased Water Permeability of the Distal Nephron

Although is principally under the control of ADH, other factors may alter although the permeability of the distal nephron to water is principally under the control of ADH, other factors may also alter permeability and decrease C_{H_2O} (see box, this page) and inhibit C_{H_2O}, e.g., glucocorticoids and some drugs (see box on this page). Hyponatremia because of impaired renal water excretion is associated with an increase in body water content.

DRUGS CAPABLE OF CAUSING HYPONATREMIA SECONDARY TO RENAL WATER RETENTION GROUPED ACCORDING TO MECHANISMS OF ACTIONS

- Increase water permeability of the nephron
  - Vasopressin (arginine or lysine) (336, 338)
  - 1-deamino, 8-D-arginine vasopressin (DDAVP)
  - Other vasopressin analogues
  - Oxytocin (330)
- Promotes ADH release
  - Barbiturates (331)
  - Carbemazepine (332)
  - Clofibrate (333)
  - Colchicine (334)
  - Isoproterenol (Isoprenaline)
  - Nicotine
  - Vincristine (335)
- Inhibits prostaglandin synthesis
  - Salicylates (339, 340)
  - Indomethacin (339)
  - Acetaminophen (Paracetamol)
  - Other nonsteroidal antiinflammatory drugs
- Potentiates action of ADH
  - Chlorpropamide (336, 337)
  - Cyclophosphamide (341, 342)

Acute Renal Insufficiency

Acute oliguric renal failure, if severe, is associated with the production of virtually no urine at all. The composition of the ECF will be altered as a direct function of input. Since water input normally exceeds solute input, dilutional hyponatremia often results. This is the case irrespective of the cause of the renal failure (chapter 48). Less severe degrees of renal failure limit free water excretion as a consequence of reduced GFR and, therefore, of reduced delivery of solute to the distal nephron (293). Hyponatremia will ensue unless appropriate adjustments are made to water intake. During recovery from acute renal failure, a polyuric (diuretic) phase frequently is seen, during which hyponatremia may occur as a result of urinary salt loss rather than water retention. This resembles primary polyuric renal failure.

Chronic Renal Failure

Chronic renal failure (CRF), likewise, reduces maximal free water clearance in proportion to the fall in GFR. The intrinsic diluting capacity of the kidney, expressed as C_{H_2O}/GFR, is well preserved even in advanced renal insufficiency (294), but since free water clearance cannot exceed 20% to 25% of GFR, the absolute water excreting capacity is severely reduced. For example, at a GFR of 5 ml/min not more than 1 ml/min (1.5 l/day) of solute-free water can be excreted (295). Free water reabsorption is more readily limited. As nephron numbers fall, the obligate solute excretion per remaining nephron increases progressively, leading to eventual isosthenuria and the inability to vary water intake without the development of hypernatremia or hyponatremia.

Congestive Cardiac Failure

Many patients with chronic heart failure become hyponatremic, despite the fact that they are edematous. The hyponatremia is a result of water retention, probably in response to reduced cardiac output, leading to a contraction of effective arterial volume and the effect this has on NaCl and water excretion. GFR decreases and proximal tubular reabsorption of NaCl increases (296). Both mannitol (297) and furosemide (298), which inhibit reabsorption in the proximal nephron, promote water excretion in cardiac failure. ADH release also contributes to water retention in these patients. ADH-like material has been identified by bioassay (299, 300) and radioimmunoassay (301) in patients with chronic heart failure. Although water diuresis may be induced in the patients with alcohol (302, 303), it is not recommended. Water is retained in dogs secondary to ligation of the thoracic inferior vena cava (296); both hypophysectomy and carotid sinus denervation reverse the effect. The ligation probably stimulates the baroreceptors to inhibit free water clearance and the denervation blocks this response.

Nephrotic Syndrome

Hyponatremia occurs in some patients with the nephrotic syndrome. Although the plasma volume is reduced, the renal response differs from that in cardiac failure in that GFR is often increased, and proximal tubular reabsorption is decreased as a result of the hypoalbuminemia and its effect in altering peritubular Starling forces (304, 305). Therefore, more distal processes must be responsible for the water retention. The association with plasma volume contraction makes it probable that ADH release is the major factor. Volume repletion with infusions of plasma improve free water clearance temporarily.

Cirrhosis of the Liver

Patients with advanced hepatic cirrhosis and fluid retention are frequently hyponatremic. As with cardiac failure and the nephrotic syndrome, this is the result of water retention in excess of Na retention. Although total plasma volume is expanded in cirrhosis (306), sequestration of some of this volume in the splanchnic venous system, hypoalbuminemia and peripheral vasodilation may lead to a reduction in effective arterial volume.

Cirrhotic patients with hyponatremia have higher plasma ADH levels (307) and lower plasma albumin (308) than those with normal water excretion, suggesting that the effective arterial volume of these patients is reduced. The ADH response is baroreceptor-mediated and ADH levels are strongly correlated with plasma norepinephrine levels—an index of sympathetic nervous activity (308, 309).

An increase in proximal tubular reabsorption of Na may contribute to the defect in urinary excretion of free water. For example, intravenous mannitol changes free water clearance from negative to positive in patients with hyponatremia and chronic liver disease (310). The relative importance of ADH stimulation and intrarenal adjustments is not known, but ADH appears to be the principal factor. However, norepinephrine and alpha-adrenergic stimulation reduce renal blood flow and GFR and increase tubular Na reabsorption (83, 111), indicating that both intrarenal and extrarenal factors act synergistically to cause retention of water.

Glucocorticoid Deficiency

Glucocorticoid deficiency is associated with a diluting defect even in the absence of mineralocorticoid deficiency. Both ADH-dependent and ADH-independent mechanisms appear to be involved. ADH levels are increased in patients with Addison's disease (311, 312) and are suppressed when glucocorticoids are given (311). Improvement in C_{H_2O} followed ethanol administration and suppression of ADH (313). Water retention and nonosmolar stimulated ADH release are accompanied by tachycardia and reduction of stroke volume in adrenalectomized, mineralocorticoid-replaced dogs (314). This response would be expected as part of a sympathetic discharge as a result of reduced effective arterial volume. Such a volume reduction may be from a direct effect on cardiac performance or by alterations in peripheral resistancer and capillary permeability.

Glucocorticoid deficiency also may directly increase collecting duct permeability (315), because ADH secretion and metabolism are normal in patients with adrenal insufficiency despite the defect in C_{H_2O}. Adrenalectomy in Brattleboro (ADH-deficient) rats reduces C_{H_2O}. Renal water handling returns to normal promptly with glucocorticoid replacement (316).

Hypothyroidism

Myxedema in the human and hypothyroidism in the rat may be associated with water retention and hyponatremia. Reduced distal delivery is a likely cause of the diluting defect; C_{H_2O} is reduced to a greater extent than is the ability to produce urine of low osmolality (317). Measures designed to increase distal delivery increase C_{H_2O} in hypothyroid humans (318) and in vasopressin-deficient rats (319). Hypothyroid rats have reduced proximal tubular reabsorption, which would tend to increase distal delivery. If this is correct, this would suggest a defect in regulating free water in the distal nephron (320, 321). A low GFR, characteristic of myxedema would tend to limit diluting capacity (322). This is unlikely to be an important factor since GFR is much more severely reduced in other conditions not associated with water retention. An independent effect of ADH has been suggested (323–325). As in other hyponatremic states, reduced effective arterial volume secondary to the circulatory effects of hypothyroidism might account for both reduced distal delivery and nonosmolar ADH release. Thyroid replacement therapy rapidly corrects the hyponatremia.

Antidiuretic Drugs

Drugs may impair water excretion in four ways: (1) by increasing permeability of the distal nephron to water by stimulating release of ADH; (2) by potentiating the action of submaximal concentrations of ADH on the collecting duct; (3) by inhibiting prostaglandin synthesis; and (4) by a direct effect on collecting duct permeability. Prostaglandins promote free water excretion by increasing distal delivery of solute and by reducing distal water reabsorption. The latter occurs because prostaglandins inhibit the effect of vasopressin (326).

The box on p. 99 lists common drugs that cause water retention by one or more of these pathways. Drugs that are promoters of ADH release may act indirectly on the pituitary or hypothalamus by stimulating a baroreceptor response to circulatory changes that act on the hypothalamus or pituitary to release ADH (231).

Chlorpropamide is of particular interest because it appears to act by enhancing the action of circulating vasopressin (327), possibly by inhibiting prostaglandin synthesis (328). It also potentiates the release of ADH (329). The drug is ineffective in patients with nephrogenic diabetes insipidus, and relatively ineffective in pituitary diabetes insipidus where ADH levels are low or absent.

Syndrome of Inappropriate ADH Secretion

ADH release is regulated in response to osmolar and nonosmolar stimuli. The latter include contraction of effective arterial volume, probably sensed via the arterial baroreceptor system. The term syndrome of inappropriate ADH secretion (SIADH) is frequently used to mean ADH release, which is unexpected in terms of plasma osmolality alone. In this discussion it is reserved for those situations where ADH secretion occurs that cannot be explained either by osmolar or baroreceptor-mediated factors (343). On careful examination, many clinical examples of SIADH turn out to be explicable in terms of nonosmolar factors (344). It is presumptuous to label these as "inappropriate". In severely volume-contracted patients, the water-retaining and pressor effects of ADH may be life saving, although the cost is dilutional hyponatremia.

Pathophysiology

The physiology of SIADH has been examined, using normal subjects given exogenous vasopressin as a model (345). Initially, water retention occurs, leading to weight gain and hyponatremia; natriuresis follows. If water intake remains high, urine output gradually increases and a new equilibrium is achieved in which urinary Na changes briskly in response to changes in input of Na or water, as in the normal situation (346). Although the initial negative Na balance means that total body Na is reduced at equilibrium, total cation is not, since K is retained. Similar effects have been noted in patients with endogenous SIADH (347, 348).

The establishment of a new equilibrium evidently represents a situation analogous to the mineralocorticoid escape phenomenon. The following mechanism is likely: during the initial phase of weight gain in response to water retention ECF volume expansion occurs and leads to natriuresis, partly a result of suppression of aldosterone release. As hyponatremia develops, however, it acts as a stimulus to aldosterone release independent of ECF volume, limiting the Na loss. This restores its capacity to regulate acid base status (349). Thus, severe hyponatremia may override volume-mediated suppression of the renin-angiotensin-aldosterone system, just as severe volume contraction may override the effect of hypoosmolality in suppressing ADH release.

Similarly, external water balance is restored by a progressive increase in urine volume as weight increases. By definition, this cannot be a result of suppression of ADH, so other factors must be responsible. There is evidence that the permeability of the collecting duct to water decreases because of a process independent of ADH (350, 351). The effect of volume expansion in increasing delivery to the distal nephron would be expected to reduce transit time through the collecting duct, diminishing osmotic backleak of water. Increases in blood flow in the vasa recta would also cause washout of medullary solute, reducing the osmotic gradient for water reabsorption. These factors combine to limit water retention and salt loss in SIADH. They are sufficiently powerful that clinical edema is rarely seen. Symptoms, when seen, are a result of acute water retention and hyponatremia.

Diagnosis. Since SIADH is neither the only nor even the most common cause of hyponatremia in pediatric practice, it should be diagnosed only when appropriate criteria have been met. The clinical criteria necessary to make the diagnosis are listed in the box on this page (352).

Treatment. The hyponatremia of SIADH is a result primarily of water retention rather than Na loss. Therefore, the appropriate treatment is water restriction. If water intake is maintained below the sum of observed urine output and estimated insensible losses, the excess water is lost and Na_P returns to normal. As ECF volume falls, the secondary changes (Na loss, K retention) are reversed. ECF composition can be maintained as long as water intake is adjusted to balance losses. Attempts to normalize plasma Na by infusing salt are self-defeating, since the administered Na is excreted promptly. Patients with neurological symptoms and signs, usually have $Na_P < 120$ mEq/l; temporary relief may be obtained by giving hypertonic saline or mannitol. Simultaneously, water intake should be restricted. Giving hypertonic saline is rarely necessary.

CRITERIA FOR DIAGNOSIS OF THE SYNDROME OF INAPPROPRIATE SECRETION OF ANTIDIURETIC HORMONE

- Urine that is not maximally dilute in the presence of hyponatremia and plasma hypoosmolality
- Normal ECF volume
- Normal renal function
- Continued sodium excretion, commensurate with intake
- Absence of antidiuretic drugs (box on p. 99)
- Absence of cardiac failure, nephrotic syndrome, chronic liver disease or hypothyroidism

HYPERNATREMIA

Hypernatremia ($Na_P > 150$ mMol/l) is much less common than hyponatremia. It may result from a primary increase in total body Na, but is much more frequently a result of abnormal renal or nonrenal water loss. The principal causes are listed in the box on p. 102.

Na Overload

Salt poisoning

The human kidney can excrete urine with a maximum concentration of about 300 mMol/l, i.e., about twice that in ECF. Since continuous hypotonic insensible losses must be taken into account, the maximum tolerated salt concentration of the diet is somewhat less than this value, which, if exceeded, must lead to hypernatremia. Infants are at increased risk resulting from high insensible water losses and a limited renal capacity to excrete Na (353–355). Even in infants, Na overload severe enough to cause hypernatremia is rare. Occasional disasters have been reported: For example, in one instance salt was substituted accidentally for sugar in the bulk preparation of infant formula; the resulting hypernatremia was severe (plasma Na >200 mMol/l in some patients) and associated with high mortality and morbidity (356). The use of hypertonic $NaHCO_3$ in the resuscitation of asphyxiated newborn infants may lead to significant hypernatremia and hypertonicity, which may predispose to intracranial hemorrhage (357). Occasional severe or even fatal hypernatremia has occurred as the result of the use of intragastric hypertonic saline as an emetic (358) or as a lavage solution (359) in the treatment of drug overdoses. Salt loading as a form of child abuse causes hypernatremia (357a).

Hyperaldosteronism

Hyperaldosteronism is another cause of hypernatremia (357a). Although the usual consequences of hyperaldosteronism are fluid retention, volume expansion, and hypertension, mild hypernatremia is occasionally seen. This probably reflects partial suppression of ADH release by volume expansion, despite the presence of ECF hypertonicity (360).

Inadequate Water Intake

If water intake is insufficient to balance obligate losses, hypernatremia will usually ensue, because Na excretion can be reduced virtually to zero while net water loss continues at about 25 ml/100 kcal (400 ml/m^2 body surface area) even in the absence of abnormal losses. In normal individuals, drinking in response to thirst prevents this form of hypernatremic dehydration, so that it is found only in the following circumstances.

Inability to Drink in Response to Thirst

Comatose or neurologically impaired patients are most at risk, since they are unable to drink when thirsty (361). An essential part of the care of such people lies in the provision of adequate water input. If cerebral edema is present or suspected this may involve walking a tightrope between twoo much and too little, as well as intensive monitoring of both intracranial and biochemical status. If cerebral edema is not considered a risk, generous water intake will allow the patient to regulate his own water balance by means of the normal renal mechanisms. Young infants are similarly vulnerable, particularly when water losses are increased by high ambient temperature or fever.

Lack of Free Access to Water

A person who lacks free access to water could be the traveller lost in the desert. However, the plight of the shipwreck survivor in an open boat on the ocean is no more enviable, since the salt concentration in seawater (Na 468, Cl 535 mEq/l) is higher than that of maximally concentrated urine; drinking it inevitably leads to progressive Na overload and hypernatremia.

Adipsia

Rare patients, usually with some form of intracranial disease, do not experience thirst in response to hypertonicity, and therefore fail to drink enough to maintain normal ECF dilution (362, 363). Most of these patients who have been adequately studied have an associated defect of ADH release and are usually classified as having essential hypernatremia (364–366).

Increased Nonrenal Water Loss

Gastrointestinal water loss as a result of diarrhea and vomiting has been discussed; other nonrenal losses occur via skin and lungs. These, when exaggerated by high ambient temperatures, pyrexia, and hyperventilation may cause net water loss and hypernatremia. Such losses alone cannot cause hypernatremia. This will occur only if they are inadequately replaced or replaced with fluid of inappropriate composition. In practice, hypernatremia is the result of increased losses and inadequate intake of water.

Increased Renal Water Loss

The capacity to conserve free water requires the presence of ADH and the capacity of the kidney to respond to the hormone. Failure of production of ADH is known as hypothalamic diabetes insipidus (DI); failure of the kidney to respond is known as vasopressin-resistant or nephrogenic DI.

Hypothalamic Diabetes Insipidus

Any disorder that interferes with synthesis or release of ADH will impair renal water conservation and expose the patient to the risk of hypernatremia; causes are found in the box on this page. Conscious patients with normal thirst perception will respond by drinking in proportion to the water loss and thus avoid severe hypertonicity unless denied access to water. In such individuals, the cardinal features are polyuria and polydipsia, often assuming enormous proportions and obliging the patient to wake repeatedly during the night to drink. Conversely, patients who are unable to maintain adequate water intake because of incompetence (coma, infancy) or lack of access to water develop severe hypernatremic dehydration. Two groups of patients are particularly likely to develop dangerous hypertonicity because of ADH deficiency: those with primary hypothalamic DI, in whom the diagnosis is often delayed and episodes of dehydration have occurred because thirst could not be satisfied, such as infants, or the sense of thirst was impaired and those in whom ADH deficiency accompanies neurological disease (trauma, tumors, encephalitis), since impairment of consciousness is a frequent associated event.

In congenital DI, cerebral damage is often present by the time diagnosis is made; there may be difficulty in deciding whether the brain damage is the cause or the consequence of the ADH deficiency. It is important to recognize that hypothalamic DI is often partial (367), in that ADH release is present but subnormal in relation to the osmolar and nonosmolar stimuli operating at the time. Many patients with partial DI can produce isotonic or slightly hypertonic urine in response to only mild ECF hypertonicity, and the resulting polyuria and polydipsia are relatively modest in degree. It follows that demonstration of the ability to elaborate urine hypertonic to plasma is not sufficient to exclude partial DI. What is required is to show that urinary concentration is inappropriately low in relation to ECF tonicity. The patient with normal renal function and an intact hypothalamic ADH release mechanism should be able to respond to dehydration (plasma osmolality >295 mOsm/kg) by producing urine of at least 800 mOsm/kg.

CAUSES OF HYPERNATREMIA

- Sodium overload
  - inappropriate IV therapy
  - salt poisoning
  - hyperaldosteronism
- Inadequate water intake
  - comatose patients
  - infants
  - inaccessibility of water (lost in desert)
  - primary adipsia
- Increased nonrenal water loss
  - gastrointestinal (diarrhea, vomiting)
  - insensible (pyrexia, high ambient temperature)
- Increased renal water loss
  - ADH deficiency (hypothalamic diabetes insipidus)
  - ADH resistance (nephrogenic diabetes insipidus)
    - chronic renal failure
    - damage to renal medulla
      - sickle cell disease
      - nephronophthisis
      - renal papillary necrosis
      - chronic pyelonephritis
    - hypokalemia
    - hypercalcemia
    - primary (idiopathic)
      - hereditary
      - sporadic
- Essential hypernatremia

Vasopressin-resistant (nephrogenic) Diabetes Insipidus

Renal water loss caused by inability of the tubule to respond to ADH may occur secondary to a variety of congenital and acquired renal diseases or as an isolated specific defect of distal tubular function. The term nephrogenic DI is commonly used to describe patients in the latter category. However, since this diagnosis can be made only after excluding structural renal disease, especially of the medulla, and since the term is linguistically unsatisfactory, it is better to use the descriptive label vasopressin(ADH)-resistant DI (VRDI) to include both primary and secondary types, as recommended by Valtin (368). Those in whom structural disease is not found should be classified as having primary or idiopathic VRDI, of sporadic or hereditary type, as appropriate. Causes of VRDI are listed in the box on this page under ADH resistance.

The clinical features of isolated VRDI are indistinguishable from those of hypothalamic DI. The distinction is made on the basis of the response to exogenous ADH or one of its analogues. Clinical aspects of DI are discussed further in chapter 26, and details of the tests used in its investigation will be found in chapter 19.

Essential Hypernatremia

The association between neurological disease and hypernatremia is not explained solely on the basis of deficient water intake. Patients have been described with intracranial lesions of various types, including histiocytosis (369), teratoma (370), postsurgical trauma (371), and infiltrative tumors involving the hypothalamus (372), who suffer from a distinctive disorder of water balance. A similar syndrome has been produced experimentally by the induction of lesions in the anteromedial hypothalamus of rats (373, 374).

The typical patient with essential hypernatremia undergoes recurrent episodes of hypernatremia in which thirst is absent. Urine osmolality varies independently of plasma osmolality, although polyuria is absent and concentrated urine is intermittently produced; these features differentiate the condition from DI. Formal investigation reveals a subnormal rise in plasma vasopressin concentration (371) with rising plasma osmolality or no rise at all (375). In contrast, ADH release is unimpaired in response to nonosmolar stimuli, such as changes in ECF volume (369), vasodilator-induced hypotension (371), and emesis (375).

The probable cause is a selective destruction of the osmoreceptor with preservation of the adjacent supraoptic and paraventricular nuclei, where ADH is synthesized. Defective or absent osmoreceptors lead to absence of thirst and osmotically mediated ADH release, while preservation of baroreceptor-mediated ADH release accounts for urinary concentration in response to nonosmolar stimuli. The existence of this curious syndrome provides strong if indirect evidence in favor of the osmoreceptor theory.

EDEMA

Pathophysiology

The balance of Starling forces between plasma and interstitium normally favors the net filtration of fluid from the capillary lumen to the interstitial space. This fluid is prevented from accumulating by the pumping action of the lymphatic system, which returns it to the circulation via the thoracic duct. The ECF, therefore, circulates from the capillaries via the interstitial space to the venous system. Edema occurs when there is interference with lymphatic function, preventing clearance of fluid from the interstitium, or when the rate of filtration of fluid from capillaries increases beyond the capacity of the lymphatics to remove it. The latter mechanism requires a change in one or more of the terms of the Starling equation describing the filtration pressure (FP), i.e., the pressure that drives fluid across the capillary walls:

$$\mathrm{FP} = (P_c - P_i) - \sigma(\pi_c - \pi_i) \qquad (1)$$

where P and π represent hydrostatic and oncotic pressures in capillaries and interstitium, respectively, and σ is the reflection coefficient of the capillary wall for albumin. Thus, an increase in the hydrostatic pressure gradient or a decrease in the oncotic pressure gradient across the capillary wall favors edema formation.

For edema to become clinically apparent, the interstitial compartment must be expanded by an amount close to 5% of body weight. In an adult this requires several liters. Such a gain in volume must occur from renal salt and water retention. Net positive salt and water balance is an invariable feature of general edema states. An altered relationship between ECF volume status and renal Na excretion is implied. Renal retention of NaCl and water may be either the cause or the consequence. The disturbance in transcapillary Starling forces that underlies the increase in interstitial volume varies, depending on the particular disease process involved. These relationships are illustrated by two simple examples. The patient with anuric renal failure who continues to ingest salt and water will initially expand his intravascular volume, since ingested fluid is absorbed into the bloodstream. The resulting hypooncotic volume expansion will lead to both an increase in P_c and a decrease in π_c, magnifying FP and causing fluid to move into the interstitial space. Such patients have generalized edema accompanied by plasma volume expansion, hypertension, and circulatory congestion.

In contrast, hypoalbuminemia in the absence of renal disease, caused, for example, by protein-losing enteropathy, leads to a reduction in π_c and an increase in FP. The resulting shift of fluid into the interstitial space causes plasma volume contraction; as discussed earlier in this chapter, this is a powerful antinatriuretic stimulus and renal salt and water retention occurs. Such patients have edema with reduced or normal blood volume, depending on the extent to which compensatory fluid retention has occurred.

Thus, two primary models of edema formation can be formulated as follows:

Model A

renal salt and water retention
circulatory volume expansion
altered Starling forces
edema

Model B

altered Starling forces
edema
circulatory volume contraction
renal salt and water retention

In practice, it is frequently difficult to be sure which of these is operating. This is an area of active research and controversy, particularly with respect to the edema of cardiac failure, cirrhosis of the liver, and the nephrotic syndrome.

Causes

Congestive Cardiac Failure

Reduction in the pumping efficiency of the heart leads directly to elevation of venous pressure and impaired arterial filling. Either of these might lead to edema formating according to one or other of the previously mentioned models.

Backward transmission of elevated central venous pressure to the capillary bed would be expected to lead directly to an increase in P_c and a consequent increase in the rate of transudation of fluid into the interstitial compartment. The resulting fall in plasma volume would then act as a stimulus to renal salt and water retention, in accordance with model B. Although venous distension leads to an increase in the total holding capacity of the circulation, the sequestration of most of the contained volume within the venous system leads to relative underfilling of the high pressure compartment, which is presumed to be the locus for sensing the "effective arterial volume."

Reversing the argument, maintenance of cardiac output in the face of impaired cardiac function is dependent on high venous filling pressure: attenuation of this pressure as a result of escape of fluid into the interstitial space is resisted by progressive renal fluid retention. This alternative or forward failure theory holds that the primary event is reduced arterial filling, leading to baroreceptor-mediated salt and water retention. The progressive expansion of ECF volume causes elevation of venous pressure, a rise in P_c and the formation of edema when the rate of filtration of fluid from the intravascular compartment to the interstitium exceeds the capacity of the lymphatics to return it to the circulation.

Distinguishing between "backward" and "forward" failure theories is extremely difficult, and the two are not mutually exclusive. Elevated venous pressure is an essential prerequisite for the development of cardiac edema (376–378), which implies that venous backpressure is a critical factor in altering the transcapillary filtration pressure, as proposed by Starling (379). The question of whether raised venous pressure is the cause or consequence of Na retention in the initiation of cardiac edema is not answerable on the basis of available evidence.

Cirrhosis of the Liver

As with cardiac failure, the edema and ascites characteristic of hepatic cirrhosis are potentially explicable in two ways. The first or traditional theory is that the primary event is sequestration of fluid in the portal venous system, the peritoneal cavity and the peripheral tissues because of alterations in Starling forces; the resulting decrease in effective blood volume leads to secondary renal salt and water retention.

According to this view, a key event is raised intrahepatic venous pressure, leading to an increase in the production of hepatic lymph (380). Because the hepatic sinusoids are freely permeable to protein (381), the rate of production of hepatic lymph is essentially hydrostatic pressure-dependent. When the increased rate of lymph production exceeds the capacity of the thoracic duct to return it to the venous system, ascites begins to form and blood volume is reduced, leading to Na retention. Effective arterial volume is also reduced by increased capacitance of the portal venous system secondary to portal hypertension. Loss of fluid from peripheral capillaries as a result of hypoalbuminemia may contribute. This hypothesis is analogous to the "backward" failure theory for edema formation in cardiac failure.

Studies reported by Lieberman and coworkers (382, 383) cast doubt on the validity of this explanation and led to the formulation of the overflow theory (384), according to which Na retention and plasma volume expansion take place before the formation of ascites and are the proximate cause of it. Numerous measurements in humans (382, 383) and experimental animals (385, 386) are consistent with this interpretation. Two main sets of observations support the overflow hypothesis: (1) measurements of plasma volume in patients actively forming ascites generally give supernormal results, indicating volume expansion rather than contraction, (2) removal of ascitic fluid by paracentesis is only followed by reaccumulation if dietary Na is provided.

The argument is bedeviled by the fact that total plasma volume is not the same as effective arterial volume, the latter being best defined as the state of fullness of the arterial compartment in relation to its holding capacity. In all the clinical and experimental situations reported, the combined effects of vasodilatation, changes in cardiac output and in capillary permeability might cause a reduction in perceived arterial volume in the presence of an increase in total or even total nonsplanchnic plasma volume.

A recent study by Bichet and coworkers (387), using plasma norepinephrine and arginine vasopressin concentrations as an index of arterial baroreceptor activity, provide strong evidence that, in those patients with cirrhosis who retain salt and water, effective arterial volume is reduced. Until more precise means of identifying and measuring effective arterial volume and its relation to total circulating volume are available, the controversy will remain unresolved.

The Nephrotic Syndrome

The association of hypoalbuminemia with edema forms part of the definition of the nephrotic syndrome. Since albumin accounts for 90% of the oncotic pressure of plasma, the latter is reduced below normal values. In the absence of other opposing changes the result will be an increase in transcapillary filtration pressure and in the rate of transudation of fluid from plasma to interstitium. If this rate exceeds the maximal rate of lymphatic return, edema will form. An essential feature of this "traditional" account of nephrotic edema is the occurrence of plasma volume contraction, which acts as a stimulus to renal salt and water retention by mechanisms discussed earlier in this chapter. Like the backward theory of cardiac failure and the traditional theory of cirrhotic edema, this explanation conforms to model B. Because of the change in transcapillary FP, a large proportion of the retained fluid "leaks" into the interstitium, attenuating the tendency to reexpand the circulating volume; the edema tends to be progressive and may become massive.

Numerous experimental observations are at variance with this explanation. Several groups have found plasma volume, measured by various techniques, to be normal or increased in at least some patients with nephrosis (388–390). Furthermore experimental reduction of plasma albumin and oncotic pressure in man (391) and laboratory animals (392–394) by plasmapheresis is followed by maintenance or even as increase in plasma volume, rather than by hypovolemia. The contrary finding that plasma volume does appear to be reduced in some nephrotic patients (395) indicates that the nephrotic syndrome may not be a physiologically homogenous entity. This suggestion is strongly supported by the work of Meltzer and coworkers (389), whose studies of renin-aldosterone profiles suggest that patients with minimal change disease are volume-contracted with nonsuppressible hyperreninemia. Patients with structural glomerular lesions are volume-expanded with low renin levels responsive to diuretics and changes in salt intake.

A number of factors might operate to resist the tendency to hypovolemia. Increased lymphatic return, probably as a consequence of increased interstitial hydrostatic pressure (396), can accommodate a substantial increase in the rate of transfer of fluid from plasma to interstitium before edema develops (397). As long as lymphatic removal keeps pace with increased filtration, plasma volume will be maintained. Additionally, increased lymph flow is associated with a fall in lymph protein concentration (397, 398); assuming that this reflects interstitial fluid protein concentration, the transcapillary oncotic pressure gradient ($\pi_c - \pi_i$) is preserved despite hypoalbuminemia.

Two processes that may contribute to the fall in interstitial protein concentration are: (1) the accelerated removal of albumin from the interstitial space that resulted from increased lymph flow and (2) the effect of hypoalbuminemia to reduce the permeability of the capillary wall to albumin, i.e., increase its reflection coefficient (394). The latter phenomenon may be modified by alterations in peripheral capillary function as a result of the underlying disease. For example, in aminonucleoside nephrosis in the rat, permeability of peripheral and glomerular capillaries to negatively charged macromolecules is increased (399). It is not known whether this is the case in the nephrotic syndrome in humans. It is possible that some of the heterogeneity observed among patients with the nephrotic syndrome is a result of different forms of glomerulonephritis that affect peripheral capillary permeability in some, but not in others. If so, those with generalized increase in capillary leak permeability to albumin would presumably have the greatest tendency to hypovolemia. Aminonucleoside nephrosis is widely considered to be a model of human minimal-change nephropathy. It is interesting to speculate that some such explanation might account for the functional differences observed by Meltzer and coworkers (389) between minimal-change disease and other glomerular lesions.

If the majority of nephrotic patients have normal or increased plasma volume, some afferent stimulus to Na retention other than hypovolemia may operate. This has not been identified. The primary abnormality of glomerular function might cause a disturbance of intrarenal hemodynamics and its control of NaCl and water reabsorption leading to glomerulotubular imbalance and fluid retention. Various humoral factors have been considered as causes of Na retention: (1) aldosterone—the failure of spironolactone to correct the edema of the nephrotic syndrome makes this an unlikely explanation and (2) natriuretic hormone—suppression of its synthesis or release has been suggested. Some evidence exists in support of this hypothesis in patients who are both uremic and nephrotic (136) compared with uremic nonnephrotic patients, but its relevance to nephrotic patients with good renal function is unknown and will remain so until the hormone can be identified and assayed at physiological concentrations.

Whatever the afferent stimulus may be, evidence points to the distal nephron as the effector site of increased Na reabsorption. Changes in GFR alone are inadequate as an explanation, since (1) in some nephrotic patients GFR is normal or increased, (2) there is no correlation between GFR and the severity of the edema state in nephrotic subjects generally, and (3) declining GFR in the absence of hypoalbuminemia is not associated with edema formation. Proximal tubular reabsorption generally is reduced rather than increased, both in experimental animals studied by micropuncture (400) and human nephrotic patients in whom proximal and distal tubular Na reabsorption were studied by diuretic blockade (401) and by clearance under maximal water diuresis (305). Bohlin and Berg (305) found a strong positive correlation between plasma albumin concentration and fractional proximal tubular Na reabsorption in children with steroid-sensitive nephrotic syndrome. This is the opposite result to that which would be expected if the proximal tubule were the site of abnormal Na retention.

It must be concluded that the mechanisms for the edema-forming state of the nephrotic syndrome is not adequately understood. In patients with minimal lesions and an abrupt onset, edema probably is secondary to circulatory hypovolemia. In those with structural glomerular lesions and more chronic course, edema occurs as a primary failure in renal excretion of NaCl and water, leading to expansion of both plasma and ISF compartments. The reason for the renal abnormality in the latter case is obscure and merits further investigation.

Acute Glomerulonephritis

In contrast to the conflicting findings in the nephrotic syndrome, circulating volume is uniformly increased in acute glomerulonephritis (AGN) (402–404), often to a clinically evident extent (chapter 49). It seems clear that the primary event in the initiation of the edema of glomerulonephritis is renal salt and water retention. The speculation that a generalized abnormality of capillary permeability might be present is not supported by experimental evidence; the protein concentration of edema fluid collected from patients with AGN is not increased (405).

Although GFR is usually decreased in AGN it is not always so, and edema may occur even when it is normal (406). In this circumstance NaCl retention cannot be explained on the basis of reduction in the filtered load alone. Further, a fall in GFR does not lead to edema formation if tubular function and its control mechanisms are intact. Regarding the question of which tubular segment is primarily responsible for the abnormally increased Na_R, no evidence is available in human AGN and results obtained in animal models are conflicting, and perhaps reflect the heterogeneity of the models.

In one series of studies of nephrotoxic serum nephritis in rats (407, 408), filtration fraction was reduced below normal, leading to a fall in efferent arteriolar oncotic pressure and a reduction in both absolute and fractional reabsorption in the proximal tubule. The increase in Na_R in this model must, therefore, take place more distally. In experimental antiglomerular basement membrane nephritis, however, filtration fraction is increased, which favors increased proximal, as well as distal, Na reabsorption (409). In a nephrotoxic model in the dog, fractional Na reabsorption in the proximal tubule is unchanged, while FE_{Na} is reduced. Much of the evidence favors the distal tubule as the principal mediator of the Na retention.

The factors mediating the increased Na reabsorption, wherever it occurs, are underdetermined. In the majority models in which filtration fraction is reduced, the effect cannot be explained on the basis of changes in efferent (postglomerular) oncotic pressure since the direction of change is such as to reduce reabsorption. Although renin levels in human poststreptococcal AGN are low in absolute terms (410), they may be high in relation to the volume-expanded state of the patient (411). This may be true in the case of plasma aldosterone levels as well. Angiotensin-II, in addition to promoting the release of aldosterone, is a powerful vasoconstrictor of glomerular vessels (412). One effect of glomerular vasoconstriction may be a reduction in the hydrostatic pressure in the postglomerular circulation. This would theoretically favor reabsorption of filtrate. Against an important role for aldosterone is the fact that hypokalemia and metabolic alkalosis, which would be predicted in a volume-expanded patient with inappropriately high aldosterone levels, are not found in AGN even when GFR is well maintained.

Alterations in the balance of the various natriuretic and antinatriuretic factors, discussed earlier in this chapter, including catecholamines, the renal nerves, intrarenal redistribution of blood flow, prostaglandins, and natriuretic hormone might all be involved in altering distal tubular function in AGN in the direction of enhanced Na_R but little evidence is available. A possible role for deficient natriuretic hormone production is suggested by the finding that rats with experimental glomerulonephritis failed to produced detectable quantities of urinary natriuretic factor, whereas the urine of normal rats consistently contained natriuretic activity following NaCl loading. Furthermore, the kidneys of nephritic rats showed no response to an extract of urine from NaCl-loaded rats, which was natriuretic when given to normal rats (413).

The edema of AGN is, therefore, a result of primary renal NaCl and water retention; redistribution of the expanded ECF is secondary as in model A. NaCl retention is a result mainly of increased distal tubular Na reabsorption, mediated by factors that are not well understood or documented, but which may include altered intrarenal hemodynamics, the renin-angiotensin-aldosterone system and natriuretic hormone.

Chronic Renal Failure

The remarkable thing about edema in CRF is its rarity. For Na excretion to be maintained in the face of severely reduced GFR, FE_{Na} must be greatly increased, an observation that led Bricker and coworkers (134, 135) to postulate that this was a hormonally mediated adaptation to CRF. The presence of a natriuretic factor in uremic, nonedematous patients and its absence in edematous nephrotic uremics (136) suggests a key role for a natriuretic factor in maintaining external salt balance in uremia. The fact that the increase in FE_{Na} can be reversed by gradual reduction of dietary Na (413a) strongly supports the interpretation that the changes in Na handling in uremia are adaptive and ultimately diet dependent. Because the kidney is chronically adapted in this way, sudden changes in salt intake in either direction are poorly tolerated. Just as an abrupt decrease in intake may lead to Na depletion, volume contraction and possible collapse, so an abrupt increase is liable to cause Na retention, volume expansion, and edema. In the absence of such changes in intake, the state of natriuretic adaptation of the nephrons usually keeps pace with the fall in GFR until uremia is far advanced. Only in the terminal phase, when the maximum adaptive capacity is exceeded, does edema occur.

Malnutrition

Severe protein energy malnutrition is frequently associated with hypoalbuminemia and edema (kwashiorkor). This is usually explained as a model B type of edema with the primary event being loss of fluid from plasma to interstitium secondary to reduced plasma oncotic pressure (414, 415). As in the nephrotic syndrome, a critical examination of the evidence reveals this to be a simplistic explanation, and many observations are at variance with it. There is no correlation between the plasma albumin concentration and the degree of edema (416). Edema may occur in malnourished children with normal plasma proteins. Resolution of edema is correlated with energy rather than protein intake; a role for K depletion, an invariable component of the syndrome, is proposed (417). The matter remains controversial (418).

One difficulty has been that the epidemiology of kwashiorkor is such that facilities for detailed physiological studies are rarely available in the field. It is likely that the edema is multifactorial and that reduced plasma oncotic pressure is not the only nor perhaps the principal cause. The importance of lymphatic function has not generally been taken into account in the analysis. A striking and invariable feature of severe malnutrition is inactivity. One way in which improved energy intake might lead to mobilization of edema is by promoting movement and muscular exertion, a powerful stimulus to lymphatic flow. Subjects, who were maintained on an inadequate diet for 6 months and lost 15% of body weight, became edematous even though plasma protein levels and plasma volume were not affected. In their diaries, they described a state of remarkable inactivity.

Lymphedema

Interruption of lymphatic flow from any region of the body leads to accumulation of fluid in the affected part. Lymphatic pumping is necessary to maintain the normal negative pressure in the interstitium (6). When this becomes positive, the compliance of the interstitial gel increases dramatically (396) and resistance to the accumulation of edema fluid is effectively lost. Lymphatic function is also essential to return the protein filtered into the interstitium to the circulation; in the absence of lymph return the ISF protein concentration will rise to eventual equilibrium with plasma. Thus, cessation of regional lymph flow leads to the development of regional edema in which the edema fluid has a high protein concentration. The causes of lymphatic obstruction are usually chronic: tissue reaction to the edema fluid, probably because of its protein content, eventually leads to fibrosis and the familiar brawny nonpitting appearance of chronic lymphedema.

Specific causes of lymphedema include malignant infiltration of regional lymph nodes or removal of lymph nodes in radical block dissection of groin or axilla, lymphatic obstruction as a result of filariasis, and hypoplasmia of lymphatic vessels, usually in the lower half of the body (Milroy's disease). Treatment includes elevation of the affected limb, pressure bandage, and occasionally surgical removal of lymphedematous tissue. Results often are unsatisfactory.

Edema Due to Drugs

Vasodilator antihypertensive drugs may cause NaCl and water retention. Sometimes this effect is sufficient to produce clinical edema. The magnitude of the effect is proportional to the magnitude of the vasodilator effect of the drug. It is most apparent with the use of diazoxide and minoxidil. The stimulus to Na retention appears to be reduction in peripheral vascular resistance, which effectively increases the holding capacity of the circulation and is perceived as a reduction in effective arterial volume. The edema is usually controlled with diuretic therapy.

Nonsteroidal antiinflammatory drugs also cause Na retention and occasionally edema. This is a result of their inhibition of prostaglandin synthetase. The renal effects of PGE_2 and PGI_2 include vasodilatation, increased blood flow and GFR, and reduction of tubular Na_R; inhibition of their synthesis is antinatriuretic (100–103). A direct mineralocorticoid effect has been postulated for some of these agents, e.g., phenylbutazone.

Estrogens, widely prescribed as oral contraceptives, may cause NaCl and water retention. The effect varies widely among different women. In some, it may limit their use. The mechanism is not clear, but may involve stimulation of antinatriuretic hormones, including aldosterone and prolactin (419).

Withdrawal of diuretics may be followed by rebound fluid retention, particularly if the drug has been taken for a long time. McGregor and de Wardener (420) propose that occult diuretic abuse is the major cause of idiopathic edema in women (421, 422). They postulate that chronic NaCl and water depletion induces an adaptive antinatriuretic state. When the diuretic is withdrawn, considerable time may elapse until adaptation to the new condition is established. The frequency with which diuretic abuse is seen is a matter of current controversy.

Treatment—a Commentary

Treatment of edema is not described in this section, as it is covered in appropriate detail in those instances where edema is likely to be a part of the clinical experience of the nephrologist (chapter 29). Treatment is changing as the pathophysiology of edema is better understood. The purpose of this section is to provide information on the mechanisms of edema formation in those conditions where edema commonly occurs, so that the reader can draw on current therapies to achieve the desired goal.

References

1. Pappenheimer JR: Passage of molecules through capillary walls. Physiol Rev 33:387, 1953.
2. Nernst W: Uber die Berechnung chemischer Gleichgewichte aus thermischen Messungen. Nachr Acad Wiss Goetingen Math Physik. Kl lla Math Physik Chem Abt. 1:1, 1906.
3. Donnan FG: Theorie der Membrangleichgewichte and Membranpotentiale bei Vorhandensein von nicht dialysierenden Elektrolyten. Ein Beitrag zur physikalisch chemischen Physiologie. Z Electrochem 17:572, 1911.
4. Manery JF: Water and electrolyte metabolism. Physiol Rev 34:334, 1954.
5. Landis EM, Pappenheimer JR: Exchange of substances through the capillary walls. In Hamilton WF, Dow P (eds): Handbook of Physiology. Washington, D.C., American Physiological Society, 1963, vol 2, p 961.
6. Guyton AC: A concept of negative interstitial pressure based on pressures in implanted perforated capsules. Circulat Res 12:399, 1963.
7. Nicoll PA, Taylor AE: Lymph formation and flow. Annu Rev Physiol 39:73, 1977.
8. Starling EH: On the absorption of fluids from the connective tissue spaces. J Physiol 19:312, 1896.
9. Guyton AC: Textbook of Medical Physiology, ed 6. Philadelphia, W. B. Saunders Co., 1981.
10. Cheek DB: Extracellular volume: its structure and measurement and the influence of age and disease. J Pediatr 58:103, 1961.
11. Comper WD, Laurent TC: Physiological function of connective tissue polysaccharides. Physiol Rev 58:225, 1978.
12. Epstein M, Saruta T: Effect of water immersion on renin-aldosterone and renal sodium handling in normal man. J Appl Physiol 31:368, 1971.
13. Epstein M: Cardiovascular and renal effects of head-out water immersion in man. Circ Res 39:619, 1976.
14. Kaczmarczyk G, Drake A, Eisele R, et al: The role of the cardiac nerves in the regulation of sodium excretion of conscious dogs. Pfluegers Arch 390:125, 1981.
15. Gillespie DS, Sandberg RL, Koike TI: Dual effect of left atrial receptors on excretion of sodium and water. Am J Physiol 225:706, 1973.
16. Wennergren G, Henrikson BA, Weiss LB, et al: Effects of stimulation of nonmedullated cardiac afferents on renal water and sodium excretion. Acta Physiol Scand 97:261, 1076.
17. Stitzer SO, Malvin RL: Right atrium and renal sodium excretion. Am J Physiol 228:184, 1975.
18. Epstein FH, Post RS, McDowell M: Effects of an arteriovenous fistula on renal haemodynamics and electrolyte excretion. J Clin Invest 32:233, 1953.
19. Taylor RR, Covell JW, Ross J Jr: Left ventricular function in experimental aorto-caval fistula with circulatory congestion and fluid retention. J Clin Invest 47:1333, 1968.
20. Guyton AC, Scanlon CJ, Armstrong GG: Effects of pressoreceptor reflex and Cushing's reflex on urinary output. Fed Proc 11:61, 1952.

21. Keeler R: Natriuresis after unilateral stimulation of carotid receptors in unanaesthetised rats. Am J Physiol 226:507, 1974.
22. Daly JJ, Roe JW, Horrocks P: A comparison of sodium excretion following the infusion of saline into systemic and portal veins in the dog. Evidence for a hepatic role in the control of sodium excretion. Clin Sci 33:481, 1967.
23. Olsson K: Further evidence for the importance of cerebrospinal fluid sodium concentration in central control of fluid balance. Acta Physiol Scand 88:183, 1973.
24. Martino JA, Earley LE: Demonstration of the role of physical factors as determinants of natriuretic response to volume expansion. J Clin Invest 46:1963, 1967.
25. Schrier RW, McDonald KM, Marshall RA, et al: Absence of natriuretic response to acute hypotonic intravascular volume expansion in dogs. Clin Sci 34:57, 1968.
26. Shrier RW, Fein RL, McNeil JS, et al: Influence of interstitial fluid volume expansion and plasma sodium concentration on the natriuretic response to volume expansion in the dog. Clin Sci 36:371, 1969.
27. Orloff J, Blake WD: Effects of concentrated salt poor albumin on metabolism and excretion of water and electrolyte in dogs. Am J Physiol 164:167, 1951.
28. Paintal AS: Vagal sensory receptors and their reflex effects. Physiol Rev 53:159, 1973.
29. Howards SS, Davis BB, Knox FG, et al: Depression of fractional sodium reabsorption by the proximal tubule of the dog without sodium diuresis. J Clin Invest 47:1561, 1968.
30. Stein JH, Osgood RW, Boonjaraern S, et al: A comparison of the segmental analysis of sodium reabsorption during Ringer's and hyperoncotic albumin infusion in the rat. J Clin Invest 52:2313, 1973.
31. Corradi A, Arendshorst WJ: Influence of renal nerves and prostaglandins in renal haemodynamic responses to elevated renal venous pressures in the rat (abstract). Fed Proc 41:1256, 1982.
31a. Francisco LL, Hoverton LG, DiBona GF: Renal nerves in the compensatory adaptation to ureteral occlusion. Am J Physiol 238:F229, 1980.
31b. Moss NG: Renal function and renal afferent and efferent nerve activity. Am J Physiol 243:F425, 1982.
32. Crawford EJ, Ludermann H: The renal response to intravenous injection of sodium chloride solutions in man. J Clin Invest 30:1456, 1951.
33. Black DAK, Platt R, Stanbury SW: Regulation of sodium excretion in normal and salt-depleted subjects. Clin Sci 9:205, 1950.
34. Rector FC Jr, van Giesen G, Kiil F, et al: Influence of expansion of extracellular volume on tubular reabsorption of sodium independent of changes in glomerular filtration rate and aldosterone activity. J Clin Invest 43:341, 1964.
35. Lindheimer MD, Lalone RC, Levinsky NG: Evidence that an acute increase in glomerular filtration has little effect on sodium excretion in the dog unless extracellular volume is expanded. J Clin Invest 46:256, 1967.
36. Dirks JH, Cirksena WJ, Berliner RW: The effect of saline infusion on sodium reabsorption by the proximal tubule of the dog. J Clin Invest 44:1160, 1965.
37. Weiner M, Wenman E, Kashgarian M, et al: Accelerated reabsorption in the proximal tubule produced by volume depletion. J Clin Invest 50:1379, 1971.
38. Burg MB: Renal handling of sodium, chloride, water, amino acids and glucose. In Brenner BM, Rector FC Jr (eds): The Kidney ed 2., 1981, p. 328.
39. Burg M, Green N: Bicarbonate transport by isolated perfused rabbit proximal convoluted tubules. Am J Physiol 233:F307, 1977.
40. Murer H, Hopfer V, Kinne R: Sodium proton antiport in brush border membrane vesicles isolated from rat small intestine and kidney. Biochem J 154:547, 1976.
41. Kinne R: Properties of the glucose transport system in the renal brush border membrane. Curr Topics Membr Transpt 8:, 1976.
42. Evers J, Murer H, Kinne R: Phenylalamine uptake in isolated renal brush border vesicles. Biochim Biophys Acta 426:598, 1976.
43. Burg M, Patlak C, Green N, et al: Organic solutes in fluid absorption by renal proximal convoluted tubules. Am J Physiol 231:627, 1976.
44. Burg MB, Orloff J: Electrical potential differences across proximal convoluted tubules. Am J Physiol 219:1714, 1970.
45. Giebisch G, Windhager E: Electrolyte transport across tubular membranes. In Orloff J, Berliner RW (eds): Handbook of Physiology. Washington, D.C., American Physiological Society, 1973, p 315.
46. Kokko J: Proximal tubule potential difference. Dependence on glucose, HCO_3 and amino acids. J Clin Invest 52:1362, 1973.
47. Diamond J, Bossert W: Standing-gradient osmotic flow. A mechanism for coupling of water and solute transport in epithelia. J Gen Physiol 50:2061, 1967.
48. Martino JA, Earley LE: Relationship between intrarenal hydrostatic pressure and haemodynamically induced changes in sodium excretion. Circ Res 23:371, 1968.
49. Brenner BM, Falchuk KH, Keimowitz RI, et al: Relationship between peritubular capillary colloid osmotic pressure and sodium reabsorption by the renal proximal tubule. Fourth Inte Congr Nephrol, Stockholm, 1969, p 324.
50. Spitzer A, Windhager EE: Effect of peritubular oncotic pressure changes on proximal tubular fluid reabsorption. Am J Physiol 218.1188, 1970.
51. Berry CA, Cogan MG: Influence of peritubular protein on solute absorption in the rabbit proximal tubule. A specific effect on Na Cl transport. J Clin Invest 68:506, 1981.
52. Berry CA: Lack of effect of peritubular protein on passive Na Cl transport in the rabbit proximal tubule. J Clin Invest 71:268, 1983.
53. de Wardener HE: The control of sodium excretion. In Orloff J, Berliner RW (eds): Handbook of Physiology. Washington, D.C., American Physiological Society, 1973, p. 677.
54. Burg M, Patlak C, Green N, et al: The role of organic solutes in fluid absorption by renal proximal convoluted tubules. Am J Physiol 231:627, 1976.
55. Ichikawa I, Hoyer JR, Seiler MW, et al: Mechanism of glomerulotubular balance in the setting of heterogeneous glomerular injury: preservation of a close functional linkage between individual nephrons and surrounding microvasculature. J Clin Invest 69:185, 1982.
56. Daugharty TM, Belleau LJ, Martino JA, et al: Interrelationship of physical factors affecting sodium reabsorption in the dog. Am J Physiol 215:1442, 1968.
57. Stein JH, Congbalay RC, Karsh DL, et al: The effect of bradykinin on proximal tubular sodium reabsorption in the dog: evidence for functional nephron heterogeneity. J Clin Invest 51:1709, 1972.
58. Lee MR: Dopamine and the kidney. Clin Sci 62:439, 1982.
59. Veress AT, Chang CK, Sonnenberg H: Effect of acute unilateral renal denervation on intrarenal haemodynamics and urinary excretion in rats before and during hypovolaemia. Clin Sci 62:457, 1982.
60. Wright FS, Briggs JP: Feedback regulation of glomerular filtration rate. Am J Physiol 233:F1, 1977.
61. Schnermann J, Ploth DW, Hermle M: Activation of tubuloglomerular feedback by chloride transport. Pfluegers Arch 362:229, 1976.
62. Stowe NT, Schnermann J: Renin-angiotensin mediation of tubulo-glomerular feedback control of filtration rate (abstract). Fed Proc 33:347, 1974.
63. Ichikawa I: Direct analysis of the effector mechanism of the tubuloglomerular feedback system. Am J Physiol 243:F447, 1982.
64. Knight TF, Weinman EJ: Renal sodium reabsorption following induction of and recovery from volume expansion. Am J Physiol 233:F416, 1977.
65. Reineck HJ, Parma R: Effect of medullary tonicity on urinary sodium excretion in the rat. J Clin Invest 69:971, 1982.
66. Sonnenberg H: Medullary collecting duct function in antidiuretic and in salt or water diuretic rats. Am J Physiol 226:501, 1974.
67. Sonnenberg H: Secretion of salt and water into the medullary collecting duct of Ringer-infused rats. Am J Physiol 228:565, 1975.
68. Shipley RE, Study RS: Factors regulating renal blood flow and urine flow following acute changes in renal artery perfusion pressure (abstract). Am J Physiol 163:750, 1950.
69. Selkurt EE: Effect of pulse pressure and mean arterial pressure modification on renal haemodynamics and electrolyte and water excretion. Circulation 4:541, 1951.
70. Fitzgibbons JP, Gennari FJ, Garfunkel HB, et al: Dependence of saline-induced natriuresis upon exposure of the kidney to the physical effects of extracellular fluid volume expansion. J Clin Invest 54:1428, 1974.
71. Osgood RW, Lameire NH, Sorkin MI, et al: Effect of aortic clamping on proximal reabsorption and sodium excretion in the rat. Am J Physiol 232:F92, 1977.
72. Gennari FJ, Lefavour GS, Caflisch CR, et al: Identification of two components in the natriuretic response to saline loading in the rat. Am J Physiol 235:F126, 1978.
73. Ichikawa I, Rennke HG, Hoyer JR, et al: Role for intrarenal mechanisms in the impaired salt excretion of experimental nephrotic syndrome. J Clin Invest 71:91, 1983.
74. Earley LE, Friedler RM: Changes in renal blood flow and possibly the intrarenal distribution of blood during the natriuresis accompanying saline loading in the dog. J Clin Invest 44:929, 1965.
75. Bruns FJ, Alexander EA, Riley AL, et al: Superficial and juxtamedullary nephron function during saline loading in the dog. J Clin Invest 53:971, 1974.
76. Banks RO: Intrarenal blood flow distribution: effect of carotid occlusion. Proc Soc Exp Biol Med 150:327, 1975.
77. Mandin H, Israelit AH, Rector FC Jr, et al: Effect of saline infusions on intrarenal distribution of glomerular filtrate and proximal reabsorption in the dog. J Clin Invest 50:514, 1971.
78. Carriere S, Boulet P, Mathieu A, et al: Isotonic saline loading and intrarenal distribution of glomerular filtration in dogs. Kidney Int 2:191, 1972.
79. Schneider EG, Lynch RE, Willis LR, et al: Single-nephron filtration rate in the dog. Am J Physiol 222:667, 1972.
80. Applegate CW, Gutman RA: Renal intracortical blood flow distribution, function and sodium excretion in response to saline loading of anesthetized and unanesthetized dogs. Pfluegers Arch 336:125, 1976.
81. Mitchell GAG: The nerve supply of the kidneys. Acta Anat 10:1, 1950.
82. Bello-Reuss E, Colindres RE, Pastoriza-Munoz E, et al: Effects of acute unilateral denervation in the rat. J Clin Invest 56:208, 1975.
83. LaGrange RG, Sloop CH, Schmid HE: Selective stimulation of renal nerves in the anaesthetised dog. Circulation Res 33:704, 1973.
84. Slick GL, Aquileva AJ, Zambraksi EJ, et al: Renal neuroadrenergic transmission. Am J Physiol 229:60, 1975.

85. Slick GL, Di Bona GF, Kaloyanides GJ: Renal sympathetic nerve activity in sodium retention of acute caval constriction. Am J Physiol 226:925, 1974.
86. Dunham EW, Zimmerman BG: Release of prostaglandin-like material from dog kidney during nerve stimulation. Am J Physiol 219:1279, 1970.
87. Zambraksi EJ, DiBona GF: Angiotensin II in antinatriuresis of low level renal nerve stimulation. Am J Physiol 231:1105, 1976.
88. DiBona GF, Zambraksi EJ, Aquilera AJ, et al: Neurogenic control of renal tubular sodium reabsorption in the dog. Circulation Res 40:(suppl I)I127, 1977.
89. DiBona GF: Neurogenic regulation of renal tubular sodium reabsorption. Am J Physiol 233:F73, 1977.
90. Moss NG: Renal function and renal afferent and efferent nerve activity. Am J Physiol 243:F425, 1982.
91. Schwartz GJ, Burg MB: Mineralocorticoid effects on cation transport by cortical collecting ducts in vitro. Am J Physiol 235:F576, 1978.
92. Ullrich KJ, Papavassiliou F: Sodium reabsorption in the papillary collecting duct of rats. Effect of adrenalectomy, low Na^+ diet, acetazolamide, HCO-3 free solutions, and amiloride. Pfluegers Arch 379:49, 1979.
93. Feldman D, Funder J, Edelman I: Subcellular mechanisms in the action of adrenal steroids. Am J Med 53:545, 1972.
94. Hierholzer K, Lange S: The effects of adrenal steroids on renal function. In MTP International Review of Science Physiology, Baltimore, University Park Press, 1974, vol 6, p 273.
95. Laragh JH, Sealey J, Brunner HR: The control of aldosterone secretion in normal and hypertensive man: abnormal renin-aldosterone patterns in low renin hypertension. Am J Med 53:649, 1972.
96. August JT, Nelson DH, Thorn GW: Response of normal subjects to large amounts of aldosterone. J Clin Invest 37:1549, 1958.
97. Young DB, McCaa RE, Pan Y-J, et al: Effectiveness of the aldosterone-sodium and potassium feedback control system. Am J Physiol 231:945, 1976.
98. Young DB, Guyton AC: Steady state aldosterone dose-response relationships. Circ Res 40:138, 1977.
99. Tannenbaum J, Splawinski JA, Oates JA, et al: Enhanced renal prostaglandin production in the dog. I. Effects on renal function. Circ Res 36:197, 1975.
100. Dunn MJ, Zambraski ED: Renal effects of drugs that inhibit prostaglandin synthesis. Kidney Intl8:609, 1980.
101. Haycock GB, Al-Dahhan J, Mak R, et al: Effect of indomethacin on clinical progress and renal function in cystinosis. Arch Dis Child 57:934, 1982.
102. Kaojarera S, Chennavasin P, Anderson, et al: Nephron site of effect of nonsteroidal antiinflammatory drugs on solute excretion in humans. Am J Physiol 244:F134, 1983.
103. Muther RS, Potter DM, Bennett WM: Aspirin-induced depression of glomerular filtration rate in normal humans: role of sodium balance. Ann Intern Med 94:317, 1981.
104. Henrich WL, Berl T, McDonald KM, et al: Angiotensin II, renal nerves and prostaglandins in renal hemodynamics during hemorrhage. Am J Physiol 235:F46, 1978.
105. Zusman RM, Keiser HR: Prostaglandin E2 biosynthesis by rabbit renomedullary interstitial cells in tissue culture. J Biol Chem 252:2069, 1977.
106. Kokko JP: Effect of prostaglandins on renal epithelial electrolyte transport. Kidney Int 19:791, 1981.
107. Jacobsen WE, Hammarsten JF, Heller BI: The effects of adrenaline upon renal function and electrolyte excretion. J Clin Invest 30:1503, 1951.
108. McDonald RH Jr, Goldsberg LI, McNay JL, et al: Effects of dopamine in man: augmentation of sodium excretion glomerular filtration rate and renal plasma flow. J Clin Invest 43:1116, 1964.
109. Lee MR: Dopamine and the kidney. Clin Sci 62:439, 1982.
110. Smythe CM, Nickel JF, Bradley SE: The effect of epinephrine (USP), l-epinephrine and l-norepinephrine on glomerular filtration rate, renal plasma flow and the urinary excretion of sodium, potassium and water in normal man. J Clin Invest 31:499, 1952.
111. Carriere S: Influence de la circulation dans la medullaire du rein sur le gradient de concentration osmolaire. Union Med Canada 95:536, 1966.
112. Eble JN: A proposed mechanism for the depressor effect of dopamine in the anaesthetized dog. J Pharm Exp Ther 145:65, 1964.
113. Bennett ED, Tighe D, Wegg W: Abolition by dopamine blockade, of the natriuretic response produced by lower-body positive pressure. Clin Sci 63:361, 1982.
114. Gill JR, Bartter FC: Adrenergic nervous system in sodium metabolism. II. Effects of guanethidine on the renal response to sodium deprivation in normal man. N Engl J Med 275:1466, 1966.
115. Alexander RW, Gill JR, Yamabe H, et al: Effect of dietary sodium and of acute saline infusion on the interrelationship between dopamine excretion and adrenergic activity in man. J Clin Invest 54:194, 1974.
116. Casson IF, Lee MR, Brownjohn AM, et al: Failure of renal dopamine response to salt loading in chronic renal disease. Brit Med J 286:503, 1983.
117. Finlay GD, Whitsett TL, Cucinell EA, et al: Augmentation of sodium and potassium excretion, glomerular filtration and renal plasma flow by levodopa. N Engl J Med 284:865, 1971.
118. Ball SG, Gunn IG, Douglas IHS: Renal handling of dopa, dopamine, norepinephrine and epinephrine in the dog. Am J Physiol 242:F56, 1982.
119. Scicli AG, Gandolfi R, Carretero OA: Site of formation of kinins in the dog nephron. Am J Physiol 234:F36, 1978.
120. Webster ME, Gilmore JP: Influence of kallidin-10 on renal function. Am J Physiol 206:714, 1964.
121. Barraclough MA, Mills IH: Effect of bradykinin on renal function. Clin Sci 28:69, 1965.
122. Stein JH, Congbalay RC, Karsh DL, et al: The effect of bradykinin on proximal tubular sodium reabsorption in the dog: evidence for functional nephron heterogeneity. J Clin Invest 51:1709, 1972.
123. McGiff JC, Terragno NA, Malik KO: Release of prostaglandin E-like substance from canine kidney by bradykinin. Circ Res 31:36, 1972.
124. Obika LFO, Mills IH: Effect of arterial infusion of prostaglandin E1 on the release of renal kallikrein. J Endocrinol 69:45P, 1976.
125. Margolius HS, Horwitz D, Geller RG: Urinary kallikrein excretion in normal man: relationship to sodium intake and sodium-retaining steroids. Circ Res 35:812, 1974.
126. de Wardener HE, Mills IH, Clapham WF, et al: Studies on the efferent mechanism of the sodium diuresis which follows the administration of intravenous saline in the dog. Clin Sci 21:249, 1961.
127. Bahlmann JS, McDonald SJ, Ventom MG, et al: The effect of urinary sodium excretion of blood volume expansion without changing the composition of blood in the dog. Clin Sci 32:403, 1967.
128. Kaloyanides GJ, Azer M: Evidence of a humoral mechanism in volume expansion natriuresis. J Clin Invest 50:1603, 1971.
129. Bengele HH, Houttuin E, Pearce JW: Volume natriuresis without renal nerves and renal vascular pressure rise in the dog. Am J Physiol 223:68, 1972.
130. Lichardus B, Nizet A: Water and sodium excretion after blood volume expansion under conditions of constant arterial, venous and plasma oncotic pressures and constant haematocrit. Clin Sci 42:701, 1972.
131. Tobian L, Coffee K, McCrea P: Evidence for a humoral factor of non-renal and non-adrenal origin which influences renal sodium excretion. Trans Assoc Am Phys 80:200, 1967.
132. Epstein M, Bricker NS, Bourgoignie JJ: Presence of a natriuretic factor in urine of normal men undergoing water immersion. Kidney Intl 13:152, 1978.
133. Pearce JW, Sonnenberg H, Veress AT, et al: Evidence for a humoral factor modifying the renal response to blood volume expansion in the rat. Can J Physiol Pharmacol 47:377, 1969.
134. Slatopolsky E, Elkan IO, Weerts C, et al: Studies on the characteristics of the control system governing sodium excretion in uremic man. J Clin Invest 47:521, 1968.
135. Bourgoignie JJ, Hwang KH, Espinel CS, et al: A natriuretic factor in the serum of patients with chronic uremia. J Clin Invest 51:1514, 1972.
136. Bourgoignie JJ, Hwang KH, Ipakchi E, et al: The presence of a natriuretic factor in urine of patients with chronic uremia; the absence of the factor in nephrotic uremic patients. J Clin Invest 53:1559, 1974.
137. Schmidt RW, Bourgoignie JJ, Bricker NS: On the adaptation in sodium excretion in chronic uremia. The effects of a "proportional reduction" of sodium intake. J Clin Invest 53:1736, 1974.
138. Nutbourne DM, Howse JD, Schrier RW, et al: The effect of expanding the blood volume of a dog on the short circuit current across an isolated frog skin incorporated in the dog's circulation. Clin Sci 38:629, 1970.
139. Buckalew VM, Martinez FJ, Green WE: The effects of dialysates and ultrafiltrates of plasma of saline loaded dogs on toad bladder sodium transport. J Clin Invest 49:926, 1970.
140. Clarkson EM, de Wardener HE: Inhibition of sodium and potassium transport in separated renal tubule fragments incubated in extracts of urine obtained from salt loaded individuals. Clin Sci 42:607, 1972.
141. Poston L, Wilkinson SP, Williams P: Sodium transport in peripheral blood leucoytes as a possible assay for natriuretic hormone. Clin Sci 6:25P, 1979.
142. Gonick HC, Kramer HJ, Paul W, et al: Circulating inhibitor of sodium-potassium activated adenosine triphosphatase after expansion of extracellular fluid volume in rats. Clin Sci Mol Med 53:329, 1977.
143. de Wardener HE, MacGregor GA, Clarkson EM, et al: Effect of sodium intake on ability of human plasma to inhibit renal Na^+-K^+ ATPase (adenosine triphosphatase) in vitro. Lancet I:411, 1981.
144. Fenton S, Clarkson EM, MacGregor GA, et al: An assay of the capacity of biological fluids to stimulate renal glucose-6-phosphate dehydrogenase (G6PD) activity in vitro as a marker of their ability to inhibit sodium-potassium dependent adenosine triphosphatase (Na^+-K^+-ATPase) activity. J Endocrinol 94:99, 1982.
145. Fine LG, Bourgoignie JJ, Weber H, et al: Enhanced end-organ responsiveness of the uremic kidney to the natriuretic factor. Kidney Intl 10:364, 1976.
145a. Atlas SA, Kleinert HD, Camargo MJ, et al: Purification, sequencing and synthesis of natriuretic and vasoactive rat atrial peptide. Nature 309:717, 1984.

145b. Saguella GA, MacGregor GA: Cardiac peptides and the control of sodium excretion. Nature 309:666, 1984.
145c. Chimosky JE, Spielman WS, Brandt MA, et al: Cardiac atria of BIO 14.6 hamsters are deficient in natriuretic factor. Science 223:820, 1984.
146. Clarkson EM, Raw SM, de Wardener HE: Two natriuretic substances in extracts of urine from normal man when salt-depleted and salt loaded. Kidney Intl 10:381, 1976.
147. Clarkson EM, Young DR, Raw SM, et al: Chemical properties, physiological action and further separation of a low molecular weight natriuretic substance in the urine of normal man. In Lichardus B, Schrier RW, Ponec J, (Eds): Hormonal Regulation of Sodium Excretion. Amsterdam, Elsevier/North Holland Biomedical Press, 1980, p. 333.
148. Gruber KA, Whitaker JM, Buckalew VM Jr: Endogenous digitalis like substance in plasma of volume expanded dogs. Nature 287:743, 1980.
149. Clarkson EM, Koutsaimanis KG, Davidman M, et al: The effect of brain extracts on urinary sodium excretion of the rat and the intracellular sodium concentration of renal tubule fragments. Clin Sci Mol Med 47:201, 1974.
150. Keeler R: Effect of hypothalamic lesions on renal excretion of sodium. Am J Physiol 197:874, 1959.
151. Lennane RJ, Peart WS, Carey RM, et al: A comparison of natriuresis after oral and intravenous sodium loading in sodium depleted rabbits: evidence for a gastrointestinal or portal monitor of sodium intake. Clin Sci Mol Med 49:433, 1975.
152. Passo SS, Thornborough JR, Rothballer AB: Hepatic receptors in control of sodium excretion in anaesthetised cats. Am J Physiol 224:373, 1973.
153. Katz AL, Lindheimer MD: Actions of hormones on the kidney. Annu Rev Physiol 39:97, 1977.
153a. Holliday MA, Kalayce MN, Harrah J: Factors that limit brain volume changes in response to acute and sustained hyper- and hyponatremia. J Clin Invest 47:1916, 1968.
153b. Kregenow FM: The response of duck erythiocytes to non hemolytic hypotomic media. Evidence for a volume controlling mechanism. J Gen Physiol 58:372, 1971.
153c. Grantham JJ, Lowe CM, Dellesega M, et al: Effect of hyptonic medium on K and Na content of proximal renal tubules. Am J Physiol 232:F42, 1977.
153d. Edelman IS, Leibman J, O'Meara MP, et al: Interrelations between serum sodium concentration, serum osmolarity and total exchangable sodium total exchangable potassium and total body water. J Clin Invest 39:1236, 1958.
154. Scholander PF: The Wonderful net. Sci Am 196(4):96, 1957.
155. Kuhn W, Ryffel K: Herstellung knozentrierte Losungen aus verdunnten durch blosse Membranewirkung: ein Modellversuch zur funcktion der niere. Ztschr Physiol Chem 276:148, 1942.
156. Wirz H, Hargitay B, Kuhn W: Lokalisation des Konzentrierungsprozesses in der Niere durch direkte Kryoscopie. Helv Pharmacol Acta 196, 1951.
157. Gottschalk CW, Mylle M: Micropuncture study of the mammalian urinary concentrating mechanism: evidence for the countercurrent hypothesis. Am J Physiol 196:927, 1959.
158. Bray G: Freezing point depression of rat kidney slices during water diuresis and antidiuresis. Am J Physiol 199:915, 1960.
159. Lassiter WE,Gottschalk CW, Mylle M: Micropuncture study of net transtubular movement of water and urea in nondiuretic mammalian kidney. Am J Physiol 200:1139, 1961.
160. Windhager EE, Giesbisch G: Micropuncture study of renal tubular transfer of sodium chloride in the rat. Am J Physiol 200:581, 1961.
161. Burg MB, Green N: Function of thick ascending limb of Henle's loop. Am J Physiol 224:659, 1973.
162. Rocha AS, Kokko JP: Sodium chloride and water transport in the medullary thick ascending limb of Henle. J Clin Invest 52:612, 1973.
163. Stephenson JL: Concentration in renal counterflow systems. Biophys J 6:537, 1966.
164. Imai M, Kokko JP: Sodium chloride, urea and water transport in the thin ascending limb of Henle: generation of osmotic gradient by passive diffusion of solute. J Clin Invest 53:393, 1974.
165. Morgan T, Berliner RW: Permeability of the loop of Henle vasa recta and collecting duct to water, urea and sodium. Am J Physiol 215:108, 1968.
166. Imai M, Kokko JP: Mechanism of sodium and chloride transport in the thin ascending limb of Henle. J Clin Invest 58:1054, 1976.
167. Imai M: Function of the thin ascending limb of Henle in rats and hamsters perfused in vivo. Am J Physiol 232:F201, 1977.
168. Windhager EE: Electrophysiological study of renal papilla of golden hamsters. Am J Physiol 206:694, 1964.
169. Jamison RL, Bennett CM, Berliner RW: Countercurrent multiplication by the thin loops of Henle. Am J Physiol 212:357, 1967.
170. Marsh DJ: Solute and water flows in thin limbs of Henle's loop in the hamster kidney. Am J Physiol 218:824, 1970.
171. Marsh DJ, Azen SP: Mechanism of Na Cl reabsorption by hamster thin ascending limb of Henle's loops. Am J Physiol 228:71, 1975.
172. Marsh DJ, Martin CM: Origin of electrical PD's in hamster thin ascending limbs of Henle's loop. Am J Physiol 232:F348, 1977.
173. Gamble JL, McKhann CF, Butler AM, et al: An economy of water in renal function referable to urea. Am J Physiol 109:139, 1934.
174. Crawford JD, Doyle AP, Probst J: Service of urea in renal water conservation. Am J Physiol 196:545, 1959.
175. Levinsky NG, Berliner RW: The role of urea in the urinary concentrating mechanism. J Clin Invest 38:741, 1959.
176. Bray GA, Preston AS: Effect of urea on urine concentration in the rat. J Clin Invest 40:1952, 1961.
177. Rabinowitz L, Thompson B, Wagman RB: Effect of acute urea administration on urinary nonurea solute concentration. Am J Physiol 221:242, 1971.
178. Edelmann CM Jr, Barnett HL, Troupkou V: Renal concentrating mechanisms in newborn infants. Effect of dietary protein and water content, role of urea, and responsiveness to antidiuretic hormone. J Clin Invest 39:1062, 1960.
179. Shannon JA: Glomerular filtration and urea excretion in relation to urine flow in dog. Am J Physiol 117:206, 1936.
180. Chasis H, Smith HW: The excretion of urea in normal man and in subjects with glomerulonephritis. J Clin Invest 17:347, 1938.
181. Klumper JD, Ullrich KJ, Hilger HH: Das Verhalten des Harnstoffs in den Sammelrohren der Saugertierniere. Pfluegers Arch 267:238, 1958.
182. Marsh DJ, Martin CM: Lack of water or urea movement from pelvic urine to pailla in hydropaenic hamsters. Miner Electrolyte Metab 3:81, 1980.
183. Stephenson JL: Concentration of urine in a central core model of the renal counterflow system. Kidney Intl 2:85, 1972.
184. Kokko JP, Rector FC: Countercurrent multiplication system without active transport in inner medulla. Kidney Intl 2:214, 1972.
185. Gottschalk CW: Osmotic concentration and dilution of the urine. Am J Med 36:670, 1964.
186. Marsh DJ, Solomon S: Analysis of electrolyte movement in thin Henle's loop of hamster papilla. Am J Physiol 208:1119, 1965.
187. de Rouffignac C, Morel F: Micropuncture study of water, electrolytes and urea movements along the loops of Henle in Psammomys. J Clin Invest 48:474, 1969.
188. Jamison RL, Buerkert J, Lacy F: A micropuncture study of Henle's thin loop in Brattleboro rats. Am J Physiol 224:180, 1973.
189. Pennell JP, Lacy FB, Jamison RJ: An in vivo study of the concentrating process in the descending limb of Henle's loop. Kidney Intl 5:337, 1974.
190. Imbert M, de Rouffignac C: Rate of sodium and urea in the renal concentrating mechanism of Psammomys obesus. Pfluegers Arch 361:107, 1976.
191. Stoner LC, Roch-Ramel F: The effects of pressure on the water permeability of the descending limb of Henle's loops of rabbits. Pfluegers Arch 382:7, 1979.
192. Bonventre JV, Lechene CP: Renal medullary concentrating process: an integrative hypothesis. Am J Physiol 239:F578, 1980.
192a. Stephenson JL, Kriz W, Jamison RL, et al: Symposium on the renal concentrating mechanism. Fed Proc 42:2377, 1983.
192b. Bonventre JV, Roman RJ, Lechene C: Effect of urea concentration of pelvic fluid on renal concentrating ability. Am J Physiol 239:F609, 1980.
192c. Oliver RE, Roy DR, Jamison RL: Urinary concentration in the papillary collecting duct of the rat. Role of the ureter. J Clin Invest 69:157, 1982.
193. du Vigneaud V: Hormones of the posterior pituitary gland: oxytocin and vasopressin. Harvey Lectures Ser 50:1, 1954–55.
194. Farini F: Diabete inspido ed opoterapia. Gazz Osped Clin 34:1135, 1913.
195. von den Velden R: Die Nierenwirkung von Hypophysenextracten beim Menschen. Berlin Klin Wchschr 50:2083, 1913.
196. Starling EH, Verney EB: The secretion of urine as studied in the isolated kidney. Proc Roy Soc London Ser B 97:321, 1924.
197. Chambers DH, Melville EV, Hare RS, et al: Regulation of the release of pituitrin by changes in the osmotic pressure of the plasma. Am J Physiol 144:311, 1945.
198. Verney EB: Absorption and excretion of water. The antidiuretic hormone. Lancet 2:739, 1946.
199. Venrey EB: The antidiuretic hormone and the factors which determine its release. Proc Roy Soc London Ser B 135:25, 1947.
200. Jewell PA, Verney EB: An experimental attempt to determine the site of the neurohypophyseal osmoreceptors in the dog. Phil Trans Roy Soc Lond Ser B 240:197, 1957.
201. Olivecrona H: Paraventricular nucleus and pituitary gland. Acta Physiol Scand (suppl) 136:1, 1957.
202. Andersson B: Regulation of water intake. Physiol Rev 58:582, 1978.
203. McKinley MJ, Denton DA, Weisinger RS: Sensors for antidiuresis and thirst-osmoreceptors or CSF sodium detectors? Brain Res 141:89, 1978.
204. Beardwell CG: Radioimmunoassay of arginine vasopressin in human plasma. J Clin Endo Metab 33:254, 1971.
205. Thrasher TN, Brown CJ, Keil LC, et al: Thirst and vasopressin release in the dog: an osmoreceptor or sodium receptor mechanism. Am J Physiol 238:R333, 1980.

206. Thrasher TN, Jones RG, Kent LC, et al: Drinking and vasopressin release during ventricular infusions of hypertonic solutions. Am J Physiol 238:R340, 1980.
207. Andersson B, Olsson K, Warner RG: Dissimilarities between the central control of thirst and the release of antidiuretic hormone (ADH). Acta Physiol Scand 71:57, 1967.
208. Olsson K: Studies on central regulation of secretion of antidiuretic hormone (ADH) in the goat. Acta Physiol Scand 77:465, 1969.
209. Olsson K: Effects of slow infusions of K Cl into the 3rd brain ventricle. Acta Physiol Scand 77:358, 1969.
210. Bie P: Osmoreceptors, vasopressin and control of renal water excretion. Physiol Rev 60:961, 1980.
211. Sladek CD, Knigge KM: Osmotic control of vasopressin release by rat hypothalamo-neurhypophyseal explants in organ culture. Endocrinology 101:1834, 1977.
212. Ishikawa S, Saito T, Yoshida S: The effect of osmotic pressure and angiotensin 11 on arginine vasopressin release from guinea pig hypothalamo-neurohypophyseal complex in organ culture. Endocrinology 106:
213. Habevich FJ: Osmoreception in the portal circulation. Fed Proc 27:1137, 1968.
214. Lydtin H: Untersuchungen uber Mechanismen der Osmo und Volumen regulation 11. Untersuchungen uber den Einfluss intravenos intraportal und oral zugefuhrter hypotoner Kochsalzlosungen auf die Diurese des Hundes. Z Gesaute Exp Med 149:193, 1969.
215. Velikanova LK, Finkinshtein ID: Osmoreceptors in the liver. Sechenov Physioll J (USSR) 45:66, 1959.
216. Robertson GL, Mahr EA, Athar S, et al: Development and clinical application of a new method for the radioimmunoassay of arginine vasopressin in human plasma. J Clin Invest 52:2340, 1974.
217. Robertson GI, Shelton RL, Athar S: The osmoregulation of vasopressin. Kidney Intl 10:25, 1976.
218. Weitman RE, Fisher DA: Log linear relationship between plasma arginine vasopressin and plasma osmolality. Am J Physiol 233:E37, 1977.
219. Rodbard D, Munson PJ: Is there an osmotic threshold for vasopressin release? Am J Physiol 234:E339, 1978.
220. Dunn FL, Brennan TJ, Nelson AE, et al: The role of blood osmolality and volume in regulating vasopressin secretion in the rat. J Clin Invest 52:3212, 1973.
221. Robertson GL, Kinney RA, Nelson AE: The effect of isoproterenol on vasopressin secretion. Endocrinology 94:(suppl) 217:A164, 1974.
222. Smythe CM, Nickel JF, Bradley SE: The effect of epinephrine (USP) l-epinephrine and l-norepinephrine on glomerular filtration rate, renal plasma flow and the urinary excretion of sodium, potassium and water in normal man. J Clin Invest 31:499, 1952.
223. Baldwin DS, Gambos EA, Chasis H: Changes in sodium and water excretion induced by epinephrine and l-norepinephrine in normotensive and hypertensive subjects. J Lab Clin Med 61:832, 1963.
224. Libermann B, Klein LA, Kleeman CR: Effect of adrenergic blocking agents on the vasopressin-inhibiting action of norepinephrine. Proc Soc Exp Biol Med 133:131, 1970.
225. Klein LA, Libermann B, Laks M, et al: Interrelated effects of antidiuretic hormone and adrenergic drugs on water metabolism. Am J Physiol 221:1657, 1971.
226. Schrier RW, Berl T: Mechanism of effect of alpha adrenergic stimulation with norepinephrine on renal water excretion. J Clin Invest 52:502, 1973.
227. Berl T, Harbottle JA, Schrier RW: Effect of alpha- and beta adrenergic stimulation with isoproterenol. J Clin Invest 53:857, 1974.
228. McDonald KM, Kuruvila KC, Aisenbrey GA, et al: Effect of alpha- and betadrenergic stimulation on renal water excretion and medullary tissue cyclic AMP in intact and diabetes insipidus rats. Kidney Intl 12:96, 1977.
229. Berl T, Cadnapaphornchai P, Harbottle JA, et al: Mechanism of suppression of vasopressin during alphaadrenergic stimulation with norepinephrine. J Clin Invest 53:219, 1974.
230. Schrier RW, Lieberman R, Ufferman RC: Mechanism of antidiuretic effect of beta adrenergic stimulation. J Clin Invest 51:97, 1972.
231. Berl T, Cadnapaphornchai P, Harbottle JA, et al: Mechanism of stimulation of vasopressin release during beta-adrenergic stimulation with isoproterenol. J Clin Invest 53:857, 1974.
232. Anderson RJ, Pluss RG, Berns AS, et al: Mechanism of effect of hypoxia renal water excretion. J Clin Invest 62:769, 1978.
233. Robertson GL: The regulation of vasopressin function in health and disease. Rec Progr Hormone Res 23:333, 1977.
234. Hayward JN, Jennings DP: Influence of sleep-waking and nociceptor-induced behavior on the activity of supraoptic neurons in the hypothalamus of the monkey. Brain Res 57:461, 1973.
235. Cadnapaphornchai P, Boykin JL, Berl T, et al: Mechanism of effect of nicotine on renal water excretion. Am J Physiol 227:1216, 1974.
236. Torres-Pinedo R, Lavastida M, Rivera CL, et al: Studies on infant diarrhea: I. A. comparison of the effects of milk feeding and intravenous therapy upon the composition and volume of the stool and urine. J Clin Invest 45:469, 1966.
237. Darrow DC: The retention of electrolyte during recovery from severe dehydration due to diarrhoea. J Pediatr 28:515, 1946.
238. Mahalanabis D, Wallace CK, Kallen RJ, et al: Water and electrolyte losses due to cholera in infants and small children. A recovery balance study. Pediatrics 45:374, 1970.
239. Darrow DC, Pratt EL, Flett J Jr, et al: Disturbances of water and electrolytes in infantile diarrhoea. Pediatrics 3:129, 1949.
240. Mann MD, Bowie MD, Hansen JKL: Total body potassium, acid-base status and serum electrolytes in acute diarrhoeal disease. S African Med J 49:709, 1975.
241. Hirschhorn N: The treatment of acute diarrhea in children. An historical and physiological perspective. Am J Clin Nutr 33:637, 1980.
242. Kildeberg P: Metabolic acidosis in infantile gastroenteritis. Acta Paediat Scand 54:155, 1965.
243. Torres-Pionedo R, Conde E, Robillard G, et al: Studies on infants diarrhea III. Changes in composition of saline and glucose-saline solutions instilled into the colon. Pediatrics 42:303, 1968.
243a. Cheek DB: Changes in total chloride and acid-base balance in gastroenteritis following treatment with large and small loads of sodium chloride. Pediatrics 17:839, 1956.
244. Katcher AL, Levitt MF, Sweet AY, et al: Alterations in fluid and electrolyte distribution and renal function in diarrhea of infancy. J Clin Invest 32:1013, 1953.
245. Oparil S, Haber E: The renin-angiotensin system. N Engl J Med 291:389, 1974.
245a. Darrow DC, Yannet H: The changes in the distribution of body water accompanying increase and decrease in extracellular electrolyte. J Clin Invest 14:266, 1935.
246. Rapoport S: Hyperosmolality and hyperelectrolytemia in pathologic conditions of childhood. Amer J Dis Child 74:682, 1947.
247. Finberg L, Harrison HE: Hypernatraemia in infants. An evaluation of the clinical and biochemical findings accompanying this state. Pediatrics 16:1, 1955.
248. Colle E, Ayoub E, Raile R: Hypertonic dehydration (hypernatraemia): the role of feedings high in solutes. Pediatrics 22:5, 1958.
249. Ahmed I, Agusto-Odutola TB: Hypernatraemia in diarrhoeal infants in Lagos. Arch Dis Child 45:97, 1970.
250. Slone D, Levin SE: Hypertonic dehydration and summer diarrhoea. S African Med J 34:209, 1960.
251. Whaley P, Walker-Smith JA: Hypernatraemia and gastroenteritis. Lancet 1:51, 1977.
252. De Young VR, Diamond EF: Possibility of iatrogenic factors responsible for hypernatraemia in dehydrated infants. JAMA 173:1806, 1960.
253. Taitz LS, Byers HD: High caloric/osmolar feeding and hypertonic dehydration in infants. Arch Dis Childh 50:610, 1975.
254. Chambers TL, Steel AE: Concentrated milk feeds and their relation to hypernatraemic dehydration of infants. Arch Dis Childh 50:610, 1975.
255. Hirschhorn N, McCarthy BJ, Ranney B, et al: Ad libitum oral glucose electrolyte therapy for acute diarrhoea in Apache children. J Pediatr 83:562, 1973.
256. Sack DA, Chowdhury AMAK, Eusof A, et al: Oral hydration in rota-virus diarrhoea: a double blind comparison of sucrose with glucose-electrolyte solution. Lancet 2:280, 1978.
257. Santosham M, Daum RS, Dillman L, et al: Oral rehydration therapy of infantile diarrhoea: a controlled study of well-nourished children hospitalised in the United States and Panama. N Engl J Med 306:1070, 1982.
258. Davies DP: Protein intake, osmolality homeostasis and renal function in infancy. Postgrad Med J 51(suppl 3):25, 1975.
259. Hirschhorn N: The treatment of acute diarrhea in children. An Historical and Physiological perspective. Am J Clin Nutr 33:637, 1980.
260. Bruck E, Abal G, Aceto T: Pathogenesis and pathophysiology of hypertonic dehydration with diarrhoea. Am J Dis Child 115:122, 1968.
261. Finberg L: The possible role of the physician in causing hypernatraemia in infants dehydrated from diarrhoea. Pediatrics 22:2, 1958.
262. Ware S: Hypernatraemia and "glucose water" (letter). Lancet 1:494, 1976.
263. Franz MN, Segar WE: The association of various factors and hypernatremic diarrhoeal dehydration. Am J Dis Child 97:298, 1959.
264. Ramirez MA, Baetrl JM, De Martinez YA, et al: The effect of potassium and protein intakes on sodium homeostasis of infants and children. J Trop Pediatr 19:275, 1973.
265. Fleming BJ, Gennth SM, Gould AB: Laxative-induced hypokalemia, sodium depletion and hyper-reninemia. Effects of potassyue and sodium replacement on the renin-angiotensin-aldosterone system. Ann Int Med 83:60, 1975.
266. Nitzan M, Zelmanovsky S: Glucose intolerance in hypernatraemic rats. Diabetes 17:597, 1968.
267. Stevenson PE, Bowyer FP: Hyperglycemia with hyperosmolal dehydration in non-diabetic infants. J Pediatr 77:818, 1970.
268. Feig PV, McCurdy KK: The hypertonic state. N Engl J Med 297:1444, 1977.
269. McDowell ME, Wolf AV, Steer O: Osmotic volumes of distribution. Idiogenic changes in osmotic pressure associated with the administration of hypertonic solutions. Am J Physiol 180:545, 1955.

270. Finberg L, Luttrell C, Redd C: Pathogenesis of lesions in the central nervous system in hypernatraemic states. II. Experimental studies of gross anatomical changes and alterations of chemical composition of the tissues. Pediatrics23: 46, 1959.
270a. Sotos JF, Dodge PR, Meara P, et al: Studies in experimental hypertonicity. I. Pathogenesis of the clinical syndrome, biochemical abnormalities and cause of death. Pediatrics 26:925, 1960.
271. Ibsen B: Treatment of shock with vasodilators measuring skin temperature on the big toe. Ten years experience in 150 cases. Dis Chest 52:425, 1967.
272. Aynsley-Green A, Pickering D: Use of central and peripheral temperature measurement in care of the critically ill child. Arch Dis Child 49:477, 1974.
273. Finberg L: Hypernatraemic dehydration. Advan Pediatr 16:325, 1969.
274. Rosenfield W, deRomana GL, Kleinman R, et al: Improving the clinical management of hypernatraemic dehydration: observations from a study of 67 infants with this disorder. Clin Pediatr 16:411, 1977.
275. Gray GM: Carbohydrate digestion and absorption. Role of the small intestine. N Engl J Med 292:1225, 1975.
276. Desjeux J-F, Tannenbaum C, Tai Y-H, et al: Effects of sugars and amino acids on sodium movement across small intestine. Am J Dis Child 131:331, 1977.
277. Nalin DR, Cash RA, Islam R, et al: Oral maintenance therapy for cholera in adults. Lancet 2:370, 1968.
278. Sack RB, Cassells J, Mitra R, et al: The use of oral replacement solutions in the treatment of cholera and other severe diarrhoeal disorders. Bull WHO 43:351, 1971.
279. Nalin DR, Cash RA: Oral or nasogastric maintenance therapy in paediatric cholera patients. J Pediatr 78:355, 1971.
280. Mahalanabis D, Sack RB, Jacobs B, et al: Use of an oral glucose-electrolyte solution in the treatment of paediatric cholera—a controlled study. J Trop Pediatr 20:82, 1974.
281. Finberg L: The role of oral electrolyte-glucose solutions in hydration for children—international and domestic aspects. J Pediatr 96:51, 1980.
282. Carey RM, Smith JR, Ortt EM: Gastrointestinal control of sodium excretion in sodium-depleted conscious rabbits. Am J Physiol 230:1504, 1976.
283. Katz MA: Hyperglycaemia-induced hyponatraemia: Calculation of expected serum sodium depression. N Engl J Med 289:843, 1973.
284. Roscoe JM, Halperin ML, Rolleston FS, et al: Hyperglycaemia-induced hyponatraemia: Metabolic considerations in calculation of serum sodium depression. Can Med Assoc J 112:452, 1975.
285. Loeb JN: The hyperosmolar state. N Engl J Med 290:1184, 1974.
286. Barlow ED, de Wardener HE: Compulsive water drinking. Q J Med 28:235, 1959.
287. Langgard H, Seith WO: Self-induced water intoxication without predisposing illness. N Engl J Med 266:378, 1962.
288. Linshaw MA, Hipp T, Gruskin A: Infantile psychogenic water drinking. J Pediatr 85:520, 1974.
289. Dugan S, Holliday MA: Water intoxication in two infants following the voluntary ingestion of excessive fluids. Pediatrics 39:418, 1967.
290. Dubrovsky SL, Grabo S, Bert T, et al: Syndrome of inappropriate secretion of antidiuretic hormone with exaggerated psychosis. Ann Intern Med 79:551, 1973.
291. Anderson B, McCann SM: The effect of hypothalamic lesions on the water uptake of the dog. Acta Physiol Scand 33:312, 1956.
292. McKuiley MJ, Denton DA, Weisinger RS: Sensors for antidiuretics and thirst — osmoreceptors or CSF sodium detectors? Brain Res 141:89, 1978.
293. Swann RC, Merrill JP: The clinical course of acute renal failure. Medicine 32:215, 1954.
294. Kleeman CR, Adams DA, Maxell MH: An evaluation of maximal water diuresis in chronic renal disease: I. Normal solute intake. J Lab Clin Med 58:169, 1961.
295. Schrier RW, Regal EM: Influence of aldosterone on sodium, water and potassium metabolism in chronic renal disease. Kidney Intl 1:156, 1972.
296. Anderson RTJ, Cadnapaphornchai P, Harbottle JA, et al: Mechanism of effect of thoracic inferior vena cava constriction on renal water excretion. J Clin Invest 54:1473, 1974.
297. Bell NH, Schedl HP, Bartter FC: An explanation for abnormal water retention and hypo-osmolality in congestive cardiac failure. Am J Med 36:351, 1964.
298. Schrier RW, Lehman D, Zacherle B, et al: Effect of furosemide on free water excretion in edematous patients with hyponatremia. Kidney Intl 3:30, 1974.
299. Stein M, Schwartz R, Mevsky LA: The antidiuretic activity of plasma of patients with hepatic cirrhosis, congestive heart failure, hypertension and other clinical disorders. J Clin Invest 33:77, 1954.
300. Yamane Y: Plasma ADH levels in patients with chronic congestive cardiac failure. Japan Circ J 32:745, 1968.
301. Szatalowicz VL, Arnold PE, Charimovitz C, et al: Radioimmunoassay of plasma arginine vasopressin in hyponatremic patients with congestive heart failure. N Engl J Med 305:263, 1981.
302. Lamdin E, Kdeeman CR, Rubin M, et al: Studies on alcohol diuresis. III. The response to ethyl alcohol in certain disease states characterised by impaired water tolerance. J Clin Invest 35:386, 1956.
303. Murdaugh HV Jr: Production of diuresis in hyponatremic edematous states with alcohol (abstract). J Clin Invest 35:726, 1956.
304. Grausz H, Lieberman R, Earley LE: Effect of plasma albumin on sodium reabsorption in patients with nephrotic syndrome. Kidney Intl 1:47, 1972.
305. Bohlin AB, Berg U: Renal water handling in minimal change nephrotic syndrome. Int J Pediatr Nephrol 6:93, 1984.
306. Liebermann FL, Ito S, Reynolds TB: Effective plasma volume in cirrhosis with ascites. J Clin Invest 48:975, 1969.
307. Bichet D, Szatalowicz V, Chaimovitx, et al: Role of vasopressin in abnormal water excretion in cirrhotic patients. Ann Int Med 96:413, 1982.
308. Bichet D, Van Putten VJ, Schrier RW: Potential role of increased sympathetic activity in impaired sodium and water excretion in cirrhosis. N Engl J Med 307:1552, 1982.
309. Lake CR, Ziegler MG, Kopin IJ: Use of plasma norepinephrine for evaluation of sympathetic neuronal function in man. Life Sci 18:1315, 1976.
310. Schedl HP, Bartter FC: An explanation for an experimental correction of the abnormal water diuresis in cirrhosis. J Clin Invest 39:248, 1960.
311. Ahmed ABJ, George BC, Gonzalez-Anvert C, et al: Increased plasma arginine vasopressin in clinical adrenocorticoid insufficiency and its inhibition by glucosteroids. J Clin Invest 46:111, 1967.
312. Aubry RH, Nankin HR, Mosis AM, et al: Measurement of osmotic threshold for vasopressin release in human subjects and its modification by cortisol. J Clin Endocrinol 25:1481, 1965.
313. Agus ZS, Goldberg M: Role of antidiuretic hormone in the abnormal water diuresis of anterior hypopituitrism in man. J Clin Invest 50:1478, 1971.
314. Boykin J, de Torrevte A, Erickson A, et al: Role of plasma vasopressin in impaired water excretion of glucocorticoid deficiency. J Clin Invest 62:738, 1978.
315. Kleeman CR, Czaczkes JW, Cutler R: Mechanisms of impaired water excretion in adrenal and pituitary insufficiency. IV. Antidiuretic hormone in primary and secondary adrenal insufficiency. J Clin Invest 43:1641, 1964.
316. Green HH, Harrington AR, Valtin H: On the role of antidiuretic hormone in the inhibition of acute water diuresis in adrenal insufficiency and the effects of gluco- and mineralocorticoids in reversing the inhibition. J Clin Invest 49:1724, 1970.
317. Di Scala VA, Kinney MJ: Effects of myxedema on the renal diluting and concentrating mechanism. Am J Med 50:325, 1971.
318. DeRubertis FR Jr, Michellis MF, Bloom ME, et al: Impaired water excretion in myxedema. Am J Med 51:41, 1971.
319. Emmanouel DS, Lindheimer MD, Katz AI: Mechanism of impaired water excretion in the hypothyroid rat. J Clin Invest 54:926, 1974.
320. Michael UF, Barenberg RL, Chavez R, et al: Renal handling of sodium and water in the hypothyroid rat: clearance and micropuncture studies. J Clin Invest 51:1405, 1972.
321. Michael UF, Kelley J, Alpert H, et al: The role of distal delivery of filtrate in the impaired renal dilution of the hypothyroid rat. Am J Physiol 230:699, 1976.
322. Young E, Little JM: Renal clearance in patients with myxedema. J Clin Endo Metab 15:343, 1955.
323. Goldberg M, Reivich M: Studies on the mechanism of hypernatraemia and impaired water excretion in myxedema. Ann Int Med 56:120, 1962.
324. Chinitz A, Turner FL: The association of primary hypothyroidysm and inappropriate secretion of antidiuretic hormone. Arch Int Med 116:871, 1965.
325. Pettinger WA, Talner L, Ferris TF: Inappropriate secretion of antidiuretic hormone due to myxedema. N Engl J Med 272:362, 1965.
326. Grantham JJ, Ordoff J: Effect of prostaglandin E, on the permeability response of the isolated collecting tubule to vasopressin, adenosine 3′, 5′ monophosphate and theophylline. J Clin Invest 47:1154, 1968.
327. Berndt WO, Miller M, Kettyle WM, et al: Potentiation of the antidiuretic action of vasopressin by chlorpropamide. Endocrinology 86:1028, 1970.
328. Zusman RM, Keiser RH, Handler JS: Chlorpropamide enhancement in vasopressin stimulated water flow in the toad bladder: role of endogenous prostaglandin E biosynthesis. Clin Res 25:452A, 1977.
329. Moses AM, Numann P, Miller M: Mechansim of chlorpropamide-induced antidiuresis in man: evidence for release of ADH and enhancement of peripheral action. Metabolism 22:59, 1973.
330. Pittman JG: Water intoxication due to oxytocin. N Engl J Med 268:481, 1963.
331. de Bodo RC, Prescott KK: The antidiuretic action of barbiturates (phenobarbitol, amytal, pentobarbitol) and the mechanism involved in this action. J Pharmacol Exp Ther 82:74, 1944.
332. Kimura T, Matsui K, Sato T, et al: Mechansim of carbemazepine (Tegretol)- induced anditiuresis: evidence for release of antidiuretic hormone and impaired excretion of water load. J Clin Endo Metab 38:356, 1974.
333. Moses AM, Howanitz J, Van Gemert M, et al: Clofibrate-induced antidiuresis. J Clin Invest 52:535, 1973.
334. Gaultier M, Bismuth C, Autret A, et al: Inappropriate antidiuresis after acute colchicine poisoning. 2 cases. Nouv Presse Med 4:3132, 1975.

335. Robertson GL, Bhoopalam N, Zelkositz LJ: Vincristine neurotoxicity and abnormal secretion of antidiuretic hormone. Arch Int Med 132:717, 1973.
336. Inglefinger JR, Hayes R: Evidence that chlorpropamide and vasopressin share a common site of action. J Clin Endo Metab 29:738, 1969.
337. Zweig SM, Ettinger B, Earley LM: Mechanism of antidiuretic action of chlorpropamide in the mammalian kidney. Am J Physiol 221:911, 1971.
338. Anderson RJ, Berl T, McDonald KM, et al: Evidence for an in vivo antagonism between vasopressin and prostaglandin in the mammalian kidney. J Clin Invest 56:420, 1975.
339. Berl T, Raz A, Wald H, et al: Prostaglandin synthesis inhibition and the action of vasopressin: studies in man and rat. Am J Physiol 232:F529, 1977.
340. Parisi M, Piccinni ZF: Aspirin potentiates the hydroosmotic effect of antidiuretic hormone in toad urinary bladder. Biochim Biophys Acta 279:209, 1972.
341. De Fronzo RA, Braime H, Colvin OM, et al: Water intoxication after cyclophosphamide therapy. Ann Int Med 78:861, 1973.
342. Steele TH, Serpick AA, Block JB: Antidiuretic response to cyclosphosphamide in man. J Pharmacol Exp Ther 185:245, 1973.
343. Berl T, Schrier RW: Water metabolism and the hypo-osmolar syndromes. In Brenner BM, Stein JH (eds): Sodium and water homeostasis. New York, Churchill-Livingstone, pp 1–23, 1978.
344. Schrier RW, Berl T: Nonosmolar factors affecting renal water excretion. N Engl J Med 292:81, 1975.
345. Schrier RW, Bichet DG: Osmotic and nonosmotic control of vasopressin release and the pathogenesis of impaired water excretion in adrenal, thyroid and edematous disorders. J Lab Clin Med 98:1, 1981.
346. Leaf A, Bartter FC, Santos RF, et al: Evidence in man that urinary electrolyte loss induced by Pitressin is a function of water retention. J Clin Invest 32:868, 1953.
347. Carter NW, Rector FC Jr, Seldin DW: Hyponatraemia in cerebral disease resulting from the inappropriate secretion of antidiuretic hormone. N Engl J Med 264:67, 1961.
348. Schwartz WB, Bennett W, Curelop S, et al: Syndrome of renal sodium loss and hyponatraemia probably resulting from inappropriate secretion of antidiuretic hormone. Am J Med 23:529, 1957.
349. Cohen JJ, Hulter HH, Smithline N, et al: The critical role of the adrenal gland in the renal regulation of acid-base equilibrium during chronic hypotonic expansion. J Clin Invest 58:1201, 1976.
350. Jaemike JR, Waterhouse C: The renal response to sustained administration of vasopressin and water in man. J Clin Endocrinol 21:231, 1961.
351. Levinsky NG, Davidson DG, Berliner RW: Changes in urine concentration during prolonged administration of vasopressin and water. Am J Physiol 196:451, 1959.
352. Bartter FC, Schwartz WB: The syndrome of inappropriate secretion of antidiuretic hormone. Am J Med 42:790, 196.
353. Dean RFA, McCance RA: The renal response of infants and adults to the administration of hypertonic solutions of sodium chloride and urea. J Physiol 109:81, 1949.
354. Janovsky M, Martivek J, Stanicova V: The distribution of sodium, chloride and fluid in the body of young infants with increased intake of Na Cl. Biol Neonate 11:261, 1967.
355. Aperia A, Broberger O, Thodenius K, et al: Developmental study of the renal response to an oral salt load in preterm infants. Acta Paediatr Scand 63:517, 1974.
356. Finberg L, Kiley J, Luttrell CN: Mass accidental salt poisoning in infancy. JAMA 184:187, 1963.
357. Simmons MA, Adcock EW, Bard H, et al: Hypernatraemia and intracranial hemorrhage in neonates. N Engl J Med 291:6, 1974.
357a. Meadows R: Munchausen syndrome by proxy—the hinterland of child abuse. Lancet 2:343, 1977.
358. Laurence BH, Hopkins BE: Hypernatraemia following a saline emetic. Med J Aust 1:1301, 1969.
359. Carter RF, Fotheringham BJ: Fatal salt poisoning due to gastric lavage with hypertonic saline. Med J Aust 1:539, 1971.
360. Robertson GL, Shelton RL, Athar S: The osmoregulation of vasopressin. Kidney Intl 10:25, 1976.
361. Zierler KL: Hyperosmolality in adults: a critical review. J Chronic Dis 7:1, 1958.
362. Hays RM, McHugh PR, Williams HE: Absence of thirst associated with hydrocephalus. N Engl J Med 269:227, 1963.
363. Travis LB, Dodge WF, Waggenor JD, et al: Defective thirst mechanism secondary to hypothalmic lesion: studies in a child with adipsia, polyphagia, obesity, and persistent hyperosmolality. J Pediat 70:915, 1967.
364. Christie SBM, Ross EJ: Ectopic pinealoma with adipsia and hypernatraemia. Brit Med J 2:669, 1968.
365. Engstrom WW, Liebman A: Chronic hyperosmolality of the body fluids with a cerebral lesion diabetes insipidus and anterior pituitary insufficiency. Am J Med 15:180, 1953.
366. Goldberg M, Weinstein G, Ades-an J, et al: Asymptomatic hypovolemic hypernatremia, a variant of essential hypernatremia. Am J Med 43:804, 1967.
367. Miller M, Dalakos T, Moses AM, et al: Recognition of partial defects in antidiuretic hormone secretion. Ann Intern Med 73:721, 1970.
368. Valtin H: Disorders of H20 balance—antidiuretic hormone (ADH). In Renal dysfunction: mechanisms involved in fluid and solute imbalance. Boston, Little, Brown and Co., p 29, 1979.
369. De Robertis FR, Michelis MF, Beck N, et al: "Essential" hypernatraemia due to ineffective osmotic and intact volume regulation of vasopressin secretion. J Clin Invest 50:97, 1971.
370. De Robertis FR, Michelis M, Davis BB: "Essential" hypernatraemia. Arch Intern Med 134:889, 1974.
371. Halter JB, Goldberg AP, Robertson GL, et al: Selective osmoreceptor dysfunction in the syndrome of chronic hypernatraemia. J Clin Endo Metab 44:609, 1977.
372. Sridhar CB, Clavert GD, Ibbertson HK: Syndrome of hypernatraemia, hypodipsia and partial diabetes insipidius: a new interpretation. J Clin Endo Metab 38:890, 1974.
373. van Gemert M, Miller M, Carey RJ, et al: Polyuria and impaired ADH release following medical preoptic lesioning in the rat. Am J Physiol 228:1293, 1975.
374. Buggy J, Johnson AK: Preoptic-hypothlamic periventricular lesions: thirst deficits and hypernatraemia. Am J Physiol 223:R44, 1977.
375. Schaff-Blass E, Robertson GL, Rosenfield RL: Chronic hypernatremia from a congenital defect in osmoregulation of thirst and vasopressin. J Pediatr 102:703, 1983.
376. Hollander WM, Judson WE: The relationship of cardiovascular and renal hemodynamic function to sodium excretion in patients with severe heart disease but without edema. J Clin Invest 35:970, 1956.
377. Friedberg CK, Lasser RP, Allen DF, et al: Production of chronic elevation of left ventricular and diastolic pressure in dogs: hemodynamic and renal studies. Circ Res 15:1, 1964.
378. Oberg B: Effects of cardiovascular reflexes on net capillary fluid transfer. Acta Physiol Scand (suppl) 229:1, 1969.
379. Starling EH: Physiological factors involved in the causation of dropsy. Lancet 1:1405, 1896.
380. Witte MH, Witte CL, Dumont AE: Progress in liver disease: physiological factors involved in the causation of cirrhotic ascites. Gastroenterology 61:742, 1971.
381. Orloff MJ: Pathogenesis and surgical treatment of intractable ascites associated with alcoholic cirrhosis. Ann N Y Acad Sci 170:213, 1970.
382. Lieberman FL, Reynolds TB: Plasma volume in cirrhosis of the liver: its relation to portal hypertension, ascites and renal failure. J Clin Invest 46:1297, 1967.
383. Liebermann, FL, Ito S, Reynolds TB: Effective plasma volume in cirrhosis with ascites. J Clin Invest 48:975, 1969.
384. Liebermann FL, Denison EK, Reynolds TB: The relationship of plasma volume, portal hypertension, ascites and renal sodium retention in cirrhosis: the overflow theory of ascites formation. Ann N Y Acad Sci 170:202, 1970.
385. Levy M: Sodium retention in dogs with cirrhosis and ascites: efferent mechanisms. Am J Physiol 233:F586, 1977.
386. Levy M, Wexler MJ: Renal sodium retention and ascites formation in dogs with experimental cirrhosis but without portal hypertension or increased splanchnic vascular capacity. J Lab Clin Med 91:520, 1978.
387. Bichet DG, Van Putten VJ, Schrier RW: Potential role of increased sympathetic activity in impaired sodium and water excretion in cirrhosis. N Engl J Med 307:1552, 1982.
388. Eisenberg S: Blood volume in persons with the nephrotic syndrome. Am J Med Sci 255:320, 1968.
389. Meltzer JI, Keim HJ, Laragh JH, et al: Nephrotic syndrome: vasoconstriction and hypervolaemic types indicated by renin-sodium profiling. Ann Int Med 91:688, 1979.
390. Dorhout Mees EJ, Roos JC, et al: Observations on oedema formation in the nephrotic syndrome in adults with minimal lesions. Am J Med 67:378, 1979.
391. Andersen SB, Rossing N: Metabolism of albumin and gamma-G-globulin during albumin infusions and plasmapheresis. Scand J Clin Lab Invest 20:183, 1967.
392. Matthews CME: Effects of plasmapheresis on albumin pools in rabbits. J Clin Invest 40:603, 1961.
393. Burgen ASV, Francombe WH: The role of plasma colloid osmotic pressure in the regulation of extracellular fluid. Proc Intl U Physiol Sci, Leiden 2:130, 1962.
394. Wraight EP: Capillary permeability to protein as a factor in the control of plasma volume. J Physiol 237:39, 1974.
395. Gur A, Adefuin PY, Siegel NJ, et al: A study of the renal handling of water in lipoid nephrosis. Ped Res 10:197, 1976.
396. Guyton AC: Interstitial fluid pressure. II. Pressure-volume curves of the interstitial space. Circ Res 16:452, 1965.
397. Zureifach BW: Capillary filtration and mechanisms of edema formation. Pfluegers Arch (suppl) 336:81, 1972.
398. Erdmann AJ, Vaughan TR, Brigham KL: Effect of increased vascular presure on lung fluid balance in unanaesthetized sheep. Circ Res 37:271, 1975.
399. Vehaskari VM, Chang CT-C, Stevens JK, et al: The effects of polycations on

vascular permeability in the rat. A proposed role for charge sites. J Clin Invest 3:1053, 1984.
400. Bernard DB, Alexander EA, Couser WG, et al: Renal sodium retention during volume expansion in experimental nephrotic syndrome. Kidney Intl 14:478, 1978.
401. Grausz H, Liebermann R, Earley L: Effect of plasma albumin on sodium reabsorption in patients with nephrotic syndrome. Kidney Intl 1:47, 1972.
402. Morita Y: Hemodynamic and electrolyte studies in acute glomerulonephritis. Clin Res 5:206, 1957.
403. Eisenberg S: Blood volume in patients with acute glomerulonephritis as determined by radioactive chromium tagged red cells. Am J Med 27:241, 1959.
404. Earle DP: Abnormalities in acute glomerulonephritis. In Metcoff J (ed): Acute Glomerulonephritis Boston, Little, Brown & Co., 1967, p. 301.
405. Warren JV, Stead EA Jr: The protein concentration of edema fluid in patients with acute glomerulonephritis. Am J Med Sci 208:618, 1944.
406. Fordham CL, Welt LG: The cardiovascular manifestation of acute glomerulonephritis: physiologic basis for treatment. Prog Cardio Dis 3:382, 1961.
407. Maddox DA, Bennett CM, Deen WM, et al: Determinants of glomerular filtration in experimental glomerulonephritis in the rat. J Clin Invest 55:305, 1975.
408. Maddox DA, Bennett CM, Deen WM, et al: Control of proximal tubule fluid reabsorption in experimental glomerulonephritis. J Clin Invest 55:1315, 1975.
409. Blantz RC, Wilson CB: Acute effects of antiglomerular basement membrane antibody on the process of glomerular filtration in the rat. J Clin Invest 58:899, 1976.
410. Powell HR, Rotenberg E, Williams AL, et al: Plasma renin activity in acute poststreptococcal glomerulonephritis and the haemolytic-uraemic syndrome. Arch Dis Child 49:802, 1974.
411. Birkenhager WH, Schalenkamp MADH, Schakekamp-Kuyken MPH, et al: Interrelations between arterial pressure, fluid volumes and plasma renin concentration in the course of acute glomerulonephritis. Lancet 1:1086, 1970.
412. Myers BP, Deen WM, Brenner BM: Effects of norepinephrine and angiotensin II on the determinants of glomerular ultrafiltration and proximal tubule fluid reabsorption in the rat. Circ Res 37:101, 1975.
413. Godon JP: Sodium and water retention in experimental glomerulonephritis: urinary natriuretic material. Nephron 14:382, 1975.
413a. Danovitch GM, Bourgoignie J, Bricker N: Reversibility of the "salt-losing" tendency of chronic renal failure. N Engl J Med 296:14, 1977.
414. Sachar LA, Horvitz A, Elman R: Studies on hypoalbuminaemia produced by protein deficient diets. I. Hypoalbuminaemia as a quantitative measure of tissue protein depletion. J Exp Med 75:453, 1942.
415. Coward DG, Whitehead RG: Experimental protein-energy malnutrition in baby baboons. Brit J Nutr 28:223, 1972.
416. Golden MHN, Golden BE, Jackson AA: Albumin and nutritional oedema. Lancet 1:114, 1980.
417. Golden MHN: Protein deficiency, energy deficiency and the oedema of malnutrition. Lancet 1:1261, 1982.
418. Fiorotto M, Nichols BL: Oedema of malnutrition (letter). Lancet 2:871, 1982.
419. Christy NP, Shaver JC: Estrogens and the kidney. Kidney Intl 6:366, 1974.
420. MacGregor GA, Markandu ND, Roulston JE, et al: Is "idiopathic" oedema idiopathic? Lancet 1:397, 1979.
421. Ferris TR, Bay WH: Idiopathic edema. In Brenner BM, Stein JH (eds): Contemporary issues in nephrology. 1. sodium and water homeostasis. New York, Churchill-Livingstone, 1973.
422. MacGregor GA, de Wardener HE: Idiopathic oedema (letter). Lancet 2:355, 1979.

CHAPTER 7

Potassium

GEORGE J. SCHWARTZ
LEONARD G. FELD

INTRODUCTION

Potassium (K) is the predominant cation in intracellular fluid (ICF). Only 2% of total body potassium (TBK) is in extracellular fluid (ECF) excluding bone (1). Because K intake is quite variable and both TBK and the concentration of K in serum (K_s) are closely regulated, controls that affect distribution and excretion overlap. Most disorders of K balance or distribution are diagnosed by deviations of K_s from normal. Hypokalemia and hyperkalemia result from alterations either in TBK or in distribution of K between ECF and ICF. This chapter describes the physiology of K homeostasis and the pathophysiology of clinical disorders of K metabolism.

NORMAL DISTRIBUTION AND TURNOVER

Total Body Potassium

TBK in adults is approximately 50 mEq/kg body weight (2, 3). Most TBK is contained in cells, primarily muscle. Infants show a more rapid increase in TBK compared with children beyond the first year of life (Fig. 7.1). The rapid increase during infancy results from rapid growth of muscle mass and from maturation of cellular composition. Intracellular K concentration, low at birth, increases to adult levels by 4 to 7 months (4). TBK increases with growth at a rate that is, after infancy, commensurate with muscle growth (2, 4, 5). There are no sex-related differences in TBK until puberty. During puberty, the increment with growth is less in girls than in boys (2–4), because girls increase adipose tissue and boys increase muscle mass at accelerated rates. TBK in adults has been estimated by whole body counting and by isotope dilution. The former method measures the naturally occurring isotope K^{40}, a gamma emitter (2, 5a). The isotope dilution method measures total exchangeable K following an intravenous injection of K^{42} (5). Compared with whole body counting, this method tends to underestimate TBK, in part because of insufficient equlibration of the isotope.

Distribution Between ICF and ECF

Normal Control

The concentration of K in ICF $(K)_i$ is 120 to 160 mEq/L. The activity of K, i.e., the concentration of K that is ionically active, is approximately 75% of its concentration in muscle (6, 7), but is lower in renal tubular cells (8). The normal $(K)_i$ is important in regulating enzyme activity, synthesis of protein and nucleic acids, transmission of impulses by excitable tissues, and regulation of K excretion by the kidney (1, 9). Normal K homeostasis is essential for growth.

The combination of high K and low Na concentrations in ICF contrast with the normal values for ECF or serum (K_s = 3.5 to 5.0 mEq/L) (Na_s = 135 to 145 mEq/L). Infants tend to have higher K_s values than children. There is an inverse relationship between K_s and gestational age in premature infants (Table 7.1) (10). K_s in serum specimens is up to 0.5 mEq/L higher than it is in plasma, because there is release of K from cells during clotting (11).

The high ratio of intracellular to extracellular K ($[K]_i/[K]_e$) is sustained primarily by the action of Na,K-adenosine triphosphatase (Na,K-ATPase) activity located in cell membranes and often described as the active Na pump. It transports three Na ions from cells in exchange for two K ions transported into cells. The Na pump has kinetic characteristics of an enzyme and is dependent on hydrolysis of ATP for energy (12).

The pump is electrogenic, creating a negative voltage inside the cell. The concentration of K in ICF exceeds that predicted from the Nernst equation (13). Increasing K intake enhances cell uptake of K because the concentration gradient across cells for K is reduced. Raising K intake also leads to enhanced secretion of K by the colon and distal portions of the nephron (14–16). Adaptation to a chronic high K intake leads to a more rapid clearing of K from ECF in both normal and anephric states (17).

The activity of Na,K-ATPase in erythrocytes (18), kidney (19, 20), and intestine (21) is low early in life. This may be a factor in the lower $(K)_i$ values observed in the first few months of life (8).

Effects of Changes in Acid-base Status

Changes in acid-base status influence the level of extracellular K (22). There is a relation between intracellular and extracellular ratios of hydrogen and K. In general, K deficiency that predisposes to metabolic alkalosis induces an intracellular acidosis (23). Metabolic disorders of acid-base regulation cause more pronounced alterations in K_s than respiratory disturbances (22).

Metabolic acidosis induced by the infusion of mineral acid (HCl, NH_4Cl) results in an outward movement of K and an elevation of K_s. Organic acids, such as lactic acid, shift extracellular K very little despite a similar depression in blood pH (24–26). In clinical practice, there is poor correlation between acidosis and K_s (26). This disparity has been attributed to the nonionic diffusion of organic acids into cells (24).

Metabolic alkalosis produced by giving $NaHCO_3$ causes K to shift into cells, with a resulting decrease in K_s; however, the changes are smaller than are the opposite changes with metabolic acidosis (22, 23). Acute changes in acid-base balance cause larger changes in plasma K than chronic states (22). Metabolic alkalosis secondary to Cl depletion lowers K_s, while ECF pH is increased and intracellular pH is decreased (23).

The concentration of bicarbonate in plasma can reciprocally affect K_s

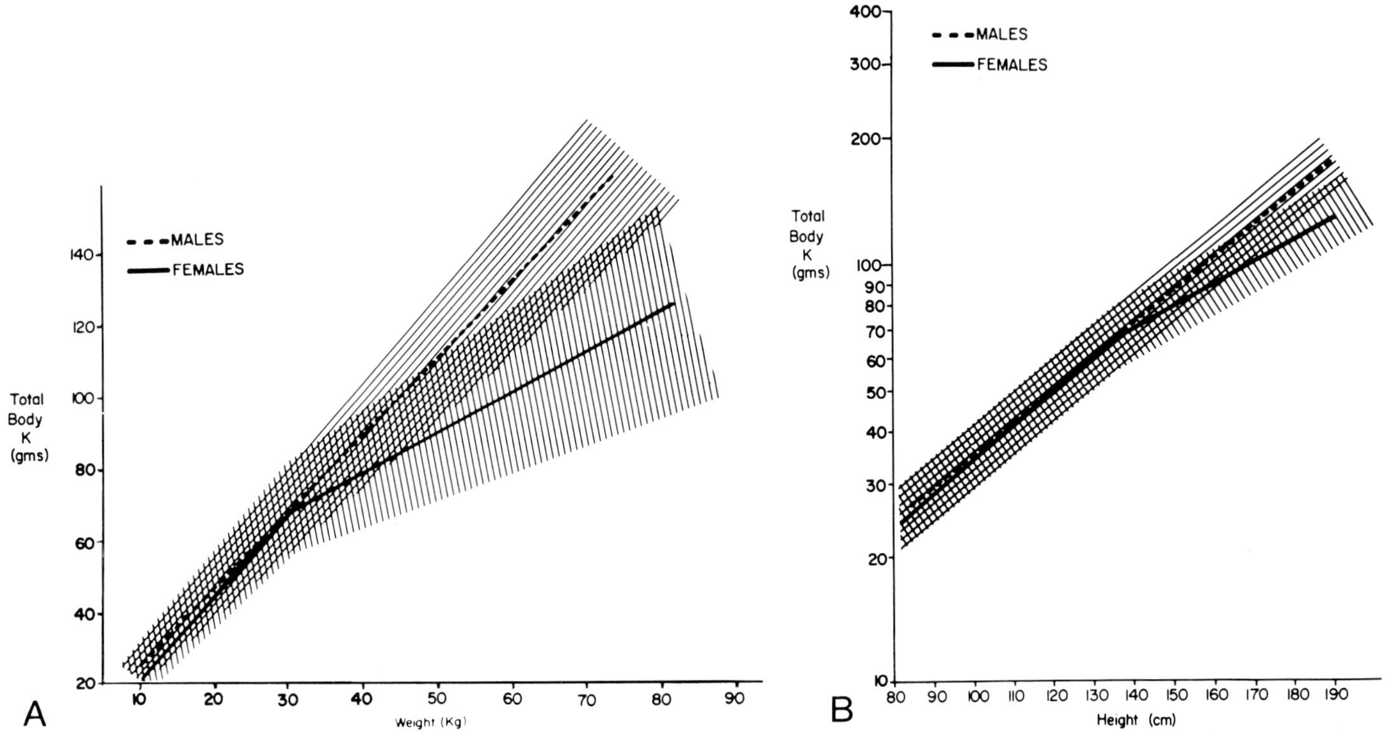

Figure 7.1. **A**, The regression lines for the mean ± 1 standard deviation for total body potassium versus weight are plotted for males and females 3 to 18 years of age. (From Flynn MA, et al: Pediatr Res 9:834, 1975.) **B**, The regression lines for the mean ± 1 standard deviation for the log of total body potassium versus height are plotted for the same population. (From Flynn MA, et al: Pediatr Res 9:834, 1975.)

Table 7.1.
Plasma Potassium Concentrations in Newborns, Infants, and Children (Mean ± Standard Deviation)

Age	Plasma K concentration (mEq/L)
Newborn[a]	
30–32	6.5 ± 0.5
33–35	5.6 ± 0.2
36–38	5.3 ± 0.3
39–41	5.1 ± 0.2
Infants[b] n = 14	
1–12 months	5.0 ± 0.5
Children[b] n = 22	
2–20 years	4.3 ± 0.4

[a] Gestational age in weeks; measurements obtained at 1 week of age. (From Sulyok E, et al: Biol Neonate 35:60, 1979.)
[b] From Schwartz GJ, Feld LG: Unpublished observations.

independent of a pH effect; raising serum bicarbonate lowers K_s (27). This may mitigate the stimulus to change K_s during acute respiratory acidosis, i.e., lowering plasma pH and elevating bicarbonate has less effect on K_s than lowering pH and bicarbonate as occurs in metabolic acidosis.

Hormonal Effects

Insulin Secretion. Insulin secretion plays an important role in the disposal of an exogenously administered K load (28–31) and on the maintenance of fasting K_s concentration within the normal range (32). An acute increase in K_s results in a twofold to threefold increase in insulin levels (28–31). Insulin stimulates the uptake of K by liver, skeletal muscle, adipose tissue, cardiac muscle, and nervous tissue (33). The mechanism for insulin-induced transcellular movement of K depends in part on its cotransport with glucose; significant K accumulates in liver with glycogen formation. However, some of the uptake of K is independent of the entry of glucose (34). The extrarenal disposal of K is impaired in insulin deficiency (32).

Adrenergic Activity. Adrenergic activity affects K movement between intracellular and extracellular compartments (35). Alpha-adrenergic stimulation directly causes the release of K from liver (36), whereas beta-2-adrenergic activity causes enhanced uptake of K by liver, skeletal muscle, and cardiac muscle (37, 38). An infusion of epinephrine causes an initial rise in K_s followed by a sustained fall (35, 39). This enhanced extrarenal translocation of K is partly independent of variations in plasma insulin concentration (35, 39–42). The beta blocker, propranolol, in large doses may cause hyperkalemia during exercise (42), probably by preventing the epinephrine-stimulated cell uptake of K (40, 42, 43).

Mineralocorticoid Hormones. Mineralocorticoid hormones stimulate uptake of K by cells. For example, the hyperkalemia that follows the administration of a KCl load to rats with adrenalectomies can be mitigated with aldosterone (44). Aldosterone administration also causes an increase in the concentration of K in saliva (45), sweat (46), and colonic fluid (47). Aldosterone and glucocorticoids stimulate colonic secretion of K following adrenalectomy (48). Under normal conditions, these extrarenal actions probably contribute little to overall K homeostasis but may be very useful in disposing of K intake and preventing hyperkalemia in the absence of renal function (49).

Intake

Intake of K varies over a wide range, from 5 to 1000 mEq/day (50). K is widely distributed in foods, particularly those that have a high cell content, fruits and meats (Table 7.2) (51), so that K intake generally is high. In adults in ranges from 50 to >500 mEq/day or 1 to 20 mEq/100 kilocalorie (kcal) of diet. This range, −2 to 20 mEq/100 kcal, is typical for children as well, since children and adults eat diets of similar

Table 7.2.
Potassium In Foods[a]

Source	Amount	Potassium (mEq)
Peaches, dried, uncooked	1 cup	39
Raisins, dried, seeded	1 cup	31
Dates, dried, cut	1 cup, pitted	29
Apricots, dried, uncooked	17 large halves	25
Figs, dried	7 medium	23
Prune juice, canned	1 cup	15
Watermelon	1 slice (6-inch diameter × 1½ inches)	15
Banana	1 medium	14
Beef round, stew meat, raw	4 oz.	14
Cantaloupe	½ (5-inch diameter)	13
Orange juice, fresh	1 cup	13
Turkey, roasted	3½ oz.	13
Milk, whole, 3.5% fat	1 cup	9
Tomato	1 cup	8

[a] Potassium in foods adapted from Pennington JAT, Church HN: Food Values of Portions Commonly Used. New York, Harper & Row, 1980.

composition. Infants fed human milk receive only 1.5 mEq/100 kcal (52). Intake provided by other mammalian milk may be 2 to 4 times this figure (cow's milk is 4.5 mEq/100 kcal).

The relation of the intake of Na to that of K (Na/K ratio) is important as well, since high Na intakes initially increase the renal loss of K. Human and all mammalian milks have a Na/K ratio of 0.6 to 0.8, i.e., K intake greater than Na. Diets rich in fruits and vegetables have low Na, high K content, hence, a low Na/K ratio. In some primitive societies, the ratio may be much less than 0.05. By contrast, diets of most western societies have a high Na content from use of salt (NaCl) in food preservation and preparation and as a condiment. This practice leads to Na/K ratios that often exceed 1.0 and may exceed 3.0 (51).

Artificial diets or parenteral fluid regimens can vary K intake from zero to any chosen level; the same is true for Na. Some parenteral fluid regimens are devoid of K and high in Na; these can lead to K deficiency. A safe minimum intake is 1.5 mEq/100 kcal of total intake unless there is adrenal insufficiency or hyperkalemia (chapter 11).

Excretion

Interpreting Excretory Patterns

The kidney is the major excretory organ for K. Normally, >90% of the K ingested daily is excreted by the kidney, which is capable of adjusting the rate of K excretion promptly in response to a wide range of intake. However, compared with Na, extreme adjustments cannot be achieved as completely or as rapidly (53). Since urinary K excretion cannot be reduced to less than 5 mEq/day, despite significant deficits in TBK, conservation is incomplete. In view of the obligatory nonrenal losses of K, the diet of the adult must contain at least 10 to 20 mEq/day K. The amount of K excreted in the urine reflects predominately dietary intake but is reduced somewhat by gastrointestinal losses and the process of body growth.

Children and adults generally excrete urine with a Na/K ratio >1.0, because their dietary intake of Na exceeds that of K. The urinary Na/K ratio ranges from one to four in infants studied in our community (Table 7.4). Infants on a milk or formula diet have Na/K ratios that are close to the ratios found in milk, i.e., 0.7 (52).

The fractional excretion of K describes K excretion as a percent of K filtered. It is determined from the following equation:

$$\frac{\text{Urinary K (mEq/L)}}{\text{Plasma K (mEq/L)}} \times \frac{\text{Plasma creatinine (mg/dl)}}{\text{Urinary creatinine (mg/dl)}} \times 100\%$$

It is usually <30% in children with normal kidney function who are on a regular diet. It may exceed 40% when mineralocorticoid response is enhanced or when kidney function is impaired.

The presence of enhanced mineralocorticoid activity frequently can be inferred from a urinary Na/K ratio <1 or a fractional excretion of K >40%. Premature infants may show urinary Na/K ratios >4 (Table 7.4), reflecting a relative hyporesponsiveness of the distal tubule and collecting duct to mineralocorticoid activity (10) and the natriuresis that occurs in the neonatal period, which is inversely proportional to gestational age. These values are estimates that may assist the clinician in establishing the presence or absence of K-wasting by the kidney.

Adaptation to Change in Intake

The kidney is capable of adapting to a chronically high K diet by increasing K secretion at various sites along the nephron. When animals are adapted to ingestion of large amounts of K, they excrete more of an acute K load per nephron than when they are on a standard K diet. This adaptation is associated with increases in the activity of Na,K-ATPase, basolateral cell membrane area, transepithelial voltage, and intracellular K (54). The final results are an increase in the ability of the distal cells to accumulate K actively and to secrete K down a more favorable electrochemical gradient into urine.

Intrarenal Mechanisms

The physiology of the renal handling of K is discussed in chapter 5. In brief, the superficial proximal convoluted tubule (SI) absorbs approximately 50% of the filtered load of K. An additional 40% is absorbed by the proximal straight tubule and loop of Henle, so that only 10% of the filtered load is present at the early distal tubule of superficial nephrons (55–57). The juxtamedullary nephrons may handle K differently, in that the delivery at the end of the descending limb of the loop of Henle is equivalent to the filtered load (49, 58, 59). K may be recycled in the medulla, being secreted from the interstitium into the proximal straight tubule and descending limb of juxtamedullary nephrons and reabsorbed in the thick ascending limb (60).

Most urinary K is derived from K secretion by the cells of the distal convoluted tubule (55) and cortical collecting duct (61). The magnitude of K secretion is determined primarily by the movement of K from cell to luminal fluid along an electrochemical gradient and by the permeability of the luminal membrane to K (9). Factors that enhance the electrochemical driving force or the permeability will favor K secretion.

An increase in delivery of solute and water to distal nephron sites augments K secretion by reducing luminal K concentration. Volume expansion and diuretics increase tubular flow rate and create a more favorable concentration gradient for K secretion (62–66).

If distal delivery of Na is accompanied by an anion that is less reabsorbable than Cl, e.g., HCO_3, sulfate, carbenicillin, the negative voltage in the lumen becomes larger, making the electrochemical forces even more favorable for K secretion (67–69).

Mineralocorticoid Effects

When mineralocorticoids are given acutely they stimulate K secretion in distal parts of the nephron by increasing the permeability of the luminal membrane to K (70). When they are given chronically, mineralocorticoids cause an increase in intracellular K (71) and stimulate Na reabsorption, which leads to a more negative transepithelial voltage (72). The long term effects enhance the electrochemical driving force favoring K secretion. Since the mineralocorticoid effect on K transport appears to precede an increase in the activity of Na,K-ATPase, K excretion is not totally under the control of this enzyme (73). Long-term administration of mineralocorticoid induces persistent kaliuresis, whereas the antinatriuretic effect is overridden in a week (74).

An acute increase in the intake of K results in an increase in cell K activity and an enhanced urinary excretion of K (8). The increase in renal cell K and transepithelial (negative) voltage enhance the electrochemical forces that favor K secretion; this response may act independently of the increased aldosterone secretion (75).

Acid-base Disturbances

Acid-base disturbances alter distal K secretion by affecting the electrochemical gradient, in particular the concentration of K in the cell. Acute metabolic or respiratory alkalosis causes a shift of K into cells. This results in enhanced K secretion into the distal tubule (8, 76–78). Conversely, the secretion of K is reduced by acidosis, probably by decreasing active uptake of K into distal tubular cells (76, 79). In clinical practice, the effects of chronic acid-base disturbances on K secretion are modified by the effects of these disturbances on ECF volume, tubular flow rate, anion delivery rate, and aldosterone excretion (see previous section) and the secondary effects may override the primary one.

Extrarenal K Excretion

Extrarenal K excretion accounts for <10% of daily intake, the percentage declining as K intake increases. Extrarenal excretion occurs mainly via the intestine. K is passively absorbed from the small intestine; final regulation of gastrointestinal K occurs in the colon (80). The rate of secretion is determined primarily by the electrical gradient generated by Na absorption (81) and is sensitive to mineralocorticoids (49). K adaptation occurs in the intestine following K loading (82) and when renal function is reduced (83).

HYPOKALEMIA AND K DEFICIENCY

Hypokalemia is defined as a plasma concentration <3.0 mEq/L. K deficiency is a loss of TBK associated with a reduction in muscle cell K concentration. Abnormalities of K deficiency appear in experimental studies when the loss of TBK is sufficient to cause a reduction in intracellular K concentration of at least 5%. Since this can only be documented by measurement of muscle intracellular K, the determination of K deficiency in clinical practice is inferred from a history predicting K losses and an associated hypokalemia, e.g., diabetic ketoacidosis, hypokalemia following a period of deficient intake or prolonged diuretic use, a urinary K of <20 mEq/L, or a low fractional excretion rate. Acute hypokalemia occurs without K deficiency only when there is a sudden internal shift, as occurs with periodic paralysis, insulin action, or alkali administration (84).

Causes

Deficient Intake

Hypokalemia and K deficiency may result from inadequate intake. Most diets contain adequate K (Table 7.2); a major exception is a high carbohydrate diet containing refined sugars or parenteral fluid regimens that are devoid of K. Diets low in K taken over weeks will result in K deficiency and hypokalemia, because of the obligatory renal and gastrointestinal losses; these will be accentuated if Na intake is high. Malnutrition, particulary kwashiorkor, is the most common setting for dietary-induced hypokalemia and K deficiency. The K deficiency is greater when the malnutrition is complicated by gastroenteritis.

Recently, infant formulas were made incorrectly so that they resulted in a deficiency of chloride. The exclusive use of these formulas for several months caused a syndrome of anorexia, failure to grow, alkalosis, and hypokalemia. Infants on special "home made" formulas also are at risk to either dietary deficiency of Cl or K, either of which may cause hypokalemia and K deficiency (86).

Causes of hypokalemia are outlined in the box below.

CAUSES OF HYPOKALEMIA

- I. Inadequate dietary intake
- II. Excessive renal losses
  - A. Diuretics
    - 1. Potent saliuretic agents
    - 2. Osmotic diuretics
    - 3. Carbonic anhydrase inhibitors
  - B. Nonreabsorbable anions (carbenicillin, pencillin)
  - C. Diabetic ketoacidosis
  - D. Mineralocorticoid excess
    - 1. Primary hyperaldosteronism
    - 2. Congenital adrenal hyperplasia
    - 3. Cushing's syndrome
    - 4. Pharmacologic use of glucocorticoids
    - 5. Excessive secretion of ACTH
    - 6. Excessive licorice or carbenoxolone ingestion
  - E. Excessive renin production
    - 1. Renal vascular hypertension
    - 2. Malignant hypertension
    - 3. Renin producing tumors
    - 4. Bartter's syndrome
  - F. Disorders of renal transport
    - 1. Renal tubular acidosis
    - 2. Fanconi's syndrome
    - 3. Amphotericin B therapy
    - 4. Recovery from acute renal failure
    - 5. Postobstructive diuresis
    - 6. Severe interstitial nephritis or chronic pyelonephritis
    - 7. Magnesium deficiency
  - G. Miscellaneous disorders
    - 1. Liddle's syndrome
    - 2. Gentamicin therapy
    - 3. Acute nonlymphocytic leukemia
- III. Excessive extrarenal losses
  - A. Gastrointestinal
    - 1. Vomiting and gastric drainage
    - 2. Diarrhea
    - 3. Villous adenoma
    - 4. Fistula or ostomy
    - 5. Ureterosigmoidostomy
    - 6. Laxative or enema abuse
    - 7. Malabsorption
    - 8. Geophagia
  - B. Integumental
    - 1. Excessive sweating
    - 2. Full thickness burns
- IV. Redistribution of potassium from extracellular fluid to intracellular fluid
  - A. Alkalosis (metabolic, respiratory)
  - B. Hypokalemic periodic paralysis
  - C. Barium poisoning
  - D. Insulin administration and excess

Renal Losses

Impermeant Anions. Renal losses in excess of intake may occur for a number of reasons and cause loss of TBK, hypokalemia, and K deficiency. Increased delivery of bicarbonate to the distal nephron increases urinary K losses (68). Other impermeant anions, e.g., probenecid-penicillin therapy, can have the same effect (67, 69, 87).

Diuretics. Hypokalemia and K deficiency may occur with the use of diuretics. Substantial kaliuresis occurs in response to a brisk diuresis induced by any agent, e.g., thiazides; loop diuretics (88), and osmotic diuretics (89). These all increase the rate of flow of tubular fluid to the distal segments of the nephron. The result can be the acute development of hypokalemia. Hypokalemia and K deficiency are infrequent in hypertensive patients on long-term diuretic therapy (90–92). However, these occur with greater frequency in edematous patients on chronic diuretic therapy. These patients, like other patients with secondary hyperaldosteronism treated with diuretics, are prone to develop K deficiency. The fraction of filtered K that is excreted is usually >30% with use of loop diuretics (93) or mannitol (89). In volume-contracted patients, secondary aldosteronism may further increase the urinary loss of K. Inhibition of carbonic anhydrase by acetazolamide causes HCO_3 wasting and an increase in the fractional excretion of K (88).

Mineralocorticoid Excess. Hypokalemia and K deficiency result from mineralocorticoid excess, either endogenous or exogenous. Primary aldosteronism is associated with hypertension, hypokalemia, metabolic alkalosis, and mild Na retention. Plasma renin activity is low (94). A similar picture is observed in patients with excess mineralocorticoid, such as corticosterone and desoxycorticosterone (DOC) (95) (chapter 33).

In children with congenital adrenal hyperplasia, 11-hydroxylase deficiency leads to a defect in synthesis of cortisol and an overproduction of ACTH, with subsequent stimulation of adrenal androgens and DOC (Fig. 7.2) (96). The 17-hydroxylase deficiency results in defective production of cortisol and adrenal sex hormones, so that there is failure of secondary sex development, as well as signs of DOC excess, hypokalemia, alkalosis, and hypertension (97). Some tumors produce an ACTH-like

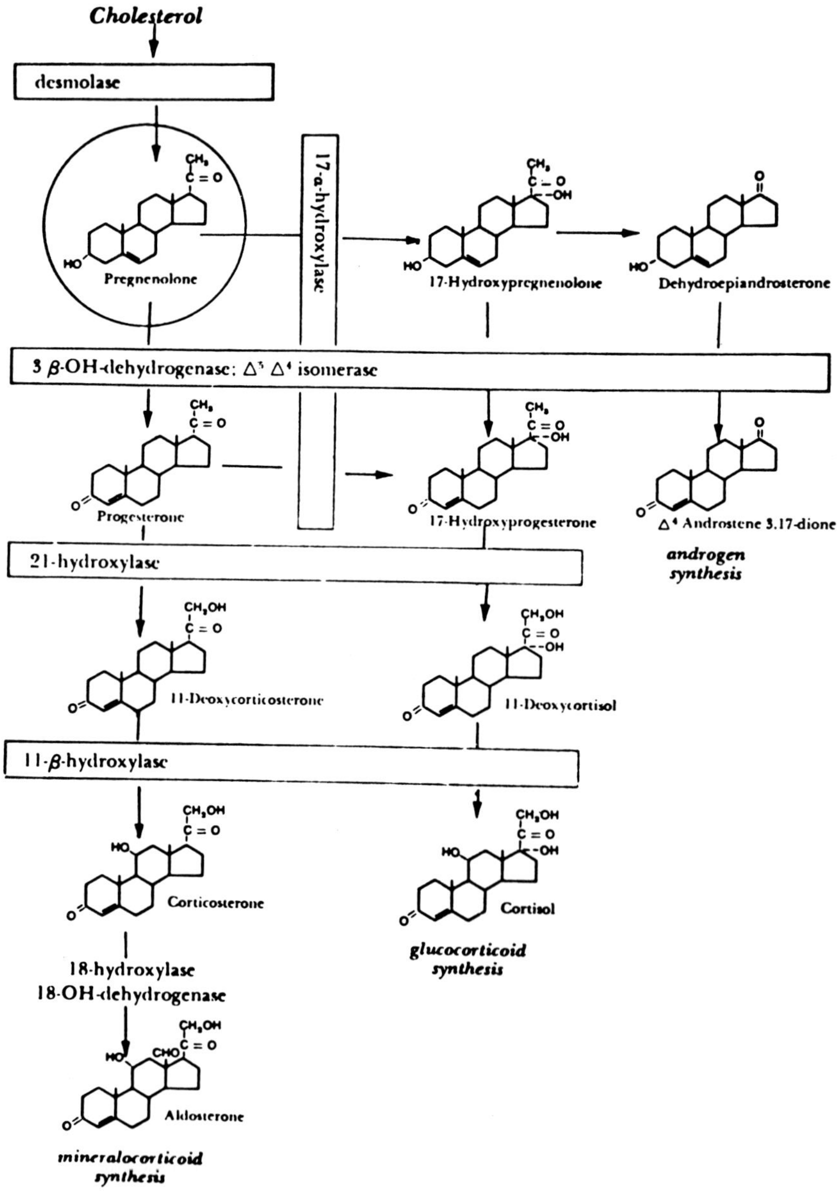

Figure 7.2. Pathways of steroid biosynthesis. (Adapted from Thomas BA (ed): Pathways of steroid biosynthesis. In The Adrenal Cortex. Kalamazoo, Mich., Upjohn Company, 1974.

substance that leads to an excessive production of cortisol, DOC, and corticosterone (98). Patients with these tumors and those with Cushing's syndrome may have hypokalemia and K deficiency. Hypokalemia and K deficiency may develop in patients producing excess DOC and in patients receiving pharmacologic doses of corticosteroids. The hypokalemia is related to the mineralocorticoid effect of such compounds. Licorice ingestion in excess can have a similar effect (98, 99).

Excess Renin. The renin-angiotensin system is a major stimulus for aldosterone production and release (100). Conditions of hyperreninemia are associated with hypokalemia and K deficiency. This resulting hyperaldosteronism occurs with malignant hypertension (101), renal artery stenosis (102), or a renin-producing tumor (hemangiopericytoma) or Wilms' tumor (103, 104). It is also usually associated with hypertension. Hyperreninemia secondary to plasma volume contraction is a factor in causing hypokalemia in diuretic therapy of edema and similar states.

Bartter's syndrome is a rare disease characterized by hyperreninemia, aldosteronism, normotension, severe hypokalemia, metabolic alkalosis, and often growth retardation (chapter 33).

Diabetes Mellitus. K deficiency is usually present in patients with diabetic ketoacidosis. Hypokalemia seldom is evident initially because of the concomitant acidosis (105); however, hypokalemia develops rapidly with insulin and glucose therapy unless K is also given. The deficiency in diabetic keotacidosis is caused by insulin deficiency, vomiting, the osmotic diuresis induced by hyperglycemia, and the increased excretion of relatively impermeant ketoacid anions.

Disorders of Renal Transport. Certain types of renal tubular acidosis (RTA) are associated with hypokalemia and K deficiency. These are characterized by acidosis, hypokalemia, and sometimes profound paralysis secondary to K deficiency. The pathophysiology varies with the different types of RTA. In the proximal form (Type II), proximal reabsorption of HCO_3 is impaired so that distal delivery of HCO_3 causes the kaliuresis. Although therapy with $NaHCO_3$ corrects the acidosis, it exacerbates distal HCO_3 delivery and enhances the kaliuresis (106). Persistent secondary aldosteronism as a result of concomitant volume depletion augments the K wasting. In the distal form (Type I), H^+ secretion in the distal tubule and collecting duct is reduced and K wasting results from both an increased tubular secretion of K and secondary aldosteronism (107) (chapter 34).

The syndrome of distal RTA may develop because of the effects of certain drugs, e.g., amphotericin B, toluene, lithium, and vitamin D. Other disorders with tubular dysfunction, e.g., pyelonephritis, interstitial nephritis, and the diuresis following successful renal transplantation, recovery from acute renal failure, and relief of urinary tract obstruction may result in hypokalemia (108).

Children with hypomagnesemia may be unable to conserve K, perhaps because of a specific transport defect. The finding of metabolic alkalosis may reflect secondary aldosteronism. Associated limitations in urinary concentrating ability and Ca excretion have been noted (109, 110).

Miscellaneous Disorders. Liddle's syndrome is a rare familial cause of hypokalemia associated with failure to thrive, Na retention, hypertension, and suppressed levels of plasma renin and aldosterone. A defect in Na transport probably affects red blood cells, as well as renal tubular cells, and may be manifested in part as a generalized increase in Na permeability across the cell membranes (111, 112) (chapter 33).

Hypokalemia and K wasting occur in association with high doses or chronic use of aminoglycosides, e.g., gentamicin and netilmicin. The decline in K_s occurs independent of changes in GFR or in other plasma electrolytes. The roles of secondary aldosteronism and of increased urinary excretion of lysosomal enzymes in contributing to the K wasting have not been established. K deficiency may potentiate aminoglycoside nephrotoxicity (113–116).

Children and adults, with various forms of leukemia and undergoing chemotherapy, may develop hypokalemia and K wasting (117). The hypokalemia is associated with high levels of lysozyme in the blood, suggesting that the renal loss of K is caused by proximal tubular damage secondary to proximal reabsorption of the lysozyme. High levels of plasma lysozyme coupled with chemotherapeutic, antibacterial, and antifungal agents, potentiate the risk of K loss. The mineralocorticoid effects of high doses of prednisone, the increased K permeability caused by amphotericin, the nonreabsorbable anion effect of penicillin and carbenicillin, contribute to the risk (118). K deficiency may occur in association with hyperthyroidism and improve with its treatment (119).

Extrarenal Losses

Gastrointestinal. In children, gastrointestinal loss is probably the most common cause of hypokalemia. Because the concentration of K in gastrointestinal fluid is usually about 10 mEq/L (120), much of the loss that leads to K deficiency must be renal. Upper gastrointestinal losses, as occur with pyloric stenosis and poor intake, lead to alkalosis, volume contraction, secondary aldosteronism, and kaliuresis. The alkalosis causes an increase in intracellular K concentration, a transient bicarbonaturia, and an increase in distal secretion of K. The reduced intake of K combined with these effects induces hypokalemia and sometimes severe K deficiency. The alkalosis usually can be repaired by giving NaCl, but sometimes it is "saline-resistant" and K and Cl are required (121, 122).

Diarrhea causes larger gastrointestinal losses of K (123). The concentration of K in stool water is generally 5 to 15 mEq/L, so that as the volume of stool water increases, the rate of stool K loss increases (120, 124). As volume contraction develops, secondary aldosteronism causes increased renal and gastrointestinal loss of K. Children with severe diarrhea and dehydration (10% to 15%) may lose 7 to 12 mEq K/kg body weight (125). The children have metabolic acidosis that often is hyperchloremic secondary to extensive losses of HCO_3 and potential alkali from the gastrointestinal tract. The acidosis may mask signs of K loss because of the marked shift of K from cells to the ECF. The tendency of K deficiency is greater in children with malnutrition, particularly those with kwashiorkor who develop gastroenteritis (126).

Large losses of K may occur in patients with gastrointestinal fistula, gastrostomy, and iliostomy, where fluid losses are large.

Ureterosigmoidostomies, in which urine is diverted into the sigmoid colon, lead to Na and Cl reabsorption in exchange for K and HCO_3, resulting in hypokalemic hyperchloremic metabolic acidosis similar to that seen in Type II RTA. Implantation of the ureter into a loop of ileum prevents this from occurring (127).

A number of conditions, common in adult patients but rare in children and adolescents, cause hypokalemia and K deficiency. These are villous adenoma (128), inappropriate laxative use (129), and licorice addiction (98, 99).

Integumental. Excessive sweating from exercise or heat stress and loss of salt may lead to volume contraction and secondary aldosteronism in patients with cystic fibrosis. The loss of K in exocrine gland secretions and in urine can result in hypokalemia (130).

Patients with full thickness burns have a large loss of ECF with secondary aldosteronism that may lead to kaliuresis and hypokalemia in the first 48 hours of the postburn period (131).

Redistribution of K

Acid-Base. Either acute metabolic or respiratory alkalosis causes a shift of K into cells in exchange for H+. The change in K concentration varies over a wide range and a simple relationship cannot be described. Usually, metabolic alkalosis is associated with both hypokalemia and decreased TBK, but the degree of K deficiency varies (121).

Periodic Paralysis. Periodic paralysis is a rare autosomal dominant disorder characterized by intermittent attacks of muscle weakness of the limbs and trunk lasting 6 to 24 hours. Patients usually become symptomatic during the first or second decade of life. The plasma K concentration falls during the attack and returns to normal during the recovery phase, indicating that K has shifted from ECF. Episodes are precipitated by a high carbohydrate/low K diet, exercise (in the postexercise phase), infection, stress, and alcohol ingestion. Acetazolamide, the carbonic anhydrase inhibitor, is effective in reversing attacks. This has led to the suggestion that the acidosis caused by acetazolamide decreases the rate of K entry into cells (132).

Insulin. Glucose administration or glucose and insulin given together cause hypokalemia. The K is taken up in the liver in association with glycogen formation and K transport into liver and muscle cells occurs independently. The clinical setting in which this can be appreciated is the management of diabetic ketoacidosis, and the effect is used in treating hyperkalemia (see p 123).

Toxins

Individuals who ingest soluble barium salts in contaminated food develop hypokalemia, paralysis, vomiting, and diarrhea. Barium induces hypokalemia by shifting K into the cells (133). Other toxic agents, such as lithium salts, antibiotics, and chemotherapy (87), have been reported to cause hypokalemia (53).

Effects

Neuromuscular

The effects of hypokalemia and K deficiency are different, but overlap (134). The clinical effects of hypokalemia are muscle weakness or paralysis, including paralysis of the diaphragm in severe cases; hyporeflexia is common. Depression, apathy, or an acute brain syndrome characterized by disorientation and confusion are reported (135). Smooth muscle dysfunction causes ileus and urinary retention. Cardiac abnormalities are characterized by depression of the ST segment, low voltage of the T wave, and appearance of a U wave. Premature atrial or ventricular contractions or atrial arrhythmias may occur.

Patients with K deficiency who receive digitalis are more likely to have increased cardiac automaticity (136). Peripheral vascular (arteriolar) dilatation during exercise may be reduced by K deficiency, leading to muscular ischemia and rhabdomyolysis (137), which can lead to shock and acute renal failure from myoglobinuria (chapter 49).

Metabolic

Hypokalemia and K deficiency impair insulin release, which may account for glucose intolerance observed with hyperaldosteronism. Chronic K deficiency retards growth. Protons, Na, and cationic amino acids may be taken up by the cells in response to K depletion. Na also is retained to produce a slight expansion of ECF volume unless ECF volume depletion is part of the underlying process causing hypokalemia (138).

Renal

Morphologic abnormalities of the kidney can be linked to K depletion. The changes in renal histology vary among species. In humans, vacuolar and degenerative changes occur in the cells of the proximal tubule. These are reversible and correlate poorly with functional alterations (139, 140). In rats, lesions in the collecting tubules are prominent and are associated with the urinary concentrating defect (138, 141). Long-standing hypokalemia may cause interstitial nephritis (140).

The most prominent functional abnormality of K deficiency nephropathy is impaired ability to concentrate urine. In rats, this is associated with a loss of hypertonicity in the medullary interstitium (141, 142). Polyuria and polydipsia resistant to exogenous administration of vasopressin is common (138). The polydipsia may be related to increased production of angiotensin II, which stimulates the thirst center (143).

K depletion leads to the retention of Na; some enters the cells and the rest remains in the ECF and, given a sufficient intake, may cause edema (8). During K depletion, Na is conserved by an increase in renal proximal reabsorption of Na. A decrease in flow rate in the distal nephron coupled with suppression of plasma aldosterone by K depletion results in conservation of K (144). Little or no change is seen in GFR (145), unless the depletion of K is prolonged or there is underlying renal disease (140).

The effect of K depletion on the renal regulation of acid-base homeostasis is not clear because maneuvers used to induce K depletion affect acid-base status independently (146). Moderate K restriction in which dietary K is replaced by Na causes minimal metabolic alkalosis (+1.8 mEq/L) in plasma HCO_3 and without an increase in mineralocorticoid production or Cl depletion. Despite the alkalosis, renal acid excretion is decreased and urinary pH is increased. Both plasma renin activity and aldosterone concentration are diminished and the reduction in acid excretion is anticipated from the decrease in plasma aldosterone. Other mechanisms are suggested to be operative in causing and maintaining the hyperbicarbonatemia. The reduction in renal excretion of acid is less than the reduction in net acid intake derived from diet and metabolism (146). K deficiency stimulates ammonia production (147) and causes a translocation of extracellular H^+ into renal cells, which may have contributed to these findings (23).

Diagnosis

The diagnosis of hypokalemia may be inferred from changes in the ECG, but should be confirmed by direct measurement of Ks. The diagnosis of K deficiency usually is made from the history and the presence of hypokalemia and alkalosis. History may document gastrointestinal or urinary tract disease, use of diuretics, or other therapeutic agents that cause hypokalemia. Aberrant behavior coupled with inappropriate drug therapy are causes in adults and may be operative in adolescents. The initial workup should establish whether blood pressure, growth, acid-base status, and GFR are appropriate for age. Abnormalities in these findings may be a clue to subtle K deficiency.

Renal K wasting is defined as a urinary excretion of K that is >40 mEq/day in hypokalemic adults. Where indicated, a test for renal K wasting is undertaken in the following manner. Na and K intake should be regulated to be equal and within 2 to 3 mEq/kg/day each. Renal K wasting is present if one of the following criteria are present: (1) urinary Na/K ratio is consistently <1 or (2) urinary K excretion exceed intake by 0.5 to 1.0 mEq/kg/day. Renal K wasting with hypertension and alkalosis suggest primary mineralocorticoid excess or primary hyperreninemia and requires investigation of the renin-angiotensin-aldosterone system. Normotensive children with alkalosis waste K in conditions of secondary aldosteronism. K is better conserved during transient cellular shifts of K. Acidosis is often seen with hypokalemia when the production of net acid or loss of base and organic anion exceeds the secondary aldosterone-stimulated increase in acid excretion, as occurs in diarrhea and RTA.

Management

Mild hypokalemia and K deficiency frequently are responsive to supplementation of the diet with foods rich in K (Table 7.2). Modest hypokalemia may be treated with oral K, either as KCl or $KHCO_3$ (or K with an organic anion), as elixir or as the wax matrix formulation, Slow-K. The latter appears to be better tolerated by children. When there is

Table 7.3.
Oral Potassium Preparations

Manufacturer	Contents
Chloride	
Kay-Ciel Elixir/Powder (Berlex)	20 mEq/15 cc
K-Lor (Abbott)	20 mEq/packet
Klorvess 10% Liquid (Dorsey)	20 mEq/15 cc
K-Lyte/Cl (Mead-Johnson)	20 mEq/tablet
Kaochlor (Warren-Teed)	20 mEq/15 cc
Kato (Ingram)	20 mEq/packet
Slow-release forms	
Slow-K (Ciba)	8 mEq/tablet
Kaon-Cl (Warren-Teed)	6.7 mEq/tablet
Klotrix (Mead-Johnson)	10 mEq/tablet
Potassium chloride with bicarbonate	
Klorvess effervescent (Dorsey)	20 mEq/packet
Potassium citrate	
Polycitra	5 mEq/5 cc
Potassium bicarbonate with citrate	
K-Lyte (Mead-Johnson)	25 mEq/tablet
Potassium gluconate	
Kaon (Warren-Teed)	5 mEq/tablet
Potassium gluconate elixir (Roxane)	20 mEq/15 cc

concomitant acidosis, as with renal tubular acidosis, the administration of K with an organic anion provides potential alkali. Elixirs of K-citrate are available and well tolerated (Table 7.3).

If renal K wasting is present, it must be determined whether that can be corrected, as is the case with some forms of toxicity or renal tubular acidosis, or whether oral K supplementation must be given long term.

Intravenous K therapy is indicated in patients with hypokalemia and neuromuscular or ECG findings or when oral administration is not practical. The concentration in parenteral fluid usually should be limited to 40 mEq/L of solution delivered at a rate not to exceed 0.5 to 1.0 mEq/kg in the first hour. Diabetic ketoacidosis and other diseases that cause large ongoing losses of K may require higher concentrations of K in parenteral fluids or higher rates of K infusion. Frequent measurement of the plasma K and serial monitoring of the ECG are indicated under these conditions.

When secondary hyperreninemia or hyperaldosteronism are underlying causes, correction of these defects is the most effective ultimate treatment.

When hypokalemia is a result of a shift in K from ECF, as occurs with alkalosis, insulin administration, or familial periodic paralysis, giving K may still be indicated. Correcting the underlying cause is important. Acetazolamide is recommended in periodic paralysis.

HYPERKALEMIA

Hyperkalemia is defined as a plasma K concentration >5.5 mEq/L (148). In infants this diagnosis is made when plasma K concentration is >6.0 mEq/L (see Table 7.1). It is a result of impaired renal excretion in the face of continued intake or redistribution of cell K to ECF. Pseudohyperkalemia may result from improper collection or storage of blood sample. It is more likely when there is leukocytosis or thrombocytosis. Too vigorous exercising of the arm or prolonged venous stasis produce pseudohyperkalemia (115).

Causes

Causes of hyperkalemia are outlined in the box on this page.

Increased Intake

Individuals with normal renal function will usually tolerate acute loads of K with little more than a transient increase in plasma K. Both increased cell uptake of K and increased renal K excretion dispose of the load. A reduction in GFR (acute renal failure) or in tubular fluid flow rate (resulting from volume depletion) interfere with the renal handling of K and may lead to hyperkalemia.

Hyperkalemia results from improper intravenous infusion, injection or infusing stored cold blood. Layering of K additives in making intravenous solutions has caused hyperkalemia. Oral K supplements or salt substitutes that include KCl may cause hyperkalemia and death (150–153).

CAUSES OF HYPERKALEMIA

I. Pseudohyperkalemia
   A. Leukocytosis
   B. Thrombocytosis
   C. Hemolysis (in vitro)
   D. Improper collection or handling of blood
II. Increased potassium load
   A. Oral potassium supplementation
   B. Intravenous administration
   C. Salt substitutes
   D. Potassium penicillin in high doses
   E. Potassium pooling in intravenous bags
   F. Stored blood
   G. Endogenous cell breakdown
      1. Trauma
      2. Intravascular hemolysis
      3. Burns
      4. Rhabdomyolysis
      5. Major surgery
      6. Total starvation
      7. Chemotherapy of lymphomas, leukemia, myeloma
III. Decreased renal potassium excretion
   A. Acute oliguric renal failure
   B. Chronic renal failure
   C. Adrenal insufficiency
      1. Hypoaldosteronism
      2. 18-OH dehydrogenase defect
      3. 21-Hydroxylase defect
   D. Hyporeninemic hypoaldosteronism
   E. Drugs
      1. Succinylcholine
      2. Arginine hydrochloride
      3. Digitalis poisoning
   F. Defective tubular secretion
      1. Sickle cell disease
      2. Systemic lupus erythematosus
      3. Renal transplantation
      4. Obstructive uropathy
      5. Interstitial nephritis
      6. Spitzer-Weinstein syndrome
      7. Low birth weight infants
   G. Potassium sparing diuretics
      1. Triamterene
      2. Spironolactone
IV. Redistribution
   A. Acidosis (metabolic or respiratory)
   B. Severe exercise with beta blockade (propranolol)
   C. Increased ECF osmolality (glucose, mannitol, saline)
   D. Hyperkalemic periodic paralysis

A large release of K into ECF from cells results from massive cell damage. Cell injury and hypercatabolic states associated with burns, surgery, crush injury, rhabdomyolysis, disseminated intravascular hemolysis, chemotherapeutic destruction of large tumors, and massive gastrointestinal or soft tissue bleeding can cause hyperkalemia (117). Rapid destruction of red blood cells, in particular in patients having hemolytic episodes, may cause hyperkalemia (154). In most cases, the release of K is short-lived, but the increase in K_s may be life-threatening, particularly if renal insufficiency, acidosis, or ECF contraction are present at the same time, as often is the case.

Decreased Excretion

Acute Renal Failure. Hyperkalemia may develop with acute oliguric renal failure. The reasons include: (1) sudden reduction in GFR, which limits the excretory capacity for K; (2) decrease in distal and collecting tubular fluid flow rate that limits K secretion; (3) insufficient time for renal and extrarenal adaptive mechanisms to develop, and (4) the association of renal failure with tissue breakdown and acidosis, which release K from cells into ECF (9, 148).

Chronic Renal Failure. In chronic renal failure, plasma K usually is maintained in the normal range by renal and extrarenal adaptive mechanisms (155) until GFR falls <10 ml/min. Renal K excretion may exceed the filtered load (fractional excretion of K >100%) when renal function is greatly reduced (156, 157); however, the capacity of surviving nephrons to adapt to an acute K load is impaired (157). In the steady state, the patient with chronic renal failure has TBK stores that are normal or low (158, 159). Intracellular K content in white cells (160) and in muscle (161) is decreased in uremic patients. It has been proposed that a uremic toxin acts to inhibit cellular Na,K-ATPase, resulting in depressed cation transport (162). The abnormality is reversed with dialysis (161, 162).

Mineralocorticoid Deficiency. Since aldosterone stimulates K secretion, its deficiency or a resistance to its effect on the target organ will cause hyperkalemia. Adrenal insufficiency or Addison's disease associated with impaired production of mineralocorticoid and glucocorticoid hormones, is characterized by salt-wasting and hyperkalemia (1, 163, 164). Patients with Addison's disease, who are on a high salt intake and maintain a high urinary flow, preserve K homeostasis with mineralocorticoid-insensitive renal mechanisms (75). However, contraction of ECF volume is frequently encountered in these patients and they are then at risk for K retention and hyperkalemia.

Hypoaldosteronism and hyporeninemia occur in older adults and are a selective deficiency of either renin or aldosterone in the absence of impaired production of glucocorticoids (165, 166). Children may be hyporeninemic and may have a similar clinical pattern (108). Patients with mild-to-moderate chronic renal insufficiency associated with primary renal interstitial disease who have hyperchloremic metabolic acidosis disproportionate to the degree of renal impairment, often have hyporeninemia (167). Nearly half the adults have diabetes mellitus, but patients having similar findings with tubulointerstitial disease, obstructive uropathy (168), sickle cell disease (169), and glomerulonephritis (170), have been described.

Resistance to Mineralocorticoid Action. Hyperkalemia results from a primary defect in renal tubular K secretion in association with normal or high levels of renin and aldosterone. The responsiveness to exogenous mineralocorticoid therapy is reduced. Children that are affected have, in addition to hyperkalemia, short stature, metabolic acidosis and hypertension, whereas GFR, Na handling, and mineralocorticoid production are normal (171, 172). Hyperkalemia secondary to a defect in tubular K secretion has been described in patients with sickle cell disease (169), systemic lupus erythematosus (173), interstitial nephritis (167), obstructive uropathy (168), and after renal transplantation (174).

Patients with high levels of plasma aldosterone and salt-wasting have pseudohypoaldosteronism (PHA) characterized by failure to gain weight, dehydration, hyponatremia, and hyperkalemia (175). These abnormalities are not sensitive to mineralocorticoid therapy but do respond to salt supplements and control of K intake (175, 176). In one patient, the activity of Na,K-ATPase in the ascending limb of the loop of Henle was low and in the proximal and distal convoluted tubules was absent (177). The condition may be a result of a delay in development of renal mechanisms for K handling, because many patients outgrow their need for supplemental salt by 2 to 4 years of age (176). On the other hand, these patients develop hyponatremia with salt restriction (chapter 33). A similar transient state of salt wasting occurs in low birth weight infants; salt wasting is very prevalent in infants <32 weeks postconceptional age (Table 7.4), but has essentially disappeared once infants have reached 36 weeks postconceptional age (178–180) (chapter 56A).

Drugs. Spironolactone, a specific inhibitor of the action of aldosterone, amiloride, and triamterene (88), can cause hyperkalemia. The latter block luminal uptake of Na into the distal tubular cell; the negative voltage in the lumen is reduced and K secretion is inhibited (181). Although these drugs may increase K_s slightly, hyperkalemia is only a problem when renal function is impaired.

Patients with diabetes, even those with normal renal function, are at risk for significant hyperkalemia, because the insulin response to the increase in plasma K is attenuated and the insulin-mediated shift in K out of ECF is blunted (182).

Redistribution of K. Hyperkalemia occurs when K intake is abruptly increased and the mechanisms for distribution of K into cells are impaired as with metabolic acidosis (183), in which the response to a hormonally-mediated shift of K from ECF is impaired. This occurs with deficiency of mineralocorticoid (184), insulin (185, 186) or epinephrine. Patients receiving beta-blockers who exercise (187) and patients given inhibitors of renin release, e.g., Captopril (188) are at risk for hyperkalemia if they are given K in amounts normally well tolerated. Patients with hyperosmolality following mannitol administration or severe hyperglycemia may become hyperkalemic by increased leakage of K from cells (189, 190). Arginine chloride, used to provoke release of growth hormone, displaces K from cells and can also cause hyperkalemia (191). Patients with familial hyperkalemic periodic paralysis become symptomatic when they exercise, are exposed to cold, or ingest K (192). Attacks have been aborted or treated with Salbutamol, a beta-2 agonist which stimulates K uptake (193).

The normal distribution of K may be altered as a side effect of drug

Table 7.4.
Urinary Potassium Excretion in Newborns, Infants, and Children (Mean ± Standard Deviation)

	Urinary sodium to potassium ratio (U_{Na^+}/U_{K^+})	Potassium excretion (mEq/kg/day)	Fractional excretion of potassium (%)
Newborns[a]			
30–32	6.2 ± 1.7	0.5 ± 0.1	25.7 ± 7.2
33–35	5.0 ± 1.8	0.4 ± 0.1	
36–38	3.4 ± 1.3	0.4 ± 0.5	
39–41	2.4 ± 1.0	0.5 ± 0.2	
Infants[b] n = 14			
1–12 months	1.1 ± 1.5	2.3 ± 1.3	16.6 ± 9.1
Children[b] n = 36			
2–20 years	1.5 ± 1.0	2.8 ± 2.4	15.4 ± 8.4

[a] Gestational age in weeks; measurements obtained at 1 week of age. (From Sulyok E, et al: Biol Neonate 35:60, 1979.)
[b] From Satlin LM, Feld LG, Schwartz GJ: Unpublished observations.

therapy. The depolarizing muscle relaxant succinylcholine causes the release of K from muscles during cellular depolarization (194). The hyperkalemia may be exaggerated if succinylcholine is used in patients suffering from burns, trauma, neuromuscular diseases, or renal failure (195). Digitalis overdose may cause hyperkalemia by inhibiting cellular Na,K-ATPase (196).

Effects

The clinical manifestations of hyperkalemia are related to the alteration in the ratio of intracellular to extracellular K with its suppressive effects on excitable tissues (depolarizing block). ECG abnormalities occur as the plasma K concentration increases to >7 mEq/L (Fig. 7.3). In general, the more rapid the development of hyperkalemia, the lower the plasma level at which cardiotoxicity develops. Initially, the T-waves become tall and peaked. As conduction becomes depressed by rising levels of plasma K, the P-R interval prolongs, the P-wave disappears, the QRS complexes widen. The AV conduction delay may cause the development of arrhythmias, such as nodal or idioventricular rhythms. A "sine wave" pattern, representing a merger of the QRS complex with the peaked T wave, is a harbinger of ventricular fibrillation or arrest.

Neuromuscular manifestations include skeletal muscle weakness and ascending flaccid paralysis. The central nervous system and muscles of respiration are usually spared.

Diagnosis

Hyperkalemia is frequently discovered before the onset of clinical symptoms. The diagnosis is made by determining K_s. Hyperkalemia suggests the existence of (1) decreased renin production, (2) decreased aldosterone production despite appropriate renin secretion (adrenal defect) or decreased response to aldosterone action, (3) markedly reduced GFR, (4) impaired renal tubular secretion, (5) insulin deficiency, (6) exogenous or endogenous load of K, (7) an abnormal shift of intracellular K to the ECF, or a combination of these (148).

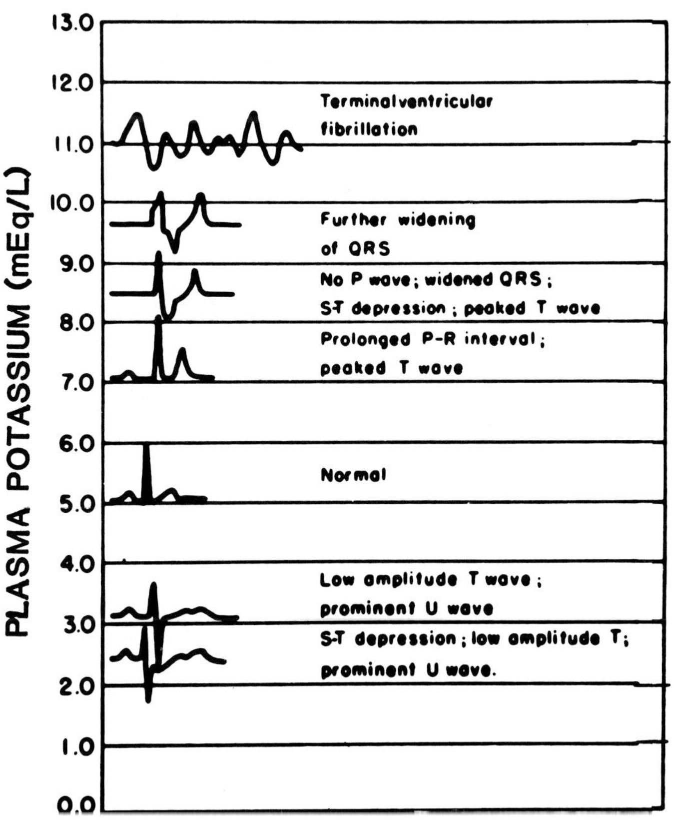

Figure 7.3. The ECG changes that occur at a given plasma potassium concentration are shown. (Adapted from Winters RW: The Body Fluids in Pediatrics. Boston, Little, Brown & Co., 1973, p 134.)

The diagnostic evaluation should include a description of growth during infancy, evidence for chronic diseases, e.g., diabetes, sickle cell disease, a history of taking medications, such as beta-blockers or digoxin. The physical examination should rule out the presence of hypertension and signs of chronic disease. Evidence for sickle cell anemia or leukemia should be sought.

Initial laboratory studies should include an ECG and an evaluation of plasma glucose, renal function, and acid-base status. An estimate of GFR from the plasma creatinine, electrolytes, glucose concentration, and a urinalysis are part of the screening procedure. Specific gravity and urinary pH may suggest other tubular disorders, RTA, or obstructive uropathy. The test for renal K wasting may be useful (p 116). Salt wasting may be identified in a patient who is mildly volume-depleted by noting the response to salt supplementation. The fractional excretion of K will be low despite hyperkalemia, either when there is a defect in the renin-angiotensin-aldosterone system or when there is a primary defect in renal tubular K excretion.

The defect in cellular K uptake is difficult to evaluate. Acute infusion of K has been used to evaluate cellular uptake in adults (148). About half of the load is excreted over 4 hours while most of the remaining half is taken up by cells. The measured increment in plasma K can be compared with that predicted to occur if all K remained extracellular. This study must be conducted with careful monitoring of plasma K concentration and ECG, but may give important information about the renin-angiotensin-aldosterone system, as well as about cellular uptake.

Management

In the treatment of hyperkalemia with major abnormalities on the ECG (Table 7.5), the immediate priority is to reverse the cardiotoxic effects with Ca at the level of the cell membrane. A 10% calcium-gluconate solution is given at a dose of 0.5 to 1.0 mg/kg intravenously over 2 to 10 minutes while monitoring with the ECG. Extreme caution should be used in patients receiving digoxin. The onset of action is within 5 minutes, but the duration is transient.

K may be transferred to the intracellular compartment with intravenous glucose (0.5 to 1.0 g/kg) given over 15 to 30 minutes, plus insulin (1 U for each 3 to 5 gram glucose). The onset of action is within 30 minutes, and the duration may exceed several hours. This maneuver is most effective in fasted or catabolic states and is not effective when glucose has been given in the immediate preceding period. In neonates, glucose should not be infused at rates >0.8 g/kg/hr. Rapid alkalinization of the plasma with $NaHCO_3$ administered at a dose of 1.5 to 2 mEq/kg over 5 to 10 minutes is helpful, particularly when acidosis is present. The action occurs within minutes and may persist for several hours. The $NaHCO_3$ should not be administered through the same intravenous line as Ca because of the likelihood of precipitating Ca carbonates in the intravenous tubing.

None of the foregoing maneuvers actually remove K from the body. The cation exchange resin, sodium polystyrene sulfonate (Kayexalate) should be administered simultaneously with the above maneuvers. The dose is 0.5 to 1.0 g/kg or it is effective and well tolerated when given as a retention enema for 15 to 30 minutes in 70% sorbitol or 10% dextrose in water (1g resin/4 ml). The sorbitol or glucose increases the amount of fluid entering the bowel lumen. The efficiency of K removal is limited and variable so that serum K concentrations should be monitored frequently. For each mEq K removed, 1 mEq of Na will be exchanged. Plasma K decreases within 1 to 2 hours.

Dialysis is required when hyperkalemia persists or renal failure is severe. This is particularly true when volume overload or edema already

Table 7.5.
Treatment of Hyperkalemia

Drug	Dose	Onset of action	Duration	Mechanism	Comments
Calcium gluconate (10%)	0.5–1.0 ml/kg	Immediate	Minutes	Antagonize membrane effects	Give IV over 2–10 minutes with continuous ECG monitoring
Sodium bicarbonate	1.0–2.0 mEq/kg	30–60 minutes	Transient (hours)	ECF expansion and intracellular uptake	Give IV over 10–30 minutes
Glucose (insulin)	0.5–1.0 gm/kg (0.1 units/kg, IV or SC)	30–60 minutes	Transient (hours)	ECF expansion, intracellular uptake and possibly increased excretion	Give IV over 15–30 minutes with insulin
Sodium polysterene sulfonate (Kayexalate)	1.0 gm/kg	60 minutes	Hours	Sodium exchanged for K in the gut to increase excretion	Give orally or per rectum diluted with 2–4 ml of sorbitol or 10% dextrose per gram of resin
Sodium chloride	0.9% NaCl, 10–20 ml/kg	30–60 minutes	Transient (hours)	ECF expansion and increased excretion	Give over 45–60 minutes

exists so that Na uptake is not desirable. Hemodialysis can remove 1 mEq K/kg/hr and can be initiated through catheters inserted into the femoral vein. The catheters may be reused up to 2 weeks. Peritoneal dialysis is less efficient than hemodialysis, but it can be performed in small infants with greater safety. Hemofiltration is used in some institutions for the rapid removal of K (chapter 51).

The management of chronic hyperkalemia, especially in chronic renal insufficiency, requires that dietary K be restricted. Patients with chronic renal failure differ in their preferences for foods that are low in K, in their extrarenal handling and disposal of K, and in their urinary flow rates and residual GFR, so that a regimen must be prescribed for individuals with these variables in mind. Rarely, supplemental oral exchange resin, i.e., Kayexalate, is required to maintain plasma K at safe levels. Children with insufficient mineralocorticoid and some with a primary tubular defect respond to fluodrocortisone acetate (0.1 to 1 mg/day). Others with renal tubular K secretory defects may respond to chlorothiazide 4 to 10 mg/kg/day, $NaHCO_3$ administration, or Na restriction (176), but treatment will be empirical unless the pathophysiology of the tubular secretory disorders is worked out in relation to K intake and the hormonal control of K distribution and excretion.

Acknowledgment

The authors wish to thank Drs. Chester M. Edelmann, Jr., Sherman Levine, Robert A. Weiss, and Frederick J. Kaskel for their helpful suggestions in the preparation of the manuscript, Ms. Amy Martinez for her technical assistance in performing the potassium analyses, and Ms. Frances Maniscalco for her secretarial assistance.

Supported by USPHS Grant #HD 13232. Dr. Feld is a postdoctoral fellow of the Kidney Disease Institute of the New York State Department of Health.

References

1. Kliger AS, Hayslett JP: Disorders of potassium balance. In Brenner BM, Stein J (eds): Acid-Base and Potassium Homeostasis. New York, Churchill-Livingstone, 1978, p 168.
2. Pierson RN Jr, Lin DHY, Phillips RA: Total body potassium in health: Effects of age, sex, height and fat. Am J Physiol 226:206, 1974.
3. Forbes GN, Lewis AM: Total sodium, potassium and chloride in adult man. J Clin Invest 35:596, 1956.
4. Flynn MA, Clark J, Reid JC, et al: A longitudinal study of total body potassium in normal children. Pediatr Res 9:834, 1975.
5. Pierson RN, Lin DHY: Measurement of body compartments in children: whole body counting and other methods. Sem Nucl Med 2:373, 1972.
5a. Corsa L, Olney JM, Steenberg RW, et al: Measurement of exchangeable potassium in man by isotope dilution. J Clin Invest 29:1280, 1950.
6. Civan MM: Intracellular activities of sodium and potassium. Am J Physiol 234:F261, 1978.
7. Maffley RH: The body fluids. In Brenner B, Rector FC (eds): The Kidney. Philadelphia, W.B. Saunders Co., 1980.
8. Khuri RM: Intracellular potassium in cells of the distal tubule. Yale J Biol Med 45:384, 1972.
9. Kunau RT Jr, Stein JH: Disorders of potassium metabolism. In Early LE, Gottschalk CW (eds): Diseases of the Kidney. Boston, Little, Brown & Co., 1979, p 1581.
10. Sulyok E, Nemeth M, Tenyi I, et al: Relationship between maturity, electrolyte balance and the function of the renin-angiotensin-aldosterone system in newborn infants. Biol Neonate 35:60, 1979.
11. Narins RG, Jones ER, Stom MC, et al: Diagnostic strategies in disorders of fluid, electrolyte and acid-base homeostasis. Am J Med 72:496, 1982.
12. Skou JC: Enzymatic basis for active transport of Na^+ and K^+ across cell membranes. Physiol Rev 45:596, 1965.
13. Thomas RC: Electrogenic sodium pump in nerve and muscle cells. Physiol Rev 52:563, 1972.
14. Finkelstein FO, Hayslett JP: Role of medullary Na-K-ATPase in renal potassium adaptation. Am J Physiol 229:524, 1975.
15. Wright FS, Streider N, Fowler HB, et al: Potassium secretion by distal tubule after potassium adaptation. Am J Physiol 221:437, 1971.
16. Fisher KA, Binder HJ, Hayslett JP: Potassium secretion by colonic mucosal cells after potassium adaptation. Am J Physiol 231:987, 1976.
17. Silva P, Brown RS, Epstein FH: Adaptation to potassium. Kidney Intl 11:466, 1977.
18. Sigstrom L, Waldenstrom J, Karlberg P: Characteristics of active sodium and potassium transport in erythrocytes of healthy infants and children. Acta Pediatr Scand 70:347, 1981.
19. Davis WD, Dixon LR: Selective postnatal development of Na^+-K^+ activated-adenosine-triphosphatase in rabbit kidneys. Proc Soc Exp Biol Med 136:95, 1971.
20. Schwartz GJ, Evan AP: Development of solute transport in rabbit proximal tubule. III Na-K-AtPase activity. Am J Physiol 246:F845, 1984.
21. Turnberg LA: Potassium transport in the human small bowel. Gut 12:811, 1971.
21a. Widdowson EM, Dickerson JWT: The effect of growth and function on the chemical composition of soft tissues. Biochem J 77:30, 1960.
22. Adrogué HJ, Madia NE: Changes in plasma potassium concentration during acute acid-base disturbances. Am J Med 71:456, 1981.
23. Adler S, Fraley DS: Potassium and intracellular pH. Kidney Intl 11:433, 1977.
24. Tobin RB: Varying role of extracellular electrolytes in metabolic acidosis and alkalosis. Am J Physiol 195:685, 1958.
25. Rogers TA, Wachenfeld AE: Effect of physiologic acids on electrolytes in rat diaphragm. Am J Physiol 193:623, 1958.
26. Fulop M: Serum potassium in lactic acidosis and ketoacidosis. N Engl J Med 300:1087, 1979.

27. Fraley DS, Adler S: Correction of hyperkalemia by bicarbonate despite constant blood pH. Kidney Intl 12:354, 1977.
28. Pettit GW, Vick RL: Contribution of pancreatic insulin to extrarenal potassium homeostasis: a two-compartmental model. Am J Physiol 226:319, 1974.
29. DeFronzo RA, Felig P, Ferrannini E, et al: Effect of gradual doses of insulin on splanchnic and peripheral potassium metabolism in man. Am J Physiol 238:E421, 1980.
30. Santeusanio F, Faloona GR, Knochel JP, et al: Evidence for a role of endogenous insulin and glucagon in the regulation of potassium homeostasis. J Lab Clin Med 81:809, 1973.
31. Pettit GW, Vick RL, Swander AM: Plasma K^+ and inulsin: change during KCl infusion in normal and nephrectomized dogs. Am J Physiol 228:107, 1975.
32. DeFronzo RA, Sherwin RS, Dillingham M, et al: Influence of basal insulin and glucagon secretion on potassium and sodium metabolism. J Clin Invest 61:472, 1978.
33. Bia MJ, DeFronzo RA: Extrarenal potassium homeostasis. Am J Physiol 240:F257, 1981.
34. Schultze RG, Nissenson AR: Potassium: physiology and pathophysiology. In Maxwell MH, Kleeman CR (eds): Clinical Disorders of Fluid and Electrolytes. New York, McGraw-Hill, 1980, p 120.
35. Vick RL, Todd EP, Leudke DW: Epinephrine induced hypokalemia: Relation to liver and skeletal muscle. J Pharmacol Exp Ther 181:139, 1972.
36. Todd EP, Vick RL: Kalemotropic effect of epinephrine: Analysis with adrenergic agonists and antagonists. Am J Physiol 220:1963, 1971.
37. Wolfe BB, Haden TK, Molinoff PB: Beta adrenergic receptors in rat liver: Effects of adrenalectomy. Proc Natl Acad Sci 73:1343, 1976.
38. Bowman WC, Nott MW: Actions of sympathomimetic amines and their antagonists on skeletal muscle. Pharm Rev 21:27, 1969.
39. D'Silva JL: The action of adrenaline on serum potassium. J Physiol (Lond) 82:893, 1934.
40. DeFronzo RA, Bia M, Birkhead G: Epinephrine and potassium homeostasis. Kidney Intl 20:83, 1981.
41. Pettit GW, Vick RL: An analysis of the contribution of the exocrine pancreas to the kalemotropic actions of catecholamines. J Pharmacol Exp Ther 190:234, 1974.
42. Carlsson E, Fellenius E, Lundborg P, et al: β-adrenoceptor blockers, plasma potassium, and exercise. Lancet 2:424, 1978.
43. Brown RS, Rowe JW, Epstein FH: Adrenergic modulation of extrarenal potassium disposal. N Engl J Med 302:431, 1980.
44. Bia MJ, Tyler KA, DeFronzo RA: Regulation of extrarenal potassium homeostasis by adrenal hormones in rats. Am J Physiol 242:F641, 1982.
45. White AG, Gordon H, Leiter L: Studies in oedema: effect of congestive heart failure on salivary electrolyte concentration. J Clin Invest 29:445, 1950.
46. Conn JW: Aldosteronism in man. Some clinical and climatological aspects. JAMA 183:775, 1963.
47. Richards P: Clinical investigation of the effects of adrenal corticosteroid excess on the colon. Lancet 1:437, 1969.
48. Bastl CP, Binder HJ, Hayslett JP: Role of glucocorticoids and aldosterone in maintenance of colonic cation transport. Am J Physiol 238:F181, 1980.
49. Alexander EA, Levinsky NG: An extrarenal mechanism of potassium adaptation. J Clin Invest 47:740, 1968.
50. Schwartz WB: Potassium and the kidney. N Engl J Med 253:601, 1955.
51. Pennington JAT, Church HN: Food values of portions commonly used. New York, Harper & Row, 1980.
52. American Academy of Pediatrics Committee on Nutrition: commentary on breast feeding and infant formulas, including proposed standards for formulas. Pediatrics 57:278, 1976.
53. Cohen JJ, Gennari FJ, Harrington JT: Disorders of Potassium Balance. In Brenner BM, Rector F (eds): The Kidney. Philadelphia, W.B. Saunders, 1980, p 911.
54. Hayslett JP, Binder HJ: Mechanism of potassium adaptation. Am J Physiol 243:F103, 1982.
55. Malnic G, Klose RM, Giebisch G: Micropuncture study of renal potassium excretion in the rat. Am J Physiol 206:674, 1964.
56. Malnic G, Klose RM, Giebisch G: Micropuncture study of distal tubular potassium and sodium transport in rat nephron. Am J Physiol 211:529, 1966.
57. Malnic G, Klose RM, Giebisch G: Microperfusion study of distal tubular potassium and sodium transfer in rat kidney. Am J Physiol 211:548, 1966.
58. Battilana CA, Dobyan DC, Lacy FN, et al: The effect of chronic potassium loading on potassium secretion by the pars recta or descending limb of the juxtamedullary nephron in the rat. J Clin Invest 62:1093, 1978.
59. Jamison RL, Lacy FN, Pennell JP, et al: Potassium secretion by the descending limb of pars recta or juxatmedullary nephron in vivo. Kidney Intl 9:323, 1976.
60. Jamison RL, Work J, Schafer JA: New pathways for potassium transport in the kidney. Am J Physiol 242:F297, 1982.
61. Grantham JJ, Burg MB, Orloff J: The nature of transtubular Na and K transport in rabbit collecting tubules. J Clin Invest 49:1815, 1970.
62. Good DW, Wright FS: Luminal influence on potassium secretion: sodium concentration and fluid flow rate. Am J Physiol 236:F192, 1979.
63. Kunau RT, Webb HL, Borman SC: Characteristics of the relationship between the flow rate of tubular fluid and potassium transport in the distal tubule of the rat. J Clin Invest 54:1488, 1974.
64. Wright FS: Sites and mechanisms of potassium transport along the renal tubule. Kidney Intl 11:415, 1977.
65. Giebisch G: Effects of flow rate and potassium intake on distal tubular potassium transfer. Am J Physiol 228:1249, 1975.
66. Reineck HJ, Osbood RW, Ferris T, et al: Potassium transport in the distal tubular collecting duct of the rat. Am J Physiol 229:1403, 1975.
67. Velazquez H, Wright FS, Good DW: Luminal influences on potassium secretion: chloride replacement with sulfate. Am J Physiol 242:F46, 1982.
68. Bank N, Schwartz WB: The influence of anion penetrating ability on urinary acidification and the excretion of titratable acid. J Clin Invest 39:1516, 1960.
69. Lipner HI, Ruzany F, Dasguptu M, et al: The behavior of carbenicillin as a nonreabsorbable anion. J Lab Clin Med 86:183, 1975.
70. Wiederholt M, Schoormans W, Fischer F, et al: Mechanism of action of aldosterone on potassium transfer in the rat kidney. Pfluegers Arch 345:159, 1973.
71. Wiederholt M, Agulian SK, Khuri RN: Intracellular potassium in the distal tubule of the adrenalectomized and aldosterone treated-rat. Pfluegers Arch 349:117, 1974.
72. Schwartz GJ, Burg MB: Mineralocorticoid effects on cation transport by cortical collecting tubules in rats. Am J Physiol 235:F576, 1978.
73. Petty KJ, Kokko JP, Marver D: Secondary effect of aldosterone on Na-K-ATPase activity in the rabbit cortical collecting tubule. J Clin Invest 68:1514, 1982.
74. August JL, Nelson DH, Thorn GW: Response of normal subjects to large amounts of aldosterone. J Clin Invest 37:1549, 1958.
75. Wingo CS, Seldin DW, Kokko JP, et al: Dietary modulation of active potassium secretion in the cortical collecting tubule of adrenalectomized rabbits. J Clin Invest 70:579, 1982.
76. Malnic G, Mello-Aires M, Giebisch G: Potassium transport across the renal distal tubular epithelium during acid-base disturbances. Am J Physiol 221:1192, 1971.
77. Gennari FJ, Goldstein MB, Schwartz WB: The nature of renal adaptation to chronic hypocapnia. J Clin Invest 51:1722, 1972.
78. Kassirer JP, Schwartz WB: The response of normal men to selective depletion of hydrochloric acid. Am J Med 40:10, 1966.
79. Boudry JF, Stoner LC, Burg MB: Effect of acid lumen pH on potassium transport in renal cortical collecting tubules. Am J Physiol 230:239, 1976.
80. Turnberg LA: Electrolyte absorption from the colon. Gut 11:1049, 1970.
81. Edmonds CJ: Transport of sodium and secretion of potassium and bicarbonate by the colon of normal and sodium-depleted rats. J Physiol (Lond.) 193:589, 1967.
82. Kashgarian M, Taylor CR, Binder HJ, et al: Amplification of cell membrane surface in potassium adaptation. Lab Invest 42:581, 1980.
83. Hayes CP Jr, McLeod MI, Robinson R: An extrarenal mechanism for the maintenance of potassium balance in severe chronic renal failure. Trans Assoc Am Physicians 80:207, 1967.
84. Kunau RT, Stein JH: Disorders of hypo- and hyperkalemia. Clin Nephrol 7:173, 1977.
85. Patrick J: Death during recovery from severe malnutrition and its possible relationship to sodium pump activity in the leukocyte. Brit Med J 1:1051, 1977.
86. Grossman H, Duggan E, McCammon S, et al: The chloride deficiency syndrome. Pediatrics 66:366, 1980.
87. Andreoli SP, Kleiman MB, Glick MR, et al: Nafcillin, pseudoproteinuria, and hypokalemic alkalosis. J Pediatr 97:841, 1980.
88. Goldberg M: The renal physiology of diuretics. In Orloff, Berliner R (eds): Handbook of Physiology. Washington, D.C., American Physiologic Society, 1973, p 1003.
89. Gennari FJ, Kassirer JP: Osmotic diuresis. N Engl J Med 291:714, 1974.
90. Lawson DH: Adverse reaction to potassium chloride. Quart J Med 43:433, 1974.
91. Kassirer JP, Harrington JT: Diuretics and potassium metabolism: A reassessment of the need, effectiveness and safety of potassium therapy. Kidney Intl 11:505, 1977.
92. Dargie HJ, Boddy K, Kennedy AC, et al: Total body potassium in long-term furosemide therapy. Is potassium supplementation necessary? Brit Med J 4:316, 1974.
93. Goldberg M, McCurdy DK, Foltz EL, et al: Effects of ethacrynic acid (a new saluretic agent) on renal diluting and concentrating mechanisms: Evidence for site of action in the loop of Henle. J Clin Invest 43:201, 1964.
94. Aitchison J, Brown JJ, Ferriss JB, et al: Quadric analysis in the preoperative distinction between patients with and without adrenocortical tumors in hypertension with aldosterone excess and low plasma renin. Am Heart J 82:660, 1971.
95. Schambelan M, Slaton PE, Biglieri EG: Mineralocorticoid production in hyperadrenocorticism: Role in pathogeneis of hypokalemic alkalosis. Am J Med 51:299, 1971
96. Eberlein WR, Bongiovanni AM: Plasma and urinary corticosteroids in the hypertensive form of congenital adrenal hyperplasia. J Biol Chem 223:85, 1956.

96a. Thomas BA (ed): Pathways of steroid biosynthesis. In The Adrenal Cortex. Kalamazoo, Mich., Upjohn Company, 1974.
97. Biglieri EG, Herron MA, Brust N: 17-Hydroxylation deficiency in man. J Clin Invest 45:1946, 1966.
98. Biglieri EG, Stockigt JF, Schambelan M: Adrenal mineralocorticoids cause hypertension. Am J Med 52:623, 1972.
99. Christy NP, Laragh JH: Pathogenesis of hypokalemic alkalosis in Cushing's Syndrome. N Engl J Med 265:1083, 1961.
100. Williams GH, Cain JP, Dluhy RG et al: Studies of the control of plasma aldosterone concentration in normal man. I. Response to posture, acute and chronic volume depletion, and sodium loading. J Clin Invest 51:1731, 1972.
101. Wrong O: Incidence of hypokalemia in severe hypertension. Brit Med J 2:419, 1961.
102. Simon M, Franklin SS, Bleifer KH, et al: Clinical characteristics of renal vascular hypertension. JAMA 220:1209, 1972.
103. Robertson TW, Kliojian A, Harding LJ, et al: Hypertension due to a renin excreting tumor. Am J Med 43:963, 1967.
104. Voute PA, Vendermeer J, Stougaard N, et al: Plasma renin activity in Wilm's tumor. Acta Endocrinol 67:197, 1971.
105. Martin H, Wertman N: Serum potassium, magnesium and calcium levels in diabetic acidosis. J Clin Invest 26:217, 1947.
106. Sebastian A, McSherry E, Morris RC Jr: Renal potassium wasting in renal tubular acidosis. J Clin Invest 50:667, 1971.
106a. Cogan MG, Rector FC Jr, Seldin DW: Acid-base disorders. In Brenner BM, Rector FC Jr (eds): The Kidney. Philadelphia, W.B. Saunders Co., 1981, p 841.
107. McSherry E, Sebastian A, Morris RC Jr: Renal tubular acidosis in infants: Several kinds, including bicarbonate wasting, classic renal tubular acidosis. J Clin Invest 51:499, 1972.
108. McSherry E: Renal tubular acidosis in childhood. Kidney Intl 20:799, 1981.
109. McCredie DA, Blair-West JR, Scoggins BA, et al: Potassium-losing nephropathy in children. Med J Australia 1:129, 1971.
110. Spencer RW, Voyce MA: Familial hypokalemia and hypomagnesemia. Acta Paediatr Scand 65:505, 1976.
111. Liddle GW, Bledsow T, Coppage WS Jr: A familial renal disorder simulating primary aldosteronism but with negligible aldosterone secretion. Trans Assoc Am Physicians 76:199, 1963.
112. Wang C, Chan TK, Yeung RTT, et al: The effect of triamterene and sodium intake on renin aldosterone and erythrocyte sodium transport in Liddle's syndrome. J Clin Endo Metab 52:1027, 1981.
113. Cronin RE, Bulger RE, Southern P, et al: Natural history of aminoglycoside nephrotoxicity in the dog. J Lab Clin Med 95:463, 1980.
114. Holmes AM, Hesling CM, Wilson TM: Drug-induced secondary hyperaldosteronism in patients with pulmonary tuberculosis. Quart J Med 39:299, 1970.
115. Bar RS, Wilson HE, Mazzaferri EL: Hypomagnesemic hypocalcemia secondary to renal magnesium wasting: A possible consequence of high-dose gentamicin therapy. Ann Intern Med 82:646, 1975.
116. Brinker KR, Bulger RE, Dobyan DC, et al: Effect of potassium depletion on gentamicin nephrotoxicity. J Lab Clin Med 98:292, 1981.
117. O'Regan S, Kaplan BS, Chesney RW, et al: Hypokalemia in children with leukemia in relapse. Am J Dis Child 130:937, 1976.
118. Stapleton FB, Nelson B, Vats TS, et al: Hypokalemia associated with antibiotic treatment. Am J Dis Child 130:1104, 1976.
119. Edmonds CJ, Smith T: Total body potassium in relation to thyroid hormones and hyperthyroidism. Clin Sci 60:311, 1981.
120. Phillips SF, Summerskill WHJ: Water and electrolytes in gastrointestinal disease. In Maxwell MM, Kleeman CR (eds): Clinical Disorders of Fluid and Electrolyte Metabolism. New York, McGraw-Hill, 1980, p 1267.
121. Kassirer JP, Schwartz WB: The response of normal man to selective depletion of hydrochloric acid. Factors in the genesis of persistent alkalosis. Am J Med 40:1018, 1966.
122. Garella S, Chazan JP, Cohen JJ: Saline resistant metabolic *alkalosis* or chloride wasting nephropathy. Ann Int Med 73:31, 1970.
123. Teree TM, Mirabel-Font E, Ortiz A, et al: Stool losses and acidosis in diarrhea disease of infancy. Pediatrics 36:704, 1965.
124. Fordtran JS: Speculations on the pathogenesis of diarrhea. Fed Proc 26:1405, 1967.
125. Darrow DC, Pratt EL, Flett J Jr, et al: Disturbances of water and electrolytes in infantile diarrhea. Pediatrics 3:129, 1949.
126. Waterlow, Alleyne: Protein Malnutrition in Children: Advances in Knowledge in the Last 10 Years. New York, Academic Press, 1971, p 25.
127. Schwartz WB, Kassirer JP: Effects of ureteral transplantations. In Strauss MB, Welt LG (eds): Disease of the Kidney. Boston, Little, Brown & Co., 1963, p 759.
128. Schrock LG, Polk HC Jr: Rectal villous adenoma producing hypokalemia. Am J Surg 40:54, 1974.
129. Flesicher N, Brown M, Graham DY, et al: Chronic laxative-induced hyperaldosteronism and hypokalemia simulating Bartter's Syndrome. Ann Int Med 70:791, 1969.
130. Gottlieb RP: Metabolic alkalosis in cystic fibrosis. J Pediatr 79:930, 1971.
131. Baxter CR: Fluid volume and electrolyte changes of the early postburn period. Clinics Plastic Surgery 1:693, 1974.
132. Streeten DHP: Periodic paralysis. In Stanbury JB, Wyngaarden JB, Frederickson DS (eds): Metabolic Basis of Inherited Disease. New York, McGraw-Hill, 1966, p 905.
133. Roza O, Berman LB: The pathophysiology of barium: Hypokalemic and cardiovascular effects. J Pharm Exp Ther 177:433, 1971.
134. Epstein FH: Signs and symptoms of electrolyte disorders. In Maxwell MM, Kleeman CR (eds): Clinical Disorders of Fluid and Electrolyte Metabolism. New York, McGraw-Hill, 1980, p 499.
135. Mitchell W, Feldman F: Neuropsychiatric aspects of hypokalemia. Can Med Assoc J 98:48, 1968.
136. Cronin RE, Knochel JP: The consequences of potassium deficiency. In Brenner BM, Stein J (eds): Acid-Base Potassium Homeostasis. New York, Churchill-Livingston, 1978, p 203.
137. Knochel JP, Schlein EM: On the mechanism of rhabdomyolysis in potassium depletion. J Clin Invest 51:1750, 1972.
138. Welt LG, Hollander W Jr, Blythe WB: The consequences of potassium depletion. J Chron Dis 11:213, 1960.
139. Relman AS, Schwartz WB: The nephropathy of potassium depletion: A clinical and pathological entity. N Engl J Med 255:195, 1956.
140. Cremer W, Bock KD: Symptoms and course of chronic hypokalemic nephropathy in man. Clin Nephrol 7:112, 1977.
141. Gottschalk CW, Mylle M, Jones NF: Osmolality of renal tubule fluid in potassium-depleted rodents. Clin Sci 29:249, 1965.
142. Manitis A, Levitin H, Beck D, et al: On the mechanism of renal concentrating ability in potassium deficiencies. J Clin Invest 39:684, 1960.
143. Berl T, Linas L, Aisenbrey GA, et al: On the mechanism of polyuria in potassium depletion: The role of polydipsia. J Clin Invest 60:620, 1977.
144. Sealey JE, Laragh JH: A proposed cybernetic system for sodium and potassium homeostasis: Coordination of aldosterone and intrarenal physical factors. Kidney Intl 6:281, 1974.
145. Schwartz WB, Relman AS: Effects of electrolyte disorders on renal structure and function. N Engl J Med 276:383, 1967.
146. Jones JW, Sebastian A, Hulter HN, et al: Systemic and renal acid-base effects of chronic dietary potassium depletion. Kidney Intl 21:402, 1982.
147. Tannen RL: Relationship of renal ammonia production and potassium homeostasis. Kidney Intl 11:453, 1977.
148. DeFronzo RA, Bia M, Smith DI: Clinical disorders of hyperkalemia. Ann Rev Med 33:521, 1982.
149. Bronson WR, DeVita TV, Carbone PP, et al: Pseudokalemia due to release of potassium from white blood cells during clotting. N Engl J Med 274:369, 1966.
150. Haddad A, Strong E: Potassium in salt substitutes. N Engl J Med 292:1082, 1975.
151. Sopko JA, Freeman RM: Salt substitutes as a source of potassium. J Am Med Assoc 238:608, 1977.
152. Williams RHP: Potassium overdosage: a potential hazard of non-rigid parenteral fluid containers. Brit Med J 1:714, 1973.
153. Bostic O, Duvernoy WFC: Hyperkalemic cardiac arrest during transfusion of stored blood. J Electrocardiol 5:407, 1972.
154. Batlle D, Itsarayoungyuen K, Arruda JAL, et al: Hyperkalemic hyperchloremic metabolic acidosis in sickle cell hemoglobinopathies. Am J Med 72:188, 1982.
155. Schultze RG, Taggart DD, Shapiro H, et al: The adaptation in potassium secretion associated with nephron reduction in the dog. J Clin Invest 50:1061, 1971.
156. Bank N, Aynedjian HS: A micropuncture study of potassium excretion by the remnant kidney. J Clin Invest 52:1480, 1973.
157. Keith NM, Burchell HB: Clinical intoxication with potassium: its occurrence in severe renal insufficiency. Am J Med Sci 217:1, 1949.
158. Mitch WE, Wilcox CS: Disorders of body fluids, sodium and potassium in chronic renal failure. Am J Med 72:536, 1982.
159. Letteri JM, Asad SN, Caselnova R, et al: Creatinine excretion and total body potassium in renal failure. Clin Nephrol 4:58, 197.
160. Patrick J, Jones NF: Cell sodium, potassium and water in uremia and the effect of regular dialysis as studied in the leucocyte. Clin Sci Mol Med 46:583, 1974.
161. Bilbrey GL, Carter NW, White MG, et al: Potassium deficiency in chronic renal failure. Kidney Intl 4:423, 1973.
162. Cole CH: Decreased ouabain-sensitive adenosine triphosphatase activity in the erythrocyte membrane of patients with chronic renal failure. Clin Sci 45:775, 1973.
163. Daughaday WH, Rendleman D: Severe symptomatic hyperkalemia in an adrenalectomized woman due to enhanced mineralocorticoid requirement. Ann Int Med 66:1197, 1967.
164. Pollen RH, Williams RH: Hyperkalemic neuromyopathy in Addison's disease. N Engl J Med 263:273, 1960.
165. Schambelan M, Stockigt JR, Biglieri EG: Isolated hypoaldosteronism in adults: A renin-deficiency syndrome. N Engl J Med 287:573, 1972.

166. DeFronzo RA: Hyperkalemia and hyporeninemic hypoaldosteronism. Kidney Intl 17:118, 1980.
167. Shambelan M, Sebastian A, Biglieri EG: Prevalence, pathogenesis and function significance of aldosterone deficiency in hyperkalemic patients with chronic renal insufficiency. Kidney Intl 17:89, 1980.
168. Batlle DC, Annuda JA, Kurtzman NA: Hyperkalemic distal tubular acidosis associated with obstructive uropathy. N Engl J Med 304:373, 1981.
169. DeFronzo RA, Taufield PA, Black H, et al: Impaired renal tubular potassium secretion in sickle cell disease. Ann Int Med 90:310, 1979.
170. Phelps KR, Lieberman RL, Oh MS, et al: Pathophysiology of the syndrome of hyporeninemic hypoaldosteronism. Metabolism 29:186, 1980.
171. Weinstein SF, Allan DME, Mendoza SA: Hyperkalemia, acidosis and short stature associated with a defect in renal potassium excretion. J Pediatr 85:355, 1974.
172. Spitzer A, Edelmann CM Jr, Goldberg LD, et al: Short stature, hyperkalemia and acidosis: A defect in renal transport of potassium. Kidney Intl 3:251, 1973.
173. DeFronzo RA, Cooke CR, Goldberg M, et al: Impaired renal tubular potassium secretion in systemic lupus erythematosus. Ann Int Med 86:268, 1977.
174. DeFronzo RA, Goldberg M, Cooke CR, et al: Investigations into the mechanisms of hyperkalemia following renal transplantation. Kidney Intl 11:357, 1977.
175. Cheek DB, Perry JW: A salt wasting syndrome in infancy. Arch Dis Child 33:252, 1958.
176. Schwartz GJ, Spitzer A: Disorders of renal transport of sodium, potassium and magnesium. In Edelmann CM (ed): Pediatric Kidney Disease. Boston, Little, Brown and Co., 1978, p 1079.
177. Bierich JR, Schmidt U: Tubular Na-K-ATPase deficiency. The cause of the congenital renal salt-losing syndrome. Eur J Pediatr 121:81, 1976.
178. Day GM, Radde IC, Balfe JW, et al: Electrolyte abnormalities in very low birth weight infants. Pediatr Res 10:522, 1972.
179. Sulyok E: The relationship between electrolyte and acid-base balance in the premature infant during early postnatal life. Biol Neonate 17:227, 1971.
180. Al-Dahhan J, Haycock GB, Chantler C, et al: Sodium homeostasis in term and preterm neonates. Arch Dis Child 58:335, 1983.
181. Giebisch G, Malnic G, Berliner RW: Renal transport and control of potassium excretion. In Brenner BM, Rector FC (eds): The Kidney. Philadelphia, W.B. Saunders Co., 1981, p 408.
182. McNay JL, Oran E: Possible predispositon of diabetic patients to hyperkalemia following administration of potassium-retaining diuretic, amiloride. Metabolism 19:58, 1970.
183. Perez GO, Oster JR, Vaamonde CA: Serum potassium concentration in acidemic states. Nephron 27:233, 1981.
184. Posner JB, Jacobs DR: Isolated analdosteronism. I. Clinical entity with manifestations of persistent hyperkalemia, periodic paralysis, salt-losing tendency and acidosis. Metabolism 13:513, 1964.
185. DeFronzo RA Sherwin RS, Felig P, et al: Nonuremic diabetic hyperkalemia. Arch Intern Med 137:842, 1979.
186. Ammon RA, May WS, Nightingale SD: Glucose-induced hyperkalemia with normal aldosterone levels. Ann Int Med 89:349, 1978.
187. Carlsson E, Fellenius E, Lundborg P, et al: β-adrenoceptor blockers, plasma potassium, and exercise. Lancet 2:424, 1978.
188. Textor SC, Bravo EL, Fouad FM, et al: Hyperkalemia in azotemic patients during angiotensin-converting enzyme inhibition and aldosterone reduction with Captopril. Am J Med 73:719, 1982.
189. Makoff DL, DaSilva JA, Rosenbaum BJ: On the mechanism of hyperkalemia due to hyperosmotic expansion with saline or mannitol. Clin Sci Mol Med 41:383, 1971.
190. Makoff DL, DaSilva JA, Rosenbaum BJ, et al: Hypertonic expansion: acid-base and electrolyte changes. Am J Physiol 218:1201, 1970.
191. Hertz P, Richardson JA: Arginine-induced hyperkalemia in renal failure patients. Arch Intern Med 130:778, 1972.
192. Pearson CM, Kalyanaraman K: Periodic paralysis. In Stanbury JB, Wyngaarden JB, Frederickson DS (eds): The Metabolic Basis of Inherited Disease. New York, McGraw-Hill Book Co., 1972, p 1181.
193. Wang P, Clausen T: The treatment of attacks in hyperkalemic familial periodic paralysis by inhalation of salbutamol. Lancet 1:221, 1976.
194. Gronett FA, Theye RA: Pathophysiology of hyperkalemia induced succinylcholine. Anesthesiology 43:89, 1975.
195. Walton JD, Farman JV: Suxamethonium hyperkalemia in uraemic neuropathy. Anaesthesia 28:666, 1973.
196. Bismuth C, Gaultier M, Conso F, et al: Hyperkalemia in acute digitalis poisoning: prognostic significance and therapeutic implications. Clin Toxicol 6:153, 1973.
197. Winters RW: The Body Fluids in Pediatrics. Boston, Little, Brown & Co., 1973, p 134.

CHAPTER 8

Acid-base Metabolism

RALPH B. DELL

INTRODUCTION

Blood pH is closely regulated between pH 7.35 and 7.45 (mean 7.40) (1). Since pH = $-\log(H^+)$ this corresponds to a narrow range of hydrogen ion (H^+) concentration—45 to 35 nEq/L, despite a large and variable input of H^+ daily. Such precise regulation is accomplished by the interaction of two different mechanisms: (1) a rapid-acting set of physiochemical or buffer mechanisms and (2) the slower-acting respiratory and renal functions that regulate the carbonic and bicarbonate buffer system. The first part of this chapter will deal with the details of how these two mechanisms operate to regulate blood pH. The second will describe the nature of H^+ intake and excretion, i.e., H^+ balance. The third defines disturbances of acid-base metabolism.

REGULATION OF pH

Buffer Mechanisms

Physical Chemistry

The Bronsted-Lowry (2, 3) definition of an acid is any molecule that can act as a proton or H^+ donor; a base is any molecule that can act as a proton or H^+ acceptor. The relationship between an acid and a base is given by the following equation:

$$Ha \rightleftarrows a^- + H^+ \tag{1}$$

where Ha is the acid capable of donating H^+ proceeding left to right and a^- is the conjugate base of Ha capable of accepting H^+ when proceeding from right to left. Acids and bases vary in the degree with which they bind H^+. Strong acids give up H^+ readily while weak acids bind H^+ tightly. For example, HCl, a strong acid, freely dissociates into H^+ and Cl^-; acetic acid, a weak acid tends not to dissociate H^+ from its base—the acetate ion—a^-.

Buffers minimize changes in pH incident to the addition of hydrogen or hydroxyl ions (4). A buffer is a weak acid and its conjugate base as shown by the following equation:

$$H^+ + a^- \rightarrow Ha \tag{2}$$

In this equation, when H^+ is increased by adding a strong acid, e.g., HCl, it reacts with the conjugate base to produce the weak acid, Ha, minimizing the change in H^+ concentration or pH.

When strong base is added to the solution, e.g., NaOH, the hydroxyl ions react with the weak acid form of the buffer pair to produce the conjugate base and water, as shown by the following equation:

$$OH^- + Ha \rightarrow a^- + HOH \tag{3}$$

Change in pH is limited by reacting the added OH^- with the H^+ from the weak acid, Ha. Buffers act to bind H^+ or OH^- and to limit changes in pH when acid or base is added.

Consider the buffer reaction (2) shown above. At equilibrium the rate of formation of Ha is equal to the rate of formation of H^+ and a^- in the reverse direction. At a steady state, the proportion of reactants (H^+ and a^-) to product (Ha) is constant. This relationship, known as the mass action law, is shown in the following equation:

$$\frac{[H^+][a^-]}{[Ha]} = K \tag{4}$$

where K is the equilibrium or dissociation constant. Strong acids have large dissociation constants, i.e., $[H^+]\cdot[a^-]$ is much larger than [Ha]; conversely, weak acids have small dissociation constants, i.e., $[H^+]\cdot[a^-]$ is much smaller than [Ha] (5), e.g., K for acetic acid is 1.6×10^{-5}. Thus, for the acetic acid-acetate buffer pair, when the concentration of a^- and Ha are 1 Mol/L, the H^+ concentration is 1.6×10^{-5} Mol/L and pH is 4.8.

Classification of Buffer Systems

The buffers in the body fluids are classified as bicarbonate and nonbicarbonate buffers. The carbonic acid-bicarbonate buffer system is directly controlled by the respiratory system and renal excretion of acid and alkali, whereas the other buffers are not (6). Hence, the bicarbonate buffer system occupies a unique position among the buffers in the body fluids, and its action appropriately is considered separately.

Table 8.1 gives the percentage of the bicarbonate buffers in plasma and erythrocyte phases of whole blood and the percentages of the various components of the nonbicarbonate buffer system in whole blood (7). The principal buffer in plasma is HCO_3^-; smaller contributions are from plasma proteins and inorganic phosphate. The principal buffer in erythrocytes is hemoglobin and oxyhemoglobin; smaller contributions are from HCO_3^- and phosphate buffers. The buffering of whole blood is approximately equally divided between HCO_3^- and nonbicarbonate buffers. Hemoglobin and oxyhemoglobin are the principal components of the nonbicarbonate buffer system and account for one third of whole blood buffering.

Table 8.1
Components of Blood Buffers

Buffer system	Buffering in whole blood (%)
Bicarbonate Buffers	
Plasma bicarbonate	35
Erythrocyte bicarbonate	18
TOTAL	53
Nonbicarbonate Buffers	
Hemoglobin and oxyhemoglobin	35
Organic phosphates	3
Inorganic phosphates	2
Plasma proteins	7
TOTAL	47

From Winters RW, Dell RB: Regulation of acid-base equilibrium. In Yamamoto WS, Brobeck JR (eds): Physiological Controls and Regulations. Philadelphia, W.B. Saunders Co., 1965.

Bicarbonate Buffer System

Buffer Reaction. The HCO_3^- buffer system is defined by the following reversible reactions:

$$CO_2 + H_2O \rightleftarrows H_2CO_3 \rightleftarrows H^+ + HCO_3^- \qquad (5)$$

Hydration reaction Dissociation reaction

The hydration reaction is the combining of the CO_2 dissolved in plasma with water to form carbonic acid, the weak acid of the HCO_3^- buffer system. This reaction rate in vitro is slow (several minutes), but the rate in vivo is markedly accelerated by carbonic anhydrase, an enzyme that is present in most tissues (8). The dissociation reaction of H_2CO_3 to H^+ and HCO_3^- is practically instantaneous. Applying the law of mass action to the HCO_3^- buffer system yields the following:

$$\frac{[H^+][HCO_3^-]}{[CO_2 + H_2CO_3]} = K \qquad (6)$$

Solving this equation for H^+ yields the following form of Henderson's equation (9):

$$[H^+] = \frac{K[CO_2 + H_2CO_3]}{[HCO_3^-]} \qquad (7)$$

Thus, the H^+ concentration of the solution is determined by the product of K and the ratio of the sum of the concentrations of dissolved CO_2 and carbonic acid to the concentration of HCO_3^- in the solution. The logarithm of this equation is the Henderson-Hasselbach equation (10):

$$pH = pK + \log \frac{[HCO_3^-]}{[CO_2 + H_2CO_3]} \qquad (8)$$

where $pH = -\log H^+$.
Thus, pH is the log of K plus the log of the ratio of HCO_3^- to the sum of dissolved CO_2 and carbonic acid.

Relationship of Dissolved CO_2 to Gaseous CO_2. Dissolved CO_2 is in equilibrium with CO_2 in the gas phase, as well as with carbonic acid. The relationship between the sum of dissolved CO_2 and the carbonic acid to the partial pressure of CO_2 in the gas phase is given by Henry's law:

$$CO_{2(d)} + H_2CO_3 = S \cdot pCO_2 \qquad (9)$$

where S, the solubility coefficient for CO_2, is 0.03 (11) (Fig. 8.1). Using Henry's law the Henderson-Hasselbalch equation becomes:

$$pH = pK' + \log \frac{HCO_3^-}{S \cdot pCO_2} \qquad (10)$$

The symbol pK′ is used instead of pK to denote the fact that the constant has been adjusted for the pH, temperature, and ionic strength of plasma (11, 12). Values for pK′ and S are 6.10 and 0.03, respectively, so that the Henderson-Hasselbalch equation becomes:

$$pH = 6.1 + \log \frac{HCO_3^-}{.03\ pCO_2} \qquad (11)$$

Buffer Properties of HCO_3^- in a Closed and Open System. The HCO_3^- buffer has unique properties that make it suitable for physiological regulation. One of these is its ability to volatilize the weak acid form of the buffer pair as CO_2. In Fig. 8.2, the normal status is shown on the left: pCO_2 is 40 torr, HCO_3^- is 24 mEq/L, pH is 7.40, and the solution is in equilibrium with a gas phase having a pCO_2 of 40 torr. When 10 mEq of H^+ are added to the solution in a closed system, i.e., no communication with a gas phase, the 10 mEq of H^+ reacts with 10 mEq of HCO_3^- to form 10 mMole H_2CO_3 so that HCO_3^- concentration falls to 14 mEq/L, dissolved CO_2 plus H_2CO_3 rises from 1.2 mMole/L to 11.2, pCO_2 from 40 (1.2/.03) to 373 (11.2/.03), and pH falls from 7.40 to 6.20.

In an open system, with an infinite gas phase whose pCO_2 remains at 40 torr, the effect is different. The 10 mEq of H^+ reacts with HCO_3^- to form 10 mMole H_2CO_3 as before, but in the open system most of the $H_2CO_3 + CO_2(d)$ formed by the buffer reaction is lost to the gas phase. At equilibrium, HCO_3^- has fallen to 14 mEq/L but $CO_2(d) + H_2CO_3$ remain at 1.2 (pCO_2 at 40 torr) and pH only falls to 7.17.

The difference between the open and closed system on the effect of the HCO_3^- buffer system's capacity to buffer added base is illustrated in Figure 8.3. When 1 mEq OH− is added to the solution on the left, in the closed system 1 mMole $CO_2(d) + H_2CO_3^-$ is consumed by the OH− to produce 1 mEq HCO_3^-. Thus, $CO_2(d) + H_2O_3$ decreases from 1.2 to 0.2 mMole/L, HCO_3^- rises from 24 to 25 mEq/L and pH increases to 8.20. When pCO_2 remains constant so that the 1 mMole H_2CO_3 consumed by buffering is replaced, HCO_3^- increases from 24 to 25 mEq/L, $CO_2(d)$ remains at 1.2 mMole/L, and pH increases from 7.40 to 7.42. The "open" system converts the HCO_3^- buffer system from a relatively poor one to one that is very effective. The continuous though variable addition of CO_2 to the system from metabolism is offset by its rapid

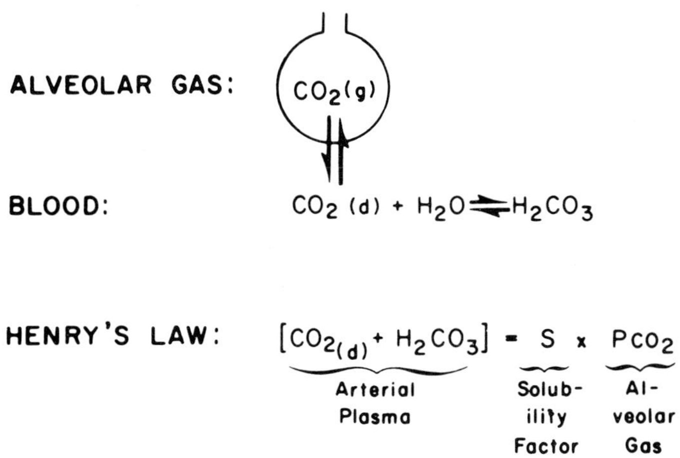

Figure 8.1. Equilibrium between CO_2 dissolved in plasma and CO_2 in alveolar gas. This equilibrium is expressed by Henry's law.

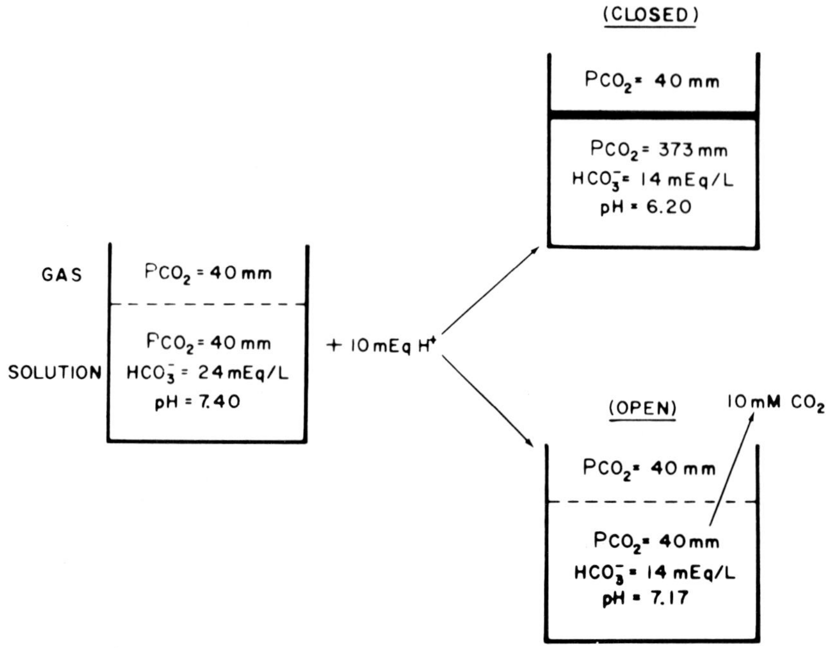

Figure 8.2. Bicarbonate buffers in an open system and in a closed system when H^+ is added.

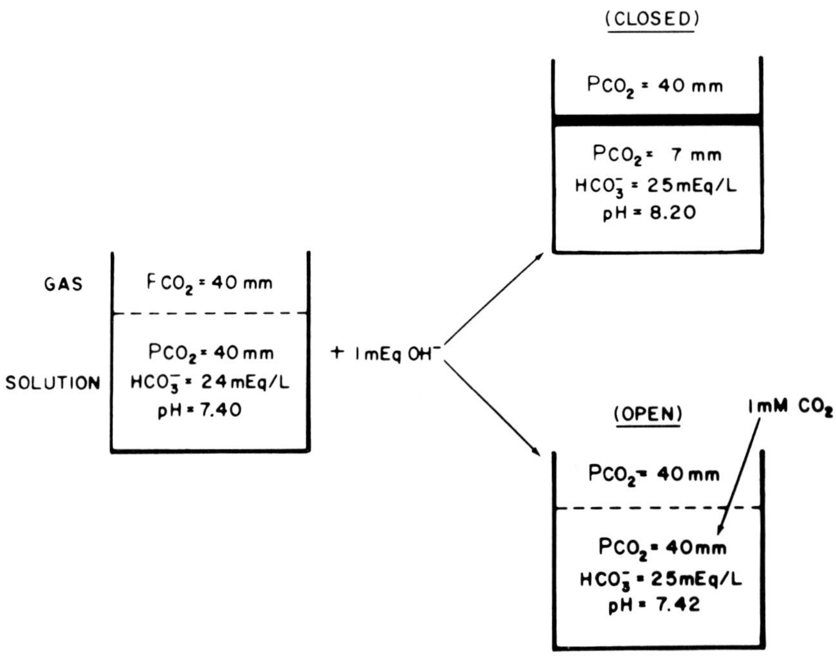

Figure 8.3. Bicarbonate buffers in an open system and in a closed system when OH^- is added.

volatilization and excretion by lungs, with little change in the concentration of HCO_3^- or other buffer systems or in pH.

Nonbicarbonate Buffer System

Nonbicarbonate buffers react with added H^+ or OH^- ion to form the conjugate acid or conjugate base, respectively:

$$H^+ + Buf^- \rightarrow HBuf \quad (12)$$

where Buf^- stands for the conjugate base form of the buffer pair and HBuf the acid form. The HCO_3^- and nonbicarbonate buffer system interact as described in Equation 13.

$$H_2CO_3 + Buf^- \rightleftarrows HCO_3^- + HBuf \quad (13)$$

The principal noncarbonate buffer system of whole blood is the hemoglobin and oxyhemoglobin system. When H^+ is added to plasma it is buffered by plasma Buf^- and HCO_3^- to form their respective conjugate acids. CO_2 thus formed diffuses readily into the erythrocyte where it is hydrated to form H_2CO_3. The newly formed H_2CO_3 reacts with erythrocyte Buf^- (equation 13) to form HBuf (HHb and $HHbO_2$) and HCO_3^-. The HCO_3^- diffuses out of the erythrocyte to replenish plasma HCO_3^-, i.e., the buffer system of erythrocytes and plasma are in equilibrium, and buffering of H^+ is distributed between them (Fig. 8.4), more than doubling the buffering capacity of plasma (13).

How this system operates is illustrated in Figure 8.5. When 10 mEq of H^+ is added to 1 liter of whole blood (Fig. 8.5, **A**), the added H^+ reacts with HCO_3^- and Buf^- to form the conjugate weak acids. The fall

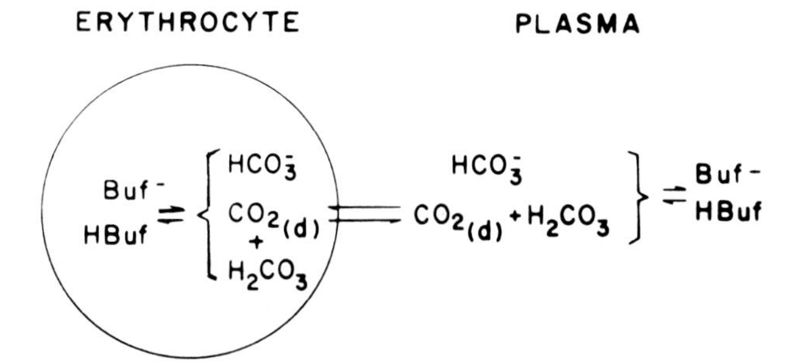

Figure 8.4. Relationships between bicarbonate and nonbicarbonate buffer systems in whole blood.

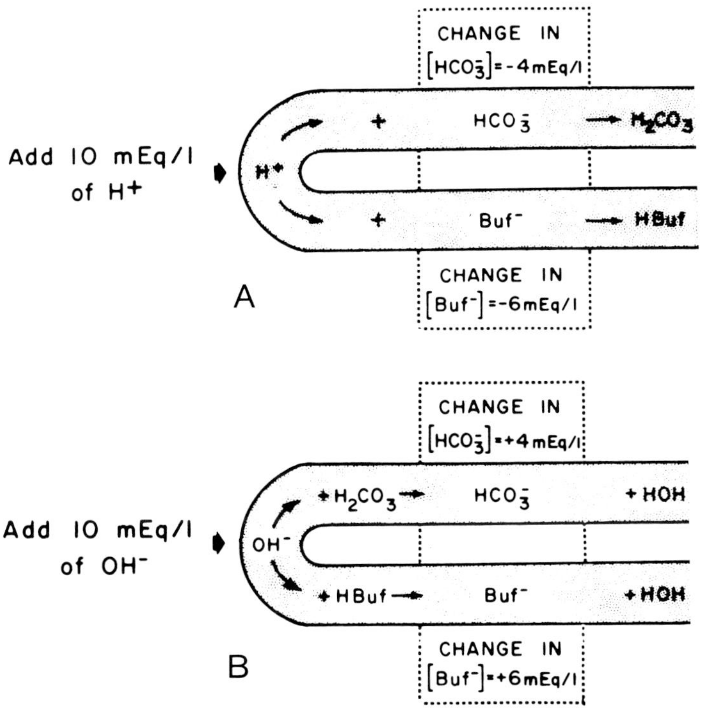

Figure 8.5. **A**, The effects of addition of H^+ or OH^- to whole blood demonstrating that the change in total conjugate base equals the amount of H^+ or OH^- added. The distribution of buffering depends on the relative amounts of Buf^- and HCO_3^- present. **B**, The effects of addition of OH^- or H^+ to whole blood demonstrating that the change in total conjugate base equals the amount of OH^- or H^+ added. The distribution of buffering depends on the relative amounts of Buf^- and HCO_3^- present.

in base concentration is equal to the amount of the H^+ added; in this example, 4 mEq is distributed to HCO_3^- and 6 mEq to Buf^-. Similarly, when 10 mEq OH^- is added (Fig. 8.5, **B**), it reacts with H_2CO_3 and HBuf to form the corresponding conjugate bases and the effect is similarly distributed—4 mEq to HCO_3^- and 6 mEq to Buf^-. The magnitude of deviation of total conjugate base concentration in whole blood from normal (whole blood buffer base) measures net addition of H^+ to, or its removal from, whole blood (14). The normal value for whole blood buffer base, when hemoglobin is 15 g/dl is 48 mEq/L:

$$BB = Buf^- + HCO_3^- \qquad (14)$$

What is of interest is the change in buffer base concentration when acid or base is added. This change has been called ΔBB or base excess (BE) (1):

$$\Delta BB = BE = \text{observed BB} - \text{normal BB} \qquad (15)$$

BE also has the units of mEq/L and normally is zero. When H^+ is added $Buf^- + HCO_3^-$ is consumed, buffer base falls, and BB becomes negative. Similarly, when OH− is added, BB rises and BE assumes a positive value. While this method increases the precision of measurement of acid-base status because it includes the contribution of hemoglobin, which varies in relation to whole blood hemoglobin concentration, in current practice, acid-base status is expressed in terms of the bicarbonate buffer system, i.e., pCO_2, pH, and plasma bicarbonate concentration.

Whole Body Buffers

Whole body buffers include interstitial and intracellular buffers, as well as blood buffers (15–17). In the interstitial fluid, bicarbonate is virtually the only buffer system since interstitial fluid has little protein. Intracellular buffers are organic and inorganic phosphate, protein, and bicarbonate. These are not in simple equilibrium with the interstitial fluid because of the transport properties of the cell wall. However, CO_2 and undissociated acid are such that buffering is distributed among the phases rapidly. Intracellular buffers are quantitatively important; they account for 55% of the total buffering capacity; ISF for 30%, blood buffers 15%, as just described. This distribution is the basis for the clinical practice of estimating alkali needs to treat acidosis as the change in plasma HCO_3^- desired × body weight = mEq alkali needed. Because production of H^+ and its excretion change rapidly, this calculation often yields a result different from the prediction.

Intracellular pH (pH_i) is difficult to measure technically and to interpret theoretically (18). However, pH_i has been estimated by intracellular electrodes (19, 20) and by the distribution of a weak acid or weak base across the cell membranes (21, 22). Both techniques yield comparable values for pH_i in various mammalian tissues of 6.7 to 7.1. Intracellular HCO_3^- concentration is 10 to 12 mEq/L and pCO_2 is 35 to 45 mm Hg. Intracellular pH is maintained by buffer mechanisms, by active H^+ extrusion, and by changes in cellular metabolism, which consume H^+ by combining them with organic anions that may then be oxidized to CO_2 and H_2O. The measurement of pH_i has been useful in experimental studies but is not used in clinical practice.

Carbon Dioxide Equilibration Curve

The buffer response of whole blood in vitro to changes in pCO_2 is quantitatively different from that of whole blood in vivo (1). The buffer response is quantitated by examining the relationship between plasma HCO_3^- and whole blood base excess to changes in pCO_2. The difference between the CO_2 equilibration curve in vitro and in vivo is illustrated in Figure 8.6 (23). The rise in plasma HCO_3^- is much greater for blood in vitro than for blood in vivo. The base excess of whole blood, however, does not fall in vitro but does fall in vivo. An understanding of this difference is important for interpreting acid-base data in acute respiratory acidosis.

When pCO_2 of whole blood is increased in vitro, CO_2 is hydrated to form carbonic acid and then is buffered by interaction with the non-bicarbonate buffer system:

$$CO_2 + H_2O \rightarrow H_2CO_3 + Buf^- \rightarrow HCO_3^- + HBuf \qquad (16)$$

For every molecule of Buf^- consumed, 1 molecule of HCO_3^- is produced. Hence, buffer base (the sum of Buf^- and HCO_3^-) remains unchanged and base excess does not change (solid lines, Fig. 8.6). However, a different relationship is found when blood is equilibrated in vivo. Normal subjects exposed to graded elevations in pco_2 reach a steady state after 45 minutes. There is a smaller rise in plasma HCO_3^- and BE falls so that at pCO_2 of 90 mm Hg, plasma HCO_3^- in vivo is 28 rather than the 32 mEq/L observed in vitro and BE in vivo is −5 rather than zero (broken lines, Fig. 8.6) (23).

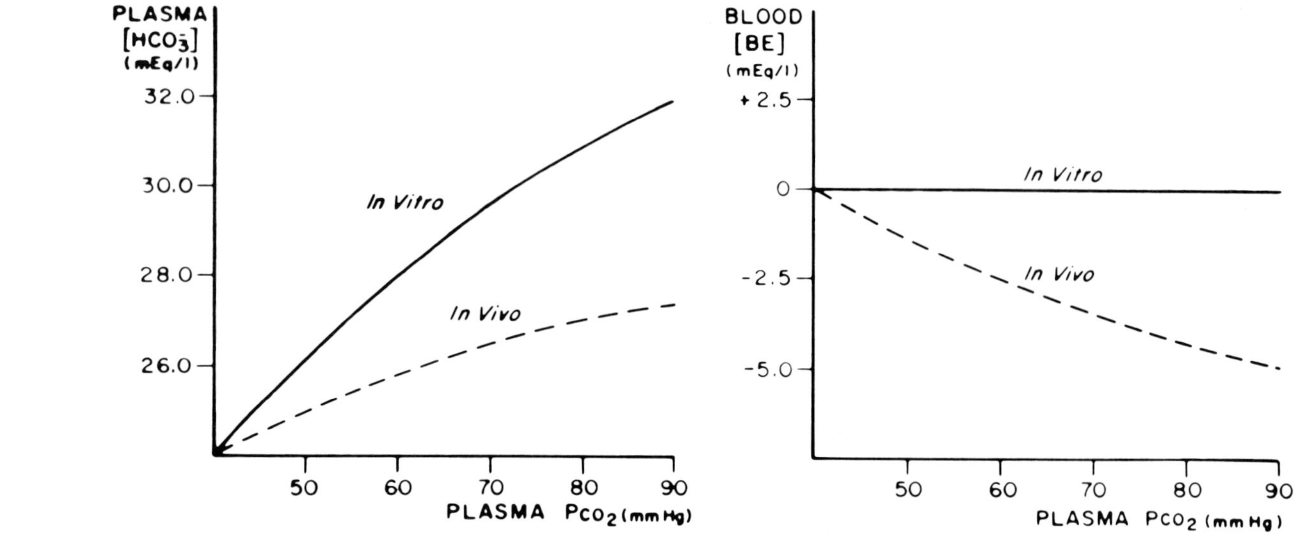

Figure 8.6. CO_2 equilibration curves in response to addition of CO_2 to plasma in vitro and in vivo. (In vivo curves from Brackett NC Jr, Cohen JJ, Schwartz WB: *N Engl J Med* 272:6, 1965.)

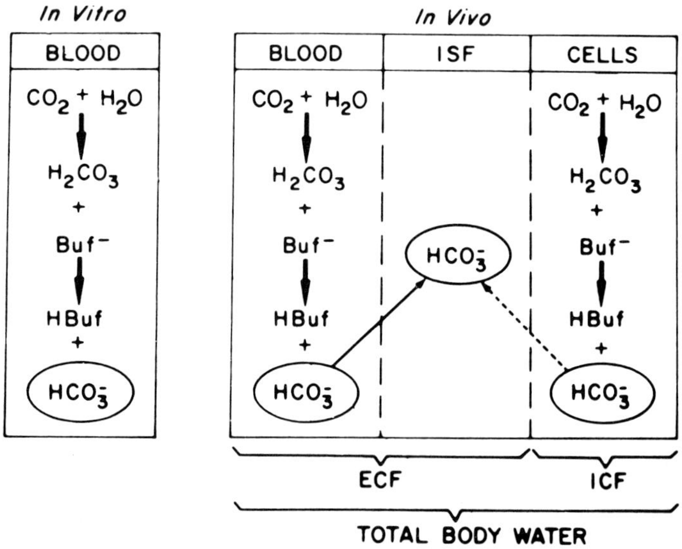

Figure 8.7. Models to explain differences between the in vitro and the in vivo equilibration curves. (From Dell RB, Winters RW: *Am J Physiol* 219:37, 1970.)

The mechanism for the difference between the in vitro and in vivo CO_2 equilibration curves may be understood by examining Figure 8.7 (24). When CO_2 is added to blood in vitro, the HCO_3^- generated by reaction with the nonbicarbonate buffer system is constrained by the walls of the tonometer and remains in the blood. However, while the same reactions occur in vivo, the HCO_3^- generated is not constrained by the capillary endothelium to remain, but diffuses down a concentration gradient into the ISF. When the acid-base status of the blood at equilibrium is examined, there is a loss of the generated HCO_3^-. Plasma HCO_3^- increases less in vivo than in vitro. Furthermore, this diffusion of HCO_3^- is a loss of total conjugate base ($HCO_3^- + Buf^-$) from the blood so that buffer base falls and base excess becomes negative. There is very little Buf^- in ISF to buffer CO_2 so most of the ISF HCO_3^- comes from plasma although a small quantity of HCO_3^- diffuses from ICF into the ISF.

The fall in BE is not great except at very high pCO_2 values but, since the fall is the result of a loss into the ISF, if its volume increases, then the loss of HCO_3^- will be greater and the fall in BE larger (24). The larger ISF volume of low birth weight infants, up to 450 ml/kg constitutes a sink for HCO_3^- that is generated by buffering in a whole blood compartment that is twice that of an adult. Therefore, the same degree of respiratory acidosis in infants will generate more HCO_3^- and have a more depressing effect on whole blood buffer base.

Physiological Mechanisms

The second set of mechanisms responsible for maintaining acid-base equilibrium is the adjustment made by the respiratory and renal systems. In contrast to the immediate effects of buffer systems, physiological adjustments occur over a longer period of time. Respiratory adjustments become discernible in minutes but require many hours to become fully developed while renal adjustments become discernible promptly but require several days to become fully operative. Respiratory adjustments control pCO_2 and, hence, the weak acid part of the HCO_3^- buffer system while the kidney operates on the HCO_3^- part of the buffer system, the so-called metabolic component of acid-base equilibrium. Since pH is proportional to the ratio of HCO_3^- to pCO_2 (from the Henderson-Hasselbalch equation), the respiratory system operates on the denominator while the kidneys regulate the enumerator.

Respiratory Regulation

The respiratory system controls arterial pCO_2 ($Paco_2$) by controlling alveolar ventilation and, hence, pCO_2 in alveolar gas ($Paco_2$). $Paco_2$ is the net result between CO_2 production and its excretion:

$$Paco_2 \propto \frac{CO_2 \text{ production}}{\text{alveolar ventilation}} \qquad (17)$$

At a steady state production of CO_2, adjustments in alveolar ventilation lead to changes in $Paco_2$ and, hence, to changes in $Paco_2$ (25). Changes in $Paco_2$ are related by Henry's law to changes in dissolved CO_2 and carbonic acid. Hence, adjustments in alveolar ventilation result directly in changes in the HCO_3^- buffer system.

Alveolar ventilation is controlled by peripheral and central chemoreceptors.

Peripheral Chemoreceptors. The peripheral chemoreceptors are in the carotid and aortic bodies and respond to changes in pH and pCO_2 and in pH of the perfusing blood; the carotid bodies are also sensitive to

pO_2 (26). The central chemoreceptors are located in the brain-stem (27) and are exquisitely sensitive to changes in pH of the cerebral ISF (28).

Steady state alveolar ventilation represents an integrative rather than additive combination of the separate effects of pH and pCO_2 on these receptors (29). The resulting effect on alveolar ventilation may be understood by considering the separate effects of pCO_2 and pH during CO_2 rebreathing and during H^+ loading with another acid.

During CO_2 rebreathing, pCO_2 rises and pH in plasma falls. Both the rise in pCO_2 and fall in pH stimulate the respiratory system to increase alveolar ventilation. Figure 8.8 shows the separate effects of pH and pCO_2 on ventilation ratio (VAR, i.e., ratio of observed to normal ventilation). The observed VAR is the sum of the effect on alveolar ventilation of decreased pH and of increased pCO_2.

On the other hand, addition of H^+ from acids other than H_2CO_3 to body fluids—metabolic acidosis—results in an immediate fall in plasma pH and HCO_3^- which stimulates the chemoreceptors to increase VAR and decrease pCO_2. The effect of pH on VAR is gradually offset; pCO_2 falls so that the final VAR is the result of stimulation, resulting from decreased pH minus inhibition because of decreased pCO_2 (Figure 8.9).

Central Chemoreceptors. The same addition of H^+ to body fluids that occurs with metabolic acidosis has a different effect on central receptors that are sensitive to pH. The drop in plasma pCO_2 is associated with a corresponding drop in CSF pCO_2. However, the drop in plasma HCO_3^- is only slowly transmitted to CSF. CSF HCO_3^- decreases slowly over several hours because the equilibrium is affected by active transport. As a result, CSF pH initially rises, inhibiting the response of the respiratory center to the peripheral stimuli. As CSF HCO_3^- falls this inhibition is removed. The final stimulus to the respiratory center is an interaction between signals derived from peripheral chemoreceptors and signals from central chemoreceptors. The peripheral receptors are responding to chemical stimuli arising directly from the blood while the central chemoreceptors are responding to changes in the CSF. The effects of the interaction between these two stimuli on respiration vary with time because of the slow rate of equilibration of CSF acid-base status with that of blood. With acute addition of H^+ to the body fluids, the major stimulus to the respiratory center arises from the low pH of the blood and is mediated by the peripheral chemoreceptors. Shortly after an acute acid load, CSF pH actually rises because the respiratory stimulus lowers pCO_2 while CSF bicarbonate is unchanged. This alkalinity inhibits the respiratory center via the central chemoreceptors. With the passage of time, CSF bicarbonate falls to a new low value and the initial inhibition is removed. With the removal of the inhibition, the full effect of the stimulus from the peripheral chemoreceptor is expressed and respiration appears to be simply a function of blood pH (30).

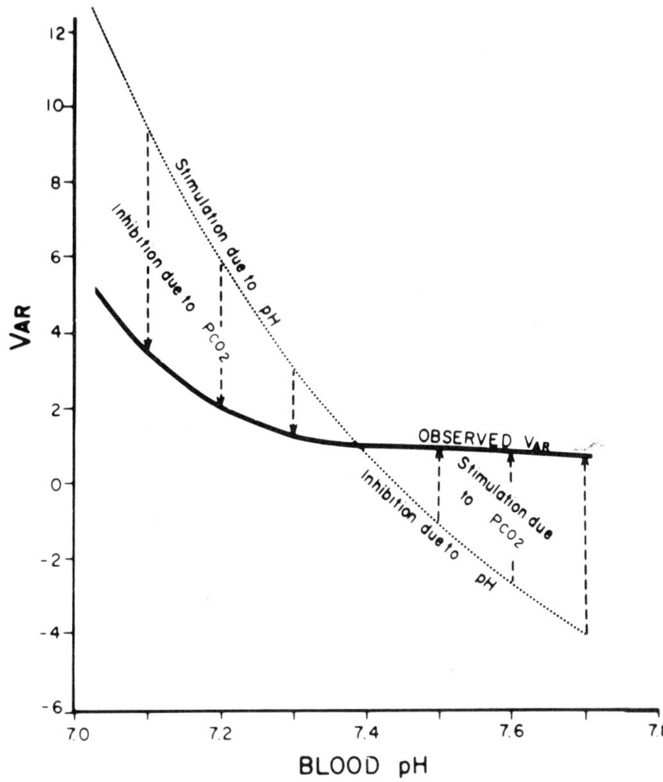

Figure 8.9. The relationship between VAR and blood pH in metabolic acid-base disturbances, showing competing effects of pH and pCO_2 on alveolar ventilation.

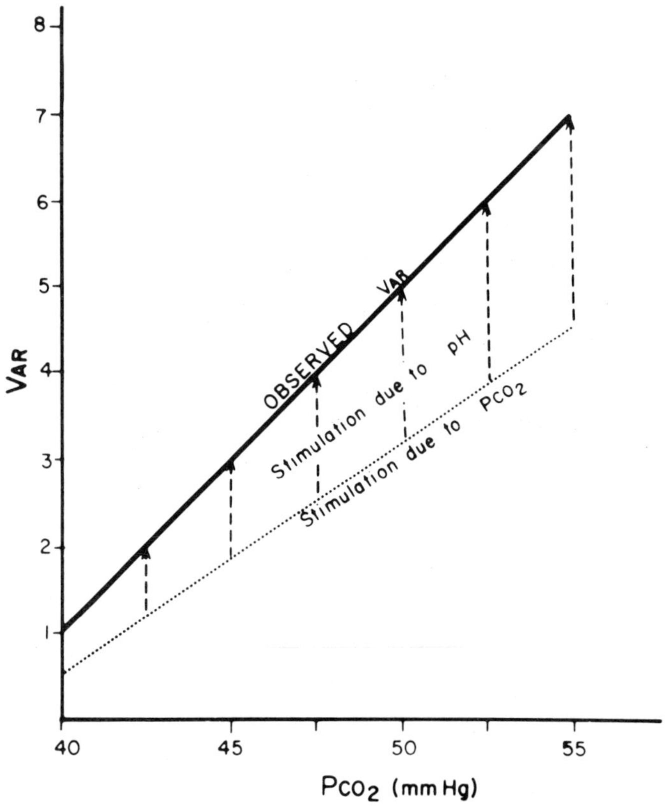

Figure 8.8. The relationship between VAR and pCO_2 during CO_2 inhalation, showing the additive effects of increased pCO_2 and low pH on alveolar ventilation.

Renal Regulation

The kidneys regulate acid-base equilibrium by regulating plasma HCO_3^- concentration. This chapter will not deal with the details of the intrarenal mechanisms responsible for this regulation (chapters 5 and 34), but rather with the kidney as a homeostatic organ responding to various stimuli by appropriate adjustment of urinary acid or base excretion.

The kidneys control plasma HCO_3^- concentration by regulating reabsorption of filtered HCO_3^- and by varying the rate of tubular secretion of H^+ (31). The renal tubular epithelium is rich in carbonic anhydrase so that CO_2 is rapidly hydrated to form carbonic acid to facilitate renal response to change in pCO_2, both general and local. When the urine is acidified, H^+ from carbonic acid is excreted while HCO_3^- that is generated is reabsorbed into renal venous plasma (32). Since urine pH does not fall to <4.5 ($10^{-1.5}$ mEq of H^+/L) the urine contains very little free H^+. Nearly all of the H^+ that is secreted is buffered by either $HPO_4^=$ to form titratable acidity (TA) and ammonia to form NH_4^+ (33, 34).

$$H^+ + HPO_4^= \rightarrow H_2PO_4^- \quad (TA) \tag{18}$$

$$H^+ + NH_3 \rightarrow NH_4^+ \quad (\text{ammonium ion}) \tag{19}$$

The sum of TA and NH_4^+ in the urine represents the total acid excretion by the kidney and is equal to the amount of new HCO_3^- formed by the kidney.

Alkalinization of the urine is accomplished by incomplete reabsorption of the filtered HCO_3^-. Some 4000 mEq of HCO_3^-/day is filtered so that failure to reabsorb only a few percent of this filtered load leads to excretion of considerable HCO_3^-, and would rapidly lower plasma HCO_3^- concentration. This occurs most commonly when alkali, e.g., $NaHCO_3$, is ingested and plasma HCO_3^- rises. The kidney's capacity to excrete HCO_3^- normally is considerable but may be limited by Na, K, and Cl depletion (35). Excretion of HCO_3^- requires some cation to accompany it so Na or K must be available. When Na is being reabsorbed avidly, e.g., in response to volume depletion, and filtered Cl^- is low, then HCO_3^- reabsorption will increase and will be excreted.

On the other hand, when H^+ is added to body fluids, as occurs in metabolic acidosis, NH_3 secretion is stimulated and buffers the secretion of H^+ so that net acid excretion is increased.

Chronic respiratory acidosis and a high pCO_2 effect a net gain in bicarbonate reabsorption so that pH changes are diminished. The converse occurs in chronic respiratory alkalosis.

NET ACID BALANCE

Balance Principle

Net acid balance, or H^+ balance, is defined as the intake of H^+ by all routes minus its output by all routes. Thus, balance is used here in the traditional sense of intake minus output. This is quite different from the usual use of the word "balance" as in the phrase "acid-base balance," which is frequently used when acid-base status is meant. In health, net acid balance (NAB) is zero so the acid-base status of the blood and body fluids is stable. The metabolic balance principle will be developed for acid-base problems and then some of its application discussed in succeeding paragraphs.

Metabolic Balance Principle

The balance method has been used for years to measure change in body composition. For example, Na balance is formulated by the following equation:

$$\begin{aligned} Na_{balance} &= Na_{oral} - Na_{urine} - Na_{stool} - Na_{sweat} \\ &= \underbrace{Na_{oral}}_{\text{intake}} - \underbrace{|Na_{urine} + Na_{stool} + Na_{sweat}|}_{\text{excretion}} \end{aligned} \tag{20}$$

All routes of intake and output can be identified and Na content of each measured independently. Na balance can be calculated. This is not the case when trying to measure H^+ balance. In this case, CO_2 production cannot be measured independently of CO_2 excretion; in fact, CO_2 production is estimated by determining CO_2 excretion and assuming zero balance when $PaCO_2$ is constant. Another feature of Na balance measurements is that Na is neither created nor destroyed by metabolic processes, so that all routes of intake and output can be identified. This is not the case with acids or bases.

For example, giving lactic acid to an individual usually results in its metabolism to CO_2 and H_2O, i.e., the acid is converted to H_2O and CO_2, which is excreted from the lungs. Giving sodium lactate results in production of base in the form of $NaHCO_3$. The metabolism of acids or bases creates uncertainties in trying to compute H^+ balance. Na, K, Cl, and N are elements that can be analyzed directly, whereas H^+ cannot. Thus, to apply the balance principle to H^+, routes of intake and output must be measured independently, taking careful account of net gains or losses by metabolism and identifying those substances in intake and output that pertain to the H^+ balance.

Acid-base Balance

Acids and bases are classified into three categories, depending on the source of production and the route of excretion, since it is these two features that determine whether the intake and output of the substances can be measured independently (36). The first category of acid is carbonic acid derived from the hydration of CO_2. Its principal route of disposition is the lung, where it is excreted as CO_2. Since CO_2 production cannot be measured independently from CO_2 eliminated, carbonic acid cannot be subjected to balance arithmetic.

The second category of acid to which the balance principle cannot be applied is the organic acids that are metabolizable by tissues to CO_2 and H_2O. Lactic acid and beta-hydroxybutyric acid are organic acids that are produced and metabolized to CO_2 and H_2O by many tissues. Because the processes of production and disposition cannot be measured separately, they also cannot be studied by the balance technique.

This leaves the third category of acids for which the principal route of elimination is the kidney, e.g., nonmetabolized and nonmetabolizable acids. These acids are called "net acids" and are capable of being studied by the balance principle. Examples of nonmetabolized acids are organic acids that escape catabolism and are excreted in the urine as the organic acid anion, e.g., beta-hydroxybutyric acid and acetoacetic acid (ketones). When the acid anion is excreted, the H^+ also must be excreted by the kidney to maintain acid-base status:

$$\underbrace{\left(HOA\right)}_{\text{metabolism}} \rightarrow \underbrace{\left(OA^-\right)}_{\text{excreted}} + + \underbrace{\left(H^+\right)}_{\text{buffered} \rightarrow \text{renal excretion}} \tag{21}$$

Nonmetabolizable acids are acids that cannot be catabolized, such as sulfuric acid, produced by the oxidation of sulfur-containing amino acids. The anions of these acids are excreted in the urine and its H^+ constitutes an acid load for the kidney. This third group of acids are nonmetabolized and nonmetabolizable acids to which the balance principle can be applied. Net acid is acid left after carbonic acid and metabolized acid production have been subtracted from the total body production of acid.

Net Acid Balance

Net acid balance (NAB) adds all sources of acid input, exogenous or metabolically derived, and subtracts acid lost. Whether a particular variable is considered as intake or output is arbitrary. What is important is the algebraic sign of the variable that denotes addition or subtraction of H^+ from the body fluids.

In the relatively simple case of Na balance, discussed previously, intake was defined as Na ingested:

$$\text{balance} = \underbrace{\left(Na_{oral}\right)}_{\text{intake}} - \underbrace{\left(Na_{feces} + Na_{urine} \quad Na_{sweat}\right)}_{\text{excretion}} \tag{22}$$

but this could just as easily, from the standpoint of the body fluids, be written as follows:

$$\text{balance} = \underbrace{([Na_{oral} - Na_{feces}])}_{\substack{\text{intake} \\ = Na^{absorbed}}} - \underbrace{([Na_{urine} + Na_{sweat}])}_{\substack{\text{excretion} \\ - Na_{urine} + Na_{sweat}}} \quad (23)$$

Thus, whether a particular route is considered, intake or excretion is largely immaterial as long as the correct algebraic sign is given to the variables. For the term "net acid balance" to include bases, the base is considered a negative acid, i.e., input of a base or potential base is considered a negative acid input.

There are a number of components that must be considered when formulating the NAB (Fig. 8.10). The first component, oral intake (37) is complicated conceptually because its effect is modified by its metabolism and, in some cases, net retention as new tissue. The pH of intake per se is immaterial in computing NAB and the titratable acidity (TA) of the intake also is immaterial if the acid in question is metabolized.

For example, 100 mMole/L lactic acid has the same TA as 100 mMole/L HCl. But, ingested lactic acid usually is oxidized to CO_2 and water and has no effect on acid-base metabolism or net acid balance, while the HCl constitutes a H^+ load that must be included as input for the NAB calculation. The most direct way to account for the H^+ burden of the diet is to measure the difference between the inorganic cations and inorganic anions. The difference is organic cation or anion and is a measure of net acid or base intake, e.g., the 100 mMole/L HCl solution has no inorganic cations and 100 mMole/L inorganic anions (Cl^-). Hence, this solution has 100 mEq/L net acid. A 100 mMole/L solution of Na-lactate has 100 mEq/L inorganic cation (Na^+), no inorganic anion and, hence, has 100 mEq/L net base when lactate is metabolized to HCO_3^-. Combining these two solutions results in a net acid intake of zero. The difference between inorganic cation and inorganic anion is called "undetermined anion" (UA) and, if positive as it is in most milk diets, is potential base, e.g., Na-lactate. It is a negative intake in computing NAB. The normal diet of adults has a negative UA and contributes acid to net acid intake (such diets have been called "acid-ash diets). UA is computed from the equation:

$$UA = (Na^+ + K^+ + Ca^{++} + Mg^{++}) - (Cl^- + 1.8P) \quad (24)$$

where P is the total phosphorus, free plus that which is bound as inorganic phosphate, of the diet and 1.8 is the average charge of phosphate at pH 7.4. It does not matter what the actual state of phosphate in the sample is because at normal pH in the body fluids, it must exist with an average charge of −1.8. Thus, if base is required to titrate the ingested phosphate to that pH, then it must be counted as net acid input (38). When the UA of the diet and of the stool are combined, the difference, diet minus stool, is the potential intake in determining NAB.

Three metabolic processes contribute to NAB by generating net acid intake (NAI): (1) sulfuric acid production by the catabolism of sulfur-containing amino acids, cysteine and methionine [39]; (2) organic anion excretion (37, 40); and (3) H^+ released by skeletal mineralization (41, 42).

The sulfur amino acids, which are not incorporated into protein but are catabolized to $SO_4^=$ yield two H^+ that will be excreted ($H^+_{SO_4^=}$). Measuring urinary sulfate identifies this component of NAI.

The second component is organic acid anion excretion, which results in the production of H^+. Organic acid is measured by extraction of all the organic acids in urine (43). Since urinary organic acids have pK values <5, they exist as anions in the urine unaccompanied by H^+ and, hence, are entered into NAB calculation as a source of H^+. A nonmetabolizable organic acid anion, e.g., hippurate, absorbed from the gastrointestinal tract and excreted in urine, is counted as acid input into the body fluids. However, hippurate contributes to the intake of UA and is counted as base or negative acid input into the body fluids. These two cancel, and NAB from the ingestion and excretion of hippurate is zero.

The third component, hydrogen ion from skeletal mineralization, is due to the fact that hydroxyapatite is solid base crystallized from neutral precursors in the body fluids. Formation of hydroxyapatite is given by the following equation:

$$\begin{aligned} &10\ CA^{++} + 4.8\ HPO_4^= + 1.2\ H_2PO_4^- \\ &\quad + 2\ H_2O \rightarrow (Ca_3PO_4)_2)_2 \cdot Ca(OH)_2 + 9.2\ H^+ \end{aligned} \quad (25)$$

so that deposition of 10 mMole Ca as hydroxyapatite results in production of 9.2 mEq H^+. This source of H^+ is determined by multiplying the Ca retained in mMole by 0.92 to give the mMole H^+ produced ($H^+_{Ca^{++}}$). Forming a base from neutral precursors leaves behind a hyrogen ion, which is an input in computing NAB (42).

Two other sources of net acid production are expansion of body fluids containing HCO_3^- and growth of soft tissues. HCO_3^- made from neutral precursors and added to total HCO_3^- entails net acid production. Usually it is small relative to other components of NAB and is ignored. However,

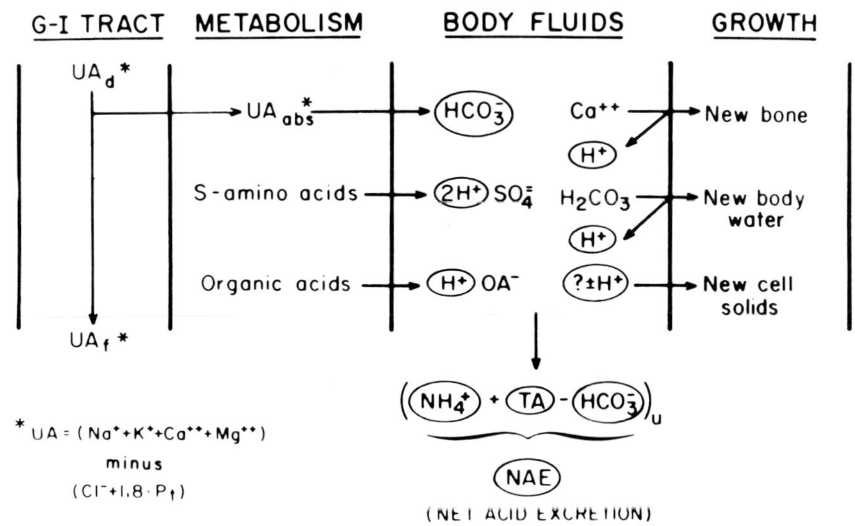

Figure 8.10. Components of NAB and their source.

when there are major changes in body fluid volume during the balance period, the HCO_3^- needed for growth should be included as acid input. Growth per se has acid-base effects through the deposition of new cell solids. However, on a day-to-day basis, the effect is small and can be ignored. In careful NAB studies on healthy, rapidly growing infants, no acid-base effect could be detected, given the errors of the measurements needed to compute NAB.

With all routes of intake of acid and base accounted for, all that is needed to calculate NAB is net acid excretion (NAE), for which there is only one route: renal NAE, which is defined by the equation:

$$NAE = TA + NH_4^+ - HCO_3^- \tag{26}$$

H^+ is not excreted as free H^+ but, instead, is buffered and excreted as either TA or NH_4^+ (p 134). NAE is determined in the urine by titration of urine to pH 7.4 at body temperature, the TA, and by ammonia measured by its release from urine made very alkaline (44).

The convention for writing the NAB equation is to place sources of H^+ on the input side and sources of base on the output side:

$$NAB = \underbrace{\left(H^+_{SO_4^=} + H^+_{Ca^{++}} + H^+_{OA^-}\right)}_{\text{input}} - \underbrace{\left((UA)_{abs} + NAE\right)}_{\text{output}} \tag{27}$$

When written in this way, all components can be expressed in a bar graph.

Even with meticulous care, measurement errors cumulate so that the final number has a standard deviation of 4.6 mEq/1000 kcal. For intake to be significantly different from excretion, it must differ by 9.2 or nearly 10 mEq/1000 kcal.

Net Acid Balance

Application of Principle

Effect of Formula Composition on New Acid Balance of Growing Infants. The major components of NAI are H^+ production from sulfuric acid production ($H^+_{SO_4}$), from bone mineralization (H^+_{Ca++}), and from excretion of organic acid ($H^+_{OA^-}$). Those of NAO are base absorption from the gastrointestinal tract (UA_{abs}) and NAE. The values of these variables have been defined in healthy growing low birth weight infants fed three different formulas (Fig. 8.11) (36). The effect of changes in these five variables among the different formulas illustrate how diet influences NAB and how the body responds to the diet differences.

Each pair of bars denotes averages for the group when receiving that formula; the left bar of the pair represents NAI and the right bar NAO. Note that there is little difference between NAI and NAO in each of the three groups, indicating that the subjects were in neutral NAB, as must be the case since the subjects were healthy growing prematurely born infants whose acid-base status was constant. Both NAI and NAO increased as the dietary protein and electrolyte increased and NAB remained neutral. This increase in NAI was the result of increases in ($H^+_{SO_4^=}$ and ($H^+_{Ca^{++}}$. The rise in ($H^+_{SO_4^=}$ was from an increase in protein ingested and a higher rate of catabolism of the sulfur-containing amino acids provided by the formula. At low intakes of protein nearly all of the sulfur-containing amino acids are used for net protein synthesis and little is catabolized, while at higher protein intakes, higher fractions of amino acids are degraded with increased sulfuric acid production.

The load of acid because of bone mineralization increases as Ca intake increases. The greatest increase in NAI is from the increase in Ca absorption and subsequent bone calcification. Changes in $H^+_{OA^-}$ contributed less.

Changing intake of protein and electrolyte changes the rate of H^+

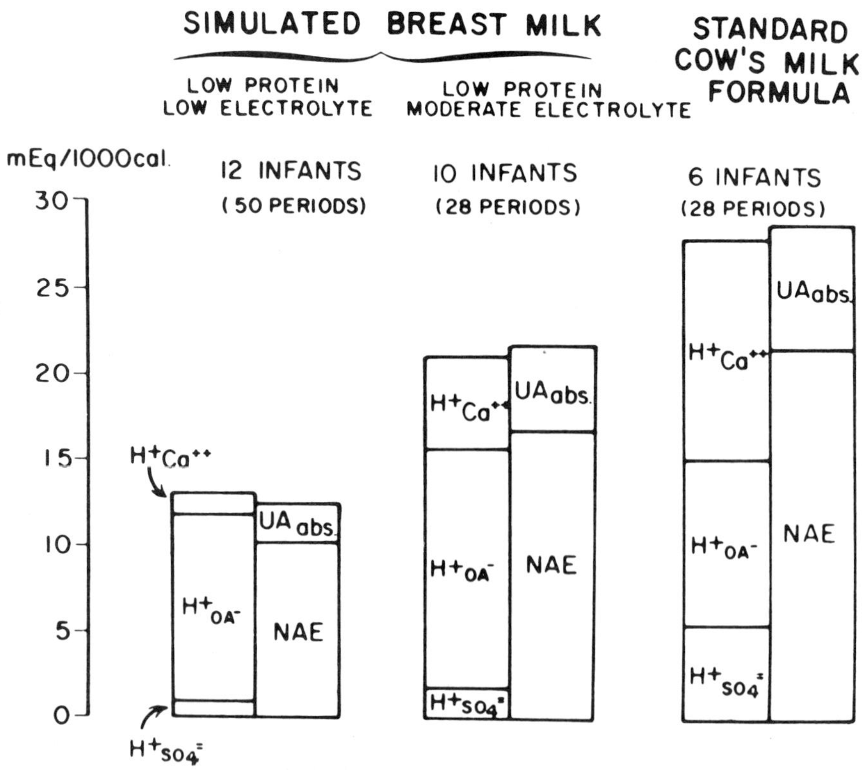

Figure 8.11. Components of NAB observed in healthy growing premature infants fed one of three different formulas.

input into the body fluids, and with this a change in NAO. Most of the change was due to a change in NAE, which increased from 10 mEq/1000 Cal when the low protein electrolyte diet was given to 22 mEq/1000 Cal. The mechanisms regulating renal acid excretion in response to change in NAI are reviewed in Chapters 5 and 29. When increases in NAE are not sufficient to match increases in NAI metabolic acidosis ensues. For example, in diabetes ketoacidosis ($H^+_{OA^-}$ increases markedly, while in gastroenteritis and acidosis, UA_{abs} becomes negative.

Regulation of Absorbed Undetermined Anion

The milk diets of infants contain relatively large amounts of potential base, in contrast to the negative UA of most adult diets. The dietary undetermined anion is greater than the fecal UA of infants receiving each of the three milk formulas (Fig. 8.12). The UA in milk is largely citrate, a metabolizable, absorbable base. Although the formulas deliver from 30 to 60 mEq/1000 kcal of UA, fecal UA increases in parallel so that the amount of UA_{abs} is a relatively small portion of the UA in the formula. If all the UA in the diet were to be absorbed, base input would exceed NAI and NAE would be negative, i.e., urine would be alkaline, which may predispose to nephrocalcinosis. Because UA_{abs} is only a small portion of the intake and UAF increases as dietary UA increases suggests that base absorption is regulated by the gastrointestinal tract of infants. Since the UA of the milk is largely citrate, which is readily absorbed and metabolized to HCO_3^-, the UA of the stool is likely to be determined by other chemical species, e.g., Ca and P.

Effects of Growth on Net Acid Balance

NAB is influenced by growth. Sulfur-containing amino acids that are incorporated into new body protein rather than being catabolized to $H^+_{SO_4^=}$ decreases the potential for net acid input. When a high protein diet is fed, $H^+_{SO_4^=}$ increases significantly. Bone growth is acidifying, since hydroxyapatite formation is the formation of a solid base from neutral precursors, creating H^+ and constituting an acid load to the body fluids. Giving more Ca and P in the formula increases the rate of formation of bone crystal and, hence, $H^+_{Ca^{++}}$. Kidney function of term infants can accommodate to this increase in NAI to excrete more net acid. Low birth weight infants develop metabolic acidosis, the late metabolic acidosis of infancy, when fed a high protein, high Ca and P formula (45, 46). The acidosis is a result, in part, of increase of the $H^+_{SO_4^=}$ and $H^+_{Ca^{++}}$ component of NAI and a limitation in NAE. A decrease in UA or an increase in $H^+_{OA^-}$ might contribute but, to date, the studies to determine these components of NAB in these infants have not been done.

The effects of growth on the components of the NAB are illustrated in Figure 8.13, which shows NAB data for healthy growing infants and healthy, nongrowing young male adults, both on a simulated breast milk

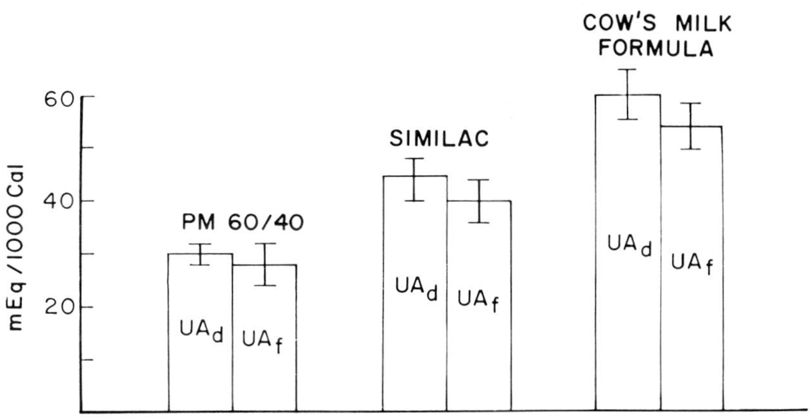

Figure 8.12. Oral and fecal UA on three different groups of healthy premature infants fed one of three different formulas.

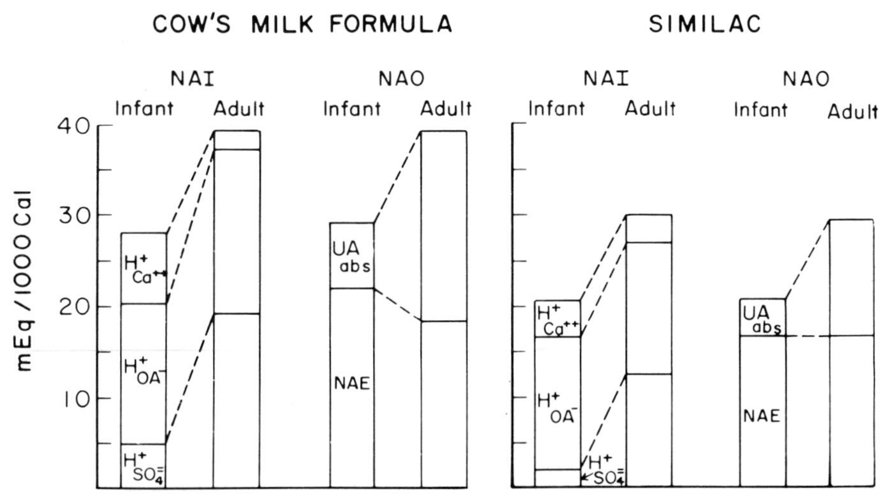

Figure 8.13. Effects on each component of NAB of growth versus no growth on two different infant formulas. The data show the comparison of each component observed in the healthy growing infant with that observed in the healthy nongrowing adult. All data are normalized to mEq per 1000 calories of intake.

formula and on cow's milk formula (47). The data were related to 1000 kcal of intake. The adults were in zero NAB. Both NAI and NAO were higher in adults than in infants. The increase in NAI was from an increase in $H^+_{SO_4^=}$. All of the ingested sulfur-containing amino acid was catabolized in the adults. There was some $H^+_{Ca^{++}}$ in the adults. Because of the large increase in dietary Ca and P a transient increase in skeletal mineralization in adults also occurred. The increase in NAO was from an increase in UA_{abs}. NAE was lower in adults than in infants because base absorption was larger. This suggests that, in the adult, the gastrointestinal tract has lost some of its ability to limit base (Ca) absorption, which may explain why the adult is so prone to the development of the milk-alkali syndrome (48).

ACID-BASE DISORDERS AND THEIR TREATMENT

Classification of Acid-Base Disorders

The four primary disturbances of acid-base equilibrium, metabolic acidosis and alkalosis and respiratory acidosis and alkalosis, are defined in terms of physiological or pathological processes (49). While each disturbance is initiated with a primary change in the respiratory or metabolic component of blood acid-base status, secondary responses in both respiration and metabolism compenstate for the primary effect, so that defining a disturbance of acid base using change in plasma HCO_3^-, whole blood base excess, and pCO_2 is neither clinically adequate or physiologically accurate. For example, metabolic acidosis is defined as a primary gain of strong acid or a primary loss of bicarbonate from the body fluids. These events result in a fall in plasma HCO_3^- concentration and pH but acidemia (low blood pH) is not synonymous with metabolic acidosis. Metabolic alkalosis arises from a primary gain of HCO_3^-; respiratory acidosis is defined as a primary decrease and respiratory alkalosis as a primary increase in alveolar ventilation resulting in either a rise or fall in pCO_2. A simple disturbance exists when there is a single etiologic factor that affects a single component of acid-base equilibrium. Often, several disturbances affect both respiratory and metabolic controls of acid-base status, leading to mixed disorders. These are affected by chronicity and by the effect the disease has upon the compensatory mechanisms.

Conceptual Framework for Analysis of Acid-Base Disturbance

In the discussion of acid-base disorders which follows, we will use a conceptual framework for analyzing acid-base disorders that aids in making a specific diagnosis, as well as in formulating therapy. This framework is as follows:

1. Definition of the primary acid base disturbance, i.e., general etiology
2. Identification of the specific etiology
3. Response of the blood buffers to the primary etiology with respect to the change in either the metabolic or respiratory component
4. Type and degree of compensation
5. Possibility of corrective mechanisms and their efficacy in correcting the primary disorder

The general etiologic factor is the primary acid-base disorder, i.e., gain or loss of fixed acid, gain or loss of CO_2. The specific etiology is the clinical disorder that causes the primary acid-base disturbance. Buffer responses are physicochemical events that react quickly to the disturbance to limit the magnitude of change in pH; compensation is a slower physiological process that tends to restore acid-base status toward normal. The possibility for, and the effectiveness of, these corrective physiological processes needs to be evaluated.

Metabolic Acidosis

Causes

Table 8.2 lists the causes of metabolic acidosis, grouped first by two general mechanisms, either a gain in fixed acid or loss of HCO_3^-. The fixed acid can be any one of a number of acids: (1) hydrochloric acid per se or hydrochloric acid derived from ammonia chloride or cationic amino acid (arginine HCl or lysine HCl) administration; (2) ketone acids—β-hydroxybutyric acid and acetoacetic acid—resulting from the incomplete oxidation of fatty acids, as seen in diabetic ketoacidosis or in starvation ketosis; (3) other organic acid anions that accumulate in the plasma in a large variety of disorders, including lactic acid acidosis, congenital organic acidosis, and as a result of intoxication with various substances, such as methyl alcohol and ethylene glycol; and (4) accumulation of the normal end products of metabolism, such as sulfate and phosphate in failure of renal acid excretion, such as occurs in CRF.

Loss of HCO_3^- from the ECF can occur via the kidney, as in renal tubular acidosis or renal carbonic anhydrase inhibition, or via the GI tract as in diarrhea or small bowel drainage. Since secretions of the small intestine beyond the pylorus contain HCO_3^-, loss of these secretions by vomiting, drainage, or diarrhea, will lead to a loss of base and can cause metabolic acidosis.

Buffer Reactions

The buffer reactions to loading with strong acid involve both the HCO_3^- and the nonbicarbonate buffer systems as follows:

$$H^+X^- + HCO_3^- \rightarrow H_2CO_3 + X^- \qquad (28)$$

$$H^+X^- + Buf^- \rightarrow HBuf + X^- \qquad (29)$$

The result is a fall in conjugate base concentration and production of the corresponding weak acids. This fall can be quantitated by measuring plasma HCO_3^- concentration or by measuring whole blood base excess. The weak acid form of the bicarbonate buffer system, H_2CO_3, is excreted as CO_2 from the lungs, so that H_2CO_3 does not accumulate.

A primary loss of HCO_3^- is buffered by interaction between the bicarbonate buffer system and the nonbicarbonate buffer system in which CO_2 generated by metabolism is hydrated to form carbonic acid, which then reacts with the conjugate bases of the nonbicarbonate buffer system to generated bicarbonate. The loss of bicarbonate with a consequent fall in plasma HCO_3^- concentration is the driving force for the reaction:

$$H_2CO_3 + Buf^- \rightarrow HBuf + HCO_3^- \qquad (30)$$

Again, the result is that both plasma HCO_3^- concentration and whole blood bases excess fall.

Table 8.2
Causes of Metabolic Acidosis

General mechanism	Specific mechanism	Example
Gain of strong acid by ECF	Gain of exogenous acid (HCl)	NH_4Cl acidosis
	Incomplete oxidation of fat (ketone body acids)	Diabetic or starvation ketoacidosis
	Incomplete oxidation of carbohydrate (lactic acid)	Lactic acidosis
	Gain of H_2SO_4, H_3PO_4, and organic acids	Uremic acidosis
Loss of HCO_3^- from ECF	Via the kidney	Renal tubular acidosis
	Via the GI tract	Diarrheal acidosis

When a strong acid is buffered HCO_3^- is lost through buffer reaction and the acid anion accumulates. The anion pattern of the plasma is characterized by a low HCO_3^- concentration and a high concentration of X^-, i.e., there is a reciprocal increase in X^- with the fall in HCO_3^-. Except when X^- is Cl^-, there will be an increase in the undetermined anion fraction of plasma. Undetermined anion is estimated by the R fraction, also called the residual fraction. The plasma R fraction is computed as follows:

$$R = Na^+ - [HCO_3^- + Cl^-] \tag{31}$$

The normal value for the R is 11 mEq/L, i.e.,

$$R = 140 - (24 + 105) = 11 \text{ mEq/L} \tag{32}$$

R normally varies from 5 to 15 mEq/L with accumulation of acetoacetate, lactate, and other organic anions. Loss of HCO_3^- from body fluids is accompanied by an accumulation of Cl^- and the R fraction does not rise. Thus, the R fraction is useful as a step in determining the cause for the metabolic acidosis. If the R fraction is not elevated, then the metabolic acidosis is a result either of loading with HCl or a loss of HCO_3^-.

If the R fraction is elevated, there is an accumulation of acid anion in plasma. The renal threshold for ketone bodies is low so that any significant increase in plasma concentration of β-hydroxybutyric or acetoacetic acid will be reflected by detectable amounts of ketones. One can suspect diabetic ketoacidosis, starvation, or other causes of incomplete fatty acid oxidation as the cause of the metabolic acidosis. Similarly, an increased R fraction and an elevated BUN would indicate renal failure. An elevated R fraction in the absence of ketonuria or an elevated BUN would indicate the accumulation of an organic acid anion, such as lactate (as in lactic acid acidosis), or glycolate (as in ethylene glycol ingestion), or some other anion as in the rare forms of congenital acidosis. Complete history and age of the patient will aid in the specific diagnosis of metabolic acidosis characterized by an elevated R fraction in the absence of ketonuria and an elevated BUN.

Respiratory Compensation

Since the primary event in metabolic acidosis causes a change in the metabolic component of acid-base equilibrium, the compensatory change occurs first in the respiratory component. Specifically, there is an increase in alveolar ventilation with a decrease in pCO_2.

The time course for complete respiratory compensation is quite long, requiring several hours to 1 or 2 days. Induction of sustained metabolic acidosis in unanesthetized trained dogs (Fig. 8.14) (50) causes an abrupt lowering of plasma HCO_3^- concentration and a discernible lowering of pCO_2. However, 6 to 8 hours was required for pCO_2 to reach steady state values because the central chemoreceptors are separated from blood by the blood-brain barrier (30). As bicarbonate crosses this barrier by active transport, pCO_2 reaches a steady state. Plasma HCO_3^- is low, with induction of acidosis, blood pH is also low and stimulates the peripheral chemoreceptors to increase alveolar ventilation and lower pCO_2. In the cerebral ISF, HCO_3^- concentration has not yet fallen from normal, pCO_2 is low resulting from peripheral drive and pH is high. The central chemoreceptors counter the stimulation of the respiratory center. As HCO_3^- concentration of cerebral ISF attains equilibrium with plasma HCO_3^-, CSF pH comes to a new equilibrium, the central chemoreceptor inhibition of the respiratory center is removed, and the respiratory compensation becomes fully manifest (51).

When this occurs, blood pH is higher than if no compensation had occurred but still is not normal. The degree of respiratory compensation for sustained metabolic acidosis in 60 children with uncomplicated, untreated metabolic acidosis is illustrated in Figure 8.15 (52). The degree

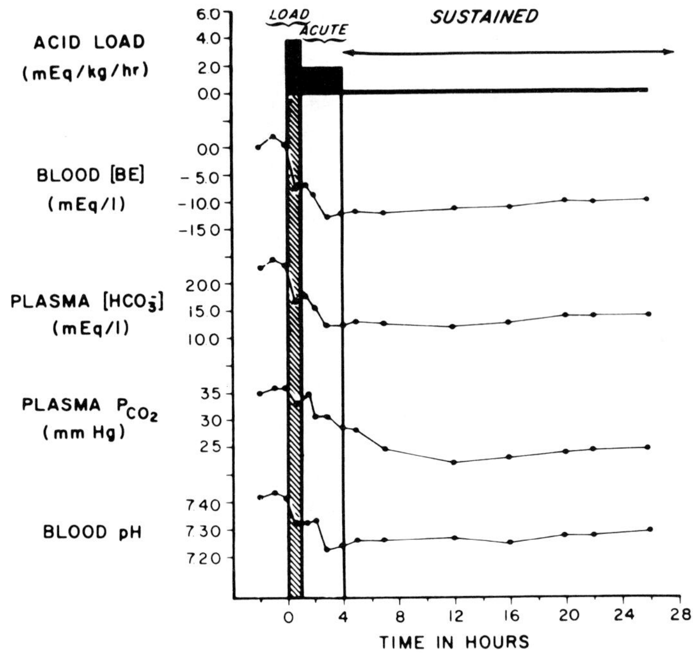

Figure 8.14. Time course of development of respiratory compensation in experimentally induced metabolic acidosis in the dog. (Asch MJ, et al: *J Lab Clin Med* 73:610, 1969.)

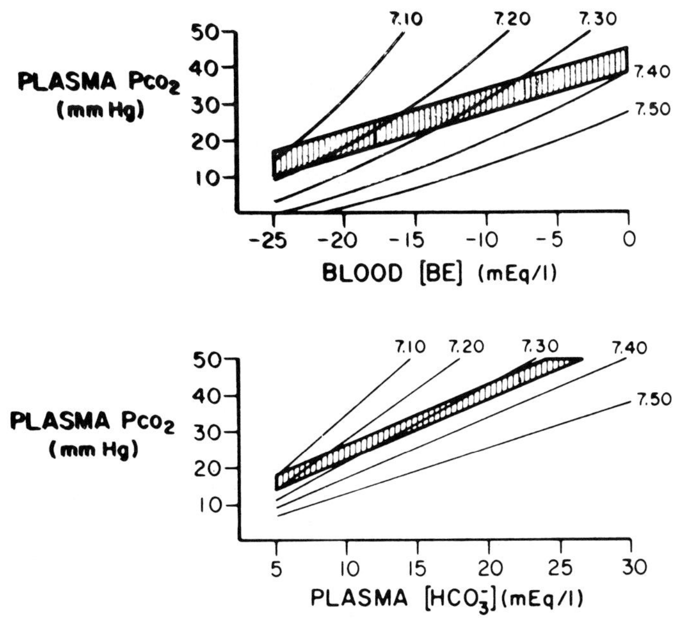

Figure 8.15. The 95% confidence limits for expected acid-base displacement in uncomplicated metabolic acidosis. (Albert MS, et al: *Ann Intern Med* 66:312, 1967.)

of fall in pCO_2 and the confidence limits for the responses are quite predictable for a given decline in either plasma HCO_3^- concentration or in blood base excess. For example, if the initial plasma HCO_3^- concentration is 10 mEq/L, the pCO_2 is predicted to be 22 ± 2.2 mm Hg. If pCO_2 is above this range and the acidosis has been present for >24 hours, the patient probably has some limitation in the ability to lower pCO_2 appropriately. On the other hand, if pCO_2 is lower than expected, there is likely to be a mixed acid-base disturbance, with the patient's respiratory center receiving two independent stimuli to increase alveolar ventilation. This results in the observed pCO_2 being below the predicted for uncomplicated metabolic acidosis. Such a mixed disturbance frequently occurs in children <4 years of age with salicylate poisoning where both metabolic acidosis and respiratory alkalosis are present (53, 54). The fall in pCO_2 (Fig. 8.15) is not sufficient to restore blood pH to normal except in mild metabolic acidosis, so that any patient with metabolic acidosis and a normal pH has some independent stimulus to the respiratory center, causing a lower then expected pCO_2.

The lag in respiratory response with development of metabolic acidosis occurs during recovery but is opposite in direction (55). If plasma HCO_3^- concentration is abruptly raised to normal values, central chemoreceptors will continue to stimulate the respiratory center until HCO_3^- concentration of the cerebral ISF rises to normal. In the face of a continuing respiratory drive, pCO_2 will remain low; at normal plasma HCO_3^- concentration, blood pH will be above normal. If blood pH abruptly becomes alkaline, the patient may suffer adverse consequences, such as convulsion or coma. Therefore, it is prudent to provide base correction at a rate that aims at restoring pH toward normal rather than restoring plasma HCO_3^- concentration to normal. When pH is close to normal, the increased alveolar ventilation will slowly abate, pCO_2 will rise and plasma HCO_3^- can rise slowly to normal, either by renal excretion of net acid or by provision of exogenous base if necessary.

Renal Response and Therapy

Metabolic acidosis due to retention of acid may be corrected by the renal excretion of net acid, with the consequent production of new HCO_3^- for the body fluids, or by the metabolism of the anion if it is an organic anion that is metabolized; if it is a fixed anion, i.e., chloride, it is excreted with net acid. Metabolic acidosis from a loss of HCO_3^- is corrected by an increase in renal excretion of TA and NH_4 to generate new HCO_3^-.

In diabetic ketoacidosis, new HCO_3^- is generated by the kidneys but when insulin is provided the ketoacid anions in body fluids are metabolized to CO_2 and H_2O with the production of HCO_3^-, as shown in the following reaction:

$$H_2CO_3 + OA^- \rightarrow HCO_3^- + \underset{\swarrow \text{ metabolized to } CO_2 \text{ and } H_2O}{HOA} \quad (33)$$

In diabetic ketoacidosis, as oxidation of fatty acids to CO_2 and H_2O occurs, there are two sources of HCO_3^-, renal and metabolic. Only modest amounts of exogenous base are recommended in treating the metabolic acidosis of diabetes.

Metabolic acidosis secondary to diarrheal dehydration, where there has been loss of HCO_3^- and there is little metabolizable anion, can only be treated by providing potential base. This may be in the form of Na and K bicarbonate, i.e., (Na + K > Cl), or as NaCl, in which case Cl is excreted as NH_4Cl and new base is generated. For treatment recommendations see Chapter 11.

Metabolic Alkalosis

Etiology

Table 8.3 lists the causes of metabolic alkalosis. There are two general mechanisms: a gain of HCO_3^- or a loss of acid from the ECF. The gain of HCO_3^- can result from administration of HCO_3^- or from oxidation of organic anions with subsequent production of HCO_3^-. Loss of acid is a result of loss of HCl in gastric fluid from obstructive vomiting or to excretion of H^+ by the kidneys during diuretic therapy.

Mechanisms responsible for the production of metabolic alkalosis need to be distinguished from mechanisms that prevent the kidney from excreting the increased amount of base. The kidneys have an enormous capacity to excrete HCO_3^- and can easily excrete extra base unless other mechanisms prevent the excretion of HCO_3^-. For example, it is virtually impossible to cause sustained metabolic alkalosis by oral loading with $NaHCO_3$ because ECF volume is expanded, so the renal excretion of Na^+ as HCO_3^- matches input (56). If there is concurrent impairment in renal function causing Na retention in the presence of volume expansion, metabolic alkalosis will result. In the setting of ECF volume contraction or Na and Cl depletion in which Na is retained, alkali given without Cl can cause metabolic alkalosis (57, 58).

Table 8.3
Causes of Metabolic Alkalosis

General mechanism	Specific mechanism	Example
Gain of HCO_3^- by ECF	Gain of exogenous HCO_3^-	Ingestion or infusion of HCO_3^-
	Oxidation of salts of organic acids	Ingestion or infusion of lactate, citrate, or acetate
Loss of acid from ECF	Loss of HCl	Vomiting of gastric juice
	Loss of H^+ via the kidney	Diuretic therapy; K^+ depletion
	Extrarenal transfer of H^+ to ICF	K^+ depletion

When hydrochloric acid is lost from the stomach, HCO_3^- is added to the body fluids on an equimolar basis with the hydrochloric acid that is lost. The extra HCO_3^- may be excreted as $NaHCO_3$ until ECF volume contraction and Na depletion occur. Then, the extra HCO_3^- is excreted with K and K depletion results. With both Na and K depletion, both cations are avidly conserved by the kidney and HCO_3^- is reabsorbed with either, since Cl has been lost (57, 59). If NaCl and water are provided and ECF volume is expanded, the excess cation is excreted with HCO_3^- and the alkalosis is quickly corrected (60).

Mineralocorticoid excess operates by the same general mechanism, i.e., sodium is reabsorbed with HCO_3^- in the presence of potassium depletion. It is not clear whether the enhanced HCO_3^- reabsorption or, more fundamentally, increased hydrogen ion secretion by the distal tubule is due to increased circulating hormone or K depletion or some other factor (61). What is clear is that in the case of mineralocorticoid excess, the alkalosis persists even with provision of NaCl, i.e., there is a saline diuresis with continuation of the metabolic alkalosis (62).

The strong association of potassium deficiency with metabolic alkalosis has been thought to be causally related to the alkalosis (63, 64). Giving $NaHCO_3$ to K-deficient rats leads to renal absorption of HCO_3^- (65); K-deficiency is necessary for induction of metabolic alkalosis in mineralocorticoid excess (64, 65). These experiments in rats are difficult to interpret because of the many factors that are present during the development of the metabolic alkalosis, in addition to simple K depletion. There are experiments (66) which point to an extrarenal renal mechanism in which potassium loss from the cells is accompanied by uptake of sodium and hydrogen ion from the ECF causing an alkalosis, but these observations have not been confirmed in larger animals. While the causal role of potassium depletion in metabolic alkalosis may be in dispute, it is clear the metabolic alkalosis does cause K depletion since renal excretion of HCO_3^- results in K loss leading to K depletion (57) (chapter 7).

Buffer Reaction

When metabolic alkalosis results from loss of gastric acid, the hydrogen ion secreted by the gastric mucosa comes from water, leaving behind hyroxyl ion to be buffered in the ECF as follows:

$$OH^- + H_2CO_3 \rightarrow HCO_3^- + H_2O \quad (34)$$

$$OH^- + HBuf \rightarrow Buf^- + H_2O \quad (35)$$

These reactions result in an increase in conjugate base concentration, which is detected by a rise in plasma HCO_3^- and by a rise in base excess, i.e., there is a rise in both HCO_3^- and nonbicarbonate conjugate bases.

Respiratory Compensation

Metabolic alkalosis results in a decrease in alveolar ventilation leading to a rise in pCO_2. In metabolic alkalosis, compensation is limited by the hypoxia that necessarily accompanies alveolar hypoventilation.

Figure 8.16 illustrates the relationship between pCO_2 and both plasma HCO_3^- concentration and whole blood base excess. The 95% confidence bands are derived from studies on alkalotic patients, most of whom were infants with pyloric stenosis (40). The 95% confidence region for respiratory compensation in metabolic alkalosis is quite high, indicating that the relationship between degree of alkalosis and the degree of rise in pCO_2 is not as predictable as in metabolic acidosis (Figure 8.15). Thus, it is more difficult to detect a mixed disturbance when one of the primary factors is metabolic alkalosis. At a plasma HCO_3^- concentration of 50 mEq/L, pCO_2 can rise from 52 to 68 torr with pH ranging from 7.48 to 7.40. If no compensation had occurred and pCO_2^- remained at 40 torr, then pH would rise to 7.72. Thus, even though limited and variable, the respiratory compensation that does occur limits the rise in plasma pH because of metabolic alkalosis.

Correction

Metabolic alkalosis is corrected by the renal excretion of HCO_3^-, which brings the buffer base concentration of whole blood back to normal levels. When Na is readily available, metabolic alkalosis is readily corrected. However, the renal excretion of HCO_3^- is limited when ECF volume (NaCl) or K are deficient, so that urine is acid and, therefore, devoid of HCO_3^- even though plasma HCO_3^- is elevated. This paradoxical aciduria is a result of the cation depletion. Providing NaCl or KCl quickly restores renal HCO_3^- excretion. Because K depletion usually is present with metabolic alkalosis, it is generally prudent to give both Na and KCl. Despite the controversy surrounding the question of whether K depletion is causally related to the metabolic alkalosis or not, the fact remains that K depletion is nearly always present in metabolic alkalosis and should be treated. Acidifying salts (arginine hydrochloride, lysine hydrochloride, or ammonium chloride) have been used with good results in the treatment of severe metabolic alkalosis. Concern has been expressed about the possibility of causing ammonia toxicity with ammonium chloride but this has not occurred (40).

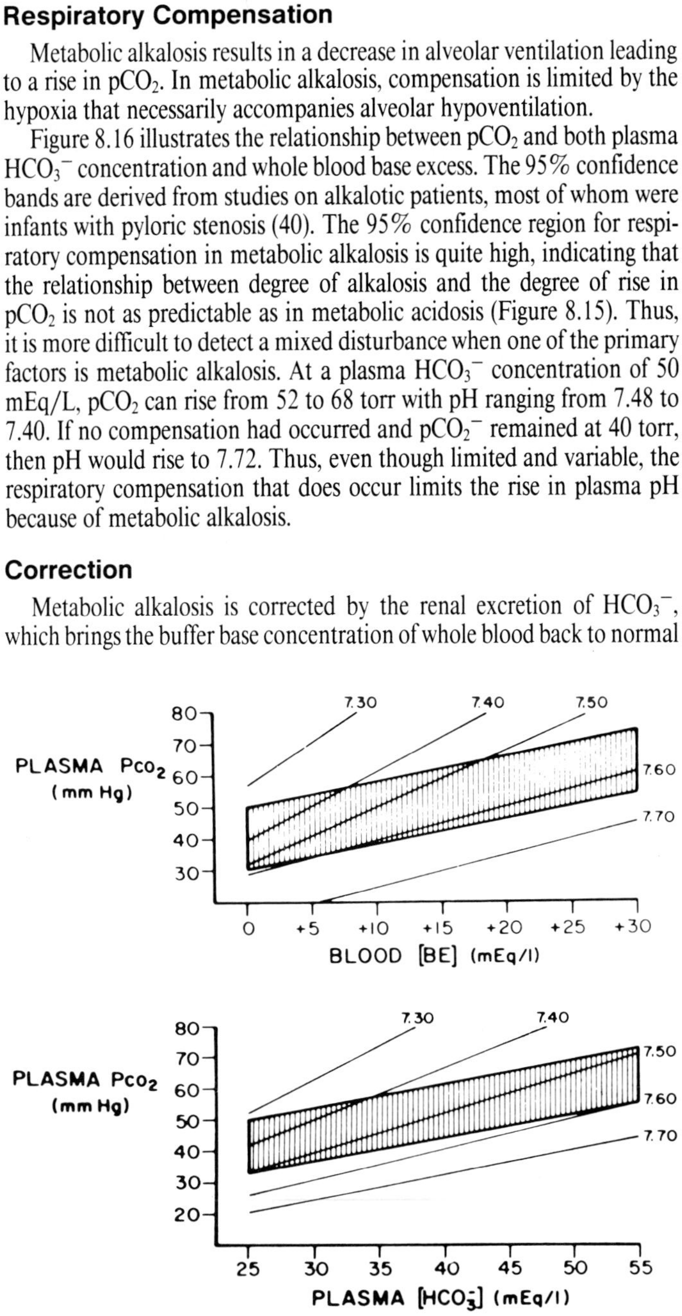

Figure 8.16. The 95% confidence limits for expected acid-base displacement in uncomplicated metabolic alkalosis. (Kildeberg P: *Clinical Acid-Base Physiology. Studies in Neonates, Infants and Young Children*, Copenhagen, Munkssgaard, 1968.)

Respiratory Acidosis

Etiology

Respiratory acidosis results from primary reduction in alveolar ventilation (Table 8.4). Any of three sites in the respiratory system can be the cause: (1) central nervous system depression caused by disease or drugs; (2) airway or lung disease resulting in decreased ventilation or impaired gaseous diffusion; and (3) chest wall disease as a result of structural or functional abnormalities of the chest wall, leading to a loss of the bellows action of the lung. The reduction in alveolar ventilation, with ongoing CO_2 production, leads to an accumulation of CO_2, a rise in pCO_2, and respiratory acidosis.

Buffer Reaction

The buffer reaction for CO_2 retention involves hydration of the CO_2 to H_2CO_3 and buffering by the interaction reaction;

$$CO_2 + H_2O \rightarrow H_2CO_3 + Buf^- \rightarrow HBuf + HCO_3^- \quad (36)$$

As noted earlier in this chapter, the HCO_3^- generated by this reaction in whole blood diffuses into the ISF so that plasma HCO_3^- does not rise as much as predicted by the above equation and base excess falls. Figure 8.17 shows the in vivo buffer response to an acute rise in pCO_2, which has been studied in healthy adult male volunteers (67). The 95% confidence limits in this figure are applicable only to acute disturbances (duration <12 hours) since, with the passage of time, renal compensation becomes apparent (69).

Table 8.4
Causes of Respiratory Acidosis

Site of respiratory system	Mechanism	Effect
Central nervous system	Depression of respiratory center (disease, certain drugs)	
Airways or lungs	Decreased ventilation or diffusion (intrinsic lung or airway disease)	Decrease in alveolar ventilation
Chest wall	Loss of bellows action (structural or functional abnormalities of chest or muscles)	

Compensation

Compensation for respiratory acidosis is renal excretion of hydrogen ion discernible in 12 to 24 hours, but is complete only after several days. Plasma HCO_3^- rises because hydrogen ion excretion is augmented and new HCO_3^- is generated.

Children with cystic fibrosis who were in a steady state of hypercapnia for at least 3 days (68) have renal compensatory responses shown in Figure 8.18. Ninety-five percent confidence limits for the plasma HCO_3^- and base excess as a function of plasma pCO_2 are shown. The compensatory response limits the fall in pH to 7.35 until pCO_2 exceeds 70 torr and to 7.31 when pCO_2 exceeds 100 torr. The confidence limits are useful in identifying patients that have a mixed acid-base disturbance when the hypercapnia is relatively stable. If the pCO_2 is changing it is not possible to predict the expected degree of compensation. However, serial studies of blood acid-base status usually will provide the information needed to diagnose a mixed disturbance.

Correction of respiratory acidosis obviously requires correction of the defect in the respiratory system causing the disturbance. Frequently this is not possible. Abruptly lowering pCO_2 to normal from a chronically elevated value will cause a shift in pH to alkalosis, since plasma HCO_3^- concentration is high. Such an abrupt shift may cause cardiac arrhythmias and seizures and should be avoided. The renal excretion of HCO_3^- in response to a lowering of pCO_2 entails excretion of Na or K; NaCl and KCl should be provided. Since patients with chronic hypercapnia often have congestive heart failure and often are treated with diuretics, such patients may have volume and cation depletion and limited ability to excrete HCO_3^-, a feature that leads to the persistence of metabolic compensation for the respiratory acidosis (see metabolic alkalosis).

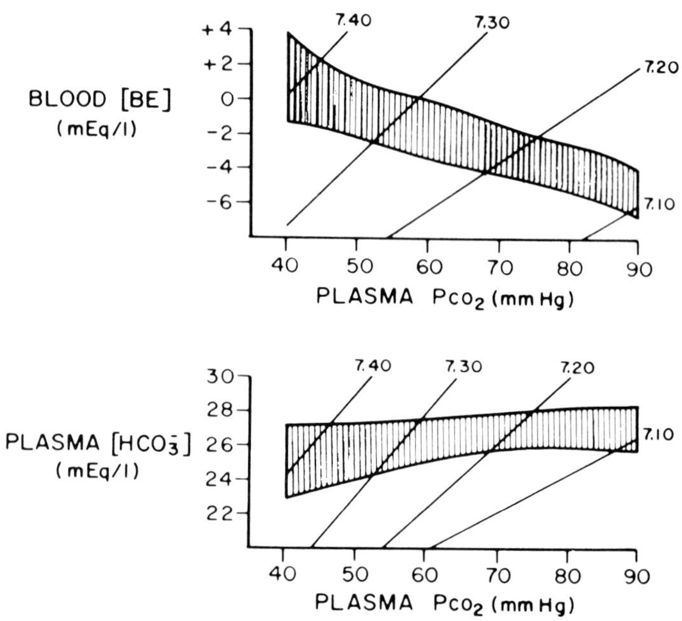

Figure 8.17. The 95% confidence limits for expected acid-base displacement in uncomplicated acute respiratory acidosis. (From Brackett NC Jr, Cohen JJ, Schwartz WB: *N Engl J Med* 272:6, 1965.)

Respiratory Alkalosis

Cause

Table 8.5 lists causes of an increase in alveolar ventilation that leads to a fall in pCO_2 and respiratory alkalosis. A common cause is hysterical hyperventilation. Hypoxia stimulates the peripheral chemoreceptors to increase alveolar ventilation and can lead to respiratory alkalosis. There are intrathoracic stretch receptors that can be stimulated by patchy bronchopneumonia or other focal pulmonary diseases that cause an increase in alveolar ventilation. Respiratory alkalosis occurs in severe hepatic failure for reasons that are not understood. During pregnancy pCO_2 is lower, presumably a result of stimulation of the respiratory center by progesterone.

Buffer Reaction

The decrease in pCO_2 leads to a decrease in carbonic acid via the hydration reaction, a decrease that is buffered by the nonbicarbonate buffer system:

$$HCO_3^- + HBuf \rightarrow Buf^- + H_2CO_3 \rightarrow \overset{\overset{\text{lost}}{\uparrow}}{CO_2} + H_2O \quad (37)$$

Just as in respiratory acidosis, HCO_3^- moves from the cerebral ISF to the plasma compartment over time, partially offsetting the fall in plasma

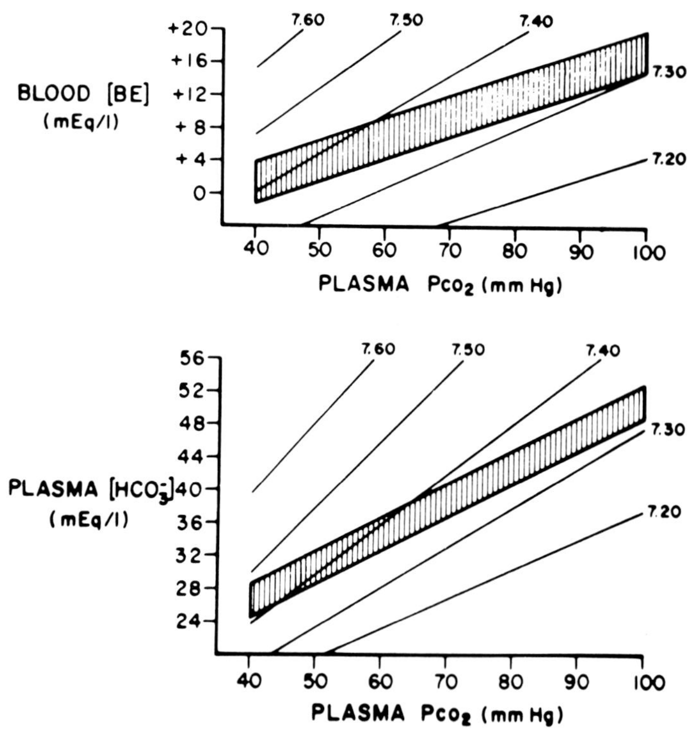

Figure 8.18. The 95% confidence limits for expected acid-base displacement in uncomplicated sustained respiratory acidosis. (From Engel K, Kildeberg P, Winters RW: *Scand J Clin Lab Invest* 23:5, 1969.)

Table 8.5
Causes of Respiratory Alkalosis

Site of respiratory system	Mechanism	Effect
Central nervous system	Primary stimulation of respiratory center (emotion, certain drugs)	
Peripheral chemoreceptors	Reflect stimulation of respiratory center (hypoxemia)	Increase in alveolar ventilation
Intrathoracic stretch receptors	Reflex stimulation of respiratory center (localized pulmonary disease)	

HCO_3^- because of the decreased pCO_2. The net result is a higher plasma HCO_3^- concentration than one would expect from studies of blood in vitro (70). Base excess rises rather than remaining at zero. However, the in vivo response is close to the in vitro response, because there is an accumulation of organic acid, particularly lactic acid, in the ECF. This organic acid production titrates down the conjugate bases of plasma, brings HCO_3^- down to the expected in vitro response, and blunts the rise in base excess.

Compensation

Renal compensation in respiratory alkalosis involves the excretion of HCO_3^-, provided there is not a concomitant cation and water deficit to limit the capacity of the kidney to excrete HCO_3^-. The time course for the renal response is similar to respiratory acidosis: it is discernible in 6 to 12 hours and complete in $1\frac{1}{2}$ to 3 days. The complete response appears to be to restore blood pH to normal. Sustained respiratory alkalosis occurs in normal individuals during exposure to high altitude when hypoxia is the driving stimulus and during pregnancy as a result of progesterone stimulation of the respiratory center. No treatment is needed. For hysterical hyperventilation and tetany, rebreathing in a closed bag sustains pCO_2 and provides correction.

References

1. Siggaard-Andersen O: The Acid-Base Status of the Blood, ed 4. Baltimore, Williams & Wilkins, 1974.
2. Brønsted JN: The acid basic function of molecules and its dependency on the electric charge type. J Phys Chem 30:777, 1926.
3. Lowry TM: The uniqueness of hydrogen. J Soc Chem Indust 42:43, 1923.
4. Van Slyke DD: On the measurement of buffer values and on the relationship of buffer value to the dissociation constant of the buffer and the concentration and reaction of the buffer solution. J Biol Chem 52:525, 1922.
5. Edsall JT, Wyman J: Thermodynamics, Electrostatics and the Biological Significance of the Properties of Matter. New York, Academic Press, 1966, vol 1.
6. Henderson LJ: The Fitness of the Environment: An Inquiry into the Biological Significance of the Properties of Matter. 1913, reprinted Boston, Beacon Press, 1958.
7. Winters RW, Dell RB: Regulation of acid-base equilibrium. In Yamamoto WS, Brobeck JR (eds): Physiological Controls and Regulations. Philadelphia, W.B. Saunders Co., 1965.
8. Roughton FJW: Transport of oxygen and carbon dioxide. In Fenn WO, Rahn H (eds): Handbook of Physiology. Washington, D.C., American Physiological Society, 1964.
9. Henderson LJ: The theory of neutrality regulation in the animal organism. Am J Physiol 21:427, 1908.
10. Hasselbalch KA: Die Berechnung der Wasserstoffzahl des Blutes aus der freien und gebundenen Kohlensaure desselben, und die Sauerstoffbindung des Blutes als Funktion der Wasserstoffzahl. Biochem Z 78:112, 1916–1917.
11. Van Slyke DD, Sendroy J Jr, Hastings AB, et al: Studies of gas and electrolyte equilibria in blood. X. The solubility of carbon dioxide at 38°C in water, salt solution, serum, and blood cells. J Biol Chem 28:765. 1928.
12. Severinghaus JW: Blood gas concentration. In Fenn WO, Rahn H (eds): Handbook of Physiology. Washington, D.C., American Physiological Society, 1964.
13. Van Slyke DD, Wu H, McLean FC: Studies of gas and electrolyte equilibria in blood. V. Factors controlling the electrolyte and water distribution in the blood. J Biol Chem 56:765, 1923.
14. Singer RB, Hastings AB: Improved clinical method for estimation of disturbances of acid-base balance of human blood. Medicine 27:223, 1948.
15. Pitts RF: Physiology of the Kidney and Body Fluids. Chicago, Year Book Medical Publishers, 1974.
16. Schwartz WB, Jensen RL, Relman AS: Disposition of acid administration to sodium depleted subjects: Renal response and role of whole body buffers. J Clin Invest 33:587, 1954.
17. Schwartz WB, Orning KJ, Porter R: The internal distribution of hydrogen ions with varying degrees of metabolic acidosis. J Clin Invest 36:373, 1957.
18. Waddell WJ, Bates RG: Intracellular pH. Physiol Rev 49:258, 1969.
19. Caldwell PC: Intracellular pH. Int Rev Cytol 5:229, 1956.
20. Carter NW: Intracellular pH. Kidney Int 1:341, 1972.
21. Waddell WJ, Butler TC: Calculation of intracellular pH from the distribution of 5,5-dimethyl-2,4-oxazolidinedione (DMO). Application to skeletal muscle of the dog. J Clin Invest 38:720, 1959.
22. Adler S: The simultaneous determination of muscle pH using a weak acid and weak base. J Clin Invest 51:256, 1972.
23. Brackett NC Jr, Cohen JJ, Schwartz WB: Carbon dioxide titration curve of normal man. Effect of increasing degrees of acute hypercapnia on acid-base equilibrium. N Engl J Med 272:6, 1965.
24. Dell RB, Winters RW: A model for the in vivo CO_2 equilibration curve. Am J Physiol 219:37, 1970.
25. Comroe JH Jr: Physiology of Respiration. Chicago, Year Book Medical Publishers, 1965.
26. Purves MJ: The Peripheral Arterial Chemoreceptors. London, Cambridge University Press, 1975.
27. Mitchell RA, Loeschcke HH, Maission WH, et al: Respiratory responses mediated through superficial chemosensitive areas on the medulla. J Appl Physiol 18:523, 1963.
28. Papperheimer JR: The ionic composition of cerebral extracellular fluid and its relation to control of breathing. Harvey Lect 61:71, 1967.
29. Gray JS: Pulmonary Ventilation and Its Physiological Regulation. Springfield, Ill., Charles C Thomas, 1950.
30. Mitchell RA, Carman CT, Severinghaus JW, et al: Stability of cerebrospinal fluid pH in chronic acid-base disturbances in blood. J Appl Physiol 20:443, 1965.
31. Warnock DG, Rector FC Jr: Proton secretion by the kidney. Ann Rev Physiol 41:117, 1979.
32. Rector FC Jr, Carter NW, Seldin DW: The mechanism of bicarbonate reabsorption in the proximal and distal tubules of the kidney. J Clin Invest 44:278, 1965.
33. Schiess WA, Ayer JL, Lotspeich WD, et al: The renal regulation of acid-base balance in man. II. Factors affecting the excretion of titratable acid by the normal human subject. J Clin Invest 27:57, 1948.
34. Sartorius OW, Roemmelt JC, Pitts RF: The renal regulation of acid-base balance in man. IV. The nature of the renal compensation in ammonium chloride acidosis. J Clin Invest 28:423, 1949.
35. Schwartz WB, Cohen JJ: The nature of the renal response to chronic disorders of acid-base equilibrium. Am J Med 64:417, 1978.
36. Kildeberg P, Engel K, Winters RW: Balance of net acid in growing infants. Endogenous and transintestinal aspects. Acta Paediatr Scand. 58:321, 1969.
37. Lennon EJ, Lemann J Jr, Litzow JR: The effects of diet and stool composition on the net external acid balance of normal subjects. J Clin Invest 45:1601, 1966.
38. Lennon EJ, Lemann J Jr, Relman AS: The effects of phosphoproteins on acid balance in normal subjects. J Clin Invest 41:637, 1962.
39. Lemann J Jr, Relman AS: The relation of sulfur metabolism to acid-base balance and electrolyte excretion: the effects of dl-methionine in normal man. J Clin Invest 38:2215, 1959.
40. Kildeberg P: Clinical Acid-base Physiology. Studies in Neonates, Infants and Young Children. Copenhagen, Munkssgaard, 1968.
41. Raaflaub J: Uber die Basizitat der Knochenmineralien. Experientia 17:443, 1961.
42. Relman AS, Lennon EJ, Lemann J Jr: Endogenous production of fixed acid and the measurement of the net balance of acid in normal subjects. J Clin Invest 40:1621, 1961.
43. Kesner L, Yao T-T, Dell RB: Determination of total organic acids in urine by extraction with organic solvents. Clin Chem 19:593, 1973.
44. Jørgensen K: Titrimetric determination of the net excretion of acid-base in urine. Scand J Clin Lab Invest 9:287, 1957.
45. Kildeberg P: Disturbances of hydrogen ion balance occurring in premature infants: II. Late metabolic acidosis. Acta Paediatr Scand 53:517, 1967.
46. Kildeberg P, Winters RW: Infant feeding and blood acid-base status. Pediatrics 49:801, 1972.
47. Winters RW: Net acid balance in the growing organism: Theoretical formulation and practical utility. Presented at the Ross Symposium Meetings, Nutritional Goals for Low-Birth-Weight infants, Tarpon Springs, Fla., 1980.
48. McMillan DE, Freeman RB: The milk alkali syndrome: A study of the acute disorder with comments on the development of the chronic condition. Medicine 44:485, 1965.
49. Winters RW: Terminology of acid-base disorders. Ann Int Med 63:873, 1965.
50. Asch MJ, Dell RB, Williams GS, et al: Time course for development of respiratory compensation in metabolic acidosis. J Lab Clin Med 73:610, 1969.
51. Albert MS, Rahill WJ, Vega L, et al: Acid-base changes in cerebrospinal fluid of infants with metabolic acidosis. N Engl J Med 274:719, 1966.
52. Albert MS, Dell RB, Winters RW: Quantitative displacement of acid-base equilibrium in metabolic acidosis. Ann Intern Med 66:312, 1967.
53. Winters RW, White JS, Hughes MC et al: Disturbances of acid-base equilibrium in salicylate intoxication. *Pediatrics* 23:260, 1959.
54. Winters RW: Salicylate intoxication in infants and children. Pediatr Clin N Am 6:281, 1959.
55. Winters RW, Lowder JA, Ordway NK: Observations on carbon dioxide tension during recovery from metabolic acidosis. J Clin Invest 37:640, 1958.
56. van Goidsenhoven GMT, Gray OV, Price AV et al: The effect of prolonged administration of large doses of sodium bicarbonate in man. Clin Sci 13:383, 1954.

57. Kassirer JP, Schwartz WB: The response of normal man to selective depletion of hydrochloric acids. Factors in the genesis of persistent gastric alkalosis. Am J Med 40:10, 1966.
58. Schwartz WB, Chen JJ: The nature of the renal response to chronic disorders of acid-base equilibrium. Am J Med 64:417, 1978.
59. Needle MA, Kaloyanides GJ, Schwartz WB: The effects of selective depletion of hydrochloric acid on acid-base and electrolyte equilibrium. J Clin Invest 43:1836, 1964.
60. Kassirer JP, Schwartz WB: Correction of metabolic alkalosis in man without repair of the potassium deficit. Am J Med 40:19, 1966.
61. Seldin DW, Rector FC Jr: The generation and maintenance of metabolic alkalosis. Kidney Intl 1:306, 1972.
62. DeGraeff J, Struyvenberg A, Lameijer LDF: The role of chloride in hypokalemic alkalosis. Balance studies in man. Am J Med 37:778, 1964.
63. Berliner RW, Kennedy TJ Jr, Orloff J: Relationship between acidification of the urine and potassium metabolism. Effect of carbonic anhydrase inhibition on potassium excretion. Am J Med 11:274, 1951.
64. Cooke RW, Segar WE, Cheek DB, et al: The extrarenal correction of alkalosis associated with potassium deficiency. J Clin Invest 31:798, 1952.
65. Giebisch A, MacLeod MB, Pitts RF: Effect of adrenal steroids on renal tubular reabsorption of bicarbonate. Am J Physiol 183:377, 1955.
66. Grollman AP, Gamble JL Jr: Metabolic alkalosis, a specific effect of adrenocortical hormones. Am J Physiol 196:135, 1959.
67. Brackett NC Jr, Cohen JJ, Schwartz WB: Carbon dioxide titration curve of normal man. Effect of increasing degrees of acute hypercapnia on acid-base equilibrium. N Engl J Med 272:6, 1965.
68. Engel K, Dell RB, Rahill WJ, et al: Quantitative displacement of acid-base equilibrium in chronic respiratory acidosis. J Appl Physiol 23:288, 1968.
69. Schwartz WB, Brackett NC Jr, Cohen JJ: The response of extracellular hydrogen ion concentration to graded degrees of chronic hypercapnia: The physiological limits of the defense of pH. J Clin Invest 44:291, 1965.
70. Engel K, Kildeberg P, Winters RW: Quantitative displacement of blood acid-base status in acute hypocapnia. Scand J Clin Lab Invest 23:5, 1969.

CHAPTER 9

Calcium, Phosphorus, and Magnesium

RUSSELL W. CHESNEY
SHERMINE DABBAGH

INTRODUCTION

This chapter is concerned with the major mineral ions, calcium (Ca), phosphorus (P), and magnesium (Mg), which are found principally in the mineral phase of bone and, to a lesser extent, in body fluids. Mineral metabolism is the term used to define the interactions of these minerals. Three sites of regulation of their metabolism, i.e., bone, intestine, kidney, and three hormones: parathyroid (PTH), calcitonin (CT), and 1,25(OH$_2$-vitamin—calcitriol), modulate their plasma pool size, absorption, and excretion.

Physiologic Functions

The regulation of these minerals is required to maintain stable concentration or pool size of each in the extracellular fluid (ECF) and in cell fluid.

Ca is maintained in plasma at a concentration of 9 to 10 mg/dl (2.25 to 2.50 mMole/L) as total Ca, approximately 50% of which is ionized or nonprotein-bound (1). The Ca level has the biological role of assuring stability of neural membranes and the neuromuscular junction, as well as regulating the contractile proteins, including skeletal and cardiac muscle. Ca also is a "second messenger" for a myriad of enzymatic reactions.

P is maintained in plasma at concentrations of 3.0 to 7.5 mg/dl depending on the age of an individual (1) (Table 9.1). Virtually all phosphorus is in the form of an inorganic anion, phosphate, but its concentration in plasma is expressed in terms of elemental phosphorus. Phosphate is the reactive group in several classes of compounds: the high energy phosphate bond group, e.g., adenosine triphosphate (ATP) and nucleotides involved in synthetic reactions deoxyribonucleic acid (DNA), ribonucleic acid (RNA, phosphorylated glycolytic compounds, and acylphosphatases (2)) and in phosphoproteins where, in enzymes, phosphorylation and dephosphorylation often regulate enzyme activity. It is present in phospholipids, which are major constituents of plasma membranes that modulate membrane activity. A substantial pool of inorganic phosphate is found in the ECF and within all cells, particularly in certain subcellular fractions (mitochondria and nucleus), where it is used in phosphorylation steps. The third phosphate, which binds to adenosine 5′-diphosphate (ADP) by an ester linkage, can arise only from this inorganic phosphate pool. Inorganic phosphate is essential for life, since it is the high-energy P bond that does not derive from other organic phosphorylated compounds. Finally, most of the P in the body (80% to 85%) along with 99% of the body Ca are found in the mineral phase of bone in the form of hydroxyapatite [$Ca_{10}(PO_4)_6(OH)_2$], octacalcium P, and amorphous CaP (3).

Mg is maintained at a concentration of 1.8 to 2.4 mg/dl in plasma. Mg along with K are the main intracellular cations; the plasma level of Mg often does not reflect body stores (4). The level of Mg within the cell is approximately 10 times that in plasma. A principal role of Mg is to stabilize the electrically excitable membranes. It is also an important cofactor in many enzymatic processes and acts to increase the affinity of many receptors to the binding of agonists (5). However, as with Ca and P, most Mg is located within bone, where it is part of the mineral phase. This Mg is bound to bone in that Mg depletion caused by diuretics or in conjunction with cirrhosis does not lower bone Mg content (4). As with Ca, a large fraction of blood Mg (25%) is bound to protein, the remainder is ultrafilterable.

Body Stores and Regulation

The main site of regulation of plasma concentration and body store of each divalent ion differs. The body stores of Ca and P are regulated by a variety of physiological mechanisms; PTH and vitamin D play

Dr. Chesney is recipient of a Research Career Development Award KO4-AM00421. Dr. Dabbagh is supported by the Stetler Research Fund for Women Physicians. Supported in part by USPHS Grant AM 31982.

Table 9.1
Factors That May Regulate 25(OH)D-1α-hydroxylase (1α-hydroxylase) Activity

Factor	Probability of regulation
PTH	Strong
Ca^{+} concentration	Strong
P anion concentration	Strong
intracellular	
intramitochondrial	
circulating level	
Vitamin D status	Strong
excess	
deficiency	
H^{+} concentration	Not established
K^{+} concentration	Nil
Sex steroids	True in Avian species
estrogens	
androgens	
Prolactin	Not established
GH	Not established
Glucocorticoids	Conflicting results
Insulin	Moderate evidence
Heavy metals	Indirect
Cd	
Sr	
Pb	

Adapted from DeLuca HF: *Nutr Rev* 37:161, 1979; Fraser DR: Physiol Rev 60:551, 1980.

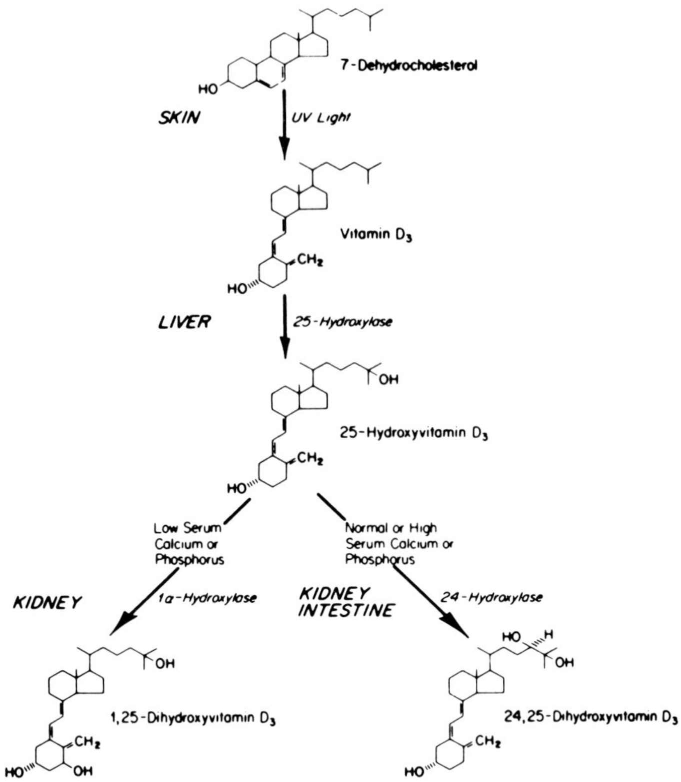

Figure 9.1. The metabolism of vitamin D showing the pathway from 7-dehydrocholesterol to $1,25(OH)_2D_3$ and $24,25(OH)_2D_3$. (Reprinted with permission from Kumar R, Riggs BL: *Mayo Clin Pract* 56:327, 1981.)

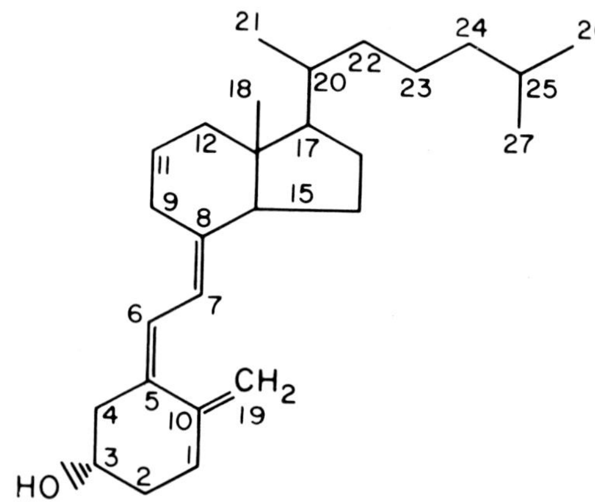

Figure 9.2. The vitamin D secosteroid, showing the carbons where major hydroxylations occur.

important roles, whereas CT is less important. Plasma Ca is regulated at the gastrointestinal (GI) tract or gut, and P is regulated in the kidney. The absorption of Ca throughout the duodenum, jejunum, ileum, and colon is under the control of $1,25(OH)_2D$. Only a small portion of filtered Ca is regulated by the kidney (6). Plasma Ca also is affected by exchange with bone Ca.

Factors regulating the intestinal absorption of P are relatively unimportant. Renal filtration and reabsorption are the major mechanisms for maintaining ECF and body stores of this anion (1, 2). Regulation of plasma phosphorus also is affected by exchange with bone and with cell P.

Mg body stores are regulated both at the level of the gut and the kidney; vitamin D and PTH are not important regulators of Mg.

Vitamin D. The main regulator of Ca and P absorption from the gut and renal reabsorption is the vitamin D-endocrine system (6, 7). Vitamin D_3 or cholecalciferol is produced by the photolysis of 7-dehydrocholesterol in the skin and by thermal conversion from previtamin D_3 (Fig. 9.1). Vitamin D_3 is transported in blood to the liver by a specific vitamin D-binding protein (DBP) of molecular weight 52,000 daltons. A hepatic microsomal enzyme adds a hydroxyl group to carbon-25 of vitamin D, from which the compound 25(OH)vitamin D_3 is produced. There is little feedback inhibition of 25-hydroxylase activity by either vitamin D_3 or 25(OH)D, as shown by the fact that animals or patients with hypervitaminosis-D have extraordinarily high values of 25(OH)D (9). In hepatic perfusion experiments, the hepatic venous output of 25(OH)D is similar, whether 25(OH)D, $1,25(OH)_2D$, or 24,25(OH)D is administered before the experiment. The 25(OH)D is transported readily to the kidney by DBP, because the affinity of this protein for 25(OH)D is greater than it is for vitamin D_3.

Within the first two segments of the proximal tubular cell of the kidney are two major hydroxylase enzymes: 25(OH)D-1α-hydroxylase and 25(OH)D-24-hydroxylase (10). The first enzyme, 1α-hydroxylase, resides within the mitochondria and appears to be a mixed function mono-oxygenase that incorporates molecular oxygen at the 1α position on the A-ring (Fig. 9.2) (6, 11). The factors regulating the activity of this enzyme are listed in Table 9.1. The enzyme also has been found in the placenta of humans and other mammals. This may be responsible for the high serum levels of $1,25(OH)_2D$ found during pregnancy (12).

The second converting enzyme synthesizes $24,25(OH)_2D$ from 25(OH)D. It also is located in the kidney and functions in inverse fashion to 1α-hydroxylase activity. Thus, the converting enzyme is activated to produce $24,25(OH)_2D$ whenever serum Ca and P values are normal, when iPTH is normal, or if excess vitamin D_2, D_3, or 25(OH)D are given. This major metabolite of 25(OH)D also is made in the intestine and in bone, but the kidney is the predominant site of its production.

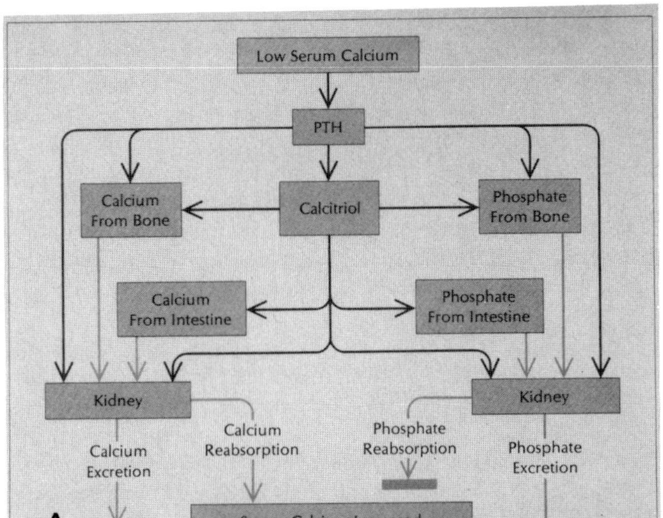

Figure 9.3. Factors regulating calcium and phosphate homeostasis. **A**, Upper physiological consequences of a reduction in serum calcium; **B**, physiological consequences of a reduction in serum phosphate. (Reprinted with permission) Deluca, HF: *Hosp Prac* 15:57, 1980.)

The vitamin D-endocrine system directly regulates the intake, distribution, and excretion of Ca and P in a feedback system (Fig. 9.3, *A* and *B*). Hypocalcemia, in which ionized Ca falls, increases release of PTH which, in turn, stimulates renal 1α-hydroxylase activity to synthesize $1,25(OH)_2D$. This interacts with receptors in the intestine and stimulates active transport of Ca and P from the lumen of the gut into the bloodstream. The active transport appears to be mediated by $1,25(OH)_2D$-dependent, DNA-directed protein synthesis. This $1,25(OH)_2D$ also acts with PTH to promote active bone resorption and release of both Ca and P from previously mineralized osteoid (6, 10). The net result is increased Ca and P in the ECF, but the higher iPTH levels cause an increase in urinary P excretion. Thus, on balance, serum Ca is higher and P remains the same.

The now higher level of Ca suppresses PTH secretion, and $1,25(OH)_2D$ synthesis declines. The synthesis of $1,25(OH)_2D$ is tightly regulated by this feedback loop. Since it is made at one site (the renal cortex) and is transported to other sites, where it is active (intestine and bone), it is considered a hormone (6, 10). If PTH secretion is impaired, as it is in hypoparathyroidism, or if the biological activity of PTH is impaired, as it is in pseudohypoparathyroidism, serum Ca values will remain low and serum P high. The synthesis of $1,25(OH)_2D$ likewise will be attenuated so that gut transport is limited and bone resorption is not stimulated.

The vitamin D endocrine system also is regulated by change in serum P (Fig. 9.3, *B*). Hypophosphatemia does not stimulate PTH secretion, but it does stimulate renal synthesis of $1,25(OH)_2D$. This results in augmented intestinal Ca and P absorption. The renal tubule, in turn, excretes Ca and retains P, because PTH values are normal or low. Accordingly, serum P concentrations increase to normal, which then slows down $1,25(OH)_2D$ synthesis. The mechanism of this augmented synthesis with hypophosphatemia is not certain; apparently it does not involve 1α-hydroxylase activation by PTH (9). Higher $1,25(OH)_2D$ values occur with hypophosphatemia without increased PTH secretion or in thyroparathyroidectomized animals (6, 10).

BONE, THE RESERVOIR OF MINERALS

Physiology of Bone

The human skeleton is composed of a collagen-containing organic matrix on which a crystalline mineral phase is deposited. The strength and structural properties of osseous tissue are influenced by its compressive strength, tensile properties, and resiliency. These properties are affected by change in the formation of the organic matrix, rate of deposition or resorption of the mineral phase, or by the cells which form and remodel bone (14). The mineral phase of bone in the body (hydroxyapatite, octacalcium P, and amorphous CaP) contains most of the content of the three major minerals (3). Therefore, these bone pools must be measured to estimate the total body Ca, P, or Mg. Physiological events that occur at the bone cell membrane, e.g., deposition or release of mineral, directly affect whole body mineral metabolism. Changes in bone cell metabolism are the mechanisms by which bone is depleted of minerals (15, 16).

Although bone deposition and resorption occur constantly, the rate of turnover is variable (3). Most hydroxyapatite is "deep" within the bone trabeculum and thus inaccessible to rapid exchange. The compartment of bone Ca, which is rapidly exchangeable with Ca in the ECF, is smaller (17). This rapidly exchangeable pool is composed of Ca in the hydration layer of newly formed, but incomplete hydroxyapatite crystals and of amorphous CaP (1, 3, 18).

Various models of bone exchange have been proposed with the use of tracers. However, the problem of measurement of pools is confounded by variable rates of exchange between readily accessible and less accessible pools in different anatomic sites, leading to underestimation. When the turnover of trabecular bone is rapid, a single radio-labeled Ca ion may exchange several times; thus, exchange is overestimated.

Bone resorption of these minerals is clearly integrated with their intestinal and renal handling. When dietary Ca intake is low, bone resorption will maintain serum Ca concentration from the pool of bone Ca. However, with prolonged Ca deficiency it does this at the expense of the strength and tensile properties of bone. This same is true when dietary P is inadequate.

In the normal individual, when Ca intake is increased, fractional Ca absorption falls and fecal Ca content rises; bone Ca does not change greatly (5, 6, 10, 18). Excessive dietary P intake does not alter serum P appreciably, since renal tubular P excretion is enhanced.

A detailed discussion of factors regulating organic matrix synthesis, bone mineralization, osteoblast and osteoclast function and their potential origin from bone marrow macrophages, as well as the putative role of the vitamin K-dependent bone protein, osteocalcin, is beyond the task of this chapter (17, 19–21). Nonetheless, the concept should be borne in mind that bone is a large but incompletely exchangeable pool of the major divalent minerals.

Hormonal Regulation of Bone Calcium and Phosphorus

Each of the three major hormones, vitamin D, PTH, and CT, affects bone mineral deposition, resorption, and turnover rate; these hormone interactions are integrated into a complex feedback loop. PTH is essential for normal mineralization of bone. In the absence of PTH, or following parathyroidectomy, osteomalacia develops (9, 10). Turnover of Ca and P in bone is low (9). In hyperparathyroidism (either primary or secondary), there is increased osteoclastic activity, subperiosteal erosion, and loss of bone mineral. Turnover of Ca and P in bone is high (3, 9). However, low PTH values cause reduced $1,25(OH)_2D$ production and high PTH values stimulate it, so that some of the PTH effects on bone are related to its effect on $1,25(OH)_2D$. PTH and $1,25(OH)_2D$ act in concert to regulate bone resorption as well (3, 5, 7, 17, 20).

With deficiency of vitamin D, circulating 25(OH)D levels are low (22). Levels of $1,25(OH)_2D$ are normal or near-normal but osteomalacia develops (22). Levels of $1,25(OH)_2D$ are relatively reduced in view of hypocalcemia, hypophosphatemia, and high PTH, which normally cause levels to increase (23). Bone turnover rates are decreased by pharmacological doses of $1,25(OH)_2D$ in normal rats; bone matrix synthesis is decreased and bone resorption is increased (20). Bone turnover rate is reduced in osteomalacia as a result of vitamin D deficiency and increased after therapy with vitamin D.

Calcitonin prevents bone resorption and slows turnover rates (11, 18). It is therapeutically indicated in hypercalcemia and after the increased bone turnover of Ca and P that follows bed rest or immobilization and in Paget's disease. The hormonal regulation of bone and ECF, Ca, and P is most likely a result of changes in the ECF concentrations of these minerals. Minute-to-minute changes in ECF Ca and P are modulated by changes in the intestinal and renal handling of the minerals and bone deposition and resorption.

RENAL HANDLING OF MINERALS

Calcium and Phosphorus

The renal handling of Ca is not as important as intestinal absorption in terms of the whole body economy of Ca (2, 18); the renal regulation of the vitamin D system is $1,25(OH)_2D$ formation. Its level regulates intestinal Ca absorption and renal P excretion. $1,25(OH)_2D$ formation is regulated by PTH, which is the most important hormone affecting renal handling of Ca and P. Nonetheless, many other factors influence the final concentration of Ca in the urine.

Renal regulation of Ca transport has been reviewed recently (24). Ionized Ca and Ca complexed to anions, e.g. citrate, P, a fraction that is approximately 0.6 of the plasma concentration is filtered. Usually, 98% of the filtered load is reabsorbed; of this, 60% is reabsorbed in the proximal convoluted tubule, 20% in the loop of Henle, and 10% in the distal convoluted tubule. The rest is taken up by the collecting system.

The mechanisms of Ca reabsorption are different at each of these sites. In the convoluted tubule, Ca is reabsorbed proportionally, along with Na and H_2O, so that the concentration of Ca differs little from that in the ultrafiltrate of plasma (25). This reabsorption of Ca may be passive, but recent evidence, using microperfusion techniques and brush-border uptake studies, suggest an active component of uptake (26). Ca may be absorbed in excess of Na in the straight portion of the proximal tubule (21) but it is in the loop of Henle that the greatest dissociation between Ca and Na absorption occurs (27). Thiazide diuretics promote Ca absorption at this site, while also promoting a NaCl diuresis (27). On the other hand, furosemide acting promotes both Ca and Na excretion at the thick cortical ascending limb (28). It is open to question whether transport of Ca in the ascending limb is active or voltage-dependent (from the net positive luminal potential difference (PD)). However, the influence of PTH is to augment Ca absorption at this site, which suggests that this component is active since PTH does not alter the PD (24). Although 9% of Ca is absorbed in the distal tubule, the mechanism of transport is not established. Finally, from 3% to 10% of filtered Ca is absorbed in the collecting duct, mainly in "granular" rather than "light" segments of the collecting tubule.

Various hormones, organic solutes, and pharmacological agents influence urinary Ca handling. Salt loading acting results in excessive Ca excretion at the proximal tubule (24). P depletion also results in hypercalcuria, and this is a feature of the P depletion syndrome in man (15). PTH and cyclic adenosine monophosphate (cAMP) probably increase proximal Ca excretion, but enhance distal and collecting tubule absorption to such an extent that the net effect is to augment Ca reabsorption (21). CT augments Ca excretion, probably at the medullary portion of the thick ascending limb. As mentioned, $1,25(OH)_2D$ enhances Ca reabsorption, probably at a distal nephron site by an uncertain mechanism (6).

The diabetic state, as well as glucose and insulin administration (particularly if given chronically), result in hypercalcuria (24, 29). An explanation for this paradox is that glucose and insulin alter many electrolytes in terms of their renal excretory patterns (30). The effects of thiazides and furosemide have been mentioned. Any mechanism of action of these agents must involve three known characteristics of renal tubular Ca transport: Ca traversing the luminal membrane is aided by the electronegativity of the interior of the cell in relation to the lumen; Ca must be pumped out of the cell at the basolateral membrane because the chemical and electrical gradient do not favor passive movement across this second membrane surface; and the mitochondrion has an intracellular pool that may greatly influence the net transtubular reabsorption of Ca (and P); the level of Ca within this subcellular organelle is as much as 10^{-3}M which is higher than that within the cytoplasm.

The most important regulator of serum P in the face of a varying intake is control of renal P excretion. This control is regulated by a number of hormones and other factors, which are described in this section. The renal mechanisms affecting P excretion are complex and act at different sites. Approximately 90% of P in the plasma is filtered; only the Ca and P microcrystals are not filtered and remain in the blood. Most of the filtered P is reabsorbed in the proximal nephron, 70% in the convoluted tubule, 15% in the pars recta, and 5 to 15% in sites beyond the proximal tubules available for micropuncture (31). Reabsorption at these sites is more sensitive to control and hence may be important in regulating serum and body P pool size.

Mechanism of Phosphorus Reabsorption

Proximal tubule P transport is active, i.e., it occurs against an electrical and chemical gradient across the brush border of the luminal membrane surface (32). The energy for this active transport is derived from Na going down its chemical gradient into cell and then being pumped out at the basal-lateral surface by the activity of Na,K-ATPase (2). Agents that affect activity of this enzyme, e.g., ouabain, block P reabsorption.

Saline expansion also reduces P reabsorption at this site. While the mechanism is not clear, ionized Ca decreases and this leads to PTH secretion and phosphaturia. The phosphaturia of saline expansion is blocked by a total parathyroidectomy. Reabsorption of P by the pars recta and distal nephron also is sensitive to PTH; reabsorption is nearly complete in the absence of circulating PTH (33).

P secretion by the tubule occurs in lower vertebrates (snakes, fish, frogs, and so on), but has not been unequivocally demonstrated in higher mammals, including man (34). P clearance may exceed the filtered load after acute infusion of large amounts of P and this may represent tubular secretion by deep nephrons unavailable for micropuncture.

Control of Phosphorus Reabsorption

Parathyroid Hormone

Among the various agents that affect reabsorption of P by the nephron, PTH is the most important. It acts on the proximal convoluted tubule, the pars recta, and the distal nephron (33). PTH acts by binding to its receptor on the antiluminal membrane and increasing the activity of the adenylate cyclase system. This, in turn, increases the intracellular concentrations of cAMP (5, 16). The increase in cAMP activates a luminal (brush border) membrane protein kinase, phosphorylates membrane proteins, and depresses P reabsorption (35). Adding cAMP or its more soluble analog, dibutryl cAMP to brush border preparations, simulates the actions of PTH, including its action to depress P transport (36). The kidney must be exposed to either PTH or cAMP for at least one hour before either the phosphaturic effect is evident or before P uptake by the brush-border vesicles is demonstrated. Neither PTH nor cAMP inhibit glucose or Na accumulation into brush-border vesicles (37).

Calcitonin

CT promotes phosphaturia regardless of serum Ca level, GFR, or the plasma concentration of P. The mechanism for this effect is not known (2). This phosphaturia may be mediated in part by hypocalcemia, which is induced by CT with a consequent rise in PTH. However, since CT lowers serum P in thyroparathyroidectomized animals, another mechanism also must be operative. Although there are receptors for CT in the renal tubule, the relation of these receptors to the phosphaturic effect of CT is not established.

Vitamin D

Vitamin D influences renal P transport in several ways. Both enhanced reabsorption and augmented excretion occur after administration of vitamin D analogs. The infusion of vitamin D analogs enhances reabsorption under some conditions, (37) but $1,25(OH)_2D$ is phosphaturic; in vitro it is without effect (37, 40). These discrepancies may be explained by such factors as whether the vitamin D analog is given acutely or chronically, the animal is vitamin D-deficient or replete, or the serum Ca is normal. The accumulation of P by isolated chick renal cells and rabbit brush-border membranes is greater if $1,25(OH)_2D$, but not other analogs, is given to vitamin D-deficient deficient animals; cells from vitamin D-replete animals were not stimulated (37).

Phosphate reabsorption is decreased in hypoparathyroidism following correction of hypocalcemia (38). On the other hand, the acute intraarterial infusion of Ca enhances P reabsorption in animals (39). Urinary P excretion decreases in thyroparathyroidectomized rats when they are given $1,25(OH)_2D$ (40). This effect may be related to the calcemia effect of vitamin D similar to the findings in hypoparathyroid man (38), i.e., raising serum Ca, except when it is strictly intrarenal, and decreases reabsorption.

The dietary intake of P affects the way that PTH, vitamin D, or Ca govern the reabsorption of P (41). When dietary intake of P is reduced (the "P-depleted state"), little is excreted in the urine, and the phosphaturic response to PTH is blunted (42). This response is expressed at the brush-border membrane where P accumulation by vesicles is increased (43). This blunting of the phosphaturic effect of PTH by a low P diet is reversed if $1,25(OH)_2D$ is given (43). These effects may be related to the regulation of renal P transport by either serum or intracellular Ca concentration. The phosphaturic effect of P loading observed in thyroparathyroidectomized rats is reduced if hypocalcuria is prevented by infusing Ca (44).

Glucose

Glucose and P transport are similar; both are taken up more avidly in the first portion of the proximal tubules, both have saturation kinetics, and the transport of each is Na dependent (45). Both glucose and galactose infusion augment P excretion. Glucose competitively inhibits renal tubular P reabsorption in vivo (46). Glucose infusion, which causes glucosuria depresses P reabsorption by 20% (46). Phloridzin, which blocks glucose reabsorption, increases P reabsorption (47). Galactose and fructose infusions inhibit P reabsorption in humans (48). Ouabain and other cardiac glycosides, which block Na,K-ATPase activity, inhibit P reabsorption (49). The renal transport of both organic solutes occurs independently of the action of insulin (50).

In the P-depleted state, the tubular maximum (Tm) glucose falls, as further evidence of competition. When PTH is given to dogs, their Tm-glucose rises, while phosphaturia ensues (51). Glucose and P share a common carrier. It is not clear whether both compounds compete for a common energy source (45); however, increasing glucose reabsorption depresses P reabsorption and increases P excretion.

Amino Acids

Amino acids, like glucose and P, are also reabsorbed in the first portion of the proximal tubule. Amino acid reabsorption is often Na dependent; the accumulation of many amino acids by brush-border membrane vesicles depends on an external Na gradient (52). The interaction between amino acids and P reabsorption (53), like that between glucose and P, may be related to competition for a common energy source.

Other Hormones

Other hormones influence the renal handling of P, e.g., growth hormone, vasopressin, thyroxine, glucagon, insulin, glucocorticoids, estrogens, and catecholamines (54).

Growth hormone (GH) increases P reabsorption, and plasma P of acromegalic subjects is higher than normal. Both GFR and $TmPO_4$/GFR are increased after human GH administration in man (55). Decreased excretion is noted 3 hours after a dose of GH in rats. The mechanism of this action of GH may involve enhanced Na reabsorption, insulin release, or synthesis of $1,25(OH)_2D$. GH does not appear to play a role in the renal adaption to P depletion (54).

Hypophosphatemia and phosphaturia are common findings in glucocorticoid excess. This effect is not related to mineralocorticoid activity (9). The increased clearance of P is independent of PTH secretion, since it is present in hypoparathyroidism (53). The mechanism of the glucocorticoid effect involves reduction of Na dependent P transport by the brush-border surface (56, 57), particularly by increasing Na/H exchange and by augmenting renal gluconeogenesis.

Other Compounds

The administration of lithium will blunt the phosphaturic effect of PTH (58). Lithium not only blocks the induction of the adenylate cyclase-cAMP system in the renal tubule in response to PTH, but blocks the phosphaturic effect that occurs when cAMP is infused. Lithium may act in this way by replacing Na and blocking Na dependent P transport.

Most diuretics (osmotic agents, mercurial diuretics, acetazolamide, thiazides, and loop diuretics) induce phosphaturia (59). K-sparing agents do not. Carbonic anhydrase inhibitors are the most potent. They impair bicarbonate reabsorption and urine pH increases, so that the ratio of

HPO_4 to H_2PO_4 is increased; the more polar (HPO_4) ion is less permeable and is less well reabsorbed (60). This effect is dependent on the pH of urine, not on PTH (61). Acetazolamide also increases the phosphaturic effect of PTH by increasing cAMP production (62). Ethacrynic acid and furosemide do not alter cAMP levels, but do cause phosphaturia.

Relief of unilateral ureteral obstruction leads to increased reabsorption of P but decreased reabsorption of Na and H_2O (32), providing evidence for a dissociation between the renal handling of Na and P in this condition. Although extracellular volume expansion enhances P excretion, this effect is blunted in an obstructed kidney. The hypophosphaturia may be related to enhanced uptake by the proximal tubule and decreased Na reabsorption distally (2).

On the other hand, compensatory phosphaturia occurs after unilateral nephrectomy in rats. The increase in the fractional excretion of P occurs despite thyroparathyroidectomy and under constant PTH infusion, indicating that this effect is not PTH-dependent (63).

Magnesium

Mg is the second most common intracellular electrolyte and the fourth most abundant cation in the body. More than half the total body Mg is in bone, with most of the balance in soft tissues, particularly muscle. Less than 1% is in the ECF. The plasma Mg concentration in man is 1.7 to 2.3 mg/100 ml (1.4 to 2.0 mEq/L or 0.7 to 1.0 mMole/L). Plasma Mg exists as a free ion (55% to 65%), a complex with P, oxalate, and other anions (20% to 30%), and it is protein-bound (64). Thus, 80% is ultrafilterable.

Usually, serum and tissue Mg correlate, but they may become dissociated, as in renal failure (65), where reduced muscle Mg has been associated with normal serum, erythrocyte, and bone Mg levels. This suggests that muscle Mg is the most freely exchangeable and thus the first to fall during Mg depletion. However, muscle Mg content has also been shown to vary directly with muscle K levels and independently of other body Mg stores (66). Serum Mg does not consistently reflect muscle Mg concentration, though serum and bone Mg levels do correlate. Bone and ECF Mg are the major body pools affected either by excess or deficiency of Mg, whereas muscle Mg tends to reflect changes in total body K. Twenty-five percent to 65% of Mg is absorbed in the small bowel, particularly in the ileum; the kidney appears to be the major regulator of its metabolism. (Mg salts are poorly absorbed.) There is no convincing evidence that intestinal absorption is physiologically regulated. Vitamin D may enhance intestinal Mg absorption in vitamin D-deficient animals, but not in the normal animals (67). An obligatory secretory loss from the gut is also present (68).

Renal Handling of Magnesium

The major excretory pathway for Mg is renal, and both oral and intravenous loads are rapidly eliminated (69). Regulation of excretion in man is determined both by filtration and reabsorption; approximately 1800 mg Mg is filtered daily, but only 3% to 5% of the filtered load is excreted (70). The hormonal controls regulating excretion are not well defined.

The ultrafilterable portion of plasma Mg, 70% to 80%, consists of free and complexed Mg. Ultrafilterability is not affected by Mg excess or deficiency (71). The many factors that may influence glomerular ultrafilterability, such as saline infusions, hypercalcemia, acidosis, P depletion, and diuretics, are not well investigated.

Mg has an unusual concentration profile along the proximal convoluted tubule, its concentration rises to 1.5 to 2.0 times that of the filtered Mg (72). Fractional Mg reabsorption in the proximal tubule is 20 to 30% of the filtered load, or half that of Na or Ca (73). Tubular fluid/ultrafilterable Mg concentration (TF/UF Mg) is unaffected by volume expansion, diuretics, metabolic acidosis and alkalosis, or changes in the plasma Ca and inorganic P in the dog (74).

Mg reabsorption is also dependent on intraluminal Mg concentration. However, the proximal tubule epithelium is comparatively impermeable to the ion under normal conditions. Diffusional backflux plays a limited role in net Mg reabsorption with hydropenia (73), suggesting that its reabsorption is largely a unidirectional process of efflux. The role of the S_3 segment of the proximal tubule remains unclear.

The loop of Henle is the major site of Mg reabsorption (75). In the rat, 50% to 60% of the filtered load is reabsorbed between the late proximal tubule and the early distal tubule. There is an increase in the TF/UF Mg in the descending limb of the loop of Henle secondary to the abstraction of water brought about by the hyperosmotic medullary solute concentration gradient (76). Consequently, the ascending limb of the loop is the major site for Mg reabsorption.

The loop of Henle is also relatively impermeable to the backflux of Mg into tubule fluid. The loop has a remarkable capacity to increase its ability to reabsorb Mg as the luminal Mg concentration is increased from 0 to 10 mEq/L. The fractional reabsorption is about 80% of the delivered load into the loop of Henle at any luminal Mg concentration (77), whereas elevation of plasma concentration results in a decrease in the absolute and fractional Mg reabsorption, i.e., hypermagnesemia retards Mg reabsorption in the loop by inhibiting its transport at the peritubular membrane. Hypercalcemia inhibits Mg reabsorption, suggesting a Mg/Ca interaction on the contraluminal side of the ascending limb that is not directly related to NaCl reabsorption. It is of interest that furosemide proportionately inhibits transport of Na, Ca, and Mg, but there is a slightly relative inhibition of absolute Mg and Ca transport vs Na (78).

The nature of Mg reabsorption in the ascending limb remains unclear. It could be voltage-dependent (73, 79), in which case active Cl^- reabsorption would be a major driving force for the reabsorption of Mg and inhibition by loop diuretics. On the other hand, separate mechanisms for the transport of Mg could exist, which could be Na-dependent or Na-independent. Further study of the ascending thick limb of the loop is required to clarify the underlying mechanism.

The distal convoluted tubule reabsorbs approximately 2% to 5% of filtered Mg by a load-dependent process (77). As Mg delivery to the distal tubule is increased by high concentration in the perfusate or by inhibition of more proximal reabsorption by furosemide, the absolute reabsorption of Mg increases with enhanced Mg delivery. However, distal Mg reabsorption is close to capacity, as the fractional Mg reabsorption falls rapidly with the increased load. The nature of the mechanisms involved in this segment are unclear. Little or no backflux is observed (77), and transport in the distal tubule is unidirectional.

All studies suggest that the collecting ductules and duct play a limited role in the homeostasis of Mg and may account for the reabsorption of less than 1% to 3% of the filtered load (74). No Mg reabsorption occurs in the papillary collecting duct of the young rat (80).

The secretion of Mg into renal tubules has been proposed but probably plays no major role in the homeostasis of this cation. A 10% to 15% increase over the filtered load in distal tubular Mg suggests the possibility of secretion (81). The data in rats are contradictory. Net Mg secretion with a fractional excretion rate of 150% during chronic Mg infusion, which increases the serum concentration, has been observed (82, 83). In another study, the fractional excretion of Mg was never more than 97% in the rat (84).

The Tm for Mg has been suggested (85). In dogs infused with $MgCl_2$, the maximum reabsorption rate was 140 μg/min/kg at a filtered load of 280 μg/min. The Tm relationship seems to have considerable splay, and its maximum value is appropriately altered by factors that change Mg excretion, such as PTH, Ca, and volume expansion. However, micropuncture studies do not support a Tm-limited system (86). The apparent Tm for Mg may be a fortuitous composite of increasing proximal tubule reabsorption, whereas loop reabsorption declines progressively with increasing hypermagnesemia. The concept of Tm was studied in normal, hyperparathyroid, and hypoparathyroid subjects infused with $MgCl_2$ and demonstrated a Tm for Mg of 1.3 to 1.4 mg/100 ml glomerular filtrate/1.73m^2 in all subjects. This would suggest the existence of a Tm-limited system for Mg transport in man (87).

Factors Affecting the Renal Handling of Mg

Although the control of renal Mg handling is not well understood, several factors are known to play roles (88, 89).

Urinary Mg excretion is increased by acute intravenous Mg infusion. Micropuncture studies show that absolute Mg reabsorption increases in the proximal tubule as the concentration of ultrafilterable Mg rises (87). However, free-flow studies (86) demonstrate that hypermagnesemia reduces the fractional reabsorption of Na and water in the proximal tubule and that the absolute Mg reabsorption does not increase greatly in that segment. In the loop of Henle, both absolute and fractional reabsorption are reduced in hypermagnesemia (87), which would account for the magnesuria that accompanies Mg excess. Similarly, fractional reabsorption is depressed in the distal tubule.

The kidney responds to hypomagnesemia and Mg deficiency by conserving this cation (89). The ascending limb of the loop is the major site at which reabsorption is enhanced. When Mg-deficient rats are given acute infusions of Mg to double their serum Mg, Mg excretion increases to values similar to those observed in normal control animals at comparable serum Mg levels. Absolute Mg reabsorption increases in the loop, but remains below normal, suggesting persistence of a cellular defect not corrected by acute infusions of Mg or a resetting of the reabsorptive mechanism. Further, proximal reabsorption remains unchanged and unaffected by acute Mg repletion. Distal tubular Mg reabsorption is limited during depletion and increases to levels comparable to those observed in normal rats after acute supplementation with Mg.

Hypercalcemia inhibits tubular Mg reabsorption. Fractional excretion of Mg rises at a faster rate than that of Ca. The infusion of Ca causes an increase in the urinary excretion of Na and Mg, despite maneuvers that acutely reduce GFR and filtered loads of Na and Mg (85, 88). Proximal TF/UF Mg and early distal TF/UF Mg remain unchanged. Early distal TF/UF Mg increases and Mg delivery rises by 30 to 40%, indicating inhibition in the loop. Absolute distal reabsorption is modestly increased because of the increased delivered load, but is readily overwhelmed by the high Mg load (90).

Generally, hypocalcemia, as occurs in hypoparathyroidism, may reduce Mg excretion.

The effect of P depletion is species-specific (91). In dogs and humans, a modest increase is found in urinary Mg without changes in the plasma Mg. However, in the rat, both hypo- and hypermagnesiuria occur. The magnitude of magnesiuria is related to the degree of hypophosphatemia and is not affected by lowering Ca intake. The magnesiuria is secondary to decreased reabsorption and does not seem to be related to PTH. Consequently, the P-depleted rat develops negative Mg balance. Infusions of saline augment the excretion of Mg by reducing its tubular reabsorption (88). Although Mg excretion increases with Na+ excretion during saline infusion, the levels of urinary Mg are dependent on the magnitude of saliuresis when GFR is acutely reduced. However, infusion of hyperoncotic albumin into dogs fails to increase the renal excretion of Mg, suggesting that volume expansion with saline decreases the distal tubular reabsorption of Mg.

Diuretics, including the organic mercurials, furosemide, ethacrynic acid, and osmotics, such as mannitol and urea, result in marked increases in urinary Mg excretion by inhibiting loop reabsorption (92). Loop diuretics inhibit active chloride transport within the thick ascending loop of Henle. The inhibition may result either from a decrease of transepithelial potential difference, which could provide the driving force for Mg reabsorption, or, alternatively, a direct effect on Mg transport. Osmotic diuretics decrease the contact-time concentration gradient for Mg, resulting in the delivered load distally. Thiazide diuretics frequently result in a mild magnesiuria, which is opposite to their effect on Ca (93). Little is known concerning the effect of distal K-sparing diuretics on Mg reabsorption, but they tend to be minor.

Acute metabolic acidosis does not alter Mg excretion (94). Acute respiratory acidosis significantly increases the absolute, but not the fractional, excretion of Mg. Acute metabolic alkalosis significantly reduces the absolute and fractional excretion of Mg. Furthermore, there is an increase in the fractional Mg delivery to the end descending limb of the juxtamedullary nephron, but not to the end-accessible proximal tubule of the superficial nephron.

The importance of PTH in renal homeostasis of Mg is not known with certainty. Initial observations suggest that excess PTH causes an increase in urinary excretion of Mg (95). Interpretation of these data is difficult because of the associated hypercalcemia, which by itself could bring about the same effect. Other studies indicate that PTH decreases fractional Mg excretion in toto (85). In thyroparathyroidectomized Mg-deficient rats, the administration of PTH does not alter Mg transport capacity, but results in enhanced transport in acutely hypermagnesemic-deficient rats (96), suggesting the depressed transport capacity in the loop of Henle is independent of intraluminal delivery and circulating PTH.

On the other hand, the golden hamster shows a striking sensitivity to the effect of PTH in the handling of Mg (97). After thyroparathyroidectomy, approximately 20% of the filtered load is excreted. Administration of PTH further reduces the fractional excretion of Mg. The infusion of cAMP or dibutyrl-cAMP mimics this effect. Calcitonin appears to exert a marked stimulatory effect on Mg reabsorption, presumably by enhancing its reabsorption by the thick ascending limb of the loop of Henle. This effect is demonstrated in thyroparathyroidectomized nondiuretic rats and is observed in the whole kidney and isolated tubule preparations (98). Further, it is independent of PTH, but is contingent on a decline in serum Ca (99). Prevention of hypocalcemia by $CaCl_2$ infusions results in loop function that is comparable to animals that do not receive the hormone.

Other hormones also seem to affect the renal handling of Mg (88). GH exerts an effect opposite to that of PTH, mainly increasing the fractional excretion of both Mg and Ca. Hypomagnesemia and slight magnesiuria are observed in hyperthyroidism. Conversely, hypothyroid patients have increased serum Mg and decreased urinary Mg; treatment restores these abnormalities to normal. Acute administration of glucocorticoids or mineralocorticoids has no effect on Mg excretion. However, chronic mineralocorticoid administration can cause an increase in Mg excretion, which may be related to volume expansion. Salt restriction corrects the increase in cation excretion. Finally, glucagon decreases the absolute and fractional excretion of Mg, associated with the well-known increase in the fractional excretions of Na and P (100). This effect is independent of PTH and calcitonin.

The role of vitamin D in Mg homeostasis remains a mystery. When the relationship between plasma concentrations of $1{,}25(OH)_2D$ and net intestinal Ca, P, and Mg absorption in healthy volunteers was evaluated (101), net intestinal Ca absorption was positively correlated to plasma concentration of the active metabolite of vitamin D. However, there was no correlation between Mg and P absorption and plasma $1{,}25(OH)_2D_3$. On the other hand, in uremic patients, the malabsorption of Mg in the intestine was restored to normal after the administration of $1{,}25(OH)_2D_3$

(102). The role of vitamin D on the renal handling of this cation remains uncertain.

COMPLICATIONS

Hypercalcemic Disorders

Although several clinical conditions may result in hypercalcemia, the features of these disorders are similar. Hypercalcemia is characterized by anorexia, vomiting, fever, polydipsia, polyuria, constipation, lethargy, headache, and irritability (18). Other findings are hypertension, growth failure, nephrocalcinosis, stone formation, and band keratopathy of the limbus of the eyes. (Familial or inherited conditions resulting in hypercalcemia are discussed in chapter 25.) Other conditions that cause hypercalcemia are noted in Table 9.2.

Sarcoidosis

The hypercalcemia of sarcoidosis is similar to the pattern found in hypervitaminosis-D, in that patients appear to have an increased sensitivity to vitamin D. Recent reports indicate that the serum levels of $1,25(OH)_2D$ were elevated, particularly in relation to the serum Ca concentration. The iPTH value is reduced, indicating that the production of $1,25(OH)_2D$ is independent of serum Ca levels and PTH (103–105). The elevation of $1,25(OH)_2D$ occurs despite normal levels of 25(OH)D and $24,25(OH)_2D$ (Fig. 9.4). An important finding is that an adult with sarcoidosis and bilateral nephrectomy also has elevated $1,25(OH)_2D$ serum values, indicating that extrarenal synthesis of the metabolite may occur in this syndrome (103). It has been suggested that sarcoid granulomas produce $1,25(OH)_2D$; this has now been demonstrated in tissue from eight patients (103a, 103b).

Hypercalcemia occurs in 2% to 50% of cases of sarcoidosis; normocalcemic patients with this disorder have increased intestinal absorption of Ca (104). Following vitamin D ingestion, serum $1,25(OH)_2D$ and

Table 9.2
Conditions that Cause Hypercalcemic Disorders of Childhood

Disorder	Condition
Idiopathic hypercalcemia	Williams' syndrome with elfin facies
Hyperparathyroidism	Adenoma at birth
	Hyperplasia—multiple endocrine neoplasia syndrome (MEN II) familial
Hypercalcemic hypocalcuria or benign familial hypercalcemia	
Associated with malignancy	Acute lymphocytic leukemia with leukopenia and bone invasion
	Burkett's lymphoma—lymphocytic production of osteoclast-activating factor and prostaglandin production
Granulomatous disease	Sarcoidosis
	Tuberculosis
	Histoplasmosis
Thyrotoxicosis	Vitamin D intoxication
	Milk alkali syndrome
	Immbolization—particularly in heavy adolescent males
	Thiazides

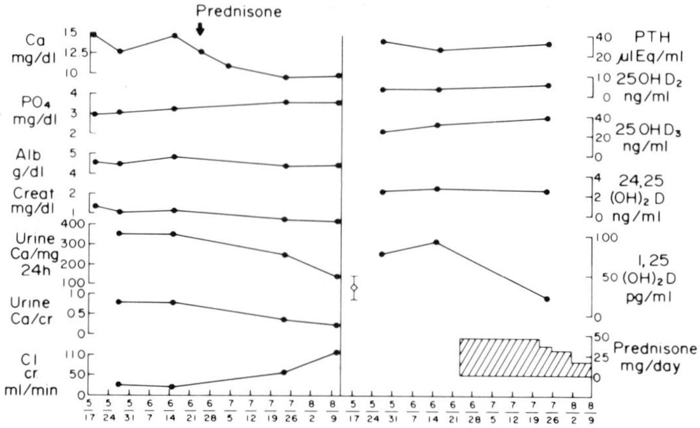

Figure 9.4. The effect of prednisone therapy on the serum and urinary calcium excretion, calcium/creatinine ratio, creatinine clearance and $1,25(OH)_2D$ concentration in a girl with sarcoidosis. (Reprinted with permission from Chesney RW: *J Pediatr* 98:919, 1981).

intestinal Ca absorption in these patients is greater than that observed in normal individuals. There is a positive correlation between serum $1,25(OH)_2D$ values and serum Ca concentration (103, 105).

Administration of prednisone or other glucocorticoids to patients with hypercalcemic sarcoidosis reverses the hypercalcemia and hypercalciuria. Creatinine clearance also increases and steroids block the intestinal hyperabsorption of calcium by reducing the circulating level of $1,25(OH)_2D$ (103–106). Glucocorticoids diminish granuloma size and may reduce levels of $1,25(OH)_2D$ by this means.

Hypercalcuria and Hypercalcemia

Hypercalcuria and, less frequently, hypercalcemia are complications of prolonged bed rest and immobilization that follow fractures, burns, or paralysis from any cause (18, 107, 108). The condition is particularly prevalent in adolescent males, who have a rapid turnover rate of bone with release of Ca. The increased serum and urinary Ca levels arise from bone, because there is increased bone resorption; bone formation rate is not greatly altered (108). The cause of the increase in bone resorption is not clear. PTH values vary, whereas they would predictably be suppressed in response to hypercalcemia. Those patients who have normal or high iPTH values may have increased resorption for this reason. Parathyroidectomy prevents increased bone resorption after immobilization (109), while vitamin D values generally are normal. One can speculate that, in adolescent males, where $1,25(OH)_2D$ values are normally 40 to 90 pg/ml (vs 20 to 40 in adults), both enhanced intestinal Ca absorption and bone turnover could occur. Dietary Ca restriction may actually increase urinary Ca excretion, possibly by increasing PTH secretion or $1,25(OH)_2D$ production (109).

Detection and Treatment

Immobilized patients may be monitored by determining the urinary Ca to creatinine ratio ($U^{Ca/Cr}$) in a random urine sample (107). This ratio is less than 0.15 in normal states; values greater than 0.4 indicate a risk for the development of hypercalcemia. Hypercalcemia is defined as a serum value of >11.0 mg/dl.

Therapy of acute hypercalcemia includes intravenous NaCl, NaCl excretion by giving isotonic saline (20 mg/kg/hr) for 1 to 4 hours and furosemide at 20 to 40 mg. Sodium sulfate and P infusions should not be given because they may cause soft tissue calcification. Glucocorticoids, mithramycin, and calcitonin have been used to treat hypercalcemia (105, 107), but, of these, only calcitonin directly inhibits bone resorption. The dose is 200 MRC units of calcitonin. Daily prednisone may be necessary to lower serum Ca, but both act within a few days. Physical therapy is of little benefit since hypercalcemia persists until the patient is ambulatory.

Hyperparathyroidism

Primary hyperparathyroidism is extremely rare in children. It occurs with multiple endocrine adenoma (MEA) syndromes (110). Parathyroid hyperplasia occurs with familial hypocalcuric hypercalcemia (FHH); in infants with this condition, it may present with life-threatening hypercalcemia (chapter 25).

The hypercalcemia, hypercalciuria, and stone formation observed in primary hyperparathyroidism are related to elevated concentrations of plasma $1,25(OH)_2D$ (111, 112). Patients with primary hyperparathyroidism and renal stones have increased intestinal absorption of an oral Ca load, hypercalciuria, and $1,25(OH)_2D$ values of 90 ± 19 pg/ml. Patients free of stones have normal intestinal Ca absorption, lower urinary Ca excretion, and $1,25(OH)_2D$ value of 57 ± 13 pg/ml. Accordingly, two subpopulations are identified: stone formers with high $1,25(OH)_2D$ values and nonstone-formers without comparable elevations of this vitamin D metabolite (111). High $1,25(OH)_2D$ are observed in patients with primary hyperparathyroidism and osteitis fibrosa, which may persist for some time despite parathyroidectomy (112). The fall in $1,25(OH)_2D$ levels and healing of the PTH-induced bone lesions appears to coincide with the reversal of hypophosphatemia. Surgery is the usual mode of therapy.

Tumoral Calcinosis

In tumoral calcinosis there is evidence for abnormal vitamin D metabolism and renal handling of O (113, 114). Tumor calcinosis is characterized by deposits of amorphous Ca-P near the joints. Hyperphosphatemia is common; hypercalcemia is uncommon so that the calcinosis results from the high Ca and P product secondary to hyperphosphatemia. Serum $1,25(OH)_2D$ values are elevated and iPTH concentrations are normal. Intestinal Ca absorption and urinary Ca excretions are elevated. Therapy with P-binding agents may benefit by preventing further calcifications, but may not cause existing lesions to regress.

Milk Alkali Syndrome

This condition is uncommon in children and occurs when a patient ingests large amounts of milk and absorbs alkali that generates HCO_3, so that alkalosis and an alkaline urine result. CaP phosphate crystals precipitate within the nephron. Patients may develop chronic hypercalcemia and renal failure, usually characterized by polyuria (110).

Malignancy

The usual tumors associated with hypercalcemia of malignancy are carcinoma of the breast, lung, kidney, or cervix, as well as multiple myeloma, but these are rarely encountered in children (115, 116). Hypercalcemia may occur in acute lymphocytic leukemia early in the course of the disease when the white cell count is low. It is not reported when the white blood cell count is high (116, 117). Patients with hypercalcemia of malignancy can be treated with glucocorticoids or mithramycin, but appropriate therapy of the underlying malignancy is indicated.

Miscellaneous Causes

Other conditions associated with hypercalcemia are hyperthyroidism and adrenal insufficiency. Glucocorticoids inhibit intestinal Ca absorption (18). This may account for the development of hypercalcemia with glucocorticoid insufficiency and is corrected with replacement therapy. Hypercalcemia associated with hyperthyroidism is seldom clinically troublesome.

Hypocalcemia

Hypocalcemia occurs in acquired and hereditary diseases (Table 9.3). It may be the main manifestation, as in hypoparathyroidism, or merely one of many abnormalities, as in CRFG. Ionized Ca is low and symptoms of neuromuscular irritability may develop (78). Symptoms are not well correlated with the degree of hypocalcemia; factors which affect ionized Ca, e.g., acid base status, serum albumin, and serum P concentration are also important.

Hypoparathyroidism

Hypoparathyroidism occurs either with decreased secretion or reduced peripheral action of PTH. The common cause of hypoparathyroidism is decreased secretion. This includes removal with thyroid surgery (3) in association with the CES and the DiGeorge syndrome (118). Iron deposition, as a complication of transfusion therapy in thalassemia major or hypoplastic anemia, may be associated with decreased PTH secretion (18).

The signs and symptoms of hypocalcemia and hyperphosphatemia

Table 9.3
Acquired and Hereditary Conditions Associated with Hypocalcemic Disorders of Childhood

Disorder	Condition
Hypoalbuminemia	
Parathyroid hormone system alterations	Hypoparathyroidism
	Postsurgery
	Infiltration with iron, tumor or lymphocytes
	Idiopathic: congenital, inherited or later onset
	Candida endocrinopathy syndrome (CES) with mucocutaneous candidiasis
	Pseudohypoparathyroidism: numerous phenotypic forms
	Hypomagnesiemia: impaired gut absorption
	excessive renal wasting
	diarrhea
Vitamin D system abnormalities	Reduced intake
	Reduced sunlight exposure
	Reduced absorption—intestinal disorders
	Hepatocellular disorders which impair absorption and 25(OH)D synthesis and enterohepatic circulation
	Augmented metabolism of 25(OH)D to inactive polar metabolites by phenobarbital, phenyl hydantoins, ethanol, etc.
	Accelerated urinary losses of 25(OH)D—nephrotic syndrome
	Decreased production of calcitriol—renal disease or autosomal recessive vitamin D-dependent rickets
	End-organ unresponsiveness to calcitriol with rickets; sometimes with alopecia
Abrupt fall in serum calcium	Pancreatitis
	Rhabdomyolysis
	Acute renal failure

range from parasthesia to muscle cramps, carpopedal spasms, severe tetany, laryngeal stridor, and convulsions (18). With long-standing hypoparathyroidism, intracranial calcifications are visible on skull x-ray films in approximately 20% of patients (118), which may result in a Parkinson-like syndrome when these calcifications are in the basal ganglia. Other features include papilledema, increased intracranial pressure, ectodermal abnormalities of the nails and hair, and lenticular cataracts (18). Abnormalities in dentition occur frequently in children. Depending on the age of onset of hypoparathyroidism, one may find abnormalities in dentin and root formation or dental hypoplasia (18).

Hypocalcemia in hypoparathyroidism results from deficiency in PTH and the resultant failure to mobilize bone Ca and from the effects of hyperphosphatemia, i.e., reduced renal 1α-hydroxylation of 25-hydrocycholecalciferol, resulting in decreased levels of 1,25$(OH)_2D_3$ (120). The treatment of hypoparathyroidism in the absence of hormone replacement therapy is vitamin D in some form, with or without supplemental Ca. Therapy with the 1α-hydroxy analogs avoids the problems of using the large doses of vitamin D_2 or D_3 required to overcome the defect in 1α-hydroxylation. Nine children have been successfully treated for 29 treatment years with 1,25$(OH)_2D_3$ (0.025 μg/kg/day), and episodes of hypercalcemia were few (121). When hypercalcemia occurs during treatment, using 1α-hydroxy analogs, it is readily controlled by discontinuing therapy because these compounds have a short half-life.

Although therapy with 1,25$(OH)_2D_3$ bypasses the block in 1α-hydroxylase activity, 25(OH)D therapy has been used successfully in correcting the hypocalcemia of 21 adults with hypoparathyroidism (122). The doses required to maintain normocalcemia (50 to 300 μg daily) are about 5% to 10% the dose required when vitamin D_2 is used.

Vitamin D Dietary Deficiency

Osteomalacia and rickets are disorders of calcification. In osteomalacia, there is a failure to mineralize newly formed ostoid. In rickets, a disease of childhood, the growth plate at the epiphyses is involved. There is defective calcification of cartilage, delayed maturation of the cellular sequence, and disorganization of the arrangement of cartilage cells, resulting in thickening of the epiphyseal plate.

Before 1920, nutritional rickets and osteomalacia were major public health problems, especially in industrial cities in the temperate zones. Recognizing the antirachitic properties of light and cod liver oil and owing to the universal supplementation of milk with either vitamin D_2 or D_3, vitamin D deficiency is now uncommon in the United States. However, it continues to be a health problem in developing countries. Furthermore, a new population at risk was emerged, which includes Asian immigrants and their children in England with their unique dietary and social customs (123), housebound and elderly subjects (124), and low birth weight premature infants (125). The latter group have hypocalcemia, hypophosphatemia, elevated iPTH levels, and multiple fractures. It tends to occur between the ages of 8 to 12 weeks in rapidly growing infants (126). Most infants are fed low-P formulas, such as breast milk; 25(OH)D levels are low, while 1,25$(OH)_2D_3$ levels are normal or elevated (126).

The chemical findings in rickets and osteomalacia include hypocalcemia, hypophosphatemia, increased serum alkaline phosphatase hyperparathyroidism (18, 127). Scriver (127) divided the evolution of vitamin D deficiency in infancy into 3 stages. In stage 1, serum Ca tends to be low, serum phosphorus normal, and aminoaciduria is absent. If the disorder is unrecognized, progression to stage 2 occurs in which phosphaturia ensues, with resultant hypophosphatemia and aminoaciduria. Serum Ca tends to return to normal, with an increase in serum alkaline phosphatase, presumably related to increased PTH secretion and increased bone turnover. Stage 3 is characterized by hypocalcemia, persistent hypophosphatemia, and aminoaciduria. It was formerly believed that PTH alone is responsible for aminoaciduria (127). However, recent studies fail to demonstrate that the hormone is the sole culprit (128). Other factors, such as calcitonin or reduced intracellular Ca, may be responsible.

The characteristic skeletal disturbance in vitamin D deficiency is osteomalacia, which literally means soft bones. The malacic bone is subject to distortion in shape and to fracture. In the first year of life, the most rapidly growing bones are the cranium, wrists, and ribs. Hence, nutritional rickets leads to widened cranial sutures, frontal bossing, craniotabes, rachitic rosary, Harrison's groove, and enlargement of the wrists (18). Dental eruption is delayed (18). There is severe muscular hypotonia and weakness. After 1 year, the deformities are most severe about the legs because of their rapid growth and weight-bearing function, resulting in genu varum or genu valgum, coxa vera, and rachitic saber shins (18). Radiologically, the ends of growing metaphyses are frayed or irregular. The diaphyseal cortex is thin. Secondary hyperparathyroid bone changes, such as subperiosteal erosions, may be present (129). In adults, bone cysts, phalangeal lesions, and pseudofractures are more common (129).

In a typical patient with vitamin D deficiency, levels of vitamin D_2D_3, 25$(OH)D_3$, and 24,25$(OH)_2$ are low or undetectable (23). Levels of 1,25$(OH)_2D_3$ are maintained in the normal range because of a host of modulators that are known to stimulate 1α-hydroxylation and which include hypocalcemia, hypophosphatemia, and elevated iPTH levels. Consequently, it has been suggested that the absence of 24,25$(OH)_2D_3$ is responsible for the osteomalacia of nutritional vitamin D deficiency (22). However, the "normal" level of 1,25$(OH)_2D_3$ should be considered low for the degree of hypocalcemia.

Treatment of nutritional deficienty consists of the oral administration of 1500 to 5000 IU ergocalciferol, which usually results in demonstrable radiological healing within 2 to 4 weeks. In patients with poor compliance, a single large parenteral dose may be indicated. However, it may incur a mild risk of hypercalcemia because of poorly understood differences in individual responses.

Rickets

Vitamin D-dependent Rickets. Hereditary vitamin D dependency (or pseudovitamin D deficiency) is a distinct, rare, autosomal recessive disorder with clinical features of the advanced stage of vitamin deficiency despite intake of adequate amounts of the vitamin (130, 131). Prominent signs are usually evident before 6 months of age. Features include hypocalcemia, often with tetany or convulsions, hypophosphatemia, marked elevation of the alkaline phosphatase activity, skeletal deformities, generalized aminoaciduria, and elevated immunoreactive PTH levels. In addition to severe radiological changes, these patients have severe hypoplasia of the enamel (Table 9.4).

In contrast to nutritional vitamin D deficiency, patients with vitamin D-dependent rickets, Type I, have a low circulating 1,25$(OH)_2D_3$ levels (132). Although not yet proved by direct tissue analysis, the underlying abnormality may be a defect in the 1α-hydroxylase enzyme system in the renal tubule. An animal model of this disease has been reported that may provide a better understanding of the underlying defect (133).

Large doses of vitamin D result in normalization of the biochemical disturbances and healing of the radiological abnormalities. The dose required is 100,000 to 300,000 U daily. Fraser and coworkers (134) report that 1000 IU/kg body weight/day is an appropriate starting dose of vitamin D_2 or D_3. More recently, they reported that small doses of 1,25$(OH)_2D_3$ (0.5 to 1.0 μg/day) could completely reverse the abnor-

Table 9.4
Features and Laboratory Findings in Hypocalcemic Forms of Rickets

	25(OH)D-deficient	Vitamin D-dependent	Vitamin D-dependent (Type II)[a]
Age of onset	9–12 months	3–6 months	3–6 months
Inheritance	None	Autosomal recessive	Autosomal recessive (often consanguinity)
Rickets	Yes	Yes	Yes
Hypocalcemia	Yes	Yes	Yes
Hypophosphatemia	Yes	Yes	Yes
Aminoaciduria	Yes	Yes	Yes
Elevated iPTH level	Yes	Yes	Yes
Intestinal calcium malabsorption	Yes	Yes	Yes
Muscle weakness	Yes	Yes	Yes
Alopecia	No	No	Common
Serum 25(OH)D (nl = 30 ± 5 ng/ml)	Very low	Normal	Normal (except in 1 case)
Serum $1,25(OH)_2D$ (nl = 20–80 pg/ml)	30–50 pg/ml (normal)	3–9 pg/ml (very low)	150–300 pg/ml (very high)
Proposed defect	Deficient intake of D or lack of sunshine	Abnormal conversion of 25(OH)D to $1,25(OH)_2D$; ? impaired 1α-hydroxylase activity	Refractoriness of target organs to calcitriol

[a] Not responsive to calcitriol.

Table 9.5
Responses to Treatment of Hypocalcemic Forms of Rickets

Daily treatment	25(OH)D-deficient	Vitamin D-dependent	Vitamin D-dependent (Type II)[a]
10 μgm of vitamin D_2 or D_3	Curative	No response	No response
1–2 μgm of calcitriol	Curative	Curative	No response
2500 μgm (100,000 units) of vitamin D_2 or D_3	Hypercalcemia	May be curative	May be curative
6 μgm of calcitriol	Hypercalcemia	Hypercalcemia	Curative in some cases

[a] Not responsive to calcitriol.

malities (132). A small number of patients with a disorder resembling vitamin D-dependency show high circulating concentrations of $1,25(OH)_2D_3$ and thus are characterized as having vitamin D-dependent rickets, type II (135, 136). These patients do not improve with physiological doses of vitamin D, suggesting an end-organ resistance. Children with this disorder exhibit alopecia by the end of the first year of life (136). The molecular basis of the defect is not clear. Recently, defective nuclear uptake of tritiated $1,25(OH)_2D_3$ demonstrated in skin fibroblasts cultured from affected kindreds (137). A similar defect in the intestine or bone could account for the resistance to vitamin D.

These patients achieve normal Ca homeostasis with high doses of $1,25(OH)_2D_3$ that are 20 to 50 times higher than those normally used in other disorders (135–137). Circulating levels of $1,25(OH)_2D_3$ as high as 100 times normal are required to overcome end-organ resistance (Table 9.5).

Anticonvulsant Therapy and Osteomalacia

Cases of rickets and osteomalacia have been reported in patients with epilepsy since 1968 (138, 139). The common factor is the intake of anticonvulsant medications, which are potent inducers of hepatic microsomal mixed-oxidase activity. The clinical abnormalities are those of rickets: hypocalcemia, elevated serum alkaline phosphatase, reduced serum $25(OH)D_3$ levels, and radiological changes of rickets or osteomalacia.

Phenobarbital and hydantoins enhance the conversion of 25(OH)D to more polar, but biologically inactive, compounds (140). Levels of $1,25(OH)_2D$ are normal or increased (141). Anticonvulsant drugs also may have direct effects on bone metabolism independent of their effects on vitamin D, e.g., diphenylhydantoin alters ion transport across cell membranes (142).

There are a number of predisposing risk factors that contribute to the occurrence and severity, e.g., drug dose, duration of therapy, vitamin D intake, sunlight exposure, coexisting diseases, and physical activity (143, 144). If there is overt disease, treatment consists of replacement of vitamin D_2 or D_3 in doses of 2000 to 4000 IU/day in combination with Ca (400 mg/day) per os as a supplement (145).

Magnesium Metabolism Disorders

Hypermagnesemia

This is usually iatrogenic, and impaired renal function is the most common prerequisite for its development. It is prone to occur in conjunction with the use of Mg containing antacids, cathartics, or enemas; it also occurs with parenteral alimentation when Mg is given intravenously. As renal failure progresses, the fractional excretion of Mg rises parallel with the rise in fractional excretion of Na. Serum Mg is normal in early CRF and rises when GFR is <30 ml/min (146). The diseased kidney is capable of maintaining Mg homeostasis until the inulin clearance is <10 ml/min (147).

Total body Mg is increased in CRF (148). Bone shows the greatest increase. Erythrocyte Mg also is increased, and muscle Mg is sometimes increased. Hypermagnesemia accompanies acute renal failure; however, with recovery and diuresis, Mg is lost and hypomagnesemia may develop and have serious consequences, e.g., cardiac arrhythmias and arrest (68).

Other causes of hypermagnesemia include parenteral administration in the therapy of toxemia and adrenal insufficiency, hypothyroidism, and lithium intoxication (148). Mg-containing enemes have caused hypermagnesemia in patients with normal renal function. However, these patients had bowel perforations that led to lethal transperitoneal absorption of the ion. Finally, hypermagnesemia has been noted in infants born to preeclamptic mothers treated with $MgSO_4$ (149). The signs and symptoms of hypermagnesemia occur when plasma levels are >4 mEq/L (148). They include depression of the central nervous system, impaired nerve conduction, and diminution or loss of deep tendon reflexes. Paralysis and respiratory depression develops with severe hypermagnesemia (150). Mentation may remain normal during these periods, but coma occurs when levels exceed 12 mEq/L (151). The cardiovascular effects (148, 152) include hypotension, tachycardia followed by bradycardia, heart block with associated ECG changes (prolonged PR interval, increased QRS duration, and cardiac arrest at levels that exceed 15 mEq/L). Mg dilates blood vessels and causes sympathetic blockade; it has cardiotoxic effects, depressing cardiac output, all of which contribute to the development of hypotension.

Immediate but transient reversal of signs may be effected by Ca. Cessation of Mg administration is necessary. Peritoneal or hemodialysis may be necessary to reduce the levels (148).

Hypomagnesemia

Mg depletion is a common clinical disorder that is frequently overlooked because of the complex clinical setting and associated electrolyte disturbances observed in these patients. The clinician must rely on measurements of serum Mg as a guide to body stores, as well as extracellular Mg.

Experimental Mg depletion in man produces an alteration in Ca metabolism (68). Ca balance studies reveal the development of hypocalcemia (153–158). The pathophysiology behind the development of hypocalcemia in hypomagnesemia is not known. When measured, these patients may have undetectable or normal PTH levels, which seem to be inappropriately low for the degree of hypocalcemia. There is evidence to suggest that the decreased Mg levels interfere with the secretion of PTH (157) and possibly with its synthesis (156). After the administration of intravenous Mg to a Mg-depleted patient, serum iPTH rises within 2 minutes (157), an effect too rapid to represent a change in PTH biosynthesis. Further, after the initial surge, the PTH level rises slowly to normal over several days, suggesting an improvement in its biosynthesis (156).

Reports of end-organ resistance to exogenous PTH in some patients with hypomagnesemia (153) conflict with those in which a calcemic response to the hormone is evident (158). Anast and coworkers demonstrated an abrupt increase in urinary cAMP in response to pharmacologic doses of exogenous PTH. However, this does not preclude the possibility that the parathyroid adenylate cyclase system, which involves the secretory process of PTH, may be selectively affected by hypomagnesemia.

Finally, hypomagnesemia affects the concentration of K. K deficiency in skeletal muscle is evident in rats made Mg-deficient (159). When the animal is Mg-depleted, there is inability to maintain a normal K concentration gradient across cell membrane. Moreover, the defect in K metabolism corrects upon repletion of Mg.

Causes of Hypomagnesemia

Defective Gastrointestinal Absorption of Magnesium. Several patients have been described with isolated GI defect in Mg absorption (160, 161). The defect is familial and is treated with oral supplements of Mg. If these supplements are discontinued, severe hypomagnesemia ensues, accompanied by hypocalcemia, hypokalemia, hypernatremia, and hyperphosphatemia. PTH, calcitonin, and 25-hydroxycholecalciferol levels remain normal. Urinary excretion of Mg is markedly decreased and most patients present with tetany.

Hypomagnesemia has been described in a number of patients with small bowel disease (162), including regional enteritis, ulcerative colitis, small bowel resection, and generalized malabsorption syndromes. Kwashiorkor has also been associated with hypomagnesemia (163).

Renal Magnesium Wasting. In 1966, 3 adult patients were described with a hereditary disorder characterized by renal Mg-wasting despite severe hypomagnesemia and hypokalemia (164). Furthermore, when these patients were placed on a low-Mg diet, they failed to conserve Mg, excreting 41 to 51 mg/day. Moreover, there was no other associated tubular dysfunction. However, renal Mg-wasting is not a specific entity, as it can be found in a variety of other clinical settings. Booth and coworkers (165) described the defect in association with aminoaciduria, glucosuria, and failure to thrive.

Evans and coworkers (166) described 2 patients with a history of tetany hypocalcemia and renal wasting of Mg, with evidence of medullary nephrocalcinosis and decreased GFR. In a review of the literature, nephrocalcinosis of unknown cause was found in 50% of the reported patients, with slow progression to renal failure. The location of the tubular disorder is not clear. By renal biopsy, neither the proximal nor the distal tubules are affected. There may be a defect in the concentration gradient between intracellular and extracellular and K ions (167).

Other causes of renal Mg-wasting include diuretics, aminoglycoside therapy, cis-platinum, hyperaldosteronism, hyperthyroidism, hypercalciuric or salt-wasting states, Bartter's syndrome, and inappropriate secretion of antidiuretic hormone (162).

Signs and Symptoms of Hypomagnesemia

The hypomagnesemia syndrome is characterized by personality change, tremors, fasciculations, spontaneous carpopedal spasm, and generalized spasticity (68). Premature ventricular beats and dysrhythmias are possible. Some patients become apathetic and depressed. Seizures and coma may occur if the deficiency is severe. The mechanisms responsible for the central nervous and cardiovascular symptoms are not fully understood, but may be related to the importance of Mg in several enzyme systems. The associated hypocalcemia and hypokalemia may contribute to the symptoms.

Treatment

Most patients with hypomagnesemia can be treated with a normal diet, unless ongoing GI or renal losses are the underlying cause. It is necessary to check renal function before supplementing Mg. Whenever possible, intravenous replacement should be avoided in small children because of the danger of hypotension. For children weighing 4 to 7 kg, a safe initial dose is 0.5 ml of 50% $MgSO_4$ (2 mEq Mg) given intramuscularly. Heavier children may be given 1.0 ml of 50% $MgSO_4$. Most patients with chronic hypomagnesemia can tolerate an oral dose (in the form of Mg) of 250 to 500 mg (12.5 to 25 mEq Mg) 4 times/day without the development of diarrhea (168).

References

1. Clayton B: Table of normal values adjusted for age. In Pediatric Chemical Pathology. London, Blackwell Scientific Publ, 1982, p. 146.
2. Chesney RW: Phosphaturic syndromes. In Gonick H (ed): Renal Tubular Disorders. Marcel Dekker Inc., 1985, p. 201.
3. Raisz LG: Bone metabolism and calcium regulation. In Avioli LV, Karne SM (eds): Metabolic Bone Disease. New York, Academic Press, 1977, vol 1, p 1.
4. Cohen L, Kitzes R: Relationship of bone and plasma magnesium in magnesium-deficient cirrhosis patients. Israel J Med Sci 18:679, 1982.
5. Farfel Z, Salomon M, Bourne HR: Genetic investigation of adenylate cyclase: mutations in mouse and man. Ann Rev Pharmacol Toxicol 21:251, 1981.
6. DeLuca HF: The vitamin D system in the regulation of calcium and phosphorus metabolism. W. O. Atwater memorial lecture. Nutr Rev 37:161, 1979.
7. Norman AW, Henry HL, Malluche HH: 24R,25-Dihydroxyvitamin D_3 and 1α-dihydroxyvitamin D_3 are both indispensable for calcium and phosphorus homeostasis. Life Sci 27:229, 1980.
8. Kumar R, Riggs BL: Vitamin D in the therapy of disorders of calcium and phosphorus metabolism. Mayo Clin Proc 56:327, 1981.
9. Chesney RW: Current clinical applications of vitamin D metabolite research. In Urist MR (ed): Clinical Orthopaedics and Related Research. Philadelphia, J.B. Lippincott, 1981, p 285.
10. Norman AW, Schaefer K, von Herrath D, et al (eds): Vitamin D: Chemical, Biochemical and Clinical Endocrinology of Calcium Metabolism. New York, Walter de Gruyter, 1982.
11. Fraser DR: Regulation of the metabolism of vitamin D. Physiol Rev 60:551, 1980.
12. Kumar R, Cohen WR, Silva P, et al: Elevated 1,25-dihydroxyvitamin D plasma levels in normal human pregnancy and lactation. J Clin Invest 63:342, 1979.
13. DeLuca HF: The vitamin D hormonal system: implications for bone disease. Hosp Practice 15:57, 1980.
14. Root AW, Harrison HE: Recent advances in calcium metabolism. I. Mechanisms of calcium homeostasis. J Pediatr 88:1, 1976.
15. Lotz M, Zisman E, Bartter FC: Evidence of a phosphorus-depletion syndrome in man. N Engl J Med 278:409, 1968.
16. Chesney RW, Dabbagh S: Disorders of tubular transport related to calcium and phosphorus metabolism. In Holliday M, Vernier R, Barratt TM (eds): Pediatric Nephrology, ed 2. Baltimore, Williams & Wilkins. (In press.)
17. Fox J, Heath H III: Parathyroid, renal and skeletal responses to induced hypocalcemia in the dog. Am J Physiol 242:E287, 1982.
18. Harrison HE, Harrison HC: Disorders of Calcium and Phosphate Metabolism in Childhood and Adolescence, Philadelphia, W.B. Saunders Co., 1979, p 53.
19. Menanteau J, Neuman WF, Neuman MW: A study of bone proteins which can prevent hydroxyapatite formation. Metab Bone Dis Rel Res 4:157, 1982.
20. Hock JM, Kream BE, Raisz LG: Autoradiographic study of the effect of 1,25-dihydroxyvitamin D_3 on bone matrix synthesis in vitamin D-replete rats. Calcif Tissue Int 32:347, 1982.
21. Plachot JJ, Bailly du Bois M, Halpern S, et al: In vitro action of 1,25-dihydroxycholecalciferol and 24,25-dihydroxycholecalciferol on matrix organization and mineral distribution in rabbit growth plate. Metab Bone Dis Rel Res 4:135, 1982.
22. Rasmussen H, Baron R, Broadus A, et al: $1,25(OH)_2D_3$ is not the only metabolite involved in the pathogenesis of osteomalacia. Am J Med 69:360, 1980.
23. Chesney RW, Zimmerman J, Hamstra AJ, et al: Vitamin D metabolite concentrations in vitamin D deficiency: Are calcitriol levels normal? Am J Dis Child 135:1025, 1981.
24. Suki WN, Rouse D: Mechanisms of calcium transport. Mineral Electrolyte Metab 5:175, 1981.
25. Edwards BR, Sutton RAL, Dirks JH: Effect of calcium infusion on renal tubular absorption in the dog. Am J Physiol 227:13, 1973.
26. Ullrich KJ, Rumrich G, Kloss S: Active Ca^{++} reabsorption in the proximal tubule of the rat kidney. Pfluegers Arch 364:223, 1976.
27. Wong NLM, Quamme GA, Dirks JH: Effect of chlorothiazide on renal calcium and magnesium handling in the hamster. Canad J Physiol Pharmacol 60:1160, 1982.
28. Bordeau JE, Buss SL, Vurek GG: Inhibition of calcium absorption in the cortical thick ascending limb of Henle's loop by furosemide. J Pharmacol Exper Ther 221:815, 1982.
29. Hough S, Russell JE, Teitelbaum SL, et al: Calcium homeostasis in chronic streptozotocin-induced diabetes mellitus in the rat. Am J Physiol 242:E451, 1982.
30. DeFronzo RA, Goldberg M, Agus ZS: The effect of glucose and insulin on renal electrolyte transport. J Clin Invest 58:83, 1976.
31. Amiel C: Sites of renal tubular reabsorption of phosphate. In Massry SG, Fleisch H (eds): The Renal Handling of Phosphate. New York, Plenum Press, 1980, p 39.
32. Lang F: Renal handling of calcium and phosphate. Klin Wochenschr 58:985, 1980.
33. Knox FG, Osswald H, Marchand GR, et al: Phosphate transport along the tubule. Am J Physiol 233:F261, 1977.
34. Schneider EG, Hanson RC, Childers JW, et al: Is phosphate secreted by the kidney? In Massry SG, Fleisch H (eds): The Renal Handling of Phosphate. New York, Plenum Press, 1980, p 59.
35. Shlatz LJ, Schwartz IL, Kinne-Saffran E, et al: Distribution of parathyroid hormone-stimulated adenylate cyclase in plasma membranes of cells of the kidney cortex. J Membr Biol 24:131, 1975.
36. Lau K, Goldfarb S, Goldberg M: The effects of parathyroid hormone on renal phosphate handling. In Massry SG, Fleisch H (eds): The Renal Handling of Phosphate. New York, Plenum Press, 1980, p 115.
37. Liang CT, Barnes J, Balakir R, et al: In vitro stimulation of phosphate uptake in isolated chick renal cells by 1,25-dihydroxycholecalciferol. Proc Natl Acad Sci USA 79:3532, 1982.
38. Eisenberg E: Effects of serum calcium level and parathyroid extract on phosphate and calcium excretion in hypoparathyroid patients. J Clin Invest 44:942, 1965.
39. Lavender AR, Pullman TN: Changes in inorganic phosphate excretion induced by renal arterial infusion of calcium. Am J Physiol 205:1025, 1963.
40. Bonjour JP, Fleisch H: Calcium supply and renal handling of phosphate. Min Electrolyte Metab 3:261, 1980.
41. Tröhler U, Bonjour JP, Fleisch H: Inorganic phosphate homeostasis: Renal adaptation to the dietary intake in intact and thyroparathyroidectomized rats. J Clin Invest 57:264, 1976.
42. Bonjour JP, Tröhler U, Preston C, et al: Parathyroid hormone and renal handling of Pi: Effect of dietary Pi and diphosphonates. Am J Physiol 234:F497, 1978.
43. Stoll R, Kinne R, Murer H: Effect of dietary phosphate intake on phosphate transport by isolated rat renal brush border vesicles. Biochem J 180:465, 1979.
44. Frick A, Dursasin I: Maximal reabsorptive capacity for inorganic phosphate (Tm_{Pi}) in the absence of parathyroid hormone in the rat: Decrease of the Tm_{Pi} during prolonged administration of phosphate and the role of calcium. Pfluegers Arch 377:9, 1978.
45. Ginsburg JN: Effect of glucose and free fatty acid on phosphate transport in dog kidney. Am J Physiol 222:1153, 1972.
46. Pitts RF, Alexander RS: The renal reabsorptive mechanism for inorganic phosphate in normal and acidotic dogs. Am J Physiol 142:648, 1944.
47. Cohen JJ, Berglund E, Lotspeich WD: Renal tubular reabsorption of acetoacetate, inorganic sulfate and inorganic phosphate in the dog as affected by glucose and phloridzin. Am J Physiol 184:91, 1956.
48. Segal S, Thier S, Fox M, et al: Inhibitory effect of sugars on amino acid accumulation by slices of rat kidney cortex. Biochim Biophys Acta 65:567, 1962.
49. Csaky TZ, Prachnamboli K, Eiseman B, et al: The effect of digitalis on the renal tubular transport of glucose in normal and heartless dogs. J Pharmacol Exp Ther 150:275, 1964.
50. Saudek CD, Boulter PR, Knopp RH, et al: Sodium retention accompanying treatment of diabetes mellitus. Diabetes 23:240, 1974.
51. Harter HR, Mercado A, Rutherford WE, et al: Effects of phosphate depletion and parathyroid hormone on renal glucose reabsorption. Am J Physiol 227:1422, 1974.
52. Rozen R, Tenenhouse HS, Scriver CR: Taurine transport in renal brush-border membrane vesicles. Biochem J 180:245, 1979.
53. Drummond KN, Michael AF: Specificity of the inhibition of tubular phosphate reabsorption by certain amino acids. Nature 201:1333, 1964.
54. Ritz E, Kreusser W, Bommer J: Effects of hormones other than parathyroid hormones on renal handling of phosphate. In Massry SG, Fleisch H (eds): The Renal Handling of Phosphate. New York, Plenum Press, 1980, p 137.
55. Corvilain J, Abramov W: Some effects of human growth hormone on renal hemodynamics and on tubular phosphate transport in man. J Clin Invest 41:1230, 1962.
56. Turner ST, Kiebzak GM, Dousa TP: Mechanism of glucocorticoid effect on renal transport of phosphate. Am J Physiol 243:C227, 1982.
57. Freiberg JM, Kinsella J, Sacktor B: Glucocorticoids increase the Na^+-H^+ exchange and decrease the Na^+ gradient-dependent phosphate-uptake systems in renal brush border membrane vesicles. Proc Natl Acad Sci USA 79:4932, 1982.
58. Arruda JAL, Richardson JM, Wolfson JA, et al: Lithium administration and phosphate excretion. Am J Physiol 231:1140, 1976.
59. Martinez-Maldonado M, Eknoyan G: Role of extracellular fluid volume expansion and diuretics in renal handling of phosphate. In Massry SG, Fleisch H (eds): The Renal Handling of Phosphate. New York, Plenum Press, 1980, p 265.
60. Puschett JB, Goldberg M: The relationship between the renal handling of phosphate and bicarbonate in man. J Lab Clin Med 73:965, 1969.
61. Beck LH, Goldberg M: Effects of acetazolamide and parathyroidectomy on renal transport of sodium, calcium and phosphate. Am J Physiol 224:1136, 1973.
62. Rodriguez HJ, Walls J, Yates J, et al: Effect of acetazolamide on the urinary

excretion of cyclic AMP and on the activity of renal adenyl cyclase. J Clin Invest 53:122, 1974.
63. Lehne C, Coe FL: Compensatory phosphaturia after unilateral nephrectomy in the rat. Am J Physiol 231:1625, 1976.
64. Walser M: Divalent cations: Physicochemical state in glomerular filtrate and urine and renal excretion. In Orloff J, Berliner RW (eds): Handbook of Physiology. Washington D.C., American Physiological Society, 1973, p 555.
65. Lim P, Jacob E: Magnesium status in chronic uremic patients. Nephron 9:300, 1972.
66. Alfrey AC, Miller NL, Butkus D: Evaluation of body magnesium stores. J Lab Clin Med 84:153, 1974.
67. Brickman AS, Hartenbower DL, Norman AW, et al: Action of $1,25(OH)_2$- and $1\alpha(OH)$-vitamin D_3 on magnesium metabolism in man. Clin Res 23:315A, 1975.
68. Shiels ME: Experimental human magnesium depletion. Medicine 48:61, 1969.
69. Heaton FW, Parson FM: The metabolic effect of high magnesium intake. Clin Sci 21:273, 1961.
70. Massry SG, Seelig MS: Hypomagnesemia and hypermagnesemia. Clin Nephrol 7:147, 1977.
71. Carney SL, Wong NL, Quamme GA, et al: Effect of magnesium deficiency on renal magnesium and calcium transport in the rat. J Clin Invest 65:180, 1980.
72. Morel F, Roinel N, Le Grimellec C: Electron probe analysis of tubular fluid composition. Nephron 6:350, 1969.
73. Quamme GA, Dirks JH: Magnesium transport in the nephron. Am J Physiol 239:F393, 1980.
74. Quamme GA, Wong NLM, Dirks JH, et al: Magnesium handling in the dog kidney: A micropuncture study. Pfluegers Arch 377:95, 1978.
75. Wen SF, Evanson RL, Dirks JH: Micropuncture study of magnesium transport in proximal and distal tubule of the dog. Am J Physiol 219:570, 1970.
76. Brunette MG, Vigenault N, Carriere S: Micropuncture study of magnesium transport along the nephron in the young rat. Am J Physiol 227:891, 1974.
77. Quamme GA, Dirks JH: Effect of intraluminal and contraluminal magnesium on magnesium and calcium transfer in the rat nephron. Am J Physiol 238:F187, 1980.
78. Quamme GA: Effect of intraluminal furosemide on calcium and magnesium transport in the loop of Henle and the role of PTH. Kidney Int 14:642, 1978.
79. Shareghi GR, Agus ZS: Magnesium transport in the rabbit cortical thick ascending limb (CTAL). Clin Res 27:430A, 1979.
80. Brunette MG, Vigneault N, Carriere S: Micropuncture study of renal magnesium transport in magnesium-loaded rats. Am J Physiol 229:1695, 1975.
81. Wen SF, Wong NLM, Dirks JH: Evidence for renal magnesium secretion during magnesium infusion in the dog. Am J Physiol 220:33, 1971.
82. Averill CM, Heaton FW: The renal handling of magnesium. Clin Sci 31:353, 1960.
83. Le Grimellec CN, Roinel N, Morel F: Simultaneous Mg, Ca, P, K, Na and Cl analysis in rat tubular fluid. II. During acute Mg plasma loading. Plfuegers Arch 340:197, 1973.
84. Alfredson KS, Walser M: Is magnesium secreted by the rat renal tubule? Nephron 7:241, 1971.
85. Massry SG, Coburn JW, Kleeman CR: Renal handling of magnesium in the dog. Am J Physiol 216:1460, 1969.
86. Wong NLM, Quamme GA, Dirks JH: Tubular maximum reabsorptive capacity for magnesium in the dog (abstract). Kidney Int 16:658, 1979.
87. Rude RK, Bethune JE, Singer FR: Renal tubular maximum for magnesium in normal, hyperparathyroid and hypoparathyroid man. J Clin Endo Metab 51:1425, 1980.
88. Massry SG, Coburn JW: The hormonal and non-hormonal control of renal excretion of calcium and magnesium. Nephron 10:66, 1973.
89. Sutton RAL, Dirks JH: Renal handling of calcium, phosphate and magnesium. In Brenner RM, Rector FC Jr (eds): The Kidney, ed 2. Philadelphia, W.B. Saunders, 1981, p 551.
90. Le Grimellec C, Roinel N, Morel F: Simultaneous Mg, Ca, P, K, Na and Cl analysis in rat tubular fluid. III. During acute Ca plasma loading. Pfluegers Arch 346:171, 1974.
91. Massry SG, Brautbar N: The interrelationship between phosphate and magnesium metabolism. Adv Exp Med Biol 128:51, 1980.
92. Dirks JH, Quamme GA: Renal magnesium transport and the effects of hypermagnesemia, hypercalcemia, body magnesium stores and parathyroid hormone. Adv Exp Med Biol 128:41, 1980.
93. Yendt ER, Cohanin M: Prevention of calcium stores with thiazides. Kidney Intl 13:397, 1978.
94. Roy DR, Blorech KL, Jamison RL: Effects of acute acid-base disturbances on renal tubule reabsorption of magnesium in the rat. Am J Physiol 243:F197, 1982.
95. Heaton FW: The parathyroid glands and magnesium metabolism in the rat. Clin Sci 28:543, 1955.
96. Quamme GA, Carney SL, Wong NLM, et al: Effect of parathyroid hormone on renal calcium and magnesium reabsorption in magnesium-deficient rats. Pfluegers Arch 386:59, 1980.
97. Brunatowska MA, Harris CA, Sutton RAL, et al: Effects of PTH and cAMP on renal handling of calcium, magnesium and phosphate in the hamster. Am J Physiol 233:F514, 1977.
98. Poujeol P, Touvay C, Roinel N, et al: Stimulation of renal magnesium reabsorption by calcitonin in the rat. Am J Physiol 239:F524, 1980.
99. Quamme GA: Effect of calcitonin on calcium and magnesium transport in rat nephron. Am J Physiol 238:E573, 1980.
100. Bailly C, Arniel C: Effect of glucagon on magnesium renal reabsorption in the rat. Pfluegers Arch 392:360, 1982.
101. Ruggiero M, Brunese M, Morelli S, et al: Plasma 1,25-hydroxycholecalciferol concentrations and net intestinal calcium, phosphate and magnesium absorption in man. Boll Soc Ital Biol Sper 57:791, 1981.
102. Schmulen AC, Lerman M, Pak CYC, et al: Effect of $1,25(OH)_2D_3$ on jejunal absorption of magnesium in patients with chronic renal failure. Am J Physiol 238:G349, 1980.
103. Barbour GL, Coburn JW, Norman AW, et al: Nonrenal hypercalcemia in sarcoidosis. Clin Res 28:46A, 1980.
103a. Mason RS, Frankel T, Chan Y-L, et al: Vitamin D conversion by sarcoid lymph node homogenate. Ann Intern Med 100:59, 1984.
103b. Adams JS, Sharma OP, Gacad MA, et al: Metabolism of 25-hydroxyvitamin D_3 by cultured pulmonary alveolar macrophages in sarcoidosis. J Clin Invest 72:1856, 1983.
104. Bell NH: Hypercalcemic and hypocalcemic disorders: Diagnosis and treatment. Nephron 23:147, 1979.
105. Chesney RW, Rosen JF, Hamstra AJ, et al: The use of serum 1,25-dihydroxyvitamin D (calcitriol) concentrations in the clinical assessment of demineralizing disorders in children. In Cohn D, Talmadge RV, Matthews JL (eds): Calcium-Regulating Hormones. Rotterdam, Excerpta Medica, 1981, p 252.
106. O'Regan S, Chesney RW, Hamstra AJ, et al: Reduced serum $1,25(OH)_2$-vitamin D levels in adolescents with systemic lupus erythematosus. Acta Pediatr Scand 68:109, 1979.
107. Conley SB, Shackelford GD, Robson AM: Severe immobilization hypercalcemia, renal insufficiency and calcification. Pediatrics 63:142, 1979.
108. Burkhart JM, Jowsey J: Parathyroid and thyroid hormones in the development of immobilization osteoporosis. Endocrinology 81:1053, 1967.
109. Conaway HH, Waite LC, Kenny AD: Immobilization and bone mass in rats: Effects of parathyroidectomy and acetazolamide. Calcif Tissue Res 11:323, 1973.
110. Potts JT Jr: Disorders of parathyroid glands. In Isselbacher KJ, et al (eds): Harrison's Principles of Internal Medicine, ed 9. New York, McGraw-Hill Book Co., 1980, p 1832.
111. Broadus AE, Horst RL, Lang R, et al: The importance of circulating 1,25-dihydroxyvitamin D in the pathogenesis of hypercalcuria and renal-stone formation in primary hyperparathyroidism. N Engl J Med 302:421, 1980.
112. Gonzalez-Villapundo C, Porath A, Berelowitz M, et al: Vitamin D metabolism during recovery from severe osteitis fibrosa cystica of primary hyperparathyroidism. J Clin Endo Metab 51:1180, 1980.
113. Prince MJ, Schaefer PC, Goldsmith RS, et al: Hyperphosphatemic tumoral calcinosis: association with elevation of serum 1,25-dihydroxycholecalciferol concentrations. Ann Intern Med 96:586, 1982.
114. Zerwekh JE, Sanders LA, Townsend J, et al: Tumoral calcinosis: evidence for concurrent defects in renal tubular phosphorus transport and 1,25-dihydroxycholecalciferol synthesis. Calif Tissue Int 32:1, 1980.
115. Chesney RW, Simpson DP, Wen SF: Effects of tumor on fluid and electrolytes. In Garnick MB, Rieselbach RE (eds): Cancer and the Kidney. Philadelphia, Lea & Febiger, 1981, p 534.
116. O'Regan S, Kaplan BS, Chesney RW, et al: Hypokalemia in childhood leukemia in relapse. Am J Dis Child 130:937, 1976.
117. Coe FL, Favus MJ, Kathpalia SC, et al: Calcium and phosphorus metabolism in cancer: Hypercalcemic nephropathy. In Garnick MB, Rieselbach RE (eds): Cancer and the Kidney. Philadelphia, Lea & Febiger, 1982, p 427.
118. Nusynowitz ML, Frame B, Kolb FO: The spectrum of the hypoparathyroid states. Medicine 55:105, 1976.
119. Schneider AB, Sherwood LM: Pathogenesis and management of hypoparathyroidism and other hypocalcemic disorders. Metabolism 24:871, 1975.
120. Parfitt AM: The actions of parathyroid hormone on bone: relation to bone remodelling and turnover, calcium homeostasis and metabolic bone disease. II. PTH and bone cells: bone turnover and plasma calcium regulation. Metabolism 25:909, 1976.
121. Rosen JF, Markowitz ME, Smith CH, et al: 1,25-Dihydroxyvitamin D_3-treated hypoparathyroidism: 29 patient years in nine children. Pediatr Res 14:484, 1980.
122. Parfitt AM: Adult hypoparathyroidism treated with calcifediol. Arch Intern Med 138:874, 1978.
123. Arneil GC, Crosbie JC: Infantile rickets returns to Glasgow. Lancet 2:423, 1963.
124. Dent CE, Smith R: Nutritional osteomalacia. Q J Med 38:195, 1969.
125. Kulkarni PB, Hall RT, Rhodes PG, et al: Rickets in very low-birth-weight infants. J Pediatr 96:250, 1980.

Table 10B-1.
Summary Of Endocrine Changes In Malnutrition, Stress, And Renal Failure

	Malnutrition	Stress	Renal failure
Growth Hormone	↑	↑	↑
Somatomedin	↓	?	↓
Insulin			
Concentration	↓	↑	↓
Sensitivity	↓	↓	↓
Adrenocorticoids	±	↑	±
Thyroxin	↓	↑	↓
Catecholamines	±	↑	±
ADH	±	↑	

question arises as to whether these changes result simply from decreased intake, which is well documented in patients with CRF, or whether they are a more direct consequence of renal failure.

If the hormonal and resultant metabolic alterations are a consequence, simply, of decreased intake, it is necessary to postulate that renal failure per se suppresses appetite. Although release of a specific appetite suppressant by a damaged kidney cannot be excluded, appetite suppression by one or more of the many nitrogenous waste products which accumulates with renal failure seems more likely. Alternatively, the possibility must be considered that appetite suppression, reduced physical activity, and growth failure characteristic of patients with CRF are a result of the hormonal alterations. Because these alterations are the same as those associated with fasting or chronic malnutrition, this seems less likely.

Whether the hormonal changes associated with CRF are primary or secondary, growth failure may be an important part of adaptation to renal failure. Growth failure may be protective in patients with suboptimal renal function. In the face of compromised renal function, growth necessitates an increase in all metabolic processes and an overall increase in metabolic end products, which, in turn, cannot be eliminated (see also chapter 49).

Failure to understand the precise relationship between growth failure and compromised renal function may explain the lack of enthusiasm on the part of some for reversing the growth failure. If growth failure is a protective or adaptive mechanism, its reversal, particularly in a patient who is not a candidate for renal transplantation, could be detrimental. On the other hand, severe growth failure has adverse psychological effects. Thus, even if the adverse physiological effects of growth failure could be discounted, which may not be the case (20), growth failure undoubtedly affects "quality of life." Nevertheless, attempts to reverse the growth failure should be made within the context of the adaptive response to compromised renal function.

In addition to growth failure, patients with suboptimal renal function generally have high plasma concentrations of various nitrogenous waste products. Both plasma and muscle free amino acid patterns are usually deranged but these derangements are at least partially reversible with appropriate dietary management (21). Glucose concentration usually is not abnormal, although there is insulin resistance (22). In many patients, the plasma concentration of several lipid fractions is elevated along with an unusual distribution of these lipids among the lipoprotein fractions (23). Some of these changes may result from carnitine deficiency, i.e., decreased incorporation of fatty acids into mitochondria for oxidation; however, it is unlikely that carnitine deficiency is the sole explanation.

The patient with severe growth retardation secondary to chronic renal insufficiency may also have structural and functional changes in other organ systems. These changes are the same as those observed following prolonged malnutrition and have the same implications for nutritional rehabilitation of the patient with renal insufficiency as they do for rehabilitation of the malnourished or chronically starved individual.

Nutritional regimens for patients with compromised renal function, either with or without growth failure, should be designed to minimize production of nitrogenous waste products. This can be done in a number of ways. Limiting total protein intake or limiting intake of protein to those of high quality, i.e., those proteins with a high ratio of essential to nonessential amino acids, have been the most frequently used techniques. Supplementation of a limited protein intake with either a mixture of essential amino acids or a mixture of the ketoacid analogs of the essential amino acids may permit delivery of sufficient precursors to improve nutritional status (24, 25). Some advocate limiting protein intake of patients with advanced renal failure entirely to one of these preparations. The basis for use of these mixtures initially was based on the concept that provision of either essential amino acids or their organic acid analogs permits endogenous production of both essential and nonessential amino acids from nitrogenous waste products (26). Alternatively, keto-leucine may exert a direct nitrogen-sparing effect. If successful, this maneuver results in availability of sufficient essential, as well as nonessential amino acids for normal protein synthesis. Certainly, it is possible to decrease plasma urea concentrations with these regimens. However, if appreciable growth occurs, deficiency of one or more of the nonessential amino acids may develop.

Although some disease states (e.g., pulmonary disease and cardiac disease) are associated with increased energy requirements, this does not seem to be the case with renal insufficiency. In one study, patients with CRF grew at or near normal velocity when the recommended dietary allowance (RDA) of calories and protein for height was provided (26), but the degree of growth retardation did not improve significantly. In another study, giving an energy intake >80% to 100% RDA for calories did not further affect growth (28). In some instances giving supplemental calories in excess causes obesity.

References

1. Cahill GF: Starvation in man. N Engl J Med 282:668, 1970.
2. Brasel JA: Endocrine adaptation to malnutrition. Pediatr Res 14:1299, 1980.
3. Eigler N, Sacca L, Sherwin RS: Synergistic interactions of physiologic increments of glucagon, epinephrine, and cortisol in the dog. J Clin Invest 63:114, 1979.
4. Smith SR, Bledsoe T, Chhetri MK: Cortisol metabolism and the pituitary-adrenal axis in the adult with protein calorie malnutrition. J Clin Endo Metab 40:43, 1975.
5. Samuel AM, Kadival GV, Patel BD, et al: Adrenocorticoids and corticosteroid binding globulins in protein calorie malnutrition. Am J Clin Nutr 29:889, 1976.
6. Kerr DS, Stevens MCG, Robinson HM: Fasting metabolism in infants. I. Effect of severe undernutrition on energy and protein utilization. Metabolism 27:411, 1978.
7. Kerr DS, Stevens MCG, Picou DIM: Fasting metabolism in infants. II. The effect of severe undernutrition and infusion of alanine on glucose production estimated with $U^{13}C$ glucose. Metabolism 27:831–848, 1978.
8. Patrick J: Death during recovery from severe malnutrition and its possible relationship to sodium pump activity in the leukocyte. Brit Med J 1:1051, 1977.
9. Pertshuck MJ, Forster J, Buzby GP, et al: The treatment of anorexia nervosa with total parenteral nutrition. Biol Psychiatry 16:539–550, 1981.
10. Moore FD: The Metabolic Care of the Surgical Patient. Philadelphia, W.B. Saunders Co., 1959.
11. Knutrud O: The water and electrolyte metabolism in the newborn child after major surgery. Oslo, Universitetsforlaget, 1965.
12. Hinton P, Littlejohn S, Allison SP, et al: Insulin and glucose to reduce catabolic response to injury in burned patients. Lancet 1:767, 1971.
13. Robin AP, Greenwood MRC, Askanazi J, et al: Influence of total parenteral nutrition on tissue lipoprotein lipase activity during chronic and acute illness. Ann Surg 194:681, 1981.
14. Blackburn GL, Flatt GP, Clowes GHA, et al: Peripheral intravenous feeding with isotonic amino acid solution. Am J Surg 125:447, 1973.
15. Cerra FB, Mazuski JE, Chute MD, et al: Branched chain metabolic support. Ann Surg 199:286, 1984.
16. Gamble JL: Physiologic information gained from studies on the life raft ration. Harvey Lect 42:247, 1946.
17. Wolfe BM, Culebras JM, Sim AJW, et al: Substrate interaction in intravenous feeding:

Comparative effects of carbohydrate and fat on amino acid utilization in fasting man. Ann Surg 186:518–540, 1977.
18. Jeejeebhoy KN, Anderson GH, Nakhooda AF, et al: Metabolic studies in total parenteral nutrition with lipid in man. J Clin Invest 57:125–136, 1976.
19. Holliday MA, Chantler C: Metabolic and nutritional factors in children with renal insufficiency. Kidney Intl 14:306, 1978.
20. Waterlow JC: Note on the assessment and classification of protein-energy malnutrition in children. Lancet 2:87, 1973.
21. Alvestrand A, Bergstrom J, Furst P, et al: Effect of essential amino acid supplementation on muscle and plasma free amino acids in chronic uremia. Kidney Intl 14:323–329, 1978.
22. Mak RHK, Haycock GB, Chantler C: Glucose intolerance in children with chronic renal failure. Kidney Intl 24:S22, 1983.
23. Pennisi AJ, Heuser ET, Mickey MR, et al: Hyperlipidemia in pediatric hemodialysis and renal transplant patients: Associated with coronary artery disease. Am J Dis Child 130:957, 1976.
24. Kopple JD, Swendseid ME: Nitrogen balance and plasma amino acid levels in uremic patients fed an essential amino acid diet. Am J Clin Nutr 27:806, 1974.
25. Walser M, Coulter AW, Dighe S: The effect of ketoanalogues of essential amino acids in severe chronic uremia. J Clin Invest 52:678, 1973.
26. Chantler C: Nutritional therapy in children with chronic renal failure. Am J Clin Nutr 33:1682, 1980.
27. Mitch WE, Abras E, Walser M: Long-term effects of a new ketoacid-amino acid supplement in patients with chronic renal failure. Kidney Intl 22:48, 1982.
28. Arnold WC, Danford D, Holliday MA: Effects of calorie supplementation on growth in children with uremia. Kidney Intl 24:205, 1983.

10C RENAL FUNCTION IN MALNOURISHED CHILDREN

GEORGE A. O. ALLEYNE

INTRODUCTION

Malnutrition in children causes a variety of metabolic and physiological changes. Some of these changes are primary, i.e., a direct result of lack of nutrient intake, and others represent an adaptation or failure of adaptation to protein, energy, or micronutrient deficiency (1). These changes may significantly modify the expression and outcome of renal disease, and are therefore considered in detail in this section.

The anecdotal association of swelling with hunger and malnutrition goes back to Biblical times, but it was the occurrence of edema in malnourished adults that first focused serious attention on the role of the kidney in malnutrition (2). Kwashiorkor, the childhood malnutrition syndrome with edema, obviously must be associated with disturbances of salt and water metabolism, but it soon came to be recognized that marasmus, the wasting form of malnutrition, also had significant abnormalities of renal function.

The functional and morphological abnormalities will be described, as well as their relationship to the genesis of some of the clinical features of malnutrition and their possible importance in therapy.

RENAL HEMODYNAMICS

Several studies have shown that glomerular filtration rate (GFR) and renal plasma flow (RPF) are reduced irrespective of the clinical type of malnutrition. On full clinical recovery both measurements return approximately to the values found in normal children (3–5). Table 10C.1 shows data from two series, which demonstrate that in renal clearances of inulin and para-aminohippuric acid (PAH). Studies in which creatinine clearances were done indicated lower absolute values for GFR, but there was still a reduction with malnutrition (6).

The fact that GFR and RPF return to normal indicates that there is no permanent structural damage in the kidney. Cardiac output, blood pressure, and peripheral blood flow are reduced in malnourished children (3, 7, 8). When these children have gastroenteritis, there is a close relationship between systolic blood pressure and inulin and PAH clearances (9). Klahr and Alleyne (10, 11) have reviewed the factors that might contribute to the reduction in GFR and suggest that there is no single entity responsible. Although systolic blood pressure is low, plasma

Table 10C-1.
Inulin and PAH Clearances in Malnourished (Kwashiorkor) Children in Absolute Values and as a Percentage of the Values Found in Children who had Recovered

CIn	CPAH	CIn	CPAH
(Malnourished)		(As a percentage of normal)	
42.9[a]	184.0[a]	44	52
28.9[b]	130.4[b]	45	44

[a] Values given in ml/min/m^3 of weight.
[b] Values given in ml/min/m^2 of surface area.

proteins are reduced and the diminished oncotic pressure should favor increased filtration. There is also the possibility that a decrease in ultrafiltration coefficient, such as accompanies hypoproteinemia, may contribute to a decrease in GFR as it does in rats (12). The reduction in GFR is not of the magnitude to produce any increase in nitrogen retention. Indeed, because of reduced protein intake and decreased muscle mass, plasma urea and creatinine concentrations are lower in malnourished children.

TUBULAR FUNCTION

It is a constant finding that malnourished children produce a dilute urine and cannot concentrate it to the same degree as healthy children (5, 13). In some, there is a loss of the diurnal rhythm, and the urine shows no peak in osmolality at night. In Jamaican malnourished children the mean urine osmolality was 238 mOsm/kg on admission and 459 mOsm/kg on recovery. When pitressin tannate was given intramuscularly, there was an increase in urine concentration in both groups of children, but it was still less than in the malnourished ones (Table 10C.2). Similar data have also been shown from Uganda (13).

The cause of the concentrating defect is almost certainly a lack of medullary solute. If there were impaired loop transport, both dilution and concentration should be affected, but at least in adult malnutrition, this does not occur. McCance and coworkers (13) have shown that administration of urea to malnourished children leads to an increase in the ability to concentrate the urine. An improvement in maximum urine concentration has been shown in normal subjects taking a low protein diet who were fed urea (14) and in protein-depleted rats given urea supplements. In the rats, the increased urine concentration was associated with an increase in urea concentration in renal papillary structures (15).

Blood pH and plasma bicarbonate concentration in malnourished children are usually normal, but the children are unable to excrete an acid load (5). In seven children studied by Smith (16), the minimum urine pH was 6.28 after an ammonium chloride load, compared with a value of 5.36 after recovery. Subsequent studies in Jamaica confirmed these findings (5) and showed that total hydrogen ion excretion after ammonium chloride increased progressively with recovery from malnutrition. Low levels of titratable acid were a constant finding and ammonium excretion as a fraction of total hydrogen ion excreted tended to be higher in malnutrition than on recovery, although the absolute ammonium excretion was reduced.

The cause of the acidification defect is not clear. The reduction in the titratable acid is a result both of the failure to acidify and the reduced availability of buffer, principally phosphate (17). The reduced ammonia production may be a result of a combination of hemodynamic and metabolic factors. The increased contribution of ammonium to acid excretion in malnutrition could be the result of potassium depletion (18–20), which has been shown to be associated with increased renal ammoniagenic capacity at least in animals (21). Florid renal tubular acidosis occurs infrequently in malnutrition and clears with recovery.

Table 10C-2.
Urine Concentrating Capacity of Jamaican Children While Malnourished and After Recovery[a]

Children (N = 15)	Urine osmolality (mOsm/kg)	
	Control	After 1 U pitressin IM
Malnourished	238 ± 37	476 ± 37
Recovered	459 ± 59	690 ± 41

[a] Values are means ± SEM for the 15 observations.

CLINICAL SEQUELAE OF CHANGES IN RENAL FUNCTION

The changes in GFR or RPF per se may have no immediate sequelae, but the sum total of the renal disturbances could contribute to some of the clinical aspects of malnutrition. One of the noticeable features of severe malnutrition is generalized edema, which implies sodium retention. Frequently, total body water (TBW) and extracellular fluid are increased in edematous malnourished children (22–24). The same claim was made for marasmic children, but Patrick and coworkers (25) reviewed the data on body water and showed that it was normal in marasmus and increased only when the children were placed on a high energy intake (25). In the first two weeks of the recovery phase, TBW increased and then fell steadily with recovery. These data may simply reflect the slowness of recovery of the renal function. With institution of feeding and increased sodium and water intakes, it is likely that TBW will increase if there is impaired renal function. The distribution of the body water will obviously depend on the relative intakes of salt and water intake.

In one series of eight nonedematous children who were studied sequentially, there were three who had repeated measurements within 2 weeks of admission; in two, there was <10% increase in the GFR (26). It has been emphasized that high sodium intakes in the recovery phase of malnutrition may lead to cardiac failure (27, 28). Nichols and coworkers (29) on the basis of careful balance studies have shown that the malnourished child is in a similar state to one with immature renal function in whom there is a solute diuresis causing obligatory losses of sodium (29). In spite of this obligatory sodium loss, the kidney still does not have the capacity to cope with markedly increased sodium and water intake.

The most significant functional disturbance is the inability to concentrate urine. This may be the reason why diarrhea is so dangerous in malnourished children and is best illustrated by the data in Table 10C.3. A normal child of 9.0 kg with a dietary intake that provides a solute load of 144 mOsm can pass urine with an osmolality of about 300 mOsm/kg. A malnourished child of about the same weight may pass a urine of a slightly lower osmolality because, in general, the insensible water loss is usually less (29).

The clinical observation is that malnourished children normally have polyuria and hyposthenuria. If a normal child has a fecal loss of 250 ml, urine needs to be concentrated to about 700 mOsm/kg to remain in water balance with the same intake. This degree of urine concentration is quite within the child's capacity. However, for a malnourished child in the same situation, a urine concentration of about 600 mOsm/kg would be required, which is virtually impossible. The actual situation is that the child, even under this kind of stress, passes urine concentrated

Table 10C-3.
Theoretical Water Balance in a Normal and a Malnourished Child: Effect of Diarrhea

	Normal (Diarrhea)		Malnourished (Diarrhea)	
Weight (kg)	9.0	9.0	9.0	9.0
Intake (ml)	900	900	900	900
Solute load (mOsm)	144	144	144	144
Insensible loss (ml)	450	450	400	400
Diarrhea loss (ml)	–	250	–	250
Urine volume (ml)	450	200	500	250
Urine osmolality (mOsm/kg)	320	720	288	576

to no more than 300 mOsm/kg. To excrete 144 mOsm of solute at a concentration of 300 mOsm/kg he needs a urine volume of 480 ml, which would lead to a total water deficit of 230 ml. This inability to concentrate urine partly explains why the combination of diarrhea and malnutrition together account for so many deaths.

EFFECT OF MALNUTRITION ON RENAL DEVELOPMENT AND MORPHOLOGY

With malnutrition, the kidney in general wastes much less than other tissues (30). It is only in very severe malnutrition that the weights of the kidneys are less than in relatively well nourished children (31). There are also no major changes in electrolyte composition of the kidney in malnutrition (32).

Renal histology has not shown any specific lesion characteristic of malnutrition. Autopsy studies show capsular epithelial cell swelling and, on occasion, cortical calcinosis (33, 34). The most detailed histological study on renal biopsies has shown cloudy swelling of tubular cells and occasional increased glomerular cellularity (35), all of which disappear with recovery. The idea that there are minor glomerular lesions in malnutrition is supported by the finding of increased protein concentration in the urine of severely ill children (36). There was more proteinuria in children with kwashiorkor than with marasmus; really severe proteinuria was a sign of a bad prognosis. The authors proposed that the proteinuria is glomerular rather than tubular because of the absence of globulins, particularly the beta-2 globulins. Proteinuria disappeared as clinical recovery occurred.

LONG TERM RENAL SEQUELAE OF MALNUTRITION

There is no direct evidence that malnutrition leads to increased prevalence of chronic renal disease in later life. It is attractive to theorize that the increased prevalence of chronic renal disease in adults in the developing world is somehow linked to malnutrition and not only to parasitic infectious diseases. However, there are no good supporting data. What is needed is a follow-up of adults who have been documented as being malnourished as children to determine if there is evidence of incipient or established renal disease.

References

1. Alleyne GAO, Hay RW, Picou DI, et al: Protein-energy Malnutrition, London, Edward Arnold, 1977.
2. McCance RA: Studies in undernutrition, Wuppertal 1946–1949. Medical Research Council (Britain), Special Report series No. 275. H.M. Stationery Office, 1951.
3. Kerpel-Fronius E, Varga F, Kun K, et al: The relationship between circulation and kidney function in infantile dehydration and malnutrition. Acta Med Acad Sci Hung 5:27, 1954.
4. Gordillo A, Soto RA, Metcoff J, et al: Intracellular composition and homeostatic mechanisms in severe chronic infantile malnutrition. III. Renal adjustments. Pediatrics 20:303, 1957.
5. Alleyne GAO: The effect of severe protein calorie malnutrition on the renal function of Jamaican children. Pediatrics 39:400, 1967.
6. Arroyave G, Wilson D, Behar M, et al: Serum and urinary creatinine in children with severe protein malnutrition. Am J Clin Nutr 9:176, 1961.
7. Alleyne GAO: Cardiac function in severely malnourished Jamaican children. Clin Sci 30:553, 1966.
8. Brooke OG, Harris M, Salvosa C: The response of malnourished babies to cold. J Physiol 233:75, 1973.
9. Garrow JG, Smith R, Ward EE: Electrolyte Metabolism in Severe Infantile Malnutrition. Oxford, Pergamon Press, 1968.
10. Klahr S, Alleyne GAO: Effects of chronic protein-calorie malnutrition on the kidney. Kidney Intl 3:129, 1973.
11. Klahr S, Alleyne GAO: Nutrition and the kidney. In Suki WS, Eknoyan G (eds): The Kidney in Systemic Disease. New York, John Wiley & Sons, 1981.
12. Baylis C, Ichikawa I, Willis WT, et al: Dynamics of glomerular ultrafiltration. IX. Effects of plasma protein concentration. Am J Physiol 232:F58, 1977.
13. McCance RA, Crowne RS, Hall TS: The effect of malnutrition and food habits on the concentrating power of the kidney. Clin Sci 37:471, 1969.
14. Levinsky NG, Berliner RW: The role of urea in the urine concentrating mechanism. J Clin Invest 38:741, 1959.
15. Pennel JP, Sanjana V, Frey NR, et al: The effect of urea infusion on the urinary concentrating mechanism in protein depleted rats. J Clin Invest 55:399, 1975.
16. Smith R: Urinary acidification defect in chronic infantile malnutrition. Lancet 1:764, 1959.
17. Waterlow JC, Wills VA: Balance studies in malnourished Jamaican infants. I. Absorption and retention of nitrogen and phosphorus. Brit J Nutr 14:183, 1960.
18. Smith R, Waterlow JC: Total exchangeable potassium in infantile malnutrition. Lancet 1:147, 1960.
19. Garrow JS: Total body potassium in kwashiorkor and marasmus. Lancet 2:455, 1965.
20. Alleyne GAO, Millward DJ, Scullard GH: Total body potassium, muscle electrolytes and glycogen in malnourished children. J Pediatr 76:75, 1970.
21. Tannen RL: Relationship of renal ammonium production and potassium homeostasis. Kidney Intl 11:453, 1976.
22. Smith R: Total body water in malnourished infants. Clin Sci 19:275, 1960.
23. Brinkman GL, Bowie MD, Friis-Hansen B, et al: Body water composition in kwashiorkor before and after loss of edema. Pediatrics 36:94, 1965.
24. Alleyne GAO: Studies on total body potassium in infantile malnutrition. The relation to body fluid spaces and urinary creatinine. Clin Sci 34:199, 1968.
25. Patrick J, Reeds PJ, Jackson AA, et al: Total body water in malnutrition: The possible role of energy intake. Brit J Nutr 39:417, 1978.
26. Alleyne GAO: Renal and cardiac function in severely malnourished Jamaican children. Dissertation, London, 1965.
27. Viteri F, Behar M, Arroyave G, et al: Clinical aspects of protein malnutrition. In Munro HN, Allison JB (eds): Mammalian Protein Metabolism New York, Academic Press, 1964, vol 2, p 523.
28. Wharton BA, Howells GR, McCance RA: Cardiac failure in kwashiorkor. Lancet 2:384, 1967.
29. Nichols BL, Alvarado J, Rodriguez J, et al: Therapeutic implications of electrolyte water and nitrogen losses during recovery from protein calorie malnutrition. J Pediatr 84:759, 1974.
30. Waterlow JC, Cravioto J, Stephen JML: Protein malnutrition in man. Adv Protein Chem 15:131, 1960.
31. Morrison EY, Alleyne GAO: Malnutrition, kidney size and composition. Arch Latinoam Nutr 26:7, 1970.
32. Alleyne GAO, Holladay D, Waterlow JC, et al: Chemical composition of organs of children who died from malnutrition. Brit J Nutr 23:783, 1969.
33. Bras J, Waterlow JC, De Pass E: Further observations on the liver pancreas and kidney in malnourished infants and children. The relation of certain histopathological changes in the pancreas and those in liver and kidney. West Ind Med J 6:33, 1957.
34. Stirling GA: Renal pathology in malnourished infants. Arch Dis Childh 37:378, 1962.
35. Dayal RS, Lathra UK, Kalra K, et al: Renal biopsy in malnourished children. Indian Pediatr 7:596, 1970.
36. Said A, El-Hawary MFS, Sakr R, et al: Protein-calorie malnutrition in Egypt. Immuno-electrophoretic studies on urinary proteins. Am J Clin Nutr 26:1355, 1973.

CHAPTER 11

FLUID AND NUTRITION THERAPY

From the Perspective of Body Composition

MALCOLM A. HOLLIDAY

INTRODUCTION

Fluid and nutrition therapy traditionally is conceived to maintain or restore body composition to normal. The replacement of normal or abnormal losses of water and electrolyte to maintain body composition is maintenance therapy. Similarly, the replacement of substrate (carbohydrate, fat, protein, and vitamins) used in metabolism is maintenance therapy. Usually, average values for maintenance therapy can be used. When this is not the case, e.g., in renal failure, maintenance therapy must be adjusted accordingly. It may be half of average, but it is not half of maintenance as is often stated. Deficit therapy is that used to restore established losses. A decreased circulating volume is the most obvious and urgent deficit to correct. Specific deficits of water, NaCl, K, and alkali are other examples; correcting malnutrition is another form of deficit therapy.

Two models for planning fluid and nutrition therapy were described in Chapter 1, Fig 1.2: (1) the input-ECF-output model, and (2) the intake-body composition-excretion model. The latter is more obviously applicable to fluid and nutrition therapy, since intake provided by prescription affects body composition; excretion should appropriately respond to change in composition so that balance is preserved or a desired change in body composition occurs. The first—the input-ECF-output model—uses the composition of ECF (plasma) and urine as measured in the laboratory and intake data to derive an estimate of the exchanges that take place between cells and ECF and the net retention of fluid and electrolyte.

The controls over electrolyte, water, acid-base balance, and mineral metabolism are described in detail in Chapters 6 to 9, and nutrient requirements are described in Chapter 10.

The concept of deficit therapy was developed in the early part of this century and was the sole function of parenteral fluid therapy initially. Experience with replacement of body fluids lost as a result of diarrhea was first reported by Thomas Latta in 1831 in treatment of victims of cholera (1). His therapy was well conceived and very successful, as he himself notes:

> . . . A female, aged 50, very destitute, but previously in good health, was seized with cholera in its most violent form, and by half-past nine was reduced to a most hopeless state. The pulse was quite gone, even in the axilla, and strength so much exhausted, that I had resolved not to try the effects of the injection, conceiving the poor woman's case to be hopeless, and that the failure of the experiment might afford the prejudiced and the illiberal an opportunity to stigmatise the practice; however, I at length thought I would give her a chance, and in the presence of Drs. Lewins and Craigie, and Messrs. Sibson and Peterson, I injected one hundred and twenty ounces, when like the effects of magic, instead of the pallid aspect of one whom death had sealed as his own, the vital tide was restored, and life and vivacity returned; but diarrhoea recurred, and in three hours she again sunk. One hundred and twenty ounces more were injected with the same good effects. In this case 330 ounces were so used in twelve hours, when reaction was completely re-established; and in forty-eight hours she smoked her pipe free from distemper."

However, the importance of his therapy was lost until the early years of this century when the value of replacement therapy, i.e., the restoration of ECF volume lost as a result of infantile diarrhea was rediscovered (2). Attempts in 1917 to reverse the high mortality of infants with diarrheal dehydration, by infusing $NaHCO_3$ solution to correct the acidosis, were unsuccessful. Although the acidosis was corrected, the mortality remained >80% (3). Shortly afterward, nine infants with diarrheal dehydration were successfully treated by giving them isotonic NaCl solution intraperitoneally. This experience established the value of restoring ECF volume to normal and showed that Cl as well as Na was important to achieve this goal (2).

The concept of maintenance parenteral fluid therapy developed more slowly. As parenteral fluid therapy was extended from a single injection of fluid to correct a deficit to therapy over several days, the value of giving patients free water, glucose, and some NaCl parenterally in place of oral intake was appreciated. The effect of simple fasting on body fluid volume and composition was detailed by Gamble in 1923 (4). From this work, the basis for a maintenance regimen was developed. Darrow, linking the loss of K noted in diarrheal disease, with the reduction of K in muscle in experimental K deficiency, recognized the value of K in parenteral fluid therapy both as replacement and maintenance (5). The concept of maintenance therapy was introduced to describe the fluid, electrolyte (Na, Cl, and K), and glucose needed to replace concurrent losses of body fluids to prevent change in body fluid composition.

Restoration of body composition to normal also is accomplished by diuretics and dialysis. Diuretics remove edema fluid; dialysis and ultrafiltration remove electrolyte and other products whose retention distorts body composition and function. Body composition in these instances is restored by "removal" therapy.

This chapter reviews methods for quantifying and evaluating fluid and nutrition therapy for maintenance and deficit therapy and comments on the use of diuretics and dialysis.

MAINTENANCE THERAPY

Maintenance therapy was developed into formulations to equal or exceed anticipated losses. The losses of water, NaCl, and K that accompanied fasting were predominately renal excretory losses. The effect of giving glucose to fasting adults was to reduce losses of water, NaCl, and K. The study by Gamble during World War II to define ideal rations for life-raft survivors showed that glucose paid its way (6) (Fig. 11.1). The effect of glucose was better understood when the metabolic response to starvation was described. Giving glucose prevented response to fasting that used amino acids as substrate for gluconeogenesis (7).

Talbott and his colleagues showed that maintenance requirements could be effectively met by giving an excess of fluid and electrolyte over minimum losses. The model they described anticipated that "homeostatic mechanisms," i.e., mechanisms for excreting excess, were intact and would maintain normal body composition in response to excess intake. This approach made the problem of planning parenteral fluid therapy simpler by establishing averages well within the generous "homeostatic limits" for the normal individual. The effects of specific diseases to narrow or change these limits, because the disease affected homeostatic mechanisms, was appreciated and specific recommendations were made that were tailored to these diseases, e.g., renal disease and nephrogenic diabetes insipidus (8).

Adults

The average recommendations for water, NaCl, and K for adults are given in Table 11.1. The controls that regulate excretion are the subjects of Chapters 6 to 8. When disease impairs these controls, the average still may suffice. In some instances, more than the average may be needed; in other cases, the minimum or close to it may best match loss because controls to excrete the excess are lost. Replacement of losses from nasogastric suction and losses that occur in salt-wasting states or renal tubular acidosis (RTA) (chapter 34) are examples of the former; reduced renal perfusion and reduced excretory capacity of end stage renal disease (ESRD) are examples of the latter.

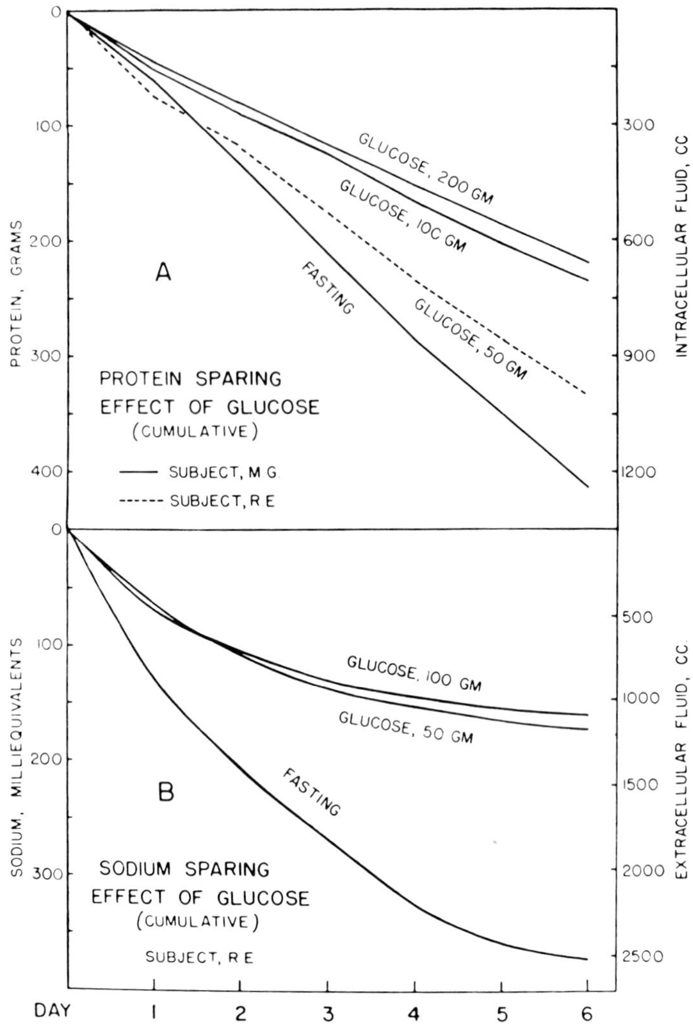

Figure 11.1. The effect of glucose on N and Na loss in normal men deprived of food. (From Gamble J: *Harvey Lect Ser* 42:247, 1946.)

Table 11.1.
Maintenance Requirements for Adults

	Minimum	Average	Supplemental
Free water (ml/da)	500–1000[a]	2000–3000	(replacement)[b]
NaCl (mEq/da)	0 plus[c]	60–90	(0.45–0.9% saline)[d]
K (mEq/da)	0 plus[e]	40–60	80–120[f]
Glucose (g/da)	100–150[g]	100–150[g]	≫200[h]

[a] For oliguria of renal failure; poor perfusion; SIADH.
[b] Excess free water to replace losses in diabetes insipidus or nephrogenic diabetes insipidus; oral replacement or replacement by nasogastric tube is recommended.
[c] In hypertension heart failure or renal failure with ECF volume overload no NaCl is needed.
[d] Replacement of GI or other losses, 0.45 to 0.9% saline often is appropriate.
[e] With hyperkalemia no K is needed. Hyperkalemia may be a result of renal failure, aldosterone deficiency, including the adrenogenital syndrome, rhabdomyolysis, or severe acidosis.
[f] To treat K deficiency.
[g] To suppress gluconeogenesis, the maintenance water given as 5% glucose meets requirement.
[h] In stress with insulin resistance or to meet total calorie needs; in the first instance, insulin (0.2 U/g glucose) may be needed.

Failure to anticipate these exceptions and to adjust therapy accordingly leads to needless and sometimes harmful morbidity in critical care medicine. For example, care in tailoring NaCl intake to excretory capacity reduces the incidence of ECF volume overload and its consequences, edema, hypertension, heart failure, or pulmonary edema. Adjustment of water intake to avoid hyponatremia or, less commonly, hypernatremia reduces the potential for their adverse effects. In their more obvious forms, both hypo- and hypernatremia cause brain injury and convulsions. The consequences of lesser degrees of hyponatremia have never been examined and generally are treated as inconsequential; however, hyponatremia can and should be avoided. Hypernatremia, similarly, should be avoided. The fact that we observe no obvious harm from hyponatremia seems poor justification for allowing it to develop when elaborate physiological controls so successfully avoid its occurrence in normal individuals in the face of extreme changes in salt and water intake. The complexity of the controls that sustain the concentration of Na within such a narrow range, despite great changes in intake of water and NaCl, argues that the maintenance of normal Na concentration in ECF, itself has important survival value (chapter 6).

Sodium Chloride

The selection of average, minimal, or supplemental NaCl intake usually can be made from clinical evaluation of the state of ECF volume and renal excretory capacity. Reevaluation of the status of the effective plasma and interstitial fluid (ISF) volume is important in appraising the correctness of the original decision. Before maintenance therapy can be projected in some special cases, deficits of ECF have to be corrected. The range for maintenance NaCl is from zero to intakes 5 to 10 times recommendation. During parenteral fluid therapy when NaCl and water requirements are average, the average maintenance intake for NaCl is met when the maintenance water requirement is given as 0.2% to 0.3% NaCl; when requirement exceeds the average because of NaCl losses, the additional NaCl usually is given as 0.45% to 0.9% NaCl. When no NaCl should be given, maintenance water requirement is given as dextrose and water.

Water

The selection of average minimal or supplemental free water intake also can be made from clinical observations. Giving free water in excess of excretory capacity causes dilutional hyponatremia. Excretory capacity is reduced when ECF volume is contracted or ESRD limits free excretion; it is also reduced in the presence of head injuries, obtunded states, increased intrathoracic pressure imposed by mechanical respirators, and the syndrome of inappropriate secretion of antidiuretic hormone (SIADH). When any of these occur, minimum free water is indicated.

Giving inadequate free water causes hypernatremia. This occurs in obtunded patients whose water intake is restricted inadvertently, particularly if they are undergoing an osmotic diuresis (chapter 6).

Potassium

The minimum requirement for K in normal adults is that required to replace obligatory renal and nonrenal losses, usually this is small when compared with the average intake.

For those individuals who have no excretory capacity or who are at risk to hyperkalemia for other causes, withholding K altogether may be appropriate. For individuals who lack excretory capacity but are wasted and are made anabolic by nutritional support, or who are K-deficient and are able to replenish cell K losses, the provision of K in carefully measured amounts monitored by following K_s is appropriate.

When none of these conditions are present, giving K at average levels is safe. For those with renal K wasting from aggressive diuretic therapy or from renal injury secondary to amphotericin, it is safer to give K at relatively steady rates rather than in bolus injections. Practical problems of venous sclerosis or acute hyperkalemia arise from high concentrations of K in infusion fluids that are improperly mixed, from injecting concentrated KCl into the burette of a delivery system, or from using "high-K" solutions to flush the tubing.

Acid-base

Acid-base status in adults usually is governed by internal metabolic events; variations in net acid intake per se are seldom causes of disturbance in ECF acid-base status. In the usual metabolic state, net acid input from metabolism is 1 mEq/kg/day for adults (chapter 34). Net acid intake is neutral or slightly negative. With conventional intakes and normal metabolism, acid-base status is preserved because net acid excretion balances input (metabolism plus intake). The reserve to increase net acid or base excretion is considerable (chapter 8). Therefore, no maintenance therapy for alkali is needed. When organic acid input is greatly increased, as in lactic or other organic acidemias, when losses of alkaline gastrointestinal fluid are copious, or when either RTA or CRF decrease the capacity to excrete net acid input, maintenance alkali is needed (Na + K) − Cl should be sufficient to maintain total CO_2 as normal. Loss of acid, leading to alkalosis, occurs when HCl is removed from the stomach or when NaCl is removed and is replaced with $NaHCO_3$. In both instances, ECF volume contraction is present. Giving Cl as NaCl to replace losses suffices.

Calcium and Phosphorus

Ca is infrequently given with intravenous solutions as "maintenance calcium." At concentrations suitable to deliver the daily recommended levels, Ca in intravenous solutions often precipitates. Furthermore, the control of serum Ca is regulated by many factors that affect distribution of Ca between bone and ECF so that short term intake usually is not important in the maintenance of serum Ca. Similarly, P generally is not included in maintenance fluid therapy. Both Ca and P are given intravenously with parenteral nutrition therapy. The recommended intake of Ca is 3 to 6 mg/kg/day, of P 10 to 20 mg/kg/day for parenteral fluid therapy (9). These intakes are inadequate for long term therapy.

Carbohydrate and Calories

Carbohydrate provides glucose as substrate for brain, red cells, and a few other specialized tissues; of these, the brain is the largest by far. For adults, this requirement is met by 100 to 150 g glucose/day. When 5% dextrose is used to meet the average maintenance requirements for water (2 to 3 L/day) this amount of glucose is provided. The 340 to 510 kcal derived from this glucose prevents ketosis, but is below maintenance calories.

For hospitalized women, maintenance calories are approximately 2000 kcal/day and for men are approximately 2500 kcal/day, i.e., about 35 kcal/kg/day for each. Calorie intake may be increased by changing the dextrose concentration of the maintenance fluids from 5% to 12.5%, the maximum concentration that can be given in peripheral veins without causing sclerosis. Forty to 50 ml/kg/day of 12.5% dextrose will deliver about 20 kcal/kg/day or between 60% to 70% maintenance calories. This is sufficient to prevent significant malnutrition in previously well-nourished patients treated for short-term illnesses. Giving calories at maintenance level means giving supplemental calories as intravenous fat or delivery of hypertonic dextrose through a central line or larger volumes of 12.5% glucose through a peripheral line; when more calories are given amino acids should be given as parenteral nutrition therapy. Some type of enteral feeding usually can be used instead; when this is practical, it is recommended.

Protein

The recommended intake for average biological value protein is 0.8 g/kg/day for both men and women, which, when delivered with recommended calorie intake, is 8% to 10% of calories as protein (10). It is not common practice to attempt to give this amount as amino acids parenterally unless long-term parenteral nutrition therapy or treatment of malnutrition is deemed desirable. This is usually done when the need for parenteral fluid therapy exceeds 5 to 10 days or when there are clinical signs of malnutrition. The range of calories as amino acids has varied between 10% to 20% of total calories given when partial or fully adequate parenteral nutrition therapy is planned; there is little reason to recommend amino acid intakes that are >12% of calories as amino acids. For patients with CRF, 8% calories as amino acids is recommended (11).

Infants and Children

The maintenance fluid and nutritional needs of infants and children tend to vary as a function of metabolic activity. Deficit therapy usually is expressed in relation to body weight. Metabolic activity of infants and children traditionally has been expressed as a function of body surface area. Traditionally, parenteral fluid therapy is related to 1 m^2; renal function, e.g., GFR, and renal blood flow (RBF) is related to 1.73 m^2. Metabolic activity either as basal metabolic rate (BMR) or average hospital metabolic rate (AMR) can be derived from an empirical relation that exists between body weight and BMR and AMR that is easily remembered (12). The unit of reference for AMR is 100 kcal. From 3 to 10 kg, the AMR is 100 kcal/kg. From 10 to 20 kg, the increment is 100 kcal for each 2 kg. In women from 20 to 45 kg, the increment is 100 kcal for each 5 kg, reaching a plateau at 2000 kcal (Fig. 11.2, *A*). For men the same relation, 100 kcal for each 5 kg, holds to 70 kg or 2500 kcal (Fig. 11.2, *B*). These lie between the minimum and median RDA for calories (Figs. 11.2, *A* and 2, *B*). GFR is 4 ml/100 kcal from 1 to 2 years of age or from 10 kg on (12). When the homeostatic limits for water, NaCl, and K were defined for children and adults, the limits and the averages, related to surface area, were constant. Before 1 year of age, the values are lower (Fig. 11.2, *C*). In this period energy metabolism per unit surface area varies significantly from the constant value noted after that period (Fig. 11.3). Renal function and the capacity to excrete free water is constant after 1 to 2 years of age when related to surface area. In the first year of life, renal function and free water clearance related to either 100 kcal or to surface area is less. The maximum capacity for free water intake is correspondingly reduced.

Water

The maintenance need for water is a function of energy metabolism (Table 11.2). The insensible water loss (ILW) dissipates 25% of heat

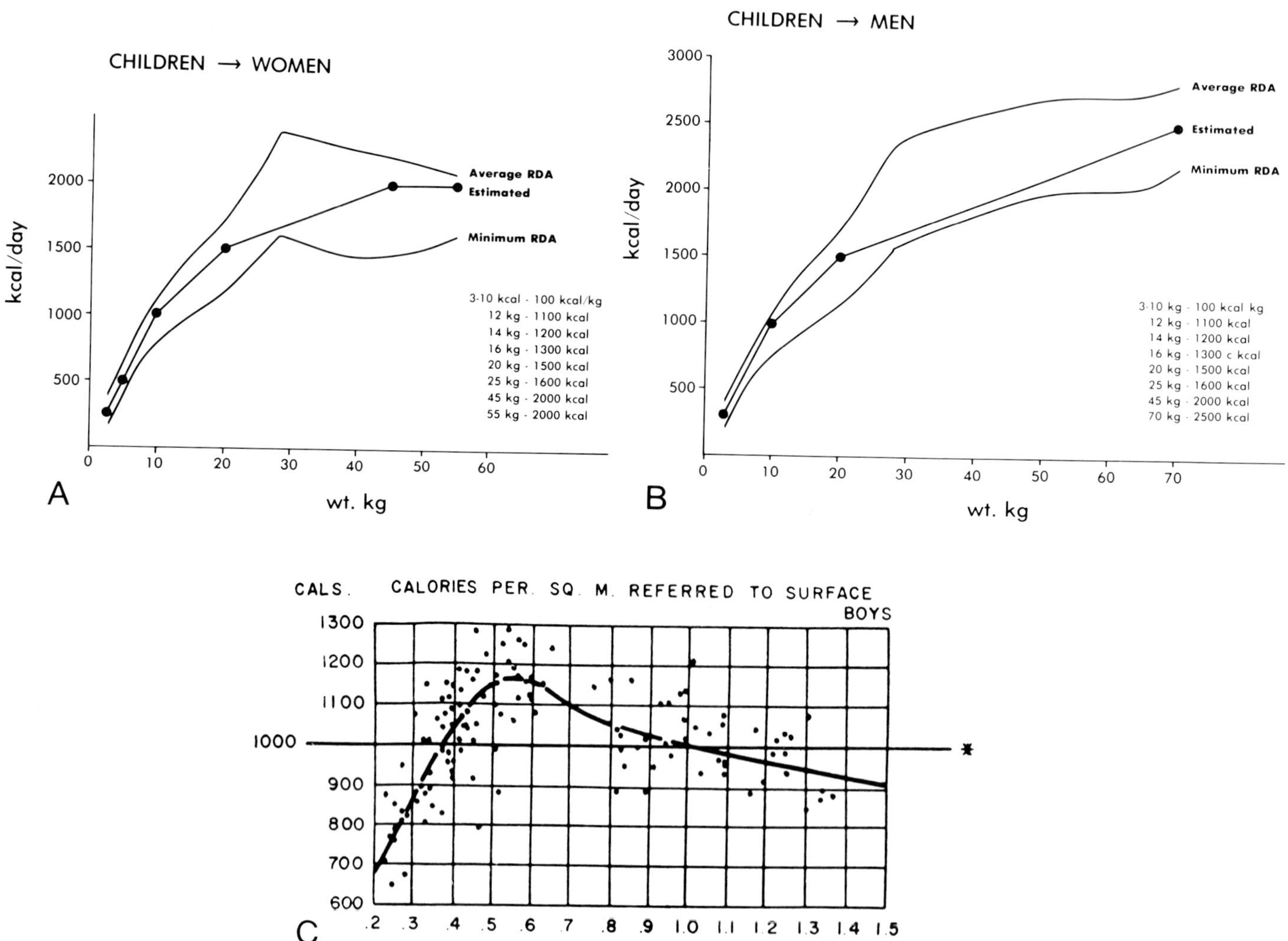

Figure 11.2. Relation of estimated calorie expenditure for hospitalized patients with the RDA average and minimum. **A**, Women; **B**, Men; **C**, Infants. (From Latta T: *Lancet* 2:274, 1965; Bier DM, et al: *Diabetes* 26:1016, 1977.)

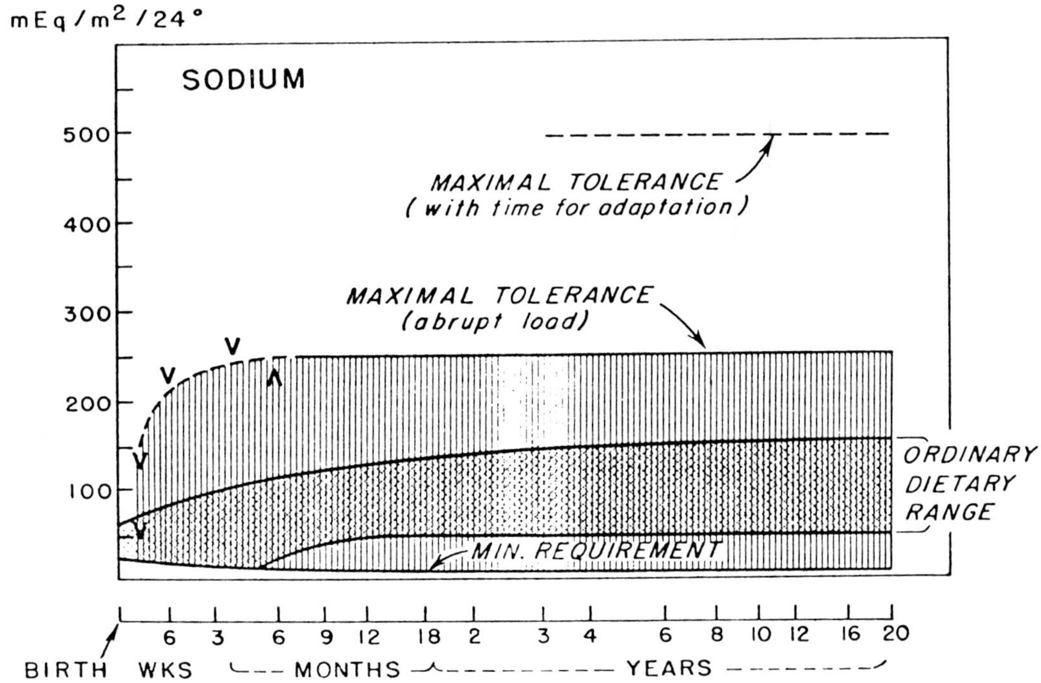

Figure 11.3. Homeostatic limits to maintenance Na requirement from infancy through maturity related to surface area. (From Talbott NB, et al: *N Engl J Med* 248:1100, 1953.)

Table 11.2.
Maintenance Water and Electrolyte Requirement per 100 kcal

Water	Anuria	Minimal	Average	Exceptional
IWL[a]	40	40	40	0–80[b]
Water of oxidation[c]	−15	−15	−15	−15
Urinary water excretion	0	25[d]	75	>75[e]
GI fluid loss (as measured)	—	—	—	
	25	50	100	
NaCl mEq/100 kcal	0	[f]	3	[g]
K	0	[f]	2	[g]

[a] 25% calories dissipated by IWL; 0.58 kcal/g water = 40 ml/100 kcal.
[b] Minimal with certain mechanical respirators; increased with dry heat application.
[c] Water derived from oxidation of carbohydrate and fat to yield 100 kcal.
[d] When average solute load is excreted at 1200 to 1400 mOsm/kg.
[e] When urinary free water or NaCl plus high water loss is due to tubular dysfunction.
[f] Depending on status, may be zero.
[g] Depending on concurrent losses.

production or calorie expenditure under a wide variety of clinical conditions. The IWL/100 kcal, accordingly, is derived from this relation and the heat dissipated by evaporation of 1 g water, 0.58 kcal, as follows:

$$\text{IWL/100 kcal} = \frac{0.25 \times 100}{0.58} = 40 \text{ g or ml} \qquad (1)$$

The water of oxidation is water yielded in the metabolic process of carbohydrate and fat oxidation. For each 100 kcal derived from oxidation, 15 g or ml of water result.

Urinary water loss (UWL) is the volume of urine anticipated when average maintenance is given. If urinary solute excretion is average then the urine is isoosmotic, 300 mOsm/kg and urine volume equals C_{Osm}. This projection gives room for higher or lower solute loads to be excreted as concentrated or dilute urine, respectively. It also provides excess water to replace extra nonrenal losses of water (12).

When the renal response to water intake is impaired so that urine is excreted at maximal concentration, the maximum rate of water excretion is 25 ml/100 kcal and the total maintenance requirement is half of average. When there is obligatory polyuria, intake must be adjusted to excretion (chapter 6).

Sodium Chloride and Potassium

It is convenient to define average recommended NaCl and K intakes in relation to fluid administered, because maintenance fluids usually are made to a consistent concentration and the recommendations fit well within the ranges of tolerance (Table 11.2). Exceptions require solutions of different composition, e.g., as described for adults (Table 11.2).

When plasma is used to replace copious losses of pleural or peritoneal protein-rich fluid in newborns, the Cl content of this replacement plasma may be inadequate, owing to the dilution of plasma with Na citrate. Contraction alkalosis results. Giving extra (0.9%) NaCl will correct the Cl deficiency (chapter 8).

Carbohydrate, Calories, and Protein

The maintenance requirement for glucose is proportional to brain metabolism which, from term birth on, is proportional to brain size (13) (Table 11.3). Brain metabolism in the neonate is proportionally greater; therefore, the quantity of glucose needed to prevent ketosis and gluconeogenesis is correspondingly increased (14). The high calorie intake and the high percentage of calories provided as carbohydrate in human milk provides the carbohydrate used in brain metabolism under normal feeding conditions.

The relation of the maintenance requirement for calories in infants and children to body weight has been described (p. 176). During the first 4 months of life a significant fraction of calorie intake is stored as body fat. Meeting the RDA is necessary for this normal gain in body fat to occur; it is also important in using dietary protein to support a gain in

Table 11.3.
Glucose Requirement Related to Brain Size and Body Weight

Body weight (kg)	Brain weight (gm)	Glucose needed (gm/da)	(gm/kg/da)
3.5	475	35	10
5.5	650	48	8.5
11.0	1045	78	7
19.0	1235	92	5
30.0	1350	100	3
50.0	1360	101	2
70.0	1400	103	1.5

Table 11.4.
Solutions Used to Replace ECF Volume

Solutions	Na	Cl	K	Glucose
IV				
0.9% saline	154	154	0	—
Ringers lactate	130	109	4	—
0.45% saline (l L) + 50 mM $NaHCO_3$	121	73	—	—[a]
Oral rehydration				
WHO	90	80	20	2%
Commercial—Pedialyte-RS[R]	60	60	15	2.5%

[a] May have 5% glucose.

muscle protein during this period. Growth in stature is sensitive to calorie intake throughout childhood. When calorie intake is provided by parenteral or enteral nutrition, change in weight is a useful guide. When it is given for long periods, growth in stature and change in skinfold thickness are reliable signs of adequacy.

The normal requirement for protein is influenced by the calories available (chapter 10). With adequate calorie intake, infants will grow normally when given 1.4 g/kg/day or 5% to 6% of calories as protein, which is comparable in quality to human milk protein (15). However, it has been the practice to recommend 2.5 to 3.0 g/kg/day of protein for infants and children on parenteral nutrition regimens (16), i.e., 12 to 15% of calories are provided as protein (chapter 10).

Calcium and Phosphorus

The recommended intake for Ca for both infants and children on parenteral nutrition therapy is 20 to 80 mg/kg/day (10). The broad range is necessary to deal with the uncertainty of compatibility of Ca with P salts in intravenous solutions; Ca as gluconate may be incompatible at the higher levels when P is used in solutions. On the other hand, infants rapidly mineralizing bone may need Ca at higher levels and P or alkali may have to be omitted from alternate solutions so that Ca can be given. The recommended intake for P is 25 to 40 mg/kg/day. The lower figure for P corresponds to that recommended for infant formulas (17), the higher figure for parenteral nutrition (16). The Ca:P ratio should be 2:1 when formulas are given to growing children, and at least 1:1 when formulas are given to children and adults.

Special Cases

Although homeostatic mechanisms usually regulate excretion to balance intake when it is given in excess of minimum, some conditions call for water intake that is minimal. When this happens, it is usually appropriate to reduce the maintenance intake of NaCl and K proportionally, or more. Often the conditions which call for reduced water intake also call for limitation or omission of NaCl and K, e.g., renal failure. When poor perfusion secondary to ECF contraction is the reason, rapid expansion of ECF with appropriate NaCl solutions (Table 11.4) is indicated.

When urine output exceeds average, as often occurs with recovery from acute renal failure, it may be difficult to distinguish between the diuresis that is delivering excess ECF and that which results from tubular dysfunction. If the latter, it is important to provide water and electrolytes that match those in urine. If there is uncertainty, it is recommended that input be reduced to two-thirds of urinary losses (chapter 48) and that weight and ECF volume status be monitored closely.

When nonrenal losses are significant, e.g., gastrointestinal losses, these are replaced with appropriate solutions. Renal losses of water, as occur in diabetes insipidus or nephrogenic diabetes insipidus, are difficult to replace with intravenous solutions. Because in this disorder urine is hypotonic with a high free water clearance, which increases as fluid is given intravenously in the amounts required, either as 2.5% glucose or 0.45% saline, it may be impossible to replace free water losses in this manner. It is recommended that free water to replace urinary losses in these patients be given by nasogastric tube, if oral intake is impractical.

Patients who are oliguric and require fluid in excess of minimum to deliver adequate calories, can only remove that fluid by dialysis. This may require special supplementation (See Chapter 50 C).

Patients with hemoglobinemia, myoglobinemia, hyperphosphatemia, and drug toxicity are given isotonic saline (20 ml/kg) and mannitol (1 g/kg) as a bolus to promote a saline and osmotic diuresis. Thereafter, it is recommended that urine volume be replaced with 2% mannitol and 0.45% NaCl to sustain the diuresis, albeit at a declining rate, for 6 to 24 hours, since the intake of NaCl and mannitol will be less than its excretion. Diuretics can be used concurrently but should not be used alone in a way that will induce dehydration.

DEFICIT THERAPY FOR ADULTS, CHILDREN, AND INFANTS

Deficit therapy usually is related to body weight. While it is practical to combine maintenance and deficit therapy into a single solution, it is often safer, when replacing deficits or losses of ECF, to have separate lines for these purposes. For other deficits, e.g., K and alkali, therapy can be given concurrently; for calories and protein, parenteral nutrition must be planned.

Sodium Chloride and Water

The replacement of deficits of ECF with NaCl and water is the most obvious and important form of replacement therapy. Usually the net loss is isotonic, so that intravenous replacement also should be isotonic or slightly hypotonic with respect to NaCl and should be given in 1 to 4 hours. Oral rehydration solution (ORS) is strongly recommended for the treatment of diarrheal dehydration. Usually this is given in doses of 75 to 100 ml/kg in 8 hours and less thereafter. The NaCl concentration (60 to 90 mEq/L) and the K (15 to 30 mEq/L) are slightly hypotonic. Continued losses may be more hypotonic. Therefore, it is recommended that free water be given alternately with ORS. The Na concentration, which is less than Ringer's solution, provides for free water to replace gastrointestinal and renal losses; the exchange of K for Na also adds Na to ECF from cells. The same ORS regimen is equally effective in treatment of isotonic, hypotonic, and hypertonic dehydration (18) (chapter 6).

Intravenous therapy for ECF volume contraction usually requires 20 to 100 ml/kg of an appropriate solution (Table 11.5). When clinical responses can be observed closely, intravenous replacement of up to 100 mg/kg should be completed in 4 hours. Under less ideal conditions or with oral rehydration solution, replacement of ECF deficits should take

Table 11.5.
Range of Deficits of ECF Volume in Children with Varying Degrees of Dehydration

Dehydration	Deficit
Mild	30–50 ml/kg
Moderate	40–80 ml/kg
Severe	60–120 ml/kg
Capillary damage	120–200 ml/kg

no more than 8 hours. The quantity recommended is related to body weight for all sized individuals and is scaled to estimated deficits, because ECF volume is a relatively consistent fraction of body weight after the neonatal period.

Patients who have hypotension or poor perfusion as a result of circulatory failure and circulatory hypovolemia should respond to therapy as described, unless they displace fluid into the extravascular or interstitial fluid (ISF) space. This occurs in burn patients, those with nephrotic syndrome in acute relapse, and patients with septic shock. They are treated with isotonic Ringer's lactate solution or a comparable saline-bicarbonate solution (Table 11.4) until circulation and blood pressure are sustained. For patients with septic shock or similar states, where there is a general capillary leak, the amount of isotonic fluid required may be as much as 200 ml/kg; the resulting edema may be massive. With recovery and redistribution of fluid from ISF space back to the circulation, a saline diuresis will occur. If renal failure is a coincident complication, as it may be, dialysis with removal of fluid by ultrafiltration is required. The initial goal of therapy is circulatory support and edema formation is a secondary result. The later goal is the expeditious removal of edema fluid. If colloid solutions are used to treat the hypoalbuminemia associated with capillary leak, the reabsorption of so much colloid may increase the risk for pulmonary edema. When fluid rich in protein is being replaced with plasma, Cl deficiency may develop because plasma is diluted with Na citrate.

Potassium

Replacement of K deficits overlaps with meeting maintenance K requirements. Because K deficiency is a deficiency of intracellular K brought about by a variety of metabolic events associated with other abnormalities, its magnitude cannot be estimated and its repair must proceed as the other metabolic events are reversed. Its replacement often is attended by release of Na from cells. As little as 1 mEq/kg of K will reverse the acute effects of hypokalemia and K deficiency; 2 to 4 mEq/kg/day, or twice the usual maintenance (4 mEq/100 kcal/day) suffices in most instances (chapter 7) to correct hypokalemia and moderate K deficiency. Often, its correction in acute deficiency coincides with correction of acid-base disorders, e.g., diabetic ketoacidosis (chapters 7 and 8). Chronic K deficiency often is a sign of a renal endocrine (adrenal) or metabolic disorder or is the consequence of drug toxicity affecting renal tubular function or mineralocorticoid action (diuretics or cancer chemotherapeutic agents) (chapters 33 and 34) or hyper-reninemic hypertension (chapter 47). K is like many other nutrients: taken in excess, renal regulation usually assures restoration of body composition to normal. Abnormalities affecting regulation are special cases (chapters 7 and 33).

Calories and Protein

The replacement of calories and protein is the treatment for malnutrition. Experience with dietary-induced malnutrition in infants emphasizes the need first to repair electrolyte and mineral imbalance and prompt but restrained replacement of substrate, i.e., glucose and amino acids, until cell metabolism is normalized. Early rapid nutritional rehabilitation of severely malnourished children is associated with death (19). Consequently, it is recommended practice to replace electrolytes over 2 to 3 days before aggressive nutritional rehabilitation is started. Nutritional rehabilitation is most efficiently achieved by giving calories well in excess of maintenance, usually 120% to 180% of maintenance (20). When achieved by oral feedings, this usually assures a corresponding increase in protein and other nutrients that more than meet requirements. Appreciating this need shortens the period required to restore weight-for-height to normal in severely malnourished infants from several months to 3 to 4 weeks. The calories are used to restore body fat, and both calories and protein are used to restore muscle mass. These measures also reverse the adverse effects of malnutrition on renal function (chapter 10C).

Practical Problems

Renal and gastrointestinal function regulates excretion, to assure retention or balance of many other nutrients, e.g., Ca, P, Mg, and trace minerals, when intake is adequate. Metabolism assures retention and balance of substrates and vitamins. Renal and gastrointestinal function control retention and balance of water, electrolyte, minerals, and trace minerals. When parenteral nutrition is used for extended periods, there are advantages to providing Ca, Mg, and trace minerals in a partial diet by the oral route, if that is practical.

When voluntary intake of diet is insufficient, supplements or formulas, specially constructed to support nutritional rehabilitation, may help. Provision of complete formulas by nasogastric tube overnight is very helpful in some instances, although these should be introduced slowly over 2 to 3 days to avoid overload and intolerance. Obstipation, when present, should be corrected first.

In patients with malnutrition and CRF or ESRD who are on dialysis, it is important to limit those nutrients whose retention in the face of excess intake depends on renal excretory function. Currently, no suitable commercial formula is available for oral or tube feeding. Ideal intakes have the following specifications: (1) calorie density 1 to 1.5 kcal/ml; (2) NaCl intake adjusted to renal losses plus 0.13 mEq/ml fluid removed by ultrafiltration; (3) K intake, 2 mEq/100 kcal, adjusted where appropriate; (4) P intake 25 mg/100 kcal; (5) Ca intake adjusted so that the ratio of Ca:P intake in mg is 2:1 (molar ratio 1.6:1); and (6) protein intake 2 g/100 kcal (8% of calories as protein).

DIURETICS, DIALYSIS, AND ULTRAFILTRATION REMOVAL THERAPY

The use of diuretics and other measures to reduce edema is covered in Chapter 29 and the use of dialysis or ultrafiltration to remove input not excreted is covered in Chapters 48 and 50. These are mentioned now to complete the development of the intake-body composition model described in Chapter 1 as it applies to fluid, electrolyte, and nutrition therapy. Under most conditions, the intake for maintenance and replacement exceeds requirement, and excretion leads to an appropriate balance. As excretory function is impaired, this response is compromised.

Edema in nephrosis forms either in response to reduced perfusion or to impaired glomerular function. In acute relapse with poor perfusion, ECF volume expansion may be indicated; otherwise NaCl restriction is indicated. The capacity to regulate NaCl and water excretion is impaired; the capacity to regulate K, H^+, and P excretion may be. Dietary intake often is decreased and the malnutrition that may result often is obscured by intractable edema. Specifically designed feedings, which allow adjustment of NaCl and water intake to tolerance, may be helpful.

The reduced excretory function of patients with CRF, including those with ESRD on dialysis, imposes a responsibility to adjust intake to meet requirements with as little excess as is practical. While it has been the practice to avoid restrictive diets for patients on dialysis, experience had led to the conclusion that dialysis as removal therapy has significant limitations. Lowering dietary NaCl, K, and P are important aspects of therapy. Restriction of fluid is not indicated unless hyponatremia is a problem because free water intake is dictated by NaCl intake. In dealing with the necessity to remove fluid by dialysis in infants given formulas low in NaCl and high in free water, it is important to give NaCl proportional to the free water that will be ultrafiltered (0.13 mEq/ml). The calorie requirements for patients on dialysis appear to be no more than RDA. Intakes <80% of RDA are associated with poor growth and reduced skinfold thickness. Protein requirements for adults on dialysis are increased; an intake of 1.2 g/kg/day (12% to 15% calories as protein) is recommended for adults on CAPD to maintain N balance and BUN at satisfactory level; slightly less is recommended for adults on hemodialysis. This is a 50% increase over the RDA. A comparable but no greater increase is recommended for infants and children (chapters 49 and 50).

References

1. Latta T: Relative to the treatment of cholera by the copious injection of aqueous and saline fluids into the vein. Lancet 2:274, 1965.
2. Blackfan KD, Maxcy KF: The intraperitoneal injection of saline solution. Am J Dis Child 15:19, 1918.
3. Schloss OM, Stetson RE: The occurrence of acidosis with severe diarrhea. Am J Dis Child 13:28, 1917.
4. Gamble JL, Ross SG, Tisdall FF: The metabolism of fixed base during fasting. J Biol Chem 57:663, 1923.
5. Darrow DC: Retention of electrolyte during recovery from severe dehydration due to diarrhea. J Pediatr 28:515, 1946.
6. Gamble JL: Physiological information from studies on the life raft ration. Harvey Lect Ser 42:247, 1946.
7. Cahill GF, Herrera MG, Morgan AP, et al: Hormone fuel interrelationships during fasting. J Clin Invest 45:1751, 1966.
8. Talbott NB, Crawford JD, Butler AM: Homeostatic limits to safe parenteral fluid therapy. N Engl J Med 248:1100, 1953.
9. Meng HC: Parenteral nutrition, principles, nutrient requirements, techniques and clinical application. In Schneider HA, Anderson CE, Coursin DB (eds): Nutritional Support of Medical Practice, ed 2. Philadelphia, Harper & Row, 1983, p 203.
10. Food and Nutrition Board Committee on Dietary Allowances, Recommended Dietary Allowances, ed 9. Washington, D.C., National Academy of Science, 1980.
11. Holliday MA, Wassner S, Ramirez J: Intravenous nutrition in uremic children with protein energy malnutrition. Am J Clin Nutr 31:1854, 1978.
12. Holliday MA, Segar WE: The maintenance need for water in parenteral fluid therapy. Pediatrics 19:823, 1957.
13. Bier DM, Leak RD, Haymond MW, et al: Measurement of "true" glucose production rates in infants and children. Diabetes 26:1016, 1977.
14. Holliday MA: Metabolic rate and organ size during growth from infancy to maturity. Pediatrics 47:169, 1971.
15. Foman SJ, Thomas SN, Filer LJ, et al: Food composition and growth of normal infants fed milk based formulas. Acta Paediat Scan (suppl 223):1, 1971.
16. Heird WC, Winters RW: Parenteral nutrition—Pediatrics. In Schneider HA, Anderson CE, Coursin DB (eds): Nutritional Support of Medical Practice, ed 2. Philadelphia, Harper & Row, 1983, p 230.
17. American Academy of Pediatrics, Committee on Nutrition: Commentary on breast feeding and infant formulas, including proposed standards for formulas. Pediatrics 57:278, 1976.
18. Cleary TG, Cleary KR, Dupont HL, et al: The relationship of oral rehydration solution to hypernatremia in infantile diarrhea. J Pediatr 99:739, 1981.
19. Patrick J: Death during recovery from severe malnutrition and its possible relationship to sodium pump activity in the leukocyte. Brit Med J 1:1051, 1977.
20. Ashworth A: Energy balance and growth. Experience in treating children with malnutrition. Kidney Intl 14:301, 1978.

3

Basic Mechanisms

CHAPTER 12

Genetic Aspects of Renal Disease

AARON L. FRIEDMAN
ENID F. GILBERT
JOHN M. OPITZ

The kidney may be involved in various hereditary or genetic conditions. To facilitate discussion, a number of terms and concepts are defined. Genetic disorders generally fall into three categories: (1) monogenic disorders—conditions that are inherited through a single gene and follow Mendelian inheritance patterns; (2) chromosomal disorders—conditions that result from abnormal chromosome structure or number; and (3) multifactorial disorders—conditions that seem to have a genetic component but do not follow Mendelian inheritance patterns and have no chromosomal abnormalities.

Genetic heterogeneity refers to the concept that a specific clinical appearance or manifestation may have more than one etiology. For example, distal renal tubular acidosis may be a solitary defect of the distal tubule or part of a generalized renal lesion such as obstructive uropathy.

Within monogenic disorders, three major modes of inheritance are discussed—autosomal dominant, autosomal recessive, and X-linked. *Autosomal dominant* refers to a condition that is manifest in heterozygotes and generally transmitted from one generation to the next. About half of the offspring of an affected individual are also affected. In renal disease, a classic autosomal dominant condition is adult polycystic kidney disease. *Penetrance* refers to the percent of individuals carrying the mutant gene who manifest the autosomal dominant condition. *Expressivity* refers to the severity of involvement. For example, excluding new mutations, tuberous sclerosis may demonstrate complete penetrance with all involved individuals demonstrating at least one manifestation of the condition. However, the expressivity may vary from mild skin involvement to severe seizure disorders, mental retardation, and numerous visceral hamartomas.

Autosomal recessive refers to an inheritance pattern in which expression of the mutant gene occurs in a homozygous state (both mutant genes present). This means that both parents are heterozygotes, each having one mutant gene. Males and females are equally involved. Heterozygote parents have a one in four chance of producing an involved (homozygous) child. Uninvolved children have a two in three chance of being carriers.

X-linked conditions are those in which the mutant gene is on the X-chromosome. In this hereditary pattern, an unaffected or mildly affected female transmits the condition to male offspring with a 50% chance of transmission. Males are hemizygotes, because they have only one X chromosome; therefore, they will manifest the condition. If it is not a lethal condition, the involved male will transmit the gene to all of his daughters, all of whom will be carriers. Male-to-male transmission rules out X-linked inheritance. In female carriers, half of the female offspring may become carriers and half of the male offspring may be involved.

In evaluating renal disease in hereditary or genetic conditions, it is clear that even with etiologically well-defined entities, great variability exists in penetrance and expressivity. Further, within more broadly defined syndromes, genetic heterogeneity may explain differences in manifestations.

Renal involvement in "genetic" disease may be divided into two broad categories. One category includes the metabolic and tubular disorders such as renal tubular acidosis, diabetes insipidus, and Fanconi syndromes. These will be covered in section VIII. The disorders discussed in this chapter primarily will be parenchymal anomalies.

Although many types of parenchymal anomalies may be seen in the disorders covered in this chapter, two predominate. The first has been termed "pluricystic" or "micromulticystic" kidney disease (1, 2). This involves gross or microscopic cysts originating from the glomerulus (2, 3) or less commonly from other portions of the nephron (Fig. 12.1). When microcysts are associated with proliferative involution or sclerosis, the term cystic infantile nephrosclerosis has been used.

More frequently recognized as part of a malformation syndrome is the cystic dysplastic kidney (Fig. 12.2). Such kidneys show the histological evidence of impaired early development with the full-blown picture, including primitive ducts and nest of metaplastic cartilage. The intriguing hypothesis is that incidental or pluricystic changes develop after the completion of nephrogenesis, while dysplastic changes occur early in development and represent a more severe impairment of normal renal architecture. This hypothesis is difficult to verify fully, since primitive ducts and metaplastic cartilage are not always present.

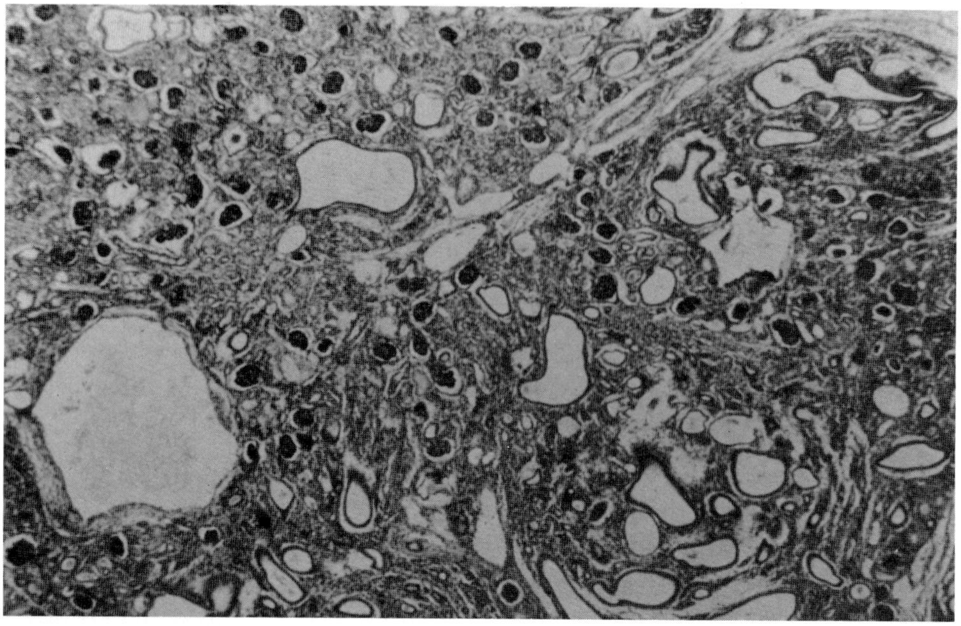

Figure 12.1. Microscopic section of micromulticystic kidney in trisomy-13 syndrome, with tubular and glomerular cysts of varying sizes. (Hematoxylin-eosin stain X100.)

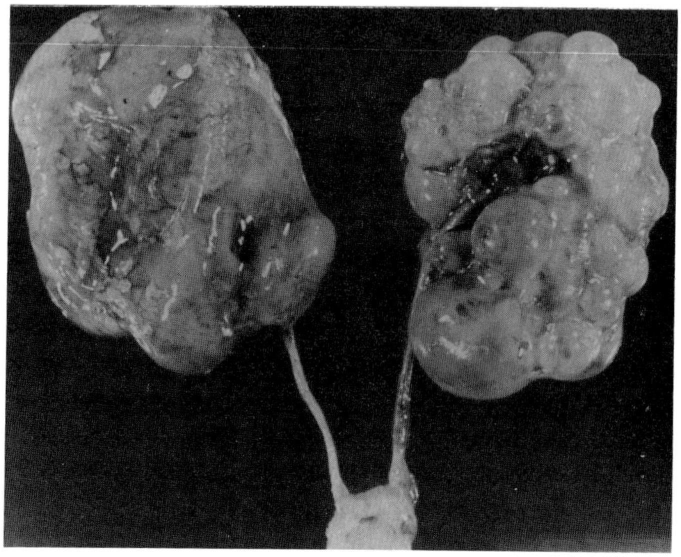

Figure 12.2. Gross appearance of bilateral cystic-dysplastic kidneys with irregular-sized cysts.

We have divided the chapter into two general areas—renal involvement with chromosomal aberrations and renal involvement with Mendelian mutation.

CHROMOSOMAL ABERRATIONS

Trisomy-21 Syndrome

The kidney is not usually involved in patients with trisomy-21. Some abnormalities have been reported and include uteropelvic junction obstruction and hydronephrosis. Renal dysplasia, nodular renal blastoma, and cystic malformation of collecting tubules with immature glomeruli have also been described (4, 5). Functionally, significant abnormalities are rare.

Trisomy-18 Syndrome

In the trisomy-18 syndrome, renal and urologic anomalies are quite common. As reviewed by Warkany and coworkers (6) in 84 cases of trisomy-18: 11% had cystic kidneys, 21% had horseshoe kidneys, 9% had renal duplication, 7% had renal dysplasia or agenesis, 3% had renal ectopy, 3% had glomerulosclerosis, and 17% had ureteral duplication. Microscopically, findings include glomerulosclerosis and cystic tubules often lined with primitive epithelium. Interestingly, many of the microscopic changes are similar to those observed in children with congenital heart disease (7). The microscopic cystic changes are associated with sclerotic changes similar to infantile glomerulosclerosis (8). Another unusual finding is the presence of nests of undifferentiated metanephric blastema (9, 10).

Trisomy-13 Syndrome

As in trisomy-18, a wide variety of renal abnormalities have been observed in trisomy-13 syndrome. Specifically, cystic kidney (6), including a description of adult type polycystic kidneys (11) are reported. Other anomalies include renal or ureteral duplication, as well as unilateral renal agenesis and urethral stenosis (12). Also described are accessory renal arteries and veins (13).

The most consistent finding in trisomy-13 is excessive fetal lobulations with cystic glomerular and tubular change (14), generally confined to the cortex. Severe cystic dysplasia of the kidneys has also been seen (14), perhaps associated with drug abuse. Lastly, hydronephrosis has also been noted (12, 15).

Other Chromosomal Defects

At least three other rare trisomy defects have been associated with renal defects. Full trisomy of the C group autosomes first described only in abortuses and was eventually reported in a living infant. That infant had bilateral cystic dysplastic kidneys (16). Further, trisomy-C mosaicism with a normal cell line has been associated with ureterovesical reflux and hydronephrosis (17, 18).

Trisomy-8 patients, in particular those who manifest the Warkany syndrome, have a high incidence of renal anomalies. In 75% of cases reviewed by Riccardi (19), severe renal or urologic abnormalities were present. These included obstructive uropathy and presumed secondary chronic interstitial nephritis.

An infant with trisomy-9 has been reported whose findings included microscopic cysts (20). A case of 46, XX, $2q^+$ has been observed with

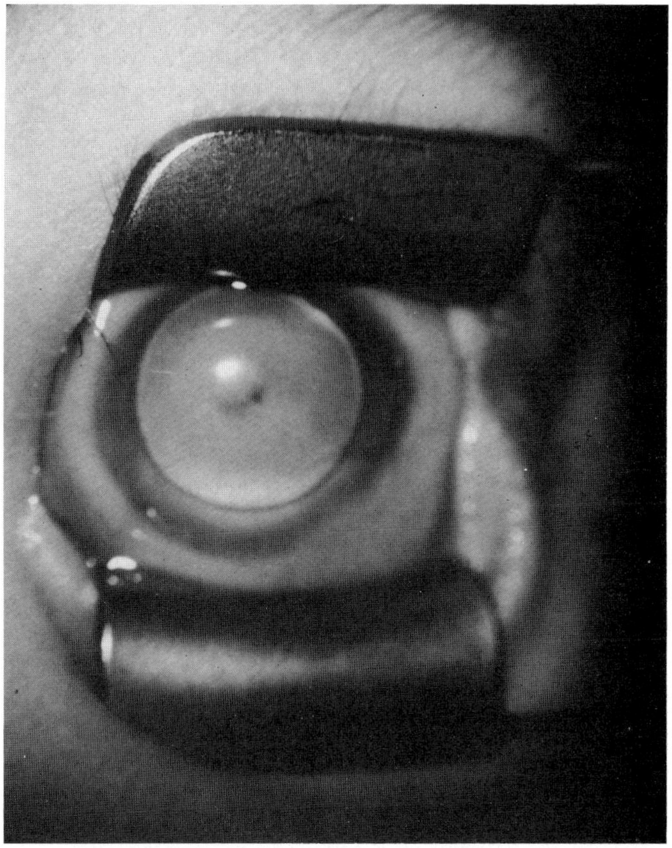

Figure 12.3. Sporadic aniridia with 11p⁻—general appearance. Note "large" pupils from lack of iris material.

microcystic kidney disease, and bilateral cortical nephroblastomatosis has been noted with $18q^-$ syndrome (14).

In the Ullrich-Turner syndrome, a sex chromosome defect, a high incidence of renal malformations has been observed. These malformations include duplications of kidneys and ureters, malrotations, horseshoe kidneys, unilateral agenesis, hypoplasia, and dysplasia (21–23).

Finally, mention should be made of the association of Wilms tumor with sporadic aniridia and $11p^-$ syndrome (Fig. 12.3). The high incidence of Wilms tumor with sporadic aniridia has been known for quite some time. However, some have speculated that those with sporadic aniridia at greatest risk are those with chromosomal aberration of $11p^-$ (24–26). Riccardi and coworkers (27) have recently reported Wilms tumor with sporadic aniridia and normal chromosomes. The Wilms tumor that develops in patients with $11p^-$ appears histologically similar to that in typical Wilms patients. The evaluation, follow-up, and ultimate prognosis of $11p^-$ patients remains to be clarified.

MENDELIAN MUTATION

Renal abnormalities are found in a great many malformation syndromes. Table 12.1 is a compilation of a number of malformation syndromes and includes the inheritance pattern and renal lesion associated with the syndrome. The rest of this chapter will discuss some of the syndromes noted in the table, with particular emphasis on common anomalies or those that present unique challenges to the nephrologist and urologist. Other common inherited malformation syndromes are discussed elsewhere in this textbook: cystic disorders (chapter 23) and tubular and metabolic defects (Section VIII). Gilbert and Opitz (14) have divided renal involvement in malformation syndromes into that associated with cerebral anomalies, that associated with skeletal dysplasias, and others.

CEREBRAL ANOMALIES WITH RENAL INVOLVEMENT

Zellweger Cerebro-hepato-renal Syndrome

The Zellweger syndrome is a multisystem disorder inherited as an autosomal recessive trait that is lethal in infancy. The anomalies include incomplete differentiation and range from aplasia to hyperplasia of nearly all organs of the body. The "classic" description (28–30) includes hypotonia, glaucoma, severe psychomotor retardation, epicanthic folds, large ears, liver enlargement, and evidence of liver dysfunction. Autopsy further reveals subcapsular cystic kidneys, patent ductus arteriosus, and severe CNS abnormalities. Since the early description, the wide spectrum of organ involvement has been documented (31).

Renal and urinary tract involvement has included persistence of fetal lobulation with cortical cysts of glomerular and tubular origin (32). Glomeruli in the outer cortex may be immature, probably as a result of epithelial hyperplasia. Pericystic fibrosis has been reported, as has mild mesangial thickening and even focal glomerulosclerosis. Bernstein (2) has described cystic dysplastic changes. Other findings have included albuminuria and aminoaciduria (32), horseshoe kidney, and ureteral duplication (31). The basic defect in the Zellweger syndrome remains to be elucidated. However, it appears to be a defect in mitochondrial oxidative function (33, 34), in particular an absence of catalase activity. Should a metabolic defect be definitively demonstrated, then the Zellweger syndrome may be viewed not as a developmental field defect, but rather as a developmental metabolic defect leading to dysplasias or hypoplasias, developmental arrest, and the secondary changes of metabolic insufficiency.

Smith-Lemli-Opitz (RSH) Syndrome

RSH syndrome is an autosomal recessive multiple anomaly, mental retardation syndrome. The clinical manifestations include: microcephaly, hypotonia, mental retardation, growth failure, and minor abnormalities of the extremities and face. Some males demonstrate incomplete development of external genitalia, including perineoscrotal hypospadias, cleft scrotum, cryptorchidism, or small testes. Also noted are cystic dysplasia, unilateral hypoplasia, and glomerular changes of thickened basement membrane and capillary tuft hyalinization (35).

Meckel Syndrome

Meckel syndrome is an autosomal recessive condition associated with severe central nervous system abnormalities, ocular anomalies, cleft palate, congenital heart disease, pseudohermaphrodism in males, and a variety of renal anomalies. This condition is fatal in the perinatal period or early infancy (36). The renal manifestations include hydronephrosis, cystic and dysplastic kidneys, and hypoplastic kidneys. The cystic changes are said to resemble a mild form of adult polycystic kidney associated with liver and pancreatic cysts.

Other cerebral anomaly syndromes with renal involvement are referenced in Table 12.1. These include the Goldston syndrome, Miranda syndrome, Ivemark syndrome, Lissencephaly syndrome, Ehler-Danlos, and Schwartz-Jampel syndrome.

Renal Anomalies Associated With Skeletal Dysplasia

Asphyxiating Thoracic Dystrophy (Jeune Syndrome)

This is an autosomal recessive, severely debilitating, and usually lethal condition consisting of an extremely constricted thorax, short limbs, and

Table 12.1
Renal Lesions in Malformation Syndromes

Disease	Inheritance	Renal lesion
Amyloidosis with polyneuropathy—familial	Autosomal dominant	Amyloid nephropathy (99)
Amyloidosis with nephropathy, neuropathy, and peptic ulcer—generalized	Autosomal dominant	Amyloid nephropathy (100)
Asphyxiating thoracic dystrophy (Jeune) syndrome	Autosomal recessive	Proximal and distal tubular dysfunction, mesangial thickening and sclerosis of glomeruli, cystic dysplasia, infantile polycystic type lesion with nephrotic syndrome
Bardet-Biedl syndrome	Autosomal recessive	Chronic glomerulonephritis, hydronephrosis, capsular adhesions, renal hypoplasia, unilateral glomerular dysplasia, abnormal fetal lobulations
Brachomesomelia	Sporadic	Glomerulocystic kidneys (101)
Charcot-Marie-Tooth disease with nephritis	?Autosomal recessive	Minute foci of tubular atrophy, thickened glomerular basement membranes (102)
Cockayne syndrome	Autosomal recessive	Thickened basement membranes, interstitial fibrosis, nephrosclerosis, tubular atrophy, immune complex nephritis (103)
Congenital muscular torticollis, multiple keloids, cryptorchidism, and renal dysplasia	X-linked recessive	Dysplasia, chronic pyelonephritis with hypertension (104)
Congenital microcephaly, hiatus hernia, and nephrotic syndrome	Autosomal recessive	Cystic dysplasia with focal glomerulosclerosis (105, 106)
Chondrodysplasia punctata, rhizomelic type	Autosomal recessive	Micromulticystic kidneys (107)
Crome syndrome	?Autosomal recessive	Renal tubular necrosis (108)
Ehlers-Danlos syndrome	Autosomal dominant, recessive, and X-linked forms	Multiple cysts containing serous fluid, associated cysts of liver (109)
Elejalde syndrome (acrocephalopolydactylous dysplasia)	Autosomal recessive	Cystic dysplasia (110)
Familial hydronephrosis	Autosomal dominant with variable expressivity	Unilateral or bilateral hydronephrosis with or without ureteropelvic obstruction contralateral agenesis in three cases (111, 112)
Familial intestinal malabsorption of vitamin B_{12} with nephropathy	Autosomal recessive	Mild subacute glomerulonephritis (113)
Familial Kallmann syndrome	X-linked recessive (?male-limited autosomal dominant)	Unilateral renal agenesis (114)
Familial steatosis	?Autosomal recessive	Fatty change of renal tubular epithelial cells (115)
Familial thrombocytopenia and elevated IgA levels with renal disease	?Autosomal recessive, ?X-linked recessive	Focal tubular atrophy with osmiophilic deposits beneath basement membrane (116)
G syndrome Total	Autosomal dominant Sporadic	Unilateral duplication of renal pelvis and ureters, bilateral ureteral reflux (117)
Glomerulonephritis and necrotizing angitis with emphysema and α_1-antitrypsin deficiency	Sporadic	Fibrin deposition in glomeruli (118)
Goldenhar syndrome	Sporadic	Renal pelvis, pelvic deformity, anomalous renal artery, unilateral cystic kidney (119, 120)
Goldston syndrome	Autosomal recessive	Cystic dysplasia (121)
Hereditary osteolysis with nephropathy	Autosomal dominant	Vascular nephropathy, "chronic glomerulonephritis," amyloidosis (122–124)
Herediatry onycho-osteodysplasia (nail-patella syndrome)	Autosomal dominant	Thickening of glomerular basement membranes, mesangial hypercellularity, glomerular sclerosis with tubular atrophy, and interstitial fibrosis
Hereditary renal adysplasia	Autosomal dominant (?X-linked recessive)	Unilateral agenesis with contralateral hypoplasia or dysplasia, virtually complete bilateral absence of kidneys (96)
Ivemark syndrome	Autosomal recessive	Cystic dysplasia with dysplasia of liver and pancreas (125)
Kaufman syndrome	?Autosomal recessive	Caliectasis, ureterectasia, bifurcation of renal pelvis (126)
Klippel-Trenaunay syndrome	Sporadic	Diffuse bilateral nephroblastomatosis (127)
Liban-Kozenitzky syndrome	?Autosomal recessive	Bilateral nephroblastomatosis (128, 129)
Liddle syndrome (pseudohyperaldosteronism)	Autosomal dominant	Tubular defect with reabsorption of sodium and excretion of potassium in the absence of mineralocorticoids (130)
Lipodystrophy Partial . . .	Sporadic or ?autosomal dominant with variable expressivity	Nephropathy of Henoch-Schonlein purpura, chronic glomerulonephritis, pyelonephritis, acute glomerulonephritis, proliferative or membranoproliferative glomerulonephritis

Table 12.1—*Continued*

Disease	Inheritance	Renal lesion
Lissencephaly syndrome	?Autosomal recessive	Unilateral agenesis, cystic kidneys, ?type, micromulticystic kidneys (131)
Lowe syndrome (oculocerebro-renal syndrome)	X-linked recessive	Convoluted tubular defect, glomerular nephropathy
Male pseudohermaphroditism, renal disease and Wilms tumor	No familial cases	Rapidly progressive glomerulonephritis, malignant nephrosclerosis, Wilms tumor (132)
Majewski short-rib polydactyly syndrome	Autosomal recessive	Cystic dysplasia (133)
Meckel syndrome	Autosomal recessive	Hypoplasia, adult polycystic type lesion with gigantic renal enlargement, vascular anomalies, hydronephrosis, dysplastic kidneys, malformations in shape, associated cysts of liver and pancreas
Miranda syndrome	Autosomal recessive	Cystic dysplasia with dysplasia of liver (134)
Myotonic dystrophy and polycystic kidney disease	Autosomal dominant	Adult polycystic lesion (135)
Oro-facial-digital syndrome	Autosomal dominant	Adult type polycystic kidneys, glomerulocystic kidneys (136, 137)
Ozer syndrome	?Autosomal recessive	Proteinuria and aminoaciduria, no pathological examination (138)
Peutz-Jeghers syndrome with polycystic kidney disease	Autosomal dominant	Adult polycystic type lesion (139)
Polycystic hepatopancreatic, epididymal, renal cystic disease with thoracic polydystrophy	Sporadic	Cystic dysplasia (140)
Prune belly syndrome	Inheritance unknown; ?unstable autosomal or X-linked premutation	Developmental dysplasia of smooth muscle of urinary tract, hydroureters and hydronephrosis, urethral or bladder neck obstruction, renal dysplasia
Pseudohypoaldosteronism	?Autosomal recessive	Unresponsiveness of renal tubule to mineralocorticoids, sclerosis of 20–25% of glomeruli, and dilatation of subcapsular tubules (141)
Renal dysplasia-familial	Autosomal recessive	Cystic dysplasia (142, 143)
Renal-retinal dysplasia:		
Isolated	Autosomal recessive	Cystic dysplasia
With cerebellar dysgenesis	Autosomal recessive	Cystic dysplasia, posterior urethral valves
With iminoglycinuria or with glycinuria	Autosomal recessive	Lesion resembling nephronophthisis with or without hepatic fibrosis
Saldino-Noonan short-rib polydactyl syndrome	Autosomal recessive	Cystic dysplasia, hypoplasia of ureters (144)
Smith-Lemli-Opitz (RSH) syndrome	Autosomal recessive	Cystic dysplasia, vascular malformations of renal artery, unilateral hypoplasia, nephrosclerosis
Schwartz-Jampel syndrome	?Autosomal recessive	Micromulticystic kidneys (145)
Sporadic aniridia, $11p^-$ syndrome	Sporadic (?Autosomal dominant)	Wilms tumor
Thyrotoxicosis and renal disease	Sporadic	Subacute proliferative glomerulonephritis with immunoglobulin deposits (146)
Tuberous sclerosis	Autosomal recessive	Papillary cysts, adult polycystic type lesion, hamartomas (13, 147, 148)
Urticaria, deafness and amyloid nephropathy (Muckle-Wells syndrome)	Autosomal dominant	Amyloid nephropathy (149)
VATER association	Sporadic	Renal dysplasia or agenesis, persistent urachus, renal ectopia, hypospadias, caudally displaced, dysplastic penis
von Hippel-Lindau disease	Autosomal dominant	Adult polycystic type lesion, cystic dysplasia, renal adenomas or hypernephromas, associated pancreatic cysts (150, 151)
Wiedemann-Beckwith syndrome	Usually sporadic familial cases: ?delayed mutation of an unstable premutated autosomal gene	Enlarged kidneys, persistent glomerulogenesis, diffuse bilateral nephroblastomatosis, metanephric hamartomas, hydronephrosis and hydroureters, Wilms tumor, duplication of collecting system
Winter syndrome	Autosomal recessive	Unilateral agenesis or hypoplasia, bilateral agenesis (152)
Wiskott-Aldrich syndrome	X-linked recessive	Interstitial nephritis immune complex glomerulonephritis (153)
Wohltman-Caglar syndrome	Sporadic	Juxtaglomerular hyperplasia (154, 155)

X-ray changes of the pelvis (37). Glomerular lesions ranging from mild mesangial thickening and sclerosis of glomerular tufts to decreased creatinine clearance to uremia have been described in this syndrome (37–39). Also reported are proximal tubule defects resembling Fanconi syndrome with uricosuria, phosphaturia, and aminoaciduria, and distal tubule defects, particularly impaired concentrating ability (39, 40). In one case, cystic dysplasia with uteropelvic junction obstruction has been noted (40). Finally, Bernstein has described varied and complex forms of cystic dysplasia in infants with the Jeune syndrome (2). No single explanation for the variety of renal lesions in this syndrome has been put forth.

Hereditary Onycho-osteodysplasia (Nail-Patella Syndrome)

This autosomal dominant condition, which is linked to the gene locus for ABO blood groups, has renal disease as a feature in approximately 40% of involved patients. Some 10% of patients with the syndrome die of renal failure (41). The clinical features include: dysplastic changes of fingers and toenails, hypoplasia or absence of the patella, and malformations of the radial capitellum and iliac wings (so-called iliac horns). The predominant renal defect is proteinuria (42, 43), which can lead to the nephrotic syndrome. Hematuria, cylinduria, and hypertension may also occur. Histologically, the early changes show thickening of the capillary walls (44, 45) with glomerular basement membrane changes. These changes have been well described (45–47) and consist of irregularly thickened and lucent lamina densa with collagen fibers within the basement membrane. Immunofluorescence may show a nonspecific focal distribution of IgM or complement, especially if focal areas of sclerosis are present. Progression of the renal lesion leads to segmental sclerosis, cortical atrophy, and eventually chronic nephritis.

Table 12.1 contains other skeletal dysplasias with associated renal abnormalities. These include hereditary osteolysis with nephropathy, the rhizomelic form of chondrodysplasia punctata, Majewski short-rib polydactyly syndrome, Elejalde syndrome, and familial Kallman syndrome.

Tuberous Sclerosis

Tuberous sclerosis is an autosomal dominant disorder characterized by skin manifestations, particularly angiofibromata, harmatomas of the central nervous system with intracerebral calcifications and harmatomas of the viscera. Mental retardation and epilepsy also may be seen.

The renal lesions of tuberous sclerosis may be among the first noted (48). Two major types of renal lesion have been described. The most common lesions are angiomyolipomatous harmatomas, which may be single or multiple and involve one or both kidneys. These are not dissimilar from harmatomas that appear in other viscera. The other type of lesion is cystic. The cysts are lined by an epithelium with a "piled-on" appearance, forming papillary and polypoid masses protruding into the cystic space (49). Bernstein and Kissane (5) have suggested that the epithelial lining of these cysts resembles proximal tubule cells. Potter (50), however, has shown that cysts are derived from all nephon segments. The clinical appearance resembles adult polycystic kidney disease, and Kissane (51) has noted adult polycystic kidney disease in patients with tuberous sclerosis.

The clinical manifestations of the renal lesions of tuberous sclerosis are varied. They may include renal enlargement, hematuria, hypertension, and, on rare occasions, renal insufficiency (48).

Von Hippel-Lindau Disease

Cerebellar angiomatosis, visceral lesions, and retinal angiomata characterize the autosomal dominant disorder of von Hippel-Lindau disease. Visceral involvement most frequently includes renal and/or pancreatic cysts. Cyst formation seems to occur in the fetus and eventually may progress during adult life to benign tumors or even malignant neoplasms (52). Gibson (53) has suggested that the cysts have neoplastic potential.

Other Renal-Associated Disorders

Prune Belly Syndrome

The prune belly syndrome (triad syndrome, Eagle-Barrett) consists of deficiency or absence of abdominal musculature, urinary tract abnormalities, and cryptorchidism (Fig. 12.4) (54–56). In the typical case, the urologic abnormalities consist of ectatic, elongated, and tortuous ureters with an enlarged bladder. There is often dilatation of the collecting system and frequently a "bulging" proximal urethra, with hypoplasia or absence of the prostate. Renal dysplasia or hypoplasia is a consistent finding.

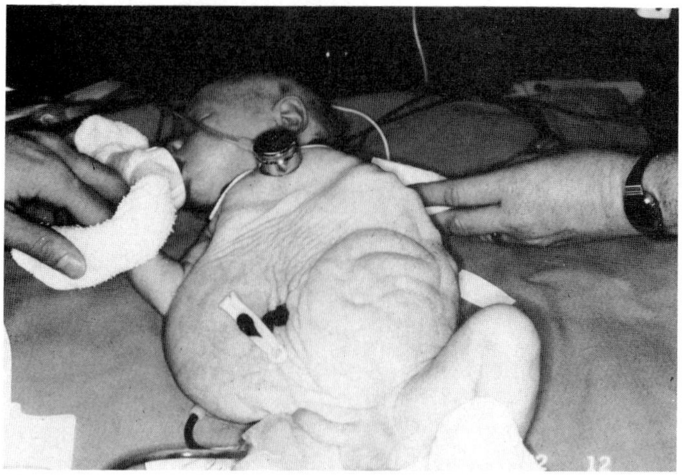

Figure 12.4. Prune belly syndrome. General appearance of child with prune belly syndrome. Note the wrinkled (prune) appearance of the abdomen as a result of lack of abdominal musculature.

The etiology and pathogenesis of the prune belly syndrome has raised considerable controversy. Straub and Spranger (57) reviewed the two major hypotheses of pathogenesis. They are an early (sixth to tenth week of development) mesenchymal developmental arrest versus the sequelae of intrauterine obstruction of proximal urethra leading to urinary tract and abdominal distension. Straub and Spranger conclude that the weight of evidence leans heavily toward the developmental defect theory as delineated by Opitz (58) and Spranger (59).

The explanation of the etiology of prune belly syndrome is not merely of academic interest. Aggressive management has been advocated and successfully used by some (60–63). This success, in fact, has been one of the arguments for the obstruction hypothesis. However, a majority of those involved in the treatment of prune belly syndrome advocate a more conservative approach (64–66). The clinical course is variable, with approximately 20% of patients dying in the neonatal period. However, the long-term, sometimes poor prognosis appears identical regardless of aggressive or cautious therapy. This is probably a result of the primary atonic nature of the bladder and ureters in these patients. This atony makes urinary stasis a constant feature. Intraluminal pressures are not high, and pressure-induced changes in renal function are not a major concern. Preservation of infection-free urine will help maintain renal function.

Oculo-cerebro-renal Syndrome of Lowe

This is a familial disorder generally viewed as X-linked recessive in origin with the features of mental retardation, glaucoma, cataracts, and the renal lesion of the Fanconi syndrome (Fig. 12.5) (67). A glomerular lesion with basement membrane thickening, foot process effacement, interstitial and glomerular fibrosis, and tubular basement membrane thickening has been described (68).

Bardet-Biedl Syndrome (Laurence-Moon-Bardet-Biedl Syndrome)

This autosomal recessive condition first described by Bardet (69) and Biedl (70) is manifested by retinitis pigmentosa, obesity, mental retar-

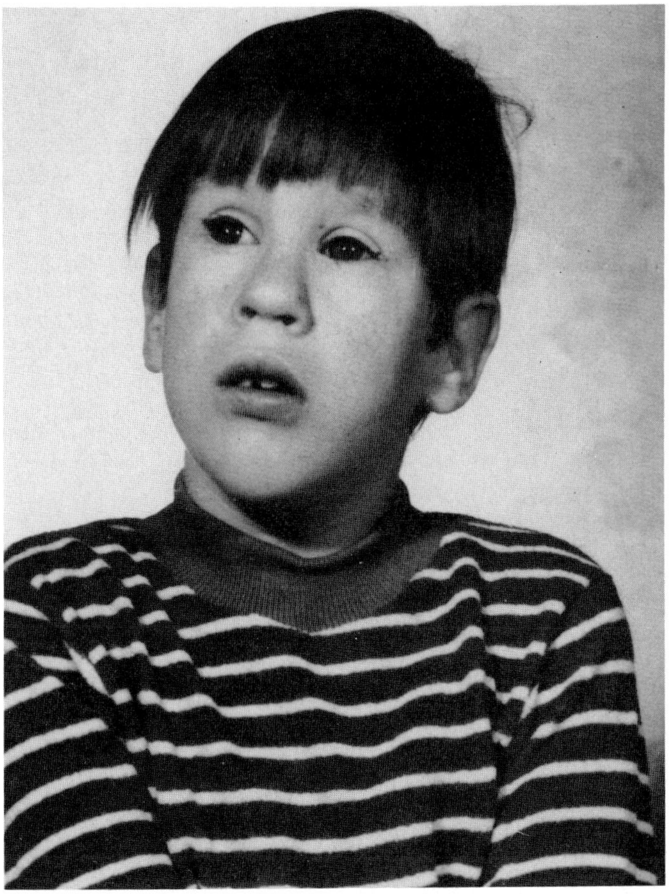

Figure 12.5. Lowe's syndrome. Typical facies of patient with Lowe's syndrome.

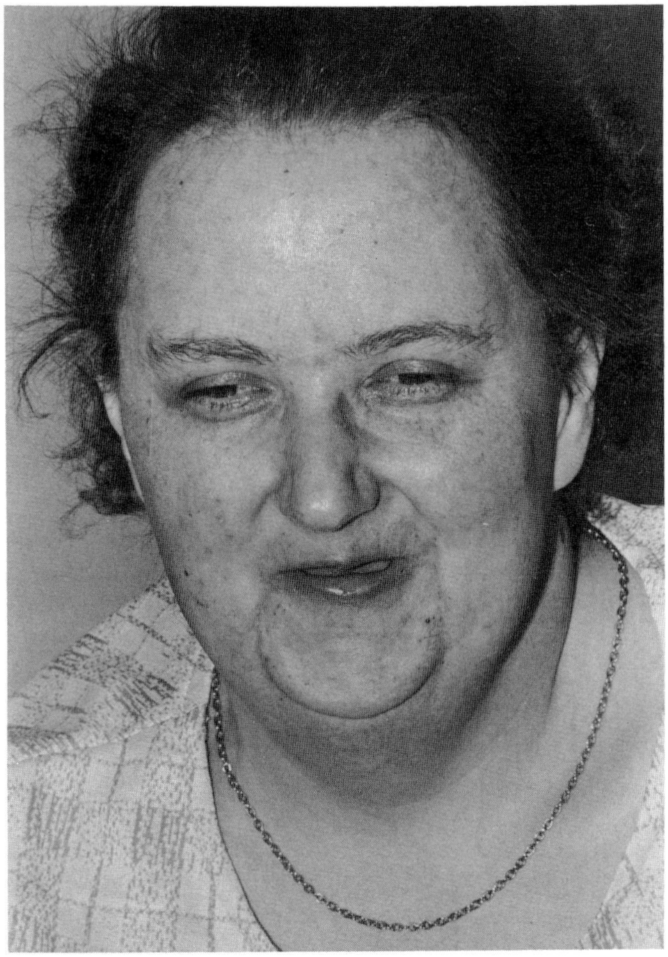

Figure 12.6. Bardet-Biedl—general appearance. Note hirsuitism, a frequent feature.

dation, polydactyly/syndactyly, and hypogenitalism (Fig. 12.6). The renal lesions in this syndrome were initially reviewed by McLaughlin and Shanklin (71) and Nadgini and coworkers (72). They documented chronic glomerulonephritis, hydronephrosis, interstitial nephritis, and nephrosclerosis. Further amplification was provided by Hurley and coworkers (73). In nine patients, they found small kidneys with a prolonged nephrogram phase, decreased concentration of contrast medium, and calyceal distortion on urographic examination. Histologically, there was evidence of mesangeal proliferation and sclerosis with cystic changes in tubules (cortical and medullary) and chronic interstitial nephritis. No immunofluorescent changes have been noted. Recently, Tieder and coworkers (74) reviewed the renal involvement in Bardet-Biedl emphasizing tubulointerstitial disease with polyuria and polydipsia, as the early signs of renal dysfunction. In the McLoughlin, Hurley, and Tieder series, renal disease was a major cause of morbidity and mortality. Further, Tieder and coworkers suggest the renal disease be considered a cardinal feature of the disorder.

Renal-retinal Dysplasia

Renal-retinal dysplasia is a diverse group of genetically determined conditions where some families show retinal blindness with severe renal disease (75–81). Lesions described include hypoplasia/dysplasia, cystic disease, iminoglycinuria, glycinuria, and a lesion similar to juvenile nephronophthisis. Dekebon (82) reports a family with mental retardation, cerebellar malformation, retinal blindness, and renal disease. Opitz and Gilbert (14) point out that the photoreceptors of the retina, development of the vermis, and completion of renal development all occur at about 32 weeks gestation. It is therefore possible that a single defect (enzymatic?) may explain the dysplasia of kidney, retina, and perhaps cerebellum.

VATER association

The VATER association is an acronym for a concurrence of congenital anomalies: V, vertebral; A, anal; TE, tracheoesophageal fistula; and R, renal or radial (83, 84). Cardiac and genital anomalies have also been recognized as part of the VATER. This association seems to originate from an early disruption of normal embryology (before the thirty-fifth day of gestation). No clear genetic or environmental factor has been elucidated, and the cases appear sporadic. At least one report of chromosomal aberration with the VATER association has been reported (85). It remains undecided whether a single developmental defect can explain the association or whether the VATER is a true malformation syndrome with two or more developmental field defects.

A wide variety of renal anomalies has been reported. These are renal agenesis, renal ectopia, cystic dysplasia, ureteropelvic junction obstruction, and vesicoureteral reflux (86). Other genitourinary anomalies include persistent urachus, hypospadias, and dysplastic caudally displaced penis. In a review of the urologic complications of VATER association, Uehling and coworkers (86) point out that despite multiple serious anomalies that must be addressed early in life, the genitourinary abnormalities are common in the VATER association. Further, these abnormalities are often persistent and may be very important to the long-term outcome of the patient. Of the 23 patients reviewed by Uehling and coworkers 21 had renal or urologic anomalies—9 with vesicoureteral reflux, 7 with renal agenesis, 5 with hydronephrosis secondary to ureteropelvic junction obstruction, and 5 with crossed fused ectopia. Two patients died in the immediate neonatal period, and 13 required at least one urologic procedure. Three patients required hemodialysis, and one patient received a successful renal transplantation. Most clearly, patients with the VATER association represent a challenge to nephrologists and urologists.

Wiedemann-Beckwith Syndrome

The Wiedemann-Beckwith syndrome consists of macroglossia, gigantism, neonatal hypoglycemia, organomegaly, and predisposition to malignant tumors (Fig. 12.7) (87, 88). The tumors include Wilms tumor, adrenocortical carcinoma, hepatoblastoma, gliobastoma, and brainstem glioma. The renal anomalies include large kidneys, bilateral nephroblastoma, hydronephrosis, hydroureter and collection system duplication (88). Most cases are sporadic with an occasional report of familial cases.

Lipodystrophy

This heterogeneous group of disorders is characterized by progressive atrophy of fat tissue. Renal abnormalities have been reported in total and partial lipodystrophy. The renal lesions are reviewed along with other aspects of total and partial lipodystrophy by Senior and Gellis (89). The descriptions of the renal involvement include pyelonephritis, Henoch-Schonlein purpura, proteinuria, nephrotic syndrome, and fulminant acute glomerulonephritis. More recently, membranoproliferative glomerulonephritis has been described as closely associated with partial lipodystrophy (90, 91). The lesion is most often type II membranoproliferative glomerulonephritis with low C_3 levels and the presence of C_3 Nef (92). How the fat abnormalities, complement profile changes, and glomerulonephritis are associated remains unclear.

Male pseudohermaphroditism, Renal Disease, and Wilms Tumor

This unusual tripart condition described by Denys and coworkers (93) and Drash and coworkers (94) includes ambiguous genitalia, rapidly progressive glomerulonephritis, and the development of Wilms tumor. The condition also results in chronic renal failure. Kissane (5) reports the occurrence of pseudohermaphroditism and progressive glomerulonephritis with Wilms tumor. One hypothesis suggests that, during embryogenesis, a disorder of nephron development and pseudohermaphroditism develops simultaneously which may have teratogenic potential (95).

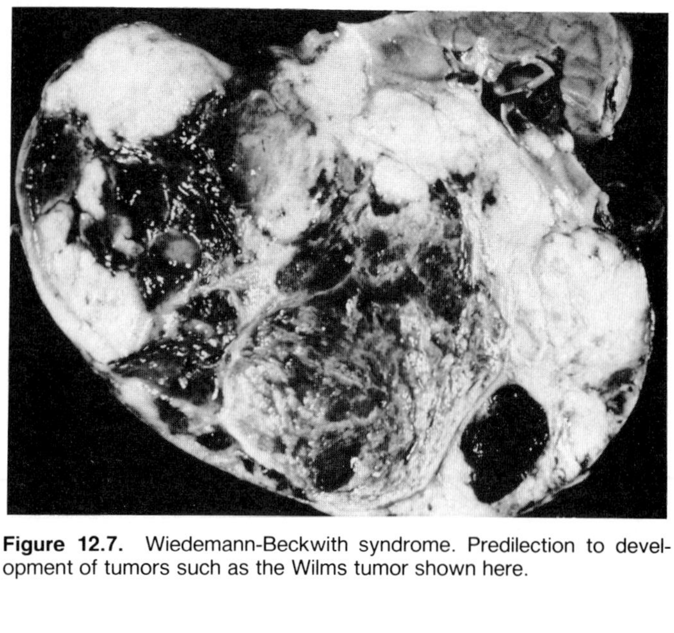

Figure 12.7. Wiedemann-Beckwith syndrome. Predilection to development of tumors such as the Wilms tumor shown here.

Renal Agenesis and Related Topics

The complexity of renal agenesis has been reviewed by Buchta and coworkers (96) and Opitz and Gilbert (14). Buchta and coworkers distinguished what they believed to be a sporadic entity termed bilateral renal agenesis (BRA) (97, 98) from an apparently autosomal dominant trait that they termed hereditary renal adysplasia (HRA). Adysplasia refers to the combination of agenesis and dysplasia with asymmetry frequently seen in this condition. The important distinction between BRA and HRA is that there is no evidence of kidneys or ureters in BRA, while in HRA, there is some vestige of renal tissue.

In Buchta's scheme, BRA was viewed as a nonspecific developmental field defect that conformed to a Potter field (14). Buchta points out that BRA has a frequency of about 1 in 4000 and low familial occurrence. Thus, the empiric recurrence risk was estimated at less than 1%. Further, since BRA was considered sporadic and HRA an autosomal dominant trait, it was felt that renal evaluation of first-degree relatives was necessary with HRA but not BRA.

Unfortunately, clarity of concept has not persisted because of mounting evidence of a relationship between BRA, HRA, and URA (unilateral renal agenesis). As carefully reviewed by Opitz and Gilbert (14), BRA, HRA, and URA have been reported to occur within the same family and even among first-degree relatives. The genetic explanation for the apparent nonpenetrance and variable expressivity seen in this complexity of conditions remains unclear. Nonetheless, it seems reasonable to study relatives of patients with BRA, HRA, and URA, although the optimal method of investigation—IVP, renal ultrasound, or computed axial tomography—also is uncertain.

References

1. Bernstein J: Morphology of inherited renal developmental abnormalities. Birth Defects 6/3:9, 1970.
2. Bernstein J, Brough AJ, McAdams AJ: The renal lesion in syndromes of multiple congenital malformations. Birth Defects 10/16:35, 1973.
3. Bartman J, Barraclough G: Cystic dysplasia of the kidneys studied by microdissection in a case of 13–15 trisomy. J Pathol Bact 89:233, 1965.
4. Ozer FL: Kidney malformations in mongolism. Birth Defects 10/4:189, 1974.
5. Bernstein J, Kissane J: Hereditary disorders of the kidney. In Perspective in Pediatric Pathology. Chicago, Year Book Medical Publishers, Inc., 1973.
6. Warkany J, Passarge E, Smith LB: Congenital malformations in autosomal trisomy syndromes. Am J Dis Child 112:502, 1966.
7. Marden PM, Walker WA: A new generalized connective tissue syndrome. Am J Dis Child 112:225, 1966.
8. Bernstein J, Meyer R: Parenchymal maldevelopment of the kidney. In Brennemann-Kelley (ed): Practice of Pediatrics. Hagerstown, Md., Harper & Row, 1967.
9. Uchida IA, Bowman JM, Wang HC: The 18-trisomy syndrome. N Engl J Med 266:1198, 1962.
10. Bove KE, Koffler H, McAdams AJ: Nodular renal blastema: Definition and possible significance. Cancer 24:323, 1969.
11. Osathanondh V, Potter EL: Pathogenesis of polycystic kidneys. Arch Pathol 77:459, 1964.
12. Townes PL, Dehart GK Jr, Hecht F, et al: Trisomy 13–15 in a male infant. J Pediatr 60:528, 1962.
13. Mottet NK, Jensen H: The anomalous embryonic development associated with trisomy 13–15. Am J Clin Pathol 43:334, 1965.
14. Gilbert E, Opitz J: Renal involvement in genetic-hereditary malformation syndromes. In Hamburgerr J, Cronier J, Grunfeld JP (eds): Nephrology. New York, Wiley-Flammarian, 1979, p 909.
15. Smith DW, Patau K, Therman E, et al: The D_1 trisomy syndrome. J Pediatr 62:326, 1963.
16. Juberg RC, Gilbert EF, Salisbury RS: Trisomy C in an infant with polycystic kidneys and other malformations. J Pediatr 76:598, 1970.
17. Casperson T, Lindsten J, Zech L, et al: Four patients with trisomy 8 identified by the fluorescence and Giemsa banding techniques. J Med Genet 9:1, 1972.

18. Crandall BF, Bass HN, Marchy SM: The trisomy 8 syndrome: Two additional mosaic cases. J Med Genet 11:393, 1974.
19. Riccardi VM: Trisomy 8: An international study of 70 patients. Birth Defects 13/3c:171, 1977.
20. Bowen P, Ying KL, Chung GSH: Trisomy 9 mosaicism in a newborn infant with multiple malformations. J Pediatr 85:95, 1974.
21. De La Chapelle A: Cytogenetical and clinical observations in female gonadal dysgenesis. Acta Endocrinol 65 (suppl):1, 1962.
22. Lindsten J: The nature and origin of X chromosome aberrations in Turner's syndrome. Stockholm, Almquist & Wiksell, 1963.
23. Miller JQ: Lissencephaly in two siblings. Neurology 13:841, 1963.
24. Yunis JJ, Ramsay NKC: Familial occurrence of the aniridia-Wilms tumor syndrome with deletion 11p13–14.1. J Pediatr 96:1027, 1980.
25. Riccardi VM, Sujowsky E, Smith AC, et al: Chromosomal imbalance in aniridia-Wilms tumor association: 11p interstitial deletion. Pediatrics 61:604, 1978.
26. Hittner HM, Riccardi VM, Francke U: Aniridia caused by a heritable chromosome 11 deletion. Ophthalmology 86:1173, 1979.
27. Riccardi VM, Hittner HM, Strong LI et al: Wilms tumor with aniridia/iris dysplasia and apparently normal chromosomes. J Pediatr 100:574, 1982.
28. Bowen P, Lee CSN, Zeilweger H, et al: A familial syndrome of multiple congenital defects. Bull J Hopkins Hosp 114:402, 1964.
29. Smith DW, Opitz JM, Inhorn SL: A syndrome of multiple developmental defects, including polycystic kidneys and intrahepatic biliary dysgenesis in two siblings. J Pediatr 67:617, 1965.
30. Passarge E, McAdams AJ: Cerebro-hepato-renal syndrome. J Pediatr 71:691, 1967.
31. Friedman A, Betzhold J, Hong R et al: Clinicopathologic conference: A three-month-old infant with failure to thrive, hepatomegaly and neurological impairment. Am J Med Gent 7:171, 1980.
32. Gilchrist KW, Gilbert EF, Goldfarb S, et al: Studies of malformation syndromes of man XIB. The cerebro-hepato-renal syndrome of Zellweger comparative pathology. Europ J Pediatr 121:99, 1976.
33. Vesmold H, Brauser B, Herzog V, et al: Deficiency of peroxisomes, catalase and cytochrome-B: A genetic defect of oxygen metabolism? Pediatr Res 9:861, 1975.
34. Vesmold HT, Brenner HJ, Herzog V, et al: A metabolic disorder similar to Zellweger syndrome with hepatic acatalasia absence of peroxisomes, altered content and redox state of cytochromes and infantile cirrhosis with hemosiderosis. Europ J Pediatr 124:261, 1977.
35. Opitz JM, Zellweger H, Shannon WR, et al: The RSH syndrome. Birth Defects 5/2:43, 1969.
36. Opitz JM, Frias JL, Gutenberger JE, et al: The G syndrome of multiple congenital anomalies. Birth Defects 5/2:167, 1969.
37. Edelson PJ, Spackman TJ, Belliveau RE, et al: A renal lesion in asphyxiating thoracic dysplasia. Birth Defects 10/16:51, 1974.
38. Gross W: Ein Fall von Agenesie der linken Lunge. Beitr Pathol Anat 37:487, 1905.
39. Herdman RC, Langer LO: The thoracic asphyxiant dystrophy and renal disease. Am J Dis Child 116:192, 1968.
40. Shokeir MHK, Houston CS, Awen CF: Asphyxiating thoracic chondrodystrophy: Association with renal disease and evidence for possible heterozygous expression. J Med Genet 8:107, 1971.
41. Simila S, Vesa L, Wazy-Hockert O: Hereditary onycho-osteodysplasia (the nail-patella syndrome) with nephrosis-like renal disease in a newborn boy. Pediatrics 46:61, 1970.
42. Del Pozo E, Lapp H: Ultrastructure of the kidney in the nephropathy of the nail-patella syndrome. Am J Clin Pathol 54:845, 1970.
43. Finn R, Carruthers JA: Genetic aspects of hydronephrosis associated with renal agenesis. Brit J Urol 46:351, 1974.
44. Bennett WM, Musgrave JE, Campbell RA, et al: The nephropathy of nail-patella syndrome. Clinicopathologic analysis of 11 kindred. Am J Med 54:304, 1973.
45. Ben-Bassat M, Cohen L, Rosenfeld J: The glomerular basement membrane in the nail-patella syndrome. Arch Pathol 92:350, 1971.
46. Del Pozo E, Lapp H: Ultrastructure of the kidney in the nephropathy of the nail-patella syndrome. Am J Clin Pathol 54:845, 1970.
47. Morita T, Laughlin LO, Kawano K, et al: Nail-patella syndrome: Light and electron microscopic studies of the kidney. Arch Int Med 131:271, 1973.
48. Gonzalez-Angulo A, Alford BR, Greenberg SD: Tuberous sclerosis: an otolaryngic diagnosis. Arch Otolaryng 80:193, 1966.
49. Stapleton FB, Johnson D, Kaplan GW, et al: The cystic renal lesion in tuberous sclerosis. J Pediatr 97:574, 1980.
50. Potter EL: Normal and Abnormal Development of the Kidney. Chicago, Year Book Medical Publishers, Inc., 1972, p 201.
51. Kissane J: Congenital anomalies. In Pathology of Infancy and Childhood, ed 2, St. Louis, The C.V. Mosby Co., 1975, p 577.
52. Isaac F, Schoen F, Walker P: An unusual case of Lindau's disease; cystic disease of the kidneys and pancreas with renal and cerebellar tumors. Am J Roentgenol 75:912, 1956.
53. Gibson T: Interrelationship of renal cysts and tumors: report of three cases. J Urol (Baltimore) 71:241, 1954.
54. Parker RW: Absence of abdominal muscles in an infant. Lancet 1:1252, 1895.
55. Eagle JF, Barrett GS: Congenital deficiency of abdominal musculature with associated genitourinary abnormalities: A syndrome; report of nine cases. Pediatrics 6:721, 1950.
56. Nunn N, Stephens FD: The triad syndrome: A composite anomaly of the abdominal wall, urinary system and testes. J Urol 86:782, 1961.
57. Straub E, Spranger J: Etiology and pathogenesis of the prune belly syndrome. Kidney Intl. 20:695, 1981.
58. Opitz JM: The development field concept in clinical genetics. Birth Defects 15:107, 1979.
59. Spranger J: Developmental terms: Some proposals. Europ J Pediatr 113:1, 1979.
60. McGovern JH, Marshall VF: Congenital deficiency of the abdominal musculature and obstructive uropathy. Surg Gynecol Obstet 108:289, 1959.
61. Spence HM, Allen T: Congenital absence of abdominal musculature: Urological aspects. JAMA 187:814, 1964.
62. Hendren WH: Restoration of function in the severely decompensated ureter. In Johnston JH, Scholtmeijer RJ (eds): Problems in Paediatric Urology. Amsterdam, Excerpta Medica, 1972, p 1.
63. Rabinowitz R, Barkin M, Schillinger JF, et al: Urinary tract reconstruction in prune belly syndrome. J Urol. 119:333, 1978.
64. Williams DI: The prune belly syndrome. In Williams DI (ed): Urology in Childhood. New York, Springer, 1974, p 230.
65. Duckett JW: The prune-belly syndrome. In Kelalis PP, King LR (eds): Clinical Pediatric Urology. Philadelphia, W.B. Saunders, 1976, p 376.
66. Johnston JH: Prune belly syndrome. In Eckstein HB, Hohenfellner R, Williams DI (eds): Surgical Pediatric Urology. Stuttgart, Thieme, 1977, p 239.
67. Lowe CU, Terrey M, MacLachlan EA: Organic aciduria, decreased renal ammonia production, hydrophthalmos and mental retardation. Am J Dis Child 83:164, 1952.
68. Witzleben CL, Schoen EJ, Tu WH, et al: Progressive morphologic renal changes in the oculo-cerebro-renal syndrome of Lowe. Am J Med 44:319, 1968.
69. Bardet G: Sur un syndomre d'obésité infantile avec polydactylie et rétinite pigmentaire. (Contribution à l'étude des formes cliniques de l'obésité hypophysaire). Thèse Méd 479, Paris, 1920.
70. Biedl A: Geschwister mit adiposo-genitaler Distrophie. Dtsch Med Wschr 48:1630, 1922.
71. McLoughlin TG, Shanklin DR: Pathology of Laurence-Moon-Bardet-Biedl syndrome. J Pathol Bact 93:65, 1967.
72. Nadjini B, Flanagan MJ, Christian JR: Laurence-Moon-Biedl syndrome associated with multiple genitourinary anomalies. Am J Dis Child 117:352, 1969.
73. Morrison-Hurley R, Dery P, Nogrady MB et al: The renal lesion of Laurence-Moon-Biedl syndrome. J Pediatr 87:206, 1975.
74. Tieder M, Levy M, Gubler MC, et al: Renal abnormalities in the Bardet-Biedl syndrome. Intl J Pediatr Nephrol 3:199, 1982.
75. Dekaban AS: Familial occurrence of congenital retinal blindness and developmental renal lesions. J Genet Hum 17:289, 1969.
76. Loken AC, Hanssen O, Halvorsen S, et al: Hereditary renal dysplasia and blindness. Acta Paediatr Scand 50:177, 1961.
77. Sarles HE, Rodin AE, Poduska PR, et al: Herediatry nephritis, retinitis pigmentosa and chromosomal abnormalities. Am J Med 45:312, 1968.
78. Senior B, Friedmann AI, Braudo JL: Juvenile familial nephropathy with tapetoretinal degeneration. Am J Ophthal 52:625, 1961.
79. Bennett WM, Simon NM, Krill AE, et al: Cystic disease of the renal medulla associated with retinitis pigmentosa and imino acid abnormalities. Clin Nephrol 4:25, 1975.
80. Reiss D, Porath U, Schreier K: Nephronophthise mit tapetoretinaler Degeneration und Glycinurie bei 2 Brudern (eine weitere familiare Nephropathie). Arch Kinderheilk 183:23, 1971.
81. Biochis H, Passwell J, David R, et al: Congenital hepatic fibrosis and nephronophthisis: A family study. Quart J Med 42:221, 1973.
82. Dekaban AS: Hereditary syndrome of congenital retinal blindness (Leber), polycystic kidneys and maldevelopment of the brain. Am J Ophthal 68:1029, 1969.
83. Quan L, Smith DW: The VATER association—Vertebral defects, Anal atresia, T-E fistula with esophageal atresia, Radial and Renal dysplasia: A spectrum of associated defects. J Pediatr 82:104, 1973.
84. Say B, Gerald PS: A new polydactylyl/imperforate-anus/vertebral-anomalies syndrome? Lancet 2:688, 1968.
85. McNeal RM, Francke V: Congenital anomalies including the VATER association in a patient with a del(6) deletion. J Pediatr 91:957, 1977.
86. Uehling DT, Gilbert E, Chesney RW: Urologic implications of the VATER association. J Urol 129:352, 1983.
87. Beckwith JB: Macroglossia, omphalocele, adrenal cytomegaly, gigantism and hyperplastic visceromegaly. Birth Defects 5/2:188, 1969.
88. Kosseff AL, Herrmann J, Gilbert EF, et al: Studies of malformation syndromes of

man XXIX: the Wiedemann-Beckwith syndrome: Clinical, genetic and pathogenic studies of 12 cases. Europ J Pediatr 123:139, 1976.
89. Senior B, Gellis SS: The syndromes of total lipodystrophy and of partial lipodystrophy. Pediatrics 33:592, 1964.
90. Ljunghall, S, Fgellstrom KE, Wibell L: Partial lipodystrophy and chronic hypocomplementemic glomerulonephritis. Acta Med Scand 195:493, 1974.
91. Peters DK, Charlesworth JA, Sissons JGP, et al: Mesangiocapillary nephritis, partial lipodystrophy and hypocomplementemia. Lancet 2:535, 1973.
92. Sisson JGP, West RJ, Fallows J, et al: The complement abnormalities of lipodystrophy. N Engl J Med 294:461, 1976.
93. Denys P, Malvuas P, Van Den Berhe H, et al: Association d'un syndrome anatomophathologique, de pseudohermaphrodisme masculin, d'une tumeur de Wilms, d'une néphropathie parenchymateuse et d'un mosaicisms XX/XY. Arch Franc Pediatr 24:729, 1967.
94. Drash A, Sherman F, Hartmann WH, et al: A syndrome of pseudohermaphroditism, Wilms tumor, hypertension and degenerative renal disease. J Pediatr 76:585, 1970.
95. Boraka AY, Papadopoulo ZC, Chandra RS, et al: Pseudohermaphroditism, nephron disorders and Wilms tumor. A unifying concept. Pediatrics 54:366, 1974.
96. Buchta RM, Viseskul C, Gilbert EF, et al: Familial bilateral renal agenesis and hereditary renal adysplasia. Z Kinderheilk 115:111, 1973.
97. Arends NW: Bilateral renal agenesis in siblings. J Am Osteopath Assn 56:681, 1957.
98. Rosenfeld L: Renal agenesis (questions and answers). JAMA 170:1247, 1959.
99. Andrade C: A peculiar form of peripheral nephropathy. Familial atypical generalized amyloidosis with special involvement of the peripheral nerves. Brain 75:408, 1952.
100. Van Hallen MW, Frohlich JA, Davis JR: Inherited predisposition to generalized amyloidosis. Neurology 19:10, 1969.
101. Langer LO, Nishino R, Yamaguchi A, et al: Brachymesomelia-renal syndrome. Am J Med Genet 15:57–65, 1983.
102. Lemieux G, Neemeh JA: Charcot-Marie-Tooth disease and nephritis. Canad Med Ass J 97:1193, 1967.
103. Higgenbottom M, Cursowold, WR, Jones KL, et al: The cockayne syndrome: An evaluation of hypertension and studies of renal pathology. Pediatrics 64:929, 1979.
104. Goeminne L: A new probably X-linked inherited syndrome: Congenital muscular torticollis, multiple keloids, cryptorchidism and renal dysplasia. Acta Genet Med 17:439, 1967.
105. Galloway WH, Mowat AP: Congenital microcephaly with hiatus hernia and nephrotic syndrome in two siblings. J Med Genet 5:319, 1968.
106. Shapiro LR, Duncan PA, Farnsworth PB, et al: Congenital microcephaly, hiatus hernia and nephritis syndrome: An autosomal recessive syndrome. Birth Defects 12/5:275, 1976.
107. Gilbert EF, Opitz JM, Spranger JW, et al: Chondrodysplasia punctata-rhizomelic form. Pathologic and radiologic studies of three infants. Europ J Pediatr 123:89, 1976.
108. Crome L, Duckett S, Franklin AW: Congenital cataracts, renal tubular necrosis and encephalopathy in two sisters. Arch Dis Childh 38:505, 1963.
109. Imahori S, Bannerman RM, Graf CJ, et al: Ehlers-Danlos syndrome with multiple arterial lesions. Am J Med 47:967, 1969.
110. Elejalde R, Giraldo C, Jimenez R, et al: Acrocephalopolydactylous dysplasia XIII. Birth Defects 13:53, 1977.
111. Lelong M, Alagille D, Philippe A, et al: Diabete salin par insensibilite congenitale du tubule a l'aldosterone: "pseudohypoadrenocorticisme." Rev Franc Clin Biol 5:558, 1960.
112. Grosse FR, Kaveggia L, Opitz JM: Familial hydronephrosis. Z Kinderheilk 114:313, 1973.
113. Mohamed SD, McKay E, Galloway WH: Juvenile familial megaloblastic anemia due to selective malabsorption of vitamin B_{12}. Quart J Med 35:433, 1966.
114. Wegenke JE, Uehling DT, Wear JB, Jr, et al: Familial Kallmann syndrome with unilateral renal aplasia. Clin Genet 7:368, 1975.
115. Rasanen O, Korhonen M, Simila S, et al: Fatal familial steatosis of the liver and kidney in two siblings. Z Kinderheilk 110:267, 1971.
116. Gutenberger J, Trygstad CW, Stiehm ER, et al: Familial thrombocytopenia, elevated serum IgA levels and renal disease: a report of a kindred. Am J Med 49:729, 1970.
117. Gilbert EF, Viseskul C, Mossman HW, et al: The pathologic anatomy of the G syndrome. Z Kinderheilk 111:290, 1972.
118. Miller I, Kuschner M: Alpha-1-antitrypsin deficiency, emphysema, necrotizing angitis and glomerulonephritis. Am J Med 46:615, 1969.
119. Gorlin RJ, Jue KL, Jacobsen U, et al: Oculoauriculovertebral dysplasia. J Pediatr 63:991, 1963.
120. Caramia G, Di Battista C, Botticelli A: La sindrome di Goldenhar. Descrizione di un caso con malformazioni cardiovascolari, agenesia del polmone destro e situs viscerum inversus. Minerva Pediatr 22:362, 1976.
121. Bowen P, Lee CSN, Zellweger H: A familial syndrome of multiple congenital defects. Bull J Hopkins Hosp 114:402, 1964.
122. Joseph R, Nezelof C, Guerard L, et al: Acroosteolyse idiopathique familiale: renseignements fournis par la biopsie. Sem Hop Ann Pediatr 35:82, 1959.
123. Marie J, Leveque G, Lyon G, et al: Acroosteolyse essentielle compliquee d'insuffisance renal d'evolution fatale. Presse Med 71:249, 1963.
124. Kleinsorge H: Akroosteolytische Ersheinungen der Osteomalacie. Fortschr Geburtsh Rontgenstr 73:471, 1950.
125. Ivemark BI, Oldfelt V, Zetterstrom R: Familial dysplasia of kidneys, liver and pancreas: A probably genetically determined syndrome. Acta Paediatr Scand 48:1, 1959.
126. Kaufman RL, McAlister WH, Ho CK, et al: Family studies in congenital heart disease. VI. The association of severe obstructive left heart lesion, vertebral and renal anomalies; a second family. Birth Defects 10/7:93, 1974.
127. Mankad VN, Gray GF, Miller DR: Bilateral nephroblastomatosis and Klippel-Trenaunay syndrome. Cancer 33:1462, 1974.
128. Perlman M, Goldberg GM, Barziv J, et al: Renal hamartomas and nephroblastomatosis with fetal gigantism: a familial syndrome. J Pediatr 83:414, 1973.
129. Perlman M, Levin M, Wittels B: Syndrome of fetal gigantism, renal hamartomas and nephroblastomatosis with Wilms tumor. Cancer 35:1212, 1975.
130. Liddle GW, Bledsoe T, Cuppage WS: A familial renal disorder simulating primary aldosteronism but with negligible aldosterone secretion. Trans Assoc Am Phys 76:199, 1963.
131. Dieker H, Edwards RH, ZuRhein G, et al: The lissencephaly syndrome. Birth Defects 5/2:53, 1969.
132. Drash A, Sherman F, Hartmann WH, et al: A syndrome of pseudohermaphroditism, Wilms tumor, hypertension and degenerative renal disease. J Pediatr 76:585, 1970.
133. Somer A, Mulne A, Cordero L: The Majewski syndrome. A case report (abstract). Birth Defects 13/3B:252, 1977.
134. Miranda D, Schinella RA, Finegold MJ: Familial renal dysplasia. Arch Pathol 93:483, 1972.
135. Emery AEH, Oleesky S, Williams, RT: Myotonic dystrophy and polycystic disease of the kidneys. J Med Genet 4:26, 1967.
136. Doege TC, Thuline HC, Priest JH, et al: Studies of a family with the oral-facial-digital syndrome. N Engl J Med 271:1073, 1964.
137. Tucker CC, Finley SC, Tucker ES, et al: Oral-facial-digital syndrome, with polycystic kidneys and liver: Pathological and cytogenetic studies. J Med Genet 3:145, 1966.
138. Ozer FL: A possible "new" syndrome with eye and renal abnormalities. Birth Defects 10/4:168, 1974.
139. Kieselstein M, Herman G, Wahrman J, et al: Mucocutaneous pigmentation and intestinal polyposis (Peutz-Jeghers syndrome) in a family of Iraqi Jews with polycystic kidney disease with a chromosome study. Israel J. Med Sci 5:81, 1969.
140. Leclerc JP, Canet J, Lancret P, et al: Polykystose hepatopancreato-epididymo-renale et polydystrophie thoracique neo-natales. Etude anatomo-clinique d'une observation. Arch Franc Pediatr 28:425, 1971.
141. Royer P, Bonnette J, Mathieu H, et al: Pseudo-hypoaldosteronisme. Ann Pediatr 10:596, 1963.
142. Lundin PM, Olow I: Polycystic kidneys in newborns, infants and children. Acta Paediatr Scand 50:185, 1961.
143. Harley LM, Chen Y, Rattner WH; Prune belly syndrome. J Urol (Baltimore) 108:174, 1972.
144. Orr LM: Familial (?) hydronephrosis. Urologists Correspondence Club Letter, August 4, 1961.
145. Osathanondh V, Potter EL: Pathogenesis of polycystic kidneys. Arch Pathol 77:459, 1964.
146. Wochner RD, Silverman D, Germuth J, et al: An apparently hereditary syndrome of throtoxicosis, renal disease and absent frontal sinuses. Clin Res 17:530, 1969.
147. Gonzales-Angulo A, Alford BR, Greenberg SD: Tuberous sclerosis: An otolaryngic diagnosis. Arch Otolaryngol 80:193, 1964.
148. Stapleton FB, Johnson D, Kaplan GW, et al: The cystic renal lesion in tuberous sclerosis. J Pediatr 97:574, 1980.
149. Muckle TJ, Wells M: Urticaria, deafness and amyloidosis: A new heredo-familial syndrome. Quart J Med 31:235, 1961.
150. Tonning HO, Warren RF, Barrie HJ: Familial haemangiomata of the cerebellum; report of three cases in a family of four. J Neurosurg 9:124, 1952.
151. Gibson T: Interrelationship of renal cysts and tumors; report of three cases. J Urol (Baltimore) 71:241, 1954.
152. Winter JSD, Kohn G, Mellman WJ, et al: A familial syndrome of renal, genital and middle ear anomalies. J Pediatr 72:88, 1968.
153. Spitler LE, Wray RB, Maserman S, et al: Nephropathy of the Wiskott-Aldrich syndrome. Pediatrics 66:391, 1980.
154. Wohltman H, Cagler M, Hartroft PM, et al: Juxtaglomerular hyperplasia and elevated renin in a normotensive infant with high serum sodium and chloride but normal potassium. Am J Pathol 62:16a, 1971.
155. Bernstein J, Kissane JM: Hereditary disorders of the kidney. In Rosenberg HS, Bolande RP (eds): Perspectives in Pediatric Pathology. Chicago, Year Book Medical, 1973, vol. 1, p 117.

CHAPTER 13

Immunological Processes in Kidney Disease

FREDERICK G. GERMUTH[a]
EUGENE RODRIGUEZ

Immunological mechanisms play a prominent role in a wide variety of human kidney diseases. Experimental models have been developed that mimic many of these diseases. To discuss such models it will be necessary to review some pertinent aspects of basic immunology.

BASIC IMMUNOLOGICAL PROCESSES

Antigen

Molecules that act as antigens show two capacities: (1) the ability to stimulate antibody formation and (2) the ability to react with antibody. Although these capacities are readily separated conceptually and may occasionally be separated in experimental work, most naturally occurring antigens display both properties.

Basic to both roles of antigen is the concept of the antigenic determinant—a region on a molecule with which antibody can react. This region is relatively large when compared to the area involved in most chemical bonds. A number of studies have shown that the determinant group corresponds to an area of five to seven amino acid or monosaccharide groups.

In terms of the ability of a molecule to stimulate antibody formation, it has been shown that it must have determinant groups of definite (rigid) structure and have more than one determinant group. Since the groups are of such large size, this means that only relatively large molecules ($\geq$1000 daltons) are able to cause antibody formation. The molecule must also have determinants that are foreign to the antibody-forming mechanisms of the host. However, it should be noted that modification of native molecules (by physical, chemical, or enzymatic means) may expose hidden antigenic determinants or generate "foreign" antigenic determinants on host molecules and thus give rise to auto-antibodies.

The number of determinant groups (valence) will influence the consequences of the reaction of antigen with antibody. A molecule with one determinant group (univalent hapten) can react with antibody, but since it cannot cross link with other antibody molecules it cannot cause precipitation, agglutination, or activation of the complement system.

[a]Deceased, 1984.

Most naturally occurring antigens have a number of antigenic determinants, which correlates closely with the size of the molecule. With most proteins, the structure of each of these determinants is distinct. With polysaccharides, a given molecule may contain several repetitions of the same determinant.

Antibodies

In contrast to the wide variety of molecular structures that serve as antigens, antibodies are members of a structurally, and therefore antigenically, closely related family. The basic unit of the immunoglobulin molecule is a four chain structure, consisting of two light chains ($\sim$25,000 daltons) and two heavy chains ($\sim$50,000 daltons) held together by disulfide bonds and noncovalent interactions. Whereas IgG, IgD, and IgE each has only one of these basic structures, IgA may have two or more and IgM almost always has five of the basic structures. In these polymeric molecules, disulphide bonds and a polypeptide called the J-chain hold the monomers together. In addition, in polymers of IgA present in the external secretions, another polypeptide, called the secretory component, is present. While the light chains of molecules of all five classes are the same (being either kappa or lambda for each molecule), each class has a distinct heavy chain, so that antibodies specific for these chains allow recognization of the various classes by, for example, immunofluorescence techniques. The different structures of the heavy chains are also responsible for the varying characteristics of the immunoglobulins. In terms of renal disease, one of the most important of these properties is the ability to activate the complement system by the "classical pathway," which is restricted to IgM and some IgG antibodies.

Each antibody combining site is made up of the amino terminal ends of a heavy and a light chain. Thus, each monomeric antibody molecule (IgG, IgD, IgE, and monomeric IgA) has two combining sites, while polymers (IgM, polymeric IgA) have multiples of two sites—ten for IgM, four for dimeric IgA, and so on.

In Vitro Ag-Ab Reactions

Since most naturally occurring antigens and all antibodies have more than one reactive group (determinant or combining site), these reagents can combine with one another in varying proportions, depending on the ratio in which they are mixed. As shown in Figure 13.1, this property can give rise to complexes of antibody and antigen with widely varying properties. The figure represents a precipitin curve in which increasing amounts of antigen are added to a constant amount of antibody. While a continuous spectrum of antigen-antibody complexes are formed, for purposes of this discussion we have divided this spectrum into three classes. Class III complexes are the largest in size and thus are removed from the supernatant fluid by ordinary centrifugal forces. Class II complexes, which are formed in the presence of larger amounts of antigen, are too small to be precipitated by ordinary centrifugal forces, but are relatively complex in structure. Class I complexes, which contain a higher proportion of antigen, are even smaller and simpler in structure. The latter two are referred to as soluble immune complexes.

In addition to the ratio in which antigens and antibodies are mixed, immune complex size (class) is influenced by a number of factors: (1) size of the antigen molecule, (2) size of the antibody molecule, which is a function of immunoglobulin class, (3) firmness of binding of antibody to antigen (avidity), and (4) interaction of complexes with other systems, e.g., complement or rheumatoid factors may increase size of complexes.

Antigen size can vary over an enormous range—from molecules as small as 1000 daltons to viruses that may be many millions in molecular weight. In contrast, antibody molecular weight is restricted by the limited classes of immunoglobulins to a range between 160,000 and about 900,000 daltons. With large antigens and large antibody molecules, it may be impossible to form Class I complexes regardless of the ratio in which antigen and antibody are mixed.

Antibody avidity is a measure of the firmness with which antibody binds to antigen. It is determined by the number of antigenic determinants that the antibody molecules in a given serum can recognize on the antigen molecule and by how well the antibody combining sites fit themselves to the various antigenic determinants. Since both the number of antigenic determinants recognized and the "goodness-of-fit" between antigenic determinant and combining site generally increase with time after immunization, a gradual rise in avidity usually occurs with time. If two antigens share some, but not all, antigenic determinants (i.e., are cross-reacting antigens) antibody to one of them will show a lower avidity in its reaction with the other (heterologous) antigen, than with the antigen which stimulated its formation.

Both complement (in particular C1, *vide infra*) and rheumatoid factors can combine with soluble immune complexes to increase their size and thus change their solubility properties. In contrast to this effect, complement has been shown to be able to solubilize insoluble complexes by interposing itself into the antigen-antibody matrix.

The Complement System

The complement system consists of nine serum proteins that can be triggered by antigen-antibody complexes to participate in a cascade of coupled enzymatic reactions, resulting in the release of biologically active molecules and the possible death and destruction of cellular elements. The classical pathway, which involves all of these components, can be initiated by most antibodies of the IgG class and by IgM antibodies. The sequence of action of the complement components involves a recognization step in which C1 recognizes sites on the antibody molecules; reactions involving C1, C4, and C2 in which a so-called C3-convertase is formed (activation step); and a sequence of reactions involving the remaining six components, termed the effector stage, which results in the release of anaphylatoxins (substances capable of increasing vascular permeability and contracting smooth muscles), chemotactic factors (substances capable of attracting leukocytes), generation of immune adher-

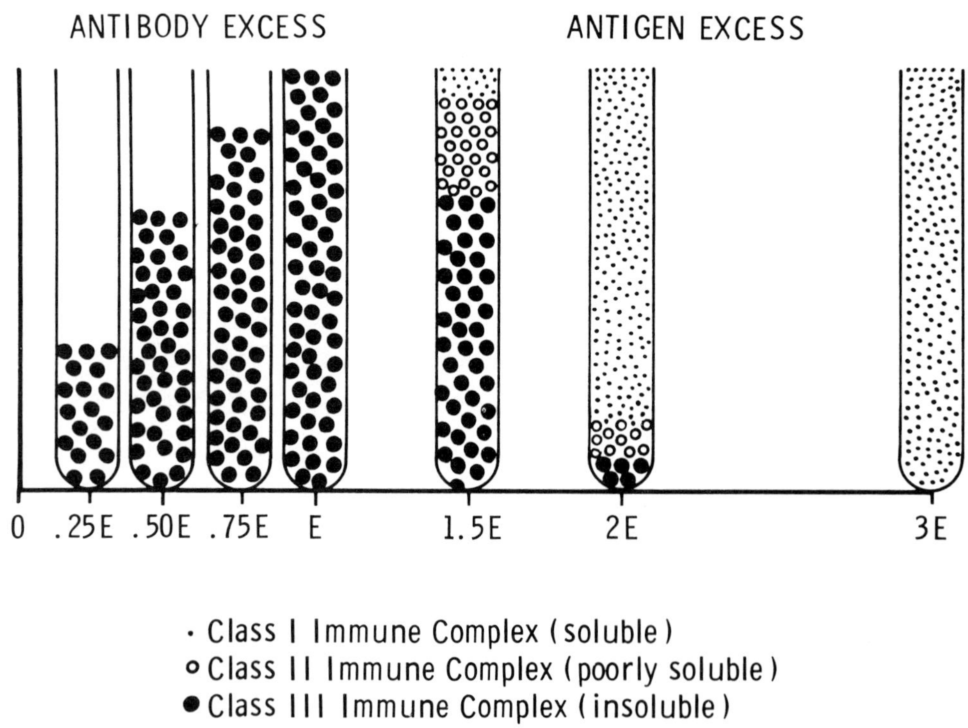

Figure 13.1. Reaction of antibody of the IgG class with its homologous antigen (MW, about 70,000 daltons). The figure represents a series of test tubes, each containing the same amount of antibody, to each of which a different quantity of antigen has been added. The antigen amounts are indicated along the abscissa, relative to E, the amount of antigen required for maximum precipitation of the antibody. The relative amounts of the different classes of immune complexes that are formed in each test tube are indicated by the volumes occupied by the appropriate symbols, which are identified below the figure. (From Germuth FG, Rodriguez E: Immunopathology of the Renal Glomerulus. Boston, Little, Brown & Co., 1973.)

ance activity (in which materials which have a portion of the C3 molecule (C3b) attached can interact with cells (monocytes, lymphocytes, polymorphonuclear leukocytes, and erythrocytes, which have receptors for C3b on their surface); and a membrane attack system (C5 through C9) that can penetrate the cell membrane of cells on which (or in the vicinity of which) the activating antigen-antibody reaction has taken place, rendering the cells susceptible to osmotic lysis.

In the alternate pathway of complement activation, the effector stage remains the same but a different C3-convertase is generated and the recognization step is initiated by different triggers—immune complexes of any immunoglobulin class, including those incapable of activating complement via the classical pathway, e.g., IgA; and cell wall materials of certain bacteria (lipopolysaccharides) and yeasts (zymosan). This pathway involves C3b and proteins designated as B, D, and properdin in the generation of the alternative C3-convertase, by-passing the need for C1, 4, and 2. The role of C3b in both the classical and alternative pathways provides a feedback amplification mechanism for complement activation by either pathway. It should be noted that localization of properdin in kidney specimens by immunofluorescence techniques provides good evidence for the presence of activation of complement by the alternative pathway.

Finally, some degree of interaction between the complement system and the coagulation system has been suspected for a long time. While it is now known that thrombin and plasmin, activated *via* the coagulation system, may in turn activate C1 and C3, the role that this mechanism may play in immunological disease is unclear.

Cell-Mediated Reactions

In addition to so-called humoral mechanisms of immunity, dependent on circulating antibodies, cell-mediated mechanisms of immunity, dependent on sensitized leukocytes, play a major role in protection from certain infections, particularly those involving viruses and intracellular pathogens. In response to such infections and other sources of antigenic exposure, T-lymphocytes become sensitized so that they respond to a second exposure to an antigen by the release of substances called lymphokines. These substances can attract macrophages to their vicinity, inhibit their migration away from that vicinity, "arm" them, i.e., increase their level of hydrolytic enzymes so that they become more efficient killers of ingested cells, and kill certain cells. In addition, such lymphocytes can release interferon, with its known antiviral activities.

While macrophages and monocytes are prominent in certain kinds of immunological kidney diseases, suggesting that cell-mediated mechanisms might be implicated, clear evidence of the importance of such mechanisms in these diseases have not yet been produced (1, 2).

In Vivo Antigen-antibody Reactions

The reaction of antibody with antigen has no effect on the antigen unless it is a virus, toxin, or enzyme, so that the mere presence of the antibody may interfere with the functioning of the antigen molecule. In order for the antigen-antibody reaction to have a biological effect, the complex must interact with some biological system. Ehrlich likened the reaction of antibody with antigen to the fitting of a key to a lock. The various mechanisms of hypersensitivity may be regarded as engines that can be started by turning the key in the lock.

Briefly, hypersensitivity reactions have been divided into five types, depending on their basic mechanisms. In Type I or anaphylactic hypersensitivity, antibody of a specific class (in man, IgE) becomes attached via its H chains to specific receptors on certain cells (mast cells and basophils). When such cell-bound antibody molecules are cross-linked by antigen, a biochemical process is initiated that leads to the release of pharmacologically active substances (histamine, serotonin, slow-reacting substance, and so on), which, by their effects on nearby tissues, bring about the symptoms of Type I allergic reactions.

In Type II (cytotoxic) reactions, the antibody is specific for antigen determinants that are part of the surface of the target cell. The cell is destroyed as a result of its interaction with antibody, either through activation of the complement system, with its membrane attack mechanism, or by the effect of "killer" lymphocytes that have receptors for the heavy chains of the antibody molecule on their surface.

In contrast to the cell-bound antibodies that are responsible for Types I and II hypersensitivity, Type III (immune complex) hypersensitivity is a result of antigen-antibody reactions occurring in the tissue spaces. A prototype of such reactions is that discovered by Maurice Arthus. The Arthus phenomenon, originally observed to follow repeated injections of antigen into the skin of experimental animals, is the result of the interaction of relatively large amounts of antigen and antibody in the vicinity of blood vessels. The result of this interaction is a vasculitis characterized by an acute inflammatory reaction including polymorphonuclear leukocytic infiltration and thrombosis of blood vessels. Experimental work has shown that both the complement system and polymorphonuclear leukocytes are required for a full-blown Arthus phenomenon (3, 4, 5). As a result of this work, the hypothesis has been suggested that complement interacts with antigen-antibody complexes formed in the vicinity of the blood vessels, generating chemotactic and anaphylactoxic factors; that polymorphonuclear leukocytes accumulate as a result; and that these cells ingest the antibody-antigen-complement complexes and release the contents of their lysosomal granules into the surrounding area. It is the enzymes contained in the released granule contents that are believed to produce the severe vascular damage characteristic of the Arthus phenomenon.

While Type I, II, and III hypersensitivity reactions are brought about by circulating antibody, i.e., are humoral or antibody mediated hypersensitivity reactions, Type IV is cell mediated and is dependent on sensitized lymphocytes (see previous paragraph).

Recently a fifth mechanism has been recognized, in which circulating antibody reacts with a component of a cell such as a hormone receptor and turns on or off the biochemical activity of that cell in an uncontrolled and unphysiological way.

As will be noted, whereas there is extensive evidence for the role of Type III mechanisms in experimental kidney disease, and mechanisms similar to those involved in Type II are also implicated, there is at present little evidence for the importance of the other three types of hypersensitivity reactions.

EXPERIMENTAL MODELS OF KIDNEY DISEASE

Experimental immunologic kidney disease can be divided into two major categories, in one of which antibodies react with antigens contained in the glomerulus (*in situ* immune complex disease) while in the other antigen-antibody complexes formed outside of the kidney become deposited in the kidney (circulating immune complex disease) (6).

In-situ Immune Complex Disease

Anti-glomerular Basement Membrane Disease

Masugi Nephritis. In Masugi nephritis (7) animals that are given injections of antiglomerular antibodies (8, 9) develop a biphasic glomerulonephritis. The primary phase is a result of the fixation of heterologous antibody to the glomerulus (8). Recent work (10, 11) has shown that the antibody is attached to the inner and outer aspects of the glomerular basement membrane (Fig. 13.2 and 13.3). In the rabbit and rat, small

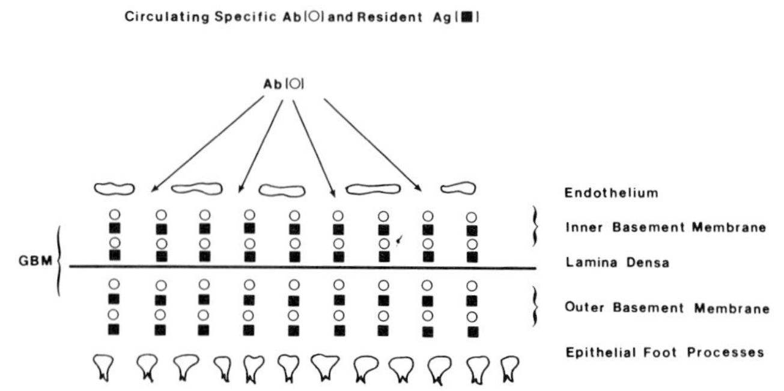

Figure 13.2. Primary phase of Masugi nephritis. Heterologous antibody attaches to resident antigen scattered diffusely through the inner and outer layers of the basement membrane. Secondary phase (not diagrammed) is a result of homologous antibody reacting with the heterologous antibody molecules.

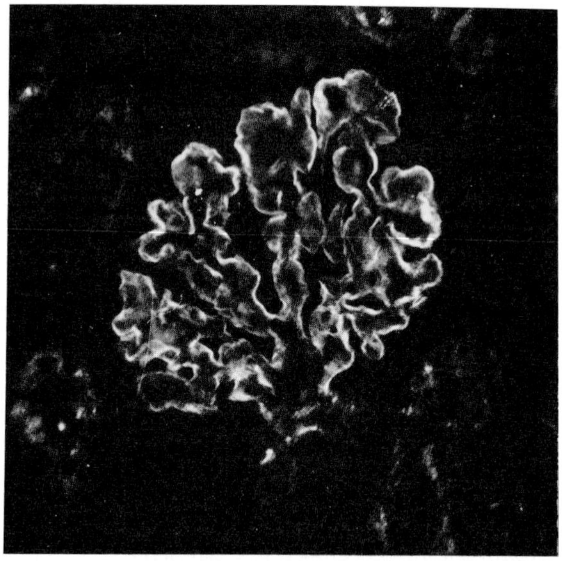

Figure 13.3. Secondary phase, Masugi nephritis. Linear deposition of rabbit IgG in the glomerulus of a rabbit developing glomerulonephritis 10 days after the injection of goat antirabbit glomerular basement membrane antibody. (Immunofluorescence microscopy, antibody specific for rabbit IgG, X200.) (From Germuth FG, Rodriguez E: Immunopathology of the Renal Glomerulus, Little, Brown & Co., 1973).

doses of heterologous mammalian antiglomerular basement membrane antibody produce a primary phase characterized by an evanescent polymorphonuclear leukocyte infiltration (12). The mild proteinuria that occurs in these animals is abrogated by depletion of polymorphonuclear leukocytes or complement (12). Large doses of heterologous antibody in the rat (12) and in the rabbit (13) may not be associated with polymorphonuclear leukocytic infiltration, even though proteinuria and azotemia are present. Since complement is detected in these lesions, they may represent the effect of the membrane attack system of complement. In the primary phase in the guinea pig with moderate doses of antibody, mild proteinuria occurs independent of complement, polymorphonuclear leukocytes and other known mediators of inflammation (14).

The secondary phase appears after a latent period of 4 or more days and follows the fixation of the host antibody (15) and complement (16) to the heterologous antibody that remains attached to the host basement membrane. In the rabbit, depending on the rate of antibody formation by the host and the amount of antibody formed, the lesions vary from glomerular hypercellularity produced by infiltration by monocytes to rapidly progressive (crescentic) glomerulonephritis associated with numerous fibrin deposits in Bowman's space and the evolution of crescents (Fig. 13.4). Little is known about the role of complement in the production of these lesions, but similar lesions can be produced in C6 deficient rabbits (13, 17). In the rat the secondary phase is characterized by a membranous type of glomerulopathy and the nephrotic syndrome (18).

Steblay Nephritis. Whereas Masugi nephritis involves injecting an animal with heterologous antiglomerular basement membrane antibody, Steblay nephritis is produced by immunizing sheep or goats with multiple injections of heterologous or homologous glomerular antigen in adjuvant, the antibodies formed going on to react with the animal's own glomerular antigens to produce an "autoimmune" glomerulonephritis (19, 20, 21, 22). The rapidity with which the lesions develop depends on whether the animals are immunized with whole glomeruli, sonicated glomerular basement membrane, or enzymatically solubilized glomerular basement membrane. The lesions are characterized by a rapidly progressive (crescentic) glomerulonephritis showing numerous polymorphonuclear leukocytes, monocytes, and occasional breaks in the continuity of the basement membrane (22). The immunofluorescence staining for IgG and C3 is linear (Fig. 13.5). Similarities between the linear staining patterns in Masugi and Steblay nephritides and human Goodpasture's syndrome led to the suggestion that the latter also is an antibasement membrane disease. It was subsequently shown that the passive transfer of human serum containing antiglomerular basement membrane antibodies (from patients with Goodpasture's disease) could produce an antiglomerular basement membrane nephritis in monkeys (23). The recent observation of the immunologic similarities between Goodpasture's and Steblay's antibodies (each showing a subendothelial linear pattern along the basement membrane) (Fig. 13.6, *A* and *B*) further confirms the similarity of the two disorders (11, 24). Although immunofluorescence studies reveal a linear staining for complement in Steblay nephritis, in Goodpasture's disease such staining may be linear, segmen-

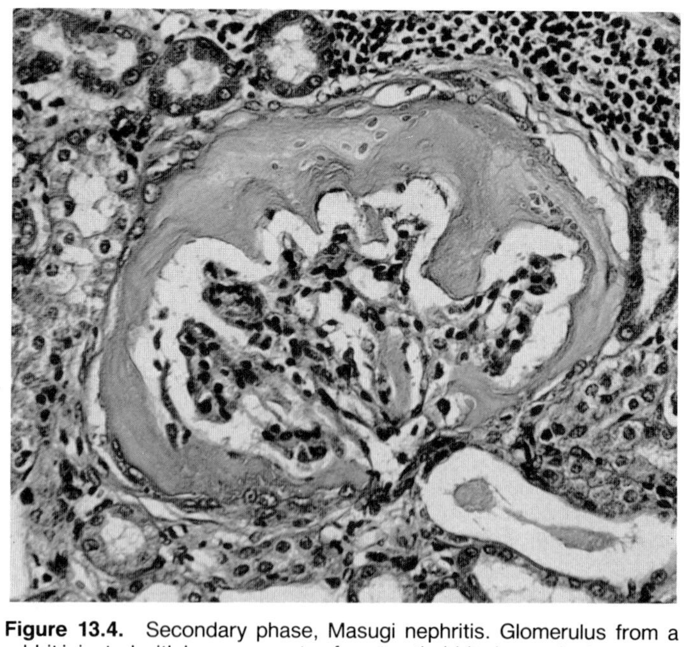

Figure 13.4. Secondary phase, Masugi nephritis. Glomerulus from a rabbit injected with large amounts of goat antirabbit glomerular basement membrane antibody 10 days before necropsy. There is significant exudation of fibrin and plasma proteins into Bowman's space, associated with localized necrosis of the glomerular loops (Hematoxylin-eosin stain; X350.) (From Germuth FG, Rodriguez E: Immunopathology of the Renal Glomerulus. Little, Brown & Co., 1973.)

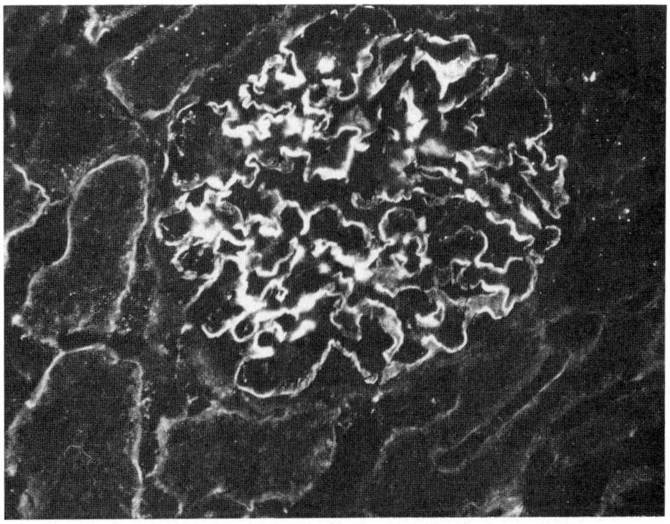

Figure 13.5. Steblay Nephritis. Linear deposition of goat IgG occurring along glomerular and tubular basement membranes. (Immunofluorescence microscopy, antibody specific for sheep IgG, X400.) (From Germuth FG, Rodriguez E: Immunopathology of the Renal Glomerulus. Little, Brown & Co., 1973.)

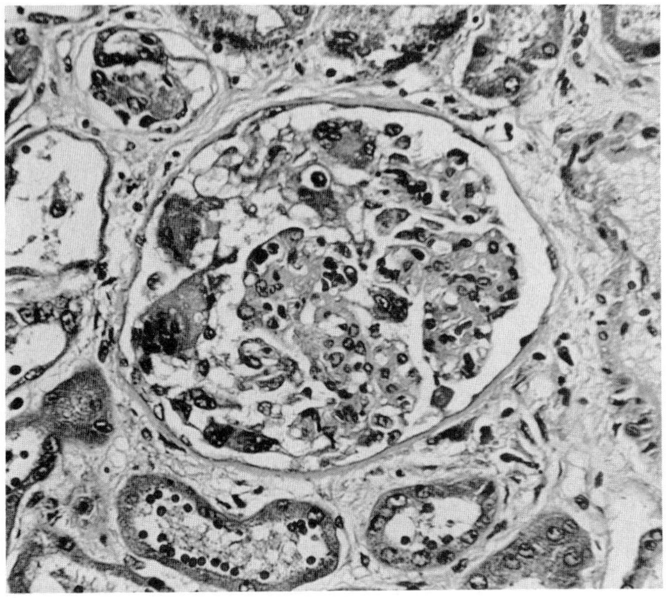

Figure 13.7. Goodpasture's disease. Renal specimen from a patient who died within one month of onset. Fragmentation of glomerular tuft associated with epithelial cell proliferation and the formation of numerous syncitial cells. (Hematoxylin-eosin stain; X350.) (From Germuth FG, Rodriguez E: Immunopathology of the Renal Glomerulus. Little, Brown & Co., 1973.)

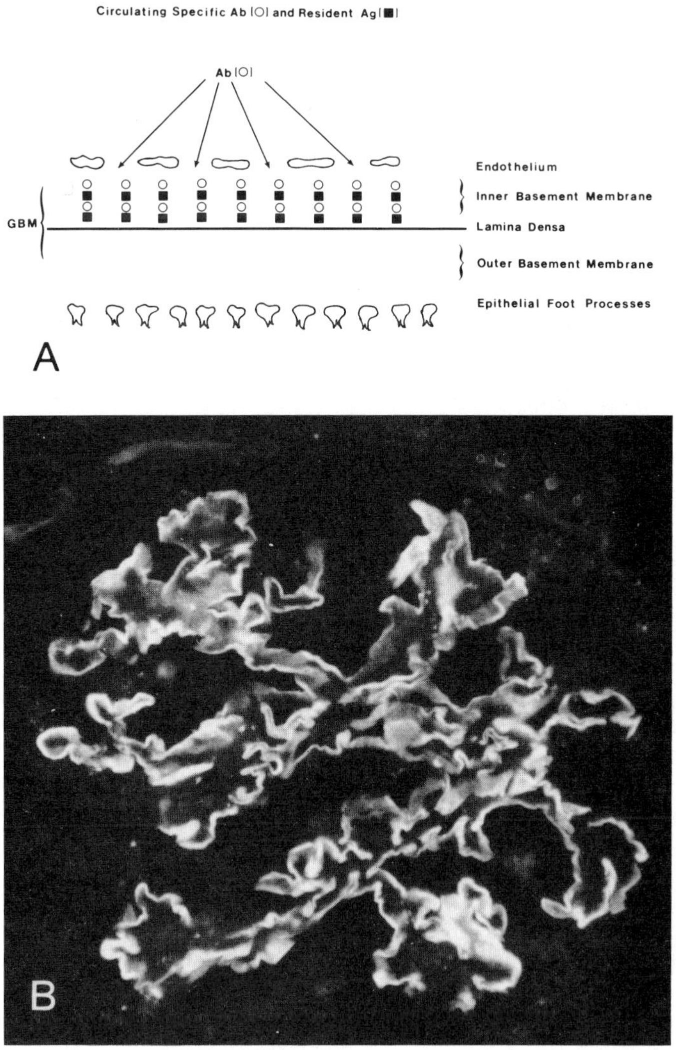

tal, or absent (6). Thus, the role of complement is not clear in the glomerular lesions of Goodpasture's disease. Steblay nephritis, as well as Goodpasture's nephritis, often show syncitial multinucleated giant epithelial cells which are almost diagnostic of these two entities (Fig. 13.7). In addition, both of these entities may be accompanied by a florid tubulointerstitial disease of the kidney in which the basement membrane stains linearly by immunofluorescence (*vide infra*).

Heymann Nephritis (Autologous Immune Complex Nephritis). Rats of certain strains immunized with rat kidney homogenate in complete Freund's adjuvant develop a chronic glomerular disease characterized by the nephrotic syndrome (25). The histology of the glomerular lesions resembles that of membranous glomerulopathy in man (26) and is characterized by subepithelial immune complex deposits producing transformation of the basement membrane. The complexes can be stained for a renal tubular brush-border antigen (Fx 1A), IgG, and C3 (27). Because of the autologous nature of the antigen and the granularity of the complexes (Fig. 13.8), Heymann nephritis was termed autologous immune complex glomerulonephritis (27, 28). It was believed to be a result of circulating antibodies capable of reacting with low serum levels of autologous renal tubular antigens and was thought to be another example of circulating immune complex disease (29). Since the disease developed in the presence of an excess of antibody, in contrast to the BSA-rabbit system that develops in antigen excess (*vide infra*), questions arose as to whether this was ordinary circulating immune complex glomerulonephritis. In a passive model of this disease (produced by

Figure 13.6. **A,** Goodpasture's disease and Steblay nephritis. Diagram showing homologous antibody reacting with resident antigen scattered diffusely throughout the inner aspect of the basement membrane. **B,** Goodpasture's disease. Renal specimen from a patient who died within 1 month of onset. Linear deposition of IgG along the glomerular loops. (Immunofluorescence microscopy, antibody specific for IgG, X400). (From Germuth FG, Rodriguez E: Immunopathology of the Renal Glomerulus. Little, Brown & Co., 1973.)

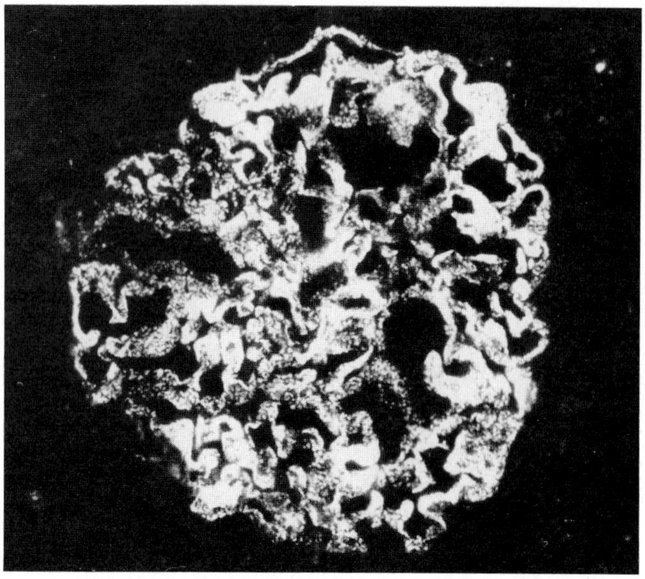

Figure 13.8. Heymann nephritis. Fourteen weeks after first injection of kidney homogenate into a Sprague Dawley rat. (Immunofluorescence microscopy, antibody specific for C3, X400). Notice thick granular deposits throughout the loops. (Courtesy of Dr. William Keene, Regional Kidney Center, Hennepin County Medical Center, Minneapolis.)

injections of heterologous antibodies to Fx 1A), it was found that immune complexes could be demonstrated along the epithelial surface of the rat glomerular basement membrane within a few minutes after the injections of antibody and that perfusion of isolated normal rat kidneys with such antibody resulted in the formation of subepithelial immune deposits. Further, Fx 1A antigen was found to be normally present in the lamina rara externa of the glomerular basement membrane. Thus, it was concluded that in this model the immune complexes were formed locally (in situ) by circulating antibody reacting with fixed antigen, rather than being formed in the circulation and being deposited in the glomeruli (30, 31). It was later shown that this mechanism of in situ immune complex formation was also applicable to the active model of autologous disease (32). In addition, antibodies eluted from the kidneys of rats with the autologous disease could be shown to localize in the characteristic subepithelial position when they were perfused into isolated normal rat kidneys (33). Presumably, an irregular distribution of the relevant antigen was responsible for the granular appearance of the deposits seen using immunofluorescence and electron microscopy (Fig. 13.9), findings which had been thought to be diagnostic of circulating immune complex disease in contrast to the linear deposits characteristic of Masugi and Steblay antiglomerular basement membrane disease in which antibody reacts with diffusely distributed antigens on the glomerular basement membrane.

Further studies of the passive Heymann nephritis model have shown that the proteinuria that begins 4 to 5 days after infusion of antibody appears to be complement dependent but not to require the presence of polymorphonuclear leukocytes (34). In the active model it has been demonstrated that the increase in glomerular capillary permeability occurs in the vicinity of the localized immune complexes (35).

Because of the evidence that this model of glomerulonephritis is a result of the reaction of antibody with a fixed antigen on the glomerular basement membrane and therefore is in essence another form of anti-basement membrane disease, it is suggested that it no longer be referred to as autologous immune complex disease, but rather be called Heymann nephritis.

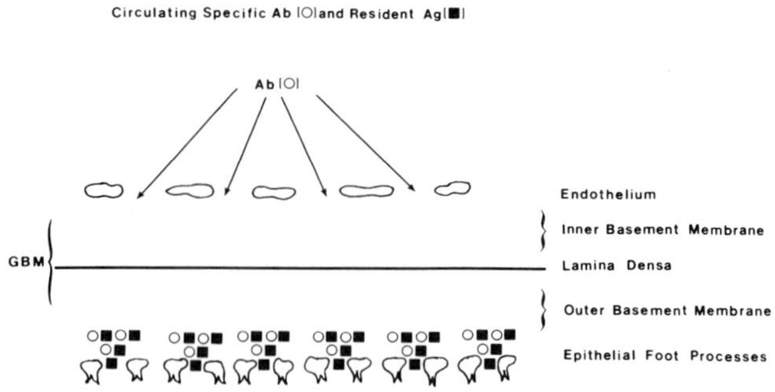

Figure 13.9. Heymann nephritis. Diagram showing homologous antibody reacting with resident antigen irregularly distributed in the outer basement membrane and epithelial cell foot processes, producing subepithelial deposits.

In-Situ Glomerular Disease Involving Nonglomerular Antigens

While the antigens involved in Masugi, Steblay, and Heymann nephritides are normally part of the glomerulus, a number of models of other in situ forms of glomerular disease have been developed in which nonglomerular antigens, fixed to or entering the glomerular basement membrane before the influx of antibody, are involved.

Endotoxin-induced Localization of DNA-anti-DNA Complexes

Injections of bacterial lipopolysaccharide endotoxins into mice are followed by the appearance of relatively low weight DNA in the circulation and subsequent formation of antibodies to DNA. In vitro studies have shown that DNA has an affinity for collagen and glomerular basement membrane, suggesting that an in situ mechanism might be responsible for the formation of DNA-antibody complexes in diseases in which such complexes are prominent (36, 37). In vivo studies in mice injected with endotoxin showed that glomerular DNA-antibody complexes could be detected before complexes appeared in the circulation, and that the circulating complexes did not contain DNA, lending support to the suggested in situ mechanism. However, a role for circulating DNA-antibody complexes could not be ruled out. The initial mesangial localization of the complexes in human and murine systemic lupus is in contrast with the in vitro localization of the DNA along the basement membrane.

Concanavalin A

The plant lectin, concanavalin A, can bind to the mannose and glucose present in the glomerular basement membrane. When concanavalin A is perfused into one kidney of rats, subsequent exposure to antibody to concanavalin A (either administered intravenously or actively formed by the perfused animal) results in a diffuse glomerulonephritis restricted to the perfused kidney. Immune complexes are found diffusely located along the inner glomerular basement membrane in the perfused kidney (38). There is thus good evidence that this represents a model of in situ immune complex disease.

In Situ Complex Formation With Lysozyme and Bovine Serum Albumin as Antigens

Using a perfusion model similar to that just described, it was found that alternate perfusions of bovine serum albumin and specific antibody, separated by perfusions of buffer, resulted in the formation of granular deposits of immune complexes along the basement membrane, in a subepithelial location (39). Similar results could be found with lysozyme, which was known to become attached to anionic sites of the basement membrane. No studies of renal function were carried out, and no microscopic evidence of glomerular damage was observed, perhaps because the experiment was terminated 3 days after perfusion to avoid complications in the interpretation of results that might be caused by an immune response to the injected materials.

Mesangial Lesions Produced by Injections of Aggregated Antigens and Appropriate Antibody

Aggregated human IgG or serum albumin injected intravenously into rabbits accumulates in the glomerular mesangium. If kidneys bearing such aggregated proteins are transplanted to normal rabbits and the latter injected with the appropriate antibody, the antibody reacts with the localized antigen, complement is localized, and an immediate polymorphonuclear leukocyte infiltration is observed. The lesion progresses to mesangial hypercellularity and increased mesangial matrix (40).

Models Dependent on the Charge Properties of Antigen or Antigen-antibody Complexes

The discovery that the glomerular basement membrane normally contains fixed negatively charged (anionic) sites, presumably heparan sulfate (41, 42), has led to investigation of a number of models of in situ complex disease in which positively charged antigen has been involved.

One model has been described wherein the perfusion of positively charged (cationized) antigen [ferritin (43) or human IgG (44)] into one kidney of rats is followed by the intravenous injection of antibody to the "planted" antigen. This protocol results in extensive proteinuria persisting for several weeks with immune complex deposits, containing the injected antigen and antibody as well as host complement, localized to the subepithelial portion of the basement membrane.

A second model involves the injection of preformed antigen-antibody complexes made from antigen and antibody molecules with selected charge properties (45). When both the antibody and antigen components of the complexes were anionic, marked subendothelial and subepithelial localization of the immune complexes was observed. However, where complexes of anionic or heterogeneous composition were employed, slight mesangial localization of the reactants was observed. Experiments were terminated 1 hour after injection; all glomeruli appeared normal.

The third kind of model involves active immunization of animals with antigens of defined charge. In one case, the kidneys of preimmunized rats were examined after two weeks of alternate injections of either cationized, anionized, or normal bovine serum albumin (46). Although no significant alterations were noted by light microscopy, it was found that the animals receiving cationic BSA showed extensive mesangial localization of complexes by immunofluorescence and electron microscopy, whereas the animals receiving anionic or native BSA (normally anionic) showed some capillary wall deposits by immunofluorescence, but not by electron microscopy. The reason for this disparity is not clear.

Another example of this kind of model involves the repeated injection into mice of dextrans varying not only in charge (anionic, neutral, and cationic) but in size (47). While this experiment is interesting in that it produced substantial deposits of IgA antibody (thus mimicking human IgA nephropathy) in the mesangium, there is no evidence that the variations in antigen size and charge could be correlated with different glomerular lesions.

CIRCULATING IMMUNE COMPLEX DISEASE

Acute Serum Sickness in Rabbits

Following the demonstration that one or two large injections of horse serum into rabbits could produce glomerular lesions (48, 49), it was shown that similar lesions could be produced using injections of purified proteins (50). It was initially suggested that the lesions might be a result of the reaction of antibody transported by mononuclear cells with antigen that had become trapped in the glomeruli. However, following the demonstration that lesions developed at the time antigen was cleared from the circulation (51) (Fig. 13.10), the possibility that soluble complexes of antigen and antibody could cause the lesions was raised. When animals were presensitized with homologous or cross-reacting antigens,

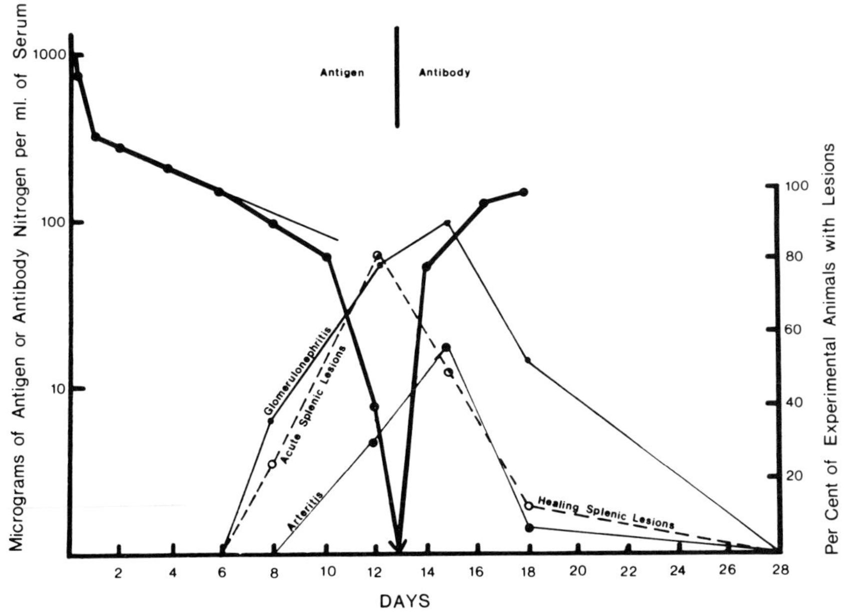

Figure 13.10. The original diagram showing the relationships between clearance of antigen, development of antibody, and the occurrence of hypersensitivity lesions of the immune complex type. The curve showing the median blood clearance of antigen and the appearance of circulating antibody is represented by the thick solid line and refers to the ordinate on the left. Values after the 13th day represent antibody. The thin solid line projected from the antigen clearance curve at the 6th day shows the course the antigen would follow in the absence of an increased elimination of antigen by antibody. The incidence of splenic lesions at various times is represented by the broken line and incidence of arteritis and glomerulonephritis by the thin solid lines. These values refer to the ordinate at the right of the figure. (From Germuth FG: J Exp Med **97**:257, 1953).

the time of elimination of a single injection of 0.5 g of BSA was shortened and so was the time of appearance of glomerulonephritis (52) (Fig. 13.11). Further evidence of the role of circulating complexes was provided by the production of glomerular lesions by the intermittent or continuous infusion of antibody into rabbits that had received an intravenous injection of antigen (53). The actual localization of host immunoglobulin (presumably antibody) at the site of the glomerular lesions in animals injected with purified proteins was demonstrated by the newly developed technique of immunofluorescence microscopy (54). Later this technique was used to show that antigen and host complement also localized at the sites of the lesions (55, 56). It should be noted, however, that deposits detected by this technique are fine and sparse and are found both in the mesangium and the loop. Electron microscopy shows small mesangial and loop deposits. Presumably, as more antibody and complement are added to the coalescing subepithelial deposits by diffusing through the glomerular basement membrane, a few large subepithelial humps are formed several days after antigen elimination (57, 58). In addition, using radiolabeled antigen, it was shown that complexes of antigen and antibody were present in the circulation at about the time when antigen was eliminated, i.e., at the time when lesions were known to occur (55). Together, these observations strengthened the concept of the glomerular lesions of serum sickness as being a result of the deposition of circulating immune complexes in the glomeruli. Further, with the onset of immune complex formation, circulating complement levels began to decline and recovered only after free antibody appeared in the circulation (59, 60) (Fig. 13.12).

The glomerular lesions of the acute-BSA rabbit system, i.e. those observed following the injection of 0.5 g bovine serum albumin in a 2 kg rabbit, consist of an accumulation of monocytes accompanied by an increase of mesangial cells, in the virtual absence of polymorphonuclear leukocytes (Fig. 13.13). The reason for the latter is not clear since the

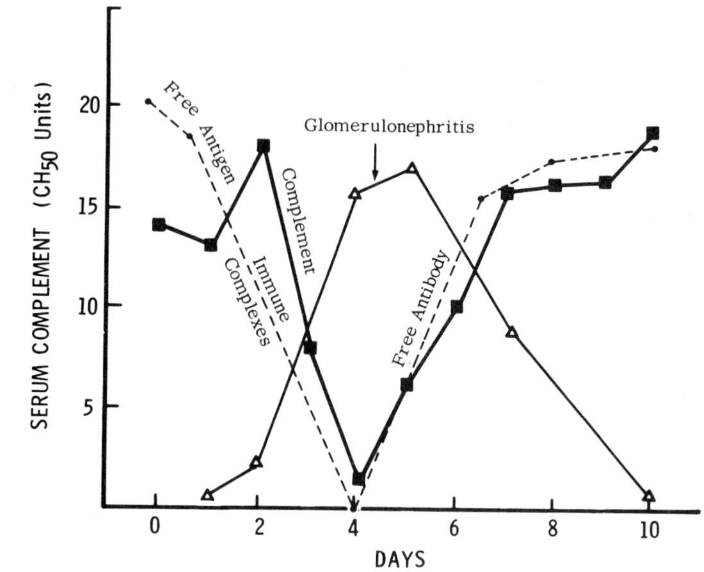

Figure 13.12. Acute BSA-rabbit system. Temporal relations among serum complement levels, antigen clearance, and the development of acute diffuse glomerulonephritis following a single injection of 0.5 gm BSA into rabbits that had previously been actively immunized with this antigen. (From Germuth FG, Rodriguez E: Immunopathology of the Renal Glomerulus. Little, Brown & Co., 1973.)

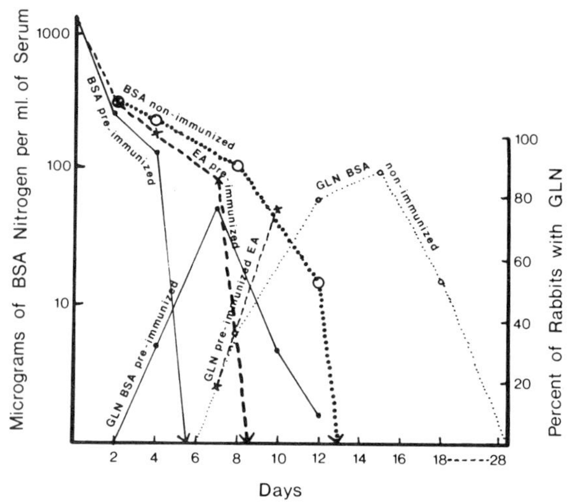

Figure 13.11. Relation of time of occurrence of glomerulonephritis to the blood clearance of bovine albumin in animals previously sensitized to bovine serum albumin, to egg albumin, and in normal unsensitized animals. The curves for the median blood clearance of bovine albumin in bovine albumin-sensitized animals (heavy solid line), in egg albumin-sensitized animals (heavy broken line), and in normal animals (heavy dotted line) begin in the upper left corner and end in arrows. Each of these curves shows three phases; an early phase of equilibration of antigen, a second phase of antigen catabolism, and a final phase of rapid elimination of antigen by newly formed antibody. The time of occurrence of glomerular lesions in each of the three groups of animals is represented by a corresponding thin line. (From Germuth FG, Pace MG, Tippett JC: J Exp Med **101:**135, 1955.)

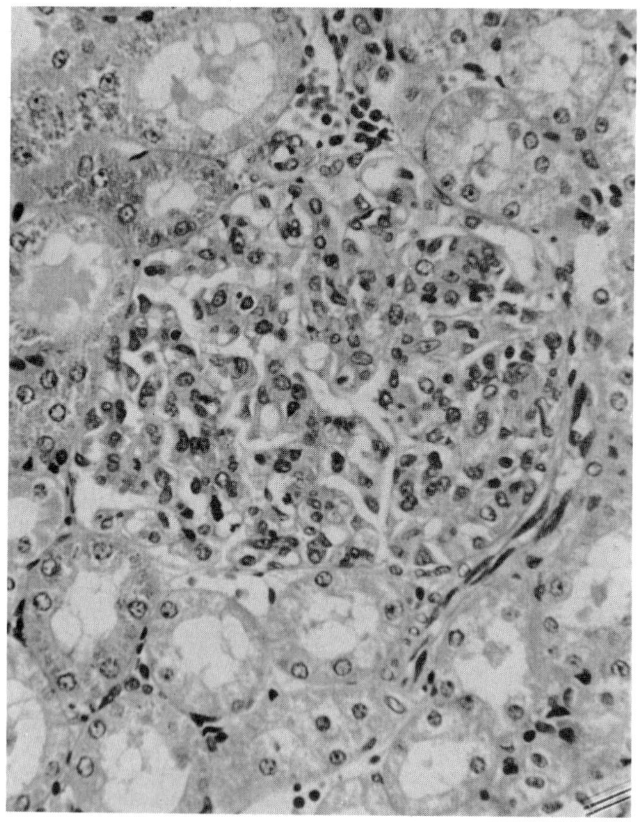

Figure 13.13. Acute BSA-rabbit system. Acute diffuse glomerulonephritis characterized by mesangial hypercellularity and infiltration by macrophages (Hematoxylin-eosin stain; X340.) (From Germuth FG, Rodriguez E: Immunopathology of the Renal Glomerulus. Little, Brown & Co., 1973.)

concomittant arteritis contains numerous polymorphonuclear leukocytes (Fig. 13.14). Depletion of macrophages by antimacrophage serum markedly inhibits the histological and physiological changes of acute serum sickness nephritis.

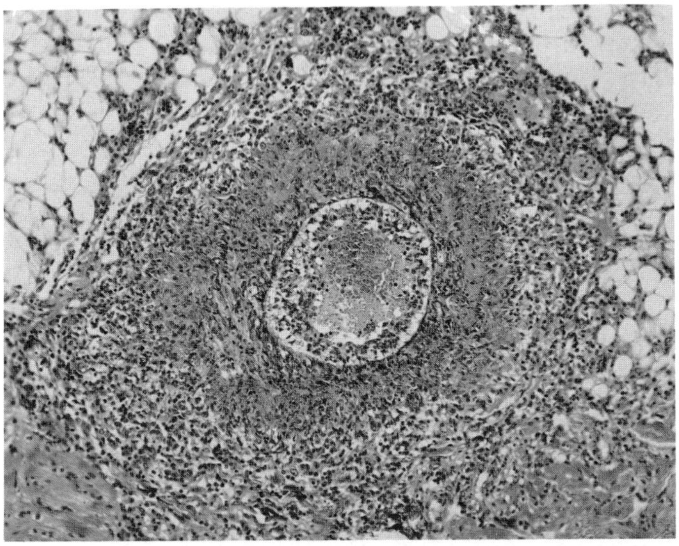

Figure 13.14. Acute BSA-rabbit system. Necrotizing arteritis (coronary artery). (Hematoxylin-eosin stain; X125.) (From Heptinstall RH, Germuth FG: Bull Johns Hopkins Hosp 100:71, 1957.)

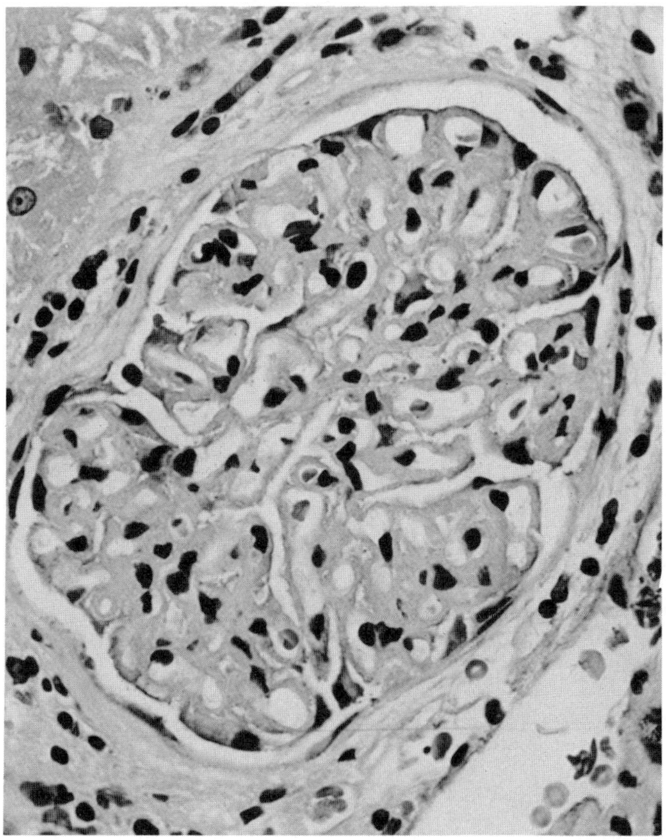

Figure 13.15. Membranous Glomerulonephritis, Stage II. Rabbit received 12.5 mg bovine serum albumin daily for a period of 32 weeks. (Hematoxylin-eosin stain; X600.) (From Germuth FG, et al: Lab Invest 37:162, 1977.)

We have recently observed that in an inbred strain of rabbits the glomerular lesions of the acute-BSA rabbit system are characterized by an abundant accumulation of polymorphonuclear leukocytes (62). One way in which the inbred strain may differ from the randomly bred animals used in all previous work is in the absence of a rheumatoid factor-like substance in the former. The role this factor may play in the production of the lesions is under investigation.

Chronic Serum Sickness

As with the acute serum sickness model, the initial experiments in the chronic model were done using horse serum as antigen. Daily injections of rabbits with small doses were found to produce progressive obliterative

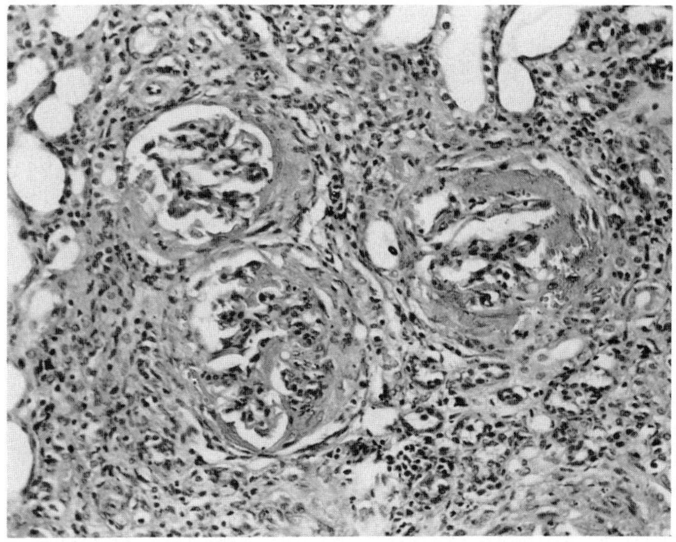

Figure 13.16. Glomerulus from a rabbit injected with 25 mg of bovine serum albumin daily and killed at 14 weeks, showing severe nitrogen retention after developing rapidly progressive glomerulonephritis. There is an organizing fibrinous transudate in Bowman's space with early crescent formation associated with marked tubular atrophy (Hematoxylin-eosin stain; X225). (From Germuth FG, et al: Johns Hopkins Med J 120:225, 1967.)

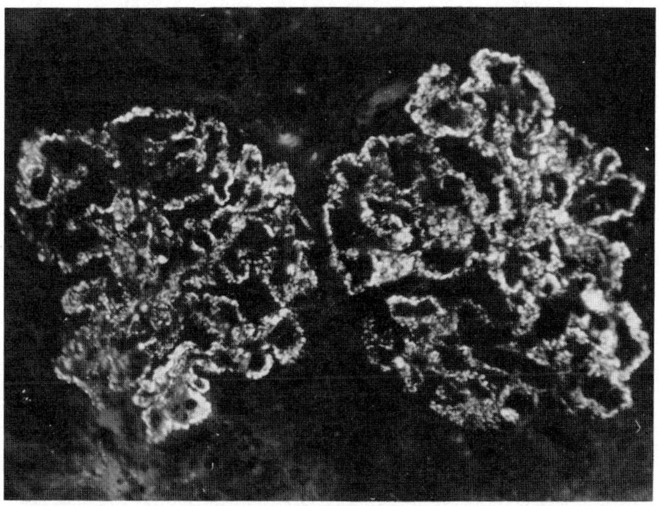

Figure 13.17. Immunofluorescence microscopy of another specimen from the animal shown in Figure 13.16. Coarsely granular deposits of rabbit IgG within the glomerular basement membrane (X320). (From Germuth FG: J Exp Med 97:257, 1953.)

glomerulonephritis associated with severe nitrogen retention in a majority of the animals. The necrotizing arteritis seen in acute serum sickness was not observed (63). Similar lesions in the absence of arteritis were obtained when animals were given weekly injections of horse serum over a 2 year period. The latter experiment was interesting in that the time of onset of glomerulonephritis coincided with a switch-over from a positive to a negative Arthus skin test, indicating that the animals developed lesions only when they were in antigen excess (64).

Use of purified serum proteins as antigens in such models produced a similar spectrum of lesions, whether the daily dose of antigen was adjusted in an attempt to maintain the rabbits in antigen excess (65) or a constant dose of antigen was used (65 addendum, 66).

In each instance the sine qua non for the development of glomerular lesions was the formation of antigen-antibody complexes in antigen excess. Large doses of antigen gave rise to rapidly progressive (crescentic) glomerulonephritis, while smaller doses of antigen produced membra-

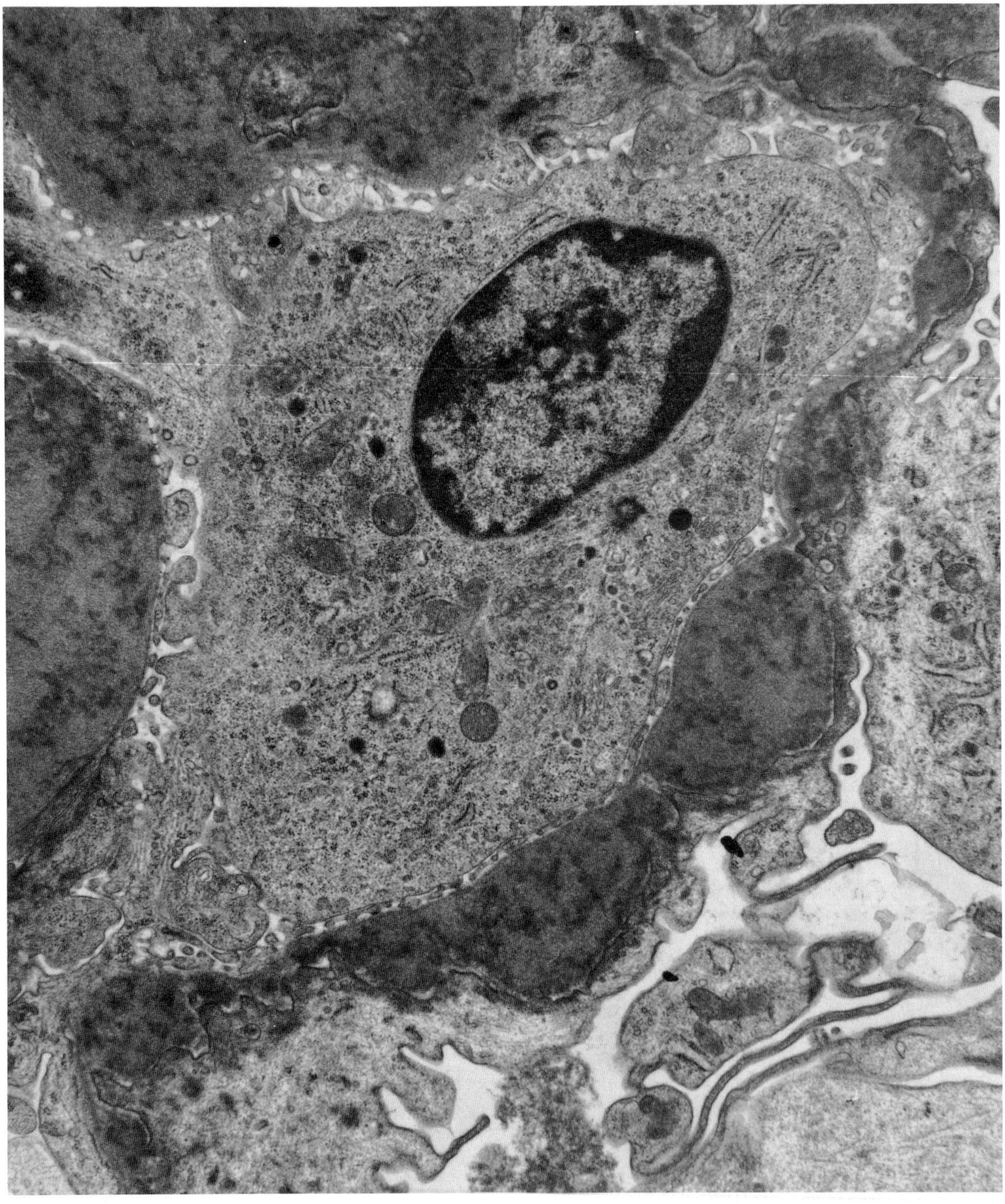

Figure 13.18. Early membranous glomerulonephritis after 32 weeks of daily administration of 12.5 mg of bovine serum albumin. Electron micrograph showing numerous large electron-dense subepithelial deposits (O) (X13,000). (From Germuth FG, et al: Lab Invest 37:162, 1977.)

nous glomerulonephritis (66, 67). By light microscopy, the rapidly progressive glomerulonephritis was associated with the accumulation of macrophages within the glomerulus, whereas the membranous glomerulonephritis was free of leukocytes (Fig. 13.15 and 13.16). Both were associated with electron dense subepithelial deposits that stained by immunofluorescence microscopy for BSA, IgG, and C3 (Fig. 13.17 and 13.18). Small traces of IgM may be seen in the membranous form after many months of antigenic stimulation. Dissolution of the subepithelial immune complex deposits can be produced by daily injections of large doses of specific antigen, showing that the deposits are indeed aggregates

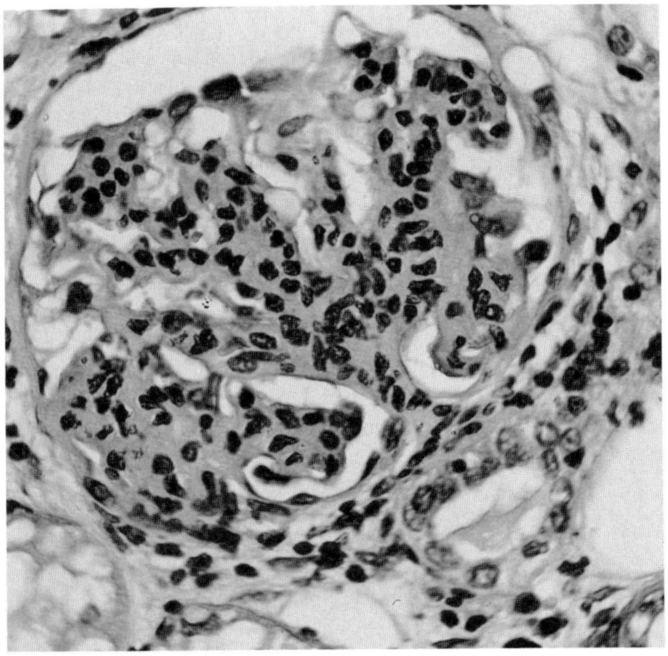

Figure 13.19. Mesangial proliferative glomerulonephritis in an animal receiving doses of antigen adjusted to the immune response for 26 weeks. (Hematoxylin-eosin stain; X500.) (From Germuth FG, et al: Lab Invest 37:162, 1977.)

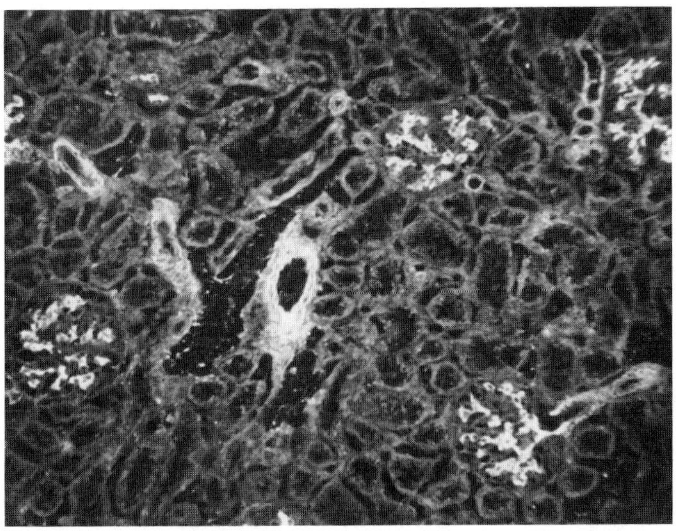

Figure 13.20. Mesangial proliferative glomerulonephritis. Massive clumps of fluorescent rabbit IgG deposits within the mesangium and contiguous arteriolar walls (X90). (From Germuth FG, Rodriguez E: Immunopathology of the Renal Glomerulus. Little, Brown & Co., 1973.)

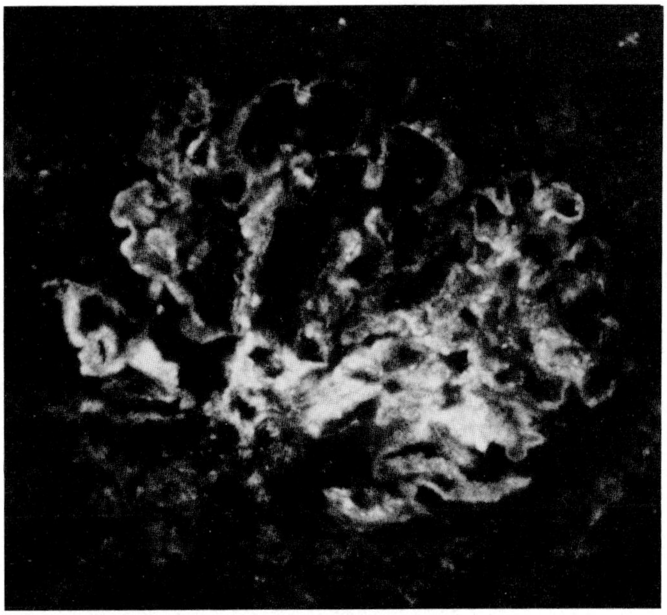

Figure 13.21. Mesangial proliferative glomerulonephritis. Same animal as shown in Figure 13.19. (Immunofluorescence microscopy, Ab for IgG, X400). (From Germuth FG, et al: Lab Invest 37:162, 1977.)

of immune complexes (68). Such a dissolution of complexes may be partly responsible for the scarcity of immune complex deposits in chronic serum sickness produced with egg albumin, to which the glomerular basement membrane is freely permeable (69, 70).

In addition to the membranous and rapidly progressive forms of glomerulonephritis, a mesangial proliferative form is found with chronic sensitization when the complex is formed at equivalence or slight antibody excess (Figs. 13.19–13.21). In this form of glomerulonephritis, the complexes are first observed in the mesangium. If immunization is further continued, the complexes are next seen in the juxtamesangial subendothelial space and later in the subendothelial portion of the peripheral loops (6).

While the majority of studies of chronic serum sickness have been carried out using rabbits, similar experiments can be performed using mice (71, 72) and rats (73). In general, results are similar to those seen in rabbits, though there does exist strain variation in susceptibility to immune complex glomerulonephritis in various species.

SPONTANEOUS ANIMAL DISEASES

Lymphocytic Choriomeningitis Virus in Mice

Of the numerous spontaneous animal diseases produced by different viruses, that resulting from infection with lymphocytic choriomeningitis virus in mice has been most extensively studied (75, 76). Neonatal mice may develop a persistent infection characterized by a sustained viremia, the magnitude of which is dependent on the mouse strain. The glomerular disease follows a progressive and characteristic course, involving first the mesangium, then the juxtamesangial subendothelial loop, and finally the subendothelial loop itself (6). By light microscopy, amorphous eosinophilic material may be seen in the aforementioned locations. It is curious that inflammation is virtually absent, although immunofluorescence studies show the presence of viral antigen, host antibody, and complement, presumably in the form of complexes. Electron dense deposits are seen in the same locations.

Murine Systemic Lupus Erythematosus

A number of mouse strains have been bred which develop a disease similar to human systemic lupus erythematosus. The strains originally developed in New Zealand [NZB and (NZB × NZW)F_1] have been most extensively studied (77). Although all develop, to a greater or lesser degree, glomerulonephritis and the serological manifestations of systemic lupus, some strains are noted for certain extrarenal features of systemic lupus, e.g., the (NZW × BXSB)F_1 strain shows a high incidence of lupus arteritis (78), while the MRL/1 strain is characterized by arthritic changes that mimic those of rheumatoid arthritis (79). It is of interest that patients with systemic lupus may show similar extrarenal manifestations either alone or accompanied by overt glomerular disease.

Based on observations that DNA and antibodies to DNA were associated with human systemic lupus (80), these materials were implicated in the murine models (81). The renal immune deposits contained C3, C1, antibodies to DNA, and antibodies to the major glycoprotein (gp 70) of murine C type viruses (81, 82).

Since the basic mechanism of these murine models of systemic lupus erythematosus are the same and since they were mostly explored using the NZB and (NZB × NZW)F_1 hybrid model, we shall concentrate on this model. As in the human disease, predominantly females are affected. Castration of the females retards the development of glomerulonephritis. In both strains of mice there exist two types of glomerulonephritis: membranous glomerulonephritis, consisting chiefly of subepithelial loop deposits stainable by immunofluorescence microscopy for IgG and C3 (13), and lupus nephritis, involving primarily the subendothelial-mesangial system (83). The mechanism of the former is not clear and published works have failed to differentiate these two forms. The incidence of membranous glomerulonephritis in the two strains of mice is approximately 6% (13).

Involvement of the subendothelial-mesangial system by complexes consisting chiefly of DNA, IgG, and C3 is seen in the large majority of the animals. The complexes are first deposited in the mesangial matrix and cells (Fig. 13.22). As more complexes are delivered to the glomerulus, the complexes in the mesangium become extensive and encroach on the glomerular capillary lumen and extend into the juxtamesangial capillary loop. Finally, the extension surrounds the inner aspect of the glomerulus, and at this time rare subepithelial deposits may be encountered. As the loops become obsolescent, the light microscopic appearance is that of glomerulosclerosis. It is noteworthy that except for the accelerated lesions in the hybrid strain, which may show areas of fibrinoid necrosis, there is little inflammatory component to murine lupus nephritis. In this respect it differs from the active lesions of human systemic lupus glomerulonephritis, which often show the presence of polymorphonuclear leukocytes and monocytes accompanying the deposits in the subendothelial-mesangial apparatus. This observation should be further explored since complexes deposited on the inner aspect of the glomerular basement membrane should be capable of generating chemotactic factors, being that they are in close proximity to the circulation.

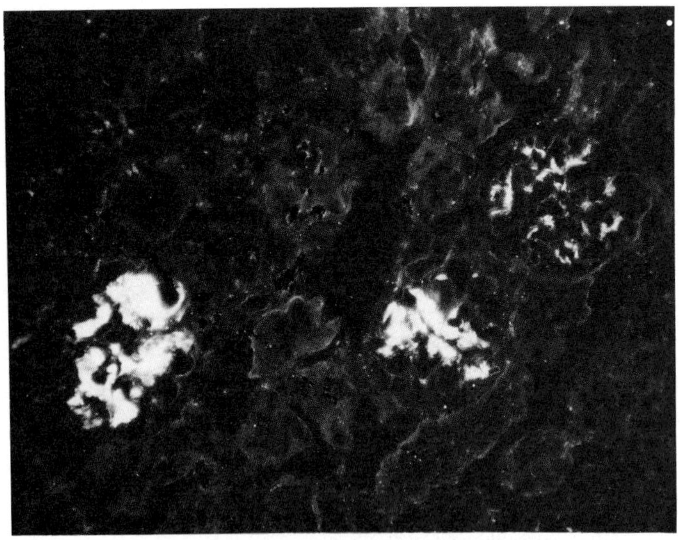

Figure 13.22. Murine lupus nephritis (NZB mouse). Varying degrees of mesangial deposition of immune complexes in all glomeruli. (Immunofluorescence microscopy, Ab specific for mouse C3 X190.) (From Germuth FG, Rodriguez E: Immunopathology of the Renal Glomerulus. Little, Brown & Co., 1973.)

In the murine models of systemic lupus erythematosus, as in the human disease, there are found a variety of immunological abnormalities, associated with antibodies capable of reacting with different antigens. It has been thought that each of these antibodies is distinct. However, it has recently been suggested, on the basis of studies with monoclonal antibodies, that in human disease the variety of immunological phenomena may be a result of cross-reactions of a limited number of antibodies (84). The murine models may provide a means of testing this hypothesis.

TUBULO-INTERSTITIAL DISEASE

Tubulo-interstitial nephritis can occur together with immune complex glomerular disease and with antibasement membrane disease. Immune complex deposits have been described along the tubular basement membrane and within the peritubular capillaries in chronic serum sickness nephritis, in which large amounts of poorly soluble complexes were produced (85). Such lesions are not uncommonly seen in human lupus nephritis (13), as well as in the nephritis of NZB mice. However, several reports suggest that the tubular alterations may occur independently of the glomerular lesions.

The first experimental model of antitubular basement membrane disease was reported in guinea pigs injected with rabbit tubular basement membrane incorporated in Freund's adjuvant. Linear deposits of IgG, tubular cell damage, and infiltration by mononuclear and giant cells characterized the lesion (86). Since that time, numerous variations of this model have been reported (87, 88). Although lesions resembling those seen in the antitubular basement membrane antibody model may be observed in some patients with antibasement membrane disease, the role of this mechanism remains unclear because the extensive glomerular damage alone might account for the tubular damage. Since mononuclear cells are involved, it has been suggested that cell-mediated immunity may play a role in some forms of tubulo-interstitial nephritis. In our own experience, the diagnosis of primary immunologically mediated tubulo-interstitial nephritis in renal biopsies has depended more on the light microscopy aspect of the lesion and the history of drug reaction rather than on immunofluorescence and electron microscopy findings.

CRITIQUE OF THE PATHOGENIC MECHANISMS INVOLVED IN IMMUNOLOGICALLY INDUCED GLOMERULONEPHRITIS

The recognition that Heymann nephritis is not, as originally suggested (27, 28), an immune complex disease, but rather represents a form of antibasement membrane disease (30, 31), has led to a reevaluation of the relative importance of the in situ and circulating immune complex mechanisms of immunologically induced glomerular disease. While some have suggested that in situ mechanisms are responsible for a variety of human and experimental diseases heretofore attributed to circulating immune complexes, an examination of the immunological and immunopathological features and tissue response in most of these diseases suggests that circulating immune complex mechanisms are of primary importance.

There is, however, considerable evidence that immunologically induced membranous glomerulopathy, in both experimental animals and man, might be a result of in situ mechanisms. This evidence is based on the aforementioned experiment showing that glomerular basement subepithelial deposits can be produced by alternating injections of antibody and antigen (39) and the inconsistent finding in humans of circulating immune complexes (89). In experimental animals receiving daily injections of small doses of antigen (12.5 mg BSA) for prolonged periods of time, membranous glomerulonephritis is found with great frequency. This appears after several months, when the decay in immune response permits a daily transient development of a low level of small immune complexes in antigen excess. Since these complexes are in equilibrium with free antibody and free antigen (Fig. 13.23), whose concentrations fluctuate daily as a consequence of the injection of antigen and the continued synthesis of antibody, the possibility presents itself that the biologically inert small complexes (Fig. 13.24) act only as a vehicle for the transport of antigen and antibody to the glomerulus.

In the other form of glomerulonephritis (rapidly progressive glomerulonephritis) observed following daily injections of antigen (25 mg BSA) this same mechanism may not be applicable. One must explain the presence of chronic inflammatory cells (macrophages), breaks in the glomerular basement membrane accompanied by the transudation of fibrin, and the formation of crescents in rapidly progressive glomerulonephritis. In membranous glomerulonephritis characterized by the in situ formation of subepithelial deposits, the lack of inflammation may be a result of the fact that any chemotactic factors formed are at a distance from the glomerular lumen. On the other hand, the inflammatory component of rapidly progressive glomerulonephritis suggests that the initial complexes are present in proximity to the circulation and are thus capable of generating chemotactic factors and that the subepithelial deposits are a consequence of a further aggregation of such complexes so that they are deposited at the interphase between the outer glomerular basement membrane and the urinary space. Electron microscopic observations showing the distribution of small amounts of complexes throughout the glomerular basement in a similar model are consistent with this hypothesis (90).

In acute serum sickness, characterized by the presence of macrophages (randomly bred rabbits) or neutrophils (JAX III inbred rabbits), the glomerulonephritis is first observed before the appearance of free antibody suggesting that an in situ mechanism is unlikely. No glomerular lesions are seen during the initial phase of immune elimination of

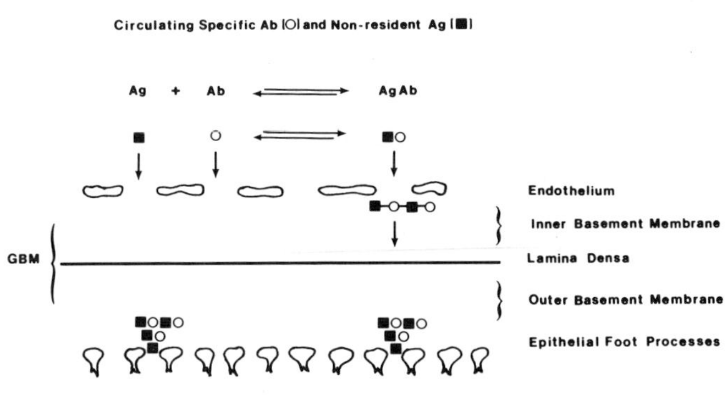

Figure 13.23. Diagram showing the possibility of two immunologic mechanisms in circulating immune complex disease associated with membranous glomerulopathy. One is the in situ mechanism, the other due to the penetration of circulating non-phlogistic small complexes into the basement membrane.

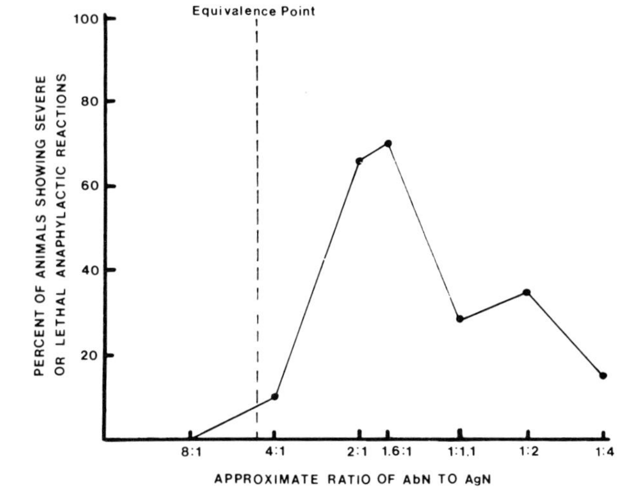

Figure 13.24. Diagram showing relative degree of biologic activity of supernatant fluids formed with increasing excess of antigen. One ml. of the appropriate concentration of BSA was added to 1 ml containing 2 mg nitrogen of antibovine serum albumin. Note the initial increase followed by a drop-off in biological activity of the supernatant fluid as the ratio of antibody to antigen decreases. (Germuth FG: Unpublished data.)

antigen, when the complexes formed are in extreme antigen excess. Studies with immune complexes of varying composition suggest that such complexes should be devoid of biologic activity (91) (Fig. 13.24). However, as such complexes are trapped by the glomerular basement membrane, complexes of greater antibody content that have phlogistic activity are formed and together they are presumably sequestered by the glomerular basement membrane, where in proximity to the circulation they generate chemotactic activity, finally ending up at the glomerular basement membrane-urinary space interphase.

Up to now one of the chief reasons for questioning the role of immune complexes in producing acute diffuse glomerulonephritis was the inability to reproduce this lesion passively by the injection of soluble immune complexes. Recently, our laboratory has shown that a model consisting of the injection of immune complexes of egg albumin and poorly avid antibody in the presence of excess antigen faithfully reproduces an acute glomerulonephritis characterized by loop deposits when visualized by immunofluorescence microscopy and subepithelial humps when examined by electron microscopy (92). The detection in the serum of these animals of free antibody, as well as small antigen-antibody complexes, raises the possibility of an in situ mechanism playing a role in this model. However, one must assume that phlogistic antigen-antibody complexes must have played a role at the level of the inner aspect of the glomerular basement membrane since the glomerular lesions are characterized by the presence of numerous polymorphonuclear leukocytes and not by membranous nephropathy. This model is made possible by the ability of egg albumin to diffuse freely across the glomerular basement membrane. Because of this, the concentration of egg albumin drops considerably in the interval between the first and subsequent injections of the immune complexes and antigen. This drop in concentration must shift the equilibrium so that an aggregation of complexes can occur in the wall of the glomerular basement membrane. It is of interest that repeated attempts to produce this model using BSA as the antigen resulted in no glomerular localization of complexes, either in the mesangium or the loop. Since BSA does not pass through the glomerular basement membrane freely and remains in the circulation in high concentrations, a similar shift in the equilibrium between larger and small complexes and free antigen and antibody may not occur.

There is additional evidence for the role of the firmness of binding of antibody to antigen (avidity) in the production of glomerulonephritis (93, 94, 95). For example, two strains of mice were selectively bred to produce low and high affinity antibodies to human serum albumin. When such animals were injected daily with sufficient antigen to maintain detectable antigen in their circulation (antigen excess), complexes were found to localize in the basement membrane in the low affinity group, but in the mesangium in the animals making high affinity antibody. While antibody affinity is one of the determinants of immune complex size (and therefore of the site of localization) it is difficult to envision how an in situ mechanism can account for these differences in complex localization. These experiments raise the possibility that in man susceptibility to nephritis depends in part on the quality of the antibody formed against the inciting antigen.

Pertinent to our understanding of various kinds of immune complex diseases (glomerulonephritis, vasculitis, valvulitis, synovitis, pleurisy, localization of complexes in the choroid plexus, interstitial pneumonitis, as may be seen in polyarteritis nodosa, and systemic lupus erythematosus) is the tendency for immune complexes to localize at the site of tissue interphases, i.e., at the boundary between a vascular region and an avascular one (e.g., glomerular basement membrane and urinary space, systemic circulation and avascular arterial media, systemic circulation and avascular valve leaflet, synovial membrane and joint space, pleural surface and pleural space, vascular choroid plexus and cerebrospinal fluid, and vascular alveolar walls and air sacs). As relatively small complexes in antigen excess pass through the tissue interphase they may aggregate into larger complexes at the edge of the interphase, as antigen is lost into the avascular space, a result of the greater mobility of the latter. This would result in the localized accumulation of immune complex aggregates, e.g., glomerular basement membrane subepithelial deposits. In support of this hypothesis, circumstances that prevent this mechanism from operating, e.g., high avidity antibody (96), antigen (97), or antibody (98) of high molecular weight, or decreased basement membrane permeability as a result of the action of cortisone (99), result in the mesangial localization of complexes.

Whereas the characteristic subepithelial deposits of active acute and chronic diffuse glomerulonephritis and glomerulopathy and of the passive model with poorly avid antibody are associated with circulating complexes varying in size up to 1×10^6 daltons, mesangial proliferative glomerulonephritis is always associated with complexes of 1×10^6 daltons or greater (100). The complexes appear to be entrapped by mesangial cells and macrophages that often accumulate in the mesangium. Microprecipitates of numerous substances, such as aggregated gamma globulin, also are entrapped in the mesangium. In experimental mesangial proliferative glomerulonephritis the complexes first appear in the mesangium. They may spread into the juxtamesangial-subendothelial loop and even completely surround the inner portion of the loop if they are delivered at a rate greater than that at which mesangium can metabolize them. Since the capacity of the mesangium may vary from one glomerulus to another, the mesangial deposition of complex is responsible for focal glomerulonephritis. Once the high molecular weight complexes or, for that matter, aggregates of IgG, are deposited in the mesangium, in situ mechanisms of free antigen or free antibody deposition may be superimposed.

A passive model, consisting of injections of mice with soluble complexes made with egg albumin and highly avid antibody faithfully reproduces this active process (96). There is no evidence for a role for in situ mechanisms in this model, since treatment of the mice with purified human rheumatoid factor deflects the complexes from the mesangium and causes cryoglobulinemia (13).

The best studied example of mesangial proliferative glomerulonephritis is the nephritis of systemic lupus erythematosus. Virtually all patients suffering from this disease show greater or lesser deposits of DNA-antibody complexes in the mesangium. If the deposits are within the inner aspect of the glomerular capillary loop, "wire-loop" lesions may appear. Subepithelial deposits are much less frequently encountered and appear to be a result of the flow of aggregates across the glomerular basement membrane. It has been found that DNA has an affinity for basement membranes and collagen. It has been proposed that in situ immune complex mechanisms are responsible for the formation of immune aggregates within the glomerulus and involved arteries. This hypothesis does not fit the facts concerning the pathogenesis of systemic lupus erythematosus, where the target organ is the mesangium and not the loops, which are only secondarily involved.

A summary of some of the characteristics of the in situ and circulating types of immune complex glomerulonephritis are shown in Table 13.1.

MECHANISMS BY WHICH IN SITU OR CIRCULATING IMMUNE COMPLEXES PRODUCE GLOMERULAR DAMAGE

The mechanism(s) by which immune complexes produce extensive glomerular damage is poorly understood. In membranous glomerulopathy the accumulation of complexes and the resultant membranous transformation of the external lamina rara alter the slit membranes. It is possible that the mere presence of this foreign material, distorting the membrane, is the cause of proteinuria. The mechanism would be similar to that seen in amyloidosis of the kidney, where massive proteinuria occurs in the absence of inflammatory cells. The role of complement in this disease is unclear.

In the acute BSA-rabbit system the proteinuria is abrogated by preventing the localization of circulating monocytes (57, 101). The role of complement has not been established in this model, although the concomittant development of arteritis appears to be complement dependent.

Because leukocytes appear to be responsible for the development of the vasculitis of the Arthus phenomenon, they have been assigned a major role in the presently popular concept that glomerular lesions are produced chiefly by the damage caused by the enzymatic contents of lysosomal granules released from such cells attracted to the site of the lesion by chemotactic factors generated by the complement system. However, glomerular lesions may be seen both in animals (lymphocytic choriomeningitis glomerulonephritis and murine lupus nephritis) and in humans (focal necrotizing glomerulonephritis of polyarteritis nodosa, Henoch-Schönlein purpura, "wire-loop" lesions of lupus nephritis, and so on) in the virtual absence of leukocytes. It is possible that the membrane attack mechanism of the complement system may be involved in such circumstances (102). However, the role of complement is far from clear, since there exist numerous studies both supporting and denying a role for complement in the various models of glomerulonephritis.

The study of immune complex–induced arteritis clearly establishes the difficulty involved in assigning responsibility for the lesions. It has been shown in the acute serum sickness model that the arteritis is dependent on the presence of polymorphonuclear leukocytes. However, it has long been appreciated by morphologists that the arteritis seen in systemic lupus erythematosus may be totally lacking in polymorphonuclear leukocytic infiltration. Indeed, this difference in morphology has helped in the past to distinguish microscopic polyarteritis nodosa from the arteritis of systemic lupus erythematosus. It is of interest that a recent report has shown that the arteritis of murine systemic lupus also lacks an appreciable polymorphonuclear leukocyte response (78).

There is no question that in numerous forms of glomerulonephritis the coagulation system plays a role (103) (chapter 15). Intravascular

Table 13.1
Animal Models of Glomerulonephritis[a]

Type of immune complex disease		Site of immune reactants	
		Mesangial-subendothelial	Subepithelial
In situ	Disease	(1) Acute nonprogressive mesangial glomerulonephritis	(6) Heymann membranous glomerulopathy (7) Immune complex glomerulopathy of the serum sickness type—in situ mechanism (see 10)
	Response	Proliferation of mesangial cells and infiltration of mesangium by leukocytes[b]	(6) and (7) Membranous transformation
	Mechanism	Localization of aggregated gamma globulin followed by Ab	(6) Reaction of noncomplexed Ab with resident antigen localized focally in outer basement membrane (7) Localization of noncomplexed Ab with Ag reaching the outer membrane interface during peaks of Ag excess (i.e., following Ag injection)
Circulating	Diseases	(2) Active and passive mesangial proliferative or focal glomerulonephritis of the serum sickness type (3) Lymphocytic choriomeningitis infection in mice (4) Murine mesangial lupus nephritis (5) Cortisone treated active diffuse glomerulonephritis of the serum sickness type (see 8)	(8) Active and passive acute diffuse glomerulonephritis of the serum sickness type (9) Rapidly progressive immune complex glomerulonephritis of the serum sickness type (10) Immune complex glomerulopathy of the serum sickness type—circulating mechanism (7 and 10 may coexist)
	Complex size	(2) and (4) Large (at least 10^6 daltons), poorly dissociable (5) Small ($<10^6$ daltons)	(8) and (9) Small ($<10^6$ daltons), readily dissociable (10) Nonpholgistic complexes in far Ag excess alone or after reaction with additional Ab
	Response	(3) and (4) Glomerulosclerosis (2) and (5) Mesangial proliferation and increase in mesangial matrix; local necrosis	(8) and (9) Mononuclear and polymorphonuclear leukocytes; membrane rupture; crescents (10) Membranous transformation
	Mechanism	Accumulation of complexes in mesangial system and subsequently in subendothelial region and finally intramembranous and subepithelial localization	Small complexes in Ag excess penetrate to outer aspect of basement membrane (at interface) while undergoing aggregation

[a] The reaction of antibody with (1) resident antigen (Steblay and primary phase of Masugi nephritis) or (2) existing antigen-antibody complexes (secondary phase of Masugi nephritis) are not included in this table. These are obviously in situ diseases in which antibodies are homogeneously localized throughout the periphery of the glomerular loop.

[b] Neutrophils or macrophages.

thrombosis is not uncommon in human glomerulonephritis and fibrin accumulation in Bowman's space leads to crescent formation. This is accompanied by the appearance of split products of fibrin in the circulation. Crescent formation is often, if not always, a result of breaks in the glomerular basement membrane produced by unknown mechanisms that play a role in both antibasement membrane disease and immune complex disease. Breaks and crescent formation, as evidence of the most severe glomerular damage, are seen most frequently in rapidly progressive (crescentic) glomerulonephritis.

As already mentioned, the role of cell-mediated immunity remains unclear, but there is increasing evidence that activated macrophages may play a role in altering the glomerular basement membrane in rapidly progressive glomerulonephritis.

It would appear then, that the mechanisms at work in producing the damaging effects of immune complexes are multifaceted and that no one simplistic theory can explain all of them. It is clear that the study of immune complex disease remains a challenge.

Although the animal experiments on the mechanism of production of immune complex lesions are provocative, to the practicing nephropathologist their implication appears puzzling in numerous situations observed through the study of renal biopsies.

We have recently made an interesting observation on the effect of IgM rheumatoid factor on the development of mesangial proliferative glomerulonephritis in the passive immune complex glomerulonephritis produced in mice with high avidity antibody (104). Injection of rheumatoid factor prevents the mesangial accumulation of complexes and is associated with cryoglobulinemia. It is well known that the latter can produce occlusive glomerulonephritis. However, under controlled conditions, treatment of immune complex disease with IgM rheumatoid factor may differentiate in situ mechanisms from circulating immune complex mechanisms in the production of glomerulonephritis and may be beneficial in the treatment of patients suffering from the latter. Theoretically, monoclonal IgM rheumatoid factors produced in large quantities may block the progression of immune complex disease, and the resultant potentially deleterious cryoglobulins, if in high concentration, could theoretically be removed by plasmaphoresis and cryogelatin (105).

Acknowledgment

The authors would like to acknowledge the assistance of Elaine T. Bauer in the preparation of the figures and Dorris A. Bowers in the typing of the manuscript.

References

1. McCluskey RT, Bhan AK: Cell mediated mechanisms in renal diseases. Kidney Intl 21 (suppl): S6, 1982.
2. Fillit HM, Zabriskie JB: Cellular immunity in glomerulonephritis. Am J Path 109:227, 1982.
3. Humphrey JH: The mechanism of Arthus reactions. I. The role of polymorphonuclear leukocytes and other factors in reversed passive Arthus reactions in rabbits. Brit J Exp Path 36:268, 1955.
4. Humphrey JH: The mechanism of Arthus reactions. II. The role of polymorphonuclear leukocytes and platelets in reversed passive reactions in the guinea pig. Brit J Exp Path 36:283, 1955.
5. Cochrane CG: Immunologic tissue injury mediated by neutrophil leukocytes. Advan Immunol 9:97, 1968.
6. Germuth FG, Rodriguez E. Immunopathology of the renal glomerulus. Boston, Little Brown & Co., 1973.
7. Masugi M: Uber die experimentelle glomerulonephritis durch das speczifische antinieren serum. Ein beitrag zur pathogenese der diffusen glomerulonephritis. Beitr Path Anat 92:429, 1934.
8. Krakower CA, Greenspon SA: Localization of the nephrotoxic antigen within the isolated renal glomerulus. Arch Path 51:629, 1951.
9. Hammer DK, Dixon FJ: Experimental glomerulonephritis. II. Immunologic events in the pathogenesis of nephrotoxic serum nephritis in the rat. J Exp Med 117:1019, 1963.
10. Fish AJ, Carmody KM, Michael AF: Spatial orientation and distribution of antigens within human glomerular basement membrane. J Lab Clin Med 94:447, 1979.
11. Schifler MS, Michael AF, Kim Y, et al: Distribution of glomerular basement membrane antigens in diseased human kidneys. Lab Invest 44:239, 1981.
12. Cochrane CG, Unanue ER, Dixon FJ: A role of polymorphonuclear leukocytes and complement in nephrotoxic nephritis. J Exp Med 122:99, 1965.
13. Germuth FG: Unpublished observations.
14. Couser WG, Stilmant MM, Jermanovich NB: Complement-independent nephrotoxic nephritis in the guinea pig. Kidney Intl 11:170, 1977.
15. Kay CF: The mechanism by which experimental nephritis is produced in rabbits injected with nephrotoxic duck serum. J Exp Med 72:559, 1940.
16. Unanue E, Dixon FJ: Experimental glomerulonephritis. IV. Participation of complement in nephrotoxic nephritis. J Exp Med 119:965, 1964.
17. Rother K, Rother U, Vassalli P, et al: Nephrotoxic serum nephritis in C6-deficient rabbits. I. Study of the second phase of the disease. J Immunol 98:965, 1967.
18. Crosson JT, Lubowitz H, Mazumdar DC, et al: The production of experimental glomerulonephritis in the rat. Arch Path 98:344, 1974.
19. Steblay RW: Glomerulonephritis induced in sheep by injections of heterologous glomerular basement membrane and Freund's complete adjuvant. J Exp Med 116:253, 1962.
20. Steblay RW: Antiglomerularbasement membrane glomerulonephritis. Am J Path 96:875, 1979.
21. Ohnuki T: Crescentic glomerulonephritis induced in the goat by immunization with homologous or heterologous glomerular basement membrane antigen. Acta Path Jap 25:319, 1975.
22. Germuth FG, Choi I-J, Taylor JJ, et al: Antibasement membrane disease. I. The glomerular lesions of Goodpasture's disease and experimental disease in sheep. Johns Hopkins Med J 131:367, 1972.
23. Lerner RA, Glassock RJ, Dixon FJ: The role of antiglomerular basement membrane antibody in the pathogenesis of human glomerulonephritis. J Exp Med 126:989, 1967.
24. Sisson S, Dysart NK, Fish AJ, et al: Localization of the Goodpasture antigen by immunoelectron microscopy. Clin Immunol Immunopath 23:414, 1982.
25. Heymann W, Hackel DB, Harwood S, et al: Production of nephrotic syndrome in rats by Freund's adjuvants and rat kidney suspension. Proc Soc Exptl Biol Med 100:660, 1959.
26. Heymann W, Kmetec EP, Wilson SGF, et al: Experimental autoimmune renal disease in rats. In Grabor P, Miescher PA (eds): Third International Symposium of Immunopathology. Basel, Schwabe, 1963, p 240.
27. Edgington TS, Glassock RJ, Dixon FJ: Autologous immune complex pathogenesis of experimental allergic glomerulonephritis. Science 155:1432, 1967.
28. Edgington TS, Glassock RJ, Dixon FJ: Autologous immune complex nephritis induced with renal tubular antigen. I. Identification and isolation of the pathogenetic antigen. J Exp Med 127:555, 1968.
29. Glassock RJ, Edgington TS, Watson JI, et al: Autologous immune complex nephritis induced with renal tubular antigen. II. The pathogenetic mechanism. J Exp Med 127:573, 1968.
30. vanDamme BJC, Fleuren GJ, Bakker WW, et al: Experimental glomerulonephritis in the rat induced by antibodies directed against tubular antigens. V. Fixed glomerular antigens in the pathogenesis of heterologous immune complex glomerulonephritis. Lab Invest 38:502, 1978.
31. Couser WG, Stanmuller DR, Stilmant MM, et al: Experimental glomerulonephritis in the isolated perfused rat kidney. J Clin Invest 62:1275, 1978.
32. Fleuren GJ, Grond J, Hoedemaeker PhJ: The pathogenetic role of free-circulating antibody in autologous immune complex glomerulonephritis. Clin Exp Immunol 41:205, 1980.
33. Neale TJ, Couser WG, Salant DJ, et al: Specific uptake of Heymann's nephritic kidney eluate by rat kidney. Studies in vivo and in isolated perfused kidneys. Lab Invest 46:450, 1982.
34. Salant DJ, Belok S, Madaio MP, et al: A new role for complement in experimental membranous nephropathy in rats. J Clin Invest 66:1339, 1980.
35. Schneeberger EE, O'Brien A, Grupe WE: Altered glomerular permeability in Munich-Wistar rats with autologous immune complex nephritis. Lab Invest 40:227, 1979.
36. Izui S, Lambert PH, Miescher PA: In vitro demonstration of a particular affinity of glomerular basement membrane and collagen for DNA. A possible basis for a local formation of DNA-anti-DNA complexes in systemic lupus erythematosus. J Exp Med 144:428, 1976.
37. Izui S, Lambert PH, Fournie GJ, et al: Features of systemic lupus erythematosus in mice injected with bacterial lipopolysaccharides. Identification of circulating DNA and renal localization of DNA-anti-DNA complexes. J Exp Med 145:1115, 1977.
38. Golbus SM, Wilson CB: Experimental glomerulonephritis induced by in situ formation of immune complexes in glomerular capillary wall. Kidney Intl 16:148, 1979.
39. Fleuren G, Grond J, Hoedemaeker PJ: In situ formation of subepithelial glomerular immune complexes in passive serum sickness. Kidney Intl 17:631, 1980.
40. Mauer SM, Sutherland DER, Howard RJ, et al: The glomerular mesangium. III. Acute immune mesangial injury: A new model of glomerulonephritis. J Exp Med 137:553, 1973.
41. Caulfield JP, Farquhar MG: Distribution of anionic sites in glomerular basement membrane: Their possible role in filtration. Proc Natl Acad Sci U.S.A. 73:1646, 1976.
42. Kanwar YS, Farquhar MG: Anionic sites in the glomerular basement membrane. In vivo and in vitro localization to the laminae rarae by cationic probes. J Cell Biol 81:137, 1976.
43. Batsford SR, Takamiya H, Vogt A: A model of in situ immune complex glomerulonephritis in the rat employing cationized ferritin. Clin Nephrol 14:211, 1980.
44. Oite T, Batsford SR, Mihatsch MJ, et al: Quantitative studies of in situ immune complex glomerulonephritis in the rat induced by planted cationized antigen. J Exp Med 155:460, 1982.
45. Gallo GR, Caulin-Glaser T, Lamm ME: Charge of circulating immune complexes as a factor in glomerular basement membrane localization in mice. J Clin Invest 67:1305, 1981.
46. Border WA, Kamil ES, Ward HJ, et al: Antigenic charge as a determinant of immune complex localization in the rat glomerulus. Lab Invest 40:442, 1981.
47. Isaacs KL, Miller F: Role of antigen size and charge in immune complex glomerulonephritis. I. Active induction of disease with dextran and its derivatives. Lab Invest 47:198, 1982.
48. Rich AR, Gregory JE: The experimental demonstration that periarteritis nodosa is a manifestation of hypersensitivity. Bull Johns Hopkins Hosp 72:65, 1943.
49. Rich AR: The pathology and pathogenesis of experimental anaphylactic glomerulonephritis in relation to human acute glomerulonephritis. Bull Johns Hopkins Hosp 98:120, 1956.
50. Hawn CVZ, Janeway CA: Histological and serological sequences in experimental hypersensitivity. J Exp Med 85:571, 1947.
51. Germuth FG: A comparative histologic and immunologic study in rabbits of induced hypersensitivity of the serum sickness type. J Exp Med 97:257, 1953.
52. Germuth FG, Pace MG, Tippett JC: Comparative histologic and immunologic studies in rabbits of induced hypersensitivity of the serum sickness type. II. The effect of sensitization to homologous and cross-reactive antigens on the rate of antigen elimination and the development of allergic lesions. J Exp Med 101:135, 1955.
53. Germuth FG, Pollack AD: The production of lesions of "serum sickness" in normal animals by the passive transfer of antibody in the presence of antigen. Bull Johns Hopkins Hosp 102:245, 1958.
54. Mellors RC, Arias-Stella J, Siegel M, et al: Analytical pathology. II. Histopathologic demonstration of glomerular localizing antibodies in experimental glomerulonephritis. Am J Path 31:687, 1955.
55. Dixon FJ, Vazquez JJ, Weigle WO, et al: The pathogenesis of serum sickness. Arch Path 65:18, 1958.
56. Knicker WT, Cochrane CG: Pathogenic factors in vascular lesions of experimental serum sickness. J Exp Med 122:83, 1965.
57. Fish AJ, Michael AF, Vernier RJ, et al: Acute serum sickness nephritis in the rabbit. An immune deposit disease. Am J Path 49:997, 1966.
58. Wilson CB, Dixon FJ: Antigen quantitation in experimental immune complex glomerulonephritis. I. Acute serum sickness. J Immunol 105:279, 1970.

59. Schwab L, Moll FC, Hall T, et al: Experimental hypersensitivity in the rabbit. Effect of inhibition of antibody formation by X-radiation or nitrogen mustard on the histologic and serologic sequences and on the behavior of serum complement following single large injections of foreign proteins. J Exp Med 91:505, 1950.
60. Rhyne MB, Germuth FG: The relationships between serum complement activity and the development of allergic lesions in rabbits. J Exp Med 114:633, 1961.
61. Holdsworth SR, Neals TJ, Wilson CB: Abrogation of immune glomerulonephritis in rabbits by anti-macrophage serum (Abstr). Kidney Intl 19:193, 1981.
62. Germuth FG: Unpublished observations.
63. McLean CR, Fitzgerald JDL, Younghusband OZ, et al: Diffuse glomerulonephritis in rabbits by small intravenous injections of horse serum. Arch Path 51:1, 1951.
64. Hamilton-Paterson JL, Henderson WG: Serum nephritis in rabbits. Brit J Exp Path 33:67, 1952.
65. Dixon FJ, Feldman JD, Vazquez JJ: Experimental glomerulonephritis. The pathogenesis of a laboratory model resembling the spectrum of human glomerulonephritis. J Exp Med 113:899, 1961.
66. Germuth FG, Senterfit LB, Pollack AD: Immune complex disease. I. Experimental acute and chronic glomerulonephritis. Johns Hopkins Med J 120:225, 1967.
67. Germuth FG, Taylor JJ, Siddiqui SY, et al: Immune complex disease. VI. Some determinants of the varieties of glomerular lesions in the chronic bovine serum-rabbit system. Lab Invest 37:162, 1977.
68. Valdes AJ, Senterfit LB, Pollack AD, et al: The effect of antigen excess on chronic immune complex glomerulonephritis. Johns Hopkins Med J 124:9, 1969.
69. Germuth FG, Valdes AJ, Taylor JJ, et al: Fatal immune complex glomerulonephritis without deposits. Johns Hopkins Med J 136:189, 1975.
70. Helin H, Rantala I, Vaisanen J, et al: Glomerulonephritis induced by high doses of ovalbumin. Studies by electron microscopy, immunofluorescence, and immuno-electron microscopy. Virchow Arch A Path Anat Histol 381:331, 1979.
71. Iskandar SS, Jenette JC, Wilkman AS, et al: Interstrain variations in nephritogenicity of heterologous protein in mice. Lab Invest 46:344, 1982.
72. McLeish KR, Gohara AF, Gunning WT III: Chronic serum sickness in the mouse. Relationship of antigen dose to glomerular pathology. Nephron 31:82, 1982.
73. Balton WK, Surgill BC: Bovine serum albumin chronic serum sickness nephropathy in rats. Brit J Exptl Path 59:167, 1978.
74. Noble B, Milgrom M, vanLiew JB, et al: Chronic serum sickness in the rat: Influence of antigen dose, route of antigen administration and strain of rat on the development of disease. Clin Exp Immunol 46:449, 1981.
75. Oldstone MBA, Dixon FJ: Pathogenesis of chronic disease associated with persistent lymphocytic choriomeningitis viral infection. I. Relationship of antibody production to disease in neonatally infected mice. J Exp Med 129:483, 1969.
76. Oldstone MBA, Dixon FJ: Pathogenesis of chronic disease associated with persistent lymphochoriomeningitis viral infection. II. Relationship of the anti-lymphocytic choriomeningitis immune response to tissue injury in chronic lymphocytic choriomeningitis disease. J Exp Med 131:1, 1970.
77. Howie JB, Helger BJ: The immunology and pathology of NZB mice. Adv Immunol 9:215, 1968.
78. Hang L, Izui S, Dixon FJ: (NZW × BXSB)F_1 hybrid. A model of acute lupus and coronary vascular disease with myocardial infarction. J Exp Med 154:216, 1981.
79. Hang L, Theofilopoulos AN, Dixon FJ: A spontaneous rheumatoid arthritis-like disease in MRL/1 mice. J Exp Med 155:1690, 1982.
80. Tan EM, Shur PH, Carr RI, et al: Deoxyribonucleic acid (DNA) and antibodies to DNA in the serum of patients with systemic lupus erythematosus. J Clin Invest 45:1732, 1966.
81. Lambert PH, Dixon FJ: Pathogenesis of the glomerulonephritis of NZB/W mice. J Exp Med 127:507, 1968.
82. Yoshiki T, Mellors RC, Strand M, et al: The viral protein envelope glycoprotein of murine leukemia virus and the pathogenesis of immune complex glomerulonephritis of New Zealand mice. J Exp Med 140:1011, 1974.
83. Comerford FR, Cohen AS, Desai RG: The evolution of the glomerular lesion in NZB mice. Lab Invest 19:643, 1968.
84. Williams RC Jr: Antibodies in systemic lupus-diversity finally simplified. J Lab Clin Med 100:161, 1982.
85. Brentjens JR, O'Connell DW, Pawlowski IB, et al: Extra-glomerular lesions associated with deposition of circulating antigen-antibody complexes in kidneys of rabbits with chronic serum sickness. Clin Immunol Immunopath 3:112, 1974.
86. Steblay RW, Rudofsky UH: Renal tubular disease and autoantibodies against tubular basement membrane induced in guinea pigs. J Immunol 107:598, 1971.
87. Sugisaki T, Klassen J, Milgron F, et al: Immunopathologic study of an autoimmune tubular and interstitial renal disease in brown Norway rats. Lab Invest 28:658, 1973.
88. Lehman DH, Wilson CB, Dixon FJ: Interstitial nephritis in rats immunized with heterologous tubular basement membrane. Kidney Intl 5:187, 1974.
89. Couser WG, Salant DJ: In situ immune complex formation and glomerular injury. Kidney Intl 17:1, 1980.
90. Andres GA, Seegal BC, Hsu KC, et al: Electron microscopic studies of experimental nephritis with ferritin-conjugated antibody. J Exp Med 117:691, 1963.
91. Ishizaka K, Campbell DH: Biological properties of soluble antigen-antibody complexes. I. Skin reactive properties. Proc Soc Exp Biol Med 97:635, 1958.
92. Germuth FG, Rodriguez E, Lorelle CA, et al: Passive immune complex glomerulonephritis in mice: Models for various lesions found in human disease. II. Low avidity complexes and diffuse proliferative glomerulonephritis with subepithelial deposits. Lab Invest 41:366, 1979.
93. Soothill JR, Steward MW: The immunopathological significance of the heterogenicity of antibody affinity. Clin Exp Immunol 9:193, 1971.
94. Steward MW, Katz FE, West NJ: The role of low affinity antibody in immune complex disease: The quantity of anti-DNA antibodies in NZB/W F_1 hybrid mice. Clin Exp Immunol 21:121, 1975.
95. Steward MW: Chronic immune complex disease in mice: The role of antibody affinity. Clin Exp Immunol 38:414, 1979.
96. Germuth FG, Rodriguez E, Lorelle CA, et al: Passive immune complex glomerulonephritis in mice: Models for various lesions found in human disease. I. High avidity complexes and mesangiopathic glomerulonephritis. Lab Invest 41:360, 1979.
97. Germuth FG, Rodriguez E, Siddiqui SY, et al: Immune complex disease. VII. Experimental mesangiopathic glomerulonephritis produced by chronic immunization with thyroglobulin. Lab Invest 38:404, 1978.
98. Dreesman GR, Germuth FG: Immune complex disease. IV. The nature of the circulating complexes associated with glomerulonephritis in the acute BSA-rabbit system. Johns Hopkins Med J 130:335, 1972.
99. Germuth FG, Valdes AJ, Senterfit LB, et al: A unique influence of cortisone on the transit of specific macromolecules across vascular walls in immune complex disease. Johns Hopkins Med J 122:137, 1968.
100. Germuth FG, Rodriguez E, Wise O: Passive immune complex glomerulonephritis in mice. III. Clearance kinetics and properties of circulating complexes. Lab Invest 46:515, 1982.
101. Lavelle KJ, Durland BD, Yum MN: The effect of antimacrophage antiserum on immune complex glomerulonephritis. J Lab Clin Med 98:195, 1981.
102. Biesecker G, Katz S, Koffler D: Renal localization of the membrane attack complex in systemic lupus erythematosus nephritis. J Exp Med 154:1779, 1981.
103. McCluskey RT, Vassalli P, Gallo G, et al: An immunofluorescent study of pathogenic mechanism in glomerular disease. J Engl J Med 274:695, 1966.
104. Germuth FG, Rodriguez E: Effect of human IgM rheumatoid factor on the glomerular site of localization of passively administered immune complexes in mice. Immunology 53:395, 1984.
105. Krakauer RS, Asunuma Y, Kawicki I, et al: Circulating immune complexes in rheumatoid arthritis. Selective removal of cryogelation with membrane filtration. Arch Intern Med 142:395, 1982.

CHAPTER 14

Microbiological Aspects of Urinary Tract Infection

GUNILLA KÄLLENIUS
R. MÖLLBY
S. B. SVENSON

URINARY TRACT PATHOGENS

The majority of urinary pathogens originate in the commensal flora of the bowel. The most common urinary pathogens in children are Gram-negative bacteria of the family *Enterobacteriaceae*, with *Escherichia coli* as the dominating species, followed by *Klebsiella*, *Enterobacter*, and *Proteus* (Table 14.1). Among the Gram-positive bacteria, the most common pathogens are streptococci, especially streptococci group D (enterococci), and staphylococci.

Although *E. coli* cause most urinary tract infections (UTI) in children without a complicating disorder of the urinary system, the usual bacterial etiology varies with age and sex of the patient (Table 36.2, chapter 36), as well as with the number of previous infections. Thus, *Proteus* is a common invader in boys (1, 2), *Staphylococcus saprophyticus* is common at puberty in girls (3), and *Klebsiella* species are seen in the newborn period. *E. coli* is common also in patients with such complications as calculus, obstruction, or neuropathic bladder, and in children with UTI.

PATHOGENIC MECHANISMS

The concept of pathogenicity in bacteria is often over-simplified in that a rigid distinction is drawn between certain bacteria considered to be pathogenic and others referred to as nonpathogenic. However, most pathogenic bacteria, for example staphylococci, streptococci, meningococci, and Hemophilus, are carried by a considerable proportion of the population without any disease at all. *E. coli* is a useful symbiotic organism in the human intestinal tract and sometimes colonizes other areas of the body as well. If, for example, it colonizes the pharynx or the bladder in patients with asymptomatic bacteriuria, the bacterium does not seem to cause any harm at all. However, in other circumstances, *E. coli* may be highly pathogenic and can cause, for example, septicemia, meningitis, peritoneal abscesses, diarrheal disease, and acute pyelonephritis.

Strains of *E. coli* isolated from such diseases have been analyzed in attempts to detect virulence factors, i.e., particular properties that virulent strains of E. coli possess in common. A number of such factors and properties have been described and statistically evaluated, but few possess absolute correlation with the capacity to cause disease (Table 14.2). Thus, certain factors are more commonly encountered among disease-producing strains than among "harmless" fecal strains from healthy donors, but they do not seem to be absolutely necessary for pathogenicity. In such cases there only may be covariation between the factor studied and the real pathogenic factor(s). This is particularly likely to be the case when it is difficult to determine the biological significance of the factor studied.

The best characterized virulence factors of *E. coli* are the enterotoxins and, in some cases, adhesion factors. These virulence factors appear more commonly in certain serotypes, i.e., bacteria carrying certain surface antigens, but this does not mean that the surface antigens other than the adhesins are important for the development of the diarrheal disease. A more probable explanation for the prevalence of certain "enterotoxigenic" serotypes of *E. coli* is that uptake of virulence plasmids is more common in strains of these serotypes. This hypothesis is valid for the uptake of certain resistance plasmids, but has not been proven for plasmids coding for such virulence factors as enterotoxins and adhesins.

Properties of *E. coli* that Cause Urinary Tract Infections

E. coli is the best studied urinary tract pathogen. There has been much discussion over the mechanisms involved in the pathogenesis of UTI caused by *E. coli*. The prevalence theory advocates that UTI is caused

Table 14.1.
Urinary Pathogens

Bacteria	Bacteria
Gram-negative rods	Gram-positive cocci
Enterobacteriaceae *Escherichia coli*	Micrococcadeae
	Staphylococcus aureus
Proteus spp	*Staphylococcus saprophyticus*
Klebsiella spp	*Staphylococcus epidermidis*
Citrobacter spp "coliforms"	
Enterobacter spp	
Pseudomonadaceae	Streptococcaceae *Streptococcus faecalis* (Enterococci) (Lancefield group D)
Pseudomonas spp	*Streptococcus agalactiae* (Lancefield group B)
	Fungi Candida sp

Table 14.2.
Factors Associated with the Virulence of Uropathogenic *E. coli*

Factor
Possession of certain O-serotypes
Amount of K-antigens
Possession of certain K-antigens
Resistance to serum bactericidal activity
Hemolytic activity
Requirement for opsonization
Temperature-sensitive growth
Colicin-V production
Adherence to human uroepithelium
P-fimbriae

From Möllby R, Källenius G, Korhonen TK, et al: Infection 11:68, 1983.

by any strain of *E. coli* that happens to have colonized the intestinal tract. The theory of special pathogenicity considers that only some strains with certain properties are able to cause infection. As will be shown, certain bacterial factors are more common among *E. coli* that cause UTI than in common *E. coli*.

Surface Antigens

In the host-parasite interrelationship in bacterial infections the host's defense mechanisms are mainly directed against targets on the surface of the invading bacteria. Therefore, a number of bacterial surface structures, commonly referred to as surface antigens, have been studied in detail. Among these are the lipopolysaccharide in the outer membrane (LPS or endotoxin), the acidic capsular polysaccharides surrounding the bacterium (K-antigen), mobile flagella (H-antigen), and adhesive structures (fimbriae or pili) (Table 14.3).

O-antigens. The outer membrane of Gram-negative bacteria consists of phospholipids, outer membrane proteins (OMP), and varying amounts of LPS (Fig. 14.1). This LPS is toxic to animals and is often referred to as endotoxin. The lipid part (Lipid A) of the LPS toxin is necessary for the toxic activity. The polysaccharide part of the molecule consists of a small constant region (core) and an outer part (O-polysaccharide), which is built up of repeating oligosaccharide units. These repeating units vary in their chemical structure among different strains of *E. coli*, giving rise to the different O-serotypes. At present more than 150 different O-serotypes of *E. coli* are recognized (4). Certain O-serotypes are more common among strains of *E. coli* that cause UTI (Table 36.4, chapter

Table 14.3.
Surface antigens of *E. coli*

Lipopolysaccharide (LPS, endotoxin, contains the O-antigen)
Capsular material (K-antigen)
Flagellae (H-antigen)
Fimbriae (pili)
Outer membrane proteins (OMP)
Peptidoglycan (murein, cell wall)

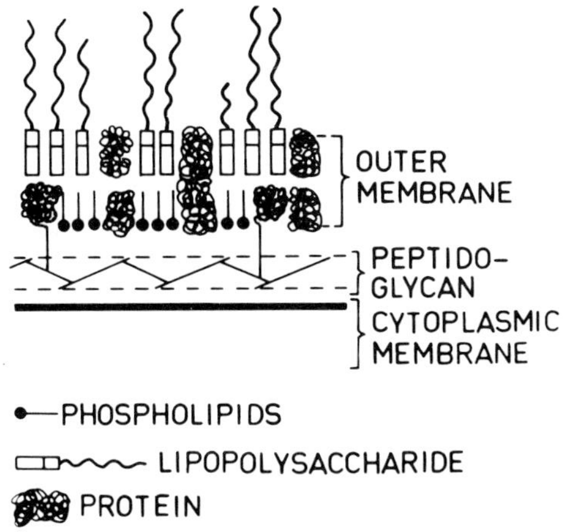

Figure 14.1. Schematic structure of Gram-negative cell envelope.

36), but it has not been proven that certain types of LPS (endotoxins) are more toxic than others.

One probable explanation may be that certain *E. coli* O-serotypes take up virulence plasmids more easily than others, as suggested for enterotoxin producing *E. coli*. If the relevant virulence factor(s) is coded on the chromosome, this gene possibly covariates with the gene that codes for the respective O-serotype. The clonal theory is based on such a hypothesis, which says that originally a few strains had all the necessary genes that coded for the UTI virulence factors, and the progeny of these strains then spread over the world. In support of this theory a number of common characters have, in fact, been detected in many *E. coli* urinary tract pathogens (5).

K-antigens. *E. coli* produce a number of capsular polysaccharides (K-antigens) and over 100 different antigenic types are recognized. Of these, only a few (K1, K2, K3, K5, K12, and K13) are common in pathogenic strains that are involved in upper tract infection.

Although there is a lack in the knowledge why these capsular polysaccharides contribute to the virulence of urinary tract pathogens, some hypotheses have been advanced. These capsular polysaccharides all contain anionic residues that render the outer surface not only strongly hydrophilic but also negatively charged. This is likely to contribute to the general virulence property of these bacterial capsules, as a result of an increase in the resistance against phagocytosis by electrostatic repulsion.

Adhesins. During the last decade there has been an increasing interest in bacterial adhesion in relation to virulence. It is self-evident that all infections on mucosal surfaces must contain an element of interaction between the host's mucosal cell surface and the bacterial surface. If this were not the case the infecting organism would be swept away in the normal flow of urine and mucosal secretions (6, 7).

In the adhesion of bacterial cells to mucosal cell surfaces, both nonspecific (hydrophobic interaction) and specific factors (receptor recognition) are involved. Several specific bacterial binding factors have been studied and they have all been found to be associated with bacterial fimbriae (pil) (Fig. 14.3).

Fimbriae. Fimbriae were first studied by Duguid (8), who observed the hairlike structures on bacteria and correlated them with the ability of the same bacteria to adhere to erythrocytes of different species, i.e., to cause hemagglutination. The same bacterial structures were later also observed by Brinton, who named them pili (9). Some of these fimbriae are coded by chromosomal genes and others by plasmids.

Fimbriae are hairlike structures that are built up by repeating protein molecules. These proteins recognize specific receptor molecules on the surface of the host cell membrane. Such receptor molecules are, in the case of *E. coli*, often of carbohydrate nature, e.g., the carbohydrate portion of glycolipids or glycoproteins. For this reason, fimbriae are sometimes called bacterial lectins.

Type 1 fimbriae, also called common fimbriae, are known to bind to D-mannose residues and are also referred to as D-mannose–sensitive (MS) fimbriae. Although type 1 fimbriae render the bacterium highly adhesive to a number of cells, their role in *E. coli* pathogenesis is still under dispute. One argument is their frequent appearance in most strains of *E. coli*. Furthermore, they are reported to bind to certain glycoproteins, e.g., Tamm-Horsfall protein, in the urine mucus, which would tend to enhance bacterial clearance (10). Finally, type 1 fimbriae facilitate the interaction between the bacterium and phagocytes and thus render it more susceptible to phagocytosis (11).

Of the mannose-resistant (MR) fimbriae, only the P-fimbriae are connected with bacterial virulence in the urinary tract. The P-fimbriae were originally so named because of their selective occurrence on strains of *E. coli* isolated from children with primary acute pyelonephritis (Table 14.4) and their specific binding to glycolipids associated with the P blood group system (12). P-fimbriae were primarily recognized on *E. coli*. They make it possible for the bacterium to adhere to uroepithelial cells and to cause agglutination of erythrocytes from particular species, including human cells. This selectivity was shown to be a result of the specific receptor molecule of these fimbriae, i.e., the disaccharide residue α-D-Galp-(1-4)-β-D-Galp of the P blood group antigens (13). These glycolipids occur only in certain species, but in practically all humans. Only a small number (about 70 individuals in the world) are known to lack these antigens. These receptor structures are present on many kinds of human cells, including erythrocytes, uroepithelial cells, and intestinal epithelium.

P-fimbriae are built up by protein subunits in a helical structure. The molecular weight of each subunit can vary from 16 to 23 kD. They all cross-react to a considerable extent, although 6 antigenic variants are known (14). The genes coding for the phenotypic expression of P-fimbriae are chromosomal. This is in contrast to several other MR-fimbriae that are plasmid-associated. Thus, P-fimbriation is a stable property of the strain and is not easily lost or transferred to other strains, as plasmic-born properties may be. The fimbriae occur in ordinary "UTI serotypes" of *E. coli*.

P-fimbriated *E. coli* are found in practically all cases of acute pyelonephritis in children, while their occurrence is more rare in other types of UTI (Table 14.4). Children with P-fimbriated *E. coli* in the urine are also colonized with the same strain in the intestinal tract, as well as in the periurethral area. This finding supports the idea that P-fimbriated *E. coli* first colonize the intestine, then advance up into the urinary tract by virtue of their adhesive ability (15). P-fimbriated *E. coli* have been used in experimental ascending infections in baboons and rhesus monkeys, animals that also carry the specific receptor structures. These studies indicate that P-fimbriae are necessary for such infections to occur and that the infection can be prevented through active immunization against purified P-fimbriae. Furthermore, the course of the infection is considerably delayed by simultaneous administration of synthesized soluble receptor analogs (16). Such studies point to new prophylactic/therapeutic measures against upper UTI.

Table 14.4.
Detection of P-fimbriae in clinical isolates of *E. coli* from children with various forms of UTI

Type of UTI	Positive/Total (%)
Pyelonephritis	34/35 (97) ($p < 0.01$)
Cystitis	5/26 (19) ($p < 0.05$)
Asymptomatic bacteriuria	5/36 (14)
Faeces strains from healthy	6/82 (7)

Modified from Möllby R, Källenius G, Korhonen TK, et al: Infection 11:68, 1983.

Others. The flagellae, which render the bacterium motile, may be involved in the pathogenesis of *E. coli* by enabling the bacteria to be spread more easily, perhaps up the catheter tubing.

The sensitivity to serum bactericidal factors (serum bacterial sensitivity) has been studied on urinary isolates of *E. coli*. Strains involved in upper UTI are more resistant than strains from lower UTI and from *E. coli* strains in general (17). This is only a statistical and not an absolute correlation.

Toxins

Hemolysins. Strains of *E. coli* are known to be hemolytic, i.e., they produce a clear "halo" around bacterial colonies on blood agar plates. Several different hemolysins have been reported, but only one has been closely studied (18). Strains that cause UTI are more often hemolytic than others, but the pathogenic significance of this finding is not clear. However, through the use of genetically changed strains, it has been shown that hemolysin is a definite virulence factor in the development of intraabdominal abscesses by *E. coli* (19). So far, corresponding experiments have not been successful for UTI. It may be that membrane-damaging toxins like hemolysins might contribute to the damage of mucosal epithelial cells, especially in the bladder. Furthermore, such toxins may impair the function of lymphocytes and other cells involved in the defense mechanisms of the body (20).

Other Toxins. A dermonecrotic toxin, which causes necrosis on injection into the skin of rabbits or guinea pigs, and cytotoxins (proteins that damage cells in culture, e.g., green monkey kidney cells) have been reported (21). To date, these toxins have not been associated with UTI, but they might participate in the local destruction of bladder and kidney tissue.

Pathogenesis of Upper Urinary Tract Infections

It is generally agreed that colonization of the intestine and the periurethral area precedes UTI. If the bacterial strain possesses the necessary virulence factors, it may then ascend in the urinary tract and eventually cause pyelonephritis. Certain "clones" of virulent strains have been shown to exist and when spread the frequency of pyelonephritis increases. Nosocomial spread of a pyelonephritogenic *E. coli* clone in a neonatal ward has been reported (22). The best characterized virulence factor of such pyelonephritogenic *E. coli* are the P-fimbriae (15).

The infectious process is thought to proceed as follows:

1. The child becomes infected orally with a pyelonephritogenic strain of *E. coli* and a colonization of the intestine and the periurethral area follows, probably partly mediated by P-fimbriae.

2. The ascending infection to the bladder also probably is related to adhesive abilities, but in cases with cystitis adhesins other than P-fimbriae may be more relevant.

3. Subsequently, ascent to the ureter occurs by transport of bacteria through turbulent flow or via minor vesicoureteral reflux.

4. P-fimbriae–mediated adhesion of the bacteria to the lower ureter subsequently induces a ureteritis with endotoxin-induced blockage of the neurotransmission and functional ureteral obstruction.

5. This event leads to an increased pressure in the ureter and the renal pelvis, which causes obstructive changes of the renal papilla and pyelotubular backflow.

6. Further bacterial attachment by P-fimbriae to epithelial cells of the tubuli promotes local bacterial replication followed by tissue damage caused by toxins and possibly free radicals of phagocyte cells. Tissue invasion occurs and an acute pyelonephritis ensues (16, 23).

Other Bacteria

The pathogenicity of bacteria other than *E. coli* has been studied very little. For Proteus species the mobility mediated by flagella has been attributed to the high frequency of these bacteria in catheterized patients. Studies to determine the adhesive abilities of Proteus strains that cause UTI in young boys have been noncontributory.

Klebsiella are well known to be highly capsulated, which may contribute to their resistance to the defense mechanisms of the body.

Staphylococci have long been considered of little significance as a cause of UTI. However, during the 1970s a particular species among the subgroup of coagulase-negative staphylococci, *Staphylococcus saprophyticus*, was shown to be an important cause of UTI in young females (24). Pure cultures of coagulase-negative staphylococci also were found in children in 3% of cases with symptomatic UTI (3). The majority of infections were observed in girls from ages 11 to 16 years, with signs of renal involvement in several cases. *S. saprophyticus* has been little studied as to pathogenic mechanisms. The bacterium produces hemolysin in about 50% of isolated strains (20). In contrast to other staphylococcal species, *S. saprophyticus* exhibits a marked tropism for the urinary tract. In vitro studies further show that this species agglutinates sheep erythrocytes and adheres better to human uroepithelial cells than to other epithelial cells of human origin. *S. saprophyticus* is not known to be pathogenic in other organ systems (25).

IMMUNOLOGY

Humoral Immune Response

Circulating Antibody

Humoral antibodies may be elicited against various targets on the *E. coli* surface. Since antibodies to O-antigens are detected easily, a large number of studies have been performed on the O-antibody response in patients with UTI caused by *E. coli*. Antibodies directed against the O-antigens, as estimated by the passive hemagglutination method (26) and the enzyme-linked immunosorbent assay (ELISA) (27), appear in the serum of patients who have clinical signs of renal involvement. Therefore, determination of serum antibody titers to O-antigens has been suggested as a method of localizing the infection. However, such determinations are of little clinical value in the individual patient, since these antibodies do not appear until several days after the onset of disease (27), and also requires knowledge of the O-serotype of the infecting strain. Elevated anti-O-antibody titers in a symptom-free patient may reflect previous *E. coli* infections (UTI as well as other sites). Accordingly, such measurements should not be used as an indication of a "silent" renal infection.

Serum antibodies are rarely induced by the capsular K-antigens of the *E. coli* involved in UTI. This is particularly true for the K-antigens that are most common among the *E. coli* clones (K1, L2, K5, and K12) that cause upper UTI. These *E. coli* clones possess K-antigens, which are of low immunogenicity and which also may mask other bacterial surface antigens (the O-antigens and outer membrane protein antigens). The rationale for the low immunogenicity of these K-antigens is that some of them are structurally related to human cell surface structures, e.g., certain gangliosides (28). This low immunogenicity helps the bacteria to escape recognition by the host. The capsular polysaccharides, which are common among the *E. coli* clones that are uropathogenic, all have high negative charge that may enable the bacteria to resist host defense mechanisms like phagocytosis. Serum antibodies against P-fimbriae are found in patients with acute pyelonephritis.

Local Antibody Response

Antibodies to *E. coli* O-antigens can be found in the urine of patients with acute pyelonephritis (27). The antibodies are primarily of the secretory IgA type, indicating local origin; IgG antibodies also are present, which are likely to be of humoral origin.

Since many bacterial surface antigens are likely to induce antibody responses, it is not surprising that antibody-coated bacteria are found in the urine. In 1974, Thomas and Jones and their colleagues reported that antibody-coated bacteria were found in the urine of patients with kidney infections, but not in the urine of patients with bladder infection (29). They suggested that determination of antibody-coated bacteria would be of aid in diagnosis. In children, however, the results in most studies have been found to be inaccurate (30).

Protective Effect of Antibodies Against Urinary Tract Infections

Preimmunization with homologous and heterologous *E. coli* has been reported to protect against experimental hematogenous infections in rabbits (31) and in an experimental model of UTI in rats (32). The protective effect was attributed to antibodies to the O and K antigens. Also in an infection model in the rat, passive transfer of urine from immunized rats protected against infection (32). Immunization with purified P-fimbriae protected against ascending pyelonephritis in the monkey (33). However, the protective significance of serum and urinary antibodies of similar specificities in human UTI has still to be determined.

Cell-mediated Immune Response

Suppression of cell-mediated immune responses has been demonstrated in the early phase of acute pyelonephritis in children (34, 35). In rats (36, 37) and monkeys (38), introduction of live *E. coli* bacteria into the kidney induces suppression of the cellular response; in the rat, the suppression has been a result of circulating T-suppressor cells (37). The biological significance of these mechanisms is unclear, but a suppressed immunological response may be one of the factors contributing to the susceptibility of the human kidney to infection.

Immunological Mechanisms in Renal Scarring

The mechanisms that lead to the development of pyelonephritic scarring after acute renal infection are not well defined. Several immune mechanisms have been proposed. Bacterial antigens that persist in the kidney, shared antigens between *E. coli* and renal tissue, and alterations in kidney tissue that expose new antigens have been suggested to be involved in destruction of the kidney. However, so far, none of these mechanisms have been shown to play a critical role in the development of renal scarring. Rather, current data from experimental animal studies suggest that infiltration of the kidney by polymorphonuclear leukocytes (PMNL) plays a more important role in the events leading to kidney injury. In a study by Shimamura (39) of acute pyelonephritis in rats, ablation of the granulocytic response with nitrogen mustard showed that the absence of PMNL in the infected kidney prevented renal damage despite the presence of many bacteria. Moreover, treatment of rats with colchicin (depression of leukocyte motility) or with cyclophosphamide (induction of neutropenia) reduced the acute inflammatory response and also the renal parenchymal destruction and scarring (40).

On contact of phagocytes with bacteria, a phagocytic respiratory burst occurs; the bacteria are endocytosed, and concurrently the phagocytes respond by releasing superoxide and other toxic oxygen radicals together with lysozomal enzymes (41). The free radical superoxide or its metabolites, hydrogen peroxide, hydroxyl radical, or singlet oxygen, are all toxic not only to the bacteria but also to granulocytes and other surrounding cells. The general toxicity of the radicals released during phagocytosis might be responsible, at least in part, for the renal tubular cell death and renal scarring following pyelonephritis (42).

Several investigators have reported an increase of antibodies that react with the Tamm-Horsfall protein during the acute phase of pyelonephritis (43). This not well-defined glycoprotein is normally formed in the distal loop of Henle and is excreted in the urine. The clinical significance of antibodies with such reactivity is as yet unsettled. In the presence of renal scarring, the titer elevation of antibody titer against Tamm-Horsfall protein is less obvious (44).

DIAGNOSTIC METHODS

The presence of bacteria in the urine is the main criterion of a UTI. Other commonly used diagnostic signs (chapter 36) may give supportive evidence. Counts of 10^5 or more organisms of one species per ml of fresh uncentrifuged voided midstream urine are usually accepted as an indication of UTI (45). Repeated cultures increase the chances of correct diagnosis. The commonly used level of 10^5 organisms per ml is, however, a statistically defined limit; lower counts of certain pathogens may be significant (46, 47).

Collection and Transport of Urine Samples

Midstream collection of urine is the preferred method for most children who can cooperate. Voided urine usually contains contaminating bacteria from the urethra, the periurethral area, and vagina. Before the sample is taken the urethral meatus of girls may be cleansed with water, and the preputial fold of small boys must be irrigated with water. Antiseptic substances may reduce the apparent number of bacteria in the urine and should not be used. In infants a plastic bag with adhesive lips is often used for collection of urine. It is preferable that the child is closely observed or be seated on the knee of a nurse, and that the specimen is removed immediately after it has been passed.

In small children, the prepuce and periurethral area are often heavily contaminated by Gram-negative bacteria (48) and even repeated cultures may give doubtful results. Suprapubic bladder aspiration may then be justified. It is easy to perform, safe, can be used in general practice, and in hospital. It is particularly suitable for infants. Aspiration should be done when the bladder is palpable, usually 1 hour or more after the child last voided. After the skin has been properly disinfected, the bladder is punctured 1.5 cm above the symphysis pubis. Local anesthesia is not essential. The urine should be aspirated slowly and the site compressed for a short while after the needle has been withdrawn. The failure rate is low, and, if urine is not obtained at the first puncture, it is usually obtained at a second attempt after allowing more time for the bladder to fill.

Catheterization of the bladder may introduce infection, at least in patients with a history of recurring infections, and usually should not be considered in children.

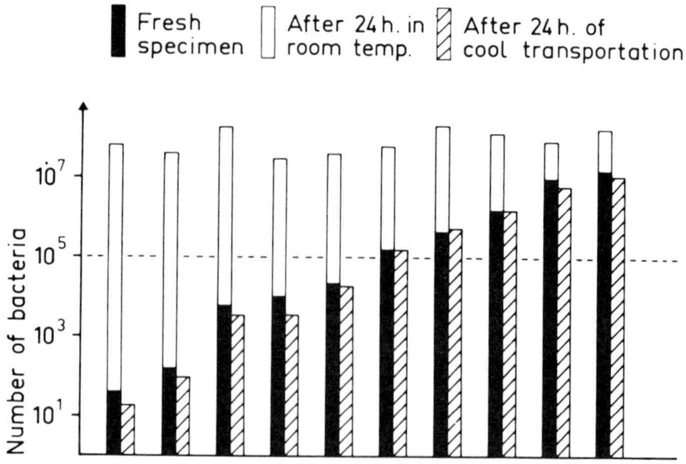

Figure 14.2. The concentration of bacteria in urine specimens before and after 24 hour at room temperature and after 24 hour at +4° C. Dotted line represents the limit for significant bacteriuria. (From Kallings LO: *Lakartidningen* 65(suppl): 30, 1968.)

Urine samples should be kept at 4° C to avoid multiplication of bacteria. Ideally the specimen should be sent to the laboratory immediately, but it can be kept at 4° C for a short period without significant alteration in the numbers of bacteria (Fig. 14.2).

Culture of Urinary Bacteria

Although quantitative urine culture yields extra information, it is time-consuming and consequently a number of semiquantitative methods have been introduced. The semiquantitative method used by most laboratories is the so-called standard loop technique. This method is based on the use of a calibrated loop that deposits a known amount of urine on the culture medium.

During the last decade the dip inoculation technique has been introduced as a method for bacteriological screening and for quantification of bacteriuria (49). One advantage of the dipslide technique is that the time between sampling and culture of specimens may be reduced. Group B streptococci may need more than overnight incubation to become visible on the dipslide (50). The practice of incubating dipslide at room temperature is not recommended, since several bacteria, especially streptococci, grow poorly at temperatures below 37° C. Subculturing from the slide is not recommended.

Chemical Methods

Bacteriological methods have the advantage of identifying the infecting organisms. However, for screening purposes a variety of chemical tests have been introduced to replace the conventional bacteriological tests. All except the nitrite test (51) give unacceptably high false-negative rates.

The nitrite test depends on the reduction of urinary nitrate by bacteria. The specificity of this test is high, more than 99.5%, while the sensitivity is lower, about 70%, since not all types bacteria, e.g., staphylococci and streptococci, reduce nitrate.

Choice of Method

The value of a test depends on the type of patients who are examined. For purposes of screening for bacteriuria, e.g., in those with recurrent symptom-free infections, one or a combination of two chemical tests may have a sufficiently high predictive value. On the other hand, in a selected population of children who are at high risk of kidney damage, such as small children with febrile UTI, the sensitivity of the test is of

Nitrite test → negative → dipslide → negative-no further steps
↘ positive ↘ positive
↘ ↙
conventional culture
for biotyping and determination
of antibiotic resistance
pattern

Figure 14.3. Suggested route of examination for UTI.

utmost importance. For most purposes a combination of the nitrite test and the dipslide test gives the required information. With a positive result, they can be combined with conventional bacteriological culture for biotyping the infecting strain and for determination of its antibiotic resistance pattern (Fig. 14.3). In cases with strong clinical signs of upper UTI or with proven kidney damage, a conventional culture should be performed from the outset.

ANTIMICROBIAL SUSCEPTIBILITY

Tests

The sensitivity of an organism may be determined by the tube dilution method, in which identical inocula are incubated in tubes of medium containing different concentrations of the drug, or by the more convenient agar dilution method. For routine purposes, most laboratories use diffusion tests because they are simple, rapid, and economical. These tests employ standardized filter paper discs impregnated with fixed amounts of antimicrobial drugs and then dried. Bacteria are seeded on the surface of an agar plate and several different drug-impregnated discs are then placed on the surface of the agar. The plates are incubated for 18 to 24 hours and the diameter of the zone around the disc showing no growth is then measured. The diameter of this zone of inhibition indicates whether the organism under scrutiny has high, intermediate, or inadequate sensitivity to the drug in question.

These tests should be performed by personnel trained in bacteriology. A dipslide technique has been advocated as a suitable alternative for susceptibility testing in general practice. However, when the dipslide technique is carried out by inexperienced personnel, the results are unacceptable (52).

Antimicrobial Agents

The mode of action of antibiotics is essentially the same whether it is against Gram-positive or Gram-negative organisms (Table 14.5). However, there is a difference in antibiotic penetrability comparing Gram-positive and Gram-negative organisms. This, in turn, depends on differences in the respective cell wall structure. The Gram-positive organism has a cell wall that contains a strong rigid layer of mucopeptides, whereas in the Gram-negative bacteria lipopolysaccharides, phospholipids, and proteins form an outer membrane (Fig. 14.1). At low concentrations, penicillin G is more effective against Gram-positive than against Gram-negative organisms, which is probably a result of the fact that penicillin G does not penetrate efficiently through the outer membrane of the Gram-negative bacterial cells. Ampicillin and cephalosporins can penetrate through the outer membrane of Gram-negative bacteria and thus may be used also against Gram-negative organisms.

Some of the synergistic and antagonistic effects of various antibiotic combinations can be explained and predicted through their mechanisms of action. For example, penicillin, which affects the peptidoglycan cell wall synthesis, is antagonized by drugs that interfere with protein synthesis.

Table 14.5.
Mechanisms of Action of Antimicrobial Agents

Antimicrobial agents	Example of drug
Effect on DNA replication	Nalidixic acid
Effect on RNA transcription	Rifampicin
Effect on RNA translation (protein synthesis)	Aminoglycosides (streptomycin, gentamicin), chloramphenicol, tetracycline
Interference with the metabolism of bacteria	Sulphonamide, trimethoprim
Effect on synthesis of bacterial cell wall of bacteria	Penicillins, cephalosporins
Direct effect on cytoplasmic membrane	Polymyxins

Table 14.6.
Molecular Mechanisms for Development of Antimicrobial Resistance

Induction of already existing, previously silent genetic elements (chromosomes or plasmids)
Mutation of genetic material
Acquisition of new genetic material (e.g., plasmids)

Table 14.7.
Bacterial Defense Mechanisms against Antimicrobial Agents

Mechanism	Example of drug
Alteration of permeability to the antibiotic changes of capsule, outer membrane, and so on	Methicillin
Changes in the target site of the antimicrobial agent (e.g., DNA polymerase, RNA polymerase, and so on)	Nalidixic acid Streptomycin
Change in metabolism	Sulphonamides
Destruction or modification of antibiotics (e.g., by β-lactamases)	Penicillins Cephalosporins Aminoglycosides

Antibiotic Resistance

Several antimicrobial agents reach effective concentrations in the urine (Table 36.13). The susceptibility of urinary tract pathogens to these agents depends on their intrinsic resistance, e.g., Gram-negative bacteria to penicillins, or on acquired resistance (Table 14.6) (53). The term drug resistance ordinarily refers to acquired changes that may be brought about either by mutation, which alters a chromosomal genetic element, or by acquisition of new non-chromosomal genetic element, or by acquisition of new nonchromosomal genes. Such nonchromosomal genes are often carried on self-replicating genetic units known as plasmids. Furthermore, genes coding for antibiotic resistance can be present in certain specialized fragments of DNA known as transposons that can be transposed from one plasmid or chromosome to another.

These new genetic elements code for changes in the bacteria that render them resistant to one or more antibiotic drugs (Table 14.7). For example, resistance to penicillins occurs when bacteria form plasmid-coded beta-lactamases, i.e., enzymes that cleave the beta-lactam ring of penicillins. Resistance to the aminoglycoside antibiotics is determined by the presence of plasmid-coded enzymes that modify the antibiotic in the outer confines of the cell, thereby preventing its transport to its target of action, the ribosome. The genetic determinants of resistance to most of the clinically significant antibiotics are commonly carried by plasmids.

Resistance-plasmids or R-factors are members of the broad group of plasmids that allow rapid spread of multiple antibiotic resistance (53, 54). The frequent exposure of a human population to a variety of antibiotics has led to a higher incidence of R-plasmids in the intestinal enterobacteria. It should be noted that antibiotics do not induce, but select for R-plasmids. Such plasmids have been found even in strains of bacteria that were stored before the use of antibiotics. The resistance patterns of various bacteria are known to almost mirror the general policy for antibiotic usage in a certain area. Because of this, certain drugs should be voluntarily "saved" for very resistant strains.

Therapy

In first-time symptomatic infections, most infecting strains are sensitive to a wide range of antimicrobial drugs. The choice of therapy, therefore, is mostly dependent on other factors, such as side effects and cost. In patients with recurrent infections who need repeated short courses or long-term prophylaxis, the risk of drug resistance is higher, since antibiotics act as a powerful selective factor in the spread of resistant bacteria. For these reasons, agents to which resistance develops rapidly should be avoided.

The agent chosen should also be as widely effective against the likely pathogens as possible and should have a minimal effect on the commensal flora of the bowel flora and other sites. The two agents that have been used most successfully for long-term prophylaxis are nitrofurantoin and trimethoprimsulphamethoxazole (chapter 38).

Long-term therapy requires periodic bacteriological reassessment and sensitivity tests on the flora isolated to indicate when changes in therapy are required.

References

1. Winberg J, Andersen HJ, Bergström T, et al: Epidemiology of symptomatic urinary tract infection in childhood. Acta Paediatr Scand 252(suppl):1, 1974.
2. Hallet RJ, Pead L, Maskell R: Urinary infection in boys. A three-year prospective study. Lancet 2:1107, 1976.
3. Hermansson G, Bollgren I, Bergström T, et al: Coagulase negative staphylococci as a cause of symptomatic urinary infections in children. J Pediatr 84:807, 1974.
4. Orskov I, Orskov F, Jann B, et al: Serology, chemistry, and genetics of O and K antigens of *Escherichia coli*. Bacteriol Rev 41:667, 1977.
5. Väisänen-Rhen V, Elo J, Väisänen E, et al: P-fimbriated clones among uropathogenic *Escherichia coli* strains. Infect Immun 43:149, 1984.
6. Svanborg-Edén C, Hanson LA, Jodal U, et al: Variable adherence to normal human urinary tract epithelial cells of *Escherichia coli* strains associated with various forms of urinary tract infections. Lancet 2:490, 1976.
7. Beachey EH: Bacterial Adherence. Receptors and Recognition, series B, London and New York, Chapman and Hall, vol 6, 1980.
8. Duguid JP, Smith IW, Dempster G, et al: Non-flagellar filamentous appendages ("fimbriae") and haemagglutinating activity in Bacterium coli. J Path Bacteriol 70:335, 1955.
9. Brinton CC: The structure, function, synthesis and genetic control of bacterial pili and a molecular model for DNA and RNA transport in gram negative bacteria. Trans NY Acad Sci 27:1003, 1965.
10. Orskov I, Ference A, Orskov F: Tamm-Horsfall protein or uromucoid is the normal urinary slime that traps type 1 fimbriated *Escherichia coli*. Lancet 1:887, 1980.
11. Bar-Shavit Z, Ofek I, Goldman R, et al: Mannose residues on phagocytes as receptors for the attachment of *Escherichia coli* and *Salmonella typhi*. Biochem Biophys Res Commun 78:455, 1977.
12. Källenius G, Svenson SB, Möllby R, et al: Carbohydrate receptor structures recognized by uropathogenic *E. coli*. Scand J Inf Dis 33(suppl):52, 1982.
13. Källenius G, Svenson SB, Möllby R, et al: Structure of carbohydrate part of receptor on human uroepithelial cells for pyelonephritogenic *E coli*. Lancet 2:604, 1981.
14. Rhen M, Klemm P, Wahlström E, et al: P-fimbriae of *Escherichia coli*: Immunoprotein-chemical characterization of fimbriae from two pyelonephritogenic strains. FEMS Microbiol Lett 18:233, 1983.
15. Svenson SB, Källenius G, Korhonen TK, et al: Initiation of clinical pyelonephritis—The role of P-fimbriae mediated bacterial adhesion. Contr Nephrol 39:252, 1984.
16. Roberts JA, Kack B, Källenius G, et al: Receptors for pyelonephritogenic *Escherichia coli* in primates. J Invest Urol 131:163, 1984.
17. Olling S, Hanson LA, Holmgren J, et al: The bactericidal effect of normal human serum on *E. coli* strains from normals and from patients with urinary tract infections. Infection 1:24, 1973.
18. Rennie RP, Freer JH, Arbuthnott JP: The kinetics of erythrocyte lysis by *Escherichia coli* haemolysin. J Med Microbiol 7:189, 1974.
19. Welch RA, Dellinger EP, Minshem B, Falkow S: Haemolysin contributes to virulence of extra-intestinal *E. coli* infections. Nature 294:665, 1981.
20. Möllby R: Isolation and properties of membrane damaging toxins. In Adlam C, Easmon CSF (eds): *Staphylococci and Staphylococcal Infections*. London, Academic Press Inc., 1983, vol 2, p 619.
21. Konowalchuk J, Speirs JI, Stavric S: Vero response to a cytotoxin of *Escherichia coli*. Infect Immun 18:775, 1977.
22. Tullus K, Hörlin K, Svenson SB, et al: Epidemic outbreaks of acute pyelonephritis caused by nosocomial spread of P-fimbriated *E. coli* in children. J Infect Dis 150:728, 1984.
23. Källenius G, Svenson SB, Hultberg H, et al: P-fimbriae of pyelonephritogenic *E. coli*: Significance for reflux and renal scarring—A hypothesis. Infection 11:73, 1983.
24. Mabeck CE: Significance of coagulase-negative staphylococcal bacteriuria. Lancet 2:1150, 1969.
25. Mårdh PA, Colleen S, Hovelius B: Attachment of bacteria to exfoliated cells from the urogenital tract. Invest Urol 16:322, 1978/79.
26. Winberg J, Anderson HJ, Hanson LA, et al: Studies of urinary tract infections in infancy and childhood. I. Antibody response in different types of urinary tract infections caused by coliform bacteria. Brit Med J 2:524, 1963.
27. Sohl Akerlund A, Ahlstedt S, Hanson LA, et al: Antibody responses in urine and serum against *Escherichia coli* O antigen in childhood urinary tract infection. Acta Path Microbiol Scand 87:29, 1979.
28. Finne J, Leinonen M, Mäkelä PH: Antigenic similarities between brain components and bacteria causing meningitis. Lancet 2:355, 1983.
29. Thomas V, Shelokov A, Forland M: Antibody-coated bacteria in the urine and the site of urinary tract infection. N Engl J Med 290:588, 1974.28.
30. Forsum U, Hjelm E, Jonsell G: Antibody coated bacteria in the urine of children with urinary tract infection. Acta Paediatr Scand 65:639, 1976.
31. Kaijser B, Olling S: Experimental haematogenous pyelonephritis due to *E. coli* in rabbits: the antibody response and its protective capacity. J Infect Dis 128:41, 1973.
32. Kaijser B, Larsson P, Olling S: Protection against ascending *Escherichia coli* pyelonephritis in rats and significance of local immunity. Infect Immun 20:78, 1978.
33. Roberts JA, Hardaway K, Kaack B, et al: Prevention of pyelonephritis by immunization with P-fimbriae. J Urol (In press.)
34. Janas T, Vesikari T, Hällström O, et al: Suppressed lymphocyte mitogen responsiveness in urinary tract infections of children and its correlation to pyelonephritis. Acta Paediatr Scand 68:501, 1979.
35. Ahlstedt S, Hagberg M, Jodal U, et al: Cell-mediated immune parameters in children with pyelonephritis caused by *Escherichia coli*. Progr Allergy 33:289, 1983.
36. Williams TW, Friedlander AM, Lyons JM, et al: Cellular immunity in pyelonephritis: Identification of suppressor cell activity of spleen cells in response to concanavalin A and inhibition of lymphocyte-mediated L cell cytotoxicity. J Immunol 116:778, 1976.
37. Miller T, Scott L, Stewart E, et al: Modification by suppressor cells and serum factors of the cell-mediated immune response in experimental pyelonephritis. J Clin Invest 61:964, 1978.
38. Roberts JA, Domingue GJ, Martin LN, et al: Immunology of pyelonephritis in the primate model: Live versus heat-killed bacteria. Kidney Intl 19:297, 1981.
39. Shimamura T: Mechanisms of renal tissue destruction in an experimental acute pyelonephritis. Exp Molec Pathol 34:34, 1981.
40. Bille J, Glauser MP: Protection against chronic pyelonephritis in rats by suppression of acute suppuration: Effect of colchicine and neutropenia. J Infect Dis 146:220, 1982.
41. McCord JM, Wong K: Phagocyte-produced free radicals: rôles in cytotoxicity and inflammation. In Fitzsimons DW (ed): Oxygen-free Radicals and Tissue Damage. Amsterdam, North Holland: Elsevier/Excerpta, 1979, p 343.
42. Roberts JA, Roth JK Jr, Domingue G, et al: Immunology of pyelonephritis in the primate model. V. Effect of superoxide dismutase. J Urol 128:1394, 1982.
43. Fasth A, Hanson LA, Jodal U, et al: Auto-antibodies to Tamm Horsfall protein associated with urinary tract infection in girls. J Pediatr 95:54, 1979.
44. Fasth A, Bjure J, Herrström M, et al: Autoantibodies to Tamm Horsfall glycoprotein in children with renal damage associated with urinary tract infections. Acta Paediatr Scand 69:709, 1980.
45. Kass EH, Finland M: Asymptomatic infection of the urinary tract. Trans Assoc Am Physic 69:56, 1956.
46. Stamm WE, Counts GW, Ruming KR, et al: Diagnosis of coliform infection in acutely dysuric women. N Engl J Med 307:463, 1982.
47. Bollgren I, Engström CF, Hammarlind M, et al: Low urinary counts of P-fimbriated

Escherichia coli in children with presumed acute pyelonephritis. Arch Dis Childh 59:102, 1984.
48. Bollgren I, Winberg J: The periurethral aerobic bacterial flora in healthy boys and girls. Acta Paediatr Scand 65:74, 1976.
49. Arneil GC, McAllister TA, Kay P: Measurement of bacteriuria by plane dipslide culture. Lancet 2:94, 1973.
50. Jokipii AMM, Jokipii L: Recognition of group B streptococci in dip-slide cultures of urine. J Clin Microbiol 10:218, 1979.
51. Schaus R: Griess' nitrate test in diagnosis of urinary infections. JAMA 161:528, 1956.
52. Dornbusch K, Lindeberg B, Nord C-E, et al: Bacteriuria diagnosis and antibiotic susceptibility testing in a group practice by dipslide techniques. Chemotherapy 25:227, 1979.
53. Novick RP: Extrachromosomal inheritance in bacteria. Bacteriol Rev 33:210, 1969.
54. Davies JE, Rownd R: Transmissible multiple drug resistance in Enterobacteriaceae. Science 176:758, 1972.

CHAPTER **15**

The Coagulation System in Experimental and Human Renal Disease

KENNETH MILLER

COAGULATION

Although activation of the coagulation system is demonstrable in some experimental or human renal diseases, its precise role as a mediator of glomerular or vascular injury remains to be defined (1–3). Clearly, if such a role for the coagulation system could be identified, the therapeutic implications would be significant. In this chapter, we will review the pertinent experimental and human studies in an attempt to provide insight into how alterations in the clotting system impact on kidney diseases. The potential role of agents available to inhibit one or more of the mediator systems involved in the coagulation process in human renal diseases will also be explored. Currently, our understanding of the role of hemostatic mechanisms in renal disease is based primarily on morphological, histochemical, radioisotopic, or serological abnormalities.

Several existing experimental models of renal injury are used to provide insight into the role of the coagulation system as a mediator of glomerular or vascular injury.

EXPERIMENTAL RENAL DISEASE

Immune Mediated Experimental Renal Diseases

Immune injury to the kidney is usually produced by one of two mechanisms: (1) the action of antibodies directed against antigens within the basement membrane [anti-glomerular basement membrane (GBM) nephritis, nephrotoxic nephritis (NTN), or *Masugi nephritis* (MN)] and (2) by the action of circulating or in situ antigen-antibody complexes on the kidney (acute or chronic serum sickness) Heymann-type autologous immune complex (AIC) nephritis (chapter 13).

Anti-glomerular Basement Membrane Nephritis

Modification of the glomerular cell proliferation and the degree of fibrin deposition with anticoagulants (heparin and warfarin) administered before or simultaneously with the infusion of nephrotoxic serum provided the initial support for the possible role of the coagulation system in anti-GBM nephritis (1, 4). Accentuation of the lesions with enhanced crescent formation and fibrin deposition could be achieved by blockade of the fibrinolytic system using either epsilonaminocaproic acid (EACA) or transaminoethyl-cyclohexane carboxylic acid (+ −AMCHA) (5). Prior administration of heparin, however, afforded protection to the glomeruli. Defibrinating animals with *Arvin* (Ancrod, malayan pit viper venom extract), which cleaves A-fibrinopeptides from the fibrinogen molecule also modified or reversed the glomerular lesions with subsequent improvement in renal function. However, urinary protein excretion was unaffected and the immune deposits of IgG and C_3 remained unchanged. Arvin was equally effective either administered during the heterologous phase or autologous phase of nephrotoxic serum nephritis (6–8). The rapid clearance of the fibrin-related antigens (FRA) suggested that alternative mechanisms for fibrin removal existed. Subsequent studies have proposed that circulating monocytes/macrophages via phagocytosis or perhaps other cells (platelets or leukocytes) via the release of secretory products, may result in the deposition or removal of fibrin within glomeruli or along the vascular endothelial surface (9).

Other studies, however, have cast doubt as to the importance of the coagulation system as a mediator of glomerular injury in anti-GBM nephritis. In the mouse, heparin was ineffectual in modifying the lesion or degree of fibrin deposition. Urokinase, a plasminogen activator, decreased the degree of fibrinogen-related antigen deposition, but had no impact on the basement membrane lesions (10). Subsequent studies in rat and New Zealand white rabbits also failed to show a protective effect from heparin therapy. Indeed, in both these animal models, high dose anticoagulant therapy resulted in a more severe histologic picture (11, 12). Urinary excretion of fibrin-related antigens correlated with the severity of the glomerular lesions and were not altered by heparin therapy. This would lend support to the suggestion that alternative pathways of fibrin (FRA) formation and clearance exist. Additionally, it should be pointed out that the doses of heparin and warfarin employed in all these studies would be therapeutically impractical in humans, resulting in a significant bleeding diathesis (1). Ancrod, however, appears to have some therapeutic attraction because it effectively modifies the lesion regardless of the time of administration, provided, of course, that renal function is only minimally impaired when this agent is infused (6–8). Scattered reports of Ancrod infusion into patients with immune complex glomerulonephritis or hyperacute renal allograft rejection by one group of investigators has shown promising results. Other purported mechanisms by which Arvin may act include the stimulation of either endothelial prostacyclin or plasminogen activator activity (13–15).

The platelets's role in anti-GBM nephritis, if any, is probably limited (1, 16). Selective depletion of platelets, by platelet antisera did not inhibit the development of the autologous phase of NTS (18). Fibrin-mediated damage, inclusive of crescent formation, was also uneffected by platelet depletion despite decreased protein excretion. Thromboxane A2, however, may cause glomerular injury, at least in the rat anti-GBM model. Administration of a thromboxane synthetase inhibitor, *OKY-1581*, before or during the infusion NTS prevented decrements in glomerular filtration rate (GFR) at 1, 2, and 3 hours while the administration of HK-38 or HK-85, other thromboxane synthetase inhibitors, prevented a decline in GFR at 2 and 3 hours. Conversely, ibuprofen, a cycloxygenase inhibitor, not only failed to prevent the decrements in GFR and renal blood flow (RBF) at 1 and 2 hours after NTS infusion but actually attenuated the partial recovery of GFR and effective RBF at 3 hours (19).

ACUTE AND CHRONIC IMMUNE COMPLEX DISEASE

Administration of either bovine serum albumin (BSA) to presensitized thorotrast-treated rabbits or the administration of soluble antigen-antibody complexes into rabbits may result in cortical necrosis (20). Heparin prevents the development of cortical necrosis, if given within 4 hours after the injection of BSA, suggesting a role for the coagulation system in this model. Prolongation of the partial thromboplastin time (PTT) with decreased plasma levels of factors IX, XI, and XII and equivocal changes in clottable fibrinogen, presumably a result of IgE induced activation of the basophil, was demonstrable in a subsequent study (21). Basophil degranulation can cause the release of mediators such as histamine and platelet-aggregating factor (PAF), resulting in platelet aggregation and release of platelet constituents. Neutrophils, however, also contain substances that can activate the coagulation, fibrinolytic, and kallikrein-kinin systems.

Subsequent studies, employing a variety of animal models have provided conflicting data. Heparin was effective in some studies but not in others. One plasminogen activator (urokinase) was ineffective in modifying the glomerular lesions while another plasminogen activator, streptokinase, was efficacious (12, 22–24). Arvin, however, was beneficial in chronic immune complex disease (25). In the NZB-NZW mouse immune complex disease model, the prototype of systemic lupus erythmatosus (SLE) in man, daily heparin administration modified the renal lesion and improved animal survival. Warfarin was of no value (1).

Ambiguity also exists as to the platelet's role in either acute or chronic immune complex disease. Earlier studies in rabbits demonstrated that vasoactive constituents of platelets were responsible for the enhanced localization of circulating immune complexes. The administration of chlorpheneramine maleate or methylsergide maleate (histamine and serotonin antagonists) prevented antigen antibody deposition. Depleting the animals of platelets also achieved these results (26, 27). Conversely, both dipyridamole and salicylaldoxime (antiplatelet drugs) proved ineffective in modifying the BSA or horse serum induced renal lesions despite evidence for platelet mediated injury (enhanced platelet factor 4 release or shortening of the stypven clotting time of platelet-rich plasma) (28). In autologous immune complex (AIC) disease in the rat, administration of any of a number of antiplatelet drugs, for example, acetylsalicylic acid (aspirin), cyproheptadine (periactin), indomethacin, ticlopridine, or a fibrinolytic inhibitor (batroxobin) proved ineffective in altering the course of the disease. Dipyridamole, did reduce protein excretion, but had no impact on the histologic lesions (19, 29, 30). In yet another immune complex disease model induced by the administration of Habu snake venom, neither platelet depletion, nor prostacyclin or dipyridamole administration proved beneficial, whereas aspirin in a dose of 10 mg/kg actually accentuated the proliferative changes (31, 32). In chronic AIC disease, cyproheptadine appeared to delay the onset of the disease and to reduce to the amount of proteinuria (29).

Whether any of the animal data can be extrapolated to predict outcome in a variety of human diseases is unclear. Certainly, species differences, particularly with respect to the ratio of platelet constitutents may have some bearing on the response to the agents employed in either the AIC or CIC animal models. Human platelets lack histamine which raises serious doubt as to the effectiveness of antihistamines in any immune complex disease in man (33, 34). Currently available data would suggest that neither anticoagulants, fibrinolytic inhibitors nor antiplatelet drugs will consistently alter the course of immune complex disorders.

GENERALIZED SCHWARTZMAN REACTION

The generalized Schwartzman reaction (GSR) is felt to be the prototype of disseminated intravascular coagulation in man. The development of bilateral renal cortical necrosis following two identical injections of endotoxin spaced 20 to 24 hours apart is unique to the rabbit (35). The initial dose of endotoxin is termed the preparatory dose, while the second injection is termed the provocative dose. Following the first injection, there is activation of the coagulation system, followed by a decline in the white blood cell and platelet counts with reduced fibrinolytic activity. In addition, there is enhanced arteriolar smooth muscle responsiveness to catecholamines. All of the above effects may resolve spontaneously provided that the provocative dose is withheld. The preparatory dose of endotoxin may be substituted by either RES blockade (thoratrast or trypan blue injection) (36) or by infusing EACA (decrease fibrinolytic activity) (37), cortisone, or norepinephrine (altered arteriolar smooth muscle response) (38–40). Utilization of pregnant animals also substitutes for the first dose of endotoxin (fibrinolytic activity diminished) (41, 42). The rat, for example, does not develop the GSR except when pregnant (42). Exposure of subendothelial vascular elements by endotoxin damages the vascular endothelium. This is probably the initial site of injury in the GSR. The presence of circulating endothelial cells and electron microscopic evidence of increased mitotic activity of endothelial cells were observed following the initial dose of endotoxin (43–45). Plasminogen activator synthesis is also impaired by the endothelial cell injury induced by the preparatory endotoxin injection. Further endothelial injury resulting from the provocative dose depletes the remaining vascular plasminogen activator resulting in renal cortical necrosis (46). Platelet subendothelial interaction allows for the adhesion and aggregation of platelets with the release of mediators such as adenosine diphosphate (ADP), serotonin, thromboxane A_2 (TxA_2), and beta thromboglobulin (BTG) with subsequent fibrin formation (47). The unilateral endotoxin perfusion model in which one systemic injection of endotoxin causes cortical necrosis in the endotoxin perfused kidney lends support to the concept of primary endothelial injury (48). Pretreatment of animals with anticoagulants does not prevent the endothelial damage.

The platelet's role is inferred from studies in which the GSR was prevented by pretreating animals with antiplatelet agents or by depleting the animal of platelets with antisera (49, 50). A diffusable substance contained within the platelet was shown to inhibit renal cortical fibrinolytic activity suggesting that platelet destruction was the mechanism responsible for inhibiting glomerular lysis (51). Conversely, neither FRA formation nor fibrin deposition was prevented by making rabbits thrombocytopenic with neuraminidase (52). Dipyridamole's protective effect may in part be mediated through its ability to inhibit lymphokine activity and release (53). Leukocytes can also release mediators such as PAF, acidic mucosubstance, or lysosomal cationic protein, which can cleave fibrin monomers causing paracoagulation of soluble fibrin monomer complexes (54, 55). Thromboplastin-like material and an antiheparin factor are also found in leukocytes (1).

The fibrinolytic system also appears to play a prominent role in the production of the GSR. Thrombin infusion results in renal cortical necrosis when EACA is injected (56). Polymyxin B (a fibrinolytic inhibitor), however, did not substitute for the preparatory dose of endotoxin (57). Liquoid (sodium polyanethol sulfate), an agent with anticoagulant and anticomplementary activity, produces a GSR-like glomerular injury with loss of glomerular fibrinolysis, which is reversible with urokinase or heparin (58). Heparin, however, did not affect the plasma fibrinogen level, platelet count, or C_3 levels, in this model despite histologic improvement (59). Liquoid also causes renal impairment in animals depleted of leukocytes or platelets, probably via activation of the extrinsic coagulation pathway (60).

Although the GSR or a GSR-like disease can develop in the absence of factor XII, factor VII, or fibrinogen, most investigators feel that the coagulation and fibrinolytic systems play crucial roles in the production of the GSR (1). Manipulations of these systems, through the use of anticoagulants, fibrinolytic activators (urokinase, streptokinase), or Arvin may prevent or modify the GSR. Platelets, leukocytes, the complement cascade, and the sympathetic nervous system, however, may be equally important. Whether this experimental model is truly representative of DIC in man still remains to be determined.

A model of ischemic renal failure was developed in the rat to investigate the relationship between intrarenal activation of the coagulation system and impaired renal function (61, 62). Intracortical fibrin deposition was essentially uneffected by high dose heparin administration alone (500 μ/100 gm) or in combination with antiplatelet serum. No improvement in GFR was observed. In this experimental renal failure model, no causal relationship appears to exist between the observed hemostatic abnormalities and the impaired renal function.

HUMAN RENAL DISEASE

In this section we will attempt to define the role of the coagulation system in human renal diseases. The value of therapeutic agents that impact on hemostatic function in modifying or reversing the lesions (glomerular or vascular) will also be explored. One can no longer infer that fibrin deposition implies activation of the clotting process because there are thrombin independent mechanisms by which fibrin formation and clearance can occur such as via the release of proteases from leukocytes or the release of other vasoactive substances from platelets (1, 2, 63). For example, the principle cell involved in crescent formation in various types of rapidly progressive glomerulonephritis, is thought to be the macrophage. This cell may be responsible for fibroblast proliferation or alternatively the macrophage may act as a phagocytic cell for clearing fibrinogen/fibrin complexes. FRA deposition in crescents is quite pronounced, yet neither factor VIII antigen nor platelet antigen is present (Fig. 15.1) (1, 64, 65). In anaphylactoid purpura, mesangial fibrin deposition occurs without factor VIII or platelet antigen deposition. Conversely, in the hemolytic uremic syndrome (HUS) and related disorders, factor VIII, platelet antigen, and fibrin deposition apparently occur in similar sites, (capillary loops or along vascular endothelial surfaces) (Fig. 15.2) (1, 87). However, therapeutic manipulations of the coagulation cascade in the latter disorders have met with equivocal results (chapter 27) (Fig. 15.2) (1, 64, 65).

FIBRINOLYSIS AND THE KIDNEY

Clearance of fibrinogen/fibrin-related antigens can occur as a result of phagocytosis (circulating monocytes or epithelial or mesangial cells) or via activation of the fibrinolytic system (1, 66). Kidney endothelial cells produce a plasminogen activator, urokinase in vitro (67). Activator activity appears to exist within the glomeruli and blood vessels. The relative concentration of urokinase in the cortex or medulla, however, is unknown. No apparent relationship between glomerular fibrinolytic activity and glomerular fibrin deposition was demonstrable in a variety of renal diseases (68). However, absent cortical fibrinolytic activity has been observed in renal ischemia, sickle cell disease, HUS, and acute homograft rejection (1, 69–71). In the latter disorder, fibrin antigen deposition was absent. In sickle cell disease, an inhibitor of urokinase was found, whereas in HUS a plasma inhibitor of renal cortical fibrinolysis was isolated, which appeared to be dialyzable (70, 71). In acute poststreptococcal GN, clear-cut evidence of activation of the coagulation system with subsequent fibrinolysis was observed by fibrinogen chromatography in which high molecular weight fibrin derivatives were found during the acute phase of the illness with fibrin-degradation products (FDP-X) found during the recovery phase (72). These FRA derivatives, however, could have arisen from the actions of nonthrombin-mediated pathways, e.g., leukocyte elastase, which can clear fibrinogen, factor VIII, and factor XIII (3).

FACTOR XIII AND RENAL DISEASE

Fibrin-stabilizing factor (FSF) or its active subunit is elevated in patients with chronic renal disease and in one study correlated with serum triglyceride levels (73). FSF may be important in the genesis of atherosclerosis, a process accelerated in the patient with chronic renal failure. In Henoch-Schonlein purpura, factor XIII levels were decreased in patients with a protracted clinical course (increased incidence of GI or renal complications). Return of factor XIII levels to normal was associated with recovery (74, 75).

FIBRIN-RELATED ANTIGENS IN THE SERUM AND URINE

In the experimental animal models, a correlation between FRA deposition, urinary FRA excretion, and the severity of the histological lesion appears to exist (11). However, in humans the data is equivocal. Although elevated serum FRA levels may be indicative of either disease activity or of the severity of the renal lesion, activation of hemostatic mechanisms may not be the sole reason for the elevated FDP levels (76). Additionally,

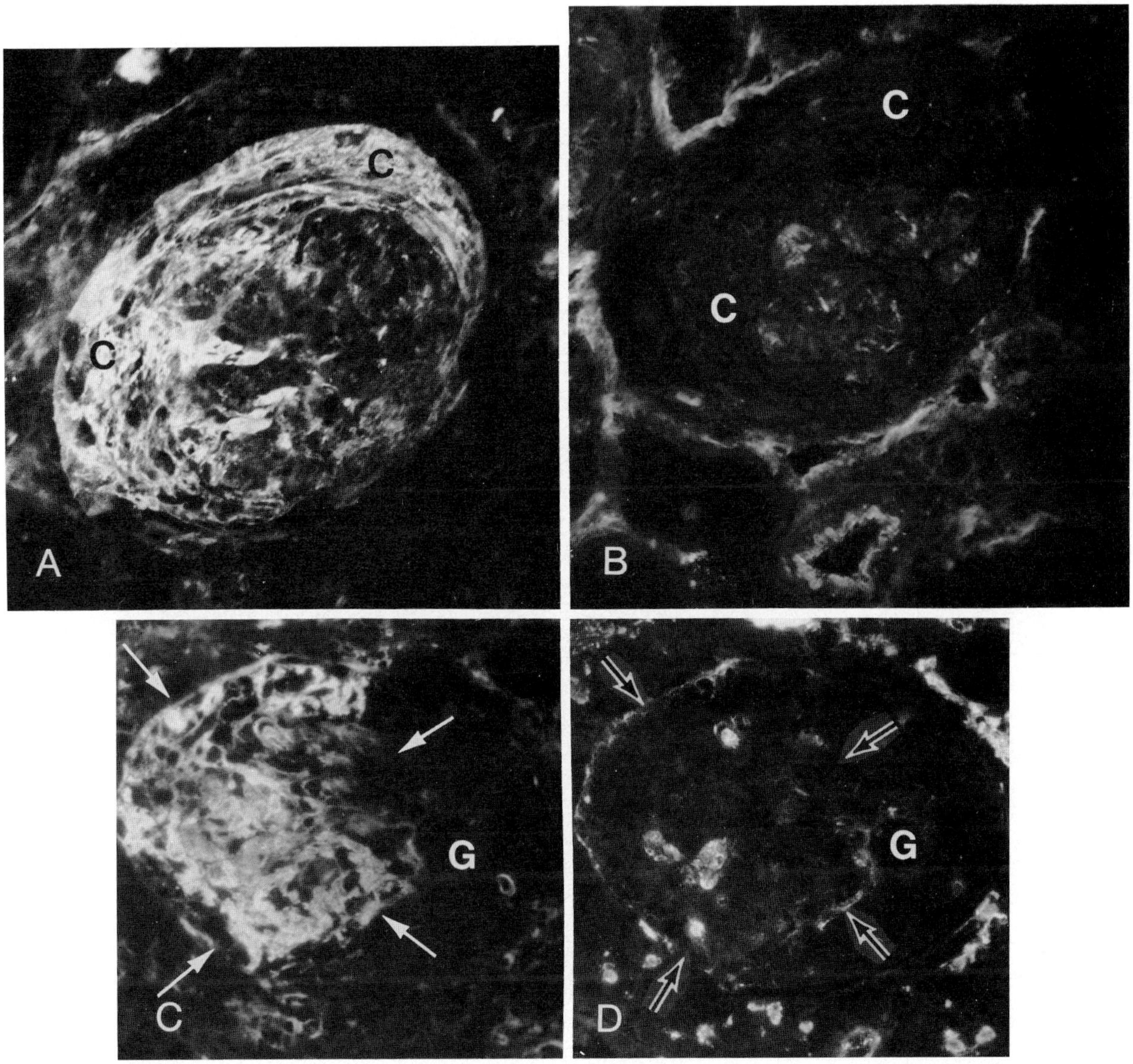

Figure 15.1. Immunofluorescent microscopy of a glomerulus from a patient with rapidly progressive glomerulonephritis. **A.** The arrows enclose a crescent containing large amounts of fibrin. The glomerulus (G) is negative. **B.** The same glomerulus shown in A, showing absence of antihemophilic factor (Factor VIII) in the crescent.

Goodpasture's syndrome with crescentric glomerulonephritis. **C.** Staining of fibrin within a crescent. **D.** The same glomerulus showing absence of platelet antigen(s) within the crescent (arrows) and minimal reaction within the glomerulus (G) (X1300).

(**A** and **B** from Miller K and Michael AF, Coagulation and the Kidney. In McIntosh RM, Guggenhein SJ, Schrier RM (eds) Kidney Disease: Hematologic and Vascular Problems, New York, John Wiley and Sons, Inc., 1977. **C** and **D** from Miller K, Dresner IG, Michael AF. Kidney Int 18:472, 1980. All with permission.)

extra renal vascular sites and tissue lysis also increase serum FRA levels. Finally, in renal failure, impaired elimination could also result in elevated serum FRA, fibrinopeptide A, (beta 15–42 antigen), and fragment E (77). Elevated serum FRA levels are also seen in a variety of unrelated renal disease, such as SLE, poststreptococal glomerulonephritis, rapidly progressive nephritis, anaphylactoid purpura, HUS, nephrotic syndrome, hypertensive patients with focal sclerosis, renal failure, and membranous nephropathy (1, 78, 79).

Several mechanisms are proposed for the elevated fibrin/fibrinogen-related antigens found in the urine (Table 15.1). Most workers believe that elevated urinary FRA levels are not indicative of intrarenal activation of the coagulation system. A poor correlation was observed when histological assessment of renal biopsy material by light microscopy, immunofluorescent and electron microscopy was compared to urinary FRA excretion (1, 80–82). Some investigators have found an association between urinary protein and urinary FDP levels, while others contend that the basic mechanism for FDP appearance in the urine is differential filtration of FDP levels from the blood through a damaged GBM (1, 79, 83). The presence of the D-dimer in urine suggests that cross-linked fibrin formed is lysed by plasmin. High values of D-dimer in the urine are believed to be indicative of intrarenal generation and were observed in some patients with acute glomerulonephritis HSP, mesangial proliferative nephritis, and membranoproliferative glomerulonephritis (MPGN) (84). Intense staining of cross-linked fibrin was observed in glomeruli, crescents, and vessels in HUS and disseminated intravascular coagulation (DIC) (85). The mechanism of cross-liked fibrin formation, however, is unknown. Factor VIII and FRA deposition occurred in similar sites to that of cross-linked fibrin and correlated with the degree

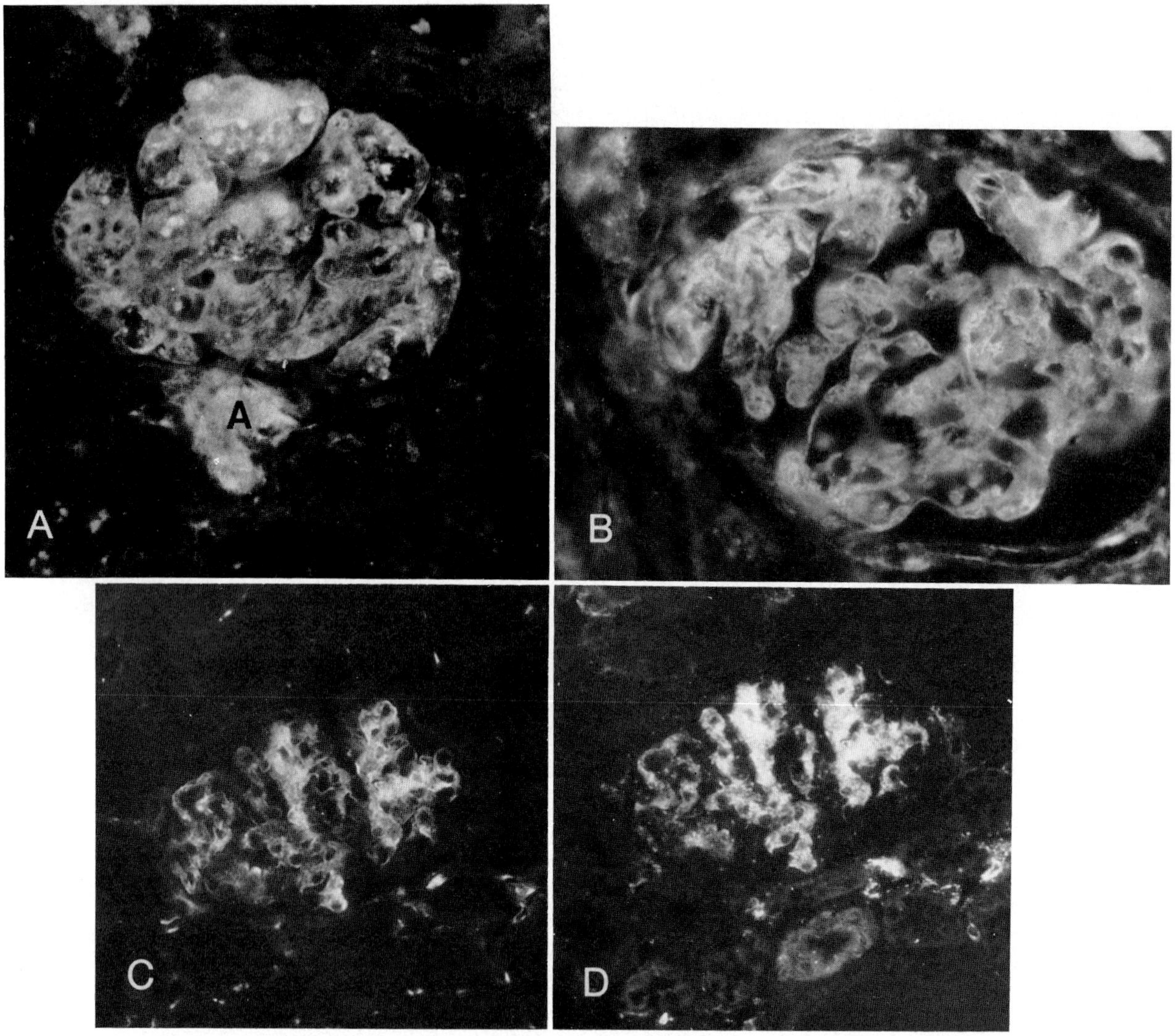

Figure 15.2. A–D. Hemolytic-uremic syndrome. **A.** Immunofluorescent photomicrographs of glomerulus showing fibrin deposited in vessels and along GBM. **B.** Same glomerulus as in A showing reaction with antihemophylic factor (Factor VIII) in same loci. **C.** Anti-fibrin related antigen within glomerular capillaries and the endothelium and mesangium. **D.** Platelet antigen is present within three capillaries of the same glomerulus (X900). (A and B from Miller K and Michael AF. Coagulation and the kidney. In McIntosh RM, Guggenheim SJ, Schrier RW (eds), Kidney Disease: Hematologic and Vascular Problems. New York, John Wiley and Sons, Inc., 1977. **C** and **D** from Miller K, Dresner IG, Michael AF. Localization of platelet antigens in human kidney disease. Kidney Int 18:472, 1980. All with permission.)

Table 15.1.
Mechanisms of FRA Appearance in the Urine

Filtration of FRA from blood secondary to:
Increased serum FRA level
Increased glomerular permeability
Impaired tubular function
Lower urinary tract fibrinolysis of previously filtered fibrinogen or FRA
Intraglomerular lysis of fibrin deposited in the kidney or lysis of circulating fibrinogen
Through the action of non-thrombin induced mechanisms (Proteases)

Modified from Miller K, Michael AF: Coagulation and the Kidney. In McIntosh RM, et al (eds): Kidney Disease: *Hematologic and Vascular Problems*. New York, John Wiley and Sons, 1977.

of renal damage. Another group found similar sites of deposition for FRA and FDP-E in the glomeruli of patients with SLE, membranous nephropathy, and active nephritis (86). There was no association between FRA and FDP-E deposits in patients with less active disease. The relationship of FDP-E to other coagulation factors was not defined. Further investigative work is necessary to better correlate the immunopathological findings with alterations in serum or urine FRA levels, other coagulation parameters, and disease activity. Until these issues are resolved, one should use agents such as Arvin, heparin, urokinase, or streptokinase rather judiciously.

FACTOR VIII AND THE KIDNEY

Factor VIII coagulant activity (fVIIIc) levels appeared to segregate patients with acute glomerulonephritis and initially normal renal function into two distinct groups. Those patients who had elevated fVIIIc activity progressed to renal failure several years later, whereas those patients with normal fVIIIc activity had no sequelae. Vascular endothelial injury is proposed as the cause of these findings because the endothelial cell was the major site of factor VIII synthesis (112). Conversely, fVIIIc levels are also increased in children with minimal change nephrotic syndrome, a condition associated with neither cellular proliferation nor progression to renal failure. Furthermore, the observation that patients with von Willebrand's disease (absent fVIIIc) and glomerulonephritis can progress to renal failure would also appear to dampen the results of the previously aforementioned study (3, 87). Finally, there are nonrenal related disorders in which tissue breakdown and repair occur where plasma factor VIII levels are elevated. Factor VIII levels are also elevated in renal failure, as are factors I, V, and the antiplasmins (3).

Immunofluorescent studies involving factor VIII antigen have revealed factor VIII, FRA, or platelet antigen deposition in the same loci in HUS, scleroderma, acute homograft rejection, postpartum renal failure, malignant hypertension, and MPGN (endothelial lining, capillary loops, or arterioles) (64, 65). IgM is often found in the same sites, suggesting an immune basis for endothelial injury with subsequent activation of the coagulation system. The discordant deposition of FRA, factor VIII, or platelet antigen in rapidly progressive nephritis or Henoch-Schönlein purpura would suggest that nonhemostatic pathways exist for FRA deposition. Clearly, further work is necessary to precisely define the role of factor VIII (coagulant or antigen) in the production of glomerular or vascular injury.

THE PLATELET AND KIDNEY DISEASE

During the past decade, evidence has accumulated that is supportive of a prominent role for the platelet or its constitutents as mediators of glomerular injury in human renal disease. The modalities used to investigate the platelet's role as a mediator of glomerular injury are outlined in Table 15.2. It is now well established that immune complexes (circulating or formed locally) play a major role in the pathogenesis of glomerular injury. How platelets or their constituents participate in these immune processes is not clearly delineated. At present, the best available data comes from platelet turnover and sequestration studies, from measurement of plasma or intraplatelet constituents, or from the detection of platelets or platelet components in renal biopsy material by immunofluorescence or electron microscopy.

Kinetic studies of platelet survival by several investigators have documented shortened survival in a variety of glomerular disorders (88–90). In one study, platelet survival was decreased in HUS, MPGN, renal allograft rejection, glomerulosclerosis, diffuse proliferation nephritis, and occasionally in diabetic nephropathy, while concommitantly obtained, fibrinogen and plasminogen survivals were usually normal (Table 15.3) (88). These workers also noted that bilateral nephrectomy normalized platelet survival in patients with glomerulosclerosis or proliferative nephritis. A correlation between the degree of platelet consumption and the severity of the vascular endothelial lesion was also observed. However, these investigators saw no improvement in renal function when patients with MPGN were given antiplatelet agents (ASA or dipyridamole) and anticoagulants (heparin) despite some improvement in platelet survival. Shortened platelet survival was also observed in acute mesangioproliferative nephritis. Intraglomerular platelet aggregation and clotting were presumed to be responsible for the observed proliferative changes (89). In SLE, immune complexes were felt to activate platelets causing intracellular proliferation with subsequent glomerulosclerosis (90). Platelets can produce a smooth muscle proliferating factor perhaps as a result of platelet endothelial interaction (1, 2). Smooth muscle cells, in turn, are capable of inhibiting fibrinolysis, thereby contributing to the severity of the histological changes seen in human glomerular diseases (1). Increased renal uptake of labeled platelets in chronic glomerulonephritis or in HUS, however, could not be demonstrated by other investigators (91, 92). Perhaps the sensitivity of the techniques used were not adequate to detect a process that could be slow in evolving or intermittent in nature.

Table 15.2.
Platelet Abnormalities in Human Glomerulonephritis

Morphological studies demonstrating platelets or platelet constituents in glomeruli
Circulating platelet abnormality
Thrombocytopenia
Functional abnormalities, e.g., altered aggregation
Altered levels of platelet constituents
Decreased survival
Kidney sequestration

Modified from Miller K, Michael AF: Coagulation and the Kidney. In McIntosh RM, et al (eds): Kidney Disease: *Hematologic and Vascular Problems*. New York, John Wiley and Sons, 1977.

Table 15.3.
Platelet and Fibrinogen Survival in Renal Disease

Renal disease	Number studied	Number with decreased platelet survival	Fibrinogen half-life
Anephric	6	1	Normal
HUS	7	7	Decreased
Crescentic GN	8	2	Normal
MPGN	11	11	Normal
Diabetes	7	3	Normal
Glomerulosclerosis	5	5	Normal
Tubulointerstitial	12	2	Normal
Transplant			
< 6 months	8	8	Decreased
> 6 months	5	1	Normal

Modified from Miller K, Michael AF: Coagulation and the Kidney. In McIntosh RM, et al (eds): Kidney Disease: Hematologic and Vascular Problems. New York, John Wiley and Sons, 1977 and George CRP, et al: *N Engl J Med* 291(21): 1111, 1974.

Evidence suggestive of the platelet's role in glomerulonephritis has also come from platelet aggregation studies. ADP and collagen enhanced aggregation were observed in patients with Alport's syndrome (four of six patients), minimal change nephrotic syndrome (six of eight patients), patients with secondary nephrotic syndrome of varied causes (eleven of fourteen), and patients with acute glomerulonephritis (eleven of twenty-one). Five patients (two with SLE and three with poststreptococcal nephritis) had normal aggregation studies suggesting that the enhanced aggregation observed in Alport's syndrome, nephrotic syndrome, and acute glomerulonephritis occurred via a nonimmune mediated mechanism (93). Enhanced aggregation was reported in diabetic nephropathy as well (94). One investigator observed abnormal aggregation studies only in patients with nephrotic syndrome (3). The platelet "hyperaggregability" commonly observed in patients with primary or secondary nephrotic syndrome may be a reflection of reduced albumin levels, decreased serum calcium levels, elevated cholesterol, or hyperbetalipoproteinemia (95–98).

Other investigators employing a platelet aggregation test (PAT) observed considerable quantities of platelet aggregating material only in patients with glomerular diseases carrying a poor prognosis (membranous glomerulonephritis, FSGN, MPGN, PAN, and SLE) (99). In patients with a relatively good prognosis (minimal change nephrotic syndrome, focal or mesangial proliferative nephritis, or HSP), PAT levels were not different from controls. A good correlation between PAT and platelet serotonin levels existed for patients with SLE and other primary glomerulonephritides. Decreased intraplatelet serotonin and elevated plasma serotonin levels were observed only in disorders in which progression to renal failure occurred (SLE, MPGN, PAN, MN, or focal segmental sclerosis) (100, 101). Measurement of plasma levels of other platelet constituent proteins such as platelet factor 4 (PF4) or BTG may be of limited value because, when GFR is decreased the plasma level of these proteins is consistently elevated. Therapeutic doses of aspirin, however, had no effect on the clinical course of those disorders with abnormal platelet aggregation despite improvement in platelet function (102). In patients with thrombovascular disease, platelet survival was unaffected by ASA therapy.

Morphological demonstration of platelet fragments or constituents have also shed some light on the possible role of the platelet in glomerular injury. The presence of platelet aggregates by electron microscopy in nephrotic syndrome observed by one investigator has not been confirmed in subsequent studies (103). More recent work has identified by immunohistochemical techniques, localization of platelet antigen along the endothelium, or as vascular plugs in HUS, MPGN, diabetic nephropathy, and other nephridites (65). Deposition of FRA usually occurred in the same loci as the platelet antigen(s) except in anaphylactoid purpura, crescentic glomerulonephritis (Goodpasture's syndrome), and MPGN (Fig. 15.1 and 15.2). Subsequent studies have demonstrated PF4 antigen and platelet-related membrane antigen(s) only in glomerular diseases with a poor outcome (101).

However, the demonstration of the platelet's presence does not represent concrete proof that platelet-mediated injury is occuring. Only in MPGN have studies been performed to evaluate the role of antiplatelet drugs alone or in conjunction with anticoagulants. In the one study employing antiplatelet agents alone (dipyridamole, 225 mg, and aspirin, 975 mg/d) progression to end-stage renal disease was slowed, and renal function was better maintained (104). In another study performed over a 2-year period, during which patients were initially randomized (year 1) into a nontreatment group or a treatment group (warfarin and dipyridamole), renal function was better preserved during the treatment year. Bleeding, however, was a frequent complication (105). The role of antiplatelet agents in the microangiopathic disorders is presented in Chapter 27.

NEPHROTIC SYNDROME

Both arterial and venous thromboembolic events are recognized complications of the nephrotic syndrome (106–108). Common sites include pulmonary veins, deep leg veins, and renal veins (chapter 26e). A slight male predeliction apparently exists. Thromboembolic events appear to occur with increased frequency in focal sclerosis, membranous, and membranoproliferative GN. A variety of coagulation disorders have been suggested to explain this increased propensity for thromboembotic complications (Table 15.4) (109, 110).

Remission of the disease clearly reduces the risk of thrombosis, since clotting factor synthesis returns to normal and the urinary loss of clotting factors ceases. The "hyperaggregability" of the platelets resolves with normalization of the serum albumin, calcium, and cholesterol (95–98). However, for those patients with thrombi, therapy with anticoagulants, fibrinolytic agents, or Ancrod, have met with varying success (13, 106, 107, 111, 112). The duration of therapy for oral anticoagulants in renal vein thrombosis is currently not resolved. Antiplatelet drugs have been of equivocal benefit. The role of anticoagulants as adjuctive therapy for renal venous thrombosis aside from conservative measures (hydration, treatment of shock, or inciting disorders) is still controversial (113).

The role of anticoagulants, fibrinolytic inhibitors or antiplatelet therapy in other renal diseases such as rapidly progressive nephritis is also controversial (1, 3, 114–116). Studies to date have been poorly controlled and have included a multiplicity of renal diseases associated with rapidly progressive glomerulonephritis (117–119). Bleeding complications have been significant and extensive glomerular scarring and fibrosis have often occurred despite therapy (116–118). Since immunosuppressive agents have often been given in conjunction with anticoagulants or antiplatelet drugs, the independent value of anticoagulants was not assessed. In postinfectious crescentic glomerulonephritis in children such "cocktail therapy" afforded no real benefit (118). Although alterations in hemostatic mechanisms are found in a variety of renal diseases, the role of anticoagulants, fibrinolytic inhibitors and antiplatelet drugs or Arvin, alone, or in combination (with their inherent risks) remains unresolved.

Table 15.4.
Coagulation Abnormalities in Nephrotic Syndrome

A—Factors Implicated in Thrombotic Diathesis
Increased Factor VIII (activity and antigen)
Increased Factor V
Increased Fibrinogen (activity and antigen)
Increased Factor XIII Subunit A
Increased II, VII, IX, I
Antiplasmins
A) Alpha 2 macroglobulin
B) Alpha 1 antitrypsin
Thrombocytosis
Deficiency of Plasminogen
Deficiency of Antithrombin III
Increased Platelet Prostaglandin Endoperoxide Formation
"Platelet Hyperactivity"
*B—Factor Deficiencies Seen in Nephrotic Syndrome**
Factor VII
Factor IX
Factor X
Factor XI
Factor XII

* Not associated with Bleeding Diathesis.

Acknowledgments

Media Services Department, Lutheran General Hospital, Larry Windland, Resource Support, Health Science Associate/Cardiovascular Dis., Merck Sharp & Dohme, Teresa Trejo, secretarial support.

References

1. Miller K, Michael AF: Coagulation and the kidney. In McIntosh RM, Guggenheim SJ, Schrier RW (eds): Kidney Disease: Hematologic and Vascular Problems. New York, John Wiley and Sons, Inc., 1977.
2. Camerson JS: Glomerulonephritis: current problems and understanding. J Lab Clin Med 99(6):755, 1982.
3. Andrassy K, Ritz E, Mauerhoff T, et al: What is the evidence for activated coagulation in glomerulonephritis? Am J Nephrol 2:293, 1982.
4. Vassalli P, McCluskey RT: The pathogenetic role of the coagulation process in glomerular diseases of immunologic origin. In Hamburger J, Crosnier J, Maxwell MH (eds): Advances in Nephrology. Chicago, Year Book Medical Publishers, Inc., 1971, vol 1, p 47.
5. Watanabe T, Tanaka K: The role of coagulation and fibrinolysis in the development of rabbit masugi nephritis. Acta Path Jap 26(2):147, 1976.
6. Naish P, Penn GB, Evans DJ, et al: The effect of defibrination of nephrotoxic serum nephritis in rabbits. Clin Sci 42:643, 1972.
7. Thomson NM, Simpson IJ, Peters DK: A quantitative evaluation of anticoagulants in experimental nephrotoxic nephritis. Clin Exp Immunol 19:301, 1975.
8. Thomson NM, Moran J, Simpson IJ, et al: Defibrination with ancrod in nephrotoxic nephritis in rabbits. Kidney Intl 10:343, 1976.
9. Atkins RC, Holdsworth SR, Glascow EF, et al: The macrophage in human rapidly progressive nephritis. Lancet 1:830, 1976.

10. Briggs JD, Kwaan HC, Potter EV: The role of fibrinogen in renal disease. III. Fibrinolytic and anticoagulant treatment of nephrotoxic serum nephritis in mice. J Lab Clin Med 74:715, 1969.
11. Bone JM, Valdes AJ, Germuth GF Jr, et al: Heparin therapy in anti-basement membrane nephritis. Kidney Intl 8:72, 1975.
12. Border WA, Wilson CB, Dixon FJ: Failure of heparin to affect two types of experimental glomerulonephritis in rabbits. Kidney Intl 8:140, 1975.
13. Dosekun AK, Pollak VE, Glas-Greenwalt P, et al: Ancrod in systemic lupus erythematosus with thrombosis: clinical and fibrinolysis effects. Arch Int Med 144:37, 1984.
14. Pollak VE, Glueck HI, Weiss MA, et al: Defibrination with ancrod in glomerulonephritis: effects on clinical and histologic findings and on blood coagulation. Am J Nephrol 2:195, 1982.
15. Dosekun AK, First MR, Chandran KG, et al: Successful treatment by defibrination with ancrod in a patient with hyperacute renal allograft failure and a deficiency of plasma prostacyclin stimulating factor. Clin Nephrol 18:101, 1982.
16. Lavelle KJ, Ransdell BA, Kleit SA: The influence of selective thrombocytopenia on nephrotoxic nephritis. J Lab Clin Med 87:967, 1976.
17. Ogawa S, Naruse T: Effects of various antiplatelet drugs and a defibrinating agent on experimental glomerulonephritis in rats. J Lab Clin Med 99:428, 1982.
18. Sindrey M, Marshall TL, Naish P: Quantitative assessment of the effects of platelet depletion in the autologous phase of nephrotoxic serum nephritis. Clin Exp Immunol 36:90, 1979.
19. Lianos EA, Andres GA, Dunn MJ: Glomerular prostaglandin and thromboxane synthesis in rat nephrotoxic serum nephritis. J Clin Invest 72:1439, 1983.
20. Lee L: Antigen-antibody reaction in the pathogenesis of bilateral renal cortical necrosis. J Exp Med 117:365, 1963.
21. Pinckard RN, Tanigawa C, Halonen M: IgE-induced blood coagulation alterations in the rabbits: consumption of coagulation factor XII, XI and IX in vivo. J Immunol 115:525, 1975.
22. Humair L, Potter EV, Kwaan HC: The role of fibrinogen in renal disease. I. Production of experimental lesions in mice. The role of fibrinogen in renal diseases. II. Effect of anticoagulants and urokinase on experimental lesions in mice. J Lab Clin Invest 74:60, 1969.
23. Salmon J, Lambert PH, Louis J: Pathogenesis of the intravascular coagulation syndrome induced by immunological reactions. Thromb Diath Haemorrh 45:161, 1971.
24. Baliah T, Drummond KN: The effect of anticoagulation on serum sickness nephritis in rabbits. Proc Soc Exp Biol Med 140:329, 1972.
25. Thomson NM, Simpson IJ, Evans DJ, et al: Defibrination with ancrod in experimental chronic immune complex nephritis. Clin Exp Immunol 20:527, 1975.
26. Kniker WT, Cochrane CG: The localization of circulating immune complexes in experimental serum sickness. J Exp Med 127:119, 1967.
27. Kniker WT: Modulation of the inflammatory response in vivo: prevention or amelioration of immune complex disease. In Lepow I, Ward PA (eds): Inflammation: Mechanisms and Control. New York, Academic Press, 1972, p 335.
28. Wardle EN: A study of intravascular coagulation in immune complex glomerulonephritis by use of ^{131}I-labelled fibrinogen and ^{125}I-labelled antigen. Clin Sci Mol Med 43:35, 1973.
29. Bolton WK, Spargo BS, Lewis EJ: Chronic autologous immune complex glomerulopathy: effect of cyproheptadine. J Lab Clin Med 83:695, 1974.
30. Kupor LR, Lowance DC, McPhaul JJ: Single and multiple drug therapy in autologous immune complex nephritis in rats. J Lab Clin Med 87:27, 1976.
31. Cattell V: Focal mesangial proliferative glomerulonephritis in the rat caused by habu snake venom: the role of platelets. Brit J Exp Path 60:201, 1979.
32. Cattell V, Mehotra A: Focal mesangial proliferative glomerulonephritis in the rat caused by habu venom: the effect of antiplatelet agents. Brit J Exp Path 61:310, 1980.
33. Humphrey JH, Jaques R: The histamine and serotonin content of the platelets and polymorphonuclear leukocytes in various species. J Physiology (London) 124:305, 1954.
34. Calkins J, Lane KP, LoSasso B, et al: Comparative study of platelet aggregation in various species. J Med 5:292, 1974.
35. McKay DG: Vessel wall and thrombogenesis—endotoxin. Thromb Diath Haemorrh 29:11, 1973.
36. Good RA, Thomas L: Studies on the generalized Shwartzman reaction. II. The production of bilateral cortical necrosis of the kidneys by a single injection of bacterial toxin in rabbits previously treated with thorotrast or trypan blue. J Exp Med 96:625, 1952.
37. Phillips LL, Margaretten W, McKay DG: Changes in the fibrinolytic enzyme system following intravascular coagulation induced by thrombin and endotoxin. Am J Obst Gynec 100:319, 1968.
38. Shen SM-C, Rapaport SI: Increased fibrinogen consumption following endotoxin injection in cortisone-treated rabbits. Proc Soc Exp Biol Med 145:851, 1974.
39. Latour J-G, Prejean JB, Margaretten W: Corticosteroids and the generalized Shwartzman reaction. Am J Path 65:189, 1971.
40. McKay DG, Merriam JC: Vascular changes induced by bacterial endotoxin during generalized Shwartzman reaction. AMA Arch Path 69:524, 1960.
41. Rodriquez-Erdmann F: Studies on the pathogenesis of the generalized Shwartzman reaction. I. Alterations in the coagulation system during the generalized Shwartzman reaction of the pregnant rabbit. II. Role played by experimentally induced fibrinolysis. III. Trigger mechanisms for the activation of the prothrombin molecule. Thromb Diath Haemorrh 12:453, 1964.
42. Bergstein JM, Hoyer JR, Michael AF: Glomerular fibrinolytic activity following endotoxin-induced glomerular fibrin deposition in the pregnant rat. Am J Path 75:195, 1974.
43. Gaynor E, Bouvier C, Spaet TH: Vascular lesions: possible pathogenetic basis of the generalized Shwartzman reaction. Science 170:986, 1970.
44. Gaynor E: Increased mitotic activity in rabbit endothelium after endotoxin. Lab Invest 24:318, 1971.
45. Stewart GJ, Anderson MJ: An ultrastructural study of endotoxin induced damage in rabbit mesenteric arteries. Brit J Exp Path 52:75, 1971.
46. Bergstein JM, Michael AF: Renal cortical fibrinolytic activity in the rabbit following one or two doses of endotoxin. Thromb Diath Haemorrh 28:27, 1973.
47. Sundsmo JS, Fair DS: Relationships among the complement, kinin, coagulation, and fibrinolytic systems. Springer Semin Immunopath 6:231, 1983.
48. Raij L, Michael AF: Unilateral schwartzman reaction: induction of cortical necrosis in one kidney following in vivo perfusion with endotoxin. Kidney Intl 12:1291, 1977.
49. Gurewich V, Lipinski B, Wetmore R: Inhibition of intravascular fibrin deposition by dipyridamole in experimental animals. Blood 45:569, 1975.
50. Margaretten W, McKay DG: The role of the platelet and leukocyte in disseminated intravascular coagulation caused by bacterial endotoxin. Thromb Diath Haemorrh 36S:151, 1969.
51. Bergstein JM: Platelet inhibition of renal cortical fibrinolytic activity in the rabbit. Lab Invest 35:171, 1976.
52. Lipinski B, Gurewich V: The effect of leukopenia versus thrombocytopenia on endotoxin induced intravascular coagulation. Throm Res 8:403, 1976.
53. Coeugniet E, Soeberg B, Dirksen A, et al: Intervention of dipyridamole and acetylsalicylic acid in the development of thrombosis in cell-mediated immune reactions: possible mechanism of action. Thromb Diath Haemorrh 34:861, 1975.
54. Kociba GJ, Griesmer RA: Disseminated intravascular coagulation induced with leukocyte procoagulant. Am J Path 69:407, 1972.
55. Horn RG: Session III. Biological responses. Evidence for participation of granulocytes in the pathogenesis of the generalized shwartzman reaction: A review. J Infect Dis 128:S134, 1973.
56. Margaretten W, Zunker HO, McKay DG: Production of the generalized Shwartzman reaction in pregnant rats by intravenous infusion of thrombin. Lab Invest 3:552, 1964.
57. Bergstein JM, Michael AF: Effect of polymyxin B and endotoxin on renal cortical fibrinolytic activity in the rabbit. Am J Path 71:113, 1973.
58. Urizar RE, Sherer G, Tartaglia A, et al: Disseminated intravascular coagulation induced by liquoid in the rat. Lab Invest 32:270, 1975.
59. Urizar RE, Sherer G, Tartaglia A, et al: Disseminated intravascular coagulation induced by liquoid in the rat. II. Effect of heparin on hematologic and complement abnormalities and renal lesions studies by light, fluorescence, and electron microscopy. Lab Invest 34:510, 1976.
60. Skjorten F, Evensen SA: Disseminated intravascular coagulation induced by normal, thrombocytopenic and granulocytopenic rabbits. Light and electron microscopy studies. Thromb Diath Haemorrh 27:377, 1972.
61. Losonczy G, Harsing L: Simultaneous activation of coagulation and fibrinolysis after severe renal ischemia in rats. Nephron 32:180, 1982.
62. Losonczy G: Intrarenal blood coagulation induced by ischemia in rats. Heparin and thrombocytopenia does not prevent the intracortical fibrin formation. Thromb Res 34:87, 1984.
64. Hoyer JR, Michael AF, Hoyer LW: Immunofluorescent localization of antihemophilic factor antigen and fibrinogen in human renal diseases. J Clin Invest 53:1375, 1974.
65. Miller K, Dresner IG, Michael AF: Localization of platelet antigens in human kidney disease. Kidney Intl 18:472, 1980.
66. Wardle EN: Fibrin in renal disease: functional considerations. Clin Neph 2:85, 1974.
67. Bernik MB, Kwaan HC: Origin of fibrinolytic activity in cultures of the human kidney. J Lab Clin Med 70:650, 1967.
68. Bergstein JM, Michael AF: Cortical fibrinolytic activity in normal and diseased human kidneys. J Lab Clin Med 79:701, 1972.
69. Bergstein JM, Michael AF: Glomerular plasminogen activator activity in renal homograft rejection. Trans 17:443, 1974.

70. Bergstein JM, Kuederli U, Bang NU: Plasma inhibitor of glomerular fibrinolysis in the hemolytic-uremic syndrome. Am J Med 73:322, 1982.
71. Kwaan HC, Green D: The inhibitors of fibrinolysis in sickle cell disease. Thromb Diath Haemorrh 53S:236, 1973.
72. Alkjaersig NK, Fletcher AP, Lewis ML, et al: Pathophysiological response of the blood coagulation system in acute glomerulonephritis. Kidney Intl 10:319, 1976.
73. Carmassi F, Mariani G, Palla R, et al: Coagulation factor XIII in patients with acute and chronic renal disease. Nephron 25:179, 1980.
74. Yoshioka K, Miyata H, Maki S: Significance of decreased factor XIII in Henoch-Schonlein purpura. Acta Ped J 22(1):51, 1980.
75. Dalens B, Travade P, Labbe A, et al: Diagnostic and prognostic value of fibrin stabilizing factor in Schonlein-Henoch syndrome. Arch Dis Childh 58:12, 1983.
76. Plow EF, Edington TS: An alternative pathway for fibrinolysis. I. The cleavage of fibrinogen by leukocyte proteases at physiology pH. J Clin Invest 56:30, 1975.
77. Lane DA, Ireland H, Knight I, et al: The significance of fibrinogen derivatives in plasma in human renal failure. Brit J Haemat 56:251, 1984.
78. Stiehm ER, Trygstad CW: Split products of fibrin in human renal disease. Am J Med 46:774, 1969.
79. Ekert H, Barratt TM, Chantler C, et al: Immunologically reactive equivalents of fibrinogen in sera and urine of children with renal disease. Arch Dis Childh 47:90, 1982.
80. Iio A, Rutherford WE, Wochner RD, et al: The roles of renal catabolism and uremia in modifying the clearance of fibrinogen and its degradative fragments D and E. J Lab Clin Med 87:934, 1976.
81. Naish P, Evans DJ, Peters DK: Urinary fibrinogen derivative excretion and intra-glomerular fibrin deposition in glomerulonephritis. Brit Med J 1:544, 1974.
82. Loschiavo C, Previato G, Valvo E, et al: Clinical significance of urinary fibrinogen degradation products. Nephron 28:200, 1981.
83. Uttley WS, Maxwell H, Cash JD: Fibrin/fibrinogen degradation products in children with renal disease. Arch Dis Childh 49:137, 1984.
84. Yoshioka K, Iscki T, Akano N, et al: Urinary fibrinogen and fibrin fragments in children with renal disease. Nephron 32:135, 1982.
85. Kamitsuji H, Kusumoto K, Taira K, et al: Localization of intrarenal cross-linked fibrin in children with various renal diseases. Nephron 35:94, 1983.
86. Nagai T, Kawai C: Fibrinogen and FDP-E antigen deposits in nephritic kidneys. Nephron 21:16, 1978.
87. Ambruso C, Drante D, McIntosh R, et al: F VIII and renal disease. Ann Int Med 87:636, 1977.
88. George CRP, Slichter SJ, Quadracci LJ, et al: A kinetic evaluation of hemostatsis in renal disease. N Engl J Med 291(21):111, 1974.
89. Carruthers, Ralfs I, Gimlette T, Finn R: Platelet survival in acute proliferative glomerulonephritis. Clin Sci Mol Med 47:507, 1974.
90. Clark WF, Lewis ML, Cameron JS, et al: Intrarenal platelet consumption in the diffuse proliferative nephritis of systemic lupus erythematosus. Clin Sci Mol Med 49:237, 1975.
91. Katz J, Krawitz S, Sachs PV, et al: Platelet erythrocyte and fibrinogen kinetics in hemolytic uremic syndrome of infancy. J Pediatr 83:739, 1973.
92. Rigby RJ, Driedger BD, Reid D, et al: Failure to demonstrate renal uptake of labelled platelets in chronic glomerulonephritis. Clin Sci 59:147, 1980.
93. Bang NU, Trygstad CW, Schroeder JE, et al: Enhanced platelet function in glomerular renal disease. J Lab Clin Med 81:651, 1973.
94. Kwaan HC, Colwell JA, Gray S, et al: Increased platelet aggregation in diabetes mellitus. J Lab Clin Med 80:236, 1972.
95. Schieppati A, Dodesini P, Benigni A, et al: The metabolism of arachidonic acid by platelets in nephrotic syndrome. Kidney Intl 25:671, 1984.
96. Stuart MJ, Gerrard JM, White JG: The influence of albumin and calcium on human platelet arachidonic acid metabolism. Blood 55:418, 1980.
97. Stuart MJ, Spitzer RE, Nelson DA, et al: Nephrotic syndrome: increased platelet prostaglandin endoperoxide formation, hyperaggregability, and reduced platelet life span. Reversal following remission. Pediatr Res 14:1078, 1980.
98. Andrassy K, Ritz E, Bommer J: Hypercoagulability in the nephrotic syndrome. Klin Wochen 58:1029, 1980.
99. Kasai N, Parbtani A, Cameron J, et al: Platelet aggregating immune complexes and intraplatelet serotonin in idiopathic glomerulonephritis and systemic lupus. Clin Exp Immunol 43:64, 1981.
100. Parbtani A, Cameron JS: Platelet and plasma serotonin concentrations in glomerulonephritis, I. Thromb Res 15:109, 1979.
101. Parbtani A, Frampton G, Cameron JS: Platelet and plasma serotonin concentrations in glomerulonephritis, II. Clin Neph 14(3):112, 1980.
102. Trygstad CW, Bang NU, Heidenreich RO, et al: A controlled trial of aspirin in childhood glomerular disorders. Thromb Diath Haemorrh 30:12, 1973.
103. Duffy JL, Cinque T, Grishwin E et al: Intraglomerular fibrin platelet aggregation and subendothelial deposits in lipoid nephrosis. J Clin Invest 49:251, 1974.
104. Donadio JV Jr, Anderson CF, Mitchell JC, et al: Membranoproliferative glomerulonephritis: a prospective clinical trial of platelet-inhibitor therapy. N Engl J Med 310:1421, 1984.
105. Zimmerman SW, Mourthy AV, Dreher WH, et al: Prospective trial of warfarin and dipyridamole in patients with membranoproliferative glomerulonephritis. Am J Med 75:920, 1983.
106. Llach F: Nephrotic syndrome, hypercoagulability, and thromboembolic complications other than renal vein thrombosis. In Renal Vein Thrombosis. Mt. Kisco, N. Y., Futura Publishing Co., 1983, p 177.
107. Cameron JS: Coagulation and thromboembolic complications in the nephrotic syndrome. In Grunfeld JP, Maxwell MH (eds): Advances in Nephrology. Chicago, Year Book Medical Publishers, Inc., 1984, vol 13, p 75.
108. Sullivan MJ III, Hough DR, Agodoa LCY: Peripheral arterial thrombosis due to the nephrotic syndrome: the clinical spectrum. South Med J 76(8):1011, 1983.
109. Vaziri ND: Nephrotic syndrome and coagulation and fibrinolytic abnormalities. Am J Neph 3(1):1, 1983.
110. Lau SO, Tkachuck JY, Hasegawa DK, et al: Plasminogen and antithrombin III deficiencies in the childhood nephrotic syndrome associated wtih plasminogenuria and antithrombinuria. J Pediatr 96:309, 1980.
111. Ross DL, Lubowitz H: Anticoagulation in renal vein thrombosis. Arch Int Med 138:1349, 1978.
112. Crowley JP, Matarese RA, Quevedo SF, et al: Fibrinolytic therapy for bilateral renal vein thrombosis. Arch Int Med 144:159, 1984.
113. Reimold EW, Wittel RA: Renal venous thrombosis in children: changes in management. South Med J 76(10):1277, 1983.
114. Bergstein JM: Anticoagulant therapy in human renal disease. Int J Pediatr Neph 2(1):1, 1981.
115. Kincaid-Smith P: Anticoagulants are of value in the treatment of renal disease. Am J Kid Dis 3(4):299, 1984.
116. Border WA: Anticoagulants are of little value in the treatment of renal disease. Am J. Kid Dis 3(4):308, 1984.
117. Fye KH, Hancock D, Moutsopoulos H, et al: Low-dosage heparin in rapidly progressive glomerulonephritis. Arch Int Med 136:995, 1976.
118. Roy S III, Murphy WM, Arant BS Jr: Poststreptococcal crescenteric glomerulonephritis in children: comparison of quintuple therapy versus supportive care. J Pediatr 98(3):403, 1981.
119. Savage JM,, Postlethwaite RJ, Lendon M, et al: Combined immunosuppressive and anticoagulant treatment in children with glomerulonephritis and declining renal function. Int J Pediatr Neph 3(3):167, 1982.

CHAPTER 16 Vasoactive Hormones

16A Renin-angiotensin System

WOLFGANG RAUH

INTRODUCTION

In 1898, Tigerstedt and Bergmann (1) demonstrated that an extract of rabbit kidney raised arterial blood pressure when injected into another rabbit. They called the active principle "renin." There was, however, little interest in the role of renin until 1934, when it was demonstrated that renal artery occlusion could cause chronic hypertension (2). This landmark experiment stimulated a research effort that has now identified the various components of the renin-angiotensin-aldosterone system (RAAS) and partially clarified its role in regulating blood pressure and salt and water balance.

RENIN

Renin is secreted by the renal juxtaglomerular cells located in the wall of the afferent arteriole, which is contiguous with the macula densa portion of the distal tubule of the same nephron (Fig. 16.1). The active form of renin is a glycoprotein enzyme with a molecular weight of 35,000 to 40,000. Its amino acid composition has been determined (3). Renin is an acidic protease that is related to other acidic proteases such as pepsin and cathepsin D. Its half-life in the circulation is 20 to 60 minutes; its volume of distribution is not known. Enzymes similar to kidney renin (iso-renins) are present in extrarenal tissue such as the brain, the submaxillary gland, the uterus, and the arterial wall (4–7).

Several inactive forms of renin with a higher molecular weight of 43,000 to 140,000 have been found in the kidney and in the plasma of various species (8–10). High molecular weight renin has been considered a zymogen of renin (prorenin), but the relationship of the active and the inactive forms or renin remains unsettled. Inactive renin is probably released from the kidney together with active renin, the relative proportions varying with the stimulus for renin release (10). Acidification, prolonged storage at −4 °F, and exposure to proteolytic enzyme result in an increase of active renin in human plasma (8–13). High molecular weight renin may comprise a large portion of total plasma renin in certain conditions, such as pregnancy or long-standing diabetes, but the physiological and pathophysiological significance of the inactive forms of renin remain to be elucidated (10, 14). The activity of renin may be modulated by one or more renin inhibitors (15) and activators (16), but their existence remains in serious question (14–16).

Angiotensinogen

Angiotensinogen, the natural protein substrate of renin, is synthesized by the liver. Human angiotensinogen has been purified (17). Angiotensinogen is a glycoprotein with a molecular weight of around 65,000. Information about the regulation of its synthesis and release is scanty. Adrenocortical steroids, estrogens, and angiotensin-II stimulate angiotensinogen production (18–20). Plasma levels of angiotensinogen may be important because its concentration is one of the determinants of the rate of angiotensin formation.

Angiotensin

After renin is released into the circulation it cleaves angiotensinogen to produce a decapeptide, angiotensin-I. The converting enzyme, a dipeptidylcarboxypeptidase found mainly in the lungs but also in other organs and in the circulating plasma, removes the carboxyl terminal His-Leu from angiotensin-I to produce the octapeptide angiotensin-II, the potent vasoconstrictor and stimulus of aldosterone production. It exerts the primary physiological effects of the RAAS, although both angiotensin-I and smaller fragments of angiotensin-II, in particular the heptapeptide des-ASP-angiotensin (angiotensin-III), also may have direct effects (14, 19, 21). Angiotensin-II is inactivated by a series of peptidase enzymes, angiotensinases, present in most tissues and in high concentrations in red blood cells.

The major components of the renin-angiotensin system (RAS) are depicted in Figure 16.2. Beyond its vasoconstrictive effects on smooth

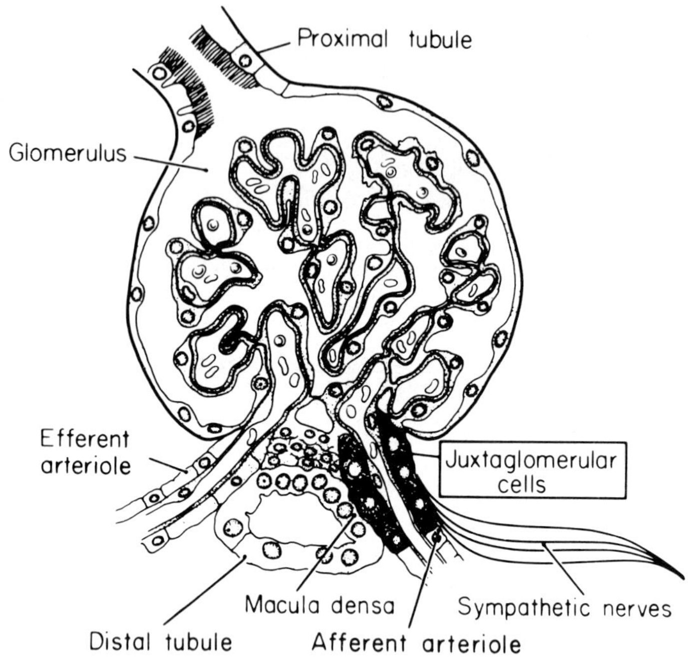

Figure 16.1. The juxtaglomerular apparatus.

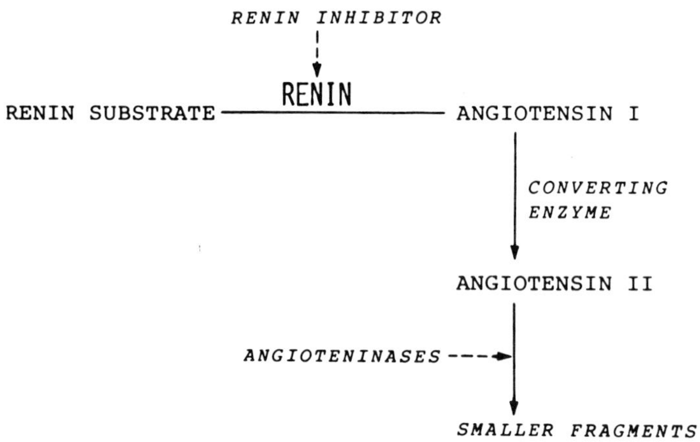

Figure 16.2. Components of the renin-angiotensin system.

muscle and its stimulation of the adrenal cortex, angiotensin-II acts within the central nervous system at the adrenergic nerve endings and the adrenal medulla (14, 22–25). This action amplifies its vasoconstrictive effect on the peripheral vascular system. Within the brain, angiotensin-II stimulates sympathetic vasomotor discharge; at the adrenergic nerve endings it stimulates norepinephrine synthesis and release; in the adrenal medulla, it stimulates release of catecholamines.

Angiotensin-II also acts centrally to induce thirst (25, 26); the increase in water intake augments the action of the hormone on other volume-expanding mechanisms. The presence of renin-like enzymes in arterial wall tissue has led to the attractive hypothesis that locally generated angiotensin-II might be responsible for facilitating adrenergic transmission (24, 27).

In addition, angiotensin-II has been shown to have pharmacological, metabolic, and biochemical effects in the genital tract, the gastrointestinal tract, and in other organs of several species (28).

Control of Renin Secretion

There is abundant evidence that the release of renin from juxtaglomerular cells can be affected by a number of factors that include the baroreceptor mechanism, macula densa mechanism, sympathetic nervous system, plasma potassium concentration, and vasoactive hormones (angiotensin-II, vasopressin, and prostaglandins).

A reduction of arterial pressure at the site of the juxtaglomerular apparatus increases renin release, but it is not clear how this signal is perceived, e.g., by sensing a reduction of stretch or of the transmural pressure gradient (28). This baroreceptor mechanism accounts for the release of renin whenever renal arterial pressure is lowered, either as part of generalized systemic hypotension or localized renal hypotension, e.g., partial clamping of the renal artery (the Goldblatt model). Angiotensin-II that is generated from the baroreceptor-mediated release of renin causes vasoconstriction and acts on the adrenal gland to stimulate the biosynthesis of aldosterone (29). Aldosterone increases renal tubular sodium reabsorption, thereby increasing plasma volume and dampening the release of renin (Fig. 16.3) (29a).

Another site involved in the regulation of renin secretion is the macula densa, which responds to changes in sodium chloride delivery to the distal tubule. Exact definition of the signals perceived, e.g., the tubular sodium load, the sodium chloride flux, and the concentration gradient across the epithelial layer or others, is still a matter of debate (30–32).

Vander (33) presented evidence that a decrease in the load of sodium delivered to the macula densa portion of the distal tubule stimulates renin release. This could explain the effects of plasma volume depletion, wherein increased proximal tubular reabsorption would allow a smaller volume of fluid with a lower sodium concentration to reach the distal tubule. A large number of animal experiments and clinical data support this hypothesis.

On the other hand, Thurau and coworkers (30, 31) showed that increasing sodium chloride concentration within the distal tubule, such as by the action of a diuretic, increases renin release. Micropuncture experiments indicate that a mechanism exists to control nephron glomerular filtration rate in accordance with the concentration of sodium chloride in the macula densa segment of the tubules (31, 32). It has been suggested that in this tubuloglomerular feedback mechanism the RAS in the juxtaglomerular apparatus acts as a local humoral mediator between the signal perceived at the macula densa and the hemodynamic response at the glomerulus (31). Plasma renin activity in the circulating plasma may not always reflect the activity of the intrarenal RAS. This could explain some of the discrepant views regarding the macula densa control of the RAS.

There is now agreement that the sympathetic nervous system plays a key role in the control of renin secretion, mainly by promoting renin release through beta-adrenergic receptor stimulation (22, 28, 33). The effects of this stimulation probably are mediated by 3′5′-cyclic adenosine monophosphate (cAMP) (34). Increased sympathetic activity may be responsible for the rise in plasma renin with exercise and with stress; this may play a role in the hemodynamic response to upright posture and hemorrhage (14, 35).

Increased plasma potassium inhibits renin secretion; however, in man, the effect of potassium seems to be of little consequence (14, 28).

While angiotensin-II and vasopressin inhibit renin secretion (14, 29), prostaglandins may be important mediators of renin release (chapter 16B). A variety of other hormones, such as ACTH, somatostatin, and glucagon may affect renin, but it is questionable if they have a physiological role in the regulation of the RAS. It has been suggested that alterations in net calcium flux in the juxtaglomerular cells represent a final pathway for all stimuli of renin release (14). Increased intracellular calcium inhibits and decreased intracellular calcium increases renin release. These findings, however, remain controversial (22).

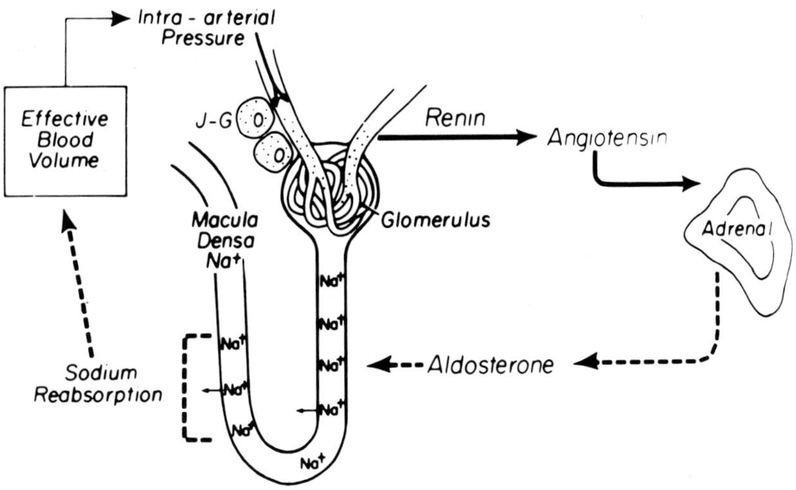

Figure 16.3. Control of renin release by the baroreceptor mechanism. (From Kaplan NM: Curable hypertension. In Stollerman G (ed): Advances in Internal Medicine. Chicago, Year Book Medical Publishers, vol 15, 1969.)

Renin and Renal Function

The RAS is usually regarded as exerting its major effects via circulating hormones (36). It has been suggested (37) that renin also might play a part in the intrarenal regulation of kidney function. All the components of the RAS are present in the kidney (38). The mechanisms of the supposed renal action of locally produced angiotensin remain unclear.

There is evidence for a local sodium-retaining effect of angiotensin-II in the kidney (38). Angiotensin-II may exert "tubular" effects by various mechanisms. One possibility is that by its vasoconstrictor effect angiotensin alters hydrostatic pressure in the peritubular circulation. Hydrostatic and oncotic forces are important determinants of the rate at which sodium and water are reabsorbed by the renal tubule (39). Another possibility is that angiotensin-II modifies sodium and water excretion by constriction and reduction of flow in the vasa recta circulation of the renal medulla (40).

Angiotensin-II also may directly influence the metabolic processes responsible for the reabsorption of sodium by the renal tubule (38). From its position in the juxtaglomerular cells, renin seems ideally placed to alter filtration and flow by constriction of afferent or efferent glomerular vessels. Goormaghtigh (36) and others have suggested that renin acts in this way. It also has been proposed that the macula densa is involved in a tubuloglomerular control mechanism (30, 32). The intrarenal RAS may play a role in the process whereby blood flow and filtration remain relatively constant when arterial pressure changes (31, 41). However, this concept of renin-angiotensin as a major factor in the renal autoregulation is controverted (38).

It is possible that redistribution of renal blood flow between cortical and juxtamedullary nephrons has profound effects on glomerular filtration and tubular reabsorption inasmuch as juxtamedullary glomeruli appear to retain sodium more than cortical nephrons do (38). The evidence that renin is responsible for diversion of intrarenal blood flow is circumstantial (42). An angiotensin-sensitive vascular bypass between afferent and efferent arteriole in the juxtamedullary glomeruli has not been widely accepted (38).

Activation of the intrarenal RAS has been proposed as being a mechanism for the pathogenesis of acute renal failure (42) (chapter 48), e.g., the RAS appears to play a role in the induction of acute renal failure with uranyl nitrate (43), whereas its role in the induction of acute renal failure by glycerol is disputed (43, 44).

In summary, there is scanty direct evidence and a great deal of indirect evidence that renin and angiotensin are involved in the physiological and pathological control of renal function. The intrarenal RAS is probably integrated in a complex system of vasoactive hormones, including kinins and prostaglandins, which also have been shown to influence kidney function by various mechanisms (45, 46).

DEVELOPMENTAL ASPECTS OF THE RENIN-ANGIOTENSIN-ALDOSTERONE SYSTEM

The human kidney is capable of producing appreciable amounts of renin from the twentieth week of gestation (47). The RAAS is greater in infants and children than it is in adults (48–51). The highest levels of plasma renin activity, angiotensin-II, and aldosterone in the plasma have been found in the neonatal period, especially in premature infants. A variety of explanations have been considered, such as the influence of blood pressure (51, 52), sodium balance (53), proximal and distal tubular function (54), mineralocorticoid unresponsiveness (55), number of angiotensin-II receptors (56), sympathetic nervous system (57), prostaglandins (58), and kinins (59).

From a functional view, the increased levels of plasma renin activity may be a result of the presence of stimuli that enhance the synthesis of this enzyme, or it might be the result of a poorly developed feedback. In the newborn, plasma renin activity changes appropriately in response to various stimuli (54). Renin suppression following sodium load, however, appears incomplete in the neonatal period; suppression becomes more effective during infancy, reflecting immaturity of the feedback system in the newborn (54). The low sodium intake and the deposition of sodium with growth may create a continuous stimulation for renin release. This, in turn, increases the amount of circulating angiotensin that stimulates the production of aldosterone, thereby enhancing tubular reabsorption of sodium.

In premature infants, around 2 to 4 weeks of age, salt wasting has been observed in the presence of a marked elevation of plasma renin activity (PRA) (chapters 6 and 54). During this period, the glomerular filtration rate (GFR) in the superficial nephrons increases disproportionately, creating a tendency toward sodium loss that further stimulates renin release (60). When aldosterone production is insufficient (60) or the distal tubule is unable to respond adequately to mineralocorticoids (55), renal loss of sodium and hyponatremia ensue. Later in the postnatal development, reabsorption or sodium in the proximal and distal tubule

Table 16A.1.
Clinical Conditions Affecting Renin Levels

Decreased PRA	Increased PRA
Expanded fluid volume	Shrunken fluid volume
Salt loads, oral or intravenous	Salt deprivation
Primary salt retention (Liddle's syndrome)	Fluid losses
Mineralocorticoid excess	Diuretic-induced
Primary aldosteronism	Gastrointestinal losses
Congenital adrenal hyperplasia (11-hydroxylase deficiency)	Hemorrhage
Licorice excess	Salt-wasting renal disease
Deoxycorticosterone (DOC), 18-hydroxy-DOC excess	Decreased effective plasma volume
Catecholamine deficiency	Upright posture
Autonomic dysfunction	Adrenal insufficiency
Beta-adrenergic blockers	Congenital adrenal hyperplasia (21-hydroxylase deficiency)
Hyperkalemia	Cirrhosis with ascites
Decrease of renal tissue	Nephrotic syndrome
Hyporeninemic hypoaldosteronism	Decreased renal perfusion pressure
Chronic renal disease	Therapy with peripheral vasodilators
Unknown	Renovascular hypertension
Low renin hypertension	Accelerated malignant hypertension
	Renal disease
	Catecholamine excess
	Pheochromocytoma
	Stress: hypoglycemia, trauma
	Exercise
	Hyperthyroidism
	Hypokalemia
	Increased renin substrate
	Pregnancy
	Estrogen therapy
	Autonomous renin hypersecretion
	Renin-secreting tumors

rises, resulting in a progressive diminution of renin release and, consequently, in a decrease in aldosterone production.

This concept of a causal link between the RAAS and the sodium balance of the growing infant, however, does not exclude other developmental factors, such as changing hormonal or neural control, that contribute to the observed decrease in the activity of the RAAS.

Renin Measurements

For clinical purposes, the state of the RAS is usually evaluated by measuring the PRA. In principle, PRA measurements involve autoincubation of pH-stabilized plasma under defined conditions and radioimmunological estimation of angiotensin-I generated (14). Since, in this method, renin acts on endogenous angiotensinogen, changes in the concentration of the latter contribute to the angiotensin-I formation rate. There are a number of technical problems that still have not been worked out to the satisfaction of the experts, and disagreement persists as to the best procedure (61). The most important clinical conditions affecting PRA levels and the factors involved are listed on Table 16A.1.

Interpretation of PRA levels requires careful consideration of the clinical conditions. Nomograms relating PRA to sodium excretion have been established (62). In children, age-appropriate control values should be used for comparison (48–51).

The measurement of plasma renin concentration (PRC) involves the addition of exogenous angiotensinogen. Techniques to measure concentrations of circulating angiotensin-I and angiotensin-II are available. However, the procedures are technically tedious and tricky and, since the values correlate well with the more easily and widely performed assays of renin activity, neither circulating angiotensin-I nor angiotensin-II is commonly measured in clinical practice.

Pharmacological Blockade of Angiotensin

Pharmacological means of blocking the action or production of angiotensin-II have been developed, which have both diagnostic and therapeutic roles.

Saralasin (Sar^1Ala^8-Angiotensin-II) is a competitive angiotensin-II antagonist, which has been found to be a valuable tool to characterize angiotensin-II receptors in various organs and to detect the presence of renin-dependent hypertension (63). Its usefulness may be limited because of its antagonistic effect under certain conditions. There is only limited experience in the use of saralasin in children (64).

The oral converting enzyme inhibitor captopril, which blocks the conversion of angiotensin-I to angiotensin-II, may be of greater value in the treatment of serious arterial hypertension (65, 66) than as a diagnostic tool for hyper-reninemic hypertension.

References

1. Tigerstedt R, Bergman PG: Niere und Kreislauf. Scand Arch Physiol 8:223, 1898.
2. Goldblatt H, Lynch J, Hanzal RF, et al: Studies in experimental hypertension. I. The production of persistent elevation of systolic blood pressure by means of renal ischemia. J Exp Med 59:347, 1934.
3. Inagami T, Murakami K: Pure renin: isolation from hog kidney and characterization. J Biol. Chem 252:2978, 1977.
4. Ferris TF, Gorden P, Mulrow PJ: Rabbit uterus as a source of renin. Am J Physiol 212:698, 1967.
5. Menzie JW, Michelakis AM, Yoshida H: Sympathetic nervous system and renin release from submaxillary glands and kidneys. Am J Physiol 6:1281, 1974.
6. Ganten D, Schelling P, Vecsei P, et al: Iso-renin of extrarenal origin. The tissue angiotensinogenase systems. Am J Med 60:760, 1976.
7. Hayduk K, Ganten D, Boucher R, et al: Arterial and urinary renin activity. In Genest J, Koiw E (eds): Hypertension 1972. Berlin, Springer-Verlag, 1972, p 435.
8. Day RP, Luetscher JA: Biochemical properties of big renin extracted from human plasma. J Clin Endocrinol Metab 40:1085, 1975.
9. Boyd GW: An inactive higher molecular weight renin in normal subjects and hypertensive patients. Lancet 1:215, 1977.
10. Derkx FHM, v Gool J, Wenting GJ, et al: Inactive renin in human plasma. Lancet 2:496, 1976.
11. Sealey JE, Moon C, Laragh JH, et al: Plasma prorenin: Cryoactivation and relationship to renin substrate in normal subjects. Am J Med 61:731, 1976.
12. Sealey JE, Atlas SA, Laragh JH, et al: Human urinary kallikrein converts inactive to active renin and is a possible physiological activator of renin. Nature 275:144, 1978.
13. Atlas SA, Sealey JE, Laragh JH: Dependency of acid and cryoactivation of inactive plasma renin or prior activation of a neutral serum protease. Kidney Intl 12:495, 1977.
14. Kaplan NM: The renin-angiotensin system. In Kaplan NM (ed): Clinical Hypertension, ed 2. Baltimore, Williams and Wilkins Co., 1978, p 178.
15. Derkx FHM, Tan-Tjiong HL, Schalekamp MADH: Endogenous activator of plasma inactive renin. Lancet 2:218, 1978.
16. Poulsen K: Round table discussion on inactive renins. Fifth Scientific Meeting, International Society Hypertension, Paris, June 12–14, 1978.
17. Tewksbury DA, Frome WL, Dumas, ML: Characterization of human angiotensinogen. J Biol Chem 253:3817, 1978.
18. Page JH, Mc Cubbin JW (eds): Renal Hypertension. Chicago, Year Book Medical Publishers, 1968.
19. Peach M: Renin-angiotensin system: biochemistry and mechanism of action. Physiol Rev 57:313, 1977.
20. Reid IA, Morris BJ, and Ganong WF: The renin-angiotensin system. Ann Rev Physiol 40:377, 1978.
21. Goodfriend TL: Receptors for angiotensins. In Genest J, Koiw E, Kuchel O (eds): Hypertension. New York, McGraw-Hill Book Co. 1977, p 173.
22. Vecsei P, Hackenthal E, Ganten D: The renin-angiotensin-aldosterone system, past, present and future. Klin Wchnschr. 56(suppl):5, 1978.

23. Malik KU, Nasjletti A: Facilitation of adrenergic transmission by locally generated angiotensin II in rat mesenteric arteries. Circ Res 38:26, 1976.
24. Ganten D, Kusumoto M, Constantopoulos G, et al: Iso-renin, electrolytes and catecholamines in dog brain: possible interrelationship. Life Sci 12:1, 1973.
25. Ganten D, Stock G: Humoral and neurohormonal aspects of blood pressure regulation: focus on angiotensin. Klin Wchnschr 56(suppl 1):31, 1978.
26. Fitzsimons JT: The physiological basis of thirst. Kidney Intl 10:3, 1976.
27. Schwartz J, Bloch R, Velly J: Relations between renin, aldosterone and experimental hypertension in rats. Canad M A J 90:243, 1964.
28. Davis JO, Freeman RH: Mechanisms regulating renin release. Physiol Rev 56:1, 1976.
29. Kaplan N, Bartter FC: The effect of ACTH, renin, angiotensin II, and various precursors on biosynthesis of aldosterone by adrenal slices. J Clin Invest 41:715, 1962.
29a. Kaplan NM: Curable hypertension. In Stollerman G (ed): Advances in Internal Medicine. Chicago, Year Book Medical Publishers, 1969, vol 15.
30. Thurau K, Schnermann J: Die Natrium-Konzentration an den Maculadensa-Zellen als regulierender Faktor für das Glomerulumfiltrat. Klin Wchnschr 43:410, 1965.
31. Thurau K, Mason J: The internal function of the juxtaglomerular apparaturs. MTP-Internat. Rev. of Science, Physiology Ser. 1; 6. In Thurau K (ed): Kidney and Urinary Tract Physiol. London, Butterworth, 1974, p 357.
32. Schnermann J, Briggs J: Concentration-dependent sodium chloride transport as the signal in feedback control of glomerular filtration rate. Kidney Intl 22(suppl 12): S82, 1982.
33. Vander AJ: Control of renin release. Physiol Rev 47:359, 1967.
34. Hofbauer KG, Konrads A, Schwarz K, et al: Role of cyclic AMP in the regulation of renin release from the isolated perfused rat kidney. Klin Wchnschr 56(suppl. 1):51, 1978.
35. Zanchetti A: Renin and the sympathetic nervous system. Verh Dtsch Ges Inn Med 80:129, 1974.
36. Goormaghtigh N: Facts in favor of endocrine function of the renal arterioles. J Path Bacteriol 57:392, 1945.
37. Peart WS: Intra-renal factors in renin release. Contr Nephrol 12:5, 1978.
38. Brown JJ, Chinn RH, Gavras H, et al: Renin and renal function. In Genest J, Koiw E (eds): Hypertension-72. New York, Springer-Verlag, 1972, p 81.
39. Falcvok HH, Brenner BM, Tadokoro M, et al: Oncotic and hydrostatic pressure in peritubular capillaries and fluid reabsorption by proximal tubule. Am J Physiol 220:1427, 1971.
40. Lever AF: The vasa recta and countercurrent multiplication. Acta Med Scand 178 (suppl. 434): 1965.
41. Navar LG, Bell PD, Burke TJ: Role of a macula densa feedback mechanism as a mediator of renal autoregulation. Kidney Intl 22(suppl 12):S157, 1982.
42. Brown JJ, Gleadle RI, Lawson VW, et al: Renin and acute renal failure; Studies in man. Brit Med J 1:253, 1970.
43. Mendelson FAO: Angiotensin II: evidence for its role as an intrarenal hormone. Kidney Intl 22(suppl 12):S78, 1982.
44. Flamembaum W: Pathophysiology of acute renal failure. Arch Int Med 131:911, 1973.
45. Itzkovitz HD, Mc Giff JC: Hormonal regulation of the renal circulation. Circ Res (suppl 1)34:1, 1974.
46. Carretero OA, Scicli AG: The renal kallikrein-kinin system in human and in experimental hypertension. Klin Wchnsch 56(suppl I):113, 1978
47. Molteni A, Rahill WJ, Koo JH: Evidence for a vasopressor substance (renin) in human fetal kidneys. Lab Invest 30:115, 1974.
48. Dillon MJ, Ryness JM: Plasma renin activity and aldosterone concentration in children. Brit Med J 4:316, 1975.
49. Sassard J, Sann L, Vincent M, et al: Plasma renin activity in normal subjects from infancy to puberty. J Clin Endocrinol Metab 40:524, 1975.
50. Giovannelli G: Plasma renin activity in normal children. J Pediatr 91:847, 1977.
51. van Acker KJ, Scharpe SL, Deprettere AJR, et al: Renin-angiotensin-aldesterone system in the healthy infant and child. Kidney Intl 16:196, 1979.
52. Broughton Pipkin F, Smales ORC, O'Callaghan MJ: Renin and angiotensin levels in children. Arch Dis Childh 56:298, 1981.
53. Aperia A, Broberger O, Herin P, et al: Sodium excretion in relation to sodium intake and aldosterone excretion in newborn pre-term and full-term infants. Acta Paediatr Scand 68:813, 1977.
54. Spitzer A: The role of the kidney in sodium homeostasis during meturation. Kidney Intl 21:539, 1982.
55. Kowarski A, Katz H, Migeon CJ: Plasma aldosterone concentration in normal subjects from infancy to adulthood. J Clin Endocrinol Metab 38:489, 1974.
56. Pernollet MG, Devynck MA, Macdonald GJ, et al: Plasma renin activity and adrenal angiotensin II receptors in fetal, newborn, adult and pregnant rabbits. Biol Neonate 36:119, 1979.
57. Vincent M, Dessart Y, Annat G, et al: Plasma renin activity, aldosterone and dopamine-β-hydroxylase activity as a function of age in normal children. Pediatr Res 14:894, 1980.
58. Joppich R, Häuser I: Urinary prostacyclin and thromboxane A_2 metabolites in preterm and full-term infants in relation to plasma renin activity and blood pressure. Biol Neonate 42:179, 1982.
59. Mills IH: The renal kallikrein-kinin system and sodium excretion. Quart J Exp Physiol 67:393, 1982.
60. Sulyok E, Nemeth M, Tenyi IF, et al: Relationship between maturity, electrolyte balance and the function of the renin-angiotensin-aldosterone system in newborn infants. Biol Neonate 35:60, 1979.
61. Bangham DR, Robertson I, Robertson JIS, et al: An international collaborative study of renin assay. Establishment of the international reference preparation of human renin. Clin Sci Mol Med 48:135S, 1975.
62. Laragh JH, Sealey JE, Sommers SC: Patterns of adrenal secretion and urinary excretion of aldosterone and plasma renin activity in normal and hypertensive subjects. Circ Res 18(suppl):158, 1966.
63. Streeten DHP, Anderson GH, Freiberg JM, et al: Use of the angiotensin II antagonist (Saralasin) in the recognition of "angiotensinogenic" hypertension. N Engl J Med 292:657, 1975.
64. Favre L, Boerth RC, Braren V, et al: Angiotensin II blockade by saralasin in the evaluation of hypertension in children. Kidney Intl 15(suppl 9):75, 1979.
65. Johnston CI, Millar JA, Mc Grath BP, et al: Longterm effects of Captopril (SQ 14 225) on blood pressure and hormone levels in essential hypertension. Lancet 2:493, 1979.
66. Oberfield SE, Case DB, Levine LS, et al: Use of oral angiotensin I—converting enzyme inhibitor (captopril) in childhood malignant hypertension. J Pediatr 95:641, 1979.

16B Prostaglandins (Arachidonate Cascade)

HANNSJÖRG W. SEYBERTH

INTRODUCTION

Biological activity attributed to the prostaglandins was first discovered by the American physicians Kurzrok and Lieb. In 1930, they published the observation that artificial insemination caused contraction of the uterus. A few years later, the pharmacologists Goldblatt in England and von Euler in Sweden independently discovered that human semen contained a factor that could contract smooth muscle and reduce blood pressure when injected intravenously into animals (1, 2). von Euler characterized the active products of the sheep seminal vesicles and "prostate glands" as fatty acids and provisionally named them prostaglandins (3). Twenty-five years later, Bergström and Sjovall (4) isolated the first of the two classical prostaglandin series, PGE and PGF. Subsequently, their structures were elucidated in a series of investigations by Bergström and colleagues (5). In 1964, von Dorp and coworkers and Bergström and associates independently achieved the biosynthesis of PGE_2 from arachidonate (6, 7).

In 1960, Muirhead and coworkers (8) demonstrated the existence of a substance in the renal medulla with antihypertensive properties and Hickler and associates (9) isolated unsaturated, hydroxylated fatty acids with vasodepressor activity. Subsequently, PGE_2, $PGF_{2\alpha}$, and PGA_2 were identified from rabbit renal medulla by gas chromatography mass spectrometry (10), after which the kidney was recognized as one of the richest sources of prostaglandin synthesis activity. Direct and indirect evidence has established that PGE_2 and PGI_2 play important roles as local mediators and modulators of renal blood flow (RBF) and water and electrolyte balance. Other oxygenated metabolites of arachidonic acid that are collectively termed eicosanoids, such as $PGF_{2\alpha}$, PGD_2, TXB_2, hydroxyeicosatetraenoic acids (HETE) and leukotrienes, can be synthesized by renal tissue; however, their definitive function remains to be elucidated.

THE ARACHIDONATE CASCADE

Biosynthesis

Arachidonate metabolites are not stored in any tissue or fluid of the mammalian organism, except seminal fluid. Their biological effects are achieved by de novo synthesis of highly labile compounds that are quickly metabolized and thereby inactivated. Arachidonate, the predominant substrate of PG synthesis, is an essential fatty acid with 20 carbon atoms and four double bonds (C20:4γ6). Dihomo-γ-linolenate (C20:3ω6), the precursor of the monoenoic prostaglandins, e.g., PGE_1 and $PGF_{1\alpha}$, is present in much smaller amounts. Eicosapentaenoic acid (C20:5ω6), a major substrate of prostaglandin synthesis in marine animals, is the precursor of the triene prostaglandins.

The abundance of arachidonate is esterified to cellular lipids, predominantly in phospholipids or triglycerides. The rate-limiting step in the release of arachidonic acid is the activity of a calcium-dependent phosphatide acyl hydrolase, most likely involving a phospholipase A_2 (11). Cleavage is stimulated by such different agents and conditions as hormones, sympathetic nerve stimulation, mechanical stimulation, ischemia, and hyperosmolality. Antiinflammatory steroids appear to reduce prostaglandin biosynthesis by lowering the availability of arachidonate to the PG-cyclo-oxygenase as a result of the formation of a peptide, such as macrocortin or lipomodulin, which inhibits the release of arachidonate from phospholipids (12, 13). Once released, arachidonic acid is rapidly metabolized to oxygenated products by two distinct enzymatic pathways, cyclo-oxygenase and lipoxygenase.

The Cyclo-oxygenase Pathway

This has been much more extensively studied than the lipoxygenase pathway (Fig. 16.4) (14). The cyclo-oxygenase enzyme complex is located in the microsomal fraction of most mammalian cells with the exception of red cells. The synthetase complex converts arachidonate to the endoperoxide intermediate PGG by hydroperoxidation at C-11, by cycling and subsequent introduction of a hydroperoxy group at C-15 (15). PGG_2 is converted to PGH_2 by a peroxidase reaction. These two endoperoxide intermediates are chemically unstable, with half-lives of 5 minutes at 37 in aqueous solutions and are metabolized enzymatically and nonenzymatically into PGE_2, $PGF_{2\alpha}$, and PGD_2. PGA_2, PGB_2, and PGC_2 are chemically formed from PGE_2 during extraction procedures and do not occur biologically.

Furthermore, the endoperoxide PGH_2 is also metabolized into two unstable and biologically highly active compounds with structures that differ from those of the primary prostaglandins. One of these is thromboxane A_2 (TxA_2) formed by the enzyme thromboxane synthetase, first isolated from platelets (16). TxA_2 has a short half-life of about 30 seconds at 37° C and pH 7.5 and contains an oxane ring instead of the cyclopentane ring of the prostaglandins. Its more stable breakdown product is TxB_2. The other route of metabolism of PGH_2 leads to prostacyclin (PGI_2), which is also very unstable with a half-life of 3 minutes at 37° C and pH 7.5 (17). The PGI_2 synthetase was first discovered in the vessel wall with the highest activity in the endothelium. PGI_2 has a double-ring structure closed by an oxygen bridge between carbon 6 and 9. It breaks

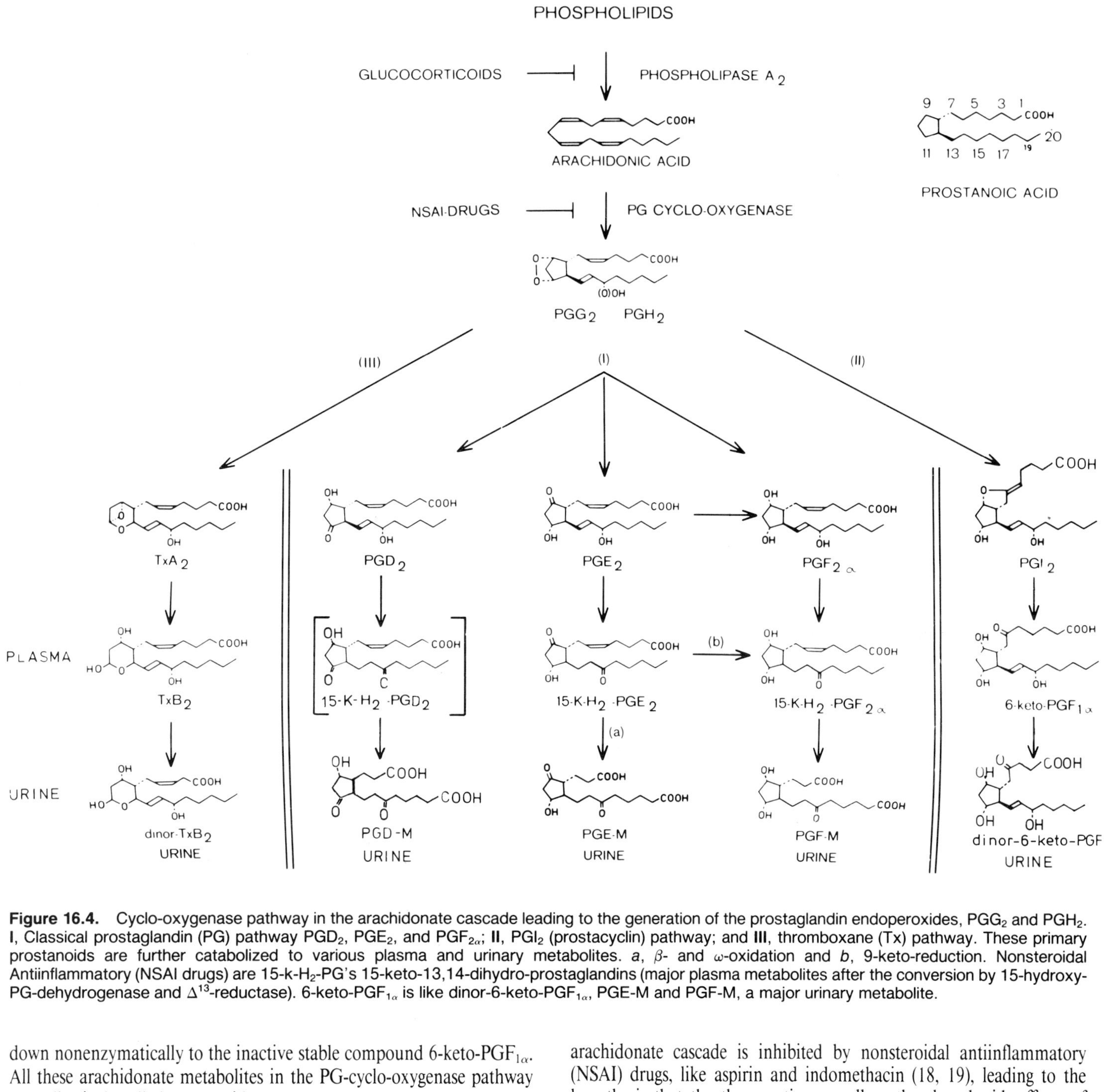

Figure 16.4. Cyclo-oxygenase pathway in the arachidonate cascade leading to the generation of the prostaglandin endoperoxides, PGG_2 and PGH_2. **I**, Classical prostaglandin (PG) pathway PGD_2, PGE_2, and $PGF_{2\alpha}$; **II**, PGI_2 (prostacyclin) pathway; and **III**, thromboxane (Tx) pathway. These primary prostanoids are further catabolized to various plasma and urinary metabolites. *a*, β- and ω-oxidation and *b*, 9-keto-reduction. Nonsteroidal Antiinflammatory (NSAI drugs) are 15-k-H_2-PG's 15-keto-13,14-dihydro-prostaglandins (major plasma metabolites after the conversion by 15-hydroxy-PG-dehydrogenase and Δ^{13}-reductase). 6-keto-$PGF_{1\alpha}$ is like dinor-6-keto-$PGF_{1\alpha}$, PGE-M and PGF-M, a major urinary metabolite.

down nonenzymatically to the inactive stable compound 6-keto-$PGF_{1\alpha}$. All these arachidonate metabolites in the PG-cyclo-oxygenase pathway are collectively called prostanoids.

While each tissue seems to be able to synthesize the PG-endoperoxides PGG_2 and PGH_2, the fate of these precursors in the various tissues depends on several factors. One of these factors is the enzymatic make-up of the tissue. There is significant variation of the different isomerases from tissue to tissue. For example, lung and spleen are able to synthesize the whole range of prostanoids in contrast to platelets and arterial endothelium that produce mainly TxA_2 and PGI_2, respectively. The formation of all these products of the cyclo-oxygenase pathway in the arachidonate cascade is inhibited by nonsteroidal antiinflammatory (NSAI) drugs, like aspirin and indomethacin (18, 19), leading to the hypothesis that the therapeutic, as well as the shared, side-effects of nonsteroidal drugs are related to inhibition of PG biosynthesis.

The Lipoxygenase Pathway

This is generally not affected by NSAI drugs and leads to the formation of eicosanoids, which are noncyclized hydroxyacids. As a result of incomplete cyclo-oxygenase reaction, an 11- and a 15-HETE may be formed. In addition, the synthesis of 12-HETE in platelets and 5-HETE in polymorphonuclear leukocytes by a separate lipoxygenase was described (20, 21). The 5-lipoxygenase in leukocytes gives rise to a family of compounds containing a conjugated triene structure, named leukotrienes (LT) (22).

Leukotriene A_4 (LTA_4) is a 5,6-epoxide of arachidonate, which can be converted to the 5,12-dihydroxy acid (LTB_4) with strong chemotactic properties. On the other hand, the addition of glutathione to LTA_4 by glutathione-S-transferase leads to the formation of LTC_4 (23). The removal of glutamate from LTC_4 by γ-glutamyl transpeptidase yields LTD_4, which is further metabolized to LTE_4 with the loss of glycine. The latest member of this cascade to be discovered is LTF_4, which is formed to a γ-glutamyl-cysteinyl derivative from LTE_4 (24). These lipid-peptide structures account for the biological activity of slow reactivity substances (SRS) released in immediate hypersensitivity reactions and are thought to contribute to the bronchoconstriction seen in anaphylactic respiratory disease. Leukotriene formation also has been identified in macropahges, mastocytoma cells, lung, spleen, skin, arteries, and in the kidney (25). The role of these very potent eicosanoids in renal physiology and pathophysiology remains to be investigated.

Metabolism

An efficient mechanism exists for preventing systemic effects of arachidonate metabolites. Such activities in certain vascular beds, for example, in the lung and in the liver, can clear the systemic circulation from these biologically potent mediators effectively by a single passage through these organs (26). Therefore, the cardiovascular and other systems are protected from prolonged exposure to these compounds, which would otherwise result in such events as shock and intravascular aggregation of platelets and leukocytes.

Prostaglandins

The so-called primary prostaglandins PGF_2, $PGF_{2\alpha}$, and PGD_2 are metabolized by enzymes that are widely distributed in the body and are present in spleen, renal cortex and papillae, intestine, liver, and, most important, in the lung. The initial, relatively rapid oxidation step of the 15-hydroxy group to the corresponding ketone is performed by a 15-hydroxy-PG-dehydrogenase (Fig. 16.4). These 15-keto compounds are then reduced to the 13,14-dihydro derivatives by a Δ^{13}-PG-reductase (27).

At this state of metabolism the prostaglandins already have lost most of their biological activity. The β- and ω-oxidation of the prostaglandin side chains proceeds more slowly, with some accumulation of the 15-keto-13,14-dihydro-compounds in the circulation. The more polar β- and ω-oxidation products are then excreted in the urine as major metabolites.

Besides many others, the major urinary metabolites of the E-prostaglandins is, for example, 7α-dihydroxy-5,11-diketotetranorprostane-1,16-dioic acid (PGE-M), while one of the F-prostaglandins is 5α,7α-dihydroxy-11-ketotetranorprostane-1,16-dioic acid (PGF-M) (Fig. 16.4). Similar metabolic pathways have also been described for TxA_2 and PGI_2, although a significant portion of these prostanoids are decomposed nonenzymatically by a hydrolytic reaction to inactive TxB_2 and 6-keto-$PGF_{1\alpha}$, respectively. The major urinary metabolite of TxA_2 is dinor-TxB_2, indicating β-oxidation before renal excretion, while PGI_2 and 6-keto-$PGF_{1\alpha}$ are, in part, subjected to β-oxidation and 15-keto-dehydrogenation, leading to the urinary excretion of dinor-6-keto-$PGF_{1\alpha}$ and dinor-6,15-diketo-$PGF_{1\alpha}$ besides 6-keto-$PGF_{1\alpha}$ as major urinary metabolites of PGI_2 (28–30).

Renal Prostaglandin Metabolism

The kidney has a high capacity of synthesizing prostaglandins. The formation of each of the different members of the prostanoid family (PGE_2, $PGF_{2\alpha}$, PGD_2, PGI_2, TxA_2) has been demonstrated in the kidney. Anatomically, the cyclo-oxygenase-containing cells in the kidney have been localized by immunofluorescence procedures. Prostaglandin synthesis takes place in the epithelial cells, medullary interstitial cells, parietal layer of Bowman's capsule and mesangial cells of the glomerulus (31–33).

There are marked differences in the total amounts of prostanoids synthesized in different regions of the kidney. The PG-synthesis in the medulla and in the papilla is four times higher than in the cortex. The main site in the papilla is the collecting ducts and interstitial cells. The major prostaglandins there are PGE_2 and $PGF_{2\alpha}$. In the cortex and outer medulla, PG synthesis is primarily located in vascular tissue that produces predominantly PGI_2 (34). Thromboxane synthesis takes place principally in response to pathological states, e.g., ureteral obstruction, glycerol-induced acute renal failure, and partial renal venous occlusion determined from animal studies (35). These observations indicate that mechanisms are available to shift from one synthetase pathway to the other in the PG-endoperoxide metabolism in response to changing conditions.

The kidney also possesses enzymatic activities for all steps in PG catabolism (31, 32). Four types of enzymes have been found in the high speed supernatant of kidney homogenates:

(1) A highly specific 15-hydroxy-PG-dehydrogenase (type I) is most abundant in the proximal and distal tubules of the cortex. This enzyme may play a major role in the intrarenal regulation of prostaglandin activities.

(2) A less specific PG-dehydrogenase (type II) catalyzes the reversible conversion of hydroxy and keto groups at both C-9 and C-15 and previously was called 9-keto-PG-reductase. This enzyme converts PGE_2 to $PGF_{2\alpha}$. The conversion of PGD_2 to urinary $PGF_{2\alpha}$ metabolites is regulated by yet another enzyme. The type II dehydrogenase is present in both cortex and medulla and is NADP-dependent. Its activity has been related to salt balance in the rabbit (36).

(3) A Δ^{13}-PG-reductase is present in close association with the type I dehydrogenase but has not been studied in detail in the kidney.

(4) A converting enzyme, 9-hydroxy-PG-dehydrogenase that changes F- to E-prostaglandins is located in the cortex. The presence of β- and ω-oxidation is universally distributed throughout the body and is found in the kidney in cortical microsomes.

Relatively little is known about the renal disposition of prostaglandins. Labeled PGE_2 and $PGF_{2\alpha}$ injected intravenously are almost exclusively excreted as metabolites in both man and experimental animals. None of the injected parent compounds is recovered in urine. Inasmuch as PGE_2 and $PGF_{2\alpha}$ are found occurring naturally in the urine of several species, including man, it seems likely that these primary prostaglandins are of renal origin (37). Prostaglandins are subjected to probenecid-sensitive secretion by the tubules (31, 38); they can be reabsorbed to some extent in the proximal tubule and in the loop of Henle. Prostaglandins released from within the kidney are recovered intact either in venous blood or in urine. Both the urinary excretion rate of PGE_2 and $PGF_{2\alpha}$ and their plasma level determined in the renal venous effluent have become useful indices of intrarenal PG biosynthesis. PGI_2, the major component in the renal vascular tissue of the cortex, as well as its more stable hydrolysis product 6-keto-$PGF_{1\alpha}$, do not show up to an appreciable extent in the urine under physiological conditions. Presumably PGI_2 is degraded rapidly at its place of synthesis by the renal cortex before it can reach tubular fluid. Under certain stress situations elevated urinary 6-keto-$PGF_{1\alpha}$ levels represent systemic rather than renal PGI_2 production (39).

PHYSIOLOGICAL ACTION

Vascular Wall and Platelet Prostanoids

In most species and in most vascular beds, PGE, PGD_2, and PGI_2 are potent vasodilators, whereas $PGF_{2\alpha}$ and particularly TxA_2 are potent vasoconstrictors. PGI_2 is produced by endothelial cells; it is a potent vasodilator and inhibits platelet aggregation as well. TxA_2, on the other hand, is produced by platelets; it is a potent vasoconstrictor and stimulates platelet aggregation as well. These observations have led to the conclusion that such a balance of opposing agonists is an important means for preserving vascular homeostasis (40).

Vascular damage causes platelet deposition, but not necessarily thrombosis. When the injury is minor, a platelet thrombus is formed, which then breaks away from the vessel wall to be washed away by the circulation. This sequence is in accordance with the distribution of PGI_2 synthetase, for it is abundant in the intima and decreases in activity progressively from the intima to the adventitia. In contrast, the proaggregating elements, like collagen, increase from the subendothelium to the adventitia. Platelets adhering to the intact vessel wall generate PG-endoperoxides close to the endothelial surface, thus providing the direct precursor of PGI_2 in addition to PGG_2 and PGH_2 synthesized by the vessel wall itself, a so-called endoperoxide steal phenomenon (Fig. 16.5). The potent stimulatory effect of PGI_2 on the adenylate cyclase of platelets will increase cAMP levels inside the platelets and as a consequence inhibit Ca^{++} release and platelet aggregation. In contrast, an endothelial defect will unmask the collagen texture of the vessel wall. Platelets will adhere to this defect. Collagen will induce a Ca^{++}-mediated release of arachidonate from platelet phospholipids. The generated PG-endoperoxides can now primarily be converted to TxA_2, which causes platelet aggregation. The concomitant rise of Ca^{++} concentration in the cytosol will stimulate further release of arachidonic acid, thus maintaining the generation of the proaggregatory-mediator TxA_2. Although this concept has been challenged by others (41–43), this view appears quite helpful as a working hypothesis, for example, in the understanding of the pathophysiology of vascular diseases and in the application of antithrombotic agents as will be outlined.

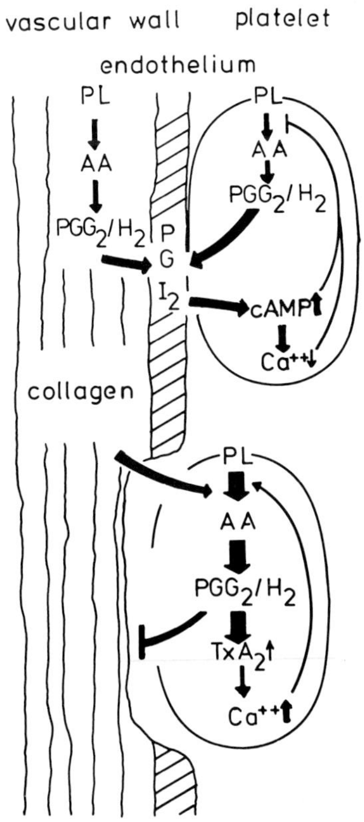

Figure 16.5. Arachidonate metabolism in vascular wall and platelets with and without endothelial defect. *PL*, phospholipids; *AA*, arachidonic acid; *cAMP*, cyclic AMP; *PGG₂/H₂*, cyclic prostaglandin endoperoxides; and *TxA₂*, thromboxane A₂.

Prostaglandins as Circulating Hormones

Generally, prostaglandins are not considered to be circulating hormones. Once synthesized, they interact with specific receptors on adjacent structures and undergo rapid metabolism. Nevertheless, three prostaglandins, PGA_2, PGI_2, and 6-keto-PGE_1, all with potent vasodilatory activity and with a low pulmonary metabolic clearance rate, have been proposed as potential antihypertensive circulating hormones. The latter two also have been proposed as circulating anticoagulant hormones (44, 45).

PGA_2 levels in stored plasma from normal man, measured by an immunoreactive method, have been reported (46), but no PGA_2 was detected in plasma analyzed by mass spectrometry (47), which is capable of detecting concentrations as low as 5 pg/ml. Presumably PGA_2 in the first instance had arisen from nonenzymatic dehydration of PGE_2 during storage or sample preparation. Currently, it appears that normal plasma does not contain significant levels of PGA_2.

After the discovery that circulating PGI_2, unlike PGE_2 and $PGF_{2\alpha}$, can pass through the lung unchanged, the proposition that PGI_2 is a circulating hormone was triggered (44). Furthermore, it was observed that pulmonary vascular tissue continuously releases PGI_2 into the circulation (45). This substance, a potent vasodilator and inhibitor of platelet aggregation could then act on the arterial side of the circulation. If this proved to be the case, its deficiency would have important implications in blood pressure control and thromboembolic disorders. However, the rate of PGI_2 secretion into the circulation, as derived from the urinary excretion rates of PGI_2 metabolites, is considered to be low in healthy man (48). This conclusion is supported by the finding that the plasma level of 6-keto-$PGF_{1\alpha}$ is in the low pg/ml range when advanced analytical technology is employed (30, 49). These levels correspond to PGI_2 plasma concentrations that are one-tenth the minimal level needed to inhibit platelet function.

These findings, however, do not exclude the possibility that levels of PGI_2 at the site of the endothelium may reach higher and physiologically effective concentrations. Furthermore, there remain methodological difficulties when chemically extracting labile mediators, such as PGI_2 and its metabolites, from a complex biological matrix like plasma, in which covalent binding to some proteins may occur. Finally, circulating levels, in the ng/ml range, of PGI-like material have been detected by the blood super-perfused bioassay (50).

The great discrepancy between bioassay and chemical analysis when measuring plasma levels of PGI_2 and 6-keto-$PGF_{1\alpha}$, respectively, also has led to the suggestion that PGI_2 might be converted to a more stable but still biologically active metabolite, such as 6-keto-PGE_1, formed by the enzyme 9-hydroxy-PG-dehydrogenase (51). This conversion might provide an explanation for the prolonged effect of the unstable PGI_2 in various biological systems. However, this does not seem likely either. Mass spectrometric studies of the metabolic disposition of PGI_2 in man have failed to detect metabolites with 6-keto-PGE structure; further, infusion of synthetic PGI_2 into humans does not result in accumulation of 6-keto-PGE_1 in plasma (29, 52). Thus, at present the whole issue about prostanoids as circulating hormones remains controversial.

Renal Hemodynamics

There is general acceptance of the role of prostanoids in the regulation and modulation of perfusion of various organs. In the kidney and most other organs of most species, PGI_2, PGE_2, and PGD_2 are vasodilators, whereas TxA_2 and, to a lesser degree, $PGF_{2\alpha}$ are vasoconstrictors. Infusion of the vasodilators into the renal artery increases RBF. These are pharmacological effects, because these substances under physiological conditions do not reach receptors of the kidney via the renal artery. However, by infusing arachidonic acid, the precursor of PG synthesis into the renal artery of the dog, a dose-related increase in RBF occurs (53). This renal effect of arachidonate is inhibited by a PG synthesis inhibitor, indicating that endogenously synthesized prostaglandins play a role in the regulation of renal hemodynamics. Indomethacin given to anesthetized and laparatomized dog causes a marked fall in RBF (54, 55), but later studies, in which indomethacin given to unanesthetized animals (56) showed no effect on RBF, led to the conclusion that trauma and stress influence the action of prostaglandins in maintaining GFR and RBF (33, 57–59). Today, it is believed that vasoconstrictors stimulate the renal synthesis of vasodilatory prostaglandins, thus attenuating hormonal-mediated renal vasoconstriction.

There are numerous disease states that show a reduction of RBF and GFR following cyclo-oxygenase inhibition. These include congestive heart failure, decompensated hepatic cirrhosis, nephrotic syndrome, volume depletion secondary to diuretics, gastrointestinal fluid loss, extensive burns, and hemorrhagic shock (33, 56, 59). The common feature of all these is a reduced circulatory volume associated with marked increase in PRA and adrenergic tone. As long as the primary cause of renal hypoperfusion exists, the kidney function will remain extremely sensitive to any PG synthetase inhibitor. More recent studies in preterm infants who have symptomatic patent ductus arteriosus (sPDA) treated for long periods with indomethacin have demonstrated that vasodilatory prostaglandins are important in maintaining renal function in stress situations (60). With a patent ductus arteriosus, the circulatory volume is insufficient because there is significant aortic runoff (up to 30% of the left ventricular output) across the ductus. This leads to renal hypoperfusion, particularly if the infants are kept on restricted fluid intake and diuretic therapy with furosemide which, in addition, is a marked stimulus for renin release (Fig. 16.6). The enhanced vasoconstrictor activity of angiotensin-II is counterbalanced by vasodilatory prostaglandins, such as PGI_2 and PGE_2. The kidney becomes dependent on its PG-biosynthesis remaining intact. Consequently, introduction of indomethacin therapy for ductal closure will cause a drop in renal perfusion and function. Once the ductus has been constricted, an effective circulatory volume can be established with readjustment of PRA toward normal levels. Under this more physiological condition, renal function can recover despite continued indomethacin therapy.

The predominance of vasodilatory prostaglandins, which protect renal perfusion, can be reversed by chronic ureteral obstruction to a predominance of the vasoconstrictor, TxA_2 (35). This finding led to the hypothesis that the intense vasoconstriction observed during chronic ureteral obstruction is a result of TxA production. This hypothesis has been reinforced since imidazole, a relatively specific thromboxane synthetase inhibitor, attenuates the vasoconstriction that occurs during ureteral obstruction. This example indicates that PG synthesis inhibition, which also inhibits the synthesis of TxA_2, may increase RBF. The overall biochemical and humoral activities influencing kidney function before PG inhibition and the character of the inhibitor significantly influence the effect on RBF.

Sodium Excretion

Arachidonic acid, PGE_2, PGI_2, or PGD_2 can cause natriuresis in a variety of experimental conditions, leading to the suggestion that most prostaglandins are natriuretic (61). However, these agents also increase RBF, an effect which induces natriuresis. PG synthesis inhibitors experimentally either reduce sodium excretion, have no effect, or even increase it. Some of the PG synthesis inhibitors have an intrinsic PG unrelated mineralocorticoid-like activity. Differences in the experimental design, e.g., anesthesia, previous sodium intake, control urinary output, or even the time point of the observation, influence the results. Studies with isolated tubular structures in which these factors are controlled still does not lead to a conclusive answer (61, 62). In one study in which PGE_2, the most likely natriuretic factor, was applied to the interstitial side of isolated collecting tubules, sodium reabsorption was inhibited. However, that observation was not reproduced in other studies. Despite these discrepancies, considerable evidence indicates that in humans various NSAI drugs lead to significant sodium retention.

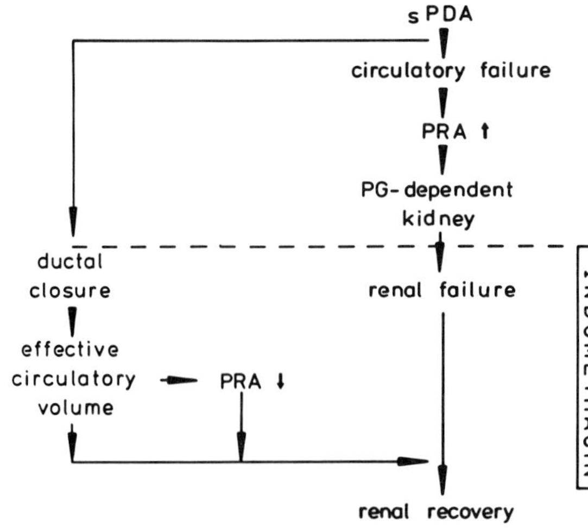

Figure 16.6. Possible mechanisms involved in deterioration and recovery of renal function in infants with patent ductus arteriosus before and during prolonged indomethacin therapy (7 days).

INTERACTION WITH OTHER HUMORAL SYSTEMS

The Vasopressin System

Renal prostaglandins also are involved in water excretion. The collecting tubule cell and the renal medullary interstitial cell synthesize prostaglandins. Although there is evidence that prostaglandins directly affect water transport, most of their effects are observed when vasopressin is present (33, 61, 63, 64), e.g., PGE_1 antagonizes vasopressin-mediated water transport in the toad bladder and in the rabbit's isolated perfused collecting duct (65). PG synthesis inhibitors in vitro and in vivo reverse this effect (63, 64).

The currently favored hypothesis to explain this action is that renal prostaglandins, e.g., PGE_2, interfere with vasopressin-stimulated cAMP synthesis. A second antagonistic effect is mediated by PG-induced increases in renal medullary blood flow, which has a "washout" effect on the medullary interstitial hypertonicity. On the other hand, vasopressin is a potent stimulator of intrarenal PG synthesis through its effect on phospholipid deacylation. Thus, a negative feedback loop operates, in which renal prostaglandins modulate the vasopressin effect on the kidney (Fig. 16.7) (65). While PG synthesis inhibition may increase renal sensitivity to vasopressin, the reverse has been proposed in nephrogenic diabetes insipidus-like states, including those induced by lithium or hypercalcemia. In these, urinary PG excretion is increased (63).

The Renin-Angiotensin System

The interactions between renal prostaglandins and the RAS were first appreciated when it was shown that intrarenal infusion of angiotensin-II gives rise to PGE-like activity in the renal venous blood (66) and that

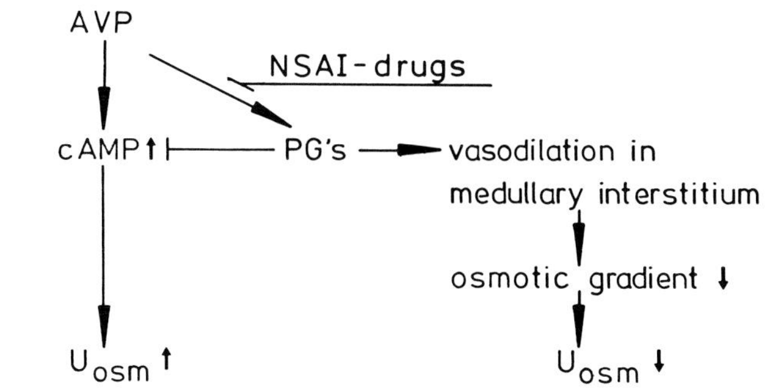

Figure 16.7. Negative feedback-modulation of vasopressin effects by vasodilatory prostaglandins in the kidney and the site of inhibitory action of NSAI drugs. *AVP*, arginine-vasopressin; *cAMP*, cyclic AMP: *NSAI drugs*, nonsteroidal antiinflammatory drugs; *PG's*, vasodilatory prostaglandins, e.g., PGE_2; and U_{osm}, urinary osmolality.

indomethacin treatment lowers the PR in man (67). Since then, numerous studies in isolated cell preparations, isolated perfused kidney, and in vivo studies in experimental animals and man have defined a complex interrelation between renal PG synthesis and the renin-angiotensin system (33, 68).

Angiotensin-II mediates intrarenal prostaglandin release, since PGE levels in urine increase after angiotensin-II is given to humans (37). This effect appears to be independent of the vasoconstricting effect of angiotensin because angiotensin-II directly stimulates PGE_2 release from renal medullary interstitial cells and human vascular endothelial cells in vitro (61, 69).

Although renal prostaglandins in humans appear to stimulate renin release and since inhibition of PG synthesis blocks renin release, there is debate as to which renal prostaglandin is the mediator of renin release, a process most likely mediated by intracellular cAMP accumulation (33). Quite a few prostaglandins have some renin-releasing activity, e.g., PGI_2, PGE_1, PGE_2, PGD_2, $PGF_{2\alpha}$, and some metabolites like 13,14-dihydro-PGE_2 and 6-keto-PGE_1 (70, 74). Recently, special emphasis has been put on PGI_2 as a local modulator of renin release (68, 75). However, in some states of high renin activity, e.g., prematurity and Bartter's syndrome, urinary excretion rates of 6-keto-$PGF_{1\alpha}$, the major chemical breakdown compound of PGI_2 (39) are not significantly increased. On the other hand, urinary excretion rates of 6-keto-$PGF_{1\alpha}$ is questioned as a reliable index of intrarenal PGI_2 synthesis.

Of the three recognized mechanisms for stimulating renin release, the baroreceptor, macula densa, and sympathetic stimulation, the first two depend on prostaglandins (62, 76, 77), whereas the sympathetic stimulation does not (68, 78). This should be kept in mind, since in severe sodium or volume depletion or circulatory failure, inhibition of PG synthesis with its renin-lowering effect might be overridden by the simultaneously increased sympathetic tonus.

Other Humoral Systems

There is a relatively well-studied relationship between the renal kallikrein-kinin system and the prostaglandins. Kininogen, the substrate, and bradykinin, the biologically active component of the kallikrein-kinin system, activate prostaglandin synthesis by the stimulation of the deacylation reaction, leading to a quite selective liberation of arachidonic acid from phospholipids (phospholipase A_2 reaction), the rate-limiting step in overall prostanoid production (79, 80). The effects of kinins on renal function, such as promoting vasodilatation and excretory function, appeared to be, at least in part, mediated by renal prostaglandins, such as PGE_2 and PGI_2 (51, 79). The involvement of prostaglandins in the control of renal kallikrein activity is less clear. In general, the physiological role of these relationships between the two endocrine systems are presently not well understood, particularly if one considers the even more complex interaction with a third system, the renin-angiotensin system (62, 79).

Most criteria have been met to prove that renal prostaglandins mediate the biological process within the kidney that leads to the production of erythropoietin (81). Major stimuli for erythropoietin release are ischemia, hypoxic and anemic hypoxia, and pathophysiological states that stimulate renal prostaglandin release as well. There is evidence that renal prostaglandins, e.g., PGI_2 and the E prostaglandins, interact directly via a cAMP-mediated activation of phospholipase A_2 with erythropoietin-producing renal cells independent of their vascular actions (81, 82).

The interaction of PGE_2 with the sympathetic nervous sytem as proposed by Hedqvist (83) will be discussed elsehwere in this book.

DRUGS AFFECTING ARACHIDONATE METABOLISM

More and more therapeutic agents are known to interfere with eicosanoid production and metabolism. Of major interest in the scope of this book are NSAI drugs, antithrombotic agents, diuretics, and various antihypertensive drugs.

Nonsteroidal Antiinflammatory Drugs

Following the discovery of Vane and others (18, 84), that aspirin and indomethacin inhibit prostaglandin biosynthesis, the use of these and related drugs has become widespread in studies on the role of prostaglandins in physiology and disease. It is important to realize, however, that the experimental background for their use in clinical situations as prostaglandin synthesis inhibitors, particularly in pediatrics, has not been thoroughly investigated. Dose- and time-response relationships are lacking for most indications. These nonsteroidal agents have several other actions apart from the reversible inhibition of the PG-cyclo-oxygenase. For example, indomethacin inhibits the 15-hydroxy-PG-dehydrogenase, the arachidonate release and the renal tubular transport of prostaglandins (59, 84). In some systems it also inhibits the lipoxygenase pathway of arachidonate metabolism and cAMP degradation (phosphodiesterase inhibition).

However, as judged from drug level monitoring, the plasma level of indomethacin that effectively inhibits PG synthesis in various pediatric age groups (85), is between 0.5 to 1.0 μg/ml, 4 to 10 hr postdosing. This is far below its inhibitory concentration for other enzyme systems (86). Indomethacin plasma levels in the therapeutic range cause adverse side effects, e.g., an increased renal sensitivity to vasopressin, leading to oliguria, weight gain, and hyponatremia; a marked drop in PRA and secondary hypoaldosteronism associated with hyperkalemia; and a decline in GFR and RBF. The latter may cause transient renal failure in situations where renal damage or circulatory failure already exist (59, 60). These effects are not specific for indomethacin, but are characteristic for all PG synthesis inhibitors, e.g., ibuprofen, napoxen, meclofenamate, and others. The possible exception is sulindac, which is thought to be inactivated in the kidney before it reaches the renal PG cyclo-oxygenase (87).

Antithrombotic Agents

The prototype of these drugs is aspirin (acetylsalicylic acid). Aspirin has a different mode of inhibiting PG cyclo-oxygenase activity. It acetylates the enzyme complex in a covalent manner (42). This acetylation permanently inactivates PG cyclo-oxygenase in platelets, since they are incapable of protein synthesis and, therefore, cannot produce a new active enzyme complex like other tissues, such as the vascular wall. In practical terms this means that a single dose of aspirin will inhibit the platelet cyclo-oxygenase for the lifespan of platelets (about 10 days) without significant inhibitory effects on PGI_2 synthetase in the endothelium. This pharmacological intervention will shift the balance from the proaggregatory TxA_2 generation toward the antiaggregatory PGI_2 production.

These considerations led to the suggestion of lowering the conventional aspirin dose in antithrombotic therapy from 1500 to 325 mg/day for adults, that means about 4 to 5 mg/kg bodyweight/day (43). Apart from tailoring an aspirin dose specific for platelet cyclo-oxygenase, an alternative approach has been offered with the development of specific inhibitors of thromboxane synthetase, like the imidazole derivative, dazoxiben (88), which is presently under clinical investigation in various cardiovascular and renal diseases. In experimental studies in rats, thromboxane inhibitors block the effect of high protein diets to accelerate loss of renal function in chronic renal failure (88a).

Diuretics and Antihypertensive Drugs

The pharmacological action of furosemide, the prototype of the loop diuretics to enhance PG action, has been studied extensively. Several lines of evidence show that the extradiuretic effects of furosemide to increase RBF, to cause renin release, and to increase peripheral venous capacitance are mediated by the prostaglandins (89). In vitro studies in rabbit and rat kidneys have shown that furosemide inhibits 15-hydroxy-PG-dehydrogenase and 9-keto-PG-reductase, the enzymes responsible for PG inactivation. The concentrations of furosemide used to produce the inhibition of these enzymes were much higher than those achieved in vivo in humans.

The currently most accepted view is that furosemide stimulates renal PG synthesis by releasing arachidonic acid from the precursor pool rather than altering PG metabolism. Other loop diuretics, such as ethacrynic acid and bumetanide, also cause a rise in RBF followed by a secondary increase in urine flow and sodium excretion. This effect is associated with prostaglandin release and can be reduced by indomethacin. In contrast, equimolar concentrations of chlorothiazide and hydrochlorothiazide had none of these effects (90, 91). There is indirect evidence that the PG-mediated vasodilatory effect of furosemide is not limited to the renal vascular bed. A positive relationship between furosemide dose and the incidence of patent ductus arteriosus was observed in preterm infants, raising concern about its use in that age group (92). In a different situation the effect of various antihypertensive drugs, e.g., beta-receptor blocking agents, hydralazine, minoxidil, and captopril are thought to act, in part, by increasing release of vasodilatory prostaglandins (90, 93).

ASSAYS AND ASSESSMENT OF PROSTAGLANDIN ACTIVITY

The major problem that has confronted investigators in prostaglandin research has been assay accuracy and reliability. The difficulties in analyzing small quantities of these biologically, highly active compounds are reflected by the numerous methods applied.

Assays

Bioassay

One of the first methods used and one that is still quite important for discovering unstable intermediates, as well as providing an on-line method for monitoring prostaglandin release, is the cascade bioassay. This assay, which played an important role in defining the function of renal prostaglandins (66), is not as sensitive as other methods; its utility is reduced by its low sample capacity and by the fact that identification of a prostaglandin requires other analytical techniques.

Radioimmunoassay

The radioimmunoassay is quite simple, more sensitive, and possibly more specific than the bioassay. A large number of these assays measuring primary prostaglandins, metabolites, prostaglandin analogues, and most recently leukotrienes, has been developed. However, there are many serious drawbacks to the use of radioimmunoassays. These assays measure the displacement of radioactive molecules from the binding sites of the antibody and displacement can be caused by factors unrelated to the compound being assayed (94). Secondly, the antiserum used sometimes has low specificity. These difficulties may lead to serious errors in reported prostaglandin levels in plasma and urine (27, 30, 61, 94). They can be safely used only in combination with rigorous sample purification, using highly specific monoclonal antibodies, and verification with other analytical procedures.

Mass Spectrometry

Quantitative mass spectrometry is used widely because of its high specificity (27). Its use has increased with the introduction of capillary column gas chromatography in mass spectrometric analysis of prostaglandins (95). This type of assay is the reference method, since it combines quantification with analysis of the specific chemical structure.

The disadvantages of this method had been the expensive equipment and low sensitivity when compared with radioimmunoassays. The latter limitations have been overcome by the combination of capillary column gas chromatography with negative ion chemical ionization mass spectrometry. These modifications allow the measurement of several prostaglandins in the same run (prostanoid profile) and sensitivity is increased a hundred-fold.

Sample Handling

Sample handling can cause unrealistically high prostanoid levels. Venous stasis or irritation by the tip of the needle might release PGI_2 from the vascular endothelium; platelets and white cells may release significant quantities of prostanoids and other eicosanoids during sample preparation. Consequently, samples should be obtained without the use of a tourniquet and with a minimum of trauma. Plasma rather than serum must be obtained and the anticoagulant, e.g., sodium citrate, should contain indomethacin or another inhibitor of PG cyclo-oxygenase. Even with these precautions, peripheral plasma concentrations often are not very meaningful because the plasma levels of primary prostaglandins and their short-lived metabolites do not reflect the rate of endogenous synthesis in vivo in tissue and organs, because of the rapid fluctuations with which they are released into the circulation (27). Determining a major metabolite in a 24-hour urine collection will provide more information about renal prostaglandin production and turnover. In certain experimental situations, rapid changes in prostanoid metabolism can be detected by frequent sampling of the venous effluent of a specific organ, like the ischemic kidney. Tissue levels are less desirable, because prostaglandins are released immediately during preparation of the tissue.

Assessment of PG Activity

The great advantage of obtaining urinary excretion rates of PGE_2 and $PGF_{2\alpha}$ is that the output is a useful index of intrarenal prostaglandin biosynthesis. The simultaneous determination of primary prostaglandins and metabolites in urine provides an integrated and noninvasive method of monitoring renal and systemic (total body) prostaglandin production. This method is useful in the clinical setting (27, 30, 96). However, this approach too has its shortcomings. Prostanoid excretion rates may be influenced by urine flow, postrenal contamination of urine, e.g., by semen in adult males, and urinary excretion of prostanoids, which are weak acids, may be influenced by urine pH. Excretion rates should be normalized for time and surface area for comparison among different age groups. No significant differences among different stages of development and age groups have been noticed when data are expressed in this way (96, 97).

ROLE OF PROSTAGLANDINS IN RENAL AND VASCULAR DISEASES

Increased Prostaglandin Production

One of the most relevant observations in renal prostaglandin research has been the efficacy of indomethacin treatment of patients with Bartter's syndrome (67) (chapter 34). Subsequently, the observed increase in urinary excretion rates of PGE_2 reflect overproduction of renal prostaglandins reported in adults (98, 99) and children (Fig. 16.7) with Bartter's syndrome. All patients reacted favorably to indomethacin therapy; this proved more effective and better tolerated in children than aspirin treatment.

Initially, it was thought that excess renal PGE_2 synthesis was the most proximal defect in the pathogenesis of Bartter's syndrome. Recently it was postulated that defective Cl reabsorption in the ascending limb of Henle's loop is the primary defect (100). According to this hypothesis, Cl loss triggers a distal tubular K wasting secondary to overproduction of renal prostaglandins, renin, and aldosterone. This increased renal PG production appears to be a consequence of K deficiency, since K loss secondary to abuse of diuretics, habitual vomiting, or renal Mg wasting triggers excess renal PG production. Urinary PG excretion rates, therefore, are not specific for the diagnosis of Bartter's syndrome; the interpretation of increased PG excretion in cases of K deficiency requires a search for the cause of K loss.

Interestingly, a syndrome with increased NaCl retention, decreased renal Cl clearance, renal tubular acidosis (RTA), hypertension, and low-to-undetectable urinary PGE_2 levels, has been reported (101). This syndrome appears to be diametrically opposite to Bartter's syndrome. The most effective intervention is the introduction of furosemide therapy, which corrects the abnormalities, including the high fractional distal Cl rebsorption; urinary excretion of PGE_2 also is increased (chapter 34).

Two extrarenal features reported in patients with Bartter's syndrome are reduced responsiveness of blood pressure to angiotensin-II and norepinephrine (99) and a defect in platelet aggregation (102). Both defects are alleviated by indomethacin therapy or by antibodies against PGI_2. Reports of elevated levels of immunreactive 6-keto-$PGF_{1\alpha}$ in urine (1–3) and high plasma levels of the antiaggregatory and vasodilatory 6-keto-PGE_1 (104) have not been confirmed by mass spectrometric assays. Neither the urinary excretion of 6-keto-$PGF_{1\alpha}$ (Fig. 16.8) or dinor-6-keto-$PGF_{1\alpha}$ (105), nor the plasma level of 6-keto-PGE_1 (106) is elevated in patients with Bartter's syndrome. The high PGE-M excretion rates in half the children and adults with Bartter's syndrome (98, 99) might indicate that excess prostaglandin-E is a factor in the systemic effects in some patients with this syndrome.

Other renal diseases in which increased urinary excretion of prostanoids has been reported are renal diabetes insipidus (idiopathic or induced by lithium therapy), nephrocalcinosis, renal dysfunction in cirrhosis with ascitis, systemic lupus erythematosus, renal allograft rejection, and various other forms of chronic renal diseases. It remains to be clarified whether this increased prostanoid production is related to the pathogenesis of the disease or, more likely, to a secondary phenomenon to conserve adequate kidney function.

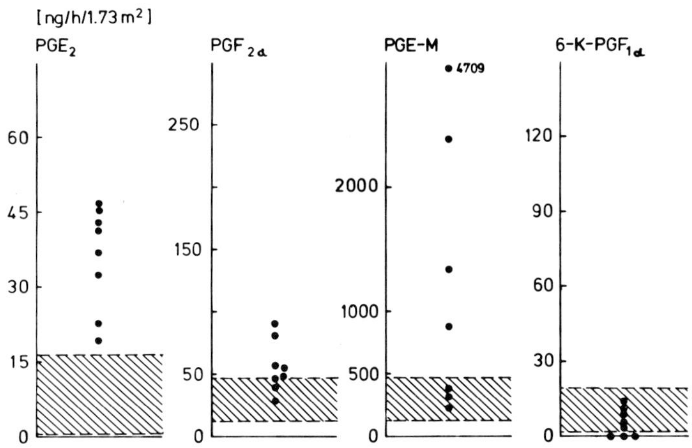

Figure 16.8. Urinary excretion of primary prostaglandins, PGE_2 and $PGF_{2\alpha}$ (indices of renal PG-synthesis) and PG-metabolites, PGE-M and 6-keto-$PGF_{1\alpha}$ (indices of total body turnover) in children with Bartter's syndrome-like symptomatology between 3 months and 11 years (median 4 years). The shaded areas indicate mean ± SD from 30 normal children of various age groups (PGE_2: 8.7 ± 7.9 ng/h/1.73m², $PGF_{2\alpha}$: 30.4 ± 17.2, PGE-M: 310.0 ± 173.5, 6-keto-$PGF_{1\alpha}$: 10.7 ± 8.4).

There are only a few reported cases of increased systemic or total body production of prostaglandins in circulatory or vascular diseases. These have included increased systemic PGI_2 release, presumed to be secondary to the artificially ventilated lung of preterm infants who have a tendency for persistent ductus arteriosus (107), and in patients with diffuse atherosclerosis releasing increased amounts of PGI_2 to compensate for an increased tendency to platelet aggregation in the vascular bed (30).

Deficient Prostaglandin Production

A major challenge in prostaglandin research has been whether a deficiency of vasodilatory prostaglandins contributes to arterial hypertension. There is, however, still no convincing evidence for such a defect (61). There might be a decreased production of PGI_2 in hypertension associated with pregnancy (108). In the hemolytic uremic syndrome and thrombotic thrombocytopenic purpura, a defect in the generation of PGI_2 may be involved in the vascular catastrophe of these diseases (108). However, the effect of PGI_2 infusions at the various stages of these diseases has been equivocal.

The technical problems encountered in prostaglandin analysis that make it difficult to demonstrate prostaglandin overproduction are even greater when attempting to demonstrate prostaglandin deficiency. In spite of these analytical difficulties, prostaglandins and their derivatives are being used as replacement therapy and as pharmacological agents, like the antiaggregatory PGI_2 in cardiopulmonary bypass with charcoal hemoperfusion and hemodialysis and in ischemic heart disease. PGE_1 is being used in peripheral vascular diseases and congenital heart lesions where well being depends on maintaining a patent ductus arteriosus.

Acknowledgment

This work was supported by the Deutsche Forschungsgemeinschaft (Grant No. Se 263). Dr. Seyberth is the recipient of a Heisenberg stipend from the Deutsche Forschungsgemeinschaft.

References

1. Moncada S, Flower RJ, Vane JR: Prostaglandins, prostacyclin, and thromboxane A_2. Gillman AG, Goodman LS, Gillman A (eds): The Pharmacological Basis of Therapeutics, ed. 6. New York, MacMillan Publishing Company, 1980.

2. Oates JA: The 1982 Nobel Prize in physiology or medicine. Science 218:765, 1982.
3. von Euler US: Über die spezifische blutdrucksenkende Substanz des menschlichen Prostata- und Samenblasensekretes. Klin Wchnschr 33:1182, 1935.
4. Bergström S, Sjövall J: The isolation of prostaglandin E from sheep prostate glands. Acta Chem Scand 14:1701, 1960.
5. Bergström S, Ryhage R, Samuelsson B, et al: Prostaglandins and related factors. J Biol Chem 238:3555, 1963.
6. Van Dorp DA, Beerthius RK, Nugteren DH, et al. The biosynthesis of prostaglandins. Biochim Biophys Acta 90:204, 1964.
7. Bergström S, Danielsson H, Samuelsson B: The enzymatic formation of prostaglandin E_2 from arachidonic acid. Prostaglandins and related factors. Biochim Biophys Acta 90:207, 1964.
8. Muirhead EE, Stirman JA, Jones F: Renal autoexplanation and protection against renoprival hypertensive cardiovascular disease and hemolysis. J Clin Invest 39:266, 1960.
9. Hickler RB, Lauler DP, Saravis CA, et al: Vasodepressor lipid from the renal medulla. Canad M A J 90:280, 1964.
10. Lee JB, Crowshaw K, Takman BH, et al: The identification of prostaglandin E_2, $F_{2\alpha}$ and A_2. Biochem J 105:1251, 1967.
11. Lands WEM, Samuelsson B: Phospholipid precursors of prostaglandins. Biochim Biophys Acta 164:426, 1968.
12. Hong SL, Levine L: Inhibition of Arachidonic acid release from cells as the biochemical action of antiinflammatory corticosteroids. Proc Natl Acad Sci USA 73:1730, 1976.
13. Flower RJ, Blackwell GJ: Anti-inflammatory steroids induce biosynthesis of a phospholipase A_2 inhibitor which prevents prostaglandin generation. Nature 278:456, 1979.
14. Samuelsson B, Hammarström S, Borgeat P: Pathways of arachidonic acid metabolism. Adv Inflam Res 1:405, 1979.
15. Hamberg M, Samuelsson B: Detection and isolation of an endoperoxide intermediate in prostaglandin biosynthesis. Proc Natl Acad Sci USA 70:899, 1973.
16. Hamberg M, Svensson J, Samuelsson B: Thromboxanes: a new group of biologically active compounds derived from prostaglandin endoperoxides. Proc Natl Acad Sci USA 72:2994, 1975.
17. Moncada S, Gryglewski R, Bunting S. et al: An enzyme isolated from arteries transforms prostaglandin endoperoxides to an unstable substance that inhibits platelet aggregation. Nature 263:663, 1976.
18. Vane JR: Inhibition of prostaglandin synthesis as a mechanism of action for aspirin-like drugs. Nature 231:232, 1971.
19. Smith JB, Willis AL: Aspirin selectively inhibits prostaglandin production in human platelets. Nature 231:235, 1971.
20. Hamberg M, Samuelsson B: Prostaglandin endoperoxides. Novel transformations of arachidonic acid in human platelets. Proc Natl Acad Sci USA 71:3400, 1974.
21. Borgeat P, Hamberg M, Samuelsson B: Transformation of arachidonic acid and homo-γ-linolenic acid by rabbit polymorphonuclear leukocytes. J Biol Chem 251:7816, 1976.
22. Murphy RC, Hammarström S, Samuelsson B: Leukotriene C: a slow-reacting substance from murine mastocytoma cells. Proc Natl Acad Sci USA 76:4275, 1979.
23. Hammarström S: Leukotrienes. Ann Rev Biochem 52:355, 1983.
24. Samuelsson B: Leukotrienes: a new class of mediators of immediate hypersensitivity reactions and inflammation. In: Adv Prostaglandin Thromboxane Leukotriene Res 11:10, 1983.
25. Van Praag D, Farber SJ: Biosynthesis of cyclooxagenase and lipooxygenase metabolites of arachidonic acid by rabbit renal microsomes. Prostaglandins Leukotrienes Med 12:29, 1983.
26. Ferreira SH, Vane JR: Prostaglandins: their disappearance from and release into the circulation. Nature 216:868, 1967.
27. Samuelsson B, Granström E, Green K, et al: Prostaglandins. Ann Rev Biochem 44:669, 1975.
28. Roberts LJ, Sweetman BJ, Oates JA: Metabolism of thromboxane B_2 in man. J Biol Chem 256:8384, 1981.
29. Brash AR, Jackson EK, Saggese CA, et al: Metabolic disposition of prostacyclin in humans. J Pharmacol Exp Ther 226:78, 1983.
30. FitzGerald GA, Pedersen AK, Patrono C: Analysis of prostacyclin and thromboxane biosynthesis in cardiovascular disease. Circulation 67:1174, 1983.
31. Änggård E, Oliw E: Formation and metabolism of prostaglandins in the kidney. Kidney Int 19:771, 1981.
32. Sun FF, Taylor BM, McGuire JC, et al: Metabolism of prostaglandins in the kidney. Kidney Int 19:760, 1981.
33. Levenson DJ, Simmons CE, Brenner BM: Arachidonic acid metabolism, prostaglandins and the kidney. Am J Med 72:354, 1982.
34. Whorton AR, Smigel M, Oates JA, et al: Regional differences in prostacyclin formation by the kidney. Prostacyclin is a major prostaglandin of renal cortex. Biochim Biophys Acta 529:176, 78.
35. Morrison AR, Benabe JE: Prostaglandins and vascular tone in experimental obstructive nephropathy. Kidney Int 19:786, 1981.
36. Weber PC, Larsson C, Scherer B: Prostaglandin E_2-9-ketoreductase as a mediator of salt intake-related prostaglandin-renin interaction. Nature 266:65, 1977.
37. Frölich JC, Wilson TW, Sweetman BJ, et al: Urinary prostaglandins. Identification and origin. J Clin Invest 55:763, 1975.
38. Rosenkranz B, Kitajima W, Frölich JC: Relevance of urinary 6-keto-prostaglandin $F_{1\alpha}$ determination. Kidney Int 19:755, 1981.
39. Seyberth HW, Müller H, Soeding K, et al: Urinary excretion rate of 6-keto-prostaglandin $F_{1\alpha}$ as an index of circulating prostacyclin. Adv Prostaglandin Thromboxane Leukotriene Res 11:533, 1983.
40. Moncada S, Vane JR: Arachidonic acid metabolites and the interactions between platelets and blood-vessel walls. N Engl J Med 300:1142, 1979.
41. Smith JB, Araki H, Lefer AM: Thromboxane A_2, prostacyclin and aspirin: effects on vascular tone and platelet aggregation. Circulation 62 (suppl V): 19, 1980.
42. Majerus PW: Arachidonate metabolism in vascular disorders. J Clin Invest 72:1521, 1983.
43. Marcus AJ: Aspirin as an antithrombotic medication. N Engl J Med 309:1515, 1983.
44. Dollery CT, Hensby CN: Is prostacyclin a circulating anti-coagulant? Nature 273:706, 1978.
45. Gryglewski RJ: Prostacyclin as a circulating hormone. Biochem Pharmacol 28:3161, 1979.
46. Zusman RM, Spector D, Caldwell B, et al: The effect of chronic sodium loading and sodium restriction on plasma prostaglandin A, E, And F concentrations in normal humans. J Clin Invest 52:1093, 1973.
47. Frölich JC, Sweetman BJ, Carr K, et al: Assessment of the levels of PGA_2 in human plasma by gas chromatography-mass spectrometry. Prostaglandins 10:185, 1975.
48. FitzGerald GA, Brash AR, Falardeau P, et al: Estimated rate of prostacyclin secretion into the circulation of normal man. J Clin Invest 68:1272, 1981.
49. Blari IA, Barrow SE, Waddell KA, et al: Prostacyclin is not a circulating hormone in man. Prostaglandins 23:579, 1982.
50. Neri Serneri GG, Masotti G, Poggesi L, et al: Reduced prostacyclin production in patients with different manifestations of ischemic heart disease. Am J Cardiol 49:1146, 1982.
51. McGiff JC: Prostaglandins, prostacyclin, and thromboxanes. Ann Rev Pharmacol Toxicol 21:479, 1981.
52. Jackson EK, Goodman RP, FitzGerald GA, et al: Assessment of the extent to which exogenous prostaglandin I_2 is converted to 6-keto-prostaglandin E_1 in human subjects. J Pharmacol Exp Ther 221:183, 1982.
53. Chang LCT, Splawinski JA, Oates JA, et al: Enhanced renal prostaglandin production in the dog. II. Effects on intrarenal hemodynamics. Circ Res 36:204, 1975.
54. Lonigro AJ, Itskovitz HD, Crowshaw K, et al: Dependency of renal blood flow on prostaglandin synthesis in the dog. Circ Res 32:712, 1973.
55. Herbaczynska-Cedro K, Vane JR: Contribution of intrarenal generation of prostaglandin to autoregulation of renal blood flow in the dog. Circ Res 33:428, 1973.
56. Baer PG: The contribution of prostaglandins to renal blood flow maintenance is determined by the level of activity of the renin-angiotensin system. Life Sci 28:587, 1981.
57. Schapel GJ, Seyberth HW, Sweetman BJ, et al: Reduced glomerular filtration rate associated with decrease in prostaglandin synthesis produced by indomethacin in sodium deprived humans. Circ Res 23:327A, 1981.
58. Donker AJM, Arisz L, Brentjens JRH, et al: The effect of indomethacin on kidney function and plasma renin activity in man. Nephron 17:288, 1976.
59. Dunn MJ, Zambraski EJ: Renal effects of drugs that inhibit prostaglandin synthesis. Kidney Int 18:609, 1980.
60. Seyberth HW, Rascher W, Hackenthal R, et al: Effect of prolonged indomethacin therapy on renal function and selected vasoactive hormones in very-low-birth-weight infants with symptomatic patent ductus arteriosus. J Pediatr 103:979, 1983.
61. Dunn MJ, Hood VL: Prostaglandins and the kidney. Am J Physiol 233:F169, 1977.
62. Frölich JC, Fejes-Toth G: Renal prostaglandins. Klin Wchnschr 60:1155, 1982.
63. Gross PA, Schrier RW, Anderson RJ: Prostaglandins and water metabolism: a review with emphasis on in vivo studies. Kidney Int 19:839, 1981.
64. Stokes JB: Integrated actions of renal medullary prostaglandins in the control of water excretion. Am J Physiol 240:F471, 1981.
65. Grantham JJ, Orloff J: Effect of prostaglandin E_1 on the permeability response of the isolated collecting tubule to vasopressin, adenosine 3′,5′-monophosphate, and theophylline. J Clin Invest 47:1154, 1968.
66. McGiff JC, Crowshaw K, Terrangno N, et al: Release of prostaglandin-like substance into renal venous blood in response to angiotensin II. Circ Res 27 (suppl 1):121, 1970.
67. Verberckmoes R, Van Damme B, Clement J, et al: Bartter's syndrome with hyperplasia of reno-medullary cells: successful treatment with indomethacin. Kidney Int 9:302, 1976.

68. Oates JA, Whorton R, Gerkens JF, et al: The participation of prostaglandins in the control of renin release. Fed Proc 38:72, 1979.
69. Danon A, Chang LCT, Sweetman BJ, et al: Synthesis of prostaglandins by the rat renal papilla in vitro. Mechanism of stimulation by angiotensin II. Biochim Biophys Acta 388:71, 1975.
70. Whorton AR, Misono K, Hollifield J, et al: Prostaglandins and renin release. Prostaglandins 14:1096, 1977.
71. Gerber JG, Keller RT, Nies AS: Prostaglandins and renin release: the effect of PGI_2, PGE_2 and 13,14-dihydro PGE_2 on the baroreceptor mechanism of renin release in the dog. Circ Res 44:796, 1979.
72. Whorton AR, Lazar JD, Smigel MD, et al: Prostaglandins and renin release: III effects of PGE_2, PGE_2, $PGF_{2\alpha}$, and PGD_2 on renin release from rabbit renal cortical slices. Prostaglandins 22:455, 1981.
73. Lin C-S, Iwao H, Puttkammer S, et al: Prostaglandins and renin release in vitro. Am J Physiol 240:E609, 1981.
74. Jackson EK, Herzer WA, Zimmerman JB, et al: 6-keto-prostaglandin E_1 is more potent than prostaglandin I_2 as a renal vasodilator and renin secretagogue. J Pharmacol Exp Ther 216:24, 1981.
75. Patrono C, Pugliese F, Ciabattoni G, et al: Evidence for a direct stimulatory effect of prostacyclin on renin release in man. J Clin Invest 69:231, 1982.
76. Gerber JG, Nies AS, Olsen RD: Control of canine renin release: macula densa requires prostaglandin synthesis. J Physiol 319:419, 1981.
77. Berl T, Henrich WL, Erickson AL, et al: Prostaglandins in the beta-adrenergic and baroreceptor-mediated secretion of renin. Am J Physiol 236:F472, 1979.
78. Frölich JC, Hollifield JW, Michelakis AM, et al: Reduction of plasma renin activity by inhibition of the fatty acid cyclooxygenase in human subjects. Circ Res 44:781, 1979.
79. Nasjletti A, Malik KU: Renal kinin-prostaglandin relationship: implications for renal function. Kidney Int 19:860, 1981.
80. Whorton AR, Young SL, Data JL, et al: Mechanism of bradykinin-stimulated prostacyclin synthesis in porcine aortic endothelial cells. Biochim Biophys Acta 712:79, 1982.
81. Fisher JW: Prostaglandins and kidney erythropoietin production. Nephron 25:53, 1980.
82. Nelson PK, Brookins J, Fisher JW: Erythropoietic effects of prostacyclin (PGI_2) and its metabolite 6-keto-prostaglandin $(PG)E_1$. J Pharmacol Exp Ther 226:493, 1983.
83. Hedqvist P: Basic mechanisms of prostaglandin action on autonomic neurotransmission. Ann Rev Pharmacol Toxicol 17:259, 1977.
84. Ferreira SH, Vane JR: New aspects of the mode of action of nonsteroid anti-inflammatory drugs. Ann Rev Pharmacol 14:57, 1974.
85. Seyberth HW, Knapp G, Wolf D, et al: Introduction of plasma indomethacin level monitoring and evaluation of an effective threshold level in very-low-birth-weight infants with symptomatic patent ductus arteriosus. Europ J Pediatr 141:71, 1983.
86. Flower RJ, Vane JR: Inhibition of prostaglandin biosynthesis. Biochem Pharmacol 23:1439, 1974.
87. Bunning RD, Barth WF: Sulindac. A potentially renal-sparing nonsteroidal anti-inflammatory drug. JAMA 248:2864, 1982.
88. FitzGerald GA, Brash AR, Oates JA, et al: Endogenous prostacyclin biosynthesis and platelet function during selective inhibition of thromboxane synthase in man. J Clin Invest 71:1336, 1983.
88a. Parkerson ML, Valdes A, Yates J, et al: Inhibition of thromboxane synthesis prevents progressive renal disease in rats with 5/6 nephrectomy. Kidney Int 25:251, 1984.
89. Gerber JG: Role of prostaglandins in the hemodynamic and tubular effects of furosemide. Fed Proc 42:1707, 1983.
90. Frölich JC: Prostaglandins: role in renin regulation and mediation of antihypertensive drug effects. Arch Int Pharamcodyn Ther 89:213, 1980.
91. Craven PA, DeRubertis FR: Calcium-dependent stimulation of renal medullary prostaglandin synthesis by furosemide. J Pharmacol Exp Ther 222:306, 1982.
92. Green TP, Thompson TR, Johnson DE, et al: Furosemide promotes patent ductus arteriosus in premature infants with the respiratory-distress syndrome. N Engl J Med 308:743, 1983.
93. Moore TJ, Crantz FR, Hollenberg NK, et al: Contribution of prostaglandins to the antihypertensive action of captopril in essential hypertension. Hypertension 3:168, 1981.
94. Granström E, Kindahl H: Radioimmunoassays of prostaglandins and thromboxanes. Adv Prostaglandin Thromboxane Res 5:119, 1978.
95. Erlenmaier T, Müller H, Seyberth HW: Combined capillary column gas chromatography-mass spectrometric method for the quantitative analysis of urinary prostaglandins. J Chromatogr 163:289, 1979.
96. Seyberth HW, Müller H, Erlenmaier T, et al: Mass spectrometric determination of urinary prostaglandins in preterm infants. Europ J Pharmacol 18:89, 1980.
97. Godard C, Valloton MB, Favre L: Urinary prostaglandins, vasopressin, and kallikrein excretion in healthy children from birth to adolescence. J Pediatr 100:898, 1982.
98. Gill JR, Frölich JC, Bowden RE, et al: Bartter's syndrome: a disorder characterized by high urinary prostaglandins and a depedence of hyperreninemia on prostaglandin synthesis. Am J Med 61:43, 1976.
99. Bartter FC, Gill JR, Frölich JC, et al: Prostaglandins are overproduced by the kidneys and mediate hyperreninemia in Bartter's syndrome. Trans Assoc Am Physicians 89:77, 1976.
100. Gill JR, Bartter FC: Evidence for a prostaglandin-independent defect in chloride reabsorption in the loop of Henle as a proximal cause of Bartter's syndrome. Am J Med 65:766, 1978.
101. Sanjad SA, Keenan BS, Hill LL: Renal hypoprostaglandism, hypertension, and type IV renal tubular acidosis reversed by furosemide. Ann Intern Med 99:624, 1983.
102. Stoff JS, Stemerman M, Steer M, et al: A defect in platelet aggregation in Bartter's syndrome. Am J Med 68:171, 1980.
103. Güllner H-G, Cerletti C, Bartter FC, et al: Prostacyclin overproduction in Bartter's syndrome. Lancet 2:767, 1979.
104. Clive DM, Leone D, MacIntyre DE, et al: A plasma factor resembling 6-oxo-PGE_1 inhibits aggregation in Bartter's syndrome and normal man. Circ Res 29:332A, 1981.
105. Watson ML, Gill JR, Branch RA, et al: Systemic prostaglandin I_2 synthesis is normal in patients with Bartter's syndrome. Lancet II:368, 1983.
106. Jackson EK, Goodman RP: 6-keto-prostaglandin E_2 and Bartter's syndrome. N Engl J Med 305:287, 1981.
107. Seyberth HW, Müller H, Ulmer HE, et al: Urinary excretion rates of 6-keto-$PGF_{1\alpha}$ in preterm infants recovering from respiratory distress with and without patent ductus arteriosus. Ped Res 18:520, 1984.
108. Perico N, Schiepatti A, Mecca G, et al: Prostacyclin and renal diseases. Clin Nephrol 18:111, 1982.

16C Catecholamines

WOLFGANG RASCHER

INTRODUCTION

In 1897, Abel and Crawford identified the chemical structure of epinephrine, the pressor substance of the adrenal medulla. Shortly afterward similarities between the action of epinephrine and the effect of stimulating sympathetic nerves were noted; Loewi, as well as Cannon and Uridil, in 1921 demonstrated that a sympathomimetic substance was released on stimulation of the sympathetic nerves. The chemical nature of the sympathetic transmitter, norepinephrine, was described in 1946 by Euler.

The in vivo synthesis of epinephrine from phenylalanine proposed in 1939 and demonstrated in 1947 by radioactively labelled phenylalanine given to rats, appeared as labelled epinephrine recovered from the adrenal gland. Subsequently, precursors and metabolites of norepinephrine and the enzymes involved in its biosynthesis and metabolism have been identified. The function of sympathetic neurons are now well understood. This has greatly enhanced our understanding of the role of catecholamines in various disorders and our knowledge of a variety of drugs that affect the function of the sympathetic nervous system.

The characterization of alpha- and beta-adrenergic receptors has increased our understanding of the biological responses to catecholaminergic stimulation. Identifying adrenergic receptors directly by ligand-binding studies has improved the understanding of how cells change their responsiveness to catecholamines and how these changes are related to changes in cell function. Methods for determining apparent norepinephrine release rate and clearance from plasma have further improved our ability to assess sympathetic nervous function.

THE ADRENERGIC SYSTEM

Catecholamines are chemically defined as dihydroxylated phenolic amines. The most prominent members of this family are the synaptic transmitters, norepinephrine and dopamine, and the hormone, epinephrine (Fig. 16.9). Not all catecholamines act as sympathomimetics.

Catecholamine Biosynthesis

Catecholamine synthesis occurs in the brain, sympathetic nerve endings, and chromaffin tissue, including the adrenal medulla (1). Synthesis begins when the adrenergic neuron takes up tyrosine from the extracellular fluid (ECF) and transforms it into L-dihydroxyphenylalanine (L-Dopa) by tyrosine hydroxylase. Decarboxylation converts L-Dopa to dopamine, which is then taken up by intraneuronal storage granules. Both the storage vesicle and its membrane contain dopamine-beta-hydroxylase, an enzyme that converts dopamine to norepinephrine. In the adrenal medulla, norepinephrine is methylated to epinephrine by phenylethanolamine-N-methyl-transferase. Epinephrine is the major hormone of the adrenal medulla.

Norepinephrine Release

Norepinephrine is released by nerve stimulation from the intraneuronal storage sites into the synaptic cleft and into plasma. Influx of calcium into the granules mediates catecholamine release (1).

In blood vessels there is, as well, a continuous leak of norepinephrine from the storage vesicles into the neuroplasma which, under normal conditions, is deaminated intraneuronally, so that the concentration of

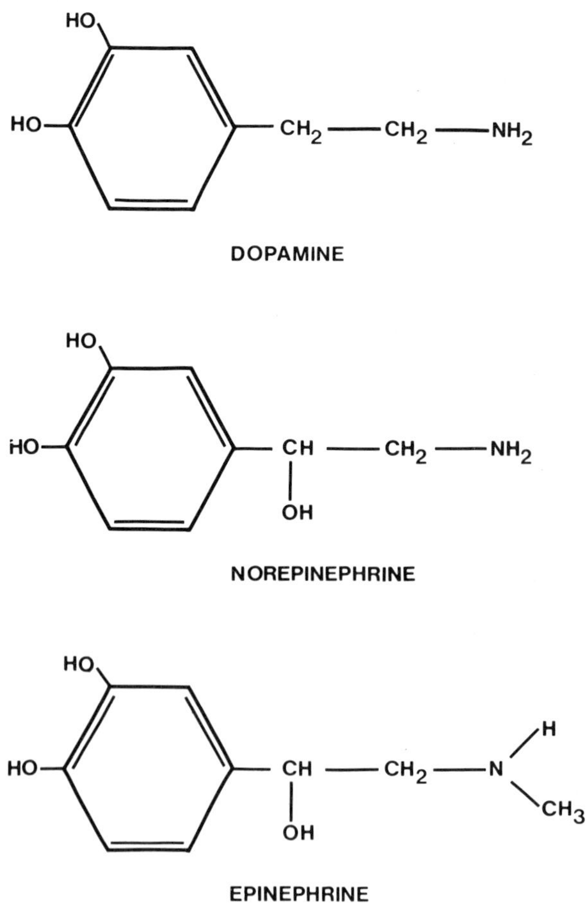

Figure 16.9. Chemical structure of the natural occurring catecholamines.

intact norepinephrine remains low. With nerve stimulation more norepinephrine is released, i.e., the storage by exocytosis along with other constituents of the storage vesicles (1).

Inactivation and Metabolism of Catecholamines

Most of the norepinephrine in the synaptic cleft, whether there by liberation from a vesicle or by reuptake into diffusion from the circulation, is inactivated by being taken up by the neuron and subsequently by the storage vesicle (2) (Fig. 16.10). The process of its uptake across the neuronal membrane is distinct from its accumulation into the storage vesicles. This active carrier system is linked to the sodium-potassium-ATPase. Inhibition of this neuronal uptake of norepinephrine augments and prolongs its effect. The carrier system is relatively nonspecific, i.e., it will transport most catecholamines into the neuron, which then are transported into the storage vesicles where they are bound by granules ready for later release.

Vascular smooth muscle cells take up a smaller fraction of norepinephrine from the synaptic cleft, which may be of little significance (Fig. 16.10) (3).

A small fraction of the catecholamines are inactivated by the enzymes monoaminoxidase (MAO) and catechol-O-methyltransferase (COMT). Both are widely distributed throughout the body; the highest concentrations are in the liver and the kidney. MAO is associated with mitochondria, including those within the adrenergic nerve terminals; COMT is in the soluble cytoplasma. Vascular smooth muscle cells take up a smaller fraction of norepinephrine into the cytoplasma, where it is converted to 3-methoxy-4-hydroxymandelic acid (VMA) (incorrectly called vanillylmandelic acid) or preferentially to 3-methoxy-4-hydroxyphenylglycol (MOPEG).

VMA is the major metabolite of catecholamines excreted into the urine. A smaller fraction of extraneuronal norepinephrine is deaminated to 3,4-dihydroxymandelic acid (DOMA) by MAO. Epinephrine metabolism overlaps considerably with that of norepinephrine, the major end-products for both compounds being MOPEG and VMA. 3-methoxy-4-hydroxyphenylacetic acid (homovanillic acid, HVA) is the major metabolite of dopamine.

Presynaptic Modulation of Norepinephrine Release

The quantity of norepinephrine liberated per unit of time from the nerve terminals depends on the activity of the nerve cells and the amount of norepinephrine released per impulse. The latter is modulated by substances at the presynaptic cell membrane, e.g., norepinephrine itself, prostaglandins, acetylcholine, and angiotensin-II.

In addition to the postsynaptic adrenergic receptors that mediate the effector organ responses there also are receptors located on the neuronal nerve terminals. Norepinephrine and other alpha-adrenergic agonists inhibit the release of new norepinephrine during nerve stimulation, whereas alpha-adrenergic antagonists enhance its stimulation-evoked release of the neurotransmitter (4). Thus, presynaptic inhibitory alpha-adrenergic receptors regulate norepinephrine release through a negative feedback mechanism mediated by itself (Fig. 16.11). These alpha-receptors differ in their relative sensitivity to various alpha-adrenergic agonists and antagonists. Therefore, a pharmacological classification of alpha-adrenergic receptors has come into use (5). The postsynaptic adrenergic receptor is called $alpha_1$; the presynaptic receptor is called $alpha_2$.

Stimulation of presynaptic $beta_2$ receptors augments the release of norepinephrine (6) in some, but not all, tissues (4, 7). This effect also occurs in blood vessels (8). Under physiological conditions, circulating epinephrine may have a greater role in this effect than locally released norepinephrine.

Prostaglandins of the E series inhibit release of norepinephrine (4, 7, 9). The prostaglandins that appear to originate from the postsynaptic nerve endings are stimulated by catecholamines (10), creating another negative feedback mechanism (9). Other substances, e.g., acetylcholine, dopamine, adenosine, histamine, serotonin, and enkephalin blunt the release of norepinephrine. However, the physiological significance of their action is not well established.

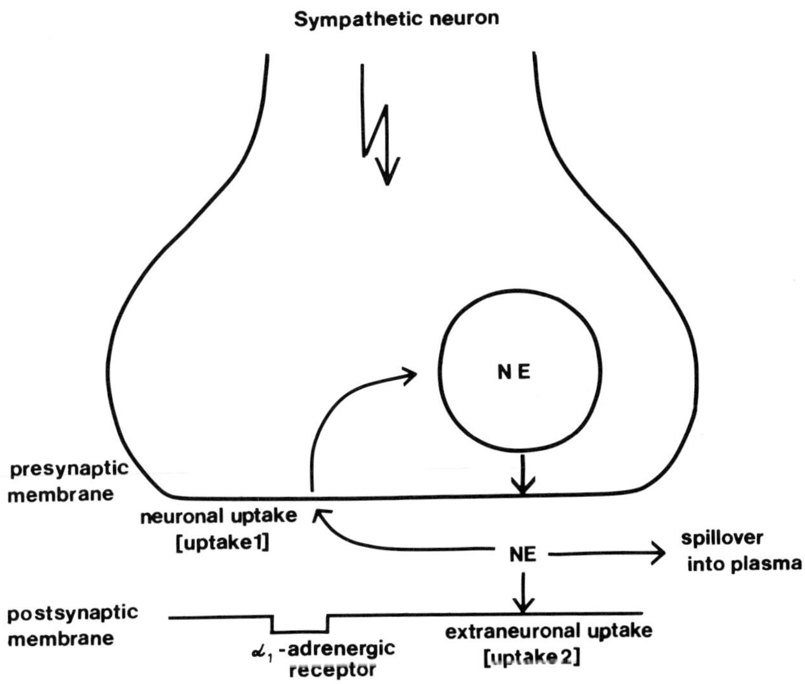

Figure 16.10. Schematic representation of the neuronal and extraneuronal uptake of norepinephrine (*NE*).

Angiotensin-II in physiological concentrations increases the release of norepinephrine by presynaptic stimulation (4, 11).

Release of Catecholamines from the Adrenal Medulla

Catecholamines are released in the adrenal medulla by exocytosis in response to cholinergic preganglionic sympathetic nerve stimulation. Both epinephrine and norepinephrine are released in response to a number of physiological stimuli, such as exercise, hypoxia, asphyxia, and hemorrhage. Insulin hypoglycemia causes a selective release of epinephrine, confirming the concept of a separate control of its release. Other agents that directly stimulate chromaffin cells and adrenergic neurons to release catecholamines include acetylcholine, histamine, nicotine, and serotonin.

PHYSIOLOGICAL ACTION

Adrenergic Receptors

Catecholamines exert their biological effects by interaction with specific receptor sites in various tissues. Norepinephrine, epinephrine, and other catecholamines cause either excitation or inhibition of smooth muscle, depending upon the site, the dose, and which catecholamine is acting. Norepinephrine is the most potent excitatory catecholamine, whereas isoproterenol is mainly inhibitory. Epinephrine is relatively potent as an excitor and as an inhibitor of smooth muscle. This classification of adrenergic receptors into alpha- and beta-receptors (12) is made by comparison of the rank order of potency of various agonists in several tissues (alpha: epinephrine > norepinephrine ≫ isoproterenol; beta: isoproterenol ≫ epinephrine > norepinephrine).

This classification has been extended so that alpha$_1$, alpha$_2$ receptors are now defined based on different sensitivities to specific agonists and antagonists (Table 16C.1). Their location is depicted in Table 16C.2 (4, 13, 14). Originally, alpha-receptors were classified anatomically as presynaptic (alpha$_2$) and postsynaptic (alpha$_1$). Postsynaptic receptors mediate vasoconstriction and presynaptic inhibit norepinephrine release. However, receptors with alpha$_2$ characteristics are located postsynaptically (15) and on nonneural tissue, such as platelets (16). Consequently, the pharmacological classification has replaced the anatomical one.

The naturally occurring catecholamines, epinephrine and norepinephrine, lack specificity for an alpha$_1$ and alpha$_2$ receptor. Similarly, beta-receptors are classified as beta$_1$ and beta$_2$ (13). Beta$_2$-receptors occur predominantly in blood vessels of skeletal muscle, in bronchial tissue and in the uterus, and stimulation dilates or relaxes these tissues. Beta$_1$-receptors are predominantly in the heart and their stimulation increases heart rate, contractility, conduction velocity, and decreases refractory period. The heart also contains beta$_2$-receptors so that beta selectivity is not absolute (17). Location and relative potency of agonists are shown in Table 16C.3.

Specific adrenergic receptors are identified in membrane preparations using radiolabelled adrenergic agonists and antagonists as ligands with high specificity and affinity for specific receptors (18, 19). These allow identification and quantification of these receptors in specific tissue preparations. Unfortunately, in clinical situations it is impossible to assay the appropriate target tissue and conclusions based on results using lymphocytes with beta-adrenergic receptors or platelets with alpha-receptors should be treated with caution. Information on biological effects should be accompanied by binding studies. In adrenergic tissue, assays of catecholamine stimulation—beta—or inhibition—alpha$_2$—of adenylatecyclase, are useful (16, 20); the second messenger for some responses to the catecholamines is cAMP.

The responses of tissues to catecholamines is modulated by hormones, e.g., glucocorticoids increase sensitivity to beta agonists. Steroids are given to mothers of potentially premature infants to prevent neonatal respiratory distress syndrome (21). They act to increase bronchial beta-adrenergic receptor response which, in turn, improves surfactant production. Glucocorticoids increase beta-adrenergic response of patients to bronchodilator therapy (22).

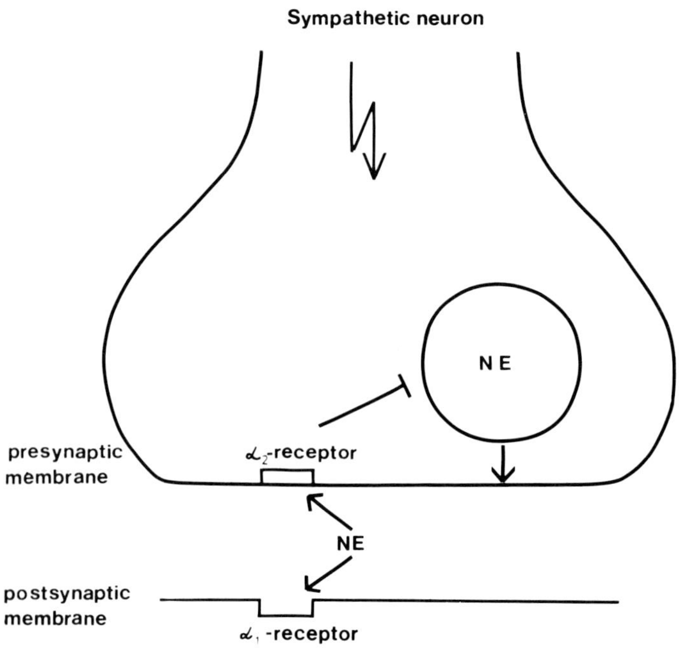

Figure 16.11. Schematic representation of presynaptic inhibition of norepinephrine (*NE*) release via alpha$_2$-adrenergic receptors.

Effect of Catecholamines on Renal Function

Renal Function

Renal adrenergic innervation regulates tubular sodium reabsorption independent of changes in renal hemodynamics (23, 24). Intrarenal

Table 16C.1.
Relative Order of Potency of Agonists and Antagonists for Alpha$_1$- and Alpha$_2$-Adrenergic Receptors

Receptors	Agonists	Antagonists
Alpha$_2$	Tramazoline > clonidine > alpha-methylnorepinephrine >	Rauwolscine > yohimbine > tolazoline >
Alpha$_2$ = alpha$_1$	Epinephrine > norepinephrine	Phentolamine >
	—	Phenoxybenzamine
Alpha$_1$	Phenylephrine > methoxamine	Prazosin

Table 16C.2.
Localization and Biological Action Mediated by Alpha$_1$- and Alpha$_2$-adrenergic Receptors

Receptor	Localization	Biological action
Alpha$_1$	Postsynaptic	Smooth muscle contraction; in central nervous system
Alpha$_2$	Presynaptic	Peripheral and central noradrenergic nerve endings (inhibition of norepinephrine release)
	Postsynaptic	Smooth muscle contraction; in the central nervous system (cardiovascular depression)
		Human fat cells (inhibition of lipolysis)
		Platelets (aggregation)

Table 16C.3.
Localization of Beta-adrenergic Receptors and the Relative Order of Potency of Various Beta-adrenergic Agonists

Localization		Relative order	
Receptor	Location	Receptor	Agonists
β_1	Heart	$\beta_1 > \beta_2$	Dobutamine, Prenalterol
β_2	Bronchial tissue		
	Peripheral blood vessels	$\beta_1 \geq \beta_2$	Orciprenaline
	Gravid uterus	$\beta_1 = \beta_2$	Isoprenaline
β_1, β_2	Central nervous system	$\beta_2 > \beta_1$	Salbutamol, Fenoterol, Terbutaline
β_2[a]	Metabolic receptors		

[a] Usually, but many unclassified.

infusion of norepinephrine causes renal vasoconstriction that is abolished by alpha-adrenergic blocking agents (25, 26). The effect of stimulating the renal nerve is the same as the effect of catecholamine infusion, i.e., RBF decreases (27). Stimulation of sympathetic nerve fibers at frequencies that do not alter renal blood flow still increases renal tubular sodium reabsorption by the proximal tubule (23), an effect to increase sodium reabsorption is independent of the effect on renal hemodynamics.

Renin Release

Renal nerve stimulation may increase renin release without altering GFR or RBF (29). Acute renal denervation decreases renin release and attenuates renin response to hemorrhage or acute volume depletion (30, 31). However, renin release in response to acute salt depletion or hypotensive hemorrhage occurs in the absence of sympathetic innervation (32); renin levels rise in patients with denervated transplanted kidneys in response to salt restriction (33). Thus, renal nerves and catecholamines influence renin release, but other mechanisms also are effective.

DRUGS AFFECTING THE CATECHOLAMINE SYSTEM

A variety of drugs interfere with the adrenergic nervous system, including various sympathomimetics, antihypertensive agents, and tricyclic antidepressants (Fig. 16.12).

Sympathomimetics

Sympathomimetics are classified as acting directly at the receptor (dopamine, epinephrine, norepinephrine, isoproterenol, and phenylephrine) or indirectly by causing a release of norepinephrine from storage granules at the nerve endings (amphetamine and tyramine).

Outside the central nervous system, dopamine acts both directly on beta$_1$-receptors of the heart and indirectly by releasing norepinephrine. In addition, dopamine acts directly on its receptors in the myocardium to increase contractility and cardiac output and in the renal and mesenteric vasculature causing vasodilation. Low doses (1 to 5 μg/kg/min) stimulate dopamine receptors, thus increasing RBF, GFR, and sodium excretion with little or no effect on cardiac output. Higher doses (5 to 10 μg/kg/min) have more pronounced beta-adrenergic stimulating effects, increasing myocardial contractility, stroke volume, and cardiac output. Higher infusion rates (10 to 20 μg/kg/min) produce alpha-adrenergic effects, with a rise in peripheral resistance and blood pressure and a fall in RBF.

Dobutamine

This synthetic derivative of isoproterenol acts directly on beta$_1$-receptors with a greater inotropic than chronotropic effect. It has little effect on peripheral vessels except when high doses are used and tachycardia and hypertension occur. Dobutamine does not interfere with dopamine receptors (34).

Clonidine

This drug enters the central nervous system and stimulates the alpha-adrenergic response in the medulla oblongata to decrease sympathetic outflow. Alpha methyldopa may act through a similar mechanism. The drug penetrates the blood-brain barrier and is metabolized in the neuron to methylnorepinephrine, which stimulates central alpha-adrenergic receptors (35).

Reserpine

This accumulates in the membrane of the storage granules and inhibits the uptake of norepinephrine and dopamine into the vesicle. By interfering with the function of the storage vesicle in the adrenergic neuron the content of norepinephrine is reduced in peripheral and central nerve endings, since cytoplasmatic norepinephrine is degraded by MAO. This action creates norepinephrine depletion in the nerve endings and a pharmacologic adrenergic blockade. Serotonin is also depleted from its storage sites by reserpine.

Guanethidine

This is an adrenergic-blocking agent with a selective action at the peripheral sympathetic nerve ending. The drug is actively transported by the amine pump into the adrenergic neuron where it binds to norepinephrine storage vesicles. Blockade of the uptake of norepinephrine into the neuron and storage vesicles leads to depletion of norepinephrine and inhibition of norepinephrine release on nerve stimulation. At the beginning of treatment, guanethidine also blocks the release of catecholamines by interfering with the action potential.

Assays for Catecholamines and Assessment of Adrenergic Function

In some diseases, such as pheochromocytoma and neuroblastoma, the measurement of catecholamines or their metabolites in urine or plasma is important in establishing the diagnosis. Catecholamines or their metabolites may have a role in many other pathological states, including thyrotoxicosis, myxedema, congestive heart failure, hypertension, and idiopathic orthostatic hypotension.

For clinical purposes, urinary catecholamine excretion can be mea-

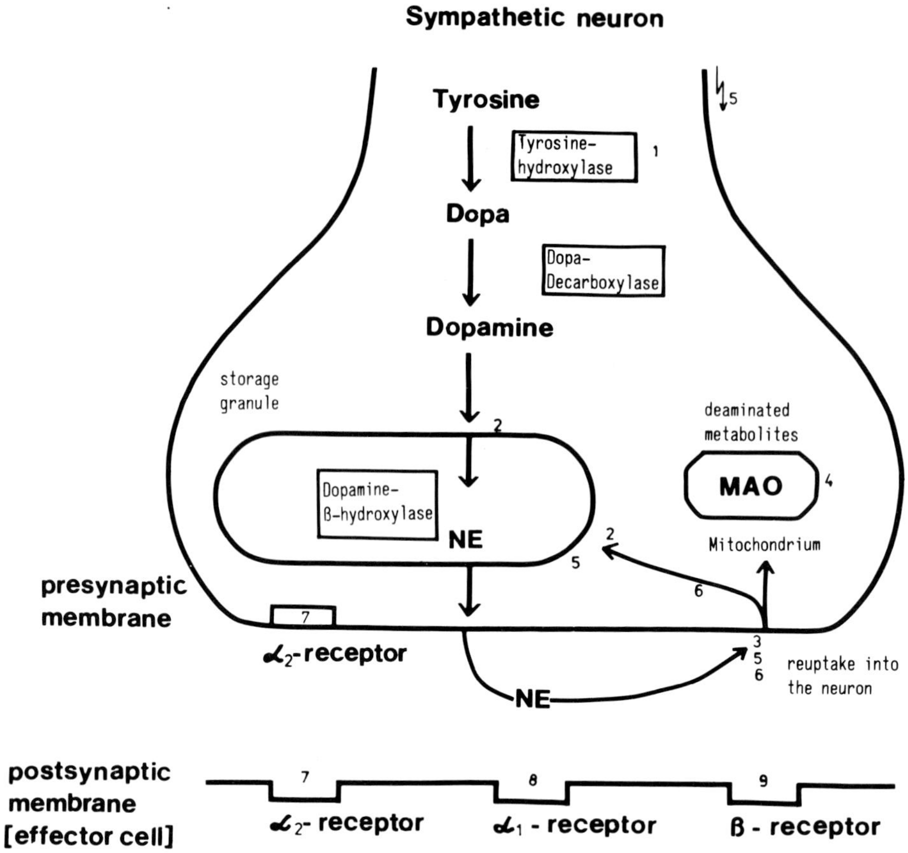

Figure 16.12. Proposed sites of action of drugs that modify synthesis, uptake, release, and action of norepinephrine (*NE*) at adrenergic nerve terminals. *1*, Inhibition of the rate limiting enzyme tyrosine hydroxylase by alpha-methyl-p-tyrosine; 2, Blockade of the active transport of dopamine and *NE* from the cytoplasma into the storage granules is thought to be the site of action of reserpine. The granules are depleted of NE and cytoplasmatic amines are deaminated by mitochondrial MAO; *3*, Blockade of active transport from the synaptic cleft to cytoplasma is thought to be the mechanism by which cocaine, imipramine, and chlorpromazine augments NE action on alpha and beta-adrenergic receptor sites; *4*, Inhibition of MAO, which leads to accumulation of the cytoplasmatic pool of *NE* is thought to be the action of tranylcypromine or nialamid; *5*, Blockade of the active transport of *NE* from the cytoplasma into the storage granule (reserpin-like) and from the synaptic cleft to cytoplasma (cocaine-like) is thought to be the action of guanethidine. Inhibition of the action potential by depolarization may explain why guanethidine exerts its initial effect on adrenergic activity before *NE* depletion; *6*, Displacement of NE from the mobile pool leading to sympathomimetic effects is thought to occur with tyramine and amphetamine (indirect sympathomimetic amines; *7*, Inhibitor of sympathetic outflow following stimulation of alpha$_2$-adrenergic receptors in the central nervous system (medulla oblongata) is thought to be the mechanism by which clonidine and alpha-methylnorepinephrine (from alpha-methyldopa) exerts its antihypertensive effect; *8*, Blockade of alpha$_1$-adrenergic receptor sites is the mechanism of action of prazosin; and *9*, Blockade of beta-adrenergic receptor sites is the mechanism of action of propranolol.

sured in 24-hour urine specimens using reliable fluorometric methods. In healthy children, free norepinephrine, epinephrine, and dopamine, as well as its metabolites, normetanephrine, metanephrine, VMA, and HVA, have been determined (36). Epinephrine and norepinephrine levels in 24-hour urine collections of newborns have been published (37). Therapy with alpha-methyldopa produces false negative elevation of urinary catecholamine excretion. It is also important to discontinue sympathomimetic agents and MAO inhibitors during urine sampling for catecholamine determination.

Reliable measurements of catecholamines in plasma require highly specific radioenzymatic assay procedures (38, 39). Plasma measurements of catecholamines are important in establishing the diagnosis of pheochromocytoma (40). Plasma norepinephrine concentration represents the spillover of norepinephrine into the plasma after release from sympathetic nerves. Assay methods assess the rate of entry of norepinephrine into plasma (norepinephrine apparent release rate) and norepinephrine clearance from plasma. This method requires infusion of tritiated L-norepinephrine with high specific activity (41). Vascular response to catecholamines can be assessed by infusion of norepinephrine (42, 43).

References

1. Axelrod J, Weinshilboum R: Catecholamines. N Engl J Med 287:237, 1972.
2. Trendelenburg U: Factors influencing the concentration of catecholamines at the receptors. In Blaschko H, Muscholl E (eds): Handbook of Experimental Pharmacology. Berlin, Springer, 1972, vol 33, p 726.
3. Vanhoutte PM: Adrenergic neuroeffector interaction in the blood vessel wall. Fed Proc 37:181, 1978.
4. Starke K: Regulation of noradrenaline release by presynaptic receptor systems. Rev Physiol Biochem Pharmacol 77:1, 1977.
5. Starke K, Langer SZ: A note on terminology for presynaptic receptors. In Langer SZ, Starke K, Dubocovich ML (eds): Presynaptic Receptors. Oxford, Pergamon Press, 1979, p 1.
6. Yamaguchi N, De Champlain J, Nadeau RA: Regulation of norepinephrine release from cardiac sympathetic fibers in the dog by presynaptic alpha- and beta-receptors. Circ Res 41:108, 1977.
7. Westfall TC: Local regulation of adrenergic neurotransmission. Physiol Rev 57:659, 1977.
8. Stjärne L, Brundin J: Beta$_2$-adrenoceptor facilitating noradrenaline secretion from human vasocontrictor nerves. Acta Physiol Scand 97:88, 1976.
9. Hedquist P: Modulating effect of prostaglandin E_2 on noradrenaline release from isolated cat spleen. Acta Physiol Scand 75:511, 1969.
10. Needleman P, Douglas JR, Jakschick B, et al: Release of renal prostaglandin by

catecholamines: relationship to renal endocrine function. J Pharmacol Exp Ther 188:453, 1974.
11. Zimmermann BG, Gomer SK, Liao JC: Action of angiotensin on vascular adrenergic nerve endings: facilitation of norepinephrine release. Fed Proc 31:1344, 1972.
12. Ahlquist PR: A study of adrenotropic receptors. Am J Physiol 153:586, 1948.
13. Lands AM, Arnold A, McAuliff JP, et al: Differentiation of receptor systems activated by sympathomimetic amines. Nature 214:597–598.
14. Berthelson S, Pettinger WA: A functional basis for classification of alpha-adrenergic receptors. Life Sci 21:595, 1977.
15. Langer SZ, Shepperson NB, Massingham R: Preferential noradrenergic innervation of alpha-adrenergic receptors in vascular smooth muscle. Hypertension 3 (suppl I):I112, 1981.
16. Lasch P, Jakobs KH: Agonistic and antagonistic effects of various alpha-adrenergic agonists in human platelets. Naunyn-Schmiedeberg's Arch Pharmacol 306:119, 1979.
17. Carlsson E, Ablad B, Brädström A, et al: Differentiated blockade of the chronotropic effects of various adrenergic stimuli in the cat heart. Life Sci 11:953, 1972.
18. Lefkowitz RJ: Direct binding studies on adrenergic receptors: biochemical, physiologic and clinical implications. Ann Intern Med 91:450, 1979.
19. Nahorski SR, Barnett DB: Biochemical assessment of adrenoceptor function and regulation: new directions and clinical relevance. Clin Sci 63:97, 1982.
20. Maguire ME, Ross EM, Gilman AG: β-adrenergic receptors: ligand binding properties and the interaction with adenylcyclase. Adv Cyc Nucleo Res 8:1, 1977.
21. Liggins GL, Howie RN: A controlled trial of antepartum glucocorticoid treatment for prevention of the respiratory distress syndrome in premature infants. Pediatr 50:515, 1972.
22. Holgate S, Baldwin GJ, Tattersfield AE: β-adrenergic agonist resistance in normal human airways. Lancet 2:375, 1977.
23. DiBona GF: Neurogenic regulation of renal tubular sodium reabsorption. Am J Physiol 233:F73, 1977.
24. Gottschalk W: Renal nerves and sodium excretion. Ann Rev Physiol 41:229, 1979.
25. Pomeranz BH, Birtch AG, Barger AC: Neural control of intrarenal blood flow. Am J Physiol 215:1067, 1968
26. Schrier RW: Effect of adrenergic nervous system and catecholamines on systemic and renal hemodynamics, sodium and water excretion and renin secretion. Kidney Intl 6:291, 1974.
27. DiSalvo J, Fell C: Changes in renal blood flow during renal nerve stimulation. Proc Soc Exp Biol Med 136:150, 1971.
28. Kim JK, Stuart LL, Schrier RW: Cathecholamines and sodium transport in the kidney. Pharmacol Rev 31:169, 1980.
29. Torretti J: Sympathetic control of renin release. Ann Rev Pharmacol Toxicol 22:167, 1982.
30. Zanchetti A, Stella A: Neural control of renin release. Clin Sci Mol Med 48:215S, 1975.
31. Gotshall RW, Davis JO, Shade RE, et al: Effect of renal denervation on renin release in sodium-depleted dogs. Am J Physiol 225:344, 1973.
32. Davis JO: The control of renin release. Am J Med 55:333, 1973.
33. Blaufox MD, Lewis EJ, Jagger P, et al: Physiologic responses to the transplanted human kidney. N Engl J Med 280:62, 1969.
34. Sonnenblick EH, Frishman WH, LeJemtel TH: Dobutamine: a synthetic cardioactive sympathetic amine. N Engl J Med 300: 17, 1979.
35. Kobinger W: Central alpha-adrenergic systems as targets for hypotensive drugs. Rev Physiol Biochem Pharmacol 81:39, 1978.
36. Schaepdryver AF, Hooft C, Delbeke MJ, et al: Urinary catecholamines and metabolites in children. J Pediatr 93:266, 1978.
37. Nakai T, Yamada R: Urinary catecholamine excretion by various age groups with special reference to clinical value of measuring catecholamines in newborns. Pediatr Res 17:456, 1983.
38. DaPrada M, Zürcher G: Simultaneous radioenzymatic determination of plasma and tissue adrenaline, noradrenaline and dopamine within the femtomole range. Life Sci 19:1161, 1976.
39. Kopin IJ: Plasma levels of norepinephrine. Ann Intern Med 88:671, 1978.
40. Bravo EL, Tarazi RC, Gifford RW, et al: Circulating and urinary catecholamines in pheochromocytoma. N Engl J Med 301:682, 1979.
41. Esler M: Assessment of sympathetic nervous function in humans from noradrenaline plasma kinetics. Clin Sci 62:247, 1982.
42. Rascher W, Schömig A, Kreye VA, et al: Diminished vascular response to norepinephrine in experimental chronic uremia. Kidney Int 21:20, 1982.
43. Skrabal F, Auböck J, Hörtnagl H: Low sodium/high potassium diet for prevention of hypertension: probable mechanisms of action. Lancet 2:895, 1981.

16D Arginine-vasopressin (Antidiuretic Hormone)

WOLFGANG RASCHER

INTRODUCTION

In 1895, Oliver and Schafer reported pressor effects of pituitary extracts; 3 years later Howell demonstrated that the pressor principle arose from the posterior lobe of the pituitary, which later was called vasopressin.

The antidiuretic action of posterior pituitary extracts was described in 1913 by von den Velden in Germany and Farini in Italy, who demonstrated that administration of these extracts to patients with diabetes insipidus decreased urine flow and increased urine osmolality. These followed the description of secretory granules in the neurons of the supraoptic and paraventricular nuclei of the hypothalamus and the synthesis of arginine vasopressin.

The most obvious physiological role for vasopressin was its antidiuretic action. Cardiovascular effects of vasopressin were elicited only by pharmacological doses many times those required for antidiuretic activity. Therefore, vasopressin, the official USP designation was called antidiuretic hormone (ADH). However, in the last few years there is renewed interest in the cardiovascular action of vasopressin and its control of

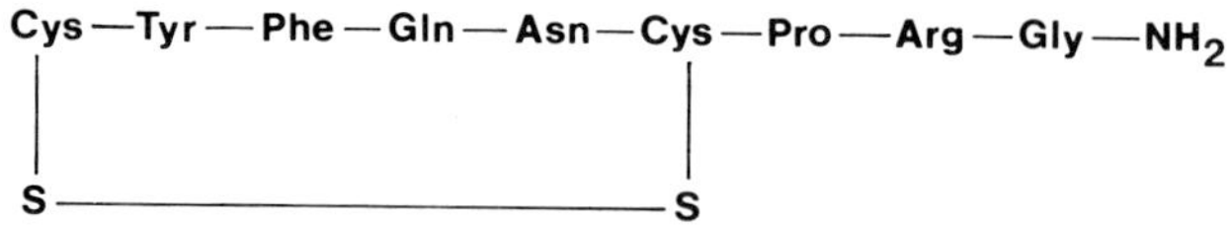

Figure 16.13. Arginine-vasopressin (AVP).

blood pressure. Vasopressin has a vasoactive function at physiological concentrations. Specific antagonists to its vasoconstrictor activity has aided in characterizing its cardiovascular effects (1, 2).

THE VASOPRESSIN SYSTEM

Arginine-vasopressin, a nonapeptide, and neurophysin-II (Fig. 16.13) are synthesized in magnocellular neurons of the supraoptic and paraventricular nuclei of the hypothalamus together (3). Neurophysin-II and vasopressin are produced as a part of a common precursor molecule packaged into secretory granules and transported via the axon to the nerve endings located in the posterior lobe of the pituitary body—the neurohypophysis. The amino acid sequence of bovine vasopressin-neurophysin-II precursor has now been deduced from cDNA prepared from hypothalamic mRNA (4). Arginine-vasopressin occurs in all mammals except the swine, in which lysine replaces arginine. Vasopressin is released into the circulation by an exocytotic process in response to osmotic and nonosmotic stimuli (5, 6). Osmoreceptors are located in the anterior part of the hypothalamus, adjacent to the supraoptic and paraventricular nuclei. Nonosmotic release of vasopressin is affected by catecholamines, acetylcholine, angiotensin-II, opioid peptides, prostaglandins, and calcium (7, 8).

Volume depletion is the other major stimulus for vasopressin release. During hypovolemia, vasopressin secretion is mediated via arterial stretch receptors, cardiac mechanoreceptors with vagal afferent limbs, and arterial baroreceptors (7, 8). Small changes in left atrial pressure stimulate secretion of vasopressin; a large decrease in blood volume or a fall in arterial blood pressure of 10 to 20 mm Hg initiates a strong stimulus for vasopressin release via the baroreceptors in the aortic arch and carotid sinus. Osmotic release of vasopressin is modulated by changes in blood volume (9–11). Contraction of blood volume enhances the sensitivity of the osmoreceptor and blood volume expansion blunts its sensitivity. During pregnancy, the threshold for vasopressin secretion is reset (12). Animal experiments suggest a pulsatile pattern of vasopressin release after osmotic stimulation (13).

Plasma vasopressin levels in normally hydrated adults, as measured by sensitive radioimmunoassays (RIA), averages 4.3 ± 0.4 pg/ml (7); in children age 1 to 18, the average is 3.3 ± 0.23 pg/ml (14). Above 1 year there is no correlation with age. In 19 infants between 1 and 12 months old plasma vasopressin levels average 5.0 ± 0.7 pg/ml, whereas newborns <1 month have higher values 8.6 ± 0.7 pg/ml, n = 62. No differences are noted between mature and premature newborns. Vaginal delivery is associated with a massive stimulation of vasopressin release (15, 16), probably secondary to increases in intracranial pressure (17).

After 12 and 24 hours of restricted water intake in adults, plasma concentration of vasopressin rises to an average of 16.0 ± 2.0 pg/ml (7). Giving water—20 ml/kg—results in suppression of plasma vasopressin to 1.5 ± 0.5 pg/ml. The relationship between plasma osmolality and vasopressin levels in children (Fig. 16.14) parallels that reported in adults. Daily plasma vasopressin levels range between 0.5 and 30 pg/ml in response to changes in the state of hydration. Stress hypotension, blood loss, pain, vomiting, or hypoxia cause vasopressin levels to increase far beyond this range to between 50 and 600 pg/ml. Pain increases plasma levels in adults (18), but not in infants (19).

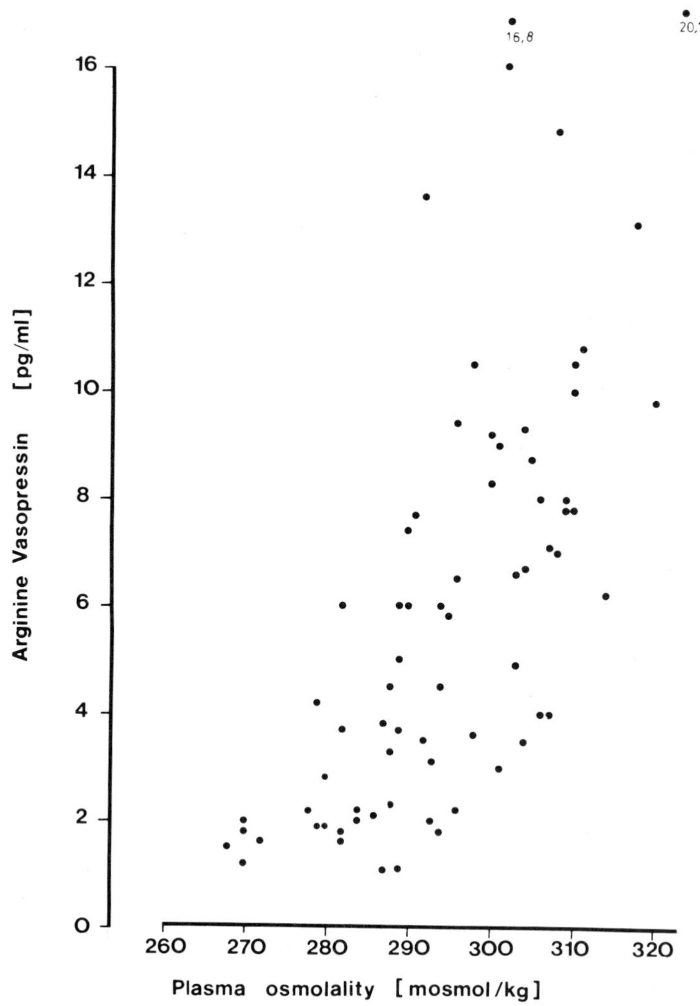

Figure 16.14. Relationship between plasma arginine-vasopressin and plasma osmolality in children older than 2 years. (From Rascher W, et al: Acta Paediatr Scand 75:111, 1986.

PHYSIOLOGICAL ACTION

Antidiuretic Effect

Vasopressin is responsible for the water homeostasis and the regulation of the osmolality of body fluids and of sodium concentration in the ECF (20). Its antidiuretic action is mediated by binding to a specific receptor located at the serosal or blood site of the collecting duct in the kidney. The hormone activates adenyl cyclase to form cAMP (21). The sequence of events after generation of cAMP is not fully understood but the tubular basement membrane of the collecting tubules become more permeable to water (22, 23).

The specific structural change in response to vasopressin is in intramembranous particle clusters in the collecting duct luminal membrane (24).

Hemodynamic Effects

In vascular tissue, vasopressin elicits a potent vasoconstrictor action after binding to a specific receptor. Stimulation of this receptor does not modify intracellular cAMP content (25). In physiological concentrations—1 to 2 pg/ml—vasopressin constricts arterioles of mesenteric vessels in the rat (26). High doses of vasopressin are necessary to increase

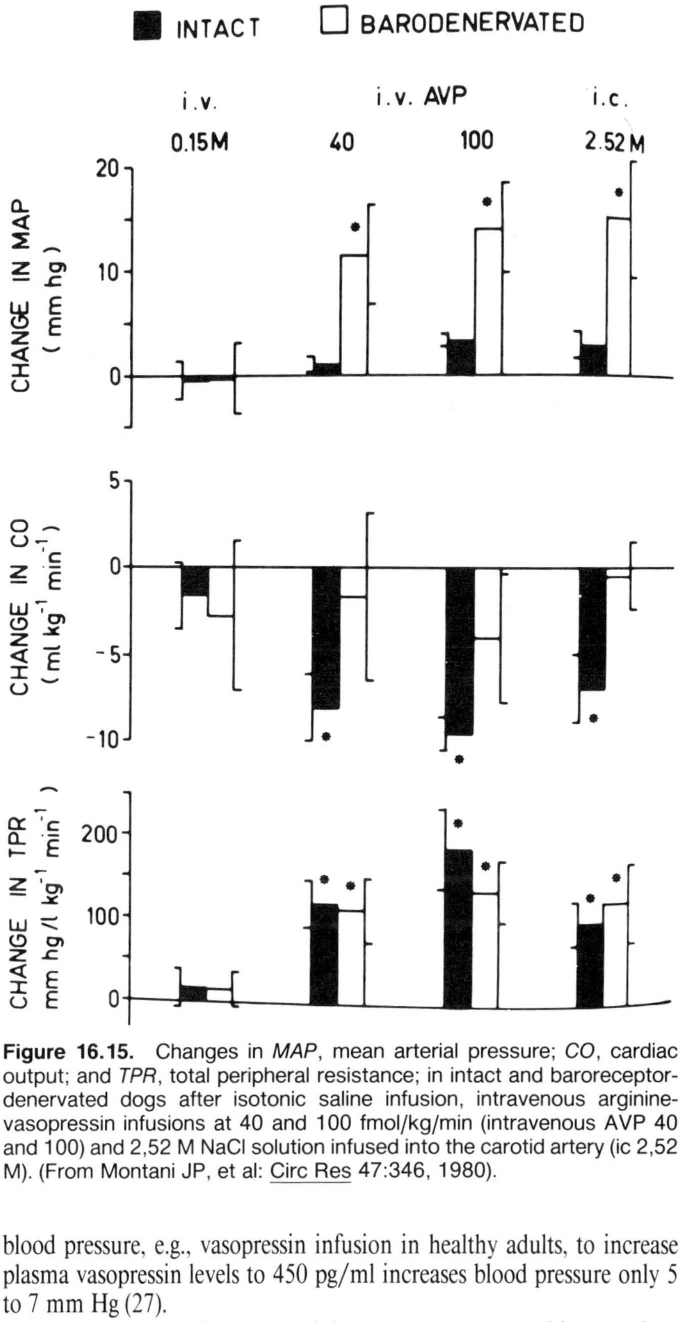

Figure 16.15. Changes in *MAP*, mean arterial pressure; *CO*, cardiac output; and *TPR*, total peripheral resistance; in intact and baroreceptor-denervated dogs after isotonic saline infusion, intravenous arginine-vasopressin infusions at 40 and 100 fmol/kg/min (intravenous AVP 40 and 100) and 2,52 M NaCl solution infused into the carotid artery (ic 2,52 M). (From Montani JP, et al: Circ Res 47:346, 1980).

blood pressure, e.g., vasopressin infusion in healthy adults, to increase plasma vasopressin levels to 450 pg/ml increases blood pressure only 5 to 7 mm Hg (27).

Despite the lack of pressor activity under normal conditions, peripheral vascular resistance in animals is significantly increased by small amounts of vasopressin in dogs and rats (28, 29). In both normal and baroreceptor-denervated dogs, total peripheral resistance rises nearly 20% from control with infusion of vasopressin to plasma levels that are <20 pg/ml. Blood pressure, however, is elevated only in the baroreceptor-denervated dogs; in intact animals, cardiac output falls instead (28) (Fig. 16.15). Vasopressin released in response to hypertonic saline produces an increase in total peripheral resistance, but does not affect arterial blood pressure, since blood pressure effects are buffered by the baroreceptor reflex mechanism (7, 28).

There are two conditions where hemodynamic effects become clinically important. One is orthostatic hypotension associated with autonomic dysfunction, called the Shy-Drager syndrome. Small doses of vasopressin to increase plasma levels between 5 to 10 pg/ml cause a rise in blood pressure (27, 30). In newborns vasopressin appears to be a significant factor in controlling blood pressure after delivery, since large amounts of vasopressin are released into the circulation; this appears to have a role in the fetal and neonatal hemodynamic response to delivery (16). Increased levels of cord plasma vasopressin in sheep fetuses are associated with severe intrauterine stress (31).

Intravenous infusion of vasopressin into fetal lambs results in a redistribution of blood flow from the gastrointestinal and peripheral circulation to the uteroplacental, myocardial, and cerebral circulation in the fetus. Since cardiovascular response to vasopressin infusion is similar to that observed during fetal hypoxia, it is suggested that vasopressin plays an important role in fetal cardiovascular response to stress, such as hypoxia (32) (see also Chapter 54).

Effects on Renal Circulation

Regional vascular beds possess different sensitivities to vasopressin. Iliac and mesenteric blood flow is sensitive, whereas RBF is minimally affected (33, 34). Moderate amounts of vasopressin do not change RBF, although it does cause a transient rise in blood pressure (35); large doses decrease RBF and low doses may actually increase it (33, 36). Maximal antidiuretic effect of vasopressin is achieved at concentrations far below those that cause renal vasoconstriction. Vasopressin in physiological doses increases GFR slightly without altering RBF (35, 37, 38), but the mechanisms responsible for the rise in GFR have not been determined. The effect of vasopressin on the distribution of RBF away from the vasa recta is disputed (39–41). A decrease of medullary blood flow would prevent dissipation of the osmotic gradient established by the countercurrent mechanism, important for the renal concentrating mechanism (39); but, in some studies this effect was not observed (40, 41).

Effects on Blood Pressure

Vasopressin at physiological plasma concentrations is a potent vasoconstrictor of mesenteric and skeletal vasculature and is one of the determinants of tissue perfusion.

Vasopressin effects on blood pressure are hardly reached under physiological conditions, since the pressor effects are greatly countered by cardiovascular reflex regulation. This counter effect to reduce cardiac output is negated in certain forms of autonomic dysfunction and in deep anesthesia.

Vasopressin levels are high during hemorrhage and have an important role in maintaining blood pressure under this condition. The rapid recovery of arterial blood pressure following hemorrhage in dogs is the result of vasopressin secretion (42). In hypovolemic states in dogs, vasopressin release is a short-term control system. It responds more rapidly (3 to 5 minutes) than the renin-angiotensin system (15 to 20 minutes), but less rapidly than the baroreceptor reflex control system, which requires only 20 seconds to achieve maximal pressor response (7). Since vasopressin is a potent vasoconstrictor agent, it has been implicated in the pathogenesis of hypertension, but its role in human hypertension is poorly defined (7, 8).

INTERACTION WITH NEURAL AND OTHER HUMORAL SYSTEMS

The counter effects of vasopressin and the baroreceptor reflex system on blood pressure have been cited in the preceding section. By contrast, small doses of vasopressin enhance vasoconstriction induced by catecholamines by sensitizing adrenergic receptor sites to the effect of adrenergic agonists (43, 44).

Catecholamines alter vasopressin release. Alpha-adrenergic stimulation enhances solute-free water excretion by suppressing vasopressin release via the baroreceptor reflex mechanisms, whereas beta-adrenergic stimulation increases vasopressin release and causes an antidiuretic response (6). Vasopressin and angiotensin-II are important mesenteric vasoconstricting agents seen with hemorrhage or hypovolemia (45, 46).

DRUGS AFFECTING THE VASOPRESSIN SYSTEM

A variety of analogues of vasopressin have different vasoconstrictor or antidiuretic activities. Substituting phenylalanine at position 2, isoleucine at position 3, or ornithine at position 8 decreases antidiuretic and enhances vasopressor activity. These substitutions have additive effects, i.e., 2-phenylalanine, 3-isoleucine, or 8-ornithine; vasotocin is the most specific vasopressor analogue known (1). Other analogues are useful as local hemostatic agents, particularly for control of esophageal bleeding.

Deamino-8-D-arginine vasopressin (DDAVP, desmopressin) is an analogue having potent and prolonged antidiuretic activity without significant cardiovascular effects (1, 2). DDAVP is now the preferred drug in treating of vasopressin-deficient diabetes insipidus. The synthesis of specific and potent antagonists of the vasoconstrictor (1, 2) or the antidiuretic activity (47, 48) of vasopressin have been reported. In the future, the antidiuretic antagonists might become useful for the treatment of hyponatremia and water retention secondary to inappropriate secretion of ADH (49).

Drugs affecting release or action of vasopressin mainly affect water homeostasis. Data on hemodynamic consequences in response to drug-induced vasopressin release are lacking. Drugs that increase vasopressin release include morphine, nicotine, clofibrate, and vincristine (50). Enhanced antidiuretic action is induced by chlorpropramide and carbamazepine.

ASSESSMENT OF VASOPRESSIN FUNCTION

Vasopressin in plasma is measured by specific and sensitive RIA procedures. Newly developed assays with appropriately documented specificity, reproducibility, and sensitivity are available. Measurements of plasma vasopressin in combination with standard stimulation tests can improve the diagnosis of disturbed vasopressin regulation and the accuracy in the differential diagnosis of polyuria (51).

Water-Deprivation Test

The water-deprivation test measures the response to deprivation of water. The following procedure is suggested: the patient is put on complete fluid restriction until 3% to 4% of body weight is lost and urine osmolality reaches a plateau. In patients with normal urine volume, this usually takes 14 to 18 hours, in polyuric patients 5 to 7 hours. Body weight and urine osmolality should be monitored at 1- to 3-hour intervals, depending on anticipated response. At the beginning and the end of the period of water restriction, blood should be drawn for measuring plasma vasopressin, serum sodium concentration, and serial urine samples measured for osmolality. Prolonged dehydration must be avoided. Patients suspected of having significant polyuria should be studied only when close supervision is possible, so that weight loss does not exceed 3% of body weight.

Hypertonic Saline Infusion Test

This study measures the acute response to the release of vasopressin in response to intravenous infusion of hypertonic saline solution. A 5% NaCl solution is infused intravenously for 2 hours at a rate of 0.04 to 0.05 ml/kg/min; blood samples for determinations of plasma osmolality and vasopressin are obtained at 30-minute intervals from a second intravenous line (51, 52). Results are evaluated by plotting plasma vasopressin as a function of concurrent plasma osmolality on the nomogram (Fig. 16.14).

Nonosmotic Vasopressin Release

Several procedures stimulate nonosmotic release of vasopressin, e.g., injecting nicotine or apomorphine (53), as well as body tilting from the horizontal to a partially upright position (54). In children, oral administration of syrup of ipecac to induce the emetic reflex has been used (55). Defects in nonosmotic vasopressin release can be differentiated from those in osmotically induced vasopressin release by these tests (55, 56).

Vasopressin Test

The response of the kidney to concentrate urine can be tested by giving vasopressin. Aqueous vasopressin, 1 u/m^2 is injected intramuscularly, and urine osmolality is monitored at hourly intervals for 3 hours. To avoid hemodynamic effects of vasopressin, DDAVP can be used instead of lysine or arginine vasopressin. DDAVP is administered intranasally in a dose of 10 μg in infants and 20 μg in children (57). Since DDAVP has a prolonged action on the kidney, fluid intake has to be restricted for 12 hours after giving DDAVP to avoid the possibility of water intoxication; some authors recommend giving vasopressin in combination with the water deprivation test.

Urinary vasopressin excretion can be measured reliably by RIA and may help to investigate the role of vasopressin in disturbed salt and water balance. Urinary vasopressin excretion rates in healthy children from birth to adolescence have been reported (58).

References

1. Manning M, Gzronka Z, Sawyer WH: Synthesis of posterior pituitary hormones and hormone analogues. In Bearwell C, Robinson G (eds): The Pituitary. Kent, England, Butterworths, 1981, p 265.
2. Sawyer WH, Grzonka Z, Manning M: Neurohypophyseal peptides: Design of tissue-specific agonists and antagonists. Mol Cell Endocrinol 22:117, 1981.
3. Walter R: Neurophysins: carriers of peptide hormones. Ann NY Acad Sci 248:1, 1975.
4. Land H, Schütz G, Schmale H: Nucleotide sequence of cloned cDNA encoding bovine arginine vasopressin-neurophysin II precursor. Nature 295:299, 1982.
5. Robertson GL: The regulation of vasopressin function in health and disease. Rec Prog Horm Res 33:333, 1977.
6. Schrier RW, Berl T, Anderson RJ: Osmotic and nonosmotic of vasopressin release. Am J Physiol 236:F321, 1979.
7. Cowley AC: Vasopressin and cardiovascular regulation. In Guyton AC, Hall JE (eds): Cardiovascular Physiology IV, International Review of Physiology. Baltimore, University Park Press, 1982, p. 89.
8. Rascher W, Lang RE, Unger Th: Vasopressin, cardiovascular regulation and hypertension. In Ganten D, Pfaff D (eds): Current Topics in Neuroendocrinology. Heidelberg, Berlin, New York, Springer, Vol 4, 1985, p. 101.
9. Dunn FJ, Brennan TJ, Nelson AE, et al: The role of blood osmolality and volume in regulating vasopressin secretion in the rat. J Clin Invest 52:3212, 1973.
10. Robertson GL, Athar S: The interaction of blood osmolality and blood volume in regulation plasma vasopressin in man. J Endocrinol Metab 42:613, 1976.
11. Quillen EW, Cowley AW: Influence of volume changes on osmolality—vasopressin relationship in conscious dogs. Am J Physiol 244:H73, 1983.
12. Dürr JA, Stamoutsos B, Lindheimer MD: Osmoregulation during pregnancy in the rat. J Clin Invest 68:337, 1981.
13. Weitzman RE, Fisher DA, Di Stefano JJ, et al: Episodic secretion of arginine vasopressin. Am J Physiol 233:E32, 1977.
14. Rascher W, Rauh W, Brandeis WE, et al: Determinants of plasma arginine-vasopressin in children. Acta Paediatr Scand 75:111, 1986.
15. Polin RW, Husain MK, James LS, et al: High vasopressin concentrations in human umbilical cord blood—lack of correlation with stress. J Perin Med 5:114, 1977.
16. Pohjavuori M, Fyhrquist F: Hemodynamic significance of vasopressin in the newborn infant. J Pediatr 97:462, 1980.
17. Hadeed AJ, Leake RD, Weitzman RE, et al: Possible mechanisms of high blood levels of vasopressin during neonatal period. J Pediatr 94:805, 1979.
18. Kentler KS, Weitzman RE, Fisher DA: The effect of pain on plasma vasopressin concentrations in man. Clin Endocrinol 8:89, 1978.

19. Waters CB, Weinberg JE, Leake RD, et al: Arginine vasopressin levels during a painful stimulus in infancy. Pediatr Res 16:569, 1982.
20. Young DB, Pan YJ, Guyton AC: Control of extracellular sodium concentration by antidiuretic hormone-thirst feedback mechanism. Am J Physiol 232:R145, 1977.
21. Dousa TP, Valtin H: Cellular actions of vasopressin in the mammalian kidney. Kidney Intl 10:46, 1976.
22. Gluck S, Al-Awqati Q: Vasopressin increases water permeability by inducing pores. Nature 284:631, 1980.
23. Morel F: Sites of hormone action in the mammalian nephron. Am J Physiol 240:F159, 1981.
24. Harmanci MC, Stern P, Kackadorian WA, et al: Vasopressin and collecting duct intramembranous particle clusters: a dose-response relationship. Am J Physiol 239:F560, 1980.
25. Penit J, Faure M, Jard S: Vasopressin and angiotensin II receptors in rat aortic smooth muscle in culture. Am J Physiol 244:E72, 1983.
26. Altura BM, Alture BT: Vascular smooth muscle and neurohypophyseal hormones. Fed Proc 36:1853, 1977.
27. Möhring J, Glänzer K, Maciel JA Jr et al: Greatly enhanced pressor response to antidiuretic hormone in patients with impaired cardiovascular reflexes due to idiopathic orthostatic hypotension. J Cardiovasc Pharmacol 2:367, 1980.
28. Montani JP, Liard JF, Schoun J, et al: Hemodynamic effects of exogenous and endogenous vasopressin at low plasma concentration in conscious dogs. Circ Res 47:346, 1980.
29. Rascher W, Lang RE, Ganten D, et al: Vasopressin in deoxycorticosterone acetate hypertension of rats: a hemodynamic analysis. J Cardiovasc Pharmacol 5:418, 1983.
30. Wagner HN, Brainwald E: The pressor effect of the antidiuretic principle of the posterior pituitary in orthostatic hypotension. J Clin Invest 35:1412, 1956.
31. De Vane GW, Naden RP, Porter JC, et al: Mechanism of arginine vasopressin release in the sheep fetus. Pediatr Res 16:504, 1982.
32. Iwamoto HS, Rudolph AM, Keil LC, et al: Hemodynamic responses to the sheep fetus to vasopressin infusion. Circ Res 44:430, 1979.
33. Schmid PG, Abboud FM, Wendling MG, et al: Regional vascular effects of vasopressin: plasma levels and circulatory responses. Am J Physiol 227:998, 1974.
34. Heyndrickx G, Boettcher D, Vatner S: Effects of angiotensin, vasopressin and methoxamine on cardiac function and blood flow distribution in conscious dogs. Am J Physiol 231:1579, 1976.
35. Smith MK, Cowley AW, Guyton AC, et al: Acute and chronic effects of vasopressin on blood pressure, electrolytes and fluid volumes. Am J Physiol 237:F232, 1979.
36. Fejes-Toth G, Magyar A, Walter J: Renal response to vasopressin after inhibition of prostaglandin synthesis. Am J Physiol 232:F416, 1977.
37. Yesberg NE, Henderson M, Budtz-Olsen OE: The effects of two analogues of arginine-vasopressin (ornithine-vasopressin and deamino-D-arginine-vasopressin) on kidney function in sheep. Q J Exp Physiol 63:179, 1978.
38. Yesberg NE, Henderson M, Budtz-Olsen OE: Inhibition by angiotensin II of some vasopressin effects on renal function in sheep. Q J Exp Physiol 64:161, 1979.
39. Thurau K, Levine DZ: The renal circulation. In Rouiller C, Miller AF (eds): The Kidney. New York, Academic Press, 1971, vol III, p 1.
40. Aukland K: Vasopressin and intrarenal blood flow distribution. Acta Physiol Scand 74:173, 1968.
41. Fisher RD, Grünfeld JP, Barger AC: Intrarenal distribution of blood flow in diabetes insipidus: role of ADH. Am J Physiol 219:1348, 1970.
42. Cowley AW, Switzer SJ, Guinn MM: Evidence and quantification of the vasopressin arterial pressure control system in the dog. Circ Res 46:58, 1980.
43. Bartelstone HJ, Nasmyth PA: Vasopressin potentiation of catecholamine actions in dog, rat, cat and rat aortic strip. Am J Physiol 208:754, 1965.
44. Erker EF, Chan WY: The site and mechanism of phenoxybenzamine potentiation of the pressor response to oxytocin and vasopressin: In vivo and isolated aortic strips studies. J Pharmacol Exp Ther 202:287, 1977.
45. McNeill JR, Stark RD, Greenway CV: Intestinal vasoconstriction after hemorrhage: roles of vasopressin and angiotensin. Am J Physiol 219:1342, 1970.
46. McNeill JR, Wilcox WC, Pang CCY: Vasopressin and angiotensin: reciprocal mechanisms controlling mesenteric conductance. Am J Physiol 232:262, 1976.
47. Manning M, Sawyer WH: Antagonists of vasopressin and antidiuretic responses to arginine vasopressin. Ann Int Med 96:520, 1982.
48. Sawyer WH, Pang PKT, Seto J, et al: Vasopressin analogs that antagonize antidiuretic responses by rats to the antidiuretic hormone. Science 212:49, 1981.
49. Robertson GL, Aycinena P, Zerbe RL: Neurogenic disorders of osmoregulation. Am J Med 72:339, 1982.
50. Narins RG, Jones ER, Stom MC, et al: Diagnostic strategies in disorders of fluid, electrolyte and acid-base homeostases. Am J Med 72:496, 1982.
51. Zerbe RL, Robertson GL: A comparison of plasma vasopressin measurements with standard indirect test in the differential diagnosis of polyuria. N Engl J Med 305:1539, 1981.
52. Kaplowitz PB, D'Ercole J, Robertson GL: Radioimmunoassay of vasopressin in familial central diabetes insipidus. J Pediatr 100:76, 1982.
53. Rowe JW, Shelton RL, Helderman JH, et al: Influence of the emetic reflex on vasopressin release in man. Kidney Intl 16:729, 1979.
54. Zerbe RL, Henry DP, Robertson GL: Vasopressin response to orthostatic hypotension. Am J Med 74:265, 1983.
55. Schaff-Blass E, Robertson GL, Rosenfield RL: Chronic hypernatremia from a congenital defect in osmoregulation of thirst and vasopressin. J Pediatr 102:703, 1983.
56. AvRuskin TW, Tang SC, Juan C: Essential hypernatraemia, antidiuretic hormone and neurophysin secretion: response to chlorpropramide. Acta Endocrinol 96:145, 1981.
57. Aronson AS, Svenningsen NW: DDAVP test for estimation of renal concentrating capacity in infants and children. Arch Dis Childh 49:654, 1974.
58. Godard C, Vallotton MB, Favre L: Urinary prostaglandins, vasopressin and kallikrein excretion in healthy children from birth to adolescence. J Pediatr 100:898, 1982.

CHAPTER 17

Drugs and The Kidney

RAYMOND D. ADELMAN
ALAN R. SINAIKO

GENERAL PRINCIPLES OF DRUG DISPOSITION

Drug therapy is an essential component in the medical management of almost all patients with renal disease. Complicated medical problems and more critically ill patients require intense pharmacological intervention. Consequently, the pediatric nephrologist must be familiar with basic principles of drug use in children and have a clear understanding of factors that influence drug response adversely in patients with compromised renal function.

This section will address the general principles of drug disposition in children and the effect of renal failure on this relationship. An added consideration in children is the impact of biological maturation on drug absorption, distribution, metabolism, and excretion, each of which undergoes dramatic change during the first year of life (Table 17.1). These changes have been reviewed in detail elsewhere (1–3).

Drug Clearance

Renal excretion plays an important role in the clearance of most drugs and their metabolic products. Hepatic metabolism is the other major route for drug clearance; pulmonary and intestinal secretion contribute to lesser degrees.

After a dose (D) of a drug is administered, it is distributed into body fluids and tissues; the concentration (C) it attains is determined by its volume of distribution (Vd):

$$C = D/Vd \tag{1}$$

Vd is derived by rearranging (1) as follows:

$$Vd = D/C \tag{2}$$

The concentration decreases in an exponential fashion, which defines the rate of clearance. For first order kinetics, the equation is the following:

$$K_{el} = \ln(C_2 - C_1)/t \tag{3}$$

Clearance of the drug is the product of the elimination constant (K_{el}) and the volume of distribution (Vd). This equation defines K_{el} in terms of clearance (Cl_T) and volume of distribution (Vd):

$$K_{el} = Cl_l/Vd \tag{4}$$

The clinical term customarily used to describe drug clearance is the plasma half-life ($T½$) defined by the equation:

$$T½ = \ln 2/K_{el} \quad \text{or} \quad .693/K_{el} \tag{5}$$

This describes the time required for the drug level to decrease to half its plasma concentration after a steady state of distribution is reached. For example, if $T½ = 2$ hours, the plasma concentration at 2 hours will be 50% of the original concentration (C_1); at 4 hours it will be 25% of C_1, and at 6 hours it will be 12.5% of C_1.

Combining equations (4) and (5) gives the following:

$$T½ = \frac{.693 \times Vd}{Cl_T} \tag{6}$$

From this it is evident that the plasma half-life of a drug is directly related to its volume of distribution (Vd) and inversely related to its total clearance (Cl_T).

When a drug has been administered for a sufficient period of time to establish steady-state conditions in which the dose administered equals the amount of drug cleared over a given period, the steady-state concentration (C_{SS}) of the drug is primarily dependent on the rate of drug clearance as expressed by the following equation:

$$C_{SS} = D/Cl_T \tag{7}$$

The dose needed to achieve steady state is defined in terms of C_{SS}, Vd and $T½$.

$$D = \frac{C_{SS} \times Vd \times .693}{T½} \tag{8}$$

The terms Vd and $T½$ often are known or can be derived from following the response of plasma concentration (C) over time to a single dose (D). From these data and knowing the C_{SS} level desired, the steady-state dose can be calculated.

Renal Clearance

Renal clearance (box on p. 253) of a drug occurs by glomerular filtration, renal tubular transport, or both pathways. For drugs that rely predominantly on the kidney for excretion, clearance is correlated with glomerular filtration rate (GFR). This is true whether the drug is cleared predominantly by renal tubular transport or glomerular filtration, since both filtration and tubular secretion decrease proportionately as renal mass and renal blood flow (RBF) decline in severe kidney disease.

This principle is represented in Figure 17.1 (4). As creatinine clearance

Table 17.1.
Maturation of Physiological Variables that Determine Drug Disposition

Aspect of drug disposition	Physiological variable	Representative values				
		Premature	Newborn	1 Year	Adult	Examples
Absorption oral	Gastric acid secretion (mEq/kg/h)	—	.015	—	0.2	Penicillin G—increased bioavailability in newborns
	Gastric emptying time (minutes)	—	87	—	65	Phenobarbital—slow rate of absorption in newborns
	Intestinal peristalsis	↓[a]	↓[a]	↔		Phenobarbital-slow rate of absorption in newborns
Absorption intramuscular	Regional muscular blood flow	[b]	[b]	↔		Digoxin, gentamicin—erratic absorption in newborns
Distribution	Total body water (% total body weight)	87	79	67	60	
	Extracellular water (% total body weight)	62	45	27	20	Amikacin, ticarcillin—increased distribution volumes in young subjects
	Adipose tissue (% total body weight)	3	12	23	12–25	
	Total serum proteins (g/dl)	5.9	6.0	6.4	7.2	
	Serum albumin (g/dl)	3.7	4.5	4.9	4.9	Sulfadiazine—decreased serum drug protein binding in newborns
Metabolism	Sulfation		↔	↔	—	Acetaminophen—predominantly sulfated in infants
	Glucuronidation	↓	↓	↔	—	Chloramphenicol—delayed elimination in prematures and newborns
	Mixed-function oxidase	↓	↓	↔	—	Theophylline—decreased rate of metabolism in newborns
Elimination	Glomerular filtration (ml/min/m^2)	5	15	50	70	Gentamicin—delayed elimination in newborns
	Tubular anion secretion (PAH clearance—ml/min/1.73 m^2)	—	50	245	380	Furosemide—delayed elimination in newborns

From Green TP, Mirkin BL: Clinical pharmokinetics: Pediatric consideration. In Benet LZ, Gambertoglio JG, Massoud N (eds): The Pharmokinetic Basis of Drug Treatment. New York, Raven Press, 1982. (With permission.)
[a] Peristalsis tends to be slow and irregular in premature and newborn infants.
[b] Muscular blood flow appears to be more labile in very young subjects.

Renal Excretion of Frequently Used Drugs

I. Glomerular Filtration
  A. Aminoglycosides
  B. Vancomycin
  C. Digoxin
  D. Flucytosine
II. Tubular Secretion
  A. Organic Acids
    1. Penicillins
    2. Cephalosporins
    3. Furosemide
    4. Thiazide diuretics
    5. Methotrexate
  B. Organic Bases
    1. Procainamide
    2. Triamterene

decreases, drug serum half-life begins to increase. However, it is not until renal function has decreased to approximately 50% of normal that serum half-life becomes sufficiently prolonged to require any modification in drug dosage. As residual renal function deteriorates further, renal drug clearance declines more precipitously so that failure to reduce drug dosage or to extend drug-dosing intervals will result in excessive plasma drug concentrations and increase the potential for toxicity.

Renal proximal tubular organic acid and base transport systems control drug extraction from plasma and secretion into the urine. Because they share a common tubular transport system, when more than one organic acid is present, they compete for tubular transport and excretion (5). For instance, the simultaneous administration of the organic acids probenecid and penicillin enhance the therapeutic effectiveness of penicillin by reducing its rate of renal tubular clearance as a result of competition with probenecid for excretion.

This principle also influences drug excretion in the patient with uremia

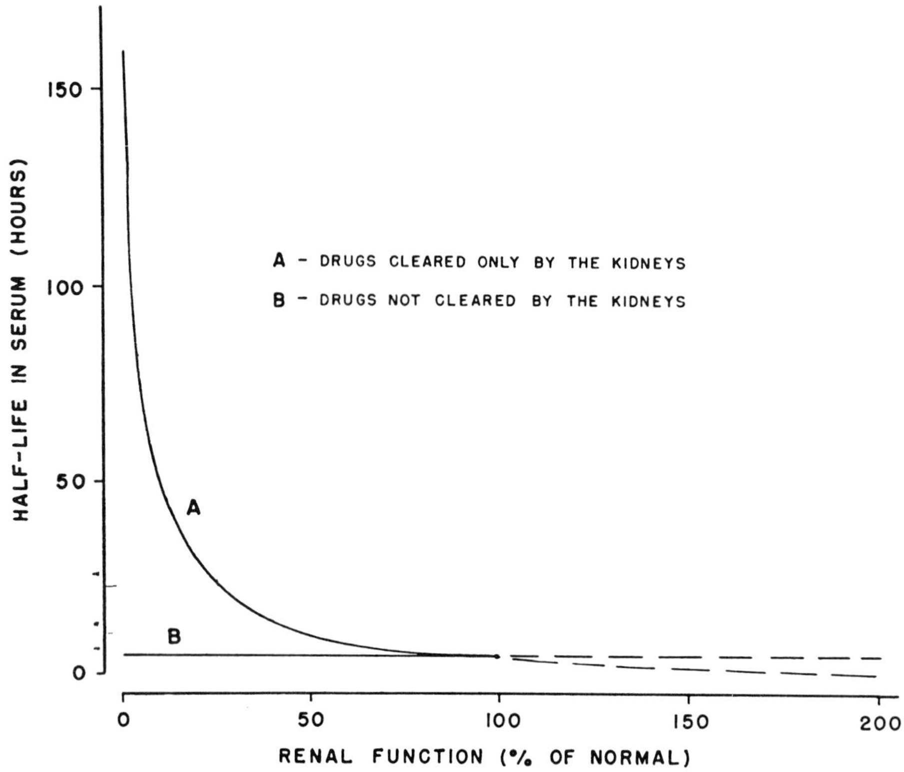

Figure 17.1. Influence of renal function on serum half-life for drugs cleared entirely by the kidney vs drugs cleared by other routes. (From Kunin CM, Finland M (eds): J Clin Invest 38:1509, 1959.)

as endogenous organic acids that accumulate during renal failure compete (5) with drugs for tubular transport site. Experimentally it has been shown that a dialyzable humoral agent, present in the serum of patients in renal failure, depresses uptake of the organic acid para-aminohippurate (PAH) in isolated rabbit renal tubules (6). Other studies in dogs (7) and humans (8) have shown a linear relationship between the degree of uremia and renal tubular clearance of the organic acid, furosemide.

The renal tubular extraction of organic bases does not appear to be similarly affected in renal failure (7, 9). For these drugs, clearance remains proportional to GFR.

Hepatic Clearance

The relationships established in Figure 17.1 suggest that decreasing renal function should not significantly affect drugs that are dependent on hepatic metabolism for clearance. However, hepatic clearance can be adversely influenced in renal failure by specific alteration of a number of independent metabolic processes, including oxidation, reduction, glucuronide and sulfate conjugation, acetylation, and ester hydrolysis (10). Ester hydrolysis and acetylation appear to be reduced in renal failure, whereas conjugation reactions and oxidation are unchanged.

Certain drugs, such as propranolol, are cleared to a significant degree after oral administration by the "first-pass effect" in which hepatic drug extraction from the portal circulation reduces the amount of drug reaching the systemic circulation following absorption from the gut (11). Renal failure inhibits this effect, thereby increasing serum drug levels above those observed with normal renal function (12). However, with continued dosing, serum levels revert back to those usually anticipated so that drug dosing adjustments may be required only during the initial stages of therapy (13).

Drugs that are cleared entirely by hepatic metabolism may continue to exert a pharmacological effect when active metabolites are produced and retained in renal failure. Biotransformation of the parent drug by the liver produces metabolic products that are generally more polar and less lipid-soluble, each of which enhances renal secretion. The pharmacological activity of these metabolites is usually so much lower than the parent compound that their biological effect can be ignored. However, the metabolic products of some drugs can exert a substantial independent or additive effect on the response elicited by the parent compound (box above) (14). For these specific drugs, dosage should be monitored closely in renal failure, with the understanding that clinical response may be the most reliable determinant in individualizing dosing regimens.

Drugs Cleared by Formation of Active Metabolites

- Allopurinol
- Cephalothin
- Cefotaxime
- Diazepam
- Imiprimine
- Meperidine

Some drugs are cleared by both renal and hepatic pathways, i.e., renal excretion may predominate when kidney function is normal but hepatic metabolism compensates in renal failure. For example, cimetidine is cleared under normal conditions by the kidney (15). However, even when GFR falls to <10 ml/min, plasma half-life does not increase above twice normal unless severe hepatic disease also develops.

Drug-protein Binding

Renal failure has a significant impact on the binding of drugs to plasma proteins (box above). Although a slight reduction in total serum

Drugs with Decreased Protein Binding in Uremia
Diazoxide
Phenytoin
Salicylate
Amphoterocin B
Warfarin
Phenobarbital
Furosemide

proteins also may occur under these conditions, this decrease is not substantial enough to affect drug-protein binding (DPB). The concentration of albumin remains in molar excess of drug concentrations, and there does not appear to be an inherent functional defect in the serum albumin (16). A more likely explanation is that this effect is related to drug displacement by organic acids (6), fatty acids (17), or peptides (18) that accumulate in patients with renal failure.

Interference with DPB can severely reduce total circulating drug levels but not necessarily diminish clinical response. The lower total drug concentration does not accurately reflect the concentration of free or unbound drug, i.e., that fraction of drug reacting with tissues to yield a specific clinical response.

The principle can be explained as follows: (1) drugs circulate in the intravascular space in two forms, a free fraction dissolved in plasma water and a fraction bound to plasma proteins; (2) only the free fraction equilibrates with body tissues and fluids to elicit a pharmacological response; (3) the concentration of free drug does not increase when DPB decreases, because the hepatic clearance maintains free drug at previous steady-state levels (19); (4) because laboratory analyses measure the total concentration of circulating drug without distinguishing between free and bound forms, the reduction in drug levels observed in renal failure represents only a decrease in the fraction of bound drug. Therefore, increasing drug doses solely to restore plasma drug concentrations to usual therapeutic levels, i.e., in uremic patients experiencing an otherwise satisfactory clincal response, is likely to accentuate drug toxicity. A widely recognized example of the effect of reduced DPB on clinical therapeutic management is the anticonvulsant, phenytoin, in which the absolute amount of free drug in plasma remains unchanged in patients with renal failure despite significant reductions in total drug concentration (20).

Adverse drug reactions have been reported with greater frequency and therapeutic response may be exaggerated in patients with altered DPB even when drug doses are not increased (21, 22). This may result from a wider range of serum drug concentrations, i.e., higher peak and lower trough levels, despite administration of usual drug doses (23). This can be avoided by decreasing the amount of drug administered per dose and the interval between dosing while maintaining a constant total daily dose so that peak and nadir concentrations are adjusted toward the mean without altering steady-state concentrations.

Clearance During Dialysis

Patients receiving chronic drug therapy may require modification of their drug-dosing schedules during periods of hemodialysis. Drug clearance during dialysis is dependent on individual drug disposition characteristics. In drugs that are distributed primarily in body water and cleared by glomerular filtration, such as the aminoglycosides, hemodialysis clearance rates usually are high. In contrast, a drug such as phenytoin, which is subject to a high degree of protein binding, is less likely to undergo substantial dialysis clearance (24). Factors inherent in the dialysis membrane itself may influence clearance. Thus, filtration of high molecular weight drugs, such as vancomycin, is minimal despite a low degree of serum protein binding and a high glomerular clearance.

To restore therapeutic drug levels after a dialysis, the amount of drug cleared by the dialyzer is calculated and replaced; dialysis clearance is calculated from the V_d and plasma drug levels obtained at the start and finish of the dialysis, using the following equation:

$$D = V_d(C_{pre} - V_{post}) \tag{9}$$

where D represents the replacement dosage,
C_{pre} the predialysis, and
C_{post} the postdialysis plasma drug concentration.

Drug clearance is more accurately calculated by measuring plasma drug levels during dialysis and applying the following equation:

$$Cl_{HD} = Q\frac{A - V}{A} \tag{10}$$

where Cl_{HD} represents clearance,
Q the dialyzer blood flow,
A the arterial, and
V the venous or return plasma drug concentration.

This equation can be used only when blood and dialysate flow are stable, so that the drug does not accumulate on the dialyzer side of the membrane.

Peritoneal dialysis is a significantly less efficient method of drug clearance, not only for short term dialysis but also in patients managed with continuous ambulatory peritoneal dialysis (CAPD). Peritoneal dialysate clearance is calculated by the following equation:

$$Cl_{PD} = \frac{C_D V}{P} \tag{11}$$

where C_D represents drug concentration in the dialysis fluid,
V volume of the dialysate, and
P the plasma drug concentration at midpoint of the the dialysis.

Drug clearance by CAPD has been determined for vancomycin (25), tobramycin (26), gentamicin (27), cefazolin, and cephalexin (28). In each case, peritoneal clearance after parenteral administration was 20% or less of total drug clearance. In contrast to the low rate of drug clearance *into* the peritoneal cavity, transfer of drug *from* the peritoneal fluid into the vascular compartment is very fast (25, 27). Approximately 65% of gentamicin or vancomycin is absorbed by intraperitoneal administration during CAPD, resulting in serum concentrations well within the therapeutic range.

The implications from these studies are apparent. Unlike the situation during hemodialysis, adjustments in drug dose are not required in patients treated with peritoneal dialysis. Peritoneal infections are less effectively treated when drug administration is only systemic. Serum drug levels in renal failure must be monitored closely when antibiotics are administered intraperitoneally because of the potential for development of toxic drug levels. Although drug levels may be lower with this route of administration, aminoglycoside toxicity cannot be neglected and even may be more likely under conditions in which constant therapeutic serum levels are maintained than when usual peak and trough conditions prevail, as during normal renal function (29).

CLINICAL MANAGEMENT OF DRUG THERAPY

Based on the previous discussion, certain generalizations can be made regarding drug administration to patients with compromised renal function.

1. The usual loading dose for almost all drugs can be given with the initial drug dose. Drug accumulation to toxic concentrations does not occur until the patient has received multiple doses.

2. Drugs that are cleared by routes other than renal, except those drugs producing active metabolites, can be used without dose modifications.
3. Drugs cleared by the kidney require careful monitoring of serum drug concentrations.
4. Drugs with significant protein binding should be monitored closely for therapeutic effect because serum levels may be misleading.

The ongoing development of laboratory analytical techniques for drug measurement is providing important methodology for monitoring drug therapy. For almost all drugs dependent on the kidney for clearance, it should be possible to provide effective therapy while minimizing the risk of drug toxicity. However, incorporation of drug measurements into patient management requires an understanding of laboratory data provided.

Most drug measurements are made with high pressure liquid chromatography systems or specific antibody techniques that have proven to be accurate and reliable. In contrast, measurement of antibiotic concentrations with microbiological assay systems can yield falsely elevated drug levels when active metabolites, produced by hepatic biotransformation, are present (30). Another important potential source of error involves the actual mechanics of serum drug measurement, including accuracy of drug administration before sample collection, accurate timing of sample collection for kinetic analysis, and handlng of blood samples by the clinical laboratory (31). Provided that each step is carried out with precision, pharmacokinetic constants can be developed easily, using published computer programs (32).

Use of Diuretics

Diuretics are widely used in patients with renal disease to treat fluid retention and hypertension. Because these agents act on the luminal side of the nephron (33), diuretic response is related directly to the amount of drug excreted via the tubular organic acid transport system. As renal function deteriorates, the effectiveness of thiazides and loop diuretics decreases accordingly (34).

Hydrochlorothiazide

The serum half-life of hydrochlorothiazide is approximately 5 hours in adults with normal renal function (35). A typical pattern of serum concentration and urinary excretion of hydrochlorothiazide in a child is represented in Figure 17.2 (36). Peak serum concentrations can be expected between 2 and 4 hours after oral dosing. Peak urinary drug excretion was observed between 4 and 8 hours, but a significant amount of hydrochlorothiazide was present in the urine for up to 12 hours. These data support the recommendation that thiazides need not be administered more often than every two half-lives, i.e., approximately every 12 hours, and confirm previous studies in adults showing that thiazide-dosing regimens more frequent than twice daily only minimally increase the 24-hour excretion of water and electrolytes (37).

The effect of renal failure on serum hydrochlorothiazide concentrations is shown in Figure 17.3 (36). In this group of children, serum drug levels are highly correlated with serum creatinine ($r = 0.91$). The hydrochlorothiazide concentration was independent over a wide dose range when GFR is >50 ml/min. However, when renal function was <50 ml/min, hydrochlorothiazide excretion decreases and serum drug levels are related directly to dose. Despite these dramatic changes in drug concentration, serum uric acid does not increase significantly.

Loop Diuretics

The most potent diuretic agents are the loop diuretics, named for their site of action at the thick ascending loop of Henle. At the present time, furosemide is the member of this class of drugs most widely used. Ethacrynic acid has been used infrequently in pediatric patients, following earlier reports of association of its use with ototoxicity. Newer loop

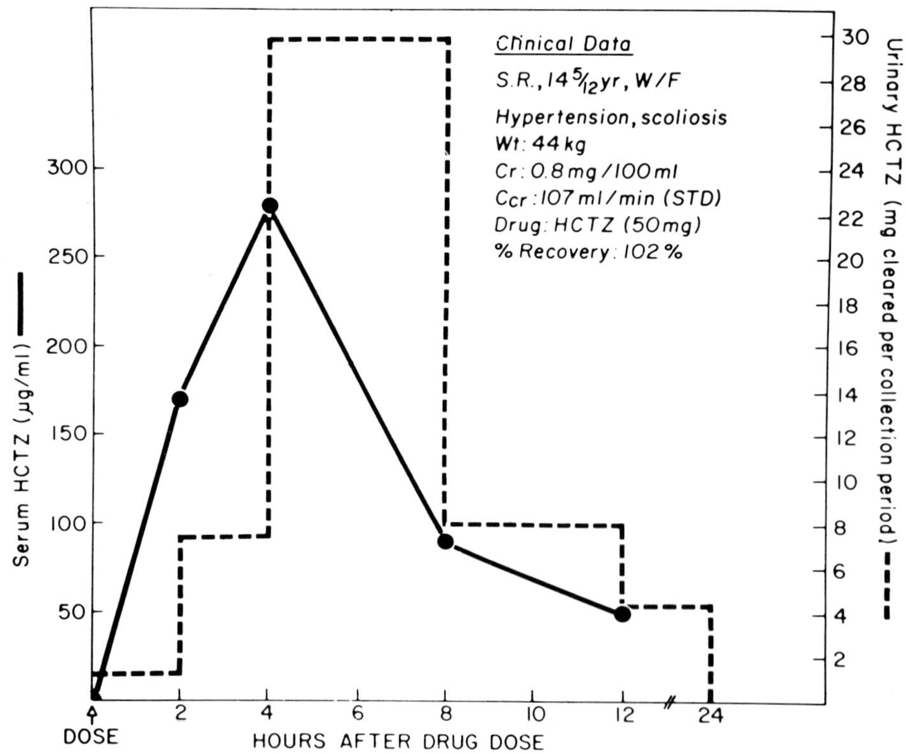

Figure 17.2. Pattern of serum drug concentration and renal excretion for hydrochlorothiazide in a patient with normal renal function. (From Mirkin BL, Sinaiko AR: Unpublished data.)

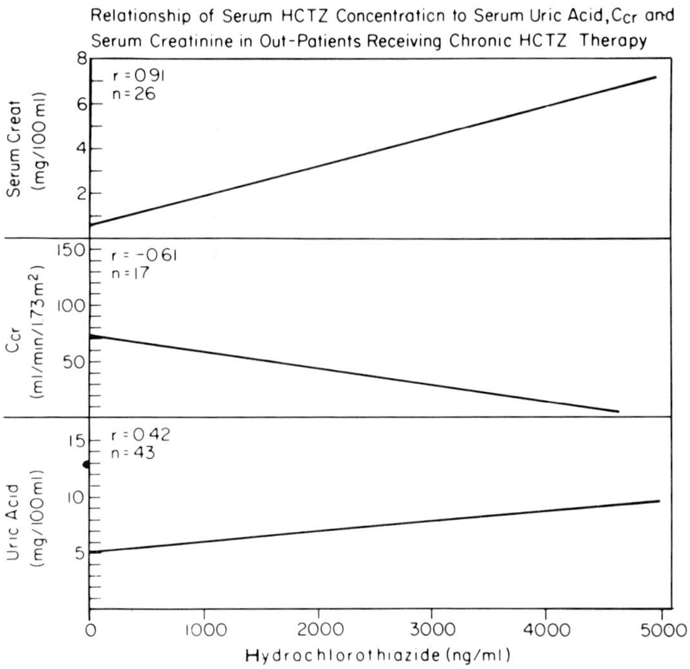

Figure 17.3. Influence of renal function on serum hydrochlorothiazide concentration. (From Mirkin BL, Sinaiko AR: Unpublished data.).

diuretics, such as bumetanide, do not offer any major advantage over furosemide, although with added experience one or another of these drugs may prove to be superior (38).

In contrast to the thiazide diuretics, the response to furosemide is more intense and occurs over a shorter period of time. The half-life of furosemide is approximately 1 hour in normal adults (39), implying that the drug is cleared rapidly and the diuretic effect is complete within a few hours. The bioavailability of furosemide after oral administration varies considerably among individuals (40). Nevertheless, it is possible to attain maximal diuresis in a given patient by increasing the oral dose to reach drug levels similar to those observed after intravenous dosing.

Because the diuretic effect is dependent on the amount of furosemide delivered to the luminal side of the tubule, the diuretic response in renal failure is altered by reduction in renal function and competition with other organic acids for renal excretion at tubular organic acid transport sites. As a result, diuresis in uremic patients does not reach the response observed with equivalent drug doses in patients with normal renal function, and takes place over a longer period of time. Although patients in renal failure respond more vigorously after intravenous furosemide than after oral administration, this occurs because of the higher concentrations delivered to the renal tubule. Patients with severe renal failure should be able to achieve a maximal diuretic response to furosemide with higher oral drug doses.

Patients with severe proteinuria and nephrotic syndrome constitute a particularly difficult group to treat with diuretics. Although a reduction in vascular volume may contribute to a concomitant reduction in diuretic response, the proteinuria itself may exert an inhibitory influence on drug-mediated diuresis. In studies of rats with aminonucleoside nephrosis, positive correlation was found between urine protein concentration and percent of bound furosemide (41). Because diuretic response is directly related to the concentration of the unbound drug in the urine, water and chloride excretion was inversely related to urinary protein excretion. A similar relationship is likely to occur in humans and may account for some of the resistance to furosemide therapy in nephrotic patients.

It has been our clinical practice to initiate diuretic therapy with a thiazide in patients with creatinine clearance >50 ml/min and to reserve furosemide for patients with a greater degree of renal failure. Fewer patients will require potassium supplementation with thiazides than with loop diuretics, which cause a high degree of potassium excretion in almost all cases. The use of a single diuretic agent is preferred. However, in cases that are refractory to usual diuretic management because of severe renal failure or nephrotic syndrome, the addition of a thiazide (42) or metolazone (43) to furosemide therapy may be beneficial (42) because the diuretic action of each occurs at separate loci in the distal renal tubule.

Antiinfective Agents (Table 17.2)

Penicillin

The penicillin antibiotics traditionally have been treated as a single class of drugs because of the similarity of their beta-lactam chemical

Table 17.2.
Antiinfective agents in renal disease

Drug	Clearance	Need to Adjust in Renal Failure	Comments
Penicillins			
Amoxicillin	R[a] and H[b]	Yes	Reduction in dose with severe renal failure
Ampicillin	R and H	Yes	
Penicillin G	R and H	Yes	
Nafcillin	H	No	
Dicloxacillin	R and H	No	
Carbenicillin	R	Yes	
Ticarcillin	R	Yes	
Azlocillin	R and H	Yes	Capacity for clearance saturated at high doses
Piperacillin	R and H	Yes	
Mezlocillin	R and H	Yes	
Cephalosporins			
Cephalexin	R	Yes	Reduction in dose with severe renal failure
Cefaclor	R	Yes	
Cefazolin	R	Yes	
Cephradine	R	Yes	
Cephalothin	R and H	Yes	
Cefamandol	R and H	Yes	
Cephapirin	R and H	Yes	
Moxalactam	R	Yes	
Cefotaxime	R and H	Yes	
Cefoperazone	Biliary	No	
Aminoglycosides			
Streptomycin	R	Yes	High potential for toxicity; pharmacokinetic analysis essential in renal failure
Gentamicin	R	Yes	
Tobramycin	R	Yes	
Kanamycin	R	Yes	
Amikacin	R	Yes	
Netilmicin	R	Yes	
Vancomycin	R	Yes	Treat as aminoglycoside
Trimethoprim	R	Yes	
Antiviral			
Acyclovir	R	Yes	Kinetic analysis indicated
Antifungal			
Flucytosine	R	Yes	Kinetic analysis indicated; decreased protein binding results in lower serum levels in renal failure
Amphoterocin B	H?	No	

[a] Renal.
[b] Hepatic.

nucleus. Despite the major molecular modifications that have been made to create penicillins with broader therapeutic indications, each of these agents, except nafcillin, relies primarily on the renal tubular organic acid transport system for clearance. However, there are other characteristics specific to certain members within this group.

Penicillin G is cleared primarily by renal tubular transport in patients with normal renal function. A modest percentage of clearance also occurs via hepatic metabolism, and, coupled with the wide therapeutic index for penicillin G, this permits the use of usual doses until renal function decreases to low levels (43). In contrast, other penicillins, e.g., carbenicillin (44), ticarcillin (45), and ampicillin (46), are cleared almost entirely by the kidney and require dosage reductions in renal failure; nafcillin can be administered independent of renal function because it is cleared almost entirely by hepatic biotransformation (47).

The new acylureidopenicillins—mezlocillin, piperacillin, and azlocillin—have been used primarily to treat Pseudomonas infections. Each of these drugs is dependent on renal clearance for elimination from the body. But unlike other beta-lactam antibiotics, these particular penicillins are characterized by dose-related pharmacokinetics (48). Capacity-limited clearance mechanisms dictate that as the drug dosage is increased there is a concomitant increase in the serum elimination half-life, serum drug concentration, and area under the concentration-time curve. With piperacillin, the capacity-limiting factor appears to be renal tubular excretion, since dose dependency could not be demonstrated in patients with severe renal failure (49). In contrast, mezlocillin elimination kinetics are dose dependent only in anuric patients, suggesting that the capacity-limiting factor for elimination is nonrenal in origin (50).

Cephalosporins

The cephalosporin antibiotics are similar in many ways to the penicillins. They are cleared primarily by the organic acid renal tubular transport system but some are also cleared by hepatic biotransformation. Because of their broad therapeutic index, dosage usually can be reduced in patients with renal failure without the added necessity of monitoring drug concentrations.

Cefazolin is an example of a cephalosporin that relies entirely on the kidney for elimination. Studies in children (51) have shown that serum half-life is related directly to creatinine clearance, following the pattern demonstrated in Figure 17.1. In contrast, cephalothin represents a cephalosporin that is cleared via renal and hepatic mechanisms. In normal children, the serum half-life is extremely rapid (18.6 minutes) (52). As the serum half-life increases in renal failure, the contribution of hepatic metabolism permits this drug to be given in the same fashion as Penicillin G, so that only modest adjustments in dose need to be made.

The newest group of cephalosporins, the so-called third generation cephalosporins, also offer a spectrum of drug-clearance mechanisms. Moxalactam is excreted almost entirely by the kidney; therefore, it is not surprising that the serum half-life in children with renal failure is 5 to 9 times longer than that in children with normal renal function (53). Cefotaxime is cleared in the same manner as cephalothin, i.e., by hepatic and renal mechanisms. Although serum half-life is inversely related to creatinine clearance, hepatic metabolism in renal failure is sufficient enough to permit the use of usual dosing regimens until GFR falls to approximately 5 ml/min (54). Cefoperazone is cleared primarily by the liver with a small percentage recovered from urine; however, it is not cleared by hepatic biotransformation. Biliary excretion appears to be the major route of elimination, and drug levels in bile are reported to be many times higher than in serum (55).

Aminoglycosides

Certain drugs require close monitoring because of a narrow therapeutic ratio and high potential for toxicity. Primary among these are aminoglycoside antibiotics and vancomycin, each of which has been associated with nephrotoxicity and ototoxicity. Although the use of aminoglycoside serum drug levels in patients with normal renal function may be of limited usefulness, drug level monitoring should be an integral component of management in children with renal failure.

Antifungal and Antiviral Agents

The use of antifungal and antiviral agents has increased dramatically in response to the growing number of patients receiving immunosuppressive therapy, particularly under conditions of kidney, liver, and bone marrow transplantation. Amphotericin B continues to be the mainstay of antifungal therapy; <10% of the drug is cleared in normal subjects. Patients with renal failure have lower total serum drug levels but this does not indicate that higher amphotericin B doses should be administered. The situation with this drug is similar to that described with phenytoin; lower total serum levels represent a reduction in protein-bound drug and normal concentration of unbound (or pharmacologically active) drug; therefore, doses of amphotericin B should not be adjusted in renal failure (56). In contrast, flucytosine, the other commonly used antifungal agent, is dependent almost entirely on the kidney for elimination and requires significant dosing modification in renal failure.

The antiviral agent acyclovir is now widely used to treat viral infections in transplant patients. The major route of clearance is via the kidney. As might be expected, clearance is lowest during infancy but approximates adult clearance rates by 1 year of age (57). In adults with renal failure, the serum half-life increases to approximately 6 times normal so that a significant reduction in dosage is required (58, 59).

TOXIC NEPHROPATHY

Introduction

This section focuses on the various clinical manifestations and pathophysiological mechanisms of drug-associated renal injury. Examples of acute and chronic renal injury as a result of common drugs will be discussed; additional information can be found in several comprehensive reviews (59–61). Much information has been drawn from experience with adults; the extent to which these data are applicable in children is, in many instances, unknown.

The apparent incidence of drug-related renal injury is related to the thoroughness of monitoring and the criteria used for defining nephrotoxicity. Approximately 5% to 10% of nephrology consultations involve drug-related renal injury (62). In cases of acute renal failure, 20% to 25% are secondary to drugs (59, 63); the most common agents are the aminoglycosides and cancer chemotherapeutic drugs.

The kidney is particularly susceptible to toxins because it has a generous blood supply, a large endothelial surface area, and high intracellular and intraluminal drug concentrations that relate to secretory and reabsorptive activities. Other features that contribute to susceptibility to renal injury include the high drug concentrations in the medulla because of the countercurrent system, and the low pH achieved in the tubular fluid in the distal nephron. The mechanisms by which renal injury is induced include vascular, obstructive, immunological, inflammatory, and metabolic. Highly metabolically active tissues, such as the proximal tubule, are especially vulnerable to toxic injury.

For the clinician, it is useful to describe toxic nephropathies according to clinical syndromes (box on p. 259). An individual agent may have more than one clinical presentation and the presentation may vary in severity because other therapeutic or toxic agents are also present. For example, gentamicin nephrotoxicity in humans is enhanced when cephalothin is given concomitantly (64) and in dogs with the use of furosemide

(65). Polybrominated biphenyl products in contaminated meats markedly potentiate chloroform-induced nephrotoxicity in mice (66). Rats pretreated with gentamicin are more susceptible to mercuric chloride nephrotoxicity, while rats pretreated with mercuric chloride are resistant to gentamicin nephrotoxicity (67).

Drugs causing acute renal failure in humans are listed in the box below. The most common agents are the aminoglycosides, amphotericin B, cisplatinum, and radiocontrast agents.

Aminoglycosides

Prevalence of Toxicity

The aminoglycosides are widely used antibiotics with known ototoxicity and nephrotoxicity. The clinical and pathological changes resulting from aminoglycoside use have been studied extensively. The incidence of nephrotoxicity varies according to the dose, duration, method of treatment, the individual aminoglycoside used, and the presence of various risk factors. Anderson (63) reported that 30% of cases of nonoliguric acute renal failure were a result of aminoglycoside use. The prevalence of significant elevation of serum creatinine (Cr_s) in patients receiving aminoglycosides varies between 1.5% and 25% (64, 68–70); 11 of 27 adults had reduced GFR, as measured by ^{125}I iothalamate clearance, but only 1 had an elevated Cr_s (71). Although children are generally thought to be less susceptible to aminoglycoside nephrotoxicity, this may not be the case. Therapy in neonates is shorter; changes in Cr_s are more readily overlooked because initially they are lower (71). Another factor may be the underlying disease; children with cystic fibrosis, given aminoglycosides in usual doses, have lower serum levels (72). The incidence of nephrotoxicity in infants and children, is probably the same as it is in adults (70–78).

Clinical Presentations in Toxic Nephropathies

- Acute renal failure
- Nephrotic syndrome
- Fluid and electrolyte abnormalities
- Chronic renal failure

Risk

The risk for nephrotoxicity in patients appears to be increased in the presence of underlying renal disease (79), sodium depletion (80), acidosis

Toxic Nephropathy

I. Acute renal failure
  - A. Nephrotoxic renal failure
    - Antibiotics
      - Aminoglycosides
      - Amphotericin B
      - Polymyxin and colistimethate
      - Cephalosporins
      - Tetracyclines
    - Metals
      - Mercury
      - Arsenic
      - Platinum
      - Bismuth
      - Lead
    - Organic Solvents
    - Other Causes
      - Acetaminophen
      - Iodinated-contrast agents
      - Pigment nephropathy
      - Cyclosporin
      - Lithium
      - Nonsteroidal antiinflammatory agents
  - B. Obstructive uropathies
    - Hyperuricemic acute renal failure
    - Methotrexate
    - Acute Oxalate Nephropathy
  - C. Acute glomerulonephritis/polyarteritis
    - Organic solvents
    - Penicillins
    - Drug abuse (heroin, amphetamine)
  - D. Acute interstitial nephritis
    - Penicillins (methicillin, ampicillin, nafcillin)
    - Sulfonamides/furosemide/thiazides
    - Nonsteroidal antiinflammatory agents

II. Chronic renal failure
  - Analgesic nephropathy
  - Radiation nephritis
  - Lead
  - Arsenic
  - Cisplatinum
  - Obstructive uropathy

III. Nephrotic syndrome
  - A. Heavy metals
    - Mercury
    - Gold
    - Bismuth
    - Thallium
  - B. Anticonvulsants
  - C. Other
    - Heroin
    - Penicillamine
    - Probenecid
    - Captopril
    - Lithium
    - Nonsteroid antiinflammatory agents

IV. Fluid and electrolyte abnormalities
  - A. Impaired water excretion
    - Vincristine
    - Carbamazepine
    - Cyclophosphamide
  - B. Impaired renal concentration
    - Lithium
    - Demeclocycline
    - Outdated tetracycline
    - Amphotericin
    - Aminoglycoside
  - C. Renal tubular acidosis (and Fanconi's syndrome)
    - Acetazolamide
    - Outdated tetracycline
    - Amphotericin B
    - Gentamicin
    - Lead
    - Bismuth
    - Lithium
    - Cyclosporin
  - D. Electrolyte wasting
    - Aminoglycoside
    - Amphotericin B
    - Polymyxin and colistimethate
    - Cisplatinum

(81), and with the concurrent use of certain other drugs: amphotericin B (82), clindamycin (83), cephalothin (84–86), cisplatinum (87), and furosemide (65, 88). Furosemide may enhance aminoglycoside nephrotoxicity by causing volume depletion. Several studies in humans have demonstrated an increased risk to gentamicin nephrotoxicity when cephalothin is also being given (86–88). Cephalosporins, except for cephaloglycin, appear to protect against gentamicin-induced nephrotoxicity in animal studies (89, 90).

Clinical Signs

The clinical manifestations of nephrotoxicity range from slight elevation of Cr_s, proteinuria, diminished urinary concentrating ability, and enzymuria (77), to acute oliguric or, more commonly, nonoliguric renal failure (63). Pitressin-resistant hyposthenuria may occur. The renal failure may be severe enough to require dialysis therapy; generally this is not the case, i.e., the renal failure is reversible, although recovery may take months. Elevation in Cr_s may not occur until several days after the aminoglycoside has been discontinued (65, 91). Severe proximal tubular dysfunction, e.g., hypokalemia, hypomagnesemia, and hypocalcemia associated with renal potassium and magnesium wasting, and inappropriately low immunoreactive parathormone levels are reported (92–94). We have seen Fanconi's syndrome develop in infants and children receiving aminoglycosides (95).

Pathology

The pathology of gentamicin nephrotoxicity is patchy proximal tubular necrosis, interstitial fibrosis, and tubular dilatation. Myeloid bodies are present within cytosomes and mitochondrial swelling and vacuolization are observed by electron microscopy (96) (Figure 17.4).

Histopathological changes in animals include the presence of cytosomes with myelin-like figures, mitochondrial swelling, and acute tubular necrosis. Tubular regeneration may occur in the rat and dog despite continued administration of aminoglycoside (97, 98).

Renal Metabolism

Aminoglycosides are excreted by glomerular filtration largely intact. Proximal tubular reabsorption (99) occurs following aminoglycoside binding to anionic phospholipids in the brush border (100). Binding is saturable, dose related, varies in avidity with the number of free amino groups (101), and is competitive with other aminoglycosides and other polycationic substances. After pinocytosis, aminoglycoside-containing endocytic vesicles fuse with intracellular lysosomes (102) and induce lysosomal dysfunction (103). A phospholipidosis ensues, with marked accumulation of phosphatidylinositol and phosphatidic acid (104) and with diminished activities of phosphatidylinositol-C phospholipase (105) and phospholipase-A (106).

Mechanism for Renal Injury

The mechanism by which aminoglycosides induce renal injury is not clear (107). Aminoglycosides concentrate in renal tissue, especially the cortex (108). Despite similar tissue levels, the various aminoglycosides differ considerably in their nephrotoxicity (109). Gentamicin is much more nephrotoxic to dogs than netilmicin, yet both drugs cause comparable changes in lysosomal morphology and in urinary activities of lysosomal hydrolases (110). Possible mechanisms for aminoglycoside nephrotoxicity include altered permeability or breakage of lysosomes that may result in the discharge of hydrolytic enzymes. There is increased activity of lysosomal enzymes in urine. Also there are marked decreases in renal mitochondrial oxidative phosphorylation (111).

Another mechanism is a decrease in ultrafiltration coefficient (K_f) (112). Improvement in K_f and also in glomerular plasma flow following the use of captopril suggests that the renin angiotensin system is affected

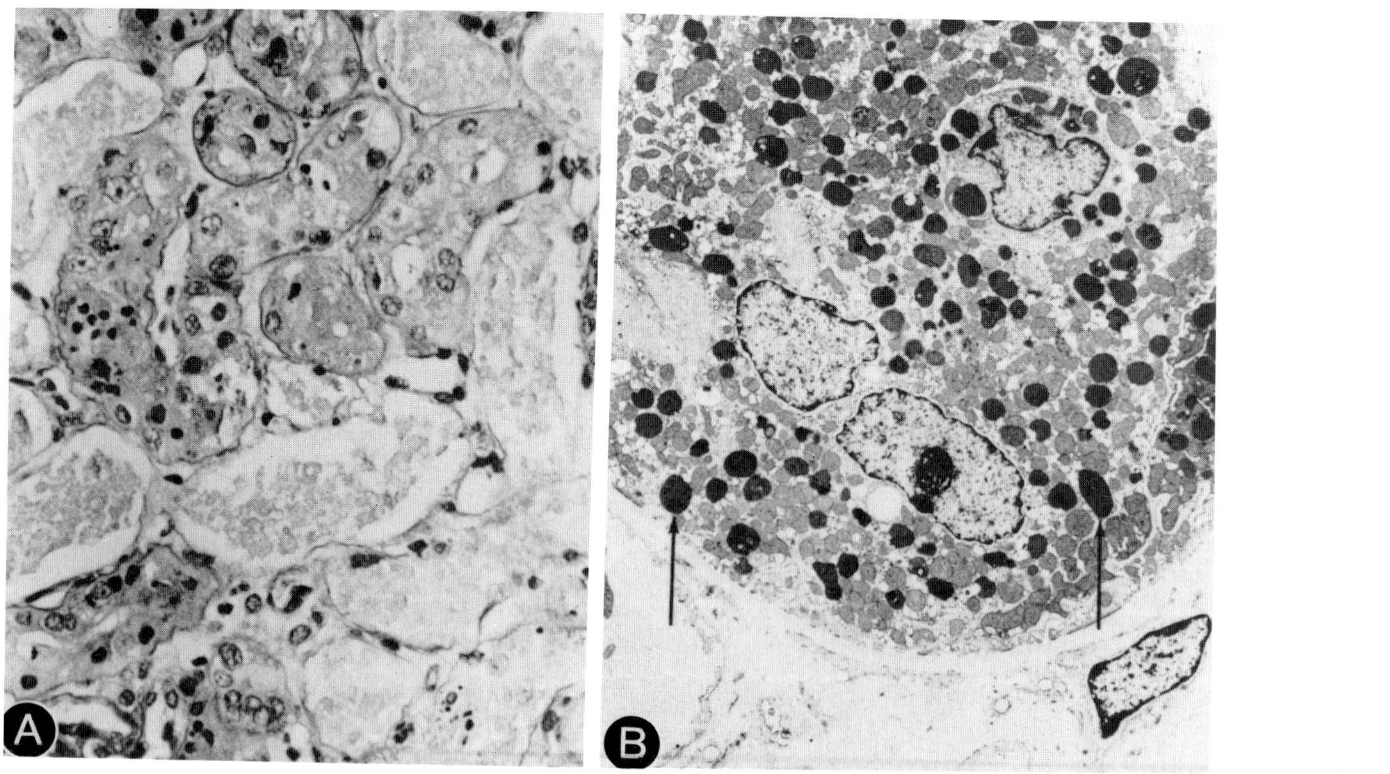

Figure 17.4. *A*, Acute tubular necrosis in a patient receiving gentamicin. *B*, Myeloid bodies (*arrows*) are present within large cytosegrosomes and mitochondria are swollen.

(113). Gentamicin causes (114) a reduction in endothelial cell pore size and number, which may correspond to the observed reduction in K_f.

Prevention

Nephrotoxicity can be decreased by following several measures. Aminoglycosides should be used only when less nephrotoxic agents are unsuitable. Cr_s levels should be monitored closely during and up to 72 hours following cessation of therapy. Volume depletion should be avoided. Although it may be helpful to monitor serum drug levels, nephrotoxicity attributed to elevated peak and trough levels (115) probably are secondary to prior reduction in renal function rather than the converse. In animal models there is no relationship between peak serum aminoglycoside levels and nephrotoxicity (116) and acute renal failure can occur in some patients with "safe" therapeutic levels (117). The management of aminoglycoside-induced acute renal failure is largely supportive.

Amphotericin B

Amphotericin B, used in treating systemic mycoses, often affects renal function. The drug causes a dose-related decrease in the clearance of inulin and PAH, which can progress to acute nonoliguric renal failure (118). Proteinuria, hematuria, and cylinduria occur. Tubular dysfunction (renal tubular acidosis, hypokalemia and renal potassium wasting, and a vasopressin-resistant hyposthenuria) is common (119). There may be a chronic moderate reduction in GFR. In some patients receiving large doses, irreversible renal failure has occurred (120). Intratubular calcium deposits, interstitial edema and fibrosis, periglomerular fibrosis, and proximal tubular necrosis (121, 122) occur, as well as focal vacuolization of medial smooth muscle cells in the arteries, secondary to afferent arteriolar vasoconstriction (123, 124).

Amphotericin may increase solute permeability of plasma membranes by interacting with membrane-bound sterols (125), leading to renal tubular acidosis, renal potassium wasting, and polyuria. Sodium bicarbonate given to rats protects against amphotericin nephrotoxicity (126).

Patients receiving amphotericin B require close monitoring of Cr_s and electrolytes. Although mannitol markedly reduces amphotericin nephrotoxicity in dogs (124), its usefulness in humans has not been well established (127).

Polymyxin, Colistin, and Other Antibiotics

Polymyxin and colistin are associated with a high incidence of nephrotoxicity that appears related to dose and duration of treatment (128, 129). Twenty percent of patients receiving colistin had adverse reactions, including decreased GFR, hematuria, proteinuria, and cylindruria; 2% had acute renal failure secondary to acute tubular necrosis (129). The risk of nephrotoxicity increased when colistin was given to patients with preexisting renal disease (128) and in conjunction with cephalothin (129, 130). Colistin overdose has caused acute renal failure, neuroparalysis, and death (131). Generally, renal insufficiency is reversible, but Cr_s may continue to rise 7 to 10 days after therapy is discontinued (129). Hypokalemia, hyponatremia, hypocalcemia, and renal sodium and potassium wasting occur in patients receiving polymyxin, especially in those who are also receiving cephalothin (130).

Nephrotoxicity associated with the use of cephalosporins alone is uncommon, except for cephaloridine (84). Some reports of acute renal failure solely a result of cephalothin are more suggestive of acute hypersensitivity (132). Risk factors for nephrotoxicity include preexisting renal disease or the concurrent use of aminoglycosides (64, 132). Nephrotoxicity appears to be related to renal cortical transport and high intracellular accumulation of the drug within the kidney (133). Less nephrotoxicity occurs in rabbits after blocking its cellular uptake with probenicid and in newborn rabbits, because the transport system is immature (134).

Tetracyclines are associated with azotemia, but primarily as a consequence of impaired amino acid utilization (135). A defect in concentrating ability occurs with demeclocycline therapy (136) and, in cirrhotic patients, reversible acute renal failure (137). Fanconi's syndrome, associated with vacuolization of the distal tubule and hydropic degeneration of the proximal epithelium, may occur with use of outdated tetracycline, presumably a result of the degradation products, anhydrotetracycline and epianhydrotetracycline (138). Potassium wasting may be severe (139).

Vancomycin, which has had a resurgence in use, especially in the management of staphylococcal shunt infections and peritonitis, appears to cause less nephrotoxicity (140) than formerly reported (141).

Significant nephrotoxicity with co-trimoxazol therapy is probably unusual (142); elevated Cr_s may reflect the effect of competition between trimethoprim and creatinine for renal secretory sites.

Cisplatinum

Cisplatinum, an inorganic complex of platinum used in the treatment of solid tumors, is frequently associated with a dose-related nephrotoxicity (126). Mild reversible nephrotoxicity occurs in 25% to 60% of patients given a single dose of 50 to 100 mg/m^2 (143). When larger does or multiple treatment courses are employed, the incidence of nephrotoxicity rises and profound, often irreversible, decreases in GFR result (144). Baum and coworkers (145) reported a 44% incidence of renal toxicity in children given cisplatinum doses of 130 mg/m^2 surface area. Preexisting renal disease and the concurrent use of other nephrotoxic drugs, such as the aminoglycosides, may increase the risk; mannitol may reduce the risk (87, 146, 147). Renal failure may be oliguric or nonoliguric and be associated with proteinuria, cylindruria, and elevated serum creatinine values, which generally peak at 1 to 2 weeks (148). Recovery usually occurs by 3 to 4 weeks but may be delayed for months or be incomplete. A persistent decrease in GFR is reported in cisplatinum-treated patients who had been observed for 24 months (144).

Significant hypomagnesemia and marked renal magnesium wasting that may last for months, has been reported in many patients treated with cisplatinum. Hypokalemia, hypocalcemia, and renal potassium wasting may also occur (147, 149).

The histological findings in cisplatinum nephrotoxicity include necrosis of the proximal and distal convoluted tubules and the collecting duct (144, 148) along with interstitial fibrosis. Phagolysosomes filled with flocculent material have been demonstrated by electron microscopy (144).

The mechanism of cisplatinum-induced renal injury is not known. Cisplatinum is taken up primarily by the liver; only 3% of injected labeling cisplatinum is localized to the kidney (150). Its renal clearance exceeds inulin clearance, suggesting cisplatinum is actively secreted by the kidney (151). Micropuncture studies indicate that cisplatinum reduces single nephron GFR and causes significant tubular fluid backleak as well (152). Rats given cisplatinum have a decrease in protein bound sulfhydryl groups, especially in mitochondrial and cytosolic fractions (151, 153).

The incidence and clinical severity of cisplatinum nephrotoxicity is lowered by continuous infusion of cisplatinum (154), saline prehydration (155), and mannitol diuresis (146, 148). Equal protection appears to be conferred either by furosemide or mannitol diuresis (156). Nephrotoxicity is reduced by a combination of hydration, furosemide, and mannitol therapy (157). Ozols et al (158) recently reported impressive protection against nephrotoxicity in 15 of 17 adults receiving high-dose cisplatinum

(200 mg/m^2 body surface area) in hypertonic saline who were given normal saline to expand extracellular fluid volume.

Radiocontrast

The incidence of radiocontrast-induced renal injury is reported low, ranging from 0.15% (159) to 0.8% (160). Most reports, however, do not include acceptable renal assessment before and after use of radiocontrast agents. In a retrospective study by Van Zee (160), where Cr_s levels were followed, the incidence of acute renal failure was 4.8%. There is a high incidence of acute renal failure following angiography especially in patients with preexisting azotemia (161, 162).

Risk factors for radiocontrast nephrotoxicity include volume depletion, preexisting renal disease, diabetes, and proteinuria (159–163). Patients with both diabetes mellitus and renal insufficiency are at extremely high risk (160).

Radiocontrast-induced acute renal failure is usually oliguric and generally resolves in a few days to a few weeks. Kidneys of neonates with radiocontrast nephropathy may appear cystic by ultrasound (164). The prognosis in the absence of underlying disease is generally good; however, irreversible renal failure has occurred, especially when there has been preexisting renal insufficiency (160). The histological findings in radiocontrast nephrotoxicity include proximal tubular epithelial cell vacuolization, and focal or diffuse proximal tubular and medullary necrosis (165, 166). Electron microscopy demonstrates engorged capillaries, cytoplasmic vacuolization of glomerular endothelium, and swelling of proximal tubular epithelial cells and their brush borders (165).

The pathophysiological mechanisms postulated for radiocontrast-induced acute renal failure include intratubular precipitation of Tamm-Horsfall protein (163), vascular constriction and decrease in RBF (165), acute hypersensitivity (167), volume depletion (168), and direct cell toxicity with proximal tubular and medullary necrosis (165). Nephrotoxicity appears to be related both to the inorganic iodide moiety and the nonhalogenated organic molecule (165), as well as to the hypertonicity of contrast (169). GFR was most severely reduced in young rabbits given radiocontrast of high osmolality (169). The incidence and severity of radiocontrast-induced acute renal failure can be reduced by avoiding volume depletion with adequate hydration (170), by replacement of urinary losses, and by prudent use of radiocontrast agents, especially in patients at high risk (171).

Mercury

Mercury is found in laxatives, fungicides, merthiolate ear irrigants, Calomel, and in food and water through industrial contamination (59). Inorganic but not elemental mercury is readily absorbed by the gastrointestinal tract and causes severe gastroenteritis and shock. The renal injury ranges from hematuria, proteinuria, glycosuria, aminoaciduria, and cylindruria to oliguric acute renal failure (59, 172). The nephrotic syndrome, as well, has been associated with organic mercurial diuretics (173, 174).

Mercury is concentrated in the proximal convoluted tubule, loop of Henle, and collecting duct. Mercury forms mercaptide bonds to sulfhydryl groups. The pathophysiology largely derived from animal studies, includes proximal tubular necrosis, tubular obstruction, backleak of glomerular filtrate, a change in glomerular ultrafiltration coefficient (175), and decreased cortical perfusion. Patients with preexisting renal disease appear to be at higher risk for nephrotoxicity, perhaps a result of increased systemic accumulation of mercury (173).

Therapy is supportive and includes lavage or emesis, chelation with BAL, N-acetyl penicillamine therapy, and dialysis.

Chronic low-dose exposure to organic and inorganic mercury, as with mercury-containing skin ointments, may lead to proteinuria and nephrotic syndrome (176–179). Glomeruli may be normal (176) or show membranous and proliferative changes (177–179). Recovery generally has occurred after elimination of mercury or with the use of steroids. Steroid therapy has induced remission in patients with normal glomeruli and in those with membranous changes. Whether remission might have occurred without therapy is not known.

Lead

Lead poisoning may occur following ingestion of lead-containing paints, soil, newsprint, and alcohol, by the inhalation of vapors from tetraethyl lead in gasoline, and from burning lead paint or battery casings (180, 181). Chisholm (182) noted that 40% of children with acute lead intoxication developed a clinical picture of acute proximal tubular dysfunction or Fanconi's syndrome, associated with generalized aminoaciduria, bicarbonaturia, phosphaturia, and glycosuria, often without impairment of GFR. This occurred more commonly with severe clinical manifestations of lead intoxication.

Lead poisoning causes cloudy swelling, mitochondrial swelling, and eosinophilic, dense-staining intranuclear inclusion bodies in the proximal tubule (183). Lead has a strong affinity for mitochondrial membranes. Diminished respiratory and phosphorylative activities in the kidney have been demonstrated in vitro, perhaps due to enzyme or substrate complexes with lead (184).

Exposure to lead-contaminated water (183, 185–187) may lead to acute or long-term hypertension, proteinuria, and renal insufficiency. Emerson (185) followed 400 Australian adults treated as children between 1920 and 1935 for lead poisoning; 108 of the 165 who had died by the time of follow-up had died with CRF or hypertension, which appeared to be a result of lead toxicity. The bone-lead content in those patients with idiopathic renal failure exceeded levels in a comparable group of patients with chronic nephritis of known etiology (185, 186). Tepper (187), however, did not report an increased incidence of CRF or hypertension in 42 adults treated during childhood in Boston for acute plumbism. It is postulated that the Australian patients may have had more prolonged lead exposure and greater body lead stores (188). Hyporeninemic hypoaldosteronism characterized by sodium wasting, hyperkalemia, and renal tubular acidosis has been reported with chronic lead poisoning (189).

The kidneys in chronic lead poisoning are granular and contracted. There is focal and diffuse interstitial fibrosis, tubular atrophy and dilatation, loss of cortical tissue, and periglomerular fibrosis (188).

The diagnosis of lead poisoning is made by increased serum or urinary lead levels. Urinary coproporphyrins may be increased; a hypochromic, microcytic anemia is present and lead may be seen on x-ray films in the gastrointestinal tract or bones. A diagnosis of chronic lead poisoning is made when lead is mobilized and excreted in urine after EDTA therapy (180, 190). Lead poisoning is treated with EDTA, BAL, or penicillamine (190).

Arsenic

Arsenic is present in many herbicides and pesticides and may be ingested or inhaled as a result of industrial or environmental exposure. Neonatal death has occurred following maternal intoxication (191). Symptoms of arsenic poisoning include vomiting, diarrhea, abdominal pain, severe intravascular hemolysis, and encephalopathy (192). Renal injury may range from pyuria, hematuria, and proteinuria, with a mild decrease in GFR to acute oliguric renal failure (193). Renal insufficiency may be permanent. An intense catabolic state may lead to marked hyperkalemia and azotemia (192). Kidneys are contracted; the proximal convoluted tubule is degenerated and necrotic. Pigmented casts may be present along with interstitial inflammation. Chronic changes include glomerular sclerosis, tubular atrophy, and interstitial fibrosis (192). Arsenic binds to sulfhydryl groups and impairs enzyme function. There also may be sludging within the renal circulation, related to presence of red cell debris from severe hemolysis (192). Therapy includes emesis or lavage, BAL chelation, and supportive dialysis.

Bismuth

Bismuth nephrotoxicity is now seen rarely. Acute renal failure has been reported in children with oral, intramuscular, or suppository administration of bismuth (194). Renal manifestations also include hypertension, proteinuria, hematuria, pyuria, and Fanconi's syndrome. Nephrotic syndrome, leading to CRF has occurred (195). Proximal tubular necrosis, tubular dilatation, and interstitial inflammation as well as refractile, spherical, brownish, PAS-positive intracytoplasmic and intranuclear inclusion bodies are observed in renal tubule epithelial cells (194).

Gold

Proteinuria occurs in 1% to 3% of patients given gold therapy for rheumatoid arthritis (196); the nephrotic syndrome occurs in 0.2%. Renal histopathology reveals a membranous glomerulopathy with granular deposits of IgG and IgM. Gold appears as filamentous and granular material in the proximal tubular and mesangial cells, but not in the subepithelial deposits of the glomerular basement membrane. Gold is taken up by mitochondria, which become swollen, and by autophagosomes (196, 197).

Organic Solvents

Carbon tetrachloride, commonly used as a cleaning agent and industrial solvent, can cause hepatic and renal failure. It is absorbed by inhalation, cutaneously, or by ingestion. Gastrointestinal tract absorption appears to be facilitated by alcohol. Clinical features of carbon tetrachloride ingestion include vomiting, abdominal pain, convulsions, coma, and jaundice, followed in 24 to 48 hours by oliguric acute renal failure associated with hematuria, proteinuria, casts, and renal tubular cells. Carbon tetrachloride is a direct nephrotoxin. Metabolites of carbon tetrachloride bind covalently to renal and liver tissue. The amount of binding, in animal studies, parallels the extent of tissue injury (198). Proximal tubule cells are swollen and contain vacuoles of neutral fat (199). There later follows an inflammatory reaction with lymphocytic infiltration. Treatment is supportive. Sulfhydryl compounds, such as methionine and cysteine, may be helpful (200). Recovery is usually complete but may take several months (201).

Trichlorethylene is an anesthetic agent which is also used as a solvent for dry cleaning. Abusive sniffing can cause jaundice, proteinuria, and occasionally acute oliguric renal failure that necessitates dialysis (202).

Intensive exposure to hydrocarbons also has been speculated as a cause of immune-mediated human renal disease. Six of 8 patients with Goodpasture's syndrome (antiglomerular basement membrane disease) had extensive exposure to hydrocarbons, often the vapor or mist of heated solvents (203). Increased exposure also was noted in patients with chronic glomerulonephritis (204) and crescentic proliferative glomerulonephritis (205). N,N^{1}-diacetylbenzidine causes crescenic glomerulonephritis in rats (205, 207). It is postulated that pulmonary exposure to volatile hydrocarbons induces antibody formation to alveolar basement membrane that crossreacts with glomerular basement membrane, leading to pulmonary and renal disease.

Heroin

Acute glomerulonephritis (208) and focal segmental glomerular sclerosis (209) have been reported in association with heroin abuse. The extent to which heroin per se contributes to renal disease is unclear, because of the concurrent use of other drugs, the probable presence of heroin contaminants, and the frequency of coexisting systemic illnesses. Patients with acute glomerulonephritis have had the nephrotic syndrome, bacterial endocarditis, or hepatitis; half had renal insufficiency. Renal histology has revealed PAS-positive material in the mesangium, focal nodular deposits containing IgG, IgM, and C_3 within glomerular capillary loops, and electron-dense glomerular basement membrane deposits, often in association with "virus-like" inclusions in endothelial cell cytoplasm (208).

Amphetamines

Amphetamine abuse is associated with a clinical and histological picture indistinguishable from polyarteritis (210). Patients may be asymptomatic or have fever, weight loss, joint involvement, rash, and abdominal pain. Renal findings include proteinuria, hematuria, hypertension, and normal-to-markedly decreased renal function. Renal angiography demonstrates tiny aneurysms of medium and small vessels. Histologically, there is fibrinoid necrosis of the intima and media with cellular infiltrate, including eosinophils.

Acetaminophen

Acetaminophen overdosage leads to severe hepatic injury that may be associated with acute renal failure, proteinuria and hematuria. Clinical features include nausea, vomiting, jaundice, and oliguria. Renal histopathology reveals loss of the brush border, mitochondrial injury, and sloughing of cells (211, 212). Acetaminophen nephrotoxicity may be related to chemically reactive metabolites, such as P-aminophenol or N-acetylimidoquinone, which preferentially bind to renal glutathione (212, 213). However, with large doses of acetaminophen or with glutathione deficiency, the metabolites covalently bind to renal macromolecules to cause tubular cell necrosis. The metabolites largely result from hepatic sulfation and glucuronidation via a microsomal cytochrome P-450 oxygenase system. Cobalt inhibition of cytochrome P-450 synthesis appears to protect against hepatic and renal injury. There is also evidence that the kidney has the potential to generate reactive acetaminophen metabolites (214).

Provision of cysteamine and methionine increase glutathione and appear to reduce renal and hepatic injury when given within 10 hours of ingestion (214). N-acetyl cystine (216), a derivative of cystine, also appears to be helpful for management of acute ingestion (216). Chronic acetaminophen abuse, which is cumulative, dose related, and potentiated by dehydration, may lead to nephrotoxicity, with a picture of analgesic nephropathy.

Methotrexate

Methotrexate is a chemotherapeutic agent that acts by binding nearly irreversibly to dihydrofolate reductase within cells. Its toxicity is related to the level of free drug and duration of exposure. The major route of clearance is renal. Methotrexate, a weak organic acid with a pKa of 4.7, is less soluble at acid pH and may precipitate in renal tubular fluid. The 7-hydroxy and D-glutamate metabolites are even less soluble than methotrexate and are capable of precipitation in tubular fluid. Nephrotoxicity is not common with lower-dose methotrexate but occurs with high-dose therapy, i.e., 1 to 15 g/m^2. The incidence of methotrexate nephrotoxicity is reduced with hydration and alkalinization; in one study, the incidence of nephrotoxicity fell from 47% to 15% with alkalinization and hydration (217). The incidence of nephrotoxicity in children who are well hydrated may be lower (218). Hydration and alkalinization do not appear to affect the pharmacokinetics of methotrexate (219).

The clinical manifestations of methotrexate nephrotoxicity include flank pain, hypertension, and nonoliguric or oliguric acute renal failure.

Renal histology may demonstrate the presence of methotrexate-containing precipitates in renal tubular lumina (217), or the presence of proximal tubule necrosis associated with dilated tubules and interstitial injury (220). Postulated pathophysiological mechanisms of methotrexate nephrotoxicity include intraluminal precipitation, a direct toxic effect on the tubules, and a decrease in glomerular perfusion (221). Acute renal failure with high-dose methotrexate therapy can occur without evidence of precipitation (220). With high-dose methotrexate therapy, i.e., 7.5 g/m^2 in children who were well hydrated but not receiving alkali, inulin clearance decreased 51% in 40 hours. Systemic toxicity appeared to be related to high serum levels in those patients with profoundly decreased inulin clearance. A significant number of children developed hypertension as well (221).

Citrovorum factor helps to reduce the nonrenal and toxic effects of high serum methotrexate levels (222). Even when citrovorum factor is given with methotrexate renal failure accounts for 20% of deaths in patients given high-dose methotrexate. Neither peritoneal nor hemodialysis are very effective in reducing levels of methotrexate, because it is protein-bound and has an apparent large volume of distribution (220).

Urate Nephropathy

Acute hyperuricemic renal failure occurs with lymphoma, leukemia, and other myeloproliferative conditions, most commonly as a consequence of cytolytic chemotherapy (223). Increased delivery of uric acid to tubular urine is by glomerular filtration and tubule secretion (224). Extremely high concentrations of uric acid are achieved in the lumina of the distal tubules and collecting ducts (225).

The clinical manifestations of urate nephropathy include nausea, vomiting, and flank or abdominal pain, which may be colicky in nature. Serum uric acid levels may exceed 20 mg/dl; acute renal failure may occur at values as low as 12 mg/dl (223). Hyperphosphatemia, with serum phosphate levels >10 mg/dl, is common. Urinalysis may show uric acid crystals. The ratio of uric acid to creatinine clearance usually exceeds 1.0 (226). With ultrasonography, the lesion is echo-dense in the renal papillae (Fig. 17.5). With an hippurate scan, a prolonged third phase is compatible with obstruction.

The primary pathophysiological mechanism for acute urate nephropathy is intrarenal obstruction in the distal tubule and collecting duct following precipitation of uric acid (224). Rarely, extrarenal ureteric obstruction occurs secondary to uric acid calculi (223). Uric acid with a pKa of 5.75 readily precipitates in the distal tubule and collecting duct when urine is acid and concentrated.

Crystals of uric acid undergo phagocytosis by epithelial cells in the collecting ducts, leading to giant cell formation (227). The tubular basement membrane may be disrupted and crystalline substances extruded into the interstitium to cause a foreign body reaction and inflammation. Tubular atrophy with dilatation, and interstitial and periglomerular fibrosis may occur.

Assuring a high urinary flow rate and alkalinization of urine, using either sodium bicarbonate or a carbonic anhydrase inhibitor, has reduced the incidence of urate nephropathy during chemotherapy (224, 228). Protection from urate nephropathy in rats is due more to high tubular fluid flow rate; alkalinization plays a lesser role (229). The use of the xanthine oxidase inhibitor, allopurinol, several days before chemotherapy, reduces the production of uric acid (230). Supportive hemodialysis may be indicated with acute renal failure or in the presence of extremely high serum levels of uric acid or phosphate (223, 231). Uric acid clearance is considerably greater with hemodialysis compared with peritoneal dialysis.

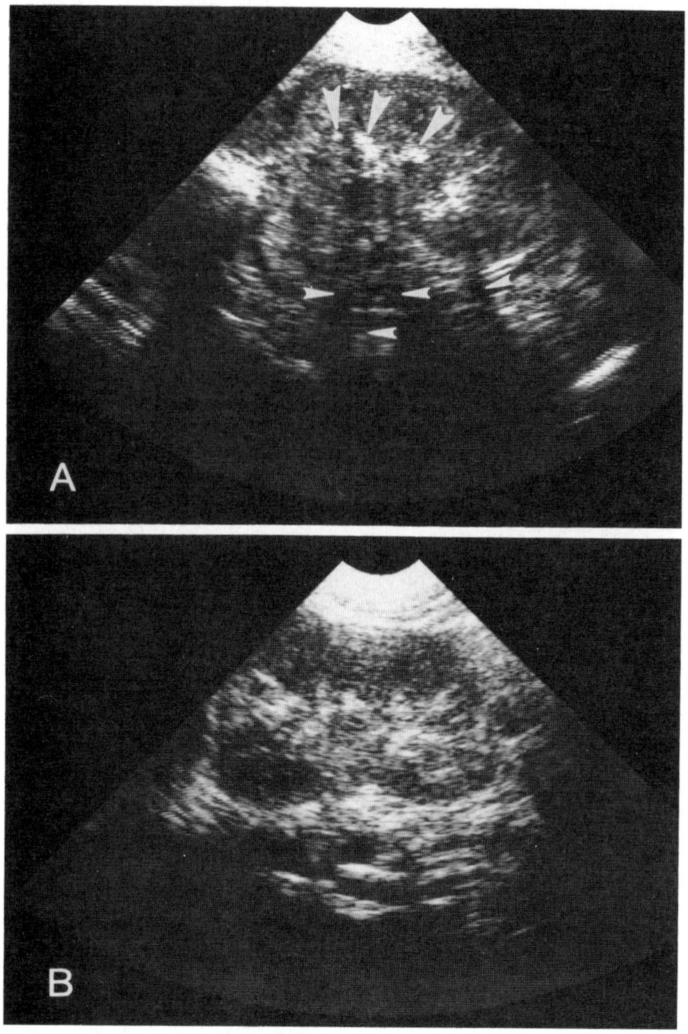

Figure 17.5. *A*, Acoustic shadowing (*small arrows*) from urate deposits (*large arrows*) within the collecting ducts in a patient with acute renal failure as a result of urate nephropathy. *B*, Normal ultrasound in same patient 18-days later.

Penicillins

Interstitial nephritis may account for 3% of patients with acute renal failure (232, 233). Several drugs have been associated with acute interstitial nephritis; the penicillins, probably because of widespread use, are the most often implicated (234–239). The common clinical presentation is fever, morbilliform rash, and gross or microscopic hematuria. Fever usually is the first sign; appearing after defervescence of the original fever, rash or hematuria may follow. This triad occurs in 10% to 40% of cases (233); nephrotic syndrome also may occur (239). Associated findings include proteinuria, pyuria, anemia, eosinophilia, and eosinophiliuria. Tubular dysfunction (aminoaciduria, glycosuria, decreased tubular reabsorption of phosphate, polyuria, and hyperchloremic acidosis) may occur. IgE may be elevated (239). The kidneys are enlarged and the gallium scan is intensely positive (233). Symptoms generally occur after 1 to 2 weeks of therapy, but they may appear as early as 1 day or as late as 6 weeks. Renal failure may be oliguric or nonoliguric. Crossreactivity has been reported (234).

Focal or diffuse interstitial inflammatory infiltrates, consisting of aggregates of plasma cells, eosinophils, lymphocytes, neutrophils, and occasionally histiocytes, in close contact with tubular basement mem-

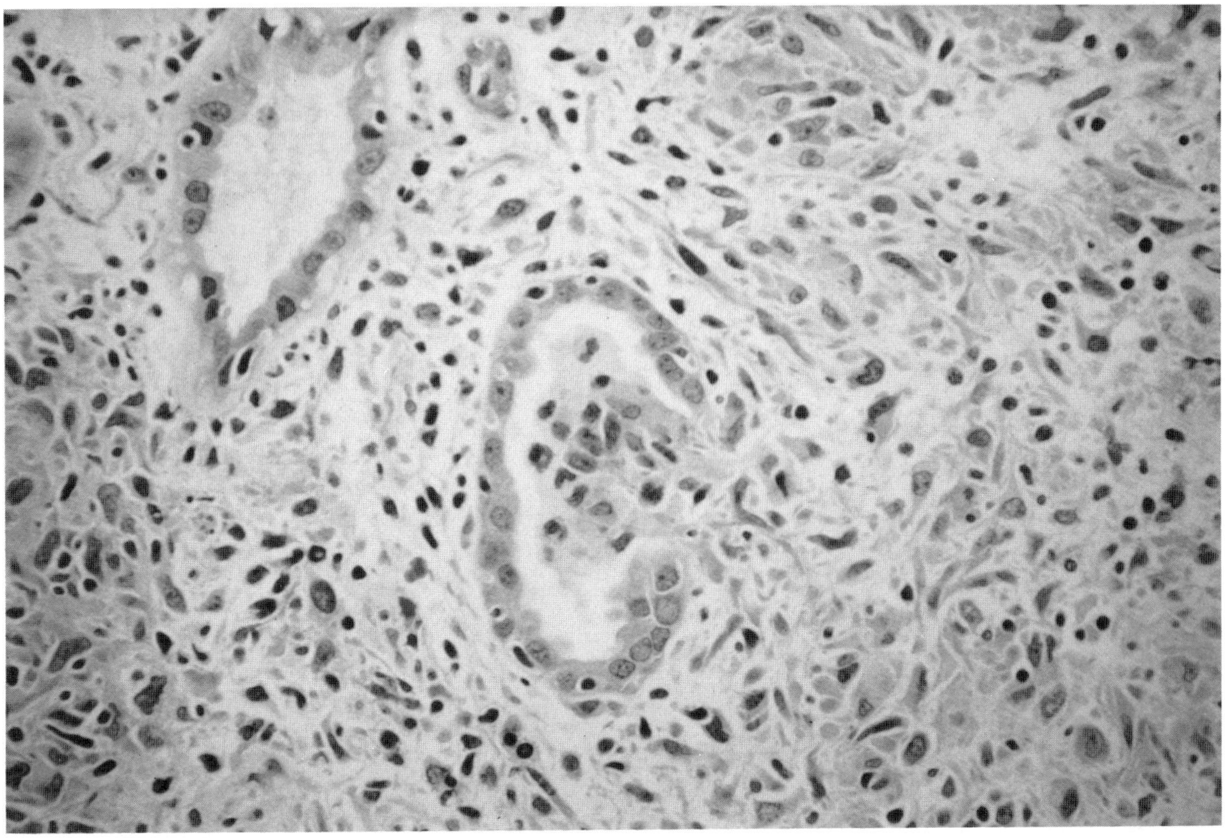

Figure 17.6. Acute interstitial nephritis with an infiltrate consisting of plasma cells, eosinophils and lymphocytes, interstitial edema and fibrosis, and tubular atrophy with necrosis.

brane, are characteristic (Fig. 17.6). Tubular atrophy and necrosis with thickening of tubular basement membrane, interstitial edema, and fibrosis may be present (240). The distal tubules are especially affected. The glomeruli are usually normal and immunofluorescence is usually negative.

The pathophysiology of methicillin acute interstitial nephritis has been studied by Baldwin et al (234) and Border et al (236). The Baldwin group reported linear staining of glomerular and tubular basement membrane with fluorescein-labelled antibody to fixed dimethoxyphenyl-penicilloyl hapten. Border's group demonstrated linear deposits of IgG, C_3, and methicillin antigen along tubular basement membrane and the presence of circulating antitubular basement membrane antibodies. Delayed hypersensitivity also may be involved. Guinea pigs previously given bovine gamma globulin developed acute interstitial nephritis with negative immunofluorescence on a second exposure to bovine albumin (233).

Management is usually supportive, with discontinuation of the drug. Dialysis may be indicated. Corticosteroid therapy may hasten recovery; whether such therapy affects ultimate renal function is unclear. Pusey et al (232) noted a diuresis or fall in Cr_s by 72 hours in patients given intravenous methylprednisolone and full recovery of renal function. In patients treated with oral prednisone there was a more rapid return of Cr_s to normal (237). In the combined series, 87% of treated patients recovered normal renal function compared with 37% of untreated patients. The prognosis in children may be better. All the children reported by Ellis et al (239) recovered renal function within 4 months.

Diuretics

Sulfonamide-derived diuretics, such as the thiazides and furosemide, have been implicated in acute interstitial nephritis (241, 242). Interstitial nephritis should be suspected in patients receiving these diuretics when renal function declines more rapidly than is characteristic of the underlying pathological process.

Lithium

Lithium therapy is frequently associated with a reversible, vasopressin-resistant concentrating defect (243). In some patients on long-term therapy, renal function may decrease (244). Minimal change nephrotic syndrome (245), acute renal failure (246), and renal tubular acidosis (247) also have been reported. Chronic tubular interstitial nephritis, sclerotic glomeruli, dilated tubules, interstitial fibrosis, microcystic changes and abnormalities of epithelial cells are described (244).

Cyclosporin A

Cyclosporin A is associated with significant nephrotoxicity. Seven of 16 patients developed nephrotoxicity after allogenic marrow transplantation (248); 3 had severe acute renal failure associated with hemolysis, fluid retention, proteinuria, and hematuria. Renal histology was similar to that in hemolytic uremic syndrome with thrombi containing fibrin and platelets occluding capillary tufts and arterioles. Proximal and distal tubular necrosis also were observed along with interstitial edema, fibrosis, and mesangial sclerosis. Similar findings had been reported in rabbits given cyclosporin A (249). The incidence of nephrotoxicity secondary to cyclosporin A is unclear; some report no major impairment in renal function and others report 80% (248, 250–252). The incidence may be dose related or obfuscated by concomitant allograft rejection. Sibley and coworkers (253) report that nephrotoxicity can be distinguished from rejection histologically (253), although not all investigators agree. Nephrotoxicity is more frequent with trough drug levels >400 ng/ml (254) and appears to be relatively low in renal allograft recipients receiving low-dose cyclosporin therapy (255). Although 15 of 19 cardiac transplant patients (250) had some elevation in Cr_s and 2 required hemodialysis, renal function improved when the dose was reduced or the drug discontinued. However, inulin clearance was still significantly reduced and hypertension was common in heart transplant patients after more than 1 year of treatment, despite dose reduction (256). Hypertension, often severe, is common with cyclosporin (257); generally, it responds well to captopril therapy. Hyperkalemia with type 4 renal tubular acidosis was reported in 16% of renal allograft recipients treated with cyclosporin (258). The concurrent use of aminoglycosides, amphotericin, and acyclovir with cyclosporin A appears to enhance its nephrotoxicity (259).

Nonsteroidal Antiinflammatory Drugs

Acute interstitial nephritis has been associated with use of nonsteroidal antiinflammatory agents (260–263). Characteristically, after prolonged drug use, patients present with acute renal failure or the nephrotic syndrome. Hematuria, rash, fever, eosinophilia and eosinophiliuria are often absent. Acute interstitial nephritis, including renal eosinophilia, is common. The interstitial infiltrates of patients studied with T and B cell-specific staining were composed exclusively of T lymphocytes. Glomeruli usually are normal by light microscopy. Immunofluorescent staining is minimal to absent and electron microscopy shows only fusion of podocytes. Recovery generally occurs following discontinuation of the drug. Steroid therapy may benefit some patients (260, 262, 263).

Nonsteroidal antiinflammatory drugs may cause a more acute form of renal injury, characterized primarily by a decline in creatinine or inulin clearance and oliguria (264–267), in patients in whom RBF and GFR are dependent on intact renal cyclo-oxygenase activity and renal synthesis of vasodilator prostaglandins. Such prostaglandins modulate renal vascular tone in the presence of vasoconstrictor stimuli, such as angiotensin-II. Hence, in clinical conditions characterized by ineffective renal perfusion, such as the nephrotic syndrome, cirrhosis, or renal ischemia, cyclo-oxygenase inhibition by nonsteroidal antiinflammatory drugs can cause acute and severe declines in RBF and GFR.

In premature infants given indomethacin for treatment of persistent patent ductus arteriosus (265), GFR declined by 27% and free water clearance by 66%. Close to half of low birth weight infants given indomethacin (0.4 mg/kg) increased Cr_s to levels of 1.5 mg/dl or more. Inulin clearance fell 33% in premature infants given 0.2 to 0.6 mg/kg of indomethacin (267). Renal function generally returns to pretreatment values 1 to 2 weeks after discontinuation of therapy.

Other Drugs

Penicillamine is a chelating agent which has been associated with proteinuria and nephrotic syndrome in 7% to 20% of patients (268–270). Renal histology is compatible with a membranous glomerulopathy. Light microscopic findings may be minimal. Electron dense deposits in the outer layer of glomerular basement membrane are associated with IgG and complement deposits (Fig. 17.7).

The pathophysiology of penicillamine-induced nephrotic syndrome appears to involve circulating immune complexes. Antibodies to penicillamine have been detected in the circulation (271). Proteinuria generally remits with cessation of therapy.

The nephrotic syndrome also has been reported with tridione (272, 273), probenecid (274), and phenindione (275), with remission following discontinuation of drug therapy.

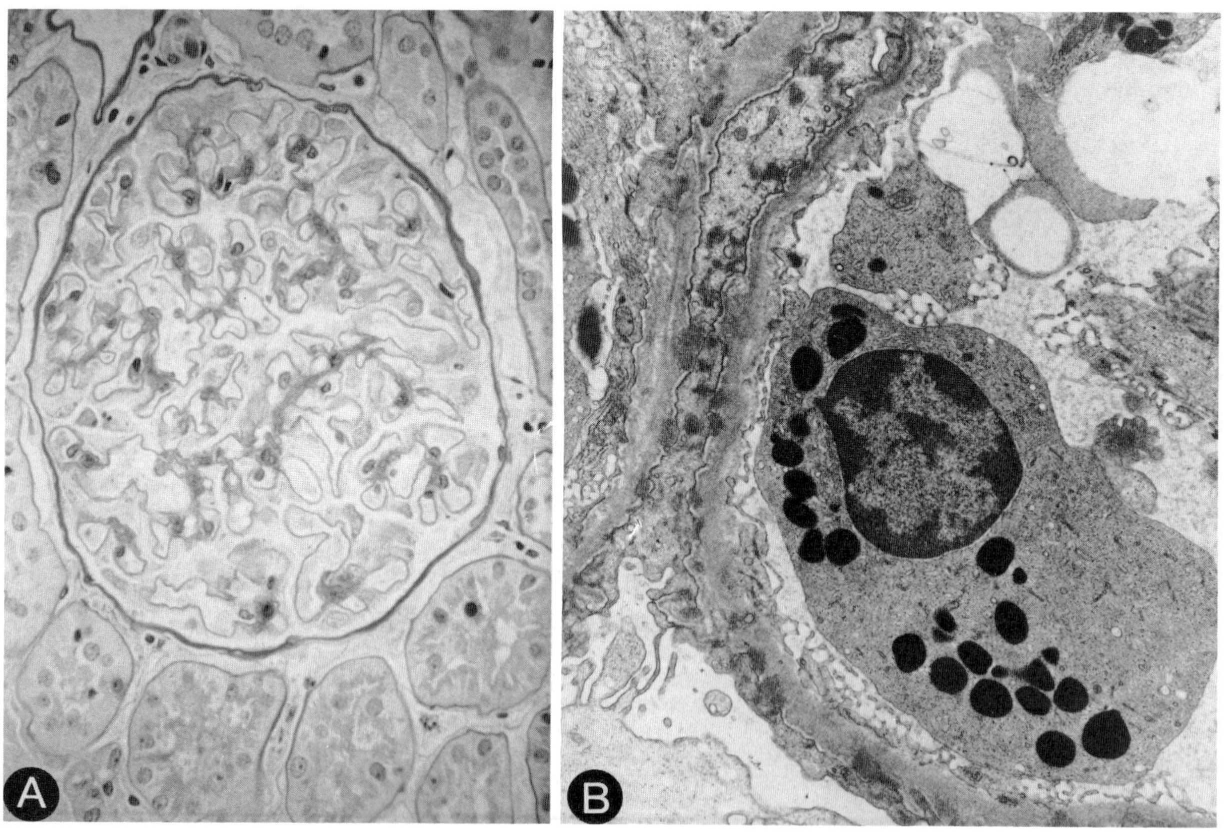

Figure 17.7. *A*, Membranous glomerulopathy in a patient receiving penicillamine. *B*, Electron dense deposits are present in the glomerular basement membrane.

Hypercalciuria and nephrocalcinosis (276) have been reported in infants receiving large doses of furosemide for management of chronic lung disease. Careful monitoring of urinary calcium excretion is indicated in these patients.

References

1. Green TP, Mirkin BL: Clinical pharmacokinetics: Pediatric considerations. In Benet LZ, Gambertoglio JG, Massoud N (eds): The Pharmacokinetic Basis of Drug Treatment. New York, Raven Press, 1982.
2. Shirkey AC: Drug administration with special emphasis on techniques and problems related to infants and children. In Shirkey HC (ed): Pediatric Therapy. St. Louis, The C.V. Mosby Co., 1972, p 14.
3. Morselli PL, Franco-Morselli R, Bossi L: Clinical pharmacokinetics in newborns and infants. Clin Pharmacokinet 5:485, 1980.
4. Kunin CM, Finland M: Persistence of antibiotics in blood of patients with acute renal failure. III. Penicillin, streptomycin, erythromycin and kanamycin. J Clin Invest 38:1509, 1959.
5. Kramer B, Selgison H, Baltrush H, et al: The isolation of several aromatic acids from the hemodialysis fluids of uremic patients. Clin Chim Acta 11:363, 1965.
6. Preuss HG, Massry SG, Maher JF, et al: Effects of uremic sera on renal tubular p-aminohippurate transport. Nephron 3:265, 1966.
7. Rose HJ, Pruit AW, McNay JL: Effect of experimental azotemia on renal clearance of furosemide in the dog. J Pharmacol Exptl Therap 196:238, 1976.
8. Rose HJ, O'Malley K, Pruitt AW: Repression of renal clearance of furosemide in man by azotemia. Clin Pharmacol Therap 21:141, 1977.
9. Bourke E, Frindt G, Preuss H, et al: Studies with uraemic serum on the renal transport of hippurates and tetraethylammonium in the rabbit and rat: Effects of oral neomycin. Clin Sci 38:41, 1970.
10. Reidenburg MR: The biotransformation of drugs in renal failure. Am J Med 62:484, 1977.
11. Shand DG, Rangno RG: The disposition of propranolol. I. Elimination during oral absorption in man. Pharmacology 7:159, 1972.
12. Lowenthal DT, Briggs WA, Gibson TP, et al: Pharmacokinetics of oral propranolol in chronic renal disease. Clin Pharmacol Therap 16:761, 1974.
13. Wood AJJ, Vestal RS, Spannuth CL, et al: Propranolol disposition in renal failure. Brit J Pharmacol 10:562, 1980.
14. Drayer DE: Pharmacologically active drug metabolites: Therapeutic and toxic activities, plasma and urine data in man, accumulation in renal failure. Clin Pharmacokinet 1:426, 1976.
15. Schentag JJ, Cerra FB, Calleri GM, et al: Age, disease and cimetidine disposition in healthy subjects and chronically ill patients. Clin Pharmacol Therap 29:737, 1981.
16. Kinniburgh DW, Boyd ND: Phenytoin binding to partially purified albumin in renal disease. Clin Pharmacol Therap 29:203, 1981.
17. Reidenberg MM: The binding of drugs to plasma proteins from patients with poor renal function. Clin Pharmacokinet 1:121, 1976.
18. Kinniburgh DW, Boyd ND: Isolation of peptides from uremic plasma that inhibits phenytoin binding to normal plasma proteins. Clin Pharmacol Therap 30:276, 1981.
19. Wilkinson GR, Shand DG: A physiological approach to hepatic drug clearance. Clin Pharmacol Therap 18:377, 1975.
20. Gugler R, Shoeman DW, Huffman DH, et al: Pharmacokinetics of drugs in patients with the nephrotic syndrome. J Clin Invest 55:1182, 1975.
21. Boston Collaborative Drug Surveillance Program. Diphenylhydantoin side effects and serum albumin levels. Clin Pharmacol Therap 14:529, 1973.
22. Pearson RM, Breckenridge AM: Renal function, protein binding and pharmacologic response to diazoxide. Brit J Clin Pharmacol 3:169, 1976.
23. Levy G: Effect of plasma protein binding of drugs on duration and intensity of pharmacologic activity. J Pharmaceut Sci 65:1264, 1976.
24. Gwilt PR, Perrier D: Plasma protein binding and distribution characteristics of drugs as indices of their hemodialyzability. Clin Pharmacol Therap 24:154, 1978.
25. Bunke CM, Aronoff GR, Brier ME, et al: Vancomycin kinetics during continuous ambulatory peritoneal dialysis. Clin Pharmacol Exptl Therap 34:631, 1983.
26. Bunke CM, Aronoff GR, Brier ME, et al: Tobramycin kinetics during continuous ambulatory peritoneal dialysis. Clin Pharmacol Therap 34:110, 1983.
27. Somani P, Shapiro RS, Stockard H, et al: Unidirectional absorption of gentamicin from the peritoneum during continuous ambulatory peritoneal dialysis. Clin Pharmacol Therap 32:113, 1982.
28. Bunke CM, Aronoff GR, Brier ME, et al: Cefazolin and cephalexin kinetics in continuous ambulatory peritoneal dialysis. Clin Pharmacol Therap 33:66, 1983.
29. Keating MJ, Bodley GP, Valdivraso M, et al: A randomized comparative trial of three aminoglycosides. Medicine 58:159, 1979.
30. Doluisio JT: Clinical pharmacokinetics of cefotaxime in patients with normal and reduced renal function. Rev Infect Dis 4(suppl):5333, 1982.
31. Green TP, Mirkin BL, Peterson PK, et al: Serum tobramycin level monitoring in young patients with normal renal function. Clin Pharmacokinet (In press).
32. Green TP, Mirkin BL: A method for the bedside application of first-order pharmacokinetics in therapeutic management. Therap Drug Monitoring 2:323, 1980.
33. Green TP, Mirkin BL: Determinants of the diuretic response to furosemide in infants with congestive heart failure. Pediat Cardiol 3:47, 1982.
34. Odlind B, Baerman B: Renal tubular secretion and effects of furosemide. Clin Pharmacol Therap 27:784, 1980.
35. Cooper MJ, Anders M, Sinaiko AR, et al: Application of HPLC to the study of the disposition of hydrochlorothiazide in adults and children. In Dixon P, Gray L, Kiu C (eds): High Pressure Liquid Chromatography in Clinical Chemistry. New York, Academic Press, 1984, p 175.
36. Mirkin B, Sinaiko A, Cooper, M, et al: Hydrochlorothiazide therapy in hypertensive and renal insufficient children: Elimination kinetics and metabolic effects. Pediatr Res 11:418, 1977.
37. Murphy J, Casey W, Lasagna L: The effect of dosage regimen on the diuretic efficacy of chlorothiazide in human subjects. J Pharmacol Exptl Therap 134:286, 1961.
38. Brater DC, Chennavasin P, Day B, et al: Bumetanide and furosemide. Clin Pharmacol Therap 34:207, 1983.
39. Cutler RE, Forrey AW, Christofer TG, et al: Pharmacokinetics of furosemide in normal subjects and functionally anephric patients. Clin Pharmacol Therap 15:588, 1974.
40. Brater DC, Seiwell R, Anderson S, et al: Absorption and disposition of furosemide in congestive heart failure. Kidney Intl 22:171, 1982.
41. Green TP, Mirkin BL: Resistance of proteinuric rats to furosemide: Urinary drug protein binding as a determinant of drug effect. Life Sci 26:623, 1980.
42. Wollam GL, Tarazi RC, Bravo EL, et al: Diuretic potency of combined hydrochlorothiazide and furosemide therapy in patients with azotemia. Am J Med 72:929, 1982.

42a. Arnold WC: Efficacy of metolazone and furosemide in children with furosemide resistant edema. Pediatrics 74:872, 1984.

43. Bryan CS, Stone WJ: Comparably massive penicillin G therapy in renal failure. Ann Intern Med 82:189, 1964.
44. Latos DL, Bryan CS, Stone WJ: Carbenicillin therapy in patients with normal and impaired renal function. Clin Pharmacol Therap 17:692, 1975.
45. Parry MF, Neu HC: Pharmacokinetics of ticarcillin in patients with abnormal renal function. J Infectious Dis 133:46, 1976.
46. Jusko WJ, Lewis GP, Schmitt GW: Ampicillin and hetacillin pharmacokinetics in normal and anephric subjects. Clin Pharmacol Therap 14:90, 1973.
47. Diaz CR, Kane JG, Parker RH, et al: Pharmacokinetics of nafcillin in patients with renal failure. Antimicrob Agents Chemo 12:98, 1977.
48. Bergan T: Overview of acylureidopenicillin pharmacokinetics. Scand J Infect Dis 29(suppl):33, 1981.
49. Aronoff GR, Sloan RS, Brier ME, et al: The effect of piperacillin dose on elimination kinetics in renal impairment. Europ J Clin Pharmacol 24:543, 1983.
50. Aronoff GR, Sloan RS, Stanish RA, et al: Mezlocillin dose dependent elimination kinetics in renal impairment. Europ J Clin Pharmacol 21:505, 1982.
51. Hiner LB, Baluarte HJ, Polinsky MS, et al: Cefazolin in children with renal insufficiency. J Pediatr 96:335, 1980.
52. Roelwicz TF, Mirkin BL, Cooper MJ, et al: Metabolic disposition of cephalothin and deacetylcephalothin in chidren and adults: Comparison of high-performance liquid chromatographic and microbial assay procedures. Clin Pharmacol Therap 22:928, 1977.
53. Kaplan SL, Berry PL, Mason EO, et al: Pharmacokinetics of moxalactam in anuric children and during hemodialysis. *Pediatr Pharmacol* 3:29, 1983.
54. Ings RMJ, Fillastre JP, Godin M, et al: The pharmacokinetics of cefotaxime and its metabolites in subjects with normal and impaired renal function. Rev Infect Dis 4(suppl):5379, 1982.
55. Greenfield RA, Gerber AM, Craig WA: Pharmacokinetics of cefoperazone in patients with normal and impaired hepatic and renal function. Rev Infect Dis 5(suppl):S127, 1983.
56. Morgan DJ, Ching MS, Raymond K, et al: Elimination of amphotericin B in impaired renal function. Clin Pharmacol Therap 34:248, 1983.
57. Blum MR, Liao SHT, De Miranda P: Overview of acyclovir pharmacokinetic disposition in adults and children. Am J Med (Acyclovir Symposium) 73:186, 1982.
58. Laskin OL, Longstreth JA, Whelton A, et al: Effect of renal failure on the pharmacokinetics of acyclovir. Am J Med (Acyclovir Symposium) 73:197, 1982.
59. Porter GA, Bennett WM: Toxic nephropathies. In Brenner BM, Rector FC Jr (eds): The Kidney. Philadelphia, W B. Saunders Co., 1981, p 2049.
60. Anderson RJ, Schrier RW: Clinical use of drugs in patients with kidney and liver disease. Philadelphia, W.B. Saunders, 1981.

61. Porter GA, Bennett WM: Nephrotoxic acute renal failure due to common drugs. Am J Physiol 241:F1, 1981.
62. Maher JF, Nolph KD, Bryan CW, et al: Etiology and distribution of renal disease in central Missouri. Missouri Med 69:799, 1972.
63. Anderson FJ, Linas SL, Berns AS, et al: Non-oliguric acute renal failure. N Engl J Med 296:1134, 1977.
64. Wade JC, Smith CR, Petty BG, et al: Cephalothin plus an aminoglycoside is more nephrotoxic than methicillin plus an aminoglycoside. Lancet 2:604, 1978.
65. Adelman RD, Spangler WL, Beasom F, et al: Furosemide enhancement of experimental gentamicin nephrotoxicity: Comparison of functional and morphological changes with activities of urinary enzymes. J Infect Dis 140:342, 1979.
66. Klune WM, Hook JB: Polybrominated biphenyl induced potentiation of chloroform toxicity. Toxicol Appl Pharmacol 45:861, 1978.
67. Luft PC, Yum MN, Kleit S: The effect of concomitant mercuric chloride to gentamicin on kidney function and structure on the rat. J Lab Clin Med 89:622, 1977.
68. Smith CR, Boughman KL, Edwards CQ, et al: Controlled comparison of amikacin and gentamicin. N Engl J Med 296:349, 1977.
69. Smith CR, Lipsky J, Laskin O, et al: Double-blind comparison of the nephrotoxicity and auditory toxicity of gentamicin and tobramycin. J Engl J Med 302:1106, 1980.
70. Bendush CL, Weber R: Tobramycin sulfate: A summary of worldwide experience from clinical trials. J Infect Dis 134(suppl):S219, 1976.
71. Keys TF, Kurtz SB, Jones JD, et al: Renal toxicity during therapy with gentamicin or tobramycin. Mayo Clin Proc 56:556, 1981.
72. Michalsen H, Bergan T: Pharmacokinetics of netilmicin in children with and without Cystic Fibrosis. Antimicrob Agents Chemo 19:1029, 1981.
73. Feldman H, Guignard JP: Plasma creatinine in the first month of life. Arch Dis Childh 57:123, 1982.
74. Faden H, Deshpande G, Gros N: Renal and auditory toxic effects of Amikacin in children with cancer. Am J Dis Child 136:223, 1982.
75. Elinder G, Aperia A: Development of glomerular filtration rate and excretion of B_2 microglobulin in neonates during gentamicin treatment. Acta Paediat Scand 72:219, 1983.
76. Adelman RD, Zakauddin S: Urinary enzyme activities in children and neonates receiving gentamicin therapy. Develop Pharmacol Therap 1:325, 1980.
77. Adelman RD, Halsted CC, Jordan GW, et al: Use of urinary enzyme activities in the early detection of aminoglycoside nephrotoxicity. Proc West Pharmacol Soc, 24:261, 1981.
78. Adelman RD: Aminoglycoside nephrotoxicity: Clinical and experimental observations. In Strauss J (ed): Pediatric Nephrology. (In Press.)
79. Lane AZ, Wright GE, Blair DC: Otoxicity and nephrotoxicity of amikacin. Am J Med 62:911, 1977.
80. Bennett WM, Hartnett NM, Gilbert D, et al: Effect of sodium intake on gentamicin nephrotoxicity in the rat. Proc Soc Exptl Biol Med 151:736, 1976.
81. Hsu CH, Kurtz TW, Easterling RE, et al: Potentiation of gentamicin nephrotoxicity by metabolic acidosis. Proc Soc Exptl Biol Med 146:894, 1974.
82. Churchill DN, Seely J: Nephrotoxicity associated with combined gentamicin-amphotericin B therapy. Nephron 19:176, 1977.
83. Butkus DC, de Torrente A, Terman DS: Renal failure following gentamicin and combination with clindamycin. Nephron 17:307, 1976.
84. Kleinknecht D, Ganeval D, Droz D: Acute renal failure after high doses of gentamicin and cephalothin. Lancet 1:1129, 1973.
85. Babrow SN, Jaffe E, Young RC: Anuria and acute tubular necrosis associated with gentamicin and cephalothin. JAMA 222:1546, 1972.
86. Plager JE: Association of renal injury with combined cephalothin-gentamicin therapy among patients severely ill with malignant disease. Cancer 37:1937, 1976.
87. Dentino ME, Luft FC, Yum MN, et al: Long term effect of cis-diammine dichloride platinum on renal function and structure in man. Cancer 41:1274, 1978.
88. Adelman RD, Spangler WL, Beasom F, et al: Furosemide enhancement of netilmicin nephrotoxicity in dogs. J Antimicrob Chemo 7:431, 1981.
89. Bendirdjian JP, Prime DJ, Browning MC, et al: Additive nephrotoxicity of cephalosporins and aminoglycosides in the rabbit. J Pharmacol Exptl Therap 218:681, 1981.
90. Luft FC, Patel V, Yum MN, et al: The nephrotoxicity of cephalosporin-gentamicin combinations in rats. Antimicrob Agents Chemo 9:831, 1976.
91. Gary NE, Buzzeo L, Salaki J, et al: Gentamicin associated acute renal failure. Arch Intern Med 136:1101, 1976.
92. Holmes AM, Hesling CM, Wilson TM: Drug-induced secondary hyperaldosteronism in patients with pulmonary tuberculosis. Quart J Med 39:299, 1970.
93. Patel R, Savage A: Symptomatic hypomagnesemia associated with gentamicin therapy. Nephron 23:50, 1979.
94. Bar RS, Wilson HE, Mazzaferri EL: Hypomagnesemic hypocalcemia secondary to renal magnesium wasting: a possible consequence of high dose gentamicin therapy. Ann Inter Med 82:646, 1975.
95. Russo J, Adelman RD: Gentamicin induced Fanconi syndrome. J Pediatr 96:151, 1980.
96. Bennett WM, Gilbert DN, Houghton D, et al: Gentamicin nephrotoxicity—morphologic and pharmacologic features. West J Med 126:65, 1977.
97. Spangler WL, Adelman RD, Conzelman GM, et al: Gentamicin nephrotoxicity in the dog: Sequential light and electron microscopy. Vet Pathol 17:206, 1980.
98. Gilbert DN, Houghton DC, Bennett WM, et al: Reversibility of gentamicin nephrotoxicity in rats: Recovery during continued drug administration. Proc Soc Exptl Biol Med 160:99, 1979.
99. Chiu P, Brown A, Miller G, et al: Renal extraction of gentamicin in anesthetized dogs. Antimicrob Agents Chemo 10:277, 1976.
100. Just M, Erdmann G, Habermann E: The renal handling of poly-basic drugs. I. Gentamicin and aprotinin in intact animals. Naunyn-Schmiedeberg Arch Pharmacol 300:57, 1977.
101. Luft FC, Kleit SA: Renal parenchymal accumulation of aminoglycoside antibiotics in rats. J Infect Dis 130:656, 1974.
102. Silverblatt FJ, Kuehn C: Autoradiography of gentamicin uptake by the rat proximal tubule cell. Kidney Intl 15:335, 1979.
103. Morin JP, Viotte G, Vandewalle A, et al: Gentamicin induced nephrotoxicity. A cell biology approach. Kidney Intl 18:583, 1980.
104. Knauss TC, Weinberg JM, Humes HD: Alterations in renal cortical phospholipid content induced by gentamicin: time course, specificity and subcellular localization. Am J Physiol 244:F535, 1983.
105. Lipsky JJ, Leitman PS: Aminoglycoside inhibition of a renal phosphatidylinositol phospholipase C. J Pharmacol Exptl Therap 220:287, 1982.
106. Carlier MB, Laurent G, Claes PJ, et al: Inhibition of lysosomal phospholipases by aminoglycoside antibiotics: *in vitro* comparative studies. Antimicrob Agents Chemo 23:440, 1983.
107. Patel V, Luft FC, Yum MN, et al: Enzymuria in gentamicin-induced kidney damage. Antimicrob Agents Chemo 7:364, 1975.
108. Luft FC, Kleit SA: Renal parenchymal accumulation of aminoglycoside antibiotics in rats. J Infect Dis 130:656, 1974.
109. Ormsby A, Plamp C, Bennett W, et al: Comparison of the nephrotoxic potential of gentamicin, tobramycin and netilmicin in the rat. Clin Res 26:141A, 1978.
110. Adelman RD, Conzelman G, Spangler W, et al: Comparative nephrotoxicity of gentamicin and netilmicin: Functional and morphological correlations with urinary enzyme activities. Curr Probl Clin Biochem 9:166, 1979.
111. Hsu CH, Kurtz TW, Easterling RE, et al: Potentiation of gentamicin nephrotoxicity by metabolic acidosis. Proc Soc Exptl Biol Med 146:894, 1974.
112. Baylis C, Rennke HR, Brenner B: Mechanisms of the defect in glomerular ultrafiltration associated with gentamicin administration. Kidney Intl 12:344, 1977.
113. Schor N, Ichikawa I, Rennke HG, et al: Pathophysiology of altered glomerular function in aminoglycoside treated rats. Kidney Intl 19:288, 1981.
114. Avasthi PS, Evan AP, Huser JW, et al: Effect of gentamicin on glomerular ultrastructure. J Lab Clin Med 98:444, 1981.
115. Dahlgren JG, Anderson ET, Hewlitt WL: Gentamicin blood levels: A guide to nephrotoxicity. Antimicrob Agents Chemo 8:58, 1975.
116. Plamp CE, Bennett WM, Gilbert DN, et al: The effect of dosage regimen on experimental gentamicin toxicity: Dissociation of peak serum levels from renal failure. Clin Res 26:125A, 1978.
117. Bennett WM, Gilbert DN, Houghton D, et al: Gentamicin nephrotoxicity—morphologic and pharmacologic features. West J Med 126:65, 1977.
118. Bennett JE: Chemotherapy of systemic mycoses. N Engl J Med 290:30, 1974.
119. Douglas JB, Healy JK: Nephrotoxic effects of amphotericin B, including renal tubular acidosis. Am J Med 46:154, 1969.
120. Takacs FJ, Tomkiewicz ZM, Merrill JP: Amphotericin B nephrotoxicity with irreversible renal failure. Ann Intern Med 59:716, 1963.
121. Butler WT, Bennett JE, Alling DW, et al: Nephrotoxicity of amphotericin B: Early and late effects in 81 patients. Ann Intern Med 61:175, 1964.
122. Bhathena DB, Bullock WE, Nuttall CE, et al: The effects of amphotericin B therapy on the intrarenal vasculature and renal tubules in man. Clin Nephrol 9:103, 1978.
123. Jose PA, Eisner GM, Hollerman CE, et al: Acute renal effects of amphotericin B. Proc Soc Exptl Biol Med 137:224, 1971.
124. Butler WT, Hill GJ, Szwed CF, et al: Amphotericin B renal toxicity in the dog. J Pharmacol Exptl Therap 143:47, 1964.
125. Andreoli TE: On the anatomy of amphotericin B—cholesterol pores in lipid bilayer membranes. Kidney Intl 4:337, 1973.
126. Gouge TH, Andriole VT: An experimental model of amphotericin B nephrotoxicity with renal tubular acidosis. J Lab Clin Med 78:713, 1971.
127. Bullock WE, Luke RG, Nuttall CE, et al: Can mannitol reduce amphotericin B nephrotoxicity. Antimicrob Agents Chemo 10:555, 1976.
128. Jawetz E: Polymyxin, colistin and bacitracin. Pediatr Clin No Am 8:1057, 1961.
129. Koch-Weser J, Sidel V, Federman ER, et al: Adverse effects of sodium colistimethate. Ann Intern Med 72:857, 1970.

130. Rodriguez V, Green S, Bodey GP: Serum electrolyte abnormalities associated with the administration of polymyxin B in febrile leukemic patients. Clin Pharmacol Therap 11:106, 1970.
131. Ryan KJ, Schainuck LI, Hickman RO, et al: Colistimethate toxicity: report of a fatal case in a previously healthy child. JAMA 207:2099, 1969.
132. Engle JE, Drago J, Carlin B, et al: Reversible acute renal failure after cephalothin. Ann Intern Med 83:232, 1975.
133. Tune BM: Relationship between the transport and toxicity of cephalosporins in the kidney. J Infect Dis 132:189, 1975.
134. Wold JS, Joost RR, Owen NV: Nephrotoxicity of cephaloridine in newborn rabbits: role of the renal anionic transport system. J Pharmacol Exptl Therap 210:778, 1977.
135. Shils ME: Renal disease and the metabolic effects of tetracycline. Ann Intern Med 58:389, 1963.
136. Singer I, Rotenberg D: Demeclocycline-induced nephrogenic diabetes insipidus. In-vivo and in-vitro studies. Ann Intern Med 79:679, 1973.
137. Carrilho F, Bosch J, Arroyo V, et al: Renal failure associated with demeclocycline in cirrhosis. Ann Intern Med 87:195, 1977.
138. Benitz KF, Diermeier HF: Renal toxicity of tetracycline degradation products. Proc Soc Exptl Biol Med 115:930, 1964.
139. Fulop M, Drapkin A: Potassium depleting syndrome secondary to nephropathy apparently caused by "outdated tetracycline." N Engl J Med 272:986, 1965.
140. Hook EW, Johnson WD: Vancomycin therapy of bacterial endocarditis. Am J Med 65:411, 1978.
141. Waisbren BA, Kleinerman L, Skemp J, et al: Comparative clinical effectiveness and toxicity of vancomycin, ristocetin and kanamycin. Arch Intern Med 106:179, 1960.
142. Lawson DH, Jick H: Adverse reactions to cotrimoxazole in hospitalized medical patients. Am J Med Sci 275:53, 1978.
143. Kovach JS, Moertel CG, Schutt AJ, et al: Phase II study of cisdiamminedichloroplatinum (NSC-119875) in advanced carcinoma of the large bowel. Cancer Chemotherapy Rept 57:337, 1973.
144. Dentino ME, Luft FC, Yum MN, et al: Long term effect of cisdiamminedichloride platinum (CDDP) on renal function and structure in man. Cancer 41:1274, 1978.
145. Baum ES, Gaynon P, Greenberg L, et al: Phase II trial of cisplatinum in refractory childhood cancer. Children's Cancer Study Group Report. Cancer Treat Rept 65:815, 1981.
146. Hayes DM, Cvitkovic E, Golbey RB, et al: High dose cis-platinum diammine dichloride: amelioration of renal toxicity by mannitol diuresis. Cancer 39:1372, 1977.
147. Blachley JD, Hill JB: Renal and electrolyte disturbances associated with cisplatin. Ann Intern Med 95:628, 1981.
148. Gonzalez-Vitale JC, Hayes DM, Cvitkoviv E, et al: The renal pathology in clinical trials of cis-platinum (II) and diamminedichloride. Cancer 39:1362, 1977.
149. Schilsky RL, Anderson TM: Hypomagnesemia and renal magnesium wasting in patients receiving cisplatin. Ann Intern Med 90:929, 1979.
150. Lange RC, Spencer RP, Harder HC: The antitumor agent cis-Pt $(NH_3)2CL_2$: Distribution studies and dose calculations for ^{193m}Pt and 193M^{Pt}. J Nuclear Med 14:191, 1973.
151. Weiner MW, Jacobs C: Mechanism of cisplatin nephrotoxicity. Fed Proc 42:2974, 1983.
152. Chopra S, Kaufman JS, Jones TW, et al: Cis-diammine dichloro platinum-induced acute renal failure in the rat. Kidney Intl 21:54, 1982.
153. Levi J, Jacobs C, Kalman SM, et al: Mechanism of cisplatinum nephrotoxicity 1. Effects of sulfhydryl groups in rat kidneys. J Pharmacol Exptl Therap 213:545, 1980.
154. Jacobs C, Bertino JR, Foffinet DR, et al: 24 hour infusion of cisplatinum in head and neck cancers. Cancer 24:2135, 1978.
155. Stark JJ, Howell SBL: Nephrotoxicity of cisplatinum (II) dichlorodiammine. Clin Pharmacol Therap 23:461, 1978.
156. Ostrow S, Egorin MJ, Hahn D, et al: High dose cisplatin therapy using mannitol versus furosemide diuresis: Comparative pharmacokinetics and toxicity. Cancer Treatment Rept 68:73, 1981.
157. Chiuten D, Vogl S, Kaplan B, et al: Is there cumulative or delayed toxicity from cis-platinum. Cancer 52:211, 1983.
158. Ozols RF, Corden BJ, Jacob J, et al: High dose cisplatinum in hypertonic saline. Ann Intern Med 100:19, 1984.
159. Byrd L, Sherman RL: Radiocontrast-induced acute renal failure. Medicine 58:270, 1979.
160. Van Zee BE, Hoy WE, Talley TE, et al: Renal injury associated with intravenous pyelography in nondiabetic and diabetic patients. Ann Intern Med 89:51, 1978.
161. Swartz RD, Rubin JE, Leeming BW, et al: Renal failure following major angiography. Am J Med 65:31, 1978.
162. D'Elia JA, Gleason RE, Alday M, et al: Nephrotoxicity from angiographic contrast media. A Prospective Study. Am J Med 72:719, 1982.
163. Berdon WE, Schwartz RH, Becker J, et al: Tamm-Horsfall proteinuria; its relationship to prolonged nephrogram in infants and children with acute renal failure, following intravenous urography, and in adults with multiple myeloma. Radiology 92:714, 1969.
164. Avner ED, Ellis D, Jaffe R, et al: Neonatal radiocontrast nephropathy simulating infantile polycystic kidney disease. J Pediatr 100:85, 1982.
165. Lasser EC, Lee SH, Fisher E, et al: Some further pertinent considerations regarding the comparative toxicity of contrast materials for the dog kidney. Radiology 78:240, 1962.
166. Gruskin AB, Oetliker OH, Wolfish NM, et al: Effect of angiography on renal function and histology in infants and piglets. J Pediatr 76:41, 1970.
167. Borra S, Hawkins D, Duguid W, et al: Acute renal failure and nephrotic syndrome after angiocardiography with meglumine diatrizoate. N Engl J Med 284:592, 1971.
168. Bennett WM: Am J Med 69:767, 1980.
169. Harvey LA, Caldicott WJH, Kuruc A: The effect of contrast media on immature renal function. Radiology 148:429, 1983.
170. Eisenberg RL, Bank WD, Hedglock MW: Renal failure after major angiography. Am J Med 68:43, 1980.
171. Shafi T, Chou SY, Porush JG, et al: Infusion intravenous pyelography and renal function. Effects in patients with chronic renal insufficiency. Arch Intern Med 138:1218, 1978.
172. Clarkson TW: The pharmacology of mercury compounds. Ann Rev Pharmacol 12:375, 1972.
173. Freeman RB, Maher JF, Schreiner GE, et al: Renal tubular necrosis due to nephrotoxicity of organic mercurial diuretics. Ann Intern Med 57:34, 1962.
174. Burston J, Darmady EM, Stranack F: Nephrosis due to mercurial diuretics. Brit Med J 1:1277, 1958.
175. Stein JH, Lifschitz MD, Barnes LD: Current concepts on the pathophysiology of acute renal failure. Am J Physiol 234:F171, 1978.
176. Felton JS, Kahn E, Salick B, et al: Heavy metal poisoning: Mercury and lead. Ann Intern Med 76:779, 1972.
177. Strunge P: Nephrotic syndrome caused by a seed disinfectant. J Occupat Med 12:178, 1970.
178. Kimbumamusoke JW, Davies DR, Huh MSK: Membranous nephropathy due to skin lightening cream. Brit Med J 2:646, 1974.
179. Becker CG, Becker EF, Maher JF, et al: Nephrotic syndrome after contact with mercury. A report of five cases, three after the use of ammoniated mercury ointment. Arch Intern Med 110:178, 1962.
180. Haley T: Saturnism, pediatric and adult lead poisoning. Clin Toxicol 4:11, 1971.
181. Hammond P: Exposure of humans to lead. Ann Rev Pharmacol Toxicol 17:197, 1977.
182. Chisholm: Aminoaciduria as a manifestation of lead intoxication. J Pediatr 60:1, 1962.
183. Morgan J: Nephropathy in lead poisoning. Archiv Intern Med 118:17, 1966.
184. Nechay Br, Saunders JP: Inhibitory characteristics of lead chloride in sodium- and potassium-dependent adenosine triphosphatase preparations derived from kidney, brain, and heart of several species. J Toxicol Environ Health 4:147, 1978.
185. Emerson B: Chronic lead nephropathy. Kidney Intl 4:1, 1973.
186. Henderson DA: The aetiology of chronic nephritis in Queensland. Med J Austral 45(1):377, 1958.
187. Tepper LB: Renal function subsequent to childhood plumbism. Archiv Environ Health 7:82, 1963.
188. Inglis JA, Henderson DA, Emmerson BT: The pathology and pathogenesis of chronic lead nephropathy occurring in Queensland. J Pathol 124:65, 1978.
189. Sandstead HH, Michelakis AM, Temple TE: Lead intoxication: its effects on the renin aldosterone response to sodium deprivation. Archiv Environ Health 20:356, 1970.
190. Weeden R: Detection and treatment of occupational lead nephropathy. Archiv Intern Med 139:53, 1979.
191. Lugo G, Cassady G, Palmisano P: Acute maternal arsenic intoxication with neonatal death. Am J Dis Child 117:328, 1969.
192. Wilkinson SP, McHugh P, Horsley S, et al: Arsine toxicity aboard the Asia freighter. Brit Med J 3:559, 1975.
193. Uldall PR, Khan HA, Ennis JE, et al: Renal damage from industrial arsenic poisoning. Brit J Indust Med 27:372, 1970.
194. Urizar R, Vernier RL: Bismuth nephropathy. JAMA 198:187, 1966.
195. Beattie JW: Nephrotic syndrome following sodium bismuth tartrate therapy in rheumatoid arthritis. Ann Rheum Dis 12:144, 1953.
196. Silverberg DS, Kidd EG, Schnitka TK, et al: Gold nephropathy: A clinical and pathologic study. Arth Rheum 13:812, 1970.
197. Tubbs RR, Valenzuela R, McCormack LJ, et al: Gold nephropathy. N Engl J Med 296:1413, 1977.
198. Jennings RB: Fatal fulminant acute carbon tetrachloride poisoning. Archiv Pathol 59:269, 1955.
199. Moon HD: The pathology of fatal carbon tetrachloride poisoning with special

reference to the histogenesis of the hepatic and renal lesions. Am J Pathol 26:1041, 1950.
200. Arena JM: The treatment of poisoning. CIBA Clinical Symposium. 30:3, 1978.
201. Sirota JH: Carbon tetrachloride poisoning in man; the mechanism of renal failure and recovery. J Clin Invest 28:1412, 1949.
202. Baerg RD, Kimberg DV: Centrilobular hepatic necrosis and acute renal failure in "solvent sniffers." Ann Intern Med 73:713, 1970.
203. Bierne GJ, Brennan JT: Glomerulonephritis associated with hydrocarbon solvents. Arch Environ Health 25:365, 1972.
204. Lagrue G: Hydrocarbon exposure and chronic glomerulonephritis (Letter). Lancet 1:1191, 1976.
205. Zimmerman SW, Groehler K, Beirne GJ: Hydrocarbon exposure and chronic glomerulonephritis. Lancet 2:199, 1975.
206. Klavis G, Drommer W: Goodpasture—Syndrome und Benzineinwirkung. Arch Toxikol 26:40, 1970.
207. Harman JW: Chronic glomerulonephritis and the nephrotic syndrome induced in rats with N,N[1]-diacetylbenzidine. J Pathol 104:119, 1972.
208. Eknoyan G, Gyorkey F, Dichaso C, et al: Renal involvement in drug abuse. Archiv Intern Med 132:801, 1973.
209. Rao TKS, Nicastri AD, Friedman EA: Renal consequences of narcotic abuse. Adv Nephrol 8:261, 1978.
210. Citron BP, Halpern M, McCarron M, et al: Necrotizing angiitis associated with drug abuse. N Engl J Med 283:1003, 1970.
211. Kleinman JG, Breitenfield RV, Roth DA: Acute renal failure associated with acetaminophen ingestion: Report of a case and review of the literature. Clin Nephrol 14:201, 1980.
212. McMurty RJ, Snodgrass WR, Mitchell JR: Renal necrosis, glutathione depletion and convalent binding after acetaminophen. J Toxicol Appl Pharmacol 46:87, 1978.
213. Calder IC, Yong AC, Wood RA, et al: The nephrotoxicity of p-aminophenol. II. The effect of metabolic inhibitors and inducers. Chem Biol Interactions 27:245, 1979.
214. Mudge GH: Analgesic Nephropathy: Renal drug distribution and metabolism. In Porter G (ed): Nephrotoxic Mechanisms of Drugs and Environmental Toxins. New York, Plenum Press, 1982, p 209.
215. Prescott LF, Park J, Sutherland GR, et al: Methionine and penicillamine in the treatment of paracetamol poisoning. Lancet 2:109, 1976.
216. Piperno E, Bersenbruegge DA: Reversal of experimental paracetamol toxicosis with N-acetylcysteine. Lancet 2:738, 1976.
217. Pitman SW, Frei E: Weekly methotrexate—calcium leucovorin rescue: effect of alkalinization on nephrotoxicity: pharmacokinetics in the CNS and use in CNS non-Hodgkin's lymphoma. Cancer Treatment Rept 61:695, 1977.
218. Jaffe N, Traggis D: Toxicity of high dose methotrexate (NSC-740) and citrovorum factor (NSC-3590) in osteogenic sarcoma. Cancer Chemo Rept (Part 3) 6:31, 1975.
219. Romolo JL, Goldberg NH, Honde KR, et al: Effect of hydration on plasma methotrexate levels. Cancer Treatment Rept 61:1393, 1977.
220. Ahmed S, Shan F, Bleyer WA: Methotrexate induced renal failure and ineffectiveness of peritoneal dialysis. Arch Intern Med 138:1146, 1978.
221. Link DA, Fosburg MT, Ingelfinger JR, et al: Renal toxicity of high dose methotrexate. Pediatr Res 10:455, 1976.
222. Pitman SW, Parker LM, Tattersall MHN, et al: Clinical trials of high dose methotrexate (NSC-740) with citrovorum factor (NSC-3590)—toxicologic and therapeutic observations. Cancer Chemotherapy Rept (Part 3) 6:43, 1975.
223. Kjellstrand CM, Campbell DC II, von Hartitzseh B, et al: Hyperuricemic acute renal failure. Arch Intern Med 133:349, 1974.
224. Reiselbach RE, Bentzel CJ, Cotlove E, et al: Uric acid excretion and renal function in the acute hyperuricemia of leukemia. Am J Med 37:872, 1964.
225. Frei EC, Benzel C, Reiselbach C, et al: Renal complications of neoplastic disease. J Chronic Dis 16:757, 1963.
226. Kelton J, Kelley WN, Holmes EW: A rapid method for the diagnosis of acute uric acid nephropathy. Arch Intern Med 138:612, 1978.
227. Kanwar YS, Manaligod JR: Leukemia urate nephropathy. Arch Pathol 99:467, 1975.
228. Engle JE, Steele TH: Variations of urate excretion with urine flow in normal man. Nephron 16:50, 1976.
229. Conger JD, Falk SA: Intrarenal dynamics in the pathogenesis and prevention of acute urate nephropathy. J Clin Invest 59:786, 1977.
230. Krakoff IH, Murphy ML: Hyperuricemia in neoplastic disease in children: Prevention with allopurinol, a xanthine oxidase inhibitor. Pediatrics 41:52, 1968.
231. Steinberg SM, Galon MA, Lazarus JM, et al: Hemodialysis for acute anuric uric acid nephropathy. Am J Dis Child 129:956, 1975.
232. Pusey CD, Saltissi D, Bloodworth L, et al: Drug associated acute interstitial nephritis: Clinical and pathological features and the response to high dose steroid therapy. Quart J Med 206:194, 1983.
233. Linton AL, Clark WF, Driedger AA, et al: Acute interstitial nephritis due to drugs. Review of the literature with a report of nine cases. Ann Intern Med 93:735, 1980.
234. Baldwin DS, Levine BB, McCluskey RT, et al: Renal failure and interstitial nephritis due to penicillin and methicillin. N Engl J Med 279:1245, 1968.
235. Gilbert DN, Gourley R, d'Agostino A, et al: Interstitial nephritis due to methicillin, penicillin and ampicillin. Ann Aller 28:378, 1970.
236. Border WA, Lehman DH, Egan JD, et al: Antitubular basement-membrane antibodies in methicillin-associated interstitial nephritis. N Engl J Med 291:381, 1974.
237. Galpin JE, Schinaberger JH, Stanley TM, et al: Acute interstitial nephritis due to methicillin. Am J Med 65:756, 1978.
238. Ruley EJ, Lisi LM: Interstitial nephritis and renal failure due to ampicillin. J Pediatr 84:878, 1974.
239. Ellis D, Fried WA, Yunis EJ, et al: Acute interstitial nephritis in children: a report of 13 cases and review of the literature. Pediatrics 67:862, 1981.
240. Ooi BS, Jao W, Frist MR, et al: Acute interstitial nephritis. A clinical and pathological study based on renal biopsies. Am J Med 59:614, 1975.
241. Lyons H, Pinn VW, Cortell S, et al: Allergic interstitial nephritis causing reversible renal failure in four patients with idiopathic nephrotic syndrome. N Engl J Med 288:124, 1973.
242. Fuller TJ, Barcenas CG, White MG: Diuretic-induced interstitial nephritis. JAMA 235:1998, 1976.
243. Vestergaard P, Amdisin A: Lithium treatment and kidney function. Acta Psychiat Scand 63:333, 1981.
244. Aurell M, Svalander C, Wallin L, et al: Renal function and biopsy findings in patients on long term lithium treatment. Kidney Intl 20:663, 1981.
245. Richman AV, Masco HL, Rifkin SI, et al: Minimal change disease and the nephrotic syndrome associated with lithium therapy. Ann Intern Med 92:70, 1980.
246. Deas N, Hacken AG: Oliguric acute renal failure complicating lithium carbonate therapy. Nephron 10:246, 1972.
247. Miller PD, Dubovsky SL, McDonald KM, et al: Hypocalciuric effect of lithium in man. Min Elect Metab 1:3, 1978.
248. Shulman H, Striker G, Deeg HJ, et al: Nephrotoxicity of cyclosporin A after allogenic marrow transplantation: glomerular thromboses and tubular injury. J Engl J Med 305:1392, 1981.
249. Neild GH, Ivory K, Williams DG: Cortical infarction in rabbits with serum sickness following cyclosporine therapy. First International Congress on Cyclosporine. Houston, Texas, May, 1983.
250. Greenburg A, Egel J, Thompson ON, et al: Renal failure in heart transplant patients receiving cyclosporin A (abstract). Clin Res 31:429A, 1983.
251. Gratwohl A, Muller M, Osterwalder B, et al: Nephrotoxicity of cyclosporin A in bone marrow transplant recipients. Lancet 2:635, 1981.
252. Powell-Jackson PR, Young B, Calne RY, et al: Nephrotoxicity of parenterally administered cyclosporine after orthotopic liver transplantation. Transplantation 36:505, 1983.
253. Sibley RK, Ferguson RM, Sutherland DE, et al: Morphology of cyclosporine nephrotoxicity and of acute rejection in cyclosporine-prednisone immunosuppressed renal allograft recipients. Transplantation Proc, 1983.
254. Bennett WM, Pulliam JP: Cyclosporine nephrotoxicity. Ann Intern Med 99:851, 1983.
255. Fine RN, Terasaki PI, Ettenger RB, et al: Renal transplantation update. Ann Intern Med 100:246, 1984.
256. Moran M, Newton L, Perlroth M, et al: Cyclosporin nephrotoxicity in man. Kidney Intl 25:346 A, 1984.
257. Joss DV, Barrett AJ, Kendra JR, et al: Hypertension and convulsions in children receiving cyclosporin A (letter). Lancet 1:906, 1982.
258. Adu D, Turney J, Michael J, et al: Hyperkalemia in cyclosporin treated renal allograft recipients. Lancet 2:370, 1983.
259. Whiting PH, Simpson JG: The enhancement of cyclosporin A induced nephrotoxicity by gentamicin. Biochem Pharmacol 32:2025, 1983.
260. Brezin JH, Katz SM, Schwartz AB, et al: Reversible renal failure and nephrotic syndrome associated with nonsteroidal antiinflammatory drugs. N Engl J Med 301:1271, 1979.
261. Gary NE, Dodelson R, Eisinger RP: Indomethacin associated renal failure. Am J Med 69:135, 1980.
262. Finkelstein A, Fraley DS, Stachura I, et al: Fenoprofen nephropathy: Lipoid nephrosis and interstitial nephritis. A possible T-lymphocyte disorder. Am J Med 72:81, 1982.
263. Curt GA, Kaldany A, Whitley LG, et al: Reversible rapidly progressive renal failure with nephrotic syndrome due to fenoprofen calcium. Ann Intern Med 92:72, 1980.
264. Ciabattoni G, Cheotti Ga, Pierucci A, et al: Effects of sulindac and ibuprofen in patients with chronic glomerular disease. Evidence for the dependence of renal function on prostacyclin. N Engl J Med 310:279, 1984.
265. Cifuentes RF, Olley PM, Balfe JW, et al: Indomethacin and renal function in premature infants with persistent patent ductus arteriosus. J Pediatr 95: 583, 1979.

266. Halliday HL, Hirata T, Brady JP: Indomethacin therapy for large patent ductus arteriosus in the very low birth weight infant: Results and complications. Pediatrics 64:154, 1979.
267. Catterton Z, Sellers B, Gray B: Inulin clearance in the premature infant receiving indomethacin. J Pediatr 96:737, 1980.
268. Rosenberg LE, Hayslett JP: Nephrotoxic effects of penicillamine in cystinuria. JAMA 201:128, 1967.
269. Bacon PA, Tribe CR, MacKenzie JC, et al: Penicillamine nephropathy in rheumatoid arthritis. Quart J Med 180:661, 1976.
270. Dische FE, Swinson DR, Hamilton EBD, et al: Immunopathology of penicillamine induced glomerular disease. J Rheumatol 3:145, 1976.
271. Lachmann PJ: Nephrotic syndrome from penicillamine. Postgrad Med J 44(suppl):23, 1968.
272. Barnett HL, Simmons DJ, Wells RE: Nephrotic syndrome occurring during Tridione therapy. Am J Med 4:760, 1948.
273. Heyman W: Nephrotic syndrome after use of trimethadione and paramethadione in petit mal. JAMA 202:893, 1967.
274. Hertz P, Yager H, Richardson JA: Probenecid-induced nephrotic syndrome. Archiv Pathol 94:241, 1972.
275. Tait GB: Nephropathy during phenindione therapy. Lancet 2:1198, 1960.
276. Hufnagle KG, Khan SN, Penn D, et al: Renal calcifications: A complication of long-term furosemide therapy in preterm infants. Pediatrics 70:360, 1982.

4

Methods of Evaluation

CHAPTER **18**

Clinical Evaluation

T. MARTIN BARRATT
CYRIL CHANTLER

PRESENTATION

The presence of a kidney disorder may be signaled by obvious changes in urine composition and volume or by disordered micturition. However, in many cases, serious renal disease may be present with complaints apparently unrelated to the urinary tract or unaccompanied by any symptoms at all. The possibility of renal disease should be considered in any sick child, particularly in an infant, as the presentation in early life is often nonspecific and encompassed by the generic term "failure to thrive."

ABNORMALITIES OF URINE APPEARANCE

Hematuria

The addition of even a small amount of blood to urine results in obvious macroscopic hematuria. If the bleeding is brisk the urine is red and may even contain clots, but usually the pigment changes to the browner color of acid hematin. However, apparently normal-looking urine may have an abnormal concentration of erythrocytes, microscopic hematuria. Hematuria must be distinguished from hemoglobinuria and myoglobinuria; porphyria also may cause reddish-brown discoloration of the urine, as may the ingestion of beetroot and certain food-coloring materials (1).

The blood may originate from the glomeruli or from the urinary tract, and a urological disorder, particularly tumor, hydronephrosis, or stone, must always be eliminated by careful intravenous urography (IVU) even if there is obvious evidence of glomerular disease. Blood in the initial part of the urinary stream suggests a urethral origin of the bleeding; terminal hematuria points to a bladder cause, particularly if associated with suprapubic pain or disturbance of micturition. However, in most affected children, hematuria has its origin in the upper urinary tract and endoscopy is not necessary as a routine investigation unless it is accompanied by lower tract symptoms.

If hematuria is persistent and accompanied by heavy proteinuria or reduced renal function, it is usually necessary to proceed to renal biopsy to define the glomerular lesion. Isolated hematuria of presumed glomerular origin, provided familial cases are excluded, is usually benign, and generally does not require to be further characterized by renal histology.

Cloudy or Offensive Urine

Cloudy, offensive urine suggests the possibility of a urinary tract infection (UTI). However, normal concentrated urine, when cooled, forms a precipitate of calcium phosphate; conversely, significant bacteriuria may be present without obvious macroscopic abnormality. Thus, the diagnosis of UTI must be confirmed by microscopy and culture of a properly collected urine sample.

Stone or Gravel

The passage of stone or gravel is a rare event in childhood. The usual variety of stone in the United Kingdom is composed of struvite (magnesium ammonium phosphate) with organic matrix and is generally associated with a Proteus UTI rather than with metabolic disturbances. Because of their soft character, such stones, when passed, may be described as a discharge or as resembling toothpaste.

ABNORMALITIES OF URINE VOLUME

Oligoanuria

Anuria is the complete suppression of urine formation; oliguria is the passage of an insufficient volume of urine to maintain homeostasis, usually taken to be <500 ml/24 hr/1.73m2 surface area, which in infants approximates 1.0 ml/hr/kg body weight. Urine volume in breast-fed, full-term babies averages 20 ml/24 hr in the first 2 days of life, rising to 200 ml by the tenth day (2). In newborn infants, 92% pass urine within the first 24 hours and 98% do so within 48 hours of birth (3). Oliguria may represent the physiological response of a healthy kidney to inadequate perfusion, parenchymal renal disease, or obstruction of the urinary passages.

Polyuria

Polyuria results from an excessive intake of fluid, a failure of release of antidiuretic hormone (ADH), osmotic diuresis, or renal resistance to the action of ADH. The distinction between primary polydipsia and primary polyuria may be inferred from the relative osmolality of plasma and urine and the response to controlled water deprivation; the distinction between pituitary and renal causes of polyuria may be made by the plasma arginine-vasopressin concentration and the urinary response to des-D-amino-arginine vasopressin (DDAVP).

It is difficult to define the threshold for polyuria with precision, but it usually does not become apparent as a clinical symptom unless the urine is persistently hypotonic to plasma. Under these circumstances, there is increased thirst (polydipsia) and infants in particular are exposed to the risk of dehydration. The principal renal lesions that result in ADH-resistant polyuria of this severity are nephrogenic diabetes insipidus, cystinosis, distal renal tubular acidosis, Bartter's syndrome, obstructive nephropathy, and medullary cystic disease.

Disturbances of Bladder Function

Incontinence and Enuresis

Daytime urinary continence is usually achieved by the age of 3 years, but 10% of boys still have occasional nocturnal enuresis at 5 years and 5% at 7 years. The development of incontinence in a child who has previously been dry suggests that a new element may have been introduced, either a psychological factor or UTI. Diurnal incontinence necessitates careful evaluation of the urinary tract but the yield from the investigation of children with uncomplicated nocturnal enuresis by IVU or endoscopy is low. Persistent dribbling incontinence associated with otherwise apparently normal micturition suggests an ectopic ureter opening below the bladder neck and should provoke careful review of the IVU for evidence of a duplex system. The possibility of a neuropathic bladder should be considered in all incontinent children.

Dysuria and Frequency

Pain on passage of urine and frequency of micturition point to urethritis or cystitis, usually a consequence of bacterial infection of the urine. However, dysuria may also be a consequence of vulvovaginitis in girls and balanitis in boys.

Abnormalities of Urinary Stream

A poor urinary stream in a male infant, particularly associated with a full bladder, strongly suggests a posterior urethral valve, and observation of the urinary stream is an integral part of the physical examination of a child suspected of having a urinary disorder. A poor stream may also be the consequence of the defective function of a neuropathic bladder. Retention of urine is an uncommon problem in childhood and demands expert urological attention to exclude tumor, stone, neuropathic bladder, ureterocele, or other congenital anomaly.

Urinary Tract Infection

The diagnosis of UTI must be rigorously confirmed by urine culture, for all affected children need some form of renal imaging to exclude an underlying urological abnormality. All children with a documented UTI should have renal imaging with ultrasound, a ^{99m}Tc-dimercaptosuccinic acid (DMSA) scan, or IVU. Younger children should also have a micturating cystourethrogram (MCU), but this may be deferred in older children unless there is an abnormality on renal imaging or the infections are recurrent.

Local Symptoms

In addition to the local symptoms of frequency, dysuria, suprapubic pain, and acquired incontinence characteristic of cystitis, involvement of the upper urinary tract and renal parenchyma (pyelonephritis) is suggested by loin pain and fever, sometimes with rigors.

Systemic Symptoms

In young children, and especially in infants, UTI may present with vague nonspecific symptoms that do not immediately point to the urinary tract: vomiting, refusal of feeds, diarrhea, failure to thrive, fever, dehydration, and jaundice of an obstructive pattern (4).

Abnormalities of Salt and Water Balance

Dehydration

Pure water depletion, resulting for example from defects of urine concentration, is associated, particularly in infants, with feeding difficulties and fever. If there is no concomitant salt depletion, the extracellular fluid (ECF) volume may be relatively well maintained with the brunt of the fluid depletion being borne by the intracellular fluid (ICF) compartment, in which case the principal symptom is thirst. With salt depletion as well, ECF volume will be depleted, resulting in hypotension and sensations of fatigue and faintness. Chronic salt-wasting is often associated with an increased salt appetite and a preference for savory rather than sweet foods.

Edema

ECF expansion results in edema, often first evident as swelling of the eyelids and sometimes mistaken for an allergic phenomenon; more severe generalized edema is associated with abdominal swelling as a result of ascites.

There are two distinct renal mechanisms of edema formation. In the first, characteristic of the acute nephritic syndrome and renal failure, there is a primary failure to excrete salt and water, with the result that the edema is accompanied by expansion of the intravascular volume, hypertension, and pulmonary congestion. In the second, as in the nephrotic syndrome, edema results from hypoproteinemia, the diminished colloid osmotic pressure of the plasma leading to a seepage of fluid from the intravascular into the interstitial compartment with the contraction of the plasma volume secondarily causing salt and water retention. Hypoproteinemic edema is more gravity-dependent than the edema of renal failure and may be accompanied by symptoms of faintness and abdominal pain attributable to hypovolemia.

Hypertension

In its early stages hypertension is asymptomatic, but may be discovered during routine examination or as part of the follow-up program of a child known to have renal disease. Unfortunately, recording a child's blood pressure, although an integral part of the routine examination, is frequently omitted, with severe hypertension not being diagnosed until a late stage. Such children may present with convulsions or coma and usually have a prolonged history of headaches and occasionally visual symptoms as well. Facial palsy is a well-established complication of severe hypertension in children (5). The complaint of headache in a child demands careful evaluation of the blood pressure.

Chronic Renal Failure

Uremia

The symptoms associated with uremia are vague ill-health, lassitude, anorexia, and vomiting. Although it is now rare for a child to reach such a condition without medical attention, an occasional case presenting with apparent acute renal failure will in fact be found to have a chronic uremic state.

Growth Failure

Growth failure is a frequent consequence of renal disease. It is most severe in children with congenital renal disease and impaired function from early life. All short children should be carefully evaluated for the presence of renal disease. If the growth retardation is a consequence of chronic renal failure, the plasma creatinine concentration usually will be evaluated, but may be only marginally so in young children with congenital renal disorders and diminished muscle bulk.

Osteodystrophy

The development of osteodystrophy, with bone pain, deformity (particularly knock-knees) or waddling gait, or the presence of unexplained rickets, may be the first clue to the presence of renal disease, either chronic renal failure or a tubular disorder.

Neurological Symptoms

Rarely, renal disease may present with convulsions, resulting from hypertension, hypocalcemia, or uremia.

Respiratory Symptoms

Breathlessness, particularly if worse on recumbency, may be a result of pulmonary edema and require urgent treatment. Hyperventilation (Kussmaul respiration) may be a consequence of the severe metabolic acidosis that usually accompanies advanced uremia.

Anemia

A greyish-yellow pallor is a feature of the uremic state and sometimes anemia is the first diagnosis in a child with chronic renal failure. Children with medullary cystic disease may develop anemia early in the course of the disease to a degree disproportionate to the severity of the impairment of renal function.

Screening Programs

Renal disease is frequently asymptomatic and may come to light as a consequence of routine examination or screening programs. It should not be assumed, however, that the natural history of a disorder detected by screening is necessarily the same as if the disorder had presented in a symptomatic manner nor that it requires the same protocol of investigation and treatment. For example, is asymptomatic bacteriuria the same disorder as a symptomatic UTI (6)?

Antenatal Ultrasound

The widespread use of a diagnostic ultrasound in contemporary obstetric practice has led to the recognition of fetal hydronephrosis in a number of instances, and attempts have been made to minimize the renal damage by premature delivery or intrauterine surgery (7). Doubtless, this is a very interesting field for future development, but considerable caution should be advised at the present time in proferring prognoses for renal function or recommendations for treatment in such cases.

Routine Neonatal Examination

The routine examination of the neonate must include abdominal palpation, which may reveal evidence of renal disease, e.g., renal masses resulting from tumor, hydronephrosis, cystic disease, or venous thrombosis. The presence of renal agenesis or severe dysplasia should be suspected if there is a history of oligohydramnios with associated compression deformities, i.e., crumpled ears, Potter facies, talipes, dislocated hips, and pulmonary hypoplasia (sometimes with pneumothorax) (8). The absent abdominal wall syndrome (prune belly) is associated with bilateral cryptorchidism and a wide range of urological disorders. There is an increased incidence of renal anomalies in association with other congenital defects, particularly of the cardiovascular system, gastrointestinal tract (especially imperforate anus), genital anomalies, and possibly also with a single umbilical artery.

Urine Screening Programs

Because of the association between UTI, vesicoureteral reflux, and renal scarring, a large number of investigations have been directed at the role of screening for bacteriuria to prevent renal damage (9). As some 5% of school girls will at some stage develop bacteriuria, the yield of such surveys is large, but it is by no means established that the widespread application of screening will reduce the incidence of end-stage renal failure in the female population.

Routine Biochemical Evaluation

The kidney may be involved in a wide variety of multisystem disorders. With the advent of the multichannel autoanalyzer, the serendipitous discovery of occult renal disease in sick children is now a not infrequent occurrence.

HISTORY

The detailed history will, of course, be different in individual patients, but certain general points must be elicited in all cases.

Family History

Genetic factors are relevant in a wide variety of renal diseases. A detailed family history is of importance for several reasons. It may contain the clue to the diagnosis in the individual patient, it may point to the possibility of previously unrecognized renal disease in other family members, and it may carry implications for genetic counselling. It is good practice to elicit the family tree for the case records.

Autosomal recessive disorders are usually self-evident though may have escaped notice, such as with the milder forms of "infantile" polycystic disease, or with as yet less severe disease in younger siblings, e.g., in families with medullary cystic disease or cystinosis. X-linked recessive disorders may be revealed only by close inquiry, perhaps a history in previous generations of the loss of male infant relative of a mother of a child with nephrogenic diabetes insipidus, though sometimes a hint may be given by the mother herself if there is mild heterozygote expression of the disorder (10). Polygenic inheritance may be operative in the etiology of vesicoureteral reflux; first-degree relatives have a 10% chance of being affected with the disorder (11).

Of all the familial conditions, Alport's syndrome and other forms of familial hematuria can be the most elusive, for they may be lost among the many other children with isolated hematuria of good prognosis. There is a marked difference in expression of the severity of the disorder in the two sexes, so that the mother may be only minimally affected. Deafness may be a clue, but urinalysis should be done in all first-degree relatives of children with unexplained hematuria (12).

Perinatal History

The role of obstetric ultrasound in the diagnosis of fetal hydronephrosis and the significance of oligohydramnios has been described already. An edematous placenta, more than 25% of the child's birth weight, is a feature of the congenital nephrotic syndrome; maternal infection, particularly syphilis, must be considered in the differential diagnosis of that disorder. Perinatal asphyxia, particularly if associated with macroscopic hematuria, may have been responsible for renal venous thrombosis and should be considered in the differential diagnosis of an older child with renal scarring, particularly if there is no suggestion of vesicoureteral reflux. Umbilical arterial catheterization may cause vascular damage and subsequent hypertension (13). In the neonatal period and early childhood, unexplained episodes of fever or dehydration may have been a result of undiagnosed UTI; feeding difficulties are frequent in the history of children with congenital renal disorders.

General Medical History

In view of the frequent involvement of the kidney or urinary tract in syndromes of congenital malformation or multisystem disorders, attention must be paid to all aspects of the child's medical history. Attendance at the department of otolaryngology for deafness may be a pointer to Alport's syndrome; at the ophthalmology department a diagnosis of retinitis pigmentosa may suggest medullary cystic disease (14). The orthopedic department may be involved because of bony deformity as a result of osteodystrophy, slipped femoral capital epiphysis, or Perthe's disease, the last more common with renal abnormalities even without renal failure (15). Renal involvement may be part of a multisystem disorder, such as systemic lupus erythematosus, juvenile rheumatoid arthritis, or other vasculitic disorders. Drug nephrotoxicity may arise in many different groups of patients, particularly from antibiotics, diuretics, and anticancer drugs. In a major children's hospital, the nephrologist may find himself as much involved with internal as with external referrals and must be familiar with the renal complications of systemic disorders and iatrogenic problems.

Micturition

A detailed inquiry into urination is always appropriate, i.e., the volume and nature of the urine passed, whether there has even been hematuria or episodes of frequency and dysuria, the nature of the urinary stream, the frequency of micturition, and the ages at which daytime and nighttime urinary continence were achieved.

Dietary History

A review of nutrition and feeding problems, beginning with the neonatal period, should be undertaken. Whether the child was breast or bottle-fed, episodes of vomiting or anorexia, thirst, dietary preferences, particularly if for savory or salty foods are important. For children with growth retardation or renal failure, a formal assessment of protein, energy, and other nutrient intake should be undertaken by a dietitian versed in the problems of renal disease in childhood.

PSYCHOSOCIAL EVALUATION

Many children with renal disease come from families with severe social problems. Some disorders, for example, nephritis secondary to skin sepsis, are more common in deprived social classes. However, more important is the effect that social circumstances have on the ability of the family to cope with such minor urinary symptoms as enuresis, or to participate in the major upheaval of a renal replacement program. The involvement of a skilled social worker is essential in all cases. The commitment of the family to the child must be assessed. If the disease is congenital, particularly if prolonged hospitalization has been required or an inappropriate pessimistic prognosis given, there may be problems arising from inadequate mother-child bonding, and the opinion of a family-oriented child psychiatrist is often helpful.

The impact of the disease on the child's emotional and intellectual progress must be assessed. In general, renal disease does not retard cognitive development, though there may be some delay if renal failure is severe in early life (16). A more common feature is emotional immaturity amounting to infantilism as a consequence of growth retardation, eliciting a response from society more appropriate to the child's size than chronological age. Later, toward puberty, there always will be concern as to whether or when dialysis and transplantation will be necessary. It is in this context that an appropriate educational program must be worked out. A detailed educational history should be obtained and communication with the school authorities established.

Skills in this area, as much as in experience in organic renal disease in childhood, distinguish the competent pediatric nephrologist from his "adult" colleague.

PHYSICAL EXAMINATION

General Appearance

The demeanor of the child should be observed, e.g., whether happy or sad, alert or somnolent, well-kempt or dishevelled. Evidence of anemia should be sought, and pigmentation suggestive of uremia noted.

Inspection of the skin may reveal the maculopapular purpuric rash of the Henoch-Schönlein syndrome, typically most severe on the buttocks, elbows, and feet, or the skin lesions of systemic lupus erythematosus in butterfly distribution across the nose and on the cheeks. Angiokeratoma points to Fabry's disease, and café-au-lait spots to neurofibromatosis, which is occasionally associated with renal artery stenosis and hypertension (17). Dystrophic nails suggest the possibility of the nail-patella syndrome.

Growth and Nutrition

Proper assessment of the growth of the child necessitates accurate measurement of height with a stadiometer and weight with scales accurate to 0.1%, together with charts of height and weight percentiles appropriate for the child's age, race, and sex.

An impression should be formed of muscle bulk and body fat, but nutritional status is difficult to assess. The relationship between weight and height may underestimate the degree of loss of muscle tissue, as there is often subclinical expansion of ECF (18). Triceps skinfold thickness probably is a reflection of body fat.

Hydration

The distribution of water between ICF and ECF is determined by osmotic forces. Sodium and its attendant anion are the principal determinants of ECF osmolality. Therefore, in states of salt and water depletion it is mainly ECF that is diminished, whereas with pure water depletion it is ICF volume that is decreased. Conversely, with pure water excess, ICF is expanded, whereas salt and water overload increases ECF. The partition of ECF between interstitial and intravascular compartments is determined by the plasma colloid osmotic pressure, venous pressure, and the integrity of the capillary wall.

Consideration should first be given to total body water and its partition between ECF and ICF, thence to ECF and its partition between intravascular and interstitial compartments, thence to intravascular volume and circulatory status.

Total Body Water

There is no simple clinical estimate of total body water, though some clues may be obtained from a review of recent changes in body weight, which largely reflect changes in total body water. In isotonic states, dehydration of moderate severity implies a deficit of total body water of some 5% and severe dehydration a deficit of 10%.

Extracellular Fluid

Changes in ECF volume are easier to detect than changes in ICF volume, though edema is not clinically evident until ECF has been expanded by some 10%. Expansion of the interstitial compartment results in peripheral edema, easiest detected in the pretibial region, and of the intravascular compartment in hypertension, raised central venous pressure (CVP), and pulmonary edema. Conversely, contraction of the interstitial compartment causes diminished skin turgor and a reduction of the intravascular compartment (hypovolemia) results in hypotension and circulatory failure with a low CVP. Occult hypovolemia may be revealed by noting an exaggerated fall in blood pressure on standing.

Circulatory Status

Hypotension and poor peripheral perfusion, characterized by cold extremities and a gap between skin and rectal temperature >2°C, indicate poor cardiac output. If the CVP is low, then hypovolemia is the cause, but if the CVP is raised, the problem is cardiac in origin. It follows from this and from what has been said in the previous section that assessment of the CVP is an important observation. In the older child, inspection of the jugular venous pulse in the semirecumbent position may be helpful, but it is often not possible to be confident of the situation in a younger child. Cardiac size on chest x-ray films may be a helpful pointer, but in the sick child under intensive care, formal CVP monitoring is usually essential.

Cardiorespiratory System

Pulse. The pulses should be examined, and rate, rhythm, and volume recorded. The femoral pulses always should be palpated for coarctation may present with renal failure or hypertension.

Blood Pressure. Frequent observation of the blood pressure is an integral part of the management of the child with renal disease. It is one of the more difficult aspects of the physical examination and should not be delegated to a junior nurse. Technical aspects of measuring the blood pressure are very important, and are considered in Chapter 46, along with standards of blood pressure for age. Convenient approximations for the 95th percentile for systolic and diastolic blood pressures can be taken as: age 1 to 5 years 115/75 mm Hg, 5 to 10 years 125/80 mm Hg, and 10 to 15 years 135/85 mm Hg [19].

Precordium. Cardiomegaly may reflect volume overload or longstanding hypertension. Murmurs may indicate a congenital cardiac anomaly that might be the seat of subacute bacterial endocarditis or may simply reflect the high output state arising from anemia. Pericarditis with rub is a feature of a severe uremic state.

Lungs. Adequacy of ventilation should be assessed clinically by cyanosis, but the anemia that accompanies uremia may mask desaturation; if there is any doubt, particularly with incipient or actual pulmonary edema, blood gas analysis is essential. Hyperventilation suggests metabolic acidosis. A rapid respiration rate with recession is a pointer to pulmonary edema. The lungs should be examined in the conventional manner, and the most important physical sign is the diffuse fine crepitations at both lung bases that suggest pulmonary edema.

Abdomen

Distension. Abdominal distension in relation to renal disease may be a consequence of ascites, of renal enlargement because of hydronephrosis or tumor, or of retention of urine in the bladder. The absent abdominal wall musculature, characteristic of the prune belly syndrome and a consequence of intrauterine abdominal distension, is obvious in infancy. This is sometimes less evident in older children or in cases of partial absence and may be revealed only by asking the recumbent child to fold his arms across the chest and raise the shoulders off the bed. In affected cases, upward movement of the umbilicus will be observed.

Renal Enlargement. Detection of renal enlargement by palpation is a skilled physical maneuver. The kidneys can be palpated in a healthy neonate but not in an older child. Palpable enlargement of the kidneys has the following characteristics: the mass can be lifted from the loin and, in contrast to the spleen, it is possible to get above the mass; there is not much movement of the mass with respiration, and it is resonant to percussion anteriorly because the bowel intervenes. Some inferences can be drawn from the nature of the mass, though it is difficult to distinguish clinically between the firm enlargement of polycystic disease and tumor or, in an infant, between the soft enlargement of hydronephrosis and multicystic kidney.

Hepatosplenomegaly. The causes of hepatic enlargement are legion, but splenomegaly in association with renal disease has a more restricted differential diagnosis, suggesting a multisystem disorder, such as systemic lupus erythematosus or juvenile rheumatoid arthritis, an infection such as bacterial endocarditis or shunt nephritis, a neoplastic process perhaps complicated by uric acid nephropathy, or hypersplenism as a consequence of the hepatic fibrosis associated with "infantile" polycystic disease.

Bladder. Enlargement of the bladder should be sought by palpation and percussion. If detected, the child should be asked to pass urine and reexamined. It is sometimes difficult to detect bladder enlargement in the neonate when the umbilical cord is still in situ; if in doubt, an ultrasound scan will quickly resolve the issue. In cases of retention of urine, a rectal examination is necessary to exclude a pelvic mass.

Genitalia. Often, examination of the genitalia is omitted by the nephrologist, if not by the urologist. The position of the urethral meatus must be ascertained in both sexes; anomalies are common. However, hypospadias is only rarely associated with upper tract anomalies. Bilateral cryptorchidism is a feature of the prune belly syndrome. Male pseudohermaphroditism with cryptorchidism is a component of the interesting syndrome associated with nephroblastoma and glomerular disease (20). Female pseudohermaphroditism suggests the possibility of adrenal hyperplasia with salt wasting.

Nervous System

Neurological Examination. A careful examination of the central nervous system is always appropriate, particularly in children with severe hypertension, multisystem disorders, and in acute intensive care situations. In the peripheral nervous system, minor defects of motor function or sensation in the lower limbs may be the only pointer to a spinal abnormality responsible for a neuropathic bladder.

Eyes. The eyes offer many clues in the evaluation of renal disease, and the assistance of an experienced pediatric ophthalmologist is helpful. Scleral calcification may be a consequence of hypercalcemia or uncontrolled hyperphosphatemia. The crystal deposits in the cornea characteristic of cystinosis are best detected by slit lamp examination, but the earliest manifestation of the disorder is a peripheral retinal pigmentary disorder (21).

Alport's syndrome may be associated with keratoconus or, more commonly, with a macular abnormality (22). Buphthalmos is a feature of Lowe's syndrome. Aniridia is accompanied by an increased incidence of nephroblastoma. Iridocyclitis may complicate juvenile rheumatoid arthritis and associated amyloid nephropathy or may be found in association with idiopathic interstitial nephritis. Cataracts occur in many disorders, among which galactosemia and fructosemia may be noted for their association with renal tubular dysfunction. Posterior lenticular opacities may be a consequence of long term corticosteroid therapy and with careful examination are quite common though rarely give rise to visual handicap (23).

Examination of the fundus may reveal the ravages of hypertension with arterial narrowing, hemorrhages, exudates, and papilledema. Papilledema is also the major sign of raised intracranial pressure, as for example with cerebral edema in acutely ill children. Reye's syndrome is one of many examples in which cerebral edema may be associated with acute tubular necrosis (24). Diabetic retinopathy tends to parallel nephropathy, but is rarely observed in childhood. Taptoretinal degeneration is found in some cases of medullary cystic disease (14), and retinitis pigmentosa is characteristic of the Laurence-Moon-Bardet-Biedl syndrome, in which renal failure consequent on medullary dysplasia is the principal cause of early death (25).

Ears. Deformities of the external ear may result from oligohydramnios (8) and even in its absence are reputed to be associated with renal anomalies. High-tone deafness is characteristic of Alport's syndrome and may be of very insidious onset, detectable at first only by audiography (22). Nerve deafness is also associated with some cases of distal renal tubular acidosis and with the syndrome of nephrosis and hypoparathyroidism. Deafness may be a consequence of the previous administration of gentamicin, particularly in the neonatal period, or of high doses of frusemide.

Musculoskeletal System

Skeleton. The classical features of rickets may be a consequence of the early osteomalacic phase of uremic osteodystrophy or of renal tubular disease. Wrists and costochondral junctions are typical sites for epiphyseal swelling to be prominent. Comparison of height and arm span, as well as of sitting and standing height may reveal skeletal disproportion. Knock-knee is common with osteodystrophy and should be quantified by measuring the intermalleolar distance. Congenital dislocation of the hips is common in infants with renal disease and should be sought with great care.

Deformities of the spine, such as meningomyelocele, are obvious but subtle signs, such as a patch of pigmentation or tuft of hair, may be pointers to an underlying spinal dysraphism responsible for a neuropathic bladder. Sacral agenesis, in particular, is very easily overlooked. Unequal leg growth may be a consequence of a spinal abnormality. Hemihypertrophy is occasionally associated with nephroblastoma (with or without the Beckwith-Wiedemann syndrome) or with medullary sponge kidney.

Joints. Arthropathy is a classic feature of systemic lupus erythematosus and the Henoch-Schönlein syndrome. It is occasionally observed in some children with idiopathic membranous nephropathy (26). Juvenile rheumatoid arthritis may be complicated by amyloid or interstitial nephritis or associated with drug nephrotoxicity. The Lesch-Nyhan syndrome may present as a renal disorder, either as calculi or renal failure in infancy, and may be associated with a gouty arthropathy affecting, for example, the interphalangeal joints (27).

URINALYSIS

Careful urinalysis is essential in every case, and facilities for dipstick testing and microscopy of fresh urine should be available both in the clinic and on the ward.

Routine Testing

Urine samples should be tested routinely for protein, blood, and sugar, with the use of commercially available dipsticks.

Protein

Proteinuria is now most conveniently detected by the protein-error-of-indicators principle with Albustix (Ames Company). These are strips impregnated with tetrabromphenol blue buffered with citrate. Protein binds with the dye, and causes a color change from yellow to green by displacement of the transformation range of the indicator. False positive results may be obtained in urine of high pH or when contaminated with quarternary ammonium salts, such as chlorhexidine, otherwise there is a good correlation between the Albustix reading and the urine albumin concentration (28); the sensitivity to other proteins is less.

Occasionally, protein is formed in the urine when the child is in the upright posture, but not while recumbent. Such postural proteinuria may be confirmed by protein-free overnight urine and does not indicate renal disease. It is obviously important to exclude such a postural effect before investigating a child with proteinuria more extensively.

Blood

The detection of blood in the urine is most conveniently undertaken with Hemastix (Ames Company). These strips are impregnated with a buffered mixture of an organic peroxide and tetramethylbenzidine. The peroxidase-like activity of hemoglobin, myoglobin, and some of their degradation products catalyzes the oxidation of the dye to a blue derivative. The system is more sensitive to free hemoglobin and myoglobin than to intact erythrocytes. It gives an indication of the amount of free hemoglobin present, and the minimum concentration of erythrocytes detectable cannot be specified, as the degree of hemolysis is variable. However, the test is sensitive, and positive results should be confirmed by microscopy of the urine (29).

Glucose

Clinistix (Ames Company) detects the presence of glucose in urine by a glucose oxidase-peroxidase-linked reaction. The system is sensitive to a concentration of about 0.5 mMol/L but is inhibited to some degree by glutathione and other substances in the urine, so that the trace amounts of glucose present in normal urine are below the threshold of the test. Modifications of the system that overcome inhibitory factors can be used to detect the subnormal urine glucose concentrations characteristic of UTI (30).

Multistix (Ames Company)

Strips for routine tests combine the above methods with systems for measuring urine osmolality (based on the change of pKa of certain polyelectrolytes in relation to ionic concentration), pH (with a double indicator principle), ketones, bilirubin, urobilinogen, and nitrite (31).

Microscopy

Careful microscopy of unspun fresh urine samples in a Fuchs-Rosenthal counting chamber should be standard practice.

Erythrocytes

In health, there is less than 1 erythrocyte/μl urine. In the past, following the work of Addis (32), considerable attention was paid to quantitation of erythrocyte excretion rates. Normal children excrete <240,000 erythrocytes/12 hours (33, 34). However, in children with hematuria there is such marked temporal variation in erythrocyte excretion rates that such precise quantitation is superfluous.

The presence of red cell or granular casts indicates hematuria of glomerular origin. Erythrocytes originating from the glomerulus also have a characteristic appearance on phase-contrast microscopy (35).

Leukocytes

Many authors have reported white cell excretion rates in normal children. Stansfield (36) put the upper limit at 10 leukocytes/μl, but in neonates higher values may be observed—up to 25 in boys and 50 in girls (37). Epithelial cells, which are prominent in the urine of neonates, should be distinguished from leukocytes by their large size and polygonal shape.

Casts

Casts are solid cylindrical structures formed by the precipitation of debris in the renal tubules. Complicated schemes for the classification of casts have given way to a simple view that coarse granular casts are essentially a consequence of hematuria of glomerular origin and broad hyaline casts the consequence of the heavy proteinuria of the nephrotic syndrome. The concurrence of both types of casts, sometimes seen in a mixed nephritic-nephrotic syndrome, is described as a telescoped urinary sediment.

Crystals

Triple phosphate and calcium oxalate crystals may be seen in normal urine, though the latter are of course more prominent in hyperoxaluria. Experienced microscopists can recognize microcrystals of cystine, uric acid, dihydroxyadenine, orotic acid, and such drugs as suphadiazine.

Organisms

Bacteria usually can be detected easily by microscopy of infected urine. Yeasts also can be seen, particularly with *Candida albicans* infection.

Urine Concentration

The urinary osmolality is the relevant parameter of urinary concentration, the specific gravity, correlates so poorly with osmolality that it should be abandoned in routine urine analysis. The refractive index, being another colligative property of urine, is closely related to osmolality. This is easily measured with a refractometer, a simple piece of equipment essential in the ward laboratory of the Renal Service. An overnight urine, particularly in the younger child, usually will be maximally concentrated (>870 mOsm/L) in children >2 years (38). Measurement of osmolality on such samples frequently can eliminate the possibility of a defect in urine concentration, and should be done before embarking on more elaborate tests.

References

1. Rubin MI, Baliah T: Urine and urinalysis. In Rubin MI, Barratt TM (eds): Pediatric Nephrology, ed 1. Baltimore, Williams & Wilkins, 1975, p 84.
2. Thomson J: Observations on the urine of the newborn infant. Arch Dis Child 19:169, 1944.
3. Sherry SN, Kramer I: The time of passage of the first urine by the newborn infant. J Pediatr 46:158, 1955.
4. Smellie JM, Hodson CJ, Edwards D, et al: Clinical and radiological features of urinary infection in childhood. Br Med J 2:1222, 1964.
5. Still JL, Cottom D: Severe hypertension in children. Arch Dis Child 42:34, 1967.
6. Cardiff Oxford Bacteriuria Study Group: Sequelae of covert bacteriuria in schoolgirls. Lancet 1:881, 1978.
7. Harrison MR, Golbus MM, Filly RA, et al: Fetal surgery for congenital hydronephrosis. N Engl J Med 306:591, 1982.
8. Potter EL: Bilateral renal agenesis. J Pediatr 29:68, 1946.
9. Kunin CM, Deutscher R, Paquin AJ: Urinary tract infection in school children: an epidemiologic, clinical and laboratory study. Medicine (Baltimore). 43:91, 1964.
10. Culpepper RM, Herbert SC, Andreoli TE: Nephrogenic diabetes insipidus. In Stanbury JB (eds): The Metabolic Basis of Inherited Disease, ed 5. New York, McGraw-Hill, 1983, p 1867.
11. de Vargas A, Evans K, Ransley P, et al: A family study of vesico-ureteric reflux. J Med Genet 15:85, 1978.
12. Yoshikawa N, White RHR, Cameron AH: Familial hematuria: clinico-pathological correlations. Clin Nephrol 17:172, 1982.
13. Adelman R: Neonatal hypertension. Pediatr Clin North Am 25:99, 1978.
14. Senior B, Friedmann AI, Braudo JL: Juvenile familial nephropathy with tapetoretinal degeneration. A new oculorenal dystrophy. Am J Opthalmol 52:625, 1961.
15. Catterall A, Lloyd-Roberts GC, Wynne-Davies R: Association of Perthes' disease with congenital anomalies of genitourinary tract and inguinal region. Lancet 1:996, 1971.
16. Rotundo A, Nevins TE, Lipton, et al: Progressive encephalopathy in children with chronic renal failure in infancy. Kidney Intl 21:486, 1982.
17. Grad E, Rance CP: Bilateral renal artery stenosis in association with neurofibromatosis: report of two cases. J Pediatr 80:804, 1972.
18. Jones RW, Rigden SP, Barratt TM, et al: The effects of chronic renal failure in infancy on growth, nutritional status and body composition. Pediat Res 16:784, 1982.
19. Blumental S, Epps RP, Heavenrich R, et al: Report of task force on blood pressure control in children. Pediatrics 58 (suppl):797, 1977.
20. Drash A, Sherman F, Hartmann WH, et al: A syndrome of pseudohermaphroditism, hypertension, and degenerative renal disease. J Pediatr 78:497, 1971.
21. Wong VG, Lietman PS, Seegmiller JE: Alterations of pigment epithelium in cystinosis. Arch Opthalmol (Chicago) 77:361, 1967.
22. Gubler M, Levy M, Broyer M, et al: Alport's syndrome. A report of 58 cases and a review of the literature. Am J Med 70:493, 1981.
23. Brocklebank JT, Harcourt RB, Meadow SR: Corticosteroid-induced cataracts in idiopathic nephrotic syndrome. Arch Dis Child 53:30, 1982.
24. Nicholls S, Gill D, Craske J: Reye's syndrome associated with acute tubular necrosis. Arch Dis Child 50:960, 1975.
25. Bluett NH, Chantler C, Singer JD, et al: Congenital renal abnormalities in the Laurence-Moon-Biedl syndrome. Arch Dis Child 52:968, 1977.
26. Habib R, Kleinkrecht C: Membranous nephropathy. In Rubin MI, Barratt TM (eds): Pediatric Nephrology, ed 1. Baltimore, Williams & Wilkins, 1975, p 515.
27. Holland PC, Dillon MJ, Pincott et al: Hypoxanthine guanine phosphoribosyl transferase deficiency presenting as gout and renal failure in infancy. Arch Dis Child 1983. (In press.)
28. Barratt TM: Assessment of renal function in children. In Apley J (ed) Modern Trends in Paediatrics, ed 4. London, Butterworths, 1974, p. 181.
29. Dodge WF, West EF, Smith EH, et al: Proteinuria and hematuria in school children. Epidemiology and early natural history. J Pediatr 88:327, 1976.
30. Scherstén B, Dahlqvist A, Fritz H, et al: Screening for bacteriuria with a test paper for glucose. JAMA 204:205, 1968.
31. Ames reagent test. Technical information manual. Ames Co, 1982.
32. Addis T: Glomerulonephritis: Diagnosis and Treatment. New York, MacMillan, 1949.
33. Lyttle JD: The Addis count in normal children. J Clin Invest 12:87, 1933.
34. Snoke AW: The normal Addis count in children. J Pediatr 12:473, 1938.
35. Fairley KF, Birch DF: Hematuria: a simple method for identifying glomerular bleeding. Kidney Intl 21:105, 1982.
36. Stansfield JM: The measurement and meaning of pyuria. Arch Dis Child 37:257, 1982.
37. Lincoln K, Winberg J: Studies of urinary tract infections in infancy and childhood. III. Quantative estimation of cellular excretion in unselected neonates. Acta Paediatr Scand 53:447, 1964.
38. Edelmann CM, Barnett HL, Boichis H, et al: A standardized test of renal concentrating capacity in children. Am J Dis Child 114:639, 1967.

CHAPTER 19 Laboratory Evaluation

CYRIL CHANTLER
T. M. BARRATT

INTRODUCTION

Pediatric nephrology is primarily a clinical discipline, but the physician who has undertaken the responsibility for children with kidney disease requires a thorough knowledge of the analytical techniques used in the laboratory, including their methodology, precision, and sources of error. In this chapter techniques necessary for routine clinical practice are discussed in detail, whereas those more appropriate to clinical research are only briefly mentioned. The guiding principle is that the diagnosis be established with sufficient precision to ensure appropriate clinical management, with the minimum of disturbance to the child, and with the maximum economy in the use of health service resources.

Blood Tests

Children hate clinical procedures in general and blood tests in particular. The association of hospitals with painful investigations can come to dominate their attitudes toward doctors and nurses and interfere with their cooperation with the essential elements of management. The following principles should be stated: keep blood tests to a minimum; take only the smallest sample necessary, especially from babies (capillary samples are suitable for most purposes and should be used if venipuncture appears difficult); never tell a child that it will not hurt, but, rather, that the pain will not last for long; encourage the mother or father to be present to comfort the child; ask for help if venipuncture is difficult—success is not a matter of honor; take time to ensure that the arrangements are satisfactory, that the child is warm, properly held, and with sufficient distractions to occupy his attention and imagination. Even the simple tests of renal function make substantial demands on nursing time and require the informed cooperation of trained pediatric nursing staff.

Urine Collection

Some tests depend on the collection of an accurately timed urine specimen; this is a major source of error. Suitably accurate urine collections often are possible with the use of collecting bags applied to the perineum, provided close nursing supervision is available so that the bags are emptied as soon as possible after micturition. A useful way to achieve this is to drain the bag with a catheter attached to a low-pressure suction pump (1). Short-time collections under diuretic conditions are more suitable for measuring clearance. A high urine flow is established by the child initially drinking 20 ml water/kg and replacing urine losses with an equivalent volume of oral fluids. With this regimen, 3 to 4 separate voidings are usually obtained over a 2-hour period; the final answer can be calculated as the average of each separate period, and some measure of confidence in the timing thereby obtained (2). Incomplete bladder emptying may be a problem, particularly in babies. When this is true, a 24-hour urine collection may be better but losses are common and catheterization for a short collection period may be preferred. A gross check on the adequacy of a 24-hour collection may be obtained from the estimation of creatinine excretion, which should be $0.14 + 0.04 \times$ age (yr) $\pm$ 0.03 (SD) mMol/kg/day ($15 + 0.5 \times$ age (yr) $\pm$ 3 mg/kg/day) (3) (1 mMol creatinine = 111 mg). However, the 95% confidence limits are wide, and losses up to 30% may pass unnoticed. In practice, a timed urine collection is often unnecessary, for many aspects of renal function can be inferred from plasma concentrations alone, from urine/plasma concentration ratios, or from the relationship between the concentration of a substance in the urine to that of creatinine.

Preservation and storage of urine specimens with thiomersalyl or sodium azide in a final concentration of 1:10,000 and storage at 4° C is adequate for most purposes.

Interpretation of Results

The result of any test may be interpreted in relation to normal, i.e., the probability that it would be found in the population of healthy children of appropriate age, size, and sexual maturity. Functional tests or excretory rates should be related to some measure of body size; body weight, surface area, or calorie expenditure are commonly used. Surface area (SA) is used in describing glomerular filtration rate (GFR) because GFR varies least when expressed per unit SA over the period from 1 year of age to maturity (4). Metabolic rate, energy consumption, and food intake are also relatively constant in relation to SA after the first year of life (5). The problem of reference standards is discussed by Tanner (6). Other possibilities are extracellular fluid (ECF) volume (7) and total body water (TBW) (8). There are difficulties inherent in the estimation of SA, but the nomogram presented by Haycock et al (9) is satisfactory for that purpose (Fig. 19.1). Estimating calorie expenditure from body weight is described in Chapter 11.

STANDARD LABORATORY INVESTIGATIONS

The following values for plasma concentrations in children are taken from Clayton et al (10), unless otherwise stated.

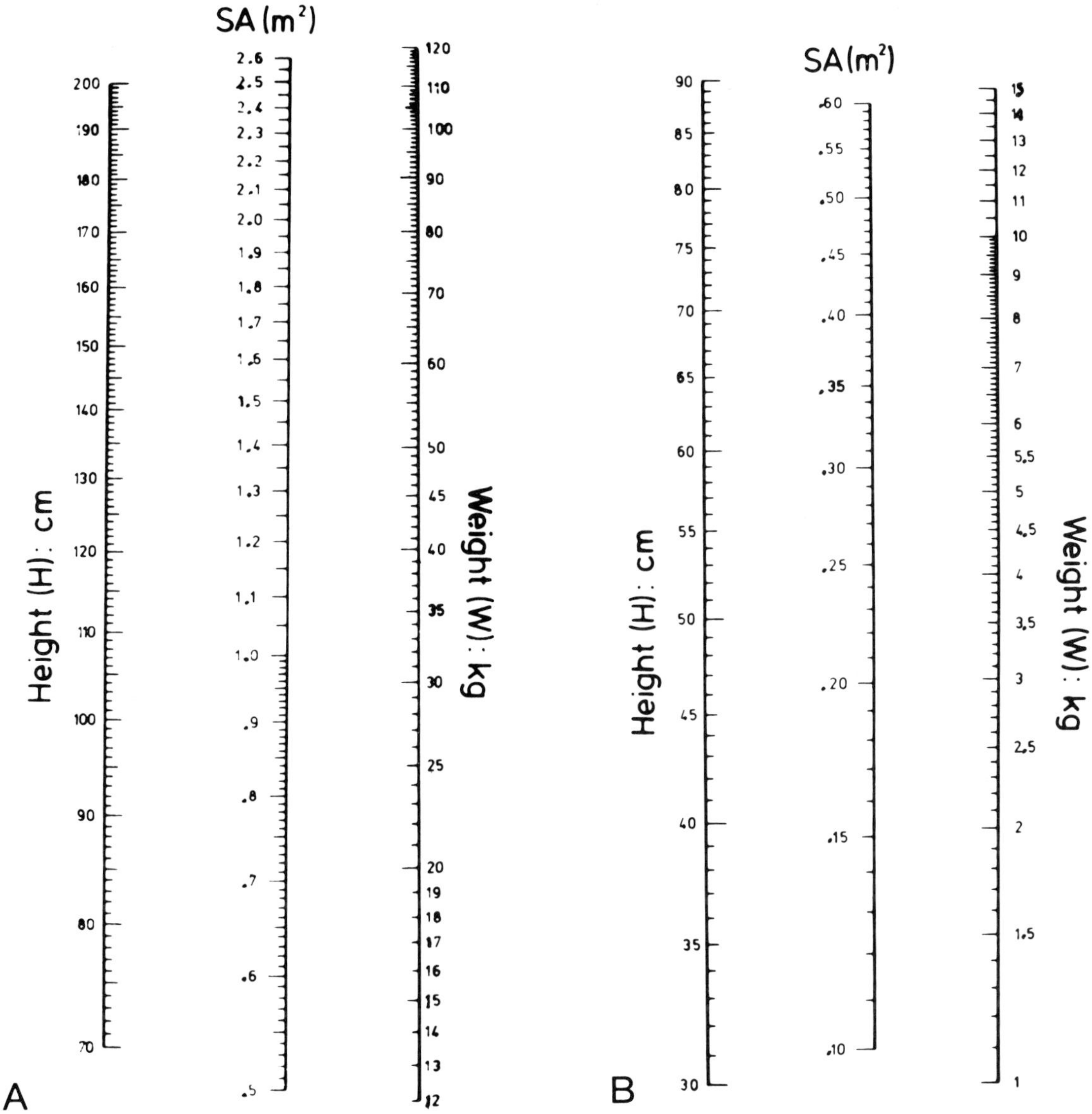

Figure 19.1. Nomogram representing the relationship between height, weight and surface area (A older children, B infants). (Reproduced with permission from Haycock et al. *J Pediatr* 93:62, 1978.)

Electrolytes

Sodium

For Na the normal plasma concentration (P_{Na}) is 135 to 145 mEq/L. The amount of NaCl in the body determines ECF volume and osmolarity, and its maintenance is critical to life (chapter 6). The capacity of the kidney to respond to change in NaCl intake is considerable: adults can maintain balance with intakes ranging from 2 to 1000 mEq/day (11) while infants can achieve balance on as little as 0.3 mEq/kg/day (12). The limits of tolerance are reduced in renal insufficiency (13) (chapter 49).

Hyponatremia. A low P_{Na} implies a dilution of body solute, either a result of sodium loss with a reduction in plasma volume or retention of water and an expansion of plasma volume (Table 19.1). Loss of NaCl associated with ECF volume depletion and circulatory inadequacy results in water retention secondary to antidiuretic hormone (ADH) secretion or renal failure. Urine Na concentration (U_{Na}) is low in both circumstances initially and the urine is concentrated with a high urea nitrogen (UN) urine/plasma (U/P) ratio. Hyponatremia secondary to plasma volume contraction and interstitial volume expansion may be encountered in children with the nephrotic syndrome in relapse. In acute renal failure the continued intake of water leads to overexpansion of ECF and hyponatremia. This occurs frequently in neonates with unsuspected renal insufficiency. Inappropriate ADH secretion is a rare, and often inappropriately diagnosed, cause of hyponatremia. The urine is hyperosmolar with respect to plasma; the expansion of ECF volume leads to a natriuresis (Chapter 6).

Hyponatremia also occurs with renal NaCl wasting, particularly in low birth weight infants and infants with obstructive uropathy or renal dysplasia. Occasionally it is misdiagnosed as congenital adrenal hyperplasia.

Spurious hyponatremia may result from hyperlipidemia or severe hyperproteinemia, but this is rare in children because the lipidemia or excess proteinemia must exceed 5 g/dl to cause a significant effect.

Hypernatremia. A raised P_{Na} is encountered in diarrheal dehydration and in infants with diabetes insipidus of pituitary or renal origin, when the hyposthenuria is accompanied by an inability to satisfy thirst. Infants with diffuse renal disease, especially those with cystinosis, dysplasia, or medullary cystic disease may have an obligatory vasopressin-resistant hyposthenuria which simulates nephrogenic diabetes insipidus (14). Ex-

Table 19.1.
Clinical Interpretation of Hyponatremia

Urine sodium (meq/L)	Urea urine: plasma ratio	Effective plasma volume	ECF volume	Clinical disorder
<10	>10	Low	Variable	Prerenal failure with "appropriate" ADH secretion or extrarenal Na losses
>10	<10	High	Increased	Renal failure with water intake exceeding Na
>10	Variable	Low	Normal or reduced	Renal Na wasting
>10	>10	High	Increased	Inappropriate ADH secretion

cessive water loss in infants with diarrhea in association with a high solute intake from unmodified cow's milk may cause hypernatremic dehydration. Rarely, hypernatremia is caused by a failure of normal thirst control (15) or by poisoning with salt (16).

Urinary Sodium Excretion. Na excretion in the steady state reflects dietary intake. The 24-hour urine Na excretion provides little information concerning renal function but acts as a check on the dietary history. In acute renal failure (ARF) the measurement of urine Na and UN concentrations is valuable in distinguishing between prerenal failure and established tubular necrosis (chapter 48). Specimens should be obtained before diuretics are administered. A low U_{Na} (<10 mEq/L) and a high UN:U/P ratio (>10) implies prerenal failure. The best discriminator is the fractional excretion of Na (FE_{Na}): a value <2.5% indicates prerenal failure (17). FE_{Na} is the proportion of filtered Na ($F_{Na} = P_{Na} \times GFR$) that is excreted ($U_{Na}V$) and is calculated from a random specimen of urine and plasma utilizing the creatinine clearance ($U_{Cr}V/P_{Cr}$) as an estimate of GFR:

$$FE_{Na} = \frac{U_{Na}V}{P_{Na} \times \dfrac{U_{Cr}V}{P_{Cr}}} \times 100 = \frac{U_{Na} \times P_{Cr}}{P_{Na} \times U_{Cr}} \times 100 \quad (1)$$

where U_{Cr} and P_{Cr} are the urine and plasma creatinine concentrations and V is the urine flow rate.

Potassium

For K the normal plasma concentration (P_K) is 3.5 to 4.5 mEq/L. The maintenance of body and ECF K is related to hormonal control, disease, and drugs more than it is to K intake. In adults, normal tolerance limits are 20 to 1000 mEq/day.

Hyperkalemia. A raised P_K may be a result of excessive intake in chronic renal failure (CRF), particularly in dialysis patients where the tolerance limits in adults are between 30 to 100 mEq/day (18). The smaller muscle mass of children and the potential for higher K intakes in relation to body weight increases the liability to hyperkalemia. Acidosis or increased catabolism as a result of intercurrent infection or inadequate energy intake also may result in hyperkalemia. Primary hypoaldosteronism and hyporeninemia cause hyperkalemia and acidosis. A common cause of spurious hyperkalemia is hemolysis due to an inappropriately collected blood sample.

Hypokalemia. K loss occurs with renal tubular disorders, e.g., Fanconi's syndrome, or renal tubular acidosis (RTA), and with hyperreninemia and hyperaldosteronism (chapters 7 and 33).

Chloride

For Cl the normal plasma concentration (P_{Cl}) is 100 to 107 mEq/L. Na, Cl, and H^+ balances are interdependent. Losses and gains of Na are usually accompanied by proportional changes in Cl. Cl is retained if bicarbonate is lost, as occurs with renal bicarbonate wastage or H^+ retention. Cl is depleted when gastric hydrochloric acid is lost, when diuretics specifically block active Cl reabsorption, or when there is bicarbonate retention, as in respiratory acidosis. In the first, bicarbonate is retained in lieu of Cl; in the last, the converse is true.

Hypochloremia. Low P_{Cl} is either associated with hyponatremia or with bicarbonate retention, as occurs with metabolic alkalosis or respiratory acidosis.

Hyperchloremia. High P_{Cl} is associated with either hypernatremia or metabolic acidosis secondary to loss of bicarbonate, as occurs with RTA and with some forms of diarrhea, or with retention of H^+ that neutralizes bicarbonate, as occurs when renal ammonia production is impaired. Retention of organic, phosphoric, or sulfuric acid does not affect Cl concentration in ECF.

Bicarbonate

The normal plasma standard bicarbonate concentration in infants is 18 to 22 mEq/L and children 20 to 26 mEq/L. Bicarbonate is commonly measured as total CO_2 ($(CO_2)t$) in plasma allowed to equilibrate with air with some loss of CO_2 (19). The result is a value for total CO_2 that is 1 to 3 mEq/L less than true $(CO_2)t$ obtained from blood gas analysis by acid extraction. Standard bicarbonate reconstitutes the total CO_2 by equilibrating it with a pCO_2 of 40 torr, the normal pCO_2 of blood. Standard bicarbonate can be derived from blood pH and pCO_2, either by nomogram or calculation. It does not reflect the actual bicarbonate if there was crying, breathholding, hyperventilation, stasis of blood, or poor perfusion of the sampling site when the sample was obtained.

Hypobicarbonatemia. Loss of bicarbonate occurs when acid is added to ECF or when carbonic acid is excreted, as occurs with hyperventilation. If low, it is usually because net acid input exceeds net acid excretion. This occurs when bicarbonate is lost in urine or gastrointestinal tract, or when H^+ generated by metabolism, e.g., lactic acid, is retained. When hypobicarbonatemia is associated with a low plasma pH, a metabolic acidosis can be inferred, but if associated with a normal to high pH there is a respiratory alkalosis.

Hypobicarbonatemia may represent a mixed acid-base disturbance, e.g., a metabolic acidosis with a lesser degree of respiratory alkalosis, as may occur with vomiting and ketosis. Salicylate intoxication results in a mixed metabolic acidosis and respiratory alkalosis in which hypobicarbonatemia may be extreme (Chapter 8).

Hyperbicarbonatemia. Retention of buffer base occurs when bicarbonate reabsorption in the renal tubule is increased, as occurs whenever Cl is lost or pH is decreased by retention of carbon dioxide in response to respiratory acidosis.

Anion Gap. The sum of the plasma concentrations of Na plus K exceeds the concentration of Cl plus bicarbonate in normal individuals by 9 to 13 mEq/L. This "anion gap" is usually balanced by the negative charges on plasma proteins. Metabolic acidosis associated with an increased anion gap suggests the accumulation of other anions—sulfate or phosphate in renal failure (20), lactate in lactic acidosis, and ketoacids (beta-hydroxybutyrate and acetoacetate) in ketosis of diabetes and other inborn errors of metabolism. The ingestion of poisons, such as salicylate, ethylene glycol (oxalate), methanol (formate), or paraldehyde, cause profound acidosis because the anions are retained as acids and because metabolism is affected. The most common cause of an increased anion gap is the accumulation of lactic acid due to shock. It is associated with an increase above the normal 10:1 molar ratio between lactate and pyruvate (lactate 1.0 mEq/L:pyruvate 0.1 mEq/L).

Minerals

Calcium

For Ca the normal plasma concentration (P_{Ca}) is 8.5 to 10.5 mg/dl (2.13 to 2.62 mMol/L) in younger children, and 9.0 to 10.5 mg/dl (2.26 to 2.62 mMol/L) after 9 years of age (1 mMol/L = 4 mg/dl). Only 50% of total P_{Ca} is ionized and that fraction is physiologically the most important. In patients with hypoalbuminemia the protein bound fraction is reduced. To correct for this, the measured P_{Ca} is adjusted by 0.09 mg/dl (0.023 mMol/L) for every 0.1 g/dl that the plasma albumin is <4.6 g/dl; values >4.6 g/dl should be correspondingly reduced. Venous occlusion causes a local increase in plasma protein concentration, and can raise total plasma Ca by as much as 1.6 mg/dl (0.4 mMol/L) (21). Similarly dehydration in nephrogenic diabetes insipidus can lead to an erroneous diagnosis of a renal concentrating defect as a result of hypercalcemia if an allowance is not made for the total plasma protein concentration. Acidosis increases and alkalosis decreases the ionized fraction.

Hypocalcemia. A low ionized P_{Ca} causes tetany. It occurs with hypoparathyroidism, dietary Ca or vitamin D deficiency, alkalosis, or with infusions that chelate or bind P_{Ca}, such as ethylenediaminotetracetic acid (EDTA) or phosphate (22).

Hypercalcemia. A raised P_{Ca} may result from vitamin D toxicity or hyperparathyroidism. If severe, it may result in arrhythmias, convulsions, and brain damage. Lesser degrees of hypercalcemia over long periods depresses the urinary concentrating mechanism and may cause nephrocalcinosis.

Hypercalcemia and hyperphosphatemia occurring coincidentally may lead to soft tissue calcification. A Ca and P product that is >60 mg/dl (>4.85 mMol/L) is considered capable of causing this. Children seem less susceptible than adults.

Hypercalciuria. Ca excretion in the urine in excess of 4 mg/kg/day (0.25 mg/mg Cr) in infants and children is considered to be hypercalciuria (3, 23–25). It occurs in response to vitamin D toxicity and is associated with hematuria in children who are prone to stone formation. While a 24-hour urine is desirable, a spot fasting urine analyzed for Ca and Cr is a satisfactory screening method.

Magnesium

The normal plasma concentration (P_{Mg}) is 1.78 to 2.41 mg/dl (0.73 to 0.99 mMol/L ; 1 mMol/L = 2.4 mg/dl). Most dietary Mg is lost in the feces and only a third is excreted in the urine. Only 1% of body Mg is extracellular.

Hypomagnesemia. A low P_{Mg} occurs in neonatal tetany, with dietary deficiency or increased gastrointestinal loss, with primary aldosteronism, hypoparathyroidism, diuretic therapy, hypercalcemia, and rarely in CRF (26–28). Renal Mg wasting may be secondary to drugs (26) or to a renal tubular defect (29) and may be associated with hypokalemia in a variant of Bartter's syndrome (30) (chapter 33). Hypomagnesemia also may be associated with increased parathyroid hormone (PTH) secretion with hypercalciuria (27). The upper limit (mean + 2SD) for urinary Mg excretion in British children was found to be 4.4 mg/kg/day (0.18 mMol/kg/day (3).

Hypermagnesemia. Hypermagnesemia may occur in acute renal failure or with Addison's disease; usually it is iatrogenic in origin.

Phosphorus

For phosphorus the normal fasting plasma concentration in neonates is 3.7 to 8.6 mg/dl (1.2 to 2.8 mMol/L), in children aged 1 year 3.4 to 5.9 mg/dl (1.1 to 1.9 mMol/L) for older children see Table II (1 mMol/L = 3.1 mg/dl). Plasma inorganic phosphorus concentration (P_{Pi}) is high in infants and decreases through childhood; values for boys remain higher than for girls until after puberty (31) (Table 19.2). The serum Pi tends to be higher than that of plasma as a result of loss from cells, and it is a less satisfactory measurement.

Assessment of the urinary excretion of phosphate ($U_{Pi}V$) is complex (32, 33). The fractional excretion of phosphate (FE_{Pi}) is derived in the same way as the FE_{Na} (equation 2). The percent tubular reabsorption (TR_{Pi} %) is derived by equation 3:

$$FE_{Pi} = \frac{U_{Pi}}{P_{Pi}} \times \frac{P_{Cr}}{U_{Cr}} \quad (2)$$

$$TR_{Pi}\ (\%) = (1 - FE_{Pi}) \times 100 \quad (3)$$

The relationship between phosphorus excretion and plasma concentration is shown in Figure 19.2. As Pi rises, a threshold is reached and Pi appears in the urine but reabsorption continues to increase until a

Table 19.2.
Normal Values for Plasma Phosphorus (P_{Pi}), Tubular Reabsorption of Phosphate (TRP), and Renal Threshold Phosphate Concentration ($TmPo_4$/GFR) (32)

Age (years)			7–9	9–11	11–13	13–15	15–17	Adult
Plasma inorganic phosphate (mg/dl)	Girls	Mean	4.3	4.2	4.1	3.8	3.6	3.6
		±2SD	3.6–5.0	3.4–5.1	3.3–4.0	3.0–4.6	2.9–4.2	2.6–4.6
	Boys	Mean	4.3	4.4	4.3	4.2	3.8	3.6
		±2SD	3.6–5.1	3.5–5.3	3.5–5.2	3.2–5.2	2.8–4.8	2.6–4.6
TRP % [100 × (1 − CPO_4/Ccr)]	Girls	Mean	94	93	93	93	90	90
		Range	86–97	83–98	79–98	84–98	84–96	81–96
	Boys	Mean	94	93	93	92	90	88
		Range	89–98	85–97	83–97	85–97	85–95	81–95
$TmPO_4$/GFR (mg/100 mlGF)	Girls	Mean	6.1	5.8	5.6	4.9	4.2	3.6
		Range	4.6–7.7	4.3–7.7	3.5–7.6	3.3–6.6	3.0–5.4	2.6–4.8
	Boys	Mean	5.9	5.7	5.5	5.3	4.5	3.2
		Range	4.5–7.3	4.0–7.3	4.0–7.0	3.5–6.8	3.5–5.9	2.1–4.3

mg/dl × 0.323 = mmol/L.

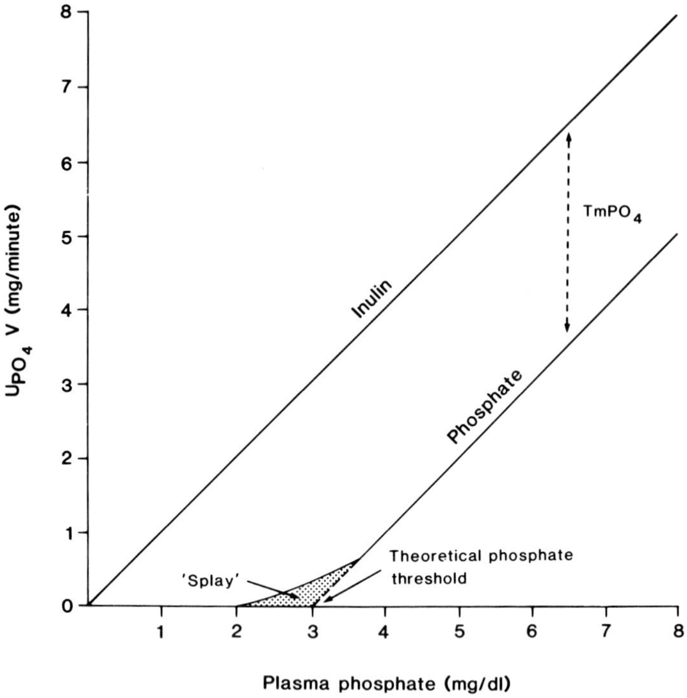

Figure 19.2. Relationship between urine excretion ($U_{Pi}V$) and plasma concentration of phosphate (P_{Pi}). At raised levels of P_{Pi} (>4 mg/dl in this example), the slope of the line relating $U_{Pi}V$ to P_{Pi} is parallel to filtered Pi, showing that when Pi is raised above this level all the Pi filtered is excreted. The vertical distance between the two lines represents the maximal tubular capacity for phosphorus reabsorption (TmPi). Extrapolation to zero excretion gives the theoretical phosphate threshold. Adapted from Bijvoet (33). Renal Handling of Phosphate, New York, Plenum Press, 1980.)

maximum tubular reabsorption capacity (Tm_{Pi}) is reached, after which all further Pi filtered is excreted. This increase in Pi excretion, reflected in the curved portion at the line, is referred to as splay. In ordinary circumstances, there is Pi in the urine so that plasma Pi is above threshold. A theoretical threshold can be derived by extrapolation of the linear part the curve representing Pi excretion to intercept the abscissa in Figure 19.2, which equals Tm_{Pi}:

$$Tm_{Pi} = P_{Pi}\ (\text{threshold}) \times GFR \qquad (4)$$

$$P_{Pi}\ (\text{threshold}) = Tm_{Pi}/GFR \qquad (5)$$

The theoretical phosphate threshold (Tm_{Pi}/GFR) is the most informative index of renal tubular phosphate handling for evaluating primary parathyroid disorders. Fractional excretion (FE_{Pi}) is influenced by variations in the dietary Pi intake and GFR, as well as by Pi threshold, whereas Tm_{Pi}/GFR is relatively insensitive to changes in intake or GFR.

The classical method of measuring Tm_{Pi}/GFR is to infuse phosphate until the linear part of the excretion/plasma concentration curve is identified. Bijvoet (31) has demonstrated that splay is proportional to Tm_{Pi}/GFR and that Tm_{Pi}/GFR can be derived in a fasting subject from phosphate and creatinine concentrations in a urine specimen obtained over a 2- to 3-hour period and a concomitant P_{Pi} (33). The urine collections should be obtained between 8 AM and 10 AM and the Pi obtained at midpoint. TR_{Pi} is derived from equation 3. Tm_{Pi}/GFR is obtained using the nomogram given in Figure 19.3 (34). The relationship between Tm_{Pi}/GFR, FE_{Pi}, and plasma Pi has not been well established in children. Data derived from normal children using the adult nomogram are given in Table 19.3 (32). The method is not applicable to infants, where splay is not known and caution is necessary in applying the method in CRF where splay is uncertain. Both Tm_{Pi}/GFR and FE_{Pi} are useful methods for assessing the role of secondary hyperparathyroidism in children with CRF (35) (chapter 49). Tm_{Pi}/GFR is the preferred test of tubular function in children with suspected proximal tubular dysfunction or primary parathyroid disorders.

Nitrogenous Substances

Urea

The normal plasma concentration of urea in infants on human milk is 15 to 30 mg/dl (2.5 to 5.0 mMol/L), on cow's milk 20 to 43 mg/dl (3.3 to 7.2 mMol/L; 1 mMol/L = 6 mg/dl). Urea is distributed throughout the body water. Blood urea concentration is about 14% less than plasma. Urea is filtered at the glomerulus and a variable amount is reabsorbed by the tubules. The concentration of urea in the plasma reflects the rate of production of urea and its clearance (36). Urea nitrogen (UN) is a convenient term beacuse it easily relates to nitrogen in diet or metabolism (1 mg UN = 2.1 mg urea).

While the clearance of urea is proportional to GFR, the rate of excretion is independent. As the GFR falls, urea clearance declines and plasma urea concentration rises (Figure 19.4). When urea production is constant its concentration is a reciprocal function of GFR. Protein intake influences P_{UN} by influencing UN production; if urea clearance is reduced to 25% of normal then P_{UN} increases 3- to 4-fold. If the protein intake is reduced from 75 to 25 g/day the P_{UN} is reduced to one third of its previous value. Because P_{UN} is affected both by net protein catabolism and by clearance, its use as a measure of renal function is limited (37). Urea clearance increases with urine flow as back diffusion of urea from the tubules is reduced (38). The dependence of urea clearance on urine flow accounts for the raised P_{UN} that occurs in conditions of oliguria without reduction in GFR, e.g., in the nephrotic syndrome. When urine flow exceeds 2 ml/min/1.73 m^2 the urea clearance is about 70% of the GFR. When GFR is <15 ml/min/1.73 m^2 the mean of the simultaneously determined urea and creatinine clearances approximates the GFR, as measured by inulin clearance (Figure 19.5) (38, 39).

Creatinine

Metabolism. (For normal values see Table 19.3). Creatinine is formed from creatine; 98% of the total body creatine is in skeletal muscle; 2% of creatine is converted each day to creatinine and excreted in the urine. Creatinine excretion is proportional to muscle mass and is relatively constant in an individual from day to day. A high meat diet containing creatine results in an increase in creatinine pool and in creatinine excretion of 10% to 26% (45). Children with reduced muscle mass have a lower creatinine excretion than would be predicted from their weight (3, 44) (Chapter 1).

Plasma creatinine. Methods for the determination of plasma creatinine concentration (P_{Cr}) depend on its reaction with alkaline picrate. Other chromogens in plasma also react with picrate (43). "True" P_{Cr} is measured by adsorption and elution from "Fuller's earth" or a cation exchange resin (46) or by high pressure liquid chromatography. Noncreatinine chromogens account for about 25% of the total chromogen in adult plasma; they have a low renal clearance and do not accumulate in renal failure. There are no differences in noncreatinine chromogen level between children and adults (47). Therefore, in children with normal renal function and low true P_{Cr}, the noncreatinine chromogens contribute up to 50% of the total. While specific methods are desirable, especially in infants (46), they require more work to achieve satisfactory accuracy and none has been automated. Current automated methods (48) measure some noncreatinine chromogen; P_{Cr} measured in this way overestimates

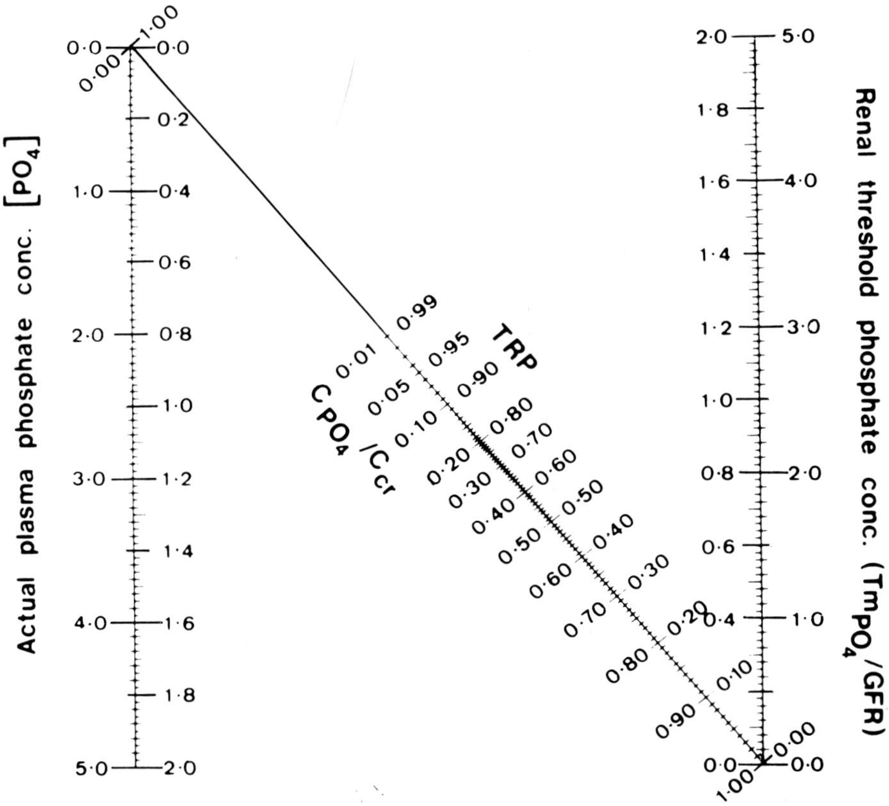

Figure 19.3. Nomogram for the derivation of the renal threshold concentration for phosphorus. (Reproduced with permission from Walton and Bijvoet (34). Lancet 2:309, 1975.)

Table 19.3.
Plasma Creatinine Levels at Different Ages (40–45)

Age	Height (cm)	True plasma creatinine (mg/dl)	
		Mean	Range (±2SD)
Cord blood		0.75	0.51–0.99
0–2 weeks	50	0.50	0.34–0.66
2–26 weeks	60	0.39	0.23–0.55
26 weeks – 1 year	70	0.32	0.18–0.46
2 years	87	0.32	0.20–0.44
4 years	101	0.37	0.25–0.49
6 years	114	0.43	0.27–0.59
8 years	126	0.48	0.31–0.65
10 years	137	0.52	0.34–0.70
12 years	147	0.59	0.41–0.78
Adult male	174	0.97	0.72–1.22
Adult female	163	0.77	0.53–1.01

Conversion factor μMol/L = mg/dl × 88.4.

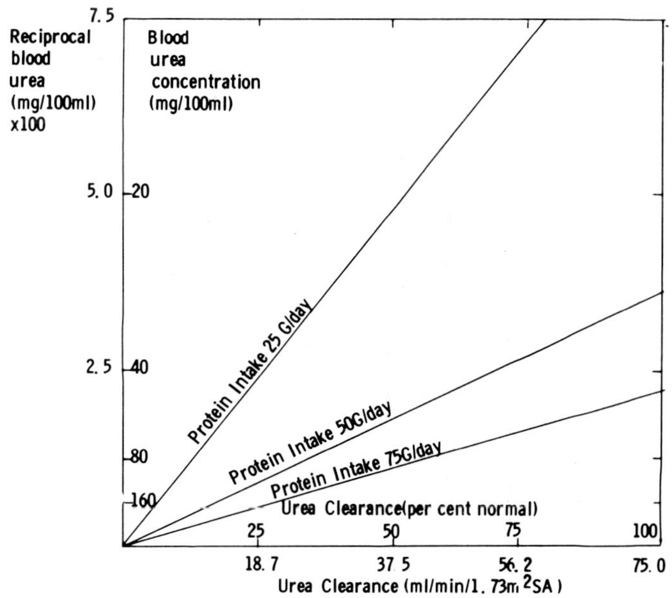

Figure 19.4. Plasma urea concentration on different protein intakes in patients with three different levels of renal function in a child of 0.77 m^2SA. Assumptions are that fecal nitrogen plus non urea urinary nitrogen excretion is equal to 2.5 g/day and that nitrogen balance is zero (37).

"true" P_{Cr} by 0.15 ± 0.13 (SD) mg/dl (12.4 ± 11 μMol/L; 1 mg/dl = 88 μMol/L) (49). Other automated methods measure the rate of production of color during incubation with picrate and are more specific and reproducible, although interference with noncreatinine chromogens is still a problem (50, 51). The coefficient of variation is 2.6% to 4.4% (52).

The normal values for P_{Cr} for children of different age and height (Table 19.3) were determined by a rate-reaction method. Values using the Technicon autoanalyzer (53) are slightly higher (0.15 mg/dl).

Cord blood P_{Cr} or P_{Cr} at birth reflects the level in the mother before delivery; it declines during the first week of life and thereafter is relatively stable until 8 years of age. Its tendency is to fall slowly as renal function increases (54) and to rise after the age of 2 years as muscle mass relative

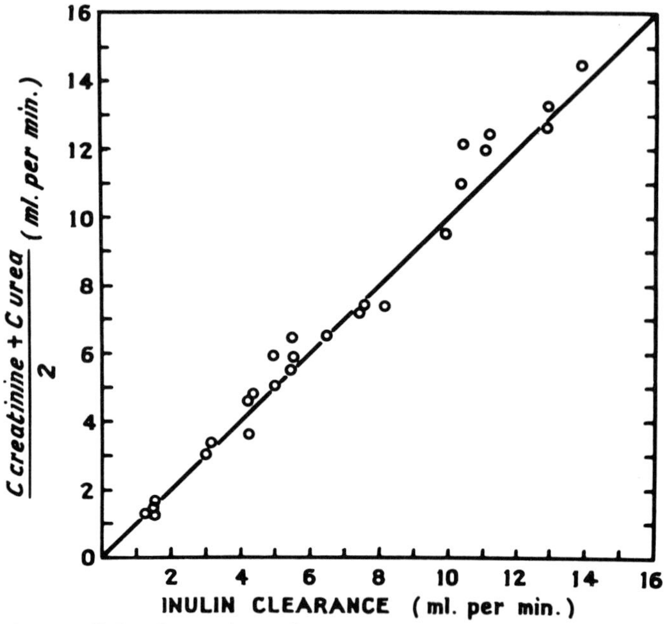

Figure 19.5. Comparison of the mean of the urea and creatinine clearances and inulin clearance in CRF. Reproduced with permission from Lavender et al (38). Lancet 2:1216, 1969.)

to C_{Cr} increases. Values in preterm infants are determined by gestational rather than postnatal age, as intrauterine and extrauterine maturation appear to occur at the same rate (54). After the fourth day of extrauterine life, P_{Cr} is 0.40 mg/dl (range 0.14 to 0.70) in infants with gestational ages between 30 and 40 weeks at birth (51). Higher values were obtained by Trompeter et al, using a different rate reaction method: 0.64 mg/dl (range 0.36 to 1.05) (54). The specificity and accuracy of the method is particularly important in this age group because the low values of true P_{Cr} magnify any measurement error.

Creatinine production and excretion ($U_{Cr}V$) are proportional to muscle mass (44) and GFR is proportional to SA. P_{Cr} is proportional to creatinine production and inversely proportional to clearance:

$$C_{Cr} = \frac{U_{Cr}V}{P_{Cr}} \tag{6}$$

therefore,

$$P_{Cr} = U_{Cr}V/GFR \tag{7}$$

In healthy children >2 years of age, P_{Cr} increases in proportion with height (Ht) because creatinine production, i.e., $U_{Cr}V$, is proportional to muscle mass and body weight (Wt), and C_{Cr} to SA (42). As a result, C_{Cr}/SA can be predicted from P_{Cr} and height (equation 8).

$$C_{Cr}/SA = Ht/P_{Cr} \times k \tag{8}$$

When P_{Cr} is expressed in mg/dl and Ht in cm, $k = 0.55$. (55). When true P_{Cr} is expressed in μMol/L, $k = 40$ (52).

The prediction of GFR in children from the height and P_{Cr} is more accurate than from the 24-hour C_{Cr} (49) because the inaccuracies of the estimation of muscle mass from height (56) are less than the inaccuracies of the 24-hour urine collection. This method is not suitable when GFR is changing rapidly, so that the production and excretion of creatinine are not equal, or if height is modified by disease, e.g., spina bifida, or if muscle mass is reduced. The normal range of P_{Cr} for children at different ages is wide (Table 19.3) and a single measurement has limitations in determining whether an individual child has a normal GFR. However,

Table 19.4.
GFR at Different Ages Adjusted to 1.73 m² (4, 57, 58)

Age	GFR (ml/min/1.73m² SA) mean	range (±2SD)
Premature	47	29–65
2–8 days	38	26–60
4–28 days	48	28–68
35–95 days	58	30–86
1–5.9 mo	77	41–103
6–11.9 mo	103	49–157
12–19 mo	127	63–191
2–12 years	127	89–165
Adult males	131	88–174
Adult females	117	87–147

the 24-hour endogenous clearance is no more useful in this respect and all methods of measuring GFR in clinical practice are imprecise. Moreover, the normal range of GFR itself is wide (Table 19.4). The Ht/P_{Cr} method is accurate in predicting GFR in children with reduced function, and change of GFR >19 ml/min/1.73m² can be detected within 95% confidence (52).

The rate of progression of renal failure in individual children can be derived either from the slope of the regression line of the plot of $1/P_{Cr}$ against time (60) or other empirical equations (61) (Chapter 49).

Clearance. C_{Cr}, first used to estimate GFR by Rehberg (62), is not a true measure of GFR. Creatinine is secreted by renal tubules so that C_{Cr} exceeds C_{in} by 20 ± 20% (63) and P_{Cr} often includes nonspecific chromogen. These deviations fortuitously cancel each other so that the C_{Cr}, where P_{Cr} includes chromogen and C_{in} is normal, is close to C_{in} (64).

In renal failure, the level of noncreatinine chromogens in the plasma is relatively constant while the concentration of P_{Cr} rises; the secretion of Cr increases progressively so that C_{Cr} overestimates GFR by 50% to 200%. In one study C_{Cr} was in the normal range in 42% of patients with minimal reduction in GFR (61–70 ml/min/1.73m²) and 23% of those with moderate reductions (51 to 60 ml/min/1.73m²) (65).

The 24-hour C_{Cr} of true creatinine is 113 ml/min/1.73m² (range 94 to 142) in healthy children aged 3 to 13 years (41); the coefficient of variation of repeated estimates in the same individual is 11.6% (66). Thus, two estimates of creatinine clearance could differ by at least 31% for a change to be identified with 95% confidence. Part of this variation is a result of inaccurately timed urine collections. Collections over 1 to 2 hours during a water diuresis are more reliable (2, 67).

In summary, the estimate of GFR from P_{Cr} and height is the most useful method in clinical practice and is superior to the measurement of C_{Cr} using a 24-hour period for collecting urine. Estimates of GFR that are more accurate than the 24-hour C_{Cr} are obtained from the 1- to 2-hour C_{Cr} during diuresis. However, tubular secretion of Cr is variable and increases as GFR declines; this renders C_{Cr} unsuitable for the precise measure of GFR in patients with reduced function.

MEASUREMENT OF RENAL FUNCTION

Glomerular Filtration Rate

The GFR is the most important measure of renal function in clinical practice because it determines the filtered load presented to the renal tubules and, thus, the flexibility of the renal response to homeostatic requirements. Furthermore, the decline in GFR is the principal functional abnormality underlying CRF. Its accurate measurement is important in detecting renal disease and in monitoring its progress and the response to treatment. However, following a reduction in functional renal mass, the remainder of the kidney hypertrophies. Accordingly, a substantial amount of damage must occur before it is reflected by a fall in GFR below the normal range (68), which in any case is wide (Table 19.4).

Inulin

The requirements of a substance for measurement of GFR are that it should not be bound to plasma proteins, be completely filterable at the glomerulus, be neither reabsorbed nor secreted by the tubules, be physiologically inert, and its concentration in plasma and urine should be easily determined (4). Apart from inulin, all substances presently in use fail to some extent to meet these requirements.

Properties. Inulin is a fructose polymer obtained from the dahlia or chicory, with an average molecular weight of 5100 dl and an Einstein-Stokes radius of 15Å, rather higher than suggested by its molecular weight as a result of asymmetry. Inulin preparations are not homogenous. They contain low molecular weight polyfructosans that may be reabsorbed by the tubules. Special precautions have to be taken to exclude these fragments from the assay and to prevent interference by either plasma glucose or fructose (68).

Automated methods for measuring plasma and urine inulin are available (69, 70) and have a coefficient of variation of about 1% (69, 70). Inulin is insoluble in cold water, which is a nuisance, but polyfructosan-S, a synthetic fructan of smaller molecular size, is an excellent alternative (71). The clearance of inulin is believed to equal the GFR in adults (4) and in children with renal disease (72).

Consideration of the relative clearance of dextrans of varying molecular size (73, 74) suggests that the infant glomerulus is relatively less permeable to macromolecules than is the adult and that significant exclusion from the glomerular filtrate occurs with an Einstein-Stokes radius of <20Å, which is only marginally greater than that of inulin. A comparison of creatinine, inulin, and iothalamate clearance in preterm infants shows a ratio of inulin to iothalamate of 0.5 at 28 weeks gestational age, but the ratio approaches unity at term (75). The creatinine clearance in this study was significantly less than the inulin clearance, possibly because of interference from noncreatinine chromogens in plasma; when true creatinine was measured the mean creatinine clearance in full-term neonates at 6 days was 36 ml/min/1.73m^2 (76), which is similar to the inulin clearance values given in Table 19.4.

The inference that inulin is unsuitable as measure of GFR in preterm infants has been disputed (77). With the possible exception of preterm babies, the clearance of inulin is taken as the standard to which all other methods of estimating GFR should be compared.

Clearance. The measurement of inulin clearance (UV/P) requires constant intravenous infusion, preferably by pump, and accurately timed urine collections. A priming dose of 50 mg/kg of inulin is given to raise the ECF concentration to about 0.25 mg/ml. An infusion is continued at a rate that will maintain the plasma concentration at this level (0.25 × estimated GFR, mg/min) (59).

After a period of 30 minutes for equilibration, the plasma concentration should remain reasonably constant, although full equilibration probably takes much longer (78). At equilibrium, the concentration of inulin in venous plasma is the same as that in arterial plasma, and venous plasma samples can be used to determine the clearance. Collection of spontaneously voided samples without bladder catheterization is possible; 3 to 4 collection periods of 20 to 30 minute duration during a moderate water diuresis should yield UV values that have a coefficient of variation of <10%. Plasma samples obtained at the estimated mid-point of each collection period also should agree within 10%.

As inulin is neither secreted nor reabsorbed by the tubules filtration and excretion rates are identical. The filtration rate of any substance freely filtered at the glomerulus is equal to the GFR multiplied by the plasma concentration; the excretion rate is the urinary concentration multiplied by the flow rate thus:

$$\text{GFR} \times P_{in} = U_{in} \times V \quad (9)$$

where P_{in} and U_{in} represent the plasma and urine concentration of inulin, respectively, V is the urine flow rate, and

$$\text{GFR} = U_{in}/P_{in} \times V \quad (10)$$

Certain precautions are necessary to obtain accurate and reproducible measurements of inulin clearance. Fluctuations in plasma concentration result in arteriovenous concentration gradients and invalidate the assumption that the arterial concentration is the same as the venous concentration. The urine flow rate should be constant: alterations cause changes in the volume and concentration in the extrarenal urinary tract and affect the clearance measurements (6). A large "dead space" in some children with obstructive uropathy renders the technique unsuitable for such patients. In small infants, blood sampling may be accompanied by a fall in urine flow because of secretion of ADH (79) so that such disturbance should be reduced to a minimum. The coefficient of variation of repeated measurements of inulin clearance is about 8% (80, 81). About a quarter to a half of this variation is analytical; with modern methodology the coefficient of variation is probably about 5%. In children, the difficulty of obtaining accurately timed urine collections by spontaneous voiding is likely to increase this variation so that catheterization may be preferred.

The complexities of the classical inulin clearance method render it unsuitable for children except when an exact measurement of GFR is required. For day to day practice, easier and less traumatic ways of measuring GFR are available.

Constant Infusion without Urine Collection. If, after a loading dose, inulin infusion is continued until the plasma level is constant, then infusion and excretion rates are the same; the UV/P clearance is equal to the rate of infusion (I) divided by the plasma concentration (82).

$$\text{GFR} = UV/P \quad (11)$$

$$UV = I \quad (12)$$

$$\text{GFR} = I/P \quad (13)$$

An estimate of the volume of distribution of inulin and GFR is required in advance to select the correct loading dose and rate of infusion. An incorrect estimate will delay the attainment of constant plasma levels (83). The gap between the initial and the plateau concentration is traversed with a half-life equal to that of injected inulin and will be only 95% complete after 5 half-lives have elapsed—a matter of many hours, particularly in infants in whom inulin half-life is long. An inaccurate estimate of the required loading dose or infusion rate, particularly if the GFR is low, may lead to a considerable inaccuracy in the apparent GFR and the failure to achieve equilibrium may not be detected as the trend in plasma concentration is small. Thus, too large a bolus loading dose, with equilibration still proceeding when the plasma concentration though apparently constant is still falling, will underestimate GFR. A loading dose that is too small with a slowly rising plasma concentration during infusion, will lead to an overestimate of GFR (84). However, properly performed, the technique provides accurate measurements of GFR that correlate well with the UV/P method (84). Substances other than inulin, such as Na-iothalamate or Cr-EDTA, which are excreted by glomerular filtration, may be substituted, but the need for a constant intravenous infusion is a disadvantage of the method.

Plasma Clearance

The GFR may be estimated from the rate of fall in the plasma concentration following intravenous injection of a substance provided it is rapidly equilibrated within its volume of distribution and thereafter removed from the body only by glomerular filtration, without secretion or reabsorption by the tubules, and has negligible extrarenal clearance (80). Following the single intravenous injection, plasma concentration is plotted as a function of time (Fig. 19.6). After equilibration, about 90 minutes after injection in the example shown, the falling plasma concentration curve can be described by a single exponential; a straight line is obtained by plotting this portion of the curve on semilogarithmic paper. By extrapolating this line back to zero time (T_0), a theoretical estimate of the plasma concentration (P_0) at T_0 is obtained and the half-life ($T_{\frac{1}{2}}$) read from the graph as the time taken for P_o to fall to $P_o/2$. Dividing the amount injected by P_0, a theoretical estimate of the volume of distribution of the substance (VD) is obtained. The clearance is calculated by inserting these values into the following formula:

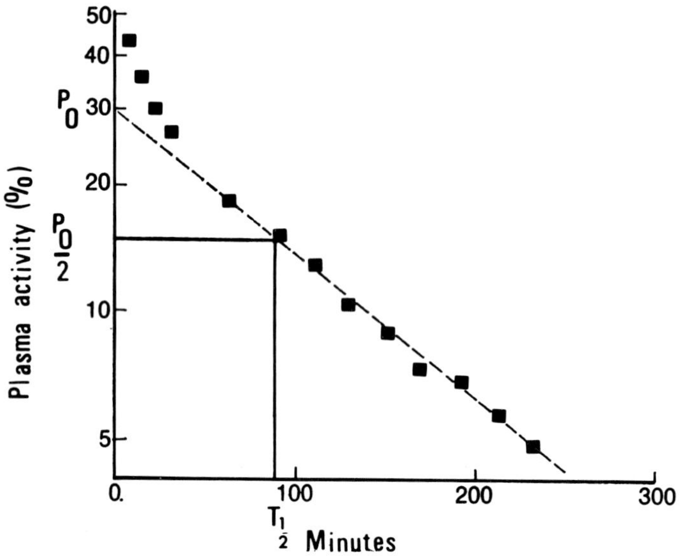

Figure 19.6. Plasma concentration of ^{51}Cr EDTA (on a logarithmic scale) as a function of time after intravenous injection in a healthy individual. (Adapted with permission from Chantler C et al (92). Clin Sci 37:169, 1969.)

$$C = VD \times 0.693/T_{\frac{1}{2}} \qquad (14)$$

where C = clearance (ml/minute), VD = volume of distribution (ml); and $T_{\frac{1}{2}}$ = half-life (minutes).

The formal proof of this clearance equation is given by Newman et al (85).

Mixing does not occur instantaneously and, therefore, certain errors are inherent in the single exponential analysis. VD always will be an overestimate of the true volume of distribution. It is assumed that during equilibration the plasma concentration can be represented by the extrapolation of the monoexponential part of the plasma disappearance curve to T_0. The actual plasma concentration during this period (Fig. 19.7) is higher and, therefore, more of the substance is cleared from the plasma than is allowed for by the analysis, so that P_0 is underestimated and VD overestimated. Further, the plasma concentration is assumed to be representative of the concentration throughout the interstitial fluid whereas after equilibration the concentration is lower in plasma because the plasma is cleared by the kidney. This underestimate of interstitial fluid concentration again leads to an overestimate of the VD.

Attempts have been made to allow for equilibration delay by resolving the falling plasma concentration curve into two exponentials (Fig. 19.7) (86, 87), one related to renal clearance (curve N) and the other to

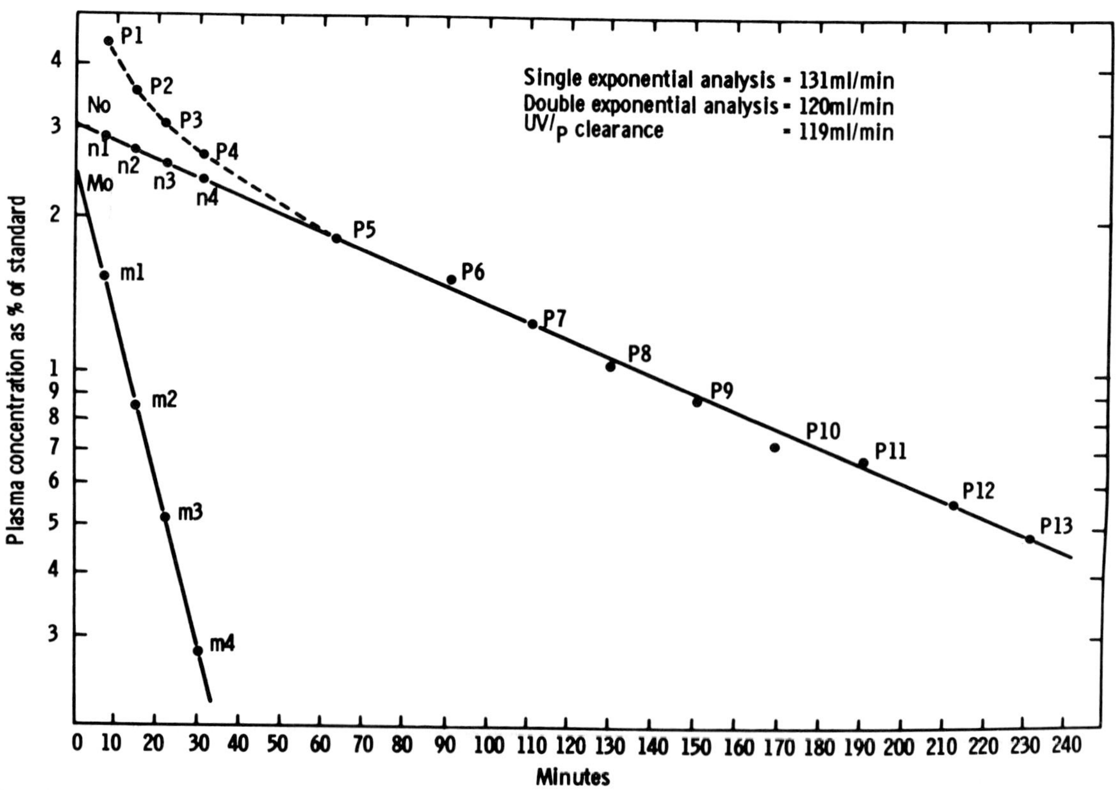

Figure 19.7. Double exponential analysis of the rate of fall of plasma concentration of ^{51}Cr EDTA. Clearance values obtained using both single and double exponential analysis as well as the UV/P clearance from 4 collection periods, are given.

exchange between plasma and interstitial fluid (curve M). Exponential M is obtained by subtracting values for N_1 to N_4 from P_1 to P_4. The clearance may now be calculated as:

$$C = I \times 0.693/M_o\ T_{\frac{1}{2}}\ (M) + N_o\ T_{\frac{1}{2}}\ (N) \qquad (15)$$

where I = dose injected (cpm); M_o = y intercept of slope M (cpm/ml); N_o = y intercept of slope N (cpm/ml); $T_{\frac{1}{2}}$ (M) = half-time of slope M; and $T_{\frac{1}{2}}$(N) = half-time of slope N.

The double exponential analysis is more accurate but requires 3 blood samples at approximately 10, 20, and 30 minutes after injection and a further 2 or 3 samples between 90 and 240 minutes, whereas the single exponential analysis only requires the last 3 samples. The clearance value from the single exponential analysis is relatively insensitive to errors in the determination of the slope, since these tend to be compensated by similar errors in the theoretical volume of distribution (88).

The magnitude of the overestimate of clearance inherent in the single exponential analysis has been investigated using chromium-51 diaminotetra-acetic acid (^{51}Cr-EDTA) (66). The mean ratio of the UV/P clearance to the single exponential clearance in 61 individuals of all ages with a GFR from 10 to 140 ml/min/1.73m^{2}SA was 0.77 + 0.07 (SD). Therefore, the UV/P clearance can be derived by multiplying the single exponential clearance by 0.77; this estimate has a 95% confidence limit of ± 17%. In view of the minimal requirement for blood samples and the reproducibility of the technique, the single exponential analysis is suitable for use in children.

When gross edema or pleural effusions are present, the falling plasma concentration cannot be described by a single exponential and the methods are invalid (87). In renal failure (GFR <20 ml/min), the amount of the substance not equilibrated by 90 minutes is proportionally greater and, therefore, blood sampling has to continue to 5 hours or more in order to identify the final exponential correctly (89). With normal function the higher the GFR the greater the overestimate produced by the single exponential method. It is, therefore, not suitable for the accurate assessment of above-average GFR. Capillary blood samples can be used in small infants if venipuncture is difficult (90). The coefficient of variation of the single exponential method is 3.9% (66). Thus, two estimates in the same individual that differ by more than 11% have a 95% probability of representing a real change in GFR. Results with double exponential analysis are equally good (91).

Various substances have been used as markers for plasma clearance methods of measuring GFR. ^{51}Cr-EDTA has a renal clearance that is 5% less than the simultaneously determined inulin clearance (92) probably because of some protein binding of chromium eluted from the EDTA. Na-iothalamate clearance is similar to inulin clearance (93) and can be assayed readily after incorporation of ^{125}I into its structure. During storage some autoradiolysis may occur and the free iodine liberated may lead to falsely low clearance estimates (94). The radiation dose with both ^{125}I-sodium-iothalamate (95) and with ^{51}Cr-EDTA is small, amounting to about 0.25 millirads to the kidneys per test, which is about equivalent to that received daily from natural sources. However, stable iodine attached to the sodium-iothalamate can also be assayed accurately, using fluorescent activation analysis, and thus avoid additional radiation (67, 96).

Other chelates of EDTA or its related compound DTPA are suitable; ^{99m}Tc-DTPA is particularly useful as it is widely used for dynamic renal scintigraphy and a measurement of total GFR and individual kidney function rate can be obtained during the same test (97). Inulin equilibrates too slowly within its volume of distribution in adults and is difficult to measure at low concentration.

The practical aspects of GFR estimation from the plasma clearance are as follows. ^{51}Cr-EDTA (0.5 μCi/kg body weight in 5% dextrose) or ^{125}I-sodium-iothalamate (0.3 μCi/kg/body weight in saline) is administered by rapid intravenous injection. A history of iodine sensitivity should be elicited before using iothalamate, and iodine uptake by the thyroid should be blocked with 2 drops of Lugol solution the night before the test. It is essential that no extravasation occurs during the injection, that the exact dose administered is determined by weighing the syringe before and after injection, and that the exact time of time of injection is recorded. An accurate dilution of the injected solution is made by diluting 100 μl to 50 ml. This serves as the counting standard. Two or three heparinized venous blood samples, to provide 0.5 to 2 ml plasma, are taken between 100 and 200 minutes after injection, and again the exact time is noted. Plasma activities are plotted against time on semilogarithmic paper so the P_0 and $T_{\frac{1}{2}}$ can be derived. VD and plasma clearance (C) are calculated as described above.

In order to relate C to GFR, it is necessary to apply certain correction factors. For ^{51}Cr-EDTA, the clearance should be multiplied by 1.05 to allow for the discrepancy with inulin clearance; for single exponential analysis, multiply by 1.07 to allow for the use of venous rather than arterial samples, and by 0.77 to allow for the overestimate in clearance inherent in single exponential analysis, amounting to a composite correction factor of 0.87 (66).

In summary, the plasma clearance method, using a single exponential analysis, provides an accurate reproducible method of measuring GFR in children without the need to collect urine samples. The method is particularly valuable in children with obstructive uropathy where suitably timed urine collections are not possible. It is more reproducible than the 24-hour endogenous creatinine clearance or the assessment of GFR from the plasma concentration alone, and is particularly valuable in detecting mild reductions in GFR. Figure 19.8 demonstrates the comparison between the creatinine clearance and the ^{51}Cr-EDTA slope in a child with Henoch-Schönlein nephritis; a steady fall in GFR is apparent from the slope clearance method, which is not demonstrated by following C_{Cr}.

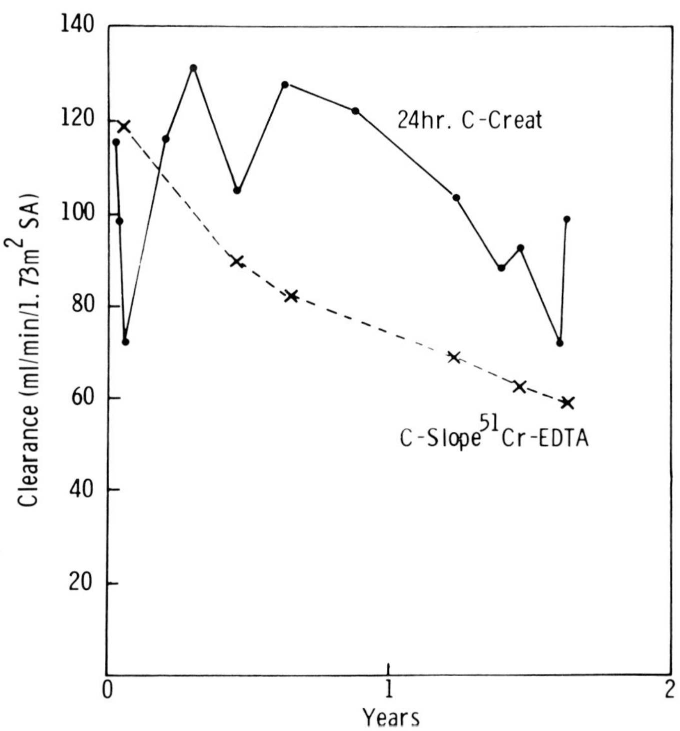

Figure 19.8. Estimates of GFR by single exponential analysis of the plasma clearance of ^{51}Cr-EDTA and creatinine clearance in a 14 year old boy with Henoch-Schönlein nephritis. (Reproduced with permission from Chantler and Barratt (66). Arch Dis Childh 47:613, 1972.)

Renal Plasma Flow

PAH Clearance

In the adult with normal renal function, about 92% of the total plasma flow to the kidney passes through functioning excretory tissue. This fraction is termed the effective renal plasma flow (ERPF) and can be measured by the clearance of para-aminohippuric acid (PAH), which is secreted by the renal tubules. At low plasma concentration, the extraction of PAH from the blood flowing through the kidney is almost complete (98). The ratio of GFR to ERPF is termed the filtration fraction. Some of the blood from the juxtamedullary glomeruli passes directly into the vasa recta without perfusing the proximal tubular cells and the PAH in this blood thus escapes secretion. When medullary blood flow is increased in relation to cortical blood flow, PAH clearance gives a greater underestimate of RPF.

For example, incomplete extraction of PAH accounts for the low ERPF and high filtration fraction in newborns as estimated from PAH clearance (99). Doubts concerning the validity of ERPF measurements using PAH clearance also affect the significance attributable to filtration fraction determinations in renal disease (100). As renal function declines, the fall in the ERPF is mirrored by a fall in the GFR and, therefore, PAH clearance is not generally measured in clinical practice. Accurate measurement of ERPF from PAH clearance requires an estimation of PAH extraction by renal vein catheterization and, therefore, is unsuitable for clinical practice as are other such methods of determining RBF, such as renal washout studies using inert gases (101).

Normal values for ERPF measured as the PAH clearance in adults, given by Smith (68), were 654 ± 163 ml/min/1.73m^{2}SA in males and 592 ± 153 in females; in infants aged 8 days to 3 months, mean plasma flow was 68 ml/min/1.73m^{2}SA and in those aged 5 months to 10 months of age the mean was 91 (99).

Ortho-iodohippurate (hippuran) is a reliable substitute for PAH in the measurement of ERPF. By labeling the compound with either ^{125}I or ^{131}I its concentration can be measured easily and accurately. The clearance of ^{125}I or ^{131}I-hippuran is slightly less than that of PAH by classical techniques (102), as a result of differences in protein binding (103). The ERPF can be derived from a double exponential analysis of the falling plasma concentration curve following a single intravenous injection of ^{131}I or ^{125}I-hippuran (104). The single injection clearance is 5% less than the classical PAH clearance but the correlation is excellent over a wide range of renal function. Using different radioactive tracers it is possible to measure both GFR and ERPF in a single test, for example by combining ^{125}I-hippuran with either ^{51}Cr-EDTA or with ^{131}I-sodium-iothalamate. However, all the criticisms of the single injection method, when considering GFR measurements, are relevant to this technique with ever greater force becuase the rapid clearance with the short half-life of the falling plasma concentration curve magnifies the inherent errors of the method. For example, the venous concentration cannot be taken as an accurate measure of the arterial concentration. For this reason, attempts to simplify the single-injection method, so that only one exponential is analyzed have not proved successful (105, 106). However, the double exponential analysis method has been applied in children (107).

Estimation of Individual Kidney Function

The rate of uptake of ^{131}I-hippuran by the kidneys may be measured by surface counters with separate collimators placed over the kidneys. The measurement of individual kidney ERPF is improved by the subtraction of blood background activity, assessed from the prior injection of ^{131}I-human albumin. The results obtained are comparable to split renal function studies using ureteral catheterization (113). The techniques are applicable to children of all ages (114), though some difficulties arise in positioning the collimators accurately over the kidneys in infants.

Dynamic renal scintigraphy is discussed in chapter 20. Analysis of the uptake and excretion of ^{99m}Tc-DTPA by the kidney, using a gamma camera, enables the total GFR (which can be measured during the same test) to be apportioned between each kidney (115). A similar and reliable assessment of individual kidney function can be obtained following the injection of ^{99m}Tc-dimercaptosuccinic acid (DMSA), which is taken up by the tubules. The ratio of uptake between the two kidneys, which is a function of ERPF and renal mass, correlates well with the individual contribution of each kidney to the total GFR (111). The development of radioisotope techniques for measuring individual renal function (109, 110) has rendered divided renal function studies by ureteral catheterization obsolete.

Proteinuria

Urinary Total Protein

Protein is present in normal urine; 32 plasma proteins have been detected (112) along with a complex array of glycoproteins (113) and other locally secreted proteins and enzymes, such as alanine aminopeptidases (114–116). In view of such heterogeneity, estimates of total urinary protein are of doubtful value and are often very dependent upon the methodology, particularly at low concentration. Albumin constitutes about one-quarter to one-half of the total urinary non-dialyzable solids and excretion rates from 6 to 31 mg/day in healthy adults have been reported (117). The distinction between normal and pathological urine is thus quantitative. Pathological proteinuria may be a result of increased glomerular permeability (glomerular proteinuria) or decreased tubular reabsorption of proteins normally present in glomerular filtrate (tubular proteinuria), though other mechanisms are possible, such as the production of abnormal plasma proteins that are then filtered (Fig. 19.9).

Glomerular Proteinuria

Albumin Excretion. The glomerulus is an ultrafilter that may become leaky, blocked, or both. Measurement of leak provides a valuable means of detecting glomerular disease in its early stages and also of evaluating its natural history and response to therapy. The most sensitive parameter of leak is the sieving coefficient (relative concentration in glomerular filtrate and plasma water) of a molecule of a size that is normally just restrained by the glomerular filter. For this purpose, the albumin/creatinine clearance ratio is the most suitable approximation for clinical use (117). It has the advantage that, being a clearance ratio, it is independent of urine flow rate and thus may be estimated on a random urine specimen and concomitant blood sample.

$$C_A = U_A V / P_A \qquad (16)$$

$$C_{Cr} = U_{Cr} V / P_{Cr} \qquad (17)$$

$$C_A / C_{Cr} = (U_A / P_A)/(U_{Cr} / P_{Cr}) \qquad (18)$$

where U_A, P_A, C_A = urine concentration, plasma concentration, and clearance of albumin.

Most of the variation in C_A/C_{Cr} is due to the urine concentration term, for the range of the variation of plasma concentration is much less. Hence, C_A/C_{Cr} may be predicted with reasonable confidence from the urine albumin/creatinine concentration ratio, U_A/U_{Cr}, measured on a random urine sample (117). Albumin is measured by immunochemical methods.

Normal values are given in Table 19.5. For convenience, a U_A/U_{Cr} (mg/mg) <0.1 is considered normal, 0.1 to 1.0 slight, 0.1 to 1.0 moderate

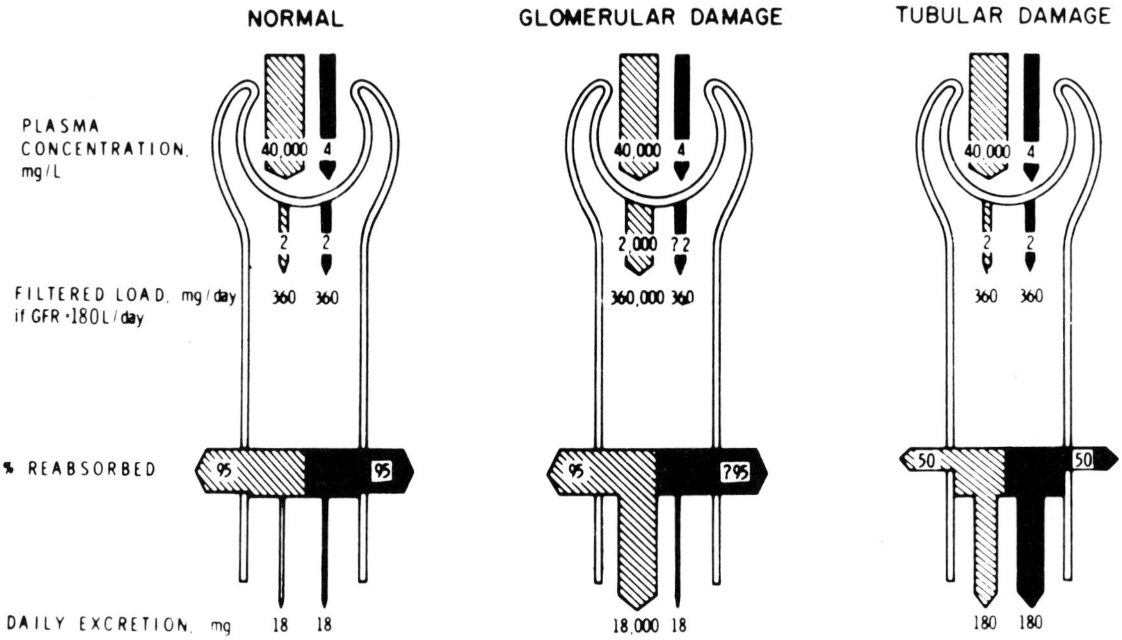

Figure 19.9. Schematic diagram illustrating two basic mechanisms which can cause proteinuria; increased glomerular permeability with no change in tubular reabsorption of protein and/or impaired tubular reabsorption of normally filtered proteins. (Adapted with permission from Heinemann H et al (116). Am J Med 56:71, 1974.)

Table 19.5.
Albumin (117) and Lysozyme (128) Excretion: Mean and SD Calculated on Log-Transformed Data

Age		Albumin			Lysozyme		
		PA (g/dl)	CA/CCr ×10⁴	UA/UCr (mg/mg)	PL (mg/dl)	CL/CCr ×10⁴	UL/UCr μg/mg
	Mean	4.0	0.11	0.08	1.4	16	4.8
Neonates	±2SD	3.6–4.5	0.03–0.40	0.02–0.39	0.9–2.3	5–54	1.2–19
	Mean			0.08			1.8
1 yr	±2SD			0.02–0.32			0.1–23
	Mean			0.03			0.4
2–12 yr	±2SD			0.01–0.15			0.1–5
	Mean	4.8	0.03	0.02	1.4	6	0.9
Adult	±2SD	3.4–6.6	0.01–0.09	0.01–0.05	1.1–1.7	0.5–>4	0.1–14

PA: plasma albumin concentration; CA: albumin clearance; UA: urine albumin concentration; PL: plasma lysozyme concentration; CL: lysozyme clearance; UL: urine lysozyme concentration; CCr: creatinine clearance; UCr: urine creatinine concentration.

and >10 heavy proteinuria. These methods have substantial theoretical and practical advantages over the more commonly used total protein excretion, where more than 300 mg protein in a 24-hour collection is regarded as abnormal (118). Children with orthostatic proteinuria (chapter 18) rarely excrete >1g protein/24 hours, though intermittent protein excretion rates up to 0.5 g/hour (12 g/24 hours) have been recorded (119).

Selectivity. Selectivity is expressed by the relative clearance of individual macromolecules of different molecular size (120). By measuring several serum and urinary proteins (121) it is possible to define glomerular permeability over a wide range of molecular size. Nephrotic patients with minimal renal histological abnormality have more selective proteinuria than patients with proliferative or membranous lesions (122).

Selectivity is conveniently assessed by the ratio of the clearances of two proteins of differing molecular size. Albumin or transferrin (123) and IgG are suitable proteins and the selectivity is calculated as:

$$\text{Selectivity} = (U_{IgG}/P_{IgG})/(U_A/P_A) \qquad (19)$$

where U_{IgG}, P_{IgG} = urine, plasma concentration of IgG; and U_A, P_A = urine, plasma concentration of albumin.

If proteinuria is only mild (U_A/U_{Cr} <1.0) then conclusions regarding size selectivity glomerular permeability are invalid because the assumption that tubular protein reabsorption is negligible is no longer held. Selectivity has been used in the nephrotic syndrome to predict the response to steroid therapy (124). An IgG/albumin clearance ratio of <10% predicts steroid responsiveness >20%, steroid resistance (Fig. 19.10). In practice, the measurement of selectivity is limited in value because the decision to undertake a trial of corticosteroids is often taken on other grounds and poor selectivity does not exclude the possibility of steroid responsiveness.

Tubular Proteinuria

The proteinuria of patients with renal tubular disorders is qualitatively different from that of patients with glomerular disease. The major constituents on electrophoresis are alpha- and beta-globulins rather than albumin. There may be a high proportion of peptides of low molecular

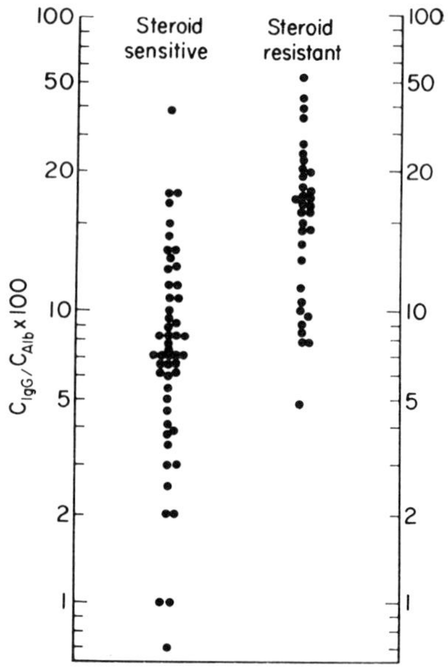

Figure 19.10. Selectivity of proteinuria expressed as the IgG/albumin clearance ratio (%) in 84 children with heavy proteinuria. (Reproduced with permission from Barratt T M and Macaulay D: Renal Disease, ed. 3. Oxford, Blackwell Scientific Publications, 1972, p. 805.)

weight and their excretion is due to failure of reabsorption and catabolism by the proximal tubule of proteins normally present in the glomerular filtrate (125–127).

Lysozyme has a molecular weight of 15,000 dl and is attractive as a representative small protein because of its ease of estimation by the lysis of susceptible bacteria (127). Data for normal children have been published (Table 19.5) (128). The interpretation of results are limited in the neonate because the lysozyme molecule may be too large to be freely filterable by the neonatal glomerulus (73), and in children with CRF, as filtration and catabolism by the renal tubules is the principal catabolic fate for lysozyme, the plasma concentration may be high and saturate the reabsorptive capacity of the residual nephrons with an increase in lysozyme excretion which is not necessarily a result of tubular dysfunction (129).

β_2-microglobulin (molecular weight 11,800 dl) is synthesized by most human cells. Tumor cells and lymphocytes are major sites of production (130). It is cleared by glomerular filtration and is reabsorbed or catabolized by tubular cells (131). Urinary concentration in the adult is <350 μg/L. Plasma concentration increases either because of increased production in inflammatory or malignant disease or because of a reduced GFR. The plasma concentration has been used with some success as an easy though relatively inaccurate method of assessing GFR (132, 133).

Tubular disease is associated with a marked increase in urinary β_2-microglobulin excretion. Increased urinary β_2-microglobulin, for example, is used in the detection of cadmium toxicity or in the early stages of Balkan nephropathy (130). The maturation of proximal tubular function in the infant has been studied by examining the fractional excretion of β_2-microglobulin in infants and children. Fractional excretion falls from 1.6% in the neonate to 0.05% by 21 months of age (132, 133).

Tubular Function

The proximal nephron is responsible for the bulk of reabsorption of water, electrolytes, glucose, amino acids and small molecular weight proteins. The presence of proximal tubular dysfunction usually can be inferred from a tendency to hyponatremia, hypokalemia, generalized aminoaciduria, bicarbonate wasting with renal tubular acidosis, glycosuria, and hyperphosphaturia with hypophosphatemia. Thus, examination of blood and urine usually will detect significant proximal tubular dysfunction, whereas distal tubular function is assessed by measuring urinary concentrating and acidifying capacity.

Proximal Tubular Tests

Sodium Reabsorption. The volume of Na and water reabsorbed by the proximal tubule can be estimated by the following study. During maximal water diuresis the distal nephron is effectively impermeable to water. Under these conditions, the urine volume is determined by the volume of fluid that emerges from the proximal tubule; the expression V/GFR equals the fraction of glomerular filtrate that is not reabsorbed by the proximal tubule. Expressed as a fraction of GFR, derived from creatinine clearance, proximal Na reabsorption is estimated by equation 20 when the data are obtained during a maximal water diuresis:

$$V/GFR = V/(U_{Cr}V/P_{Cr}) = P_{Cr}/U_{Cr} \qquad (20)$$

It is important to ensure that the water diuresis is maximal. Measurements should be considered only when urine osmolalities are <75 mOsm/L. An oral water load of 20 ml/kg or 800 ml/m^{2}SA and replacement of urine losses with an equal amount of oral water for up to 4 hours is required to achieve these conditions.

The function of the distal nephron may be examined by measuring relative clearance of Na and water to creatinine during a hypotonic saline diuresis. Distal NaCl reabsorption is derived from the rate of generation of solute-free water (CH_2O) (135); the method has been used in a number of clinical studies (136, 137) (Chapter 33).

Glucose Reabsorption. The renal glucose threshold is the plasma glucose concentration at which significant amounts of glucose appear in the urine. The presence of glucose in the urine (>10 mg/dl, 0.5 mMol/L) must be interpreted in relation to the simultaneously determined

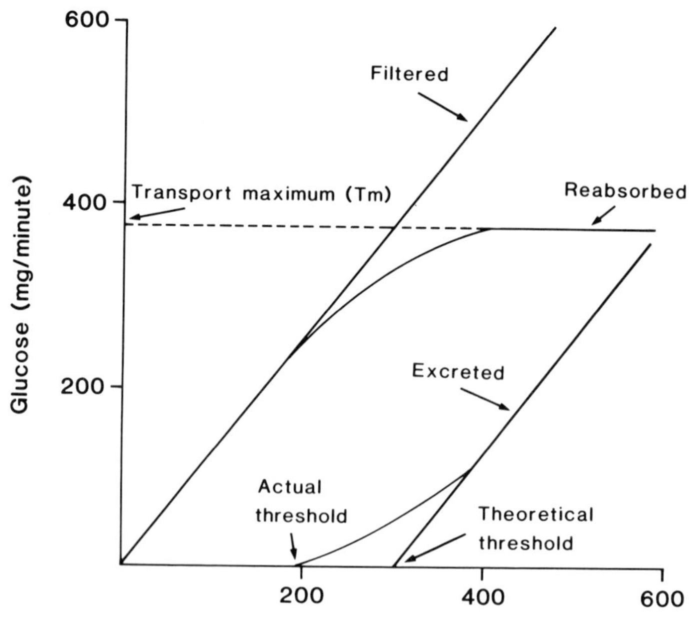

Figure 19.11. Glucose titration curve in a normal man. The line for glucose filtered is calculated from GFR × plasma glucose and the GFR is assumed to be 125 ml/min. The curve for glucose reabsorbed is derived by subtracting glucose excreted from glucose filtered. TmG is 375 mg/min. The actual threshold is 180 mg/dl whereas the theoretical threshold ignoring splay is 300 mg/dl. (1 mMol/l = 18 mg/dl).

plasma glucose concentration. If this is <116 mg/dl (6 mMol/L) there is incomplete tubular reabsorption of glucose, i.e., a renal glucosuria.

Renal glucosuria may be further characterized by measuring the tubular maximum reabsorption (Tm_G). If glucose is infused, the plasma glucose concentration (P_G) and, hence, filtered glucose (GFR × P_G) rise, the tubular glucose reabsorption (filtered glucose − excreted glucose: GFR × P_G − U_GV) rises to a plateau (Fig. 19.11). The normal range of Tm_G is 375 ± 80 mg/min/1.73m.[2] When corrected for GFR it is the same for all ages (138, 139). In theory, glucose will appear in the urine only when plasma glucose is 300 mg/dl, i.e., the point where tubular reabsorptive capacity is saturated. In practice, the titration curve exhibits a splay and glucose appears in the urine before the tubular reabsorptive capacity is saturated. Estimates of Tm_G are difficult to obtain and are rarely of any clinical value. A reduction in Tm_G as a result of tubular disease is associated with a reduction in threshold to renal glucosuria, which is useful for detecting proximal tubular dysfunction, as in Fanconi's syndrome (Chapter 30). Renal glucosuria also may be an isolated defect that is sometimes congenital, sometimes familial, and is benign. In one variety of isolated renal glucosuria Tm_G is reduced, with a proportional reduction in threshold, while in another variety Tm_G is normal but splay is increased (140).

Aminoaciduria. Free L-amino acids are reabsorbed from the glomerular filtrate by transport systems (141, 142) that may be at fault individually, as in specific aminoaciduria (chapter 31) or generally, as in Fanconi's syndrome (chapter 30). Measurement of urinary total alpha amino nitrogen (143) is of little value except when it is done to look for diffuse proximal injury, e.g., Fanconi's syndrome. Screening by thin layer chromatography (144) is useful but accurate quantitative data for deriving clearance values requires the measurement of amino acids and of GFR by appropriate quantitative techniques (chapter 31).

Clearances in healthy adults, which, in ml/min, approximately correspond to percentage of filtered load excreted, are <1.0 ml/min for alanine, arginine, glutamine, isoleucine, leucine, ornithine, proline, and valine; 1.0 to 3.0 ml/min for lysine, methionine, phenylalanine, serine, tryptophan, threonine, and tyrosine; and 2.0 to 8.0 ml/min for cystine, asparagine, glycine, and histidine (146). There is an increased excretion of free amino acids in the normal young child (145), particularly of the iminoglycine group (141). Data on the quantitative excretions, clearances, and tubular reabsorption of free amino acids throughout childhood have been published (147–149).

Urinary Acidification

Tests for renal acidification are done when renal tubular acidosis (RTA) is suspected (chapter 34). Hydrogen ion secreted by the proximal tubule neutralizes filtered bicarbonate to form carbonic acid, which on reabsorption reconstitutes bicarbonate. Distal tubular fluid usually is nearly free of bicarbonate and pH is approximately 6. Net hydrogen ion secretion may take place, and is buffered as titratable acid and ammonium ion. The urinary pH is determined by these steps. Measurement of urine pH and its relationship to plasma bicarbonate concentration usually will determine whether RTA is present.

Urine pH. Urine pH is measured in a fresh sample, using a pH meter. Urinary tract infection, particularly with a urea-splitting organism forming NH_3, invalidates any estimate of pH. Fasting urine of most infants and children is acid. If the child is not acidotic and pH is <5.3, RTA is highly unlikely. This simple screening test should always be done before more elaborate tests for acidification are undertaken.

Bicarbonate Threshold. The bicarbonate threshold is the plasma bicarbonate at which bicarbonate appears in the urine; if bicarbonate in urine exceeds 1 mEq/L, urine pH rises above 6.1 (Fig. 19.12) (150–153) The determintion of bicarbonate threshold is required to identify the

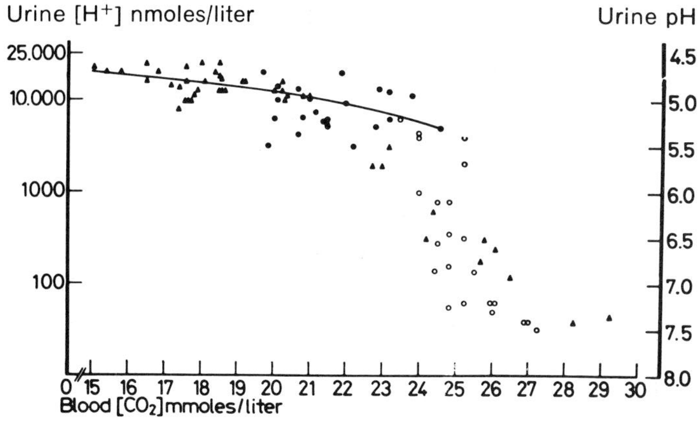

Figure 19.12. Urinary (H^+) as a function of blood (tCO_2) in children. Two points are plotted for each subject, a control value derived from control blood, and the mean of the two control urines (open symbols) and a post-NH_4Cl value derived from the test blood and the mean of the urine between the third and fifth hours (closed symbols). (Reproduced with permission from Edelmann et al (150). Pediatr Res 1:452, 1967.)

defect in proximal tubular bicarbonate reabsorption that underlies proximal RTA (154). A child with proximal RTA may have a low plasma bicarbonate and an acid urine. The threshold is identified by raising the plasma bicarbonate by infusing bicarbonate in a stepwise fashion until urine pH is >6.0. Alternatively, if the child is on bicarbonate therapy, therapy can be withheld and urine pH observed as the plasma bicarbonate falls. The test is positive if urine pH >5.3 when plasma bicarbonate is below the normal threshold.

Ammonium Chloride Response. Giving ammonium chloride results in metabolic acidosis (Table 19.6); this is done as a standard challenge of renal acidification (150, 155). The test is done by measuring two baseline urine specimens and then giving NH_4Cl orally in fruit juice. Each urine thereafter is collected at approximately one-hour intervals for the next 6 hours and urine pH, titratable acidity, and ammonium are measured. A blood sample taken at 3 to 4 hours after giving NH_4Cl ensures that a metabolic acidosis has been induced. Blood sampling is more frequent if the plasma bicarbonate threshold is to be identified. The amount of NH_4Cl used has varied in different studies. Edelmann et al (150) used two dose levels of 75 mMol (4 g) and 150 mMol (8g) per m^2SA. The urine pH should fall to 5.3 or less after the ammonium chloride, but the lower dose may sometimes be insufficient to achieve this. Ammonium chloride should not be administered to children with uremia, liver disease, or defects of urea synthesis.

Urine pCO_2. The distal acidification mechanism is studied by measuring urinary pCO_2 following bicarbonate loading (157). When CO_2 is generated by hydrogen ion secretion into tubular fluid containing bicarbonate the urinary pCO_2 increases to levels that are >30 torr above plasma pCO_2. In children with distal RTA there is little difference in plasma and urinary pCO_2 under these conditions. The test is done by giving 3 mEq/kg $NaHCO_3$ to raise urine pH >7.4. Provided a concentrated urine is obtained, normal children can be reliably distinguished from those with distal RTA. Suitably concentrated urine may be achieved by water deprivation or administering 20 μg DDAVP intranasally 2 hours after the sodium bicarbonate administration. The test is not valid if a renal concentrating defect exists in conjunction with the acidification defect. Normal children were found to have a urine − blood pCO_2 difference of 40 torr (range 16 to 66) while children with distal RTA had a difference of 1 mm Hg (range −9 to +8) (158).

In summary, the diagnosis of distal RTA can be made with a high

Table 19.6.
The Renal Response to Acute Ammonium Chloride Acidosis at Two Dose Levels of 75 and 150 mEq/m² SA (150)

NH_4Cl Dose		Control Periods		Hours after Administration of NH_4Cl				
		1	2	1	2	3	4	5
75 mEq/m²SA	Urine pH	6.46 (5.1–7.7)	6.51 (5.2–7.4)	5.33 (4.9–6.1)	5.16 (4.8–5.9)	5.11 (4.7–5.9)	5.15 (4.7–6.0)	5.11 (4.7–5.9)
	TA	15 (0–37)	16 (0–39)	41 (11–85)	46 (19–71)	48 (26–70)	49 (30–70)	51 (31–88)
	$UV_{NH_4^+}$	21 (9–57)	27 (8–89)	57 (22–118)	60 (29–109)	65 (30–115)	63 (29–85)	68 (27–111)
	UV_{H^+}	28 (0–74)	29 (0–80)	97 (32–203)	105 (51–175)	113 (56–174)	110 (59–148)	119 (60–168)
	Blood pH		7.41 (7.35–7.48)			7.36 (7.29–7.45)		
	Plasma tCO_2		25.1 (23.5–27.2)			21.6 (19.4–24.6)		
150 mEq/m²SA	Urine pH	6.00 (5.1–7.3)	6.50 (5.5–7.4)	5.11 (4.7–5.9)	4.92 (4.6–5.8)	4.85 (4.6–5.3)	4.85 (4.6–5.2)	4.95 (4.6–5.9)
	TA	18 (3–26)	11 (0–23)	34 (18–65)	46 (27–78)	51 (28–73)	54 (40–77)	53 (35–73)
	$UV_{NH_4^+}$	24 (15–35)	24 (13–45)	66 (38–129)	73 (33–136)	74 (42–105)	79 (58–106)	80 (62–89)
	UV_{H^+}	31 (0–67)	14 (0.68)	100 (61–168)	119 (78–181)	125 (91–157)	133 (100–157)	133 (115–155)
	Blood pH		7.41 (7.38–7.51)			7.27 (7.19–7.36)		
	Plasma tCO_2		25.7 (23.0–29.2)			18.4 (15.1–21.5)		

The results given are the mean with the observed range in parentheses. TA, titratable acidity (μEq/min/1.73m²SA); $UV_{NH_4^+}$, urine ammonium excretion (μEq/min/1.73m²SA); $UV_{H^+} = TA + UV_{NH_4^+} - UV_{HCO_3} -$ (μEq/min/1.73m²SA).

level of probability by comparing the urine pH and the plasma bicarbonate. If urine is <5.3 and the plasma bicarbonate is normal, an acidification defect is excluded. If the plasma bicarbonate is below normal and the urine pH is >5.3, a defect exists (chapter 34).

Urinary Concentrating Capacity

Defects in urinary concentrating mechanisms are of 2 types: (1) a defect in the ability to concentrate urine much above plasma osmolality (<400 mOsm/L), and (2) a defect in the ability to concentrate urine to plasma osmolality (<250 mOsm/L), i.e., hyposthenuria. The first is characteristic of CRF, sickle cell disease, and heavy glycosuria associated with diabetes mellitus. In patients with CRF and sickle cell disease, neither polydipsia nor polyuria are clinical complaints; with heavy glycosuria, the osmotic diuresis precludes forming concentrated urine (chapters 5 and 6). Hyposthenuria ($U_{osm} < P_{osm}$) is characteristic of vasopressin-deficient diabetes insipidus and vasopressin-resistant diabetes insipidus, including the hereditary form of nephrogenic diabetes insipidus (chapter 35) and the vasopressin-resistant form of diabetes insipidus associated with renal medullary disease, e.g., medullary cystic disease, or obstructive uropathy (chapter 49). In patients with diabetes insipidus, the hyposthenuria is resistant to water deprivation but responsive to ADH. In patients with vasopressin-resistent hyposthenuria, the hyposthenuria is resistant to water deprivation and to ADH.

Urine Osmolality. Most children pass a concentrated urine in the early morning; U_{osm} should be checked on a fresh specimen before embarking on more complicated tests. U_{osm} >800 mOsm/L excludes a significant concentrating defect. If P_{osm} is >290 mOsm/L and the urine is not concentrated, a concentration defect exists. While tests of specific gravity (SG) correlate with U_{osm}, SG often does not discriminate between hyposthenuria and isosthenuria (isotonic urine). When tests of concentrating capacity are being done, U_{osm} not SG should be measured.

Water Deprivation. In response to water deprivation, normal children aged 2 to 16 years achieve a U_{osm} of 1089 + 110 (SD) mOsm/L (159). In the standardized test no fluid is administered after a normal lunch though a dry supper is allowed. The bladder is emptied at about 8 PM and all the urine passed subsequently until 8 AM is pooled and the osmolality measured. If marked polyuria and polydypsia are clinically evident, the child should be weighed at intervals throughout the test (it is terminated if the weight loss is 3% or more). In such circumstances, it is often safer to deprive the child of water through the day when closer observation is likely. Plasma osmolality can be measured at the end of the test to confirm that an adequate stimulus to urine concentration has been achieved.

The magnitude of the urinary response to water deprivation or vasopressin depends in part on urea excretion (and, hence, dietary protein intake). This effect is particularly evident in babies on low protein milk feeds (160). Here, the ability to concentrate the urine in response to water deprivation is reduced due to the low urea excretion, but the urinary concentration of non-urea solute is similar to that in older children (161).

Vasopressin. Failure to concentrate the urine in response to water deprivation may be due to lack of ADH or resistance to its action. The alternatives may be discriminated by the administration of DDAVP (20 μg intranasally; 10 μg in infants) (162). This test should be carried out in a water-depleted state to avoid the danger of water intoxication in young infants.

References

1. Al-Dahhan J, Haycock GB, Chantler C, et al: Sodium homeostasis in mature and immature neonates. I. Renal aspects. Arch Dis Child 58:335, 1983.
2. Arant BS, Edelmann CM, Spitzer A: The congruence of creatinine and inulin clearances in children; use of the Technicon Autoanalyzer. J Pediatr 81:559, 1972.

3. Ghazali S, Barratt TM: Urine calcium excretion in children. Arch Dis Child 49:97, 1974.
4. Smith HW: The Kidney: Structure and Function in Health and Disease. New York, Oxford University Press, 1951.
5. Holliday MA: Body composition and energy needs during growth. In Faulkner F, Tanner JM. (eds): Human Growth New York, Plenum Publishers, 1978, vol 2.
6. Tanner JM: Fallacy of per weight and per surface area standards and their relation to spurious correlation. J Appl Physiol 2:1, 1949.
7. Friis Hansen B: Body water compartments in children; changes during growth and related changes in body composition. Pediatrics 28:169, 1961.
8. McCance RA, Widdowson EM: The correct physiological basis on which to compare infant and adult renal function. Lancet 2:860, 1952.
9. Haycock GB, Schwartz GJ, Wisotsky DH: Geometric method for measuring body surface area; a height weight formula validated in infants, children and adults. J Pediatr 93:62, 1978.
10. Clayton BE, Jenkins P, Round JM: Paediatric Chemical Pathology. Oxford, London, Blackwell Scientific Publications, 1980, p 1.
11. Tobian L: The relationship of salt to hypertension. Am J Clin Nutr 32:115, 1974.
12. Biancani F, Rappaport R, Balsan S, et al: L'épreuve de restriction sodée chez l'enfant normal. Etude de la conservation rénale du sodium et des variations de la tetrahydro-aldosterone urinaire. Arch Franc Pediatr 29:609, 1972.
13. Slatopoulsky E, Ekkan IO, Werts C, et al: Studies on the characteristics of the control system governing sodium excretion in uremic man. J Clin Invest 47:521, 1968.
14. Holliday MA, Egan TJ, Morris CR: Pitressin resistant hyposthenuria in chronic renal disease. Am J Med 42:378, 1967.
15. Robertson GL, Aycinena P, Zerbe RL: Neurogenic disorders of osmoregulation. Am J Med 72:339, 1982.
16. Rogers D, Tripp J, Bentovim A, et al: Non-accidental poisoning; an extended syndrome of child abuse. Brit Med J 1:793, 1976.
17. Mathew OP, Jones AS, James E et al: Neonatal renal failure, usefulness of diagnostic indices. Pediatrics 65:57, 1980.
18. Van Ypersele de Stihou C: Potassium homeostasis in renal failure. Kidney Int 11:491, 1977.
19. Van Slyke DD, Neill JM: The determination of gases in blood by vacuum extraction and manometric measurement. J Biol Chem 61:523, 1924.
20. Michalk D, Manz F, Muller Wiefel DE, et al: Renal handling of inorganic sulphate in children with chronic kidney disorders. Mineral Electrolyte Metab 8:255, 1982.
21. Berry EM, Gupta MM, Turner SJ et al: Variations in plasma calcium with induced changes in plasma specific gravity, total protein and albumin. Brit Med J 11:640, 1973.
22. Herbert LA, Lemann J, Peterson JR, et al: Studies on the mechanism by which phosphate infusion lowers serum calcium concentration. J Clin Invest 45:1886, 1966.
23. Knapp EL: Factors influencing urinary excretion of calcium in normal persons. J Clin Invest 26:182, 1947.
24. Paunier L, Borgeaud M, Wyss M: Urinary excretion of magnesium and calcium in normal children. Helv Paediat Acta 25:577, 1970.
25. Royer P: Explorations biologiques due métabolisme calcique chez l'enfant. Helv Paediatr Acta 16:230, 1961.
26. Bar RS, Wilson HE, Mazzaferri EL: Hypomagnesemic hypocalcaemia secondary to renal magnesium wasting. Ann Int Med 82:646, 1975.
27. Manz F, Schärer K, Janka P, et al: Renal magnesium wasting, incomplete renal tubular acidosis, hypercalciuria and nephrocalcinosis in siblings. Eur J Pediatr 128:67, 1978.
28. Ghazali S, Hallet RJ, Barratt TM: Hypomagnesemia in uraemic infants. J Pediatr 81:747, 1972.
29. Booth BE, Johanson A: Hypomagnesemia due to renal tubular defect in the reabsorption of magnesium. J Pediatr 84:350, 1974.
30. Paunier L, Sizonenko PC: Asymptomatic chronic hypomagnesemia and hypokalemia in a child: cell membrane disease? J Paediatr 88:51, 1976.
31. Round JM: Plasma calcium, magnesium, phosphorus and alkaline phosphatase levels in normal British school children. Brit Med J 3:137, 1973.
32. Kruse K, Kracht U, Gopfert G: Renal threshold phosphate concentration ($TmPO_4$/GFR). Arch Dis Child 57:212, 1982.
33. Bijvoet OLM: Indices for the measurement of the renal handling of phosphate. In Massry SG, Fleish H (eds): Renal Handling of Phosphate. New York, Plenum Med Book Co, 1980.
34. Walton RJ, Bijvoet OLM: Nomogram for the derivation of renal threshold phosphate concentration. Lancet 2:309, 1975.
35. Mak RHK, Turner C, Haycock GB, et al: Control of secondary hyperparathyroidism in children with chronic renal failure by reducing dietary phosphate intake and using phosphate binders. (Submitted for publication.)
36. Addis T: The ratio between the urea content of the urine and of the blood after the administration of large quantities of urea. An approximate index of the quantity of actively functioning kidney tissue. J Urol 1:263, 1917.
37. Möller E, McIntosh JF, Van Slyke DD: Studies of urea secretion. II. Relationship between urine volume and the rate of urea excretion by normal adults. J Clin Invest 6:427, 1928.
38. Lavender S, Hilton PJ, Jones NF: The measurement of glomerular filtration rate in renal disease. Lancet 2:1216, 1969.
39. Lubowitz H, Spatopoulsky E, Shankel S, et al: Glomerular filtration rate determination in patients with chronic renal disease. J Am Med Ass 199:252, 1967.
40. Kuhlback B, Pasternack A, Laniola K, et al: Serum creatine and creatinine in children and adolescents. Scand J Clin Lab Invest 22:37, 1968.
41. Winberg J: The 24-hour true endogenous creatinine clearance in infants and children without renal disease. Acta Paediatr Scand 48:443, 1959.
42. Donckerwolcke RAMG, Sander PC, Van Stekelenberg J, et al: Serum creatinine values in healthy children. Acta Paediatr Scand 59:399, 1970.
43. Doolan PD, Alpon EL, Theil GB: A clinical appraisal of the plasma concentration and endogenous clearance of creatinine. Am J Med 32:65, 1962.
44. Cheek DB: Human Growth. Philadelphia, Lea and Febiger, 1968, p 741.
45. Edwards KDG, Whyte HM: Plasma creatinine level and creatinine clearance as tests of renal function. Austral Ann Med 8:218, 1959.
46. Stoten A: A micromethod for creatinine using resin to remove interfering substances. J Med Lab Tech 25:240, 1968.
47. Dodge WF, Travis LB, Daeschner CW: Comparison of endogenous creatinine clearance with inulin clearance. Am J Dis Child 113:683, 1967.
48. Counahan R, Chantler C, Ghazali S, et al: Estimation of glomerular filtration rate from plasma creatinine concentration in children. Arch Dis Childh 51:875, 1976.
50. Chasson AL, Grady HJ, Stanley MA: Determination of creatinine by means of automatic analysis. Am J Clin Path 35:83, 1981.
51. Feldman A, Guignard JP: Plasma creatinine in the first month of life. Arch Dis Childh 57:123, 1981.
52. Morris MC, Allanby CW, Toseland P, et al: Evaluation of a height/plasma creatinine formula in the measurement of glomerular filtration rate. Arch Dis Childh 57:611, 1981.
53. Schwartz GJ, Haycock GB, Spitzer A: Plasma creatinine and urea concentration in children; normal values for age and sex. J Pediatr 88:828, 1976.
54. Trompeter RS, Al-Dahhan J, Haycock, et al: Normal values for plasma creatinine concentration related to maturity in normal and preterm infants. Int J Pediatr Nephrol 4:145, 1983.
55. Schwartz GJ, Haycock GB, Edelmann CM, et al: A simple estimate of glomerular filtration rate in children derived from body length and plasma creatinine. J Pediatr 58:259, 1976.
56. Cheek DB, Habicht JP, Berrall J, et al: Protein-calorie malnutrition and the significance of cell mass relative to body length. Am J Clin Nutr 30:851, 1977.
57. Barnett HL, Hare K, McNamara H, et al: Measurement of glomerular filtration rate in premature infants. J Clin Invest 32:691, 1948.
58. Edelmann CM, Bernstein J: In Barnett HL (ed): Pediatrics. New York, Appleton-Century Crofts, 1968, p 1332.
59. Smith HW, Golding W, Chasis H, et al: The application of saturation methods to the study of glomerular and tubular function in the human kidney. J Mt Sinai Hosp 10:59, 1943.
60. Mitch WE, Walser M: A simple method for estimating progression of chronic renal failure. Lancet 2:1326, 1976.
61. Gretz N, Manz F, Strauch M: Predictability of the progression to chronic renal failure. Kidney Int 24(suppl 15):52, 1983.
62. Rehberg PB: Studies on renal function. 1. Rate of filtration and reabsorption in the human kidney. Biochem J 20:447, 1926.
63. Shannon JA: The renal excretion of creatinine in man. J Clin Invest 14:403, 1935.
64. Brod J, Sirota JH: The renal clearance of endogenous creatinine in man. J Clin Invest 27:645, 1948.
65. Kim KE, Onesti G, Ramirez O, et al: Creatinine clearance in renal disease, a reappraisal. Brit Med J 4:11, 1969.
66. Chantler C, Barratt TM: Estmation of glomerular filtration rate from the plasma clearance of 51-chromium edetic acid. Arch Dis Childh 47:613, 1972.
67. Mak RHK, Al-Dahhan JA, Azzopardi D, et al: Measurement of glomerular filtration rate in children after renal transplantation. Kidney Int 23:410, 1983.
68. Smith HW: Principles of Renal Physiology. New York, Oxford University Press, 1956.
69. Rose GA: Measurement of GFR by inulin clearance without urine collections. Brit Med J 2:91, 1969.
70. Dawborn JW: Application of Hevrovsky's inulin method to automatic analysis. Clin Chem Acta 12:63, 1965.
71. Hart O: Ein neues inulinahnliches polyfructose-saccharid. Klin Wchnschr 41:769, 1963.
72. Mattar G, Barnett HL, McNamara HL, et al: Measurement of glomerular filtration rate in children with kidney disease. J. Clin Invest 31:938, 1952.
73. Arturson G, Groth T, Grotte G: Human glomerular membrane porosity and filtration pressure: dextran clearance analyzed by theoretical models. Clin Sci 40:137, 1971.

74. Arturson G, Gramath K, Grotte G: Intravascular persistence and renal clearance of dextran of different molecular sizes in normal children. Arch Dis Child 41:168, 1966.
75. Al-Dahhan J, Haycock G, Stimmler, et al: Glomerular permeability in the premature infant; restricted filtration of inulin. Int J Paediatr Nephrol 2:125, 1981.
76. Sertal H, Scopes J: Rates of creatinine excretion in babies less than one week of age. Arch Dis Childh 48:717, 1973.
77. Coulthard MG, Ruddock V: Validation of inulin as a marker for glomerular filtration in preterm babies. Kidney Int 23:407, 1983.
78. Schwartz IL, Breed ES, Maxwell MH: Comparison of the volume of distribution, renal and extrarenal clearances of inulin and mannitol in man. J Clin Invest 29:517, 1950.
79. Ames RG: Urinary water excretion and neurohypophyseal function in fullterm and premature infants shortly after birth. Pediatrics. 12:272, 1953.
80. Smith HW, Goldring W, Chasis H: The measurement of the tubular excretory mass effective blood flow and filtration rate in the normal human kidney. J Clin Invest 17:263, 1938.
81. Davies HF, Schock NW: The variation of measurement of inulin and diodrast tests of kidney function. J Clin Invest 29:491, 1950.
82. Berger EY, Farber SJ, Earle DP: Comparison of the constant infusion and urine collection techniques for the measurement of renal function. J Clin Invest 27:710, 1948.
83. Cole BAR, Giangiacoma J, Ingelfinger JR, et al: Measurement of renal function without urine collection. Evaluation of the constant infusion technique for determination of inulin and PAH clearances. Pediatr Res 6:415, 1972.
84. Coulthard MG: Comparison of methods of measuring renal function in pre-term babies using insulin. J Pediatr 102:923, 1984.
85. Newman EV, Bordley J, Winternitz J: The interrelationships of glomerular filtration rate (mannitol clearance), extracellular fluid volume, surface area of the body and plasma concentration of mannitol. A definition of extracellular fluid clearance determined by following the plasma concentration after a single injection of mannitol. Bull Johns Hopk Hosp 75:253, 1944.
86. Dominguez R, Corcoran AC, Page IH: Mannitol: kinetics of distribution, excretion and utilization in human beings. J Lab Clin Med 32:1192, 1947.
87. Sapirstein LA, Viat DG, Mandel MJ, et al: Volume of distribution and clearances of intravenously injected creatinine in the dog. Am J Physiol 181:330, 1955.
88. Chantler C: The Measurement of GFR in Children Using ^{51}Cr-Edetic Acid. MD Thesis, University of Cambridge, 1973.
89. Maisey MN, Ogg CS, Cameron JS: Measuring glomerular filtration rate. Lancet 1:735, 1969.
90. Brochner-Mortensen J, Christoffersen J: Single injection ^{51}Cr-EDTA plasma clearance determination in children using capillary blood samples. Scand J Clin Lab Invest 37:631, 1977.
91. Elwood CM, Sigman EM: The measurement of glomerular filtration rate in man by iothalamate-I^{125} and iodopyracet I^{131}. Circulation 36:441, 1967.
92. Chantler C, Garnett ES, Parsons V, et al: Glomerular filtration rate in man by single injection method using ^{51}Cr-EDTA. Clin Sci 37:169, 1969.
93. Maher FT, Tauxe WN: Renal clearances in man of pharmaceuticals containing radioactive iodine. Influence of plasma binding. J Am Med Ass 207:97, 1969.
94. Bianchi C, Hegesippe E, Meozzi A, et al: The effect of autoradiolysis on renal clearances of I^{131}-labeled hypaque and hippuran. Minerva Nucleare 9:152, 1965.
95. Cohen ML, Smith FG, Mindell RS, et al: A simple reliable method of measuring glomerular filtration rate using single low dose sodium iothalamate. Pediatrics 43:407, 1969.
96. Moss A, Kauffman L, Nelson JA: Fluorescent excitation analysis. A new method of in vitro iodine determination. Invest Radiol 7:335, 1972.
97. Hilson AJW, Mistry RD, Maisey MN: ^{99m}Tc-DTPA for the measurement of glomerular filtration rate. Brit J Radiol 49:794, 1976.
98. Wolff AV: Total renal blood flow at any urine flow or extraction fraction. Am J Physiol 133:469, 1941.
99. Calcagno PL, Rubin MI: Renal extraction of paraaminohippurate in infants and children. J Clin Invest 42:1632, 1963.
100. Bradley SW, Bradley GP, Tyson CI, et al: Renal function in renal disease. Am J Med 9:766, 1950.
101. Gruskin AB, Auerbach VA, Black IFS: Intrarenal blood flow in children with normal kidneys and congenital heart disease. Changes attributable to angiography. Pediatr Res 8:561, 1974.
102. Tauxe WN, Burbank MKJ, Maher FT, et al: Renal clearances of radioactive orthoiodoohippurate and diatrozoate. Mayo Clin Proc 39:761, 1964.
103. Maher FT, Tauxe WN: Renal clearance in man of pharmaceuticals containing radio iodine; influence of protein binding. J Am Med Ass 207:97, 1969.
104. Farmer CF, Tauxe WN, Maher FT, et al: Measurement of renal function with radioiodinated diatrizoate and oiodohippurate. Am J Clin Path 47:9, 1967.
105. Blaufox MD, Merrill JP: Simplified hippuran clearance. Nephron 3:274, 1966.
106. Truniger B, Donath A, Kappeler M: Simplified clearance techniques. Helv Med Acta 34:116, 1968.
107. Cohen ML, Patel JK, Baxter DL: External monitoring and plasma disappearance for the determination of renal function, comparison of effective renal plasma flow and glomerular filtration rate. Pediatrics 48:377, 1971.
108. Brown NJG, Britton KE: The renogram and its quantitation. Brit J Urol 41(suppl 15), 1969.
109. Johnston JH, Irving IM: Experiences with radioisotopic renography in children. Arch Dis Childh 42:583, 1967.
110. Maisey MN, Ogg CS: Advances in the use of radionuclides in clinical nephrology. In Jones NF, Peters DK (eds): Recent Advances in Renal Medicine. London, Churchill-Livingstone, 1982.
111. Bingham JB, Maisey WN, Joyce MRI, et al: Use of ^{99m}-DMSA as a static renal imaging agent. Contrib Nephrol 11:95, 1978.
112. Berggard I: Plasma proteins in normal human urine. In Manuel Y, Revillard JP, Betuel H (eds): Proteins in Normal and Pathological Urine. Basel, Karger, 1970, p 7.
113. Bourillon R: Glycoproteins, glycopeptides and other carbohydrate complexes of normal human urine. In Manuel Y, Revillard JP, Betuel H (eds): Proteins in Normal and Pathological Urine. Basel, Karger, 1970, p 20.
114. Mondorf AW, Breier J, Mendus J, et al: The effect of aminoglycosides on proximal tubular membranes of human kidney. Europ J Clin Pharmacol 13:133, 1978.
115. Hardwicke J, Cameron JS, Harrison JF, et al Proteinuria studied by clearances of individual macromolecules. In Manuel Y, Revillard JP, Betuel H (eds): Proteins in Normal and Pathological Urine. Basel, Karger, 1970, p 111.
116. Heinemann HO, Maack TM, Sherman RL: Proteinuria: combined chemical and basic science seminar. Am J Med 56:71, 1974.
117. Barratt TM, McLaine PN, Soothill JF: Albumin excretion as a measure of glomerular dysfunction in children. Arch Dis Child 45:496, 1970.
118. Wagner MG, Smith FG, Tinglof BO, et al: Epidemiology of proteinuria. J Pediatr 73:825, 1968.
119. Vehaskari VM: Orthostatic proteinuria. Arch Dis Childh 57:729, 1982.
120. Hardwicke J, Cameron JS, Harrison JRF, et al: Proteinuria studied by clearances of individual macromolecules. In Manuel Y, Revillard JP, Betuel H (eds): Proteins in Normal and Pathological Urine. Basel, Karger, 1970.
121. Soothill JF: The estimation of eight serum proteins by gel diffusion precipitin technique. J Lab Clin Med 59:859, 1962.
122. Blainey JF, Brewer DB, Hardwicke J, et al: The nephrotic syndrome. Diagnosis by renal biopsy and biochemical and immunological analysis related to the response to steroid therapy. Quart J Med 29:235, 1960.
123. Cameron JS, Blandford G: The simple assessment of permeability in heavy proteinuria. Lancet 2:242, 1966.
124. Barratt TM, Macaulay D: Renal disease in childhood. In Black DAK (ed): Renal Disease, ed 3. Oxford, Blackwell Scientific Publications, 1972, p 805.
125. Butler EA, Flynn FV: The proteinuria of renal tubular disorders. Lancet 2:978, 1958.
126. Harrison JF, Blainey JD: Low molecular weight proteinuria in chronic renal disease. Clin Sci 33:381, 1967.
127. Harrison JF, Lunt GS, Scott P, et al: Urinary lysozyme ribonuclease and low molecular weight protein in renal disease. Lancet 1:371, 1968.
128. Barratt TM, Crawford R: Lysozyme excretion as a measure of renal tubular dysfunction in children. Clin Sci 39:457, 1970.
129. Carone FA, Peterson DR, Oparil S, et al: Renal tubular transport and catabolism of proteins and peptides. Kidney Int 16:271, 1979.
130. Revillard JP, Wibell L, Hall PW: Beta$_2$-microglobulin. In Renal Diseases. Uppsala, Sweden, Phadedoc Diagnostic Communications, Pharmacia Diagnostics A B, 1979.
131. Wibell L: Studies on beta$_2$-microglobulin in patients and normal subjects. Acta Clin Belg 31(suppl 8):14, 1976.
132. van Oort A, Monnens L, van Munster P: Beta$_2$-microglobulin in renal disorders with special reference to the hepatorenal syndrome. Nephron 27:62, 1981.
133. Hall PW, Ricaneli ES: Renal handling of beta$_2$-microglobulin in renal disorders with special reference to the hepatorenal syndrome. Nephron 27:62, 1981.
134. Donaldson M, Haycock G, Chantler C: Urinary beta$_2$-microglobulin in children with renal disease. (Submitted for publication).
135. Danovitch GM, Bricker: Influence of volume expansion on NaCl reabsorption in the diluting segments of the nephron; a study using clearance methods. Kidney Int 10:229, 1976.
136. Rodriquez-Soriano J, Vallo A, Castillo G, et al: Renal handling of water and sodium in infancy and childhood. A study using clearance methods during hypotonic saline diuresis. Kidney Int 20:700, 1981.
137. Haycock GB, Al-Dahhan J, Mak RHK, et al: Effect of indomethacin on clinical progress and renal function in cystinosis. Arch Dis Childh 57:934, 1982.
138. Smith HW: The Kidney: Structure and Function in Health and Disease. New York, Oxford University Press, 1951.
139. Arant BS: Developmental patterns of renal functional maturation compared in the human neonate. J Pediatr 92:705, 1978.
140. Brodehl J: Renal glucosuria. In Edelman CM (ed): Pediatric Kidney Disease. Boston, Little, Brown & Co, 1978, p 1036.

141. Scriver CR: Amino acid transport in the mammalian kidney. In Nyhan WL (ed): Amino Acid Metabolism and Genetic Variation. New York, McGraw Hill, 1967, p 327.
142. Young JA, Freedman BS: Renal tubular transport for amino acids. Clin Chem 17:245, 1971.
143. Childs B: Urinary excretion of free alpha amino acid nitrogen by normal infants and children. Proc Soc Exp Biol Med 81:225, 1952.
144. Saifer A: Rapid screening methods for the detection of inherited and acquired amino acidopathies. Adv Clin Chem 14:145, 1971.
145. Woolf LI, Norman AP: The urinary excretion of amino acids and sugars in early infancy. J Pediatr 50:271, 1957.
146. Cusworth DC, Dent CE: Renal clearances of endogenous amino acids in normal adults and in patients with amino aciduria. Biochem J 74:550, 1960.
147. O'Brien D, Butterfield LJ: Further studies on renal tubular conservation of free amino acids in early infancy. Arch Dis Childh 38:437, 1963.
148. Scriver CR, Davies E: Endogenous renal clearance rates of free amino acids in prepubertal children. Pediatrics 36:592, 1965.
149. Brodehl J, Gellissen K: Endogenous renal transport of free amino acids in infancy and childhood. Pediatrics 42:395, 1968.
150. Edelman CM, Boichis H, Rodriguez-Soriano J, et al: The renal response of children to acute ammonium chloride acidosis. Pediatr Res 1:452, 1967.
151. Pitts RF, Ayer JL, Schiess WA: The renal regulation of acid base balance in man. III. The reabsorption and excretion of bicarbonate. J Clin Invest 28:35, 1949.
152. Pukerson M, Lubowitz H, White RW, et al: On the influence of extracellular fluid volume expansion on bicarbonate reabsorption in the rat. J Clin Invest 48:1754, 1967.
153. Rodriguez-Soriano J, Edelmann CM: Renal tubular acidosis. Ann Rev Med 20:363, 1969.
154. Rodriguez-Soriano J, Boichis H, Edelmann CM: Bicarbonate reabsorption and hydrogen ion excretion in children with renal tubular acidosis. J Pediatr 71:802, 1967.
155. Wrong O, Davies HEF: The excretion of acid in renal disease. Quart J Med 28:249, 1959.
156. Halperin ML: Pathogenesis of type 1 (distal) renal tubular acidosis: reevaluation of diagnostic criteria. Ann Roy Coll Phys Surg Can 7:103, 1975.
157. Kennedy TJ, Orloff J, Berliner RW: Significance of carbon dioxide tension in urine. Am J Physiol 169:596, 1952.
158. Donckerwolcke RA, Valk C, Van Wijngaarden-Pentermann, et al: The diagnostic value of urine to blood carbon dioxide tension gradient for the assessment of distal tubular hydrogen secretion in paediatric patients with renal tubular disorders. Clin Nephrol 1983. (In Press.)
159. Edelmann CM, Barnett HL, Troupkou V: A standardized test of renal concentrating capacity in infants and children. Am J Dis Child 114:639, 1967.
160. Edelmann CM, Barnett HL, Troupkou V: Renal concentrating mechanisms in newborn infants. Effect of dietary protein and water content, role of urea and responsiveness to antidiuretic hormone. J Clin Invest 39:1062, 1960.
161. Edelmann CM, Barnett HL, Stark H: Effect of urea on concentration of urinary non-urea solute in premature infants. J Appl Physiol 21:1021, 1966.
162. Aronson AS, Svenningsen NW: dDAVP test for estimation of renal concentrating capacity in infants and children. Arch Dis Childh 49:654, 1974.

CHAPTER 20

Imaging the Urinary Tract

ISKY GORDON

INTRODUCTION

The urinary system is not readily accessible to clinical examination, and therefore emphasis has always been placed on tests of renal function and imaging methods to provide the necessary information. Until recently the intravenous urogram (IVU) was the principal source of information about the upper urinary tract while the micturating cystourethrogram (MCU) provided images of the lower urinary tract. Technical advances have altered this, and a reappraisal of all imaging methods is in progress. With the assembly of other imaging modalities, the number of IVU required has decreased significantly, yet in the complex case it may be the IVU that allows the overall perspective of the case to be maintained.

Abdominal ultrasound provides anatomical information without exposure to ionizing radiation, is noninvasive, and is frequently the most appropriate initial examination. Radioisotopes offer the opportunity of studying renal pathophysiology with low radiation doses and only minimal trauma. Computed tomography (CT) scanning has only a limited role in the provision of anatomical information of the urinary tract in children. Aortography with selective renal arteriography provides great detail but is invasive and, therefore, has limited indications.

In building up the overall clinical picture, the integration of the clinical and laboratory data with the imaging results is essential. The IVU, ultrasound, and radioisotope scan depend on different phenomena and, therefore, provide different information about the kidneys and urinary tract (Table 20.1). For this reason, the clinician must be very explicit about the questions asked so that the appropriate examination can be undertaken. Communication between radiologist and clinician assumes ever greater importance.

IMAGING TECHNIQUES

Radiography
Plain Film and IVU

The plain abdominal radiograph is essential before every IVU; small calculi may be overlooked on ultrasound and also after intravenous (IV) contrast. The spine warrants careful examination and, with renal failure, the femoral epiphyses may slip or renal osteodystrophy may become apparent.

Physiology. The IV contrast medium used may be either a high osmolar solution, e.g., diatrizoate (Hypaque or Renograffin) or iothalamate (Conray), or one of the newer low osmolar contrast media; both are <3% plasma-bound (1) and their renal clearance approximates that of inulin (2, 3). There is no tubular handling of the contrast medium and with good renal function there is negligible extrarenal clearance (4). The nephrogram is, therefore, dependent on glomerular filtration. However, once the contrast is in the tubules, the density of the nephrogram depends on fluid reabsorption. A high urine flow rate results in rapid washing out of the contrast from the renal pelvis, whereas dehydration results in a reduced urine flow rate and tends to intensify the nephrogram. On the other hand, contrast medium constitutes an osmotic load which decreases water reabsorption from the tubules and so counterbalances the dehydration effect.

Contrast. New contrast materials have been developed that are nonionic and, therefore, are less active osmotically. They have many advantages, especially in the ill child or in renal failure, since the high osmolality of conventional contrast media affects capillary endothelium, vasomotor tone, and the circulatory blood volume (5). Conventional contrast media are ionic monomeric triiodinated derivatives of benzoic acid prepared as the sodium or methylglucamine salt or a mixture of both. In solution, this contrast ionizes into two particles, the cation, which is ineffective as a contrast, and an iodinated benzoate anion. The osmolality is proportional to the number of particles in solution; with monomeric media the iodine:particle ratio is 3:2. The new low osmolar contrast media have an iodine:particle ratio of 3:1. In theory, use of the low osmolar contrast should halve the osmotic load yet in practice the reduction is even greater, to about one-third, because of aggregation of molecules in solution. Current clinical studies show a reduction in side effects using the new low-osmolar contrast in adults (6). The viscosity of the new contrast agents, if warmed to body temperature, are generally lower or the same as conventional contrast (7). The advantages of these new contrast agents, iohexol (Omnipaque), iopamidol (Niopam), ioxaglate (Hexabrix), lie in the reduction of side effects, and the strong impression that still requires proof of an improved safety factor (8). They all are more expensive than the conventional contrast agents.

Technique. Fluid and food should be withheld for approximately 2 to 3 hours before the investigation. Excessive dehydration causes an unhappy uncooperative child and, in the presence of chronic renal failure (CRF), may be harmful. A small enema may be useful (9). The contrast must always be given intravenously; intramuscular or subcutaneous injection must be avoided. The usual dose is 2 ml/kg body weight using media with low iodine concentration, e.g., Hypaque 45% or Conray

Table 20.1.
Imaging the Kidney[a]

	Small kidney	Ectopic kidney	Focal scar	Obstruction	Vascular pathology
IVU	+	+	±	+	−
US	+	−	−	+	−
DMSA	++	++	++	−	++
DTPA	+	+	±	++	+

[a] +, High detection rate; −, Low detection rate.

280; the maximum dose suggested is 3 ml/kg. Either the sodium or methylglucamine salt can be used.

Within a minute of the injection children are given a fizzy drink, and babies and toddlers are given a bottle to suck. If adequate visualization is not obtained with the first radiograph at 4 to 5 minutes, then a renal window view at 7 to 10 minutes is useful (10). In this view, the x-ray tube is angled 35° toward the feet and is centered on the xiphoid sternum (Fig. 20.1). Following these two radiographs of the renal areas, a full length film between 15 to 20 minutes should include the base of the bladder and the kidneys.

Unless an abnormality has been detected, the examination is terminated at this stage in children <4 years of age; if the child will micturate, a coned postmicturition view of the bladder is a useful adjunct. When dilatation of the collecting system has been revealed, the exact level of the obstruction must be discovered and may require delayed images for up to 18 hours. Poor visualization of the kidney in the neonatal period also warrants delayed radiographs. Tomography is now less frequently used since children with poor renal function are no longer examined in the first instance by IVU; an isotope examination and ultrasound are carried out instead.

If the IVU is not the first examination carried out, but follows on the abdominal ultrasound and radioisotope scan, then the examination can be tailored to the specific clinical problems that the individual child presents. This results in fewer radiographs and a lower radiation dose.

Indications. The IVU remains the best investigation if detailed anatomy of the renal parenchyma or pelvicalyceal system is required. It also provides a good basis for assessing renal growth. The size of normal kidneys on IVU has been established by Hodson et al (11), who related renal length to the patient's age and weight, and by Eklof and Ringertz (12), who established normal values in relation to vertebral length.

Following acute renal failure in the first 3 months of life, an IVU carried out at follow-up may aid in distinguishing between medullary necrosis and renal vein thrombosis. A normal ^{99m}Tc-DMSA scan may be seen following medullary necrosis, but the IVU, in spite of showing normal-sized kidneys, reveals the loss of the calyceal fornix and the pooling of contrast in the parenchyma which establishes the diagnosis (Fig. 20.2). When the problem is a duplex kidney the IVU is the examination of choice, but may need to be followed by other imaging (Fig. 20.3). An IVU is helpful when a small kidney is discovered by other techniques (Table 20.2).

There are some contraindications to an IVU. The kidneys may not be adequately visualized within 48 hours of birth despite normal renal function; for this reason, an emergency IVU at this age is contraindicated (13). The osmotic load of relatively large doses of contrast material in a neonate may aggravate dehydration and renal failure and may also be a contributory factor in the pathogenesis of renal venous thrombosis or medullary necrosis. Children with severe defects of urinary concentration, such as nephrogenic diabetes insipidus, are particularly vulnerable to the dehydrating effect of the osmotic load of contrast. Other contraindications to an IVU include a past history of allergy, especially to contrast medium, and the presence of severe hypertension. Urgent or emergency IVUs are rarely required, for the ability of the ultrasound to demonstrate the renal anatomy allows the IVU to be undertaken under calmer conditions. Acute obstructive uropathy, however, still requires an emergency IVU following the ultrasound examination.

Micturating Cystourethrogram

The MCU is the definitive method of assessing the lower urinary tract, but also may reveal upper tract detail if vesicoureteric reflux (VUR) is present.

Technique. An x-ray table with an overhead tube allows free mobility of the radiologist, nurse, and parent so that the child does not feel caught between the large mobile overhead image intensifier and the table top and maximum cooperation is obtained. Contrast is introduced via a catheter, either a 6- or 8-French gauge. The contrast used is generally 20% strength. The bladder either may be filled via gravity, using an inverted contrast bottle at a fixed height above the table top, or injected slowly with a 50 ml syringe; the small catheter size prevents too rapid filling of the bladder (14). Sedation rarely is necessary, and a parent should always accompany the child. An MCU under general anesthesia may not provide satisfactory information about VUR during micturition, and should be avoided if possible. In all boys, the urethra must be demonstrated; this is best done in the oblique projection. The bladder must be visualized when full, during and after micturition. Oblique views to show the vesicoureteric junction during micturition are important.

Indications. An MCU is indicated with a urinary tract infection (UTI) in all children <5 years of age; when there is ureteric dilatation, as VUR may be the cause; when a small kidney is discovered; with hematuria accompanied by lower urinary tract symptomatology; and with renal failure of undetermined cause (Fig. 20.4). Radioisotope cystograms can be carried out in all followup studies and may be useful as a screening procedure for the child with a UTI.

Antegrade Pyelogram

This investigation should be carried out only by an experienced operator. It is done either in theater immediately prior to surgery or may be the basis for urodynamic studies, a procedure that requires considerable expertise. The purpose is to determine the level of obstruction in the collecting system when this is not apparent from less invasive procedures. It may be combined with pressure flow measurements to determine the physiological significance of an apparently obstructive abnormality (Fig. 20.5) (15).

Retrograde Pyelogram

This examination has a limited role in pediatric urology. The major indication is when there is poor visualization of the collecting systems on IVU with the patient in renal failure, in whom the ultrasound fails to show significant ureteric dilatation, the MCU does not show reflux, and the isotope studies fail to reveal the cause of the renal failure. Occasionally, when the anatomy is uncertain despite numerous other imaging modalities, a retrograde is helpful.

Cutaneous Diversion Studies

When a diversionary procedure has been undertaken, contrast studies may be carried out by catheterization of the stoma. Nephrostograms, ureterostograms, and loopograms are the most common procedures. These examinations are done in the postoperative period to demonstrate adequate urinary drainage by the diversion, or to delineate anatomical detail of the urinary tract.

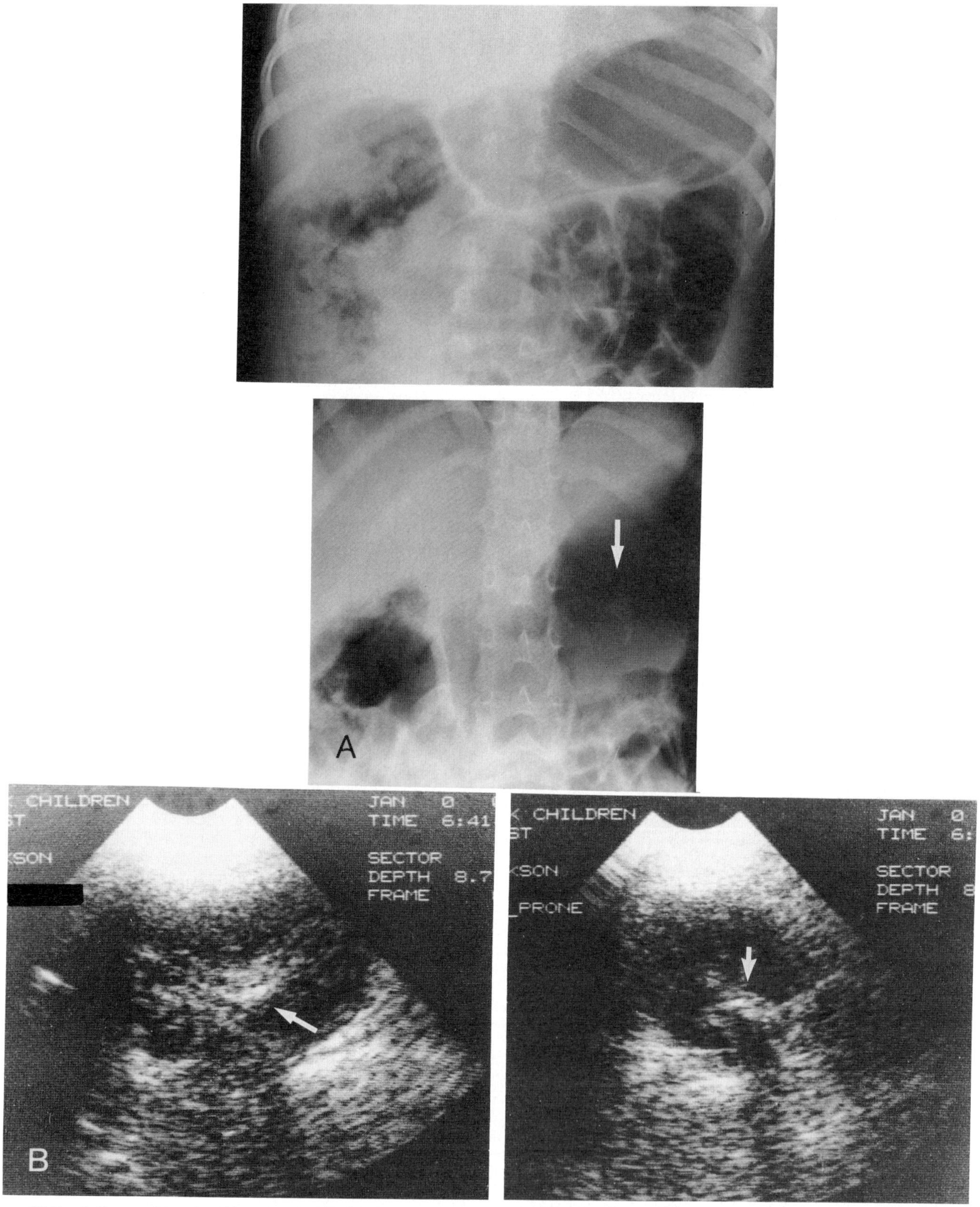

Figure 20.1. A 6-year-old male with recurrent UTI and left loin pain. **A,** This shows the radiograph of the renal areas that are normal (*top*); the bottom image is the "renal window view" showing the left renal calculus. **B,** This is the ultrasound examination. The longitudinal prone view on the *left* shows the echo-dense area with a weak acoustic shadow, which is also seen on the transverse scan (*arrows*).

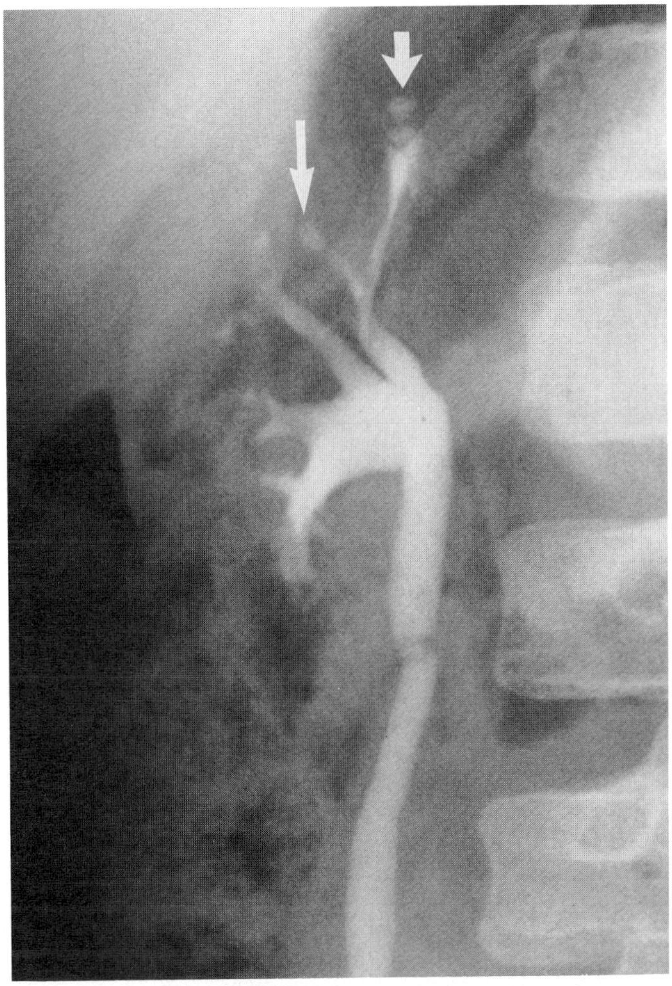

Figure 20.2. This 7-year-old male had suffered severe diarrhea and vomiting in the neonatal period following which he went into acute renal failure. His recovery was rapid but he was later noted to have polyuria. The IVU shows pooling of contrast in the renal parenchyme outside the calyceal fornix. All the calyces are abnormal and "cut off." These are the features of medullary necrosis.

Arteriography

This invasive investigation, with its high radiation dose, should be reserved for special clinical situations. When used judiciously, it is an invaluable asset, with the ability to demonstrate detailed anatomy but potential complications must be borne in mind (16, 17).

Technique. Arteriography should be carried out only by a skilled operator with pediatric experience, using the smallest catheter compatible with obtaining adequate results. Selective renal arteriography with magnification is important. Small doses of intraarterial contrast should be used; this may be further aided by using digital vascular imaging (DVI). Cut films with a rapid changer are essential, and cineradiography is inadequate.

Indications. The investigation of hypertension is a major indication for arteriography (chapter 47). Analysis of a renal mass in an anomalous kidney which is solid on ultrasound, or bilateral masses, may require arteriography to assess the feasibility of surgery, e.g., partial nephrectomy. Nevertheless, a biopsy is essential, since the histology of a renal mass cannot be predicted with confidence from the arteriographic appearances (18). Trauma complicated by persistent hematuria or hypertension, may necessitate arteriography preoperatively. The ability of the arteriogram to display the detailed anatomy of the arterial tree is helpful in the diagnosis of polyarteritis; there are characteristic appearances of both the macroscopic and microscopic forms of this disease. The splanchnic vessels, including the hepatic arteries, must also be visualized (Fig. 20.3, *B*). Arteriography is necessary before interventional procedures, e.g., embolization for A-V malformations or arterial dilatation for stenosis (Fig. 20.6).

CT Scanning

CT scanning provides excellent anatomical details and the equipment is now more readily available, but since patient cooperation is required, sedation or anaesthesia is frequently used.

Indications. Mass lesions especially in the pelvis and also in the suprarenal area remain the major indication. Ultrasound is highly accurate in the diagnosis of obstructive uropathy, renal mass lesions, and for small kidneys. Although CT scanning has been advocated in the infantile polycystic kidney by certain authors, the value of ultrasound cannot be too highly recommended in cystic disease of the kidney. This examination has no place in hypertension or suspected arterial lesions. The role of CT in trauma is not controversial with certain centres being impressed with its value.

Bone Radiography

In patients with CRF there is a need to monitor the development of renal osteodystrophy. High quality radiographs are required, necessitating the use of a fine focus x-ray tube, magnification, and a combination of a high quality x-ray film with an appropriate screen. We use a 0.03 mm focal spot with magnification X2 and an appropriate x-ray film/screen (Fig. 20.4).

Ultrasound

Ultrasound provides a noninvasive examination which should now be available in all units responsible for the care of children with kidney disease (19–22). It does not involve the use of ionizing radiation. The examination is independent of function, but provides anatomical detail of the retroperitoneal and intraabdominal structures.

There are three types of basic ultrasound equipment. Real-time ultrasound is gaining popularity in pediatrics because of the ease of use and accuracy. It permits visualization of movement of an organ, e.g., cardiac or bowel motion. A problem arises in the neonate when prone renal ultrasound is necessary; this can be overcome with the use of a "water bath." Linear array ultrasound equipment is popular among obstetricians but the disadvantage for children is the physical size of the transducer. This equipment also provides dynamic images, but the quality of the image in infants is not as good as that obtainable with real-time equipment. Static grey-scale ultrasound still provides the best anatomical detail because of the high quality resolution, but its static nature may not allow adequate distinction between a mass and bowel containing feces. Computers have been linked to the real-time ultrasound equipment in an attempt to quantify renal volume and make accurate measurement of anatomical detail.

The ability to delineate normal and abnormal anatomy is directly related to the skill of the ultrasonographer, who must be experienced in examining children and fully conversant with the spectrum of disease in childhood. The cooperation of the child is necessary; therefore, a quiet environment geared to children, and a skilled operator, are essential for good results. The major drawbacks of ultrasound are the problems presented by the unskilled operator and the difficulty in making accurate comparisons of small changes on sequential abdominal ultrasound examinations.

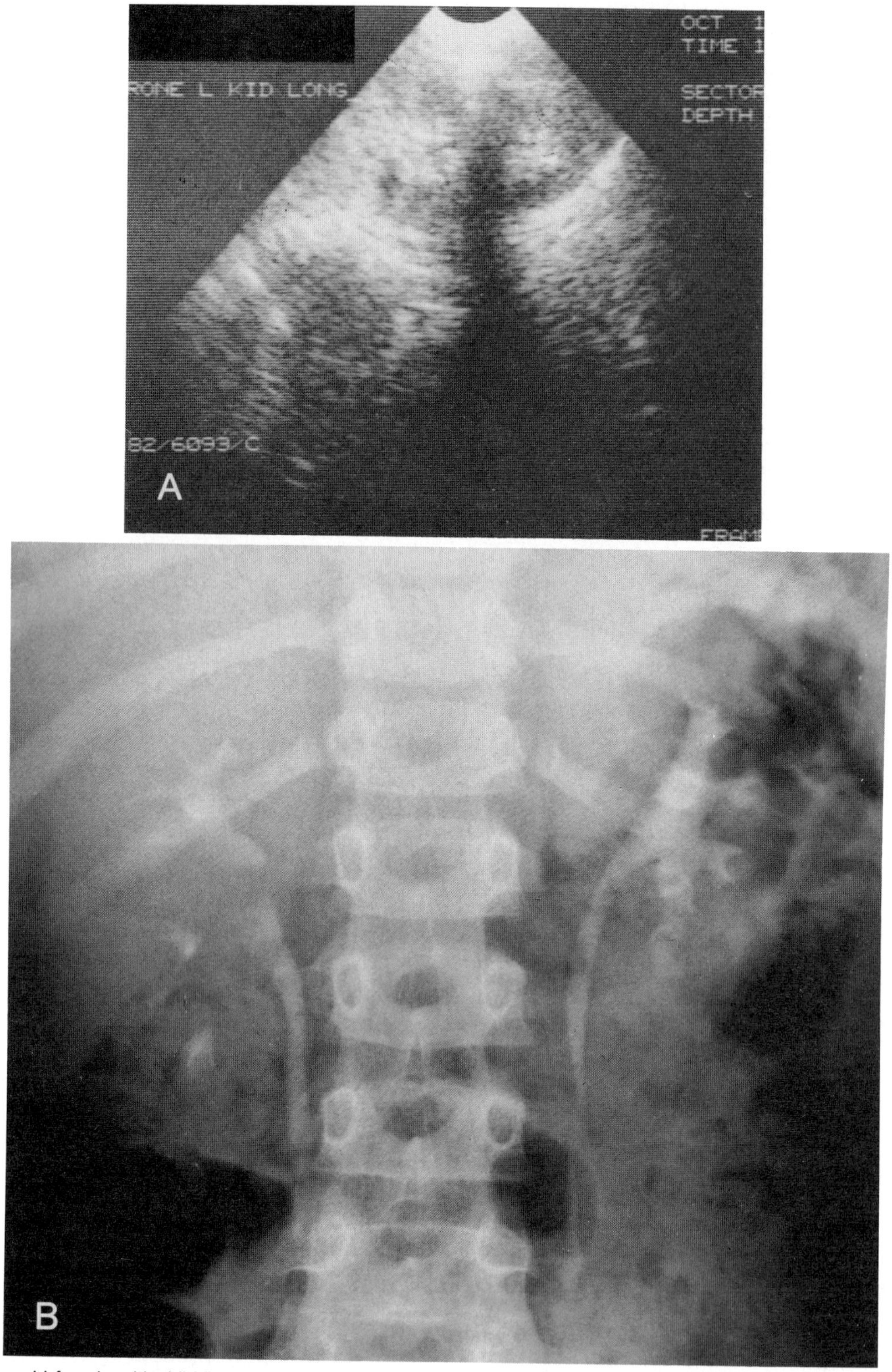

Figure 20.3. A 4-year-old female with dribbling incontinence. **A,** The ultrasound examination was not helpful, showing a normal left kidney. The ^{99m}Tc-DMSA scan showed two normally shaped kidneys but the left kidney contributed less than 45% of overall function, suggesting pathology. **B,** This shows a normal right kidney. The left kidney has an abnormal axis with the uppermost calyces lying lateral to the lower calyces and the left renal pelvis displaced laterally. At surgery the upper pole of the left duplex kidney was found draining into the vagina.

It would be ideal if pediatricians had their own mobile ultrasound units, so that examination of the kidneys would represent an extension of the physical examination, in much the same way that the stethoscope permits auscultation of the cardiac cycle. Present circumstances fall short of this, but an ultrasound should be the first examination before a renal isotope scan or IVU if the kidneys need to be visualized.

If an abdominal mass is present, the ultrasound can define its origin and nature, and determine whether it is renal or nonrenal, cystic or solid.

Table 20.2.
The Small Kidney on IVU

	Outline		Calyces				Parenchymal loss		Ureter	
	Smooth	Irregular	Normal	Blunt	Clubbed	Spidery	Global	Focal	Normal	Dilated
Dysplasia		+			+		+	+		+
Reflux		+		+			+	+	+	+
Renal venous thrombosis		+		+			+	+	+	
Medullary necrosis	+			+			+		+	
Postobstructive changes	+				+		+			+
Main renal artery stenosis	+					+	+		+	
Intrarenal arteriopathy		+	+		+			+	+	

If the mass is solid, then the possibility that it may be malignant should be considered and its spread sought with the ultrasound, including examination of the liver and inferior vena cava. Calculi cause acoustic shadows and thus have a characteristic appearance, but must be differentiated from rib shadows (Fig. 20.1 and 7). The kidney in the neonate differs from that of the older child, since there is a clear distinction between the renal cortex and medulla. This may be so marked that to the unskilled observer the medulla appears transonic, suggesting the diagnosis of multiple cysts (Fig. 20.8). The dilated ureter containing urine may be detected readily, especially in the pelvis when the bladder is full (Fig. 20.9). This is an important part of a full ultrasound examination, which may also provide valuable information on the thickness of the bladder wall, and on the completeness of a bladder emptying with micturition.

Radioisotopes

Renal pathophysiology can be assessed either by dynamic scans (23), using ^{99m}Tc-diaminotetraethylpentacetic acid (DTPA) or ^{123}I-hippuran, or by static scans using ^{99m}Tc-dimercaptosuccinic acid (DMSA) (24). Uptake and excretion of the isotope is detected by a gamma camera; probe renogram systems are now obsolete in pediatrics.

Dynamic Scan

Physiology. The parameters that can be measured are the rate of uptake of the isotope by the kidney from the blood (uptake phase), the time taken for the isotope to pass through the kidney into the renal pelvis and ureter (transit time), and the rate at which the isotope leaves the kidney (excretory phase). The isotope is not completely cleared by the kidney from the blood immediately after injection so that uptake by the kidney continues for the duration of the examination at a rate proportional to the plasma concentration and GFR (using DTPA). During the first 3 minutes after injection of the isotope the excretion has yet to begin, so that the uptake phase can be analyzed independently. After this time, there is a more complex situation with the isotope leaving the renal parenchyma and entering the renal pelvis and ureter simultaneously with continued uptake.

The extraction of ^{99m}Tc-DTPA by glomerular filtration during each passage of blood through the kidney is about 20%. ^{123}I-hippuran is actively excreted by the proximal tubules as well as being filtered by the glomerulus; the extraction factor is >80% during each passage through the kidney. The high extraction is an advantage, but the cost of ^{123}I and its limited availability are reasons why its use is mainly confined to patients with severe renal failure, where visualization with DTPA is poor.

With ^{99m}Tc-DTPA, analysis of the kidney region during the uptake phase enables differential renal function to be assessed (25). If the procedure is coupled with a blood sample at 20 minutes then individual kidney GFR (IKGFR) estimation is possible (26). Analysis of the renal parenchymal area separate from the renal pelvis allows both whole kidney transit time and renal parenchymal transit time to be calculated. This may be useful in patients suspected of having urinary obstruction but is still being evaluated. The technique of parenchymal transit time analysis is difficult and prone to error in children, due to the small size of the kidneys. Analysis of the excretory phase provides information about possible urinary obstruction.

In the presence of suspected obstruction of the renal pelvis or ureter, furosemide can be used to assess drainage by inducing a diuresis. Furosemide was first used in cases of possible pelviureteric junction (PUJ) obstruction to distinguish an obstructed dilated renal pelvis from a nonobstructed one; however, it is now widely used whenever there is dilatation of the collecting system (Fig. 20.5) (27). Caution must be exercised in interpreting the response of a urinary system to furosemide if there is poor renal function or gross dilatation of the collecting system. The diuretic excretion index of obstruction, using DTPA, is not applicable to children (28, 29). If furosemide is not used, voiding views 60 minutes after the injection of DTPA may be used to demonstrate VUR, this being the indirect radioisotope cystogram (Fig. 20.10).

A complete ^{99m}Tc-DTPA scan, therefore, provides images of the functioning renal parenchyma, renal pelves, and bladder. Normally, the ureters are not visualized. Analysis of the data provides differential renal function and IKGFR, transit time data, and either the response to furosemide or an assessment of VUR.

Indications. A DTPA scan is indicated if there is suspected unilateral renal disease or obstruction, especially prior to surgery. Sequential scans with an abdominal ultrasound examination are the most satisfactory way of monitoring long-term individual renal function and structure. When VUR is being followed up, voiding views are essential.

Static Scan

Physiology. Dimercaptosuccinic acid (DMSA) is loosely bound to proteins in the plasma and is handled by the kidney like chlormeridrin. It attaches to the proximal convoluted tubules and is incorporated into them by binding to sulfhydryl groups. Only 10% is excreted in the urine. The images thus obtained reflect renal cortical mass. The scan should be done 2 hours or more after the IV injection. Posterior and both oblique projections should be obtained routinely. Anterior views, including the bladder, are essential when only one kidney appears to be present.

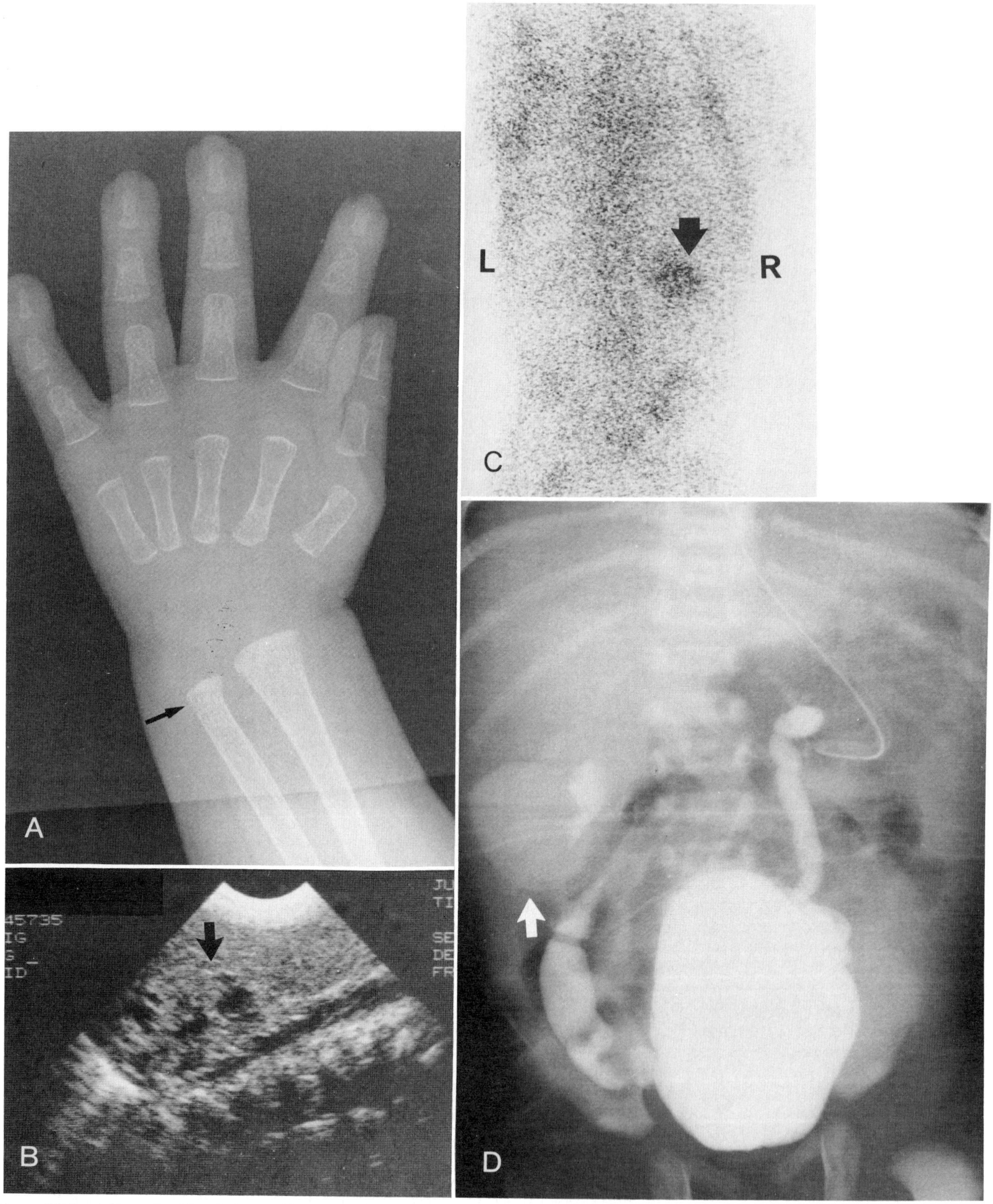

Figure 20.4. A 3-month-old male born with an imperforate anus was referred with an elevated serum creatinine. The magnified radiograph of the hand, **A,** reveals a coarse trabecular pattern; subperiosteal bone resorption (*arrow*) is noted, confirming the renal osteodystrophy of chronic renal failure. The ultrasound examination, **B,** right longitudinal, showed a very bright echonephrogram in a generally small kidney. The ^{99m}Tc-DMSA scan, **C,** shows a high background activity at 6 hours with the isotope accumulating in the bone marrow. A small nubbin of renal tissue is seen on the right (*arrow*). **D,** This is the MCU where bilateral VUR is noted with a very small left kidney. Note the colostomy over the right kidney (*arrow*).

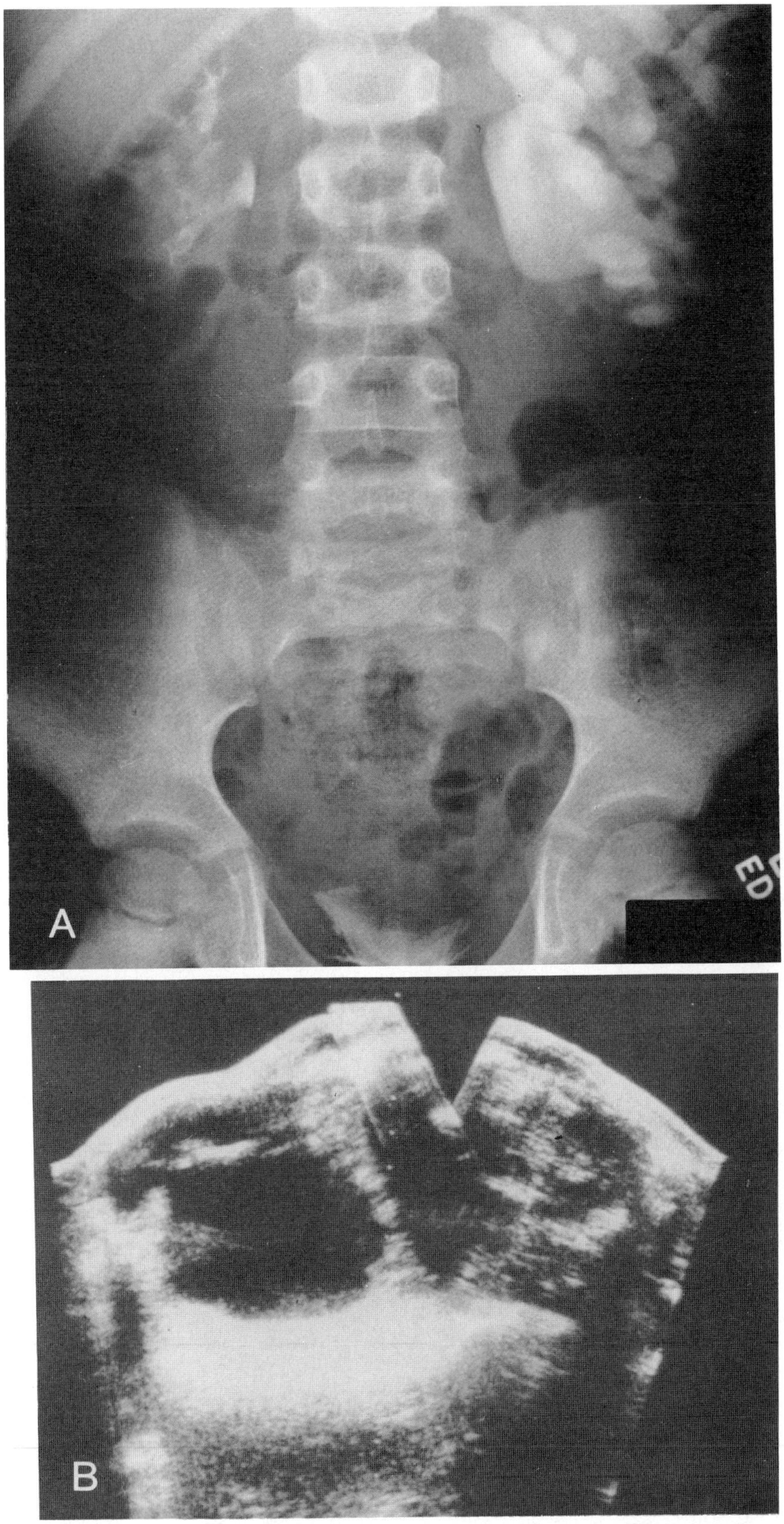

Figure 20.5. A 12-year-old male presented with intermittent left loin pain. The IVU, **A,** shows evidence of a full left renal pelvis and calyces after micturition. The abdominal ultrasound, **B,** confirmed the left hydronephrosis. **C,** A ^{99m}Tc-DTPA scan preoperatively failed to show drainage of isotope from the renal pelvis. **D** and **E,** Two years after surgery, after new attacks of loin pain, the repeat ^{99m}Tc-DTPA scan again showed evidence of poor drainage after furosemide. **F,** An antegrade pyelogram confirmed the presence of a recovery PUJ obstruction.

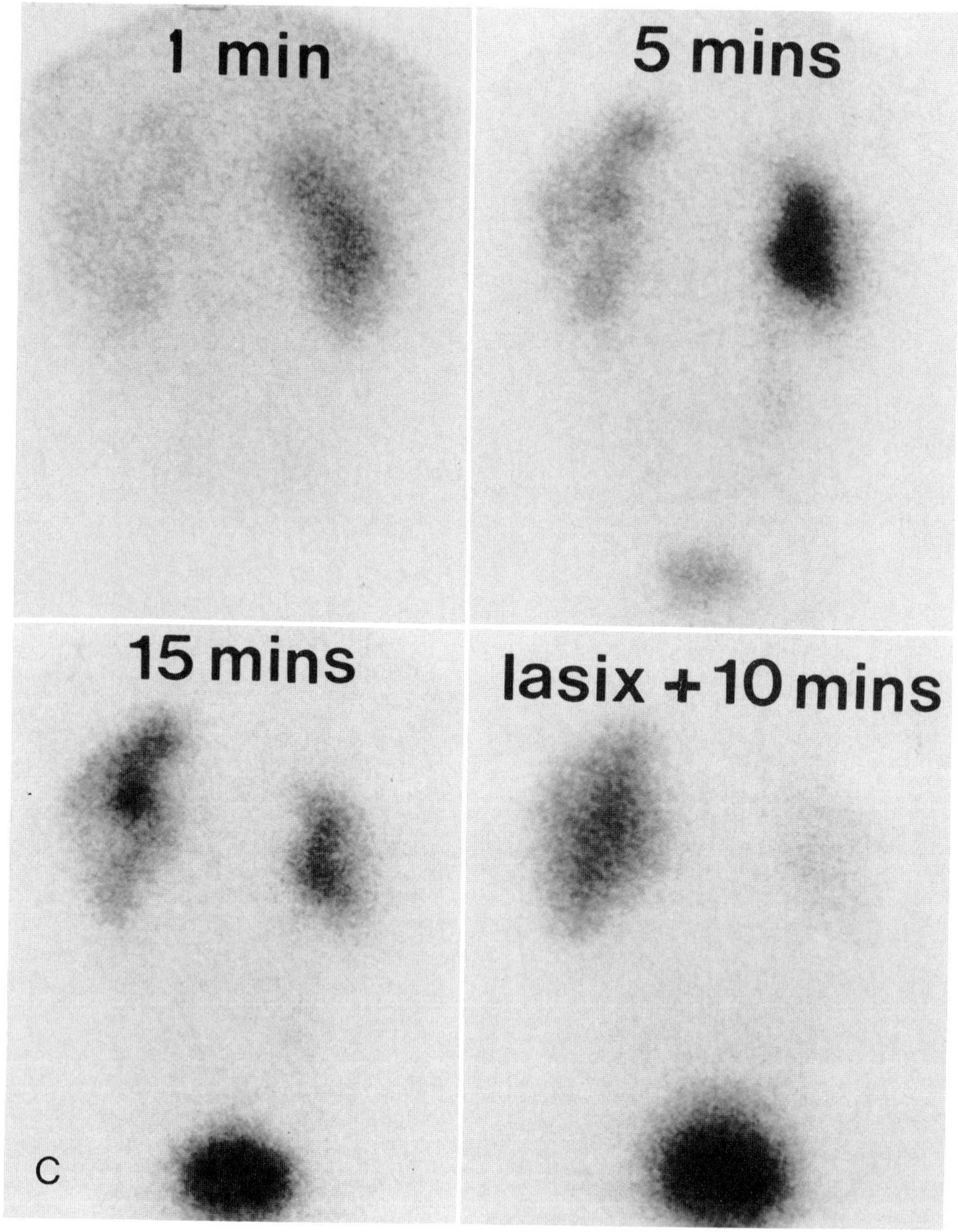

Figure 20.5 C

Absolute quantitation of the kidneys 6 hours after injection has been described, but the full potential of this technique is being assessed.

Indications. A DMSA scan is indicated when only one kidney has been identified and doubt exists about the presence of a second kidney (23). In the presence of an ectopic kidney this may be the examination of choice (Fig. 20.11). It can be used to assess differential function, particularly to establish whether a kidney is worth conserving, or whether nephrectomy is appropriate. Caution must be exercised in the presence of obstruction, since recoverability cannot be assessed. With more equal renal function, a dynamic DTPA scan with IKGFR determination is the more accurate method. In children with hypertension, segmental areas of poor function due to ischemia, which may be the cause of renin-dependent hypertension, can be detected by diminished DMSA uptake (Fig. 20.12). With VUR, the DMSA scan is the most sensitive technique for the detection of renal scarring (Fig. 20.13) (30).

A normal DMSA scan (including both posterior oblique projections) effectively excludes significant focal renal parenchymal pathology (31). With VUR it excludes scars, with hypertension it excludes most renovascular causes with the notable exception of main renal artery stenosis. In children suffering from polyartcritis and other vasculitides, the DMSA scan has proved a sensitive indicator of renal parenchyman areas of hypoperfusion consequent upon small artery disease (Fig. 20.14).

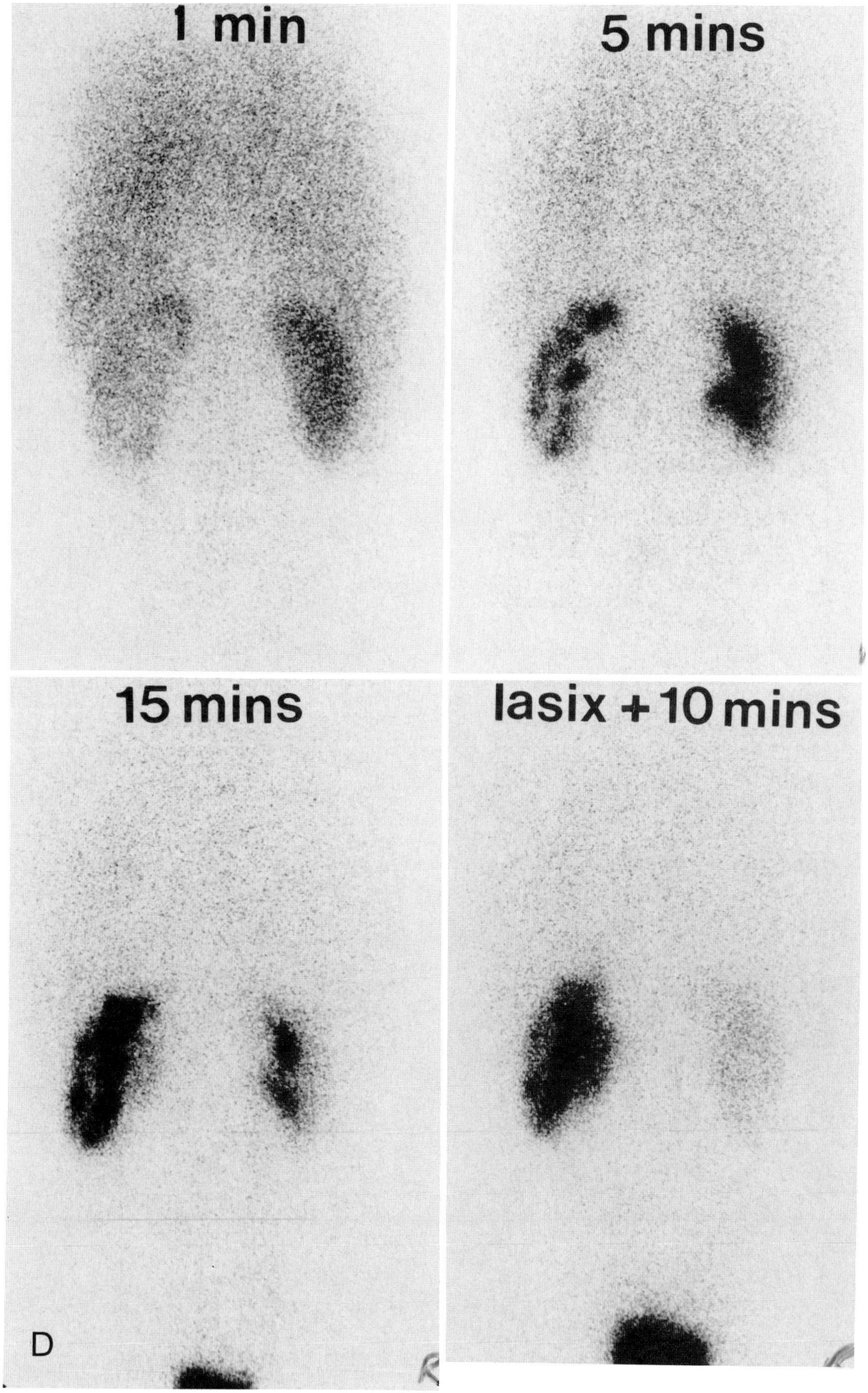

Figure 20.5 D

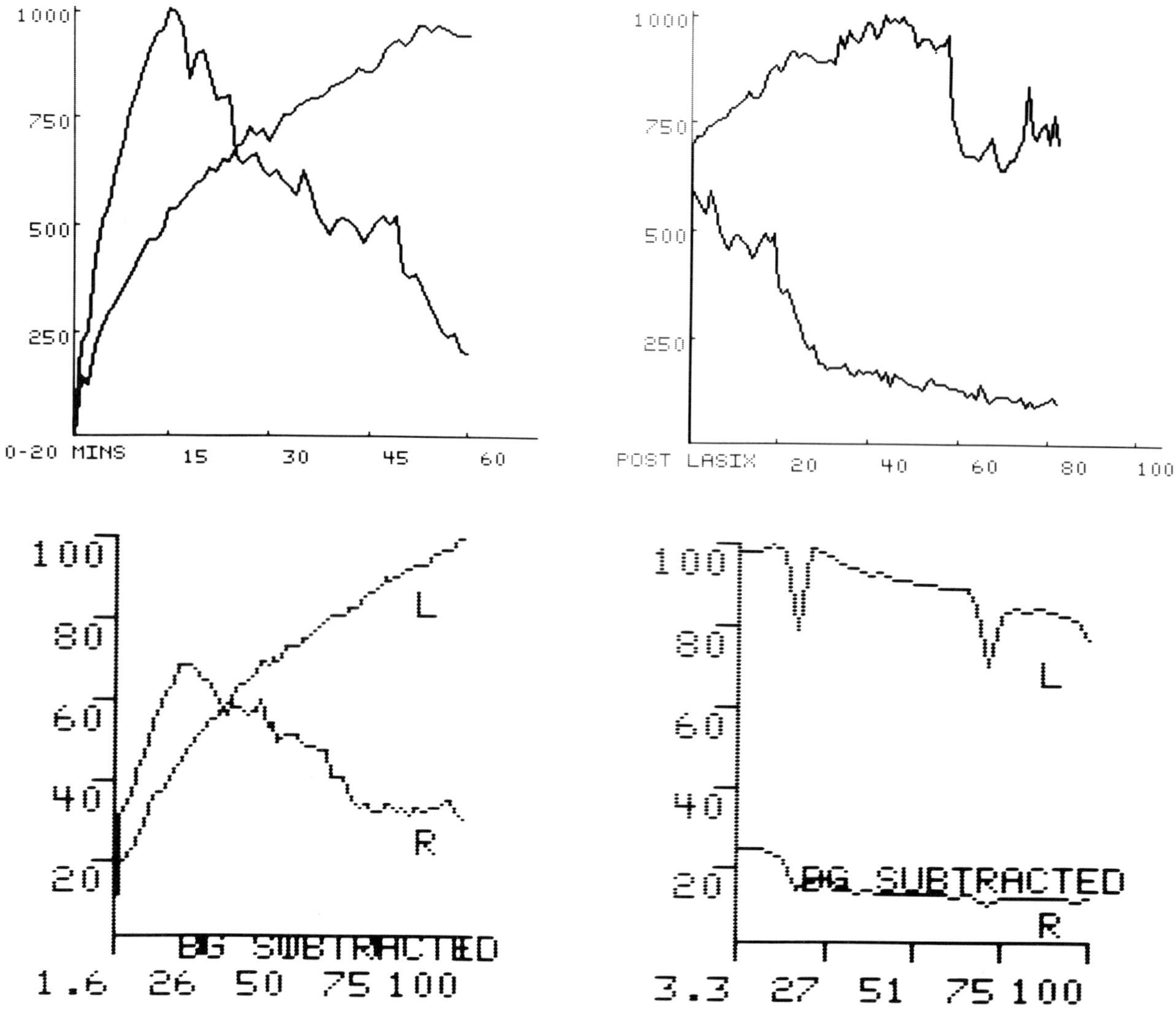

E

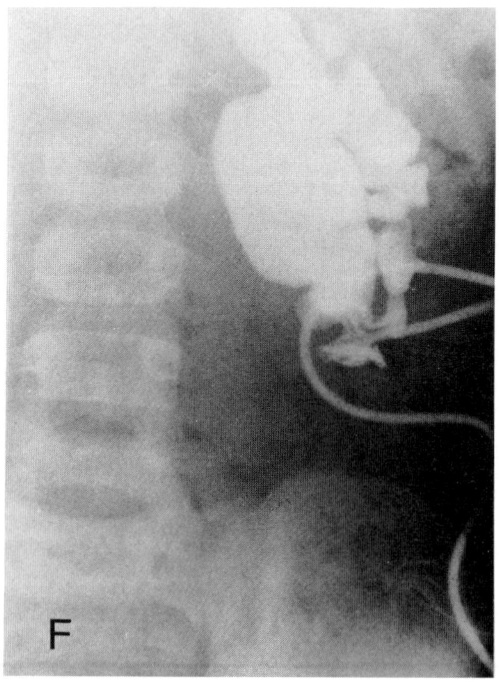

Figure 20.5 E,F

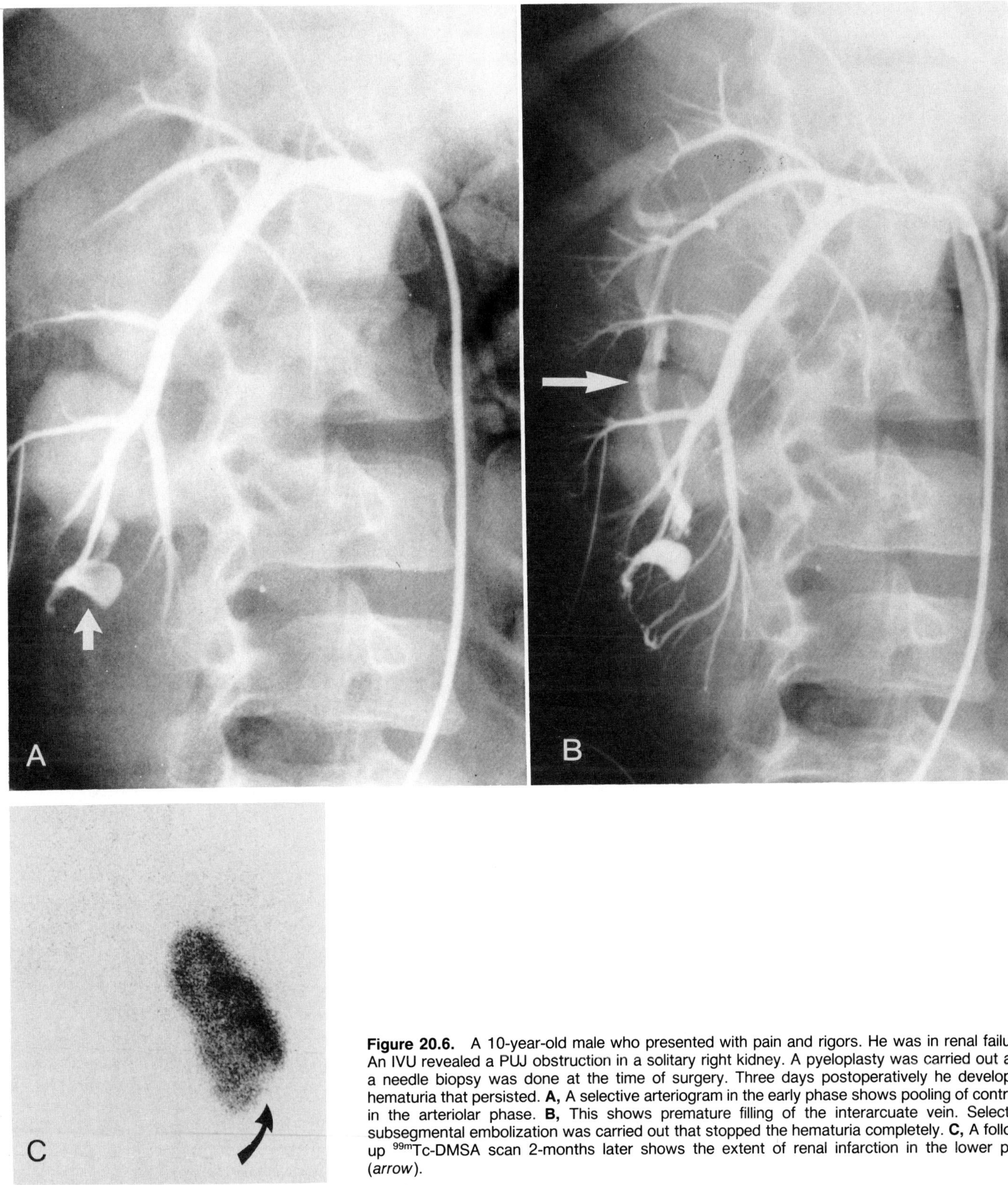

Figure 20.6. A 10-year-old male who presented with pain and rigors. He was in renal failure. An IVU revealed a PUJ obstruction in a solitary right kidney. A pyeloplasty was carried out and a needle biopsy was done at the time of surgery. Three days postoperatively he developed hematuria that persisted. **A,** A selective arteriogram in the early phase shows pooling of contrast in the arteriolar phase. **B,** This shows premature filling of the interarcuate vein. Selective subsegmental embolization was carried out that stopped the hematuria completely. **C,** A follow-up ^{99m}Tc-DMSA scan 2-months later shows the extent of renal infarction in the lower pole (*arrow*).

Radioisotope Cystogram

Direct Radioisotope Cystogram. The technique is similar to the MCU and requires bladder catheterization, draining the urine off, instilling ^{99m}Tc-pertechnetate (500 μCi) then running in normal saline until the bladder is full, when micturition should occur (32). The entire procedure is carried out in front of, or on top of, the gamma camera linked to a computer system. Both renal areas and the bladder are kept in the field of view. The residual volume after micturition can be estimated. The advantages of this technique are mainly the low radiation exposure compared with a conventional MCU, the dose being reduced by a factor of 20 (33). It does, however, require a catheter so that the circumstances of micturition are unphysiological.

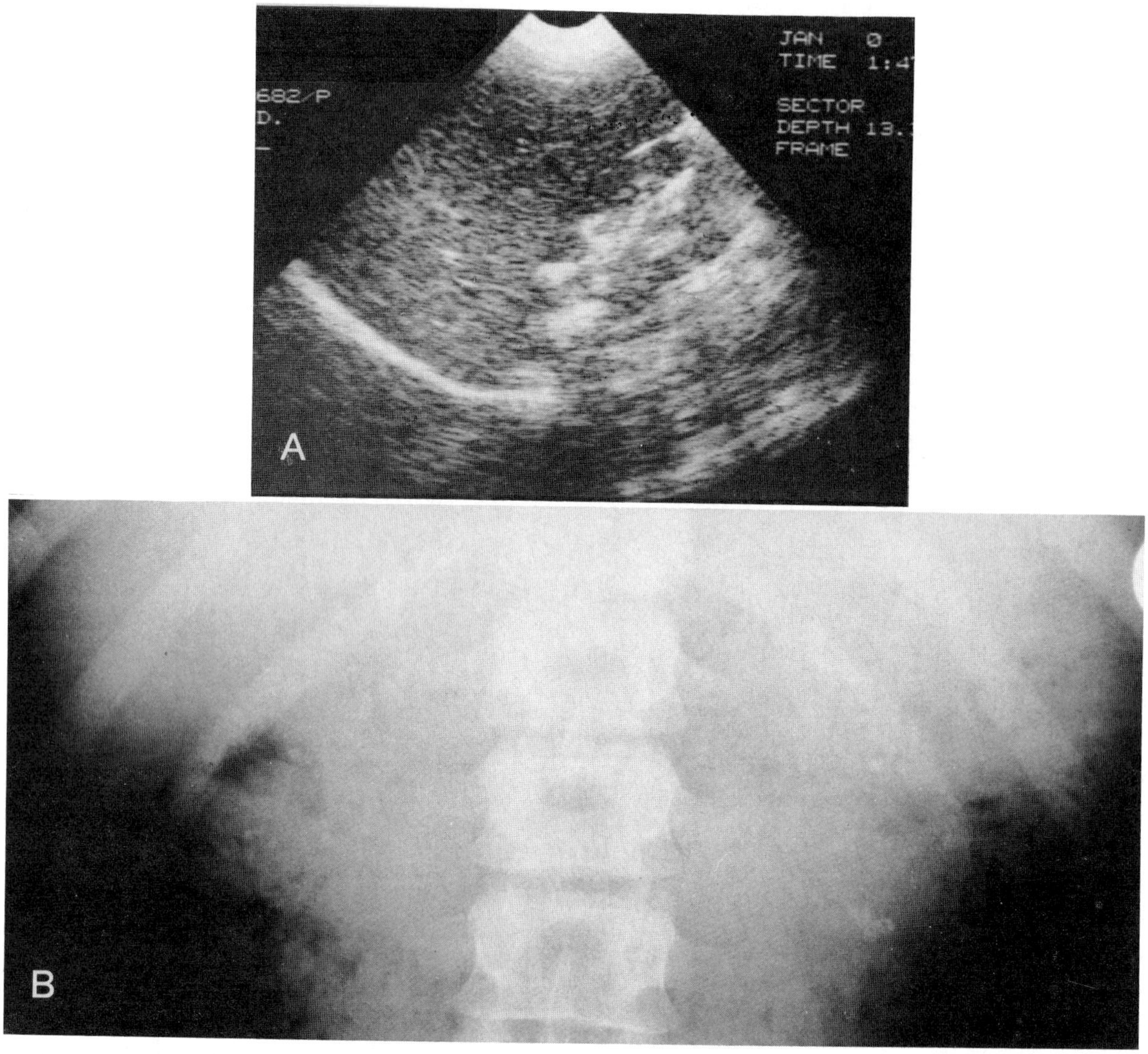

Figure 20.7. **A,** A longitudinal ultrasound scan of the right kidney shows very bright medullae with acoustic shadows. **B,** The plain radiograph confirms the nephrocalcinosis, in this child as a result of distal renal tubular acidosis. Ultrasound is often more sensitive than radiographs in the detection of nephrocalcinosis.

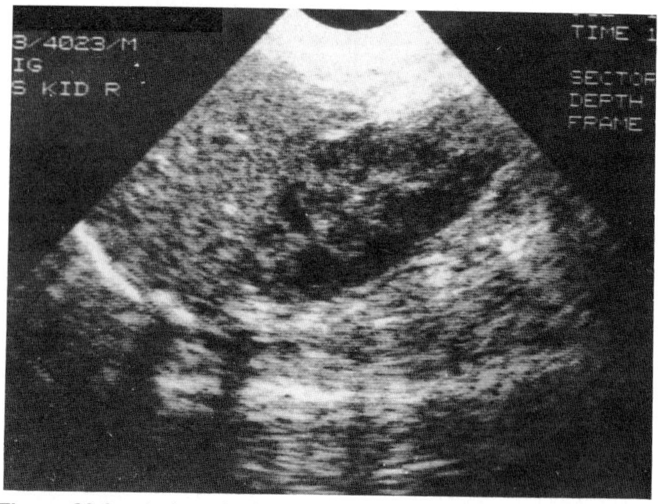

Figure 20.8. A 1-week-old neonate underwent an abdominal ultrasound because of associated congenital abnormalities. The bright cortex with relatively transonic medulla in normal-sized kidneys are well seen in this longitudinal scan. This is the appearance of a normal kidney in the first 3 months of life.

Indirect Radioisotope Cystogram. Thirty to 60 minutes after the IV injection of ^{99m}Tc-DTPA, when most of the isotope is in the bladder (Fig. 20.10) and little remains in the kidneys, the child is asked to void in front of the gamma camera. Voiding views are more accurate than the MCU in detecting reflux (34, 35). The advantages are that it involves only the radiation dose of the routine DTPA scan, is noninvasive, does not require bladder catheterization, and is physiological. The disadvantages lie in the fact that the child must be cooperative, i.e., toilet-trained and over the age of 3 to 4 years; secondly, VUR will only be detectable on the voiding phase, since the filling of the bladder is from the kidneys. When there is a high urine flow rate, e.g., after the administration of furosemide or in an overhydrated child, VUR may not be detected (36). Since these circumstances may be necessary for certain ^{99m}Tc-DTPA scans, a conflict in methodology may be inevitable if the indirect cystogram is combined with a complete DTPA scan using furosemide.

Indications. When VUR has been documented by MCU, subsequent evaluation should be carried out by an isotope cystogram rather than a repeat MCU. The isotope cystogram alone is insufficient as a primary investigation since it may diagnose VUR accurately but it fails to provide essential anatomical detail of the vesicoureteric junction and bladder

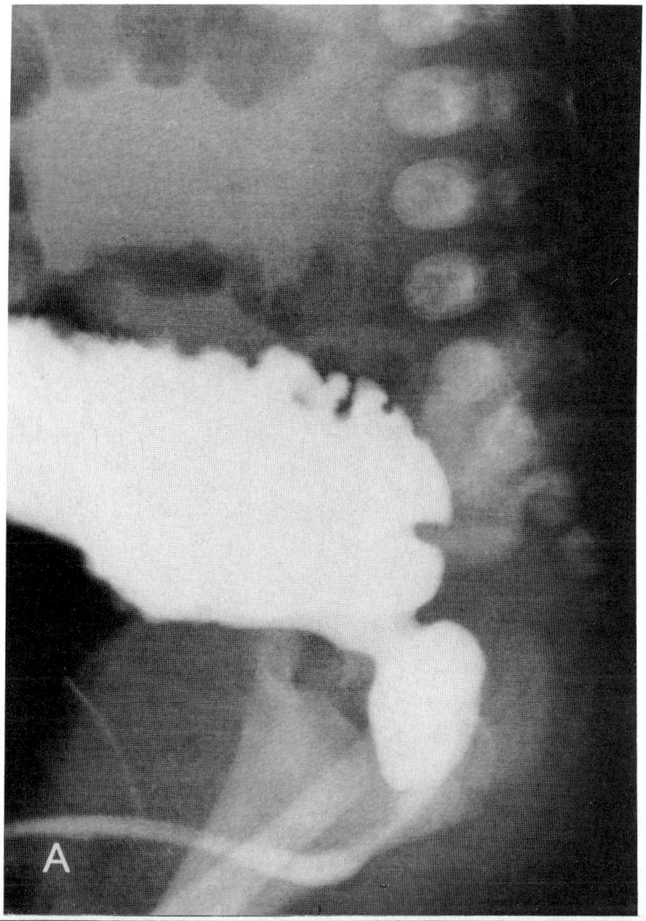

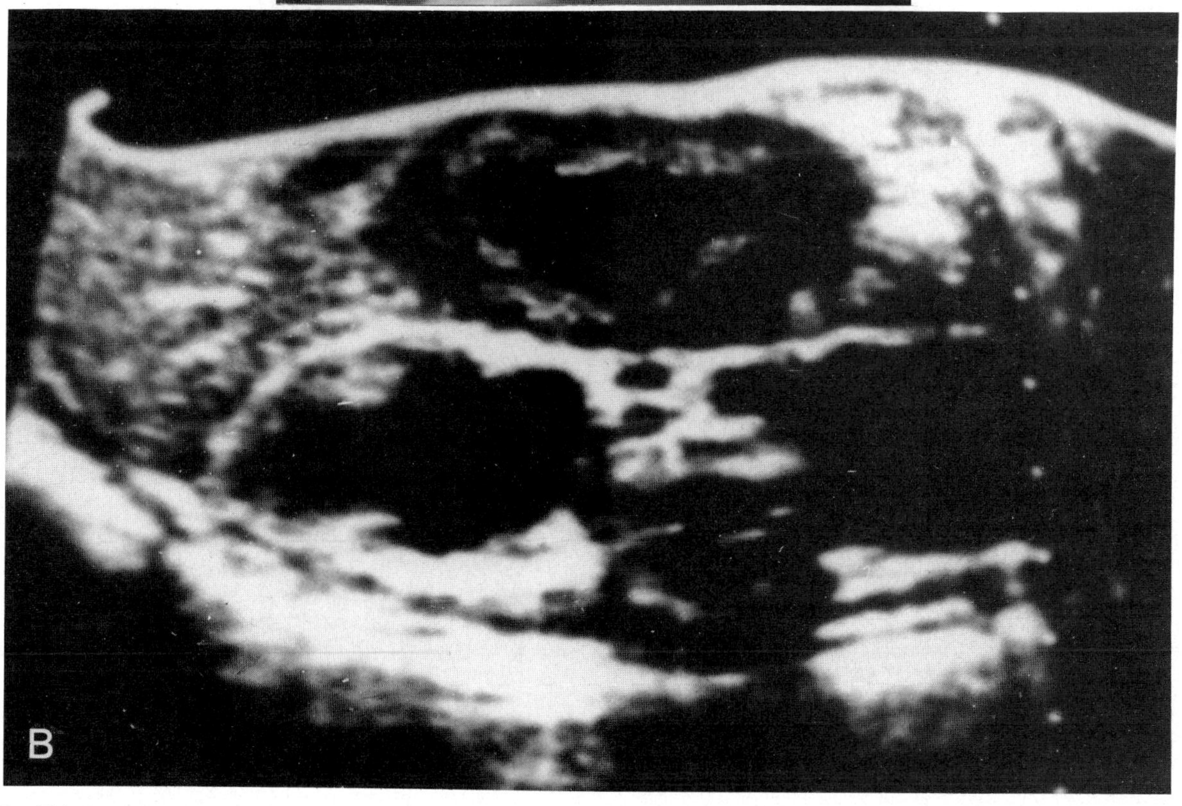

Figure 20.9. This neonate was vomiting and septicemic with a palpable bladder. **A,** The MCU showed a trabeculated bladder with typical posterior urethral valves. **B,** The transverse ultrasound scan through the bladder revealed a thick-walled bladder with dilated tortuous ureters behind the bladder. **C,** The transverse prone ultrasound through the kidneys showed a more massive right-sided hydronephrosis (*arrow*). **D,** Following treatment of the infection and valve resection, this boy was followed with ^{99m}Tc-DTPA scans. **E,** The isotope accumulates progressively in both kidneys with the right kidney contributing 65% to overall function. Drainage is seen after furosemide.

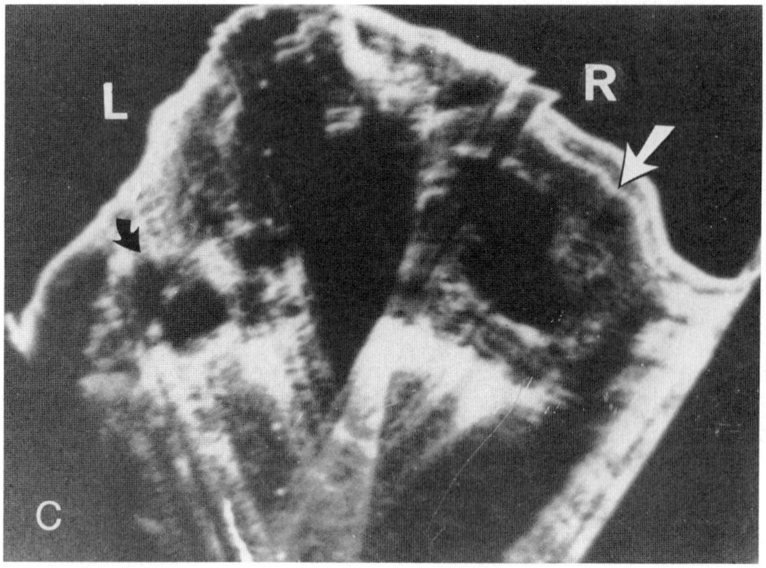

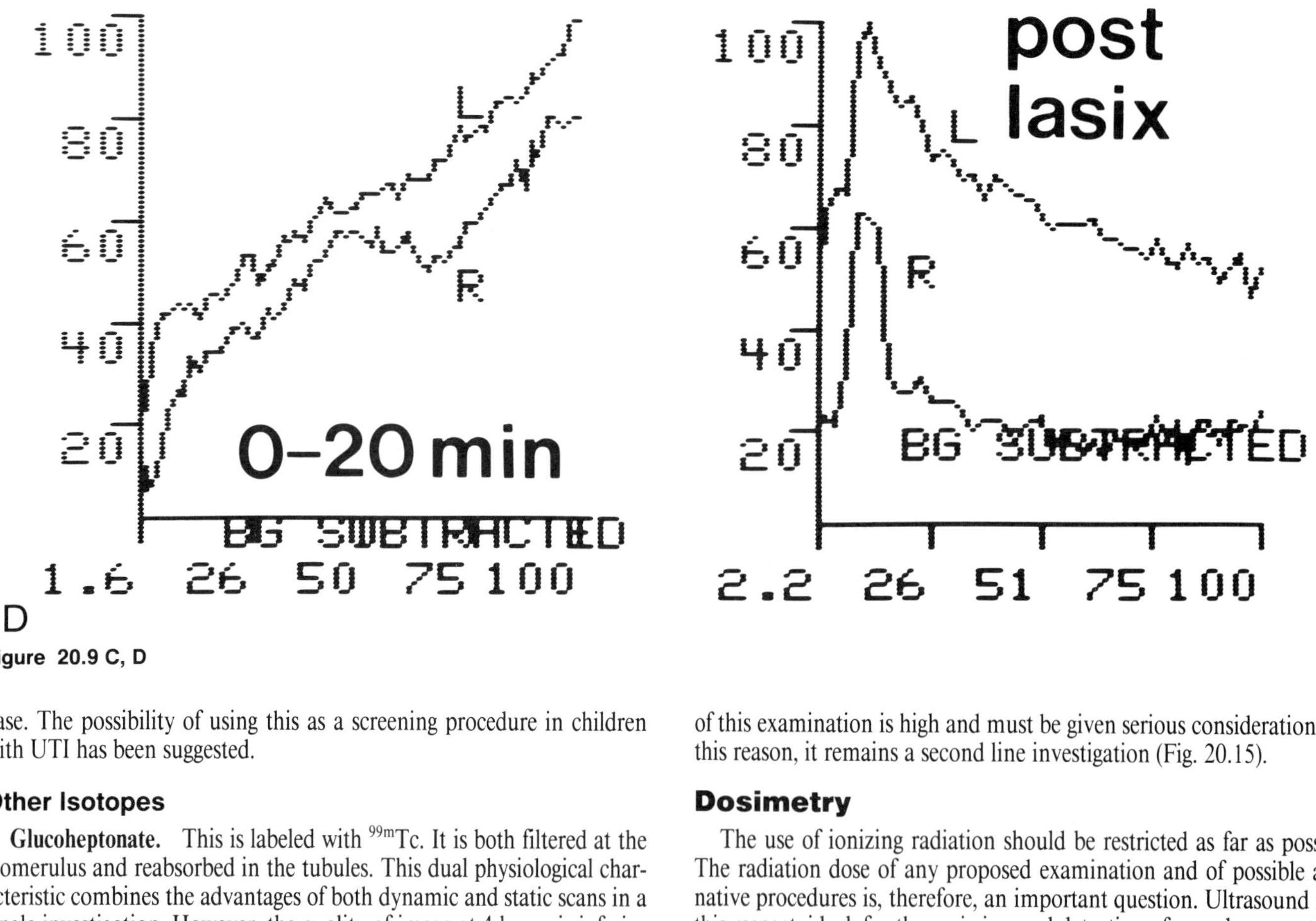

Figure 20.9 C, D

base. The possibility of using this as a screening procedure in children with UTI has been suggested.

Other Isotopes

Glucoheptonate. This is labeled with ^{99m}Tc. It is both filtered at the glomerulus and reabsorbed in the tubules. This dual physiological characteristic combines the advantages of both dynamic and static scans in a single investigation. However, the quality of image at 4 hours is inferior to ^{99m}Tc-DMSA and the early phase does not allow estimation of GFR a result of the tubular uptake. It is considered a useful radiopharmaceutical where DMSA is not freely available (37).

^{111}Indium White Blood Cells. ^{111}Indium white blood cells (^{111}In-WBC) technique allows labeling of either autologous or donor WBC with ^{111}In and reinjection. Images are obtained at 4 and 24 hours, which allows physiological monitoring of the leukocytes. It has proved valuable in difficult cases of occult infection, especially perinephric abscesses and renal carbuncles as a second line investigation (38). The radiation dose of this examination is high and must be given serious consideration. For this reason, it remains a second line investigation (Fig. 20.15).

Dosimetry

The use of ionizing radiation should be restricted as far as possible. The radiation dose of any proposed examination and of possible alternative procedures is, therefore, an important question. Ultrasound is, in this respect, ideal, for the emission and detection of sound waves at high frequency does not involve ionizing radiation and no tissue damage has yet been attributed to it.

Radiography

The x-rays are emitted from a point source, pass into the patient, and those that leave the patient are detected on the x-ray film or seen on the TV monitor. This means that the skin surface closest to the x-ray tube received the highest radiation dose. Organs within the field of view receive a dose proportional to their size and depth within the body. There

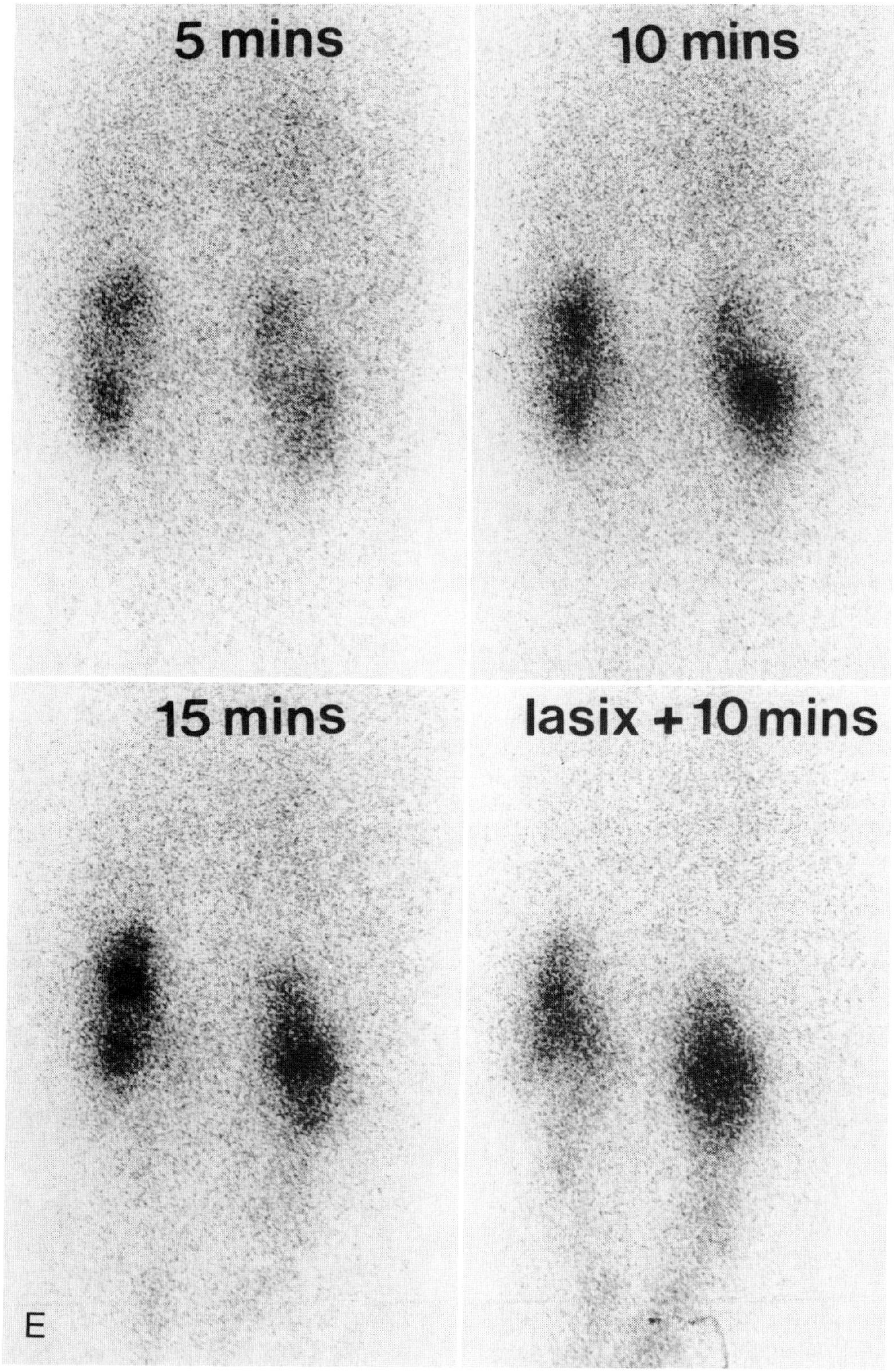

Figure 20.9 E

is also a dose to the whole body from absorbed radiation (Table 20.3); with conventional cystography, exposure is high. With a CT scan, only a narrow slice (3 to 13 mm) of the patient receives radiation, but at a high level. Again, the skin closest to the x-ray source receives the highest dose and the organs closest to the detectors receive the lowest.

Radioisotopes

A small amount of tracer is labeled with an isotope, which emits gamma radiation. Each radioisotope emits gamma rays at a well-defined energy level and has a characteristic half-life, e.g., ^{99m}Tc emits gamma rays at 140 KeV and has a half-life of 6 hours, whereas ^{123}I emits gamma

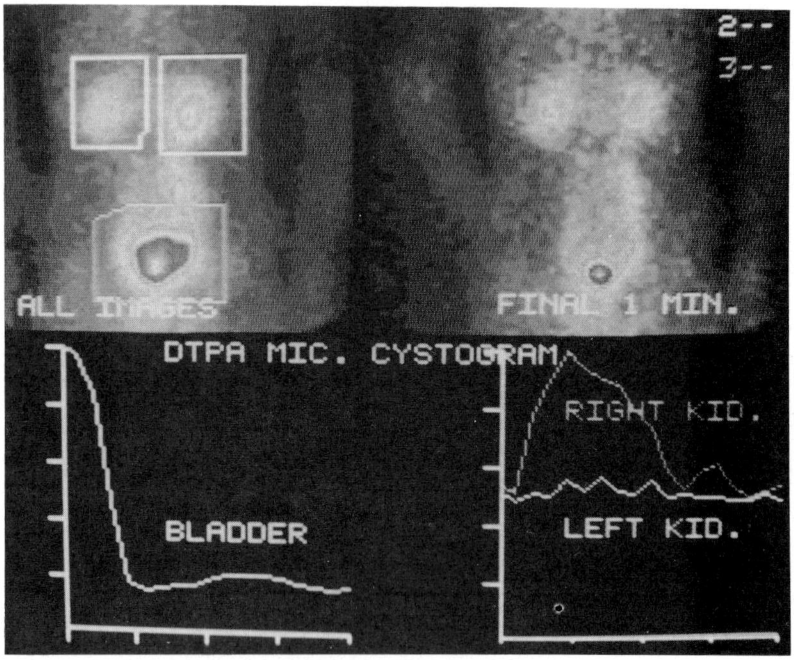

Figure 20.10. One-hour after the IV injection of ^{99m}Tc-DTPA, this 4-year-old male micturated while standing in front of the gamma camera. He was known to have bilateral vesicoureteric reflux. The top image shows all the frames accumulated in the computer summated with regions of interest generated over each kidney and the bladder. The curves from each region are shown in the lower half and right-sided VUR is clearly demonstrated.

rays of 159 KeV and has a half-life of 12.5 hours. Since these are injected into the blood, the radiation dose must be calculated for the target organ, i.e., the organ in which the tracer is concentrated. In a dynamic scan using ^{99m}Tc-DTPA or ^{123}I-hippuran the target organ is the bladder since the uptake, transit, and excretion through the kidney is very rapid (Table 20.4). In the static scan using ^{99m}Tc-DMSA the target organ is the kidney, since the isotope is fixed in the proximal convoluted tubules (Table 20.5). To calculate the radiation dose, not only must the physical half-life of the isotope be known but the biological half-life must be assessed, e.g., in dynamic renal scans with normal function the biological half-life will be far shorter than the physical half-life. In the bladder, exposure is markedly influenced by the frequency of micturition. It must be stressed that pure gamma-emitting isotopes should be used since this minimizes useless tissue dose (Tables 20.3-5).

Conclusion

It is difficult to compare radiation exposure from x-rays directly with radioisotopes, but some close approximations can be given (Tables 20.3-5). There are national idiosyncrasies in the assessment of the risks so that in certain countries the use of DMSA is severely curtailed because of the relatively high kidney radiation dose. However, the DMSA scan provides specific information that is not available by any other technique that has as low a radiation and is as non-invasive.

> The implication of the review of biological effects in human beings is that any amount of radiation, no matter how small, has a deleterious effect even if it is not detectable. This conclusion is based on the assumption of a linear non-threshold dose effect model which has been adopted by the national and international bodies as the most conservative basis for risk estimates. Perhaps it would be easier to provide a firm lower limit, e.g., 1 to 10 rems, below which no radiation effect has been observed . . . at any specific dose we are left with the useful concept of the lowest practicable dose (39).

This philosophy requires that the clinicians should have some reasonable expectation that the gain for the individual patient in using a procedure in nuclear medicine will exceed potential risks.

> Nuclear medicine can provide the pediatrician with valuable clinical information about the sick child that is uniquely available with this technique. The methods can be considered entirely safe with the employment of appropriate radiopharmaceuticals, equipment, highly qualified personnel and, above all, the selection of proper patients by the physician (39).

Table 20.3.
Dosimetry (Radiography)

	Age (years)			
	1	5	10	15
Maximum skin dose (rads)				
IVU (4 films)	0.2	0.3	0.5	0.8
Angiography (20 films)	1.4	3.0	4.8	7.5
Fluoroscopy (4 min)	3.2	4.8	6.8	8.8
Mean whole body dose (rads)				
IVU (4 films)	0.03	0.04	0.06	0.07
Angiography (20 films)	0.03	0.06	0.06	0.06
Fluoroscopy (4 min)	0.15	0.20	0.20	0.20

From James AW, et al: In Paediatric Nuclear Medicine, ed 1. Philadelphia, W. B. Saunders, 1974.

Table 20.4.
^{99m}Technetium-DTPA: Radiation Dose

Age (years)	Newborn	1	5	10	15	Adult
Weight (kg)	3.5	12	20	33	55	70
Administered radioactivity (mCi)	0.28	0.60	0.87	1.2	1.7	2.0
Dose per μCi given (rads)						
Bladder	1.4	1.0	1.0	0.96	0.9	0.90
Kidney	0.11	0.09	0.09	0.08	0.09	0.08
Whole Body	0.047	0.037	0.037	0.035	0.035	0.032

From James AW, et al: In Paediatric Nephrology, ed 1. Philadelphia, W. B. Saunders, 1974.

Table 20.5.
Radiation Dose from DTPA and DMSA in Adults[a]

	^{99m}Tc-DTPA μGy/mBq	^{99m}Tc-DMSA μGy/mBq
Kidney	11.4	168
Bladder	150	76
Whole Body	4.3	4.3

From Bingham JB Maisey NM: Brit J Radiol 51: 599, 1979.
[a] Units: μGy/mBq, micrograys/megabequarel; 1 Gy (gray), 10^{-1} rad; 1 Bq (Bequarel), 27×10^{-12} Ci.

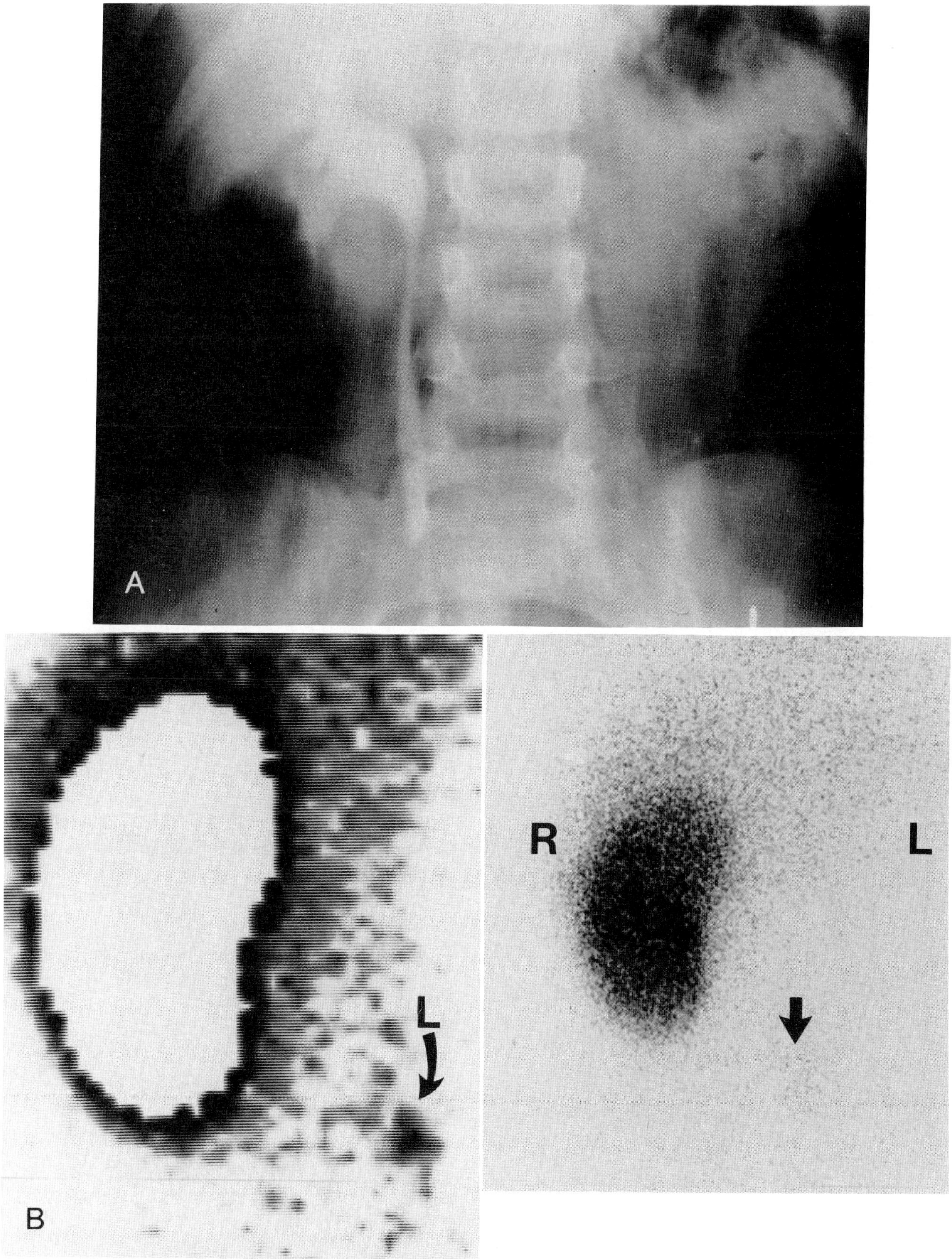

Figure 20.11. A 5-year-old female with intermittently diurnal incontinence. The abdominal ultrasound revealed a single right kidney, but no abnormality was seen behind the bladder. **A,** The tomographic cut of the IVU shows a normal right kidney. No left kidney is seen. **B,** The ^{99m}Tc-DMSA scan shows a normal right kidney with a small area of increased uptake of isotope low on the left (*arrow*). The image on the left is a computer manipulation in which only isotope activity between 5% and 20% of peak activity is displayed. This technique masks out the normal kidney and also subtracts a small amount of background activity, permitting clear visualization of the small ectopic left kidney (*arrow*).

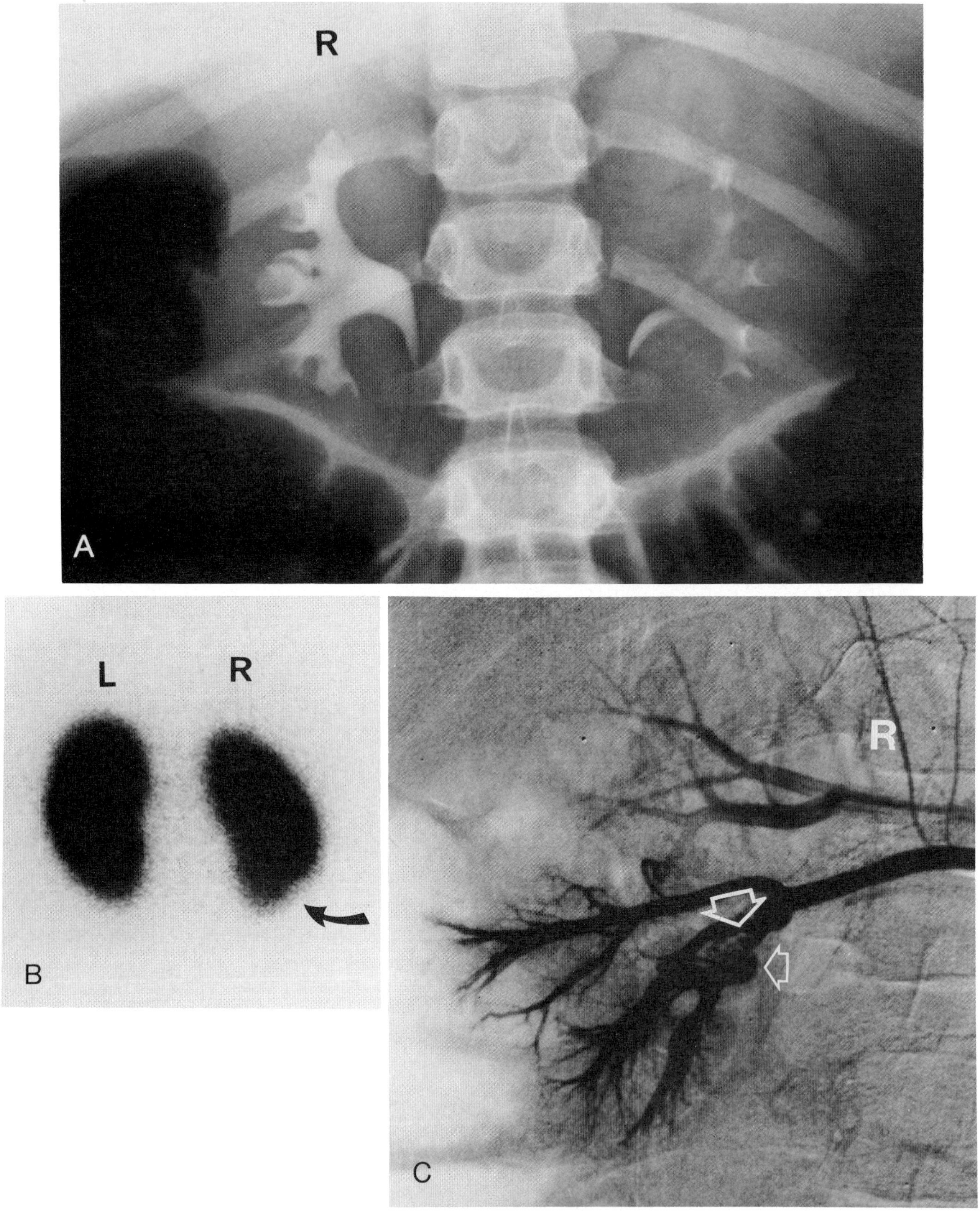

Figure 20.12. An 8-year-old female was found to be hypertensive with raised peripheral plasma renin levels. **A,** The abdominal ultrasound was normal as was the IVU. **B,** The ^{99m}Tc-DMSA scan shows a focal decrease in the activity in the lower pole of the right kidney (*arrow*). **C,** The selective renal arteriogram showed a single abnormality in the lower pole of the right kidney with narrowing of a single intrarenal artery, distal dilatation, and corkscrew collaterals (*arrows*). The selective renal vein renin estimation confirmed that the lower pole of the right kidney was driving the hypertension. A partial nephrectomy cured the hypertension and histology revealed evidence of fibromuscular hyperplasia.

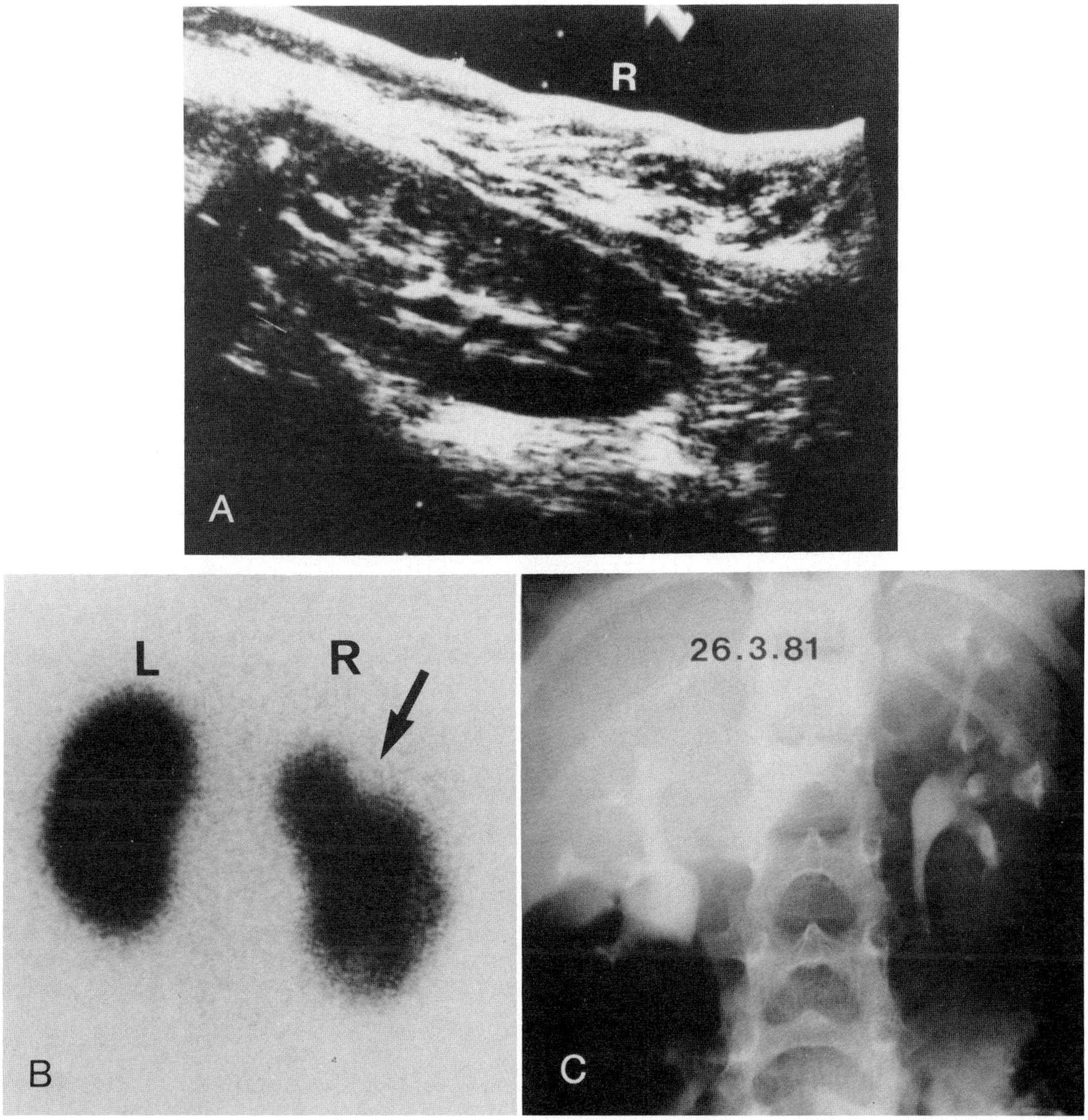

Figure 20.13. A 7-year-old male presented with a UTI and became septicemic and shocked. Following intensive antibiotic therapy he made an uneventful recovery. An MCU was normal. **A,** The abdominal ultrasound during the acute illness and subsequently have been normal. **B,** The ^{99m}Tc-DMSA scan shows a normal left kidney and a photon deficient area in the right upper pole. Subsequent DMSA scans 2-years later confirm the presence of the scar. The IVU at the time of the acute illness was normal as was the follow-up IVU, **C,** 18 months later. This confirms the increased sensitivity of the ^{99m}Tc-DMSA scan in the detection of renal scars.

CLINICAL PROBLEM

The Neonate

Attention can be drawn to the urinary tract in the neonatal period for a variety of reasons, e.g., anorectal anomaly, an abdominal mass, or poor urine output, but there still are essentially only two questions of clinical relevance. Those questions are the following: (1) Are there two kidneys and, if so, what is their function? (2) Is there dilatation of the collecting systems and, if so, is there obstruction? However, there are certain important aspects of imaging the urinary tract of the neonate that act as guidelines no matter what the indication for the investigations may be.

The function of the neonatal kidney is immature compared with that of older children or adults. GFR and renal plasma flow are low and renal vascular resistance is high, especially in the outer cortical zones, so that there is a preferential distribution of renal blood flow to the juxtamedullary region. Proximal tubular reabsorptive capacity is poorly developed. As a consequence, there is greater dependence on distal sodium reabsorption to maintain Na balance, with a much higher plasma renin activity and aldosterone concentration than in the adult. These factors militate against satisfactory visualization with an IVU and complicate interpretation of DTPA scans (40, 44) (Fig. 20.16). Furthermore, there is difficulty in disposing of a sodium load (42). Consequently, there is a greater risk of volume overload with inappropriate intravenous therapy or with the osmotic load of contrast material. Urinary concentrating capacity is less well developed (43); therefore, obligatory water loss with an osmotic load of contrast is greater, predisposing to subsequent dehydration. Fluid deprivation before an IVU is unfortunately still practiced so that the neonate may arrive dehydrated for this examination, which further adds to the morbidity (Fig. 20.10).

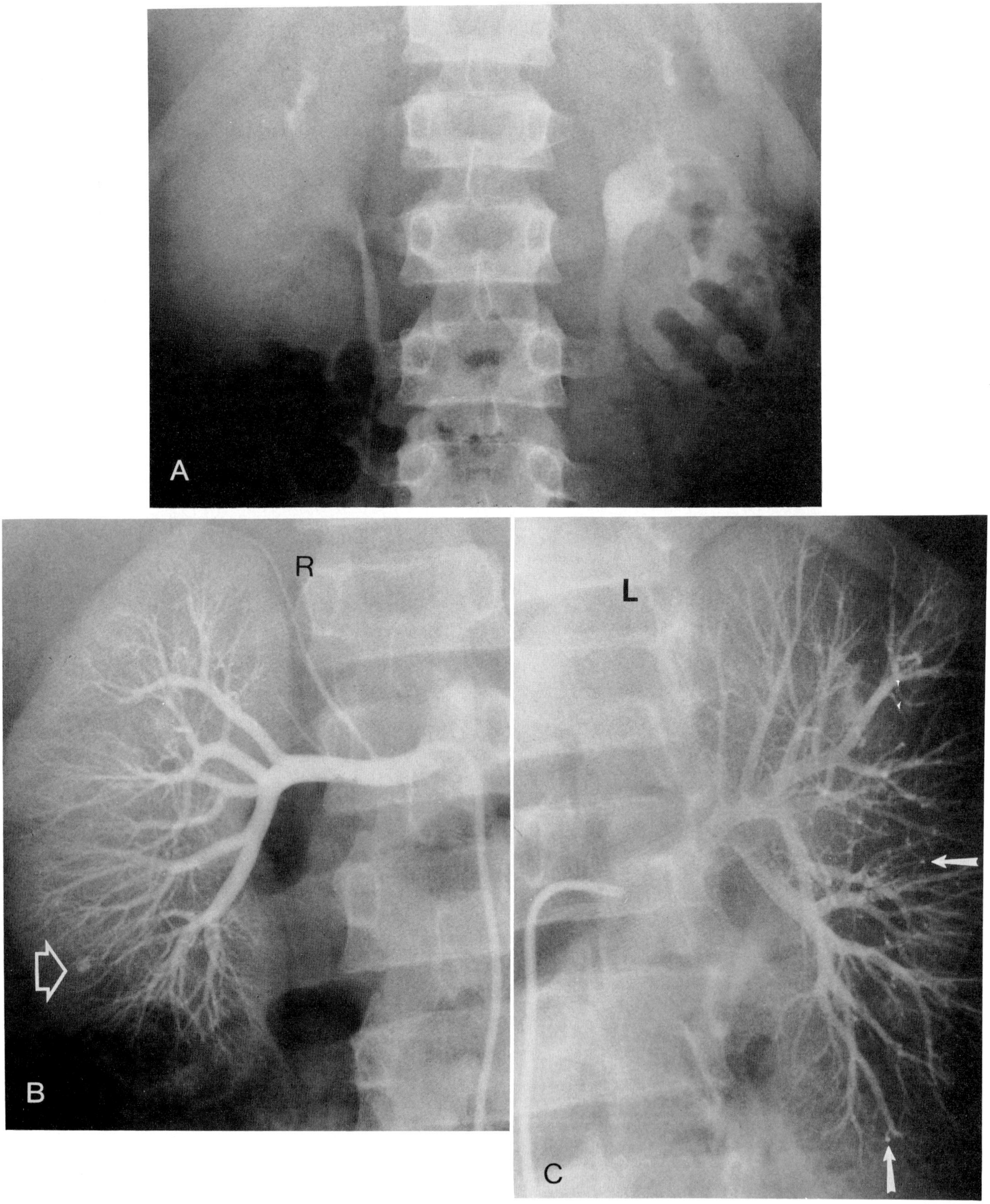

Figure 20.14. A 5-year-old male presented with ill health, a high ESR, fever, and microscopic hematuria. **A,** The IVU was normal. The ^{99m}Tc-DMSA scan showed patchy uptake in both kidneys. **B,** Selective renal arteriography showed a microaneurysm on the right (*arrow*). **C,** The selective left renal arteriogram showed abrupt cut-off of the peripheral vessels on the frontal projection and also on the oblique view, as very small microaneurysms were also present (*arrows*). These features suggest polyarteritis nodosa.

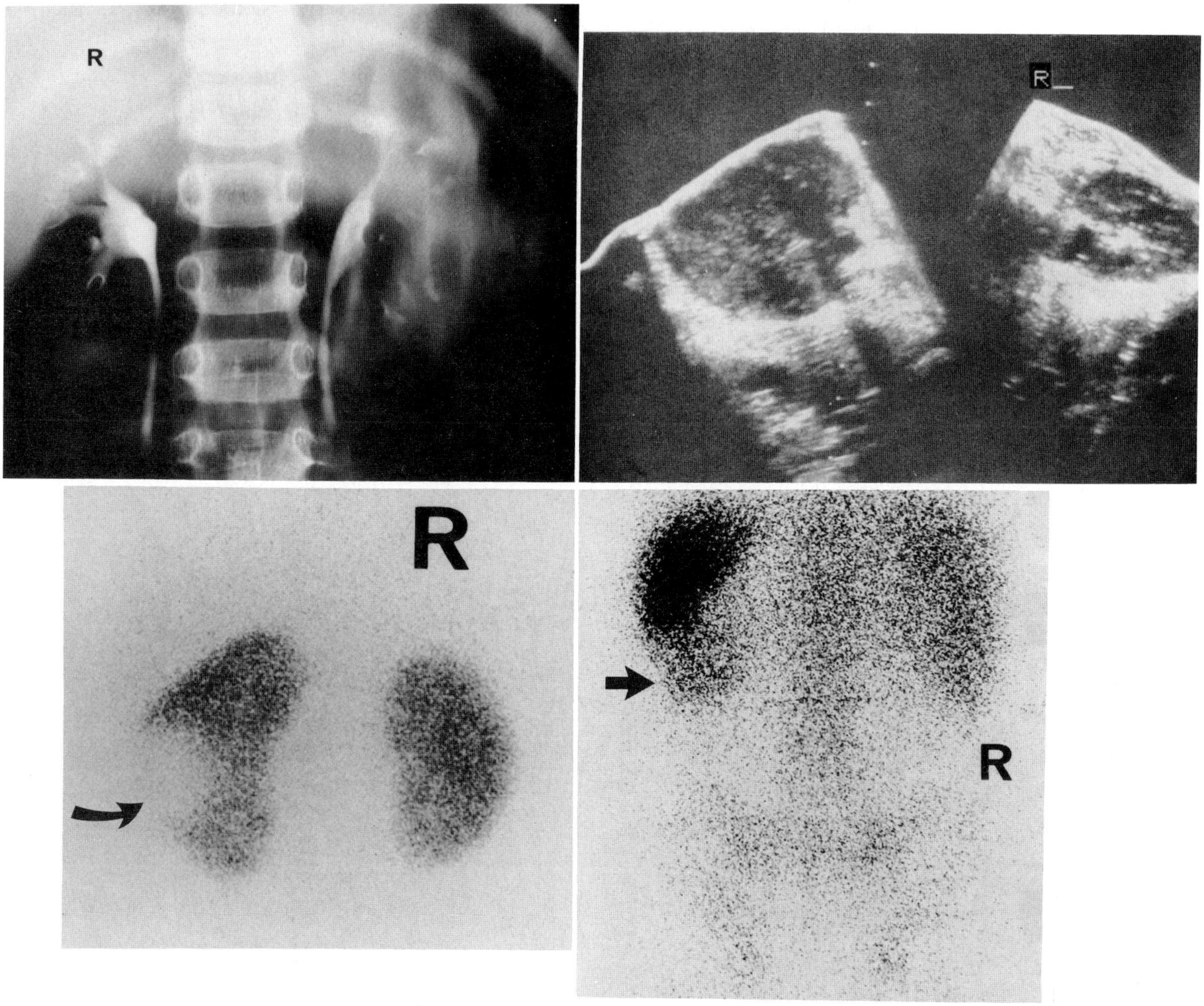

Figure 20.15. A 6-year-old boy presented with rigors, fever, and general malaise. The urine was normal. The IVU (tomographic cut, *top left*) shows a normal right kidney and an enlarged left kidney with the calyces in the mid- and lower zones being compressed. The transverse ultrasound scan (*top right*) showed a normal right kidney with a diffusely enlarged left kidney but no focal abnormality. The ^{99m}Tc-DMSA scan (*bottom left*) showed a well defined photon-deficient area in the lower pole of the left kidney (*arrow*). The ^{111}In-WBC scan (*bottom right*) showed focal accumulation of the isotope below the spleen (*arrow*). These two normal areas on the isotope scans could be superimposed strongly supporting the diagnosis of a renal carbuncle. The child responded to intensive antibiotic therapy.

An IVU requires an injection of up to 3 ml/kg of an osmotically active substance with a high sodium content. The new non-ionic contrast media with 30% iodine should be used whenever possible. Even so, the contrast may be detrimental to an immature kidney, particularly if it has been exposed to any insult, e.g., anoxia. An IVU in the neonatal period may cause severe metabolic upset and certain pathological states may be aggravated by the contrast medium, particularly with renal venous thrombosis or medullary necrosis. Even in normal neonates, an IVU may fail to outline the kidneys, especially in the first 48 hours of life. These factors suggest that there is no place for an IVU within the first 2 to 3 days of life, but if it is undertaken there may be no visualization of the kidneys during the first few hours, and delayed images at 6, 12, and 18 hours may be necessary. An IVU should not be carried out in the neonate with sepsis or renal failure.

An abdominal ultrasound should always be the first line of investigation (44). Certain basic questions are usually answered. Are both kidneys present? Are they normal in size? Do they have a normal echogenic pattern? Is there dilatation of the collecting system? What is the state of the bladder and the bladder base?

The next mode of investigation depends on the clinical problem and the result of the ultrasound examination. The two main options are a radioisotope scan or an MCU. The latter is indicated when there is renal failure with ureteric dilatation. Under these circumstances obstruction must be distinguished from reflux. An MCU in the neonate needs to be well orchestrated so that appropriate catheter management ensues if an obstructive lesion is found (Fig. 20.9). If the neonate has deficient abdominal wall musculature (prune belly syndrome) an MCU should be avoided in the neonatal period if possible, since an infection in this grossly dilated urinary tract may prove serious. Investigation of this type of child should be the province of specialized units.

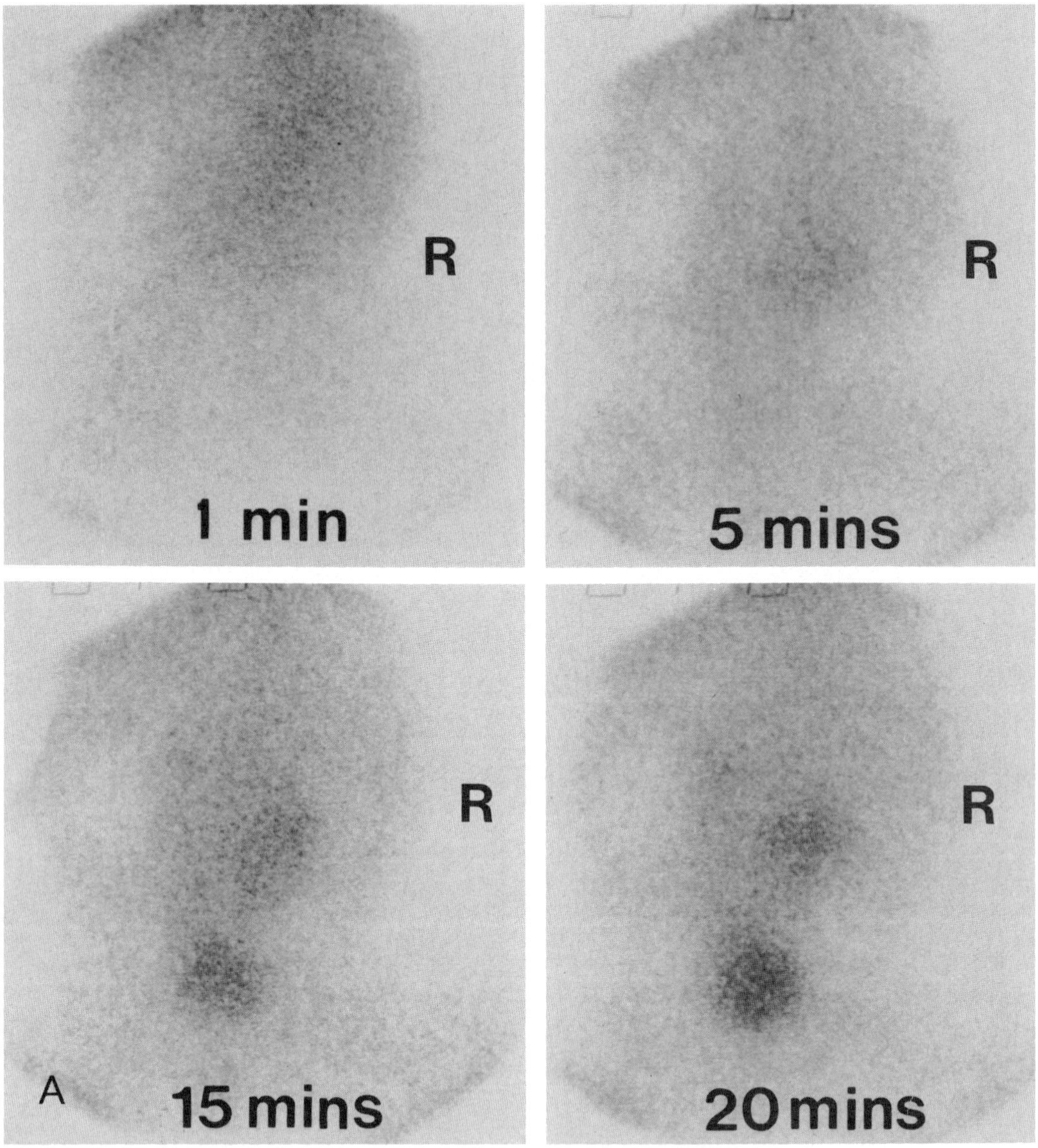

Figure 20.16. A neonate was found to have an abdominal mass at birth. An ultrasound suggested that the mass was a multicystic kidney on the left. **A,** A ^{99m}Tc-DTPA scan was carried out on the first day of life, which showed slow progressive uptake of the tracer in the right kidney with isotope in the bladder by 15 minutes. **B,** A follow-up ^{99m}Tc-DTPA scan was performed 6 days later, which showed normal renal function on the right with isotope in the bladder by 5 minutes. **C,** The curves generated from regions of interest drawn around the heart and right kidney show the poor renal extraction of isotope on the first scan with a poor right renal curve. The follow-up scan shows normal curves. This is a dramatic reflection of transitional nephrology and explains why functional studies are difficult to interpret.

Urinary Tract Infection

UTI is a common condition and the imaging that such children may undergo is important in terms of discomfort, radiation exposure, and resource utilization. There is, therefore, a need to select those patients in whom the probable yield from diagnostic imaging is significant. Also, an effort must be made not to overburden the radiology department nor overinvestigate the child, but at the same time not to overlook treatable pathology or long-term complications (45, 46).

There is controversy about the appropriate investigation of UTI, which will continue until more information is available from the newer modes of imaging and a better understanding of the pathogenesis of the disorder and its complications is reached. The role of diagnostic imaging is to reveal those abnormalities that require surgery, to identify those children with the potential for renal damage, to identify those children with renal scarring at risk of the long-term complications of hypertension or CRF, and to monitor progress and the results of surgery.

At the outset one must consider the age of the child (Table 20.6). Children <5 years of both sexes are at risk of renal damage with UTI and VUR and need full investigation. Over 5 years, UTI rarely leads to renal damage if the kidney was previously normal, even if reflux is present (47). In boys, there is a possibility of bladder outflow obstruction, and, therefore, a UTI usually requires an MCU, but in girls >5 years an experienced ultrasonographer will provide sufficient information with the demonstration of normal kidneys, no dilated ureter, and an empty bladder following micturition.

With the first documented UTI, all children require some form of imaging. This should consist of a plain abdominal radiograph to exclude urinary calculi and an abdominal ultrasound of the kidneys and bladder (48) (Fig. 20.1). If these investigations are normal, then further investi-

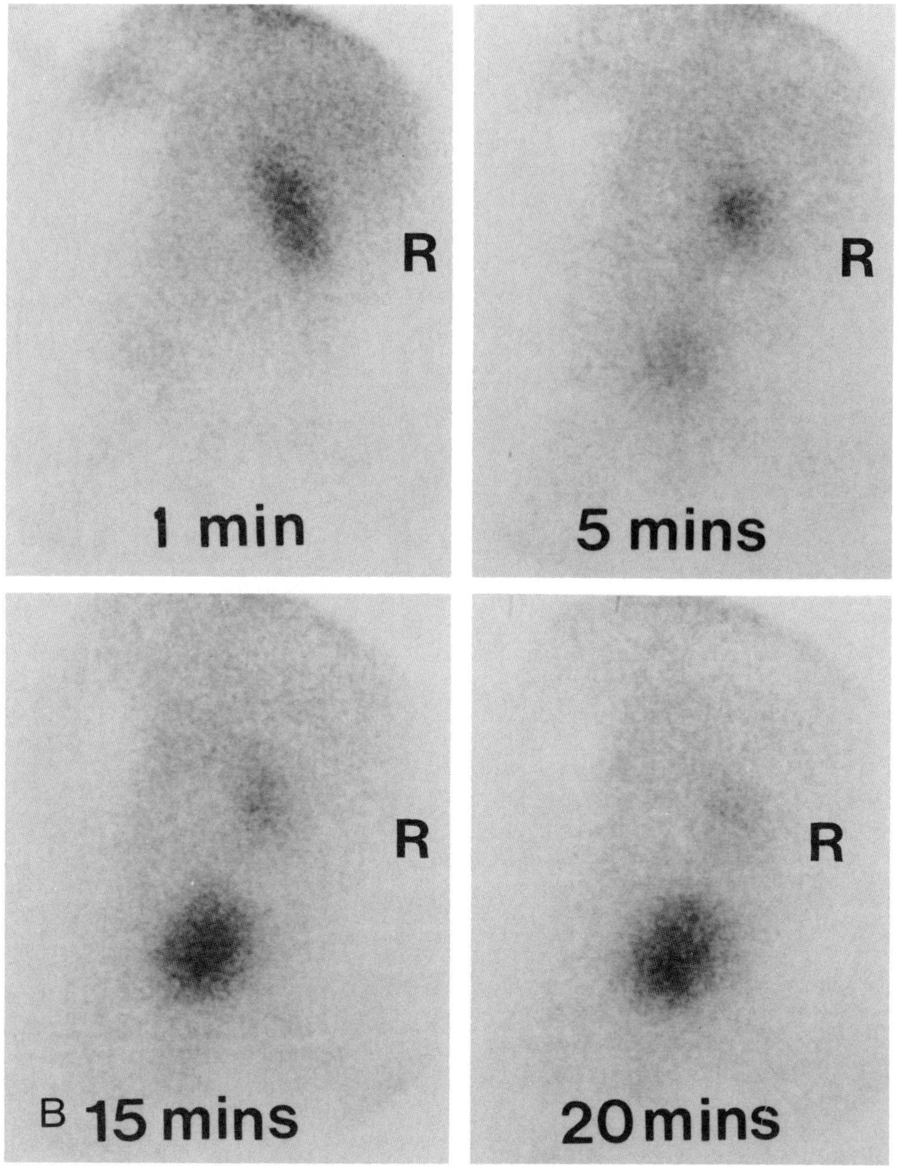

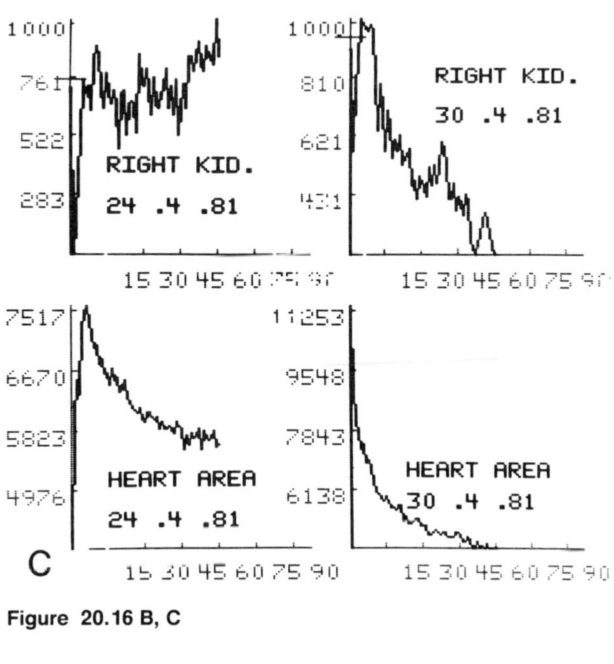

Figure 20.16 B, C

gations should be instigated only if a second UTI occurs, at which time a DMSA scan should be done. An MCU is required after the initial UTI has subsided in children <5 years of age to exclude VUR. In children >5 years of age, an MCU need be done only if the episodes of UTI are recurrent. When an abnormal kidney is found on either ultrasound (49) or DMSA scan then an MCU should be obtained together with an IVU and a DTPA scan (Fig. 20.4), irrespective of the age of the child. The purpose of the DTPA scan is to obtain an estimate of IKGFR for long-term follow-up; the MCU is to assess VUR.

All children in whom VUR has been detected require follow-up, irrespective of age. Many children will be placed on long-term antibiotic prophylaxis, and the cessation of VUR is an indication to stop this treatment. Reevaluation for VUR should be done preferably with a radioisotope cystogram. For children <4 years of age, i.e., not toilet-trained, the direct radionuclide cystogram is required; for older children, micturating views following IV ^{99m}Tc-DTPA will suffice. If ureteric reimplantation has been undertaken, then a ^{99m}Tc-DTPA scan is essential to ensure that no obstruction has resulted following surgery and also that reflux has been cured.

When renal scarring is found, long-term follow-up (after UTI and VUR have ceased) is necessary because of the increased incidence of

Table 20.6.
Investigations on First Documented UTI

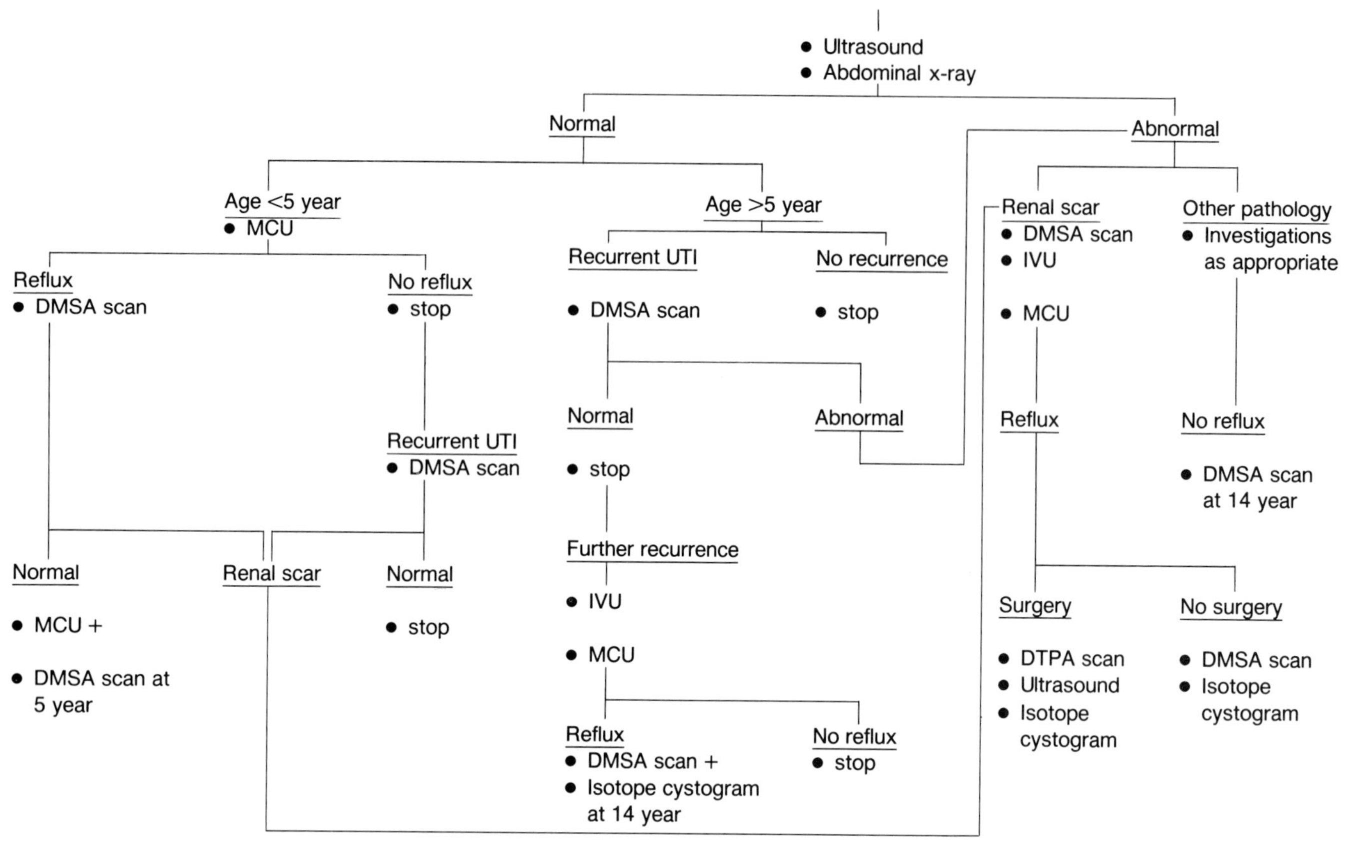

hypertension and the occasional development of CRF. These children require regular, although infrequent, imaging. Ultrasound plus a ^{99m}Tc-DMSA scan every 2 to 4 years is probably adequate, or a ^{99m}Tc-DTPA scan can be combined with IKGFR measurements and micturating views.

In recent years, pediatric ultrasonographers and nuclear medicine specialists have combined to question the accepted techniques of IVU and MCU for the investigation of UTI, and the scheme presented represents but one contemporary view. However, this is a dynamic field, which is in a constant state of evolution, and as new experimental information comes to light and the prospective clinical trials draw to a close, there will be a need to reevaluate the protocol for investigation. Schemes for imaging of children with UTI and VUR should not be regarded as definitive (Table 20.6).

Renal infection may be secondary to bacteremia or septicemia. In this case, the clinical setting is that of a very ill child with a tender loin and leukocytosis. The urinalysis does not necessarily show a UTI. The IVU changes are those of a big kidney that does not concentrate the contrast well with compression of the calyces. The renal outlines may be lost with scoliosis concave to the tender side, if unilateral. The ultrasound shows a large echographically bright kidney compared with the opposite side, or it may be normal. The ^{99m}Tc-DMSA scan allows the poorly functioning areas to be demonstrated clearly. Progress of the condition can be monitored by ultrasound and ^{99m}Tc-DMSA scans. In the infant who has recovered, a limited IVU may be undertaken if acute renal failure complicated the infection, to ensure that medullary necrosis has not ensued (Fig. 20.15).

Obstruction

The rigorous definition of urinary obstruction remains elusive. It has been defined by pressure/flow measurements in the renal pelvis showing a rise of >22 mm Hg with a flow of 10 ml/min (50), a progressive increase of isotope in the collecting systems following IV furosemide during a ^{99m}Tc-DTPA scan (27), or the appearance of a dilated collecting system on IVU that does not drain after furosemide. Other definitions have been used, but the problem is that one test is compared with a second and there are no absolute criteria on which to validate the results.

Diagnosis

When there is an acute obstruction, the clinical story is usually that of loin pain and an IVU during the acute episode shows a delayed dense nephrogram with contrast, subsequently accumulating in the dilated collecting system. With a delayed film, the level of the obstruction usually can be judged, for the contrast collects proximally. In such circumstances, the diagnosis is not in doubt. This is, however, a rather uncommon presentation for obstruction in childhood, for the lesions, being usually congenital in origin, are generally of long-standing and only partial in degree (Fig. 20.5).

A common presentation is with vague abdominal pain or UTI. When certain congenital renal abnormalities are discovered in association with a dilated collecting system, the diagnosis can be inferred with confidence, for example, a duplex collecting system with an ectopic ureterocele and a dilated ureter draining the upper moiety.

Diagnostic difficulties arise in two groups of children. First, in those with vague abdominal symptoms who have dilated renal pelvis on IVU, the question arises whether the dilatation is secondary to an obstruction at the PUJ or is merely a manifestation of a floppy extrarenal pelvis. The second group of patients is those in whom dilated collecting systems persist after urological surgery for presumed obstruction. Commonly, there is diminished renal function in these patients, as for example following urethral valve resection or reimplantation of an obstructive megaureter, but rarely following pyeloplasty for PUJ obstruction. In such circumstances, the collecting system may be placed under stress by promoting a diuresis. The passage of the isotope through the kidney is delayed, and by deconvolution analysis the transit time can be determined, either as the whole kidney (50) transit time, or, if a suitable area can be identified, the parenchymal transit time (51). Alternatively, obstruction can be defined by measuring the pressure in the renal pelvis during antegrade perfusion.

These two tests, the radioisotope dynamic renal scan with furosemide and antegrade pressure-flow measurements, are the only accepted means of diagnosing obstruction. When there is good renal function associated with the pelvic dilatation, either test is adequate. However, when the kidney has poor function, neither is reliable in excluding obstruction. The more severe the dilatation of the ureter the more unreliable are these two tests because of the difficulty in allowing for the capacious urinary reservoir.

Using the dynamic isotope scan and furosemide, one may confidently exclude PUJ obstruction if there is an adequate response. Failure to obtain an adequate response in the presence of good renal function is suggestive of an obstruction. No single investigation is foolproof, the intermittent nature of some PUJ obstructions means that there will always be a group of children who remain in the group "equivocal."

Long-term Follow-up

All children who have had urinary obstruction relieved need long-term follow-up. Inevitably some degree of renal damage with dilatation of the collecting system remains. The ^{99m}Tc-DTPA scan with furosemide is the most convenient test, for it provides IKGFR, parenchymal transit time, whole kidney transit time, and the response to furosemide. When done sequentially, both preoperatively and at regular intervals postoperatively, the best comparative data about the function of each individual kidney will be obtained and deterioration detected rapidly. Ultrasound is less reliable, as the degree of dilatation of the collecting system varies during the day and with the urine flow rate.

Abdominal Mass

The discovery of an abdominal mass in a child always raises the possibility of malignancy. For this reason, no time should be lost in ensuring an adequate examination.

Differential Diagnosis

A renal mass may result from an obstruction, usually at the PUJ, and is transonic on ultrasound; a cystic change, either multicystic or polycystic; a tumor, particularly nephroblastoma and mesoblastic nephroma; or xanthogranulomatous pyelonephritis. Nonrenal masses to be considered may arise from the bladder, as obstruction to outflow or tumor; adrenal, as neuroblastoma, pheochromocytoma or other adrenal tumor, or adrenal hemorrhage; retroperitoneal, as teratoma, small round cell tumor, or lymphoma; gut, as mesenteric or duplication cyst, or lymphoma; liver, such tumors as hamartoma, hepatoblastoma, or secondaries; or ovary, as cyst or teratoma.

Imaging Protocol

Once a mass has been detected imaging must be undertaken immediately. The aims of imaging are to determine from which organ it originates; to determine if the mass is solid, suggesting tumor, or cystic; and to ascertain, if the mass is solid, the local extent and the possibility of involvement of other organs, particularly liver, inferior vena cava, and lymph nodes. The combination of high quality ultrasound with a plain abdominal x-ray and chest x-ray is the foundation. The ultrasound will differentiate between a transonic mass (almost always benign) and solid masses (frequently malignant). When a solid lesion is found then spread of disease within the abdomen must be sought. The ultrasound frequently identifies the origin in the mass. The plain abdominal film may reveal calcification, e.g., with neuroblastoma, dermoid, or Wilms' tumor.

When a solid mass is found then a posteroanterior and lateral chest x-ray are essential to exclude secondary deposits. A limited IVU is also indicated since distinction between a neuroblastoma and nephroblastoma may be very difficult on ultrasound but critical for management.

If a solid lesion is diagnosed in one kidney then histological confirmation of the suspected diagnosis must be undertaken. Solid intrarenal lesions on ultrasound necessitate an IVU and also a careful ultrasound examination of the contralateral kidney. Arteriography is limited to those cases with solid lesions in both kidneys (bilateral nephroblastoma) or with a mass in a single, horseshoe, or a crossed-fused ectopic kidney. A CT scan is very helpful in difficult cases.

An example of a benign mass that is solid on ultrasound is infantile polycystic kidney; in this case, both kidneys are usually enlarged, and delayed images on the IVU are usually diagnostic. Tuberous sclerosis also may give bilateral solid masses. If the renal mass is transonic, the inference is that there is a collection of fluid and urinary obstruction must be considered. Other possibilities are adult polycystic disease and tuberous sclerosis. Both these conditions are bilateral. Tuberous sclerosis rarely presents as an abdominal mass and may have mixed echogenic pattern, depending on age (52).

Neonate

The commonest abdominal mass in an otherwise healthy neonate is a multicystic kidney (Fig. 20.17), but other renal masses include infantile polycystic disease, "adult" polycystic disease with infantile presentation (usually bilateral), an obstructive uropathy (commonly at the PUJ), gross dilatation without obstruction (prune belly syndrome), and tumor (mesoblastic nephroma). Extrarenal masses include neuroblastoma, teratoma, and mesenteric cyst among other causes. In a sick neonate, either with sepsis or renal failure, an abdominal mass may be a result of renal venous thrombosis, medullary necrosis, acute hematogenous pyelonephritis, an obstructive uropathy, or adrenal hemorrhage (which may coexist with venous thrombosis). The first investigation is an ultrasound, which establishes whether the mass is renal or extrarenal. A transonic renal mass may be due to obstructive uropathy, a dilated nonobstructive collecting system, a multicystic kidney, or adult polycystic disease in infancy. A solid renal mass may be a mesoblastic nephroma, hypernephroma, infantile polycystic kidneys, renal venous thrombosis (Fig. 20.18), an acute septic kidney, or a neuroblastoma. With a multicystic kidney, careful attention must be focused on the opposite kidney, which determines the prognosis. The ultrasound may be able to give a definitive diagnosis in certain situations, such as multicystic kidney, but does not offer information in respect to function.

Functional details about the kidneys are now required. A ^{99m}Tc-DTPA is indicated when obstructive uropathy, venous thrombosis, multicystic kidney (Fig. 20.16), or prune belly syndrome is suspected. When the suggested ultrasound diagnosis is polycystic disease or an extrarenal mass, then an IVU without dehydration is appropriate. If a renal tumor is suspected at this age, a ^{99m}Tc-DMSA scan is adequate since Wilms'

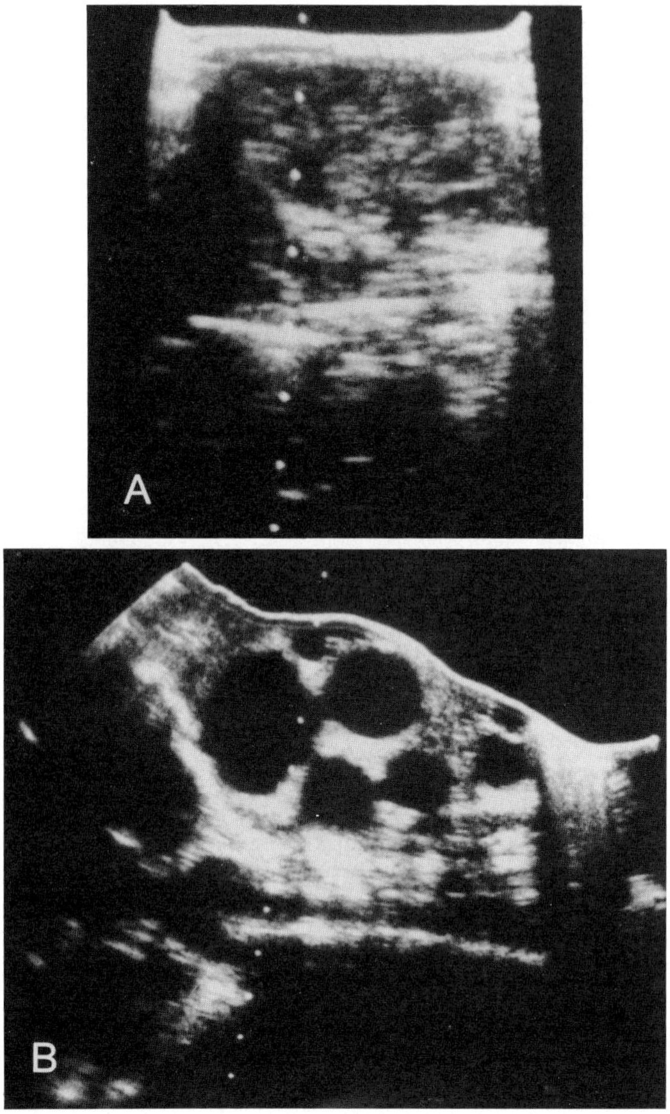

Figure 20.17. This neonate was found to have an abdominal mass after delivery. The ultrasound scan reveals one normal kidney. The mass is noted to contain multiple transonic areas, none of which are in communication. This appearance is typical of a multicystic kidney. A functional study must be carried out to assess the opposite kidney.

tumors are very rare in the neonate. The more probable diagnosis is a mesoblastic nephroma, which takes up the ^{99m}Tc-DMSA. An MCU is required if the collecting systems are dilated, but must be carefully integrated with the overall urological management of the case.

Scarred Kidney

The sensitivity with which an abnormality in the kidney may be detected depends on the technique of imaging used (Table 20.1). An apparently normal kidney on IVU and ultrasound may turn out on the DMSA scan to have a scar. On the other hand, the IVU may be more informative about the pathogenesis of what appears on the DMSA scan to be a small kidney (Fig. 20.18) because of the calyceal detail provided (Fig. 20.18) (Table 20.2).

Intravenous Urogram

A normal kidney is characterized by a smooth outline, with indentations between draining calyces due to fetal lobulation. The length of the kidney measures approximately 3 to $3\frac{1}{2}$ vertebral bodies, including the intervening disc spaces. The calyceal fornices describe a line roughly parallel to the renal outline and show the delicate architecture of a fornix with a cup. The axis of the kidney is such that the upper pole calyces are medial to those of the lower pole, with almost as much renal parenchyma in the upper as in the lower pole. A scar results in loss of renal parenchyma and focal depression of the renal outline which, in the upper pole, results in a more medial location of the calyces, i.e., the calyces are too close to the spine. The calyx itself is abnormal, with loss of the delicate architecture and clubbing of the fornix to some degree.

A small kidney has a reduced long axis, i.e., less than 3 vertebral bodies in length, and may or may not be associated with focal scarring or calyceal abnormality, depending on the etiology. When a small kidney is present and no VUR is seen on MCU, the IVU offers the best possibility of distinguishing the various causes (Table 20.1). When there is focal pathology of the renal parenchyma with loss of renal substance, then the renal outline (if in profile) may be lost on the IVU since the distinction between perinephric fat and contrast in the kidney is lost. The loss of the renal outline is of prime importance in detecting pathology. However, overlying colonic content or the use of the wrong exposure factors may obscure the renal outline. Furthermore, the preservation of the outline does not exclude pathology in that portion of the kidney that is not on the periphery of the particular view. Therefore, it can be concluded that though a high quality IVU demonstrating pathology is a rewarding examination, a normal examination does not exclude a significant scar.

Ultrasound

There are certain areas that are difficult to visualize adequately with ultrasound, particularly the upper pole of the left kidney, which may be hidden behind the twelfth rib posteriorly and behind the stomach anteriorly. With real-time ultrasound on line to a computer it is now becoming feasible to measure overall renal volume. Ultrasound may detect the small kidney (48), renal calculi, the dilated collecting system, and also give a view of the echo pattern of the renal cortex relative to the medulla. When pathology is detected, it is usually a true positive result; however, when the ultrasound examination reveals two normal kidneys, significant renal scarring, renovascular disease, or a duplex system cannot be excluded. Failure of ultrasound to demonstrate the presence of a kidney does not necessarily mean there is no kidney present. The suggestion of an absent kidney on ultrasound should be followed by a ^{99m}Tc-DMSA scan.

DMSA Scan

The ^{99m}Tc-DMSA scan is the most reliable technique for detecting focal renal disease (31). Diagnoses that are readily made include the small kidney, renal scarring, renal ectopia, horseshoe kidney, and intrarenal vascular disease. Focal areas of decreased function may be seen immediately after UTI, which is some instances returns to normal but in others is followed by a scar. The limitation of the DMSA is its inability to define the etiology of a small kidney (Table II) or of photon-deficient areas.

^{99m}Tc-DTPA Scan

The ^{99m}Tc-DTPA scan offers the least amount of anatomical information, but is the most accurate in the assessment of individual renal function.

Hypertension

Primary (essential) hypertension is a rare finding in children with severe hypertension, but is common in those with mild or borderline hypertension (53). The most common cause of severe hypertension is

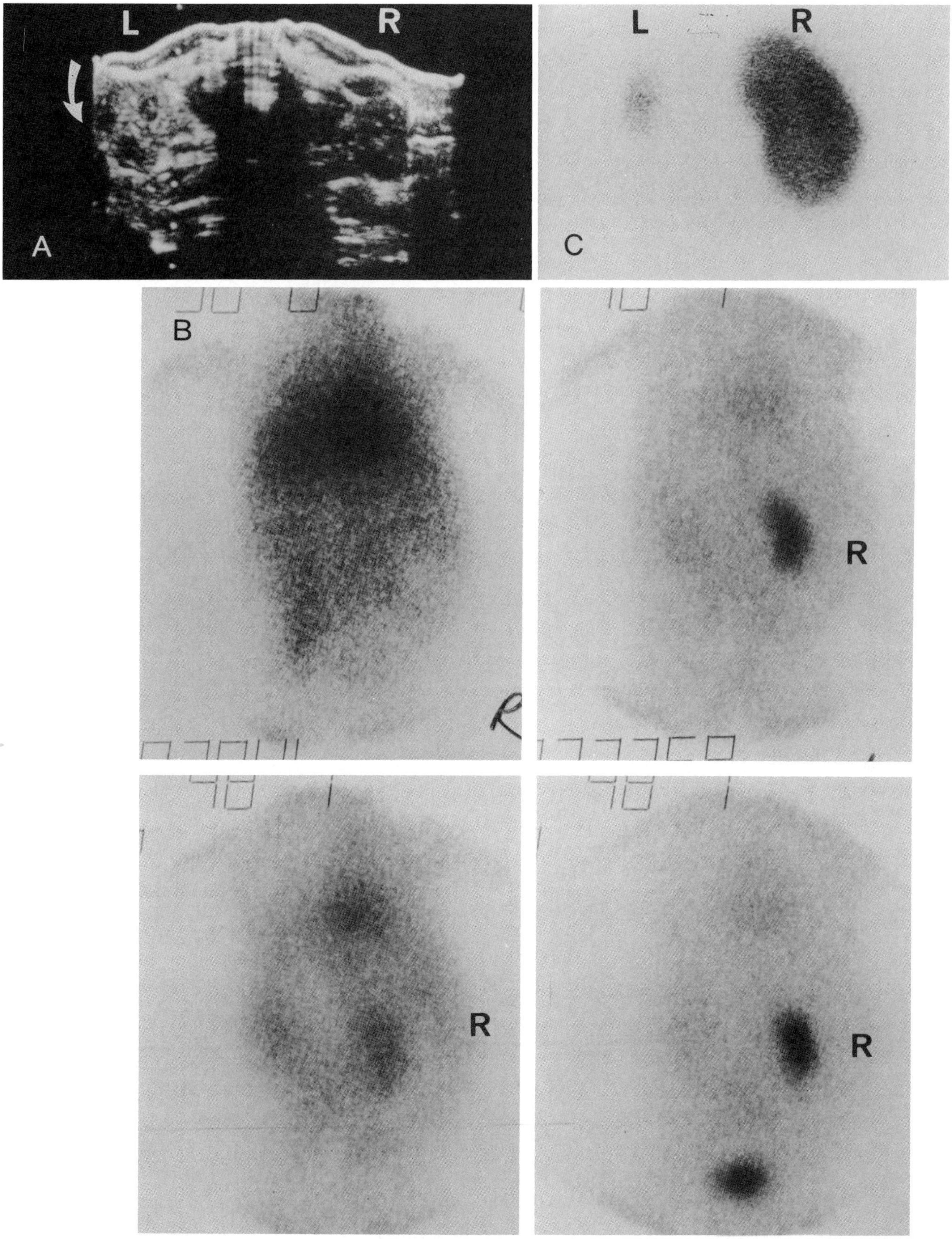

Figure 20.18. A neonate had a stormy delivery and required intensive resuscitation; subsequently he developed hematuria and a palpable left kidney. **A,** The transverse prone ultrasound shows a large bright kidney (*arrow*). **B,** A ^{99m}Tc-DTPA scan, at the age of 6 days, showed a normal right kidney and a poorly functioning left kidney, which was still palpable. **C,** A follow-up ^{99m}Tc-DMSA scan 3 years later revealed a normal right kidney that contributed 95% to overall function and a small shrunken left kidney, confirming the diagnosis of renal venous thrombosis.

renal disease. Severe or sustained hypertension needs prompt investigation directed at discovering both the cause and assessment of the complications of the raised blood pressure. The latter relies mainly on clinical examination and radiology offers help in assessing the heart and central nervous system.

Imaging plays an important role in diagnosis, the aim being to define renal anatomy. If a small or a scarred kidney is found, the underlying cause of this abnormality must be sought. If two normal-sized kidneys with smooth outlines are found, renal arterial pathology may be the underlying cause of the hypertension. The routine should be an abdominal ultrasound and ^{99m}Tc-DMSA scan. These two examinations will pick up the small kidney, the renal scar (31), the dilated collecting system, and intrarenal arterial disease (30). If both these examinations are normal, the only diagnoses that have not been excluded are abdominal aortic coarctation or main renal artery stenosis (54).

The IVU is no longer the crucial investigation in the hypertensive child nor should it be the first imaging procedure undertaken. Rapid sequence films should be discouraged since they involve a high radiation dose and are a very crude method of detecting renal perfusion. There are many series of renal hypertension tension with a normal IVU (55–57), and others with a pick-up rate of renal abnormalities between 24% (58, 59) to 65% (60). Dynamic renal scans have a variable pick-up rate reported in the literature, and ^{99m}Tc-DTPA scans in children have proved disappointing (61). ^{123}I-hippuran with the higher extraction fraction is theoretically a better agent to use when looking for main renal artery stenosis.

Vascular studies should be carried out in children in whom no diagnosis is established on ultrasound and ^{99m}Tc-DMSA or in whom the only abnormality is on ^{99m}Tc-DMSA scan, since these children may warrant angioplasty or surgical treatment.

Before arteriography, digital vascular imaging (DVI) should be undertaken to delineate the aorta and main renal arteries. Vascular studies include both venous sampling, including segmental renal venous sampling for renin determination, and arteriography. These two examinations are complementary and are generally performed as one combined procedure, the venous sampling being done first. Aortography must not be undertaken until the hypertension is well controlled. Selective renal artery injections are required (54). A team approach to this investigation is essential if maximum information is to be obtained (Fig. 20.12).

References

1. Sigman EM, Elwood CM, Knox F: The measurement of glomerular filtration rate in man with sodium iothalamate ^{131}I (Conray). J Nucl Med 7:60, 1966.
2. Bianchi C, Coli A, Gallucci L, et al: The measurement of glomerular filtration rate in children by ^{131}I hypaque and external counting. J Nucl Biol Med 11:144, 1967.
3. Cohen ML, Smith FG, Mandell RS, et al: A simple, reliable method of measuring glomerular filtration rate using single, low dose sodium iothalamate ^{131}I. Pediatrics 43:407, 1969.
4. Grainger RG: Formulation and clinical introduction of low osmolar contrast medium. In Proceedings of Symposium on Iopamidol, Oxford, 1982. Franklyn Scientific Projects, London, 1983, p 1078.
5. Grainger RC: Osmolality of intravascular radiological contrast media. Brit J Radiol 53:739, 1980.
6. Partridge JB, Robinson PJ, Turnbull CM, et al: Clinical cardiovascular experiences with iopamidol: a new non-ionic contrast media. Clin Radiol 32:451, 1981.
7. Dawson P, Grainger RC, Pitfield J: The new low osmolar contrast media. A simple guide. Clin Radiol 34:221, 1983.
8. Lasser EC, Lang JH, Hamblin AE, et al: Activation systems in contrast idiosyncrasy. Invest Radiol 15 (suppl):2, 1980.
9. Gordon I: Renal diagnostic imaging. In Williams DI, Johnston JH (eds): Paediatric Urology, ed 2. London, Butterworth, 1982, p 11.
10. Lucas A: The window view of the renal area in infants and children. Radiography 45:216, 1979.
11. Hodson CJ, Drewe JA, Karn MN, et al: Renal size in normal children, a radiological study during life. Arch Dis Childh 35:616, 1962.
12. Eklof O, Ringertz H: Kidney size in children. A method of assessment. Acta Radiol Diagn 17:617, 1976.
13. Gordon I: Renal diagnostic imaging. In Williams DI, Johnston JH (eds): Paediatric Urology, ed 2. London, Butterworth, 1982, p 23.
14. Johnston JH, Harrison N: Investigation of bladder function. In Williams DI, Johnston JH (eds): Paediatric Urology, ed 2. London, Butterworth, 1982, p 216.
15. Liebowitz RL: Post-operative Paediatric Uroradiology. New York, Appleton-Century-Crofts, 1981.
16. Kirks DR, Fritz CR, Harwood-Nash DC: Paediatric abdominal angiography, a practical guide to catheter selection, flow rates and contrast doses, Pediat Radiol 5:19, 1976.
17. Stanley P: In Stanley P (ed): Pediatric Angiography, Baltimore, Williams & Wilkins, 1982, p 11.
18. Pritchard J, Gordon I: Retroperitoneum. N Engl J Med 305:285, 1981.
19. Haller JO, Schneider MD. In Haller JO, Schneider MD (eds): Pediatric Ultrasound. Chicago, Year Book Publishers, 1980.
20. Berger PE, Munschauer RW, Kuhn JP: Computed tomography and ultrasound of renal and perirenal diseases in infants and children. Pediat Radiol 9:91, 1980.
21. Shan KJ: Beckwith-Wiedemann syndrome: role of ultrasound in its management. Clin Radiol 34:313, 1983.
22. Chrispin AR, Gordon I, Hall CM, et al: In Diagnostic Imaging of the Kidney and Urinary Tract in Children. Berlin, Springer International, 1980, p 19.
23. Britton KE, Maisey MN: Renal radionuclide studies. In Britton K, Maisey MN, Gilday D (eds): Clinical Nuclear Medicine. London, Chapman & Hall, p 68.
24. Bingham JB, Maisey MN: An evaluation of the use of ^{99m}Tc-dimercaptosuccinic acid (DMSA) as a static renal imaging agent. Brit J Radiol 51:599, 1979.
25. Pieretti R, Gilday D, Jeffs R: Differential kidney scans in paediatric urology. Urology 4:665, 1974.
26. Piepsz A, Denis R, Ham R, et al: A simple method for measuring separate glomerular filtration rate using a single injection of ^{99m}Tc-DTPA and the scintillation camera. J Pediatr 93:769, 1978.
27. Koff SA, Thrall JH, Keyes JW: Assessment of hydroureteronephrosis in children using diuretic radionuclide urography. J Urol 123:531, 1980.
28. O'Reilly PH, Testa HJ, Lawson RS, et al: Diuresis renography in equivocal urinary tract obstruction. Brit J Urol 50:76, 1978.
29. Gordon I: Use of frusemide-DTPA scans in distinguishing dilatation with obstruction from dilatation without obstruction in paediatrics. Brit Nucl Med Soc Meeting, 1981, (abstract).
30. Vivian G, Stringer D, deBruyn R, et al: ^{99m}Tc-DMSA scans in renovascular hypertension in children. Proc Third World Congress Nuclear Med Biol Paris, France, Pergamon IV, 1982, p 2663.
31. Merrick MV, Uttley WAS, Wild SR: The detection of pyelonephritic scarring in children by radioisotope imaging. Brit J Radiol 53:544, 1980.
32. Conway JJ, Kruglik GD: Effectiveness of direct and indirect radionuclide cystography in detecting vesico-ureteric reflux. J Nucl Med 17:81, 1976.
33. Rothwell DL, Constable AR, Albrecht M: Radionuclide cystography in the investigation of vesico-ureteric reflux in children. Lancet 1:1072, 1977.
34. Pollet JE, Sharp PF, Smith FW: Radionuclide imaging for vesico-renal reflux using intravenous ^{99m}Tc-DTPA. Pediatr Radiol 8:165, 1979.
35. Hedman PJK, Kempi V, Voss H: Measurement of vesico-ureteric reflux with intravenous ^{99m}Tc-DTPA compared to radiographic cystography. Radiology 126:205, 1978.
36. Cremin BJ: Observations on vesico-ureteric reflux and intrarenal reflux. A review and survey of material. Clin Radiol 30:607, 1979.
37. Gilday D: Special clinical problems in paediatrics. In Britton K, Maisey NM, Gilday DP (eds): Clinical Nuclear Medicine. London, Chapman and Hall, 1983, p 163.
38. Goden CJ, Tsai SH, Smith SJ, et al: Diagnostic strategy in evaluation of renal abscess. Urology 18:535, 1981.
39. James AW, Wagner HN, Cooke RE: In Paediatric Nuclear Medicine, ed 1. Philadelphia, W. B. Saunders, 1974.
40. Fowler CL, Torrado A, Guignard JP: Single injection clearance in the neonate. Biol Neonate 35:321, 1979.
41. Strauss J, Daniel SS, James LS: Post-natal adjustments in renal function. Pediatrics 68:802, 1981.
42. Aperia A, Broberger O, Elinder G, et al: Post-natal development of renal function in preterm and full term infants. Acta Pediat Scand 70:183, 1981.
43. Edelmann CM, Barnett HL, Troupkov V: Renal concentrating mechanism in newborn infants. J Clin Invest 39:1062, 1960.
44. Athey PA, Carpenter RJ, Hadlock FP, et al: Ultrasonic demonstration of ectopic ureterocoele. Paediatrics 71:568, 1983.
45. Saxcna SR, Lawrence BM, Shaw DG: The justification for early radiological investigation of urinary tract in children. Lancet 2:403, 1975.

46. Asscher WA: Sequelae of urinary tract infection. In The Challenge of Urinary Tract Infections. London, Academic Press, 1980, p 122.
47. Cardiff-Oxford Bacteriuria Study Group. The sequelae of urinary tract infections in schoolgirls. A four-year follow-up study. Lancet 1:889, 1978.
48. Jequier S, Borges M, Forbes P, et al: The value of ultrasound examination as a screening procedure in first documented urinary tract infection in children. Pediat Radiol 13:173, 1983.
49. Christophe C, Bogaert C, Spehl M, et al: Ultrasound of pyelonephritis. Pediatrics 13:173, 1983.
50. Piepsz A, Ham HP, Erbsman F, et al: A cooperative study on the clinical value of dynamic renal scanning with deconvolutional analysis. Brit J Radiol 55:419, 1982.
51. Whitfield HN, Britton KE, Hendry WF, et al: The distinction between obstructive uropathy and nephropathy by radioisotope transit times. Brit J Urol 50:433, 1978.
52. Avni EF, Szliwowski H, Spehl M, et al: A spectrum of renal involvement in tuberous sclerosis. Pediatrics 13:174, 1983.
53. Leumann EP: Blood pressure and hypertension in childhood and adolescence. Ergeb Inn Med Kinderheilk 43:109, 1979.
54. Stringer DA, deBruyn R, Dillon MJ, et al: Comparison of aortography, renal vein renin sampling, radionuclide scans, ultrasound and the IVU in the investigation of childhood renovascular hypertension. Brit J Radiol 57:111, 1983.
55. Rance CP, Arbus GS, Balfe JW: Persistent systemic hypertension in infants and children. Pediat Clin N Am 21:801, 1974.
56. Clayman AA, Bookstein JJ: The role of renal arteriography in paediatric hypertension. Radiology 108:107, 1973.
57. Korobkin M, Perloff DL, Palububsjas AJ: Renal arteriography in the evaluation of unexplained hypertension in children and adolescents. J Pediatr 88:388, 1976.
58. Stanley JC, Fry WJ: Surgical treatment of renovascular hypertension. Arch Surg 112:1291, 1977.
59. Broyer M, Bacri JL, Royer P: Renal forms of hypertension in children. Report on 238 cases. In Giovanelli G, New MI, Gorini S (eds): Hypertension in Children and Adolescents. New York, Raven Press, 1981, p 161.
60. Stanley P, Gyepes MT, Olson DL: Renovascular hypertension in children and adolescents. Radiology 129:123, 1978.
61. Gordon I, de Bruyn R, Stringer DA, et al: Technetium-^{99m}-DMSA scan. A sensitive index of renal perfusion in hypertension. In Jewkes R, Constable AR, Brown NJR, et al (eds): Radionuclides in Nephrology. Proceedings of the SVI Int Symposium, New York, Academic Press, 1981, p 205.

CHAPTER 21

Renal Biopsy in Children

ALFONSO CAMPOS
ROBERT L. VERNIER

Percutaneous renal biopsy was introduced in 1944 by Alwall (1) and first used systematically in the study of kidney disease by Iversen and Brun (2). Modification of the original technique and introduction of the modified Franklin-Silverman needle (3) led to application of the method throughout the world, and renal biopsy is now a safe and essential part of the management of patients with renal disease. The technique offers invaluable aid in the diagnosis, and has contributed to the understanding of the causes, pathogenesis, natural history, and forms of treatment in many kidney diseases. Its value depends on the type of disease, the adequacy and quality of preparation of the sample, and the availability of a competent and experienced pathologist. We present our views on renal biopsy, including indications, contraindications, evaluation and preparation of the patient, imaging methods, actual biopsy technique, and possible complications. Although not intended to provide a detailed pathological analysis, a brief review of the methods used in interpretation of renal biopsy specimens is also presented.

INDICATIONS

There are differences in opinion regarding the indications for a renal biopsy, but in any case, the potential benefits to the patient must outweigh the risks involved. We believe that a kidney biopsy should be done whenever evaluation of the renal tissue is likely to provide better understanding of the disease process and will facilitate optimal planning of therapy and aid in establishing a prognosis.

Hematuria

Microscopic hematuria is a common isolated finding in otherwise asymptomatic patients, and in many instances, it is transient (4, 5). Because acute poststreptococcal glomerulonephritis (APSGN) is still one of the most common causes of transient microscopic hematuria, it remains an important differential consideration, especially in children. Evidence of streptococcal infection with elevated anti-DNAase B titer or streptozyme test and transient hypocomplementemia strongly suggest the diagnosis. If the clinical course is compatible with APSGN, a biopsy is usually not indicated. Idiopathic hypercalciuria should also be considered in the differential diagnosis of microscopic hematuria; an elevated urinary calcium: creatinine ratio will give a clue to the correct diagnosis (6, 7).

Other studies of persistent hematuria should also be selected to rule out urinary tract infection (UTI), chronic glomerulonephritis, renal cystic disease, anatomic abnormalities, familial nephritis, lithiasis, hematologic disorders, and bleeding diatheses (8). All black children with hematuria should be evaluated for sickle cell trait or disease. Cystoscopy should not be part of the routine evaluation of microscopic hematuria in children, because it is unlikely to provide sufficient useful information to justify the trauma and the risk of general anesthesia. Cystoscopy is more useful in those patients with gross hematuria, dysuria, and sterile urine cultures. If, after the initial studies, the cause of hematuria is still uncertain, regular follow-up is all that is indicated provided that proteinuria is absent and the renal function and blood pressure are normal.

Should the isolated microscopic hematuria persist for more than a year, it may be important to know, for reasons of insurability, military service, organ donation, parental anxiety, and soon, whether the patient has a potentially serious disease. Under these circumstances, examination of a kidney biopsy specimen may allow definitive diagnosis of important diseases, such as IgA nephropathy or hereditary nephritis, and provide important prognostic information (9, 10). In these circumstances, the finding of "normal kidney" after thorough study may also have important implications for selected patients.

Microscopic hematuria associated with proteinuria almost invariably signals acute or chronic glomerulonephritis. Detection of a low serum complement narrows the differential diagnosis (11). Unless there is strong evidence for APSGN, renal biopsy is usually indicated.

Macroscopic hematuria in the adult patient usually suggests urinary tract malignancy, lithiasis, or infection. In children and young adults, however, IgA-IgG nephropathy is the single most common cause of intermittent gross hematuria (chapter 26D).

Proteinuria

Asymptomatic proteinuria is a common finding in the pediatric population (5, 12). Although most often proteinuria is intermittent, some children may develop persistent proteinuria. If hematuria is excluded and the renal function, radiographic studies, serum complement, and blood pressure are normal, intermittent proteinuria, even though substantial (0.5–1.0 gm/day), is not usually associated with definable histological glomerular abnormalities (12), therefore, renal biopsy is not indicated.

In the older child and young adult, the most frequent cause of persistent asymptomatic proteinuria is orthostatic proteinuria, a normal variant that should be ruled out in the initial evaluation (13). Fixed or persistent orthostatic proteinuria has been found to be of no major significance in young adults (13). However, similar long-term follow-up data does not exist in large numbers of children and there remains some concern about fixed orthostatic proteinuria as an early marker of significant renal disease. However, renal biopsy findings in a small group of these patients revealed no significant or consistent abnormalities (14) and therefore biopsy may not be indicated, but rather continued clinical observation.

Persistent proteinuria is often the first sign of many diseases and should be investigated. It may represent congenital anomalies, reflux nephropathy, renal cystic disease, hereditary nephritis, membrano proliferative glomerulonephritis (MPGN), focal sclerosis, membranous nephropathy, or subclinical nephrotic syndrome (8).

Evaluation of a child with persistent asymptomatic proteinuria should include 24-hour urine protein excretion, creatinine clearances, serum complement levels, serum total proteins and albumin, cholesterol, urine cultures, and radiographic studies. If urine cultures are negative and no anatomic abnormalities are detected, renal biopsy may be helpful in the patient with persistence of significant proteinuria (arbitrarily, duration of more than 6 months or excretion of more than 1 gram/24 hours), in the presence of hypertension, hematuria, impaired renal function, or unexplained hypocomplementemia.

Nephrotic Syndrome

Nephrotic syndrome (NS) is characterized by severe proteinuria and subsequent hypoalbuminemia, edema, and hyperlipidemia and is associated with a wide spectrum of pathological changes, ranging from minimal change disease, focal sclerosis, and mesangial proliferation, to MPGN and membranous nephropathy (chapters 26 and 28). It may be primary or idiopathic or secondary to systemic diseases such as SLE, Henoch-Schönlein nephritis, diabetes, familial nephritis, amyloidosis, malignancies or drugs (15, 16, 17).

Primary nephrotic syndrome accounts for over 90% of the cases diagnosed in children (15, 16, 17), with minimal change disease being by far the most common pathological lesion. Clinical, laboratory, and therapeutic correlations in idiopathic NS allows a reasonable prediction of minimal change disease versus the other histopathological types (16, 17). Based on the experience of the past 30 years, the indication for renal biopsy in children with the nephrotic syndrome have changed markedly and include the following relatively restricted groups of the total population:

1. The nephrotic child in the first year of life (chapter 26F).
2. The older child with nephrotic syndrome. Since the percentage incidence of the minimal lesion and steroid responsive disease decreases sharply after age 8, this older population of children is more likely to present the wide range of histological lesions seen in adults with NS and renal biopsy is more likely to be helpful in the development of an optimal therapeutic plan.
3. The child with demonstrated resistance to a 6 to 8 week course of adrenocorticosteroid therapy.
4. The child with the frequently relapsing or steroid dependent course, who may be a candidate for cytotoxic therapy.
5. The child with any unusual clinical or laboratory manifestation such as hypertension, hypocomplementemia, gross hematuria, or persistently abnormal renal function.

Glomerulonephritis

With the exception of typical APSGN, renal biopsy is often indicated to establish the diagnosis and to reveal the extent and the specifics of the histopathology of the kidney in the child with either clinically acute or chronic glomerulonephritis. Since the available therapy for glomerulonephritis in all its forms is controversial and potentially harmful (chapter 29), careful study of the renal tissue and quantitative assessment of the type and extent of the injury is usually a necessary step in consideration of therapy of glomerulonephritis.

In the glomerulonephritis associated with systemic manifestations, such as Henoch-Schönlein's purpura, the vast majority of children recover with supportive care alone. The higher risk group for chronic renal injury and progression to renal failure includes those older than 7 years of age and those with nephritic/nephrotic syndrome (18). The presence of glomerular crescents have been described as a poor prognostic sign and such patients may be candidates for various therapies that can only be considered experimental at this time.

Systemic lupus erythematosus (chapter 28B) is frequently associated with glomerulonephritis, which is the major cause of mortality in this disease. The correlations of clinical and laboratory manifestations with the severity and form of the glomerular lesions are imperfect and numerous exceptions have been reported (19, 20). In addition, the glomerular lesions found in a given patient at any time in the course, frequently undergo transition to another histopathological varient during subsequent exacerbations (21, 22). The assessment of the pathological renal changes and the systematic scoring of both the acute and chronic glomerular and interstitial lesions (22, 23) may allow a more intelligent and effective utilization of available therapy. Thus most investigators advocate judicial use of sequential renal biopsy specimens in the management of this chronic renal disease.

Acute Renal Failure

The differential diagnosis of acute renal failure (ARF) includes a variety of disorders, but with the proper use of clinical, laboratory, and radiological techniques, the etiology can usually be identified in the majority of cases (24). Patients in whom the diagnosis of acute tubular necrosis can be confidently made do not require a kidney biopsy. However, this may not be an easy task and it is not unusual to find an unsuspected etiology through renal biopsy of patients with ARF (24, 25). This is emphasized by a study of unselected adult patients with ARF in whom biopsy findings influenced the choice of medical therapy in 20% of patients (26). However, the conditions that cause ARF in children are different than the ones in adults and no similar study is available in regard to pediatric patients with ARF.

In general, the indications for renal biopsy in ARF include the following: (1) when the cause of ARF is in doubt after full investigation, (2) severe oligoanuria lasting more than 2 to 3 weeks, (3) the presence of extra renal manifestation of a more diffuse disease, and (4) to exclude the possibility of acute interstitial nephritis in those patients who require continued therapy with the alleged etiologic medication (27).

Before performing a biopsy in acute renal failure, careful attention must be given to correction of hypertension, uremia, thrombocytopenia, and bleeding diathesis. This may require the use of hemodialysis with protamine reversal, infusion of cryoprecipitate (28), platelet transfusions, and antihypertensive therapy.

Renal Transplants

Several reports have described the utility and safety of percutaneous biopsy of renal transplants (29, 30, 31, 32, 33, 34, 35) and biopsy of renal allograft are increasingly recognized as an important method in the management of transplant recipients (chapter 52). Although the percutaneous biopsy of a solitary native kidney entails unacceptable risks, those risks do not seem to apply to the transplanted kidney, which is located superficially in the iliac fossa. The incidence of gross hematuria, perirenal hematoma, and other potential complications are equal to or less than those associated with open surgical biopsies of transplanted kidneys (36). Moreover, the biopsy sample usually provides more representative information of changes occurring throughout the kidney (31). Renal biopsy specimens are helpful in allowing a more precise diagnosis of renal dysfunction, especially rejection (31, 32), evaluation of prolonged post operative oligoanuria (37), proteinuria/hematuria (28), glomerulopathy associated with infections (38), diagnosis of recurrence of original disease (39, 40), the de novo development of glomerulonephritis (41), and cyclosporine nephrotoxicity (42).

The diagnosis and treatment of an acute rejection reaction is paramount in the case of renal transplants. Unfortunately, the clinical signs and symptoms of rejection can be mimicked by many other conditions (31). Although a number of tests have been developed with the aim of diagnosing early rejection (43), none has proven entirely satisfactory since they are either too time-consuming or they are not sufficiently specific. Many centers therefore rely on kidney biopsies to decide the best management for the patient with a putative rejection episode (31, 32, 44), leading in a significant number of cases to a diagnosis of "no rejection" (31, 32). Moreover, in cases in which the diagnosis of rejection is made, the biopsy is helpful in predicting not only the outcome, but also the reversibility of the lesions, therefore avoiding unnecessary immunosuppressive therapy that could lead to infection and increased mortality (31, 32, 33, 36).

CONTRAINDICATIONS

Absolute contraindications for a percutaneous kidney biopsy include bleeding diathesis, anticoagulation therapy, and a solitary kidney, with an exception to the latter being the solitary allograft. Intrarenal infection and perinephric abscess are also contraindications because of the risk of causing septicemia. Percutaneous renal biopsy should not be considered for patients with mass lesions.

Relative contraindications include severe azotemia and hypertension, because they increase the risk of bleeding (45, 46). If the kidney biopsy is indicated on solid grounds, the benefit of the procedure should not be denied to these patients and steps should be taken to decrease the uremia and control the high blood pressure (see patient preparation). Although some authors recommend kidney biopsy in patients with end-stage renal failure (47, 48) we believe that small, fibrotic, and scarred kidneys are more likely to bleed after the procedure. In addition, the yield of information that might change the management of the patient is likely to be minimal (49). Should biopsy in end-stage renal disease (ESRD) patients be necessary, an open biopsy may be used. Open biopsy should be done when indicated for patients with abnormalities of kidney fusion and position, marked hydronephrosis, and renal cystic diseases.

Lack of cooperation may be thought to be a contraindication for percutaneous renal biopsy, especially in young children. However, with reassurance, good sedation and technical skills, a percutaneous kidney biopsy in these patients is as successful and safe as in older children and adults (46, 50).

EVALUATION AND PREPARATION

The indications and possible value of the renal biopsy in management must be discussed with the patient or the parents of the child. The possible complications should be discussed and informed consent obtained. A detailed explanation of the procedure usually relieves the anxiety of the patient. The older child should be given the opportunity to practice his or her role in the procedure before the biopsy, rehearsing the breathing pattern recommended for safe advancement of the needle. Younger children may need simple reassurance, and the presence of the parents during the procedure may ease the child's anxiety.

A detailed medical history should be obtained, with special attention to evidence of bleeding disorders. In the physical examination, skeletal abnormalities or local skin disorders that might preclude placing the patient in the prone position must be ruled out. The blood pressure should be normal and excessive edema resolved. Adequate preparation also includes use of dialysis for correction of severe uremic abnormalities, blood or platelet transfusions for anemia or thrombocytopenia, and cryoprecipitate for prolonged bleeding time (28). Should hemodialysis be necessary, reversal of heparin induced bleeding diathesis with protamine would be indicated. The necessary laboratory studies include a complete blood and platelet count, prothrombin and partial thromboplastin times, and serum creatinine measurements. A urinalysis is performed to obtain baseline information for the evaluation of postprocedure hematuria. The urine should be sterile. Study of the size, configuration, and location of the kidneys is mandatory.

Patients are given nothing by mouth for 4 to 8 hours before the procedure. Sedation is given 30 to 60 minutes beforehand, but oversedation must be avoided because, except in the very young child, the patient's cooperation in suspending breathing is necessary. In children, we use meperidine hydrochloride (Demerol) 1–2 mg per kilogram and promethazine hydrochloride (Phenergan) 1 mg per kilogram or pentobarbital sodium (Nembutal) intramuscularly. In adults, meperidine and local anesthesia are usually adequate.

LOCATION METHODS

Accurate location of the kidney is essential to the success of a renal biopsy. Several methods, such as radiography (51, 52), fluoroscopy (53, 54), radio nuclide imaging (55), ultrasound (56, 57, 58), and CT scan (59) have been used for this purpose. The original method needle touch directed percutaneous biopsy has many advocates, including ourselves.

As long as an experienced operator is doing the percutaneous biopsy, the rates of success and complications are surprisingly similar, regardless of the method used for location of the kidney (53). It is best that the operator be allowed to choose the method with which he feels more confident.

Fluoroscopy

In this method, the kidneys are visualized after intravenous injection of contrast medium. The advantage of the method is real-time imaging. The disadvantages are the radiation exposure of the patient and operating room staff, the longer operating time and higher costs, and the possibility of significant allergic and toxic reactions to the contrast medium. The method should not be used in patients with renal failure (serum creatinine level >2 mg per deciliter), because opacification will be poor and because there is a significantly increased risk of acute renal failure after injection of contrast medium in patients whose renal function is already compromised.

With the patient prone, the skin is cleaned, and, using an aseptic technique, a radiopaque marker is placed on the patient's back and moved, under fluoroscopic observation, until it is over the desired puncture site. The biopsy needle is then inserted and advanced toward the kidney during fluoroscopic monitoring. Once the needle has reached the renal cortex, both will move together. The actual biopsy procedure is then carried out.

Radiography

Since 1955, we have used either an intravenous pyelogram (IVP) or a tomogram for locating the kidneys and have had very little operative morbidity. The patient is placed prone with a sandbag or a tight roll of blankets beneath the umbilicus between the rib cage and pelvic bones;

this eliminates lordosis and creates radiologic topography that can be transferred accurately to the patient's back by palpation of bones and by measurement. The roll also may support the kidney and prevents its movement away from the biopsy needle. The radiographic studies are done at the end of inspiration.

Ultrasound

Since its introduction in 1961 (56), the ultrasonic guidance has gained wide acceptance for biopsy location of the kidney. Many authors believe that ultrasound is the best technique for visualization of the renal tissue, since it is highly accurate, noninvasive, and requires neither contrast material nor ionizing radiation (57, 58, 60, 60A).

Initially, static A mode ultrasound was used for guidance of renal biopsy (56). Later on, a B mode scanner was used for the same purpose (57, 58) with a success rate close to 90%. More recently, ultrasonic real-time guidance using a sector scanner has been the suggested method of choice (60, 61). The advantage over the previous two methods includes the fact that the passage of the needle through the tissues can be observed on a monitor display. The method uses a needle guidance attachment with a canal through which the guiding needle and biopsy needle are inserted for the procedure itself. The patient is placed in a prone position with a bag or pillow under the abdomen for better renal fixation. The needle guiding attachment is connected to the previously sterilized scanner. The skin is prepared in a standard fashion. The kidney is then scanned, measuring its position and depth. The site for the biopsy, usually the lower pole, is then selected. (Fig. 21.1). The guiding needle is used to inject anesthesia along the pathway, the needle biopsy is then inserted into the kidney, under two dimensional real time monitoring. The scanner is then released from the needle and the actual biopsy done as will be described.

Percutaneous Kidney Biopsy Technique

We usually prefer to biopsy the left lower pole of the kidney except when splenomegaly is present. With the patient prone as described, the lumbar spinous processes, twelfth rib, posterior iliac crest, and sacrospinalis muscles are outlined on the skin with a marker pen (Fig. 21.2). Then, using the IVP or tomogram films, the distances from the lower pole of the kidney to the lumbar spinous processes and posterior iliac crest is measured and transferred to the patient's back. Usually, the biopsy site falls at the angle formed by the intersection of the twelfth rib and the lateral border of the sacrospinalis muscle, about 1 cm cephalad to the determined lower pole of the kidney.

Using an aseptic technique, the skin is cleaned and draped, and the site selected for the biopsy is infiltrated with intradermal, subcutaneous, and intramuscular injections of procaine. A small incision is made in the skin with the point of a scalpel blade. The location and depth of the kidney are then determined using an exploring needle; we recommend a long No. 22 spinal needle, which is introduced at the biopsy site, parallel to the spine, and in a slightly cephalad direction at an angle of 15° to 20°. Once the needle is in the subcutaneous tissues, it should be advanced a few millimeters with each breath, as the patient holds his breath on inspiration, to avoid renal laceration. The subcutaneous and muscle layers can be felt independently by the experienced operator, and the distinct renal mass is recognizable on contact. Occasionally, one can feel a "pop" as the needle goes through the renal capsule. More characteristically, the swinging arc of the exploring needle with each breath (Fig. 21.3) and the vibration of the needle with the pulsation of the kidney are useful indications that the needle has reached the kidney. These motions of the needle should cease if it is withdrawn a few millimeters. The probing needle is then removed while procaine is injected along the track, and the depth of the kidney is measured. It is important not to insert the biopsy needle until the kidney has been identified with reasonable certainty with the exploring needle.

Although there are many biopsy needles available, we prefer the Vim-Silverman biopsy needle as modified by Franklin. The 11.4 cm needle is used for older children and adults and for obese patients, the 15.8 cm needle is recommended. For younger children, the 7.8 cm needle is used. In using the Franklin modified Vim-Silverman needle, it is important to keep the cutting prongs in optimal condition. The Tru-Cut disposable needle (Travenol), which is available in different sizes, may also be used. The Metcoff needle (62) may be of special value for young children.

The biopsy needle is inserted along the same track, and to the same depth, as the probing needle. The needle and its stylet are slowly advanced as described until the tip penetrates the renal capsule, as determined by the characteristic movements. Then the needle is embedded about 2 mm within the kidney, the stylet is removed, and the cutting needle is inserted

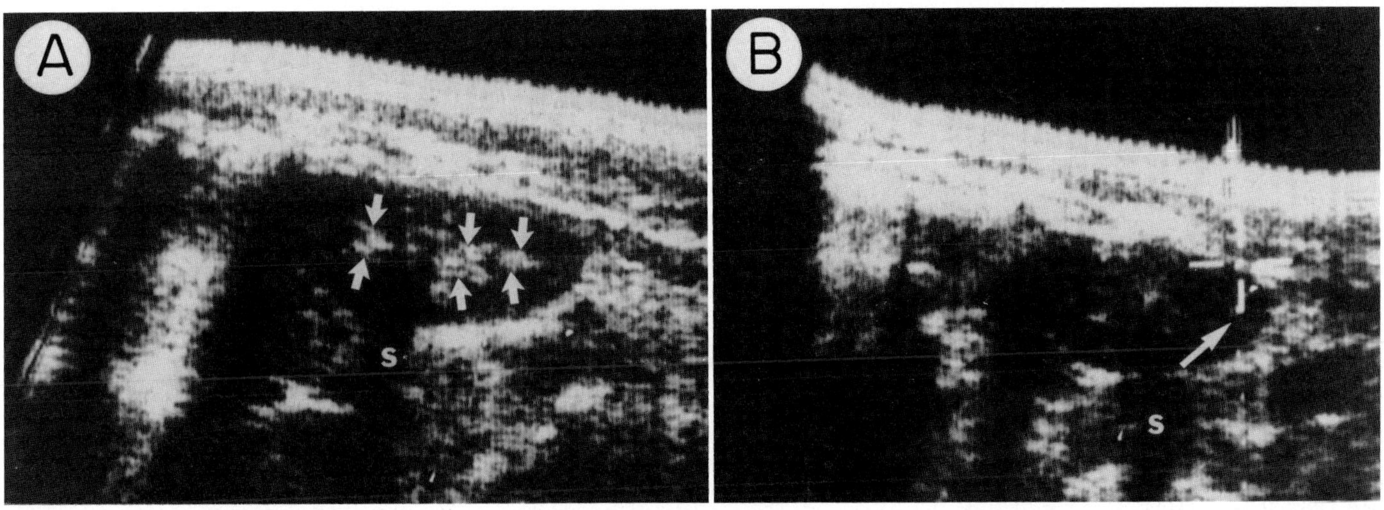

Figure 21.1. Left renal biopsy under ultrasound guidance shows twelfth rib acoustic shadow(s). **A,** Longitudinal view of greatest long axis of left kidney reveals the central echo complex (caliceal system) (*arrows*). **B,** Longitudinal view of kidney at location lateral **A** at approximate site for biopsy (*arrow*) in lower pole, distal to central echos. The superimposed electronic dots near the arrow, indicate the proposed biopsy tract on the image. (Reproduced with permission from Chan JCM, et al: *J Urol* 129:103, 1983.)

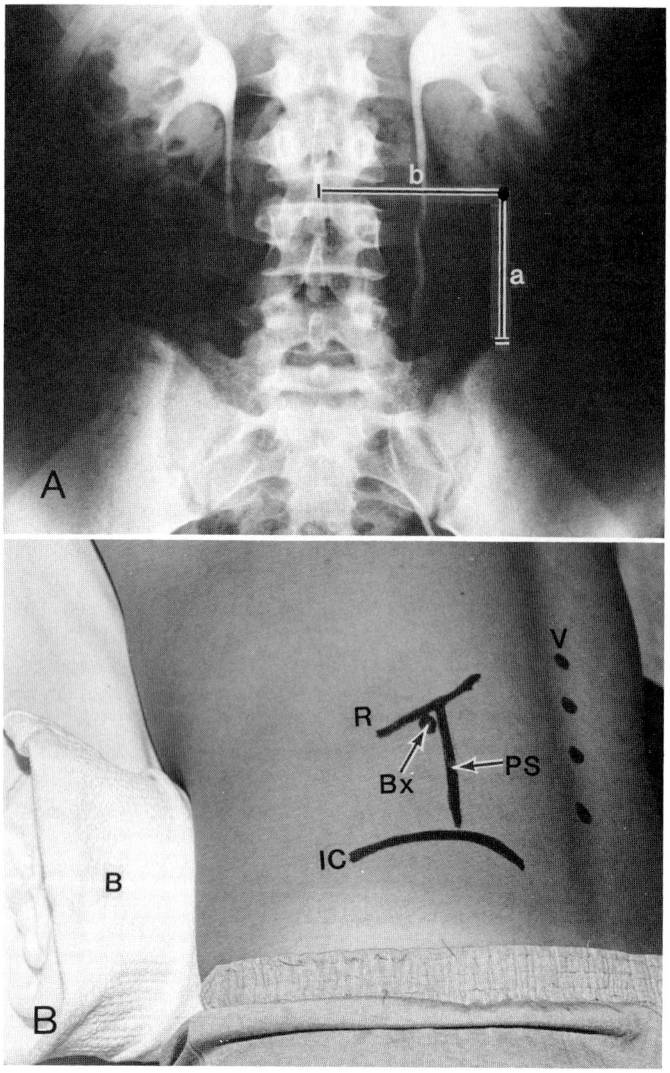

Figure 21.2. **A,** The distance (cm) from the iliac crest to the biopsy site (*a*) and the distance from the spinous process of the vertebra to the biopsy site (*b*) are measured on the intra venous urogram. **B,** These distances are transferred to the patients back and the biopsy site (*Bx*) marked. Note the position of the vertebral spines (*V*) twelfth rib (*R*) the iliac crest (*IC*), the line of the para spinus muscles (*PS*), and the position of the blanket roll (*B*) protruding from under the flank.

until a characteristic resistance is met. If resistance is not found, it means that the outer needle has not penetrated the kidney; the stylet should be replaced and the needle redirected. At the time of the actual procedure, the patient is asked to hold his/her breath at the end of inspiration. Then, in rapid sequence, with the outer needle being held with the left hand at the skin level, the cutting needle is pushed with the right hand into the kidney with a sharp, rapid movement. The inner needle is then held steady while the outer needle is advanced 1 to 1.5 cm, to cut off the tissue sample. The whole needle is rotated and removed, with the outer needle covering the cutting prongs.

In the child who is unable to cooperate, each movement of the needle should be made during the expiratory phase. If the child is sleeping, the respiration movements are usually shallow; and if the biopsy is done rapidly and skillfully, the risk of capsular tear is small.

We recommend that two biopsy cores be obtained to provide enough tissue for the different microscopic studies. Multiple attempts to puncture the kidney should be avoided, since the risk of injury probably increases

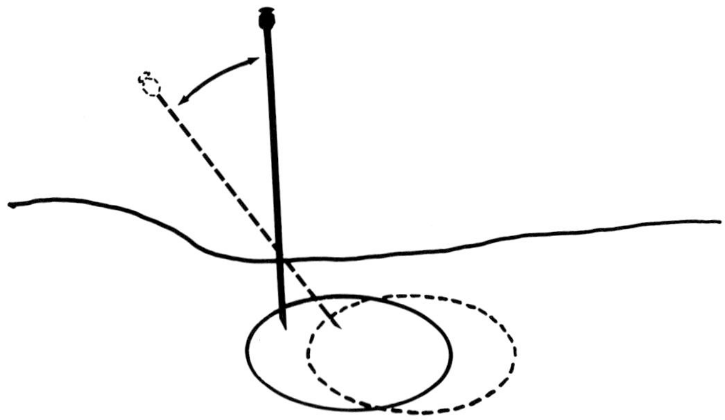

Figure 21.3. Diagram of the cephalad motion of exploratory needle (*dotted line*) as the kidney moves with inspiration.

with frustration. In the case of failure to obtain a specimen, after 3 or 4 attempts, it is usually wise to allow the patient to be observed for 24 hours, and to try again the next day.

Biopsy of Transplanted Kidneys

For biopsy of transplanted kidneys, most physicians prefer the percutaneous approach, avoiding the inherent problems of the open, surgical biopsy, which may lead to a higher frequency of complications (36). The extra peritoneal and superficial location of the allograft makes the percutaneous biopsy a simple and relatively safe procedure. In expert hands, blind percutaneous kidney transplant biopsies can be done with minimal risk of damaging the solitary kidney (34). Others, however, recommend the use of ultrasound or fluoroscopy to localize the site of biopsy (33, 36, 63).

In either case, strict attention to pre biopsy coagulation studies and good blood pressure control are mandatory. After preparation of the patient's lower abdomen, using the operative note and palpation, the kidney is localized and the patient's lower abdomen is prepared in a standard aseptic fashion. Local anesthetic is injected and a small incision made on the skin at the point of the biopsy. The cortex can be safely approached through a perpendicular plane directed towards the lateral curvature of the allograft. The needle is then advanced without difficulty until it reaches the fibrous capsule that usually surrounds the transplant. At this point, significant but steady pressure may be required to reach the kidney. The needle is advanced 0.5 to 1 cm into the renal cortex and the biopsy completed as described.

If ultrasound is used, pictures are obtained to define the allograft and surrounding tissues. Measurements are obtained for the depth of the cortex beneath the skin surface, orientation of the kidney, and the required angulation for the biopsy needle is determined.

The depth of the penetration of the needle into the kidney is measured (usually 0.5 to 1.0 cm) and the biopsy performed.

After the biopsy specimen is obtained, direct manual compression over the needle puncture site is advisable for at least 10 minutes to minimize the risk of bleeding.

Open (Surgical) Biopsy

In some centers, a surgical biopsy is the procedure of choice for obtaining renal tissue. Many surgeons who perform this procedure argue that the yield is higher under direct visualization. However, even with a surgical approach, a needle biopsy is usually required to obtain a representative specimen of cortex and outer medulla, since the scalpel may provide only superficial cortical tissue.

The main disadvantages of the surgical approach include a longer hospitalization, higher cost, added risk of general anesthesia, wound infection, and a cosmetically deforming scar. Some of the complications of an open surgical biopsy are similar to those of the percutaneous procedure. Other problems, mainly related to anesthesia and the wound infection are not seen using a percutaneous biopsy. The overall complication rate is 9% to 11% (64, 65) and deaths have been reported (66), both numbers being similar to those described with the percutaneous needle biopsy method.

Although the criteria for selection of open versus percutaneous kidney biopsy depends on the expertise available, we recommend an open biopsy for those patients with a solitary native kidney, abnormalities of kidney fusion or position, renal cystic diseases, marked hydronephrosis, for infants under 6 months of age and when attempts with the needle biopsy technique have failed.

Postprocedure Management

After the biopsy, the child is returned to his or her room and asked to remain supine in bed. Vital signs are monitored every 15 minutes for 1 hour, every 30 minutes for 2 hours, if stable, and every hour for 4 hours. If the patient condition remains satisfactory, vital signs may then be checked less frequently. Patients should be kept supine for 12 to 24 hours. All voided urine should be collected and portions kept for evaluation of hematuria. Diuresis with oral fluids, to decrease the risk of obstruction by clots, should be encouraged, and analgesics should be avoided as they may mask a complication. The abdomen should be examined frequently for the first several hours, with auscultation of the flank and abdomen to detect any arteriovenous fistula. Pain, gross hematuria, fever, tachycardia or hypotension should be reported immediately to the physician. The hemoglobin level and hematocrit should be obtained 4 to 8 hours after the procedure and before discharge. On the next day, if the child's condition is satisfactory, he or she may be discharged. Body contact sports, diving, and other vigorous physical activity should be avoided for 2 weeks.

COMPLICATIONS

Microscopic hematuria and mild abdominal and flank pain that disappear within 24 hours are common and generally not considered complications (29, 67, 68, 70). In fact, postbiopsy microscopic hematuria is present in almost 100% of the cases. Bleeding manifested by gross hematuria or perinephric hematoma occurs in 5% to 15% of cases (45, 46, 50, 71, 68, 72). The method of localization and the renal biopsy technique appear to have a small influence on these results. Approximately 1% to 3% of patients undergoing percutaneous renal biopsy require a blood transfusion (46, 54) and about 0.3% require surgical intervention. In large series, nephrectomy has been required in less than 0.05% of biopsies (73, 74). The frequency of hemorrhagic complication parallels the blood urea nitrogen level and the degree of hypertension (46, 45, 68). Usually, postoperative bleeding is apparent within 1 to 8 hours. Bleeding associated with a greater than 4% decrease in the hematocrit is likely to cause significant complications (72). Gross hematuria usually responds to conservative management such as bed rest, and subsides within 24 to 48 hours. If the gross hematuria is accompanied by clots and renal colic, intravenous fluids and analgesics are recommended. If blood loss is significant, blood transfusions should be given.

With follow-up by ultrasound or computed tomography, it has been found that perirenal hematoma is more common after biopsies than had been recognized, with an incidence of up to 85% (72, 75). Management is expectant, since in the vast majority of patients, the hematoma is self-limited and resolves spontaneously. Clinically significant hematomas occur in only 0.2 to 5% of cases (46, 68, 72, 76, 67).

Although most arteriovenous fistulas are asymptomatic, they may occur in as many as 15% of patients according to angiography findings (77). Hypertension and vasculitis are predisposing factors (46, 77, 78). Most are small and heal spontaneously within few months. Clinically significant fistulas occur in less than 1% of cases (68, 79). An arteriovenous fistula should be suspected if the patient develops hypertension, congestive heart failure, persistent or recurrent hematuria. A bruit in the abdominal or lumbar area may be present. The persistence of any of the fistula or its complications usually requires surgical or radiological repair. Infusion of epsilon aminocaproic acid may avoid the need for surgery (80). Others have reported successful control of the hemorrhage by arterial embolization with a transfemoral percutaneous catheter (81, 82).

Other rare complications are renal and perirenal infections, punctures or lacerations of other organs, such as the pancreas, liver, bowel, spleen, gallbladder, and lungs (45, 85).

Percutaneous renal biopsy is a safe diagnostic procedure with proven value through experience acquired over the past 30 years. In large series, the mortality rate is less than 0.1% (Table 21.1). When performed by experienced operators, in carefully selected patients, the usefulness of the procedure clearly outweighs the risks.

HANDLING OF TISSUE

The biopsy sample should be inspected for adequacy. With a hand lens or a dissecting microscope, glomeruli can be identified as red, flower-like blushes on the surface of the biopsy core. At least 10 glomeruli must be present to minimize sampling error.

Table 21.1
Complications of Percutaneous Renal Biopsy in Children⁺ and Adults⁺⁺

Author No.	Carvajal 890⁺ (%)	Dodge 205⁺ (%)	Edelman 200⁺ (%)	Karafin 210⁺ (%)	Alterbamakian 632⁺⁺ (%)	Brun 510⁺⁺ (%)	Diaz-Buxo 1000⁺⁺ (%)	Kark 500⁺⁺ (%)	Muth 500⁺⁺ (%)	Rosenbaum 342⁺⁺ (%)
Gross hematuria	13.4	5.0	5.0	22	5.0	7.9	6.9	5.8	3.8	2.3
Perirenal hematoma	1.0	1.4		0.9	1.5	0.2	1.4	0.6	0.4	0.9
Severe pain	2.9			6.0	4.9	7.0		3.4	0.4	0.6
Blood transfusion	1.7	1.9	1.0	1.4	0.9	2.2		0.4	0.4	2.9
AV fistula	0.7		0.5		0.3					
Fever				5.6	1.7	3.4				
Other						0.2[a]	0.8[a]	0.2[b]		0.3[b]
Nephrectomy	0	1.0	1.0	0	0.1	0	0		0	0.6
Death	0	0	0	0	0	0	0.1		0	0.6

[a] Biopsy of other organs.
[b] Sepsis.

It is no longer reasonable to study the renal biopsy specimen by light microscopy alone; arrangements must be made in advance with the pathologist and the tissue divided into portions for light, immunofluorescence, and electron microscopy. Using a sharp razor blade on a wax board, 0.5 to 1mm samples are taken from each end of the core for electron microscopy. The central core may then be either divided longitudinally for immunofluorescence and light microscopy or a second biopsy core may be obtained and the two samples divided appropriately. If little tissue is obtained, the nephrologist must decide which techniques are most likely to provide the needed information.

References

1. Alwall N: Aspiration biopsy of the kidney. Acta Med Scand 143:430, 1952.
2. Iversen P, Brun C: Aspiration biopsy of the kidney. Am J Med 11:324, 1951.
3. Muerhrcke RC, Kark RM, Pirani CL: Biopsy of the kidney in the diagnosis and management of renal disease. N Engl J Med 253:537, 1955.
4. Vehaskari VM, Rapola J, Koskimies O, et al: Microscopic hematuria in school children: epidemiologic and clinocopathologic evaluation. J Pediatr 95:676, 1979.
5. Dodge WF, West EF, Smith EH, et al: Proteinuria and hematuria in school children: epidemiology and early natural history. J Pediatr 88:327, 1976.
6. Moore ES: Hypercalciuria in children. In Berlyne GM (ed): Contributions to Nephrology. New York, Karger, 1981, vol 20.
7. Stapleton FB, Roy S, Noe HR, et al: Hypercalciuria in children with hematuria. N Engl J Med 310:1345, 1984.
8. Bergstein J: Hematuria, proteinuria and urinary tract infections. Ped Clin North Am 29:55, 1982.
9. McCoy RC, Abramowsky CR, Tisher CC: IgA nephropathy. Am J Pathol 76:123, 1974.
10. Gubler M, Levy M, Broyer M, et al: Alport's Syndrome. A Report of 58 cases and a review of the literature. Am J Med 70:493, 1981.
11. Madaio MP, Harrington JT: The diagnosis of acute glomerulonephritis. N Engl J Med 309:1299, 1983.
12. Vehaskari VM, Rapola J: Isolated proteinuria: analysis of a school-age population. J Pediatr 101:661, 1982.
13. Robinson RR: Isolated proteinuria in asymptomatic patients. Kidney Int 18:395, 1980.
14. Travis LB: Overview—with special emphasis on epidemiologic considerations. In Brenner BM, Stein JK (eds): Contemporary Issues in Nephrology. Pediatric Nephrology. New York, Churchill Livingstone, 1984, vol 12.
15. Gruppe WE: Primary nephrotic syndrome in childhood. Adv Pediatr 26:163, 1979.
16. Chung J, Habib R, White RHR: Pathology of the nephrotic syndrome in children. A report of the international study of kidney disease in children. Lancet 1:1299, 1970.
17. Habib R, Kleinknecht C: The primary nephrotic syndrome of childhood: classification and clinicopathology study of 406 cases. In Sommers SC (ed): Pathology Annual. New York, Appleton Century-Crofts, 1971.
18. Counahan R, Winterborn MH, White RHR, et al: Prognosis of Henoch-Schonlein nephritis in children. Brit Med J 2:11, 1977.
19. Eiser AR, Katz SM, Swartz C: Clinically occult diffuse proliferative lupus nephritis: an age-related phenomenon. Arch Int Med 139:1022, 1979.
20. Woolf A, Croker B, Osofsky SG, et al: Nephritis in children and young adults with systemic lupus erythematosus and normal urinary sediment. Pediatrics 64:678, 1979.
21. Platt JL, Burke BA, Fish AJ, et al: Systemic lupus erythematosus in the first two decades of life. Am J Kidney Dis 2:212, 1982.
22. Baldwin DS, Gluck MC, Lowestein J: Lupus nephritis: clinical course related to morphological forms and their transitions. Am J Med 62:12, 1977.
23. Austin HA, Muenz LR, Joyce KM, et al: Prognostic factors in lupus nephritis. Contribution of renal histologic data. Am J Med 75:382, 1983.
24. Rudnick MR, Bastl CP, Elfinbein IB, et al: The Differential Diagnosis of Acute Renal Failure. In Brenner BM, Lazarus JM (eds): Acute Renal Failure. Philadelphia, W.B. Saunders Company, 1983.
25. Wilson DM, Turner DR, Cameron JS, Value of renal biopsy in acute intrinsic renal failure. Brit Med J 2:459, 1976.
26. Mustonen J, Pasternak A, Helin H, et al: Renal biopsy in acute renal failure. Am J Nephrol 4:27, 1984.
27. Linton AL, Clark WF, Driedger AA, et al: Acute interstitial nephritis due to drugs: review of the literature with report of nine cases. Ann Int Med 93:735, 1980.
28. Janson PA, Jubelirer SJ, Weinstein MJ, et al: Treatment of the Bleeding Tendency in Uremia with Cryoprecipitate. N Engl J Med 303:1318, 1980.
29. Mauer SM, Howard RJ: Renal transplantation in children. In Edelmann Jr CM (ed): Pediatric Kidney Disease. Boston, Little, Brown & Co, 1978, vol 1.
30. Millard PR, Herbertson BM, Evans DB: Renal biopsy in clinical management of renal transplantation. Lancet i:113, 1970.
31. Matas AJ, Sibley R, Mauer M, et al: The value of needle renal allograft biopsy. A retrospective study of biopsies performed during putative rejection episodes. Ann Surg 197:226, 1983.
32. Finkelstein FO, Siegel NJ, Bastl C, et al: Kidney transplant biopsies in the diagnosis and management of acute rejection reactions. Kidney Intl 10:171, 1976.
33. Parker RA, Elliot WC, Muther RS, et al: Percutaneous aspiration biopsy of renal allografts using ultrasound localization. Urology 15:534, 1980.
34. Buselmeier TJ, Schauer RM, Mauer SM, et al: A simplified method of percutaneous allograft biopsy. Nephron 16:318, 1976.
35. Murphy GP: Percutaneous needle biopsy of human allotransplant. J Urol 107:193, 1972.
36. Pillay VK, Kurtzman NA: Percutaneous biopsy of the transplanted kidney. JAMA 226:1561, 1973.
37. Goldszer RC, Strom TB, Tilney NL: Acute Renal Failure Associated with Renal Transplantation. In Brenner BM, Lazarus JM (eds): Acute Renal Failure. Philadelphia, W.B. Saunders Co., 1983.
38. Richardson WP, Colvin RB, Cheeseman SH, et al: Glomerulopathy associated with cytomegalovirus uremia in renal allografts. N Engl J Med 305:57, 1981.
39. Leumann EP, Briner J, Largiader F: Recurrence of the original disease in the transplanted kidney. In Gruskin AB, Normal MH (eds): Pediatric Nephrology. Proceedings of the fifth International Pediatric Nephrology Symposium, 1980, The Hague, Martins Nijhoff, 1981.
40. McPhaul JJ, Lorden R, Thompson AL, et al: Nephritogenic immunopathologic mechanisms and human renal transplants: the problem of recurrent glomerulonephritis. Kidney Intl 10:135, 1976.
41. Dische FE, Hebertson BM, Melcher DH, et al: Membranous glomerulonephritis in transplanted kidneys: recurrent de novo disease in 4 patients. Clin Nephrol 15:154, 1981.
42. Sibley RK, Ferguson RM, Sutherland DER, et al: Morphology of cyclosporine nephrotoxicity and of acute rejection in cyclosporine-prednisone immunosuppressed renal allograft recipients. Transplant Proc 15(suppl 1):2836, 1983.
43. Winchester JF, Gelfand MC, Foegh ML, et al: Early indicators of renal allograft rejection. Kidney Intl 23(suppl 14):S34, 1983.
44. Tilney NL, Strom TB, Vineyard GC, et al: Factors contributing to the declining mortality rate in renal transplantation. N Engl J Med 299:1321, 1978.
45. Diaz-Buxo JA, Donadio Jr JV: Complications of percutaneous renal biopsy: an analysis of 1,000 consecutive biopsies. Clin Nephrol 4:223, 1975.
46. Carvajal HF, Travis LB, Srivastava RN, et al: Percutaneous renal biopsy in children—an analysis of complications in 890 consecutive biopsies. Texas Rep Biol Med 29:3, 1971.
47. Krapp KA, Shapiro RS, Jhunjhunwala JS: Role of Renal Biopsy in End Stage Renal Failure. Urology 12:631, 1978.
48. Curtis JJ, Rakowski TA, Argy WP, et al: Evaluation of percutaneous kidney biopsy in advanced renal failure. Nephron 17:259, 1976.
49. Paone DP, Meyer LRE: The Effect of biopsy on therapy in renal disease. Arch Int Med 141:1039, 1981.
50. Vernier RL: Kidney biopsy in the study of renal disease. Pediatr Clin North Am 7:353, 1960.
51. Colodny AH, Reckler JM: A safe, simple and reliable method for percutaneous (closed) renal biopsies in children: results in 100 consecutive patients. J Urol 113:222, 1975.
52. Muehrcke RC, Kark RM, Pirani CL: Technique of percutaneous renal biopsy in the prone position. J Urol 74:267, 1955.
53. Almkuist RD, Buckalew VM: Techniques of renal biopsy. Urol Clin North Am 6:503, 1979.
54. Edelman Sr CM, Greifer I: A Modified technique for percutaneous needle biopsy of the kidney. J Pediatr 70:81, 1967.
55. Tully RJ, Stark VJ, Hoffer PB, et al: Renal scan prior to renal biopsy—a method of renal localization. J Nucl Med 13:544, 1972.
56. Berlyne GM: Ultrasonics in renal biopsy. an aid to determination of kidney position. Lancet ii:750, 1961.
57. Goldberg BB, Pollack HM, Kellerman F: Ultrasonic localization for renal biopsy. Radiology 115:167, 1975.
58. Mailloux LV, Mossey RT, McVicar MM, et al: Ultrasonic guidance for renal biopsy. Arch Int Med 138:438, 1978.
59. Haaga JR, Alfidi RJ: Precise biopsy localization by computed tomography. Radiology 118:603, 1976
60. Saitoh M: Selective renal biopsy under ultrasonic real-time guidance. Urol Radiol 6:30, 1984.

60A. Chan JCM, Brewer WH, Still W: Renal biopsy under ultrasound guidance: 100 consecutive biopsies in children. J Urol 129:103, 1983.

61. Backman U, Lindgren PG: Percutaneous renal biopsy with real-time ultrasonography. Scand J Urol Nephrol 16:65, 1982.

62. Metcoff J: Needles for percutaneous renal biopsy in infants and children. Pediatrics 46:788, 1970.
63. Appel GB, Saltzman MJ, King DL, et al: Use of ultrasound for renal allograft biopsy. Kidney Intl 19:471, 1981.
64. Schmidt A, Baker R: Renal biopsy in children: Analysis of 61 cases of open wedge biopsy and comparison with percutaneous biopsy. J Urol 116:79, 1976.
65. Bolton WK, Vaughan Jr ED: A comparative study of open surgical and percutaneous renal biopsies. J Urol 117:696, 1977.
66. Patil L, Bailey GL, Mahoney EF: Open Renal Biopsy in Uremic Patients. Urology 3:293, 1974.
67. Dodge WF, Daeschner CW, Brennan JC, et al: Percutaneous renal biopsy in children. I. General considerations. Pediatrics 30:287, 1962.
68. Wickre LC, Golper TA: Complications of percutaneous needle biopsy of the kidney. Am J Nephrol 2:173, 1982.
69. Kark R, Muehrcke RC, Pollack VE, et al: An analysis of five hundred percutaneous renal biopsies. Arch Int Med 101:439, 1958.
70. Muth RG: The safety of percutaneous renal biopsy: An analysis of 500 consecutive cases. J Urol 94:1, 1965.
71. White RHR: Observations on percutaneous renal biopsy in children. Arch Dis Childh 38:260, 1963.
72. Rosenbaum R, Hoffsten PE, Stanley RJ, et al: Use of computerized tomography to diagnose complications of percutaneous renal biopsy. Kidney Intl 14:87, 1978.
73. Wolstenholme GEW, Cameron MP (ed): Ciba Foundation Symposium on Renal Biopsy: Clinical and pathological significance. General discussion. London, Churchill, 1961, p. 371.
74. Welt L: Questionnaire on Renal Biopsies. Cited by Kark RM, Renal Biopsy. JAMA 205:226, 1968.
75. Haber K, Asher, WM: Complications of closed renal biopsy documented by ultrasonography. Urology 8:662, 1976.
76. Slotkin EA, Medren PO: Complications of renal biopsy: incidence in 5000 reported cases. J Urol 87:13, 1962.
77. Bennett AR, Wiener SN: Intrarenal arteriovenous fistula and aneurysm. Am J Roentg 95:372, 1965.
78. DeBeukalaer MM, Schreiber MH, Dodge WF, et al: Intrarenal arteriovenous fistulas following needle biopsy of the kidney. J Pediatr 78:266, 1971.
79. Ekelund L: Arteriovenous fistulae secondary to renal biopsy. An experimental study in the rabbit. Acta Radiol (Diag) 10:218, 1970.
80. Silverberg DS, Dossetor JB, Eid TC, et al: Arteriovenous fistula and prolonged hematuria after renal biopsy: treatment with epsilon aminocaproic acid. Can Med Assoc J 110:671, 1974.
81. Silber SJ, Clark RE: Treatment of massive hemorrhage after renal biopsy with angiographic injection of clot. N Engl J Med 292:1387, 1975.
82. Bookstein JJ, Goldstein HM: Successful management of post biopsy arteriovenous fistula with selective arterial embolization. Radiology 109:535, 1973.
83. Karafin L, Kendall AR, Fleisher DS: Urologic complications in percutaneous renal biopsy in children. J Urol 103:332, 1970.
84. Alterbarmakian VK, Guthinger WP, Yakub YN, et al: Percutaneous kidney biopsies, complications and their management. Urology 18:118, 1981.
85. Brun C, Raaschou F: The results of five hundred percutaneous renal biopsies. Arch Int Med 102:716, 1958.

5

Epidemiology

CHAPTER 22

Historical, Social, and Geographical Factors: Pediatric Nephrology in an Unjust World

J. STEWART CAMERON

The title of this chapter is, of course, adapted from that of Dr. King of Nairobi, writing in the *Oxford Textbook of Medicine* on "Medicine in an Unjust World" (1). Pediatrics perhaps shows the effect of this injustice more sharply than any other field, since children are so vulnerable to their environment from the time they are conceived (5). In reading the present book it is necessary to remember that the majority of what lies within its covers originates from, and applies to, only a minority of the world's children. Table 22.1 gives the 1981 populations of the countries with more than 10 million inhabitants. Glance at the origins of the author list of this book, then compare them with the countries in Table 22.1. How many readers were aware, for example, that Indonesia is the fifth largest country in the world in terms of population, ahead of Brazil and Japan? One hardly needs remind pediatricians that the structure of these populations also is very different. Figure 22.1 exemplifies this, comparing the population structure of Madagascar in 1966 with that of the United Kingdom (UK) in 1968; 52% of the Madagascar population was <15 years of age, and 18.5% <5 years, while in the UK the corresponding figures were 23% and 8% (3). Between these extremes, many countries are in rapid transition, with falling mortalities but birth rates still very high, which leads to a rapid expansion in population, particularly in the younger age groups. Whereas a highly developed nation, such as Sweden, is in population equilibrium, with a birth and death rate approximately equal at about 12/1000 population per annum, in Sri Lanka the death rate is even lower than in Sweden (because of the higher proportion of young people and children) at only 7/1000 population/year, while the birth rate remains at 27/1000/year, although it had already fallen from 37/1000/year in 1950 (4).

Apart from a dearth of physicians investigating disease from a research point of view, it is, of course, common knowledge that the countries with the largest child populations (with the possible exception of China) have the worst provision in terms of health services. A number of countries had an annual per capita gross national product of <200 US dollars in 1979, at a time when the equivalent figure for the industrial

Table 22.1.
Countries With a Population of 10 Million or More in 1981

Country	Population (thousands) 1950	1981	Country	Population (thousands) 1950	1981
China (mainland)	547,364	1,041,532	Colombia	11,592	25,217
India	369,880	707,836	Canada	13,737	24,190
Soviet Union	180,075	267,735	Yugoslavia	16,346	22,545
United States	152,271	230,049	Romania	16,311	22,381
Indonesia	83,414	154,339	Morocco	9,343	21,590
Brazil	53,443	124,815	Algeria	8,893	19,422
Japan	83,805	117,711	Sudan	8,051	19,312
Bangladesh	44,863	90,680	Tanzania	8,313	19,233
Pakistan	39,448	90,439	Korea (Dem People's Rep)	9,740	18,317
Nigeria	33,230	79,686	China (Taiwan)	7,981	18,125
Mexico	26,715	69,608	Peru	7,988	18,119
Germany (Fed. Rep.)	49,986	61,760	Venezuela	5,139	17,913
Italy	47,105	57,173	Kenya	6,121	17,116
United Kingdom	50,363	56,020	Germany (Dem Rep)	18,388	16,771
Vietnam	27,072	55,053	Nepal	8,990	15,338
France	41,829	53,945	Czechoslovakia	12,389	15,312
Philippines	20,647	50,310	Sri Lanka	7,533	15,172
Thailand	20,042	48,787	Afghanistan	8,491	15,113
Turkey	21,122	46,673	Australia	8,267	14,817
Egypt	20,797	43,437	Malaysia	6,434	14,330
Korea (Rep)	21,147	40,430	Netherlands	10,114	14,253
Iran	16,357	39,958	Iraq	5,163	13,375
Spain	28,009	37,711	Uganda	5,522	13,222
Poland	24,824	35,925	Ghana	5,297	12,531
Burma	17,927	35,289	Mozambique	6,383	12,356
Ethiopia	16,251	29,994	Chile	6,091	11,162
Zaire	13,055	29,441	Hungary	9,338	10,738
South Africa	13,573	29,313			
Argentina	17,150	28,130			

From WHO Annual Report, Geneva, 1982.

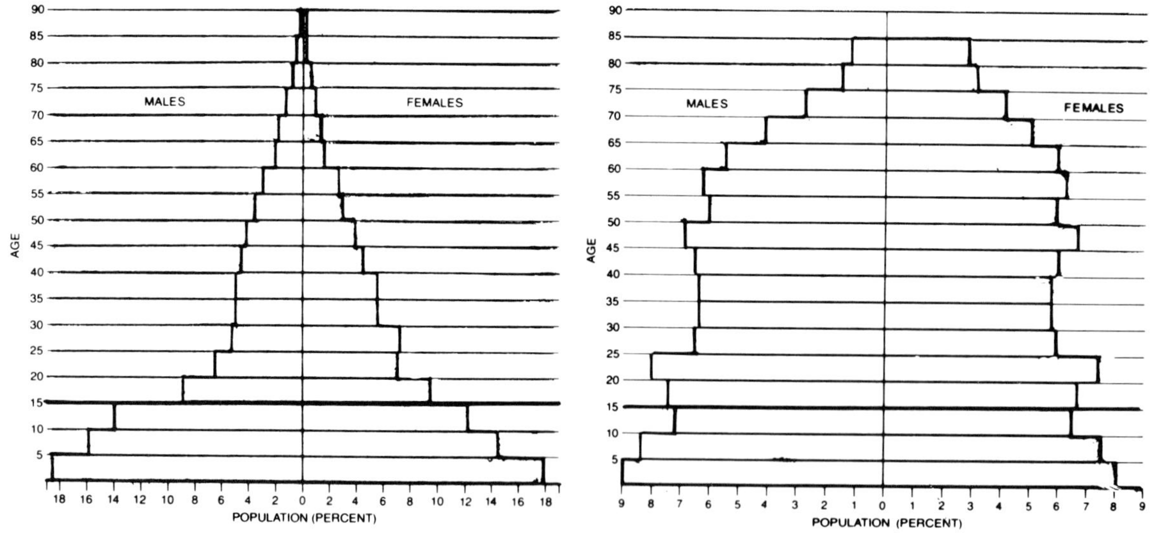

Figure 22.1. Population structure for Madagascar in 1966 (*left*) and England and Wales in 1968. Note the different scales of percentage in the two diagrams. In the English data the group over 80 have been considered as a whole. (From Taylor D: Sci Am 243:54, 1980.)

west was $9600. Life expectancy at birth for these very poor countries (with the notable exception of China and Sri Lanka) varied from 29 (Mali and Ethiopia) to 54 years (Burma); infant mortality remained around 150/1000 births in these countries, at a time when the industrialized west had achieved about 15/1000 (4). The proportion of deaths from children <5 years of age, of all deaths, was 80% in Malawi, 45% in India, 3% in the United States and 1% in Sweden, while mortality of children aged 1 to 4 years, negligible in the developed world, was as high as 49/1000 children at risk each year in Sierra Leone (5).

Table 22.2 summarizes some data from the WHO statistics for 1981,

Table 22.2.
Availability of Health Care Personnel and Clean Water Throughout the World

	Least-developed countries	Other developing countries	Developed countries
Number of countries	31	89	37
Total population (millions)	283	3,001	1,131
Safe water supply (%)	31	41	100
Population/doctor	17,000	2,700	520
Population/nurse	6,500	1,500	220
Population/any health worker[a]	2,400	500	130

Modified from Taylor D: Medicines, Health and the Poor World, London, Office of Health Economics, 1982.
[a] Including traditional birth attendants.

which deal with available health care and safe water supplies (4). Most of the world's children do not, even now, have access to safe water or any form of health care. At the same time, they are exposed to a combination of malnutrition and an environmental load of parasitic, bacterial, and viral infection which shows little sign of diminishing. In many instances, the economic and nutritional state of the children is made even worse by commerical links with the developed world (6). Finally, many children no longer grow up in a poverty-ridden rural environment, but in massive shanty towns that envelop the major cities of the poor world; some data are abstracted in Table 22.3 (7). A number of cities in the poor world are likely to top 20 million in population by the year 2000, and, at the extreme, Mexico City may well exceed 30 million.

Some of these features, such as this massive urbanization, are new, but if we look at the history of the now "developed" west we can see many resemblances to the poor world of today. Until the agricultural revolution in the 18th century, failure of the harvest and widespread starvation occurred about 1 year in 3, as English parish records attest. Laslett (7) showed that the infant mortality in the slums of the industrial early 19th century (8) was less than in the supposedly idyllic rustic environment that preceded it. Plague was an almost annual visitor to the UK until 1700 (9) and not just a feature of 1666. Leprosy and malaria were common, joined by cholera after the explosive pandemic of the 1820s. Life expectancy at birth was only 40 years in the UK, the United States, and Sweden, as recently as 1850 (4), comparable to the least developed countries today listed in Table 22.2. In 1840, 3 years after Victoria ascended the British throne, there were 19,800 deaths from scarlatina, 17,200 from typhus, and 10,400 from smallpox in England and Wales (population only 14 million in 1841). Only after 1866, following repeated cholera epidemics, did London and other major British cities get clean water. One difference was than rather than developing massive shanty towns, Britain's huge surplus population, arising when infant mortality declined, was siphoned off to populate and clear the forests and plains of North America, Australia, and New Zealand.

What impact does all this have on the type and incidence of renal disease in childhood? Data on the prevalence and incidence of diseases in children (or in adults for that matter) are difficult enough to obtain in developed countries with well-documented, literate populations, and widespread centralized health care. From the rest of the world, we can glimpse only tantalizing fragments of epidemiology that undoubtedly contain much of great interest and value. In most instances, it is impossible to sort out the different contributions of genetic, socioeconomic, infectious, climatic, and political factors and understand why there should be, or should have been, such great variations in the incidence and severity of different renal diseases in childhood.

Bladder Stones

One of the most striking features of pediatric nephrology on a world basis is the incidence of bladder stones, usually of ammonium phosphate or calcium oxalate, in children in poor countries from Turkey through the Middle East and India to the Far East (10). The incidence appears to have declined during the past 50 years in mainland China and a similar less well-documented decline in incidence seems to have occurred during the early part of the 19th century in the UK and in Europe as a whole (10). The exact cause of this decline is not clear, although it appears to follow a major change in diet from a predominantly carbohydrate base to a higher protein intake. Ironically, this type of diet seems to be associated with an increase in upper urinary tract stones in adults, to almost epidemic proportions, perhaps because of the higher associated urate production and excretion, although the stones are predominantly calcium oxalate.

Acute Renal Failure

The incidence of acute renal failure in children is extremely high in all poorly developed countries, mainly because of untreated infective diarrhea in children often debilitated by malnutrition and other infections. It is gratifying to learn that the previously high incidence of this type of disease in Mexico City (11) is now coming under control with better and earlier fluid replacement. Other local factors, such as plant toxins and venomous snakes in Africa and Asia, may also play a part in the high incidence of acute renal failure, together with a genetic predisposition to hemolysis from glucose-6-phosphate dehydrogenase deficiency, particularly in Africa.

Glomerulonephritis, Nephrotic Syndrome, and Chronic Renal Failure

It is perhaps in the question of glomerulonephritis, the nephrotic syndrome, and chronic renal failure that we have the most numerous tantalizing glimpses of data that seem to lead to important conclusions on the nature of the disease. There seems little doubt that the incidence of chronic glomerulonephritis leading to the nephrotic syndrome is much more common in tropical areas than in the developed world or in China

Table 22.3.
Populations (Millions) of Some Urban Areas 1950–2000

	1950	1975	2000 (projected)
Mexico City	2.9	10.9	31.5
Sao Paolo	2.5	9.9	26.0
Rio de Janiero	2.9	8.3	19.3
Calcutta	4.5	8.1	20.4
Bombay	2.9	7.1	19.8
Cairo	2.4	6.9	16.9
Jakarta	1.6	5.6	17.8
Manila	1.5	4.4	12.8
Bogota	0.7	3.4	9.5
Lagos	0.3	2.1	9.4
Kinshaha	0.2	2.0	7.8
Shanghai	5.8	11.5	22.1
Beijing	2.2	8.9	22.0
Tokyo-Yokohama	6.7	17.5	28.7
New York	12.3	17.0	22.3
London	10.2	10.7	12.7

From Taylor D: Medicines, Health and the Poor World. London, Office of Health Economics, 1982.

(Table 22.4). Kibukamusoke's analysis of admission data (12) from which Table 22.4 has been expanded, suggests a 50-fold higher incidence in tropical areas where malaria is endemic than in the west, but in nonmalarious tropical countries the admission rate is still 15- to 20-fold higher. Kibukamusoke has argued plausibly that the association with the nephrotic syndrome and malaria known to the ancients is mainly the result of chronic *P. malariae* infection (12), but this cannot be the only factor. Schistosomiasis (*S. mansoni*) has been suggested as another major immunogen, particularly in Brazil (13). In that country *S. hematobium* is absent, but in Eygpt there is some controversial evidence that it, too, may play a role in glomerular disease (14). In many tropical countries streptococcal glomerulonephritis is common, while in the UK it is now rare (15), along with other chronic manifestations of streptococcal disease. In the Caribbean and in Venezuela it is endemic and epidemic (16, 17). Hepatitis B carrier rate is high in many parts of the tropics (Fig. 22.2), exceeding 5% of the population. There is no doubt that hepatitis B antigenemia is associated with glomerulonephritis, usually membranous in pattern. However, in Senegal, one of the countries with the highest hepatitis B carrier rates in the world, no link between hepatitis and nephritis could be established (18). Moreover, there seemed to be no link between nephritis and malaria either (19).

Table 22.4.
World Incidence of Nephrotic Syndrome (NS)

Country	Hospital	NS admission rate (%)	Malaria
Papua	Port Moresby	>4.0	+++
Yemen	Taiz	3.0	+++
Guyana	Mackenzie	2.8	+++
	Mackenzie	0.05	–
	Demerara	0.05	–
Nigeria	Ibadan	2.4	+++
	Lagos	2.1	+++
Uganda	Mulago	2.0	+++
	Fort Portugal	1.8	+++
Senegal	Dakar	0.85	+
Rhodesia	Harare	0.7	–
	Bulawayo	0.15	–
Great Britain	S.E. Thames	0.04	–
US	L.A. County	0.03	–
	Utah	0.15	–
China	Human Med Coll	0.02	–

Modified and expanded from Kibukamusoke JW: Nephrotic Syndrome of Quartan Malaria. Bristol, Edward Arnold, 1973.

There is considerable evidence that the incidence of renal failure from glomerulonephritis has declined during the past century, both in the United States (20) and in the UK (21), from rates perhaps comparable with the nonmalarious tropics to the present level of some 70 million total population/year for males and 45 for females. In 1848, the death rate from nephritis in the UK was over 600 million/year (22). This decline in both countries has continued until recently and is confirmed by recent data from other parts of the developed world (23), but appears to have flattened off since 1970 (24). In fact, there is some suggestion that the rates for those over 60 may have increased in the past 10 years (24), while those in young adults and children still decline. It is well known that the incidence of renal failure, high in infancy, reaches a nadir of 10 to 20 million/year during childhood, with a roughly logarithmic rise from the age of 15 upward, to reach very high figures of 200 to 500

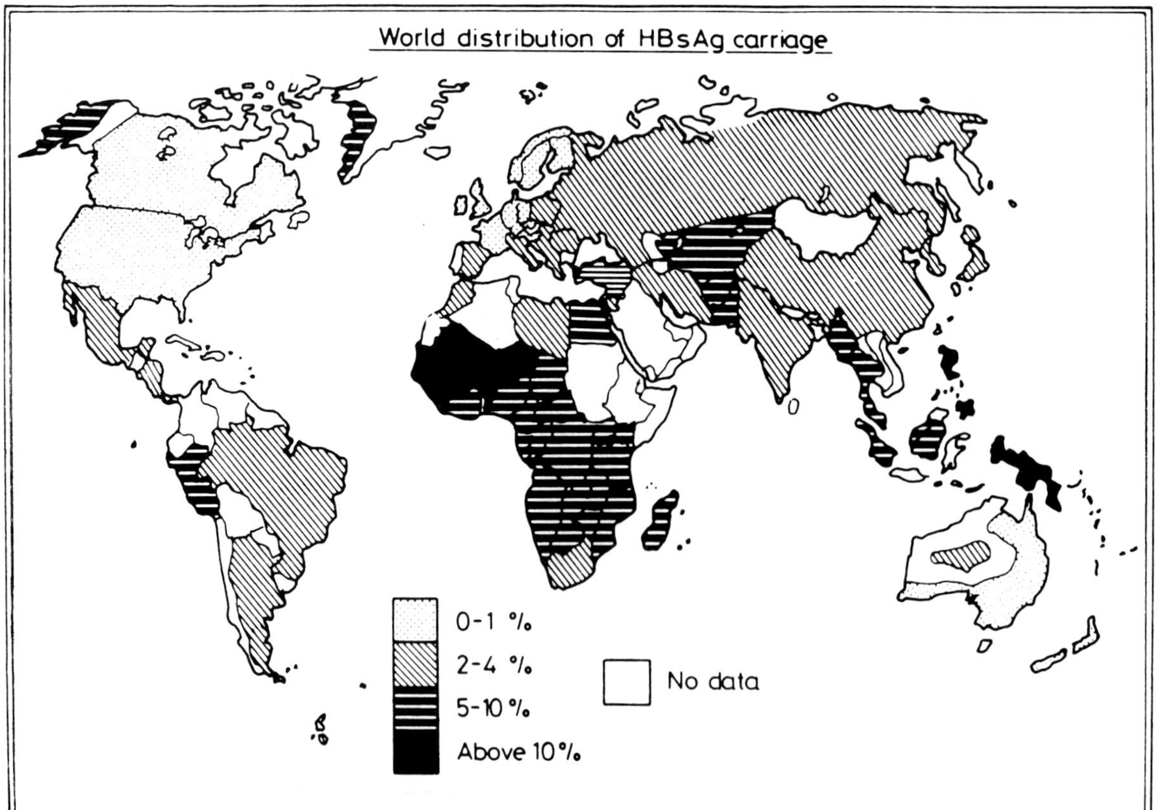

Figure 22.2. World distribution of hepatitis B carrier rates. With the exception of the Eskimo population in Alaska and Greenland, hepatitis B carriage is a tropical phenomenon and probably relates to insector vectors. (Reproduced with permisson from Williams SG: Brit Med J 286:703, 1983.)

million/year over the age of 60 (20, 23, 24). Even in the UK, within the low total incidence of chronic renal failure (about 150 million total population/year, as in most of Europe) (25), there are environmental factors strongly at work. The death rates for 1970 to 1972 from diseases of the urinary tract taken altogether show a mortality ratio (taking the whole population as 100) of 270 for 25- to 35-year olds from social class V (unskilled laborers) and only 37 from those from social class I (professional) (26). This difference persists (but with less emphasis) throughout life, being 140 and 90, respectively, for 55- to 65-year olds. There are no analyses of data for more restricted groups on renal diseases, such as glomerulonephritis, although, for example, minimal change nephrotic syndrome appears to be much more common in social class IV and V.

Even in developed countries, blacks of West African origin have a much higher incidence of renal failure at all ages (27), probably the result of essential hypertension, although the role of glomerulonephritis in this has yet to be defined. To what extent this is the result of a change from rural existence to an urban one, especially with regard to diet—above all, sodium or potassium intakes—is the subject of much debate at the moment (28). There seems little doubt, from a glance at hospital wards, that chronic renal failure associated with severe hypertension is common among young Africans in Africa, although there is no hard information on this point.

What can we make of these data? There is growing evidence of genetic factors in the susceptibility to nephritis. A number of experimental animal nephritides are genetically linked, and associations between a number of forms of human nephritis and HLA types, particularly of class 2 antigens, such as the DR series, have been described (29). Other allotypes, such as C4 and Bf complement, and the Gm immunoglobulin series, also have been implicated. It seems possible that, in situations of low antigenic exposure, as in the west, these genetic predispositions might be predominant, whereas the much higher incidence of glomerulonephritis in the poorer world may arise mainly from massive exposure to pathogens (Table 22.5).

It is possible that other factors, such as malnutrition-induced variations in immune responsiveness could play a part. The relationship of nutrition to the immune response is complex (30), but, in general, malnutrition of most types leads to a multifactorial defect in antigen clearance. Since there is evidence that the fundamental defect in nephritis-prone individuals is a relative immuno-incompetence (31), it is attractive to suppose that nutritionally-induced immuno-incompetence may contribute, as well as interactions between different infections (e.g., malaria, Epstein-Barr virus), in depressing the immune response to other pathogens.

There are also more subtle differences in the histological pattern, as well as the frequency of glomerulonephritis throughout the world. Mesangiocapillary glomerulonephritis (MCGN) is a very rare cause of the nephrotic syndrome in Japan, both in children (32) and in adults

Table 22.5.
A Hypothetical Model to Explain the Different Incidence of Glomerulonephritis in the Developed and the Poor World

	Mainly environmentally determined	→ ←	Mainly genetically determined	Total
Developed world	1		5	6
Poor world	95		5	100

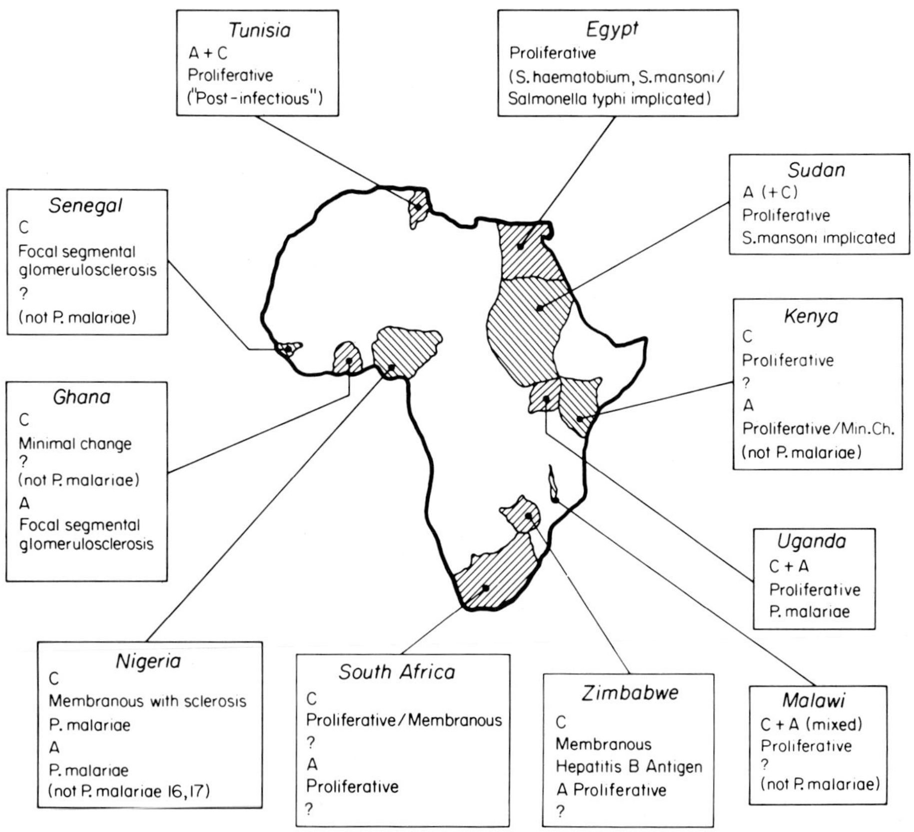

Figure 22.3. Patterns of glomerulonephritis underlying nephrotic syndromes in different parts of Africa. The major histological patterns are summarized in each box and associated etiological factors (where known or suspected) are indicated. Note that no data are available for a large part of the continent. (Reproduced with permission from Seggie J, et al: Quart J Med 43:109, 1984.)

(Arakawa M: personal communication, 1983), whereas in the West it forms a constant 10% to 12% of adults and 5% to 7% of childhood nephrotics (33), while in Iran two thirds of adult nephrotic syndromes show MCGN (34). Membranous nephropathy is much more common in nephrotic children in Japan (35) and probably Hong Kong (36) than in Europe, and all of this difference cannot be explained by hepatitis B carriage. In adults also, membranous nephropathy is particularly common in Greece, where it forms the most frequent histological pattern in nephrotic syndrome (37) and in the United States (38), particularly California. There, more than half the nephrotic adults show this histopathological appearance, whereas, in the UK it underlies less than a quarter of the cases. In adults, the pattern of IgA-associated nephropathy is the largest single biopsy group in France (18%) (39) and Italy (20%) (40) and in parts of Australia (South Australia in particular) (41), whereas it appears in only 5% of biopsies in the UK (42). Although common around the rest of the Mediterranean basin, it is distinctly uncommon in Greece (37).

Within Africa itself, there are also great variations in the histopathology found in the nephrotic syndrome. These have been well summarized by Seggie (43), from whose work, among others, Figure 22.3 is taken (12, 14, 18, 19, 44–60). Some of these variations can be equated with climatic and infectious agents, but most are as yet unexplained. Also, there are few data from Africa on the population incidence of any type of glomerulonephritis in children or adults. To date, minimal-change nephrotic syndrome has been reported with any frequency in African nephrotic children only from Ghana (60); in South Africa, it is distinctly rare in black children, although common in Indians and whites. This may represent a much higher total incidence, with an excess of nonminimal change patterns. To what extent any or all of these data represent variations in referral patterns and biopsy policy is also unknown.

There is also the enigma of systemic lupus erythematosus (SLE) with nephritis in black populations. In the United States, the Caribbean, and in the UK, black children and adults suffer SLE more frequently than their white neighbors. We calculate that our local black population, mainly of Jamaican origin, has a liability to SLE of at least 20 times the remainder of the local population, and community surveys in San Francisco and New York show how common SLE is among American black women (61, 62). Yet, in Africa, keen observers have almost been unable to find cases of SLE with or without nephritis (60, 63). It is of interest to note that in South Africa all the children with SLE were of Indian extraction. Possibly some environmental factor absent in Africa operates in the Caribbean, North America, and Britain to act on a genetic susceptibility of no significance in the country of origin. What is certain is that study of racial, national, and regional variations in the pattern of disease have much to tell us about the nature and operation of the disease process, as well as being of local value for planning purposes.

It is clear that the incidence of renal disease as a whole and renal failure in particular is much higher in the poor world than in the west. There is a linear regression between annual per capita gross national product and number of patients dialyzed and transplanted, which suggests that any country with a per capita gross national product figure <\$2000 (in 1979) is unable to afford any treatment for its citizens in renal failure by dialysis or transplantation (64). This would exclude more than two thirds of the world from any treatment, other than by diet. In this segment of the world, it is doubtful if much protein restriction would be needed!

References

1. King MH: Medicine in an unjust world. In Weatherall DJ, Ledingham JGG, Warrell DA, (eds): Oxford Textbook of Medicine. Oxford, Oxford University Press, 1983, p 3.
2. WHO Annual Report, Geneva, 1982.
3. Dadzie KKS: Economic development. Sci Am 243:54, 1980.
4. Taylor D: Medicines, Health and the Poor World. London, Office of Health Economics, 1982.
5. UNICEF: The State of the World's Children 1984. Oxford, Oxford University Press, 1963.
6. George S: How the Other Half Dies. The Real Reasons for World Hunger. London, Penguin, 1976.
7. Laslett P: The World We Have Lost. London, Methuen, 1965.
8. Engels F: The Condition of the Working Class in England (Leipzig 1845). London, Panther Books, 1969.
9. McNeill WH: Plagues and Peoples. London, Penguin, 1979.
10. Ellis H: A History of Bladder Stones. Oxford, Blackwell, 1969.
11. Gordillo-Paniagua G, Velasquez-Jones L: Acute renal failure. Ped Clin No Am 23:817, 1976.
12. Kibukamusoke JW: Nephrotic Syndrome of Quartan Malaria. Bristol, Edward Arnold, 1973.
13. Andrade ZA, Rocha H: Schistosomal glomerulopathy. Kidney Intl 16:23, 1979.
14. Ezzat E, Osman RA, Ahmet KY, et al: The association between Schistosoma haematobium infection and heavy proteinuria. Trans Roy Soc Trop Med Hyg 68:315, 1974.
15. Meadow SR: Post-streptococcal glomerulonephritis—a rare disease? Arch Dis Childh 50:379, 1975.
16. Rodriguez-Iturbe B, Gastillo L, Valbuena R, et al: Acute post-streptococcal glomerulonephritis. Recent developments. Pediatrician 8:307, 1979.
17. Poon-King T, Potter EV, Svartmen M, et al: Epidemic acute nephritis with reappearance of M-type 55 streptococci in Trinidad. Lancet 1:475, 1973.
18. Satge P, Habib R, Querum C, et al: Particularite du syndrome nephrotique chez l'enfant au Senegal. Ann de Pediatrie 5:382, 1970.
19. Morel-Maroger LJ, Saimot AG, Sloper JC, et al: "Tropical nephropathy" and "Tropical extramembranous glomerulonephritis" of unknown aetiology in Senegal. Brit Med J 1:541, 1975.
20. Kessner DM, Florey C du V: Mortality trends for acute and chronic nephritis infections of the kidney. Lancet 2:979, 1967.
21. Walters WE: Mortality trends in renal disease. Lancet 1:1091, 1968.
22. McKeown T: The Role of Medicine: Dream, Mirage or Nemesis? London, Nuffield Provincial Hospitals Trust, 1976, p 38.
23. Alderson MR: International Mortality Statistics. London, MacMillan, 1981.
24. Sorahan T, Kokoszynska R, Adams RG: Trends in mortality from nephritis and nephrosis. Lancet 1:567, 1982.
25. The Registrar General's Statistical Review of England and Wales. Part I: Tables, Medical 1950–1973. London, Her Majesty's Stationery Office, 1978.
26. Occupational Mortality, 1970–1972. London, Her Majesty's Stationery Office, 1978.
27. Rostand SG, Kirk KA, Rutsky GA, et al: Racial differences in the incidence of treatment for end-stage renal disease. N Engl J Med 306:1276, 1982.
28. Sever PS, Peart WS, Gordon D, et al: Blood pressure and its correlates in urban and tribal Africa. Lancet July 12, 1980.
29. Cameron JS, Rees AJ, Peters DK: New perspectives in glomerulonephritis. In Jones NF, Peters DK (eds): Recent Advances in Nephrology-2. London, Churchill-Livingstone, 1982.
30. Kroc Foundation Series, No. 7: In Suskind RM (ed): Malnutrition and the Immune Response. New York, Raven Press, 1977.
31. Peters DK, Lachmann PJ: Immunity deficiency in pathogenesis of glomerulonephritis. Lancet 1:59, 1974.
32. Kobayashi O: Unpublished data of the International Study of Kidney Disease in Childhood, Japan.
33. Cameron JS: Clinicopathlogical correlations in glomerular disease. In Kidney Disease—Present Status. IAP Monograph No. 20. Baltimore, Williams and Wilkins, 1979, p. 76.
34. Ipakachi E, Kashanian B, Khanmohamadi M, et al: Light microscopy proteinuria and nephrotic syndrome in Iran. Abstracts 1 to 6, Seventh Intl Congress of Nephrology, Montreal, 1978.
35. Takekoshi Y, Tanaka M, Shida N, et al: Strong association between membranous nephropathy and hepatitis B surface antigenaemia in Japanese children. Lancet 2:1065, 1978.
36. Chan WC, Tsao YC: Diffuse membranous glomerulonephritis in children. J Clin Path 19:464, 1966.
37. Vosnides G: Presented to the Hellenic Society of Nephrology, Athens, October 1982.
38. Collaborative study of the adult idiopathic nephrotic syndrome. A controlled study of short-term prednisone treatment in adults with membranous nephropathy. N Engl J Med 301:1301, 1979.
39. Berger J, Yaneva H, Nabarra B, et al: Recurrence of mesangial deposition of IgA after renal transplantation. Kidney Intl 7:232, 1975.
40. Imbasciati E, Colasanti G, Barbiano di Belgiojoso G, et al: Long-term follow-up of IgA mesangial deposits in glomerulonephritis. Proc Europ Dial Transplant Assoc 14:472, 1977.

41. Clarkson AR, Seymour AE, Thompson AJ, et al: IgA nephropathy: A syndrome of uniform morphology, diverse clinical features and uncertain prognosis. Clin Nephrol 2:459, 1977.
42. Cameron JS: The natural history of glomerulonephritis. In Black DAK, Jones NF (eds): Renal Disease, ed 4. Oxford, Blackwell Scientific Publications, 1979, p 329.
43. Seggie J, Davies PG, Ninin D, Henry J: Patterns of glomerulonephritis in Zimbabwe: survey of disease characterized by nephrotic proteinuria. Quart J Med 43:109, 1984.
44. Furman KI: Nephritis in Bantu. S African Med J 29:590, 1955.
45. Hersch C, Seftel HC, Isaacson C: The nephrotic syndrome in the Bantu. A clinicopathological study. S African Med J 36:534, 1962.
46. Hendrickse RG, Gilles HM: The nephrotic syndrome and other renal diseases in children in Western Nigeria. East African Med J 40:186, 1963.
47. Gilles HM, Hendrickse RG: Nephrosis in Nigerian children. Role of plasmodium malariae and effect of antimalarial treatment. Brit Med J 2:27, 1963.
48. Kibukamusoke JW, Hutt MSR, Wilks NE: The nephrotic syndrome in Uganda and its association with quartan malaria. Quart J Med 36:393, 1967.
49. Kibukamusoke JW, Hutt MSR: Histological features of the nephrotic syndrome associated with quartan malaria. J Clin Path 20:117, 1967.
50. Hendrickse RG, White RHR, Edington GM, et al: Quartan malarial nephrotic syndrome. Lancet 1:1143, 1972.
51. Bassily S, Farid Z, Barsoum RS, et al: Renal biopsy in schistosoma-salmonella associated nephrotic syndrome. J Tropic Med Hyg 79:256, 1976.
52. Brown KGE, Abrahams C, Meyers AM: The nephrotic syndrome in Malawian Blacks. S African Med J 52:275, 1977.
53. Barsoum RS, Bassily S, Baligh OK, et al: Renal disease in hepatosplenic schistosomiasis: A clinical pathological study. Trans Roy Soc Trop Med Hyg 71:387, 1977.
54. Beaufils H, Lebon P, Auriol M, et al: Glomerular lesions in patients with Schistosoma haemotobium infection. J Trop Geographic Med 30:183, 1978.
55. Verroust PJ, BenMaiz H, Morel-Maroger L, et al: A clinical and immunopathological study of 304 cases of glomerulonephritis in Tunisia. Europ J Clin Invest 9:75, 1979.
56. Seedat YK: Clinicopathological features of the nephrotic syndrome in the Africans and Indians of South Africa. S African J Hosp Med 5:219, 1979.
57. Hendrickse RG, Adeniyi: Quartan malarial nephrotic syndrome in children. Kidney Intl 16:64, 1979.
58. Kung'u A, Sitati SM: Glomerulonephropathies in Kenya. A histological study. E African Med J 57:525, 1980.
59. Musa AM, Abu-Asha H, Veress B: Nephrotic syndrome in Sudanese patients with schistosomiasis mansoni infection. Ann Trop Med Parasit 74:615, 1980.
60. Adu D, Anim-Addo Y, Foli AK, et al: The nephrotic syndrome in Ghana: Clincal and pathological aspects. Quart J Med 50:297, 1981.
61. Siegel M, Lee SL: The epidemiology of systemic lupus erythematosus. Sem Arthr Rheumatol 3:1, 1973.
62. Fessel J: Systemic lupus erythematosus in the community. Arch Int Med 143:1027, 1974.
63. Greenwood BM: Autoimmune diseases and parasitic infections in Nigerians. Lancet 2:380, 1968.
64. Wing AJ: Treatment of end-stage renal failure. In Jones NF, Peters DK (eds): Recent Advances in Nephrology. London, Churchill-Livingstone, 1982, p 103.

CHAPTER 23 Nephrology Around the World

INTRODUCTION

Pediatric nephrology is now an international discipline with regular meetings and conferences, and it has become apparent from discussions among colleagues that the calls of clinical practice, influenced by genetic, environmental, and social factors, vary widely in different parts of the world. The epidemiology of renal disease worldwide in childhood has not been systematically studied, so, as an alternative, a number of authorities were asked to describe the clinical spectrum of renal disease in children in their country, with particular emphasis on differences from the pattern seen in Europe and North America.

23A Argentina

NORMA N. BIBILONI

The prevalence and relative incidence of various renal diseases in Argentinian children are known only in the high density population centers, but are not established in large rural areas of the country.

HEMOLYTIC UREMIC SYNDROME

At the present time in Argentina hemolytic uremic syndrome (HUS) is the main cause of acute renal failure (ARF) during late infancy and early childhood. It is an important cause of chronic renal failure (CRF) in later childhood as well, comparable in incidence with CRF as a result of urinary tract malformations and renal hypoplasia/dysplasia. HUS is a well-established entity in pediatrics with a clear-cut picture defined by abrupt onset of microangiopathic hemolytic anemia, thrombocytopenia, and ARF. In Argentina the incidence of HUS is high: 1456 cases were reported during the period 1965–76 in comparison with only 58 cases in other countries of South America (Brazil, Chile, Colombia, El Salvador, Mexico, Panama, and Peru) (1). Among Argentinian patients a striking feature in contrast to other series is the neurological involvement, which is present in different degrees in about two thirds of the cases. HUS remains a disease of unknown etiology. It is occasionally possible to identify a precipitating factor, usually a viral infection. In Argentina a viral agent was isolated from the blood in eight patients during the acute phase (virus Portillo from the Tacaribe group) (2). More recently arenavirus antigens were found in kidney specimens from patients with HUS (3).

The brief analysis to be presented reflects the experience of the Hospital de Niños de La Plata, Buenos Aires, a general pediatric hospital with a referral base of approximately 3 million individuals in which the Nephrology Department has managed 292 children with HUS from 1969 to the present time. The data are similar to other larger series reported from Argentina (4). The mean age of the patients at onset was 12.6 ± 8.2 months with a range of 3 months to 5 years, a similar distribution to that described by Gianantonio (5). Two thirds of the patients were aged from 6 to 18 months and only 6 were over 3 years. Age over 3 years was not associated with a poor outcome, as has been reported in other series (6). The incidence was similar in the two sexes. Nearly 80% of the children belonged to middle and high socioeconomic groups, representing a very different background from the rest of the hospitalized population.

There were only three pairs of affected siblings; in them the outcome was similar to the rest of the group (7). There were no relapses apart from one patient who had twelve episodes of microangiopathic hemolytic anemia with thrombocytopenia and ARF over a period of 10 years with normal renal function in between. This relapsing case should probably be considered a different entity from endemic HUS. There were often small epidemics occurring in the course of days or few weeks. There were peaks of incidence two of three times a year, but they did not follow a seasonal pattern.

The clinical picture has been fully described by Gianantonio (4, 8). Manifestations of the prodromal phase were usually mild. One to ten days before the acute phase a previously healthy infant developed nonspecific symptoms, such as moderate fever with or without coryza and pharyngitis, vomiting, irritability, and malaise. Diarrhea was present in 93%, with bloody stools in 74% of the patients. Some children presented with colicky abdominal pain, mimicking intussusception. The acute phase was characterized by intense pallor, with ARF presenting with oliguria or anuria; convulsions or minor neurological manifestations were frequent. On some occasions hemolytic anemia was the only relevant clinical feature to be observed, but the degree of anemia did not correlate with the outcome of the disease. Thrombocytopenia was found in 93% of the children with some sort of hemorraghic feature in nearly every patient.

Renal involvement varied from slight changes expressed by microscopic hematuria present in all the patients and transient decrease in urine output, to severe degrees of ARF. Oliguria persisted for more than 4 days in 80% and for more than 7 days in 50% of the children. Arterial hypertension was detected in half of the children and was much more severe in anuric patients. It was usually controlled by water and sodium restriction or peritoneal dialysis, and hypotensive drugs were only seldom necessary.

One third of the children had one or more convulsive episodes, and 70% developed some degree of neurologic deficit during the initial oliguric period. Patients with long periods of anuria had more severe neurological manifestations. Central nervous system symptoms improved dramatically with peritoneal dialysis. Severe permanent neurological sequelae were not observed. Gianantonio found no strict correlation between the intensity of neurological involvement and the severity of renal impairment (5).

Treatment was based on supportive management of anemia and ARF. Transfusions were required in most of the patients, mainly during the first 2 weeks of illness. Early and repeated dialysis and supportive treatment led to a low mortality rate (Table 23A.1) and excellent prognosis of the acute phase. Even in patients with long periods of anuria malnutrition was minimized by high calorie protein intake and intensive dialysis. Those basic principles of treatment together with an increasingly early recognition and referral of the syndrome by general pediatricians has reduced the mortality from about 50% (1957–61) (4) to less than 5% in 1969–77 and less than 1% currently (Table 23A.1).

As time passes, it has become increasingly apparent that HUS is accompanied in many cases by long-term sequelae, with the prospect of developing CRF. One hundred and ninety-two patients have been followed up for periods ranging from 6 months to 14.6 years; the incidences of the principal sequelae of the disease, e.g. diminished glomerular filtration rate, arterial hypertension, and persistent proteinuria are given in Table 23A.2. The probability of developing chronic renal abnormalities with decreased renal function or proteinuria correlated closely with the duration of the anuric period. About 30% of the patients with less than 5 days of anuria had permanent sequelae, but they were present in 80% of cases with anuria of 10 days or more.

Table 23A.1.
Mortality from HUS[a]

Period	Number of cases	Dead	Mortality (%)
1969–77	110	6	5.4
1978–81	114	1	0.8
1981–83	68	0	0
TOTAL	292	7	2.4

[a] Mortality from HUS has declined in recent years, irrespective of the severity of the early phase of the disease, as a result of early recognition and active treatment.

Table 23A.2.
Sequelae of HUS[a]

	Acute phase	Chronic renal sequelae (CRF, hypertension, or proteinuria)
Follow-up	Not anuric: 75	4 (5.6%)
6 mo to 13.6 years	Anuric: 97	47 (49%)

[a] Sequelae were less common in the group who were not anuric in the acute phase; half of the anuric patients had some degree of residual renal impairment, as did 80% of those who were anuric for 10 days or more.

OTHER DISORDERS

Few other forms of renal disease offer regional peculiarities that deserve mention. Among the patients requiring acute dialysis the great majority belonged to the HUS group. Apart from this, there are infants or little children with intoxications, patients with sepsis who developed ARF, and some who developed complications from cardiac surgery. Among older children there are a few who are admitted with different forms of primary or secondary "anuric nephritis" (lupus nephritis, crescentic glomerulonephritis, or mesangiocapillary glomerulonephritis).

At present in Argentina, most children who present acutely with edema, hematuria, and oliguria accompanied by arterial hypertention during school age have acute poststreptococcal glomerulonephritis, with other antecedent infections being most unusual. Upper respiratory infection was present in >40% (confirmed bacteriologically in 40%) of the patients and skin infections in 30%, the latter particularly in patients from poor socioeconomic groups. Edema was the most frequent symptom at presentation. Symptomatic circulatory congestion was evident in 40% of the children admitted to the hospital, ranging from dyspnea and slight signs of pulmonary edema up to established cardiac failure. Hypertensive encephalopathy was observed in 8% of hospitalized patients. A few patients presented simultaneously with acute glomerulonephritis and chest infection, unrelated to the development of acute pulmonary congestion or edema. This group tended to have positive blood cultures. The illness is almost invariably benign and mortality near zero. The outcome of the group as a whole does not correlate at all with the site of

Table 23.3.
Nephrotic syndrome in children (1971–1983)

	No	%
Primary (177)		
Corticosteroid-sensitive	118	67
Corticosteroid-resistant	59	33
Secondary (35)		
Systemic lupus erythematosus	12	
Congenital syphilis	5	
Poststreptococcal glomerulonephritis	5	
Henoch-Schönlein syndrome	4	
Alport's syndrome	2	
Reflux nephropathy	2	
Hodgkin's disease	2	
Hemolytic uremic syndrome	1	
Pneumococcl sepsis	1	
Celiac disease	1	
TOTAL	212	

Table 23.4.
Histopathological findings in children with primary nephrotic syndrome

	No	%
Minimal-change	118	67
Mesangioproliferative glomerulonephritis	11	8
Focal segmental glomerulosclerosis	16	9
Mesangiocapillary glomerulonephritis	7	4
Membranous nephropathy	7	4
Others	15	8
TOTAL	177	100

the initial infection (throat or skin). Only a very few patients from a large population with acute poststreptococcal nephritis developed nephrotic syndrome later.

From 1971 to 1983, 212 children with the nephrotic syndrome were treated at the Hospital de Niños. Of these, 177 were primary and 118 (67%) of them responded to corticosteroids. In 35 patients the nephrotic syndrome was secondary to overt systemic disease (Table 23A.3), among which may be noted the absence of congential nephrotic syndrome, but persistence of congenital symphilis and the high frequency of lupus nephritis. The histopathological findings in children with primary nephrotic syndrome are given in Table 23.4.

References

1. Gianantonio CA: Epidemiologia de las enfermedades renales en la infancia en America Latina. Revista del Hospital de Niños de Buenos Aires 19:258, 1977.
2. Mettler NE, Gianantonio CA, Parodi A: Asilamiento del agente causal del sindrome uremico-hemolitico. Medicina 23:139, 1963.
3. Laguens RP, Cossio PM, Patin DJ et al: Presencia de antigenos de arenavirus y particulas de tipo viral en riñones de enfermos con sindrome uremico hemolitico (SUH) de la ciudad de Buenos Aires. Medicina 35:611, 1975.
4. Gianantonio CA, Vitacco M, Mendilaharzu F et al: The hemolytic-uremic syndrome. Nephron 11:174, 1973.
5. Gianantonio CA. The hemolytic-uremic syndrome. In Edelmann CM (ed): Pediatric Kidney Disease. Boston, Little, Brown and Co., 1978, p 724.
6. Tune BM, Leavitt TJ, Gribble TJ: The hemolytic-uremic syndrome in California: A review of 28 non-heparinized cases with long-term follow-up. J Pediatr 82:304, 1973.
7. Kaplan BS, Chesney RW, Drummond KN: Hemolytic-uremic syndrome in families. N Engl J Med 292:1090, 1975.
8. Gianantonio CA, Vitacco M, Mendilaharzu F et al: The hemolytic-uremic syndrome. J Pediatr 64:478, 1964.

23B Cameroon

JACOB L. NGU

The myriad of clinical afflictions of children in Cameroon is striking. It is unfortunate, though understandable, that priority in the health program has been given to those conditions that are overtly associated with either a high mortality (for example, malaria or measles) or with dramatic, emotive clinical manifestations (as in malnutrition). This relegates renal disease to the group of less pressing, though important, public health problems. The insidious onset of many forms of nephropathy, the dearth of skilled medical personnel, and infrequent routine screening of patients results in the detection of only the most obvious and advanced types of renal disease. Further, the multiplicity of pathologies in a single patient and the modulation of the clinical expression of some renal disorders by coexisting disease (e.g., parasitic infestations) may obscure the underlying renal pathology. The diagnosis made in such instances, more often than not, is that of the pathological condition with the most obvious manifestation.

In the two major hospitals in Yaounde, serving a population of about 600,000 people, there are two to three new children with renal diseases admitted each month into the combined pediatric units with a total bed capacity of 100; 75% of these children present with the nephrotic syndrome. Most of the remaining cases are those with isolated albuminuria, hematuria, hypertension, urinary tract infection, and chronic (less frequently acute) renal failure. Approximately one case of nephroblastoma per year has been recorded in the past few years. Concomitant diseases most frequently encountered are infections (parasitic, viral, and bacterial), anemia, and heart failure.

In a number of children, the diagnosis of nephropathy is delayed because of other pathologies common in this age group that may be confused with renal disease. These are kwashiorkor, allergic reactions to foods and insect bites, anemia of nutritional origin or hemoglobinopathy, and congestive heart failure. These mistakes occur particularly in rural dispensaries where the large numbers of patients make thorough clinical evaluation difficult.

In the group of nephritides attributable to immune complex damage (accounting for more than half of hospitalized renal patients) certain interesting observations have been made. Plasmodium malariae infection is rare, at least in this part of Cameroon, in contrast to *P. falciparum*, which is endemic. Thus, the *P. malariae* origin of immune complex glomerulonephritis, which has been widely documented in many tropical areas, is unusual in Cameroon. However, in Yaounde, a wide range of etiological factors in immune complex nephropathy have been identified.

Candidate antigens considered in all new cases of immune complex nephropathy admitted to hospital are hepatitis B virus, filariasis (laoisis and onchocerciasis) in >9-year group, bacterial endocarditis in some, and toxoplasmosis in a few.

About 40% of children with the nephrotic syndrome have detectable circulating hepatitis B surface antigen. Carrier rate is about 15% in this part of Cameroon (1, 2). Local preference for parenteral drug administration over the oral route, and the use of sterilizable, rather than disposable, needles and syringes is undoubtedly a major contributing factor to the high prevalence of HB virus among children with glomerulonephritis. For example, intramuscular Qunimax or parenteral antibiotics are used routinely for the treatment of children with fevers at some health care centers. The same prevalence of the virus was observed among Cameroonian adult renal patients, with the demonstrable viral antigen complexed with immunoglobulin and complement in glomeruli of renal biopsies (2).

Cameroon is endemic for filariasis. Both loiasis and onchocerciasis may cause immune complex nephropathy (3). A number of children in Yaounde with the nephrotic syndrome, particularly those .8 years of age, have overt filariasis.

The response of nephrotic syndrome in children to steroid therapy appears to differ significantly from those recorded in temperate climates. More than half of the nephrotic children, particularly those <5 years, do not respond to high doses of steroids. Of those who do, the majority are aged 8 to 12 years, with equal distribution between the sexes.

References

1. Nzoyem M: Prevalence de l'Antigene Australia (HBsAg) chez une groupe de sujets presume a haut risque et chez des donneurs de sang a l'Hopital Central de Yaounde. MD thesis, University of Yaounde, 1981.
2. Kollo B: Recerche d'une Association entre le port de l'HGsAg (Antigene Australia) et la Maladie Renale. MD thesis, University of Yaounde, 1982.
3. Ngu JL, Soothill JF: Immune-complex nephropathy. In Chandra RK (ed): Critical Reviews in Tropical Medicine. New York, Plenum Press, 1982.

23C China

JI-YUN YANG

THE EPIDEMIOLOGY AND INCIDENCE OF RENAL DISEASE

The results of an investigation on the morbidity of urinary tract diseases were reported recently (1982) (1). Among a total population of 188,697 from different areas of China, 4245 (2.3%) were found to be suffering from urinary tract diseases. The most common ones were urinary tract infection (UTI) (0.91%) and glomerulonephritis (GN) (0.49%). Because the authors used urinalysis as the screening test, there must be a possibility of further cases having been missed.

An observation from Beijing, Shanghai, and Jiangsu Province found that there were 70,692 children admitted to hospital during a 3-year period (1979–1981), of which 3,526 (5.0%) had urinary tract diseases (2). The most common were acute GN (55%), nephrotic syndrome (19%), and UTI (6.0%). In an analysis of 944 cases (including 153 autopsies) with chronic renal failure, the principal diseases found were chronic GN (diagnosed clinically in 65%, by autopsy 60%), chronic pyelonephritis (19%, 20%), hypertensive glomerulosclerosis (6.9%, 5.9%) congenital polycystic disease (3.8%, 9.2%), and lupus nephritis (1.9%, 3.9%). Tuberculosis, diabetes mellitus, and gout were occasionally found (3).

In children the causes of acute renal failure (ARF) were mainly acute GN and nephrotic syndrome (about 70%), sepsis, poisons, (such as mycetism and drugs) and epidemic hemorrhagic fever (4, 5). In adults ARF was mainly a result of sepsis, poison, shock (cardiogenic or hemorrhagic), and epidemic hemorrhagic fever (6).

GLOMERULONEPHRITIS

Histopathology

In recent years, percutaneous renal biopsy has been widely used to evaluate glomerular disease in China. The distribution of pathological diagnoses in a collected series of 1011 adults with primary glomerulonephritis from Beijing. Shanghai, and Nanking is given in Table 23C-1 (24). In 165 cases of secondary glomerular disease, the breakdown was systemic lupus erythematosus—35%, diabetes mellitus—8%, Henoch-Schönlein purpura—10%, other collagen vascular disease—6.7%, epidemic hemorrhagic fever—6.7%, schistosomiasis—4.8%, liver disease—3%, and transplants—2.4%. Of 57 children biopsied, 27 (47%) showed mesangioproliferative glomerulonephritis.

Acute glomerulonephritis

The true incidence of acute glomerulonephritis (AGN) is difficult to ascertain. This is a result of the large percentage of cases of AGN that are subclinical in nature and the host factors that account for a marked variability in attack rate. Qing-shan Hospital reported that the annual incidence of AGN in children admitted from 1972 to 1980 was 2.0 to

Table 23C.1.
Renal histology in 1011 adults with primary glomerular disease in Beijing, Shanghai, and Nanking

Disease	No.	%
Mesangioproliferative glomerulonephritis	402	40
Membranoproliferative glomerulonephritis	107	11
Membranous nephropathy	93	9.2
IgA nephropathy	86	8.5
Focal segmental glomerulosclerosis	82	8.1
Endocapillary glomerulonephritis	67	6.6
Minimal change	66	6.5
Focal proliferative glomerulonephritis	64	6.3
IgM nephropathy	17	1.7
Sclerotic glomerulonephritis	17	1.7
Crescentic glomerulonephritis	5	0.5
End-stage kidney	5	0.5

From Editorial: Chin J Int Med 23: 131, 1984.

4.3%. This implies that about one out of 300 children would suffer from AGN each year (7). According to the report from Beijing, Shanghai, and Jiangsu Province, AGN accounted for approximately 2% to 5% of all children admitted to hospital and for 55% of the patients with urinary tract disease (2). The incidence of AGN is much higher in children than in adults. From a report of Shanghai Ruijin Hospital, there were 2040 children with AGN in hospital, accounting for 4.7% of all the children admitted during the period 1953–1974, whereas in the adults with AGN there were only 227 cases (0.57% of those admitted). This report showed that 93% of the 2267 patients were less than 20 years old, and 78% were less than 10 years. Although AGN occurred all year round, 54% of the patients presented in the period September to December (2).

It has long been known that most cases of AGN have, as their prodromal diseases, respiratory tract infection and impetigo. As China is a large country, there are many factors affecting the kinds and frequency of the prodromal diseases, such as geographic environment, climate; the epidemic, social, and economic conditions; and hygienic habits. In northern China, AGN followed mainly respiratory tract infection, and in the south, impetigo. For example, in Beijing, 70% of the prodromal disease was respiratory tract infection and 15% was impetigo, whereas in Shanghai the incidence was 61% and 23% respectively (2). Recently, a decreased incidence of impetigo has been reported. At Beijing Medical College, 34% and 37% of patients with AGN first had recognized respiratory tract infection and impetigo, respectively, during the period of 1962–1964, while in the period from 1966 to 1972 the corresponding figures were 59% and 14%.

The mortality of AGN in the acute stage was 1% to 3% in the early 1950s, but has since dropped significantly and now there are almost no deaths in the acute stage. The most serious complications of AGN are circulatory congestion, hypertensive encephalopathy, and ARF. From a recent report of 1948 cases with AGN, there were 77 cases (4.2%) with severe oliguria, 47 cases (2.4%) with heart failure, 15 cases (0.7%) with ARF, and 11 (0.5%) with hypertensive encephalopathy. These complications now occur less frequently (2).

As elsewhere, AGN has a good prognosis in children. Beijing Children's Hospital reported long-term follow-up of 500 cases and found 9.4% patients with an abnormal urinalysis.

Nephrotic syndrome

The nephrotic syndrome (NS) is a relatively common disease in China. Since only a few renal biopsies were done until recently, the classification of primary nephrotic syndrome in children mainly depended on clinical evidence. According to the criteria proposed by the Nanking Forum of Pediatric Nephrologists in 1979, NS was divided into two types: simple pattern and nephritic pattern (8). This classification depended on the presence, or absence, of hematuria (>10 rbc/hpf), hypertension (for older children >130/90, for preschool children >120/80), and azotemia (NPN >50 mg%, BUN >30 mg%). In the past 3 years, experience has shown that this classification was helpful for some clinical work, but inadequate for research. Recently the criteria have been modified by some authors. They suggested that the classification should be based on the clinical and laboratory characteristics, the response to medical intervention, the course and ultimate outcome, and the renal biopsy, if possible. Thus, there are some reports about the relationship between the histological changes and clinical data and more reports about the laboratory parameters, especially immunological data. The parameters investigated have included complement (including C3 in the urine), Ig determination, erythrocyte rosette formation, lymphocyte transformation, migration inhibition test, selectivity of proteinuria, urinary FDP, lysozyme in the urine, circulating immune complexes, and urinary cytology.

Corticosteroid therapy in NS generally followed the recommendations of the International Study of Kidney Disease in Children. But some hospitals preferred a longer course (an intensive therapy of 4 to 8 weeks and then an intermittent therapy for 5 to 8 months) (8). For steroid nonresponders, a combination of immunosuppressive therapy was used (cyclophosphamide, chlorambucil, and nitrogen mustard). Some patients were also treated by traditional Chinese herbal medicine.

The mortality was quite high (about 30%) in the 1950s. With the use of corticosteroid and antibiotics, it gradually declined to 10% to 17%. Since the 1970s, with the use of immunosuppressive drugs, it was less than 3% in some areas (9). The most common complications of NS were infections and impaired growth. Hypovolemia and imbalance of electrolytes were also reported. Hypercoagulability and thrombosis were rarely reported.

Glomerulonephritis Associated with Hepatitis B

The relationship between hepatitis B and GN is an interesting subject in China. Some authors noticed that carriers of hepatitis B surface antigen (HBsAg) were much more common in children than adults. It was reported that 1.3% to 13% of the population from different areas showed a positive HBsAg (R-PHA method) and in some areas even much higher, especially in children. Beijing Children's Hospital reported that 4.4% of 436 patients with hepatitis B antigenemia showed some extrahepatic manifestations, of which kidney disease was most common (47%) (10). Wuhan Children's Hospital reported that out of 98 cases of hepatitis B, 8 patients (8.2%) showed the manifestations of GN. On the other hand, some patients with GN were positive for HBsAg. For example, Zhao (24) reported that among 106 patients with GN, 32 cases were positive for HBsAg. Another report (11) from Wuhan Medical College showed that out of 275 children with GN, 46 (17%) were associated with hepatitis B. Most of these patients had an insidious onset proteinuria, recurrent hematuria, or nephrotic syndrome. Some of them did not respond well to steroid therapy and took a chronic course. Although many authors reported their clinical data, only a few had kidney histological examination. A report of six cases from Shanghai (12) described three cases of mesangial proliferation, two cases with membranous nephropathy, and one case with endocapillary mesangial proliferation. Circulating immune-complexes positive for HBsAg were reported, but HBsAg was not detected in renal tissue.

Purpura nephritis

The incidence of renal involvement in Henoch-Schönlein syndrome (SHS) varies from 11% to 41%. This variation can be accounted for by the different criteria used to define "renal involvement," by the different methods used to detect microscopic hematuria, and the duration of follow-up (20).

Compared with AGN, fewer patients with SHS nephritis manifested edema (30%) and hypertension (20–40%) than the patients with AGN (96% and 80%, respectively) (21). In an analyses of 71 cases with purpura nephritis, four clinical patterns were reported: mild pattern (asymptomatic hematuria or abnormal Addis count), 19 cases (26%); acute nephritic syndrome, 43 cases (60%); nephrotic syndrome, 6 cases (8.5%); chronic GN and probable progression to CRF, 2 cases (2.8%) (21). Rapidly progressive GN was also reported occasionally.

According to a report of 344 patients with SHS at the acute stage, 115 cases (33%) showed renal involvement. There were 87 cases with 4.5 years of follow-up. Of these 73% of patients recovered completely, 24% of patients still had an abnormal urinalysis, one patient progressed into chronic GN and one died from rapidly progressive GN.

Traditional Chinese Herbal Medicine

It has long been known that traditional Chinese herbal medicine has a clinical effect on edema. In addition to clinical observations, some labortory investigations have also been done in the past 30 years.

Some nephrologists have treated patients with GN or NS with herbs only or have combined herbs with corticosteroid therapy. The prescription usually consists of several ingredients, but recently there is a tendency to use single ingredients. For example, some nephrologists used tripterygium wilfordin or triptergium hypoglaucum in treating patients with GN or NS (1, 13, 14). According to their experience, it was proven to have some value in idiopathic nephrotic syndrome, lupus nephritis, and SHS nephritis. Benefit has been claimed even in some patients with steroid-dependent or resistant renal disease. The side effects of these herbs include gastrointestinal symptoms (nausea, constipation, and so on), leukopenia, and occasionally menopause. Some authors (14) observed beneficial effects on Masugi nephritis in rabbits. They treated the rabbits with these herbs before immunization, and milder sclerotic and fibrotic lesions were found than in the control groups.

TUMOR

The most important kidney tumor in children is nephroblastoma (Wilm's tumor). In an analysis of 1897 cases of tumor in children 501 cases were malignant, of which Wilm's tumor (111 cases) was the second most common, only exceeded by malignant lymphoma (139 cases) in frequency (15). Although this neoplasm occurs at any age, it mainly attacks children less than 5 years old. There has been a decline in mortality during the past 30 years. During the 1950s and 1960s the patients were treated by surgical operation and irradiation, and 2 years after diagnosis the survival rate was about 30%. In the 1970s with the addition of chemotherapy (actinomycin D and vincristine) the survival rate doubled (16).

Tumors of the testes in children are rare. A recent report of 52 children with testicular tumors from Shanghai (1980) showed that 84% (37 cases) were embryonal carcinoma. Most of the patients were less than 3 years old and the youngest was only 3 months of age. The author emphasized that aggressive therapy should be used, including a radical orchiectomy with retroperitoneal lymph node dissection. After a long-term follow-up, 40% of patients were surviving and well. The other 21 cases died within 2 years from multiple metastascs.

UROLITHIASIS IN CHILDREN

In a recent report (1976) of 10,876 patients from China (including children and adults) with urological disorders there were 2424 (22%) cases with urolithiasis. Urinary stone disease occurs more frequently in the southern part of China. The report showed that in Shenyang (a city in the north) urolithiasis contributed only 4% of all urological patients, whereas in Nanjin (a city in the south) the incidence was 22% and in Zunyi (an endemic area in the south) 59% of urologic patients had urolithiasis.

Children in China used to have a high frequency of bladder stones containing uric acid. An observation in Canton (1920) (18) found that among 3492 cases of urolithiasis, bladder stones occurred in 2962 cases; 25% of these occurred in children less than 10 years old and 43% in patients less than 20 years old. In the 1950s, 44% of cases with bladder stones occurred in children (19). In the past 2 decades there has been a significant decline of bladder stones in children in China. In 1976, among the 2424 patients with stones, there were only 386 cases with bladder stones of which only 51 cases (13%) were in children (18).

OTHER KIDNEY DISEASES IN CHILDREN

UTI, lupus nephritis, and the kidney involvement in connective tissue diseases are also relatively common diseases in children in China. With the use of renal biopsy, more IgA nephropathy has been reported. In addition, hemolytic uremic syndrome, renal tubular acidosis, Fanconi's syndrome, nephrogenic diabetes insipidus, and renal vascular hypertension (nonspecific arteritis has been considered the most frequent cause) have also been reported occasionally.

DIALYSIS AND RENAL TRANSPLANTATION IN CHILDREN

Peritoneal dialysis is frequently used to treat patients with acute renal failure and poisoning. Few children have been treated by hemodialysis. In some hemodialysis units, children accounted for only 1% to 2% of the patients treated. Sometimes the doctors give uremic patients dialysate containing mannitol by a stomach tube and report some benefit.

Only a few renal transplants in older children have been done. On the other hand, an investigation of the use of double renal transplants from newborn infants to adult recipients was reported recently (22, 23).

References

1. Li Shi-mei, Li Lei-Shi, Qiu Chuan-Lu: A summary of the symposium of kidney disease. Chin J Int Med 21:619, 1982.
2. Beijing Cooperation of Children's Kidney Disease: An investigation on children's urinary tract disease. Absrtact of the symposium of Kidney Disease, Chinese Medical Association, 1982, p 5.
3. Ye Ren-Gao, Li Ying, Li Hui-Gun, et al: An analysis of the causes of chronic renal failure of 944 cases. Chin J Int Med 21:210, 1982.
4. Beijing Children's Hospital: An analysis of acute renal failure in children. Abstract of the symposium of Kidney Disease, Chinese Medical Association, 1982, p 172.
5. Zhao Song-Jie, Wu Gimg-Ging, Pang Ning, et al: An analysis of acute renal failure in children. Abstract of the symposium of Kidney Disease, Chinese Medical Association, 1982, p 175.
6. Xu Jun-Jie: An analysis of the causes and death of acute renal failure in internal medicine. Abstract of the symposium of Kidney Disease, Chinese Medical Association, 1982, p 176.
7. Hu Xiangli. An observation of acute glomerulonephritis in children (814 cases). Wuhan Med J 6:93, 1982.
8. Cooperation of Children's Kidney Diseases: A suggestion of the classification and treatment of glomerular disease in children. Chin J Pediatr 17:248, 1979.

9. Wang Pao-Lin, Li Shu-Zheng, et al: A comment on the study of glomerulonephritis and nephrotic syndrome in children. Chin J Pediatr 18:1, 1980.
10. Zeng Jun-Gua: Virus hepatitis and immunology. In Clinical Immunology of Children. Chinese Medical Association, 1982, p 30.
11. Wang Yun-Gin, Song Ming-tong: Clinical diagnosis of glomerulonephritis associated with Hepatitis B, a clinical analysis of 275 HBsAg (+) and (−) cases. Acta Acad Med Wuhan 11:19, 1982.
12. Guo Yi-Qing, Sheng Fang-Yun, Fang Li-Jun: Glomerulonephritis associated with Hepatitis B in children. Abstract of the symposium of Kidney Disease, Chinese Medical Association, 1982, p 40.
13. Li Leisni, Zhang Xun, Chen Guang-Yong, et al: Clinical study of Tripterygium Wilfordii Hook in treating GN. Chin J Int Med 20:216, 1981.
14. Abstract of Symposium of Kidney Disease, Chinese Medical Association, 1982, p 8, 83, 84, 124, 132, 134.
15. Beijing Children's Hospital: Pediatrics. People's Health Publication, Beijing, 1973, p 868.
16. Ge lin-Juan, Ji Baixing, et al: An analysis of Wilm's tumor of the last 20 years. Shanghai Medical Journal 3:402, 1980.
17. Ji Baixiang, Ge Lin-Juan, et al: Testicular tumors in children, a report of 52 cases. Chinese Journal of Surgery 18:504, 1980.
18. Wu Jie-ping, Gu Fang-Liu, Sun Chang-Ti: Urothiasis in China. Chin J Urol 1:1, 1980.
19. Ku Fang-lu: Geographical environment and urolithiasis. Chin J Surg 16:323, 1978.
20. Xin Hua Hospital: A study of glomerulonephritis associated with Schönlein-Henoch purpura, a clinical observation and follow-up of 115 cases. Shanghai Med J 1:343, 1978.
21. Yang Ji-Yun: Schonlein-Henoch Nephritis—an observation and follow-up of 71 cases. Collection of Pediatric Essays, Beijing Medical College, 1980, p 58.
22. Yu Tianlin, Liu De-Fu, Yu Xiang-Cai: The use of renal transplants from newborn to adult recipients. Chin J Org Transplant 3:53, 1982.
23. Yu Hui-Yuan, Guan De-Lin, Wang Zhi-Gang: A clinical study of renal transplants from infant to adult recipients. Chin J Org Transplant 2:1, 1981.
24. Zhao Ji-Lin: Virus Infection and glomerular disease. In Wang Po-Lin (eds): Pediatric Nephrology. Beijing, Peoples Health Publication, 1983, p 231.
25. Editorial: The renal biopsy in the diagnosis of glomerular disease. Chin J Int Med 23:131, 1984.

23D India

R. N. SRIVASTAVA

Socioeconomic and geographical factors play important roles in determining the prevalence and pattern of renal diseases in India. Climatic conditions and dietary habits vary in different parts of the country, but poverty, lack of education, poor hygienic conditions, and inadequate medical facilities are common denominators, and greatly influence the incidence, as well as outcome of renal diseases. Hereditary and genetic factors are comparatively much less important.

Acute gastroenteritis, dysentery, and streptococcal infections of throat and skin and malaria are widely prevalent and, directly or indirectly, affect the spectrum of renal diseases in children. In terms of importance the main disorders are the nephrotic syndrome, acute glomerulonephritis, acute renal failure, obstructive nephropathy, and vesical calculi. In hospital practice, there is a preponderance of acute conditions, with the patients often brought late with serious complications. The pattern of nephrotic syndrome is similar to that observed in western countries. Acute post-streptococcal glomerulonephritis is still a common condition in this country. Acute renal failure has a different etiologic spectrum from that observed in western countries.

Quartan malarial nephropathy and schistosomiasis have apparently not been reported from India. Thalassemia is widely prevalent in northern India. It is, however, not associated with significant renal involvement. Renal disease in leprosy has now been well recognized, but is rarely prominent in children. Exposure to toxic chemicals, such as mercury or lead, or possible harmful indigenous drugs, has not been reported as a cause of nephropathy in children. No endemic renal disorder, such as Balkan nephropathy or renal amyloidosis in familial mediterranean fever, is known to exist in India.

NEPHROTIC SYNDROME

Idiopathic Nephrotic Syndrome

The nephrotic syndrome constitutes the most common renal disorder in childhood, in hospital as well as in family practice, because the majority of such cases comprise frequently relapsing lipoid nephrosis or the corticosteroid resistant group. We undertook a clinicopathological study, in which renal biopsy was done in 206 consecutive cases, which showed that 96% were idiopathic, and of these 77% were of the minimal lesion variety (1). Subsequently renal biopsies have not been undertaken in uncomplicated corticosteroid sensitive patients, but the pattern appears to be similar. Mesangial proliferative, mesangiocapillary, and focal glomerulosclerosis are the main types of lesions in the "nonminimal" category, constituting about 40%, 30%, and 20%, respectively. Membranous nephropathy was seen in five cases. One of them had systemic lupus and another hepatitis B.

The majority of Indian children with lipoid nephrosis suffer from frequent relapses. In 52 patients we tried an 8-week course of cyclophosphamide along with "alternate-day" prednisone. Our results in inducing longer periods of remission with this regimen have not been as impressive as in reports from western countries. Experience with nephrotic syndrome from other centers in India has been similar to ours. Among patients with significant glomerular lesions, only about 20%, having mild mesangial proliferative lesions or focal glomerulosclerosis, have responded to prednisone but mostly followed a relapsing course. An occasional patient with mesangiocapillary glomerulonephritis has also responded to prednisone, but the majority have had progressive disease.

Secondary Nephrotic Syndrome

In less than 2% of all cases of nephrotic syndrome an underlying cause was present. We have seen five cases of congenital nephrotic syndrome and occasional examples have been reported from other centers. Renal histology in the majority showed "microcystic disease." Renal amyloidosis is rarely seen in children, although, among the conditions associated with it, tuberculosis is common in all parts of the country and juvenile rheumatoid arthritis is seen with regular frequency. In one of our patients with nephrotic syndrome, active chronic hepatitis was present, and his blood was positive for hepatitis B surface antigen. Renal biopsy showed membranous nephropathy, and abundant amounts of hepatitis B surface antigen were demonstrated in the glomeruli. Subsequently, over the past year, we have conducted a study to demonstrate hepatitis B surface antigen in the blood and glomeruli of children with steroid-resistant nephrotic syndrome. Among 19 cases, 6 with mesangiocapillary glomerulonephritis, 9 with mesangial proliferative lesions, 3 with membranous nephropathy, and 2 with crescentic glomerulonephritis, the results were negative. The carrier rate for hepatitis B surface antigenemia in the northern Indian population is reported to be about 3%, and one would expect that it might be more commonly implicated in immune complex induced renal injury.

Patients with nephrotic syndrome and serious infections, particularly peritonitis, are frequently seen. The most common organisms are *Str. pneumoniae* and *E. coli.*

ACUTE GLOMERULONEPHRITIS

Poststreptococcal Glomerulonephritis

Beta-hemolytic streptococcal infections of the throat, as well as skin, remain widely prevalent. The incidence of acute poststreptococcal glomerulonephritis and acute rheumatic fever is therefore high. The clinical profile is simlar to that reported from other parts of the world. We see a disproportionately greater number of patients with serious complications such as hypertensive encephalopathy, left ventricular failure, and anuria. In five cases crescentic glomerulonephritis was seen. All of them had a progressive course resulting in renal failure. We have not observed continued slow progression to irreversible renal damage in other cases of poststreptococcal acute glomerulonephritis.

Crescentic (Rapidly Progressive) Glomerulonephritis

Fourteen patients with crescentic glomerulonephritis have been seen in 12 years (2). Five were of poststreptococcal type, three had Henoch-Schönlein vasculitis, one had juvenile rheumatoid arthritis, and the remainder were idiopathic. In eleven cases a combination of prednisone, cyclophosphamide, and anticoagulant drugs was administered. It appeared to be beneficial in three of them where such therapy could be started early in the course of the disease. In the remainder, the outcome was poor.

ACUTE RENAL FAILURE

Acute renal failure constitutes the most important condition in pediatric nephrology in hospital practice. At this center it is responsible for approximately 20 patients per year, about 1.5% of all inpatients. The main etiological conditions are acute gastroenteritis, hemolytic uremic syndrome associated with acute dysentery, acute glomerulonephritis, intravascular hemolysis (mainly in glucose-6-phosphate dehydrogenase (G6PD) deficient subjects), and severe infections in early infancy (Table 23D.1). Liberal use of nephrotoxic drugs may be contributory in some cases. The mortality is particularly high because of the delay in instituting appropriate treatment, as well as lack of widely available dialysis facilities.

Table 23D.1.
Etiology of Acute Renal Failure[a]

Diagnosis	Cases (No.)
Acute gastroenteritis	55
Acute glomerulonephritis	36
Crescentic glomerulonephritis	12
HUS (mostly in association with bacillary dysentery)	16
Acute tubular necrosis	25
Acute intravascular hemolysis	21
Infections, septicemia	21
Obstructive nephropathy	6
Miscellaneous (fulminating hepatitis, hepatic coma, or Reye's syndrome)	15
TOTAL	207

[a] Patients with "acute on chronic" renal failure have not been included.

Acute Gastroenteritis

Acute diarrheal illness in infants, mainly seen in summer months, is common in all parts of the country, as in most other developing countries. The etiologic agents include enterotoxigenic *E. coli*, rotavirus, and enteropathogenic *E. coli*. In a significant proportion of patients, the severity of disease and lack of early rehydration lead to the development of acute renal failure. Malnutrition, anemia, and other infections may be associated. This form of renal failure has responded satisfactorily to standard treatment, and whenever necessary one peritoneal dialysis has usually been sufficient. Acute gastroenteritis used to be the most frequent cause of acute renal failure in our experience. Over the past 5 years or so such cases appear to be declining, possibly related to widespread application of oral rehydration in the management of diarrhea.

Acute Glomerulonephritis

Poststreptococcal acute glomerulonephritis with severe oliguria and azotemia has been quite frequent in our experience. Overhydration and hypertension are the more common complications. Renal function impairment takes 2 to 4 weeks to improve. Peritoneal dialysis has been necessary in a few instances. Except for patients with crescentic glomerulonephritis and an occasional patient who died of hypertensive encephalopathy and heart failure, complete recovery has followed in the rest.

Acute Dysentery, Hemolytic Uremic Syndrome, and Acute Renal Failure

During the last few years, acute dysentery has emerged as the most frequent cause of renal failure at this center. Similar observations have been reported from other parts of this country (3) and Bangladesh (4). Mostly infants and young children are affected, and they often have associated mild-to-moderate malnutrition. Dysentery is almost invariably severe and responds poorly to treatment. After 1 to 2 weeks of illness there is rapid development of oligoanuria, pallor, and drowsiness. Microscopic examination of stools shows an exudate containing numerous neutrophils and macrophages, which is characteristically observed in shigellosis. Cultures of stools are, however, positive in only about a third of the cases, showing *Shigella dysenteriae* or *Shigella flexneri* and occasionally *E. coli* or *Klebsiella* species. The low culture positivity rate is probably a result of administration of various antibiotics before the patients are referred to hospital. A marked neutrophilic leukocytosis or a leukemoid reaction is usually present, being a common feature of severe shigellosis.

Hemolytic uremic syndrome (HUS) is present in about 70% of patients with acute renal failure following dysentery. The disorder is of a particularly severe variety, usually associated with anuria for several days. We have detected evidence of disseminated intravascular coagulation in 75% of such patients. Decreased levels of serum C3, circulating immune complexes, and glomerular deposits of IgM and C3 have been found in 20%. Renal histology shows diffuse or patchy cortical necrosis in the majority, whereas a small proportion show predominant arteriolar and glomerular lesions indicative of thrombotic microangiopathy. Similar observations have been reported from Bangladesh in patients with HUS following shigellosis (5). We have managed these patients with supportive care including transfusion of fresh blood and peritoneal dialysis. The mortality is about 70%, being chiefly related to the severity of renal lesions, although late referral of the patients could also be contributory. The survivors have been observed to show persistent proteinuria and histological evidence of chronic renal damage. The pathogenesis of HUS following dysentery is not clear, but the role of endotoxin-mediated injury to renal microvasculature is probably important (4). Fluid deficit and hypovolemia do not appear to be directly responsible.

About a third of patients with acute renal failure developing after dysentery do not show the features of microangiopathic hemolysis. Renal histological changes in such cases mainly consist of tubular damage and occasional thrombi in glomeruli. These patients have a comparatively better outcome and those who survive the acute phase seem to make a complete recovery.

Intravascular Hemolysis

Acute intravascular hemolysis was responsible for renal failure in 10% of our cases. It mainly occurred in subjects with G6PD deficiency and was precipitated by the ingestion of antimalarial drugs. The characteristic features were rapid development of pallor, fatigue, passage of dark-red urine, and mild jaundice. Anemia, peripheral blood smear abnormalities suggestive of intravascular hemolysis, increased serum bilirubin, and azotemia were present. Renal failure was of "nonoliguric" type in 60%. The response to supportive treatment was very satisfactory in these cases (6). A high incidence of G6PD deficiency in the population reported as being from 2.2% to 15% and widespread use of antimalarial drugs following a resurgence of malaria in this country, make intravascular hemolysis and renal failure a particularly important condition.

Intravascular hemolysis has been implicated in two other conditions leading to acute renal failure in the adult population in this region. These are snake-bite and copper sulphate poisoning (7). Fortunately, these appear to be rare during childhood.

Other Causes of Acute Renal Failure

During neonatal period and early infancy, serious infections accounted for the majority of cases of acute renal failure. Nephrotoxic drugs, such as kanamycin and gentamycin are important contributory factors in this age group. The outcome was poor in these patients, mainly because of lack of appropriate intensive care facilities.

Acute established renal failure in minimal lesion nephrotic syndrome in relapse, frequently seen in some countries (8), has been rare in our experience, despite the fact that patients with massive edema and ascites are commonly encountered. Often such patients have associated acute respiratory or gastrointestinal infection. Major cardiovascular surgical procedures are comparatively infrequently carried out in infancy in this country, and consequently associated postoperative acute renal failure is uncommon.

CHRONIC RENAL FAILURE

Glomerulonephritis is the most common cause of chronic renal failure in our experience, followed by chronic pyelonephritis and obstructive nephropathy. Congenital anomalies, renal calculus disease, and heredofamilial nephropathies account for most of the remainder (Table 23D.2). We have managed these patients with supportive care. Long-term dialysis and renal transplantation has not been feasible as yet in the pediatric age group.

HYPERTENSION

Large scale surveys to detect hypertension in children have not been carried out in this country. A study of the causes of sustained hypertension in hospitalized children indicates that persistent glomerulonephritis and chronic pyelonephritis are the main causes (Table 23D.3).

Nonspecific Aortoarteritis (Takayasu Disease)

Nonspecific aortoarteritis is responsible for the majority of cases of renovascular hypertension (9). The disease resembles obstructive aortitis reported from Thailand. It affects older children and is about three times as common in girls as in boys. The presenting symptoms are usually related to severe hypertension, such as encephalopathy and heart failure. There usually is, however, a preceding history of vague complaints such as low grade fever, malaise, and asthenia of several months' duration. Excretory urography and isotope renogram indicate arterial involvement, which is demonstrated on aortography. The abdominal aorta is mainly

Table 23D.2.
Etiology of Chronic Renal Failure

Diagnosis	Cases (No.)
Chronic glomerulonephritis (excluding crescentic glomerulonephritis and HUS)	41
Chronic pyelonephritis	28
Obstructive nephropathy	16
Renal lithiasis	15
Congenital anomalies (neurogenic dysfunction with meningomyelocele, ectopia vesicae, prune belly syndrome, or polycystic kidney)	21
Alport's syndrome	5
Nephronophthisis	3
Congenital nephrosis	3
TOTAL	132

Table 23D.3.
Disorders Causing Persistent Hypertension

Diagnosis	Cases (No.)
Chronic glomerulonephritis	57
Chronic pyelonephritis	17
Nonspecific aortoarteritis	16
Renal lithiasis	11
Obstructive nephropathy	9
Renal artery stenosis	2
Coarctation of aorta	3
Polycystic kidneys	5
Phaeochromocytoma	2
Miscellaneous (Wilms' tumor, neuroblastoma, cyanotic heart disease, or brain tumor)	11
Essential hypertension	5
TOTAL	138

affected. Renal arterial narrowing that can be unilateral or bilateral is a chronic process leading over a period of several months or years to stenosis and complete occlusion. The diagnosis is rarely made in the early stages. Histological changes in the major vessels include thickening of adventitia by fibrocollagenous tissue, fibrosis of media with fragmentation of elastic fibres, chronic inflammatory changes, and thickening of intima.

The etiology of nonspecific aortoarteritis is not known. It has been suggested that it may represent an unusual manifestation of tuberculosis. Indirect evidence of tuberculosis, such as a positive tuberculin test, cervical, or pulmonary hilar lymphadenopathy is often present in the patients, but tubercle bacilli, giant cells, or caseation have not been demonstrated in the lesions. Antitubercular treatment and corticosteroids do not appear to offer any benefit.

URINARY TRACT CALCULI

Vesical calculus disease in children is endemic in northern and northwestern parts of the country, including Delhi. It is almost confined to preschool age boys. In India, the chief constituent of such stones has been found to be calcium oxalate and ammonium acid urate (10). Studies from a neighboring country, Afghanistan, reveal similar findings. Vesical calculus is the most common cause of admission to the surgical wards of the leading children's hospital in that country. The stones are mostly seen in young boys. They are composed of calcium oxalate and uric acid. Vesical calculi do not seem to recur after cystolithotomy.

The etiology of bladder stones disease remains obscure. Urinary tract infections are not considered to be the primary event and a metabolic abnormality has not been detected. Dietary and environmental factors are probably important. High ambient temperatures and low humidity could lead to passage of relatively more concentrated urine. A predominantly wheat-based diet (as in northern India and Afghanistan), deficiency of pyridoxine, and excessive intake of articles rich in oxalic acid have been suggested to be contributory. Bladder stones seldom occur in children with severe degrees of malnutrition. While the etiology may be multifactorial, it is well known that with overall improvement in socioeconomic conditions, vesical calculus disease declines.

CONGENITAL AND HEREDITARY NEPHROPATHIES AND RENAL TUBULAR DISORDERS

The pattern of such disorders in India is similar to that reported from western countries, and none of the conditions is unusually common. Several examples of polycystic kidneys, congenital nephrotic syndrome, Alport's syndrome, and juvenile nephronophthisis are on our records. Renal tubular disorders such as vitamin D-resistant hypophosphatemic rickets, renal tubular acidosis, renal glycosuria, and nephrogenic diabetes insipidus have also been observed. Vitamin D-deficiency rickets has become uncommon, probably as a result of widespread vitamin D supplementation, and cases of vitamin D-resistant rickets are being recognized more frequently.

COLLAGEN DISEASES

Among the various collagen diseases, only juvenile rheumatoid arthritis is commonly seen. Out of our 63 patients seen over a 12-year period, one had renal amyloidosis, and another with systemic onset variety had crescentic glomerulonephritis. In the remainder, urinary abnormalities were unremarkable, and renal biopsies were not done. The condition next in frequency was Henoch-Schönlein vasculitis. Renal involvement was of variable severity, being crescentic glomerulonephritis in three cases.

Systemic lupus erythematosus is rare in children, although common in adults. Polyarteritis, polymyositis, and systemic sclerosis have been very infrequent in our experience.

RENAL INVOLVEMENT IN PEDIATRIC DISEASES COMMON IN INDIA

A number of diseases such as tuberculosis, malaria, typhoid, and hepatitis are particularly common in India. Some others including severe degrees of malnutrition and intestinal parasitic infections are mainly seen in the pediatric age group. A form of cirrhosis of liver termed "Indian childhood cirrhosis" is almost confined to the Indian subcontinent. Among various hemoglobinopathies, thalassemia is particularly common in northern India. Varying types and degrees of renal involvement have been observed in some of these conditions but are comparatively of little significance.

Malaria and Kala Azar

Vivax malaria is endemic in most parts of the country. The falciparum variety is mainly seen in eastern hilly regions, but occasional cases are encountered in other parts. Significant glomerular involvement has not been reported in vivax malaria. Typical examples of black-water fever also appear to be rare. The main renal problem in relation to malaria is from acute intravascular hemolysis following intake of antimalarial drugs in subjects with G6PD deficiency. In eastern states of the country kala azar is widely prevalent. Glomerular involvement in leishmaniasis has been reported from Brazil, but progressive renal disease, however, does not appear to be an important feature in India.

Typhoid

Renal histological abnormalities in typhoid fever have been reported in occasional instances. A diffuse, moderately severe proliferative glomerulonephritis was observed in one of our patients with typhoid. The child had shown proteinuria and microscopic hematuria, which gradually disappeared over 6 months. We have carefully examined the urine in patients with typhoid, but the abnormalities have been unremarkable, not justifying performance of renal biopsy.

Indian Childhood Cirrhosis

A distinct form of cirrhosis of liver affecting infants is almost exclusively seen in India (11). In most cases the disorder is steadily progressive and death occurs from hepatic failure within 1 or 2 years of diagnosis. The etiology is obscure. Nutritional deficiency and infections are not important. Siblings are sometimes affected and a polygenic pattern of inheritance has been suggested. There is increased accumulation of copper in the liver, and although its pathogenesis is not known, it is believed to have an injurious effect. Circulating immune complexes and evidence of complement activation have been found in some cases. Most patients show a generalised aminoaciduria. In a study of 15 patients, we found slight proteinuria, microscopic hematuria, and reduction of creatinine clearance values. Renal biopsy showed mild mesangial proliferative lesions and prominent granular deposits of IgA, IgM, and C3 in mesangium and capillary walls. The evolution of these glomerular lesions appears to be very gradual and does not lead to clinically significant renal insufficiency.

Malnutrition

Several parameters of renal function have been found to be abnormal in severe forms of protein energy malnutrition (12). These include reduction of glomerular filtration rate and renal blood flow, generalised aminoaciduria, and impairment of maximum urinary concentration, as well as maximum acidification. The etiology of such a generalised renal dysfunction is probably multifactorial and related to deficiency of protein, potassium, magnesium, and vitamin D. The abnormalities do not appear to present serious problems in the managment of such patients and gradually improve following nutritional rehabilitation.

References

1. Srivastava RN, Mayekar G, Anand R, et al: Nephrotic syndrome in Indian children. Arch Dis Childh 50:626, 1975.
2. Srivastava RN, Choudhry VP: Rapidly progressive (crescentic) glomerulonephritis. Int J Pediatr Nephrol 1:94, 1980.
3. Raghupathy P, Date A, Shastry JCM, et al: Hemolytic uremic syndrome complicating shigella dysentery in South Indian children. Brit Med J I:1518, 1978.
4. Koster F, Levin J, Walker L, et al: Hemolytic uremic syndrome after shigellosis: Relation to endotoxemia and circulating immune complexes. N Engl J Med 298:927, 1978.
5. Koster FT, Boonpucknavig V, Sujaho S, et al: Renal histopathology in the hemolytic uremic syndrome following shigellosis. Clin Nephrol 21:126, 1984.
6. Choudhry VP, Madan N, Sood SK. Intravascular hemolysis and renal insufficiency in children with glucose-6-phosphate dehydrogenase deficiency following antimalarial therapy. Ind J Med Res 71:561, 1980.
7. Chugh KS, Singhal PC, Nath IVS, et al: Spectrum of acute renal failure in North India. J Assoc Phy India 26:147, 1978.
8. Chantler C: Renal Failure in Childhood. In Renal Disease Black D, Jones NF (eds): ed 4. Oxford, Blackwell Scientific Publications, 1979, p 832.
9. Shrivastava S, Rajani M, Chopra P, et al: Systemic hypertension and aortic obstruction in children. Europ J Pediatr 135:281, 1981.
10. Teotia M, Teotia SPS: Kidney and bladder stones in India. Postgrad Med J 53 (suppl 2):41, 1977.
11. Proceedings of workshop on Indian Childhood Cirrhosis. Indian Pediatr 19:1051, 1982.
12. Salam NMA, Mehta S, Chugh KS: Renal function in children with protein calorie malnutrition. Indian Pediatr 15:121, 1978.

23E Japan

TADASU SAKAI

Renal disease in children may present in a variety of ways or it may be covert and escape medical attention. The child who belongs to the latter category may nevertheless be as sick as the child who belongs to the former. Although there have been many advances in the field of dialysis and transplantation, there unfortunately has been little concerted effort given to initial recognition of the renal maladies that lead to end-stage renal disease.

In 1973, a program of urine screening for asymptomatic hematuria and proteinuria in school children was instituted by the Ministry of Education in Japan. Since then, we have found many cases of renal disease at an early stage as a result of this nation-wide adoption of urinary screening. However, the ultimate goal of this screening program cannot be realized until an effective treatment for the found cases is available.

Since 1974, in Kanagawa prefecture, more than 99% of school children have been screened by urinalysis, supervised by the Association of Health Services, and a special committee composed of pediatric nephrologist, school physician, school nurse, public health nurse, school board members, members of the community physicians' association, and the community health care team. Nearly one million children have been screened.

THE TEST

An early-morning urine is collected, and a simple dip-stick method is used for the detection of proteinuria and hematuria. When the urine is positive for either test, a second sample is examined in the same manner. When the urine abnormalities are persistently encountered, urine sediments are checked by microscopy and diagnostic steps instituted to determine the cause of urinary abnormalities. The first filter consists of examination of urinary protein and occult blood in early morning urine by test tape. The second filter involves confirmation of proteinuria by sulfosalicylic acid and boiling, and examination of the sediment for red blood cells, leukocytes, or casts by microscopy. The third filter consists of systematic review and physical examination by the school or private physician. The cases are classified into 3 categories: (1) "healthy," following which the child is released from the survey; (2) "follow-up," with monthly urinalysis under the supervision of a physician; (3) "medical care," leading to further evaluation by specific tests, such as serology, intravenous pyelogram, or renal biopsy to determine the etiology of the abnormal urinary findings.

RESULTS

Table 23E.1 shows the result of the annual examination of school children from 1977 to 1980 in Odawara City, Kanagawa prefecture. The introduction in Japan of urinalysis for school-age children has greatly facilitated the discovery of renal disease in asymptomatic children. Over the past 8 years at Kitasato University Hospital, we have studied 113 cases of chronic progressive renal disease, 31 of whom were found by routine urinalysis at area schools (Table 23E.2).

Membranoproliferative glomerulonephritis (MPGN) is one of the diseases that leads to chronic renal failure and has been investigated extensively during the past decade. Since the introduction of annual check-ups in Japan, including urinalysis, cases of asymptomatic MPGN

Table 23E.1.
Results of Screening Urinalysis, Odawara City, Japan (1977–1980) (No = 99,658)

	Primary school 69,692	Junior high school 29,966
First filter	826 (1.2%)	1534 (4.9%)
Second filter	120 (0.17%)	77 (0.29%)

are found more often, enabling study of the early phase of the disease. Over the past 8 years we have studied 25 children with MPGN, the diagnosis being confirmed by renal biopsy; 16 of the 25 were found by chance during routine urinalysis at school or at employment physicals.

Recently, a collaborative study of kidney diseases in children was conducted by the Ministry of Education in Japan. Renal biopsy was performed in 172 patients with no previous history of kidney disease who were suspected to have primary glomerular disease on the basis of urinalysis. They were placed in one of six categories according to hematuria and proteinuria (Fig. 23E.1). Children with asymptomatic hematuria without proteinuria tended to have minor pathological abnormalities with focal segmental lesions. In those with proteinuria and hematuria, diffuse proliferative lesions were more frequent. Renal pathology suggesting poor prognosis is not uncommon among cases with heavy proteinuria and hematuria.

For a comprehensive detection and preventive program to be fruitful and significant for the child with renal disease, it must be accurate, safe,

Table 23E.2.
Classification of Renal Disorders, Detected at School Urinalysis (Kitasato University Hospital)

Cause	Patient categories[a]				
	I	II	III	IV	V
Obstructive uropathy	8	—	2	3	1
Chronic GN with uropathy	5	1	1	3	1
Focal glomerulosclerosis	3	—	2	1	1
MPGN	17	—	1	4	9
Henoch-Schönlein GN	5	4	3	—	—
IgA nephropathy	16	—	—	1	7
SLE nephropathy	5	—	1	—	—
Medullary cystic disease	1	1	—	—	—
Rapidly progressive GN	11	5	3	—	—
Chronic GN	33	10	16	2	9
Hypoplastic kidney	9	4	2	4	3
TOTALS	113	25	31	18	31

[a] I, total number of patients; II, transplanted patients; III, chronic dialysis patients; IV, patients with renal insufficiency; V, patients detected by school urinalysis.

and economical, for both false-positive and false-negative results are harmful. The program also must be backed by an organization capable of full evaluation of the significance of abnormal results. We believe that the discovery of an asymptomatic child with renal disease is timely and important.

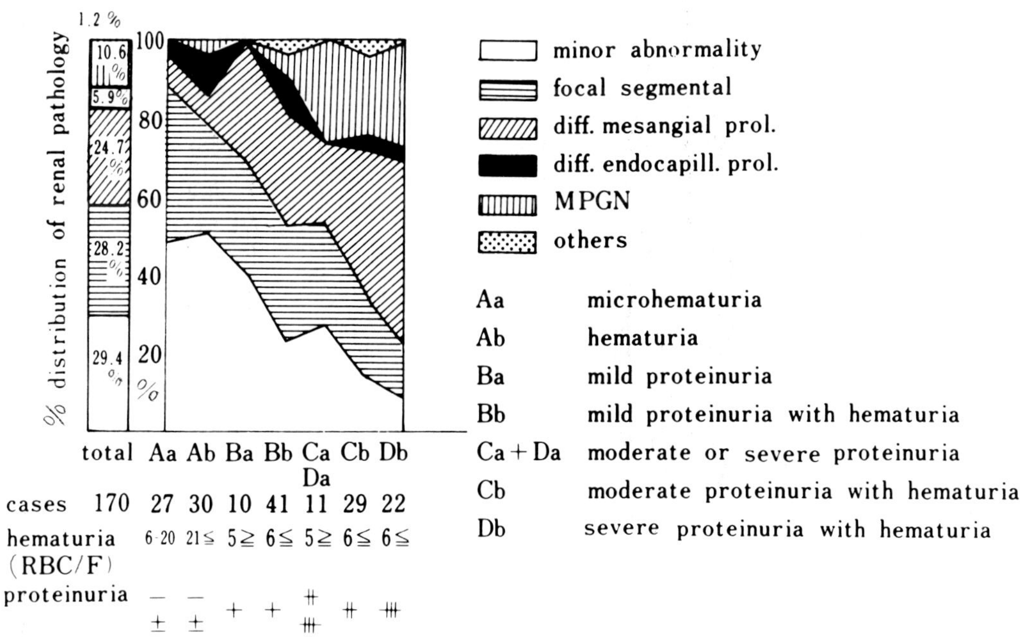

Figure 23E.1. Histopathological findings in Japanese school children suspected of having glomerulonephritis on the basis of screening urinalysis.

23F Mexico

GUSTAVO GORDILLO-PANIAGUA
RICARDO MUNOZ-ARIZPE

The following information is the 5-year experience (1977 to 1981) of the Department of Nephrology, Hospital Infantil de Mexico. The hospital is a referral center for sick children; 44% of the admissions to the Department of Nephrology came from Mexico City; the remaining children came from all over Mexico. Most of the parents were indigent peasants of low economic class, and the children were often malnourished and sometimes neglected. There were 34,070 admissions to the Hospital in this period, an average of 6814/year; 770 of these patients were admitted to the Department of Nephrology, averaging 154/year.

The main condition was a nephritic syndrome of acute onset (319 cases, an average of 64/year). Most of them (92%) were found to have poststreptococcal glomerulonephritis; 61% were males; 79% were school-age children (6 years old or more), the rest were between 2 and 5 years of age. The diagnosis of poststreptococcal disease was based on the history of previous throat infection with isolated beta-hemolytic streptococcus or scarlet fever, hypocomplementemia, and ASO titer elevation.

The high incidence of streptococcal infection is related to socioeconomic factors. Nephritogenic strains, particularly the M2T2 type of streptococcus, are frequent (1, 2). The remaining 8.2% patients presenting with a nephritic syndrome turned out to have mesangiocapillary glomerulonephritis; all were school-age children and 62% were males. The patients with acute nephritic syndrome accounted for 32% of the total number of patients admitted to the Department of Nephrology and 1.1% of all admissions to the Hospital.

Idiopathic nephrotic syndrome was diagnosed in 183 children, an average of 37/year; 58% were males, 48% were preschool-age children, and 4.3% were <2 years of age. This group accounted for 26% of the admissions to the Nephrology Department and 0.36% of all admissions to the Hospital; 84% of the patients showed a good response to prednisone therapy. The remaining 16% did not respond to corticosteroid therapy and turned out to have focal and segmental glomerulosclerosis or mesangial proliferation. Next in importance is the group of children with chronic renal failure. Of 126 patients admitted to the Nephrology Department, averaging 25/year, 50% were males, 88% were school-age children. Of the remainder, half were preschool-age children and half <2 years of age. They accounted for 17% of the admissions to the Nephrology Department and 0.3% of all the admissions to the Hospital. Of this group, 23 are under rehabilitation programs (renal transplantation, hemodialysis, chronic intermittent peritoneal dialysis, or continuous ambulatory peritoneal dialysis), while the remaining children were lost to follow-up or died in chronic uremia. Socioeconomic factors were the major determinants of the outcome.

Twenty-six patients were found to have various nephropathies secondary to systemic disease: 12 had systemic lupus erythematosus, 13 nephritis with anaphylactoid purpura, and 1 nephritis associated with dermatomyositis. This group of patients accounted for 3.2% of all admissions to the Nephrology Department; 68% were males and all but 1 were >6 years of age. Congenital malformations of the urinary tract, mainly cases of obstructive uropathy or vesicoureteric reflux, with or without infection, are admitted to the Nephrology Department for the purpose of studying their renal function or when they reach end-stage renal failure and require dialysis. There were 23 admissions in this group, averaging 4.6/year, of whom 74% were males, 13% were <2 years old, 13% of preschool age, and 57% school-age children. They accounted for 3% of the admissions of the Nephrology Department.

The diagnosis of nonbacterial tubulointerstitial nephritis was made in 11 patients, most of them secondary to aminoglycosides. Eleven patients had the diagnosis of recurrent hematuria, five had Alport's syndrome, and the remaining three had cystinosis, nephrophthisis, and renal glucosuria, respectively.

Acute renal failure secondary to severe dehydration, hypovolemic shock, sepsis, and disseminated intravascular coagulation was common in our hospital a few years ago. Recently, the incidence has decreased as a result of early hospitalization and better treatment of patients with acute diarrhea or infections. Now, the incidence of acute renal failure in the Hospital is between 5 and 10 cases/year.

References

1. Rodriguez RS: Glomerulonefritis aguda consecutiva a fiebre escarlatina causada por Streptococcus pyogenes M-2/t-2. Bol Med Hosp Inf Mex 25:1069, 1968.
2. Rodriguez RS: Acute glomerulonephritis and scarlet fever caused by Streptococcus pyogenes type 2 (M2T-2). J Infect Dis 130:315, 1974.

23G South Africa

H. M. COOVADIA

It is within a social matrix of poverty, malnutrition, and repeated infection that the renal problems of African children in southern Africa develop and emerge. There is no doubt that in general these factors affect the pattern of infections seen among black children but to what extent they have a similar influence on diseases of the kidney is unclear. There is possibly no other subcontinent in which the races are segregated so distinctly and one in which socioeconomic differences rest so clearly on color. Accordingly racial differences in renal disease often, though not always, indicate the effect indirectly of institutionalized privilege or disadvantage.

ACUTE GLOMERULONEPHRITIS

Acute glomerulonephritis accounts for roughly 2% to 5% of all admissions of African and Indian children to the pediatric wards in Durban and is therefore the commonest renal problem seen in a hospital setting. Among white South Africans the prevalence of glomerulonephritis in children is much less than among black children (1).

Poststreptococcal Glomerulonephritis

An unusual finding detected both in Johannesburg (1) and Durban is that poststreptococcal glomerulonephritis (PSGN) occurs nearly always in adequately nourished children. This association is probably not a result of chance as indicated by experimental evidence that suggests that mice on a restricted protein diet are relatively resistant to the induction of immune complex nephritis (2).

Whereas the incidence of acute glomerulonephritis has declined in developed countries and the etiology of cases has been uncertain, streptococcal infection remains almost the sole cause (>94%) of this syndrome in African children in South Africa (1, 3). In common with experience in other parts of Africa most patients develop glomerulonephritis following impetigo. The clinical course of this disease is fairly typical and the presenting features noted retrospectively for a 20-year period in Durban are summarized in Table 23G.1. White children with nephritis have similar clinical features except that edema and hypertension are less frequent and impetigo rare (1).

Studies in South Africa (1, 3) have confirmed the well-recognized and predictable nature of the disease irrespective of geographical location and have demonstrated that the tendency in the vast majority of children with PSGN is towards quick resolution and rapid recovery. A small minority of patients develop complications in the short term.

Rapidly progressive glomerulonephritis with crescents in more than 80% of glomeruli occurred in a small fraction (4 cases) of patients with PSGN (4). The clinical presentation in these children was dominated by oligoanuria in a setting of acute glomerulonephritis or nephrotic syndrome with a relentless progression to chronic renal failure (2 patients) or death (2 patients). Quadruple chemotherapy was ineffective and attended by serious complications.

The nephrotic syndrome developed in 0.3% of African children with PSGN (5). This improved or resolved over a few months. Children with PSGN who subsequently progressed to nephrosis have been found to have minimal activation of complement components in blood, particularly C3, early in their disease.

The considerable experience in South Africa, despite limitations imposed by poor follow-up, suggests that in almost all children with PSGN there are probably no long-term sequelae in childhood of this disease.

Typhoid Glomerulonephritis

Typhoid fever, which is endemic in Natal, presents as nephritis in 4% of cases and this can lead to a mistaken diagnosis of PSGN. Criteria which have been found helpful in distinguishing one from the other include a prolonged duration of edema before admission, pyrexia (>37.5%) with splenomegaly and milder consumption of C3 in those with salmonella typhi glomerulonephritis (6).

Systemic Lupus Erythematosus

Systemic lupus erythematosus (SLE) has not been reported among African children in South Africa. In a 20-year experience in Durban only five children were diagnosed as SLE (7). Although Indians accounted for only 8.2% of admissions during this period, all five children were from this community. Clinical features were similar to standard descriptions of the disease. Renal biopsies available in four, showed focal nephritis in two, diffuse proliferative nephritis with haemotoxylin bodies and "wire-loops" in one, and no changes in 1. There was no correlation between renal histology and clinical disease. All patients died despite steroid therapy. Causes of death were renal failure, uncontrolled bleeding from coagulopathy, and neurological complications.

ACUTE RENAL FAILURE AS A RESULT OF A HERBAL TOXIN

The commonest causes of acute renal failure are PSGN and tubular necrosis. Acute tubular necrosis poisoning from herbal medicines containing extracts of the tuber *Callilepis laureola* is common in Durban. The essential components of this syndrome are hypoglycaemia, centrilobular liver necrosis, and acute renal tubular necrosis. It is almost always fatal. Wainwright and co-workers have established the epidemiological, toxicological, pathological, clinical, and experimental basis of this disease (8). The nephrotoxic and hypoglycemic constituent of extracts of the tuber has been identified as a glycoside designated atractyloside. This

Table 23G.1.
Acute Glomerulonephritis in African children, Durban, 1960–1979 (N = 2765)

Volume overload (cardiac failure)	20%
Hypertensive encephalopathy	2.9%
Severe renal failure (i.e., requiring dialysis)	1.2%
Deaths	1.84%

poisoning closely resembles Reye's syndrome clinically (9), but is easily distinguished by the characteristic histopathological changes in the liver.

NEPHROTIC SYNDROME

African Children

The clinicopathological features of the nephrotic syndrome among children in southern Africa are sufficiently distinctive to require special emphasis (10, 11). Away from tropical Africa the incidence of malarial nephropathy diminishes in Malawi (12) and Zimbabwe (13) and disappears in South Africa (10). Despite the absence of the damaging effects of malaria on the kidney, there still remains in African children in southern Africa an unusual distribution of histopathological types of nephrosis that distinguishes them from children in both tropical Africa and other continents (10, 11). The disease clearly behaves differently in African children generally compared with most nonAfricans.

The rough incidence of nephrotic syndrome assessed by estimates of hospital admissions is 1.35% in Malawi (12), 0.67% in Zimbabwe (13), and 0.17% in South Africa (10). Accordingly the frequency of this disorder among blacks in southern Africa lies between that of tropical (2.4%) (13) and temperate (0.03%) countries (13).

Throughout the subcontinent only a minority of African children have minimal change while the majority have "obvious" glomerular lesions (Tables 23G.2 & 23G.3). Studies from centers other than Durban are based on small numbers and therefore conclusions derived from these have to be guarded. The major histological types of nephrosis in African children appear to vary in the different regions of southern Africa. Extramembranous is most common in Natal (Table 23G.3), focal segmental hyalinosis in the Transvaal (6 of 15 patients) (14), and diffuse mesangial proliferative in Namibia (8 of 23 patients) (15), and Zimbabwe (8 of 11 patients) (16). A recent study in Zimbabwe however showed that extramembranous lesions were most frequent and present in 7 of 17 children with nephrosis (17).

Features of nephrotic syndrome in African children from the Durban study (10, 11) are given below. The disease was seen most frequently in either preschool or late-primary school children and among adults.

Extramembranous nephropathy was followed by the different subgroups of proliferative glomerulonephritis as most common lesions among African children (Table 23G.3). Minimal change nephrotic syndrome (MCNS) (defined by light microscopy and followed for up to 2 years) differed from "classical" MCNS in two critical aspects: the lack of a predictable response to steroid and cyclophosphamide therapy and in a later peak age of presentation (7 to 8 years). The clinical presentation in this group of children, a favorable short-term outcome, immunofluorescent and electron-microscopic findings, and selectivity of proteinuria paralleled that of "classical" MCNS. The relevant clinical features at initial presentation in each histological group are indicated in Table 23G.4. Hematuria and hypertension occurred frequently and were detected in almost all the groups but renal failure was uncommon on first admission. The clinical course of patients over a period of 6 months to 10 years is presented in Figure 23G.1. It can be seen that the prognosis was fair with remissions occurring among some children in the minimal change, membranous, mesangial, and exudative proliferative groups. The overall prognosis in the other groups was less favourable with a significant morbidity as reflected by the inability of a single child to achieve remission and a small mortality.

There is no firm evidence that African children with nephrosis (including those with minimal change) respond to drugs used conventionally

Table 23G.2.
Percentage Incidence of Minimal Change in Nephrotic Syndrome

	South Africa	Zimbabwe	Namibia	Malawi
African	0–14	0	0	0
"Colored"	25	—	—	—
Indian	75	—	—	—
White	70–80	—	—	—

Data derived from Adhikari M: M. D. thesis, University of Natal, 1982; Brown KGE, et al: S Afri Med J 52:275, 1977; Van Buuren: Personal communication, 1982; Betts PR: Trans Roy Soc Trop Med Hyg 74:8, 1980; Seggie J: Personal communication, 1982.

Table 23G.3.
Histological Categories of Nephrotic Syndrome in African and Indian Children in South Africa

	African	Indian
N	104	66
No obvious lesions	(%)	(%)
Minimal change	14.4	72.7
Obvious glomerular lesions		
Extramembranous	29.8	3.1
Proliferative	40.4	12.1
Mesangial	6.7	6.0
Exudative	8.7	1.5
Endocapillary	6.7	—
Membranoproliferative	8.7	3.1
Focal	9.6	1.5
Focal glomerulosclerosis	3.9	9.1
Tropical extramembranous	5.8	—
Tropical nephropathy	1.9	1.5
Unclassified	3.8	1.5
TOTAL	100.0	100.0

Table 23G.4.
Some Clinical Features at Presentation in African Children with Nephrotic Synrome

Histological group	Peak age (yrs)	Sex	HPT[a] (%)	HEM[b] (%)	RF[c] (%)
Minimal change	>5	M > F	0	27	0
Extramembranous	>5	M > F	20	47	0
Proliferative					
Mesangial	<5	M = F	50	28.5	0
Exudative	>5	M = F	22.2	44.4	0
Endocapillary	>5	M = F	28.6	28.6	0
Membranoproliferative	<5	M > F	10	33	10
Focal	>5	M = F	20	40	0
Focal glomerulosclerosis	>5	M > F	25	0	0
Tropical extramembranous	>5	M > F	0	0	0

[a] HPT, hypertension.
[b] HEM, hematuria.
[c] RF, renal failure.

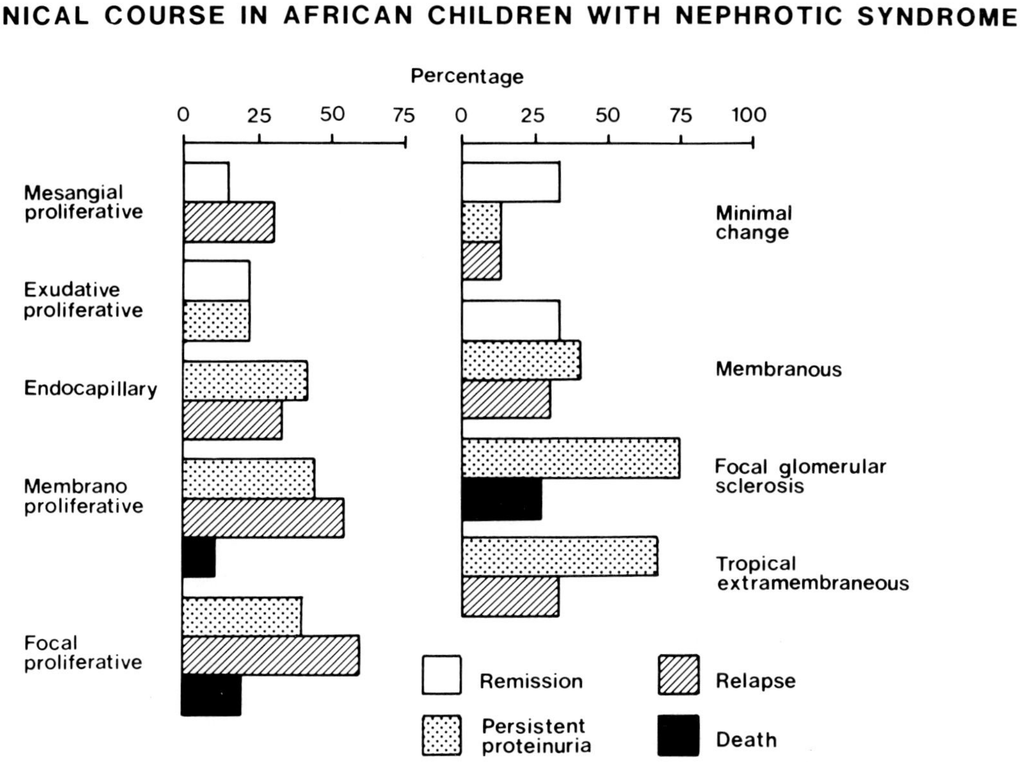

Figure 23G.1.

in this disease (i.e., steroids and cyclophosphamide). As all these drugs can have serious side effects their use is best avoided in all African children. Management is supportive with a high protein diet and diuretics. Despite intensive investigation, the cause of the disease remains unknown in many of these patients. In particular a causal link with *Schistosoma mansoni* could not be established. HBs antigen was associated with extramembranous nephropathy in our study and a strong correlation has also been established among children in Namibia (15) and Zimbabwe (17). African children therefore differed from children in other continents in relative frequency (and therefore also in their response to steroid therapy) and occasionally in the clinical behaviour of the histological types of nephrosis. They were also different from children with nephrotic syndrome in West and East Africa in the absence of malarial nephropathy, a lower incidence of the disease, and male dominance.

Non-African Children

The nephrotic syndrome in Indian South African children was similar to that in other continents (Tables 23G.2 and 23G.3). Among Indian children, the age of maximum incidence, the preponderance of males, the histological changes and their relative frequencies, and the responsiveness to steroids, cyclophosphamide and chlorambucil, resembled these features in children in the West and Asia. For students of ethnology it is of interest to note that white children with nephrotic syndrome in South Africa follow a pattern similar to the Indians while "colored" South Africans have an incidence of minimal change between these groups and blacks (Table 23G.2).

References

1. Rabinowitz L, Thompson P: Glomerulonephritis in children. Leech 49:45, 1979.
2. Reinhardt MC, Devey M, Collins M, et al: The effect of protein deficiency on the development of chronic antigen-antibody complex disease in mice. Clin Exper Immunol 44:528, 1981.
3. Hallett AF, Adhikari M, Cooper R, et al: Post streptococcal glomerulonephritis in African children. Trans Roy Soc Trop Med Hyg 71:241, 1977.
4. Dilima MG, Adhikari M, Coovadia HM: Rapidly progressive glomerulonephritis in four African children. S Afr Med J 60:829, 1981.
5. Diedericks R, Coovadia HM: Complement consumption and progression to post-streptococcal nephrotic syndrome. S Afr Med J 54:208, 1978.
6. Buka I, Coovadia HM: Typhoid glomerulonephritis. Arch Dis Child 55:305, 1980.
7. Rovers MJC, Coovadia HM: Systemic lupus erythematosus in children: report on 3 cases. S Afr Med J 60:711, 1981.
8. Wainwright J, Schonland MM: Toxic hepatitis in black patients in Natal. S Afr Med J 51:571, 1977.
9. Watson AR, Coovadia HM, Bhoola KD: The clinical syndrome of Impila (Callilepis Laureola) poisoning in children. S Afr Med J 55:290, 1979.
10. Coovadia HM, Adhikari M, Morel-Maroger L: Clinico-pathological features of the nephrotic syndrome in South African children. Quart J Med 48:77, 1979.
11. Adhikari M: Nephrotic Syndrome in African and Indian children in South Africa. M.D. thesis, University of Natal, 1982.
12. Brown KGE, Abrahams C, Meyers AM: The nephrotic syndrome in Malawian Blacks. S Afr Med J 52:275, 1977.
13. Kibukamusoke JW, Hutt MSR, Wilks NE: The nephrotic syndrome in Uganda and its association with Quartan malaria. Quart J Med 36:393, 1967.
14. Lewin JR, Jankowitz PJ, Thompson PD: The differing histology in black and white children with the nephrotic syndrome (abstract). Kidney Intl 16:88, 1979.
15. Van Buuren AJ: Personal communication, 1982.
16. Betts PR: Quoted in Hendrickse RG: Epidemiology and prevention of kidney disease in Africa. Trans Roy Soc Trop Med Hyg 74:8, 1980.
17. Seggie J: Personal communication, 1982.

23H Thailand

P. FUTRAKUL

Thailand exemplifies a developing country in the tropics, in which the differences in socioeconomic, genetic, environmental, cultural, and educational backgrounds from those of the well-developed western world explains the occurrence of unusual insults to the kidneys of children. In this so-called "third world," nutritional, infectious, and environmental factors are the major contributors intricately responsible for the development of a variety of glomerulotubular injuries. The common clinical manifestations of renal disease, e.g., acute nephritic syndrome, nephrosis, acute renal failure of tropics, and idiopathic vesical lithiasis will be discussed in brief.

ACUTE NEPHRITIC SYNDROME

Acute glomerulonephritis (AGN) following poststreptococcal infection, although now rare in the western world, is still the most common cause of classical glomerulonephritis (GN) in this region (1). In addition, a subclinical manifestation of GN has been documented frequently in association with a variety of infectious diseases, such as falciparum malaria (2, 3), dengue hemorrhagic syndrome (4, 5), diphtheria (6), trichinosis (7), and salmonellosis (8). Hypertension or edema in these cases is usually absent. Mild proteinuria and microscopic hematuria with few other cellular elements are observed in the urine in 3% to 80% of cases. The third component of serum complements (C3) is normal or only slightly decreased in all of these clinical disorders, with the exception of the dengue hemorrhagic syndrome in which severe depletion of C3 is closely related to the clinical manifestation of shock. Immune complexes are frequently detected in the blood during the acute stage of the disease. The abnormal findings in urinary sediments subside during recovery. The histopathological changes in most of these cases are mild, with mesangial hyperplasia and hypertrophy being generally noted. Hyperplasia and hypertrophy of endothelial cells may be present in some capillaries. On immunofluorescence, deposition of IgA and C3 with or without IgG is observed in the mesangial area and C3 in the wall of arterioles. Electron microscopy reveals electron dense deposits in the subendothelial and paramesangial areas and focal thickening of the basement membrane. These glomerular lesions usually resolve within 4 to 6 weeks.

The clinical course of acute nephritic syndrome associated with the infectious diseases in these children is usually benign and self-limited.

NEPHROTIC SYNDROME

The incidence of nephrotic syndrome (NS) in the developing world, as judged by hospital admission rates, is from 15 to 100 times that in developed temperate countries (9). There is no good explanation for this. However, it is likely that a defective immune response to various environmental pathogens with predisposing malnutrition potentiates the risk of chronic immunization by antigen(s) with consequent immune complex disease. The best examples are nephropathy associated with quartan malaria, leprosy, and the chronic viral antigenemia of hepatitis B. The high incidence of membranous nephropathy among the Chinese inhabitants in Hong Kong and Taiwan appears to correlate with the prevalence of chronic viral antigenemia (10, 11). The higher incidence of IgM mesangial nephropathy (54%) (12) and of the focal segmental glomerulosclerotic lesion with IgM deposits (13 to 28%) (13) among our nephrotic children may reflect the strong influence of infection in this developing area.

Blood hypercoagulability, hyperviscosity, and platelet consumption have been documented during the active proteinuric stage in most nephrotic children, both steroid-sensitive and steroid-resistant cases (14–18). This abnormal blood hemostasis and platelet activation and abnormal hemostatic mechanism is usually sustained in the steroid-resistant nephrotic patients, many of whom are destined for chronic renal insufficiency (14). Furthermore, correction of this abnormality of hemostasis and prevention of further consumption of platelets by the long-term administration of antiplatelet and anticoagulant agents, appears to improve the clinical outcome in treated children (19–22). Therefore, the hypothesis has been proposed that the activation of platelets and the related abnormal hemostatic mechanisms may be responsible, at least in part, for the development of progressive glomerulotubular injury in the severe forms of nephrosis, such as those associated with focal segmental glomerulosclerosis.

ACUTE RENAL FAILURE IN THE TROPICS

Prerenal azotemia because of fluid and electrolyte losses constitutes an important variety of acute renal failure (ARF) in this region. The precipitating causes include infective gastroenteritis, food poisoning, dysentery, typhoid fever, cholera, and necrotizing enterocolitis (23). Other infectious causes of ARF are leptospirosis (24, 25), malaria, dengue hemorrhagic shock syndrome (4), diphtheria (6), and trichinosis (7). The renal lesion in most of these cases is usually a mild mesangial proliferation with IgM, C3, and occasionally IgG deposits. Acute tubular necrosis has been documented in most cases and, occasionally, a few with severe clinical manifestation, such as prolonged shock, develop acute cortical necrosis.

Additional factors that cause ARF are animal and plant toxins. The renal lesions from snake-bite (23, 26) have been associated with wide manifestations, varying from mild proteinuria and hematuria to renal failure. All structures of the kidney can be affected. The most severe form occurs in Russell's viper bite, in which there is an extracapillary proliferative glomerulonephritis, tubular and cortical necrosis, segmental necrotizing arteritis with C3 deposits, and thrombophlebitis of the arcuate vein and its tributaries. Several factors are involved in the pathogenesis of this variety of renal failure, e.g., hypovolemia, shock, intravascular hemolysis, disseminated intravascular coagulation, and direct nephrotoxicity.

Acute tubular necrosis may follow scorpion sting, spider bite, and multiple stings by wasps or hornets. ARF also has been reported following ingestion of the raw bile of the grass carp (*Clenopharyngodon idellus*), which is tubulotoxic, a traditional Chinese way of improving visual acuity (27). In addition, ARF has been ascribed to ingestion of various herbal medicines and plant toxins, such as Callilepsis laureola, seculidaca longipedunculata, Crotalaria laburnifolia, and djenkol bean (23, 28).

IDIOPATHIC VESICAL LITHIASIS

Bladder stone has been encountered in the endemic areas in the north and northeast regions of Thailand, as well as in other countries in Southeast Asia, e.g., Burma, Laos, and Indonesia (29, 30). It occurs predominantly in children <10 years of age, with males more commonly affected than females in a ratio of 10:1. Interesting data from epidemiological surveys indicate that there are more children with stone symptoms in the village inhabitants than in the city dwellers. Village children excrete unusually high amounts of aggregated oxalate crystals, calcium, and uric acid in more concentrated urine than do city children, reflecting a defect in the inhibition of calcium stone crystallization. This is probably a result of improper feeding with rice containing low dietary phosphate and with vegetables rich in calcium oxalate content to the water-deprived village infants and children. Thus, many factors are believed to be intricately involved in the pathogenesis of bladder stone formation. A prospective, preventive program supplementing the diet with orthophosphate has yielded a fruitful result in inhibiting the crystalluria and preventing bladder stone disease in Thai children (30).

References

1. Futrakul P: Renal disease in Thai children: A tropical problem. J Med Assoc Thai 56:265, 1973.
2. Futrakul P, Boonpucknavig V, Boonpucknavig S, et al: Acute glomerulonephritis complicating plasmodium falciparum infection. Clin Pediat 13:281, 1974.
3. Sitprija V, Boonpucknavig V: Malarial nephropathy in Thailand. In Oshima K, Yoshitoshi Y, Hatano M (eds): Proceedings of the First Asian Pacific Congress Nephrology. Tokyo, Gakujutsutosho Printing Co., 1979, p 126.
4. Futrakul P, Poshyachinda V, Mitrakul C, et al: Renal involvement and reticuloendothelial system clearance in dengue hemorrhagic fever. J Med Assoc Thai 56:33, 1973.
5. Boonpucknavig V, Bhamarapravati N, Boonpucknavig S, et al: Glomerular changes in dengue hemorrhagic fever. Arch Pathol Lab Med 100:206, 1976.
6. Futrakul P, Sitprija V, Teranaparin C, et al: Diphtheria with renal failure (abstract). Fourth Colloquium in Nephrology. Hong Kong, 1981, p 44.
7. Sitprija V, Keoplung M, Boonpucknavig V, et al: Renal involvement in trichinosis. Arch Intern Med 140:544, 1980.
8. Sitprija V, Pipatanagul V, Boonpucknavig V, et al: Glomerulitis in typhoid fever. Ann Intern Med 81:210, 1974.
9. Cameron JS: The prevention of glomerulonephritis. In Proceedings of Eighth International Congress of Nephrology. Athens, S. Karger, Basel, 1981, p 321.
10. Hsa HC, Lin GJ, Chang MH, et al: Hepatitis B surface (HBs) antigenemia and pediatric membranous nephropathy (abstract). Fourth Colloquium in Nephrology. Hong Kong, 1981, p 50.
11. Chen WY, Yen TS, Hsieh BS, et al: The studies on hepatitis B surface antigen in primary glomerular lesion. Third Colloquium in Nephrology. Tokyo, 1979, p 69.
12. Tanphaichitr P, Boonpucknavig V, Boonpucknavig S: A clinicopathological correlation study of 157 Thai children with nephrotic syndrome. Proceedings of the Third Asian Congress of Pediatrics. Bangkok, 1979, p 151.
13. Sinniah R, Lee HS: Nephrotic syndrome in adults: Light, electron and immunofluorescent microscopic findings (abstract). First Asian Pacific Congress of Nephrology. Tokyo, 1979, p 5.
14. Futrakul P, Poshyachinda M, Mitrakul C: Focal sclerosing glomerulonephritis: A kinetic evaluation of hemostasis and the effect of anticoagulant therapy: a controlled study. Clin Nephrol 16:180, 1978.
15. Kendall AG, Lohmann RC, Dossetor JB: Nephrotic syndrome: a hypercoagulable state. Arch Int Med 127:1021, 1971.
16. Parbtani A, Frampton G, Cameron JS: Platelet and plasma serotonin concentrations in glomerulonephritis. II. Clin Nephrol 14:112, 1980.
17. Futrakul P, Poshychinda M: Kinetic evaluation on hemostasis in the steroid-sensitive nephrotic syndrome. J Singa Ped Soc 19:273, 1977.
18. Woo KT, Junor BJR, Salem H, et al: Beta-thromboglobulin and platelet aggregates in glomerulonephritis. Clin Nephrol 14:92, 1980.
19. Futrakul P, Poshyachinda M, Mitrakul C: Hypercoagulability in the nephrotic syndrome: Use of anticoagulation. Proceedings Eighth International Congress Nephrology. Athens, 1981, p 297.
20. Kobayashi N: Heparin and antiplatelet therapy for nephrosis and glomerulonephritis. Proceedings Third Asian Congress of Pediatrics. Bangkok, 1979, p 143.
21. Tojo S, Narita M, Koyama A, et al: Dipyridamole therapy in the nephrotic syndrome. Contrib Nephrol 9:111, 1978.
22. Woo KT, Whitworth JA, Kincaid Smith P: Effect of antiplatelet agents on circulating platelet aggregates in patients with glomerulonephritis. Thromb Res 20:663, 1980.
23. Sitprija V: The kidney in acute tropical disease. In Kibukamysoke JW (ed): Tropical Nephrology. New York, Marcel Dekker. (In press.)
24. Chugh KS, Singhal PC: Acute renal failure in the tropics. In Takeuchi T, Sugino N, Ota K (eds): Asian Manual of Nephrology. Tokyo, pp. 181–194, 1981.
25. Sitprija V, Pipatanagul V, Mertowidjojo K, et al: Pathogenesis of renal disease in leptospirosis: Clinical and experimental studies. Kidney Int 17:927, 1980.
26. Sitprija V, Boonpucknavig V: Snake venoms and nephrotoxicity. In Burn GVR, et al (eds): Handbook of Experimental Pharmacology. Berlin, Heidelberg, Springer-Verlag, 1979, p 997.
27. Chen WY, Yen TS, Cheng JT, et al: Acute renal failure due to raw bile of grass carp (Clenopharyryngodon idellus). J Med Assoc Thai 61(suppl I):63, 1978.
28. Areekul S: Djenkol bean, djenkolic acid and djenkolism. J Med Assoc Thai 62:529, 1979.
29. Sidabutan RP: Nephrolithiasis. In Takeuchi T, Sugino N, Ota K (eds): Asian Manual of Nephrology. Tokyo, Seamic, 1981, p 97.
30. Valyasevi A, Dhanamitta S: Diet and bladder stone disease. Proceedings Eleventh Congress Nutrition. Rio de Janiero, Brazil, 1978. (In press.)

231 Yugoslavia

M. POPOVIĆ-ROLOVIĆ

The epidemiology of renal diseases in Yugoslavia is similar to that in other European countries, but with certain specific features observable in a retrospective survey of about 230 patients treated annually over the past 14 years in the Nephrology Department of the University Children's Hospital of Belgrade. The incidence of primary glomerular disease is of the same order as in other European countries, except for acute post-streptococcal glomerulonephritis, which is still common, though less prevalent than in the 1960s.

Of the secondary glomerular diseases, Henoch-Schönlein nephritis is frequent, but lupus nephritis and hemolytic uremic syndrome are rare (91, 13, and 4 cases, respectively). Progressive and nonprogressive hereditary nephritis were identified in 18 and 25 families, respectively. Genetically determined disorders of the tubular transport have been seen occasionally (cystinosis in 1 and distal tubular acidosis in 2), but familial calculosis seems to be quite common. Of the 31 patients now on chronic hemodialysis, 14 had reflux nephropathy as a cause of terminal renal failure.

BALKAN NEPHROPATHY (ENDEMIC NEPHROPATHY)

Balkan nephropathy (BN) is still not a well-understood disease and does not affect children. It is a slowly progressive tubulointerstitial disease, which seems to have been noticed much earlier, but the first publication describing its features appeared in the late 1950s (1, 2).

The disease is endemic in the population of rural areas, mainly along the Danube river and its tributaries. The prevalence of BN in the most affected villages has been estimated at 10% and the mortality rate at 3.8% (3, 4). The etiology is unknown, despite an extensive search for infective or toxic agents, and immunological injury (5–8). Familial distribution of the disease is now well established but genetic studies do not suggest a specific mode of transmission (9). Of note is the increased prevalence of papillomas and carcinomas of the renal pelvis and ureters, which is 1/200, compared with 1/22,000 in nonendemic regions (10).

The kidneys are bilaterally small, weighing only 20 to 25 g. In the early phase of the disease, pathological findings consist of the focal changes of interstitial fibrosis, tubular degeneration, and atrophy. Most of the glomeruli are preserved. Interstitial changes are mainly acellular or may show mild mononuclear infiltration, whereas the focal changes progress to diffuse cortical sclerosis as the disease advances. Immunofluorescence examination for the deposition of immunoglobulins and complement components are negative (8, 11, 12). The onset of the disease is insidious in the fifth or sixth decade. Patients are usually in good condition until advanced renal failure occurs. Anemia and xanthochromia of the skin may precede renal failure. Proteinuria is mild and of a tubular pattern (13). Urinary beta-2 microglobulin concentration is high in 73% of patients and raised levels have been found in community screening in 35% of this population (14). Urinary sediment is scanty. Early in the course of the disease, while the glomerular filtration is still normal, tubular function may be impaired. The disease is slowly progressive and some patients die in their eighth decade of nonrenal causes, with their glomerular function only moderately reduced (15).

BN IN CHILDREN

BN is not a disease of childhood. In the last 22 years, none of the patients treated in the Nephrology Department of the University Children's Hospital of Belgrade (only 60 km from the most affected endemic area) had BN as a cause of disease. Screening programs to detect the disease in children have been carried out in endemic regions. Asymptomatic proteinuria and hematuria were found in the child population, with a high prevalence of 13% to 34% (16, 17). However, extensive clinical evaluation of these children offered no substantial evidence of BN.

In a recent study of 100 children, aged 3 to 15 years, offspring of affected families in the endemic villages were investigated in our hospital to evaluate their renal structure and function (17, 18). Seven children had vesicoureteral reflux and ten had developmental abnormalities of form and position (duplication—3, ectopia—1, malrotation—3, and retrocaval ureter—3). Furthermore, bladder diverticula were found in two, and one had a radiopaque silent kidney. Such a prevalence of developmental abnormalities is not easy to explain, but no control group was studied.

The possibility of an unknown etiological factor that would influence renal development does not seem a likely explanation, because adult patients with BN do not have urinary tract abnormalities. In the children with no urinary tract abnormalities, all the findings were within normal limits. Proteinuria did not exceed 180 mg/day. In three slightly elevated urine beta-2 microglobulin concentration was found, but this measurement was not repeated. In five children with urinary tract abnormalities, proteinuria, microscopic hematuria, reduced urine osmolality, and hydrogen ion excretion (after an acid load) were recorded. In nine children from the most affected families, renal biopsy was performed. Light microscopy, immunofluorescence, and electron microscopic findings were normal (8, 19).

References

1. Danilović V, Durišić M, Stojimitrović B, et al: Nephrites chroniques provoquées par intoxication au plomb par voi digestive. Presse Med 62:2039, 1957.

2. Radošević Z, Radonić M, Horvat Z: Kliničko zapažanje o endemskoj nefropatiji u Hrvatskoj. Lij Vjes 81:445, 1959.
3. Danilović V, Naumović T, Velimirović V: Učestalost endemske nefropatije kod stanovništva opštine Lazarevac. Glas Srpske akademije nauka i umetnosti CCLXXXVII. 25: 1974.
4. Velimirović D, Naumović T, Danilović V: Mortality rate of endemic nephropathy in the three most affected villages in the Lazarevac community. Proceedings of the International Symposium on Endemic Nephropathy, Bulgarian Academy of Sciences, Sofia, 1974, p 313.
5. Durišić M, Danilović V, Brnbolić A, et al: Further studies of the role of microorganisms in the etiology of Balkan nephropathy. Proceedings of the Second International Symposium on Endemic Nephropathy, Bulgarian Academy of Sciences, Sofia, 1974, p 221.
6. Apostolov K, Spasić P, Bojanić N: Evidence of viral etiology in endemic (Balkan) enphropathy. Lancet 2:1271, 1975.
7. Hall PW, Dammin GJ: Balkan nephropathy. Nephron 22:281, 1978.
8. Sindić M: Rezultati autopsijskih i biopsijskih ispitivanja bubrežnih promena u obolelih od endemske nefropatije. Thesis. Medical School, University of Belgrade, 1981.
9. Radošević Z, Mihelčić N, Radonić M, et al: Study of genetic factors in the pathogenesis of endemic nephropathy. Proceedings of the Second International Symposium on Endemic Nephropathy, Bulgarian Academy of Sciences, Sofia, 1974, p 247.
10. Petković S, Mutavdžić M, Petronić V, et al: Les tumeurs de bassinet et de l'uretère. Récherches cliniques et étiologiques. J Urol Nephrol 77:420, 1971.
11. Radontić M, Radošević Z, Zupanić V: Endemic nephropathy in Yugoslavia. *Symposium on Geographic Pathology of Renal Diseases.* Kidney, Intern Acad of Pathology, Monograph No. 6, Baltimore, Williams and Wilkins Company, 1966, p 503.
12. Hall PW, Dammin GJ, Griggs RC, et al: Investigation of chronic endemic nephropathy in Yugoslavia. II. Renal Pathology, Am J Med 39:210, 1965.
13. Radošević Z, Traeger J, Radonić M, et al: Etude électrophoretique de la proteinuries de 31 sujetes Chroates vivant en pays de nephropathy endemique. J Urol Nephrol 74:703, 1968.
14. Radovanović Z: Prilog otkrivanju endemske nefropatije u terenskim uslovima. Thesis. Medical School, University of Belgrade, 1977.
15. Velimirović D: Prilog poznavanja kliničkog toka endemske nefro-patije. Thesis. Medical School, University of Belgrade, 1984.
16. Čvorić A, Milosavljević J, Subotić Z, et al: Dobijeni rezultati istrazivanja proteinurije i renalnih funkcija dece i adolescenata iz regiona sa endemskom nefropatijom. Proceedings of the Second Symposium Pediatric Nephrology, Paris, 1971, p 181.
17. Čalić-Parišić N, Popović-Rolović M, Dukić D, et al: Rezultati ispitivanja dece iz porodica sa endemskom nefropatijom. Proceedings of the First Yugoslav Congress on Nephrology. Beograd, 1979, p 129.
18. Calić-Perišić N: Ispitivanje dece iz porodica i krajeva sa endemskom nefropatijom. III Simpozijum o Endemskoj nefropatiji, Srpska Akademija nauka i umetnosti, Beograd, knjiga 3, 1985, p 267.
19. Sindjić M, Čalić-Perišić N, Popović-Rolović M, et al: Morphologic study of kidney in children from families with endemic nephropathy. Proceedings First Yugoslav Congress on Nephrology. Beograd, 1979, p 134.

6

Congenital Disease

CHAPTER 24

Renal Cystic Diseases and Renal Dysplasia

JACK RESNICK
ROBERT L. VERNIER

The cystic diseases of the kidney include a heterogeneous group of developmental, hereditary, and acquired disorders. A recent review of 6521 consecutive autopsies in a children's hospital for the years 1949–1978 revealed various forms of renal cysts in 2% of patients (1). The authors acknowledge that autopsy records ignore the large numbers of cases of, for example, multicystic kidney disease and infantile polycystic kidney disease discovered during life; thus, the actual incidence of the cystic diseases is considerably higher than 2% but is unknown.

The terminology utilized to designate the various types of cystic and dysplastic kidney malformations is confusing. Perhaps the definitions developed by Bernstein (2) provide the most rational system of classification for clinicopathologic correlation.

Renal agenesis: absence of the kidney or a grossly identifiable metanephric structure.

Renal hypoplasia: a significant reduction of renal mass without evidence of parenchymal maldevelopment.

Renal dysplasia: abnormal parenchymal differentiation reflected by the presence of abnormal structures including primitive ducts surrounded by collars of connective tissue, metaplastic cartilage, and less specific lesions such as fetal or poorly differentiated glomeruli and tubules and cystic dilatation of tubular structures.

Aplastic kidney: a form of severe dysplasia in which the kidney is extremely small.

Multicystic kidney: a closely related form of severe dysplasia in which the kidney is enlarged and variably distorted with cysts.

Polycystic kidney: diffuse cystic changes in both kidneys without other evidence of parenchymal maldevelopment.

THE PATHOGENESIS OF CYSTIC KIDNEYS AND OTHER MALFORMATIONS

As discussed in Chapter 3, normal renal development results in the formation of about 1 million nephrons in each kidney. Theoretically, the failure of that portion of the distal nephron and collecting system derived from the ureteral bud to connect properly with the remainder of the nephron and from the S-shaped renal vesicle of the metanephros could result in a reduced number of complete nephrons or maldevelopment. However, the majority of studies of nephrons in human cystic diseases and dysplasia demonstrate continuity of the lumens along the full length of the nephron, and there is little experimental evidence in support of this theory.

Considerable evidence has been advanced by Schwarz, Stevens, and Cussen (3) to support the hypothesis that congenital malformations including hypoplasia and dysplasia, are often associated with an abnormal embryological origin of the ureteral bud. They have shown that when the position of the ureteric orifice is displaced posteriorly and laterally in the bladder trigone of infants (caudal ectopy), dysplasia, or obstructive uropathy are also common. Bernstein and Meyer (4) have demonstrated that morphological alterations mimicking primitive ductules, tubules, and glomeruli may be seen as a sequela of ischemic necrosis in newborn infants. Thus, it is likely that dysplasia and primitive structures result from a variety of injuries to the developing kidney and that hereditary factors may modify the susceptibility to the injury induced by a number of poorly defined mechansims and by urinary tract obstruction (5). The possible role of exogenous toxins and drugs in the induction of cystic malformation of the kidney will be discussed.

Renal Agenesis

Failure of development of both kidneys is almost always associated with absence of the ureters that derive from the ureteral buds and is thus a consequence of failure of induction of the metanephros. This condition occurs in about 1:6000 deliveries and is more common in male infants. The pregnancy is always associated with olighydramnios beginning about the fourteenth week of gestation when fetal urine begins to make a significant contribution to the volume of the amniotic fluid. Affected infants are usually premature, 40% are stillborn, and survival beyond a few days is unusual.

Examination of the infant reveals a characteristic facial appearance termed "Potter's facies" (6), consisting of flattening of the profile and nose, low set ears, an underdeveloped chin, and a prominent fold of skin extending from over the eye and curving medially to the inner canthus and laterally to the cheek (Fig. 24.1). These changes presumably result

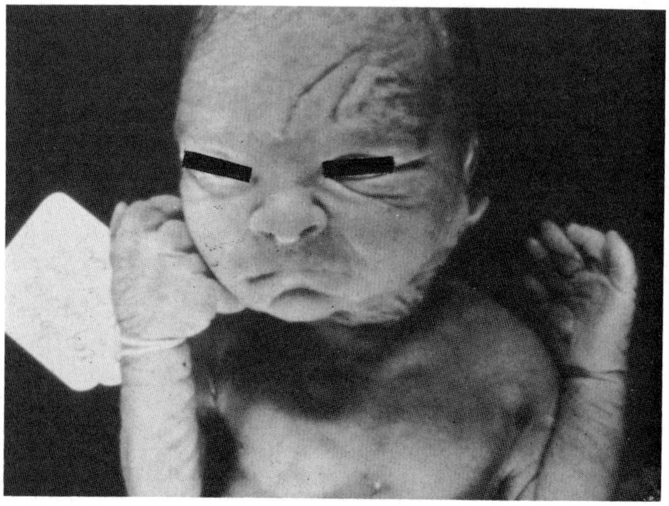

Figure 24.1. Postmortem photograph of an infant with bilateral renal agenesis, showing Potter's facies. (Courtesy of Dr. Theodore Thompson, Division of Neonatology, University of Minnesota.)

from compression of the face in the restricted space of the amnion lacking adequate fluid (olighydramnios). These infants usually die a respiratory death as a result of pulmonary hypoplasia, which is believed to also be a consequence of severe oligohydramnios. Typically, the lungs weigh about one-half the expected weight and demonstrate alveolar hypodevelopment. Other associated anomalies include clubbed feet (a positional abnormality), a single umbilical artery, absence of the vas deferens and seminal vesicles in the male and the uterus and upper vagina in females, and gastrointestinal malformations such as anal atresia or absence of the sigmoid colon and rectum.

Unilateral renal agenesis is a relatively common, usually asymptomatic condition, discovered in the course of an evaluation of another problem or in the study of families in which bilateral renal agenesis has occurred. We have described monoamniotic twins, one of whom had bilateral renal agenesis, while the other infant had a single kidney (7). In this rare circumstance the infant with bilateral renal agenesis had none of the pulmonary, facial or limb deformities usually seen, since the twin with a single kidney provided an adequate amount of amniotic fluid in their shared amniotic sac.

Although renal agenesis or dysplasia have not been considered hereditary conditions, a recent report emphasizes the value of studies of the family of index cases with bilateral renal agenesis/dysplasia (8). These authors evaluated by ultrasonography 71 parents and 40 siblings of 41 index patients with this condition and found asymptomatic renal malformations in 9% of the subjects at risk. The abnormalities included a 4.5% incidence of unilateral renal agenesis in family members, whereas the incidence in a control population of 682 adults was only 0.3%. Use of ultrasonography for evaluation of those at risk seems clearly indicated since the study showed an increased frequency of recurrence of the anomaly with subsequent pregnancies and an increased incidence of other renal malformations, such as unilateral renal agenesis, which may require more careful monitoring for detection of infection or stone formation within their solitary kidney.

Ultrasonography may also be useful in detecting bilateral renal agenesis in utero in a family at risk because of the prior delivery of an affected infant. Kaffe and coworkers (9) have described detection of severe olighydramnios and absence of renal structures at 19 to 21 weeks gestation in such a pregnancy. Based on evidence that fetal kidneys excrete small amounts of contrast material (10), intravenous pyelogram (50 ml of Renograffin® injected into the mother) demonstrated no renal structures in the fetus and no intestinal dye at 24 hours after injection of the contrast. Although the excretion of alpha feto-protein or alpha 1,4,glucosidase into the amniotic fluid should also be useful tests for fetal renal function; amniocentesis is often unsuccessful when the quantity of amniotic fluid is very small. The utilization of these tests may allow prenatal diagnosis of bilateral renal agenesis and appropriate counseling of families at risk.

Renal Hypoplasia

There is a high degree of correlation between renal weight or renal mass (volume) and height or age throughout childhood (Chapter 3). Renal hypoplasia as defined is an uncommon condition, and many of the "miniature" kidneys described in the literature were in fact dysplasic (11). Hypoplastic kidneys that are histologically normal could theoretically result from inadequate branching of the ureteral bud and a decreased number of reniculi and nephrons. The rare patients with bilateral hypoplasia described have usually presented with dehydration, as a reflection of the inability of the reduced renal mass to maintain body water homeostasis. A few infants have demonstrated renal tubular insufficiency, such as renal tubular acidosis, growth failure, cation wasting syndromes, and eventually renal failure. Fleischer (12) has described laterally displaced nipples as a sign of bilateral renal hypoplasia.

Oligonephronic hypoplasia (oligomeganephronie) is a distinctive nonfamilial form of congenital bilateral renal hypoplasia that usually leads to renal failure in infancy (13). The kidneys are small and demonstrate a reduced number of reniculi, usually less than six. The number of nephrons is greatly reduced, and each glomerulus and tubule is enlarged; the proximal tubules being 4 times larger than normal and the volume increased to about 17 times normal (14). Infants with this syndrome usually present with cyclic vomiting, fever, polyuria, and dehydration, secondary to a reduced concentrating capacity. Their glomerular filtration rate is reduced, proteinuria is usually present, and progressive renal failure develops within the first few years of life.

Renal Dysplasia (Multicystic Kidney Disease)

The term multicystic kidney is usually used to describe this condition even though all evidence suggests that the kidney is actually dysplastic, usually nonfunctional, and nearly always associated with ureteral atresia or severe obstruction. Histological examination reveals the hallmarks of dysplasia including cysts of various sizes, primitive epithelial ducts surrounded by fibromuscular collars, islands of cartilage, clusters of immature glomeruli and tubules, and regions of undifferentiated mesenchyme (Fig. 24.2).

The presenting sign of the multicystic kidney is usually a unilateral mass. Considerable enlargement may be present, and the kidney in the newborn may weigh up to several hundred grams. Although multicystic kidneys are usually unilateral, bilateral dysplasia occurs and abnormalities of the contralateral kidney may be present in 30% of patients (15). It is therefore important to search carefully for abnormalities of function or structure of the contralateral kidney before consideration of surgical removal of a multicystic kidney. Ultrasonography combined with isotopic renograms and standard renal function tests usually constitute a sufficient evaluation. Surgical removal of the unilateral mass has been advocated for many years, based on the potential risks of hypertension (16) and malignancy. The risk of malignancy is probably low, since few instances of malignancy in adults with this lesion have been described (17). The outcome is excellent in most children with the unilateral lesions.

Renal dysplasia may also result from early intrauterine obstruction and the effects of obstruction on the developing kidney. Experimentally,

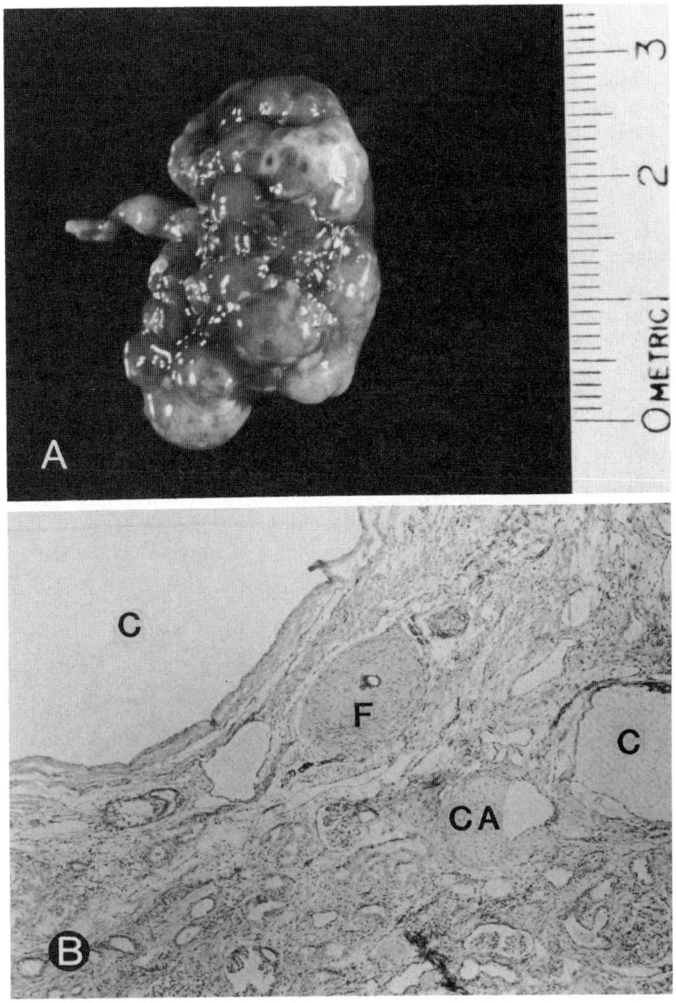

Figure 24.2. A, Photograph of a small multicystic-dysplastic kidney. The ureter (*left*) was atretic distal to the portion shown. B, Photomicrograph of a portion of a similar kidney demonstrating the characteristic pathologic features: cysts of various sizes (*C*), cartilage (*CA*), and prominent fibromuscular collars (*F*) around primitive ducts. The parenchyma is very disorganized, but a few immature glomeruli and tubules are shown. (PAS stain, X140.) (Reproduced with permission from Resnick J, Vernier RL: Clin Perinatol 8:375, 1981.)

ligation of the urethra or ureter of the lamb in early gestation has been shown to result in dysplasia and cystic malformation of the kidney (18). The previously cited studies of Schwartz, Stephens, and Cussen (3) further emphasize the importance of obstruction by lesions, such as posterior urethral valves, in the pathogenesis of renal dysplasia in man. With the increased use of ultrasonography during pregnancy, intrauterine obstructive lesions and associated dysplastic and cystic kidneys are being recognized more frequently. This new technology has resulted in many attempts to intervene with intrauterine surgery, to relieve obstruction and improve renal function of these infants. The results of intrauterine surgery have to date been disappointing (19), since with bilateral lesions, the associated renal dysplasia, olighydramnios and pulmonary hypoplasia, often result in asphyxial death at birth, even when the obstruction has been successfully relieved by intrauterine surgery. The risk/benefit ratio for the fetus at the present time seems to favor conservative management, delivery at term, careful postdelivery studies to firmly establish the nature of the obstructive lesion, and appropriate postnatal repair.

Cystic Kidney Diseases

Polycystic kidney diseases include a number of clinical, pathological, radiological, and genetic syndromes that share the feature of multiple cysts of both kidneys. These exclude "simple renal cysts" frequently seen in adults over 50 years of age, but also seen in children (20), renal cysts associated with multiple malformation syndromes, and cysts associated with renal dysplasia. The mechanism of cyst formation is poorly understood but is based on experimental studies, which demonstrate that the cysts are functioning portions of the nephron that become progressively dilated with time and may mechanically obstruct adjacent tubules. None of the theories regarding cyst formation completely explain the pathogenesis of human polycystic disease and a comprehensive review of experimental animal studies is available to the interested reader (21).

A great deal of confusion has existed in the medical literature regarding the two classic forms of polycystic disease; "infantile" polycystic kidney disease (IPKD) and "adult" polycystic kidney disease (APKD). This is apparent from many confusing statements in the literature. For example, the "poor prognosis" and "ultimate fatality" in IPKD, the contradictory opinions regarding APKD occurring in infants, and IPKD occurring in older children are repeatedly quoted. Statements regarding unilateral polycystic kidney disease (by definition there must be bilateral involvement), the relationship of polycystic kidney disease with a variety of liver diseases (congenital hepatic fibrosis, biliary duct ectasia, and polycystic hepatic disease), and the spectrum of renal cystic involvement from macroscopic cysts to renal tubular ectasia lend confusion to the literature. This section will define the two major polycystic kidney diseases (IPKD and APKD) and a separate section will discuss the medullary cystic disease—juvenile nephronophthesis complex.

DEFINITION AND CLASSIFICATION

Infantile (Recessive) Polycystic Kidney Disease

The term IPKD refers to the most common form of renal cystic disease seen in children, but unfortunately this entity is not confined to "infants." For many years this disease was regarded as ultimately fatal; however, recent experience indicates that many patients may survive to adulthood, especially those with minimal renal involvement and more severe hepatic disease (hepatic fibrosis with portal hypertension) (22). The term IPKD should be restricted to the *autosomal recessive* disease involving both kidneys (cysts or tubular ectasia) and liver (congenital hepatic fibrosis) to varying degrees. The clinical features and pathological involvement may vary between patients and within families depending on the age of presentation and the extent of involvement of each organ system.

The inheritance of IPKD is autosommal recessive when it can be ascertained. Neither parent is involved (no kidney or liver abnormalities) and other affected siblings may be detected if sufficient numbers of offspring are available for investigation. Previously, the occurrence of IPKD in a first child or a child with noninvolved siblings may have made the physician reluctant to definitively diagnose an inherited disease. However, the diagnosis assumes importance for genetic counselling because of the 25% risk in future pregnancies. IPKD can be reliably detected in utero by the ultrasonographic findings of massive nephromegally with increased echogenicity when severe renal involvement is present (23) (Fig. 24.3).

Infantile polycystic kidney disease is believed to be a developmental disorder of the branching tubular system of the kidney and a similar process involving the biliary system of the liver. Morphological studies of microdissected kidneys have revealed tubular enlargement or "tubular gigantism," involving the terminal branches of collecting tubules and saccular enlargements or diverticulum of more proximal branches (24). A variety of experimental models in animals utilizing chemicals (diphenylamine or nordihydroguaiaretic acid) result in injury to the tubular cells, possible tubular obstruction, and cyst formation; however, significant differences from the human disease remain (25, 26). Tubular dilatation has also been observed in newborn rabbits injected with steroids (27), but convincing evidence of a similar mechanism in humans is lacking. The present most acceptable hypothesis for this disease is an inherited undefined abnormality or deficiency of an enzyme essential for the normal formation and integration of the renal and hepatic tubular (ductal) system. The heterogeneity and severity of involvement in various patients may reflect different degrees of enzymatic abnormalities or other modifying factors. The autosomal recessive inheritance probably excludes exogenous toxins or drugs as the sole etiology factors in human disease.

The study of Lieberman & coworkers (23) demonstrated the variable expression of IPKD and described the presentation in infants and older children. They also showed the common association of renal disease with hepatic fibrosis and emphasized the similar features of IPKD and congenital hepatic fibrosis in the older children, but concluded that there were sufficient differences to separate the hepatic and renal involvement into two separate and distinct entities. The report by Blythe and Ockenden (28) attempted to clarify the interrelationships of the age of presentation and clinical pathological findings. They noted the constant finding of both renal tubular cystic changes and hepatic fibrosis with bile duct ectasia in varying proportions related to the age of presentation. Their somewhat rigid classification into four subgroups (Table 24.1) emphasized the findings of bilateral renal masses with severe tubular involvement and minimal hepatic involvement in neonates and young infants. In contrast, mild renal tubular disease (ectasia) and severe hepatic fibrosis were found in the older children. It is possible that the milder renal involvement escapes detection in the neonate or infant and that the hepatic disease becomes the predominant problem as the child ages. This clinical relationship between age of onset and severity of organ involvement appears to be consistent among affected individuals within the same family, although exceptions have been noted (29).

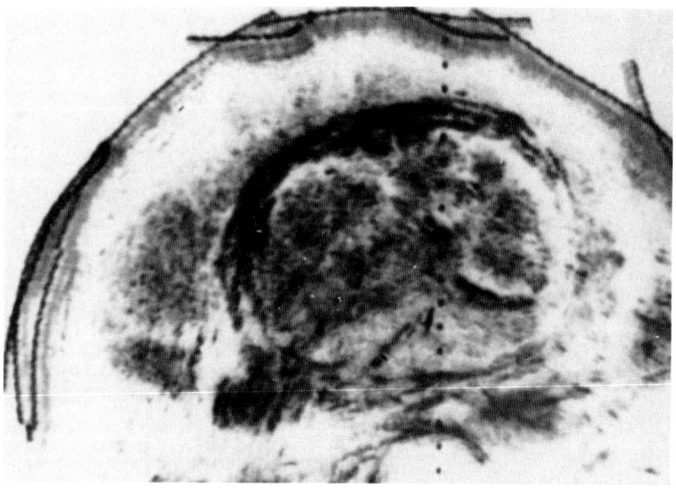

Figure 24.3. Ultrasonography demonstrating bilaterally enlarged kidneys with increased echogenicity in utero; later shown to be infantile polycystic kidney disease. (Courtesy of Dr. Hugh Williams, Department of Radiology, Children's Hospital, St. Paul, Minn.)

A recent review of a large number of children with congenital hepatic fibrosis (30) demonstrated renal cystic abnormalities in almost all patients (from classical polycystic kidneys to renal tubular ectasia). Some patients remained asymptomatic, whereas others progressed from tubular ectasia to typical IPKD with renal failure. This study appears to conclusively prove that IPKD and childhood congenital hepatic fibrosis are different spectrums of the same inherited (autosomal recessive) disease with varying severity of renal and hepatic involvement.

Clinical Presentation

The classical clinical presentation is that of a newborn infant with abdominal (renal) masses whose delivery may have been complicated by dystocia secondary to fetal abdominal enlargement or oligohydramnios, secondary to decreased intrauterine fluid production. The initial problem the clinician encounters is often respiratory distress secondary to pulmonary hypoplasia or pneumothoraces accompanied by pneumomediastinum. The pulmonary abnormalities are associated with oligohydramnios and the resultant fetal compression syndrome (31), which may include "Potter's facies" as a result of uterine compression of the fetus. These findings are more frequently seen in bilateral renal agenesis; however, they can be seen in any condition with decreased urine production (32). The pulmonary complications presumably occur because of oligohydramnios with intrauterine compression of the thorax, a decreased exchange of amniotic fluid in the tracheobronchial tree, and decreased thoracic volume, resulting from compression and elevation of the diaphragm secondary to the renal masses. The pneumothoraces and pneumomediastinum may occur spontaneously and may be a clue to underlying renal disease or may occur secondary to resuscitative efforts.

The major management problems result from respiratory distress with associated tachypnea, hypoxemia and acidosis, and early death from renal insufficiency is unusual despite varying degrees of oliguria. With vigorous respiratory support, survival for the initial critical period is possible, after which time continual pulmonary development progresses, the pulmonary problems usually decrease, and renal insufficiency then becomes the major management problem. Progressive renal insufficiency with varying degrees of oliguria, metabolic acidosis, hypervolemia, hy-

Table 24.1
Infantile (Recessive) Polycystic Kidney Disease

Type	Onset	Major clinical findings	Renal tubules "ectasia"	Hepatic fibrosis biliary duct dilatation	Prognosis
Perinatal	Birth	Huge bilateral renal masses	90%	Minimal	Renal and pulmonary death
Neonatal	1st month	Large bilateral renal masses	60%	Minimal	Progressive renal failure
Infantile	3–6 months	Large kidneys hepatosplenomegaly	25%	Moderate	Chronic renal failure and hypertension
Juvenile	Older children	Heptosplenomegaly	10%	Severe	Portal hypertension

Modified from Blythe H, Ockenden BG: J Med Genet 8:257, 1971.

pocalcemia, hyperphosphatemia, hypertension, and congestive heart failure may occur. Urinary abnormalities may include proteinuria and impaired concentrating capacity, but the urinary sediment is usually normal. With prolonged survival, the kidneys become smaller and interstitial fibrosis with tubular atrophy become more severe, leading to worsening renal function. The liver may be mildly enlarged and hepatic involvement with hepatic fibrosis is universally present in varying degrees. Despite the hepatic fibrosis, liver function studies are usually normal and esophageal varices do not usually occur until later. In atypical cases, a liver biopsy may be helpful to confirm the diagnosis of IPKD by demonstrating periductal fibrosis and biliary duct proliferation (29). Cysts in organs other than the kidneys do not occur in this form of cystic kidney disease and other malformations should make one think of other diseases.

The differential diagnosis of bilateral renal masses in the newborn infant includes in addition to IPKD, obstructive uropathy, bilateral multicystic dysplastic kidneys (discussed elsewhere), bilateral renal vein thrombosis, renal tumors (mesoblastic nephroma or nephroblastomatosis), tuberous sclerosis and a variety of other syndromes associated with polycystic kidney disease, such as cerebrohepatorenal syndrome, Jeune's asphyxiating thoracic dystrophy syndrome, autosomal trisomy syndromes (D and E), and numerous others (Chapter 12). Recently several infants with "transient nephromegally" have been described who were initially thought to have IPKD. In one case renal biopsy demonstrated tubular necrosis thought to be secondary to intravenous urographic contrast (33) and in another case (34) the etiology of the transient nephromegaly was unknown.

Confusion regarding the type of renal cystic disease present has occurred when the presentation was different from the classic description as was discussed. These cases have included older infants or children presenting with renal enlargement, congestive heart failure secondary to hypertension, or proteinuria or portal hypertension associated with congenital hepatic fibrosis and renal tubular ectasia.

Diagnostic Studies

The diagnosis can usually be confirmed by radiological investigations (35), which in the newborn reveal poorly visualized and massively enlarged kidneys with normal calyces by intravenous urography (IVU) (Fig. 24.4). Because of the poor renal excretory function, delayed (2 to 12 hours) films reveal either a mottled nephrogram as a result of contrast retention in small cysts of the cortex and medulla or a characteristic pattern of centrally radiating striations representing contrast within dilated collecting ducts. Ultrasonography will help establish the diagnosis by showing the nondilated renal pelvis (ruling out obstruction) and demonstrating a characteristic pattern of increased medullary echogenicity that results from the dilated collecting ducts and numerous small cysts (1 to 2 mm) (Fig. 24.5) (23, 36). Retrograde pyelography and renal arteriography are no longer necessary to diagnose IPKD, are potentially dangerous, and should be avoided. Computed tomography (CT) would not be expected to add new information not available from less costly studies and would add unnecessary radiation. The renal anatomy is, however, nicely demonstrated by CT, as shown in Figure 24.6. Esophageal varices in the newborn and infant are unlikely to be present because of the minimal hepatic fibrosis usually present at that age.

Radiographical studies of the older child with IPKD usually demonstrate varying degrees of renal enlargement. The IVU will reveal changes of either enlarged kidneys, with renal tubular ectasia, or small cysts resulting in a mottled nephrogram. Distortion of the pelvicalyceal system may also be seen, which may represent compression by cysts or scarring due to interstitial fibrosis. In some cases, progressive shrinkage of renal size has been noted as a result of progressive scarring and cortical atrophy (22). Delayed films may be beneficial since renal excretory function is often decreased. Ultrasonography may demonstrate larger cysts (>0.5 to 1.0 cm) and will reflect the irregular renal enlargement and pelvicalyceal distortion. The older child may demonstrate esophageal varices as a result of hepatic fibrosis and portal hypertension despite normal hepatic function.

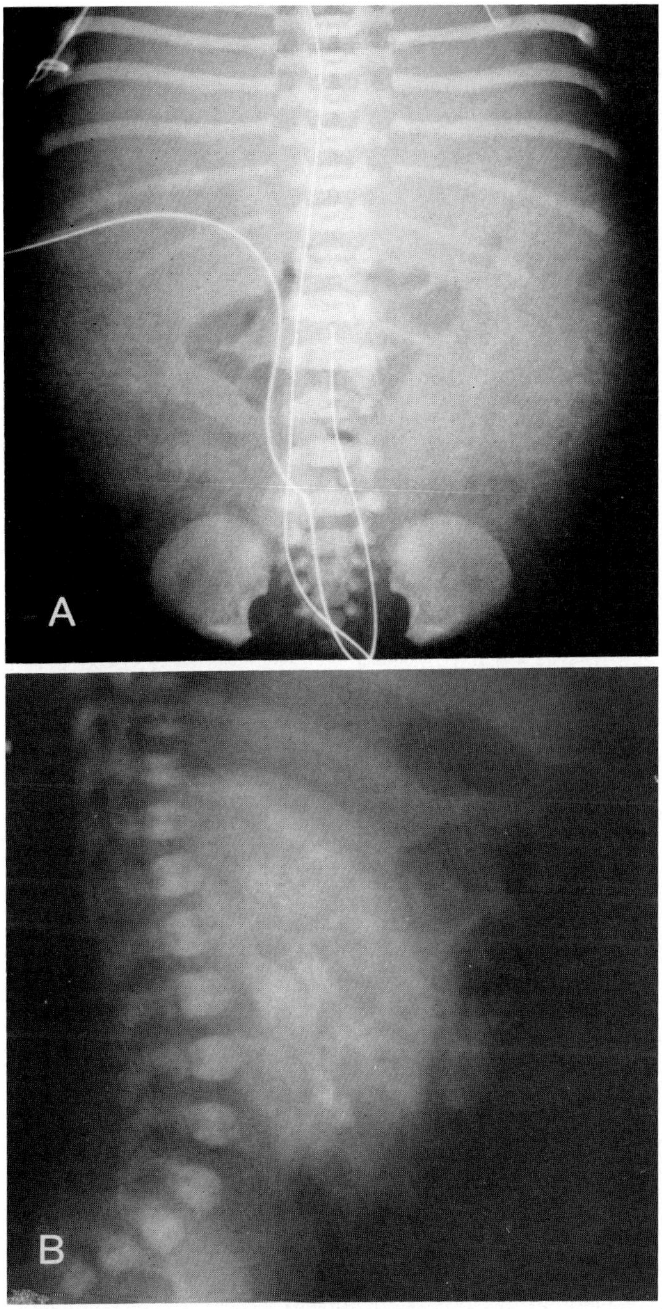

Figure 24.4. Intravenous urography in newborn infants with infantile polycystic kidney disease. **A**, Anterior posterior view. Note massive kidney that fill the abdomen and demonstrate the characteristic striations representing contrast within the dilated collecting ducts. (Courtesy of Dr. Hugh Williams, Department of Radiology, Children's Hospital, St. Paul, Minn.) **B**, Lateral view of enlarged kidney with typical centrally radiating streaks of contrast material within dilated renal tubules. (Courtesy of Dr. Jack Slivka, San Diego, Calif.)

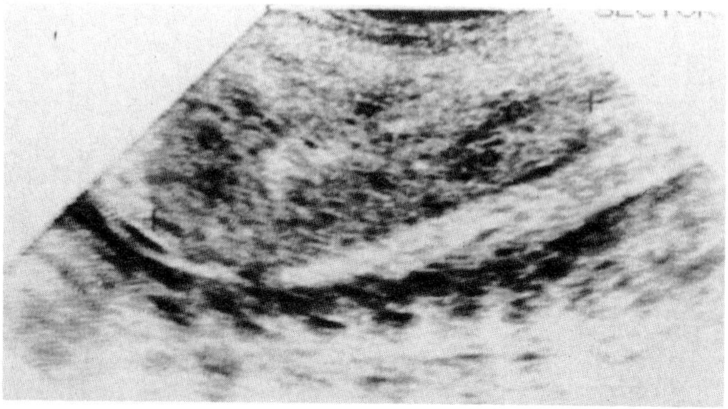

Figure 24.5. Ultrasonography (longitudinal) of left kidney of infant illustrated in Figure 24.4,**B**, showing marked nephromegaly and increased medullary echogenicity. (Courtesy of Dr. Jack Slivka, San Diego, Calif.)

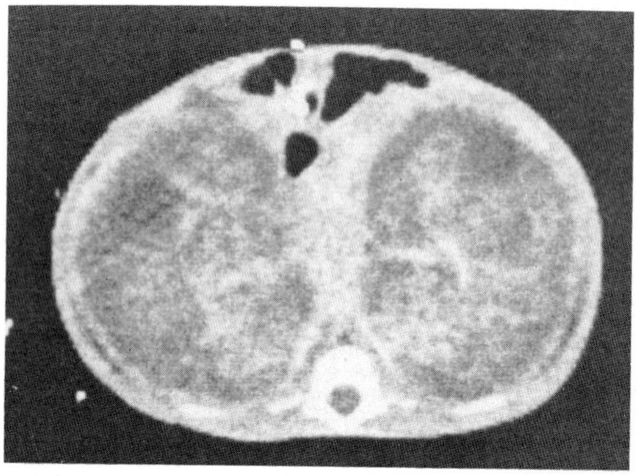

Figure 24.6. Computed tomography demonstrating bilateral massively enlarged kidneys of infantile polycystic kidney disease. (Courtesy of Dr. Hugh Williams, Children's Hospital, St. Paul, Minn.)

Pathology

Surgical renal biopsy is usually not necessary to establish the diagnosis of IPKD given modern radiological imaging modalities; however, the occasional atypical case may necessitate pathological confirmation. The infant with normal renal function (described previously) or the older child with questionable renal involvement may require renal or hepatic tissue examination. In such cases, we have performed open renal biopsies to obtain sufficient tissue to establish a diagnosis or percutaneous hepatic biopsy to demonstrate hepatic fibrosis and biliary ductal ectasia.

Pathological specimens of the kidneys invariably show medullary ductal dilatation usually associated with scattered small cortical cysts and varying degrees of tubulointerstitial fibrosis (37). The kidneys in the newborn are often massive (150 gms; 10 times normal) and demonstrate numerous small cysts over the surface. Sections cut through the kidney reveal the radial array of dilated collecting ducts extending from the medulla to the cortical surface corresponding to the striations seen radiographically (Fig. 24.7). Cystic changes in the older child are less striking, more irregular in distribution, and associated with varying degrees of scarring and tubular atrophy. The characteristic feature in these late onset cases is ectasia of the medullary tubules. The cystic tubules are lined by normal or slightly flattened cuboidal epithelial cells and later are associated with peritubular fibrosis.

Hepatic involvement consisting of periductal fibrosis and proliferation or ectasia of biliary duct epithelium (Fig. 24.8) is invariably present and, as discussed, is age related. Other organs that may show abnormalities include the pancreas (fibrosis) and pulmonary hypoplasia (newborns).

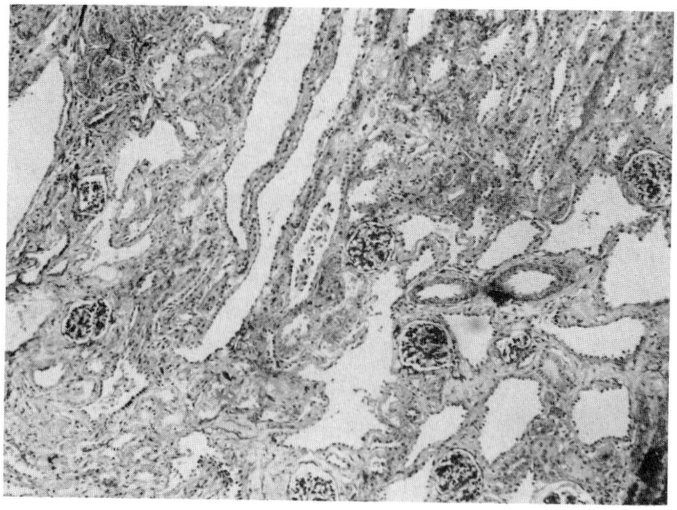

Figure 24.7. Light micrograph of a section of kidney from an infant with IPKD showing longitudinal and cross sections of dilated collecting ducts within the renal cortex. (PAS stain, X88.)

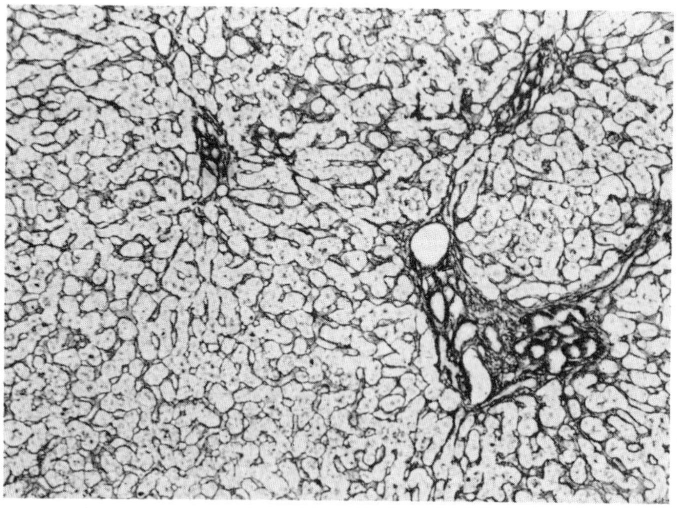

Figure 24.8. Photomicrograph of liver biopsy specimen from same patient shown in Figure 24.7, demonstrating biliary duct proliferation and marked increase in hepatic connective tissue. The liver cells are normal. (Reticulum stain, X88.)

Cysts in other organs and cerebral aneurysms are unusual and should make one consider other diagnoses such as other malformation syndromes associated with cystic kidneys (chapter 12).

Microdissection studies of newborn kidneys reveal patent nephrons with normal branching patterns and normal glomeruli. No evidence of tubular obstruction has been demonstrated (38). Tubular abnormalities must, therefore, occur either after normal intrauterine nephron formation or the abnormality of collecting duct cells does not preclude normal nephron induction. Similar mechanisms likely result in the formation of an abnormal hepatic biliary duct system.

Treatment

Treatment of IPKD in the newborn depends on prompt recognition for immediate treatment of the respiratory problems associated with pulmonary hypoplasia, and prevention of further respiratory compromise by avoiding high ventilatory pressures that may lead to pneumothoraces. The majority of newborn deaths result from pulmonary problems; however, if the infant survives the critical first week, careful management of hypertension and renal failure assume prime importance. Antihypertensive therapy is often necessary to prevent left ventricular decompensation and congestive heart failure. Management of renal failure requires meticulous attention to fluid and sodium balance to prevent dehydration (impaired-concentrating capacity) and edema and to help control hypertension. The renal failure may result in varying degrees of metabolic acidosis, hypocalcemia, hyperphosphatemia, and hypervolemia. Each of these problems must be managed with the patient's volume status carefully monitored as adjustments take place. During this time, adequate nutrition must be provided to ensure proper growth of the child. Adequate nutrition in the face of varying degrees of renal failure requires skilled nursing and dietician support. The dietician can provide special low phosphorus formulas with added calories in the form of lipids and carbohydrates, amino acid supplements, and high biological value proteins. Nasogastric tube feeding or supplemental peripheral hyperalimentation may be temporarily required during the critical early stages, but proper oral nutrition is necessary to allow the child to grow and develop optimally so that future consideration for dialysis and renal transplantation can be offered. Recurrence of the disease in transplanted kidneys has not been reported. In the older child, management of portal hypertension associated with gastrointestinal bleeding from esophageal varices is a major problem. Portal-systemic shunting when deemed necessary has been successful (30); however, the type of shunt must be carefully planned to avoid problems with future renal transplantation.

The diagnosis of IPKD is not necessarily fatal (as older texts have claimed), and the variable expression of renal and hepatic damage allows many children to survive with a reasonable quality of life before dialysis and renal transplantation are required. Careful genetic counseling must be provided to parents of affected children so that they may understand the risks for future pregnancies, the potential for prenatal diagnosis, and consideration of therapeutic abortion.

Adult (Dominant) Polycystic Kidney Disease

APKD is a bilateral, dominantly inherited disease that usually becomes manifest in the adult. There is high penetrance (nearly 100% by the seventh to eighth decade). APKD is a common cause of chronic renal failure in the adult. Unfortunately, the term "adult" type is inappropriate, since the disease may be found in children and occasionally in the newborn infant (22), although it is unlikely to be symptomatic. The genetic transmission of APKD is well recognized, and this disease may be considered a congenital abnormality, even though it is usually recognized in the adult. Although the dominant inheritance is well documented, many patients lack a positive family history. This may reflect a high spontaneous mutation rate, inadequate medical documentation, or the long latent period before symptoms occur. With the use of new, noninvasive radiological imaging modalities (CT and ultrasound), many "asymptomatic" family members are now being identified and at an earlier age than in the past (39). In the later prospective study, 18 children from 13 families were discovered to have definite APKD before age 18 (mean age 9.6 years). Two affected children were recognized in utero by ultrasound. Nine children were asymptomatic (50%), 3 were hypertensive, 2 had reduced renal function, and 10 had abnormal urinalyses at diagnosis. An additional 29 children from 22 families had suspicious minimal kidney abnormalities by ultrasonography (a few cysts or unilateral cysts). Definite APKD developed in 5 of the children followed for an additional 7 years. Thus, survey of family members at risk by ultrasonography has been shown to be a useful method for early recognition of APKD in children who may only become symptomatic many years later (40). APKD classically involves both kidneys with progressively enlarging renal cysts, hepatic cysts in 35% of patients, and cysts occasionally found in other organs (pancreas, lung, ovary, and cerebral aneurysms). The mechanism of renal cyst formation is unknown. The cysts are found as local or diffuse dilatations of any part of the nephron or collecting tubule and on microdissection studies often reveal irregular branching of the collecting tubules (38). Although polypoid and papillary epithelial cell hyperplasia has been described in specimens of advanced APKD and these lesions have been proposed as possibly obstructing tubules (41), similar lesions were not found in biopsy specimens obtained early in the course of the disease (42). The later authors demonstrated lamination of the tubular basement membranes (TBM) by electron microscopy of early renal biopsy specimens and concluded, as have others, that the fundamental lesion involves abnormal structure and compliance of the TBM. The cysts remain functional and with continual enlargement, secondary obstruction of remaining, more normal nephrons may occur.

Clinical Presentation

The clinical presentation of APKD in children is varied. Infants have usually been recognized by detection of flank or abdominal masses, although the kidneys are not often as large as found in IPKD (29). Signs or symptoms of renal disease are rare, although renal failure has been described in at least one infant (43). The "classic" presentation seen in adults of hematuria, hypertension, abdominal masses, and uremia is rarely seen in children. Some children diagnosed as APKD have been detected because of palpably enlarged kidneys, hypertension, proteinuria, hematuria (usually microscopic), or a combination of these findings (40). Urinary concentrating defects are regularly present in APKD and are thought to be an early marker in individuals genetically at risk, and are present in affected patients with normal glomerular filtration rates (44). The concentrating defect appears to be a result of an ill-defined disorder of the collecting tubules or the medullary counter-current multiplication system.

A recent report emphasizes a number of unusual aspects of this disease in children (45), including the fact that the renal enlargement is not always symmetrical. A unilateral renal mass was discovered in a girl at age 2 years. Her family history was strikingly positive for APKD in four generations. She had hematuria at age 3 years and died of a massive intracerebral bleeding from an aneurysm at age 12. Autopsy revealed bilateral cystic disease, but the right kidney weighed 1700 gm, while the left kidney was only slightly enlarged (300 gm).

Diagnostic Studies

Detection of APKD in children and young adults has improved tremendously with the use of modern radiological imaging modalities. The initial examination of a child (either clinically suspected or genetically at risk) should include an ultrasound study of the kidneys and liver to detect cysts. Ultrasound can detect cysts as small as 0.5 cm, if the patient is old enough to be cooperative (Fig. 24.9). As an initial screening device, ultrasound is ideal for there is no risk of ionizing radiation. In a child at risk, the finding of even a single renal cyst is suspicious for APKD, although simple renal cysts that are common in older adults have been observed in children (20). If a single renal cyst is observed and the parents have no demonstrable cystic disease, the diagnosis of a simple renal cyst is likely, although follow-up examinations should be performed to exclude a spontaneous genetic mutation and early asymptomatic APKD. Bilateral cystic involvement is necessary for the diagnosis of APKD, although a case thought to represent "unilateral" polycystic kidney disease is reported (46) (unfortunately no family studies were

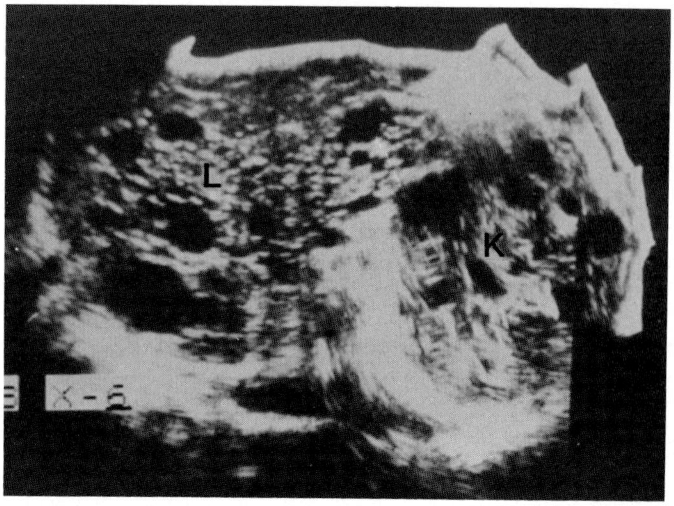

Figure 24.9. Transverse ultrasonography in a 9-year-old male originally thought to have infantile polycystic kidney disease. The field includes the enlarged left kidney (*K*) that contains numerous large cysts and the liver (*L*) that also contains several large cysts.

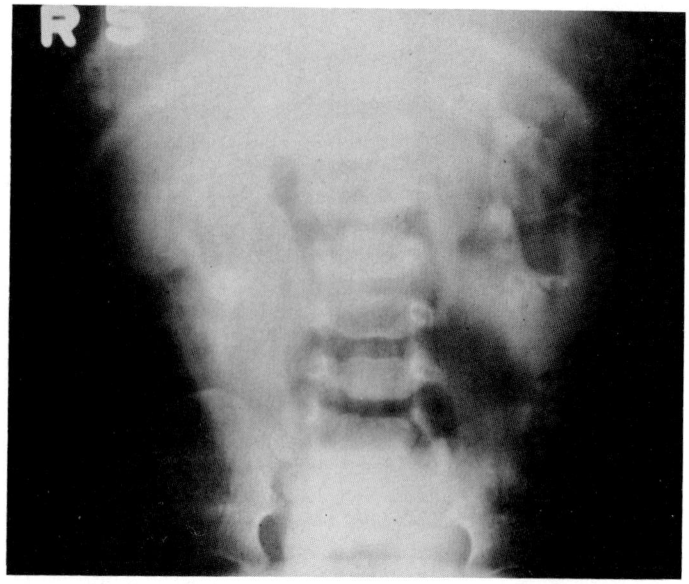

Figure 24.10. Tomogram during an intravenous urogram in a 9-month old-infant with bilateral abdominal masses, oliguria, and transient renal failure following dehydration. The kidneys are large and the collecting system is splayed. Lucent areas representing large cysts can be seen in the left kidney. Subsequent studies revealed cystic kidneys in a 9-year-old sibling and the patient's mother. (Reproduced with permission from Resnick J, Vernier RL: Clin Perinatol 8:375, 1981.)

performed), and a localized, unilateral form of cystic disease differing from APKD has been described (47).

Intravenous urography (IVU) may show a variety of abnormalities from mildly enlarged kidneys with distortion or splaying of the collecting system, giving a "spidery" appearance to massively enlarged nodular kidneys (Fig. 24.10). The lucencies of varying size within the kidneys are best seen by tomography. Unfortunately, in the early stages of the disease in children, the IVU may be normal, since the cysts may be too small to visualize.

CT scanning is an excellent method for demonstration of renal, hepatic, and other cysts (48), but is not usually necessary to establish the diagnosis. This method is costly and, in addition, exposes the child to excessive radiation. However, the method has been shown to demonstrate cysts as small as 0.3 cm and to be superior to ultrasound or nephrotomography in detecting asymptomatic individuals (48).

Renal Pathology

The gross renal pathology seen in APKD in children is that of bilateral, although often asymmetric, renal enlargement with scattered small cysts scattered over the kidney surfaces (Fig. 24.11). The cysts are unlikely to be as large or numerous as those found in adults. Microscopically, there is focal tubular dilatation, tubular cysts of varying size, and cystic dilatation of Bowman's space. As mentioned previously, cysts may be found in other organs (liver, pancreas, ovary, lungs, and cerebral aneurysms); however, hepatic fibrosis is not seen. This difference may help to differentiate APKD from IPKD in unusual circumstances. With present radiological imaging modalities, renal or hepatic biopsy specimens are not usually needed to establish the diagnosis.

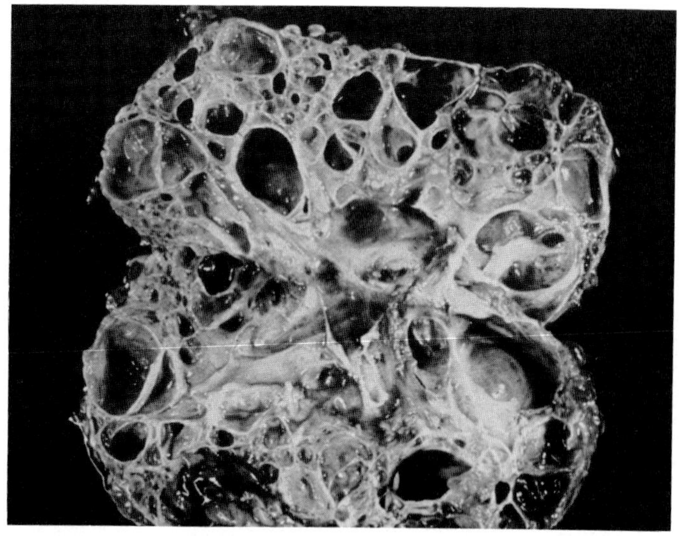

Figure 24.11. Gross appearance of adult (dominant) polycystic kidney. The kidney has been bivalved to show the gross distortion of the parenchyma by cysts of variable sizes. Kidney length, 20 cm.

Differential Diagnosis and Treatment

The differential diagnosis of APKD in the older child or teenager with a positive family history is not a problem; however, in an infant or young child, entities such as IPKD, tuberous sclerosis, or other malformation syndromes that may be associated with cystic kidneys should be considered. A similar but uncommon entity to be considered is glomerulocystic kidney disease, a condition associated with multiple small cortical cysts, early renal failure, with a negative family history of renal cystic disease (49). A positive family history or an investigation of other family members that demonstrates APKD, is confirmatory, although the possibility of a spontaneous mutation should be considered.

Treatment of APKD is nonspecific and preventative. Early and careful treatment of hypertension is important to prevent the added insult of nephrosclerosis in already diseased kidneys and to hopefully prevent rupture of possible cerebral aneurysms. Although severe renal infections (renal and perirenal abscesses and infected cysts) and renal calculi as a result of stasis of urine are common in adults, these complications are uncommon in children. Periodic monitoring of urine cultures to detect early or asymptomatic urinary tract infections should be performed in girls, and, if recurrent infections occur, prophylactic antibiotic treatment should be considered to prevent severe renal damage. Since most children will survive into adulthood before renal insufficiency occurs, discussions of dialysis and renal transplantation should be delayed until the child is mature enough to make future life and career plans to minimize psychological trauma. Genetic counseling regarding this dominantly inherited disease is essential for the parents and the affected individuals when he/she is old enough to consider marriage.

MEDULLARY CYSTIC DISEASE

Familial Juvenile Nephronophthisis Complex

Medullary cystic disease (MCD) is an important cause of end-stage renal failure in children. For example, Garel and coworkers (50) have reported that this disease was responsible for 15% (37/250) of the pediatric kidney transplantation procedures performed at the Hopital des Enfants-Malades in Paris. The disease is chronic and progressive and is characterized clinically by an insidious onset of hyposthenuria, anemia, and growth retardation. Pathologically, MCD is characterized by small kidneys with severe tubulointerstitial disease, *with or without cysts*, of the renal medulla. The terminology regarding this syndrome complex has been confusing, since it has been called both medullary cystic disease and familial juvenile nephronophthisis. Originally described in 1945 as "congenital medullary cysts of kidneys with severe refractory anemia" (51), a similar condition was termed in Europe "familial juvenile nephronophthisis" (52), and in the United States known as "cystic disease of the renal medulla" (53). An attempt at distinguishing these conditions based on mode of inheritance (dominant, recessive or sporadic), age of onset (child or adult), and presence or absence of cysts has been made by many authors; however, careful review of pathological material from juvenile nephronophthisis patients and MCD patients could not distinguish any important differences, and the authors concluded that they were identical conditions (54). The differences in terminology depend on whether or not medullary cysts can be identified (MCD) or whether only tubulointerstitial fibrosis (mainly medullary) is seen (juvenile nephronophthisis). However, the results of the review depend on the intensity of the search for cysts and whether or not small cysts (0.1 to 1.0 cm) are considered to be secondarily dilated tubules. It is also possible that some of the earlier diagnosed cases (siblings of affected patients) did not have cysts identified because the cysts may develop later in the disease. It is possible that the cysts acquired in some late patients may have had a pathogenesis similar to those recently described in patients receiving chronic hemodialysis (55). A recent review of this condition recommends the term "nephronophthisis complex" (56); however, we prefer the use of MCD despite the "absence" of cysts in some cases.

MCD can be considered to have two distinct genetic and age related forms (Table 24.2). The first is inherited as an autosomal recessive disorder and in children is frequently associated with a variety of nonrenal abnormalities (ophthalmologic, mental retardation, cerebellar ataxia, skeletal anomalies, and hepatic fibrosis). These abnormalities have been described and summarized in the recent report of Waldherr and associates (56). They include an increased incidence of red and blonde hair (possible gene linkage) in some series (57). The ophthalmologic abnormalities were initially described as tapetoretinal degeneration or retinitis pigmentosa associated with blindness (58, 59). The list of ophthalmologic abnormalities has been expanded to include colobomas, nystagmus, myopia, strabismus, hyperopia, amblyopia, and optic nerve atrophy, and one or more of these abnormalities were found in 13 of 27 children recently reported (56). The specific association of MCD with retinitis pigmentosa is referred to as renal-retinal dysplasia (60), and retinal dysfunction has been found in parents (heterozygotes) of MCD patients with electro-ophthalmologic studies (61). A high incidence of ophthalmologic abnormalities has not been seen in the adult-onset (dominantly inherited) MCD, which supports a different genetic abnormality leading to the renal changes of MCD in this form. MCD associated with congenital hepatic fibrosis was first described by Boichis and coworkers (62) in several siblings and has subsequently been found in several other families (63). This association of congenital hepatic fibrosis and renal cystic disease is also seen in IPKD (see previous section), which is easily distinguished from MCD. Skeletal anomalies, notably cone-shaped epiphyses (64), have also been noted as has mental retardation and cerebellar ataxia (64). The latter abnormalities are less frequently found than are the ophthalmologic anomalies.

The second form of MCD is an autosomal dominant condition that has its onset in adults and is not associated with other nonrenal conditions. The genetic differences have been well studied by Gardner (65), who noted that the recessive form began in childhood (age of onset 10.0 ± 1.2 years), whereas the dominant variety began in early adulthood (28.3 ± 2.4 years) and that both had similar durations of disease before death or end-stage kidney treatment was instituted. Consanguinity has often been noted in childhood cases, which suggests the recessive mode of inheritance (66). Sporadic cases have been seen in both children and adults and may reflect spontaneous mutation of a dominant gene or may reflect the statistical probability of a recessive condition being present in siblings (1 in 4). Attempts to document renal tubular abnormalities in asymptomatic parents or siblings in the childhood (recessive) disease has been occasionally reported, but convincing evidence for detection of the heterozygous (carrier) state is lacking (67). Renal biopsy in one parent demonstrated normal kidney (66). The mild concentrating defects noted in occasional parents may only reflect other renal abnormalities (i.e., pyelonephritis, tubular atrophy, or vascular disease) and are probably not related to a heterozygous MCD state.

Clinical Presentation

The clinical presentation of children with MCD is that of insidious onset of chronic renal failure with polyuria and polydypsia, anemia, and

Table 24.2
Comparison of Familial Juvenile Nephronophthisis (FJN) and Medullary Cystic Disease (MCD)

	Inheritance	Age onset (years)	Renal pathology	Associated nonrenal abnormalities
FJN	Autosomal recessive (occasional sporadic)	10 ± 1.2	Tubulointerstitial disease ± Cysts	Ophthalmologic Central nervous system Hepatic Skeletal
MCD	Autosomal dominant (occasional sporadic)	28.4 ± 2.4	Tubulointerstitial disease ± Cysts	None

growth retardation. These nonspecific signs and symptoms often lead to investigation of other organ systems (endocrine and hematopoietic) before the finding of mild to moderate uremia is noted. Other nonspecific symptoms relate to the tubular defect in concentrating capacity. Salt wasting, salt craving, and hypokalemia and weakness are occasionally also noted. The hypokalemia may be severe and may contribute to the severe polyuria, and, in some patients, normalization of the serum potassium with oral supplementation has significantly reduced the polyuria. Bone pain secondary to renal osteodystrophy may bring the patient to medical attention, and in long-standing cases secondary bony deformities and slipped capital femoral epiphyses may be present. Enuresis, secondary to polyuria, may also be the presenting symptom, and many patients have been treated with a variety of potentially harmful modalities before the proper diagnosis has been established (drug therapy, water restriction, or psychological manipulation). Edema and hypertension are uncommon until end-stage renal failure occurs, their rarity probably reflecting the salt-wasting condition. The anemia is often severe and occasionally disproportionate to the degree of renal insufficiency. The anemia may be a result of a lack of erythropoietin or other erythropoietic factors as a consequence of tubulointerstitial disease; however, this mechanism has not been carefully studied.

Laboratory and Diagnostic Studies

Laboratory studies reflect the severity of chronic renal failure with elevated BUN, creatinine, phosphorus, and hypocalcemia, when secondary hyperparathyroidism is not sufficient to maintain serum calcium. Anemia, hypokalemia, and metabolic acidosis are often noted. The urinalysis usually reveals a decreased specific gravity (hyposthenuria or isosthenuria) and mild proteinuria (usually tubular proteinuria). The urine sediment is usually normal, and hematuria and leukocyturia are usually not found. Other tubular defects, such as aminoaciduria, glucosuria, and acidification defects, have been noted early in the disease (67). The major abnormality is the tubular defect with salt wasting and inability to concentrate urine even with exogenous vasopression. Tests of urinary concentrating ability with water deprivation (8 hour) may establish the tubular defect (urinary osmolality after 8 hours >750 to 800 mosm/kg/H_2O) but should be performed with caution with frequent observation, including weighing the patient, to avoid dehydration. Individuals who are asymptomatic have been detected by maximal urinary concentrating tests, and this abnormality appears to be the earliest manifestation of MCD and is present before decreases in glomerular filtration rate (GFR) can be detected (65, 68).

Radiological studies are often unrewarding because of the poor renal function at the time of presentation. IVU usually shows only poor renal visualization and small renal outlines, but is helpful to rule out other renal diseases (i.e., hydronephrosis, atrophic pyelonephritis, cortical scarring, and so on). High dose excretory urography with tomography has occasionally demonstrated the small cysts, as cystic lucencies of the medulla without distortion of the collecting system (69). (NOTE: Caution must be exercised in performance of contrast studies in all patients with renal failure.) Reports of contrast accumulation within dilated tubules of the medulla must be regarded with caution, as these may reflect medullary sponge kidney, a benign, sporadic condition associated with opacification of the dilated papillary ducts. Retrograde pyelography has occasionally demonstrated small medullary cysts but is usually not indicated. Angiography may reveal small kidneys with cortical thinning and small medullary cysts or show nonspecific changes undistinguishable from chronic glomerulonephritis (70). The most useful technique for detection of MCD is ultrasound (50). Garel and associates (50) have described detection of a few small medullary cysts in 13 of 15 children (mean age 9.7 years) studied by sonography at the time of renal failure. The

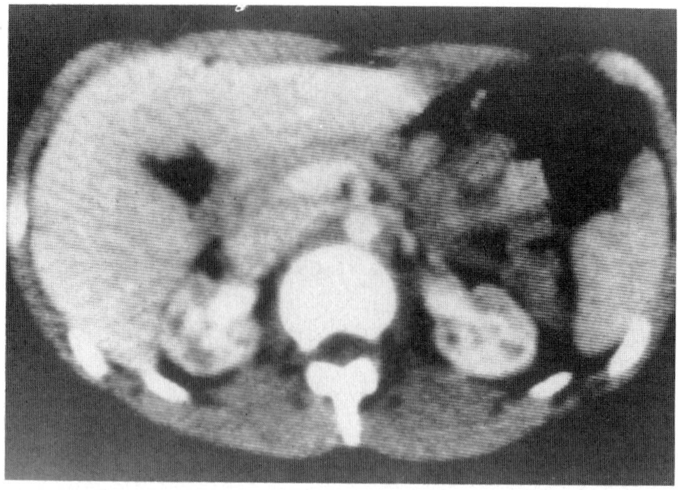

Figure 24.12. Computed tomography demonstrating small kidneys with medullary cysts bilaterally. (Courtesy of Dr. Alan Davidson, San Francisco, Calif.)

diagnostic medullary cysts are often not found by renal biopsy, and since chronic tubulointerstitial inflammation and fibrosis more often revealed by biopsy are nonspecific, these authors feel that sonography should obviate the need for biopsy in most patients. In an occasional patient the added cost and radiation of CT scanning may be justified and helpful in establishing the diagnosis (Fig. 24.12).

Renal Pathology and Pathogenesis

Typical pathology has remained the sine qua non for the diagnosis of MCD. Unfortunately, the tubulointerstitial disease usually is nonspecific, and cysts, either macroscopic or microscopic, may be present or absent. The size of the renal biopsy may reflect the ability to locate the small, scattered, medullary cysts, and a larger open biopsy may establish the diagnosis of MCD more reliably than a small needle biopsy. Early in the course of MCD the biopsy may be normal or show only scattered cystic tubules with peritubular fibrosis and thickened tubular basement membranes reflecting tubular atrophy (66, 71) (Fig. 24.13). If cysts cannot be demonstrated, these findings are nonspecific, although in the appropriate clinical setting they support the diagnosis of MCD and eliminate other pathology such as glomerular or immunologically mediated diseases. In the later stages of the disease, the kidneys are small, uniformly shrunken with atrophic parenchyma and severe tubulointerstitial fibrosis, making percutaneous biopsy difficult and potentially dangerous.

Microdissection studies have shown the cysts to be located in the collecting ducts and distal convoluted tubules, while the loops of Henle and proximal tubules were normal (71). Diverticuli of the loops of Henle were noted but were thought to be nonspecific and similar to those seen in other renal diseases. Cortical cysts have occasionally been seen in MCD but are infrequent and differ from the numerous elongated cysts seen in IPKD. The cysts are lined by simple cuboidal or flattened epithelium with fibrotic basal membranes which are often surrounded by interstitial lymphocytic infiltration (71). An unusual, homogeneous mucopolysaccharide substance had been noted surrounding many tubules (72) and recently has been identified as Tamm-Horsfall protein (THP), a specific urinary glycoprotein originating in the ascending limb of loop of Henle and distal convoluted tubule (Fig. 24.14). Interstitial localization of this protein was found in a variety of tubulointerstitial diseases, most notably in 50% of patients with MCD, and may reflect distal tubular damage and escape of THP from the tubules into the interstitium.

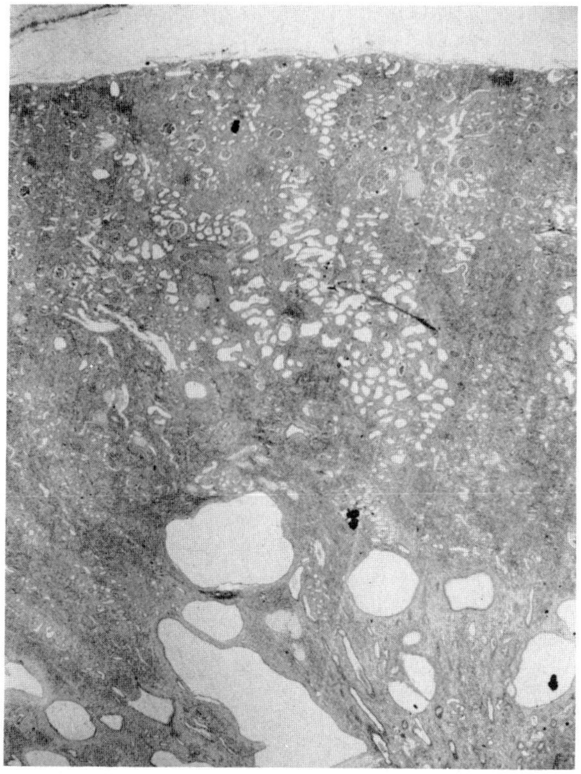

Figure 24.13. Photomicrograph of a nephrectomy specimen from a child with medullary cystic disease. The capsule is at the top of the photograph. Numerous cysts of variable size are present within the medulla. Scattered collecting ducts within the cortex are dilated. (H & E, X14.)

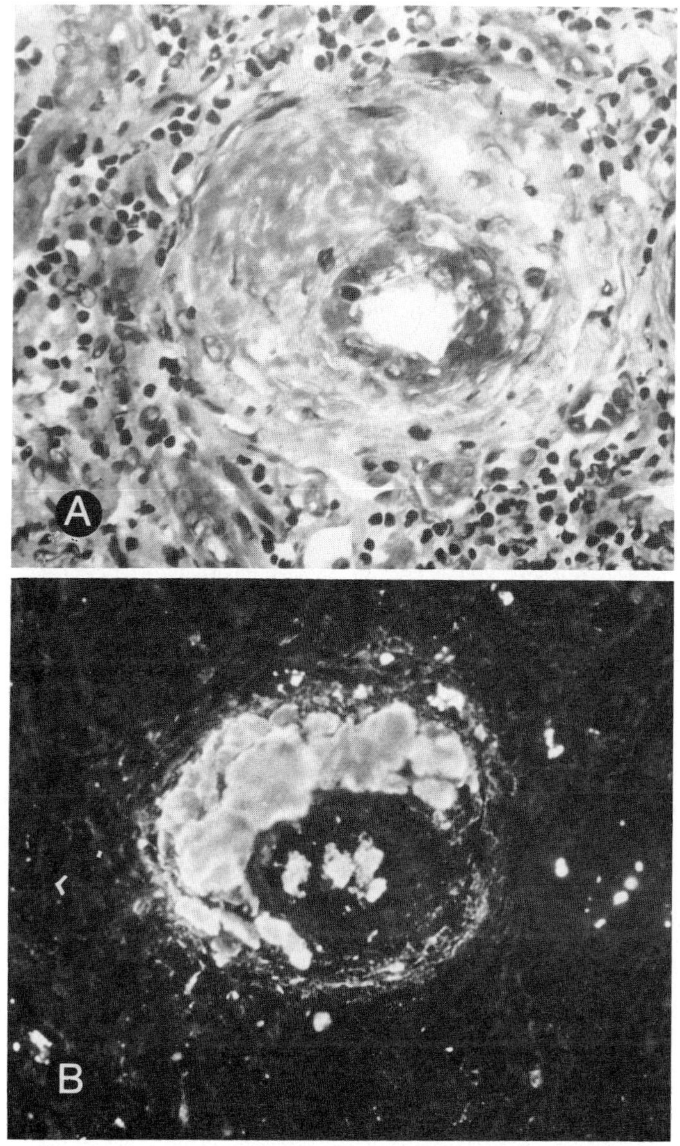

Figure 24.14. **A**, Photomicrograph of the frozen section below showing a mass of fibrillar to glassy periodic acid-Schiff stain positive material surrounding a tubule in the kidney of a patient with medullary cystic disease. Note the intense interstitial cellular infiltrate in the region. (X300.) **B**, Fluorescent photomicrograph of the same field stained with fluorescein labelled rabbit antihuman Tamm-Horsfall protein, demonstrating THP as a major component of the interstitial deposit. (X300.) (Reproduced with permission from Resnick J, Sisson S, Vernier RL: Lab Invest 38:550, 1978.)

The pathogenesis of MCD is unknown, but its genetic inheritance and association with other "dysplastic" conditions of the recessive variety is well established. The renal lesion is functionally and morphologically a tubular defect with progressive interstitial inflammation and fibrosis. Thus, a deficiency of an enzyme required to maintain the normal tubular structure or actively metabolize potential tubular toxins could possibly explain both the renal lesion and the associated nonrenal abnormalities.

In experimental animals, a large number of nephrotoxic, cyst-inducing agents have been identified, including diphenylamine, alloxan, diphenylthiazides, biphenyls, and lithium (21). A familial renal disease with pathological changes similar to MCD has been described in dogs (73) and in mice (74); however, one investigation of the mice has failed to confirm the association (75).

There has been no evidence for a circulating tubular toxin or metabolic abnormality in patients with MCD; however, the presumed genetic basis and the experimental data justify continued search for a biochemical or enzymic abnormality in these patients. The escape of THP from damaged tubules into the interstitium could provide a mechanism for chronic interstitial inflammation (immune or other); however, no direct support for such a mechanism has been provided. The differential diagnois of MCD should include a variety of diseases causing a chronic, progressive tubulointerstitial disease with minimal or no glomerular abnormalities (absence of significant proteinuria and hematuria). In the presence of a positive family history consistent with MCD or associated nonrenal abnormalities, the classical findings of polyuria, anemia, growth retardation, and renal insufficiency make the diagnosis of MCD likely. However, in less classic cases, sonography or renal biopsy may be required to make the diagnosis. Care should be taken to obtain a large enough sample of the corticomedullary region or the findings may be too nonspecific or nondiagnostic. Renal imaging studies will eliminate obstructive uropathy as a cause of tubular damage, and other entities such as dysplastic-hypoplastic kidneys (including oligomeganephronia), renal tubular acidosis, and nephrotoxic agents must be considered. Confusion with other forms of renal cystic disease, such as IPKD should be easily resolved by age of onset, renal size, and identification of large cysts; however, exclusion of late onset IPKD associated with hepatic fibrosis and tubular ectasia may require examination of a renal biopsy. In the older child or young adult with tubular ectasia on IVU, medullary sponge kidney may be considered; however, this is a nonfamilial disease in which renal failure does not occur. The radiographical findings may be similar (medullary tubular dilatation); however, medullary cysts are uncommonly seen in medullary sponge kidney. The coexistence of medullary sponge kidney in family members of patients with MCD has been reported (76) but is probably a coincidental finding.

Treatment

The treatment of patients with MCD is nonspecific and includes adequate nutrition (caloric and amino-acid supplementation) to optimize remaining growth potential, access to water to prevent dehydration, salt supplementation if salt wasting is present, and correction of metabolic acidosis. Treatment of renal osteodystrophy with adequate dietary or supplemental calcium, phosphorus restriction or binders, and appropriate vitamin D therapy is obviously indicated. No specific therapy is effective for the anemia seen in MCD, although associated dietary (iron and so on) deficits should be searched for and treated. Correction of hypokalemia by potassium supplementation may drastically improve polyuria and muscle weakness and simultaneously increase caloric intake when polydypsia decreases. All of the above therapies may help to minimize growth retardation and prevent bone pain or deformities, but the eventual course is progression to end-stage renal failure. Renal dialysis and transplantation have been successful modalities in MCD and to date there has been no evidence of recurrence of the disease in the transplanted kidney.

Family counseling and genetic counseling are important once the diagnosis is established, and careful examination of siblings with annual reevaluation of maximal urinary concentrating ability may allow early detection and early therapy for prevention of complications. Psychological counseling of the patients is an integral part of therapy because of the poor self-image associated with growth retardation and the limitation of physical activities as renal failure progresses. The use of a skilled dietician is necessary to achieve acceptance of the many medications and to achieve adequate caloric intake.

References

1. Mir S, Rapolo J, Koskimies O: Renal cysts in pediatric autopsy material. Nephron 33:189, 1983.
2. Bernstein J: The morphogenesis of renal parenchymal maldevelopment (renal dysplasia). Pediat-Clin N Am 18:395, 1971.
3. Schwarz RD, Stephens FD, Cussen LJ: The pathogenesis of renal dysplasia (3 parts). Invest Urol 19:94, 97, 101, 1981.
4. Bernstein J, Meyer R: Congenital abnormalities of the urinary system. II. Renal cortical and medullary necrosis. J Pediatr 59:657, 1961.
5. Crocker JFS, Brown DM, Vernier RL: Developmental defects of the kidney: A review of renal development and experimental studies of maldevelopment. Pediatr Clin N Am 18:355, 1971.
6. Potter EL: Bilateral absence of ureters and kidneys: A report of 50 cases. Obstet Gynecol 25:3, 1965.
7. Mauer SM, Dobrin R, Vernier RL: Unilateral and bilateral renal agenesis in monoamniotic twins. J Pediatr 84:236, 1974.
8. Roodhooft AM, Birnholz JC, Holmes LB: Familial nature of congenital absence and severe dysgenesis of both kidneys. N Engl J Med 310:1341, 1984.
9. Kaffe S, Goodmilow L, Wolker BA, et al: Prenatal diagnosis of bilateral renal agenesis. Obstet Gynecol 49:478, 1977.
10. Thomas CR, Lang EK, Lloyd FP: Fetal pyelography. A method for detecting fetal life. Obstet Gynecol 22:335, 1963.
11. Bernstein J, Meyer R: Some speculations on the nature and significance of developmentally small kidneys (renal hypoplasia). Nephron 1:137, 1964.
12. Fleischer DA: Lateral displacement of the nipples: A sign of bilateral renal hypoplasia. J Pediatr 69:806, 1966.
13. Royer P, Habib R, Mathieu H: Courtecuisse V. L'hypoplasie renale bilaterale congenital avee reduction du nombre et hypertrophie des nephrons chez lenfant. Ann Pediatr 9:133, 1962.
14. Fitterman GH, Habib R: Congenital bilateral oligonephronic renal hypoplasia with hypertrophy of nephrons (oligomeganephronie). Studies by micro dissection. Am J Clin Path 52:199, 1969.
15. Kyaw M: Roentgenologic triad of congenital multicystic kidneys. AJR 119:710, 1975.
16. Javadpour N, Dellon AL, Kumpe DA: Multilocular cystic disease in adults, imitators of renal cell carcinoma. Urology 1:596, 1973.
17. Barrett DM, Wineland RE: Renal cell carcinoma in multicystic dysplastic kidney. Urology 15:152, 1980.
18. Beck AD: The effect of intra-uterine urinary obstruction upon the development of the kidney. J Urol 105:784, 1971.
19. Harrison MR, Golbus MS, Lilly RA et al: Management of the fetus with congenital hydronephrosis. J Pediatr Surg 17:728, 1982.
20. Gordon RL, Pollack HM, Popky GL, et al: Simple serous cysts of the kidney in children. Radiology 131:357, 1979.
21. Resnick JS, Brown DM, Vernier RL: Normal development and experimental models of cystic renal disease. In Gardner KD Jr (ed): Cystic Diseases of the Kidney. New York, John Wiley & Sons, 1976, p 221.
22. Lieberman E, Salinas-Madrigal L, Gwinn JL, et al: Infantile polycystic disease of the kidneys and liver. Medicine 50:277, 1971.
23. Habif DV, Bendon WE, Yeh M: Infantile polycystic kidney disease: In-utero sonographic diagnosis. Radiology 142:475, 1982.
24. Gsathanondh V, Potter EL: Pathogenesis of polycystic kidneys: Type I due to hyperplasia of interstitial portions of collecting tubules. Ach Path 77:466, 1964.
25. Safouh M, Crocker JFS, Vernier RL: Experimental cystic disease of the kidney. Sequential, functional and morphologic studies. Lab Invest 23:392, 1970.
26. Evan AP, Gardner KD: Nephron obstruction in nondihydroguairanetic acid induced renal cystic disease. Kidney Intl 15:7, 1979.
27. Ojeda JL, Garcia-Porrero JA: Structure and development of parietal podocytes in renal glomerular cysts induced in rabbits with methylprednisolone acetate. Lab Invest 47:167, 1982.
28. Blythe H, Ockenden BG: Polycystic disease of kidneys and liver presenting in childhood. J Med Genet 8:257, 1971.
29. Resnick J, Vernier RL: Cystic disease of the kidney in the newborn infant. Clin Perinatol 8:375, 1981.
30. Alvarez F, Bernard O, Brunelle F, et al: Congential hepatic fibrosis in children. J Pediatr 99:370, 1981.
31. Swischuk LE, Richardson CJ, Nichols MM, et al: Review: Bilateral pulmonary hypoplasia in the neonate. AJR 133:1057, 1979.
32. Thomas IT, Smith DW: Oligohydramnious as a cause of the nonrenal features of Potter's syndrome including pulmonary hypoplasia. J Pediatr 84:811, 1974.
33. Avner ED, Demetrius E, Jaffe R, et al: Neonatal radiocontrast nephropathy simulating infantile polycystic kidney disease. J Pediatr 100:85, 1982.
34. Stapleton FB, Hilton S, Wilcox J, et al: Transient nephromegally simulating infantile polycystic disease of the kidneys. Pediatrics 67:554, 1981.
35. Madewell JE, Hartman DS, Lichtenstein JE: Radiological-pathological correlations in cystic disease of the kidney. Radiol Clin No Am 17:261, 1979.
36. Sanders RC: Sonographic diagnosis of polycystic kidney. AJR 135:212, 1980.
37. Bernstein JA: The morphology of renal cystic disease. In Gardner KD Jr (ed): Cystic Diseases of the Kidney. New York, John Wiley & Sons, 1976, p 40.
38. Potter EL: Normal and abnormal development of the kidneys. Chicago, Year Book Medical Publishers, 1972, p 148.
39. Gabow PA, Ikle DW, Holmes JH: Polycystic kidney disease: Prospective analysis of nonazotemic patients and family members. Ann Int Med 101:238, 1984.
40. Sedman A, Butler N, Gabow P: Adult dominant polycystic kidney disease (PKD) in children (abstract). Kidney Intl 27:55A, 1985.
41. Evan AP, Gardner KD, Bernstein J: Polypoid and papillary epithelial hyperplasia: A potential cause of ductal obstruction in adult polycystic disease. Kidney Intl 16:743, 1979.
42. Milutinovic J, Aquduo LY: Potential causes and pathogenesis in autosomal dominant polycystic kidney disease. Nephron 33:139, 1983.
43. Ross DG, Travers H: Infantile presentation in adult-type polycystic kidney disease in a large kindred. J Pediatr 87:760, 1975.
44. Martinez-Maldanado M, Yiun JJ, Eknoyan G, et al: Adult polycystic kidney disease. Studies of the defect in urine concentration. Kidney Intl 2:107, 1972.
45. Anton PA, Abramowsky CR: Adult polycystic kidney disease presenting in infancy. Report emphasizing the bilateral involvement. J Urol 128:1290, 1982.
46. Lee JKT, McClennan BL, Kissane JM: Unilateral polycystic kidney disease. AJR 130:1165, 1978.
47. Cho KJ, Thornbury JR, Bernstein J, et al: Localized cystic disease of the kidney. Angiographic-pathologic correlation. AJR 132:891, 1979.
48. Levine E, Grantham JJ: The role of computed tomography in the evaluation of adult polycystic disease. Am J Kidney Dis 1:99, 1981.
49. McAlister WH, Siegel MJK, Shackelford G, et al: Glomerulocystic disease. AJR 133:536, 1979.
50. Garel LA, Habib R, Pariente D, et al: Juvenile nephronophthisis: Sonographic appearance in children with severe uremia. Radiology 151:93, 1984.

51. Smith CH, Graham JB: Congenital medullary cysts of kidneys with severe refractory anemia. Am J Dis Child 69:369, 1945.
52. Fanconi G, Hanhant E, von Albertini A, et al: Die familiare juvenile nephronophthisis. Helv Paediatr Acta 6:1, 1951.
53. Strauss MB: Clinical and pathological aspects of cystic disease of renal medulla: Analysis of eighteen cases. Ann Int Med 57:373, 1962.
54. Strauss MB, Sommers SC: Medullary cystic disease and familial juvenile nephronophthisis. N Engl J Med 277:863, 1967.
55. Dunnill MS, Millard PR, Oliver D: Acquired cystic disease of the kidneys: A hazard of long-term intermittent maintenance haemodialysis. J Clin Path 30:868, 1977.
56. Waldherr R, Lennert T, Weber H-P, et al: The nephronophthisis complex: A clinicopathologic study in children. Virch Arch 394:235, 1982.
57. Rayfield EJ, McDonald FD: Red and blonde hair in renal medullary cystic disease. Arch Intern Med 130:72, 1972.
58. Loken AC, Hanssen O, Halvorsen J, et al: Hereditary renal dysplasia and blindness. Acta Paediatr 50:177, 1961.
59. Senior B, Friedman AI, Brando JL: Juvenile familial nephropathy with tapetoretinal degeneration. Am J Ophth 52:625, 1961.
60. Schimke RN: Hereditary renal-retinal dysplasia. *Ann Int Med* 70:735, 1969.
61. Hogewind BL, Veltkamp JJ, Polak BCP, et al: Electro-retinal abnormalities in heterozygotes of renal-retinal dysplasia. Acta Med Scand 202:323, 1977.
62. Biochis H, Passwell J, David R, et al: Congenital hepatic fibrosis and nephronophthisis. Quart J Med 42:221, 1973.
63. Mainzer F, Saldino RM, Ozonoff MD, et al: Familial nephropathy associated with retinitis pigmentosa, cerebellar ataxia, and skeletal abnormalities. Am J Med 49:556, 1970.
64. Popovie-Rolovic M, Calic-Penisic N, Bunjevacki G: Juvenile nephronopthisis associated with retinal pigmentary dystrophy, cerebellar ataxia, and skeletal abnormalities. Arch Dis Childh 51:801, 1976.
65. Gardner KD Jr: Evolution of clinical signs in adult-onset cystic disease of the renal medulla. Ann Int Med 74:47, 1971.
66. Herdman RC, Good RA, Vernier RL: Medullary cystic disease in two siblings. Am J Med 43:335, 1967.
67. Giselson N, Heinegaard D, Holmberg C-G, et al: Renal medullary cystic disease or familial juvenile nephronophthisis. A renal tubular disease. Biochemical findings in two siblings. Am J Med 48:174, 1970.
68. Kligen AS, Scheer RL: Familial disease of the renal medulla. A study of progeny in a family with medullary cystic disease. Ann Int Med 85:190, 1976.
69. Link DP, Hansen S, Plamer J: High dose excretory urography and medullary cystic disease of the kidney. AJR 133:303, 1979.
70. Mena E, Bookstein JJ, McDonald FD, et al: Angiographic findings in renal medullary cystic disease. Radiology 110:277, 1973.
71. Sherman FE, Studnicki FM, Fetterman GH: Renal lesions of familial juvenile nephronophthisis examined by microdissection. Am J Clin Path 55:391, 1971.
72. Resnick J, Sisson S, Vernier RL: Tamm-Horsfall protein. Abnormal localization in renal disease. Lab Invest 38:550, 1978.
73. Finco DR, Duncan JR, Crowell WA, et al: Familial renal disease in Norwegian elkhound dogs. Am J Vet Med 38:941, 1977.
74. Lyon MF, Hulse EV: An inherited kidney disease of mice resembling human nephronophthisis. J Med Genet 8:41, 1971.
75. Resnick JS, Vernier RL: Unpublished observations.
76. Bennett WB: Kindred coexistence of medullary sponge kidney and medullary cystic disease. Ann Int Med 85:829, 1976.

CHAPTER 25

Syndromes with a Renal Component

GIULIO GILLI
A. CAROLINE BERRY
CYRIL CHANTLER

Renal abnormalities are present at birth in a large number of conditions or develop later. The pediatrician needs to be aware of the possible involvement of the kidney in syndromes associated with dysmorphology or dysfunction in other organs. The pediatric nephrologist needs to be able to recognize the association of renal disease with abnormalities in other systems, because the generalized abnormality may be of more clinical importance and the condition may carry genetic implications.

This chapter will provide a general description of the etiology of renal malformations, as well as Tables 25.1 to 25.12, which are tables of syndromes and diseases associated with urinary tract malformations and dysfunction. Conditions have been excluded where the abnormality in other organs is secondary to renal disease or that are fully discussed elsewhere in the book, e.g., the Henoch-Schönlein syndrome. Although one reference to each condition is given, the reader should refer especially to McKusick (1), Smith (2), and Stanbury and coworkers (3) for more extensive bibliographies.

Rare components of a syndrome or associations of a disease have been placed in parentheses. Syndrome identification is frequently complicated and the genetic implications and genetic counselling are complicated and hazardous. Then it is desirable and necessary to consult an experienced dysmorphologist and clinical geneticist before discussion with parents.

ETIOLOGY OF RENAL MALFORMATIONS

The kidney is a vulnerable organ and errors in its development may occur in a large number of conditions from varying primary causes. Developmental errors may result in either hypoplasia, with its ultimate limit of aplasia or agenesis; in dysgenesis, which frequently includes cystic changes; in errors of tubular function; or in errors of position and gross structure, as in the horseshoe kidney. Renal lesions can be primary or secondary.

Renal Anomalies Secondary to Malformations Elsewhere

An obstructive lesion at any site in the renal tract will lead to destruction of renal tissue, dilation of tubules, and dysgenesis. The best example of this is the prune belly syndrome or the urethral obstruction sequence. Obstruction, probably from mid first trimester and usually secondary to urethral valve formation, leads to fetal bladder distention. This, in turn, leads to hydroureter and renal dysplasia and, at the same time, distends the abdominal wall and leads to muscle-wall deficiency and excess abdominal skin. Frequently, decompression occurs through a patent urachus or by other means, and the child is born with the findings typical of the prune belly syndrome.

Primary Renal Anomalies

Primary renal anomalies may arise as a manifestation of a generalized disorder affecting numerous other structures, an error in a developmental field complex, or a pleiotropic gene.

Generalized Disorders

Generalized disorders include chromosomal disorders, consequences of teratogens, or generalized tissue dysplasias.

Chromosomal Disorders. Chromosomal disorders, in general, cause dysgenesis of most organs, a result in part of the specific effects of those genes that are lacking (deletion syndromes) or present in excess (trisomies). They may be secondary to a nonspecific effect, possibly on the cell cycle or some other fundamental cell function, which is common to all chromosomal disorders. Renal manifestations vary. The horseshoe kidney is the hallmark of the Turner syndrome and also is frequent in the Edward syndrome (trisomy 18), whereas cystic dysplasia is more common in the Patau syndrome (trisomy 13), and anomalies of position and of the collecting system in trisomy 8 mosaicism (4). These anomalies probably reflect the interaction of the nonspecific cellular effect with the specific defects of individual genes.

A chromosomal abnormality with highly specific manifestations is deletion of band p(13) of chromosome 11. Children with this deletion have aniridia, ambiguous genitalia, mental retardation, and a 30% risk of developing Wilms' tumor (5). Why loss of this band should be specifically associated with this malignancy and no other and why it occurs only in a proportion of those with this deletion may become clearer when DNA sequencing of that chromosomal region has been achieved.

Teratogenic Agents. In general, the kidney seems less vulnerable to circulating chemicals and viruses than such organs as the heart or brain. Renal anomalies occur only rarely in the rubella embryopathy and are not associated with cytomegalovirus infection. Among teratogens, alcohol seems the most likely to cause renal dysgenesis; renal anomalies are reported in about 10% of those affected (6). They are not a feature of fetal hydantoin or fetal warfarin syndromes.

Generalized Tissue Dysplasia. A dysplasia affects a single tissue and, hence, those organs in which that tissue is of major importance. Most dysplasias, e.g., skeletal dysplasias, leave renal tissue unscathed, but there are some generalized dysplasias that affect the kidney. Beckwith syndrome is a poorly understood generalized dysplasia, probably resulting from a disturbance of growth rate. There is generalized visceromegaly with renal hypertrophy and a tendency to develop Wilms' tumor. This latter factor is not only of practical importance but also of great theoretical interest. An example of a generalized dysplasia under direct genetic control is that of tuberous sclerosis. The primary source of error is not identified but tubers may occur in numerous organs, including the kidney; occasionally the disease may present as renal cystic disease (7).

In other genetically determined disorders, the primary lesion is metabolic. Recently two siblings with glutaric acidemia type II have been reported (8). These premature newborns had a "warty dysplasia" of the cerebral cortex and microscopic abnormality of other organs; the kidneys were most dramatically affected, being exceedingly large and made up entirely of small cysts. Thus, lack of a single enzyme can give rise to major structural defects of renal tissue. This provides a clue as to the possible etiology of such disorders as infantile polycystic disease.

Developmental Field Complexes

The concept that associations of congenital malformations may be the end result of a single error that occurs in an embryonic developmental field has been well promoted by Opitz (9). He states

> A developmental field is that part of an embryo that reacts as a temporally and spatially coordinated unit to normal, localized, forces of organization and differentiation, and to surgical manipulations, gene and chromosome mutations, and the effect of certain teratogens. A developmental-field complex, then, is a group of more or less localized primary disturbances of embryonic development that originate from a single pathogenetic defect that exerts a temporally and spatially coordinated effect in a field, thus resulting in what is commonly called a (primary) malformation.

A good example is the caudal regression syndrome, which, in its most extreme form, results in the birth of an infant with sirenomelia, absent bladder, renal agenesis, absent external genitalia, imperforate anus, and lower limb abnormalities. Less severely affected infants may have renal defects, imperforate anus, and vertebral defects (2).

Another developmental field defect in which renal anomalies are an important feature is the Müllerian, Renal, Cervical Somites (MURCS) association, in which there is absence or hypoplasia of the vagina and uterus, renal agenesis or ectopy, and defects of the cervical vertebrae (2). An error of development in the very early embryo, when the cervical somites and pronephric ducts are close to one another, could explain this association.

In general, these developmental field defects are sporadic, but a few are determined by a single gene. The branchio-oto-renal syndrome is a dominantly inherited disorder with variable expression (2). The least serious manifestation is the presence of cervical or preauricular sinuses, while other gene carriers with or without the sinuses have sensorineural or conductive deafness of varying degrees. Other affected family members may have renal dysplasia of varying severity. Rather than postulating a single gene that acts in so varied a way, it is more economic to hypothesize its activity at the early embryonic stage.

Other examples that suggest a strong genetic controlling component are the occasional reports of the apparently dominant inheritance of renal agenesis with uterine anomalies (10) and some recent findings in the families of infants with the Potter syndrome. Unilateral or bilateral agenesis in 7 of 199 siblings and preliminary findings indicate that a significant number of parents have unilateral agenesis or hypoplasia (11, 12). It appears that these parents have a higher risk of having a further affected child.

Pleiotropic Genes

Although some single gene disorders affect a developmental field or give rise to multiple defects through the action of a single enzyme, there are large numbers of syndromes where the only apparent explanation is that the gene acts in a number of places (pleiotropy). The Bardet-Biedl syndrome is characterized by polydactyly, retinitis pigmentosa, obesity, hypogonadism, and renal lesions in a significant proportion of affected individuals (13) and is controlled by a single autosomal recessive gene. It is difficult at this time to suggest any mechanism that would account for such diverse effects. A number of disorders of renal tubular function have manifestations outside the kidney. Lowe syndrome is X-linked and includes cataracts and mental retardation, whereas renal tubular acidosis and sensorineural deafness arise from a single autosomal recessive gene. At present, there is no unifying explanation; however, as our knowledge increases, a rational explanation for these rather bizarre groupings of manifestations may become apparent.

ABNORMALITIES SECONDARY TO RENAL AGENESIS OR HYPOPLASIA

Renal agenesis or severe dysplasia can give rise to a series of clinical abnormalities that may be more dramatic and life-threatening than the renal anomaly that may be recognized only postmortem. The Potter syndrome (bilateral renal agenesis) is the most severe example of this group. Since fetal urine makes a considerable contribution to the amniotic fluid, renal agenesis or urethral obstruction give rise to oligohydramnios. This hinders fetal movement and results in fetal limb deformity, ranging from simple positional talipes to severe arthrogryposis. More important for fetal survival is the association of oligohydramnios, with failure of fetal lungs to mature, resulting in respiratory failure and death soon after birth. Thus, in the Potter syndrome, death is secondary to respiratory rather than renal failure.

It is possible to explain the concurrence of renal and other clinical features for a considerable number of syndromes with a renal component. In the tables that follow it is clear that many syndromes do not fit into the categories outlined. It is these conundrums that highlight our ignorance of both normal developmental processes and of the pathology of the embryo and fetus.

Table 25.1
Chromosomal Aberrations

No.	Syndrome	Main features	Urinary tract abnormality	Inheritance	Ref.
1	Trisomy 13-15, Patau	Small-for-dates, microcephaly, cleft lip and palate, digital anomalies, rocker-bottom feet, severe mental defect	Cystic and other renal anomalies in 60% of cases	—	4
2	Trisomy 16-18, Edwards	Small-for-dates, characteristic facies, overlapping fingers, foot deformities, thin ribs, muscular hypertonicity, neonatal hepatitis	Horseshoe kidney, cystic dysplasia, and duplication in 70% of cases	—	4
3	Trisomy 21, Down	Brachycephaly, epicanthal folds, protruding tongue, hypotonia, congenital heart disease	Horseshoe kidney, cystic dysplasia, and duplication in less than 10% of cases	—	14
4	Cat-eye	Coloboma, ocular hypertelorism with antimongoloid slant, anorectal anomalies	Agenesis and other anomalies in the majority of cases	—	14
5	Cri-du-chat (deletion 5p)	Severe growth and mental retardation, catlike cry, microcephaly, muscular hypotonia	Various renal anomalies	—	14
6	Deletion 11p	Aniridia, ambiguous genitalia, mental retardation	Wilms' tumour	—	4, 5
7	Other autosomal aberrations	—	Various, but not common	—	14
8	45X, Turner	Small stature, shield chest, widely spaced hypoplastic nipples, coarctation of aorta, amenorrhea	Horseshoe kidney, duplication, malrotation, and other abnormalities in 60% of cases	—	4, 14
9	47XXY, Klinefelter	Eunuchoid appearance, gynecomastia, hypergonadotropic hypogonadism, testicular atrophy, azoospermia	Rare	—	14
10	Other gonosomal aberrations	—	Various, but not common	—	15, 16

Table 25.2
Skeletal Abnormalities

No.	Syndrome	Main features	Urinary tract abnormality	Inheritance	Ref.
11	Achondrogenesis	Micromelic dwarfism, short trunk, fetal hydrops	Hydronephrosis, hydroureter, duplication of collecting system	AR	17
12	Thanatophoric dysplasia	Short-limbed dwarfism, large cranium, narrow thorax, flattened vertebral bodies, respiratory distress, hypotonia	(Hydronephrosis)	Sporadic	18
13	Short rib-polydactyly, syndromes of various types	Short-limbed dwarfism, short ribs, polydactyly, cleft lip and palate	Polycystic kidneys	AR	19
14	Chondrodysplasia punctata, rhizomelic type	Flat face, microcephaly, cataracts, short femura and humeri, stippled epiphyses	Micromulticystic kidneys	AR	20
15	Campomelic dysplasia	Anterior bowing of leg bones, abnormal facies, cleft palate	Hydroureter, hydronephrosis, hypoplasia, cystic kidneys	AR	21
16	Metatropic dysplasia	Short-limbed dwarfism, narrow thorax with short ribs, progressive kyphoscoliosis	(Bilateral hydroureter)	?AR	22
17	Chondroectodermal dysplasia, Ellis-van Creveld	Acromelic dwarfism, polydactyly, hypoplasia and dystrophy of nails and teeth, congenital heart disease	Nephrocalcinosis, glomerulosclerosis, unilateral agenesis, megaureter	AR	23, 24
18	Asphyxiating thoracic dysplasia, Jeune	Short-limbed dwarfism, narrow thorax, hypoplastic iliac wings	Tubular dysfunction, cystic dysplasia, cortical cysts, juvenile nephronophthisis, renal failure	AR	25, 26
19	(Dyssegmental dysplasia)	Short trunk and limbs, narrow thorax, defects of vertebral ossification and segmentation, cleft palate, reduced joint mobility	Hydroureter, hydronephrosis	?AR	27
20	Mesomelic dysplasia, type Robinow, fetal face	Mesomelic dwarfism, hemivertebrae, characteristic facies, hypoplastic external genitalia	Duplication, hydronephrosis	?AR; ?AD	28
21	(Brachymesomelia-renal)	Brachymesomelia of upper limbs, craniofacial dysmorphism, corneal opacities, renal anomalies	Glomerulocystic dysplasia	?	29
22	Larsen	Multiple joint dislocations, flat facies	Hydroureteronephrosis, unilateral agenesis	?AD ?AR	30, 31
23	Oto-palato-digital	Short stature, characteristic craniofacial features, cleft palate, conductive deafness, broad terminal phalanges	(Hypoplasia)	?X-linked ?AD	32
24	Dyschondrosteosis	Mesomelic dwarfism, Madelung deformity	(Nephritis)	AD	33
25	Metaphyseal chondrodysplasia, type Shwachman	Metaphyseal changes of femurs, ribs, short stature, bone marrow hypoplasia with neutropenia and thrombocytopenia, exocrine pancreatic insufficiency	Renal glycosuria, aminoaciduria, renal acidosis, nephrocalcinosis	AR	34
26	Marden-Walker	Kyphoscoliosis, joint contractures, immobile facies, blepharophimosis, growth and developmental delay	(Microcystic kidneys, mild dilatation of collecting system)	AR	35, 36
27	Trichorhinophalangeal dysplasia I, Giedion-Langer	Thin, sparse hair, bulbous nose, peripheral dysostosis	Small, scarred kidney; renal hypertension	AD	37
28	Trichorhinophalangeal dysplasia II, MEMR	Thin, sparse hair, bulbous nose, protruding ears, peripheral dysostosis, multiple cartilaginous exostoses, variable mental retardation	(Generalized aminoaciduria)	?Sporadic ?AD	38
29	Marble brain disease	Osteopetrosis, cerebral calcifications, stunted growth, peculiar facies, renal tubular acidosis	Distal tubular acidosis	AR	39
30	Osteodysplasty, Melnick-Needles	Bowing of long bones, short upper limbs, ribbon-like ribs, prominent eyes, small mandible	Hydroureteronephrosis, ureteral stenosis, dysplastic kidneys	AD; AR; X-linked	40

Table 25.2—*Continued*

No.	Syndrome	Main features	Urinary tract abnormality	Inheritance	Ref.
31	Frontometaphyseal dysplasia	Prominent supraorbital ridges, metaphyseal dysplasia, joint limitations, conductive deafness	Bilateral duplication of collecting system, ureterovesical obstruction, pyelonephritis	X-linked	41, 42
32	Craniosynostosis-radial aplasia, Baller-Gerold	Craniosynostosis, radial hypoplasia or aplasia, hand deformities	Crossed renal ectopia	?AR	43
33	Trapezoidocephaly-multiple synostoses, Antley-Bixler, acrocephalosynanky	Craniosynostosis, humeroradial synostosis, midface hypoplasia, abnormal ears; narrow chest and pelvis, digital abnormalities	Ectopia, duplication of kidney and ureter, renal hypertension	AR	44, 45
34	Acrocephalosyndactyly, type Apert	Acrocephaly, syndactyly	Cystic kidneys, hydronephrosis	AD	46
35	Acrocephalosyndactyly, type Saethre-Chotzen	Acrocephaly, facial asymmetry, brachydactyly, partial cutaneous syndactyly	Duplication of collecting system	AD	47
36	(Acrocephalosyndactyly, type Waardenburg)	Acrocephaly, hydrophthalmos, cutaneous syndactyly, cleft palate, congenital heart disease, genital anomalies	Hypospadias	?	48
37	Acrocephalopolysyndactyly, type Carpenter	Acrocephaly, brachysyndactyly of hands, polysyndactyly of feet, mental retardation	Hydronephrosis, hydroureter	AR	49, 50
38	(Acrocephalopolydactylous dysplasia, Elejalde)	Acrocephaly, hexadactyly of hands, gigantism, thick skin, visceromegaly, connective tissue hyperplasia	Cystic dysplasia	?AR	51
39	C-trigonocephaly	Trigonocephaly, polysyndactyly, abnormal ears, joint dislocations	Unilateral agenesis, hypospadias	AR	52
40	Oral-cranial-digital, Juberg-Hayward	Cleft lip/palate, microcephaly, syndactyly of toes, hypoplasia and inflexibility of thumbs	Horseshoe kidney	AR	53
41	Occipital horns, Ehlers-Danlos type IX	Symmetrical occipital bony protuberances, platyspondyly, carpal fusions, chronic diarrhea, lysyl oxidase deficiency	Obstructive uropathy	?X-linked	54
42	Frontonasal dysplasia	Median cleft face, ocular hypertelorism	Unilateral agenesis	Sporadic; ?AD; ?AR	55
43	Unilateral mandibulofacial dysostosis, Weyers-Thier	Unilateral ear and ocular abnormalities, no hair behind the affected ear, hypoplasia of malar bones	(Hypospadias)	?AR	56
44	Oculo-auriculo-vertebral dysplasia, Goldenhar-Gorlin	Asymmetrical or unilateral lesions consisting in epidermal bulboids, colobomas, anomalies of external, middle and inner ear; hemivertebrae	Unilateral agenesis, crossed ectopy, ureteral duplication	Sporadic; ?AD	57, 58
45	Klippel-Feil anomaly	Fusion of cervical vertebrae, short neck with motion limitation, low posterior hairline	Unilateral agenesis, ectopy, duplication of collecting system	Sporadic; AD	59
46	Branchio-skeletal-genital, Elsahy-Waters	Fusion of cervical vertebrae, pectus excavatum, craniofacial dysmorphism, seizures, mental retardation, hypospadias	Hypospadias	?AR	60
47	MURCS association	Müllerian duct aplasia, renal anomalies, cervicothoracic somite dysplasia	Unilateral agenesis, ectopy	Sporadic	2
48	VATER association	Vertebral anomalies, anorectal malformations, tracheoesophageal fistula with esophageal atresia, renal anomalies, radial defects	Unilateral agenesis; dysplasia, ectopy, hydronephrosis	Sporadic; multifactorial	2, 61
49	Caudal regression, sirenomelia sequence	All degrees of severity, from imperforate anus to sirenomelia	Unilateral agenesis, dysplasia, horseshoe kidney, duplications, etc.	Sporadic	2, 58
50	Spondylocostal dysostosis	Vertebral anomalies, barrel-shaped chest, rib defects, short neck	Unilateral agenesis, ectopy, hydronephrosis	AR; AD	62, 63
51	Cerebro-costo-mandibular	Cerebral maldevelopment or malfunction, severe rib defects, micrognathia	Ectopy, medullary cysts	?AR; ?AD	64
52	Onycho-osteodysplasia (nail-patella)	Dysplasia of nails and patella, iliac horns	Proteinuria, hematuria, renal insufficiency	AD	65

Table 25.2—*Continued*

No.	Syndrome	Main features	Urinary tract abnormality	Inheritance	Ref.
53	EEC	Ectrodactyly, ectodermal dysplasia, cleft lip/palate	Unilateral agenesis, hypoplasia, hydronephrosis and hydroureter, duplications	?AD; ?Sporadic	66, 67
54	Aglossia-adactyly	Hypo-aglossia, micrognathia, hypo-adactyly, cranial nerves palsy	Unilateral agenesis	Sporadic	68
55	Camptobrachydactyly	Brachydactyly of hands and feet, polydactyly, polymetatarsalia, flexion contractures of fingers, septate vagina	Urinary incontinence (?bladder neck dysmorphism)	AD	69
56	Syndactyly, type V	Metacarpal 4–5 fusion, brachydactyly, camptodactyly	Hypoplasia, bladder extrophy	AD	70
57	Schinzel-Giedion	Midface hypoplasia and other craniofacial anomalies, brachymesomelia, hypoplasia of distal phalanges, clubfeet, hypertrichosis, seizures	Hydronephrosis, hypospadias	?AR	71
58	Acro-renal, Dieker-Opitz	Various acral and renal anomalies	Unilateral agenesis, duplications	Sporadic	72
59	Acro-renal-mandibular	Ectrodactyly, hypoplastic mandible, renal anomalies	Unilateral agenesis, polycystic kidneys	?AR	73
60	Roberts, SC-phocomelia	Tetraphocomelia, cleft lip/palate, genital hypertrophy	Horseshoe kidney, polycystic kidneys	AR	74, 75
61	—	Shortened forearm and upper arm, absent or hypoplastic thumbs, flexion contractures of fingers, minor craniofacial anomalies, hearing loss	Urethral valves, bladder diverticula	?AD	76
62	REAR, Townes-Kurnit	**R**adial ray anomalies, abnormal **e**ars, **a**nal defects, **r**enal anomalies	Hypoplasia, ureterovesical reflux, urethral valves	AD	2
63	—	Radial ray aplasia, short stature, renal anomalies	Unilateral agenesis, crossed fused kidney	AD	77
64	IVIC	Radial ray hypoplasia, hearing impairment, external ophthalmoplegia, thrombocytopenia	Ectopy	AD	78
65	—	Radial hypoplasia, triphalangeal thumbs, maxillary diastema	Hypospadias	AD	79
66	Weyers oligodactyly	Ulnar ray defects with oligodactyly, antecubital pterygia, sternal anomalies, cleft lip/palate	Horseshoe kidney, ureteral duplication	Sporadic	80
67	Ulnar-mammary, Pallister	Ulnar ray defects, hypoplasia or absence of mammary glands and axillary apocrine glands	Unilateral agenesis, malrotation	AD	81
68	Poland	Unilateral aplasia of pectoralis major with ipsilateral symbrachydactyly and ipsilateral hypo-aplasia of breast and nipple	Ipsilateral agenesis, hypoplasia or duplication of collecting system	Sporadic	82
69	Rubinstein-Taybi	Broad thumbs and toes, abnormal facies, short stature, mental retardation	Various anomalies, including agenesis and duplications	Sporadic	2
70	Fanconi pancytopenia	Pancytopenia, radial ray defects, hyperpigmentation	Various anomalies, including horseshoe kidney, hydronephrosis	AR	83
71	Oral-facial-digital I, Papillon-Léage-Psaume	Oral frenula, cleft tongue/jaw/palate, hypoplasia of alar cartilages, digital malformations	Polycystic kidneys	X-linked	84
72	Hand-foot-genital	Short metacarpal I, brachymesophalangy V, short metatarsal I, phalangeal fusion of other toes, uterus anomalies	Hypospadias	?AR; ?AD	85
73	Osteolysis with nephropathy	Progressive osteolysis of carpal and tarsal bones, nephropathy	Chronic glomerulonephritis, hypertension, renal failure	Sporadic	86
74	Arthro-dento-osteodysplasia, Hajdu-Cheney	Pseudo-osteolysis of terminal phalanges, generalized osteoporosis, joint laxity, small stature, wormian bones, persistent cranial sutures, early loss of teeth	Polycystic kidneys	AD	87

Other syndromes with skeletal anomalies: 75–79, 81, 90, 91, 94, 103, 104, 106–111, 116, 121, 127, 130, 132, 138, 140, 156, 159, 167, 174–175, 185, 186, 193, 195, 198, 201, 203, 206, 218, 219, 224, 265–267, 269–271, 273, 278–281

Table 25.3
Syndromes with Aberrant Growth

No.	Syndrome	Main features	Urinary tract abnormality	Inheritance	Ref.
75	Seckel	Severe short stature, microcephaly, narrow face, beaklike protrusion of the nose	Ectopy, hypoplasia, nephritis	AR	88
76	Cerebro-oculo-facio-skeletal, Pena-Shokeir	Failure to thrive, microcephaly, microphthalmia, prominent nose, large ears, hypotonia, flexion contractures	Unilateral agenesis, horseshoe kidney, duplication of collecting system	AR	89, 90
77	Neu-Laxova	Intrauterine growth retardation, microcephaly, abnormal facies, short neck, arthrogryposis, CNS malformations	Unilateral agenesis	AR	91
78	Cockayne	Small stature, microcephaly, deafness, retinal dysplasia, photosensitivity, mental retardation	Albuminuria, glomerulonephritis, renal insufficiency	AR	92
79	Coffin-Siris	Prenatal and postnatal growth deficiency, microcephaly, abnormal facies, absent fifth fingernail and terminal phalanx, mental retardation	Unilateral agenesis, hydronephrosis, bladder diverticula	?AR	93, 94
80	Brachmann-de Lange	Prenatal and postnatal growth deficiency, dysmorphic facies, hirsutism, mental retardation	Hypoplasia, cystic dysplasia, hydronephrosis, hypospadias	Sporadic	95
81	Dubowitz	Primordial shortness of stature, microcephaly, sparse hair, peculiar facies, hypertelorism, toe syndactyly	Hypospadias	AR	96
82	MULIBREY dysplasia	Progressive growth failure, hydrocephaloid head, ocular abnormalities, muscular hypotonia, hepatomegaly	(Wilms' tumor)	AR	97
83	Noonan	Short stature, webbed neck, pulmonary stenosis, cryptorchidism, mental retardation	Polycystic kidneys, hydronephrosis, malrotation, duplication of collecting system	?AD; sporadic	98, 99
84	Russell-Silver	Short stature, craniofacial dysmorphism, asymmetry	Unilateral agenesis, pelviureteric obstruction, pyelonephritis, enlarged kidneys, hypospadias	?	100
85	Hemihypertrophy, congenital asymmetry	Partial or total asymmetry	Enlarged kidneys, nephrocalcinosis, medullary sponge kidney, tumors of kidney (and liver & adrenal glands), hypospadias	?	101, 102
86	Congenital total lipodystrophy, Seip-Berardinelli	Generalized absence of adipose tissue, accelerated growth and maturation, hirsutism, acanthosis nigricans, insulin-resistant nonketotic diabetes	Nephromegaly with splaying of collecting system, hydronephrosis, hydroureter	AR	103, 104, 105
87	Acquired total lipodystrophy, Lawrence	Progressive, generalized loss of adipose tissue, liver cirrhosis, hyperlipemia, acanthosis nigricans, insulin-resistant nonketotic diabetes	Bilateral nephromegaly with splaying collecting system, glomerular sclerosis with renal insufficiency	Sporadic	103, 104, 105
88	Partial lipodystrophy, Barraquer-Simons	Loss of adipose tissue from face and upper half of body, hypertriglyceridemia, hypocomplementemia	Mesangiocapillary glomerulonephritis	Sporadic	See chapter 26B
89	Leprechaunism	Failure to thrive, emaciation, hirsutism, endocrine disorders	Tubular ectasia, medullary calcification	?AR	106
90	Marshall-Smith	Failure to thrive, accelerated skeletal maturation, craniofacial dysmorphism, psychomotor retardation	Hydroureteronephrosis	?	107
91	Cerebral gigantism, Sotos	Acceleration of growth, acromegalic appearance, large hands and feet, characteristic facies, variable mental retardation	Urethral stricture, Wilms' tumor	Sporadic; ?AD	108
92	EMG, Beckwith-Wiedemann	Exomphalos, macroglossia, gigantism, visceromegaly	Enlarged kidneys, cystic medullary dysplasia, Wilms' tumor	Sporadic; ?multifactorial	109, 110

Other syndromes with growth disturbances: most syndromes with skeletal abnormalities and: 100, 101, 110, 111, 140, 142, 153, 169, 175–177, 180–184, 186, 188, 195, 200, 211, 217, 224, 227, 231, 238, 244, 260, 265, 272, 278, 280, 281

Table 25.4
Ocular Abnormalities

No.	Syndrome	Main features	Urinary tract abnormality	Inheritance	Ref.
93	Senior-Løken	Tapetoretinal degeneration, retinal dysplasia, renal anomalies	Nephronophthisis, renal dysplasia	AR	111, 112
94	Mainzer-Saldino	Tapetoretinal degeneration, ataxia, peripheral dysostosis, renal anomalies	Nephronophthisis	AR	113, 114
95	—	Retinal dysplasia, cataracts, cystic kidneys	Polycystic kidneys, medullary cysts	?AR	115
96	—	Fundus flavimaculatus, cystic kidneys	Polycystic kidneys	?	116
97	Aniridia-Wilms' tumor	Aniridia or iris dysplasia, Wilms' tumor, deletion of chromosome 11	Wilms' tumor	Sporadic	5, 117
98	—	Partial aniridia, congenital glaucoma, hypotonia, mild mental retardation, renal agenesis	Unilateral agenesis	?AR	118
99	Oculo-cerebro-renal, Lowe	Cataracts, hypotonia, mental retardation, renal tubular dysfunction	Proximal tubular defects	X-linked	See chapter 30
100	Oculo-cerebro-renal, McCance	Corneal opacities, nystagmus, brain abnormalities, mental retardation, failure to thrive, absence of testes, renal anomalies	Tubular dysfunction, small glomeruli, and chronic renal failure	?AR; ?X-linked	119
101	Oculo-cerebro-renal, Denys	Hydrophthalmos and secondary glaucoma, mental retardation, short stature, renal tubular dysfunction	Renal acidosis with hypercalciuria and hyperphosphaturia	?AR	120
102	Oculo-renal-cerebellar	Tapetoretinal degeneration, choreoathetosis of upper limbs, spastic diplegia, mental retardation, glomerulopathy	Glomerular sclerosis, renal failure	AR	121
103	Bardet-Biedl	Tapetoretinal degeneration, obesity, hypogenitalism, mental retardation, polydactyly	Cystic dysplasia, obstructive uropathy, renal failure	AR	13, 122
104	Biemond II	Iris coloboma, obesity, hypogenitalism, mental retardation, polydactyly	Hypospadias	?AD	123
105	Alström	Blindness, nerve deafness, obesity, diabetes mellitus	Albuminuria, renal failure	AR	124
106	Lacrimo-auricular-dento-digital	Nasolacrimal duct obstruction, cup-shaped ears, enamel dysplasia, digital malformations	Unilateral agenesis	AD	125
107	Sorsby	Pigmented macular coloboma, type B brachydactyly	Unilateral agenesis	AD	126
108	Cryptophthalmos-syndactyly, Fraser	Fused eyelids, ear anomalies, syndactylies, genital anomalies	Unilateral or bilateral agenesis, dysplasia, hypospadias	AR	2, 127
109	Lenz microphthalmia	Microphthalmia, short stature, skeletal anomalies, dental anomalies	Unilateral agenesis, dysplasia	X-linked	128
110	—	Keratoconus, cleft lip and palate, short stature, mental retardation	Double ureters	?AR	129
111	Abruzzo-Erickson	Coloboma, deafness, cleft palate, radiosynostosis, hypospadias, short stature	Horseshoe kidney, hypospadias	?AD; ?X-linked	130
112	—	Coloboma, congenital heart defect	Unilateral agenesis, ectopy, duplications, hypospadias	?Sporadic	131
113	Facio-oculo-acustico-renal	Facial abnormalities, colobomas, cataracts, perceptive deafness, proteinuria	Proteinuria	?AR	132
114	Hypertelorism-hypospadias, BBB, Opitz	Ocular hypertelorism, coloboma, hypospadias,	Hypospadias	AD	133, 134
115	Hypertelorism-dysphagia, G, Opitz-Frias	Ocular hypertelorism, dysphagia, hoarse cry	Hypospadias, ureteral reflux, duplication of pelvis and ureter	?AD; ?X-linked	135
116	HMC	Hypertelorism, microtia, cleft lip/palate/nose	Ectopy	?AR	136
117	—	Coloboma, cataracts, iris anomalies, myopia, hypertelorism, deafness, umbilical hernia, mental retardation	Proteinuria, generalized aminoaciduria	?AR	137

Other syndromes with ocular abnormalities: 14, 21, 26, 36, 43, 44, 64, 76, 78, 82, 124–127, 142, 161, 164, 169, 176, 186, 189, 194, 211, 219, 230, 234, 245, 256, 266, 270. 275, 276, 278, 281

Table 25.5
External, Middle, and Inner Ear Abnormalities

No.	Syndrome	Main features	Urinary tract abnormality	Inheritance	Ref.
118	Branchio-oto-renal, Melnick-Fraser	Branchial fistulas or cysts, preauricular pits, hearing loss, renal abnormalities	Renal dysplasia, hypoplasia, renal failure	AD	2
119	Branchio-oto-ureteral	Preauricular tags and pits, sensorineural deafness, urinary tract anomalies	Bifid renal pelvices, duplication of the ureters	AD	138
120	Oto-renal-genital, Winter	Middle ear anomalies, hearing impairment, vaginal atresia, renal anomalies	Unilateral or bilateral agenesis, dysplasia	?AR	139
121	Braun-Bayer	Deafness, bifid uvula, digital anomalies, nephrosis, urinary tract anomalies	Nephrosis, ureteral constriction, duplication of collecting system	?AR; ?X-linked	140
122	—	Sensorineural deafness, tubular acidosis	Distal tubular acidosis	AR	141
123	—	Sensorineural deafness, urinary tract abnormalities	Calyceal diverticula, attenuation of the pelvicalyceal system	AD	142
124	Alport	Nerve deafness, cataracts, hereditary nephritis	Nephritis, nephrosis	?AD; ?X-linked	See chapter 26H
125	—	Progressive deafness, cataracts, myopia, marfanoid habitus, renal disease	Proteinuria, renal insufficiency	?AD	143
126	—	Deafness, severe myopia, renal disease	Albuminuria, hematuria	?AR	144
127	—	Deafness, lens opacities, pigmentation of sun-exposed skin regions, short broad fingers, progressive arthritis, susceptibility to infections, mental retardation, renal disease	Chronic glomerulonephritis, renal failure	?X-linked	145

Other syndromes with ear abnormalities: 23, 28, 31, 33, 39, 43, 44, 61, 62, 64, 76, 78, 105, 106, 108, 111, 113, 116, 117, 168, 170, 184, 208, 216, 220, 222, 230, 250, 263, 266, 268, 271, 272, 280

Table 25.6
Visceral Abnormalities

No.	Syndrome	Main features	Urinary tract abnormality	Inheritance	Ref.
128	Cardiofacial, Cayler	Asymmetric facies when crying, cardiovascular anomalies	Various anomalies, including unilateral agenesis, ectopy, cystic dysplasia	?	146
129	Facio-cardio-renal, Eastman-Bixler	Conduction defects, endocardial fibroelastosis, characteristic facies, severe mental retardation, horseshoe kidney	Horseshoe kidney	?AR	147
130	—	Severe obstructive left heart abnormalities, vertebral anomalies, renal anomalies	Calyceal and ureteral ectasia, bifid pelvis, papillary necrosis	?AR	148
131	—	Pulmonary stenosis, congenital nephrotic syndrome	Congenital nephrotic syndrome	?AR	149
132	Potter	Abnormal facies, pulmonary hypoplasia, limb positioning defects, renal agenesis; genital, cardiac, and skeletal anomalies	Bilateral agenesis	Multifactorial	2
133	—	Spontaneous pneumothorax and/or pneumomediastinum, urinary tract anomalies	Obstructive uropathy, polycystic	Sporadic	150
134	Kartagener	Bronchiectasis, sinusitis, situs viscerum inversus	(Mesangiocapillary glomerulonephritis)	AR	151
135	Familial congenital diaphragmatic hernia	Congenital diaphragmatic hernia, respiratory distress at birth	(Various anomalies)	Multifactorial	152
136	Pyloric stenosis	Hypertrophic pylorus	Polycystic kidneys, horseshoe, hypoplasia, duplex systems, hydronephrosis	Multifactorial	153

Table 25.6—*Continued*

No.	Syndrome	Main features	Urinary tract abnormality	Inheritance	Ref.
137	—	Intrahepatic cholestasis, renal disease	Tubulointerstitial nephropathy	?AR	154
138	Arteriohepatic dysplasia, Alagille	Unusual facies, vertebral anomalies, congenital heart disease, intrahepatic biliary atresia	Unilateral agenesis, proteinuria, tubular acidosis, renal insufficiency, mesangial foam cells	?AD	155, 156
139	Caroli	Segmental saccular dilatation of intrahepatic bile ducts, cholelithiasis, often hepatic fibrosis	Medullary sponge kidneys	Sporadic	157
140	Lutz-Richner	Intrahepatic and extrahepatic biliary hyperplasia, feet malformations, failure to thrive, predisposition to infections, muscle hypotonia	Tubular dysfunction, aminoaciduria	?AR	158
141	Hepatic fibrosis	Hepatic fibrosis	Cystic dysplastic kidneys		159
142	—	Hepatic fibrosis, coloboma, growth and mental retardation, cerebral palsy	Polycystic kidneys	?AR	160
143	Baber	Congenital liver cirrhosis	Aminoaciduria	?	161
144	Familial hepatic steatosis	Neonatal hepatic steatosis	Fatty changes of renal tubular epithelial cells	?AR	162
145	—	Small liver with hepatocellular damage, splenomegaly with hypersplenism, papulosquamous dermatitis, Ig deposition in the skin	Proteinuria, membranoproliferative glomerulonephritis	?AR	163
146	—	Hepatomegaly, hepatic dysplasia, pancreatic dysplasia, renal dysplasia	Renal dysplasia, renal failure	AR	164
147	Ivemark	Spleen agenesis or hypoplasia (or polysplenia), complex cyanotic heart diseases, trilobulated left lung, gut malrotation	Unilateral agenesis, hypoplasia, fused kidneys, dysplastic kidneys, cysts, enlarged cystic kidneys	Sporadic; AR	165, 166
148	—	Chronic diarrhea, villous atrophy of small intestine, chronic pancreatitis, elevated IgE and IgA levels, dermatitis	Tubulointerstitial nephritis	?AR	167
149	Familial intestinal pseudoobstruction	Intermittent episodes of abdominal pain or distention, megaduodenum, smooth muscle degeneration	Hydronephrosis, vesicoureteral reflux, megacystis	AD	168
150	MMIH	Megacystis, microcolon, dilated small bowel, malrotation, intestinal hypoperistalsis	Megacystis, hydronephrosis, hydroureter	Sporadic	169
151	Intestinal lymphangiectasia	Protein-losing enteropathy	Nephrotic syndrome	—	170
152	Hirschsprung	Congenital megacolon	Obstructive uropathy	Multifactorial	171
153	Regional enteritis, Crohn	Abdominal pain, diarrhea, weight loss, growth retardation	Nephrotic syndrome, nephrolithiasis, hydronephrosis, hydroureter, ileovesical fistulae	—	172
154	Ulcerative colitis	Bloody diarrhea, abdominal cramps, weight loss	Nephrolithiasis	—	173
155	—	Uterovaginal duplication, hematocolpos	Unilateral agenesis	Sporadic; AD	174
156	Kaufman-McKusick	Hydrometrocolpos, polydactyly, congenital heart disease	Polycystic kidneys, hydronephrosis, bladder neck obstruction	AR	175, 176
157	Mayer-Rokitansky	Absence of vagina, various uterine anomalies, primary amenorrhea, normal ovarian function and secondary sex characteristics	Unilateral agenesis, ectopy	Sporadic; ?AR	177
158	Drash	Pseudohermaphroditism, Wilms' tumor and nephron disorders in various combinations	Wilms' tumor, nephrotic syndrome, glomerulonephritis, ectopy, duplications, etc.	Sporadic	178

Other syndromes with visceral abnormalities: 17, 36, 38, 47–49, 55, 62, 72, 82, 83, 87, 92, 112, 120, 163, 166–168, 176, 186–188, 192, 194, 202, 203, 205, 206, 212, 232, 234, 238, 240, 242, 244, 259, 260, 262, 263, 264, 270, 277, 281, 282

Table 25.7
Neurological Abnormalities

No.	Syndrome	Main features	Urinary tract abnormality	Inheritance	Ref.
159	Meckel-Gruber	Occipital encephalocele, cleft lip/palate, polydactyly, cystic dysplastic kidneys	Cystic dysplastic kidneys	AR	2
160	Goldston	Dandy-Walker malformation, cerebellar malformations, dysplastic kidneys	Cystic dysplastic kidneys	?AR	179
161	—	Brain malformations, optic atrophy, mental retardation	Cystic dysplastic kidneys	?AR	180
162	Simopoulos	Internal hydrocephalus, polydactyly, dysplastic kidneys	Cystic dysplastic kidneys	AR	181
163	Miranda	Brain malformations, renal dysplasia, liver dysplasia	Cystic dysplastic kidneys	?AR	182
164	Crome	Brain malformations, epilepsy, cataracts, renal damage	Renal tubular necrosis	AR	183
165	Miller-Dieker, lissencephaly	Incomplete brain development, microcephaly, seizures, severe mental deficiency, abnormal facies	Unilateral agenesis, cystic dysplastic kidneys	?AR	184
166	—	Microencephaly with dysmyelination, spastic cerebral palsy, seizures, severe mental retardation, biliary duct hypoplasia	Hydroureter, hydronephrosis	AR	185
167	Cerebro-hepato-renal, Zellweger	Brain malformations, severe hypotonia, craniofacial dysmorphism, chondral calcifications, limb deformities, renal anomalies, possible metabolic defect	Polycystic kidneys	AR	186, 187
168	Cerebro-hepato-renal, Passarge	Hypotonia, abnormal ears, hepatomegaly, renal cysts	Cortical cysts, hypospadias	?AR	188
169	Mitochondrial cytopathy, ragged red fibres	Ataxia, seizures, retinitis pigmentosa, ophthalmoplegia, failure to thrive, abnormal mitochondria on muscle biopsy	Glomerulosclerosis, renal failure	AR	189
170	—	Photomyoclonus, ataxia, progressive nerve deafness, mild diabetes mellitus, nephropathy	Focal nephritis	AD	190
171	Familial dysautonomia, Riley-Day	Lack of tears, insensitivity to pain, unstable temperature	Glomerulosclerosis	AR	191
172	Charcot-Marie-Tooth	Progressive peripheral neuropathy	Progressive nephropathy with focal sclerosis	?AD	192
173	Myotonic dystrophy	Myotonic dystrophy	(Polycystic kidneys)	AD	193

Other syndromes with neurological abnormalities: 29, 46, 51, 54, 57, 76, 77, 82, 94, 98–102, 140, 142, 182, 192, 194, 196, 216, 217, 219, 233–235, 250, 252, 263, 265, 267, 268, 270, 275, 276

Table 25.8
Skin, Connective Tissue, and Muscle Diseases

No.	Syndrome	Main features	Urinary tract abnormality	Inheritance	Ref.
174	Epidermolysis bullosa dystrophica	Subepidermal blisters, ulceration of mucosae, flexion contractures of fingers, osteoporosis	Hydroureteronephrosis, renal amyloid	AD; AR	194, 195
175	Rapp-Hodgkin, hypohidrotic ectodermal dysplasia	Hypohidrosis, thin hair, nail dystrophy, cleft lip and palate, short stature	Hypospadias	AD	196
176	Multiple lentigines, LEOPARD	**L**entiginosis, **E**CG abnormalities, **o**cular hypertelorism, **p**ulmonary stenosis, **a**bnormalities of genitalia, **r**etardation of growth, **d**eafness	Hypospadias, ?unilateral agenesis	AD	197, 198
177	Bloom	Telangiectatic erythema of face, photosensitivity, short stature, immunoglobulin deficiency, tendency to develop lymphoreticular malignancies	Hypospadias	AR	199
178	Mammorenal	Lateral displacement of nipples, bilateral renal hypoplasia	Bilateral hypoplasia	Sporadic	200
179	Mammorenal	Unilateral or bilateral suprannumerary breasts, ipsilateral kidney duplication	Kidney duplication	Sporadic	201
180	(Netherton)	Congenital ichthyosis, "bamboo" hair, short stature, variable mental retardation	Selective or generalized aminoaciduria	AR	202, 203
181	—	Ichthyosiform erythroderma, atrophic skin, coarse hair, short stature, mental retardation, aminoaciduria	Generalized aminoaciduria	?AR	204
182	—	Congenital ichthyosis, dwarfism, hypogonadism, spasticity, mental retardation, renal disease	Chronic pyelonephritis, glomerulosclerosis	?AR	205
183	—	Congenital ichthyosis, dwarfism, mental retardation, renal disease	Renal insufficiency	?AR	206
184	—	Congenital ichthyosis, dwarfism, neurosensory deafness, prolinuria, renal disease	Renal cysts, chronic pyelonephritis	?AR	207
185	CHILD, **c**ongenital **h**emydysplasia with **i**chthyosiform erythroderma and **l**imb **d**efects	Unilateral ichthyosiform erythroderma, ipsilateral limb defects	Ipsilateral renal agenesis, hydronephrosis, hydroureter	?X-linked; ?AR	208
186	Marfan	Arachnodactyly, joint laxity, lens subluxation, aortic dilatation	Various anomalies including ectopy and duplex systems, pyelonephritis	AD	209, 210
187	Ehlers-Danlos, cutis hyperelastica	Joint hyperextensibility, abnormal stretchability of skin, fragility of blood vessels	Various anomalies including polycystic kidneys, medullary sponge kidneys, tubular acidosis, bladder diverticula	AD; AR; X-linked	211, 212
188	Cutis laxa, generalized elastolysis	Loose skin, growth retardation, pulmonary emphysema	Bladder diverticula	AD; AR; X-linked	213
189	Pseudoxanthoma elasticum	Xanthoma-like skin lesions, diminished vision, diminished peripheral pulses, hypertension	Renal artery stenosis	AR; AD	214
190	Goeminne	Congenital muscular torticollis, multiple keloids, cryptorchidism, renal disease	Renal dysplasia, renal failure	?X-linked	215
191	Prune belly, Eagle-Barrett, early urethral obstruction sequence	Dysplasia of abdominal muscle, cryptorchidism	Renal dysplasia, hypoplasia, hydronephrosis, bladder neck obstruction, etc.	Sporadic; multifactorial	2

Other syndromes with skin abnormalities: 17, 27, 28, 38, 53, 57, 60, 67, 68, 70, 74, 81, 86, 87, 89, 127, 145, 148, 189, 192, 193, 196–199, 203, 209, 235, 263, 272, 276

Table 25.9
Hamartoses

No.	Syndrome	Main features	Urinary tract abnormality	Inheritance	Ref.
192	Tuberous sclerosis, Bourneville-Pringle	Fibrous-angiomatous skin lesions, seizures, mental deficiency, cardiovascular abnormalities	Renal hamartoma, angiomyolipoma, cystic kidneys, renal failure	AD	7, 216
193	Neurofibromatosis, von Recklinghausen	Multiple neurofibromas, cutaneous pigmentation, skeletal anomalies	Renal artery stenosis, renal hypertension	AD	217
194	von Hippel-Lindau	Angiomatous lesions of retina, brain, cystic pancreas	Hypernephroma, cystic kidneys	AD	218, 219
195	Angio-osteohypertrophy, Klippel-Trénaunay	Hemangiomas, phlebectasia, asymmetric limb hypertrophy	Urinary tract hemangiomas, (nephroblastoma), nephromegaly	Sporadic	220, 221
196	Epidermal nevus	Midfacial nevus, seizures, mental deficiency	Renal hamartoma, nephroblastoma, renal artery stenosis	Sporadic	222
197	Blue rubber bleb nevus	Rubbery, bluish to black cutaneous nevi, mucosal hemangiomas	Hypernephroma	Sporadic; AD	223
198	Focal dermal hypoplasia, Goltz-Gorlin	Atrophy and linear pigmentation of skin, papillomas of skin and mucosae, dysplastic nails, anomalies of hands and vertebrae, osteopathia striata	Horseshoe kidney	?X-linked dominant	224, 225
199	—	Leukonychia totalis, sebaceous cysts, renal calculi	Renal calculi	AD	226
200	Perlman	Large birth size, unusual facies, kidney malignancies	Renal hamartoma, nephroblastomatosis	?AR	227
201	Hall-Pallister	Hypothalamic hamartoblastoma, hypopituitarism, imperforate anus, polydactyly	Unilateral and bilateral agenesis, dysplasia, horseshoe kidney, crossed ectopy	Sporadic	228
202	Peutz-Jeghers	Intestinal polyposis, mucocutaneous pigmentation	(Polycystic kidneys)	AD	229
203	Gardner	Colon polyposis, epidermal cysts, osteomas	(Hydronephrosis)	AD	230

Other syndromes with tendency to malignancies: 70, 177

Table 25.10
Hematologic Disorders

No.	Syndrome	Main features	Urinary tract abnormality	Inheritance	Ref.
204	Elliptocytosis	Mild anemia, if any	Tubular acidosis	AD	231
205	Spherocytosis	Anemia, intermittent jaundice, splenomegaly	Polycystic kidneys	AD	232
206	Sickle cell anemia	Anemia, jaundice, hepatosplenomegaly, painful limbs with radiologic skeletal changes	Hematuria, nephrotic syndrome, glomerular fibrosis, uremia, distal tubular acidosis, calyceal clubbing	AR	233, 234
207	Familial thrombocytopenia	Bleeding tendency	Hydronephrosis	AD	235
208	—	Thrombocytopenia and macrothrombocytopathia, sensorineural deafness, nephritis	Chronic glomerulonephritis	?AD	236
209	Wiskott-Aldrich	Congenital thrombocytopenia, bloody diarrhea, eczema, recurrent infections, elevated serum IgA	Hematuria, proteinuria, nephrotic syndrome, renal failure	X-linked	237
210	Chronic granulomatous disease	Neutrophil dysfunction, recurrent bacterial infections	Cystitis	X-linked	238
211	—	Lymphopenia, T-cell deficiency, recurrent infections, photophobia, short stature	Glycosuria, focal sclerosis	?AR	239
212	DiGeorge	Absence of thymus and parathyroid glands, immunodeficiency, congenital heart defect, characteristic facies	Hydronephrosis, malrotation	Sporadic	240
213	Hemophilia A and B	Factor VIII or factor IX deficiency, bleeding episodes	Filling defects, calculi, papillary necrosis, hydronephrosis	X-linked	241
214	Meltzer	Cryoglobulinemia, renal damage	Proteinuria, hematuria, renal insufficiency	AD	242

Other syndromes with hematologic abnormalities: 64, 70, 216, 237, 246, 256, 281

Table 25.11
Endocrino-metabolic Abnormalities

No.	Syndrome	Main features	Urinary tract abnormality	Inheritance	Ref.
215	—	Thyrotoxicosis, absent frontal sinuses, renal disease	Subacute proliferative glomerulonephritis	?AR	243
216	Thyrocerebrorenal	Goiter, cerebellar ataxia, seizures, sensorineural deafness, muscle wasting, thrombocytopenia	Tubulointerstitial nephritis	?AR	244
217	Neonatal hyperparathyroidism	Respiratory distress, hypotonia, seizures, polyuria, failure to thrive	Nephrocalcinosis	AD; AR	245
218	Hyperparathyroidism	Hypercalcemia and related symptoms, osteitis fibrosa	Nephrocalcinosis, urolithiasis, salt wastage, medullary sponge kidney	AD	246, 247
219	—	Hypoparathyroidism, congenital lymphedema, brachytelephalangy	Unspecified nephropathy	?AR; ?X-linked	248
220	—	Hypoparathyroidism, nephrotic syndrome, nerve deafness	Proteinuria, steroid-resistant nephrotic syndrome, renal failure	?AR	249
221	Adrenogenital, 21-OH-ase deficiency	Virilization, adrenal insufficiency	Unilateral agenesis, ureteropelvic junction obstruction, duplications	AR	250
222	—	Abnormal steroidogenesis, hyporeninemia, hypogenitalism, renal disease, deafness	Focal nephritis, renal failure	AR	251
223	—	Adrenal insufficiency, renal disease	Renal microangiopathy, renal failure	Sporadic	252
224	Cushing	Obesity, osteoporosis, growth retardation, hypertension, etc.	Urolithiasis, adysplasia	Sporadic	253, 254
225	Aldosteronism, Conn	Hyperaldosteronism, low renin secretion, systemic hypertension	Proteinuria, impairment of urinary concentration ability		255
226	Hypoaldosteronism	Hypoaldosteronism, hyporeninemia, hyperkalemia	Distal tubular acidosis		256
227	Psuedohypoaldosteronism	Salt wasting, failure to thrive	Focal glomerular sclerosis	Sporadic; AR	257
228	Olfactogenital dysplasia, Kallmann	Anosmia, hypogonadotropic hypogonadism	Unilateral agenesis	?X-linked	258
229	Wolcott-Rallison	Infancy onset diabetes mellitus, spondyloepiphyseal dysplasia	Renal insufficiency	?AR	259
230	DIDMOAD, Wolfram	Various combinations of **di**abetes **m**ellitus, **d**iabetes **i**nsipidus, **o**ptic **a**trophy, and sensorineural **d**eafness	Hydroureter, hydronephrosis, neurogenic bladder	AR	260
231	Pseudo-vitamin D-deficiency	Hypocalcemia, hypotonia, rickets, growth retardation	Mild tubular acidosis, aminoaciduria	AR	261
232	Infantile hypercalcemia, Williams-Beuren	Hypercalcemia in infancy, abnormal facies, mental retardation, supravalvular aortic stenosis	Segmental hypoplasia, renal artery stenosis	?AD; sporadic	262, 263
233	Congenital primary hypomagnesemia	Convulsions, tetany, hypomagnesemia with secondary hypocalcemia	Nephrocalcinosis	?X-linked; ?AR	264
234	Hepatolenticular degeneration, Wilson	Ceruloplasmin deficiency, loss of copper, severe neurologic abnormalities, liver cirrhosis, ocular changes	Nephrocalcinosis, tubular acidosis, aminoaciduria	AR	265
235	Trichopoliodystrophy, Menkes	Ceruloplasmin deficiency, copper malabsorption, peculiar hair, progressive neurological impairment	Bladder diverticula, hydronephrosis, hydroureter	X-linked	266
236	Congenital chloride diarrhea	Defective intestinal transport of chloride, diarrhea, salt-water wasting	Juxtaglomerular hyperplasia, nephrocalcinosis	AR	267
237	Juvenile pernicious anemia, Imerslund	Vitamin B_{12} malabsorption, megaloblastic anemia	Proteinuria	AR	268
238	Galactosemia	Cataracts, hepatosplenomegaly, failure to thrive, variable mental retardation	Proteinuria, aminoaciduria	AR	269
239	Sucrose intolerance	Diarrhea	Urolithiasis	AR	270
240	Fructosemia	Hypoglycemia, liver cirrhosis	Tubular acidosis, proteinuria, aminoaciduria	AR	271
241	Blue diaper	Intestinal transport defect of tryptophan, hypercalcemia	Nephrocalcinosis	?AR; ?X-linked	272
242	Hypermethioninemia	Hepatic cirrhosis, pancreatic cell hyperplasia	Enlarged kidneys, aminoaciduria	AR	273
243	Cystinuria	Increased risk for mental retardation	Cystine stones	AR	274

Table 25.11—*Continued*

No.	Syndrome	Main features	Urinary tract abnormality	Inheritance	Ref.
244	Hereditary tyrosinemia	Hepatosplenomegaly, rickets, failure-to-thrive	Proteinuria, tubular dysfunction	AR	275
245	Alkaptonuria	Pigmented urine, pigmentation of sclerae, chronic arthropathy	Nephrocalcinosis	AR	276
246	Cystathioninuria	Variable mental retardation, thrombocytopenia	Urolithiasis	AR	227
247	Glycinuria	Renal colic	Renal oxalate stones	AD	278
248	Hyperoxaluria	Renal colic	Hematuria, nephrocalcinosis, uremia	AR	279
249	Familial hyperuricemia	Hyperuricemia, gout	Hereditary nephropathy, renal failure	AD	280
250	—	Hyperuricemia, ataxia, deafness, nephropathy	Renal insufficiency	?AD; ?X-linked	281
251	Phosphoribosylpyrophosphate synthetase overactivity	Hyperuricemia, gout	Urolithiasis	?AR	282
252	HGPRT deficiency, Lesch-Nyhan	Hyperuricemia, cerebral palsy, self-mutilation, mental retardation	Nephrolithiasis	X-linked	283
253	APRT deficiency	Gout	Renal impairment	AD	284
254	Xanthine-oxidase deficiency	Hypouricemia, xanthinuria	Urolithiasis	AR	285
255	Hypouricemia	Hypouricemia, hyperabsorptive hypercalciuria	Urolithiasis	?AR	286
256	Lecithin:cholesterol acyltransferase deficiency, Norum	Normochromic anemia, corneal opacities	Proteinuria, renal failure	AR	287
257	—	Mild hyper-beta-lipoproteinemia, mental retardation	Low molecular weight proteinuria	?AR; ?X-linked	288
258	Hypophosphatasia	Low alkaline phosphatase, hypercalcemia, rickets	Nephrocalcinosis	AR	289
259	Alpha$_1$-antitrypsin deficiency	Hepatic cirrhosis, chronic emphysema	Mesangiocapillary glomerulonephritis	AR	290, 291
260	Glycogenosis I, von Gierke	Hypoglycemia, hepatomegaly, growth retardation	Nephromegaly, tubular dysfunction, renal failure	AR	292
261	Glycogenosis V, McArdle	Cramping muscle pain on exertion, myoglobinuria	Acute renal failure	AR	292
262	Angiokeratoma diffusum, Fabry	Skin angioma, recurrent abdominal and limb pain	Nephritis, renal failure	X-linked	293
263	Inherited amyloidoses	Neuropathy, recurrent fever, urticaria	Renal amyloidosis	AD	294, 295
264	Familial mediterranean fever	Recurrent fever, abdominal pain	Renal amyloidosis	AR	296

Other syndromes with endocrino-metabolic abnormalities: 41, 86–89, 103–105, 157, 167, 170, 184, 201, 212, 272, 275

Table 25.12
Multiple Congenital Anomalies and Miscellaneous Syndromes

No.	Syndrome	Main features	Urinary tract abnormality	Inheritance	Ref.
265	Smith-Lemli-Opitz	Abnormal facies, failure to thrive, hypotonia at birth followed by spasticity, mental retardation, cutaneous syndactylies	Hypospadias, focal renal dysplasia	AR	2, 297
266	(N)	Characteristic facies, abnormal auricles, visual impairment, deafness, mental retardation, cryptorchidism, skeletal abnormalities	Hypospadias	?AR; ?X-linked	298
267	FG	Characteristic facies, macrocephaly, mental retardation, imperforate anus, partial agenesis of corpus callosum	(Generalized dilatation of urinary tract with stone formation)	X-linked	299
268	(—)	Congenital glaucoma, malformed ears, heart malformations, agenesis of corpus callosum, hypo-areflexia, failure to thrive	Hypospadias	?AR	300
269	Bowen-Conradi	Microcephaly, prominent nose, micrognathia, joint deformities	Horseshoe kidney, duplex collecting system	AR	301
270	—	Dandy-Walker malformation, corneal opacities, cleft lip/palate, pulmonary hypoplasia, diaphragmatic hernia, digital hypoplasia	Cystic dysplasia	AR	302
271	Rüdiger	Coarse facial features, lack of ear cartilage, bifid uvula, brachydactyly	Vesicoureteral junction obstruction	?AR	303
272	Johanson-Blizzard	Aplastic alae nasi, midline scalp defects, sensorineural deafness, oligodontia, short stature, hypothyroidism, trypsinogen deficiency	Enlarged pelvis, caliectasis, hydronephrosis	AR	304
273	Freeman-Sheldon, cranio-carpo-tarsal dysplasia	Mask-like "whistling" face, ulnar deviation of the hands, talipes equinovarus	(Kidney hypoplasia with contralateral hydronephrosis)	AD	305
274	Ochoa	Peculiar facies and gestures while smiling and crying, urinary tract abnormalities	Hydronephrosis, hydroureter, urethral valves and other abnormalities	?AD	306
275	—	Microphthalmos, cataracts, persistent tachycardia, hypertension, seizures, hyperglycinuria	Urolithiasis	?	307
276	(—)	Hydrocephalus, peculiar facies, blue sclerae, thin skin, abnormal T-cell function, familial nephrosis	Steroid-resistant nephrotic syndrome, renal failure	?AR; ?X-linked	308
277	(—)	Microcephaly, hiatus hernia, nephrotic syndrome	Albuminuria, nephrotic syndrome, microcystic dysplasia with focal sclerosis	?AR	309
278	Alcohol embryopathy	Prenatal and postnatal growth retardation, microcephaly, short palpebral fissures, retrognathia, joint contractures, mental retardation	Unilateral agenesis, hypoplasia, hydronephrosis, duplex systems and other anomalies	—	310
279	Thalidomide embryopathy	Limb defects	Agenesis, cystic dysplasia, hydronephrosis	—	311
280	Fetal trimethadione	Small for date, microcephaly, malformed ears, irregular teeth, inguinal hernia	Hypospadias	—	312
281	Congenital rubella	Small for date, microcephaly, cataracts, cardiovascular defects, hepatosplenomegaly, thrombocytopenic purpura	(Polycystic kidneys, unilateral agenesis, glomerular sclerosis, nephrocalcinosis, duplications, hypospadias)	—	313
282	Diethylstilbestrol exposure in utero	Abnormalities and neoplasms of the genital tract	Hypospadias, urethral stenosis	—	314

References

1. McKusick VA: Mendelian Inheritance in Man, ed 6. Baltimore and London, Johns Hopkins Press, 1983.
2. Smith DW: Recognizable Patterns of Human Malformation, ed 3. Philadelphia, WB Saunders Co., 1982.
3. Stanbury JB, Wyngaarden JB, Fredrickson DS, et al: Metabolic Basis of Inherited Disease, ed 5. New York, McGraw-Hill Book Co., 1983.
4. De Grouchy J, Turleau C: Clinical Atlas of Human Chromosomes, ed 2. New York, John Wiley & Sons, 1984.
5. Francke U, Holmes LB, Atkins L, et al: Aniridia-Wilms Tumour Association; evidence for specific deletion of 11p13. Cytogenet Cell Gen 24:185, 1979.
6. Beattie JO, Day RE, Cockburn F, et al: Alcohol and the fetus in the west of Scotland. Brit Med J 287:17, 1983.
7. Michel JM, Diggle JH: Two half siblings with tuberous sclerosis, polycystic kidneys and hypertension. Develop Med Child Neurol 25:239, 1983.
8. Bohm N, Uy J, Kiesling M, et al: Multiple acyl-CoA dehydrogenation deficiency (glutaric aciduria type II), congenital polycystic kidneys, and symmetric warty dysplasia of the cerebral cortex in two newborn brothers. Europ J Paediatr 139:60, 1982.
9. Opitz JM: Terminological and epistemological considerations of human malformations. In Harris H, Hirschhorn K (eds): Advances in Human Genetics. London, Plenum Press, 1979.
10. Schimke RN, King CR: Hereditary urogenital dysplasia. Clin Genet 18:417, 1980.
11. Buchta RM, Viseskul C, Gilbert EF, et al: Familial bilateral renal agenesis and hereditary renal adysplasia. Z. Kinderheilk 115:111, 1973.
12. Carter CO, Evans K, Pescia G: A family study of renal agenesis. J Med Gen 16:176, 1979.
13. Bluett NH, Chantler C, Singer JD, et al: Congenital renal abnormalities in the Laurence-Moon-Biedl syndrome. Arch Dis Child 52:968, 1978.
14. Egli F, Stalder G: Malformations of kidney and urinary tract in common chromosomal aberrations. I. Clinical studies. Humangenetik 18:1, 1973.
15. Machin GA: Urinary tract malformation in the XYY male. Clin Genet 14:370, 1978.
16. Toussi T, Halal F, Lesage R, et al: Renal hypodysplasia and unilateral ovarian agenesis in the penta-X syndrome. Am J Med Genet 6:153, 1980.
17. Schulte JM, Lenz W, Vogel M: Lethale Achondrogenesis: eine Übersicht über 56 Fälle. Klin Pädiatr 191:327, 1978.
18. Harris R, Patton JT: Achondroplasia and thanatophoric dwarfism in the newborn. Clin Genet 2:61, 1971.
19. Cherstvoy ED, Lurie IW, Shved IA, et al: Difficulties in classification of the short rib-polydactyly syndromes. Europ J Pediatr 133:57, 1980.
20. Gilbert EF, Optiz JM, Spranger JW, et al: Chondrodysplasia punctata-rhizomelic form. Pathologic and radiologic studies of three infants. Europ J Pediatr 123:89, 1976.
21. Houston CS, Opitz JM, Spranger JW, et al: The campomelic syndrome. Am J Med Genet 15:3, 1983.
22. Castel Y, Benardeau M, Dantoine G, et al: Nanisme métatropique. Ann Pédiat 21:101, 1974.
23. Blackburn M, Belliveau RE: Ellis-van Creveld syndrome. Am J Dis Child 122:267, 1971.
24. Rosemberg S, Carneiro PC, Zerbini MCN, et al: Chondroectodermal dysplasia (Ellis-van Creveld) with anomalies of CNS and urinary tract. Am J Med Genet 15:291, 1983.
25. Herdman RC, Langer LO: The thoracic asphyxiant dystrophy and renal disease. Am J Dis Child 116:192, 1968.
26. Bernstein J, Brough AJ, McAdams AJ: The renal lesion in syndromes of multiple congenital malformations. Birth Defects 10/16: 35, 1973.
27. Gruhn JG, Gorlin RJ, Langer LO: Dyssegmental dwarfism—a lethal anisospondylic camptomicromelic dwarfism. Am J Dis Child 132:382, 1978.
28. Robinow M: A syndrome's progress. Am J Dis Child 126:150, 1973.
29. Langer LO Jr, Nishino R, Yamaguchi A, et al: Brachymesomelia-renal syndrome. Am J Med Genet 15:57, 1983.
30. Silverman FN: Larsen's syndrome: congenital dislocation of the knees and other joints, distinctive facies, and, frequently, cleft palate. Ann Radiol 15:297, 1972.
31. Galvan C, Domenech E, Méndez A: Síndrome de Larsen con malformaciones asociadas. Ann Esp Pediatr 12:631, 1979.
32. Fryns JP, Michielsen P, Vinken L, et al: The otopalatodigital syndrome. Acta Paediatr Belg 31:159, 1978.
33. Funderburk SJ, Smith L, Falk RE, et al: A family with concurrent mesomelic shortening and hereditary nephritis. Birth Defects 12/6: 47, 1976.
34. Aggett PJ, Cavanagh NPC, Matthew DJ, et al: Shwachman's syndrome. A review of 21 cases. Arch Dis Childh 55:331, 1980.
35. Marden PM, Walker WA: A new generalized connective tissue syndrome. Association with multiple congenital anomalies. Am J Dis Child 112:225, 1966.
36. Jaatoul NY, Haddad NE, Khoury LA, et al: Brief clinical report and review: the Marden-Walker syndrome. Am J Med Genet 11:259, 1982.
37. Giedion A, Burdea M, Fruchter Z, et al: Autosomal-dominant transmission of the tricho-rhino-phalangeal syndrome. Report of 4 unrelated families, review of 60 cases. Helv Paediatr Acta 28:249, 1973.
38. Murachi S, Nogami H, Oki T, et al: Familial tricho-rhino-phalangeal syndrome type II. Clin Genet 19:149, 1981.
39. Ohlsson A, Stark G, Sakati N: Marble brain disease: recessive osteopetrosis, renal tubular acidosis and cerebral calcification in three Saudi Arabian families. Develop Med Child Neurol 22:72, 1980.
40. von Oeyen P, Holmes LB, Trelstad RL, et al: Omphalocele and multiple severe congenital anomalies associated with osteodysplasty. Am J Med Genet 13:453, 1982.
41. Kanemura T, Orii T, Ohtani M: Frontometaphyseal dysplasia with congenital urinary tract malformations. Clin Genet 16:399, 1979.
42. Gorlin RJ, Winger RB: Frontometaphyseal dysplasia—evidence for X-linked inheritance. Am J Med Genet 5:81, 1980.
43. Anyane-Yeboa K, Gunning L, Bloom AD: Baller-Gerold syndrome: craniosynostosis-radial aplasia syndrome. Clin Genet 17:161, 1980.
44. Allain D, Babin JP, Demarquez JL, et al: Acrocéphalo-synankie, pseudohermaphrodisme féminin et néphropathie hypertensive. Ann Pédiatr 23:277, 1976.
45. Schinzel A, Savoldelli G, Briner J, et al: Antley-Bixler syndrome in sisters: a term newborn and a prenatally diagnosed fetus. Am J Med Genet 14:139, 1983.
46. Blank CE: Apert's syndrome (a type of acrocephalosyndactyly). Observations on a British series of 39 cases. Ann Hum Genet 24:151, 1960.
47. Bartsocas CS, Weber AL, Crawford JD: Acrocephalosydactyly type III: Chotzen's syndrome. J Pediatr 77:267, 1970.
48. Waardenburg PJ: Eine merkwürdige Kombination von angeborenen Missbildungen: doppelseitiger Hydrophthalmos verbunden mit Akrozephalosyndaktylie, Herzfehler, Pseudohermaphroditismus und anderen Abweichungen. Klin Mbl Augenheilk 92:29, 1934.
49. McLoughlin TG, Krovetz LJ, Schiebler GL: Heart disease in the Laurence-Moon-Bardet-Biedl syndrome: a review and report of three brothers. J Pediatr 65:388, 1964.
50. Temtamy SA: Carpenter Syndrome: Acrocephalopolysyndactyly. An autosomal recessive syndrome. J Pediatr 69:111, 1966.
51. Elejalde R, Giraldo C, Jiménez R, et al: Acrocephalopolydactylous dysplasia. Birth Defects 13/3B: 53, 1977.
52. Antley RM, Hwang DS, Theopold W, et al: Further delineation of the C (trigonocephaly) syndrome. Am J Med Genet 9:147, 1981.
53. Juberg RC, Hayward JR: A new familial syndrome of oral, cranial, and digital anomalies. J Pediatr 74:755, 1969.
54. Lazoff SG, Rybak JJ, Parker BR, et al: Skeletal dysplasia, occipital horns, intestinal malabsorption, and obstructive uropathy—a new hereditary syndrome. Birth Defects 11/5: 71, 1975.
55. Roizenblatt J, Wajntal A, Diament AJ: Median cleft face syndrome or frontonasal dysplasia: a case report with associated kidney malformation. J Pediatr Ophthalmol Strabismus 16:16, 1979.
56. Jarrett TE, Marsh EJ, Fridman J: Unilateral mandibulofacial dysostosis (Weyers syndrome) with hypospadias and ventricular septal defect: report of case. J Am Osteopath Assoc 75:389, 1975.
57. Gorlin RJ, Jue KL, Jacobsen U, et al: Oculoauriculovertebral dysplasia. J Pediatr 63:991, 1963.
58. Russell LJ, Weaver DD, Bull MJ: The axial mesodermal dysplasia spectrum. Pediatrics 67:176, 1981.
59. Moore WB, Matthews TJ, Rabinowitz R: Genitourinary anomalies associated with Klippel-Feil syndrome. J Bone Jt Surg 57A:355, 1975.
60. Elsahy NI, Waters WR: The branchio-skeletal-genital syndrome. A new hereditary syndrome. Plast Reconstr Surg 48:542, 1971.
61. Auchterlonie IA, White MP: Recurrence of the VATER association within a sibship. Clin Genet 21:122, 1982.
62. Bonaime JL, Bonne B, Joannard A, et al: Le syndrome de dysostose spondylo-thoracique ou spondylo-costale. Etude clinique, radiologique et génétique à propos de 7 observations. Pédiatrie 33:173, 1978.
63. Casamassima AC, Morton CC, Nance WE, et al: Spondylocostal dysostosis associated with anal and urogenital anomalies in a Mennonite sibship. Am J Med Genet 8:117, 1981.
64. Silverman FN, Strefling AM, Stevenson DK, et al: Cerebrocosto-mandibular syndrome. J Pediatr 97:406, 1980.
65. Bennett WM, Musgrave JE, Campbell RA, et al: The nephropathy of the nail-patella syndrome: clinicopathologic analysis of 11 kindreds. Am J Med 54:304, 1973.
66. Preus M, Fraser FC: The lobster claw defect with ectodermal defects, cleft lip-palate, tear duct anomaly and renal anomalies. Clin Genet 4:369, 1973.
67. Rosselli D, Gulienetti R: Ectodermal dysplasia. Brit J Plast Surg 14:190, 1961.
68. Johnson GF, Robinow M: Aglossia-adactylia. Radiology 128:127, 1978.

deposit. Like normal basement membrane, the dense material is impregnated by metallic silver with methenamine silver stain and hence in such preparations cannot be distinguished (Fig. 26B.6). Its great ability to take up metallic silver is evidence that it is not an immune deposit. In some cases, the material is in a continuous linear distribution and in others such as the example in Figure 26B.6, it is segmentally distributed and of variable width producing irregular enlargement of the basement membrane (14). Dense deposits are also seen focally on the external side of Bowman's capsule; on the antiluminal side of basement membranes of the proximal convoluted tubule and, occasionally, in the mesangial matrix (7, 13), and in a subendothelial position in peritubular capillaries (15, 16). Their presence in these nonfiltering structures is evidence that they are not derived from the circulation in the same manner as are the immune complexes making up glomerular deposits in other locations. In about one-fourth of the cases there are subepithelial deposits in the form of humps (13, 14) and occasionally small, scattered subendothelial deposits are encountered. A lesion thought to be a variant of Type II with scattered, discontinuous deposits within the basement membrane has been described (38), but is probably identical with MPGN Type III.

By light microscopy, the degree of mesangial proliferation is generally less in Type II than in Type I, but mesangial interposition and double contours may be present. Using PAS stain, the basement membrane in Type II appears ribbon-like and refractile. Metallic silver deposition in silver stained preparations shows a basement membrane that may be thickened and irregular and is various shades of brown in color rather than black. Type II can be quickly distinguished from the other types by use of the fluorescent dye, Thioflavin T (39). This dye also gives positive basement membrane staining in amyloidosis and certain other gammopathies.

In Type III, electron microscopy of uranyl lead stained preparations reveals a basement membrane that is grossly irregular and frequently contains deposits (8, 40). These deposits usually differ from the intramembranous material seen in Type II in that they are globular, discontinuous, and less electron dense (Fig. 26B.7). Occasionally, in some segments of basement membrane the deposits resemble those produced by advanced membranous nephropathy. The relationship of the deposits to the basement membrane is best appreciated in the ultrastructure of silver impregnated tissue fixed only in osmium (8). With this stain, the deposits are seen to be in both subepithelial and subendothelial locations and are associated with a disrupted lamina densa (Fig. 26B.8). The deposits are usually surrounded partially or completely by newly formed basement membrane. It is the disrupted appearance of the lamina densa and the luxuriant elaboration of new basement membrane that characterizes this lesion; the membrane has a frayed, and, in more advanced lesions, fenestrated appearance. Deposits are also present in the mesangium.

By light microscopy, a distinguishing feature of Type III is that capillary wall deposits, capillary wall thickening, and mesangial interposition are characteristically segmental in distribution. On the other hand, mesangial proliferation is diffuse and is usually slight to moderate, but in a minority of cases it is marked. When there is minimal proliferation associated with thickened capillary walls,the appearance by light microscopy is that of membranous nephropathy (Fig. 26B.9). On the other hand, the light microscopic appearance may closely resemble Type I MPGN when severe proliferation and double contours are present (8).

For reasons that are not understood, in occasional patients the mesangial proliferation is focal and segmental in distribution rather than diffuse. Focal lesions were seen in 10% of our patients (41) and in 4%

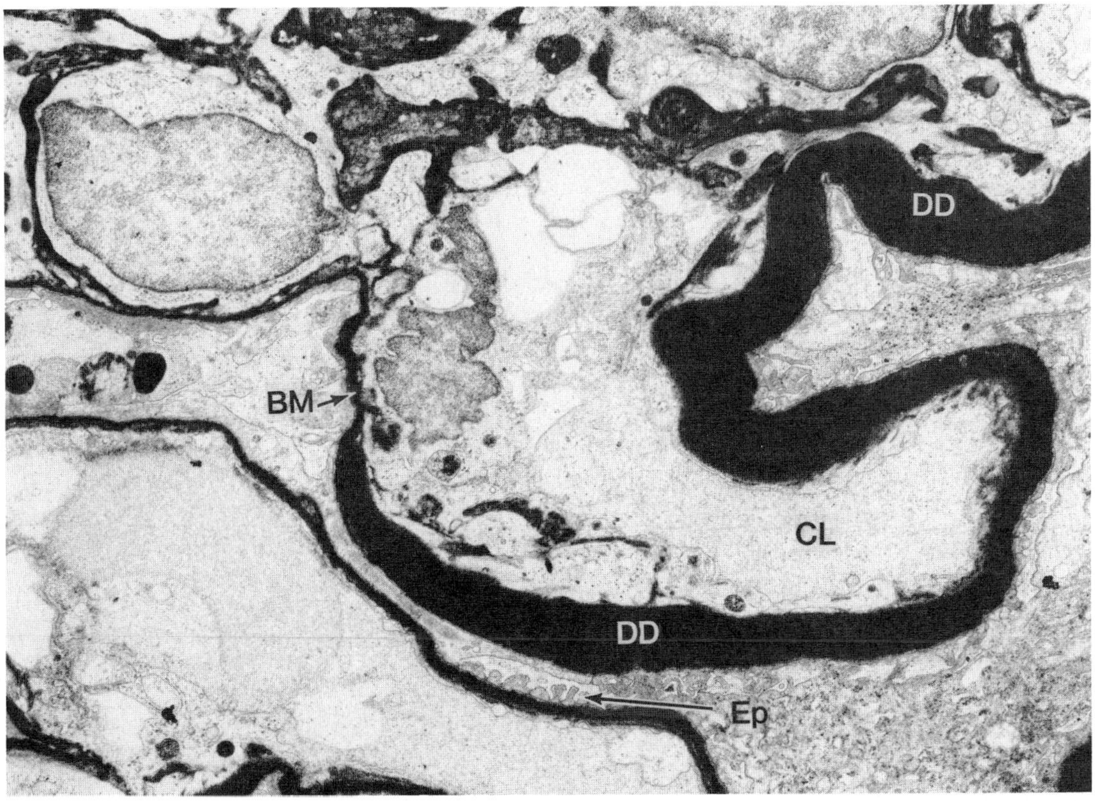

Figure 26B.6. MPGN Type II—electron micrograph of glomerular capillary stained by silver impregnation. This method of staining does not allow distinction between the bulky intramembranous material (*DD*) and the rest of the basement membrane. The portion of the membrane thickened by this material merges with normal basement membrane (*BM*). *Ep*, foot processes of epithelial cells. *CL*, capillary lumen (X6800).

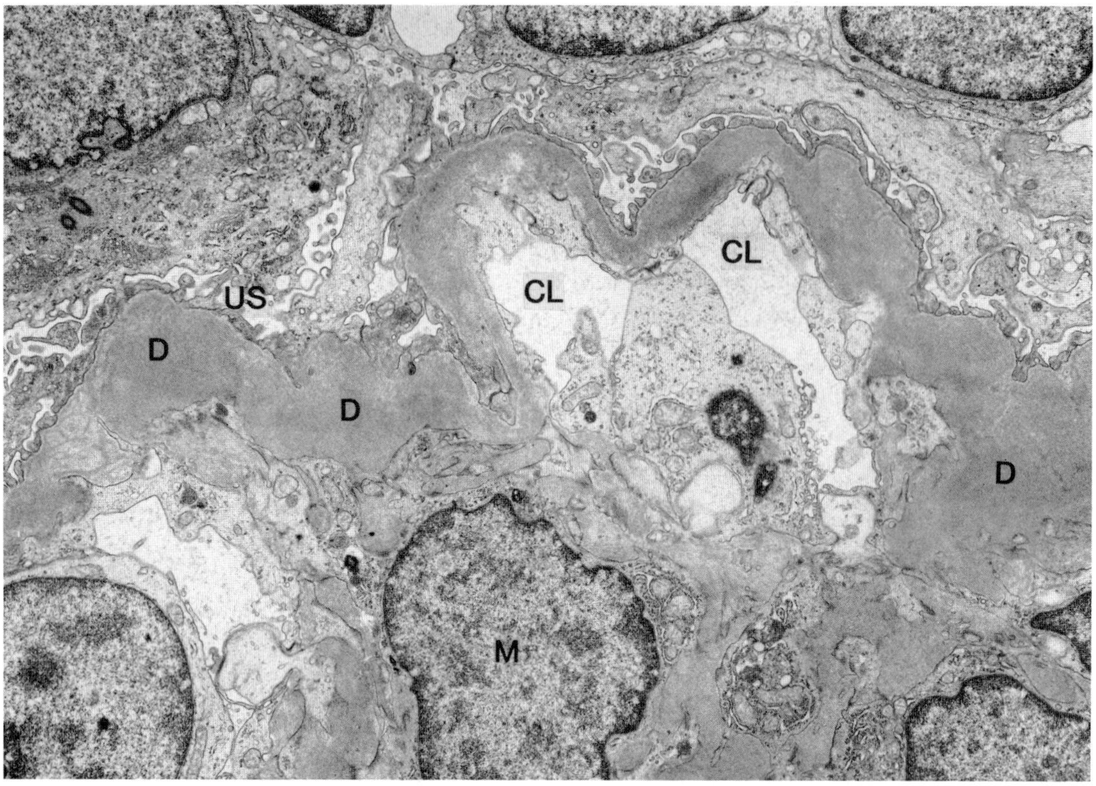

Figure 26B.7. MPGN Type III—electron micrograph of glomerular capillary stained with uranyl lead. Bulky deposits (*D*) are present in the basement membrane. This type of stain does not allow clear distinction of Type III from Type I. *CL,* capillary lumen; *M*, nucleus of mesangial cell; *US*, urinary space (X6400).

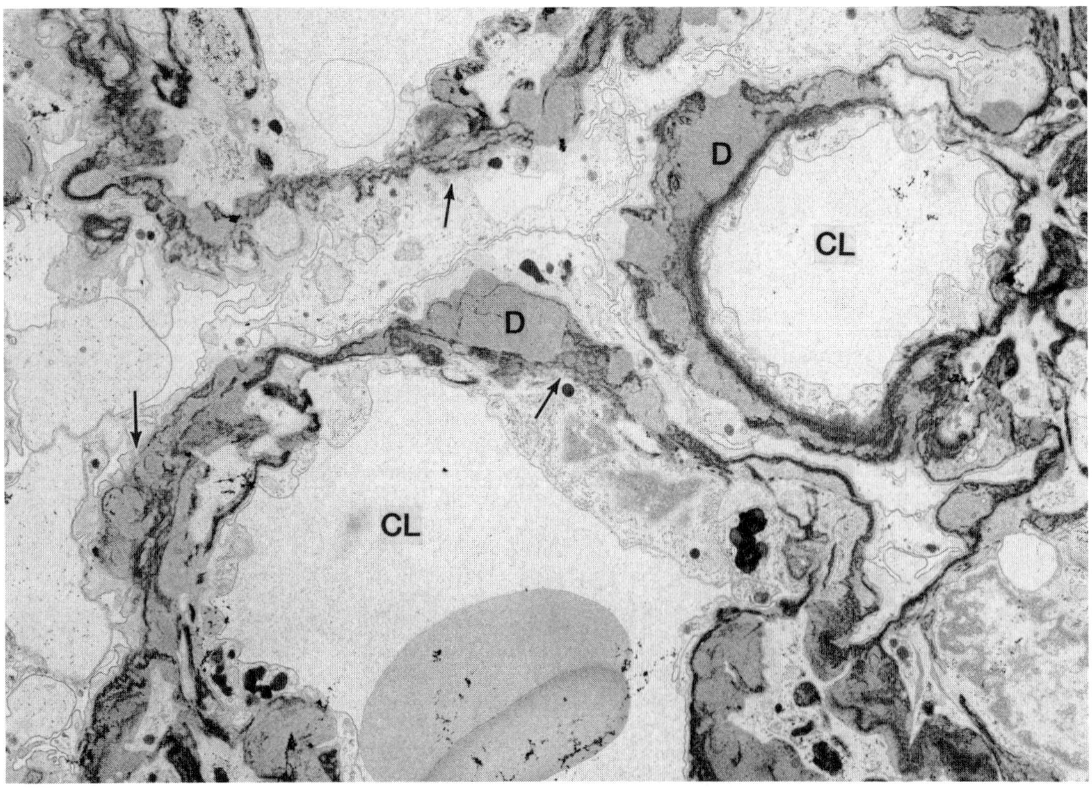

Figure 26B.8. MPGN Type III—electron micrograph of glomerular capillary stained by silver impregnation. The capillary wall deposits (*D*), stained gray by this method, are associated with newly elaborated lamina densa (*arrows*). As a result, the basement membrane appears duplicated, disrupted and frayed. *CL,* capillary lumen (X6000).

lulants (7, 10, 17). These early sporadic attempts at therapy did not, in the main, convincingly alter the course of the disease (7); untreated patients, if reported in the series, did as well as those treated. In fact, the use of high doses of prednisone several times daily for several weeks has resulted in morbidity by hemorrhage from gastric erosion and hypertensive encephalopathy (10).

In recent years, several groups have reported on the use of combinations of cytotoxic agents, corticosteroids, and anticoagulants. In addition, nonsteroidal antiinflammatory drugs, antiplatelet drugs, and prednisone alone in an alternate-day regimen or an alternate-day regimen preceded by high dose intravenous methylprednisolone have been used.

In 1972, Kincaid-Smith (52) reported that a regimen consisting of cyclophosphamide, dipyridamole, and anticoagulant given over periods of up to 4 years improved the survival of adults with MPGN whose renal function had already started to deteriorate. Two other groups have used a similar regimen in children. Robson and coworkers (53) reported success in the treatment of 4 children with a regimen similar to that of Kincaid-Smith except that azathioprine was substituted for cyclophosphamide. Chapman and coworkers (54) used the same regimen as Robson (53) but added prednisone. His group treated in this way 10 patients with diminished function for a year. There was improvement in 6, deterioration in 2, and 2 showed no change. After stopping treatment, 2 who had improved promptly deteriorated. Although only 50% improved, the authors felt that the overall result was better than that reported by others for untreated patients with disease of similar severity.

The results of two prospective randomized trials of the regimen used by Kincaid-Smith (52) have recently been reported. In one (55), nearly 40% of the treated patients dropped out because of cystitis, bone marrow depression, and bleeding complications, leaving too few to allow judgment of efficacy. In the other (56), with follow-up periods of about 2.5 years, there was no significant difference in protein excretion or creatinine clearance in the treated and control groups. The conclusion was that the triple therapy regimen was ineffective.

Indomethacin has been used alone but more successfully in combination with low doses of cyclophosphamide (57). In addition to the fall in proteinuria expected with indomethacin alone, there was also an increase in filtration rate in half of the patients. No controlled trials of this combination have been reported.

Donadio and coworkers (58) have prospectively studied the use of dipyridamole and aspirin in a double-masked prosepctive study. After 2 years, filtration rates were significantly higher in the treated than in the untreated patients without a change in protein excretion or hematuria. Platelet survival times, initially low, increased to normal in the treated group. Whether their success with this therapy is a result of a reduction in platelet activation in the glomerular capillaries is not known.

Methylprednisolone pulse therapy has also been used in MPGN. All of 8 patients so treated (59) had reduced glomerular filtration rates (average 31 ml/min/1.73M^2). Following the pulses, they were given prednisone in an alternate-day regimen for 3 to 44 months. All showed improvement in glomerular filtration rate, but function subsequently diminished in 50%. All did well who were treated within 6 months of diagnosis, whereas 3 of those who eventually deteriorated had been diagnosed 1 to 4 years before therapy was started.

Prednisone in a high dose alternate-day regimen has also been used as the only treatment in these patients. In a series of 27 patients treated by this means for periods of 2 to 15 years (24), actuarial survival was significantly better than for two series reported by others of untreated or sporadically treated patients who were very similar in their manifestations of disease at diagnosis to the treated group. Those with a poor outcome started treatment a number of years after diagnosis. In parallel with the improved survival, the morphology of functioning glomerular tissue also showed improvement in those with Types I or II. Improvement was less impressive in those with Type III, although the progression of their disease was, in most cases, halted. Subsequently, 2 more years of experience have been added to the above study and the number of patients has increased to 37. Survival remains significantly better than in the other series. The 37 have now been followed for a total of 310 patient years and three have developed end-stage disease. Uncontrollable hypertension and seizures, prominent in treated patients in the controlled trial of this therapy by the International Study of Kidney Disease in Children (60), have not been seen even though the dose of prednisone is higher than that in the trial. Growth retardation has been the main manifestation of toxicity; it has occurred when the dose of prednisone has to remain high because the patient responds slowly to the regimen or a return to high dosage is necessary because of a relapse. A number of patients who have developed a nephrotic syndrome or increased hematuria while on treatment have had these signs disappear when the alternate-day dose is increased.

In summary, judgment of the merits of the therapeutic regimen in a chronic disease with as variable a course as MPGN is difficult. From the above reports it would appear, however, that progression of the disease can be at least slowed by some therapies, but the experience is not great enough to define a regimen that is optimum. The reports do indicate, however, that if treatment is instituted early, the chance of success is enhanced, and they suggest that discontinuing or reducing the dose in a successful regimen may result in a relapse and hence the patient must be carefully followed and the regimen continued for long periods. The ease of administering the therapy and its complications, therefore, become important considerations.

The experience with renal transplantation in patients with MPGN is now large. Both Type I and Type II can recur in the graft, Type II frequently manifesting itself only by densification of the glomerular basement membrane (47). Whereas grafts have been lost because of recurrence, the frequency is not great enough to justify refusing transplantation with either cadaver or living donor kidney in the otherwise suitable recipient (61).

Membranoproliferative Glomerulonephritis Associated with Systemic Disease

MPGN, defined by glomerular morphology as mesangial proliferation, increase in mesangial matrix, and thickening and double contouring of the glomerular capillary walls, appears to be a well-defined response of the glomerulus and can be seen in a number of conditions. This morphology is said to be occasionally seen in patients with systemic lupus erythematosus, periarteritis nodosa, and Henoch-Schönlein glomerulonephritis (7). We have seen it in two patients with renal insufficiency as the result of chronic familial hemolytic uremic syndrome. The latter cases fulfilled all the morphological criteria, but there were no glomerular deposits of Ig or complement.

The most common form of MPGN associated with systemic disease is that which develops after infectious agent has been present in the circulation over a long period. In simple terms, this form results when antibodies, produced in response to the foreign antigen, combine with it and the resultant immune complexes deposit in the glomerular mesangium, producing mesangial proliferation and interposition. The most frequently cited examples are shunt nephritis with the infecting organism usually staphylococcus albus (45, 46), persistent viral hepatitis (37, 62), and visceral abscess, with or without documented bacteremia (63). Immune deposits are subendothelial and in the mesangium and hence the disease is like Type I MPGN. Hypocomplementemia with signs of activation of the classical pathway is often present (46). If elimination of the infecting agent is possible, the lesion heals but considerable scarring may result. It should be noted that not all the glomerulonephritides produced by such indolent infections have the morphology of membraneproliferative. The morphology may be that of membranous glomerulopathy (62), focal glomerulosclerosis (62), focal and segmental proliferative glomerulonephritis (63), or acute poststreptococcal glomerulonephritis (64).

References

1. West CD, McAdams AJ, McConville JM, et al: Hypocomplementemic and normocomplementemic persistent (chronic) glomerulonephritis; clinical and pathologic characteristics. J Pediatr 67:1089, 1965.
2. Gotoff SP, Fellers FX, Vawter GF, et al: The β1C globulin in childhood nephrotic syndrome. Laboratory diagnosis of progressive glomerulonephritis. N Engl J Med 273:524, 1965.
3. Ogg CS, Cameron JS, White RHR: The C3 component of complement in patients with heavy proteinuria. Lancet 2:78, 1968.
4. Churg J, Habib R, White RHR: Pathology of the nephrotic syndrome in children. A report for the International Study of Kidney Disease in Children. Lancet 1:1299, 1970.
5. Mandelenakis N, Mendoza N, Pirani CL et al: Lobular glomerulonephritis and membranoproliferative glomerulonephritis: a clinical and pathologic study based on renal biopsies. Medicine 50:319, 1971.
6. Berger J, Galle P: Depots denses du sein des basales du rein. Presse Med 71:2351, 1963.
7. Habib R, Kleinknecht C, Gubler MC, et al: Idiopathic membranoproliferative glomerulonephritis in children. Report of 105 cases. Clin Nephrol 1:194, 1973.
8. Strife CF, McEnery PT, McAdams AJ, et al: Membranoproliferative glomerulonephritis with disruption of the glomerular basement membrane. Clin Nephrol 7:65, 1977.
9. Habib R: Classification of glomerulonephritis based on morphology In Kincaid-Smith P, Mathew TH, Becker EL (eds): Glomerulonephritis: Morphology, Natural History, and Treatment. New York, John Wiley & Sons. 1973, p 17.
10. Cameron JS, Glasgow EF, Ogg CS, et al: Membranoproliferative glomerulonephritis and persistent hypocomplementemia. Brit Med J 4:7, 1970.
11. Report of International Study of Kidney Disease in Children: Nephrotic syndrome in children: prediction of histopathology from clinical and laboratory characteristics at time of diagnosis. Kidney Intl 13:159, 1978.
12. Vargas A, Thomson, KJ, Wilson D, et al: Mesangiocapillary glomerulonephritis with dense "deposits" in the basement membranes of the kidney. Clin Nephrol 5: 73, 1976.
13. Davis AE, Schneeberger EE, Grupe WE, et al: Membranoproliferative glomerulonephritis (MPGN Type I) and dense deposit disease (DDD) in children. Clin Nephrol 9:184, 1978.
14. Habib R, Gubler M-C, Loirat C, et al: Dense deposit disease: A variant of membranoproliferative glomerulonephritis. Kidney Intl 7:204, 1975.
15. Bohle A, Gartner HV, Fischback H, et al: The morphological and clinical features of membranoproliferative glomerulonephritis in adults. Virchows Arch [Pathol Anat] Histol 363:213, 1974.
16. Donadio JV Jr, Slack TK, Holley KE, et al: Idiopathic membranoproliferative (mesangiocapillary) glomerulonephritis: A clinicopathologic study. Mayo Clin Proc 54:141, 1979.
17. Herdman RC, Pickering RJ, Michael AF, et al: Chronic glomerulonephritis associated with low serum complement activity (chronic hypocomplementemic glomerulonephritis). Medicine (Baltimore) 49:207, 1970.
18. Okuda R, Watanabe Y, Tamamoto Y, et al: The origin of membranoproliferative glomerulonephritis: evidence against an origin from acute post-streptococcal nephritis. Am J Dis Child 119:291, 1970.
19. Northway JD, McAdams AJ, Forristal J, et al: A "silent" phase of hypocomplementemic persistent nephritis detectable by reduced serum β1C globulin levels. J Pediatr 74:28, 1969.
20. Cameron JS, Ogg CS, White RHR, et al: The clinical features and prognosis of patients with normocomplementemic mesangiocapillary glomerulonephritis. Clin Nephrol 1:8, 1973.
21. Sissons JGP, West RJ, Fallows J, et al: The complement abnormalities of lipodystrophy. N Engl J Med 294:461, 1976.
22. Senior B, Gellis SS: The syndromes of total lipodystrophy and partial lipodystrophy. Pediatrics 33:593, 1964.
23. Cameron JS, Ogg CS, Turner DR, et al: Mesangiocapillary glomerulonephritis and persistent hypocomplementemia. In Kincaid-Smith P, et al (eds): Glomerulonephritis: Morphology, Natural History and Treatment. New York, John Wiley & Sons, 1973, p 541.
24. McEnery PT, McAdams AJ, West CD: Membranoproliferative glomerulonephritis: Improved survival with alternate day prednisone therapy. Clin Nephrol 13:117, 1980.
25. Antoine B, Faye C: The clinical course associated with dense deposits in the kidney basement membranes. Kidney Intl 1:420, 1972.
26. Levy M, Gubler M-C, Sich M, et al: Immunopathology of membranoproliferative glomerulonephritis with subendothelial deposits (Type I MPGN). Clin Immunol Immunopathol 10:477, 1978.
27. Wyatt RJ, McAdams AJ, Forristal J, et al: Glomerular deposition of complement control proteins in acute and chronic glomerulonephritis. Kidney Intl 16:505, 1979.
28. Ooi YM, Vallota EH, West CD: Classical complement pathway activation in membranoproliferative glomerulonephritis. Kidney Intl 9:46, 1976.
29. Davis, CA, Marder H, West CD: Circulating immune complexes in membranoproliferative glomerulonephritis. Kidney Intl 20:728, 1981.
30. Border WA: Immune complex detection in glomerular disease. Nephron 24:105, 1979.
31. Daha MR, Fearon DT, Austen KF: C3 nephritic factor (C3NeF): stabilization of fluid phase and cell-bound alternative pathway convertase. J Immunol 116:1, 1976.
32. Weiler JM, Daha MR, Austen KF, et al: Control of the amplification convertase of complement by the plasma protein, β1H. Proc Natl Acad Sci USA 73:3268, 1976.
33. Daha MR, Austen KF, Fearon, DT: The incorporation of C3 nephritic factor (C3NeF) into a stabilized C3 convertase, C3bBb (C3NeF), and its release after decay of convertase function. J Immunol 119:812, 1977.
34. Charlesworth JA, Williams DG, Sheringtin, E, et al: Metabolic studies of the third component of complement and the glycine-rich beta glycoprotein in patients with hypocomplementemia. J Clin Invest 53:1578, 1974.
35. Hunsicker LG, Ruddy S, Carpenter CB, et al: Metabolism of the third complement (C3) in nephritis. N Engl J Med 287:835, 1972.
36. Perrin LH, Lambert PH, Miescher PA: Complement breakdown products in plasma from patients with systemic lupus erythematosus and patients with membranoproliferative or other glomerulonephritis. J Clin Invest 56:165, 1975.
37. McAdams AJ, McEnery PT, West CD: Mesangiocapillary glomerulonephritis: Changes in glomerular morphology with long-term alternate day prednisone therapy. J Pediatr 86:23, 1975.
38. Davis AE, Schneeberger EE, McCluskey RT, et al: Mesangial proliferative glomerulonephritis with irregular intramembranous deposits; another variant of hypocomplementemic nephritis. Am J Med 63:481, 1977.
39. Churg J, Duffy JL, Bernstein J: Identification of dense deposit disease. A report for the International Study of Kidney Diseases in Children. Arch Pathol Lab Med 103:67, 1979.
40. Anders D, Thoenes W: Basement membrane changes in membranoproliferative glomerulonephritis. A light and electron microscopic study. Virchows Arch [Pathol Anat] 369:87, 1975.
41. Strife CF, McAdams AJ, West CD: Membranoproliferative glomerulonephritis characterized by focal, segmental proliferative lesions. Clin Nephrol 18:9, 1982.
42. Abreo K, Moorthy AV: Type III membranoproliferative glomerulonephritis. Arch Pathol Lab Med 106:413, 1982.
43. Berry PL, McEnery PT, McAdams AJ, et al: Membranoproliferative glomerulonephritis in two sibships. Clin Nephrol 16:101, 1981.
44. Myers BD, Griffel B, Naveh D, et al: Membranoproliferative glomerulonephritis associated with persistent viral hepatitis. Am J Clin Pathol 59:222, 1973.
45. Michael AF, Herdman RC, Fish AJ, et al: Chronic membranoproliferative glomerulonephritis with hypocomplementemia. Transplant Proc 1:925, 1969.
46. Strife CF, McDonald BM, Ruley EJ, et al: Shunt nephritis: The nature of the serum cryoglobulins and their relation to the complement profile. J Pediatr 88:403, 1976.
47. Droz D, Nabarra B, Noel C-H, et al: Recurrence of dense deposits in transplanted kidneys. Kidney Intl 15:386, 1979.
48. Peters DK, Williams DG: Complement and mesangiocapillary glomerulonephritis role of complement deficiency in the pathogenesis of nephritis. Editorial. Nephron 13:187, 1974.
49. Nussenzweig V: Interaction between complement and immune complexes. Role of complement in containing immune complex damage. Prog Immunol 4:1044, 1980.
50. Vallota EH, Forristal J, Davis NC, et al: The C3 nephritic factor and membranoproliferative nephritis: correlation of serum levels of the nephritic factor with C3 levels, with therapy and with progression of the disease. J Pediatr 80:947, 1972.
51. Loirat C, Levy M, Peltier AP, et al: Deficiency of the second component of complement; its occurrence with membranoproliferative glomerulonephritis. Arch Pathol Lab Med 104:467, 1980.
52. Kincaid-Smith P: The treatment of chronic mesangiocapillary (membranoproliferative) glomerulonephritis with impaired renal function. Med J Aust II:587, 1972.
53. Robson AM, Cole BR, Kienstra RA, et al: Severe glomerulonephritis complicated by coagulopathy: treatment with anticoagulant and immunosuppressive drugs. J Pediatr 90:881, 1977.

54. Chapman SJ, Cameron JS, Chantler C, et al: Treatment of mesangiocapillary glomerulonephritis in children with combined immunosuppression and anticoagulation. Arch Dis Childh 55:446, 1980.
55. Tiller DJ, Clarkson AR, Mathew T, et al: A prospective randomized trial in the use of cyclophosphamide, dipyridamole and warfarin in membranous and mesangiocapillary glomerulonephritis. In Zurukzoglu W (eds): Proceedings of Eighth International Congress of Nephrology: Advances in Basic and Clinical Nephrology. Basel, S. Karger, 1981, p 345.
56. Cattran D, Charron R, Cardella C, et al: Controlled trial on mesangiocapillary glomerulonephritis (MCGN). In Eighth International Congress of Nephrology (abstracts). 1981, p 287.
57. Vanrenterghen Y, Roels L, Verberckmoes R, et al: Treatment of chronic glomerulonephritis with a combination of indomethacin and cyclophosphamide. Clin Nephrol 4:218–222, 1975.
58. Donadio JV Jr, Anderson CF, Mitchell JC, et al: Membranoproliferative glomerulonephritis (MPGN): A prospective clinical trial of platelet inhibitor therapy (abstract). Kidney Intl 23:121, 1983.
59. Rose GN, Cole BR, Robson AM: The treatment of severe glomerulonephritis in children using high dose intravenous methylprednisolone pulses. Am J Kid Dis 1:148, 1981.
60. A report of the International Study of Kidney Disease in Children: Alternate day steroid therapy in membranoproliferative glomerulonephritis: A randomized controlled clinical trial (abstract). Kidney Intl 21:150, 1982.
61. Curtis JJ, Wyatt RJ, Bhathena D, et al: Renal transplantation for patients with Type I and Type II membranoproliferative glomerulonephritis. Am J Med 66:216, 1979.
62. Knieser MR, Jenis EH, Lowenthal DT, et al: Pathogenesis of renal disease associated with viral hepatitis. Arch Pathol 97:193, 1974.
63. Beaufils M, Morel-Maroger L, Sraer J-D, et al: Acute renal failure of glomerular origin during visceral abscesses. N Engl J Med 295:185, 1976.
64. Stickler GB, Shin MH, Burke EH, et al: Diffuse glomerulonephritis associated with infected ventriculo atrial shunt. N Engl J Med 279:1077, 1968.

26C Crescentic Glomerulonephritis

GLENN H. BOCK
EDWARD J. RULEY

INTRODUCTION

Crescentic glomerulonephritis (CGN) is a histopathological entity characterized by intraglomerular extracapillary cellular proliferation. It may occur in both children and adults in response to inflammatory injuries to the glomerular capillary wall either de novo or as a manifestation of a number of distinct glomerulopathies.

The clinical syndrome of rapidly progressive glomerulonephritis, (RPGN) in which there is sudden, progressive decline in renal function with oliguria or anuria, is often associated with glomerular crescents on biopsy (1, 2). However, while glomerular crescents are frequently seen in RPGN, they are not exclusively associated with this syndrome (3). Thus there exists some confusion in both clinical practice and the literature with regard to the clinical syndromes associated with CGN. This variable clinical expression, the relatively uncommon occurrence, and the lack of controlled clinical treatment trials make prognostic and therapeutic decisions difficult. The clinical manifestations of disease processes associated with CGN, as well as current data regarding pathogenesis and treatment, are presented.

Clinical Presentation

While CGN is primarily a disease of adults, having a peak incidence in the fourth and fifth decades, it has been described in children in the first and second decades with clinical symptoms similar to those of the adult population. The clinical manifestations of CGN may mimic any acute glomerulonephritis at the time of presentation (3–5). In addition, CGN may be a histological finding associated with a number of well-described primary nephrologic and systemic diseases (6) (Table 26C.1). The percentage of glomeruli occupied by crescents statistically relates to the severity of the presenting clinical and biochemical abnormalities, although there may be great variability in individual cases.

Perhaps the best known clinical syndrome associated with CGN is RPGN, in which an acute nephritic syndrome is associated with rapidly progressing azotemia (7). In the child, RPGN often follows an acute infectious illness (Table 26C.1). While several studies have noted the association of hydrocarbon exposure and idiopathic RPGN in adults, no such reports exist for children (3). The presenting signs and symptoms of RPGN often relate to the underlying disease (i.e., poststreptococcal glomerulonephritis, anaphylactoid purpura, systemic lupus erythematosus, and so on). The largest group of pediatric patients with CGN develop their disease after a streptococcal infection (7). Many individuals first seek medical attention for the symptoms of their acute nephritis, particularly edema or gross hematuria. Hypertension on initial evaluation is more common in children than adults. The majority of patients will be anemic out of proportion to the duration or degree of their azotemia and most are oliguric.

Although the degree of clinical symptomatology does not help in predicting outcome, it is generally agreed that patients having crescents in greater than 50% to 75% of their glomeruli have a high rate of morbidity and mortality and a low expectation for the recovery of normal renal function.

Table 26C.1.
Differential Diagnoses of Glomerulonephritis in which Crescents have been Reported

Primary renal
Membranoproliferative glomerulonephritis
Types I and II
Membranous nephropathy
IgA-IgG (Berger's) nephropathy
Alport's Syndrome
Idiopathic
Type I (anti GBM antibody without pulmonary disease)
Type II (with immune complexes)
Type III (no immune complexes)
Associated with infection
Poststreptococcal glomerulonephritis
Bacterial endocarditis
Hepatitis
Other infections
Associated with systemic disorder
Systemic lupus erythematosis
Henoch-Schönlein purpura
Wegener's granulomatosis
Polyarteritis nodosa
Neoplasm (lymphoma, carcinoma)
Mixed essential cryoglobulinemia
Relapsing pancreatitis
Goodpasture's syndrome
Hydrocarbon exposure
Sarcoidosis

Pathology

The sine qua non of CGN is the glomerular crescent, a proliferative lesion appearing to arise from Bowman's capsule, which occupies the urinary space (Fig. 26C.1). The percentage of glomeruli containing crescents and the size of the crescents vary. Occasionally they are sufficiently large to compress and collapse the glomerulus. The minimum percentage of glomeruli containing crescents to fulfill the diagnosis of CGN has not been defined, although it has been proposed that the term should be reserved for individuals who have the majority of glomeruli involved and thus are at high risk for renal failure (8). The appearance of the crescent itself on light, immunofluorescent, and electron microscopy is the same regardless of etiology (9). The majority of cells that make up the crescent appear epitheloid histologically, although monocytes and granulocytes can be seen. By immunofluorescent and electron microscopy study there is fibrin deposition within and around the cells of the crescent. Older crescents appear less cellular and more fibrous (Fig. 26C.2).

The histology of the glomerular capillary loops in CGN varies. Even when compressed by the crescent, the glomerular capillary basement membrane may be preserved with insignificant intrinsic cellular proliferation, particularly in idiopathic CGN. In contrast, CGN associated with infectious or systemic diseases is commonly associated with profuse mesangial or capillary endothelial cell proliferation. Proliferation in CGN associated with poststreptococcal glomerulonephritis usually involves both mesangial and endothelial cells giving rise to a diffuse lobulation affecting all glomeruli equally. In contrast, the proliferative lesion occasionally seen in idiopathic CGN is more focal and segmental in distribution with varying stages and degrees of crescent development. All forms of CGN may be associated with necrotizing glomerular lesions. Occasionally, multinucleated giant cells are present within the glomerular tuft, and fibrin may be detected in the capillary loops in the areas of segmental necrosis.

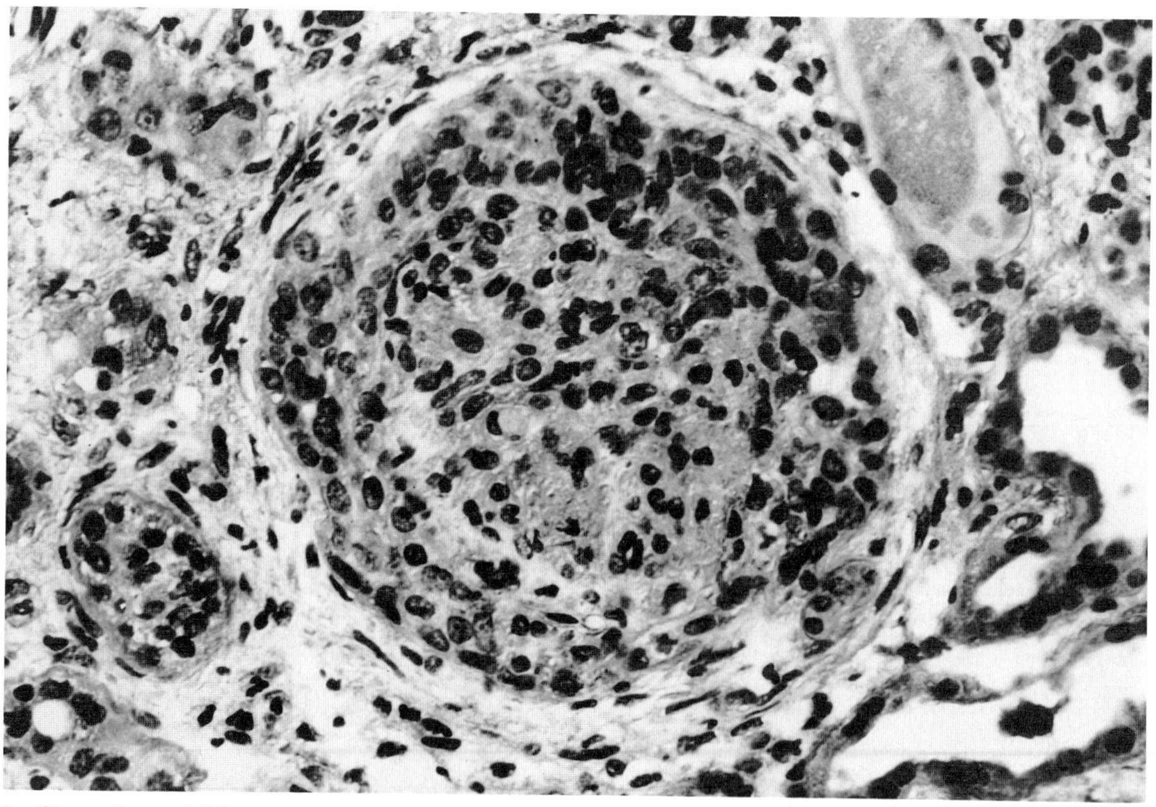

Figure 26C.1. Glomerulus containing an early proliferative crescent filling Bowman's space and compressing the glomerulus centrally. (PAS stain, X525.)

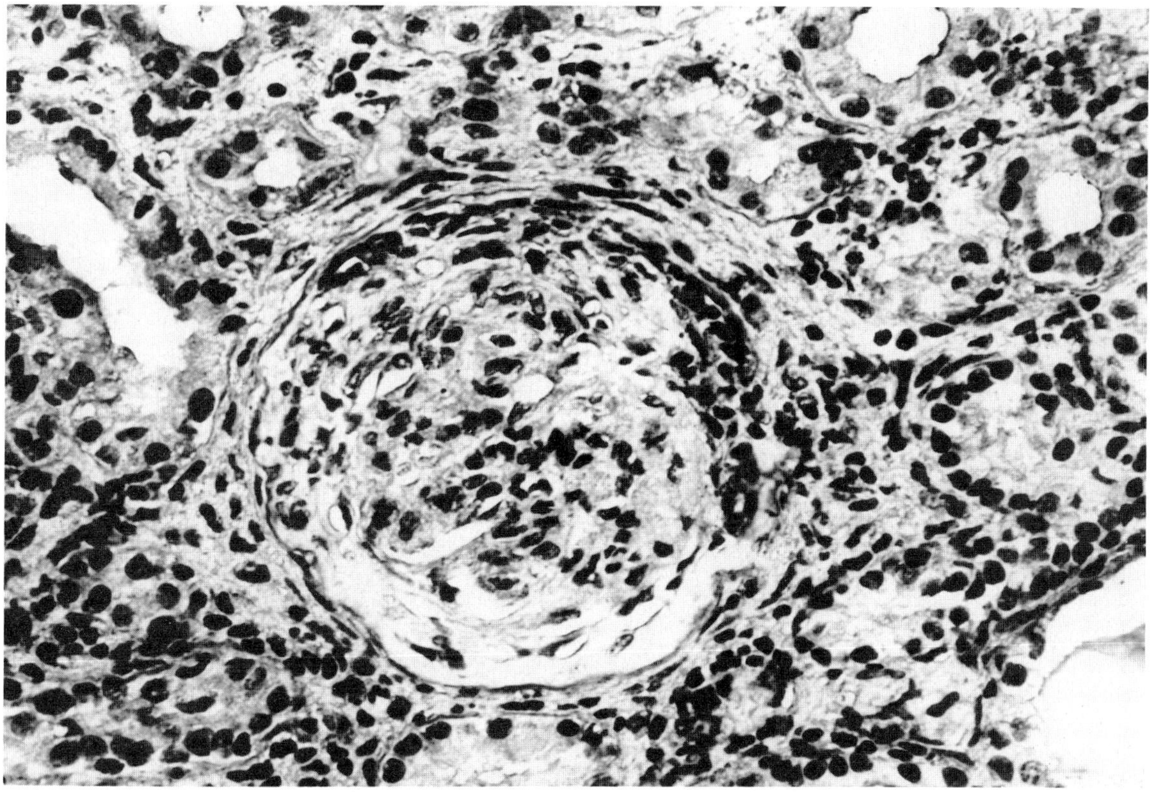

Figure 26C.2. Glomerulus with an aging fibroepithelial crescent occupying the upper half of Bowman's space. (PAS stain, X525.)

Three immunopathologic varieties of CGN (9) have been described based on the immunofluorescent findings in the glomeruli. In Type I CGN there is a uniform linear deposition of IgG along the glomerular capillary basement membrane (GBM). The deposited IgG consists of antibody directed against basement membrane antigens (10–12). Other immunoglobulins and C3 may also be present in a linear or granular pattern (9, 12). Focal linear IgG may be detected on Bowman's capsule or the tubular basement membranes in some patients. The term Goodpasture's syndrome is reserved for patients who have CGN associated with an anti-GBM antibody that also reacts with alveolar basement membrane producing pulmonary disease. The majority of individuals with Type I CGN will have anti-GBM antibody in their serum, although it may not be detectable until after nephrectomy (11, 13, 14). By electron microscopy (EM), there may be widening of the lamina rara externa, detachment of endothelial cells, and focal disruptive lesions in the GBM. Wrinkling and collapse of the capillary basement membranes may be seen in all forms of CGN, but is most prominent in patients with Type I. An important EM characteristic of Type I CGN is the absence of electron dense deposits.

Type II CGN is characterized by the finding of discrete granular deposits of IgG or C3 along the peripheral capillary loops and within the mesangium presumably a result of deposition of antigen-antibody complexes (Fig. 26C.3). IgM may be seen in the granular pattern in some patients. Ultrastructurally, electron dense deposits may be seen in a subendothelial or subepithelial distribution along the basement membrane or in the mesangium.

In Type III CGN there is sparse or absent immunoglobulin and complement deposition within the glomerulus. When present, it is usually in a globular pattern (15). Ultrastructurally, occasional patients will have subendothelial dense deposits usually associated with capillary thrombosis in isolated glomerular capillaries. These glomerular lesions are virtually indistinguishable from the microscopic form of polyarteritis

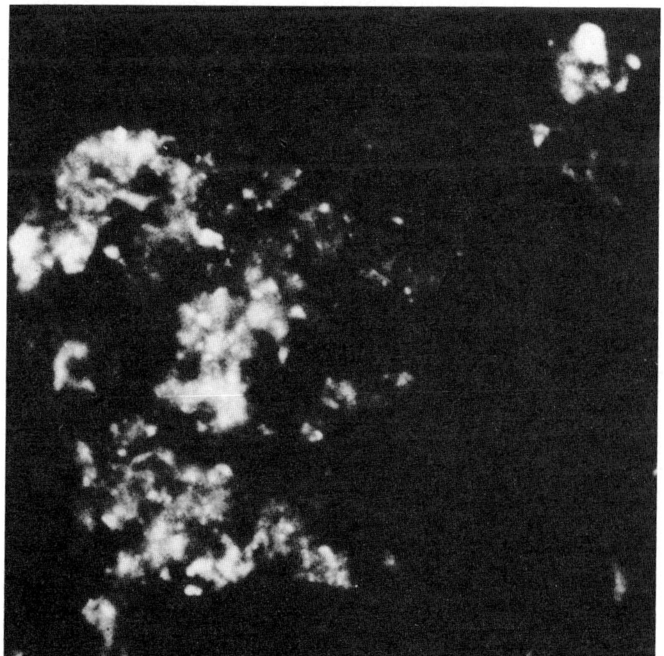

Figure 26C.3. Immunofluorescence microscopy. IgG in a coarse granular pattern with mesangial distribution in CGN (X525.)

(16). Therefore, some investigators question the existence of this form as a separate entity (17).

Interstitial involvement with edema or fibrosis tends to vary with the severity of crescent formation. It may range from normal to widespread mononuclear cell infiltration. Healing of crescents may be associated with interstitial fibrosis and scarring, particularly in the periglomerular area.

Although crescents have been noted to completely resolve, some crescentic lesions progress to complete destruction of glomerular architecture, making it difficult to recognize any of the original glomerular structures.

Pathogenesis

The following proposed mechanisms of crescent formation are based on histological, histochemical, and immunochemical observations of CGN in animals and man. Even so, the pathogenesis of CGN remains incompletely understood.

The subcategorization of CGN by immunofluorescent findings suggest at least three different specific immunopathologic insults that can produce glomerular crescents. In Type I CGN (including Goodpasture's syndrome) circulating antibodies react with native antigen(s) in the basement membrane, and subsequently initiate a severe inflammatory reaction. The specificity and pathogenicity of these antibodies have been previously demonstrated (11, 18, 19). In type II CGN, similar glomerular inflammation results from deposition of immune complexes as in post-streptococcal glomerulonephritis, the nephritis of systemic lupus erythematosus, or the nephritis of Henoch-Schönlein purpura. In addition, immune complexes can occur in the absence of these clinical entities. Finally, the microscopic form of polyarteritis may be associated with type III CGN. Absence of immune complexes, immunoglobulin, and complement deposition in the renal biopsy characterizes this variety. The mechanism of glomerular damage is unknown.

It has been proposed that these renal insults produce glomerular inflammation by cleavage of vasoactive amines and the activation of complement, with the subsequent stimulation of mesangial cell proliferation and phagocytic cell infiltration (Fig. 26C.4). The inflammatory lesion weakens the GBM, ultimately resulting in a break in its continuity through which the intravascular contents may leak. This break has been called the "focal disruptive lesion" by Min and coworkers (20) and has been proposed to represent the nidus for crescent formation. These lesions and the localized area of fibrin and cellular extravasation may sometimes be seen after careful examination of serial biopsy sections using light and electron microscopic techniques.

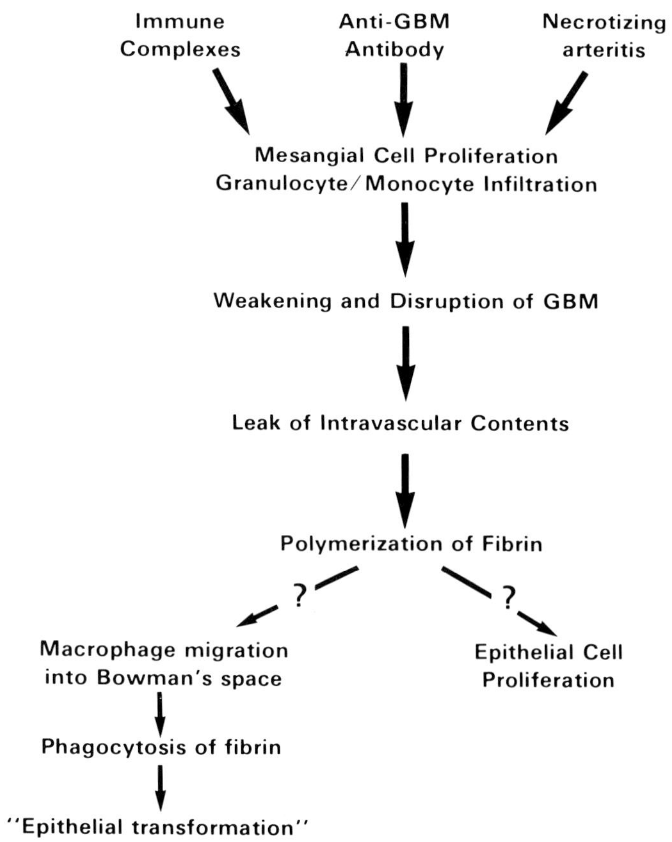

Figure 26C.4. Proposed pathophysiologic schema for CGN.

The presence of fibrin in Bowman's space in CGN is one of the most consistent findings. While inflammatory cells and fibrin can be thought of as "plugging" the break in the GBM, the leak of fibrin into the extracapillary space is considered an important event in the formation of the crescent. It has been proposed that the exuded fibrin stimulates the proliferation of the cells that form the crescent. The pathogenicity of fibrin is supported by observations that defibrination of rabbits with the coagulant fraction of Malayan pit viper venom will markedly attenuate the development of CGN if given before induction of nephrotoxic nephritis (21, 22) and diminish fibrin deposition, crescent formation, and the rise in serum creatinine if given as late as 10 days after disease induction, providing that severe renal failure has not already occurred (23).

The origin of the cells in crescents is the subject of controversy. Because of their histological appearance, it had been proposed that the crescents were derived from proliferated epithelial cells of Bowman's capsule (16, 20). More recently, studies have demonstrated the importance of monocytes in many other forms of glomerulonephritis, which has led to the hypothesis that the monocyte is an important component of the glomerular crescent (24–26). Ultrastructurally, many of the cells in the crescents from both human (27) and animal (24) kidney tissue have the prominent golgi apparati and phagolysosomes characteristic of monocytes. Furthermore, histochemical techniques have detected monocytes as cellular components in crescents from human CGN (26, 27) and animal nephrotoxic nephritis (NTN) (29). Cytogenetic study of renal transplant allograft biopsies from two males who developed CGN in the transplant and whose donors were female revealed the presence of Y bodies in 10% of the cells in the crescents (30). Since the Y body is a marker for male cells, at least part of the crescents originated from infiltrating cells of the recipient rather than from the cells of Bowman's capsule. Finally, tissue culture of glomerular cells from humans (31) and animals (28, 32) have demonstrated mononuclear-like cells from biopsies in which crescents were present. The significance of these tissue culture studies has been criticized (27) in that the source of the monocytes is uncertain. While some may have grown out of the glomerular crescent, many could have originated from infiltrated monocytes in the glomerular tuft. More recently, histochemical studies of human biopsy material suggest that monocytes are much more prominent histochemically in CGN associated with anti-GBM disease than in immune complex disease (26–27). This difference may reflect a difference in pathogenetic mechanisms.

Serial observations in rabbit NTN (28) have demonstrated that macrophage infiltration in Bowman's space follows fibrin deposition. These cells were seen to phagocytose the fibrin and undergo epithelial and giant cell transformation to form part of a crescent. A similar transformation has been suggested to occur in human CGN (31). This event is associated with a loss of histochemical staining characteristics rendering the cells undifferentiatable from epithelial cells derived from Bowman's capsule (27).

At this time it can be stated that monocytes do participate in crescent formation, although it is unclear whether their primary role is phagocytosis or crescent organization. It is of interest that monocytes have been shown to release a factor(s) that stimulates the proliferation of fibroblasts in vitro (33). Whether such factors relate to progression of the crescent to global sclerosis is subject to speculation.

Therapy and Outcome

An understanding of these proposed pathophysiological mechanisms has been used to justify three types of therapeutic strategies—immunosuppression, anticoagulants/antiaggregants, and plasmapheresis.

The use of immunosuppression is based on the mechanisms of inflammation and cellular immunity that have been purported to contribute to both the glomerular and tubulointerstitial injury in CGN. Steroids and cytotoxic agents have been used to suppress specific antibody production and attenuate humoral or cellular mechanisms of inflammation in the expectation that such an effect will interrupt the pathophysiological process.

The consistent finding of fibrin in crescents and its prominence as the crescents "age" and organize support a pathogenic role for fibrin (34). The importance of platelet participation in the pathogenesis of CGN is not clear. Although accelerated platelet turnover has been demonstrated in a number of human glomerulopathies in which crescents appear, the absence of similar findings in all forms of CGN make the role of platelets even less clear. Regardless, these and other observations have prompted trials of anticoagulation and antiaggregation agents in CGN.

The benefit of plasmapheresis in a number of renal and nonrenal immunological disorders, particularly those associated with circulating or in situ immune complexes, has led to its use in CGN. Most investigators advocate the adjunctive use of cytotoxic agents with this therapy. However, the exact mechanism whereby plasmapheresis may ameliorate certain cases of CGN and the criteria for patient selection are undetermined.

The efficacy of these regimens in pediatrics is uncertain as a result of the heterogeneity of underlying disease in reports of treated and untreated patients and the lack of follow-up in the latter. Although it has generally been accepted that recovery of renal function after PSGN is better than other underlying etiologies for CGN, a recent report of 60 patients in which 22 were children (35) presented data that recovery from CGN following PSGN is no better than the overall group statistics. In this report, patients with less than 50% crescents treated conservatively had a 30% morbidity with improvement in renal function or recovery in the remaining patients. Follow-up reports of untreated adults with CGN who have crescents in greater than 50% of their glomeruli have found sustaining kidney function over the short term in only 30% to 40% with a decrease to 20% to 30% after longer follow-up. In these reports, a poor outlook is related to the percentages of glomeruli containing crescents at onset, the presence of oliguria, the duration of disease, and the presence of tubulointerstitial involvement. Any evaluation of the efficacy of treatment must take these variables into account.

Corticosteroids and Immunosuppressive Agents

Whereas there are a number of small, uncontrolled studies of the efficacy of corticosteroid therapy in adults with CGN (36–38), similar data are lacking for this syndrome in childhood. Most reports utilize three to six "pulse" doses of intravenous methylprednisolone given over a period of 3 to 7 days, after which most patients are continued on maintenance oral corticosteroids for variable periods of time.

Understanding that groups with a tendency to respond are more likely to be reported, the data suggests an improved dialysis-independent survival rate of between 40% and 80% after pulse corticosteroid treatment. While early treatment appears to be associated with a more favorable response, life-threatening infectious complications of treatment occur more frequently in this group as well. In five children with CGN treated with three every-other-day doses of methylprednisolone (30 mg/kg/dose) (39) all survived. Four had adequate renal function as indicated by inulin clearances ranging from 84 to 135 ml/min/1.73 M^2, whereas one had renal failure requiring a kidney transplant. Since none of these four patients had evidence for PSGN that could be considered a short-lived acute illness, the authors felt the better outcome could be attributed to the corticosteroid treatment. However, the two patients with the highest follow-up inulin clearances had Henoch-Schönlein purpura, which is known to frequently resolve spontaneously. Interestingly, the patient who underwent renal transplantation had only 25% glomerular crescents at presentation, pointing out the lack of predictability of outcome in a single case by biopsy.

A variety of cytotoxic agents have been used in the treatment of CGN including azothiaprine, cyclophosphamide, and nitrogen mustard. Most patients have received these agents in combination with corticosteroids. Anand and coworkers (5) reported a group of seven children with nonstreptococcal CGN, five of whom had severe disease (greater than 50% crescents), who they treated with either prednisone alone, or in combination with cyclophosphamide or azothiaprine. In the severely affected patients three of five developed terminal renal failure and the remaining patients had reduced renal function and hypertension.

In this same study, the authors reported an additional 10 patients with CGN associated with PSGN, three of whom had greater than 60% crescents. One of these latter patients completely recovered and the other two developed terminal renal failure. Of the remaining seven patients who had 25% to 59% crescents, 43% developed terminal renal failure. Specifics of treatment in this study are, unfortunately, not stated. Other small series of combination therapy report little improvement in survival or preservation of kidney function compared to corticosteroid treatment alone.

Anticoagulants/Antiaggregates

Although the initial observations of the adjunctive use of anticoagulants and antiplatelet agents in combination with immunosuppression in CGN were encouraging, subsequent reports have been less so.

Chapman (40) treated five children with CGN associated with membranoproliferative glomerulonephritis (MPGN) (three type I and two type II) in whom there were crescents in 50% to 100% of the glomeruli. The quadruple treatment regimen used consisted of azothiaprine, prednisone, and heparin followed by warfarin. In follow-up ranging from 0.5 to 3.5 years, only 40% survived with renal function and there was a 40% mortality.

Savage and coworkers (41), using a similar regimen, which also included dipyridamole, treated a group of patients with glomerulonephritis in which were included three patients with CGN—two patients with idiopathic CGN and one with type II membranoproliferative glomerulonephritis. One patient was dialysis-dependent at onset and remained so, but follow-up was limited to several months. Of the remaining two patients, one recovered normal renal function and one (who was on dialysis at onset) had stable renal insufficiency after 1 year. In another study of RPGN in children, the authors report 13 children with variable degrees of crescent formation (10% to 100%) in which 7 had CGN in association with PSGN (7). The remaining six had CGN in association with MPGN or of unknown etiology. The patients were treated with a pot pourri of immunosuppressive and antiplatelet/anticoagulation agents. Three of four patients with CGN following PSGN who received heparin as part of their regimen survived with renal function compared to only one of three who received no heparin. The only non-PSGN patient receiving heparin survived compared to two of five surviving without heparin therapy. A recent study of adults and children with CGN of mixed etiology used a combination of oral corticosteroids, cyclophosphamide, and antiplatelet and anticoagulation agents in patients with greater than 50% crescents. Mortality in patients with 50% to 80% crescents was 33%. In patients with greater than 80% crescents it was 77% regardless of etiology.

These studies point out the heterogeneity of both patient populations and treatment regimens. All in all, there remains no convincing evidence that patient survival or recovery of kidney function is in any way improved with these agents compared to high dose intravenous corticosteroid therapy alone. Furthermore, the therapy is not benign since iatrogenic bleeding diatheses have been reported in this setting.

Plasmapheresis

A number of reports now suggest the benefit of plasmapheresis therapy combined with immunosuppression in the treatment of several disorders, including Goodpasture's syndrome and proliferative lupus erythematosus nephritis (42, 43). Recently, reports using a combination of corticosteroid, immunosuppressive, and plasmaperesis therapy have also suggested a benefit in the treatment of CGN. One study, in which nine adults with immune complex CGN were treated with repetitive plasmapheresis in combination with corticosteroids and immunosuppressives, showed an improvement in renal function in 56% of the patients treated. However, the group had great variability in the degree of crescent formation (5% to 96%) and follow-up was short (4 to 40 weeks) (43). Rifle and coworkers (44) reported a prospective randomized treatment protocol evaluating the effect of adding plasmapheresis to a regimen of steroids, immunosuppressives, and anticoagulants in a group of 14 patients with severe CGN. Two children were included in this study. Their data demonstrated improved outcome in the group treated with plasmapheresis compared to the group receiving pharmacological therapy only.

In a recent review, Glassock (45) found the use of quadruple therapy or the combination of immunosuppression and intensive plasmapheresis to be about equivalent in long-term outcome in CGN and far superior to oral prednisone and azothiaprine. Again, survival statistics for the former groups are similar to the pulse methylprednisolone data.

In addition to the equivocal evidence of an adjunctive therapeutic benefit of plasmapheresis, there is data indicating a disturbingly high incidence of life-threatening infections in patients with renal disease receiving immunosuppressive agents and plasmapheresis (46). These infections consisted of both pathogenic and opportunistic bacteria and occurred in 33% of the cases reviewed. A further consideration in the use of plasmapheresis for the pediatric patient is the difficulty of vascular access.

In conclusion, while the value of the above regimens in CGN is not clear, it is evident that all of these therapeutic modalities have a significant inherent clinical risk. In the absence of sufficiently large and well-controlled clinical studies, risk and benefit need to be carefully weighed in each individual patient before embarking on therapy.

References

1. Ellis A: Natural history of Bright's disease: Clinical, histological and experimental observations. Lancet 1:1, 1942.
2. Lewis EJ, Schwartz MM: Idiopathic crescentic glomerulonephritis. Semin Nephrol 2:193, 1982.
3. Whitworth JA, Morel-Maroger L, Mignon F, et al: The significance of extracapillary proliferation. Nephron 16:1, 1976.
4. Berine GJ, Wagnild JD, Zimmerman SW, et al: Idiopathic crescentic glomerulonephritis. Medicine 56:349, 1977.
5. Anand SK, Trygstad CW, Sharma HM, et al: Extracapillary proliferative glomerulonephritis in children. Pediatrics 56:434, 1975.
6. Spargo GH, Ordonez NG, Ringus JC: The differential diagnosis of crescentic glomerulonephritis. Hum Pathol 8:187, 1977.
7. Cunningham RJ III, Gilfoil M, Cavallo T, et al: Rapidly progressive glomerulonephritis in children: A report of 13 cases and a review of the literature. Pediatr Res 14:128, 1980.
8. Lewis EJ, Schwartz MM: Idiopathic crescentic glomerulonephritis. Semin Nephrol 2(3):193, 1982
9. McLeish KR, Yumm N, Luft FC: Rapidly progressive glomerulonephritis in adults: Clinical and histologic correlations. Clin Nephrol 10:43, 1978.
10. Lewis EJ, Cavallo T, Harrington JT, et al: An immunopathologic study of rapidly progressive glomerulonephritis in the adult. Hum Pathol 2:185, 1971.
11. Lerner RA, Glassock RJ, Dixon FJ: The role of antiglomerular basement membrane antibody in the pathogenesis of human glomerulonephritis. J Exp Med 126:989, 1967.
12. Wilson CB, Dixon FJ: Antiglomerular basement membrane antibody-induced glomerulonephritis. Kidney Intl 3:74, 1973.
13. McPhaul JJ, Dixon FJ: The presence of antiglomerular basement membrane antibodies in peripheral blood. J Immunol 103:1168, 1969.
14. McPhaul JJ, Dixon FJ: Characterization of human antiglomerular basement membrane antibodies elicited from glomerulonephritic kidneys. J Clin Invest 49:308, 1970.
15. Stilmant MM, Bolton WK, Sturgill BC, et al: Crescentic glomerulonephritis without immune deposits: Clinicopathologic features. Kidney Intl 15:184, 1979.
16. Heptinstall RH: Rapidly progressive glomerulonephritis. In Heptinstall RH (ed): Pathology of the Kidney. Boston, Little, Brown, & Co, 1974, p 371.
17. Cohen AH, Border WA, Shankel E, et al: Crescentic glomerulonephritis: Immune *vs* non-immune mechanisms. Am J Nephrol 1:78, 1981.
18. Poskitt TR: Immunologic and electron microscopic studies in Goodpasture's syndrome Am J Med 49:250, 1970.
19. Beleil VM, Coburn JW, Shinaberger JH, et al: Recurrent glomerulonephritis due to antiglomerular basement membrane-antibodies in two successive allografts. Clin Nephrol 1:377, 1973.
20. Min KW, Gyorkey F, Gyorkey P, et al: The morphogenesis of glomerular crescents in rapidly progressive glomerulonephritis. Kidney Intl 5:47, 1974.
21. Naish P, Penn GB, Evans DJ, et al: The effect of defibrination on nephrotoxic serum nephritis in rabbits. Clin Sci 42:643, 1972.
22. Thomson NM, Simpson IJ, Peters DK: A quantitative evaluation of anticoagulants in experimental nephrotoxic nephritis. Clin Exp Immunol 19:301, 1975.
23. Thomson NM, Moran J, Simpson IF, et al: Defibrination with ancrod in nephrotoxic nephritis in rabbits. Kidney Intl 10:343, 1976.
24. Magil AB, Wadsworth MB, Lowen M, et al: Monocytes and human renal glomerular disease: a quantitative evaluation. Lab Invest 44:27, 1981.
25. Monga G, Mazzucco G, di Belgiojoso GB, et al: The presence and possible role of monocyte infiltration in human chronic proliferative glomerulonephritis. Am J Pathol 94:271, 1979.
26. Harry T, Bryant D, Coles GA: The detection of monocytes in human renal biopsies: A prospective study. Clin Nephrol 18:29, 1982.
27. Magil AB, Wadsworth LD: Monocyte involvement in glomerular crescents: A histochemical and ultrastructural study. Lab Invest 47:160, 1982.
28. Thomson NM, Holdsworth SR, Glasgow EF: The macrophage in the development of experimental crescentic glomerulonephritis. Am J Pathol 94:223, 1979.
29. Holdsworth SR, Allen DE, Thomson NM, et al: Histochemistry of glomerular cells in animal models of crescentic glomerulonephritis. Pathology 12:339, 1980.
30. Schiffer MS, Michael AF: Renal cell turnover studied by Y chromosome (Y-body) staining of the transplanted human kidney. J Lab Clin Med 92:841, 1978.
31. Adkins RD, Holdsworth SR, Glasgow EF, et al: The macrophage in human rapidly progressive glomerulonephritis. Lancet 1:830, 1976.
32. Holdsworth SR, Thomson NM, Glasgow EF, et al: Tissue culture of isolated glomeruli in experimental crescentic glomerulonephritis. J Exp Med 147:98, 1978.
33. Leibovich SJ, Ross R: A macrophage-dependent factor that stimulates the proliferation of fibroblasts in vitro. Am J Pathol 84:501, 1976.
34. Hoyer JR, Michael AF, Hoyer LW: Immunofluorescent localization of antihemophilic factor antigen and fibrinogen in human renal diseases. J Clin Invest 53:1375, 1974.
35. Bhuyan UN, Dash SC, Srifastava RN, et al: Immunopathology, extent and course of glomerulonephritis with crescent formation. Clin Nephrol 18:280, 1982.
36. Bolton WK, Couser WG: Intravenous pulse methylprednisolone therapy of acute crescentic rapidly progressive glomerulonephritis. Am J Med 66:495, 1979.
37. O'Neill WM, Etheridge WB, Bloomer A: High dose corticosteroids. Their use in treating idiopathic rapidly progressive glomerulonephritis. Arch Intern Med 139:514, 1979.
38. Oredugba O, Mazumdar DC, Meyer JS, et al: Pulse methylprednisolone therapy in idiopathic rapidly progressive glomerulonephritis. Ann Int Med 92:504, 1980.
39. Cole BR, Brocklebank JT, Kienstra RA, et al: "Pulse" methylprednisolone therapy in the treatment of severe glomerulonephritis. J Pediatr 88:307, 1976.
40. Chapman SJ, Cameron JS, Chantler C, et al: Treatment of mesangiocapillary glomerulonephritis in children with combined immunosuppression and anticoagulation. Arch Dis Childh 55:446, 1980.
41. Savage JM, Postlethwaite RJ, Lendon M, et al: Combined immunosuppressive and anticoagulant treatment in children with glomerulonephritis and declining renal function. Int J Pediatr Nephrol 3:167, 1982.

42. Siegler RL, Bone RE, Morris AH: Treatment of Goodpasture's syndrome with plasma exchange and immunosuppression. Clin Pediatr 19:488, 1980.
43. Lockwood CM, Pinchins AJ, Sweny P, et al: Plasma exchange and immunosuppression in the treatment of fulminating immune complex crescentic nephritis. Lancet 1:63, 1977.
44. Rifle G, Chalopin JM, Zech P, et al: Treatment of idiopathic acute crescentic glomerulonephritis by immunosuppression and plasma exchanges. Proc EDTA 18:493, 1980.
45. Glassock RJ: Immunosuppressive treatment in the prevention of renal failure in primary glomerular diseases. Clin Exper Dial Apher 5:21, 1981.
46. Wing EJ, Bruns FJ, Fraley DS, et al: Infectious complications with plasmapheresis in rapidly progressive glomerulonephritis. JAMA 244:2423, 1980.

26D IgA Nephropathy

TYRONE MELVIN
YOUNGKI KIM

IgA nephropathy (IgAN) is a clinical/pathological entity defined by the presence of macroscopic or microscopic hematuria and mesangial IgA deposits in the absence of features diagnostic of systemic lupus erythematosus (SLE), anaphylactoid purpura, and liver disease. Since its description by Berger and coworkers (1), it has been discovered all over the world and is now recognized as one of the most common glomerular diseases in France (2), Japan (3), Australia (4), and Italy (5). It is also frequently seen in West Germany (6), Singapore (7), the Netherlands (8), Israel (9), as well as in the United States (10), Canada (11), and England (12).

It is not a benign illness as once believed. Up to 25% of patients in some series will ultimately develop renal failure (8, 13), and the process may also recur in transplanted kidneys (2, 14).

The pathogenetic events leading to this disease remain unknown, and there is no proven therapy. The last decade has, however, seen a rapid advance in understanding IgA synthesis, its role in interacting with infectious agents, and in understanding its metabolism in experimental animals and man.

Clinical Presentation

IgAN has many clinical presentations. Clarkson and coworkers (4) described a group of 50 patients in which it was manifested by the following symptoms or constellation of symptoms: macroscopic hematuria (34%), proteinuria with or without microhematuria (30%), nephrotic syndrome (6%), acute nephritis (10%), malignant hypertension (8%), chronic renal failure (6%), and acute renal failure (6%). Other studies describe large numbers of patients who were discovered to have IgAN after presentation with isolated microhematuria (5, 15). Despite the range of manifestations possible at the time of presentation, the majority of patients reported have had either intermittent gross hematuria or microhematuria with or without proteinuria. A review of 20 series comprising 1407 patients with IgAN (2–5, 8, 10–15, 15–24) reveals that the weighted mean percentage (calculated as: the number of patients with indicated clinical sign or laboratory parameter ÷ by the total number of patients × 100) of patients with gross hematuria or history of recurrent gross hematuria at diagnosis, is 45%; 8% presented with the nephrotic syndrome; 20% had hypertension and 22% decreased renal function (Fig. 26D.1).

There is a 2:1 male predominance in this disease and 9 selected series (4, 8, 11, 12, 15, 20–23) (N = 358 patients) reveal a peak incidence in late childhood through early adult life (Fig. 26D.2). Also the prevalence of upper respiratory infections (usually pharyngitis) or gastrointestinal complaints at the time of or near the time of gross hematuria is great. Sissons and coworkers (12) reported 14/15 with pharyngitis occurring near the onset of gross hematuria. Other series have also reported a significant number of patients with upper respiratory infection including Clarkson (4) (83%), and Imbasciati (5) (36%). The bacteria or viruses responsible for these clinical symptoms are not frequently known, but have included group A streptococci (23), influenza A, Epstein-Barr virus, staphylococcus aureus, and Brucellosis (4). The gross hematuria usually occurs within 48 hours (4, 23) of the onset of the upper respiratory illness, lasts 1–2 days (18), and recurs at intervals from several days (15) to several years (2). The individual episodes may occasionally last up to 2½ years.

In the interval between episodes of gross hematuria, patients (except for those with nephrotic syndrome) have normal urinalyses, persistent hematuria or persistent proteinuria or intermittent hematuria or proteinuria. In the combined series of Levy (23) and Michalk (15), 33% had normal urinalyses in between episodes of gross hematuria, 18% had intermittent hematuria and proteinuria, 21% had persistent hematuria and proteinuria, 14% isolated persistent microhematuria, and 14% persistent proteinuria (Table 26D.1).

Loin pain is another clinical symptom that is frequently seen in these patients (16). This has been reported in 36% of patients with IgAN in the series of Bennett and Kincaid-Smith (16) and in approximately 50% of the patients reported by other authors. It tends to occur at the time of gross hematuria or during an increase in microhematuria or proteinuria.

Exercise has also been reported by several investigators to exacerbate or be associated with the onset of gross hematuria (12, 15).

Although uncommon, IgAN can present as acute renal failure (4). This has been observed in association with diffuse glomerular crescents or with a morphological picture in which there are minimal glomerular lesions and associated massive glomerular bleeding (16). This presentation has also been reported in a patient in whom it was recurrent, requiring dialysis.

Natural History

The natural history of this syndrome is now recognized to be less benign than originally thought. The longest actuarial studies show that the 10-year survival is approximately 90% in the series of Kincaid-Smith and Nicholls (25) and Imbasciati (5). Less optimistic is the survival curve of Droz (2), revealing a constant mortality of 2.5%/year (Fig. 26D.3). Aside from mortality, the long-term outlook for renal function is difficult to assess because of conflicting reports. Although many studies have suggested a favorable outcome (17, 19), others have described frequent deterioration in renal function (2, 4, 8). A more difficult problem has been determining how many patients with normal renal function at diagnosis ultimately develop decreased renal function and how many with minor decreases in function progress to end-stage renal failure. Imbasciati (5) describes 22 patients with initially normal renal function (from a study population of 178) that developed decreased renal function during follow-up. Thirteen of these 22 ultimately developed end-stage renal disease. In the study of Droz (2) approximately 2.5%/year developed end-stage renal failure, paralleling the annual mortality rate.

In contrast, pediatric series (15, 23) suggest a universally good outcome. This may be a result of the progressive nature of the disease, requiring several years for renal damage to become manifest, as has been suggested by Kincaid-Smith and Nicholls (25), or alternatively it may be that IgAN with onset in childhood does in fact have a benign course. An equally difficult problem to resolve is whether patients who initially have decreased function can have both clinical and histological remissions. Evidence to date suggests that some patients may have return of renal function after an initial deterioration but the immunopathological features do not remit, e.g., mesangial IgA is always present in these patients (25) (University of Minnesota, unpublished observations).

Transplantation

Several patients with IgAN have received renal transplants for this syndrome and the recurrence of urinary abnormalities and mesangial IgA deposition is frequent. Droz (2) described 19 patients receiving transplants as a result of IgAN in whom 9 developed recurrence of mesangial IgA deposits 3 months to 3 years after transplantation. Only 1 had gross hematuria, and only 1 patient in a follow-up ranging from 2.5 to 8 years developed renal failure and that 1 was a result of chronic

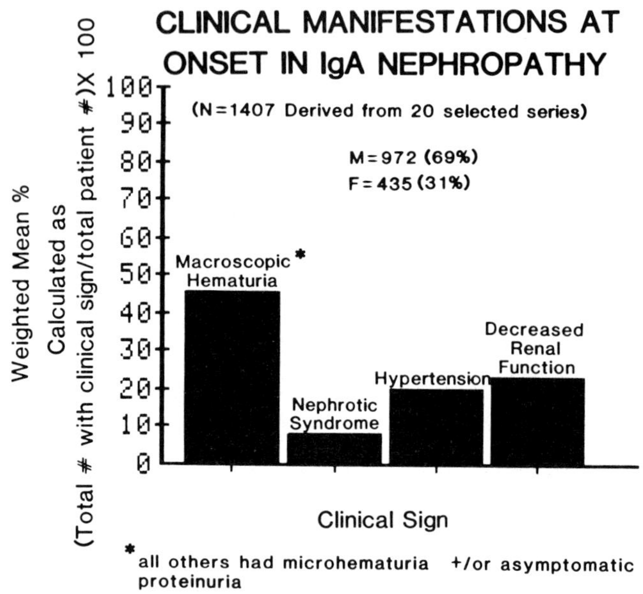

Figure 26D.1. Clinical manifestations at onset in IgA nephropathy. Bar height represents weighted mean percentage of patients with indicated sign or symptom. Data derived from references 2–5, 8, 10–13, 15–22.

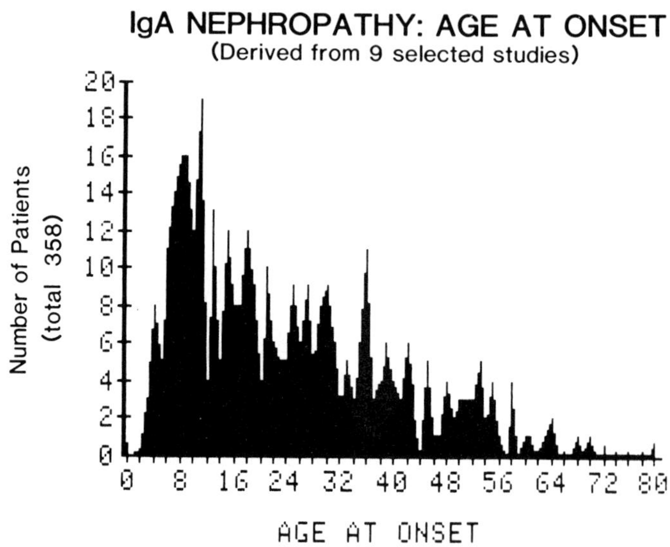

Figure 26D.2. Age at onset in IgA nephropathy. Data derived from references 4, 8, 11, 12, 15, 20–23.

Table 26D.1.
Clinicopathological Correlations in IgA Nephropathy

Disease course	Pathological group		
	Minimal glomerular lesions	Focal glomerulo-nephritis	Diffuse proliferative glomerulonephritis (focal crescents)
Remission (between attacks or at last exam)	9	6	1
Intermittent hematuria[a] and proteinuria	5	2	2
Persistent hematuria and proteinuria	2	3	5
Persistent hematuria	1	5	1
Persistent proteinuria	0	4	3

From Levy M, et al: Clin Nephrol 1:63, 1973 and Michalk D, et al: Eur J Pediatr 143:13, 1980.
[a] Patients are placed in this category even if proteinuria only occurred during episodes of gross hematuria.

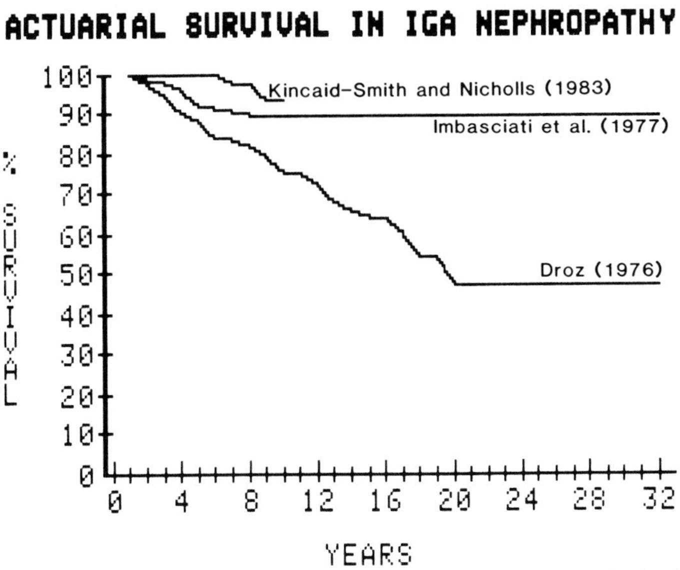

Figure 26D.3. Life table analysis of survival in IgA nephropathy. Derived from references 2, 5, 25.

rejection. Berger (14) reported 12 patients transplanted as a result of renal failure because of IgAN. In 7 there was recurrence of IgA deposits usually with urinary abnormalities, but without reduction in function. This occurred in both HLA identical, as well as in patients with only 1 HLA antigen matched, in living related, as well as cadaver donor kidneys, and in male, as well as female donor, kidneys. One unique case of an HLA-identical brother to brother kidney donor was reported by Tolkoff-Rubin (26) in which a donor kidney biopsy done at the time of transplantation revealed IgA mesangial deposits. Sabatier and coworkers (27) have also reported the occurrence of this disease in HLA identical siblings. This phenomenon raises questions about genetic factors in the etiology of this syndrome and it may explain some of what has been termed "recurrence" of the IgA deposits in transplants. Noel (28) found that the incidence of recurrence was greater if the donor was HLA identical or haploidentical compared with cadaver grafts. This lends further support to the notion of a genetic predisposition to this syndrome as does the unpublished data of Berger, noted in Sabatier (27), documenting resolution of IgA deposits in kidneys with IgA mesangial deposits which were inadvertently transplanted into patients with renal failure due to diseases other than IgAN.

Pregnancy in Patients with IgAN

The outcome of pregnancy in patients with IgAN has been favorable. Droz (2) describes 15 pregnancies (in 11 patients), 14 of which resulted in normal infants. One patient had a therapeutic abortion because of massive anasarca. This study stands in contrast to that of Whitworth (29) in which only 65% of 34 pregnancies in 20 patients with IgAN were successful. Preeclampsia developed during 62% of the pregnancies. These patients had a higher incidence of focal and segmental proliferative lesions and hyalinosis than those nonpregnant women with IgAN. Hypertension before pregnancy was a poor prognostic marker for fetal survival; however, pregnant patients described by Droz (2) had proteinuria and hypertension but all had normal infants.

Pathology

Light Microscopy

By light microscopy, three types of glomerular histological lesions can be seen in IgAN. They are minimal glomerular lesion; focal, segmental glomerulonephritis (GN); and diffuse proliferative GN.

The minimal glomerular lesion encompasses the spectrum from completely normal to a slight increase in mesangial matrix without cellular proliferation. The tubules, interstitium, and blood vessels are normal in this category. This morphological picture is present in 1% to 25% of the biopsies reviewed in the series referenced above.

Focal segmental glomerulonephritis is the most prevalent lesion, being present in 50% to 80% of biopsies. This lesion consists of focal segmental proliferation of mesangial and epithelial cells with frequent matrix increase (Fig. 26D.4, *A*). In addition, areas of fibrinoid necrosis, crescents and fibrous lesions with capsular adhesions may also be present. The less frequent lesion of focal segmental sclerosis/hyalinosis may simply reflect progression of the FSGN lesion with subsequent sclerosis and hyalinosis.

Diffuse proliferative GN is the least common lesion found in these patients. All glomeruli show diffuse mesangial proliferation and increase in mesangial matrix. Frequently, a variable degree of fibrinoid necrosis, crescent formation, or fibrous capsular lesions may be seen.

In both focal and diffuse proliferative GN, there is a relationship between the degree of crescent formation and the timing of renal biopsy. Bennett and Kincaid-Smith (20) demonstrated that if biopsies are done at or near the time of gross hematuria or when urinary erythrocyte counts are $>10^6$/ml, crescents are present in >75% of the biopsies.

Tubulointerstitial changes in most biopsies usually correlate with glomerular damage. However, Kincaid-Smith (25) described a patient with IgAN whose clinical course was characterized by oliguric acute renal failure coinciding with gross hematuria. A kidney biopsy done in this patient failed to show any significant glomerular damages. Instead, there was extensive acute tubular necrosis, most probably as a result of intratubular obstruction secondary to severe glomerular bleeding.

Vascular lesions have been noted in many series as well. Arteriosclerotic and arterioscleritic lesions have been seen in up to 33% of patients at the time of first biopsy (30). These lesions may precede the onset of hypertension and have been reported to parallel glomerular sclerosis suggesting that renal damage in some patients was a result in part of these vascular lesions.

Immunofluorescence Microscopy

The hallmark of IgAN is the presence of IgA in the glomerular mesangium as the predominant immunoglobulin (Fig. 26D.4, *B*). Review of several selected large series further define characteristics identified by immunofluorescence microscopy (2–13, 15–17, 19–22). Regardless of light histology, the distribution of IgA is always generalized (present in each glomerulus) and diffuse (throughout each glomerulus), and the intensity with which it stains is stronger than other immunoglobulins, although sometimes they may be equal. Occasionally one may also find IgA along the glomerular basement membrane. Although IgA can be the sole immunoglobulin in the glomeruli, IgG and less frequently IgM are usually found in the same location as that of IgA, but in a lesser intensity. C3 and properdin are also present in the majority of the patients, whereas C1q and C4 are usually absent. This seems to indicate the activation of the alternative complement pathway in IgAN. More recently, C9 neoantigen of the membrane attack complex of the human complement system has been also found to be present in the glomerular mesangium together with C5, C6, C7, C8, and monomeric C9 (31). Fibrin may also be present together with IgA, but its intensity is usually quite weak.

Immune deposits are detected in other areas of the kidney as well. Frasca (32) describes C3 with and without IgA, IgG, or IgM in tubulo-interstitial loci. IgA renal vascular deposits are described in some series (4, 21). IgA deposits have also been noted in cutaneous vessel walls in some patients with IgAN (33, 34). Similar findings have been noted in the vessel walls of skeletal muscle in some patients with IgAN (35).

Significant glomerular deposition of IgA can also be seen in systemic lupus erythematosus, anaphylactoid purpura, liver disease and dermatitis

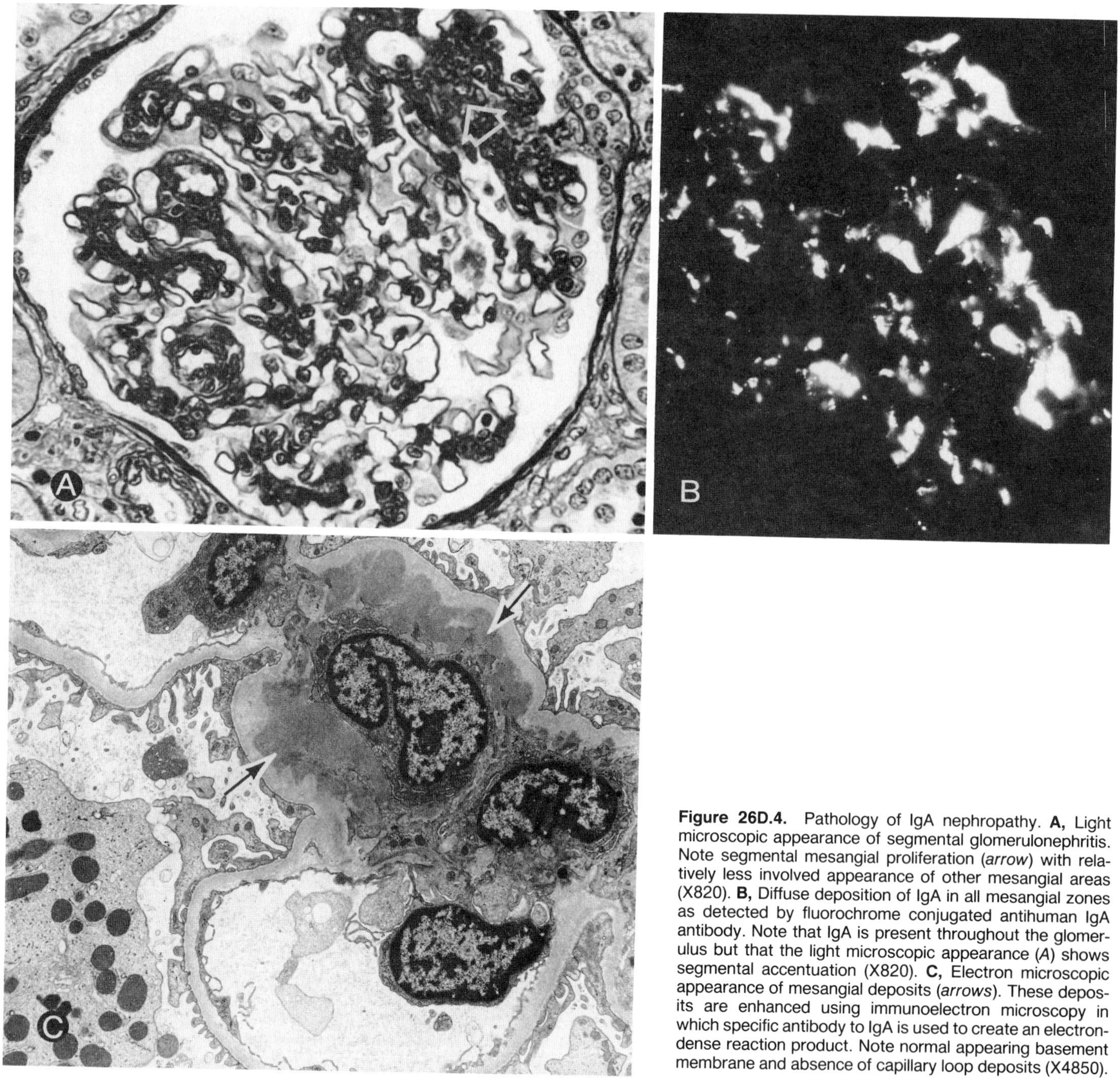

Figure 26D.4. Pathology of IgA nephropathy. **A,** Light microscopic appearance of segmental glomerulonephritis. Note segmental mesangial proliferation (*arrow*) with relatively less involved appearance of other mesangial areas (X820). **B,** Diffuse deposition of IgA in all mesangial zones as detected by fluorochrome conjugated antihuman IgA antibody. Note that IgA is present throughout the glomerulus but that the light microscopic appearance (*A*) shows segmental accentuation (X820). **C,** Electron microscopic appearance of mesangial deposits (*arrows*). These deposits are enhanced using immunoelectron microscopy in which specific antibody to IgA is used to create an electron-dense reaction product. Note normal appearing basement membrane and absence of capillary loop deposits (X4850).

herpetiformis. However, they can be easily differentiated from IgAN based on their immunofluorescent and clinical findings.

Electron Microscopy

By electron microscopy, electron-dense deposits are usually found in the mesangial area (1, 23, 36) and occasionally also in subendothelial (4), subepithelial, or intramembranous (15) loci. However, the amount of glomerular electron-dense deposits is frequently less than that of IgA detected by immunofluorescence microscopy; in some patients they may even be totally absent despite abundant presence of IgA by immunofluorescence microscopy (10). Using immunoelectron microscopy (a technique in which electron-dense deposits are enhanced by specific antisera), Dysart (37) demonstrated that IgA and C3 deposits were present in the mesangial matrix (Fig. 26D.4, *C*) and occasionally along peripheral capillary loops, along tubular basement membranes, and within the interstitial matrix. Also large amounts were present in the walls of small renal arterioles. In addition, one may find mesangial expansion with increase in mesangial cellularity or endothelial and epithelial hypertrophy.

Clinical/Pathological Correlations

Certain morphological patterns seen in IgAN nephropathy appear to be associated with different disease courses. In a combined review of 52 patients in childhood from Levy (23) and Michalk (15) (Table 26D.1) it holds, not surprisingly, that the patients with minimal glomerular lesions tend to have normal or intermittently abnormal urinary sediment between episodes of gross hematuria and at the other end of the spectrum, those with diffuse proliferative GN have persistent microhematuria and proteinuria.

In general, severe glomerular changes (e.g., high percentage of sclerosed glomeruli, crescents, or adhesions) are indicative of a worse prognosis. Tubulointerstitial damage and peripheral capillary wall changes have been specifically cited by the Southwest Pediatric Study Group (SWPSG) (21) as indicators of poor prognosis. Crescents in >30% glomeruli that persist on repeated biopsy have also shown to be poor prognostic indicators and may be associated with a particularly fulminant course (33).

Clinical features that are associated with a poor outcome include older age, hypertension, marked proteinuria, and renal impairment at presentation. One clinical feature, recurrent gross hematuria, is still contested as to its being a good or bad prognostic sign. Clarkson (4), Droz (2), and Imbasciati (5) all find it a favorable sign. Bennett and Kincaid-Smith (16) find the opposite. They have demonstrated that in patients with IgAN in whom gross hematuria or urinary erythrocyte counts exceed 10^6/ml, crescents are invariably present in biopsies done near the episode of hematuria. They had a higher incidence of renal insufficiency as well (Fig. 26D.5). Further, of these patients, those with persistent crescents on serial biopsies run a "malignant" course.

Treatment

Therapy has been uniformly unsuccessful in modifying this disease, and there are no known spontaneous clinical and immunopathological remissions. Clarkson (38) reported that the use of corticosteroids, cyclophosphamide, and anticoagulants alone or in combination did not affect the disease. Others have noted reduction in the severity of the urinary abnormalities in a few patients during corticosteroid therapy (given on an intermittent regimen) but return of urinary abnormalities after 1 to 2 years occurred in most patients. The use of plasmapheresis in one patient had no benefit. This is corroborated by Levy (23). Other therapies reported have also failed, including long-term oral penicillin or tonsillectomy (23). Clarkson (39) later reported a controlled trial of phenytoin in these patients. This agent was used because of its known effect in reducing serum IgA levels (40). Although there was a significant reduction in serum IgA, there was no significant change in any other clinical, biochemical, or pathological parameter. It has been reported recently that the phenytoin reduces the polymeric IgA fraction, although not selectively (41). Such reduction in polymeric IgA is confirmed by Coppo (42), although the quantity of IgA immune complexes did not change.

More recently, corticosteroids were used to treat patients with IgA nephropathy and nephrotic syndrome by Mustonen (43). Three patients with minimal glomerular histological changes responded with loss of nephrotic syndrome, whereas the other three with moderate to severe mesangial changes did not. Since minimal mesangial changes and IgA deposition can also be seen in steroid responsive minimal change nephrotic syndrome (44), it is not clear whether this represents minimal change nephrotic syndrome (MCNS), an incidental association of MCNS with IgAN, or a subtype of IgAN. At present all other therapeutic trials aimed at the disease itself have been unsuccessful, therefore, conservative medical management of hypertension and renal failure is the recommended approach.

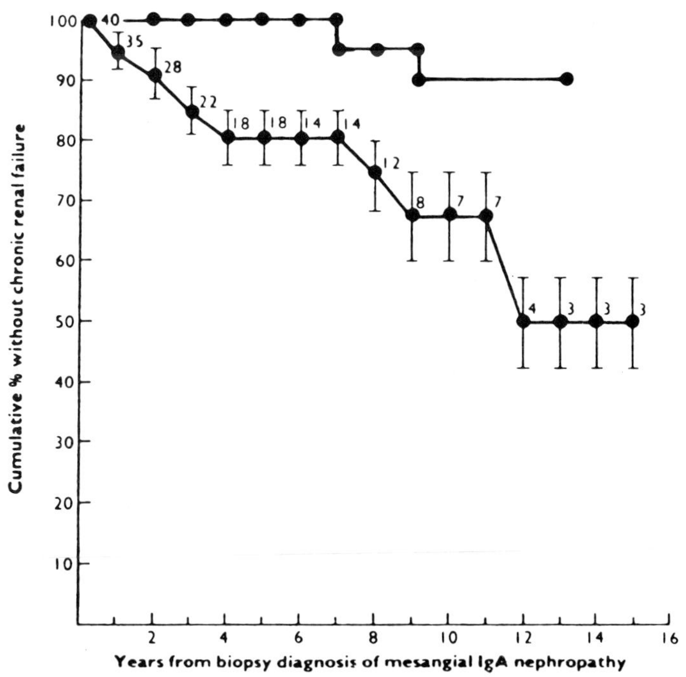

Figure 26D.5. Life table analysis of absence of renal failure. Top line represents total number of patients. The bottom line represents those with gross hematuria indicating a worse prognosis in this group. (Reprinted with permission from Kincaid-Smith P, Nicholls K: Am J Kid Dis 3(2): 98, 1983.

Etiology and Pathogenesis

Although the cause of IgA nephropathy (IgAN) remains unknown, observations regarding its pathogenesis have been made in the following three major areas: (1) identification of associated immunological abnormalities, (2) evaluation of HLA associations, and (3) development of animal models. However, many of these abnormalities and associations remain controversial, and the experimental models do not truly mimic human disease (45).

Immunological Abnormalities

It is commonly suggested that IgAN is mediated by immune complex deposition. The common immunohistological findings of mesangial IgA, C3 and less often IgG, IgM, properdin, and other complement components are consistent with this notion. Measurement of serum IgA and immune complexes have not offered conclusive support for this hypothesis, however. Elevated serum IgA levels have been reported in from 5% to 75% of patients with IgAN. It is not clear whether this broad range is a result of timing of the serum samples with respect to onset of the disease or other factors. In those studies where serial serum samples have been measured, the IgA level appears to be relatively constant for a given patient (4, 46, 48) and does not appear to correlate with the degree of hematuria (46, 47, 48), or with histological changes (4, 47). Elevations in serum IgA are also not limited to IgA nephropathy. High serum IgA levels have been reported in Henoch-Schönlein purpura and SLE (49, 72) alcoholic cirrhosis, sicca syndrome and in patients who have undergone ileojejunal bypass (50) as well. Serum IgG or IgM has been reported to be elevated also by several investigators. No consistent relationships with hematuria, histological severity, or IgA levels have been demonstrated in these studies.

Various forms of circulating IgA have been reported in IgA nephropathy. Human serum IgA consists of monomers, polymers with J chain, and secretory IgA. Eighty percent of serum IgA is monomeric in normal man (51). Lopez-Trascasa (41) and DesGeorges (52) have reported an increase in circulating polymeric IgA in patients with IgA nephropathy. These results are contradicted by others (50, 53) in which no increase in polymeric IgA was detected using similar methodologies. If true, the finding would not be unique to IgA nephropathy as several investigators have documented an increase in polymeric IgA in patients with liver disease (50, 54). This issue is further clouded by reports indicating that there is an increased in vitro synthesis of polymeric IgA when lymphoid cells from patients with IgAN and nonaffected family members (55) were cultured with pokeweed mitogen. These findings require further confirmation, since it is known that lymphocytes from normal individuals when cultured with PWM synthesize predominantly polymeric IgA (80% at 7 days) (56).

IgA_1, the major subclass of IgA in serum, is increased relative to IgA_2 in IgAN (50). However, this increase is also seen in connective tissue diseases (rheumatoid arthritis, SLE, and sicca syndrome) and chronic active liver disease as well. These findings are consistent with the predominant deposition of IgA_1 in glomeruli of these patients as reported by some investigators (57, 58).

Recently the presence of macromolecular IgA complexes ranging in size from 9 to 21S have been reported (48) and have been suggested to be causally related to the development of IgA glomerular deposits, whereas others were not able to confirm this (University of Minnesota, unpublished observations).

There are also reports of an increase in circulating IgA bearing B cells in patients with IgAN and their family members (59). However, Cosio (60) and Fiorini (61) could not demonstrate a significant increase in IgA bearing lymphocytes.

The studies of circulating IgA immune complexes in IgAN have also been difficult to evaluate because of the unavailability of the optimal assay for IgA immune complexes. With refinement of both the Raji cell radioimmunoassay (RIA) and the conglutinin binding assays, recent reports (47, 53, 62, 63) support the existence of such complexes in IgAN. Le Savre (53) has suggested that the presence of conglutinin binding immune complexes predicts recurrence in the transplanted kidney.

In addition to IgA containing immune complexes, IgG or IgM complexes have also been reported by several investigators (46, 47, 53).

Various other humoral immune abnormalities have been described including the presence of an IgA related platelet agglutinin (64), presence of cold reacting antinuclear antibodies (65), properdin deficiency and partial deficiency (66), partial deficiency of BIH (67), partial deficiency of C4 (67), and an increase in certain B cell alloantigens (68).

To determine whether IgA present in the mesangium is monomeric (90% of serum IgA is monomeric) as opposed to polymeric (IgA secreted at mucosal surface is 50% polymeric), investigators have examined the mesangium for the presence of J chain (present in polymeric immunoglobulin) and the ability of the IgA deposits to bind secretory component (SC) in vitro (only polymers will bind SC). While results of these studies are inconclusive (57, 69), there is general agreement that SC itself is not found in these deposits.

Recent reports (70) have suggested that IgA deposits eluted from kidneys of patients with IgAN react *in vitro* with their renal and tonsillar tissue but not with renal tissue from patients with HSP. IgA, eluted from renal tissue of patients with HSP did, however, react in vitro with tissue from patients with IgAN. Tonsillar tissue from patients with IgAN has been shown by another group (71) to have an increased number of IgA secreting plasma cells compared to patients with recurrent tonsillitis.

Furthermore, sporadic reports have suggested that the clearance of IgA and IgA immune complexes by neutrophils may be impaired (70). This is supported by the observation that IgA immune complexes have been detected within neutrophils from patients with IgAN (72, 73) and that plasma from these patients inhibits the migration of neutrophils in vitro.

It has been recently proposed that there is a delayed clearance of polymeric IgA containing immune complexes in IgAN (74). There are no experimental reports linking the two phenomena, but it is speculated that the decreased clearance may expose the mesangium to more of these complexes, influencing localization there.

Abnormalities in cellular immune mechanisms have been of equal interest. Evaluation of peripheral blood lymphocytes with monoclonal antibodies in patients with IgAN has shown a decrease in the suppressor/cytotoxic lymphocyte population and a relative increase in helper T lymphocytes. Egido (75) and Chatenoud and Bach (76) have found similar elevations in helper to suppressor:cytotoxic T cell ratios in these patients, but with normal to high absolute numbers of cytotoxic/suppressor cells. Sakai (77) and Egido (73) have carried these studies further by demonstrating increased IgA specific helper cell functional activity determined by coculturing the T cell population bearing receptors for the Fc portion of IgA (FcαR) with normal B cells and measuring the cells with cytoplasmic Ig that are produced. This FcαR on lymphocytes has been reported to be quantitatively abnormal in IgAN when in vitro stimulation with IgA proteins is carried out (78). An FcαR has also been identified on granulocytes and monocytes, but its potential role in IgAN is unknown.

Cagnoli (79), utilizing indirect immunofluorescent microscopy, found a normal ratio of helper to cytotoxic/suppressor cells in IgAN patients and, therefore, the variance of this ratio in IgAN remains unknown. Family members of patients when studied have had normal helper:cytotoxic/suppressor cell ratios (75).

Functional studies of suppressor T cell activity in IgAN patients have shown a decrease of suppressor activity in these patients (75, 131), whereas others have found normal suppression in their patients. Other cellular immune changes have also been documented. A factor derived from lymphocytes of patients with IgAN cultured with the mitogen concanavalin A (ConA) has been reported to increase vascular permeability (80).

These widely discrepant, often conflicting, results of immunological studies, may be in part a result of etiologic or pathogenetic heterogeneity of IgAN.

HLA Associations

Studies of HLA association in patients with IgAN and their family members have been inconclusive. While some found an association with BW35 (81), Cw1, B12, DR4 (82), DEN, or KMI alloantigen, others have not (83, 84). Of interest is the occurrence of IgAN in HLA identical siblings (26, 27).

Experimental Models

Experimental models of mesangial IgA deposition have dealt with three aspects of IgA handling: the nature of the complex deposited, the effect of interrupting hepatobiliary transport of IgA, and the nature of the antigen eliciting an IgA response.

Rifai (85) described a model in which IgA immune complexes formed in vitro or in vivo with polymeric, but not monomeric IgA, induced glomerulonephritis. IgA and C3 were present in the mesangium (detected by immunofluorescent microscopy), and focal mesangial widening was present in some glomeruli on light microscopy. Prior depletion of C3 had no effect on the deposition of IgA. Gormly (86) created cirrhosis in the rat using carbon tetrachloride and were able to show circulating immune complexes, increased serum IgA, and IgA and C3 deposits in the glomeruli. There were minimal changes at the light microscopic level, however. Melvin (87) described mesangial IgA, C3, and secretory component deposition in rats that had undergone bile duct ligation. In this study, serum IgA and C3 were markedly elevated. These last two studies have manipulated the normal transfer of polymeric IgA and polymeric IgA containing immune complexes from blood to bile. This transport is mediated via binding of polymeric IgA to secretory component on the hepatocyte surface, internalization, and transcellular transport to the bile canaliculi. This mechanism, while attractive, seems to be relatively unimportant with respect to normal IgA handling in man, (88) as well as in the mouse, although it has been suggested that a small quantitative defect might exist in this mechanism in some IgA patients based upon preliminary clearance studies in man (73). Isaacs (89) exploited the fact that certain dextran antigens elicit primarily an IgA response. They utilized parenteral immunization with neutral and sulfated dextrans and detected mesangial deposition of IgA, less frequently C3, and mesangial proliferation by light microscopy. They proposed that such carbohydrate antigens may be relevant to IgAN since many bacteria and viral products to which we are exposed are frequently carbohydrates (e.g., pneumococcus capsule). They have further characterized this model (90) demonstrating that anionic dextran antigen led to the most significant deposition and proliferation. Emancipator (91) demonstrated that oral administration of certain protein antigens in mice led to a specific IgA response and deposition of immunogen and IgA in the mesangium. No hematuria was evident and no changes were present by light microscopy.

The application of these experimental models to human disease is difficult because the metabolism of IgA in man is different than in rodents, and mesangial proliferation and macroscopic hematuria are not prominent features in any of the models.

Association with Other Diseases

IgAN has been associated with other disease entities (Table 26D.2). In a patient with mycoplasma pneumoniae pneumonia (92) treatment of the serum to remove IgA removed the fraction that bound mycoplasma, suggesting that at least some of the circulating IgA in this patient was specific for the primary pathogen. Cyclical neutropenia in one patient with recurrent apthous ulcers has been associated with macroscopic hematuria, decreased creatinine clearance, and IgA and C3 in the glomerular mesangium (93). The hematuria in this patient was recurrent, happening at times of oral ulceration and neutropenia. Other diseases include mycosis fungoides (93), leprosy (95), scleritis (96), and seronegative spondyloarthropathies (97). Many other disease processes have been reported in association with mesangial IgA deposition, but do not have characteristic clinical features of IgAN or have serological features more typical of other disease processes.

The relationship between IgAN and Henoch-Schönlein purpura is also unresolved. Several investigators have proposed that they are part of a single disease spectrum (3, 98, 99). These hypotheses have been based on similar features including recurrent hematuria following respiratory infection, elevated serum IgA, focal and segmental nature of the glomerulonephritis coexisting with generalized IgA deposition, recurrence in transplanted kidneys (100), dermal vascular IgA deposits (33, 34), and presence of circulating IgA containing immune complexes. Recently it was demonstrated that IgA eluted from HSP or IgAN cross reacted with each other. However, IgAN can be easily separated from HSP on the basis of clinical and pathological features, such as absence of systemic manifestations and small blood vessel vasculitis.

Table 26D.2.
Diseases Associated with IgA Nephropathy[a]

Disease	First author (reference) year
Mycosis fungoides	Ramirez (94) 1981
Mycoplasma pneumoniae	Kanayama (92) 1982
Cyclical neutropenia	Nash (93) 1978
Leprosy	Valles (95) 1982
Scleritis	Nomoto (96) 1980
Seronegative spondyloarthropathies	Jennette (97) 1982
	Sissons (12) 1975

[a] Many other disease processes have been reported in association with mesangial IgA deposition but do not have characteristic clinical features of IgA nephropathy or have serological features more typical of other disease processes.

References

1. Berger J, Hinglais N: Les dépôts intercapillaires d'IgA-IgG. J Urol Néphrol 74:694, 1968.
2. Droz D: Natural history of primary glomerulonephritis with mesangial deposits of IgA. Contr Nephrol 2:150, 1976.
3. Nakamoto Y, Asano Y, Dohi K, et al: Primary IgA glomerulonephritis and Schönlein-Henoch purpura nephritis: Clinicopathological and immunohistochemical characteristics. Quart J Med XLVII:495, 1978.
4. Clarkson AR, Seymour AE, Thompson AJ, et al: IgA nephropathy: A syndrome of uniform morphology, diverse clinical features and uncertain prognosis. Clin Nephrol 8:459, 1977.
5. Imbasciati E, Colosanti G, Barbiano di Belgioioso G, et al: Long term followup of IgA mesangial deposits glomerulonephritis. Proc Eur Dial Transpl Assoc 14:472, 1977.
6. Zollinger HU, Gaboardi F: Verzogerte Heilung einer diffusion intra-und extrapillären glomerulonephritis mit IgA depots. Virchows Arch (Pathol Anat) 354:349, 1979.
7. Sinniah R, Pwee HS, Lim CH: Glomerular lesions in asymptomatic microscopic hematuria discovered on routine medical examination. Clin Nephrol 5:216, 1976.
8. van der Peet J, Arisz L, Brentjens JRH, et al: The clinical course of IgA nephropathy in adults. Clin Nephrol 8:335, 1977.
9. Joshua H, Sharon Z, Gutglas E, Rosenfeld J, et al: IgA-IgG nephropathy: A clinicopathologic entity with slow evolution and favorable prognosis. AJCP 6:289, 1977.
10. Lowance DC, Mullins JD, McPhaul JJ Jr: Immunoglobulin A (IgA) associated glomerulonephritis. Kidney Intl 3:167, 1973.
11. Katz A, Underdown BJ, Minta JO, et al: Glomerulonephritis with mesangial deposits of IgA unassociated with systemic disease. CMA J 114:209, 1976.
12. Sissons JGP, Woodrow DF, Curtis JR, et al: Isolated glomerulonephritis with mesangial IgA deposits. Brit Med J 13:611, 1975.
13. Kurt Lee S-M, Rao VM, Franklin WA, et al: IgA nephropathy: Morphologic predictors of progressive renal disease. Hum Pathol 13:314, 1982.
14. Berger J, Yaneva H, Nabarra B, et al: Recurrence of mesangial deposition of IgA after renal transplantation. Kidney Intl 7:232, 1975.
15. Michalk D, Waldherr R, Seelig H, et al: Idiopathic mesangial IgA-glomerulonephritis in childhood: Description of 19 pediatric cases and review of the literature. Eur J Pediatr 143:13, 1980.
16. Bennett WM, Kincaid-Smith P: Macroscopic hematuria in mesangial IgA nephropathy: Correlation with glomerular crescents and renal dysfunction. Kidney Intl 23:393, 1983.
17. McCoy RC, Abramowsky CR, Tisher CC: IgA nephropathy. Am J Pathol 76:123, 1974.
18. Katz A, Walker JF, Landy PJ: IgA nephritis with nephrotic range proteinuria. Clin Nephrol 20:67, 1983.
19. Finlayson G, Alexander R, Juncos L, et al: Immunoglobulin A glomerulonephritis. A clinicopathologic study. Lab Invest 32:140, 1975.
20. Hood SA, Velosa JA, Holley KA, et al: IgA-IgG nephropathy: Predictive indices of progressive disease. Clin Nephrol 16:55, 1981.
21. Southwest Pediatric Study Group. A multicenter study of IgA nephropathy in children. A report of the Southwest Pediatric Nephrology Study Group. Kidney Intl 22:643, 1982.
22. Croker BP, Dawson DV, Sanfilippo F: IgA nephropathy: Correlation of clinical and histologic features. Lab Invest 48:19, 1983.
23. Levy M, Beaufils H, Gubler MC, et al: Idiopathic recurrent macroscopic hematuria and mesangial IgA-IgG deposits in children (Berger's disease). Clin Nephrol 1:63, 1973.
24. Gärtner H-V, Hönlein F, Traub U, et al: IgA-nephropathy (IgA-IgG-Nephropathy/IgA-Nephritis)—A disease entity? Virchows Arch A Path Anat Histol 385:1, 1979.
25. Kincaid-Smith P, Nicholls K: Mesangial IgA nephropathy. Am J Kidney Dis 3:90, 1983.
26. Tolkoff-Rubin NE, Cosimi AB, Fuller T, et al: IgA nephropathy in HLA-identical siblings. Transplantation 26:430, 1978.
27. Sabatier JC, Genin C, Assenat H, et al: Mesangial IgA-glomerulonephritis in HLA-identical brothers. Clin Nephrol 11:35,1979.
28. Noël LH, Descamps B, Jungers P, et al: HLA antigen in three types of glomerulonephritis. Clin Immunol Immunopath 10:19, 1978.
29. Whitworth JA, Kincaid-Smith PS, Fairley KF: The outcome of pregnancy in mesangial IgA nephropathy. In Sammour MB, et al (eds): Pregnancy Hypertension. Abbasiah, Cairo, Ain Shams University Press, 1982, p 403.
30. Feiner HD, Cabili S, Baldwin DS, et al: Intrarenal vascular sclerosis in IgA nephropathy. Clin Nephrol 18:183, 1982.
31. Falk RJ, Dalmasso AP, Kim Y, et al: Neoantigen of the polymerized ninth component of complement. Characterization of a monoclonal antibody and immunohistochemical localization in renal disease. J Clin Invest 72:560, 1983.

32. Fracsa GM, Vangelista A, Biagini G, et al: Immunological tubulo-interstitial deposits in IgA nephropathy. Kidney Intl 22:184, 1982.
33. Baart de la Faille-Kuyper EH, Kater L, Kuijten RH, et al: Occurrence of vascular IgA deposits in clinically normal skin of patients with renal disease. Kidney Intl 9:424, 1976.
34. Tsai CC, Giangiacomo J, Zuckner J: Dermal IgA deposits in Henoch-Schönlein purpura and Berger's nephritis. Lancet 1:342, 1975.
35. Tomino Y, Nomoto Y, Endoh M, et al: Deposition of IgA-dominant immune-complexes in muscular vessels from patients with IgA nephropathy. Acta Pathol Jpn 31:361, 1981.
36. Urizar RE, Michael AF, Sisson S, et al: Anaphylactoid purpura. II. Immunofluorescent and electron microscopic studies of the glomerular lesion. Lab Invest 19:437, 1968.
37. Dysart NK, Sisson S, Vernier RL: Immunoelectron microscopy of IgA nephropathy. Clin Immunol Immunopath 29:254, 1983.
38. Clarkson AR, et al: IgA nephropathy, In Massry SG, Glassock RJ (eds): Textbook of Nephrology. Baltimore, Williams and Wilkins, 1983, p 6 56.
39. Clarkson AR, Seymour AE, Woodroffe AJ, et al: Controlled trial of phenytoin therapy in IgA nephropathy. Clin Nephrol 13:215, 1980.
40. Modéer T, Tomson G, Falk O, et al: Phenytoin and IgA concentrations in plasma and saliva in epileptic children. Acta Paediatr Scand 70:373, 1981.
41. Lopez Trascasa M, Egido J, Sancho J, et al: IgA glomerulonephritis (Berger's disease): Evidence of high serum levels of polymeric IgA. Clin Exp Immunol 42:247, 1980.
42. Coppo R, Basolo B, Bulzomi MR, et al: Ineffectiveness of phenytoin treatment on IgA-containing circulating immune complexes in IgA nephropathy. Nephron 36:275, 1984.
43. Mustonen J, Pasternack A, Rantala I: The nephrotic syndrome in IgA glomerulonephritis: Response to corticosteroid therapy. Clin Nephrol 20:172, 1983.
44. Yang Y-J, Melvin T, Sibley R, et al: No evidence for a specific role of IgM in mesangial proliferation of idiopathic nephrotic syndrome. Kidney Intl 25:100, 1984.
45. Delacroix DL, Furtado-Barreira G, de Hemptinne B, et al: The liver in the IgA secretory immune system. Dogs, but not rats and rabbits, are suitable models for human studies. Hepatology 3:980, 1983.
46. Woodroffe AJ, Gormly AA, McKenzie PE, et al: Immunologic studies in IgA nephropathy. Kidney Intl 18:366, 1980.
47. Coppo R, Basolo B, Martina G, et al: Circulating immune complexes containing IgA, IgG and IgM in patients with primary IgA nephropathy and with Henoch-Schoenlein nephritis. Correlation with clinical and histologic signs of activity. Clin Nephrol 18:230, 1982.
48. Valentijn RM, Kauffmann RH, De La Riviere GB, et al: Presence of circulating macromolecular IgA in patients with hematuria due to primary IgA nephropathy. Am J Med 74:375, 1983.
49. Whitworth JA, Leibowitz S, Kennedy MC, et al: IgA and glomerular disease. Clin Nephrol 5:33, 1976.
50. Delacroix DL, Elkon KB, Geubel AP, et al: Changes in size, subclass, and metabolic properties of serum immunoglobulin A in liver diseases and in other diseases with high serum immunoglobulin A. J Clin Invest 71:358, 1983.
51. Tomasi TB, Grey HM: Structure and function of immunoglobulin A. Progr Allergy 16:81, 1972.
52. Desgeorges PT, Despont JP, Dechelette E, et al: Biochemic study of serum IgA of three patients with mesangial IgA deposits associated glomerulonephritis (Berger's disease). Kidney Intl 12:152A, 1977.
53. Lesavre PH, Digeon M, Bach JF: Analysis of circulating IgA and detection of immune complexes in primary IgA nephropathy. Clin Exp Immunol 48:61, 1982.
54. Chandy KG, Hübscher SG, Elias E, et al: Dual role of the liver in regulating circulating polymeric IgA in man: Studies on patients with liver disease. Clin Exp Immunol 52:207, 1983.
55. Egido J, Blasco R, Sancho J, et al: Increased rates of polymeric IgA synthesis by circulating lymphoid cells in IgA mesangial glomerulonephritis. Clin Exp Immunol 47:309, 1982.
56. Kutteh WH, Koopman WJ, Conley ME, et al: Production of predominantly polymeric IgA by human peripheral blood lymphocytes stimulated in vitro with mitogens. J Exp Med 152:1424, 1980.
57. Conley ME, Cooper M, Michael AF: Selective deposition of immunoglobulin A1 in immunoglobulin A nephropathy, anaphylactoid purpura nephritis, and systemic lupus erythematosus. J Clin Invest 66:1432, 1980.
58. Tomino Y, Endoh M, Nomoto Y, et al: Immunoglobulin A1 in IgA nephropathy. N Engl J Med 305:1159, 1981.
59. Sakai H, Nomoto Y, Arimori S, et al: Increase of IgA-bearing peripheral blood lymphocytes in families of patients with IgA nephropathy. Am J Clin Pathol 72:452, 1979.
60. Cosio FG, Lam S, Folami AO, et al: Immune regulation of immunoglobulin production in IgA-nephropathy. Clin Immunol Immunopath 23:403, 1982.
61. Fiorini G, Fornasieri A, Sinico R, et al: Lymphocyte populations in the peripheral blood from patients with IgA nephropathy. Nephron 31:354, 1982.
62. Doi T, Kanatsu K, Sekita K, et al: Circulating immune complexes of IgG, IgA, and IgM classes in various glomerular diseases. Nephron 32:335, 1982.
63. Kanatsu K, Doi T, Sekita K, et al: A comparative immunologic study of IgA nephropathy. Am J Kidney Dis 2:618, 1983.
64. Imai H, Nakamoto Y, Miki K, et al: Pseudothrombocytopenia and IgA-related platelet agglutinin in a patient with IgA nephritis. Nephron 34:154, 1983.
65. Nomoto Y, Sakai H: Cold-reacting antinuclear factor in sera from patients with IgA nephropathy. J Lab Clin Med 94:76, 1979.
66. Wyatt RJ, Julian BA, Galla HJ: Properdin deficiency with IgA nephropathy. N Engl J Med 305:1097, 1981.
67. Julian BA, Wyatt RJ, McMorrow RG, et al: Serum complement proteins in IgA nephropathy. Clin Nephrol 20:251, 1983.
68. Friend PS, Yunis EJ, Noreen HJ, et al: B lymphocyte determinants in immunoglobulin A nephropathy. J Immunol 123:2182, 1979.
69. Bene M-C, Faure G, Duheille J: IgA nephropathy: Characterization of the polymeric nature of mesangial deposits by in vitro binding of free secretory component. Clin Exp Immunol 47:527, 1982.
70. Tomino Y, Sakai H, Endoh M, et al: Cross-reactivity of eluted antibodies from renal tissues of patients with Henoch-Schönlein purpura nephritis and IgA nephropathy. Am J Nephrol 3:315, 1983.
71. Bene MC, Faure G, Hurault de Ligny B, et al: Immunoglobulin A nephropathy: Quantitative immunohistomorphometry of the tonsillar plasma cells evidences an inversion of the immunoglobulin A versus immunoglobulin G secreting cell balance. J Clin Invest 71:1342, 1983.
72. Egido J, Sancho J, Lorente F, et al: Inhibition of neutrophil migration by serum IgA from patients with IgA nephropathy. Clin Exp Immunol 49:709, 1982.
73. Sato M, Kinugassa E, Ideura T, et al: Phagocytic activity of polymorphonuclear leukocytes in patients with IgA nephropathy. Clin Nephrol 19:166, 1983.
74. Sancho J, Egido J, Rivera F, et al: Delayed clearance of specific polymeric IgA immune complexes in patients with IgA nephropathy. Kidney Intl 24:424A, 1983.
75. Egido J, Blasco R, Sancho J, et al: T-cell dysfunctions in IgA nephropathy: Specific abnormalities in the regulation of IgA synthesis. Clin Immunol Immunopath 26:201, 1983.
76. Chatenoud L, Bach M-A: Abnormalities of T-cell subsets in glomerulonephritis and systemic lupus erythematosus. Kidney Intl 20:267, 1981.
77. Sakai H, Endoh M, Tomino Y, et al: Increase of IgA specific helper T cells in patients with IgA nephropathy. Clin Exp Immunol 50:77, 1982.
78. Adachi M, Yodoi J, Masuda T, et al: Altered expression of lymphocyte Fc receptor in selective IgA deficiency and IgA nephropathy. J Immunol 131:1246, 1983.
79. Cagnoli L, Tabacchi P, Pasquali S, et al: T cell subset alterations in idiopathic glomerulonephritis. Clin Exp Immunol 50:70, 1982.
80. Bakker WW, Beukhof JR, van Luijk WHJ, et al: Vascular permeability increasing factor (VPF) in IgA nephropathy. Clin Nephrol 18:165, 1982.
81. Berthoux FC, Gagne A, Sabatier JC, et al: HLA-Bw35 and mesangial IgA glomerulonephritis. N Engl J Med 298:1034, 1978.
82. Fauchet R, Gueguen M, Genetet B, et al: HLA-DR antigen and IgA nephropathy (Berger's disease). N Engl J Med 302:1033, 1980.
83. Bignon JD, Houssin A, Soulillou JP, et al: HLA antigens and Berger's disease. Tissue Antigens 16:108, 1980.
84. Arnaiz-Villena A, Gonzalo A, Mampaso F, et al: HLA and IgA nephropathy in Spanish population. Tissue Antigens 17:549, 1981.
85. Rifai A, Small PA Jr, Teague PO, et al: Experimental IgA nephropathy. J Exp Med 150:1161, 1979.
86. Gormly AA, Smith PS, Seymour AE, et al: IgA glomerular deposits in experimental cirrhosis. Am J Pathol 104:50, 1981
87. Melvin T, Burke B, Michael AF, et al: Experimental IgA nephropathy in bile duct ligated rats. Clin Immunol Immunopath 27:369, 1983.
88. Delacroix DL, Hodgson HJF, McPherson A, et al: Selective transport of polymeric immunoglobulin A in bile. J Clin Invest 70:230, 1982.
89. Isaacs K, Miller F, Lane B: Experimental model for IgA nephropathy. Clin Immunol Immunpath 20:419, 1981.
90. Isaacs KL, Miller F: Role of antigen size and charge in immune complex glomerulonephritis. Lab Invest 47:198, 1982.
91. Emancipator SN, Gallo GR, Lamm ME: Experimental IgA nephropathy induced by oral immunization. J Exp Med 157:572, 1983.
92. Kanayama Y, Shiota K, Kotumi K, et al: Mycoplasma pneumoniae pneumonia associated with IgA nephropathy. Scand J Infect Dis 14:231, 1982.
93. Nash H, Binns GF, Clarkson AR, et al: Concomitant IgA nephropathy and cyclical neutropaenia. Aust N Z J Med 8:184, 1978.
94. Ramirez G, Stinson JB, Zawada ET, et al: IgA nephritis associated with mycosis fungoides. Report of two cases. Arch Intern Med 141:1287, 1981.

95. Valles M, Cantarell C, Fort J, et al: IgA nephropathy in leprosy. Arch Intern Med 142:1238, 1982.
96. Nomoto Y, Sakai H, Endoh M, et al: Scleritis and IgA nephropathy. Arch Intern Med 140:785, 1980.
97. Jennette JC, Ferguson AL, Moore MA, et al: IgA nephropathy associated with seronegative spondylarthropathies. Arthr Rheum 125:144, 1982.
98. Roy PL, Fish AJ, Vernier RL, et al: Recurrent macroscopic hematuria, focal nephritis, and mesangial deposition of immunoglobulin and complement. J Pediatr 82:767, 1973.
99. Weiss JH, Bhathena DB, Curtis JJ, et al: A possible relationship between Henoch-Schönlein syndrome and IgA nephropathy (Berger's disease). Nephron 22:582, 1978.
100. Baliah T, Kim KH, Anthone S, et al: Recurrence of Henoch-Schönlein purpura glomerulonephritis in transplanted kidneys. Transplantation 18:343, 1974.

26E Primary (Idiopathic) Nephrotic Syndrome

ROBERT L. VERNIER.

The preceding chapters and other sections that follow indicate that a nephrotic syndrome may occur in association with a larger number of distinct diseases and with varied renal pathology. The primary (idiopathic) nephrotic syndrome is, however, the major category of nephrotic syndrome occurring in children. The terminology that has been applied to this syndrome over the years has been and remains unsatisfactory; doubtless a reflection of our continued poor understanding of the fundamental etiology and the pathogenesis of the disease(s). A long list of terms, including lipoid nephrosis, childhood nephrosis, idiopathic nephrotic syndrome, minimal change-nephrotic syndrome (MCNS), nil disease, foot process disease, and steroid responsive nephrotic syndrome, has been used to describe the syndrome. Primary has the virtue of indicating "principle cause" and will suffice until improved understanding evolves. The term implies exclusion of all cases of nephrotic syndrome associated with systemic disease. However, this discussion will include children with nephrotic syndrome and histologically documented glomerular disease, including the various forms of glomerulonephritis described elsewhere, and those with biopsy proven, or assumed, minimal glomerular changes and variants.

Incidence and Prevalence

Age and Sex

Estimates of the annual incidence of the nephrotic syndrome (all forms) in children less than 16 years of age vary from 2 to 7 cases per 100,000. Schlesinger and coworkers (1) surveyed the total population (1 million) of Erie County, New York, between 1946 and 1961 and found an incidence of 2.0 and a cumulative prevalence, for that 16 year period, of 15.7 cases per 100,000 children under 16 years of age. Since about 80% of children with nephrotic syndrome have minimal glomerular abnormalities when renal biopsy is obtained, the incidence and prevalence of this condition in children under 16 years of age are about 1.6 and 13 per 100,000, respectively.

The primary nephrotic syndrome is predominantly a disease of young children. Prospective data collected by the International Study of Kidney Disease in Children (ISKDC) (2), demonstrated that 60% of children with minimal change nephrotic syndrome (MCNS) were 2 to 6 years of age. The disease is uncommon under the age of one year and decreasingly common after the age of 10 years, but has been described in old persons. Data from Cameron and coworkers (3) indicate that, whereas MCNS is found in 80% to 85% of young children with nephrotic syndrome, it accounts for only 15% to 20% of adult cases. Age, thus, becomes an important factor in the differential diagnosis of the nephrotic syndrome in a given patient. Because of this striking difference in incidence of MCNS at different ages, a histological diagnosis is usually advisable in the management of older children and adults with nephrotic syndrome.

In most large series of children with nephrotic syndrome, the ratio of males to females is about 2:1 (4, 5). It is interesting, and unexplained, that this male predominance seems to disappear in older children and adults, where the sex ratio is about 1:1 (3).

Genetic Considerations

Familial Incidence

Familial cases of the primary nephrotic syndrome occur more frequently than can be explained by chance. White (6) found affected siblings in 3.5% of patients in a survey of European centers, and Habib and Kleinknecht (5) reported that 3.3% of their 209 patients had affected siblings. Affected relatives in other generations are uncommon, but an occasional family in which one of the parents had nephrotic syndrome has been described. A number of cases in monozygotic twins, but not in dizygotic twins, have been described by Norio (7). The disease has been remarkably concordant with regard to age of onset and course in all sets of twins thus described. Norio argues that the absence of affected dizygotic twins suggests that undefined genetic rather than environmental factors are operating, since, if environmental factors were responsible, the number of affected dizygotic twins would be expected to be twice that of the incidence in monozygotic twins, since dizygotic twins are twice as common.

An increased frequency of HLA-B12 and HLA-A1/B8 have been described in several series of patients with MCNS and atopy, but has not been confirmed in other studies (8, 9). More recently a strong association of HLA-DR7 was described (10) in patients with MCNS and atopy, but further studies will be required to assess the full significance of this genetic marker.

The association of MCNS with specific atopic diseases (hay fever, asthma, and eczema) has been discussed for many years. Meadows and Sarsfield (8) have recently evaluated the clinical and selected immunological parameters in 84 children with steroid responsive nephrotic syndrome. They found an increased incidence of atopy in affected children and their first degree relatives as compared to controls and an increased incidence of positive skin tests to common antigens (e.g., house dust). Therapeutic attempts to modify the course of the disease by avoidance of sensitization to allergens were, however, unsuccessful. This controversy continues since Scharer and coworkers (9), in a study of 42 patients with MCNS, were unable to show an increased incidence of atopy, an increase in either total or allergen specific IgE, or the incidence of positive skin tests to common allergens.

Clinical Presentation

The initial clinical manifestations of the nephrotic syndrome in the vast majority of children is the appearance of edema. Infrequently, asymptomatic proteinuria may represent the prodrome and allow early discovery. It is known that some children have proteinuria for 1 to 2 months before edema becomes apparent. The edema is dependent and is expressed as puffy eyes in the morning and as swelling of the feet and legs during the day. In the early phases of the disease, the edema may fluctuate in degree and may completely disappear, to return as the disease progresses. Generalized edema, marked weight gain, ascites, and pleural effusions (anasarca) are common consequences of this progression.

Usually the child does not appear to be ill in the early stages of the disease. About one-half of children or their parents recall an upper respiratory infection that occurred before the onset of edema. Rarely the onset follows immunizations or allergic reactions, but the true significance of these preceding events is unknown. With generalized edema, abdominal pain, vomiting, or diarrhea are relatively common complaints.

The abnormal physical findings relate to the extent of edema. With anasarca and abdominal distention, respiratory distress, umbilical and inguinal hernias, and rectal prolapse may be seen. Blood pressure is usually normal in MCNS, but hypertension (>98% for age) has been described in 6% to 13% of patients in several large series (2, 4, 5). Persistent hypertension is uncommon and suggests that a histological lesion other than MCNS may be present.

Laboratory Findings

In addition to edema, the nephrotic syndrome is characterized by proteinuria (often massive), hypoproteinemia, and hyperlipidemia.

Proteinuria

Increased excretion of protein in the urine is the principal abnormality of the nephrotic syndrome and the most important diagnostic laboratory finding in the subsequent follow-up of the patient. The rate of excretion usually considered diagnostic is greater than 3 gm/1.73M^2 SA per 24 hours (see chapter 19 for discussion of normal values). For standardization, diagnostic values have been expressed as greater than 50 mg/kg/24 hrs (5) and greater than 40 mg/hr m^2 (2). However, much higher excretion rates, often exceeding 5 gm/24 hrs in very young children, are common at the time of clinical presentation. These values usually result in a "4$^+$" reading by the "Albustix®" or similar "dipstick" methods for qualitative protein excretion.

The proteinuria seen in the primary nephrotic syndrome of childhood is usually highly selective, and the urine contains a high percentage of plasma albumin. However, depending on the methods used and the series studied, the incidence of highly selective proteinuria (Chapter 19) has varied among series of patients with histologically defined MCNS from 53% to 95% (2, 11). The recent application of methods for the measurement of specific serum albumin in urine, such as radial immunodiffusion sensitive to 4 mg/100 ml, demonstrated that albuminuria could not be detected in normal adult subjects, whereas adults with MCNS excreted 250 μg albumin/minute (12). It is clear that the primary pathophysiological disturbance in MCNS is an increased permeability of the glomerular capillary wall to plasma proteins, principally serum albumin.

The observation of lipid and protein droplets in renal tubular cells in autopsy specimens by Muller (13), in the presence of well-preserved glomeruli, leads to the concept that some patients with nephrotic syndrome had a degenerative disease of the tubules or nephrosis, later termed lipoid nephrosis. It is important that we now discard this terminology, since abundant evidence exists that the tubular changes regularly seen in tissue from patients with the primary nephrotic syndrome of childhood (MCNS) are secondary to proteinuria and a glomerular leak. All available evidence indicates that the renal tubules are maximally absorbing protein in the average patient, and there is no evidence that the proteinuria seen in this disease reflects a failure of tubular reabsorption of protein.

Serum proteins

Hypoalbuminemia is another of the major characteristics of the nephrotic syndrome. Relatively severe hypoalbuminemia, <2 g/dl was noted in 91% and <1 g/dl in 38% of 136 children in one series of children (5). The level often considered essential for diagnosis is <2.5 g/dl. A decreased alpha-1 globulin, a relative or absolute increase in alpha-2 globulins, beta globulins, and fibrinogen are also typically noted. The increase in high molecular weight proteins, such as alpha-2 macroglobulin, is believed to result from selective retention of these large molecules, since normal rates of synthesis have been demonstrated (14).

Elevated levels of IgM have been recognized for some time in the primary nephrotic syndrome, but persistence of high levels during long-standing remissions has been emphasized by Giangiacomo and coworkers (15). These authors suggested that elevated levels of IgM might reflect an abnormality of T cell function that regulates conversion of IgM synthesis to IgG synthesis and persistence of accelerated IgM production during the remission of nephrotic syndrome.

The level of serum albumin reflects the sum of the rate of synthesis, the catabolic rate, and the rate of loss via the urine, gut, and perhaps tears and other secretions. It has been shown that increased synthesis of albumin is present in most nephrotic patients, but the increase in synthesis is not sufficient to maintain normal levels (16). An increased catabolism of albumin, in part by renal tubular cells, has been described

(17, 18), but remains somewhat controversial. Although significant gastrointestinal losses of serum albumin in the nephrotic syndrome have been described by several investigators, using various methods, recent studies using CR^{51}-albumin indicate that patients with MCNS have insignificant losses, whereas nephrotic patients with other glomerulopathy have significant fecal losses, comparable to those seen in patients with gastrointestinal disorders (19).

Even though hypoalbuminemia is regularly present in nephrotic children, there is no consistent relationship between the level of serum albumin, the degree of lowering of plasma blood volume, or the extent of edema. The controversy concerning blood volume in nephrotic children was emphasized by Oliver's early sequential studies (20) of 22 children with steroid responsive nephrotic syndrome, in whom only 4 showed an increase in blood volume after disappearance of the nephrotic syndrome. It now seems clear that many patients with the syndrome including some children have normal or even elevated blood volumes (21). The assumption of low plasma and blood volumes in nephrotic syndrome is logical, based upon Starling's hypothesis, and is consistent with the observed increase in renin activity, aldosterone production, and fluid retention. However, many observations fail to support this concept. These issues remain controversial, in part, because of differing methods for measurement and calculation of blood volume. It is also probable that other ill-defined volume regulating factors are involved.

For example, a recent study of patients with nephrotic syndrome, including some children, demonstrated a sustained volume mediated secretion of antidiuretic hormone, and a disturbance in this regulator was proposed as a responsible mechanism for the impaired water secretion in this disease (22). Recent studies by Bohlin and Bert (23) of 23 children with MCNS evaluated the handling of infused sodium in this population. They confirmed that edematous patients (but not proteinuric patients in a steady state) had a profound inability to excrete sodium. Because of the results of hypertonic albumin infusions and the response to furosemide, they concluded that these patients have a defect in sodium excretion, which is independent of aldosterone and involves the distal nephron, perhaps the collecting duct, as suggested by Ichikawa and coworkers (24). Further discussion of the mechanisms of edema in nephrotic children occurs in Chapter 6B.

Hyperlipidemia

Elevation of serum cholesterol, triglycerides, and total lipids, including low density lipoproteins (LDL) and very low density lipoproteins (VLDL), are a constant feature of the primary nephrotic syndrome of childhood. The serum cholesterol exceeded 400 mg% at diagnosis in two-thirds of the 398 children with MCNS described in the ISKDC study (2). The level of serum cholesterol is inversely related to the level of serum albumin in most children. The mechanism of the hyperlipidemia is complex and poorly understood. Urinary losses of albumin and of a heparin-like substance responsible for clearing of lipids are thought to be important. Increased hepatic synthesis of lipids and lipoproteins has also been demonstrated (25), and the activity of lipoprotein lipase has been shown to be decreased (26) in the nephrotic patients. Since the nephrotic syndrome is primarily a disorder of protein metabolism, it is not surprising that major disturbances of the lipoprotein carriers of lipids are also responsible for the hyperlipidemia. High levels of LDL and VLDL have been consistently noted in nephrotic plasma, but high density lipoprotein (HDL) levels are usually normal, and may be low, presumably as a consequence of urinary loss of this molecule, which has a molecular size similar to plasma albumin. It is of interest that elevated levels of serum cholesterol may persist long after the serum albumin concentration and urinary protein excretion have returned to normal (27). The persistence of serum lipid abnormalities may imply an increased risk of premature atherosclerosis in these children.

Renal Function

The glomerular filtration rate (GFR), as estimated by inulin or creatinine clearances, or level of serum creatinine level corrected for age and sex, is normal in the majority of children with primary nephrotic syndrome. However, both elevated and depressed levels may be seen in patients with histological minimal change disease. About 25% of children with MCNS have increased function (in excess of the 98th percentile) and about 30% have levels that are abnormally low at diagnosis (2). Decreased levels of renal function are often transient and probably reflect poor renal perfusion and hypovolemia. Persistent elevation of serum creatinine or reduced clearance should suggest the possibility of a glomerular lesion other than MCNS. Maximal concentrating ability and acidification are also normal in MCNS. Aminoaciduria, bicarbonateuria, and glycosuria occur in a rare child with massive proteinuria and MCNS, but these abnormalities of tubular function should raise the question of another lesion, such as focal segmental glomerulosclerosis, in which tubulointerstitial lesions are also present (28).

New insights into the alterations of renal function and glomerular permeability characteristic of the primary nephrotic syndrome have been provided by Robson and coworkers (29). These authors have measured the glomerular clearance and urinary excretion (permselectivity) of polyvinylpyrrolidone (PVP) in normal and nephrotic children. They have shown in normal children that when the molecular radius of each fraction of inert PVP is plotted against the clearance (simultaneously determined inulin clearance), small molecules have high clearances and larger PVP molecules are virtually excluded from the urine (Fig. 26E.1). Surprisingly, in nephrotic children, the relative clearance of PVP molecules equivalent in size to albumin (about 35 A radius) was not increased but rather decreased (Fig. 26E.1). In fact, the relative clearance of all PVP molecules with a radius of 35 A or less was decreased in nephrotic children. It was proposed that these findings were best explained by losses of the anionic charges in the glomerular basement membrane in the primary nephrotic syndrome, and numerous subsequent studies, which will be discussed later, support this interpretation.

Urine Sediment

In addition to protein, hyaline, granular, and cellular casts are usually found in the urine of nephrotic patients. Free lipids, doubly refractile bodies containing cholesterol, and fatty casts are also present, often in large numbers. Neither the quantity nor the quality of urinary casts or lipids are predictive of the type of histological lesion present in a child with nephrotic syndrome, nor do these features predict the future course of the patient. Microscopic hematuria has long been regarded as a useful differential laboratory sign, predictive of histology and outcome. However, in the ISKDC study about 25% of children with proved MCNS had significant hematuria at the time of diagnosis (2), and hematuria was not found to be a statistically useful predictor of outcome. Gross hematuria is, however, rare, occurring in only 1.4% of 406 cases (5). Since microscopic hematuria occurs in about 50% of patients with focal segmental glomerulosclerosis (2), persistence of this laboratory abnormality adds support for consideration of that pathologic lesion and the possible value of review of renal histology in a given patient.

Other Abnormalities of Serum and Urine

Clinical Consequences

Abnormal levels of many other serum factors occur in nephrotic patients and many of their clinical findings and complications are related to these abnormalities. It is clear that most of the pathophysiology of the nephrotic syndrome results from an abnormality of permeability of the glomerular capillaries and the leak into the urine of large amounts of

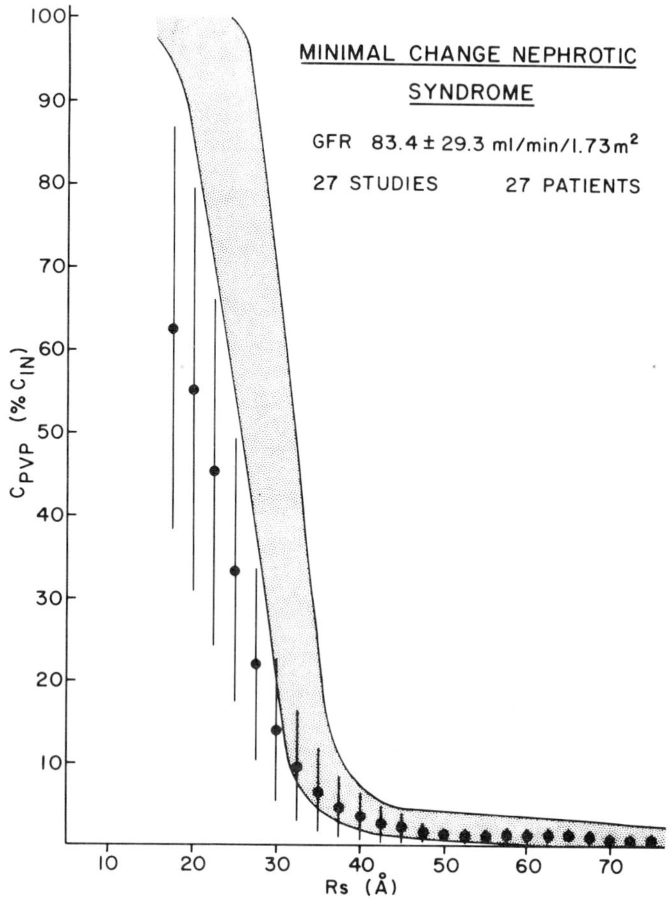

Figure 26E.1. The pattern of permselectivity to PVP observed in 27 untreated patients in relapse for MCNS. The shaded area represents the normal range of values observed in 6 healthy children; the values from the children with MCNS are depicted as the mean ± SD for each moiety of PVP shown. (Reproduced with permission from Robson AM, Cole BR: Pathologic and functional correlations in the glomerulopathies. Robson AM and Cole BR, In Cumings N, et al (eds): Immune Mechanisms in Renal Disease. New York, Plenum Medical Publishers, 1983, p 109.)

small molecular weight substances. It is useful to relate these phenomenon to the molecular weight of plasma albumin (≃68,000) and to appreciate that many of the other laboratory abnormalities are consequent to the loss into the urine of factors of similar low molecular weight (Table 26E.1). However, as we shall see, molecular weight is not the sole determinant of the permeability characteristics of a substance since glomerular clearance is also markedly influenced by the charge on the molecule. The recently recognized importance of molecular charge undoubtedly explains some of the inconsistencies of the permeability of various proteins that are involved in the pathophysiology and the complications of the nephrotic state.

Urinary Losses of Immunoproteins and Infections

Before the availability of antibiotic therapy, a high percentage of nephrotic children died of overwhelming infection involving primarily the peritoneal, pleural, and subcutaneous spaces, which became infected with pneumococci or hemolytic streptococci. Arneil's report (30) of a series of 164 children who were seen between 1929 and 1957 emphasizes the scale of the problem. Thirty-five deaths occurred in the first year of their disease and 28 of these were consequent to infection. In a 10-year follow-up from onset, infection was the principal cause of death, although renal failure became increasingly common in the later years of the study.

Table 26E.1.
Selected Serum Proteins Lost in the Urine in Nephrotic Syndrome and the Clinical Consequences

Protein	Molecular weight	Clinical consequences
Albumin	68,000	Hypoproteinemia, edema, abnormal binding of drugs, and others
Factor B	80,000 25,000	Infection, abnormalities of the alternative complement pathway
Vitamin D–binding globulin	59,000	Decreased Ca+ absorption, low ionized Ca+, osteoporosis
Thyroid-binding globulin	85,000	Functional hypothyroidism
Antithrombin III	68,000	hypercoagulability, thromboses
Factor XII	79,000	
Factor X	56,000	
Factor IX	55,000	

Complement Factors, IgG—Infection

The total hemolytic complement, C3 and C4, are normal in patients with the primary nephrotic syndrome. The low levels of C1q which have been described may reflect the loss of this protein in the urine (31). Factor B is a low molecular weight (≃80,000) protein, which is a component of the alternate pathway of complement activation (chapter 26B), critical for the opsonization of encapsulated bacteria, such as pneumococci and *E. Coli* in nonimmune individuals. McLean and coworkers (32) have shown that the plasma levels of Factor B are low in nephrotic children and that the levels of Factor B parallel the levels of plasma albumin. They also demonstrated that addition of Factor B to nephrotic plasma in vitro restored the opsonizing capacity of most nephrotic plasma and that levels of Factor B returned to normal during remission of the nephrotic syndrome. Presumably, Factor B is another of the important low molecular weight proteins that are lost in the urine in nephrotics, although urinary measurement of the factor has proved to be very difficult. A similar plasma deficiency of Factor D, another small molecular weight protein of the alternate pathway of complement, has been described (33).

It is well known that nephrotic children often have low levels of immunoglobulin G (IgG); occasionally the levels approach those of patients with Bruton's congenital agammaglobulinemia (34). Since IgG has a molecular weight of 168,000, the cause of the low levels is not believed to be urinary loss alone. There is also considerable evidence for both increased catabolism and for decreased synthesis of IgG in nephrotic patients; together these abnormalities probably explain the complex origin of low IgG levels in nephrotic patients.

Urinary Losses of Coagulation Factors, Hypercoagulability, and Thromboses

Thrombotic events are among the more serious complications occurring in nephrotic patients. Although earlier reports and speculations suggested that thrombosis of the renal veins might cause the nephrotic syndrome, the evidence now available indicates that the thromboses observed in various arteries and veins in these patients result from a hypercoagulable state that develops consequent to the nephrotic syndrome. The incidence of thromboses in nephrotic children was surveyed in European centers by Egli and coworkers (35) and of 3377 nephrotic children, 60 (1.8%) were reported to have had thromboembolic complications. Thrombosis of the inferior vena cava, renal veins, hepatic veins, pulmonary artery or pulmonary veins, femoral arteries, deep leg veins and arteries, and saggittal sinus have all been described in children with the primary nephrotic syndrome (36). In adults and older children in whom membranous nephropathy and membranoproliferative glomerulonephritis are more common, the propensity to renal vein clotting could be considered consequent to altered vascular endothelium and, in fact, the clinical incidence of renal vein thrombosis (RVT) in adults is between 5% and 10%. Asymptomatic but radiologically diagnosible clotting may be recognized in 20% to 30% of adult patients (37) and as many as 20% to 30% of adults with renal vein thrombosis develop pulmonary emboli, although the mortality rate is surprisingly low (0.5%) (37). As with adults, it is probable that thromboembolism occurs more commonly in children than is indicated by recognized clinical signs and symptoms and that RVT is an underdiagnosed problem with severe short-term and long-term consequences.

It has been recognized that hemoconcentration occurring in the renal venous blood, as a result of filtration of a portion of plasma water and high renal lymph flow, could explain the relatively high incidence of RVT. However, many additional abnormalities consequent to the nephrotic state clearly have an important role in predisposing nephrotic patients to thromboembolic complications in many vessels.

The nephrotic syndrome is characterized by profound changes in the turnover and concentrations of most plasma proteins (see previous section), including altered synthesis, turnover, and urinary losses of proteins involved in the initiation of both coagulation and fibrinolysis. Plasma fibrinogen (Factor I) is markedly increased in almost all nephrotics, probably as a consequence of increased synthesis. Excess of combined Factor VII and X, Factor VIII, and other clotting factors have also been described less consistently in nephrotic patients.

Perhaps of more importance are urinary losses of small molecular weight factors in the urine. Kauffman and coworkers (38) described low levels of plasma antithrombin III (ATIII) in nephrotic patients and demonstrated an association between plasma levels of this antithrombin factor, proteinuria, urinary losses of the protein, and plasma albumin levels. Urinary losses of both antithrombin III and plasminogen, with plasma deficiencies, have also been recognized in children with primary nephrotic syndrome (39). The decreased levels of plasminogen described are indicative of a disturbance of the fibrinolytic system and are supported by observations of deficiency of other anti-plasmin factors, such as alpha-1-antitrypsin in nephrotic patients.

Given the complexity of the disturbances of clotting and anticlotting factors described, can the propensity for thromboembolism be predicted in this disease? A recent report by Francis and coworkers (40) suggests that in adults, measurement of hematocrit, creatinine, fibrinogen, ATIII, plasminogen, and alpha 2 plasma inhibitor (α2P) levels may allow prediction of the risk of thrombosis. These authors found that elevations of fibrinogen, hematocrit, and α2P, combined with reductions of ATIII and plasminogen, predisposed to thrombosis, whereas elevations of creatinine were protective, presumably through the associated platelet dysfunction of uremia.

Renal Vein Thrombosis

The clinical syndrome of RVT may be associated with acute flank pain, renal enlargement, hematuria, unexplained deterioration of renal function, oliguria, and renal failure. However, as indicated earlier, clinical findings may be minimal and the diagnosis is often difficult to establish. The intravenous pyelogram (IVP) may show unilateral renal enlargement and "spindled" calyces because of edema of the kidney. The standard confirmatory test, venography, may be replaced by ultrasound or CT scanning, but these methods have not yet been established as superior methods.

Therapy of RVT and other thromboembolic complications of the nephrotic syndrome with anticoagulants, such as heparin, presents special problems in this disease because this highly negatively charged molecule binds to many proteins and alters their activity (chapter 15). The binding of heparin to ATIII, in the presence of low plasma levels of the latter, may theoretically have adverse effects so far as thrombin antagonism is concerned. Because of the many alterations of proteins found in the nephrotic state, stable and safe levels of anticoagulation are also difficult to achieve. Nevertheless, given the high risks of further complications, we believe that nephrotic patients with proved thrombosis should be anticoagulated until the nephrotic state remits, at which time all coagulation parameters return to normal. The observation of shortened platelet half-life in patients with focal segmental sclerosis and nephrotic syndrome and the reversal of this abnormality by antiplatelet drugs (dipyridamole) in adults (41) and children (42) may indicate the utility of combined use of antiplatelet (dipyridamole and aspirin) and anticoagulation therapy in patients with thromboembolism and nephrotic syndrome.

Thyroid Hormones and Thyroid Function

Decreased serum levels of protein-bound iodine and reduced basal metabolic rates have been recognized for many years. Current evidence suggests that the measured decreased levels of total thyroxine (T4) and total triiodothyronine (T3) found in many nephrotic patients with normal renal function reflect the loss into the urine of thyroid binding proteins or other carrier proteins, since a direct relationship between the level of these hormones and serum albumin has usually been found (43). The normal serum levels of free T4, normal thyroid-stimulating hormone (TSH) levels, and normal response of TSH levels to thyroid-releasing hormone, in most patients, also support this conclusion.

Vitamin D and Metabolites

Low plasma levels of 25 hydroxycholecalciferol (250HD$_2$) and vitamin D-binding globulin (VDBG) have been described in two series of nephrotic patients with normal renal function (44, 45). In addition, the urine of nephrotic patients contained large amounts of VDBG and injected radioactive cholecalciferol appeared in the urine of nephrotic patients as 250HD$_2$ bound to VDBG, but was not excreted by normal subjects. These findings explain the shortened half-life of 250HD$_2$ in nephrotic patients and may explain the abnormalities of mineralization of osteoid and borderline vitamin D deficiency described in occasional patients.

Pathogenesis of the Primary Nephrotic Syndrome

The cause of the primary nephrotic syndrome remains unknown. Current research focuses on numerous abnormalities of immune response that have been observed in nephrotic children for decades, including the apparent induction of relapse by exposure to inhaled allergens in rare patients, abnormalities of immunoglobulin synthesis by isolated mononuclear cells, and inhibition of lymphocyte responses to mitogens. Shalhoub (46) was among the first to outline a hypothesis that linked T cell dysfunction with MCNS. The hypothesis was derived from observations of decreased humoral antibody responses; the fact that remissions were often induced by infection with rubeola, which is known to modify cell-mediated immunity; the occurrence of MCNS in rare patients with Hodgkins disease; and the fact that drugs that modify lymphocytes and monocyte function, such as corticosteroids and alkalinating agents (cyclophosphamide and nitrogen mustard), often induced remission. Shalhoub concluded that production of a circulating chemical mediator toxic to an immunologically innocent glomerular basement membrane best explained the noted observations. Although numerous additional observations, including the frequent recurrence of nephrotic syndrome following renal transplantation and reappearance of pathologic lesions such as focal segmental glomerulosclerosis in the graft (47), support the existence of a circulating factor, the evidence (48, 49) is indirect and inconclusive.

Pathophysiology

Much of our current knowledge and ongoing research regarding the pathophysiology of the nephrotic syndrome derives from studies of experimental models of this disease. Histochemical studies of glomeruli from rats with nephrotic syndrome induced by the aminonucleoside of puromycin (PAN) were first shown to have many of the renal morphological and physiological features of MCNS. In 1970 it was shown by histochemical studies that rats with PAN had a partial loss of a highly negatively charged, sialic acid–rich substance (glomerular polyanion) that coated the glomerular epithelial cells (50). A functional basis for an electrostatic barrier to the glomerular filtration of macromolecules was firmly established in the rat by Brenner and associates (51) by the demonstration of a relatively reduced glomerular clearance of negatively charged dextran molecules, as compared with the clearance of neutrally charged molecules of the same size. Numerous cytochemical and biochemical studies (52) have demonstrated that major contributions to the electrostatic filtration barrier are provided by a network of heparan sulfate proteoglycan molecules distributed within the lamina rarae of glomerular basement membrane (GBM). These high molecular weight, negatively charged polysaccharide side chains of proteoglycans, apparently impede the filtration of negatively charged macromolecules, such as plasma albumin, which in the circulation have an isoelectric point (pI) of 5.1. Removal of heparan sulfate by enzyme digestion results in increased permeability of the GBM to albumin (53) and to larger molecules, such as ferritin (54).

Histochemical studies of patients with MCNS have demonstrated a decrease in staining of the glomerular polyanion (55). The previously discussed physiologic studies of Robson and coworkers (29) using polyvinyl pyrrolidone and more recent dextran clearance experiments by Carrie and coworkers (56) and others (57) strongly support an alteration of the electrostatic filtration barrier as the basis of the permeability abnormalities observed in the primary nephrotic syndrome in man.

Morphological studies of the glomerular electrostatic filtration barrier in normal man have revealed a remarkably orderly array of heparan sulfate proteolgycan charge sites distributed in the GBM in the low density region beneath the epithelial cells (lamina rara externa, LRE) and a less orderly array of sites in the lamina rara interna (LRI) adjacent to the endothelial cells (58) (Fig. 26E.2). Quantitative studies of these sites has revealed 23.8 ± 6.8 per 1000 nm of GMB length in the LRE of normal subjects of all ages. Preliminary studies of glomeruli from children with MCNS have demonstrated a normal number of anionic charge sites in the LRE of the GBM, but a 30% decrease in anionic sites within the LRI in this condition (59) (Fig. 26E.3).

The mechanism underlying the filtration barrier effects of heparan sulfate proteoglycans in the GBM remains uncertain. In addition to their negative charge, proteoglycans form highly viscous solutions and display complex interactions with virtually all of the other known constituents of the GBM, including the glycoproteins laminin, fibronectin, and GBM collagen. Recent studies of PAN nephrotic syndrome in rats suggest that the synthesis of heparan sulfate proteoglycan by nephrotic rats is increased twofold to threefold as compared to controls, and that failure of normal interaction of the proteoglycan with other GBM components to form the normal barrier may explain the permeability defect of that experimental model (60).

Pathology

As indicated in the introduction, the morphological changes found in patients presenting with the idiopathic nephrotic syndrome is highly variable and age related. In children the vast majority have minimal

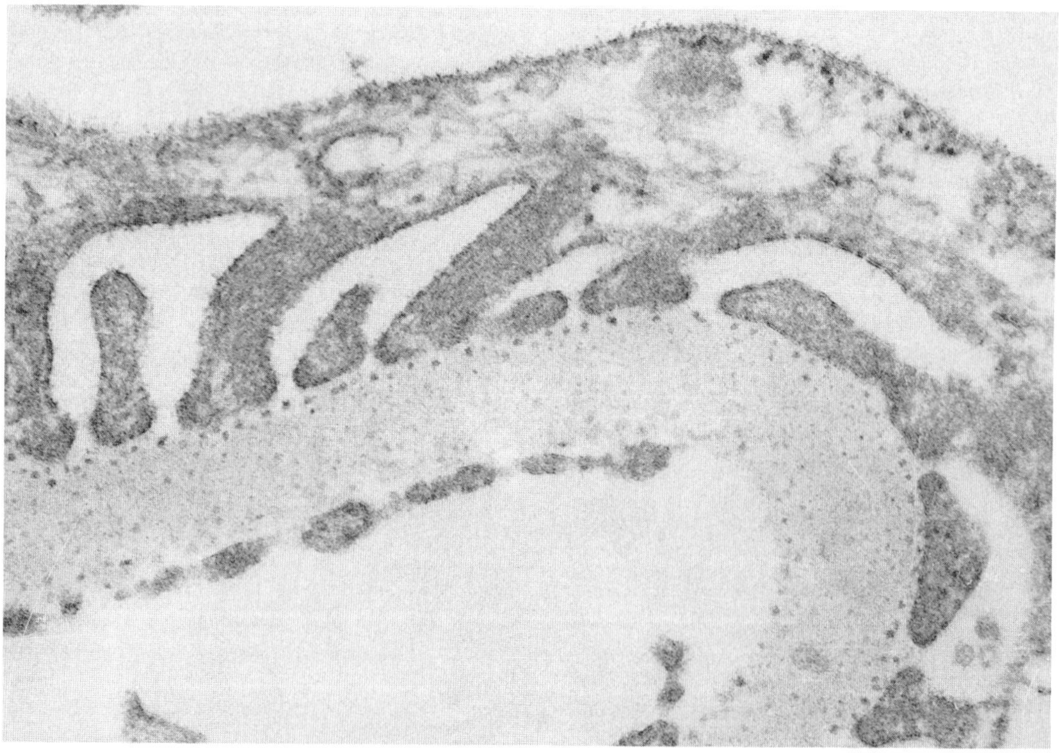

Figure 26E.2. Electron micrograph of a portion of glomerular capillary from a section of normal human kidney previously incubated in polyethyleneimine (PEI), 1200 MW, as processed as described in Vernier RL, et al: New Engl J Med 309:1001, 1983. An orderly array of punctate anionic sites, containing heparan sulfate, is labelled by the PEI within the LRE of the GBM. Less regularly distributed labelled sites are present within the lamina densa and the LRI. Note the normal epithelial cell and foot processes. (X47,500.)

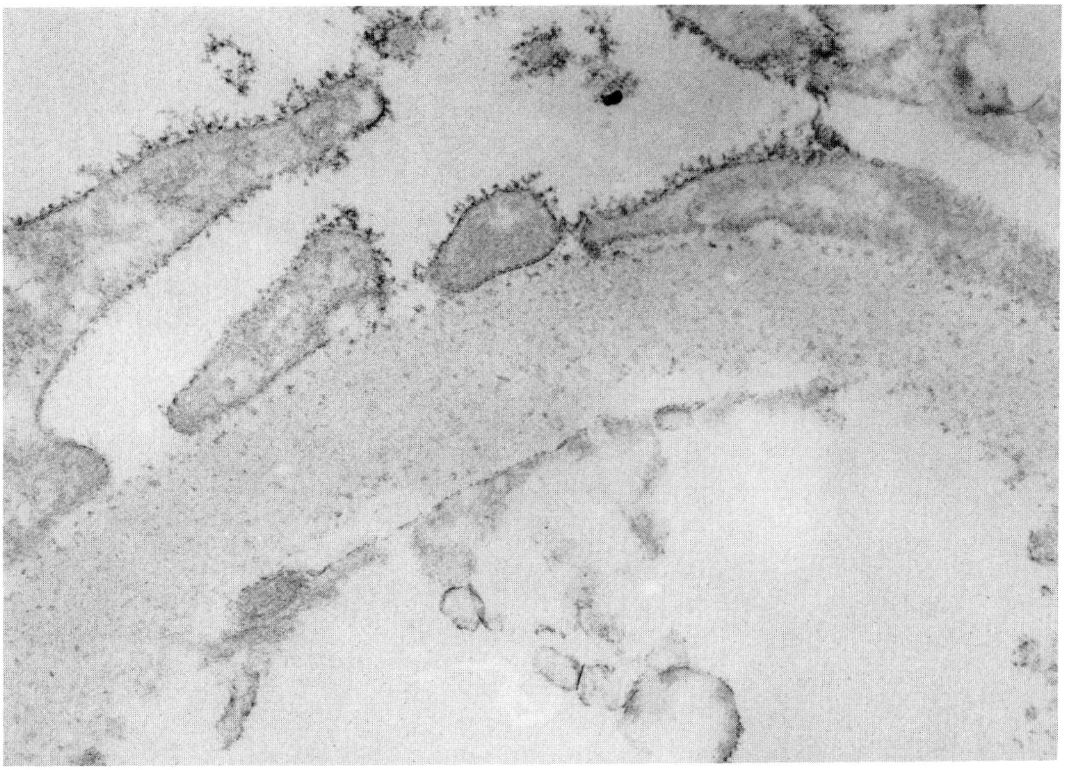

Figure 26E.3. Electron micrograph of a portion of a glomerular capillary in a section of kidney from a child with primary nephrotic syndrome, previously incubated with PEI, as indicated in Fig. 26E.2. A normal number of small punctate anionic sites labelled with PEI is distributed with the LRE. The number of labelled anionic sites within the lamina densa and the lamina rara interna is decreased, as compared to Fig. 26E.2. Note the absence of normal epithelial cell foot processes. (X47,700.)

glomerular changes (Table 26E.2). This lesion is defined as the absence of any conspicuous abnormalities by light microscopy, except for a slight and usually focal increase in number of mesangial cells and mesangial matrix. Variations in criteria for this diagnosis, allowed by some pathologists, include an occasional sclerotic glomerulus without associated tubular atrophy or with slight focal tubular atrophy. Approximately 85% of the 471 unselected children in the ISKDC study of pathology (61) demonstrated this lesion (Fig. 26E.4, *A*). The second most common lesion found in all series represents focal sclerosis, defined as glomerular sclerosis that has both a focal and segmental distribution and is associated with segmental glomerular hyalinosis, focal tubular atrophy, and interstitial inflammatory changes FSGS/H (Fig. 26E.4, *C*). The lesions may have great prognostic significance even when only one lesion is present in the biopsy specimen. Since the lesions apparently develop first in the deeper juxtamedullary glomeruli, the adequacy of the biopsy sample becomes important in establishing the pathological diagnosis. A third lesion observed less frequently, termed focal global sclerosis (FGS), consists of a totally scarred glomerulus. The significance of this lesion is debated, but most agree that more than when 5% or more of glomeruli show FGS, the therapeutic response of the patient may be altered. Mesangial proliferation, defined as three or more mesangial cells in most mesangial regions of many glomeruli (diffuse) (Fig. 26E.4, *B*), may be associated with FSGS/H and may also have independent prognostic significance.

Table 26E.2.
Incidence of Various Histological Lesions in Two Large Series of Children with Primary Nephrotic Syndrome

	Habib and Kleinknecht (310 patients)	ISKDC (471 patients unselected)
Minimal glomerular changes	67.4	84.5
Focal glomerulosclerosis	15.2	9.5
Segmental	11.3	7.5
Global	3.9	2.0
Mesangial proliferation	6.8	2.5
Other[a]	10.6	3.5

[a] Patients with unclassified lesions.

Immunofluorescence Microscopy

Immunohistochemical studies of kidney biopsy specimens in the idiopathic nephrotic syndrome do not demonstrate granular deposits of IgG or complement components along the glomerular capillaries; however, C3 and IgM are frequently present within the mesangium (Fig. 26E.5). The suggestion by several groups of investigators that mesangial deposits of IgM might predict steroid nonresponsiveness has not been supported by a recent retrospective review of 100 consecutive patients from our clinic (62) (Table 26E.3). Mesangial IgM was observed in glomeruli of 75% to 90% of patients in all of the histological categories discussed, and this finding was not useful in predicting steroid responsiveness or the eventual outcome. In that study, mesangial deposits of C3 were also common (77% to 90% of patients in each histological category) and were similarly not helpful in predicting results of therapy or outcome. Smaller percentages of patients demonstrated low intensity mesangial and linear capillary loop fluorescence patterns for IgG, IgA, and fibrin/fibrinogen, which were not significantly different from that seen in normal tissue.

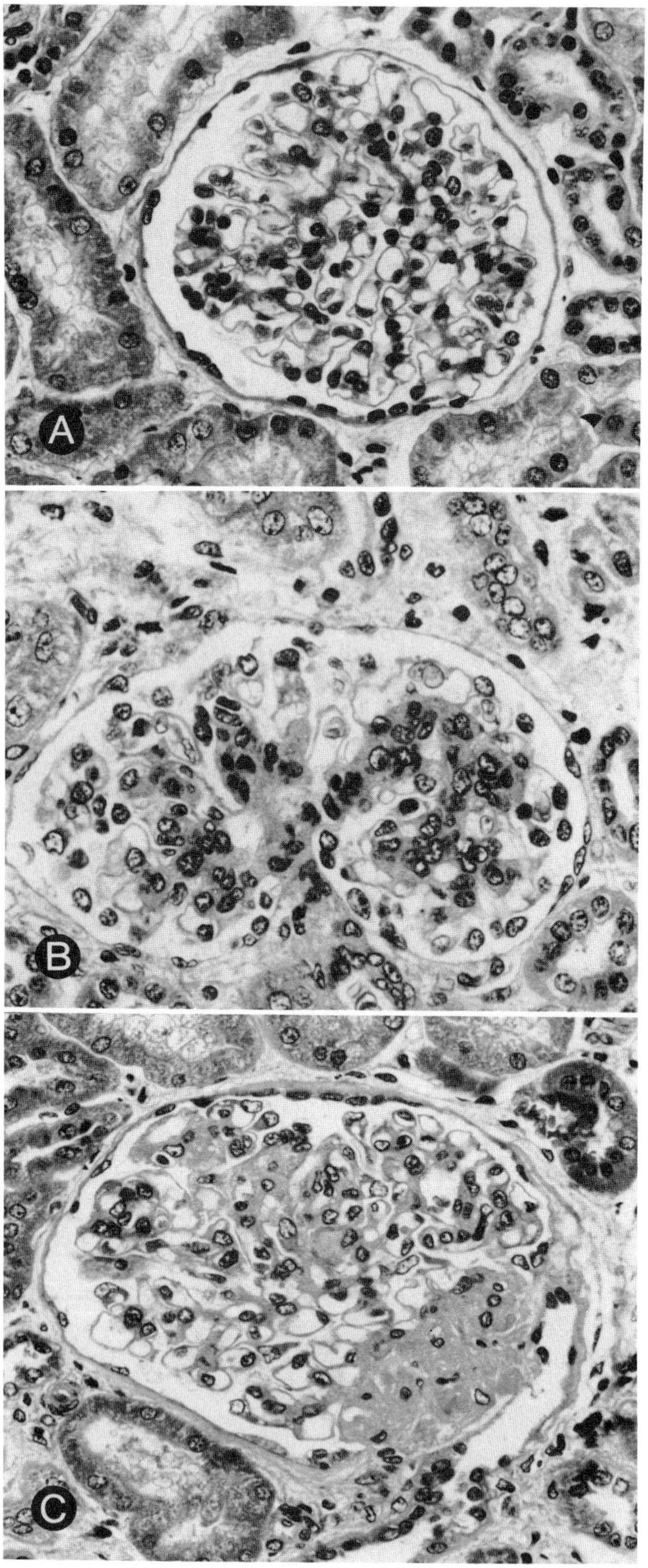

Figure 26E.4. Representative examples of the principle morphologic lesions found in children with primary nephrotic syndrome. **A**, Minimal lesion (<2 cells per mesangial zone). **B**, Mesangial proliferation (≥4 cells per mesangial zone). **C**, Focal segmental glomerulosclerosis. (Reproduced with permission from Melvin T, Sibley R, Michael AF: In Tune BM, Mendoza SA, Brenner BM, Stein JH (eds): Contemporary Issues in Nephrology. New York, Churchill-Livingstone, 1984, p 191.

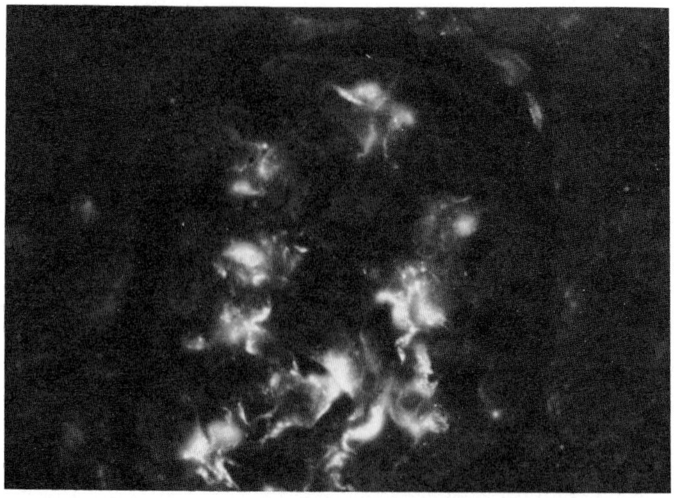

Figure 26E.5. Immunofluorescence micrograph of a glomerulus from a patient with primary nephrotic syndrome and mesangial proliferation showing distribution of IgM primarily within the mesangium. (X550.) (Reproduced with permission from Yang JY, et al: Kidney Intl 25:100, 1984.)

Table 26E.3.
Relationships Between Pathological Lesion, Presence of IgM in Glomeruli, and Initial Steroid Responsiveness in 100 Referred Patients with Primary Nephrotic Syndrome

	Pathological lesion (%)	Fluorescent microscopy IgM[a] (%)	Initially steroid responsive (%)
Minimal glomerular changes	38	89.5	94.7
Focal glomerulosclerosis			
Global	18	83.3	62
Segmental	23	85.9	23
Mesangial proliferation	12	75	45
Mesangial proliferation with focal segmental glomerulosclerosis	9	88.0	55

Adapted from Yang JY, et al: Kidney Intl 25:100, 1984.
[a] Trace to 3+ staining of glomeruli for IgM.

Electron Microscopy

In 1957 we first recognized the uniform association of extensive "fusion" or replacement of glomerular epithelial cell foot processes by a more or less continuous sheet of epithelial cytoplasm along the glomerular capillary walls in idiopathic nephrotic syndrome (63) (Fig. 26E.6). This ultrastructural abnormality remains the principal lesion seen in this condition. The extent of the foot-process lesion is correlated with the quality of protein excreted in various patients (64) and the foot-process lesion is reversible in that repeat biopsy specimens during remission have demonstrated return of the epithelial cell foot processes to a normal appearance. Variable degrees of mesangial proliferation and mesangial matrix expansion with associated electron-dense mesangial deposits are found in confirmation of similar mesangial lesions noted by light microscopy. Many nephrotic patients also demonstrate minimal widening of the lamina rara interna, but the lamina densa is typically normal and capillary loop oriented electron-dense deposits are unusual.

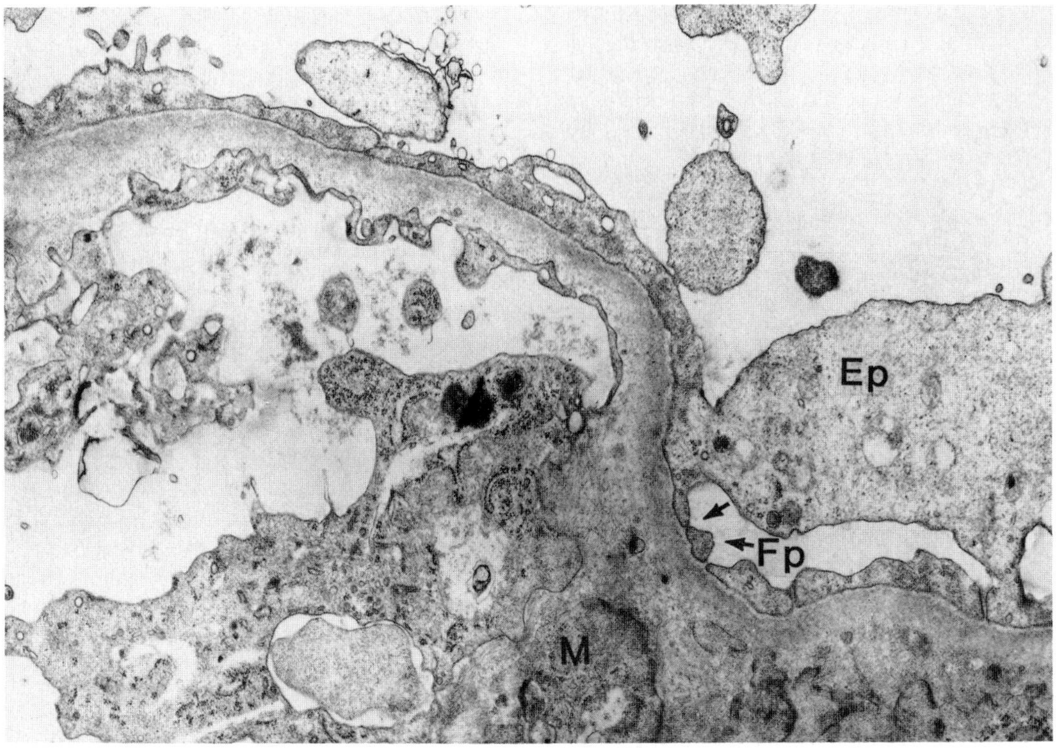

Figure 26E.6. Routine electron micrograph of a portion of a glomerulus from a child with primary nephrotic syndrome showing portions of the capillary walls and mesangium (*M*). The most striking abnormality is the nearly total coalescence of the epithelial cell (*Ep*) foot processes. Very few normal foot processes (*Fp*) and filtration slits (*arrows*) remain. (X12,500.)

Therapy and Clinical/Pathological Correlations of Therapy

Having established the diagnosis of nephrotic syndrome in a child, are there clinical characteristics of a given case that allow reasonably accurate prediction of the histopathology, the response to therapy, and ultimate outcome? These important questions were answered in the affirmative by a 1978 report of the ISKDC (2). This study compared the results of clinical-laboratory tests, renal biopsy specimens, and the response to initial treatment with prednisone in 521 children. The authors placed major emphasis on the recognition of patients in the principal diagnostic categories of MCNS, FSGS, and membranoproliferative glomerulonephritis (MPGN). It was found, for example, that 80% of patients with MCNS presented before age 6 years, whereas MPGN rarely presented before age 6 years (Fig. 26E.7). Serum levels of the complement component C3 was also confirmed to be a powerful test in discriminating between MPGN and both MCNS and FSGS, in which the levels were normal in the vast majority of patients, whereas the level was significantly low in 74% of patients with the pathology of MPGN. In fact, children with MCNS differed from those with MPGN in nearly every category tested, whereas patients with FSGS shared many features with MPGN, but had a higher frequency of hematuria and diastolic hypertension than patients with MCNS. The principal value of the multivariant analysis described in this study is the recognition of patients with MPGN who require a renal biopsy for definitive diagnosis and may be spared the risks of steroid therapy when this analysis is conducted before therapy (chapter 26B).

Having excluded the patients with MPGN by clinical analysis or renal biopsy, the subsequent response of the patients to a standard course of treatment with adrenocortical steroids has also been shown to have predictive value with regard to both the histopathology and the ultimate outcome (65). When response to therapy is defined as a 3 days or more

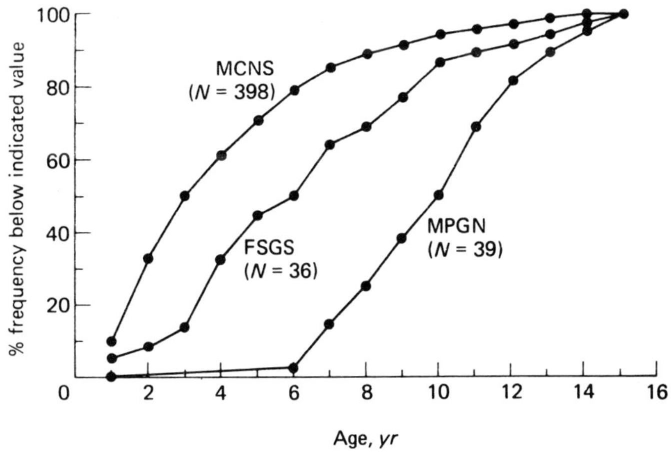

Figure 26E.7. Age at time of diagnosis of patients with MCNS, FSGS, and MPGN. Cumulative percentages are shown. Median values are MCNS—3 years, FSGS—6 years, and MPGN—10 years. (Reproduced with permission from International Study of Kidney Disease in Children: Kidney Intl 13:43, 1978.)

period of "protein free" urine (<1+ by Albustix® or <4 mg/hr/m² SA), it was found that 95% of patients with MCNS responded, whereas the response rates in patients with FSGS/H, FGS, and mesangial proliferation were 18%, 75%, and 55%, respectively. Similar results were observed in a retrospective study of 100 consecutive referred patients at the University of Minnesota (66) (Table 26E.3).

These results have culminated in recommendations and criteria for performing renal biopsies in children with nephrotic syndrome. The presence of systemic disease is an obvious indication for renal biopsy (chapter 21). The older child (>6 years) and the patient with a low serum

C3, gross hematuria, or persistent hypertension are likely to benefit from the knowledge obtained by analysis of kidney tissue. Finally, the child who fails to respond to a standard course of therapy may benefit from renal biopsy, since the recognition of lesions such as membranous glomerulopathy, FSGS/H, or diffuse mesangial proliferation cannot with certainty be predicted, and these lesions have important therapeutic implications.

Therapy

Since the therapy of glomerular disease, including the primary nephrotic syndrome is discussed in detail in Chapter 29, only brief reference to selected therapeutic issues will be made here.

The treatment of the hypovolemia, hypoalbuminemia, and edema of the nephrotic syndrome require judicious use of dietary restriction of salt and water, infusions of plasma or salt-poor albumin, or diuretics as outlined in Chapter 29. The risks of hypervolemia secondary to inappropriate use, or excessive volumes of albumin in nephrotic children requires emphasis, since often the harm of such therapy exceeds the benefits to the patient. The prompt recognition of hypertension which develops consequent to either the disease process or therapy is important and is outlined in Chapter 47.

Among the life-threatening complications that commonly occur in nephrotic patients, thrombosis has been discussed earlier and guidelines for management suggested (chapters 15 and 29). Nephrotic children are especially prone to infection for the reasons discussed earlier. The edematous subcutaneous tissues frequently become infected (cellulitis), and peritonitis remains a major cause of morbidity. A recent review of a decade's (1970–1980) experience with 351 nephrotic children revealed 24 episodes of peritonitis in 19 patients (67). As in most series, 50% of the infections were a result of *Streptococcus pneumoniae* and in an additional 25% of cases *E. Coli* were isolated. Because of the high incidence of *S. Pneumococci*, the value of polyvalent pneumococcal vaccine in nephrotic children has recently been studied, and the results demonstrate a satisfactory and protective immune response by nephrotic children, including those on steroid therapy at the time of immunization (68). It is clear that the incidence of pneumococcal peritonitis as a result of strains included in the vaccine may be reduced by immunization of nephrotic children. Urinary tract infection is also common, especially in girls with nephrotic syndrome, and some have suggested an increased incidence of vesicoureteral reflux and congential malformations of the urinary tract in these children (69). Clinicians should be aware of this increased risk in the edematous child, obtain urinalyses and urine cultures, and treat appropriately.

Corticosteroid and Cytotoxic Therapy

Although corticosteroid therapy of the primary nephrotic syndrome has been used since 1951 and is considered to be "specific" therapy by most clinicians, the fact is that this therapy is empirical; it is discouraging that the scientific basis for the remarkable success of this treatment that we have used for 35 years remains unknown. The known pharmacology, indications, choices of drugs, accepted dosage regimens, and side effects are discussed in detail in Chapter 29. It is sufficient here to emphasize the frequency of relapse in patients who respond and the correlations of the histological lesions, discussed earlier, with response to corticosteroid therapy. The actual results of current therapy of the primary nephrotic syndrome in the general populations may be best portrayed in a recent paper describing the long-term (5 to 14 years) results of a clinic that cares for essentially the entire population of effected children (114 patients) in an area of Finland (70). These results contrast strikingly with the usual experience of referral clinics (Table 26E.4). An initial response, as defined earlier, occurred in 82%, while 18% failed the initial therapy. Of the initial responders, 24% did not relapse and remained well. An additional 22% had infrequent relapses and most were symptom free for at least 3 years. However, 53% of the responders had frequent relapses, defined as two or more relapses within a 6-month period. As discussed in Chapter 29, many of these patients were treated with cytotoxic therapy, since the cumulative toxicity of reported corticosteroid therapy was intolerable. At the end of the follow-up period, 36% of these children continued to have infrequent relapses. This group of patients, and those which fail to respond, are the groups that frustrate the child, the parents, and the physician and stimulate the search for improved understanding of this frustrating disease. Many such patients have mesangial proliferation or focal segmental sclerosis/hyalinosis on renal biopsy specimens.

In the Finnish experience, 18% (20/114) of the children with primary nephrotic syndrome failed to respond to the initial course of corticosteroid therapy (Table 26E.4). Of these, the majority (13/20) eventually responded to additional corticosteroid or cytotoxic therapy, and, although a few continued to have relapses, none died of their disease during the follow-up period. The remaining 7 children (35% of the nonresponders to initial therapy; 6% of the total series) had continuous proteinuria in spite of all therapeutic efforts, and four died during the follow-up period. Most of this group had either focal segmental glomerulosclerosis/hyalinosis or mesangial proliferation on renal biopsy and progressed or likely will progress to end-stage renal failure.

Immunosuppressive and Cytotoxic Agents

The presumed mode of action, side effects, indications, and efficacy of this group of drugs in the primary nephrotic syndrome is discussed in Chapter 29. The known and potential risks of these therapies must be carefully weighed against the possible benefits in each child. Persistence with conservative and corticosteroid therapy may occasionally be the wiser choice, given the long list of serious and potentially lethal consequences of this group of drugs.

Table 26E.4.
Therapeutic Response and Outcome of 114 Unselected Children with Primary Nephrotic Syndrome

Outcome (5–14 years)	Steroid Responsive (94)			Steroid resistant (20)	
	No relapse (23)	Infrequent relapses (21)	Frequent relapses (50)	Eventual remission (13)	Continuous proteinuria (7)
Well[a]	23	19	32	11	0
Relapses	0	2	16	2	0
Continuous proteinuria	0	0	1	0	3
Dead	0	0	1 (trauma)	0	4

Adapted from Koskimies O, et al: Arch Dis Childh 57:544, 1982.
[a] Asymptomatic, protein free for 3 or more years.

Eventual Outcome—Late Recurrences

The great majority of children with the primary nephrotic syndrome eventually respond to therapy and remain well as adults. Once the child has been free of disease for 4 or more years and has reached adolescence, the disease rarely recurs. Women who have had the syndrome in childhood usually have a normal pregnancy without risk of recurrence of disease (71). However, a rare patient, free of disease for many years, may as an adult have a recurrence of nephrotic syndrome. In our experience (72), late relapses beginning 4 to 25 years after complete remission have occurred in at least 16 of 400+ patients. Fortunately, all such late recurrences have been steroid responsive and most have had minimal glomerular changes on repeated renal biopsy specimens.

Renal Transplantation—Risk of Recurrence

In 1972 Hoyer and coworkers (73) described the rapid recurrence of nephrotic syndrome and focal segmental glomerulosclerosis/hyalinosis in three renal transplant recipients whose original disease was the primary nephrotic syndrome with FSGS/H. Subsequently, other investigators have also observed a recurrence of FSGS/H in transplanted kidneys with the occasional progression of the lesions to end-stage renal failure. Although the lesion FSGS/H may occur in allografts of recipients whose original disease was unrelated to primary nephrotic syndrome or FSGS/H (74), there are compelling reasons to believe that the induction of proteinuria and the development of these renal lesions after renal transplantation results from undefined circulating factors. A review describes the experience of the University of Minnesota with renal transplantation in 25 patients (33 allografts) who developed renal failure secondary to nephrotic syndrome with focal segmental glomerulosclerosis (75). Recurrent FSGS/H was documented histologically in 9/33 allografts (27.3%). There was no significant correlation between recurrence of disease in the allograft and age at onset, duration of nephrotic syndrome, or donor source (cadaver vs living related). Histological analysis of multiple biopsy specimens of the native kidneys indicated an increased risk of recurrence of FSGS/H in the allograft in patients whose original disease was characterized by the presence of both FSGS/H and diffuse mesangial proliferation. These data suggest that the risk of recurrence of disease may be predicted by the histology of the original kidney, but the numbers of patients studied is small and confirmation of these findings is needed.

We believe that these observations on the increased risk of recurrence of disease in the allograft do not contraindicate renal transplantation in these children, since recurrence of disease is not associated with rapid graft loss in most patients, and since for these children there are few therapeutic alternatives. A rare patient who develops recurrent nephrotic syndrome following renal transplantation may have the steroid responsive form of the disease. We have described one such patient in whom a nephrotic syndrome developed 3-years following renal transplantation (76). A renal biopsy demonstrated only minimal changes, the patient responded to a standard course of prednisone therapy, was free of abnormal proteinuria within 10 days after onset of treatment, and has remained in remission without additional recurrences for more than 6 years (9½-years following transplantation).

The primary (idiopathic) nephrotic syndrome is challenging, often chronic and recurrent, and a difficult disease for the patient, his/her parents, and the physician. However, great progress in our understanding of the disease and in management have occurred in the recent past and the mortality has been markedly decreased. There are reasons to be optimistic that ongoing research may provide more effective, more specific, and less toxic therapy in the foreseeable future.

References

1. Schlesinger ER, Sulz HA, Mosher WE, et al: The nephrotic syndrome. Its incidence and implications for the community. Am J Dis Child 116:623, 1968.
2. International Study of Kidney Disease in Children. The nephrotic syndrome in children. Prediction of histopathology from clinical and laboratory characteristics at the time of diagnosis. Kidney Intl 13:43, 1978.
3. Cameron JS, Turner DR, Ogg CS, et al: The nephrotic syndrome in adults with "minimal change" glomerular lesions. Quart J Med 43:461, 1974.
4. White RHR, Glasgow EF, Mills RJ: Clinicopathological study of nephrotic syndrome in childhood. Lancet 1:1353, 1970.
5. Habib R, Kleinknecht C: The primary nephrotic syndrome of childhood. Classification and clinicopathologic study of 406 cases. In Sommers SC (ed): Pathology Annual. New York, Appleton-Century-Crofts, 1971, p 417.
6. White RHR: The familial nephrotic syndrome. I. A European survey. Clin Nephrol 1:215, 1973
7. Norio R: The nephrotic syndrome and heredity. Hum Hered 19:113, 1970.
8. Meadow SR, Sarsfield JK, Scott DG, et al: Steroid responsive nephrotic syndrome and allergy. Immunological studies. Arch Dis Child 56:517, 1981.
9. Scharer K, Wahn U, Muller-Wiefel DE, et al: Steroid responsive nephrotic syndrome and allergy. Arch Dis Child 57:401, 1982.
10. deMouzon-Cambon A, Boulsson F, Datau G, et al: HLA-DR7 in children with idiopathic nephrotic syndrome. Correlation with atopy. Tissue Antigens 17:518, 1981.
11. White RHR, Glasgow EF, Mills RJ: Clinicopathologic study of nephrotic syndrome in childhood. Lancet 1:1353, 1970.
12. Winetz JA, Robertson CR, Golbetz HV, et al: The nature of the glomerular injury in minimal change and focal sclerosing glomerulopathies. Am J Kidney Dis 1:91, 1981.
13. Muller F: Morbus brightti. Verh Otsch Pathol Ges 9:64, 1905.
14. Kluthe R, Hagemann V, Klein N: The turnover of $\alpha 2$ macroglobulin in the nephrotic syndrome. Vox Sang 12:308, 1967.
15. Giangiacomo J, Cleary RG, Cole BR, et al: Serum immunoglobulins in the nephrotic syndrome. N Engl J Med 293:8, 1975.
16. Walker WA, Ulstrom RA, Lowman JI: Albumin synthesis rates in patients with hypoproteinemia. J Pediatr 78:812, 1971
17. Gitlin D, Janeway CA, Farr LE: Studies on the metabolism of plasma proteins in the nephrotic syndrome. J Clin Invest 35:44, 1956.
18. Jensen H, Rossing N, Andersen SB, et al: Albumin metabolism in the nephrotic syndrome in adults. Clin Sci 33:445, 1967.
19. Schultze G, Ahuja S, Faber U, et al: Gastrointestinal protein loss in the nephrotic syndrome studied with Cr51-albumin. Nephron 25:227, 1980.
20. Oliver WS: Physiologic responses associated with steroid-induced diuresis in the nephrotic syndrome. J Lab Clin Med 62:449, 1963.
21. Dorhout Mees EJ, Roos JC, Boer R, et al: Observation on edema formation in the nephrotic syndrome in adults with minimal lesions. Am J Med 67:378, 1979.
22. Usberti M, Federico S, Meccarcello S, et al: Role of plasma vasopressin in the impairment of water excretion in nephrotic syndrome. Kidney Intl 25:411, 1984.
23. Bohlin AB, Berg U: Renal sodium handling in minimal change nephrotic syndrome. Arch Dis Childh 59:825, 1984.
24. Ichikawa I, Rennke HG, Hoyer JR, et al: Role for intrarenal mechanisms in the impaired salt excretion of experimental nephrotic syndrome. J Clin Invest 71:91, 1983.
25. Baxter JH, Goodman HC, Allen JC: Effects of infusions of serum albumin on serum lipids and lipoproteins in nephrosis. J Clin Invest 40:490, 1961.
26. McKenzie IFC, Nestel PJ: Studies on the turnover of triglycerides and esterified cholesterol in subjects with nephrotic syndrome. J Clin Invest 47:1685, 1968.
27. Zilleruelo G, Hsui SL, Freundlich M, et al: Persistence of serum lipid abnormalities in children with idiopathic nephrotic syndrome. J Pediatr 104:61, 1984.
28. McVicar MI, Exeni R, Susin M: Renal glycosuria, an early sign of focal segmental glomerulosclerosis. Pediatr Res 9:376, 1975.
29. Robson AM, Giangiacomo J, Kienstra R, et al: Normal glomerular permeability and its modification by minimal change nephrotic syndrome. J Clin Invest 54:510, 1974.
30. Arniel GC: 164 children with nephrosis. Lancet 2:1103, 1961.
31. Michael AF, McLean RH, Roy LP, et al: Immunologic aspects of the nephrotic syndrome. Kidney Intl 3:105, 1973.
32. McLean RH, Forsgren, A, Bjorkstein B, et al: Decreased serum factor B concentrations associated with decreased opsonization of Escherichia Coli in the idiopathic nephrotic syndrome. Pediatr Res 11:910, 1977.
33. Ballow M, Kennedy TL III, Gandio KM, et al: Serum hemolytic factor D values in children with steroid responsive idiopathic nephrotic syndrome. J Pediatr 100:192, 1982.
34. Giangiacomo J, Cleary T, Cole BR, et al: Serum immunoglobulins in the nephrotic syndrome. A possible cause of minimal change nephrotic syndrome. N Engl J Med 293:8, 1975.

35. Egli F, Einiger P, Stalder G: Thromboembolism in the nephrotic syndrome. (Abstract No. 42. Eur Soc Pediat Neph) Pediatr Res 8:903, 1974.
36. Lau SO, Bock GH, Edson JR, et al: Sagittal sinus thrombosis in the nephrotic syndrome. J Pediatr 97:984, 1980.
37. Cameron JS: Coagulation and thromboembolic complications in the nephrotic syndrome. In Bach JF, et al (eds): Advances in Nephrology. Chicago Year Book Publishers, 1984, vol 13, p 75.
38. Kauffman RH, Veltkamp JJ, Von Tilburg NH, et al: Aquired antithrombin III deficiency and thrombosis in the nephrotic syndrome. Am J Med 65, 607, 1978.
39. Lau SO, Tkachuck JY, Hasegawa DK, et al: Plasminogen and anti-thrombin III deficiencies in childhood nephrotic syndrome associated with plasminogenuria and antithrombinuria. J Pediatr 96:39, 1980.
40. Francis RB, Sandler RM, Levitan D, et al: Use of non-invasive laboratory testing in the prediction of thrombosis in the nephrotic syndrome. Am J Nephrol 4:43, 1984.
41. George GRP, Stichter SJM, Quadracci L, et al: A kinetic evaluation of hemostasis in renal disease. N Engl J Med 291:1111, 1974.
42. Futrakul P, Poshyachinda M, Mitrakul C: Focal sclerosing glomerulonephritis: A kinetic evaluation of homeostasis and the effect of anti-coagulant therapy: A controlled study. Clin Nephrol 10:180, 1978.
43. Feinstein EI, Kaptein EM, Nicolott JT, et al: Thyroid function in patients with nephrotic syndrome and normal renal function. Am J Nephrol 2-70, 1982.
44. Smith-Gayk H, Grawunder C, Tschop W, et al: 25-hydroxy-vitamin D in nephrotic syndrome. Lancet II:105, 1977.
45. Gorragry JM, Carter ND, Beer M, et al: Vitamin-D metabolism in nephrotic syndrome. Lancet II:629, 1977.
46. Shalhoub RJ: Pathogenesis of lipoid nephrosis: A disorder of T-cell function. Lancet II:556, 1974.
47. Hoyer JR, Raij L, Vernier RL, et al: Recurrence of idiopathic nephrotic syndrome after renal transplantation. Lancet 2:343, 1972.
48. Hoyer JR: Idiopathic nephrotic syndrome with minimal glomerular changes. In Brenner B, Stein J (eds): Contemporary Issues in Nephrology. New York, Churchill-Livingstone, 1982, vol 9.
49. Fillit HM, Zabriskie JB: Cellular immunity in glomerulonephritis. Am J Pathol 109:227, 1982.
50. Michael AF, Blau E, Vernier RL: Glomerular polyanion: Alterations in aminonucleoside nephrosis. Lab Invest 23:649, 1970.
51. Brenner BM, Hostetter TH, Humes HD: Molecular basis of proteinuria of glomerular origin. N Engl J Med 298:826, 1978.
52. Farquhar MG: The glomerular basement membrane: A selective macromolecular filter. In Hay ED (ed): Cell Biology of the Extracellular Matrix. New York, Plenum Press, 1981, p 335.
53. Rosenzweig LJ, Kanwar YS: Removal of sulfated (heparan sulfate) or non-sulfated (hyaluronic acid) glycosaminoglycans results in increased permeability of the glomerular basement membrane to ^{125}I bovine serum albumin. Lab Invest 47:177, 1982.
54. Kanwar YS, Linker A, Farquhar MG: Increased permeability of the glomerular basement membrane to ferritin after removal of glycosaminoglycans (heparan sulfate) by enzyme digestion. J Cell Biol 86:688, 1980.
55. Blau EB, Haas JE: Glomerular sialic acid and proteinuria in human renal disease. Lab Invest 28:477, 1973.
56. Carrie BJ, Salyer WR, Myers BD: Minimal change nephropathy: An electro-chemical disorder of the glomerular membrane. Am J Med 70:262, 1981.
57. Winetz JA, Robertson CR, Galbetz HV, et al: The nature of the glomerular injury in minimal change and focal sclerosing glomerulopathies. Am J Kidney Dis 1:91, 1981.
58. Vernier RL, Klein DJ, Sisson SP, et al: Heparan sulfate-rich anionic sites in the human glomerular basement membrane. Decreased concentration in congenital nephrotic syndrome. N Engl J Med 309:1001, 1983.
59. Mahan JD, Sisson SP, Vernier RL: Altered glomerular basement membrane (GBM) anionic sites in the minimal change nephrotic syndrome (MCNS) in man. Kidney Intl 27:119A, 1985.
60. Klein DJ, Dehnel PJ, Oegema TR, et al: Alterations in proteoglycan metabolism in the nephrotic syndrome induced by the aminonucleoside of puromycin. Lab Invest 50:543, 1984.
61. Churg J, Habib R, White RHR: Pathology of the nephrotic syndrome in children: A report of the International study of kidney disease in children. Lancet 1:1299, 1970.
62. Yang JY, Melvin T, Sibley R, et al: No evidence for specific role of IgM in mesangial proliferation of idiopathic nephrotic syndrome. Kidney Intl 25:100, 1984.
63. Farquhar MG, Vernier RL, Good RA: An electron microscopic study of the glomerulus in nephrosis, glomerulonephritis, and lupus erythematosus. J Exp Med 106:649, 1957.
64. Powell HR: Relationship between proteinuria and epithelial cell changes in minimal lesion glomerulopathy. Nephron 16:310, 1976.
65. Report of the International study of kidney disease in children. The primary nephrotic syndrome in children. Identification of patients with minimal change from initial response to prednisone. J Pediatr 98:561, 1981.
66. Melvin T, Sibley R, Michael AF: Nephrotic syndrome. In Tune BM, et al (eds): Contemporary Issues in Nephrology. New York, Churchill-Livingstone, 1984, vol 12, p 191.
67. Krensky AM, Ingelfinger JR, Grupe WE: Peritonitis in childhood nephrotic syndrome 1970–1980. Am J Dis Child 136:732, 1982.
68. Spika JS, Holsey NA, Fish AJ, et al: Serum antibody response to pneumococcal vaccine in children with nephrotic syndrome. Pediatrics 69:219, 1982.
69. Demario WJH, Krueger RP, Anderson EE: Urinary tract abnormalities in the nephrotic syndrome. Clin Pediatr 11:530, 1972.
70. Koskimies O, Vilska J, Rapola J, et al: Long-term outcome of primary nephrotic syndrome. Arch Dis Child 57:544, 1982.
71. Makker SP, Heymann W: Pregnancy in patients who have had the idiopathic nephrotic syndrome in childhood. J Pediatr 81:1140, 1972.
72. Pru C, Kjellstrand CM, Cohn RA, et al: Late recurrence of minimal lesion nephrotic syndrome. Ann Int Med 100:69, 1984.
73. Hoyer JR, Vernier RL, Simmons RL, et al: Recurrence of idiopathic nephrotic syndrome after transplantation. Lancet 2:343, 1972.
74. Cheigh JS, Mauradian J, Soliman M, et al: Focal segmental glomerulosclerosis in renal transplants. Am J Kidney Dis 2:449, 1983.
75. Maizell SE, Sibley RK, Horstman JP, et al: Incidence and significance of recurrent focal segmental glomerulosclerosis in renal allograft recipients. Transplantation 32:512, 1981.
76. Mauer SM, Hellerstein S, Cohn RA, et al: Recurrence of steroid responsive nephrotic syndrome after renal transplantation. J Pediatr 95:261, 1979.

26F Congenital Nephrotic Syndrome

JOHN D. MAHAN, JR.
ROBERT L. VERNIER

INTRODUCTION

Infants with onset of the nephrotic syndrome in the first 3 months of life have a clinical course that is different from that of children with onset of the syndrome at other ages. The designation congenital nephrotic syndrome (CNS) identifies infants of this age as a separate group, and the term congenital implies the presumed inborn basis of their disorder. The majority of reported cases of CNS are from Finland, and these children have been identified as having congenital nephrotic syndrome of the Finnish type (CNF) (1, 2). Similar cases of nephrotic infants have been reported from many other countries and every racial background, and the clinical course of affected infants appears remarkably similar regardless of ethnic background. Infants with CNS often have proteinuria at birth, although clinical evidence of disease, such as edema or poor growth, may not be apparent until somewhat later (3).

Babies with CNS present a formidable challenge to the pediatric nephrologist and merit special consideration as to their evaluation, clinical course, and management. Many important issues, such as the specificity of the renal pathology, the particular clinical/pathological features predictive of progressive renal impairment, improved methods for prevention of infection (prophylaxis), nutritional management, and optimal planning for dialysis and transplantation, and so on remain to be clearly defined.

The grim clinical course that befalls almost every infant with CNS is the reality that unites this heterogeneous group of disorders that cause the nephrotic syndrome in the newborn period and shapes the therapeutic response.

Classification

As with many renal diseases, the classification of infants with CNS has been based primarily on the pathological changes demonstrated in the kidney by renal biopsy. The majority of cases described have had cortical microcysts (see Pathology) and have been considered on the basis of this finding to represent the autosomal recessive CNF, even in the absence of evidence for Finnish ancestry. This pathological group, together with less common lesions, including diffuse mesangial sclerosis (DMS), minimal change nephrotic syndrome (MCNS), and focal segmental glomerulosclerosis (FSGS), constitute the idiopathic or primary forms of CNS occurring in infants before 3 months of age (Table 26F.1).

Several secondary causes of CNS have been identified, although the number of reported cases is small in each category. Congenital infections, such as syphilis, toxoplasmosis, and cytomegalovirus (CMV) have been associated with the nephrotic syndrome (3–5). Mercury intoxication and systemic lupus erythematosus (6, 7) have caused membranous glomerulonephritis with the nephrotic syndrome in infants less than 3 months of age. Rare newborns with Wilms' tumor, XY gonadal dysgenesis, or the nail-patella syndrome have also demonstrated the nephrotic syndrome (8, 9).

Clinical Aspects

The majority of infants with CNS display similar clinical abnormalities, regardless of the presence or absence of Finnish ancestry and resemble the large groups of Finnish infants described by Hallman and coworkers (1), Huttunen (2), and others (3, 10). In our study of 41 infants, 78% of whom had no recognized Finnish ancestry, no clinical or pathological features allowed recognition of a distinct subgroup (10). Nevertheless, review of family origins is an important aspect of the history in this disorder. It seems likely that the disease, when genetic, results from one or several distinct gene disorders, which are diffusely distributed in the population. The frequency of the disorder in the total population is unknown.

In Finland the incidence of CNS has been estimated at 1.2/10,000 births, and an autosomal recessive inheritance has been defined (11). In this circumstance, genetic counseling may be rewarding, since the disease may be recognized in utero by demonstration of elevated levels of alpha fetoprotein (AFP) in amniotic fluid.

Although the course of pregnancy is usually normal, the majority of CNS infants are born prematurely and are small for gestational age. The placenta is usually larger than normal and often weighs more than 25% of the baby's birth weight. Huttunen determined a mean ratio of placenta to infant weight of 0.43 in affected babies compared to 0.18 in normals (2). Breech presentation and fetal asphyxia are common. The cranial sutures are often wide at birth and both fontanelles are usually large and open. The cartilage of the face may be soft and very pliable, and the infants may have a small nose, wide-set eyes, and low ears. More than half of CNS infants are edematous in the first week of life, and abdominal distention with ascites soon follows in most cases. Umbilical hernias may be quite prominent.

These babies feed poorly and vomiting, from abdominal distention, and diarrhea, from gut edema, frequently hinder normal nutrition; an increased incidence of pyloric stenosis and symptomatic gastroesophageal reflux has been noted as well (10). Growth retardation becomes more

Table 26F.1.
Nephrotic Syndrome in the First 3 Months of Life

PRIMARY	
	Congenital nephrotic syndrome—Finnish ancestry; without Finnish ancestry
	Minimal change nephrotic syndrome
	Focal segmental glomerular sclerosis
	Diffuse mesangial sclerosis
SECONDARY	
	Parainfectious—Syphilis, Toxoplasmosis, CMV, Rubella, Hepatitis, and Malaria
	Toxic—Mercury
	Membranous glomerulopathy
	XY gonadal dysgenesis
	Nephroblastoma
	Nail-patella syndrome
	Hemolytic uremic syndrome

prominent during the first year of life, and complications of the persistent nephrotic state are increasingly common over time. Frequent serious bacterial infections are the rule, occurring in over 85% of the children. Thromboembolic complications from hypercoagulability affect a number of infants. Evidence of delayed development is almost uniformly present by the second year of life and seizures, generally metabolic in origin but occasionally without obvious cause, occur in 30%. Infant mortality from infection is quite common, and in Finland these babies have invariably died by 4 years of age. Progressive renal insufficiency was evident in all infants by 2 years of age in the Finnish series (2) and infants with Finnish ancestral and without Finnish ancestral forms of CNS in our experience demonstrated decreased renal function by 2 years of age and required end-stage renal disease treatment at the average age of 2 years 9 months (10).

The clinical features of the rare infants with a secondary form of CNS are similar to those with primary CNS, with additional historical factors, signs and symptoms related to specific infections, exposure, or systemic conditions. Specific diagnostic tests are important in this group, since recovery may follow recognition of a specific etiology and appropriate management.

Laboratory Findings

The typical abnormal laboratory findings of the nephrotic syndrome include significant proteinuria (>4 mg/kg/hr), hypoalbuminemia, and hypercholesterolemia. Infants with primary CNS usually have abnormal proteinuria in their initial urinalysis and when studied usually have proteinuria at birth. Rare infants have been described with initially normal urinalyses. Hematuria and leukocyturia may be present early but usually occur later in the first year of life in these babies. Renal function is always normal for age in the newborn period. Typically, these infants become hypoproteinemic and serum albumin levels of less than 1 gm/dl are the rule. Hyperlipidemia and hypogammaglobulinemia invariably occur and may be quite severe. Occasional infants may present with low T4 values on routine newborn screening and other examples of specific protein deficiencies, such as iron deficiency anemia as a result of loss of transferrin and iron in the urine, and vitamin D deficiency as a result of loss of vitamin D–binding protein and vitamin D in the urine, may be seen. Recently, attention has been focused on the hypercoagulable state of these infants; 21 of 27 infants in the Minnesota series had either a short or prolonged PTT often accompanied by a prolonged TT, consistent with an activated clotting system (10).

Proteinuria is massive and persistent from onset. Early in the course the proteinuria appears highly selective as in MCNS; several studies have demonstrated a decrease in selectivity as renal function deteriorates (12). Several reports of infants with primary CNS and normal amniotic fluid AFP determinations have been published, suggesting that abnormal proteinuria may not be present during fetal life in all infants with this disorder (13). Severe proteinuria usually persists even as renal failure develops and by 2 to 3 years of age, the biochemical alterations of chronic renal failure usually occur in surviving children.

Pathology

The variety of pathological findings seen in infants with primary CNS are less specific than previously believed (14). Early in the course of the disease and in the affected fetus, the only abnormality appears to be diffuse epithelial cell proliferation and effacement of foot processes, demonstrable by electron microscopy (15, 16) (Fig. 26F.1). In the first year of life a variable number of CNS infants may demonstrate proximal tubule cystic dilatation (microcysts), a finding noted in many older infants with noncongenital nephrotic syndrome and thus apparently a nonspecific finding (14) (Fig. 26F.2). Mesangial cell proliferation and increase in mesangial matrix, persistence of fetal glomeruli, and focal segmental sclerosis have been noted in many CNS infants in the first year of life.

Sequential morphological studies have documented increasing numbers of sclerosing glomeruli in these children with advancing age. Glomerular hyalinization and associated tubular atrophy and interstitial fibrosis become more common in the second and third year of life, resulting ultimately in end-stage chronic glomerulonephritis. Early in the disease course, immunofluorescent and electron microscopic studies have failed to demonstrate deposits of immunoproteins. Later, in the fibrosing kidney, occasional deposits of immunoglobulins may be seen in the glomerular mesangium in a nonspecific pattern (14).

In our experience, the frequency of these various pathological lesions (microcysts, mesangial proliferation, fetal glomeruli, and FSGS) was not different in infants with or without Finnish ancestry or consistent among affected siblings, and the pathological findings did not correlate with or predict the eventual outcome (14). An entirely similar incidence of pathological lesions was also observed in infants with onset of the nephrotic syndrome at 4 to 12 months of age (Table 26F.2), and again there appears to be no relationship between specific morphological features and outcome (14). Only 13 cases of the rare and apparently lethal lesion DMS have been described, and a familial incidence has been reported by Habib and coworkers (17). DMS is characterized by mesangial matrix expansion without hypercellularity and progressive sclerotic obliteration of capillary loops over time with apparent shrinkage of the glomerular tuft. Immunofluorescent and ultrastructural studies have failed to reveal any evidence of immune complexes but have demonstrated early GBM thickening and lamellation. Rare infants with MCNS or FSGS have been described, suggesting that some cases of the primary nephrotic syndrome of childhood may present within the first 3 months of life (3, 18). The different clinical course and responsiveness to treatment remain the principal differential features for eventual recognition of infants with potentially reversible FSGS or MCNS with onset in infancy.

In contrast, distinct pathological features are often present in secondary forms of CNS. Epimembranous glomerulonephritis with associated mesangial deposits containing treponemal antigen have been noted by fluorescent and electron microscopy in cases of syphilitic CNS (4). An immune-complex nephritis has been described in infants with toxoplasmosis, rubella and CMV, and the nephrotic syndrome. Epimembranous lesions have also been described with mercury intoxication and infantile systemic lupus erythematosus. Infants with XY gonadal dysgenesis and Wilms' tumor have no specific pathological renal lesions, although

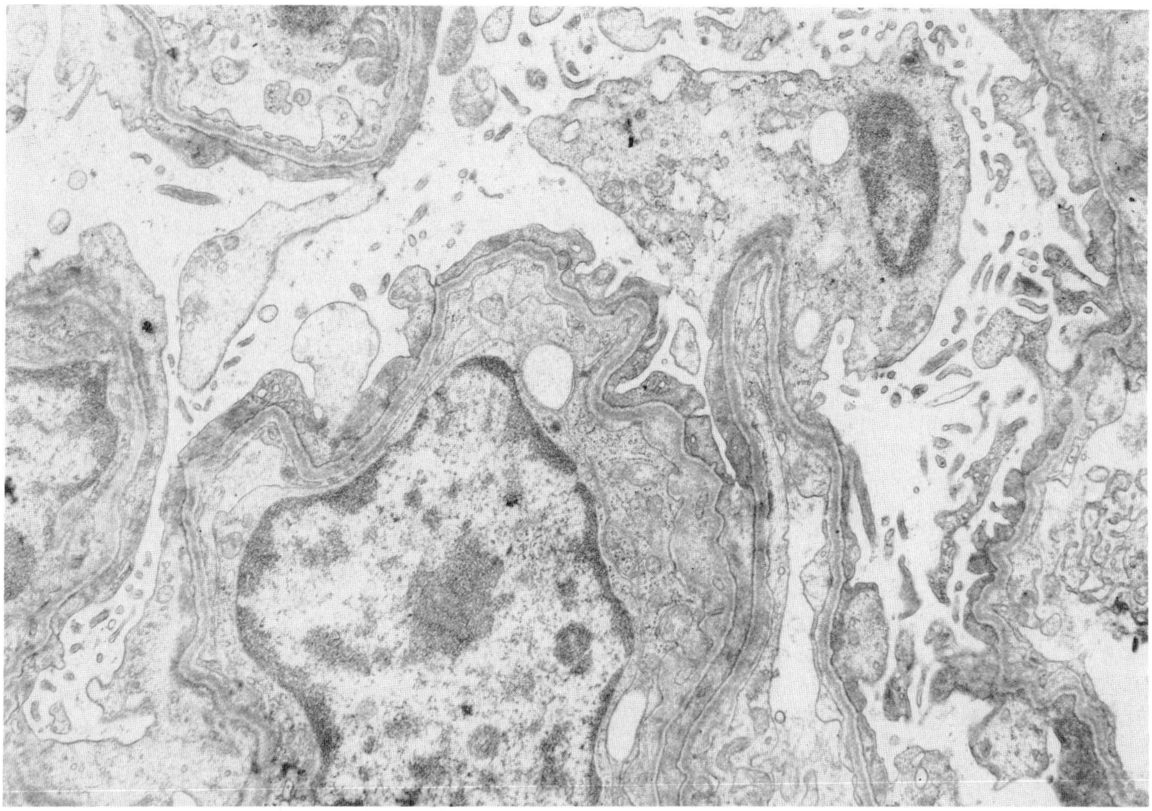

Figure 26F.1. Electron micrograph of several capillaries from a glomerulus in an infant with congenital nephrotic syndrome. The principal abnormality shown is the diffuse effacement (fusion) of the foot processes of the glomerular epithelial cells. The basement membranes are normal. (X18,000.)

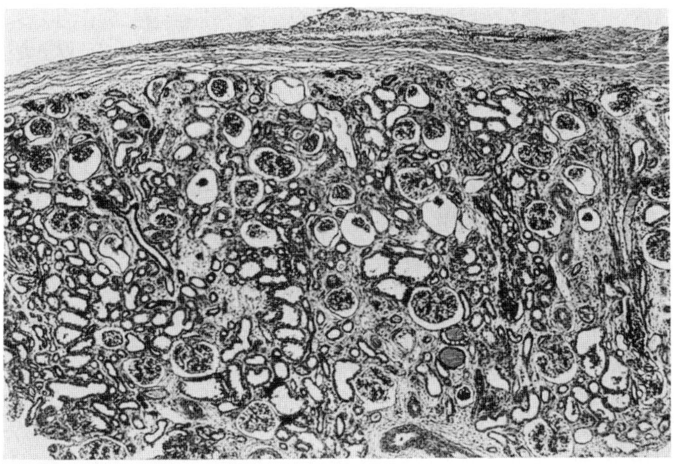

Figure 26F.2. Light micrograph of the renal cortex of an infant with congenital nephrotic syndrome demonstrating numerous dilated tubules (microcysts) and occasional dilated Bowman's spaces. (PAS stain X60.)

glomerular sclerosis appears earlier in these children than in infants with primary CNS.

Pathogenesis

The genetic basis of CNS in Finland has been well demonstrated in family studies that have documented an autosomal recessive pattern of inheritance (11). Several reports of infants without Finnish ancestry with CNS have documented a similar familial pattern of inheritance (10). The defect in these children appears to occur early in fetal life as indicated by the presence of fetal proteinuria in both groups at 16 to 18 weeks' gestation and the finding of epithelial cell foot-process effacement in the fetal tissue. There is no convincing evidence of an immune basis for these abnormalities and the primary defect more likely resides in a lack of integrity of the glomerular filter, since the initial proteinuria is glomerular in origin and is associated with normal renal tubular function. Recent studies have described the charge and size selective properties of the GBM associated with fixed negatively charged molecules located primarily in the lamina rarae (19). The demonstration of a decrease in the number of anionic sites in the lamina rara externa of the GBM in children with primary CNS supports the hypothesis that alterations in the synthesis or the maintenance of a heparan sulfate-rich proteoglycan component of the GBM and their role in integration of the GBM may result in the proteinuria seen in this disorder (Fig. 26F.3). The anionic sites in renal tubular and peritubular capillary basement membranes appear to be unaffected, and thus the abnormality of anionic sites is apparently unique to the GBM. The progressive glomerular sclerosis seen in these children may be the result of continued proteinuria and secondary damage to glomeruli, as seen in experimental models that develop focal segmental and global sclerosis with long-standing proteinuria (20). The lack of recurrence of the nephrotic syndrome following successful renal transplantation in 17 children indicates that the proposed defect in the GBM is probably not acquired as part of a systemic disorder (10). There is some evidence that the GBM in children with CNS is more immature than that of age-matched controls (21), and this finding, if confirmed, may indicate that a delay in glomerular maturation may be in part responsible for the defective GBM seen in this disorder. It is not known whether proteinuria in all infants with CNS involves alterations of GBM anionic sites and other GBM constituents, and it is possible that other mechanisms may be involved in this apparently heterogenous group of patients.

Table 26F.2.
Nephrotic Syndrome in the First Year of Life Histological Features Related to Remission

	MG (%)	MP (%)	MH (%)	Normal (%)	EP (%)	FN (%)	FSGS/H (%)	FGGS (%)	MC (%)
Remission[a] (8 patients)	50	75	0	25	37.5	13	25	50	50
No remission[b] (40 patients)	62.5	80	15	5	35	8	40	35	55
p value	NS	NS	NS	NS	NS	NS	NS	NS	NS

Adapted from Sibley RK, et al: Lab Invest 48: 12P, 1983.

MG, microglomeruli; MP, mesangial proliferation; MH, mesangial hypercellularity; EP, epithelial proliferation; FN, fibrinoid necrosis; FSGS/H, Focal segmental glomerulosclerosis and hyalinosis; FGGS, focal global glomerulosclerosis; and MC = tubular microcysts.

[a] Includes 7 children with NS onset >3 months of age, 1 with NS onset <3 months of age.

[b] Includes 1 child with NS onset >3 months of age, 39 with NS onset <3 months of age.

The lack of tubular microcysts in all affected infants with typical Finnish CNS and the common presence of this lesion in infants with CNS of apparently diverse causes and very different outcomes suggests that microcysts may result from heavy proteinuria occurring in the infant kidney (14).

Management

Appropriate management requires a definitive diagnosis in the child with CNS. Many of the secondary forms of CNS deserve specific therapy, such as antibiotics for syphillis or toxoplasmosis and immunosuppressive therapy for systemic lupus erythematosus. In concert with a careful and complete clinical and laboratory evaluation, a renal biopsy is usually a necessary diagnostic procedure. With proper control of edema and good sedation, a percutaneous renal biopsy is safe and is preferred to surgical biopsy in these infants. Although the pathological features of idiopathic CNS are not specific, examination of renal tissue in an affected infant is the ultimate means of excluding the secondary forms of CNS. In the infant with a positive family history of idiopathic CNS or an elevated level of alpha fetoprotein in amniotic fluid, early renal biopsy may be unnecessary.

Better appreciation of the natural history of children with primary CNS, the futility of steroid therapy (22), and the successful results of renal transplantation in these infants has required changes in their management over the last decade. In early reports from Finland, all children with CNS (1) died of infection, neurological deterioration, or uremia. Although rare examples of spontaneous remission (3, 10) in infants with onset of nephrotic syndrome before 3 months of life have been described, the vast majority of infants with CNS have a dismal prognosis regardless of ancestry (Finnish or not Finnish) or other clinical variables. Moreover, every reported infant with congenital onset who has remained proteinuric and has demonstrated progressive renal insufficiency over the first 2 years of life has eventually developed renal failure. The rare children who have had spontaneous remissions have demonstrated improvement (decreased proteinuria) by 14 months of age and have not had progressive renal insufficiency (10, 18). Several reports now have confirmed the futility of steroid and immunosuppressive therapy in primary CNS, and these toxic drugs should not be given, since the risk of complications is high and the likelihood of benefit low (22, 23). The thrust of all therapeutic decisions should instead be directed toward renal transplantation, which is currently the only effective therapy for primary CNS. Maximal efforts to provide optimal nutrition, control edema, prevent infection, and achieve growth are indicated in order that the natural history of the disease may be revealed in each individual infant and that the child may reach a weight and body size consistent with successful renal transplantation.

The mainstay of aggressive medical therapy involves nutritional supplementation with a high caloric, high protein, low sodium formula (such as PM 60/40®) with added polycose or medium-chain triglyceride oil, often given by nasogastric drip or gastrostomy feedings to provide at least 120 cal/kg/day. Hyperalimentation may be required for selected infants who are particularly malnourished, to enable them to become anabolic and tolerate oral feedings. Oral diuretic therapy with thiazides or furosemide and occasional serum albumin infusions should be used to allow the fluid intake necessary for good nutrition while avoiding excessive edema or ascites that predispose to infection and malabsorption. Infections are often life threatening and require prompt evaluation and specific therapy. Prophylaxis with penicillin can largely prevent *S. pneumoniae* infections and should be used (10). In children with laboratory evidence of hypercoagulability or clinical evidence of thrombosis, low dose aspirin and dipyridamole therapy should be considered to minimize the risk of major vascular thromboses. Some infants experience a "fall off" in growth despite aggressive medical treatment before the development of end-stage renal failure. These children, even with advanced uremia, often have persistent proteinuria and nephrotic syndrome. Nephrectomy may be necessary, before end-stage renal failure, in the child who is not growing despite aggressive therapy, to correct severe protein malnutrition and permit growth before planned renal transplantation. Several infants in our series with relatively well-preserved renal function (creatinine clearance ≃50% of normal), but with persistent growth failure, have demonstrated dramatic improvement in affect, appetite, and real weight gain following nephrectomy and dialysis (10). We believe that this drastic measure may allow selected infants to reach a body size consistent with successful renal transplantation. To minimize the risk of including the rare child with potential for spontaneous remission, a renal biopsy should be obtained before nephrectomy in any infant with moderate residual renal function, since the presence of glomerular sclerosis, tubular atrophy, and interstitial fibrosis are usually indicators of irreversible disease and provide valuable support for the decision of nephrectomy. Children with persistent nephrotic syndrome at the time of planned renal transplantation should also undergo nephrectomy and short-term dialysis in order that they may be anabolic and no longer hypercoagulable at the time of renal transplantation.

Our experience with renal transplantation in CNS now includes over 20 infants, has been very rewarding (10, 24) and contrasts strikingly with our prior experience (10, 21). All 17 CNS infants seen before 1971 died of infection [15], congestive heart failure [1], or cerebral hemorrhage [1]. Renal transplantation of 23 kidneys in 17 children has resulted in a 2-year patient survival of 82% and 2-year graft survival of 71%. Five children have required a second renal transplant because of rejection, and one child required a third kidney 10 years after the original renal transplant for the same indication.

The long-term results have been equally encouraging. Although one child died of disseminated varicella 11 years after his original renal transplant (with normal renal function), 14 of the 17 children are alive

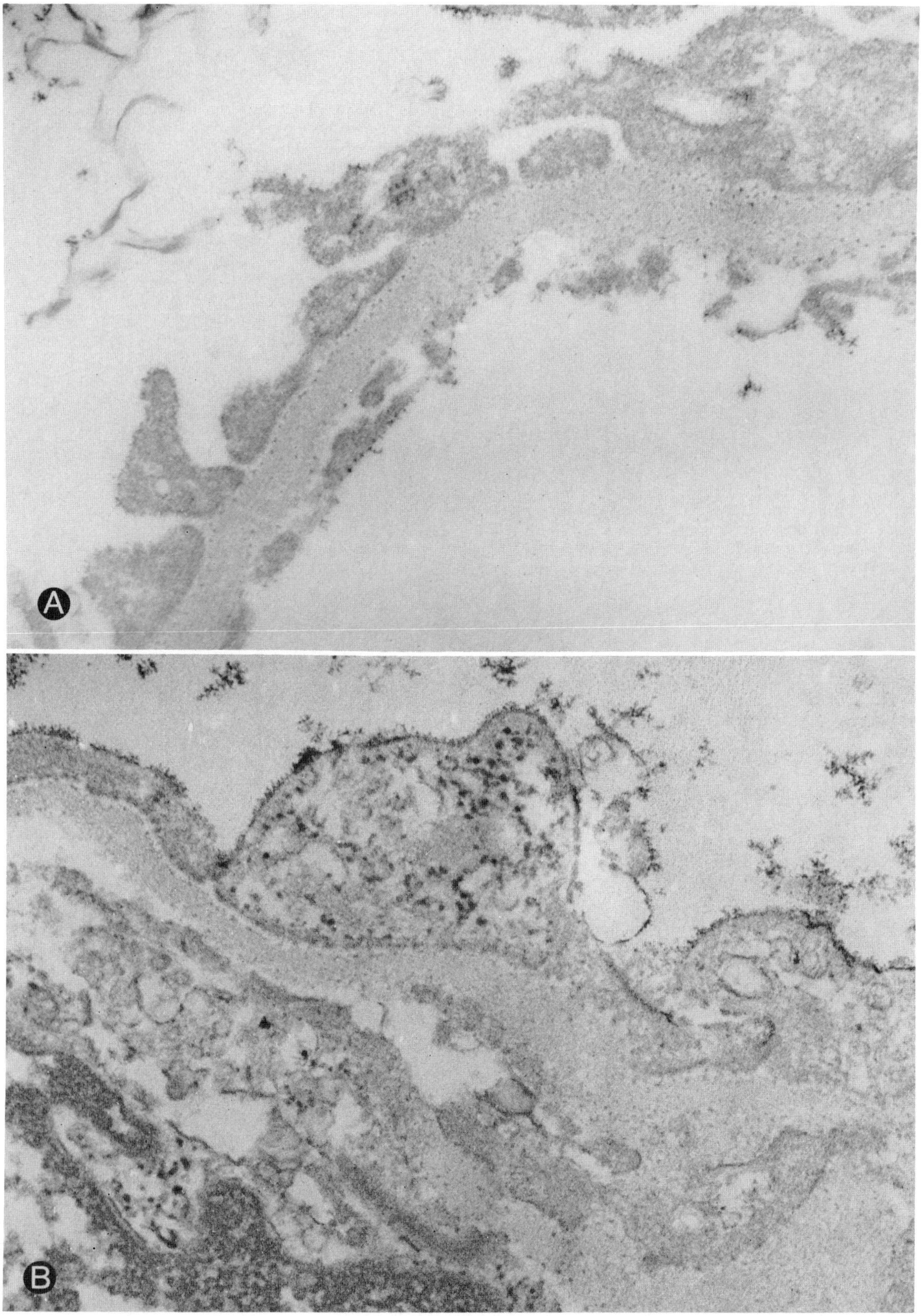

Figure 26F.3. Electron micrographs of sections of kidney incubated in the cationic polymer polyethyleneimine (PEI) MW 1200, to demonstrate anionic charge sites in the GBM. (See reference 19 for details.) **A**, Portion of the GBM from a 10-month old child with normal renal function. There is a regular array of small dots in the lamina rara externa (*LRE*) of the GBM, beneath the epithelial cell foot processes and less regular anionic sites within the GBM and lamina rara interna (*LRI*). (X50,000.) **B**, Similarly prepared section of a capillary from an infant with congenital nephrotic syndrome. Note the reduced number of irregularly spaced less distinct anionic sites in the LRE. (X50,000.)

with functioning renal allografts for a mean of 6.2 years (range 0.8 to 12 yrs) posttransplant.

All infants with continued good graft function post-transplantation have demonstrated catch-up growth. The improvement in developmental skills has been dramatic for all infants with functioning grafts and was usually evident one year after transplantation. Three-quarters of these infants have normal school and social performance posttransplantation, and those who did not progress as well had either specific handicaps pretransplantation or poor graft function posttransplantation. The growth and development data support the use of aggressive medical management and renal transplantation for the young child with CNS and indicate that primary CNS can no longer be considered a uniformly fatal disorder.

References

1. Hallman N, Norio R, Konvalainen K: Main features of the congenital nephrotic syndrome. Acta Paediatr Scand Suppl 172:75, 1967.
2. Huttunen N-P: Congenital nephrotic syndrome of Finnish type. Arch Dis Childh 51:344, 1976.
3. Hoyer JR, Anderson CE: Congenital nephrotic syndrome. Clin Perinatol 8:333, 1981.
4. Papairoannou AC, Asrow GC, Schackmell NH: Nephrotic syndrome in early infancy as a manifestation of congenital syphilis. Pediatrics 27:636, 1961.
5. Shahin B, Papadopoupou ZL, Jenis EH: Congenital nephrotic syndrome associated with congenital toxoplasmosis. J Pediatr 85:366, 1974.
6. Wilson VK, Thompson MC, Holzel A: Mercury nephrosis in young children. Brit Med J 1:359, 1952.
7. Ty A, Fine B: Membranous nephritis in infantile systemic lupus erythematosus associated with chromosomal abnormalities. Clin Nephrol 12:137, 1979.
8. Simila S, Vesa L, Wasz-Hochert O: Hereditary onycho-osteodysplasia (the Nail-Patella Syndrome) with nephrosis-like renal disease in a newborn boy. Pediatrics 461:61, 1970.
9. Gentner JM, Kanschonsky A, Gresher DW, et al: XY gonadal dysgenesis associated with the congenital nephrotic syndrome. Obstet Gynecol 35(suppl 3):665, 1980.
10. Mahan JD Jr, Mauer SM, Sibley RK, et al: Congenital nephrotic syndrome: The evolution of medical management and results of renal transplantation. J Pediatr 105:549, 1984.
11. Norio R: Heredity in the congenital nephrotic syndrome. A genetic study of 57 Finnish families with a review of reported cases. Ann Paediat Fenn 12:27, 1966.
12. Huttunen NP, Vehaskari M, Viikati M, et al: Proteinuria in congenital nephrotic syndrome of the Finnish type. Clin Nephrol 13:12, 1980.
13. Kjessler B, Johansson SGO, Sherman M, et al: Alpha-fetoprotein in antenatal diagnosis of congenital nephrosis. Lancet 1:432, 1975.
14. Sibley RK, Mahan JD, Vernier RL: Congenital and infantile nephrotic syndrome: A clinicopathologic study of 46 cases. Lab Invest 48:12P, 1983.
15. Huttunen NP, Rapola J, Vilska J, et al: Renal pathology in congenital nephrotic syndrome of Finnish type. A quantitative light microscopic study on 50 patients. Int J Ped Nephrol 1:10, 1980.
16. Autio-Hermainen H: Renal pathology of fetuses with congenital nephrotic syndrome of the Finnish type. 2. A qualitative and quantitative electron microscopic study. Acta Patho Micro Scand A89:215, 1981.
17. Habib R, Bois E: Heterogeneite des syndromes nephrotiques a debut prococe du nourrisson (Syndrome Nephrotique "Infantile"). Halv Paed Acta 28:91, 1973.
18. Anand SK, Northway JD, Vernier RL: Congenital nephrotic syndrome: Report of a patient with cystic tubular changes who recovered. J Pediatr 95:265, 1979.
19. Vernier RL, Klein DJ, Sisson SP, et al: Heparan sulfate-rich anionic sites in the human glomerular basement membrane. N Engl J Med 309:1001, 1983.
20. Brenner BM, Hostetter TH, Humes HA: Molecular basis of proteinuria of glomerular origin. N Engl J Med 298:826, 1978.
21. Autio-Harmainen H, Rapalo J: The thickness of the glomerular basement membrane in congenital nephrotic syndrome of the Finnish type. Nephron 34:48, 1983.
22. Worthen HC, Vernier RL, Good RA: Infantile nephrosis. Am J Dis Child 98:731, 1959.
23. Hoyer JR, Michael AF, Good RA, Vernier RL: The nephrotic syndrome in infancy: Clinical, morphologic and immunologic studies of four infants. Pediatrics 40:233, 1967.
24. Hoyer JR, Mauer SM, Kjellstrand CM, et al: Successful renal transplantation in 3 children with congenital nephrotic syndrome. Lancet 1:1410, 1973.

26G Membranous Glomerulonephritis

CLAIRE KLEINKNECHT
RENEE HABIB

Membranous glomerulonephritis (MGN) (also called extramembranous or epimembranous glomerulonephritis or nephropathy) is defined by its histopathological aspect: presence of contiguous subepithelial deposits on the glomerular basement membrane (GBM) and usually no significant cellular proliferation. Immunofluorescent study indicates that these deposits always contain IgG. The aspect varies according to the extent of deposits and the reaction of the GBM. Although typical cases can be diagnosed by light microscopy, particularly after silver staining, in some instances immunofluorescence or electron microscopy studies are necessary for diagnosis.

Among various types of glomerulonephritis, MGN is one of the best studied, a result in part of the fact that it can be reproduced experimentally. It is well accepted that the origin of this lesion is immunologically mediated. The mechanism of deposition is still disputed. MGN may have various associations, including some whose relationship with the renal disease has not been established.

MGN was long considered an adult disease, occurring only rarely in the child. Pediatric reports in the literature include 50 cases in the Enfants-Malades series published in 1973 (1) and other series as follows: 9 cases (2), 11 cases (3), 14 cases each (4, 5, 6), and 22 cases (7). In addition, at least 20 cases have been included in various adult series. At the present time, approximately 100 pediatric cases have been observed at Enfants-Malades, and an equal number have been reported by others.

In all series of biopsied patients, the proportion of pediatric cases of MGN is far less than that in the adult. It has been variously reported as representing 20% (8), 19% (9), and 34% (10) of nephrotic syndromes (NS) in the adult, and 2.76% (9), 1.6% (11), to 6% (1) of pediatric NS. In both populations, however, MGN may be found in the absence of NS. It has been reported to represent 15.5% (8) or 17% (9) of adult glomerulopathies; our experience would indicate 6 to 7%, whereas 6.7% was reported in a Japanese series (3). The lower proportion observed in children is partly a result of the higher frequency of other nephropathies, particularly steroid sensitive NS. The 1979 Necker Hospital series included 116 adults (12), and the Hôpital des Enfants-Malades study included 85 patients (13).

Geographical differences in the incidence of MGN are likely, but are difficult to assess, since differences in the indications for renal biopsy in nonnephrotic patients may introduce important bias.

Our present description of MGN will therefore be mainly based on a series of 96 pediatric cases followed at the Hôpital des Enfants-Malades, including those published previously (1, 13), but excluding 4 cases with systemic lupus erythematosus.

Clinical Presentation

The disease can occur at any age, including infancy (3 cases in our series were aged 2 to 11 months), without any clear predominance, although in all published series occurrence before the age of 2 years is rare. A predominance among males is clear in our series (77 boys, 74% of cases); similar findings were seen in other series (3, 4, 6), but not in all (2, 5, 7). Such a predominance also appears in cumulated adult series (10).

Onset is often covert, with the disease discovered at routine urinalysis (58 cases) or because of edema (35 cases); less often macroscopic hematuria (6 cases) leads to discovery. In a few children the onset mimics that of steroid sensitive NS, with a sudden development of diffuse edema including ascites. In some patients initial signs may suggest the diagnosis of acute glomerulonephritis because of proteinuria and hematuria found after sore throat, but hypertension and renal failure are rare.

Clinical and Laboratory Findings

Edema is almost the only clinical finding and may be absent throughout the evolution. It is more frequent near clinical onset and rarely develops later. It usually subsides within a few months, particularly in children with an apparently sudden and severe initial attack.

Proteinuria is virtually constant, although isolated hematuria has been described. It is highly variable, not only among children but also from day to day in the same child. It is considered nonselective or poorly selective in the majority of adult cases, but is selective in approximately half of pediatric cases. Evidence of clinical or laboratory NS was found at first examination in 71 children. It was generally slight, but some children had abrupt and severe onset of NS, with diffuse edema and severe drop in plasma protein and albumin, as in steroid sensitive nephrosis. In this case, it diminishes rapidly but rarely disappears before several months, even with corticosteroid therapy. In a few children (10 cases) laboratory evidence of NS appeared during the course of the disease and was often transient. The NS remitted in 70 patients within 12 to 18 months of its discovery. It persisted during the follow-up period in 16 patients, and the remainder never developed hypoproteinemia and NS.

Gross hematuria was observed in 19/96 children, most often during the first weeks or months. At variance with adult series, microscopic hematuria was frequent; it was found in 80% of cases and was often abundant, but most often disappeared during the course. Hypertension was present in four children; it was mild and transient in three, whereas it was severe and required therapy for several years before disappearing in the last child. Increased urea and creatinine at onset were rare (three cases) and never very severe. Glomerular filtration rate (GFR) returned to normal in all. Alteration in function of proximal convoluted tubules was associated with signs of glomerular alteration, either at onset (one case) or subsequently (two cases) (Table 26G.1).

Complement C3 was low in only three cases and was never below 35 mg/dl. In half the cases, a clear decrease in plasma C4 and C1q, either persistent or transient, was observed, and the mean levels in children with MGN were significantly lower than in the normal population. Plasma C5 was normal. Factor B could be decreased without evidence of severe proteinuria. Abnormal levels of complement components could persist despite prolonged clinical remission (13, 15).

In sum, the clinical signs suggest a glomerular nephropathy. Symptoms more precisely suggestive of MGN are rare aside from certain associations (presence of hepatitis B antigen, administration of drugs or toxic substances); but a covert onset, hematuria, and lowered C4 with normal C3 are highly suggestive of MGN. In any case, only renal biopsy can lead to diagnosis.

Pathogenesis

MGN has long been considered to be a perfect model of circulating immune complex-induced glomerulonephritis. It was accepted that circulating soluble, small-sized immune complexes were able to cross the GBM and to localize within the subepithelial space. This concept was supported by experimental studies. MGN could be induced in animals by the injection of either foreign serum proteins (bovine serum albumin in chronic serum sickness in rabbits) or autologous antigen (antigen derived from the brush border of proximal tubular epithelial cells or Fx 1A antigen in Heymann nephritis in rats). Some findings, however, were surprising, such as the rarity of detectable immune complexes in patients with MGN and the failure of injection of preformed immune complexes to produce MGN (10, 18).

A more recent hypothesis is that the subepithelial deposits were formed in situ by the fixation of a circulating antibody on an antigen present in the lamina rara region (16, 17). Various studies showed that the injection of antibody directed against the Fx 1A antigen produced experimental

Table 26G.1.
Clinical Evolution of Children with MGN

Status at last investigation	All patients	Patients followed for >3 years
Complete remission	44	38 (53.5%)
Mild proteinuria (<0.5 g/day)	13	7 (10%)
Isolated microscopic hematuria	1	—
Persistent proteinuria (>0.5 g/day)	20	13 (18%)
Nephrotic syndrome	9	4 (5.5%)
Renal failure	9[a]	9[a] (13%)
TOTAL	96	71 (100%)

[a] Two of these children had proximal tubular dysfunction; anti-tubular basement membrane antibodies were found in one, not done in the other.

MGN, demonstrating that Fx 1A was present in the normal capillary wall. MGN can also be induced by a foreign nonglomerular antigen capable of binding to the capillary wall. The injection of antibodies directed against this antigen planted along the GBM results in in situ formation and deposition of immune complexes. MGN has been obtained using the lectin concanavalin A as an antigen localizing in the subepithelial space without causing detectable glomerular injury by themselves, but reacting with injected antibodies to induce MGN. These models have been shown to be complement-dependent but neutrophil-independent (19).

In all instances, the penetration of either immune complexes or the antigen alone would be facilitated if they carried cationic charges (19a).

If inflammation and neutrophils seem to have no or little role in the immune reaction leading to MGN, there is some evidence, although not yet well established, for a role of cellular immunity disturbances. The possibility of inducing MGN by injection of lymphocytes taken from diseased animals is debated. Litwin (20), using Fx 1A antigens, showed skin hypersensitivity in rats associated with in vitro proliferation of lymphocytes in the presence of this antigen. Hypersensitivity to Heymann antigen has been reported by Grupe (21). Other cellular immunity alterations have been described, but whether they are specific of MGN is unknown. For example, decreased synthesis of IgG by patient lymphocytes has been reported in MGN, as well as in nephrosis.

Last, the importance of predisposing hereditary factors is likely in rats. Mercury-induced MGN can be obtained only with certain strains of rats and not in all; in man, a high incidence of HLA DR W3 in patients with MGN has been pointed out.

The mechanism of MGN in humans remains poorly understood. The fact that MGN may be associated with a variety of diseases suggests that many various antigens can be responsible. The possibly causal antigen or antibody has been detected in several instances by immunofluorescence studies, but these findings have not been convincingly confirmed. For instance, the presence of hepatitis B surface antigen in the deposits of some MGN remains controversial.

Finally, MGN can be considered to be a result of the deposition, probably in situ, either of antigens and antibodies or of antibodies to some component of the GBM, which has perhaps been modified and rendered antigenic by unrecognized phenomena. Deposit formation appears to be influenced by disturbances of the immune system (such as those induced by some drugs) and would be facilitated by hereditary factors.

Etiologies and Associations

MGN has been described in association with several disorders or medical treatments. Some are the causes of the disease; in other cases, the association does not represent a sure etiology. The main extrarenal conditions associated with MGN in our series are shown in Table 26G.2 and have been previously published (13).

Drugs and Toxic Agents

Drug-induced MGN was recently reviewed (22). Two types of drugs are implicated, heavy metals and substances having a sulfhydryl radical. Clinical manifestations appear after 6 to 12 months of treatment, without evident relationship to doses, and consist of isolated proteinuria or NS. Lesions are often focal and discrete (23) and can go unnoticed when electronic microscopy or immunofluorescence study is not made. The course is usually to recovery after stopping treatment, often after an interval of several months. The disease can reappear when treatment is restarted, or more rarely, can heal clinically despite its continuation.

The role of heavy metals has been confirmed by experimental studies. Gold salts (23) are particularly used in treatment of rheumatoid arthritis

Table 26G.2.
Extrarenal Conditions Associated with MGN in 96 Children

Condition	Children
D-penicillamine therapy	1
Hepatitis and/or circulating HBsAg[a]	18
Syphilis	1
Idiopathic thrombocytopenia	3
Myelomonocytic leukemia plus arthralgias	1
Proximal tubular dysfunction[b]	3
Sickle-cell disease (homozygotous or heterozygotous)	3
Streptococcal infection	4
Arthralgias or skin rash	5
TOTAL	39

[a] Two children had an acute hepatitis, one of them has not been investigated for blood HBsAg. In the remainder, HBsAg with or without hepatic symptoms was discovered by investigation.

[b] Two of these children were studied by IF and antitubular basement membrane antibodies were found. One child had a celiac disease and a favorable outcome. The two others developed renal failure.

and may induce MGN in humans and in animals. Proteinuria appears in approximately 10% of patients receiving such treatment, and NS in approximately 1%. Gold inclusions have been found in various parts of the kidney but not in the deposits.

MGN following ingestion of mercury salts has been observed in both children and adults, following either treatment or professional or accidental contamination. Mercury intoxication can be unrecognized in the absence of serious inquiry. This mercury-induced MGN has been the most extensively studied and its occurrence was shown to be affected by hereditary factors linked to histocompatibility antigens (24).

Other heavy metals incriminated in MGN are bismuth salts and silver salts; their responsibility has been less well demonstrated.

Among drugs with a sulfhydryl radical, D-penicillamine is most often incriminated. It is used in the treatment of rheumatoid arthritis and in the child with Wilson's disease and cystinuria. We observed one case (Table 26G.2) associated with segmental lesions and having a favorable course despite reinitiation of treatment. Gartner reported 51 cases (14), and approximately 100 others have been observed (22).

Other drugs suggested as causes are thiopronine, pyrithioxine, and 5-thiopyrodoxine (22). More recently, several cases have been reported following treatment by captopril (25); they were more often associated with an isolated proteinuria than with NS.

The mechanism of drug-induced MGN remains debated. It seems excluded that drugs act as antigens. It is possible that they induce modifications of native tissue initiating the immunological process. It is better established that they can modify the immune reactions, thus favorizing the development of autoimmune disease. Most of the drugs causing MGN can induce several extrarenal manifestations (circulating antiDNA antibodies, skin rashes, and so on) and disorders of the immune system. In humans as in animals, the susceptibility to develop drug-induced MGN differs according to the presence of various HLA antigens.

Infectious and Parasitic Diseases

Secondary or congenital syphilis can be associated with renal involvement, which often appears as abrupt NS and would seem in most cases to correspond to MGN. Some authors have found treponema antigen by immunofluorescence studies in the deposits (26) and an antibody in the kidney eluates (27). This finding suggests a mechanism of specific immune complexes. This etiology should always be sought, particularly in the infant. Early treatment by penicillin brings fast recovery. Delayed treatment can result in diffuse renal lesions and a severe course. We observed one case, an infant of 2 months with frank NS who rapidly recovered with treatment.

The association of hepatitis B (HB), or more often the chronic asymptomatic presence of the HB surface antigen (HBsAg), is by far the most frequent agent in our series. HBsAg was sought in 40 children and was found in 18. An even higher proportion was found in Japan with 11/11 children with MGN (3). The presence of HBsAg has been reported in other nephropathies, but is by far the most frequently found in MGN (15), particularly in the child. It is unlikely that these results are mere chance. Most cases observed at Enfants-Malades Hospital have already been reported, and this association has been discussed (15). A high percentage of boys is found among children having MGN associated with HBsAg (16/18 or 89%), whereas in MGN without HBsAg both sexes are affected similarly.

MGN was usually the presenting disease, and HBsAg was found at examination. In all cases, NS was present initially, often very frank, but rapidly regressing. No clinical finding appeared to distinguish MGN with HBsAg from idiopathic MGN. Symptomology was similar; the frequency of various immunoglobulins and complement fractions in the deposits appeared similar, as well as that of lowered C4 and C1q and more rarely C3. The presence of immune complexes was rare in both instances. The course of HBsAg-associated MGN was most often favorable. At last examination, eight children showed clinical recovery, three minimal proteinuria, five proteinuria and one NS. Only one developed renal failure. The prognosis thus appears favorable in MGN with HBsAg, particularly since the child having a severe course was investigated for the presence of HBsAg only after several years so that a late contamination could not be excluded.

These children often had moderately elevated transaminases, either transient or chronic. Hepatomegaly was noted in six. Liver biopsy was made in five and showed chronic active hepatitis in one, persistent hepatitis in three, and discrete fibrosis in one.

Long-term clinical recovery may coexist with the persistence of circulating HBsAg, but repeat renal biopsies showed persistence of deposits. HBsAg disappeared in only one child, while HB antibodies appeared.

Several authors have described the presence of HBsAg in extramembranous deposits seen by immunofluorescence. These results were not confirmed in our series nor in others and are presently disputed. Some authors have incriminated other hepatitis B antigens such as HBcAg (28) and, above all, HBeAg (29, 30). The few patients studied in the present series had HBc antibodies and HBeAg; the latter disappeared in one case, whereas in the other it was low during remission and had totally disappeared at time of relapse. These data are too few and too preliminary to permit any conclusion. It should also be noted that HBsAg or other hepatitis B markers are often found in family members of these children. This finding has suggested transmission during pregnancy, but in some instances the father was the carrier.

At the present time, it cannot be concluded that a hepatitis B antigen is at the origin of MGN nor which antigen might be responsible or whether the association is a result of an immune deficit favoring the development of both diseases.

Two cases of acute poststreptococcal glomerulonephritis, which developed into MGN, have been reported (31). In four children of our series, MGN appeared after streptococcal infection. A possible link between the two remains to be documented.

It is known that NS can be associated with infection by *Plasmodium malariae.* Some authors consider this nephropathy to be MGN, whereas others think they are different diseases.

MGN has also been found in association with other states, such as filariosis or hydatic disease (32).

Immunological Diseases

In systemic lupus erythematosus (SLE) the histological aspect of the renal lesion in SLE may be typical MGN. It should be remembered that MGN can be isolated and idiopathic during a long period, sometimes years, before laboratory signs of SLE appear. The prognosis (90% survival after 5 years) does not differ from that of idiopathic MGN.

We observed four patients with SLE-associated MGN. All had proteinuria with NS in three, hematuria in three, and hypertension in one. One child had clinical remission for 3 years; two remain proteinuric, one of them with hypertension. The last developed end-stage renal failure and a second renal biopsy showed signs of activity and diffuse crescents.

Association with other immune diseases has been reported. Thyroiditis (33–35), was found, often associated with the presence of thyroglobulin antibodies, which were also found in the deposits (35, 36). Guillain-Barré syndrome (37), pulmonary manifestation with clinical Goodpasture's syndrome, and mixed association of Sjögren's and Gardner-Diamond syndromes with MGN were also found (13).

In some of our cases, the onset of the disease included signs suggestive of circulating immune complexes, such as fever, rash, arthralgias, and, in two cases, tubular basement membrane antibodies (38). Three children had thrombocytopenia of varying duration. The finding of renal tubular epithelium antigen (RTE) by some authors (39, 40) has not been confirmed by others.

Malignancies

An association with cancer is more frequent in the adult (9). Carcinoma is the most frequently seen. An antigen specific to the tumor was found in the deposits, but this finding remains to be confirmed (41–43). Leukemia may also be involved (13). The association with a Wilms' tumor has been reported in the child (9), but NS in a child with nephroblastoma generally corresponds to another histological category. One child had MGN associated with an ovarian carcinoma; her renal disease remitted after surgical ablation of the tumor. (Beauvais, Hôpital Trousseau, personal communication.)

Other Associations

Other associations have been observed, such as celiac disease (one case in our series), diabetes, drepanocytosis, in which tubular epithelium antigen was incriminated, or cutaneous lymphfolliculosis. The association of renal vein thrombosis has been stressed and the role of RTE suggested, but in fact thrombosis seems the consequence and not the cause of MGN (43). This association appears to be frequent in some adult series, but most often it is latent. It was not found in our series.

Post-transplantation Membranous Glomerulonephritis

Recurrence of MGN after renal transplantation is relatively rare. However, de novo MGN on a transplanted kidney occurs rather frequently, and 61 such cases have been reported (44). Proteinuria appears at a mean of 2 years after transplantation (range 2 to 58 months). It is seen in both children and adults. It rarely appears to result in graft loss. In conclusion, MGN is observed in a large number of circumstances. Certain agents, such as drugs, syphilis, and SLE, are clearly implicated. The nature of the association is less well established in other cases. Despite the large number of associations described, the great majority of MGN remain idiopathic, with an undetermined etiology.

Pathology

Light Microscopy

By light microscopy, MGN is characterized by diffuse thickening of the glomerular capillary walls (Fig. 26G.1), with widely patent lumens

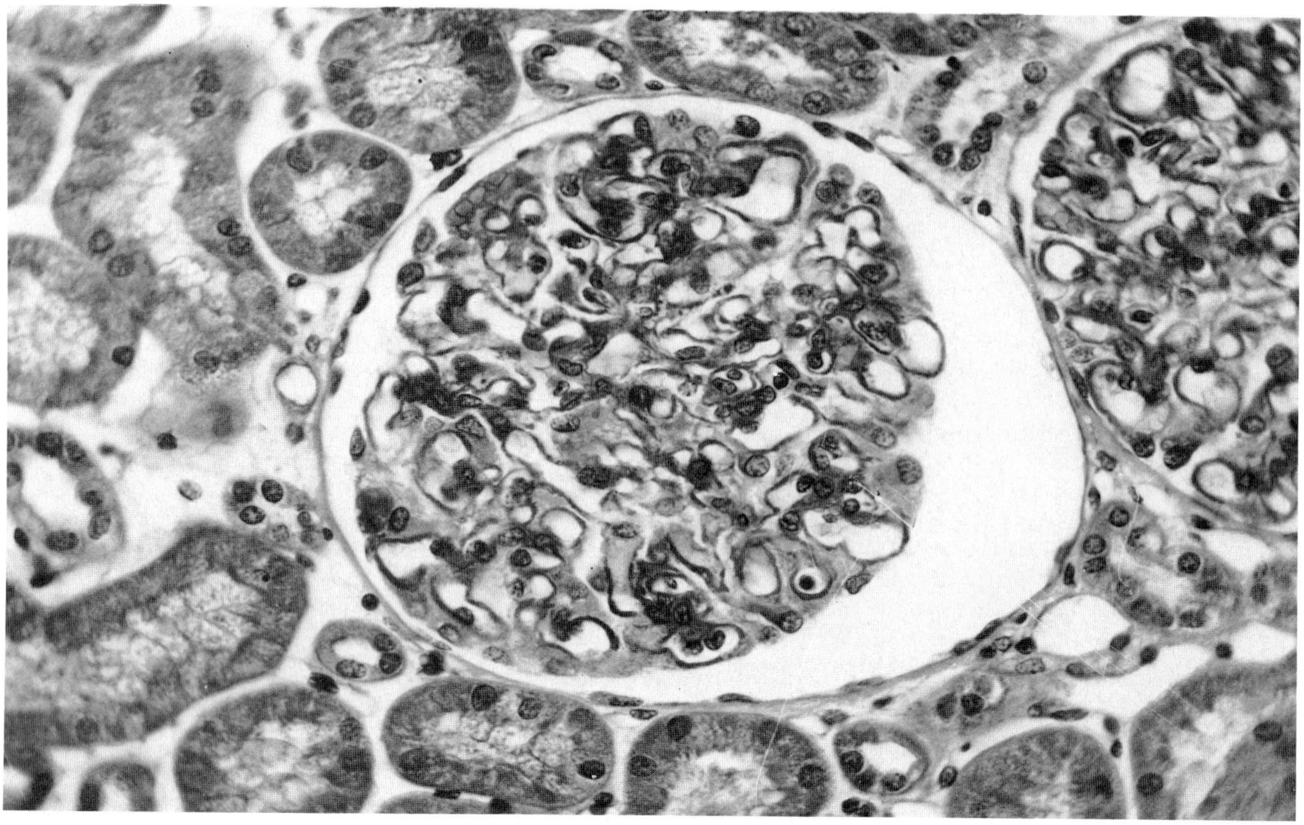

Figure 26G.1. Light microscopy, showing a regular and diffuse increase of the thickness of all the capillary walls, and the absence of mesangial proliferation.

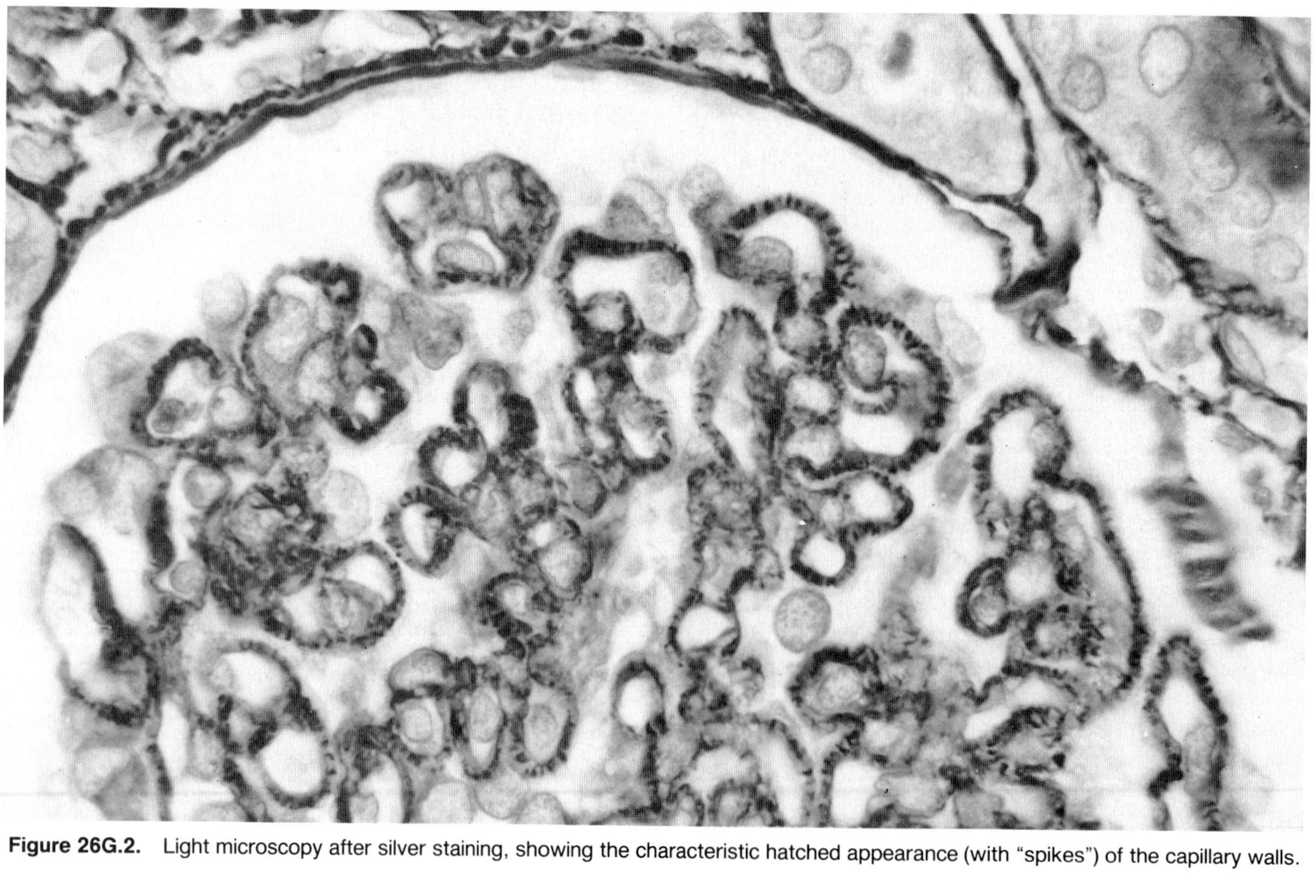

Figure 26G.2. Light microscopy after silver staining, showing the characteristic hatched appearance (with "spikes") of the capillary walls.

and marked hypertrophy of the epithelial cells. Usually there is no obvious mesangial proliferation, although morphometric studies have shown moderate mesangial hypercellularity with increased mesangial matrix material (14). In certain cases, trichrome staining shows that the thickening of the capillary walls is a result of the presence of abnormal, more or less continuous deposits on the epithelial side of the GBM. The deposits are not argyrophilic, but silver stains show argyrophilic projections arising from the glomerular basement membrane, resembling spikes. These spikes can be numerous, hence giving the wall a characteristic hatched appearance (Fig. 26G.2). On the other hand, these deposits can be spaced or occur on only some of the capillary walls. In advanced lesions, the spikes can meet and give a chainlike aspect to the capillary walls. The tubules and the interstitium are usually normal. In advanced cases some glomeruli may show superimposed lesions of segmental sclerosis or hyalinosis, tubular atrophy, and interstitial sclerosis. Epithelial crescentic proliferation appearing during the course of the disease has been reported, but is rare. Finally, in some cases the MGN lesion may be associated with cellular infiltration of the interstitium and tubular atrophy without severe glomerular lesions.

Electron Microscopy

Studies using electron microscopy (EM) have analyzed the lesions and distinguished several patterns according to the extent of the deposits and the intensity of the reaction of the basement membrane. Three (45) or four (46) types of lesions are considered to be various stages in the histological course of the disease. They are better visualized after silver staining in the EM preparation.

Stage I is considered the initial stage and includes more or less numerous deposits located beneath the foot processes, on the epithelial side of the basement membrane. MGN spikes are rare or absent, and the lamina densa remains normal.

Stage II corresponds to the classic and most common form of MGN. Subepithelial deposits are abundant and more diffuse. There are extensions of the lamina densa called spikes, also stained by silver, which appear between the deposits (Fig. 26G.3). Generally, both the deposits and the spikes are diffuse along the lamina densa. The lamina densa itself is irregular and often thin. The mesangium may contain abnormal deposits (47).

Stage III is characterized by large deposits and by lateral projections from the spikes so that the extensions of the lamina densa meet and encircle the deposits, tending to form a new layer of lamina densa on their external side. The deposits are thus progressively incorporated into the GBM, losing their density, and become difficult to distinguish. At this stage the GBM appears irregularly thickened.

Some authors have described a stage IV (46), characterized by severe alterations of the GBM, leading to successive, mixed layers of deposits and expansions of the lamina densa.

In addition, a stage V (14, 48), or a healing stage has been described in some patients who had clinically recovered (48, 49). A new lamina densa appears to have formed under the epithelial cells. The endothelial side of the GBM is irregular, with lucent areas interpreted as a trace of the deposits that have been incorporated into the GBM and that have lost their density.

The lesions are not always diffuse. There are rare forms where they remain focal (1, 50, 51), with deposits and expansions of the lamina densa visible only on some capillary walls. These forms were first considered early aspects of the disease. In fact, it appears that the lesions can remain focal while going through the same stages as the diffuse forms (1, 51).

In any case, various stages can exist at the same time and affect different capillary walls (1).

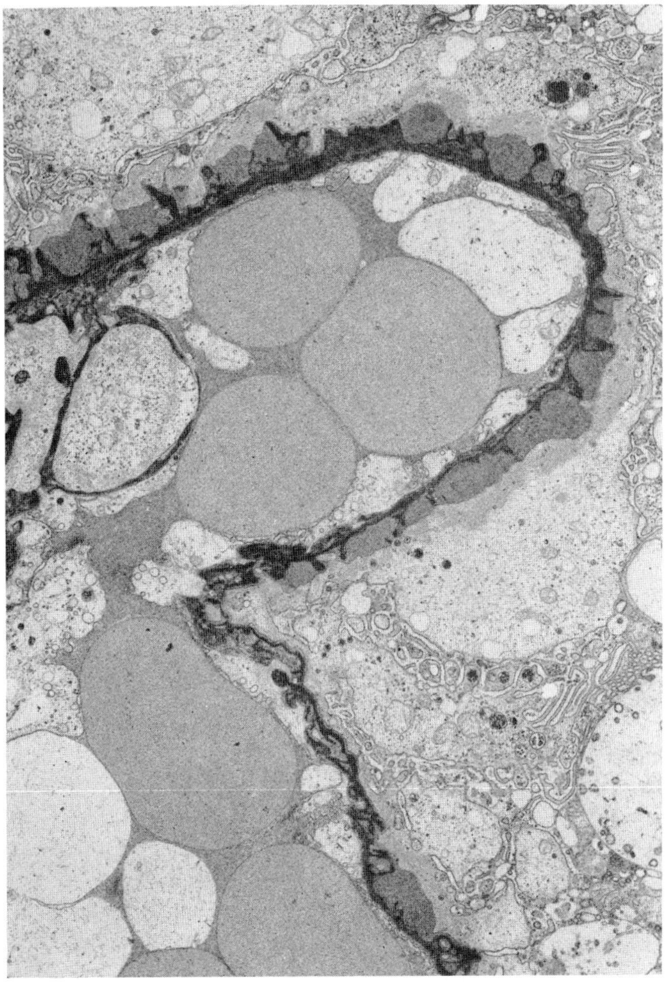

Figure 26G.3. Electron microscopy. Silver methenamine impregnation stain. (X5100.) Presence of diffuse osmiophilic, nonargyrophilic deposits located on the epithelial side of the basement membrane. They are separated by spiky projections arising from the lamina densa.

In some reports, MGN is classified into stages only by light microscopy following silver staining. In stage I, the lesions are hardly visible, while the capillary wall appears somewhat rigid but almost normal. Stage II corresponds to the hatched stage, with clearly visible spikes after silver staining. Stage III corresponds to extreme thickening of the GBM with chainlike aspects. In fact, it should be noted that these classifications can be established precisely only by the electron microscopic study that was used to describe them. It has been shown that a practically normal aspect of the GBM, which would have been classified stage I in light microscopy can correspond to more advanced stages or to a healing stage by electron microscopy (52).

Immunofluorescence

By immunofluorescence, the GBM is characteristically stained by granular fixation of anti-IgG serum of variable intensity. The granular deposits are usually of identical size and are regularly distributed along the glomerular capillary walls (pearl necklace aspect) (Fig. 26G.4). More rarely, the deposits are small and at low magnification may appear to be linear. Often in fact, the deposits vary in size and are irregularly distributed along the walls, sometimes in several layers. Rarely, the deposits are segmental, affecting only a few capillary walls. These deposits consistently fix anti-IgG serum, but can also fix anti-IgM or IgA (67% and 30% of

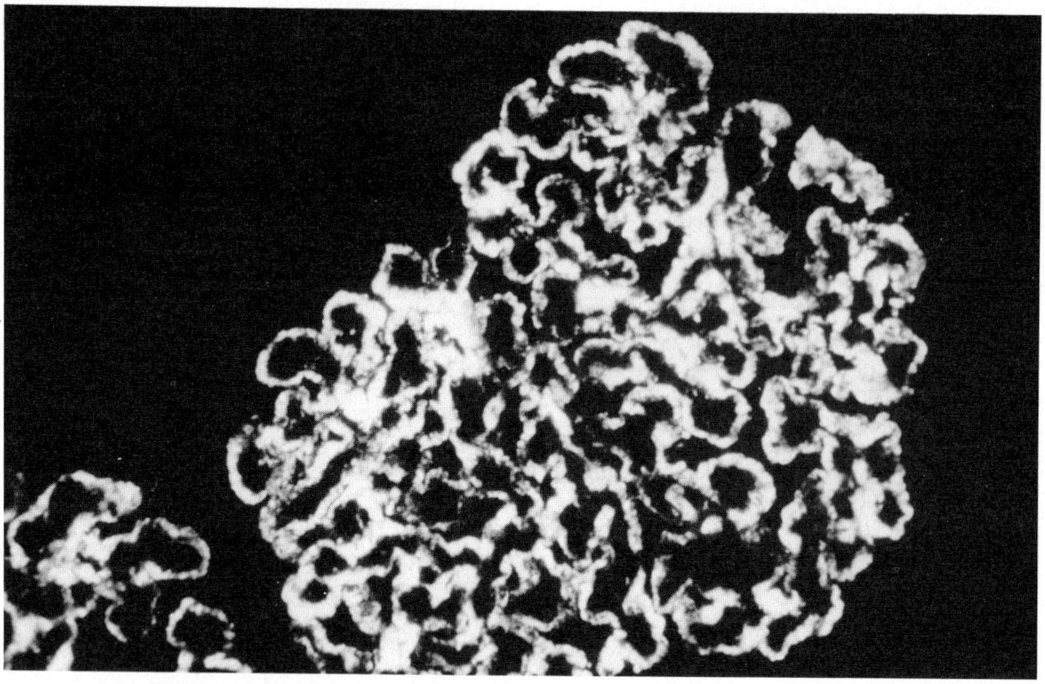

Figure 26G.4. Immunofluorescence using anti-IgG serum. Granular deposits are regularly distributed along the epithelial side of the glomerular capillary walls.

cases). They often contain C3 (78% of cases), more rarely C1q (54%), or C4 (25%). Only rarely are the C1q deposits very abundant.

The presence of all classes of immunoglobulins and of early complement components, particularly C1q and C4, has been considered as indicative of underlying SLE. In fact, they are far from exceptional in idiopathic MGN, with or without extrarenal associated conditions (13, 15).

Granular deposits of IgG along tubular basement membranes may be seen in the absence of lupus. The description of a few cases with linear deposits of IgG along the tubular basement membranes of the proximal convoluted tubules is intriguing (38).

Principles of Treatment

The effectiveness of treatment and its indications are presently controversial. Most retrospective studies, both in the adult (9, 12) and in the child (53), conclude that corticosteroids or immunodepressive agents are ineffective. Remission was usually observed after intervals of several months, whether treatment had been continued or stopped for a long time. Remission was also observed when no treatment had been given. Among the nine children in our series who progressed to renal failure, seven had received treatment. In some cases, rapid improvement of NS appeared to be linked to the administration of corticosteroids, but a similar brief course can be observed without treatment. One of the series with the most favorable prognosis (12) reports patients who never had any treatment.

The idea that no useful therapy was available has been accepted by most authors for several years. One retrospective study showed that patients treated by glucocorticoids had a more favorable outcome than untreated patients, but the two groups differed by many factors other than treatment (54).

One prospective randomized trial conducted by the colloborative Study of Adult Idiopathic Nephrotic Syndromes (55) recently led to new debates on this subject. Nephrotic adult patients with MGN, receiving a relatively short course of corticosteroids (150 or 100 mg/day every other day during 8 weeks) followed by gradual tapering over an additional 8 weeks, showed clear-cut improvement in prognosis in the treated patients, whatever the previous length of the disease. After an interval of 4 to 56 months (24 months in 43/67 patients), plasma creatinine had at least doubled in 2/34 treated patients and in 11/38 of those who received a placebo. Renal failure appeared in one treated and ten nontreated patients.

These are spectacular and convincing results, but the problem remains that the proportion of renal failure occurring after very short intervals (26%) was higher than that observed in most European series, whereas the percentage of remission at last examination was lower. It would thus appear that the patients studied in the American investigation form a population that is different from that observed in France, in particular in children. This may be in part a result of the fact that only nephrotic patients were included in the therapeutic study. It may also be supposed that the distribution of the causes of MGN may vary from one region to another, accounting for differences in prognosis and response to therapy. Since etiology remains unknown in the great majority of cases, its link with a benefit of steroids is difficult to study.

In the present status of knowledge it can be admitted that children with no or transient NS are at only slight risk of developing renal failure and do not require treatment. In children with NS of some duration, a poor outcome is rare but cannot be excluded; alternate-day steroid therapy for a few weeks has little toxicity and its possible benefit cannot be refused, keeping in mind that it does not always prevent renal deterioration. Whether longer treatment would be more beneficial has not been evaluated.

There is presently no evidence for a beneficial effect of other drugs, such as immunosuppressors, that are in addition more toxic.

Course and Prognosis

In our experience, the clinical course is highly variable but rarely severe. Of the 96 children followed during 1 to 18 years, 9 progressed to renal failure. Two (the youngest) had a tubular syndrome associated with severe tubulointerstitial alterations on renal biopsy, with antitubular basement membrane antibodies documented in one. One had severe homozygote drepanocytosis, the role of which cannot be excluded. The 6 others were 11 to 13 years of age at onset. All had NS, permanent in four. One had transient improvement, but showed severe tubulointerstitial lesions on a second renal biopsy. One, after having had NS during 7 months, had complete remission lasting 3.5 years, followed by reappearance of NS with rapid progression to renal failure. This last evolution seems exceptional, and all authors agree that the occurrence of a complete or partial remission is indicative of a good outcome. Renal failure was present after a 7-year course in one child and after less than 5 years in the others. At last examination, 44 children had no symptoms and 13 had only mild and intermittent proteinuria (<0.50 g/d). One child had isolated microscopic hematuria, 20 had persistent proteinuria, and 9 had NS. Among the latter, 5 had a course of less than 3 years.

Among the 71 children followed up for at least 3 years, 63% have no symptom or only slight proteinuria, 18% have proteinuria, 6% have NS, and 13% have renal failure.

One characteristic of our series is its favorable prognosis as compared to other series, particularly those of adults. This finding has led to a conclusion that prognosis is better in children than in adults. In fact, large variations among series in both age groups remain unexplained. In our series, among the children with unfavorable outcome, three had renal lesions in addition to MGN; the six others were 11 years of age or more at onset. Renal failure was observed in 20% of children 11 years or older and in 10% of the overall series. In other pediatric series, the percentage of renal failure is highly varied: 7/12 (58%) for Ehrenreich and coworkers (54), 29% (5), 33% (2), 27% (7), 21% (4), and 1/7 or 14% (9). The course is also highly variable in adult series, with frequency of renal failure reported as 10% (45), 33% (53), 19% (14), and 41% (55), and the proportion of patients in remission as 0 (56) to 20 to 30% (9, 12). It has been reported that the prognosis is better in females, but other series show no difference (10); in our series, renal failure was observed in 2 of 25 girls and in 7 of 71 boys, i.e., frequencies that are very close.

Given such diversity, prognostic factors are difficult to determine. In our experience, the presence and particularly the persistence of NS would indicate poor prognosis. Focal forms appear to correspond to a regressive course rather than to an early form of the disease, which will eventually become severe. The prognostic value of histological stages is variously interpreted and far from definitely established.

References

1. Habib R, Kleinknecht C, Gubler MC: Extramembranous glomerulonephritis in children: report of 50 cases. J Pediatr 82:754, 1972.
2. Olbing H, Greifer J, Bennet BP, et al: Idiopathic membranous nephropathy in children. Kidney Intl 3:381, 1973.
3. Takekoshi Y, Tanaka M, Shida N, et al: Strong association between membranous nephropathy and hepatitis-B surface antigaenemia in japanese children. Lancet 2:1065, 1978.
4. Latham P, Poucell S, Koresaar A, et al: Idiopathic membranous glomerulopathy in canadian children: a clinicopathologic study. J Pediatr 101:682, 1982.
5. Trainin EB, Boichis H, Spitzer A, et al: Idiopathic membranous nephropathy. Clinical course in children. NY State J Med 76:357, 1976.
6. Tsao YC, Chan WC, Gibson JP: Persistant proteinuria in children. Arch Dis Child 44:443, 1966.
7. Ramirez F, Brouhard BH, Travis LB, et al: Idiopathic membranous nephropathy in children. J Pediatr 101:667, 1982.
8. Barbanel C, Noel LH: Glomérulonéphrites extra-membraneuses. In J Hamburger, J Crosnier, JP Grunfeld (es): Néphrologie, Paris, Flammarion, 1979, p 499.
9. Row PG, Cameron JS, Turner DR, et al: Membranous nephropathy. Quart J Med, 44:207, 1975.
10. Coggins CH, Glassock RJ: Membranous nephropathy. Semin Nephrol 2:264, 1982.
11. International Study of Kidney Disease in Children: Nephrotic syndrome in children: prediction of histopathology from clinical and laboratory characteristics at time of diagnosis. Kidney Int 13:159, 1978.
12. Noel LH, Zanetti M, Droz D, et al: Long term prognosis for idiopathic membranous glomerulonephritis. Study of 116 untreated patients. Am J Med 66:82, 1979.
13. Kleinknecht C, Levy M, Gagnadoux MF, et al: Extramembranous with extrarenal disorders in children. Medicine 58:219, 1979.
14. Gärtner HV: Membranous glomerulonephritis. Prototype of an immune complex glomerulonephritis. In Büngeler W, Eder M, Lennert K, et al (eds): Stuttgart, New York, Gustav Fisher Verlag, 1980, p 1.
15. Kleinknecht C, Levy M, Peix A, et al: Membranous glomerulonephritis and hepatitis-B surface antigen in children. J Pediatr 95:946, 1979.
16. Glassock RJ, Edgington TS, Watson JJ: Autologous immune-complex nephritis induced with renal tubular antigen II: the pathogenetic mechanism. J Exp Med 127:573, 1968.
17. Makker SP, Moorthy B: In situ immune complex formation in isolated perfused kidney using homologous kidney. Lab Invest 44:1, 1981.
18. Cameron JS: Pathogenesis and treatment of membranous nephropathy. Kidney Intl 15:88, 1979.
19. Adler S, Salant DJ, Dittmer JE, et al: Meditation of proteinuria in membranous nephropathy due to a planted glomerular antigen. Kidney Intl 23:807, 1983.
19a. Border WA, Ward HJ, Kamil ES, et al: Induction of membranous nephropathy in rabbits by administration of an exogenous cationic antigen: demonstration of a pathogenic role for electrical charge. J Clin Invest 69:451, 1981.
20. Litwin A, Adams LE, Levy R, et al: Cellular immunity in experimental glomerulonephritis of rats II. Immunology 25:227, 1973.
21. Grupe WE: An in vitro demonstration of cellular sensitivity in experimental auto immune nephrosis in rats. Proc Soc Exp Biol Med 127:1217, 1968.
22. Fillastre JP, Mery JPh, Druet Ph: Néphropathies glomérulaires médicamenteuses. Néphrologie 4:1, 1983.
23. Törnroth T, Skrifvars B: Gold nephropathy prototype of membranous glomerulonephritis. Am J Pathol 75:573, 1974.
24. Bariety J, Druet P, Laliberte F, et al: Glomerulonephritis with γ and βIC-globulin deposits induced in rats by mercuric chloride. Am J Pathol 65:293, 1971.
25. Textor SC, Gephardt GN, Bravo EL, et al: Membranous glomerulopathy associated with captopril therapy. Am J Med 74:705, 1983.
26. Tourville DR, Burd LH, Kim DU, et al: Treponemal antigen in immunopathogenesis of syphilitic glomerulonephritis. Am J Pathol 82:479, 1976.
27. O'Regan S, Fong JSC, de Chadarevian JP, et al: Treponemal antigens in congenital and acquired syphilitic nephritis. Ann Intern Med 85:325, 1976.
28. Slusarczyk J, Michalak T, Nazarewicz-Demezer T, et al: Membranous glomerulopathy associated with hepatitis B core antigen immune complexes in children. Am J Pathol 98:29, 1980.
29. Ito H, Hattori S, Matusda I, et al: Hepatitis Be Antigen-mediated membranous glomerulonephritis. Lab Invest 44:214, 1981.
30. Takekoshi Y, Tanaka M, Miyakawa Y, et al: Free "small" and IgG-associated "large" hepatitis Be antigen in the serum and glomerular capillary walls of two patients with membranous glomerulonephritis. N Engl J Med 300:814, 1979.
31. Richet G, Fillastre JP, Morel-Maroger L, et al: Change from diffuse proliferative to membranous glomerulonephritis: serial biopsies in four cases. Kidney Intl 5:57, 1974.
32. Ibarrola AS, Sobrini B, Guisantes J, et al: Membranous glomerulonephritis secondary to hydatid disease. Am J Med 70:311, 1981.
33. Horvath F, Teague P, Gaffney EF, et al: Thyroid antigen associated immune complex glomerulonephritis in Grave's disease. Am J Med 67:901, 1979.
34. Jordan SC, Buckingham B, Sakair Olson D: Studies on immune-complex glomerulonephritis mediated by human thyroglobulin. N Engl J Med 304:1212, 1981.
35. O'Regan S, Fong JSC, Kaplan BS, et al: Thyroid antigen-antibody nephritis. Clin Immunol Immunopathol 6:341, 1976.
36. Ploth DW, Fitz A, Schnetzler D, et al: Thyroglobulin-antithyroglobulin immune complex glomerulonephritis complicating radioiodine therapy. Clin Immunol Immunopathol 9:327, 1978.
37. Talamo TS, Borochovitz D: Membranous glomerulonephritis associated with the Guillain-Barré syndrome. Am J Clin Pathol 78:563, 1982.
38. Levy M, Gagnadoux MF, Beziau A, et al: Membranous glomerulonephritis associated with anti-tubular and anti-alveolar basement membrane antibodies. Clin Nephrol 10:158, 1978.
39. Naruse J, Kitamura K, Miyakawa Y, et al: Deposition of renal tubular epithelial antigen along the glomerular capillary walls of patients with membranous glomerulonephritis. J Immunol 110:1163, 1973.
40. Ozawa T, Boedeker EA, Schorr W, et al: Immune-complex disease with unilateral renal vein thrombosis. Arch Pathol Lab Med 100:279, 1976.
41. Costanza ME, Pinn V, Schwartz RS, et al: Carcinoembryonic antigen-antibody complexes in a patient with colonic carcinoma and nephrotic syndrome. N Engl J Med 289:520, 1973.

42. Couser WG, Wagonfeld JB, Spargo BH, et al: Glomerular deposition of tumor antigen in membranous nephropathy associated with colonic carcinoma. Am J Med 57:962, 1974.
43. Lewis MG, Loughridge LW, Phillips TM: Immunological studies in nephrotic syndrome associated with extra-renal malignant disease. Lancet 2:134, 1971.
44. Wagoner RD, Stanson AW, Holley KE, et al: Renal vein thrombosis in idiopathic membranous glomerulopathy and nephrotic syndrome: incidence and significance. Kidney Int 23:368, 1983.
45. Charpentier B, Levy M: Etude coopérative des glomérulonéphrites extramembraneuses de novo sur allogreffe rénale humaine: rapport de 19 nouveaux cas sur 1550 transplantés rénaux du groupe de transplantation de l'Ile de France. Néphrologie 3:158, 1982.
46. Bariety J, Druet Ph, Lagrue G, et al: Les glomérulonéphrites "extramembraneuses". Etude morphologique en microscopie optique, électronique et immunofluorescence. Pathol Biol (Paris) 18:5, 1970.
47. Ehrenreich T, Churg J: Pathology of membranous nephropathy. In Scheldom C, Sommers E (eds): Pathology Annual New York, Appleton Century Crofts, 1968, p 145.
48. Honig C, Mouradian JA, Montoliu J, et al: Mesangial electron dense deposits in membranous nephropathy. Lab Invest 42:427, 1980.
49. Bariety J, Samarcq P, Lagrue G, et al: Evolution ultrastructurale favorable de deux cas de glomérulopathies primitives à dépôts extramembraneux diffus. Presse Med 76:2179, 1968.
50. Ozawa AG, Kinoshita Y, Morita J, et al: Resolution of membranous changes with remission of nephrotic syndrome. Tohoku J Exp Med 120:177, 1976.
51. Gaffney EF, Alexander RW, Donnelly WH: Segmental membranous glomerulonephritis. Arch Pathol Lab Med 106:409, 1982.
52. Törnroth T, Tallquist G, Pasternack A, et al: Nonprogressive, histologically mild membranous glomerulonephritis appearing in all evolutionary phases as histologically "early" membranous glomerulonephritis. Kidney Intl 14:511, 1978.
53. Kleinknecht C, Broyer M, Habib R: Steroids for idiopathic membranous nephritis. N Engl J Med 296:49, 1977.
54. Ehrenreich T, Porush JG, Churg J, et al: Treatment of idiopathic membranous nephropathy. N Engl J Med 295:741, 1976.
55. Collaborative study of the adult nephrotic syndrome: A controlled study of short-term prednisone treatment in adults with membranous nephropathy. N Engl J Med 301:1301, 1979.
56. Erwing DJ, Donadio JV, Holley KE: The clinical course of idiopathic membranous neprhopathy. Mayo Clin Proc 48:697, 1973.
57. Forland M, Spargo BH: Clinicopathological correlations in idiopathic nephrotic syndrome with membranous nephropathy. Nephron 6:498, 1969.

26H Alport's Syndrome—Hereditary Nephritis

MARIE-CLAIRE GUBLER
RENEE HABIB

Among the hereditary nephritis syndromes, Alport's syndrome (1) is an inherited renal disorder characterized by the familial occurrence in successive generations of progressive hematuric nephritis and of neural hearing loss. Usually male patients have a severe renal disease with progressive renal failure occurring before the fourth decade, whereas most females have a normal life-span. Alport's syndrome has been reported in more than 250 unrelated kindreds of all racial and geographical origins. It has been considered as the cause of end-stage renal failure in 0.6% of all patients starting renal replacement therapy in Europe (2) and in 2.3% of patients in Milliner's series (3).

Associated changes, including ocular defects, platelet abnormalities, cerebral dysfunction, polyneuropathy, hyperprolinemia, ichthyosis, and thyroid and parathyroid involvement, have been reported. In contrast to neural deafness, they affect only a few kindreds. Most of these abnormalities seem not to be part of Alport's syndrome, appearing rather as coincidental associations, complications of renal failure, or the association of extrarenal symptoms with various types of renal diseases (4). However, a relationship between ocular changes and platelet abnormalities on one hand and Alport's syndrome on the other hand has been clearly demonstrated.

Clinical Presentation

First symptoms usually occur early in life, especially in males (4–8). In our group of 58 pediatric patients (4), symptoms were detected before the age of 1 year in 14% of the children and before the age of 6 in 72% of them. However, onset may be observed later, during adulthood (9), as is generally the case in mildly affected female patients, whose disease is revealed by routine urinalysis during a pregnancy or by family screening. Macroscopic or microscopic hematuria is the major presenting symptom in most series (4–12) (Table 26H.1). It may be observed at birth (4, 5). Other presenting symptoms include proteinuria, edema, hypertension, renal failure, and deafness (4, 9, 11).

Clinical and Laboratory Findings

Renal Disease

Microscopic hematuria is present in every patient (4, 6, 7, 9) and is usually persistent. It may be intermittent in some girls and in younger males (4). Single or recurrent episodes of macroscopic hematuria are observed in about half of the patients, often occurring within 2 days following an upper respiratory tract infection. In our experience, these

Table 26H.1.
Presenting Symptoms in 58 Children (42 Males and 16 Females)

Presenting Symptoms	Males	Females
Macroscopic hematuria	12	6
Microscopic hematuria and/or proteinuria	28	10
Edema	1	
Deafness	1	0

From Hôpital Necker—Enfants-Malades' experience.

Table 26H.2.
Long-term Follow-up in 58 Children (42 Males and 16 Females)

Clinical Status	Patients		Mean age (years)
	Male	Female	
Terminal renal failure	18	2	17.3
Proteinuria >1 g/24 hrs ± nephrotic syndrome, renal failure, hypertension	15	0	14
Mild proteinuria	9	7	10
Isolated hematuria	0	7	6.9

From Hôpital Necker—Enfants-Malades' experience).

episodes are frequent during the first years of the disease and disappear after the age of 10 to 15 years. Although the duration of macroscopic hematuria usually varies from 1 to 10 days, in some instances it may persist for months (4).

Proteinuria is a common finding (4, 7, 9, 14), but is not necessarily present, and is often absent, mild, or intermittent in affected female patients. In males, proteinuria increases progressively with age, often exceeding 1 g/24 hrs after 10 to 15 years of age; development of nephrotic syndrome is not exceptional. Proteinuria in the absence of hematuria is not diagnostic for Alport's syndrome.

By intravenous pyelography (IVP), kidneys and urinary tracts are usually normal. Leucocyturia and pyuria are incidental findings.

Long-term follow-up varies according to the sex of affected patients (Table 26H.2). Most male patients progress to terminal renal failure associated with moderate hypertension, during or before the third decade (4, 9, 10, 13). Patients with this unfavorable course follow a similar pattern of mild or intermittent proteinuria in childhood, then increasing and persistent proteinuria with frequent development of nephrotic syndrome, hypertension, renal failure and terminal uremia. Conversely, most females have a mild disease. However atypical evolutions have been reported including a long-lasting course in affected males (15–17) and severe renal disease in female subjects (4, 7, 9, 18). In our series, terminal renal failure occurred in 20 patients, 18 males and 2 females between 8 and 26 years of age (Table 26H.2).

Hearing Defect

Hearing defects are not present in all affected members of a family and are more frequent in male patients. The true incidence of hearing loss is difficult to evaluate in the absence of systematic audiological studies. Cassady and coworkers (19) using audiograms found that only 25% of male patients under 19 years of age had hearing impairment.

Of the patients followed by Farboody (11), 59% had hearing loss. In our experience (4), 85% of male patients and 18% of female patients had a hearing defect detected in all cases before the age of 15 years.

The hearing defect is of the neurogenic type, is bilateral with an initial maximum hearing loss at 2000, 4000 or 8000 Hz, which is only recognized by audiometry. Serial audiological studies of males often demonstrate progression of hearing loss and extension to other frequencies. Involvement of the conversational zones may lead to considerable hearing difficulties. Hearing impairment may be temporarily compensated with hearing aids. Hearing improvement has been reported after renal transplantation in patients with Alport's syndrome, but also occurs in patients with hearing defects related to uremia. In some patients, especially in females, a mild hearing defect detected by audiometry is present throughout the lifetime.

Progression of hearing loss usually suggests a poor prognosis (4, 19). However, some reported patients are deaf without renal involvement or without progression to renal failure (13, 16).

Ocular Defects

Various types of ocular changes involving lens and retina have been described. Lenticonus anterior has been considered until recently as the most common eye abnormality found in Alport's syndrome (13, 20). It is seen as a regular, conical protrusion of the anterior part of the lens into the chamber (13, 20–22), leading to progressive disturbance of the vision. It is often associated with posterior or anterior cataract. It is seen only as a part of Alport's syndrome (22). The microspherophakia described by Sohar (23) and reported by Farboody (11) in 2 patients each, respectively, has never been observed by other authors. Histological examination of both eyes in one of Sohar's patients revealed, in fact, lenticonus anterior (24).

Various fundus lesions have occasionally been described (13). In two recent reports (25, 26) characteristic macular and perimacular changes have been recognized. They consist of bilateral densely packed whitish, yellow granulations surrounding the foveal area. They are superficially located in the retina. The fovea itself, whose reflexion is suppressed, is dark red. These lesions were present in 29 of 79 investigated subjects (26). In some patients (22) and especially in children (4) the only fundus lesion detected is the disappearance of the foveola reflex with changes in pigmentation of the macula. When macular and perimacular changes are isolated, no functional disturbance is observed (25, 26).

Ocular lesions were observed in 18 of the 41 investigated children in our series (4). Macular changes were found in 18 and lenticonus anterior was associated in 10 males. Both lesions, though inconstant, are reliable diagnostic criteria for Alport's syndrome; moreover, they seem to portend a poor prognosis (26).

Platelet Disorders

Severe platelet disorder has been reported in patients of five unrelated families (4, 18, 27, 28) and in a few subjects presenting hematuric nephritis and deafness without any family history. It is characterized by a prolonged bleeding time with severe thrombocytopenia, giant platelets, defective adherence of platelets to glass, absent or poor aggregation in response to collagen, ADP, and ristocetin. When a family study is available, the platelet abnormality is present in all patients affected with nephritis or deafness, although it is absent in nonaffected relatives. The association of these platelet abnormalities and hereditary nephritis has been termed Epstein's syndrome.

Morphological Characteristics

By light microscopy, renal findings are not specific. In young children, renal biopsy specimens show no abnormalities although increased numbers of immature glomeruli have been reported (6). With increasing age, the mesangium shows a mild and irregular excess in matrix with areas of segmental proliferation, and the capillary walls may appear thickened and irregular. Advancing glomerular disease is characterized by increasing mesangial enlargement and segmental sclerosis and hyalinosis. Tubulointerstitial changes appear early and are not related to the extent of glomerular damage (29). The presence of interstitial foam cells has often been considered as suggestive of Alport's syndrome, but these cells are frequently seen in most types of chronic glomerulonephritis (4).

Immunofluorescent study of renal tissue is usually negative (7, 14); however, occasional granular deposits of C3 or IgM are observed in some patients (4, 30). In advanced cases, focal deposits of immunoglobulins may be present along some glomerular basement membranes (GBM) and focal deposits of IgM and C3 within areas of glomerular segmental hyalinosis (4).

The characteristic morphological lesion of Alport's syndrome has been demonstrated by ultrastructural studies (4, 8, 14, 31–33). It consists of GBM thickening with irregular outer and inner contours and with splitting and splintering of the lamina densa (Fig. 26H.1). Small, round electron-dense granulations are present within the lucent zones delineated by the thin interwoven layers of lamina densa. These changes are often widespread, especially in adults, but they may be patchy and alternating with segments of normal thickness. They seem to increase on serial biopsy specimens (14, 33), at least in male patients (34). In some subjects, especially children, an extreme thinning of the lamina densa also occurs (4, 8, 12, 32, 35) (Fig. 26H.2). GBM ruptures with repair by endothelial and epithelial cells and newly formed basement membrane material may be seen. The GBM changes observed are, therefore, characterized by their irregular appearance and the association of thick, normal, and thin segments, sometimes affecting the same loops (8) (Fig. 26H.3). These lesions are present in both sexes and have been observed as early in life as 1 to 5 years (4, 8, 12, 32, 33). In a quantitative ultrastructural analysis, Rumpelt (34) observed that males had more splitting than females and that proteinuria correlated with the degree of GBM splitting.

GBM lesions therefore seem to be the hallmark of Alport's syndrome. However, no information is yet available concerning the GBM of healthy female carriers. Late occurrence of GBM changes seems possible. In 2 siblings, GBM thickening was only demonstrated on a second renal biopsy specimen obtained 8 years after the initial one (36). Moreover, in a few patients (12, 17), GBM has been found normal or thin, even in adulthood.

The specificity of the ultrastructural GBM changes has been questioned (37). Focal areas of splitting of the GBM have been observed in IgA nephropathy, in various types of immune complex glomerulonephritis, and in idiopathic nephrosis with focal and segmental glomerular sclerosis; these have no diagnostic value. By contrast, in our experience and that of others (38), widespread GBM changes are strongly suggestive of Alport's syndrome. The diagnostic value of GBM changes was highlighted by an ultrastructural study of biopsy specimens obtained in 50 of our children presenting with persistent hematuria, without IgA mesangial deposits by immunofluorescence. The characteristic GBM changes of Alport's syndrome were found in 30 of them. Subsequent clinical and genetic investigations revealed at least one criteria of Alport's syndrome in 26 of these 30 children (17).

In addition to the GBM changes, focal thickening of Bowman's capsules or tubular basement membranes may be observed. These changes are characterized by a marked bulging and splitting of the basement membrane delineating clear areas containing osmiophilic granules, droplets, or vesicular formations. These lesions are inconstant and nonspecific and are usually associated with the most severe GBM changes.

Basement membranes of lens capsule, retina, and inner ear have not been studied by electron microscopy. Epidermal basement membranes were found to be multilamellated in a family studied by Martinez-Hernandez (39) but have been normal in our experience.

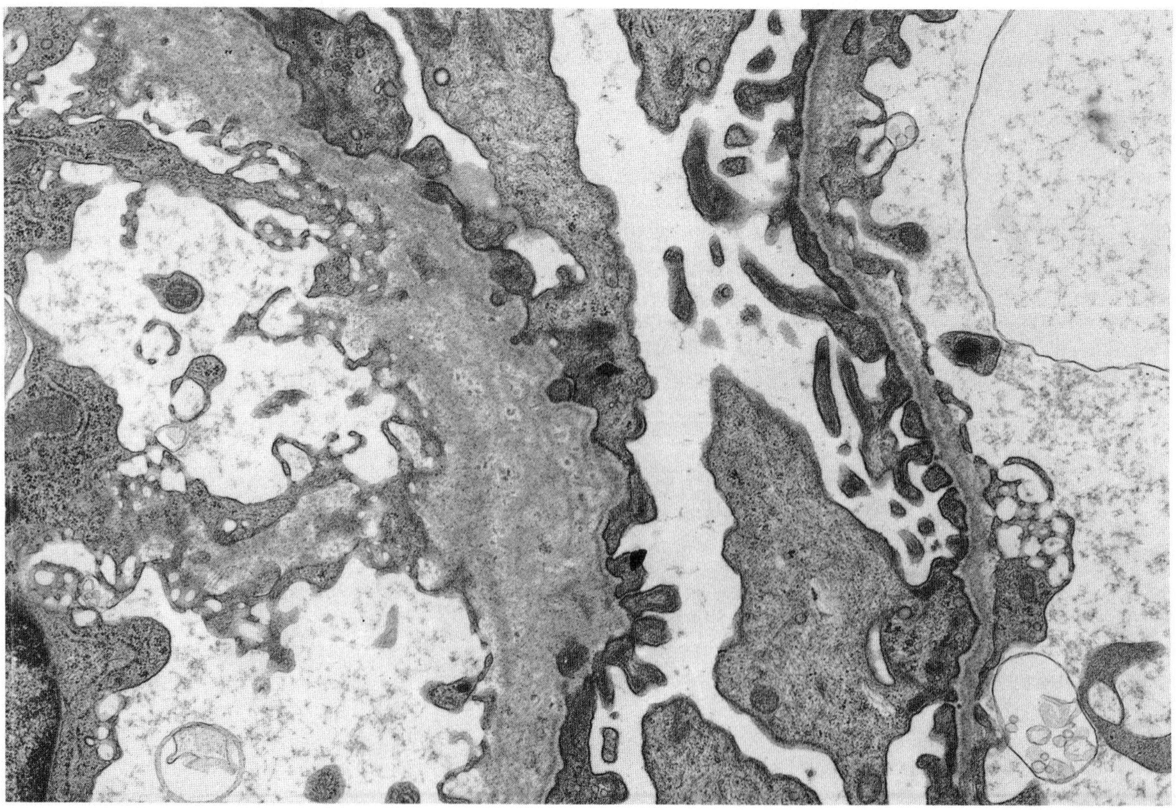

Figure 26H.1. Electron micrograph. Lead citrate and uranyl acetate stain. (X11250.) Thickened GBM showing splitting of the lamina densa and presence of granulations.

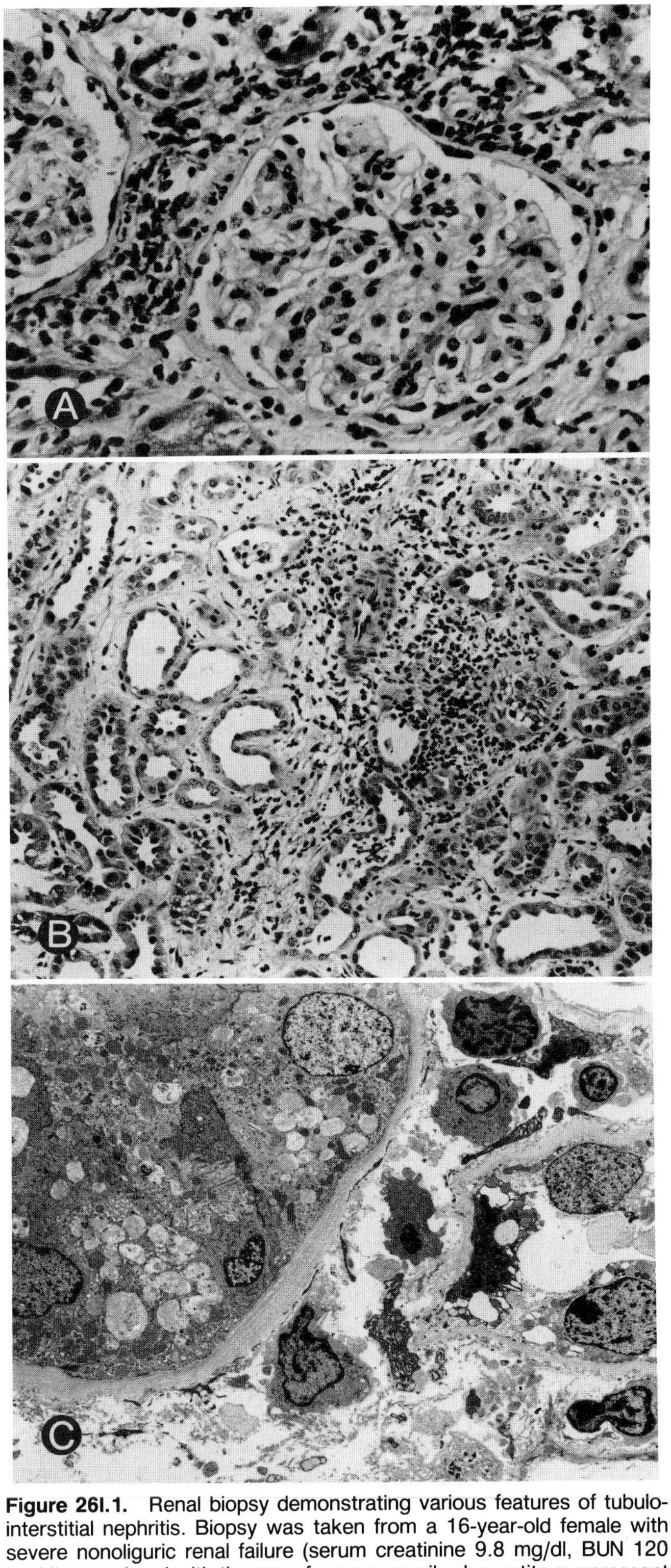

Figure 26I.1. Renal biopsy demonstrating various features of tubulointerstitial nephritis. Biopsy was taken from a 16-year-old female with severe nonoliguric renal failure (serum creatinine 9.8 mg/dl, BUN 120 mg/dl, associated with the use of a nonprescribed appetite suppressant containing caffeine and phenylpropanolamine). With discontinuation of the drug and therapy consisting of a tapering course of prednisone, renal function returned to normal within 2 months. **A,** Leukocytic infiltration is seen adjacent to a relatively normal glomerulus. (PAS stain X360.) **B,** Tubular dilatation, interstitial edema, mild fibrosis, and focal leukocytic infiltration are seen. (H & E stain X144.) **C,** Electron micrograph showing thickening and reduplication of the tubular basement membrane with edema and inflammatory cells in the interstitium. Tubular epithelial cells have many cytoplasmic vacuoles. (X2900.)

Data from adults indicates that about 5% to 30% of all nephrological consultations involve one or more nephrotoxins and about 8% to 20% of patients with acute renal failure may be secondary to drug use (1, 2). Such figures are not available in children.

The frequency of chronic TIN in the general population is also unknown. In individuals exposed to specific occupational nephrotoxins, one may be able to estimate the risk rate (3). Even after exclusion of obstructive uropathy, chronic TIN accounts from 8% to 18.7% of adult patients with end-stage kidney disease and approximates 6% to 8% in children (4–8).

Acute Tubulointerstitial Nephritis

Acute TIN was originally reported by Councilman in 1898 in 42 children who had died with scarlet fever, often complicated by diphtheria (9). In many of these patients who survived the first week of illness, interstitial round cell infiltration was described as an incidental autopsy finding, primarily in the heart and kidneys. In the late 1930s, streptococci were further implicated in such nonsuppurative tubulointerstitial lesions of children and correlated with clinical findings ranging from minimal proteinuria or hematuria to oliguric renal failure (10–15). Since then, histologically documented cases of TIN have been only sporadically reported in the pediatric population despite increased recognition in adults (4, 16, 17). Although infection-associated acute TIN is still important in children, the number of cases related to the use of nephrotoxic drugs appears to be on the increase and will probably constitute the major single etiology in the future (18). The anticipated increased use of nonsteroidal antiinflammatory agents in the treatment of juvenile rheumatoid arthritis and other childhood disorders will undoubtedly result in an increased incidence of interstitial nephritis as has been reported in adults (19–21) (chapter 28E). As shown in Table 26I.1, infections and drugs are most commonly implicated in the etiology of acute TIN. Specific etiologies identified in reported pediatric cases are noted.

Certain clinical features may strongly incriminate infection as the cause of acute TIN. Pharyngitis as a result of Group A, β-hemolytic streptococcus is more common from December through June. Evidence for infection may include fever, flank pain, exudative pharyngitis, otitis media, sinusitis, cellulitis, fasciitis, lobar pneumonia, or painful lymphadenopathy. Pathogens may be cultured from the throat, blood, sputum, urine, skin, or wounds, and the patients may have pyuria and bacteruria, leukocytosis with a left shift, and, at times, eosinophilia, anemia, and a rise in the anti-streptolysin-O, DNA-ase B, or other antibody titers to specific bacterial antigens. Other common but nonspecific symptoms may include abdominal pain, anorexia and weight loss, emesis, diarrhea, fatigue, pallor, or headache. Edema may be present in patients with extensive proteinuria. Hypertension is generally absent, but can occur in patients with severe renal failure with oliguria or fluid overload. The occurrence of progressive renal insufficiency often in the face of good urine output, along with various combinations of urinary abnormalities, such as hyposthenuria, proteinuria, hematuria, leukocyturia, glucosuria, and granular casts at the time of the symptoms, should strongly suggest the diagnosis of acute TIN (chapter 30A).

Drug-induced acute TIN has been reported in all age groups, the youngest patient being 4 months of age (18). Based on available evidence, it appears that the route of administration (by mouth, intravenous, or muscle), the dose of the antibiotic, and the duration of treatment are not the key factors in the development of acute TIN (18, 22–24). There is a suggestion that the risk is greater when drug usage is prolonged or if the

Table 26I.1.
Agents Implicated in the Cause of Acute or Chronic Tubulointerstitial Nephritis

ACUTE TIN	
INFECTIONS	**Nonsteroidal antiinflammatory agents**
Group A, β-hemolytic streptococcus[a]	Indomethacin
Toxoplasmosis[a]	Fenoprofen
Streptococcus pneumoniae[a]	Ibuprofen
Brucellosis	Naproxen
Syphilis	Tolmetin[a]
Typhoid fever	**Other drugs**
Leptospirosis	Phenytoin[a]
Infectious mononucleosis[a]	Phenobarbital
Legionnaire's disease	Phenindione[a]
? Viral[a]	Phenazone
DRUGS	Cyclosporin[a]
Antibiotics	Azathioprine
Methicillin[a]	Cimetidine
Penicillin[a]	Clofibrate
Sulfonamides[a]	? Caffeine vs. phenylpropanolamine[a]
Ampicillin[a]	Chlorthalidone
Oxacillin	Allopurinol
Carbenicillin	Glafenine[a]
Cephalothin	Thiazides
Cephalexin	Ethacrynic acid
Nitrofurantoin	Furosemide
Co-trimazole	*MISCELLANEOUS*
Rifampin	Allograft rejection[a]
Nafcillin[a]	Idiopathic[a]
Cephaloridine	High-dose irradiation
CHRONIC TIN	
UROLOGIC DISORDERS	
Urinary obstruction[a] (congenital, calculi, tumors, surgery)	Sickle cell disease[a]
	Balkan nephropathy
Vesicoureteral reflux[a]	*DRUGS*
INFECTIONS	Phenacetin/acetaminophen
Chronic pyelonephritis[a]	
Tuberculosis	Aspirin
METABOLIC/HEREDITARY	Phenylbutazone
Oxalosis[a]	Lithium
Cystinosis[a]	Cadmium
Wilson's disease[a]	Methoxyfluorane
Lesch-Nyhan syndrome[a]	*MISCELLANEOUS*
Gout	Allograft rejection[a]
Nephrocalcinosis[a] (hypercalcemic and hypercalciuric disorders)	Low-dose irradiation[a]
	Hypoxic disorders
	Hemorrhagic fever
Potassium-losing nephropathy	Heat stroke
Hyperphosphatemia	Idiopathic[a]

[a] Cases involving children.

drug is given in high doses (17, 25). Helpful clinical features, which may implicate a drug as the cause of acute TIN include an abrupt onset or recurrence of fever—often with chills, morbilliform, maculopapular, or urticarial skin rash, arthralgias, lethargy, and abdominal pain, beginning at any time but typically 1 to 8 weeks after starting the drug. Temporally related to these symptoms, one may find declining renal function with normal or decreased urine output, leukocytouria, hematuria, granular casts, and laboratory evidence for renal tubular dysfunction. In some hospitalized patients, the diagnosis of TIN may be strengthened by the absence of these symptoms and signs at an earlier time in the clinical course.

Other common pediatric disorders that can mimic the clinical presentation of acute TIN should be excluded. Unlike patients with poststreptococcal glomerulonephritis, streptococcal-associated acute TIN has no latency period and serum complement levels are normal (16, 17, 27). Furthermore, renal biopsy shows normal glomeruli and absence of immunoglobulin deposits. Unlike children with acute tubular necrosis (ATN) in whom renal failure is frequently preceded by hypotension or hypoxia, such evidence is absent in acute TIN. Moreover, histological features that may suggest ATN, such as scanty inflammatory infiltrate, prominent injury to tubular epithelium, and absence of tubular basement membrane thickening and hyaline droplets in the epithelial cytoplasm, are usually lacking (28).

Chronic Tubulointerstitial Nephritis

The most common causes of chronic TIN in children are related to obstructive genitourinary tract disorders or those associated with a high grade of vesicoureteral reflux with or without infection (pyelonephritis). Infection is no longer regarded as a necessary factor in the development of chronic TIN in children with vesicoureteral reflux, but rather it is a frequent and important additional insult that accelerates the destructive process (29–31). Although the glomeruli are not affected by the initial interstitial inflammatory process, eventually lesions identical to focal and segmental glomerulosclerosis may develop. When these glomerular, tubular, and interstitial lesions are present, along with often severe proteinuria, they are collectively known as reflux nephropathy (31, 32). In many of the disorders in Table 26I.1 associated with chronic TIN, the interstitial reaction is likely to be secondary to papillary, ductular, and tubular damage produced by various processes, which may include suppurative reactions (acute or recurrent bacterial pyelonephritis); ischemia (diabetes, sickle cell disease, or anoxic states); mechanical plus vascular injury from precipitation of drugs in these areas (phenacetin or obstructive uropathy); radiation-induced vascular and cellular injury; and metabolic disorders or toxins that interfere with the normal physiological processes of cells. Depending on the mechanism involved and severity of the underlying disorder, the morphological changes may be limited to one kidney and renal size may vary greatly. In addition, chronic TIN is a frequent nonspecific pathological finding in patients with advanced chronic renal failure from any cause, and its presence provides little information regarding the primary disorder.

Investigation

As with other disorders, a systematic evaluation of children suspected to have TIN should begin with a careful medical history. A history of recurrent urinary tract infections, with or without known vesicoureteral reflux, use of nephrotoxic drugs or exposure to toxic substances (Table 26I.1), recurrent renal colic, polyuria and polydipsia, excessive fatigue, a family history of TIN, fever, pharyngitis, lymphadenopathy, and previously available renal function tests may provide clues as to the cause and onset of the disorder. Examination of the patient may show growth retardation, hypertension, hypertensive retinopathy, or EKG evidence for left ventricular hypertrophy, rachetic changes, pallor, and joint or skin abnormalities. Such clinical signs may aid in assessing the chronicity of the disorder and in determining if it is related to a metabolic or systemic disease.

Evidence supporting the presence of renal tubular injury is usually found in the urine. In acute TIN, urinalysis may reveal hematuria, proteinuria, glucosuria, and, often, coarse or fine granular casts. Leukocytes are frequently present, and Wright's stain of the urine sediment may reveal eosinophils, particularly in drug-induced TIN (26). In patients with chronic TIN, the urinary sediment varies widely. It may be normal or show proteinuria or leukocyturia in long-standing chronic pyelonephritis; have leukocyte clumps or casts and bacteria in ongoing pyelonephritis; or contain tissue fragments in patients with papillary necrosis. The urine is frequently isosthenuric (SG $\simeq$ 1.015 or osmolality $\simeq$300 mOsm/kg).

One may then proceed with a baseline structural evaluation. Renal ultrasonography is a noninvasive means of assessing renal size, the presence of obstruction, or the presence of underlying structural abnormalities. When renal ultrasound is combined with one of the many available renal radionuclide scans, such as ^{99m}Tc-DTPA or ^{131}I-OIH, one is often able to rapidly ascertain the degree of renal function, the renal blood flow, if the disorder is acute or chronic, or if reversibility may be possible. In addition, preferential uptake of ^{67}Ga by kidneys of patients with acute TIN may have a specific diagnostic value in this disorder (4). Although studies using renal contrast media should generally be avoided in patients with severe renal failure, an intravenous pyelogram may be helpful in demonstrating papillary necrosis when it is suspected.

Since the renal tubules have diverse specialized functions that are largely responsible for the modification of the glomerular filtrate, TIN may result in many detectable plasma and urinary abnormalities. In both acute and chronic TIN, one may find evidence for proximal, distal, or combined tubular dysfunction (33). Understanding of the normal reabsorptive and secretory functions of the proximal and distal tubules (chapter 5) forms the basis for the biochemical assessment of children with TIN. TIN mainly impairs the reabsorptive function of the tubules. For the clinician, it is usually practical to measure only a few of these processes.

Proximal tubular dysfunction may be reflected by glucosuria with normal blood glucose levels; aminoaciduria detected by reacting urine containing a-amino nitrogen with 1, fluoro-2,4-dinitrobenzine and measuring the color reaction; a total reabsorption of phosphate below 80% in a 24-hour urine (TRP = 1-U/P iP/U/P creat × 100); a fractional excretion of sodium greater than 3% measured on a spot urine specimen (FE_{Na} = U/P Na/U/P creat × 100); and a total protein excretion above 300 mg/24 hours. In a few instances proteinuria can be marked, but typically it is less than 1 gm/24 hours, with β_2-microglobulin and other small molecular weight proteins comprising up to 50% of the total protein excreted (34). A ratio of urinary albumin to β_2-microglobulin <13.0 is frequently found in patients with tubular disorders (35).

Distal tubular dysfunction may be primarily responsible for the inability to concentrate the urine after withholding fluids overnight or after performing other modified tests of water deprivation (36). Unless renal function is greatly diminished, free-water clearance generally remains intact. Other tests that stress specific physiological functions of the renal tubules, such as bicarbonate and acid loading to evaluate renal tubular acidosis, and calcium loading or deprivation to evaluate hypercalciuria, are not performed routinely.

Blood chemistries are not helpful in distinguishing between acute and chronic TIN. Apart from having evidence for a variable degree of renal failure (elevated BUN and creatinine), patients with TIN frequently have a hyperchloremic metabolic acidosis suggesting renal tubular acidosis, hypocalcemia, and hyponatremia. Serum potassium and phosphorus levels are normal unless significant renal failure is present. Serum proteins are usually normal except for a small decrement in serum albumin. However, severe hypoalbuminemia and other features of the nephrotic syndrome may occasionally occur in patients with TIN (see Pathogenesis).

Serum complement levels and immunoglobulins are normal and circulating immune complexes are usually absent. In some patients with SLE having TIN in the absence of glomerular lesions, circulating immune complexes and a positive ANA titer may be present. In addition, circulating immune complexes may be found in patients with immune-mediated TIN and in patients with reflux nephropathy.

Hematological studies may reveal leukocytosis, eosinophilia, and normochromic, normocytic anemia, but no evidence of a hemolytic process or disseminated intravascular coagulopathy.

If the above studies are not helpful in determining the cause of the renal failure and associated urinary abnormalities, a renal biopsy may aid in establishing the diagnosis, in the planning of therapy, and in assessing the prognosis.

Pathogenesis and Pathophysiology of Tubulointerstitial Nephritis

The pathogenetic mechanisms responsible for TIN are largely unknown, partly because of lack of a suitable animal model for this disorder. Most of the available evidence implicates several immunological mechanisms, particularly in drug-induced acute TIN (37, 38). It has been shown by immunofluorescent techniques that the dimethoxyphenylpenicilloyl hapten group was firmly bound to the kidney tissue of a patient with methicillin-associated acute TIN (39). Hapten-protein conjugates have been found to bind to both the tubular basement membrane and glomerular basement membrane (40) or to tubular basement membrane alone (41, 42). It is thus postulated that in patients with drug-associated acute TIN, the chemotherapeutic agents form stable immunogenic conjugates with kidney protein, most commonly along the tubular basement membrane. It is further theorized that TIN will occur only in those individuals whose immune response to hapten-kidney conjugates is unusually vigorous (39). Other circumstantial evidence implicating immunologic mechanisms in patients with drug-induced TIN include the finding of an elevated serum IgE and the identification of the lymphocytes in the renal parenchyma as T-lymphocytes using monoclonal antibodies or human antithymocyte serum (21, 43, 44). In the absence of a positive immunofluorescence reaction, the tissue presence of T-lymphocytes suggests that cell-mediated immunity plays an important role in the pathogenesis of TIN in certain instances. Similarly, lymphocyte blast transformation studies may indicate an allergy or hypersensitivity to a drug or toxin (45). In addition, circulating antibodies to tubular basement membrane as shown by direct immunofluorescence techniques, have been found in rare instances of TIN in humans; this disorder is believed to represent the tubular counterpart to antiglomerular basement membrane disease (46).

Nonimmunological mechanisms may involve direct tubular injury because of a high intraluminal, intracellular, and interstitial concentration of drugs, which are excreted by the kidneys; tubular injury may then provoke interstitial inflammation and fibrosis. Thus, one should refrain from incriminating immunological mechanisms in the pathogenesis of most cases of TIN secondary to drug use.

There is little proof that immunological mechanisms are involved in infection-related acute TIN. The importance of genetic factors that may modulate an individual's response to drugs, infections, and other environmental toxins is currently unknown.

Immunological mechanisms are believed to play a major role in several conditions associated with chronic TIN. In children with high pressure vesicoureteral reflux, it has been proposed that slowly progressive injury to the renal papillae and renal tubules may render Tamm-Horsfall glycoprotein antigenic; subsequent production of antibody to this tubular protein circulates and reacts in situ (31, 47). Many humoral and cellular immunological mechanisms then interact locally and produce further damage. Bacterial infection clearly accelerates tubulointerstitial damage and scarring in young children with vesicoureteral reflux (50). The role of sequestered bacterial antigens or unusual bacteria (L-forms) in perpetuating renal lesions remains unclear. Following the acute inflammatory reaction initiated by infection, limited experimental evidence suggests that cellular immunity may be responsible for perpetuating chronic TIN (31, 48, 49).

The pathophysiology of TIN is poorly understood. Many of the functional tubular disturbances, such as proximal or distal tubular acidosis or inability to reabsorb fluid, are common to both acute and chronic TIN and can, at times, be explained on an anatomic predilection of different disorders (33). However, certain abnormalities are not readily explained. In acute TIN one frequently finds a disparity between the degree of renal failure and the amount of interstitial inflammation and tubular damage (11). This may in part explain the wide diversity in urinary signs among individual patients. Those with patchy interstitial inflammation and limited tubular injury may have few urinary sediment or tubular abnormalities, yet, depending on the degree of interstitial edema and expansion of interstitial volume, there may be a significant impediment to renal blood flow; this, combined with an obstruction to urine flow from cellular debris and casts, may result in an increased intratubular pressure and a decrease in glomerular filtration rate (51, 52). These factors, together with an impaired tubular responsiveness to antidiuretic and other hormones, may also explain the variation in the renal capacity to excrete a free-water load among patients with TIN.

The amount and quality of the proteinuria is also variable. Although tubular reabsorption of small, and, to a lesser degree, large proteins, is recognized as an important determinant of final protein excretion, tubular disorders generally do not result in nephrotic range proteinuria. Nevertheless, few patients in previous reports and an increasing number of patients with acute TIN related to use of nonsteroidal antiinflammatory agents may have combined tubular and glomerular proteinuria and nephrotic syndrome in the absence of any glomerular histological changes apart from epithelial foot process fusion (19–21). However, one cannot discount the possibility that in some patients with acute TIN glomerular dysfunction also exists. One may speculate that humoral factors, such as lymphokines, released by the local accumulation of T-lymphocytes may account for the increased basement membrane permeability to macromolecules, as is theorized to occur in minimal change disease (53).

Morphometric studies of renal tissue from patients with chronic TIN have shown a greater correlation between the serum creatinine concentration and glomerular filtration rate and loss of functional interstitial tissue, than found in acute TIN (54).

Treatment and Prognosis of Tubulointerstitial Nephritis

Management of TIN is largely supportive. Depending on the clinical setting, therapeutic measures include appropriate and expeditious treatment of infections and withdrawal of nephrotoxic agents. Surgical correction of obstructive genitourinary abnormalities may be warranted if reasonable prospects for preservation of remaining functional renal tissue exist. Temporary dialysis may be required in some instances of acute TIN, as indicated by fluid or electrolyte imbalance, but this is usually not necessary if the condition is recognized early and preventive measures are undertaken.

The use of corticosteroids or cytotoxic drugs to treat patients with TIN and nephrotic syndrome or to hasten their recovery from renal failure is controversial. Uncontrolled evidence suggests that in selected patients with idiopathic or drug-induced acute TIN, particularly those with extensive proteinuria, a beneficial effect can be derived from use of these agents (17, 26, 55). Treatment may be started at doses of prednisone of 2 mg/kg/day or cyclophosphamide, 2 mg/kg/day. Response to this treatment is generally rapid so that after 1 to 2 weeks, prednisone can be given on alternate days. All drugs can usually be stopped after 1 month of treatment.

With appropriate management, prognosis in children with infection or drug-related acute TIN is excellent with full recovery occurring from 1 week to 3 months after the onset of the disorder. In children with chronic TIN, one is generally content in arresting or delaying, rather than reversing, the progression to renal failure.

References

1. Maher JF, Nolph KD, Bryan CW, et al: Etiology and distribution of renal disease in central Missouri. Mo Med 69:799, 1972.
2. Porter GA, Bennett WM: Toxic nephropathies. In Brenner BM, Rector FC (eds): The Kidney. Philadelphia, W.B. Saunders Co., 1981, p 2047.
3. Kazantzis G: Cadmium nephropathy. Contr Nephrol 16:161, 1979.
4. Linton AL, Clark WF, Driedger AA, et al: Acute interstitial nephritis due to drugs. Ann Intern Med 93:735, 1980.
5. Hirschman GH, Wolfson M, Mosimann JE, et al: Complications of dialysis. Clin Nephrol 15:66, 1981.
6. Jacobs C, Broyer M, Brunner FP, et al: Combined report of regular dialysis and transplantation in Europe, XI, 1980. Proc EDTA 18:4, 1981.
7. Potter DE, Holliday MA, Piel CF, et al: Treatment of end-stage renal disease in children: A 15-year experience. Kidney Intl 18:103, 1980.
8. Avner ED, Harmon WE, Grupe WE, et al: Mortality of chronic hemodialysis and renal transplantation in pediatric end-stage disease. Pediatr 67:412, 1981.
9. Councilman WT: Acute interstitial nephritis. J Exp Med 3:393, 1898.
10. Brody H, Smith LW: The visceral pathology in scarlet fever and related streptococcus infections. Am J Pathol 12:373, 1936.
11. Kimmelstiel P: Acute hematogeneous interstitial nephritis. Am J Pathol 14:737, 1938.
12. Mallory GK, Keefer CS: Tissue reactions in fatal cases of streptococcus haemolyticus infections. Arch Pathol 32:334, 1941.
13. Kannerstein M: Histologic kidney changes in the common acute infectious diseases. Am J Med Sci 203:65, 1942.
14. Matthews WR: Acute hematogenous interstitial nephritis. South Med J 35:1055, 1942.
15. Melnick, PJ: Acute interstitial nephritis with uremia. Arch Pathol 36:499, 1943.
16. Knepshield JH, Carstens PHB, Gentile DE: Recovery from renal failure due to acute diffuse interstitial nephritis. Pediatrics 43:533, 1969.
17. Ellis D, Fried WA, Yunis EJ, et al: Acute interstitial nephritis in children: A report of 13 cases and review of the literature. Pediatr 67:862, 1981.
18. Sanjad SA, Haddad GG, Nassar VH: Nephropathy, an under-estimated complication of methicillin therapy. J Pediatr 84:873, 1974.
19. Brezin JH, Katz SM, Schwartz AB, et al: Reversible renal failure and nephrotic syndrome associated with non-steroidal anti-inflammatory agents. N Engl J Med 301:1271, 1979.
20. Lofgren RP, Nelson AE, Ehlers SM: Fenoprofen-induced acute interstitial nephritis presenting with nephrotic syndrome. Minn Med 64:227, 1981.
21. Finkelstein A, Fraley DS, Stachura I, et al: Fenoprofen nephropathy: Lipoid nephrosis and interstitial nephritis. Am J Med 72:81, 1982.
22. London RD: Hematuria associated with methicillin therapy. J Pediatr 70:285, 1967.
23. Woodroffe AJ, Thomson NM, Meadows R: Nephropathy associated with methicillin administration. Aust NZ J Med 4:256, 1974.
24. Chesney RW, Chesney PJ: Methicillin-associated nephritis. Clinical rarity or common entity? Clin Pediatr 15:1013, 1976.
25. Feigin RD, Van Reken DE, Pickering LK: Dosage in methicillin-associated nephropathy. J Pediatr 85:734, 1974.
26. Galpin JE, Shinaberger JH, Stanley TM, et al: Acute interstitial nephritis due to methicillin. Am J Med 65:756, 1978.
27. Haddow JE, Sher N, Gall DG: Streptococcal wound infection with evidence of widespread tissue involvement. Pediatrics 48:458, 1971.
28. Dunnill MS: Interstitial nephritis. In Dunnill MS (ed): Pathological Basis of Renal Disease. Philadelphia, W.B. Saunders Co., 1976, p 337.
29. Asscher AW: Urinary tract infection. Lancet 2:1365, 1974.
30. Winberg J, Bergstrom T, Jacobsson B: Morbidity, age and sex distribution, recurrences and renal scarring in symptomatic urinary tract infection in childhood. Kidney Intl 8:101, 1975.
31. Hodson J, Maling JMJ, McManamon PJ, et al: Reflux nephropathy. Kidney Intl 8:550, 1975.
32. Senekjian HO, Stinebaugh B, Mattishi CA, et al: Irreversible renal failure following vesicoureteral reflux. JAMA 241:160, 1979.
33. Cogan MG: Tubulointerstitial nephropathies: A pathophysiological approach. Medical Staff Conference, University of California, San Francisco. West J Med 132:134, 1980.
34. Dillard MG, Pesce AJ, Pollak VE, et al: Proteinuria and renal protein clearance in patients with renal tubular disorders. J Lab Clin Med 78:203, 1971.

35. Peterson PA, Evrin P-E, Berggard I: Differentiation of glomerular, tubular, and normal proteinuria: Determination of urinary excretion of β_2-microglobulin, albumin, and total protein. J Clin Invest 48:1189, 1969.
36. Frasier SD, Kutnik LA, Schmidt RT, et al: A water deprivation test for the diagnosis of diabetes insipidus in children. Am J Dis Child 114:157, 1967.
37. Klassen J, Andres GA, Brennan JC, et al: An immunologic renal tubular lesion in man. Clin Immunol Immunopathol 1:69, 1972.
38. Lehman DH, Wilson CB, Dixon FJ: Extraglomerular immunoglobulin deposits in human nephritis. Am J Med 58:765, 1975.
39. Baldwin DS, Levine BB, McCluskey RT, et al: Renal failure and interstitial nephritis due to penicillin and methicillin. N Engl J Med 279:1245, 1968.
40. Colvin RB, Burton JR, Hyslop NE, et al: Penicillin-associated interstitial nephritis. Ann Intern Med 81:404, 1974.
41. Border WA, Lehman DH, Egan JD, et al: Antitubular basement membrane antibodies in methicillin-associated interstitial nephritis. N Engl J Med 291:381, 1974.
42. Cogan MC, Arieff AL: Sodium wasting, acidosis, and hyperkalemia induced by methicillin interstitial nephritis. Am J Med 64:500, 1978.
43. Ooi BS, First MR, Pesce AJ, et al: IgE levels in interstitial nephritis. Lancet 1:1254, 1974.
44. Husby G, Tung KSK, Williams RC JR: Characterization of renal tissue lymphocytes in patients with interstitial nephritis. Am J Med 70:31, 1981.
45. Hyman LR, Bollow M, Knieser MR: Diphenylhydantoin interstitial nephritis. Roles of cellular and humoral immunologic injury. J Pediatr 92:915, 1978.
46. Bergstein J, Litman N: Interstitial nephritis with antitubular basement membrane antibody. N Engl J Med 292:875, 1975.
47. Hanson LA, Fasth A, Godal U: Autoantibodies to Tamm-Horsfall protein, a tool for diagnosing the level of urinary tract infection. Lancet 1:226, 1976.
48. Ransley PG, Risdon RA: Reflux nephropathy: Effects of antimicrobial therapy on the evaluation of the early pyelonephritic scar. Kidney Intl 20:733, 1981.
49. Smellie JM, Normand ICS, Katz G: Children with urinary infection: A comparison of those with and those without vesicoureteral reflux. Kidney Intl 20:717, 1981.
50. Kalmanson GM, Glassock RJ, Harwick HJ, et al: Cellular immunity in experimental pyelonephritis. Kidney Intl 8:535, 1975.
51. Oken DE: On the passive backflow theory of acute renal failure. Am J Med 58:77, 1975.
52. Bohle A, Glomb D, Grund KE, et al: Correlations between relative interstitial volume of the renal cortex and serum creatinine concentration in minimal changes with nephrotic syndrome and in focal sclerosing glomerulonephritis. Virch Arch (Pathol Anat) 376:221, 1977.
53. Shalhoub RJ: Pathogenesis of lipoid nephrosis: A disorder of T-cell function. Lancet 2:556, 1974.
54. Mackensen S, Grund KE, Sindjic M, et al: The influence of the renal cortical interstitium on the serum creatinine concentration and the serum creatinine clearance in different chronic sclerosing interstitial nephritides. Nephron 24:30, 1979.
55. Taube D, Brown A, Williams DG: Long-term impairment of suppressorcell function by cyclophosphamide in minimal-change nephropathy and its association with therapeutic response. Lancet 1:235, 1981.

CHAPTER **27**

Hemolytic Uremic Syndrome

KENNETH MILLER
YOUNGKI KIM

INTRODUCTION

The hemolytic uremic syndrome (HUS) is characterized by the classic triad of microangiopathic hemolytic anemia (MHA), thrombocytopenia (TP), and acute renal failure (ARF) (1–14). In children, it is often thought of as a discrete clinicopathological entity of unknown etiology, in which the previously mentioned constellation of findings develop following a gastrointestinal or, on occasion, a respiratory prodromal illness. Perhaps fortuitously, Gasser (15), who provided the initial descriptions of HUS, used the plural term *hamoly tisch uramische* syndrome, because HUS is, in all likelihood, both a heterogenic-heterogenous entity with several discrete clinical variants. The adult disorder is even more heterogenous.

HUS is the most common cause of ARF in children. Endothelial injury, most pronounced in the kidney, likely results from localized activation of the coagulation system with the subsequent deposition of fibrinogen or fibrin-related antigens. However, alternative pathogenetic mechanisms have recently been proposed. The same constellation of findings in HUS may be seen in several other conditions, such as thrombotic thrombocytopenic purpura (16), postpartum renal failure (17, 18), hyperacute homograft rejection (19), malignant hypertension (20, 21), scleroderma, vasculitis, and systemic lupus erythematosus (22, 23).

In the following sections, we will describe the disease in children, some of the recent developments regarding the role of various metabolites of the arachadonic acid pathway in the pathogenesis of HUS, the role of plasma infusions or plasmapheresis in the treatment of HUS, and the importance of extrarenal manifestations of HUS, which may directly impact on both morbidity and mortality.

Etiology

The search for a specific infectious agent has generally been unsuccessful. A variety of organisms, however, have been implicated with several of the miniepidemics of HUS (organism isolated or rising titers documented). These include *Coxsackie*, *ECHO*, *Adenovirus*, *Influenza*, *Salmonella typhi*, *E. coli*, and *Shigella dysenteriae* (1, 4, 24–30). In the Shigella epidemic, endotoxin was detected in 9 of 18 patients who later developed a hemolytic anemia (30). In 11 of 13 patients, circulating immune complexes were found as well. The latter investigators observed a broad spectrum of disease occurring with this epidemic ranging from uncomplicated Shigellosis to overt HUS (3.7% of the cases). In Argentina, perhaps the largest reporting center of HUS cases, a portillo virus was isolated during the acute phase of the disease in eight cases with complement fixing antibody demonstrable in an additional 36 cases (10). Additionally, isolated case reports of HUS associated with other organisms have been observed (e.g., pseudomonas, bacteroides, campylobacter, yersinia, rota virus, mumps, myxovirus, parainfluenza, and microtabiotes (1, 4, 31–36). Pyranocopolymer was also implicated as a cause of HUS, and HUS has occurred following immunizations (DPT, polio, and smallpox), ingestion of fresh apple juice, in women on oral contraceptives, in patients given antineoplastic chemotherapeutic agents, penicillin or cyclosporine, in the posttransplant patient (renal and bone marrow), and in association with other renal diseases (37–50).

Recently, the development of an HUS-like illness in association with streptococcal pneumoniae infections inclusive of pneumococcal septicema was described by several investigators. The incidence of persisting renal abnormalities following recovery from the initial illness appears to be increased in association with this possible etiological factor (51–53).

Clinical Presentation

HUS occurs primarily in infants and young children. In North America the average age of effected children is about 3 years, whereas in the southern hemisphere and in South Africa the mean age is less than 18 months (1–14, 54). Neonatal cases are rare, whereas the majority of adult cases occur either with pregnancy, following the use of oral contraceptives, or in association with essential hypertension (1–3, 40, 55, 56). The incidence and prevelance of the disease appears to be on the rise, based on the increasing number of reporting centers. Although a few centers have observed a sex predilection (female greater than male), most groups have noted an equal distribution of cases (8, 14). Rarely is HUS seen in blacks (57, 58). Several investigators have noted a seasonal variation, and others have not (1–5, 10, 12). Endemic outbreaks of HUS still apparently exist (Argentina, South Africa, and Southern California) (10, 12, 54). The reason for the latter observations are unknown.

A prodromal illness, usually gastrointestinal, proceeds the development of HUS. In one series, however, an upper respiratory illness predominated (33% of cases) (10). The gastrointestinal symptoms are usually nonspecific with vague abdominal pains, vomiting, and diarrhea (which is often bloody) predominating. However, since the initial description of five patients who were first thought to have ulcerative colitis, we have become increasingly cognizant of the protean nature of the gastrointestinal features of HUS (59). HUS can present as an acute abdominal emergency, acute appendicitis, toxic megacolon, or intussusception (60–63). In addition, cases of bowel perforation, ischemic injury with gangrene, colonic stricture, intussusception, presence of abdominal mass, and toxic megacolon are reported (1, 64, 65).

The absence of a diarrheal prodrome, however, may also have prognostic significance, since mortality rates appear to be significantly higher in these patients (14).

HUS may, on occasion, mimic acute hepatitis (66). Jaundice is seen in up to 15% to 30% of infants and children, and hepatomegaly occurs in 13% to 50% of cases (1, 5, 12). Cholilithiasis developed as a late complication in one case (67). Several studies have documented pancreatic involvement evidenced either by the development, albeit transient, of insulin-dependent diabetes mellitus during the acute phase of the disease or the histological presence of islet cell necrosis at autopsy (68–70). In addition, pericardial, myocardial, and pulmonary involvement have also been observed (71–73). Other common physical findings include fever, pallor, ecchymosis, petechaie (30% to 40%), and hypertension (40% to 50%) (1–14).

Central nervous system (CNS) involvement in HUS is quite common, varying from subtle abnormalities, such as irritability, lethargy, gait, or personality disturbances, to such profound manifestations as seizures, cortical blindness, hemiparesis, decerebrate posturing, and coma (1, 3, 10–13, 74–77). The absence of discrete neuropathological lesions in earlier reports led investigators to postulate that the neurologic manifestations were, in all likelihood, a result either of uremia, hypertensive encephalopathy, or other metabolic derangements. With the advent of computed tomography (CT), several centers have described discrete neurological abnormalities occurring in HUS patients. Among the abnormalities reported have been basal ganglion infarcts and the development of hemorrhages (often delayed), primarily in the frontal-parietal region of the brain. Concomitant with the above radiological abnormalities, a recent pathological study has demonstrated cerebral microthrombi or areas of ischemic injury or infarction (72, 78, 79).

Major CNS abnormalities have been associated with a poor prognosis and high mortality (33% to 90%). Morbidity has also been higher in patients with CNS dysfunction. Most likely, a combination of metabolic alterations (elevated CSF protein, low serum sodium, high BUN), pathological lesions, and severe hypertension contribute both to the acute mortality and high morbidity rates. However, spontaneous and complete recovery has been observed even in patients with profound neurological deficits, such as coma and cortical blindness (76, 79).

Laboratory Features

A hemolytic process characterizes the anemia of the HUS patient. Serum haptoglobin levels are depressed, serum bilirubin is elevated, and the reticulocyte count is high. Both the direct and indirect Coombs test are negative, with rare exception (80). Osmotic fragility and red cell enzyme levels are usually normal (81).

A microangiopathic process in conjunction with localized intravascular coagulation in areas of endothelial injury, following exposure to one or more noxious stimuli, is the likeliest explanation for the morphological changes seen in the RBC (tear drop cells, burr cells, helmet cells, and microspherocytes) (Fig. 27.1). The erythrocyte is believed to be damaged and fragmented by its passage through fibrin strands in the renal vasculature. Red cell survival is shortened and the abnormal red cells are removed from the circulation by the reticuloendothelial system (spleen and liver). The lifespan of infused normal red cells is also shortened (1, 81, 82). Alternative or concurrent mechanisms, however, may also exist. One theory suggests that alterations in the antioxidant status of the erythrocyte may lead to hemolysis. Another suggests that the hemolytic process occurs as the result of the exposure of hidden surface antigens by noxious agents.

Based on experimental studies in which hemolysis and cortical necrosis could be produced in animals by feeding either a choline deficient diet or a diet rich in unsaturated fats and lacking vitamin E, one investigator proposed that HUS might be a result of the absorption of peroxidized lipids. This theory now gains a sounder foundation based on some recent studies in both children and adults in which decreased levels of red cell superoxide dismutase, decreased plasma alpha tocopherol levels, decreased phosphatidyl ethanolamine levels, or increased malonyldialdehyde levels were found. The latter compound is a breakdown product of autooxidized fats (83–87).

Alternatively, exposure of an antigen—the Thomsen-Friedenreich (TF) antigen—found primarily on the erythrocyte, platelet, and glomerular endothelial cell surface, by neurominidase producing organisms, such as *S. pneumoniae*, could result in TF antigen interaction with IgM and anti-TF antibody (53, 88). This could produce both cellular agglutination and alteration, causing vascular endothelial cell damage. Whether other organisms causing an HUS-like illness produce neuromanidase remains to be elucidated.

Thrombocytopenia is another of the classic features of HUS. However, cases of HUS in which the platelet count was normal or only transiently low have also been recognized (1, 9). As opposed to red cell fragmentation that may persist for weeks to months, thrombocytopenia rarely persists beyond 2 weeks. The degree of thrombocytopenia has no prognostic significance. Platelet survival of administered random-donor platelets was shortened in HUS patients. Bone marrow specimens show normal appearing megakaryocytes. Initially, it was felt that platelet consumption occurred within the reticuloendothelial system. Subsequent studies, employing a variety of techniques, have demonstrated platelets or platelet remnants entrapped within glomerular capillaries or arteriolar vessels. Immunofluorescent studies have shown that platelet remnants were

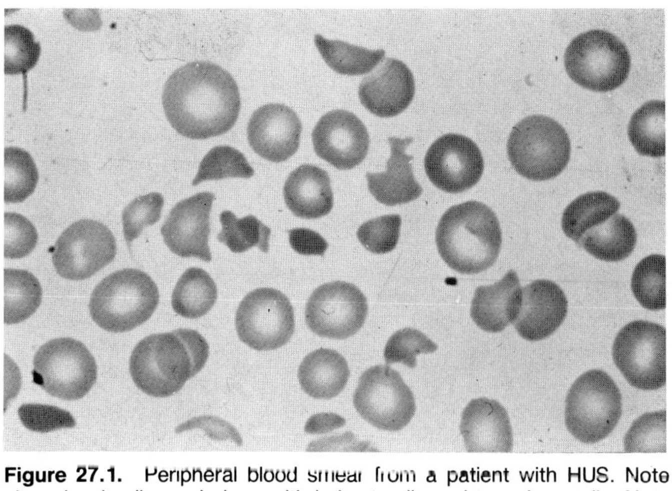

Figure 27.1. Peripheral blood smear from a patient with HUS. Note altered red cell morphology with helmet cells and tear drop cells. Note also the absence of platelets.

found in the same loci as Factor VIII and fibrin-related antigens (89). In several patients, bilateral nephrectomy resulted in normalization of the platelet count, suggesting that the kidney was the major site of platelet deposition or destruction (90, 91).

The mechanism(s) causing enhanced platelet aggregation are not well defined. Several possibilities exist (Table 27.1). Chief amongst these are the lack of a cofactor in normal plasma that prevents spontaneous platelet aggregation as seen in TTP (92, 93), the failure of vascular cells of affected patients to either elaborate a platelet-disaggregating substance presumed to be prostacyclin (PGI_2) (94, 95), an inability of the patients' plasma to stimulate PGI_2 production (96), or accelerated prostacyclin degradation (97). Alternatively, increased thromboxane generation can lead to enhanced aggregation (98). Similar mechanisms are proposed for TTP (99). Thus, metabolites of the arachadonic acid pathway may play a crucial role in the pathogenesis of HUS and TTP. Hypoalbuminemia and alpha-tocopherol deficiency also cause platelets to react more vigorously to noxious stimuli (85, 100). Localized intravascular coagulation may also be a contributing factor to the observed platelet consumption.

Alterations of the immune system in HUS have been dismissed by some, although it is quite possible that thrombotic consequences can arise from either immune complement-dependent endothelial injury or through binding of an IgG antibody present in the patient's serum to endothelial cells or platelets, resulting in aggregation and release of a variety of mediators, such as thromboxane A_2 or other vasoactive substances (101–106).

Enhanced in vitro aggregation of normal platelets by HUS patient plasma has also been demonstrated. However, antiplatelet (IgG) antibodies have not been described in HUS patients. The only report in which a common HLA marker was found is that of a family with relapsing HUS and hypocomplementemia. Each member had HLA haplotype A3B7 (107).

Conversely, several groups have purported to demonstrate impaired platelet aggregation (decreased intraplatelet nucleotides, serotonin, beta thromboglobulin, or blunted aggregation of HUS patient platelets with epinephrine ADP or collagen) (1). A recent communication, however, would suggest that platelet agglutination does not require platelet metabolism, because the aggregation process can occur in the absence of platelet cell respiration, extracellular calcium, ADP release, or arachadonic acid pathway alterations in patients with TTP (93). A defect in the processing of Factor VIII/von Willebrand factor multimers was proposed by one investigator of patients with TTP (108). Perhaps such a defect may also exist in HUS patients. Thus, it is apparent that further clarification of the mechanism(s) responsible both for the thrombocytopenia and the hemolytic anemia is necessary.

Table 27.1.
Platelet or Prostaglandin Abnormalities Observed in HUS

Increased platelet destruction
Platelet antigen or aggregates seen in the kidney (vessels-glomeruli)
Plasma platelet Factor 4 (increased)[a]
Plasma beta thromboglobulin (increased)[a]
Platelet beta thromboglobulin (BTG) (decreased)
Platelet Factor 4 (in platelets) (decreased)
Platelet activating factor (increased)[b]
Platelet aggregation (increased)[b]
Prostacyclin (decreased)
Thromboxane A_2 (increased)

Modified from Fong JSC, de Chadarevian J-P, Kaplan BS: Pediatr Clin NA 29(4):835, 1982.

[a] Also increased in renal failure.

[b] Decreased in one series—associated with decreased BTG and decreased platelet serotonin, and decreased or absent response to epinephrine, ADP, or collagen.

Table 27.2.
The Coagulation System in HUS

Coagulation factor	Abnormality
Prothrombin time	Prolonged (ocasionally)[a]
PTT	Shorter than normal[b]
Fibrin degradation products	Increased
Fibrinogen	Usually increased[c]
Antithrombin III	Usually normal[d]
Factor XI	Occasionally decreased

[a] Usually due to decreased levels of Factors II, VII, IX, X (secondary to Vitamin K deficiency).

[b] Usually due to increased levels of Factors V, VIII, IX, XI, and fibrinogen.

[c] Isolated cases of decreased fibrinogen.

[d] Ten cases of decreased levels have been reported.

Table 27.3.
Electrolyte and Metabolic Abnormalities Observed in HUS

Metabolic acidosis
Hyponatremia
Hypernatremia
Hyperkalemia
Hyperuricemia
Hypoproteinemia and hypoalbuminemia
Hyperlipidemia
Liver enzyme elevation (SGOT, SGPT, LDH, GGTP)
Hyperbilirubinemia
Hypocalcemia
Hyperphosphatemia

Aside from the occasional mention of vitamin K deficiency developing in HUS patients, coagulation factor abnormalities are either rarely or inconsistently observed (Table 27.2) (109–112). Studies from several laboratories have failed to demonstrate any evidence for disseminated intravascular coagulation (113). However, localized activation of the clotting system cannot be discounted. The presence of factor VIII, fibrinogen, or fibrin-related antigens, as well as platelet antigen within the same loci in the kidney, would lend support to this latter concept. Decreased antithrombin III (AT III) levels were noted in a patient with postpartum renal failure who appeared to improve clinically after antithrombin III concentrate administration (114). However, available data from two recent pediatric studies are at variance with each other. The discrepancy may be a result of one group having measured plasma AT III levels by immunodiffusion alone without concomitant measurement of plasma AT III activity (115, 116). Alpha-2 macroglobulin and alpha-1 antitrypsin levels and fibrin reactive antigens are often increased in HUS patients (1, 112). However, these antiplasmins are increased in other renal diseases as well. A plasma inhibitor of renal cortical fibrinolysis was demonstrated in a recent study of HUS. There appeared to be a correlation between the duration of detection of lysis inhibitor titer and the number of peritoneal dialysis treatments performed in these patients (117).

A multiplicity of electrolyte and acid-base abnormalities occur in HUS that are similar to those seen in either renal failure or with severe gastroenteritis (Table 27.3). Of particular interest is the consistent finding of hypoalbuminemia (6). To date, the cause of this abnormality has not been clearly delineated. Altered synthesis as a result of hepatocellular dysfunction (SGOT, SGPT, GGPT, LDH, and bilirubin are often increased in HUS) is one possibility, as is gastrointestinal loss as a result of an exudative enteropathy or renal loss caused by glomerular or tubular injury. Hyperlipidemia and hyperuricemia have also been reported (3, 18).

The role of the immune system in HUS is unclear. Among the most common abnormalities seen are decreased serum levels of complement components (C_1Q, C_3, C_4, CH_{50}, Factor B, Factor D) (119, 120), the presence of factor B and other breakdown products of C_3 (121, 122), high concentrations of circulating immune complexes (19, 30, 123), and the presence of C_3 nephritic factor (124). A familial form of HUS with persistent hypocomplementemia was recently reported (107). Hypocomplementemia may persist despite nephrectomy in patients with thrombotic microangiopathy (125). The finding of normal C_5 levels in several studies suggests that complement activation does not go beyond C_3 (122, 126). However, further work is clearly necessary to better define the role of the complement system in this disease. Alterations in the level of immunoglobulins (IgG, IgA, IgM) have been observed in some cases and several cases of HUS have been described in immunologically compromised children (3, 127, 128).

The radiological picture of HUS is often indistinguishable from that of patients with either ulcerative colitis, viral gastroenteritis, or intussusception (Fig. 27.2) (129–132). The diagnosis of HUS can be difficult and unduly delayed by the initial clinical presentation or by the interpretation of the radiological studies (Fig. 27.2). Meticulous attention to the initial laboratory abnormalities is, therefore, imperative. However, in view of one recent study, we must now be cognizant that laboratory studies may be normal at the onset of the prodromal illness (133). Commonly noted gastrointestinal X-ray film findings in HUS patients include submucosal edema and spasm, superficial ulcerations, areas of narrowing distention, and thumbprinting. In addition, toxic megacolon, colonic perforation, and stricture formation may occur acutely or as a late complication of HUS.

Several investigators have attempted to predict the outcome in HUS from radionuclide studies of renal function. Renogram studies in a variety of renal diseases suggested that the presence of a flat renogram or the absence of visualization on a renal scan employing ^{131}I-Hippuran was indicative of a poor renal outcome. In children with HUS, however, radionuclide renography cannot predict outcome even if more than one radioisotope is used (134, 135). Total recovery of renal function often occurs in anuric patients who fail to demonstrate any radioisotope in the kidney. Indeed, one patient voided 12 hours after her radionuclide study, which showed absent visualization and a flat execretory curve (136). Thus, radionuclide studies should be no longer be considered to predict the outcome of this disease.

Atypical HUS Variants

Several distinct familial forms of HUS have been observed. Via a questionnaire sent to reporting centers throughout the world, one group of investigators were able to identify two apparently distinct groups in which a familial incidence was noted (137). The major differences are listed in Table 27.4. Clearly, the one familial variant (Group 2) was associated with a much more severe illness as evidenced by a mortality approaching 70% and an increased incidence of renal failure. Recurrent episodes of HUS also tended to occur in this subset.

In addition, at least four families have been described in which an autosomal dominant type of inheritance was observed (138–141). Most of the patients were adults; mortality was high (70%) and end-stage renal failure occurred in 23%. Several recent studies perhaps shed some light on several of these familial variants. Reduced prostacyclin generating capacity in a proband and half of her off-spring suggested that a genetic predisposition existed, with an HUS-like disease only surfacing when exposure to a noxious agent occurred (94).

Of the cases of HUS observed in identical twins, all but one set of twins developed their illness within days to weeks of each other (142,

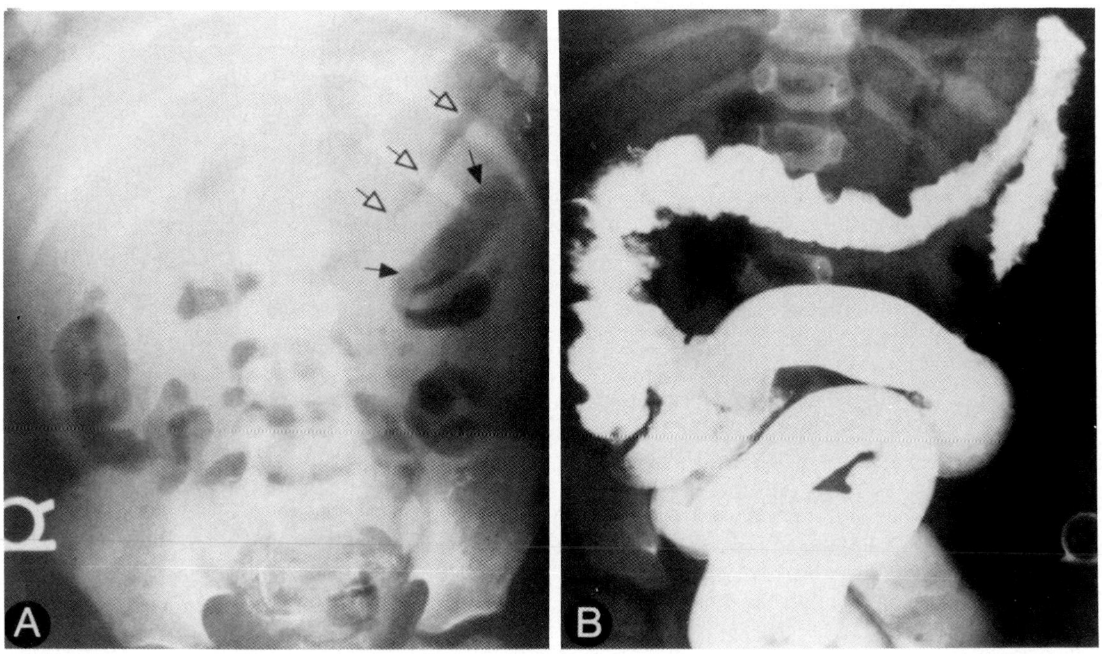

Figure 27.2.
A, Plain film of the abdomen shows thumb printing and marginal irregularities of the left transverse colon (*open arrows*), as well as a loop of small bowel (*closed arrows*).
B, Barium enema confirms submucosal edema, marginal ulcerations, and areas of spasm. The radiological changes are most marked in the left transverse colon and proximal descending colon.
(Reproduced with permission from Kirks DR: Pediatr Radiol 12:179, 1982.)

Table 27.4.
Hemolytic Uremic Syndrome in 48 Families

	Group 1	Group 2
Interval between onset in siblings	Days-weeks	More than 1 year apart
Families	29	19
Patients	58	44
Twins	7 pairs	None
Geographic distribution	Mainly in endemic areas (16/19)	Mainly in nonendemic areas (26/29)
Relapses or recurrences	None reported	5 cases
Required renal transplantations	1	2
Mortality	11/57 (19%)[a]	29/42 (69%)[a]

Modified from Kaplan BS, Thomson PD, de Chadarevian J-P: Pediatr Clin NA 23:761, 1976.
[a] Transplanted patients excluded from these calculations.

143). Complete recovery of both twins was usually the rule, with but one known exception (143). In one set of identical twins, an HUS-like illness developed in one, while a TTP-like illness developed in the other twin, suggesting perhaps that HUS and TTP are closely related disorders (142).

In addition to the familial subsets, another unique variant described is the patient with recurrent episodes of HUS. The clinical presentation is often atypical and the mortality rate is high (30%) (38). Finally, the HUS-like syndrome occurring in young women receiving oral contraceptives or in the immediate postpartum period is associated with high morbidity and mortality rates (17, 18, 40, 55, 56).

Pathology

The renal structural abnormalities in HUS result from FRA, platelet antigen, and factor VIII antigen deposition within glomerular capillaries, afferent arterioles, and interlobular arteries (89, 144). These changes may range from subtle glomerular abnormalities, evidenced only by electron microscopy particularly in milder cases, to extensive glomerular and vascular thrombosis with bilateral cortical infarction in the more severe cases (1, 3, 145–148). The typical changes usually associated with HUS depend on the severity of the disease, as well as the duration of illness before the time of biopsy. These lesions are best visualized by electron microscopy. Characteristically, one may see endothelial cell proliferation and swelling; detachment of the endothelium from the capillary basal lamina with the formation of a subendothelial space in which one may find fibrin, platelets, other cellular debris, or semilucent flocculent-like material; epithelial cell foot-process obliteration, particularly in areas of capillary damage; the presence of tactoids of fibrin-like material or depolymerized fibrin; entrapment of fragmented or crenated erythrocytes in narrowed capillary lumens; lipoid droplets or myelin figures within endothelial or mesangial cells; and splitting of capillary basement membranes as a result of either endothelial cell basa lamina formation or on occasion, mesangial interposition (Fig. 27.3).

Corresponding light microscopic features include capillary wall thickening with narrowing of the lumens or thrombosis and congestion of capillaries. Often, one will see preinfarcted or infarcted glomeruli with extensive glomerular or arteriolar thrombosis. PAS and silver methenamine stains may show an increase in fibrillar mesangial matrix-like material or varying amounts of splitting of capillary wall basement membranes. Mesangial proliferation, and, on occasion, crescent formation can also be seen (Fig. 27.3) (13, 145–148).

Arteriolar injury during the acute phase is manifested by either thrombosis with recanalization or by fibrinoid necrosis. Fibrointimal obliteration or medial fibrosis may be seen as healing occurs often with superimposed hypertensive vascular changes. Intralobular arteries are less commonly involved and usually exhibit similar morphological features. On occasion, a subintimal mucoid appearance to the vessels, similar to that seen in scleroderma, is encountered. Tubular and interstitial changes are nonspecific and include ectasia, focal to diffuse necrosis, atrophy, interstitial edema, fibrosis or inflammation.

Immunohistochemical studies have demonstrated fibrinogen, factor VIII, and platelet membrane antigen or other platelet constituents either along the endothelium of glomerular capillaries or within capillary or vessel lumina (89, 100, 114). Occasionally, occlusion of vessels is noted (Fig. 27.3). Although the kidney is usually the predominant organ involved, thrombosis and fibrinoid necrosis has been observed in other organs inclusive of brain, adrenals, spleen, liver, myocardium, and intestine (1, 3, 13, 71–73).

Studies, which have looked at the relationship between the duration of the disease before autopsy and the distribution of the microthrombi, have shown that in patients evaluated 2 months or more after the onset of HUS, abnormalities were confined primarily to the kidney. These changes included glomerular capillary narrowing, thickening of the basement membrane, tubular atrophy, and interstitial fibrosis. Hypertensive vascular changes may be present as well (10, 13).

The glomerular and vascular lesions seen in HUS of childhood, however, are not specific for this disorder alone. Similar lesions have been observed in the adult form of HUS, postpartum renal failure, microangiopathy associated with contraceptive pills, scleroderma, malignant hypertension, hyperacute and accelerated acute allograft rejection, and in TTP (13, 17–23, 145–147).

Management

None of the many therapeutic approaches that have been used, including immunosuppressive agents (steroids and vincristine) (5, 58, 149), anticoagulants (heparin) (150–152), antiplatelet drugs (dipyridamole and ASA) (153, 154), fibrinolytic activators (streptokinase and urokinase) (155–159), prostacyclin (160), defibrotide (161), plasma infusions, or plasmapheresis, have proven to be uniformly successful; most having been subsequently abandoned (162–165). In the only prospective study that compared heparin therapy to supportive care alone, no significant differences in patient survival was observed. In fact, the mortality rate was higher in the heparin treated group (166). With respect to the presumed benefit of streptokinase therapy in reducing the incidence of proteinuria and hypertension, caution must be exercised because of the significant risk of bleeding (156, 158). Furthermore, equivocal results were obtained in other series (157, 167). Antiplatelet agents (acetyl salicylic acid and dipyridamole) have received limited use with equivocal therapeutic response (126, 153, 154); however, the poor results may have been related to inappropriate aspirin dosages (168). In adults with HUS, there are reports in which the outcome was positively influenced by the early institution of protracted anticoagulant or antiplatelet therapy (56).

In all likelihood, earlier recognition of the disorder, prompt attention to the multiplicity of fluid and electrolyte problems that occur during the early phase of the disease, normalization of the blood pressure and early institution of either hemo or peritoneal dialysis have been primarily responsible for the decreased morbidity and mortality rates (1–14). Increased awareness of the potential late gastrointestinal complications may also have improved survival statistics. In Argentina, for example, acute mortality has decreased from 15% to 6% with the institution of conservative measures alone (10) (Table 27.5). Mortality rates were also higher from those series reported before 1966 (Table 27.5) (10, 169). Suffice it to say that in those studies in which an attempt was made to

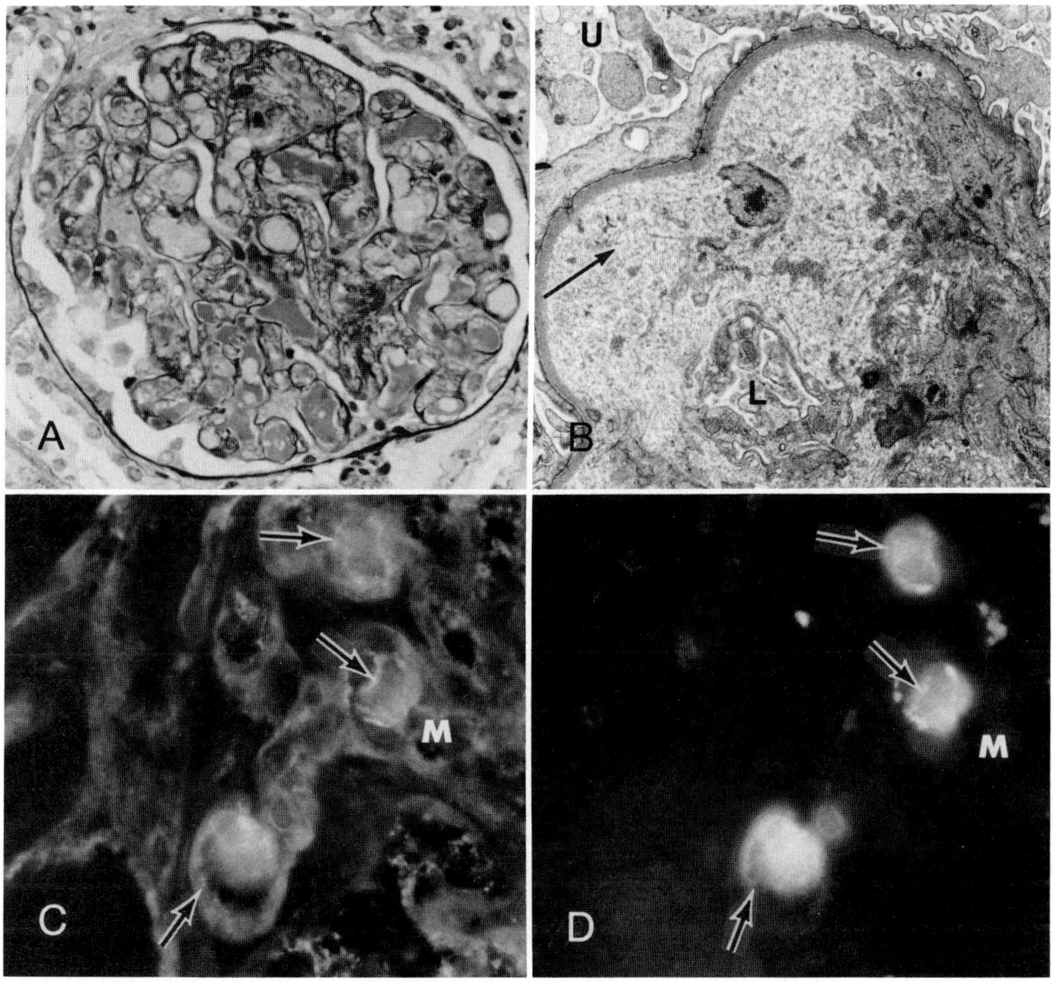

Figure 27.3. Pathological findings in HUS.
A, Light microscopy. Note the fibrin thrombi within capillary loops. (PAS X315).
B, Electron microscopy showing stripping of the endothelium from the capillary wall, with accumulation of flocculent material and cellular debris in the resulting subendothelial space (*arrow*). *L,* lumen; *U,* urinary space. (X5800.) Adapted with permission from Campos, A et al. The Kidney, 14(2):23, 1981.
C and **D**, Kidney sections stained sequentially with FITC labelled antifibrin/fibrinogen and rhodamine conjugated antiplatelet antibody. Note in **C** the presence of fibrin/fibrinogen within the glomerular capillaries (*arrows*) and mesangium (*M*); in **D** platelet antigen(s) are present in the same capillaries (*arrows*), but not in the mesangium. (Immunofluorescence microscopy X900.) (Adapted with permission from Miller K, et al: Kidney Intl 18:472, 1980.)

prospectively look at the value of drug therapy, no clear-cut benefit was demonstrated (1–14, 54, 170). The long-term, as opposed to short-term, benefit of any of the aforementioned agents remains to be established.

Presently, a great deal of attention has been focused on the possible beneficial effect of plasma infusions or plasmapheresis, with or without dialysis, on patient survival. To date, relatively few HUS patients have been studied and no controlled study has been performed (171, 172). Thus, it is too early to state whether these forms of therapy will impact on either patient morbidity or mortality.

In TTP, plasmapheresis or plasma infusions appear to benefit both the acute illness and to attentuate the disease process in patients with recurrent episodes (173–176). Currently, there is a paucity of information on the value of prostacyclin infusion. The few studies published have described variable results in both TTP and HUS (160, 177, 178). Newer agents, such as thromboxane synthetase inhibitors, cyclo-oxygenase inhibitors, prostacyclin stimulants, and phospholipase A_2, are currently under investigation.

The incidence of chronic renal disease resulting from HUS has usually been low except in Argentina where, in an early report, hypertension or chronic renal insufficiency occurred in 60% of surviving patients (10). Other reporting centers have described late renal sequelae in 6% to 24% of patients (1–14, 54, 77, 156, 167, 172, 173). Some centers have observed a direct correlation between the persistence of oliguria beyond 26 days and the development of chronic renal failure (43%) (10). However, in our series from the University of Minnesota, the duration of oligoanuria did not appear to impact on either the short-term or long-term prognosis.

Certain features, however, appear to suggest a poorer outcome. These include an atypical prodromal illness (nondiarrheal prodrome), patients with a familial predisposition, the patient with recurrent episodes, the adult HUS patient, the postpartum patient, the patient who has severe CNS involvement, the patient with persistent or recurrent thrombocytopenia, the patient with prolonged anuria, or the patient who has primarily arteriolar lesions or diffuse cortical necrosis on histological examination.

Despite the wealth of material accumulated to date on HUS, many unanswered questions remain. Yet, great improvements in the management of these patients have been made, particularly with regards to recognition of the need for early institution of dialysis and aggressive

Table 27.5.
Summary of Reported Series of HUS in Children

Source	No	Mean age (mo)	Anuria/ Oliguria (%)	Treatment[b]	Overall acute mortality (%)	Sequelae[a] (%)
Kaplan (3, 54)						
S. Africa (1962–69)	67	8	—	Heparin (8)	34[e]	11
				Dialysis		
(1968–75)	44		—	Dialysis	4.5	10
Kibel (169)						
S. Africa (1958–67)	109	10.5	34	Steroids (24)	36.8[d]	—
Monnens (155, 156)[c]	35	39		Early dialysis		
Netherlands				Heparin	5.7	24.2
	38	42	—	Early dialysis		
				Streptokinase (38)	7.8	5.7
				Heparin (38)		
Gianantonio (10)						
Argentina (1962–66)	130	12.2	100	No dialysis	15.6	60
(1967–72)	516	12.1		Early dialysis	6.2	
Tune (12)						
Stanford (1960–69)	27	54	64	Early dialysis	11.1	9.5
Lieberman (5)				Steroids (5)		
L.A., CA (1954–70)	39	—	23	Heparin (16)	20.5	—
				Dialysis		
Sorrenti (7)						
Chicago (1968–76)	19	54	50	Heparin (4)	10.5	17.6
				Early dialysis		
Bale (77)						
Utah (1972–78)	60	39	64	Early dialysis	5	7.0
Janssen (170)	20	18	75	Heparin (1)	15	10
Belgium (1957–72)				Early dialysis		
				Cortisone (1)		
Donckerwolcke (9)	49	28.3	84	Heparin (9)	16	6
Netherlands (1964–73)				Dialysis		
Riella (8)	18	64	61	Heparin (6)	0	10
Seattle (1967–73)				Cortisone/Heparin (6)		
				Dialysis		
Miller (167)[f]						
Minnesota (1972–78)	30	58	96	Streptokinase (6)	10	16
				Heparin (8)		
				Aspirin/Dipyridamole (1)		
				Corticosteroids (1)		
				Early dialysis		

[a] Presence of either hypertension, proteinuria, decreased creatinine clearance, or CNS abnormalities.
[b] Number in parentheses indicates number of patients in whom this therapy was used.
[c] Period of study not stated.
[d] Mortality rate—75% if patient was anuric.
[e] Two of 7 died when dialysis started within 48 hours, 18 of 21 died when dialysis not used or when started later in the course of the disease, 4 of the 8 children who received heparin died.
[f] Personal communication.

management of electrolyte imbalance and hypertension. The appreciation that there are several discrete subsets of HUS that may be recognized based on either clinical presentation or course, inheritance patterns, inciting agents, or laboratory abnormalities has allowed these high-risk patients to receive special and early attention. However, we must bear in mind that since HUS is indeed a syndrome, no one set of clinical features, laboratory abnormalities, or therapeutic approaches are likely to be applicable to all patients.

Acknowledgments

Media Services Department, Lutheran General Hospital; Larry Windland, Resource Support, Health Science Associate/Cardiovascular Diseases, Merck Sharp & Dohme; Teresa Trejo, secretarial support.

References

1. Fong JS, de Chadarevian JP, Kaplan BS: Hemolytic-uremic syndrome—current concepts and management. Pediatr Clin of NA 29(4):835, 1982.
2. Goldstein MH, Churg J, Strauss L, et al: Hemolytic-uremic syndrome. Nephron 23:263, 1979.
3. Kaplan BS, Thomson PD, de Chadarevian JP: The hemolytic uremic syndrome. Pediatr Clin NA 23(4):761, 1976.
4. Van Wieringen PM, Monnens LA, Schretlen ED: Haemolytic-uraemic syndrome—epidemiological and clinical study. Arch Dis Child 49(6):432, 1974.
5. Lieberman E: Hemolytic-uremic syndrome. J Pediatr 80(1):1, 1972.
6. Chesney RW, Friedman AL, Segar WE: The hemolytic-uremic syndrome in Wisconsin: experience in 22 cases. Wis Med J 79:21, 1980.
7. Sorrenti LY, Lewy PR: The hemolytic-uremic syndrome—experience at a center in the midwest. Am J Dis Child 132:59, 1978.

8. Riella MC, George CR, Hickman RO, et al: Renal microangiopathy of the hemolytic-uremic syndrome in childhood. Nephron 17:188, 1976.
9. Donckerwolcke RA, Kuyten RH, Tiddens HA: Haemolytic-uraemic syndrome. Paediatrician 4:27, 1975.
10. Gianantonio CA, Vitacco M, Mendilaharzu F, et al: The hemolytic-uremic syndrome. Nephron 11:174, 1973.
11. Brasher C, Sigler RL: The hemolytic-uremic syndrome. West J Med 134:193, 1981.
12. Tune BM, Leavitt TJ, Gribble TJ: The hemolytic uremic syndrome in California. A review of 28 non-heparinized cases with long-term follow-up. J Pediatr 82:304, 1973.
13. Campos A, Sibley R, Kim Y, et al: The hemolytic uremic syndrome. The Kidney 14(2):23, 1981.
14. Dolislager D, Tune B: The hemolytic-uremic syndrome. Am J Dis Child 122:55, 1978.
15. Gasser C, Gauthier E, Steck A, et al: Hamolytisch-Uramisch Syndrome: Bilaterale Nierenrindennekrosen bei Akuten Erworbenen Hamolytischen Anamien. Schweiz Med Wochensch 38:905, 1955.
16. Nalbadian RM, Henry RL, Bick RL: Thrombotic thrombocytopenic purpura: an extended editorial. Semin Thromb Hemost 5:216, 1976.
17. Robson JS, Martin AM, Ruckley VA, et al: Irreversible post partum renal failure. Quart J Med 37:423, 1968.
18. Segonds A, Louradour N, Suc JM, et al: Postpartum hemolytic uremic syndrome: A study of three cases with a review of the literature. Clin Neph 2(5):229, 1979.
19. Magalhaes RL, Braun WE, Straffon RA, et al: Microangiopathic hemolytic anemia in renal allotransplantation. Am J Med 58:862, 1975.
20. Tobon H: Malignant hypertension, uremia and hemolytic anemia in a patient on oral contraceptives. Obstet Gynec NY 40:681, 1972.
21. Gavras H, Oliver N, Aitchison J, et al: Abnormalities of coagulation and the development of malignant phase hypertension. Kidney Intl 8:S-252, 1975.
22. Schuette PT, Brabham AM, Eurenius K: Thrombotic thrombocytopenic purpura—A re-evaluation. So Med J 67:915, 1974.
23. Pisciotta AV, Gottschall JL: Clinical features of thrombotic thrombocytopenic purpura. Semin Thromb Hemost 5:330, 1980.
24. Ray CG, Tucker VL, Harris DJ, et al: Enteroviruses associated with the hemolytic-uremic syndrome. Pediatr 46:378, 1970.
25. Glasgow LA, Balduzzi P: Isolation of coxsackie virus group A, type 4, from a patient with hemolytic-uremic syndrome. NEJM 273:754, 1965.
26. O'Regan S, Robitaille P, Mongeau JG, et al: The hemolytic uremic syndrome associated with ECHO 22 infection. Clin Pediatr 19(2):125, 1980.
27. Davison AM, Thomson D, Robson JS: Intravascular coagulation complicating influenza A2 infection. Brit Med J 1:654, 1973.
28. Austin TW, Ray CG: Coxsackie virus group B infections and the hemolytic uremic syndrome. J Infect Dis 127(6):698, 1973.
29. McKay DB, Wahle GH Jr: Epidemic gastroenteritis due to *Escherichia coli* O 111 B_4. Archs Path 60:679, 1955.
30. Koster F, Levin J, Walker L, et al: Hemolytic-uremic syndrome after shigellosis: relation to endotoxemia and circulating immune complexes. NEJM 298(17):927, 1978.
31. Rapaport SE, Tatter D, Coeur-Barrow N, et al: Pseudomonas septicemia with intravascular clotting leading to the generalized Schwartzman reaction. NEJM 271:80, 1964.
32. Fiala M, Bauer H, Khaleeli M, et al: Dog bite, bacteroides infection, coagulopathy, renal microangiopathy. Ann Intern Med 87:248, 1977.
33. Chamovitz BN, Hartstein AI, Alexander SR, et al: Campylobacter jejuni—associated hemolytic-uremic syndrome in a mother and daughter. Pediatr 71:253, 1983.
34. Prober CG, Tune B, Hoder L: Yersinia pseudotuberculosis septicemia. Am J Dis Child 133:623, 1979.
35. Miller K: Personal Communication.
36. Mettler NE: Isolation of a microtatabiote from patients with hemolytic-uremic syndrome and thrombotic thrombocytopenic purpura and from mites in the United States. NEJM 281:1023, 1968.
37. Leavitt TJ, Merigan TC, Freeman JM: Hemolytic-uremic-like syndrome following polycarboxylate interferon induction. Am J Dis Child 121:43, 1971.
38. Kaplan BS: Hemolytic uremic syndrome with recurrent episodes: an important subset. Clin Neph 8(6):495, 1977.
39. Steele BT, Arbus GS, Rance CP: An outbreak of hemolytic uremic syndrome associated with ingestion of fresh apple juice. J Pediatr 101:963, 1982.
40. Jackson B, Clarkson AR, Seymour AE: The haemolytic uraemic syndrome and oral contraceptives. Aust NZ J Med 6:580, 1976.
41. Lyman NW, Michaelson R, Viscuso RI, et al: Mitomycin-induced hemolytic-uremic syndrome: successful treatment with corticosteroids and intense plasma exchange. Arch Intern Med 143:1617, 1983.
42. Jackson AM, Rose BD, Graff LG, et al: Thrombotic microangiopathy and renal failure associated with antineoplastic chemotherapy. Ann Intern Med 101:41, 1984.
43. Crocker J, Jones EL: Haemolytic-uraemic syndrome complicating long-term mitomycin C and 5-fluorouracil therapy for gastric carcinoma. J Clin Path 36:24, 1983.
44. McPherson AJ, Parkin JD, Hope R: Penicillin-induced haemolytic anaemia associated with microangiopathy. Aust NZ J Med 6:152, 1976.
45. Leithner C, Sinzinger J, Pohanka E, et al: Occurrence of hemolytic uremic syndrome under cyclosporine treatment: accident or possible side effect mediated by a lack of prostacyclin-stimulating plasma factor? Transplant Proceed 15(4):2787, 1983.
46. Petersen VP, Olsen TS: Late renal transplant failure due to the hemolytic-uremic syndrome. Acta Med Scand 189:377, 1971.
47. Folman R, Arbus GS, Churchill B, et al: Recurrence of the hemolytic uremic syndrome in a $3\frac{1}{2}$-year-old child, 4 months after second renal transplantation. Clin Neph 10(3):121, 1978.
48. Spruce WE, Forman SJ, Blume KG, et al: Hemolytic uremic syndrome after bone marrow transplantation. Acta Haematol 67:206, 1982.
49. de Chadarevian JP, Goodyer PR, Kaplan BS: Acute glomerulonephritis and hemolytic uremic syndrome. CMA J 123:391, 1980.
50. Dische FE, Culliford EJ, Parsons V: Haemolytic uraemic syndrome and idiopathic membranous glomerulonephritis. Brit Med J 126:1112, 1978.
51. Alon R, Adler SP, Chan JC: Hemolytic-uremic syndrome associated with streptococcus pneumoniae. Am J Dis Child 138:496, 1984.
52. Moorthy B, Makker SP: Hemolytic-uremic syndrome associated with pneumococcal sepsis. J Pediatr 95(4):558, 1979.
53. Seger R, Joller P, Baerlocher K, et al: Hemolytic-uremic syndrome associated with neuraminidase-producing microorganisms: treatment by exchange transfusion. Helv Paediat Acta 35:359, 1980.
54. Kaplan BS, Katz J, Krawitz S, et al: An analysis of the results of therapy in 67 cases of the hemolytic-uremic syndrome. J Pediatr 78(3):420, 1971.
55. Pertuiset N, Ganeval LD, Grunfeld, J-P: Acute renal failure in pregnancy: An update. Sem Neph 4:232, 1984.
56. Ponticelli C, Rivolta E, Imbasciati E, et al: Hemolytic uremic syndrome in adults. Arch Int Med 140:353, 1980.
57. Davies P: The haemolytic-uraemic syndrome. East Afr Med J 45:136, 1968.
58. Barnard PJ, Kibel M: The haemolytic-uraemic syndrome of infancy and childhood. Cent Afr J Med II:4, 1965.
59. Berman W Jr: The hemolytic-uremic syndrome: initial clinical presentation mimicking ulcerative colitis. J Pediatr 81(2):275, 1972.
60. Edmonson MB, Chesney RW: Hemolytic-uremic syndrome confused with acute appendicitis. Arch Surg 113:754, 1978.
61. Tochen ML, Campbell JR: Colitis in children with the hemolytic-uremic syndrome. J Pediatr Surg 12(2):213, 1977.
62. Whitington PF, Friedman AL, Chesney RW: Gastrointestinal disease in the hemolytic-uremic syndrome. Gastro 76:728, 1979.
63. Smith CD, Schuster SR, Gruppe WE, et al: Hemolytic-uremic syndrome: a diagnostic and therapeutic dilemma for the surgeon. J Pediatr Surg 18(6D):597, 1978.
64. Maki S, Ulda H: Hemolytic-uremic syndrome: a fatal case after operation for intussesception as a complication of upper respiratory infection. Med J Osaka Univ 19:157, 1968.
65. Sawaf H, Sharp MJ, Youn KJ, et al: Ischemic colitis and stricture after hemolytic-uremic syndrome. Pediatr 61:315, 1978.
66. Van Rhijn A, Donckerwolcke RA, Kuitjen RH, et al: Liver damage in the hemolytic-uremic syndrome. Helv Paediatr Acta 32:77, 1977.
67. Schweighofer S Jr, Primack WA, Slovis TL, et al: Cholelithiasis associated with the hemolytic-uremic syndrome. Amer J Dis Child 134:622, 1980.
68. Burns JC, Berman ER, Fagre JL, et al: Pancreatic islet cell necrosis: association with hemolytic-uremic syndrome. J Pediatr April, 582, 1982.
69. Andreoli SP, Bergstein JM: Development of insulin-dependent diabetes mellitus during the hemolytic-uremic syndrome. J Pediatr d100(4):541, 1982.
70. Adelman RD, Halsted CC, Sheikholishlam BM: Hemolytic-uremic syndrome: associated conditions. J Pediatr 97:161, 1980.
71. Ray CG, Portman JN, Stamm SJ, et al: Hemolytic-uremic syndrome and myocarditis. Amer J Dis Child 122:418, 1971.
72. Upadhyaya K, Barwick K, Fishaut M, et al: The importance of nonrenal involvement in hemolytic-uremic syndrome. Pediatr 65(1):115, 1980.
73. Utting JA, Shreeve DR: Haemolytic-uraemic syndrome in an adult with pericarditis and pleurisy. Brit Med J June 9, 1973.
74. Meadow R: Central nervous system involvement in the haemolytic uraemic syndrome. Develop Med and Child Neur 13:812, 1971.
75. Rooney JC, Anderson RM, Hopkins IJ: Clinical and pathological aspects of central nervous system involvement in the haemolytic uraemic syndrome. Austral Paediatr J 7:28, 1971.
76. Kahn SI, Tolkan SR, Kothari O, et al: Spontaneous recovery of the hemolytic uremic syndrome with prolonged renal and neurological manifestations. Nephron 32:18891, 1982.
77. Bale JRF, Brasher C, Siegler RL: CNS manifestations of the hemolytic-uremic syndrome. Amer J Dis Child 134:869, 1980.
78. Crisp DE, Siegler RL, Bale JF, et al: Hemorrhagic cerebral infarction in the hemolytic-uremic syndrome. J Pediatr 99(2):273, 1981.

79. Steele BT, Murphy N, Chuang SH, et al: Recovery from prolonged coma in hemolytic uremic syndrome. J Pediatr 102(3):402, 1983.
80. Ferris Z, Zeis PM: Coombs-positive hemolytic uremic syndrome. JAMA 235(5):521, 1976.
81. Metz J: Observations on the mechanisms of the hematological changes in the hemolytic uremic syndrome of infancy. Brit J Haemat 23(suppl):53, 1972.
82. Brain MC: The haemolytic-uraemic syndrome. Semin Hematol 6:162, 1969.
83. Patterson JM, McHenry EW: Choline and the prevention of hemorrhagic kidneys in the rat. J Biol Chem 145:207, 1942; 156:265, 1944.
84. Monserrat AJ, Ghoshal AK, Hartroft WS, et al: Lipoperoxidation in the pathogenesis of renal necrosis in choline deficient diet. Am J Path 55:163, 1969.
85. Wolman M: Etiology and pathogenesis of the hemolytic-uremic syndrome—a hypothesis. Israel J Med Scien 8(7):984, 1972.
86. Kobayashi Y, Okahata S, Tanabe K, et al: Erythrocyte superoxide dismutase activity in hemolytic uremic syndrome. Hiroshima J Med Sci 27:181, 1978.
87. O'Regan S, Chesney RW, Kaplan BS, et al: Red cell membrane abnormalities in the hemolytic-uremic syndrome. Clin Neph 15:14, 1980.
88. Klein PJ, Bulla M, Newman RA, et al: Thomsen-Friedenreich antigen in haemolytic uraemic syndrome. Lancet 1:1024, 1977.
89. Miller K, Dresner IG, Michael AF: Localization of platelet antigens in human kidney disease. Kidney Intl 18:472, 1980.
90. Alfrey AC: The renal response to vascular injury. In Brenner BM, Rector FC (eds): The Kidney Philadelphia, W. B. Saunders Co., 1976.
91. Giromini M, Hapenouza C: Prolonged survival after bilateral nephrectomy in an adult with hemolytic uremic syndrome. Lancet 2:169, 1969.
92. Remuzzi G, Misiani R, Marchesi D, et al: Haemolytic-uraemic syndrome: deficiency of plasma factor(s) regulating prostacyclin activity? Lancet 2:871, 1978.
93. Lian EC: The role of increased platelet aggregation in TTP. Semin Thromb and Hemost 6(4):401, 1980.
94. Remuzzi G, Misiani R, Marchesi D, et al: Familial deficiency of a plasma factor stimulating vascular prostacyclin activity. Throm Res 16:517, 1979.
95. Remuzzi G, Ross EC, Misiani R, et al: Prostacyclin and thrombotic microangiopathy. Semin Thromb and Hemost 6(4):391, 1980.
96. Jorgensen KA, Pedersen RS: Familial deficiency of prostacyclin production stimulating factor in the hemolytic uremic syndrome of childhood. Thromb Res 21:311, 1981.
97. Chen YC, McLeod B, Hall ER, et al: Accelerated prostacyclin degradation in thrombotic thrombocytopenic purpura. Lancet 267, 1981.
98. Remuzzi G, Livio M, Mecca G, et al: Prostacyclin and kidney disease: focus on uremia and thrombotic microangiopathy. In Lewis PJ, O'Grady J (eds): Clinical Pharmacology of Prostacyclin New York, Raven Press, 1981.
99. Naughton J, Kacich R: Thrombotic thrombocytopenic purpura. West Med 136:513, 1982.
100. Miller K: The coagulation system in experimental and human renal diseases. In Holliday M, Vernier R, Barratt T (eds): Pediatric Nephrology Baltimore, Williams & Wilkins, 1987.
101. Polley MJ, Nachman R: The human complement system in thrombin-mediated platelet function. J Exp Med 147:1713, 1978.
102. Poskitt TR, Fortwengler HP Jr, Lunskis BJ: Activation of the alternate complement pathway by autologous red cell stroma. J Exp Med 138:715, 1973.
103. Burns ER, Zucker-Franklin D: Pathologic effects of plasma from patients with thrombotic thrombocytopenic purpura on platelets and cultured vascular endothelial cells. Blood 60(4):1030, 1982.
104. Sims PJ, Boswell EB: Elevated platelet-bound IgG associated with an episode of thrombotic thrombocytopenic purpura. Blood 58(4):682, 1981.
105. Foser PA, Anderson JC: Effects of plasma from patients with thrombotic thrombocytopenic purpura (TTP) on cultured human endothelial cells. Blood 54(Suppl 1):240a, 1979.
106. Wall RT, Harker LA: The endothelium and thrombosis. Annu Rev Med 31:361, 1980.
107. Carreras L, Romero R, Requesens C, et al: Familial hypocomplementemic hemolytic uremic syndrome with HLA-A3,B7 haplotype. JAMA 245(6):602, 1981.
108. Moake JL, Rudy CK, Troll JH, et al: Unusually large plasma factor VIII: von Willebrand factor multimers in chronic relapsing thrombotic thrombocytopenic purpura. NEJM 307:1432, 1982.
109. Willoughby ML, Murphy AV, McMorris S, et al: Coagulation studies in haemolytic uraemic syndrome. Arch Dis Childh 47:766, 1972.
110. Sanchez Avalos J, Vitacco M, Molinas F, et al: Coagulation studies in the hemolytic-uremic syndrome. J Pediatr 76:538, 1970.
111. Monnens L, Kleynen F, van Munster P, et al: Coagulation studies and streptokinase therapy in the haemolytic-uraemic syndrome. Helv Paediat Acta 27:45, 1972.
112. Uttley WS: Serum levels of fibrin/fibrinogen degradation products in the haemolytic-uraemic syndrome. Arch Dis Childh 45:587, 1970.
113. Ekberg M, Holmberg L, Denneberg T: Hemolytic uremic syndrome: results of treatment with hemodialysis. Acta Paediatr Scand 66:693, 1977.
114. Brandt P, Jespersen J, Gregersen G: Postpartum haemolytic-uraemic syndrome successfully treated with antithrombin III. Brit Med J 2/1966.
115. Monnens L, de John M, van Oostrom P, et al: Anti-thrombin III levels in children with the epidemic form of hemolytic-uremic syndrome. Nephron 32:261, 1982.
116. Roth B, von Lilien T, Busch B, et al: Deficiency of antithrombin III in children with hemolytic-uremic syndrome. Euro J Pediatr 142:16, 1984.
117. Bergstein JM, Kuederli U, Bang NU: Plasma inhibitor of glomerular fibrinolysis in the hemolytic-uremic syndrome. Am J Med 73:322, 1982.
118. Kaplan BS, Gale D, Ipp T: Hyperlipidemia in the hemolytic-uremic syndrome. Pediatr 47:777, 1971.
119. Kaplan BS, Thomson PD, MacNab GM: Serum complement levels in the haemolytic uraemic syndrome. Lancet 2:1505, 1983.
120. Cameron JS, Vick R: Plasma-C_3 in haemolytic-uraemic syndrome and thrombocytopenic purpura. Lancet 2:975, 1973.
121. Kim Y, Miller K, Michael AF: Breakdown products of C_3 and Factor B in hemolytic-uremic syndrome. J Lab Clin Med 89(4):845–850, 1977.
122. Monnens L, Molenaar J, Lambert PH, et al: The complement system in hemolytic-uremic syndrome in childhood. Clin Neph 13:168, 1980.
123. Furuse A, Hattori S, Matsuda I: A case of hemolytic uremic syndrome with high concentration of circulating immune complex in the initial stage. Intl J Pediatr Neph 4(2):123, 1983.
124. Barre P, Kaplan BS, de Chadarevian JP, et al: Hemolytic uremic syndrome with hypocomplementemia, serum C_3NeF, and glomerular deposits of C_3. Arch Pathol Lab Med 101:357, 1977.
125. Gonzalo A, Mampaso F, Gallego N, et al: Hemolytic uremic syndrome with hypocomplementemia and deposits of IgM and C_3 in the involved renal tissue. Clin Neph 16:193, 1981.
126. Stuhlinger W, Kourilsky O, Smith MD, et al: Haemolytic uraemic syndrome: evidence for intravascular C_3 activation. Lancet 2:788, 1974.
127. Dubilier LD, Chadwick JA, Leddy JP: Thymic alymphoplasia associated with the hemolytic-uremic syndrome. J Pediatr 73:714, 1968.
128. Fluge G, Moe PG: Hemolytic-uremic (nephropathic) syndrome. A clinical picture unrecognized in the past? Acta Paediat Scand 56:665, 1967.
129. Kirks DR: The radiology of enteritis due to hemolytic-uremic syndrome. Pediatr Radiol 12:179, 1982.
130. Kawanami T, Bowen A, Girdany BR: Enterocolitis: prodrome of the hemolytic-uremic syndrome. Radiol 151(1):91, 1984.
131. Peterson RB, Meseroll WP, Shrage GG, et al: Radiographic findings of colitis associated with the hemolytic-uremic syndrome. Rad 118:667, 1976.
132. Bar-Ziv J, Ayoub JI, Fletcher BD: Hemolytic uremic syndrome: a case presenting with acute colitis. Pediatr Radiol 2:203, 1974.
133. Dillard RP: Hemolytic-uremic syndrome mimicking ulcerative colitis. Clin Pediatr 22(1):66, 1983.
134. Geft CH, Arbus GS: Hemolytic uremic syndrome and renal scanning. Intern J Pediatr Neph 1(2):106, 1980.
135. Campos A, Kim Y, Miller K, et al: Radionuclide studies of the kidney in children with hemolytic-uremic syndrome. Radiology 145(3):811, 1982.
136. Miller K, Cohn R, Lundeberg P, et al: Radioisotopic findings in a patient with the hemolytic uremic syndrome. Pediatr Res 13:(abstract 1142), 1979.
137. Kaplan BS, Chesney RW, Drummond KN: Hemolytic uremic syndrome in families. NEJM 292:1090, 1975.
138. Farr MJ, Roberts S, Morley AR, et al: The haemolytic-uraemic syndrome: a family study. Am J Med 44:161, 1975.
139. Hogewind BL, de la Riviere GB, van Es LA, et al: Familial occurrence of the haemolytic uraemic syndrome. Acta Med Scand 207:73, 1980.
140. Karlsberg RP, Lacher JW, Bartecchi CE: Adult hemolytic-uremic syndrome. Arch Intern Med 137:1155, 1977.
141. Perret B, Gaze H, Zinnerman A, et al: Syndrome hemolytique uremique familial non endemique: nephrectomie et transplantation. Helv Pediat Acta 34:167, 1979.
142. Hellman RM, Jackson DV, Buss DH: Thrombotic thrombocytopenic purpura and hemolytic-uremic syndrome in HLA-identical siblings. Ann Intern Med 93:283, 1980.
143. Campbell S, Carre TJ: Fatal haemolytic uraemic syndrome and idiopathic hyperlipaemia in monozygotic twins. Arch Dis Childh 40:654, 1965.
144. Hoyer JR, Michael AF, Hoyer LW: Immunofluorescent localization of antihemophilic factor antigen and fibrinogen in human renal diseases. J Clin Invest 53:1375, 1974.
145. Morel-Maroger L, Kanfer A, Solez K, et al: Prognostic importance of vascular lesions in acute renal failure with microangiopathic hemolytic anemia (hemolytic-uremic syndrome): clinicopathologic study in 20 adults. Kidney Intl 15:548, 1979.
146. Habib R, Levy M, Gagnadoux ME, et al: Prognosis of the HUS in children. Adv Neph 11:99, 1982.
147. Thoenes W, John HD: Endotheliotropic (hemolytic) nephroangiopathy and its various manifestation forms (thrombotic microangiopathy, primary malignant nephrosclerosis, hemolytic-uremic syndrome). Klin Wochnschr 58:173, 1980.

148. Shigematsu H, Dikman SH, Churg J, et al: Mesangial involvement in hemolytic-uremic syndrome. Amer J Path 85(2):349, 1976.
149. Gutterman LA, Levin DM, George BS, et al: The hemolytic-uremic syndrome: recovery after treatment with vincristine. Ann Inter Med 98(5):612, 1983.
150. Proesmans W, Eeckels R: Has heparin changed the prognosis of the hemolytic-uremic syndrome. Clin Nephrol 2(5):169, 1974.
151. Coulthard MG: An evaluation of treatment with heparin in the haemolytic-uraemic syndrome successfully treated by peritoneal dialysis. Arch Dis Childh 55:393, 1980.
152. Khanh BT, Bhathena D, Vazquez, et al: Role of heparin therapy in the outcome of adult hemolytic uremic syndrome. Nephron 16:292, 1976.
153. Arenson EB, August CS: Preliminary report: treatment of the hemolytic-uremic syndrome with aspirin and dipyridamole. J Pediatr 86(6):957, 1975.
154. O'Regan S, Chesney RW, Mongeau JG, et al: Aspirin and dipyridamole therapy in the hemolytic uremic syndrome. J Pediatr 97(3):473, 1980.
155. Monnens L, Kleynen F, van Munster P, et al: Coagulation studies and streptokinase therapy in the haemolytic-uraemic syndrome. Helv Paediat Acta 27:45, 1972.
156. Monnens L, van Collenburg J, de Jong M, et al: Treatment of the hemolytic-uremic syndrome. Helv Paediat Acta 33:321, 1978.
157. Stuart J, Winterborn MH, White RHR, et al: Thrombolytic therapy in haemolytic-uraemic syndrome. Brit Med J 3:217, 1974.
158. Powell HR, Ekert H: Streptokinase and anti-thrombotic therapy in the hemolytic-uremic syndrome. J Pediatr 84(3):345, 1974.
159. Loirat C, Beaufils F, Sonsino E, et al: Urokinase (UK) treatment for hemolytic-uremic syndrome (HUS) in childhood—A multicenter controlled trial from the French society of pediatric nephrology. Internat J Pediatr Neph 3(1):46, 1982.
160. Webster J, Rees AJ, Lewis PJ, et al: Prostacyclin deficiency in haemolytic-uraemic syndrome. Brit Med J 270:1980.
161. Bonomini V, Vangelista A, Frasca G: A new antithrombotic agent in the treatment of acute renal failure due to hemolytic-uremic syndrome and thrombotic thrombocytopenic purpura. Nephron 37:144, 1984.
162. Remuzzi G, Misiani R, Marchesi D, et al: Treatment of the hemolytic uremic syndrome with plasma. Clin Neph 12(6):279, 1979.
163. Bergada E, Torras A, Puig I, et al: Plasmapheresis-dependent recovery from recurrent hemolytic-uremic syndrome. Inter J Artif Organs 6:79, 1983.
164. Upshaw JD: Congenital deficiency of a factor in normal plasma that reverses microangiopathic hemolysis and thrombocytopenia. NEJM 298:1350, 1978.
165. Beattie TJ, Murphy AV, Willoughby MN: Plasmapheresis in the haemolytic-uraemic syndrome in children. Brit Med J 282:1667, 1981.
166. Vitacco M, Sanchez-Avalos J, Gianantonio CA: Heparin therapy in the hemolytic syndrome. J Pediatr 83:271, 1973.
167. Miller K: Personal Communication.
168. Stuart MJ, Spitzer RE, Coppe D: Abnormal platelet and vascular prostaglandin synthesis in an infant with hemolytic uremic syndrome. Pediatr 71(1):120, 1983.
169. Kibel MA, Barnard PJ: The hemolytic uremic syndrome. A survey in Southern Africa. S Afr Med J 42:692, 1968.
170. Janssen F, Potvliege PR, Vainsel M, et al: Le pronostic a court et a long terme du syndrome hemolytique et uremique. Arch Franc Ped 31:59, 1974.
171. Weyl M, Rivard GE, O'Regan S, et al: Hemolytic uremic syndrome; treatment with plasma, vitamin E and cod liver oil. Inter J Pediatr Neph 4(4):243, 1983.
172. Harden LW, Gluck RS, Salcedo JR: Simultaneous hemodialysis and exchange transfusion in hemolytic uremic syndrome. Clin Pediatr 19(9):640, 1980.
173. Pisciotto P, Rosen D, Silver H, et al: Treatment of thrombotic thrombocytopenic purpura: evaluation of plasma exchange and review of the literature. Vox Sang 45:185, 1983.
174. Richmond JM, d'Apice AJF, Whitworth JA, et al: Thrombotic thrombocytopaenic purpura and anuria: response to plasma exchange. Aust NZ J Med 19:48, 1980.
175. Dal Col A, Busnach G, Perrino ML, et al: Renal abnormalities reverted by plasma exchange in thrombotic thrombocytopenic purpura. Int J Artif Organs 6:69, 1982.
176. Frankel AE, Rubenstein MD, Wall RT: Thrombotic thrombocytopenic purpura: prolonged coma with recovery of neurologic function with intensive plasma exchange. Am J Hemat 10:387, 1981.
177. Fitzgerald GA, Maas RL, Stein R, et al: Intravenous prostacyclin in thrombotic thrombocytopenic purpura. Ann Intern Med 95(3):319, 1981.
178. Cocchetto DM, Cook L, Cato AE, et al: Rationale and proposal for use of prostacyclin in thrombotic thrombocytopenic purpura therapy. Sem Thromb and Hemostas 7(1):43, 1981.

CHAPTER 28 Renal Manifestations of Systemic Disease

28A Henoch-Schönlein Purpura

L. A. VAN ES
R. H. KAUFFMANN
R. M. VALENTIJN

INTRODUCTION

Henoch-Schönlein purpura (HSP) was probably first described by Heberden (1801) and Willan (1808). Schönlein described the association of purpura with arthralgia (1), whereas his former pupil Henoch reported on the association with gastrointestinal manifestation (2) and the renal abnormalities (3). Presently Henoch-Schönlein syndrome is recognized as a systemic small vessel vasculitis involving mainly the blood vessels of the skin, the gastrointestinal tract, the kidneys, and the joints. Platelet counts are typically normal. Because the syndrome is frequently incomplete, the term Henoch-Schönlein purpura is also used. On the basis of a presumed hypersensitivity to microorganisms, food, or drugs, the term anaphylactoid or allergic purpura was introduced. However, children with HSP are not significantly more allergic than other children. Recently it was realized that IgA antibodies may play an important role in the pathogenesis of HSP. The presence of IgA deposits in the vessel walls and the renal mesangium during the acute stage of the disease is one of the most characteristic features of HSP. The finding of IgA containing immune complexes in the circulation together with these deposits (4) suggests that circulating IgA-complexes are responsible for the development of vasculitis and glomerulonephritis in HSP.

CLINICAL MANIFESTATIONS

HSP affects mainly children between the ages of 3 and 10 years (5). In decreasing order of incidence, it also occurs in children older than 10 years, babies, adolescents, and adults. Males are affected more often (1,5:1) than females. In about two thirds of children an upper respiratory tract infection precedes the onset of HSP by 1 to 3 weeks (6). The incidence shows a seasonal variation with a peak around November to January in the northern hemisphere (7). In general, children are ill, and they frequently have an elevated body temperature, usually not higher than 38°C.

Cutaneous Manifestations

The disease starts usually with an acute and symmetrical erythematous macular rash. It may initially be restricted to the skin around the malleoli of the ankle, but usually it extends to the dorsal surface of the legs, the buttocks, and the ulnar side of the arms. It usually spares the trunk, unless it has been provoked by pressure, for instance under the waistband. Within a few hours the rash develops into pink maculopapules that are less edematous and darker. After 12 to 24 hours, the lesions become dusky red and have a diameter of 0.5 to 2 cm. They may coalesce into larger patches or ecchymoses. In the course of about 2 weeks the purpura turns from purple to brown before it disappears. The same time sequence is seen when the patients skin is stroked with a blunt rod or when the upperarm is compressed by the cuff of a sphygmomanometer; the immediate wheal is followed about 12 to 24 hours later by a purpuric lesion (8). The rash may come in crops of skin lesions that each are in the same stage of development. The purpura may also come in separate attacks, commonly not more than two or three, but in some children the attacks can recur during a period of 6 months or even longer.

In children younger than 3 years the clinical picture may be dominated by edema of the scalp, the periorbital area, the hands, and feet. The edema correlates with the activity of the vasculitis and not with the degree of proteinuria. It has also been attributed to the enteric loss of protein (9). In adults the skin lesions most frequently present as purpura, but it may also present as a papular rash, nodules, blisters, or ulcers (10).

Joint Involvement

The joints are involved in 60% to 75% of the cases. The arthralgia affects most commonly the knees and ankles and less often the wrists and fingers. The joints are painful and may be swollen because of periarticular edema, but they are not red, warm, or tender to touch as is the case in acute rheumatic fever. Joint effusions are rare. The joints are only transiently involved, and they recover without leaving residual deformity.

Gastrointestinal Manifestations

Gastrointestinal manifestations occur in about 50% of the cases and consist usually of colicky abdominal pains, melaena, or bloody diarrhea. Hematemesis occurs less frequently. These manifestations may precede the skin and joint manifestations in one fifth of the patients (11). In that situation laparotomies are frequently performed because patients may have the clinical picture of an acute abdomen. HSP may involve any portion of the gastrointestinal tract. Petechiae and ecchymoses have been observed endoscopically in the stomach, duodenum, sigmoid colon, and rectum (12). Radiologically, the jejunum and ileum are most frequently affected. The local edema and intramural hemorrhages may appear like thumb prints or pseudotumors (13). These lesions may occasionally lead to massive gastrointestinal hemorrhages (5%) or intussusception (3%), but perforation as a result of local necrosis occurs rarely. Protein-losing enteropathy and steatorrhea have also been observed (9).

Renal Manifestations

In HSP the whole clinical spectrum of glomerulonephritis may occur. Hematuria with mild or moderate proteinuria is the most common presentation (5). If proteinuria is heavy, it may lead to the nephrotic syndrome and is often accompanied by renal insufficiency. If the urine is examined regularly, microscopic hematuria is detected more often and the incidence of renal involvement may be as high as 80% of the cases or even higher (14). However, nephritis becomes clinically manifest in only 20% to 30% of unselected children. Clinical signs of renal involvement may follow or coincide with the appearance of the purpura, but rarely precedes it. The incidence of renal involvement is higher in patients with recurrent attacks of purpura (5) and in patients with abdominal manifestations (15, 16). Children with nephritis are as an average a little older.

Involvement of Other Organs

Almost any other organ can be involved in HSP. In case reports the following organs were involved: the heart (17, 18), the lungs (19, 20), the pancreas (21, 22), the parotid gland (7), the adrenals (23), the brain (24), peripheral nerves (26), and the gallbladder (27). Hepatosplenomegaly has also been reported. Although it is very attractive to assume that any blood vessel in the body can be affected by the systemic vasculitis, histological and immunofluorescence data are not currently available to confirm or refute such a supposition. Clinical or laboratory evidence of involvement of organs other than the skin, joints, gastrointestinal tract, and kidneys should raise the question of large vessel vasculitis, such as polyarteritis (chapter 28C).

PATHOLOGY

Few well-documented autopsies of fatal cases of HSP have been reported. Most of the histological documentation has been obtained by skin and kidney biopsies. The most typical lesion of HSP consist of a leukocytoclastic vasculitis, which is characterized by a transmural and perivascular infiltration with polymorphonuclear leukocytes, histiocytes, and sometimes eosinophils in association with fibrinoid necrosis, nuclear debris, and extravasation of erythrocytes (Fig. 28A.1). This lesion is frequently found in the superficial postcapillary venules of the skin. In studies of individual cases it has also been reported in the capillaries and arterioles of the lungs, the esophagus, the stomach, the duodenum (19), the jejunum (27), the ileum, the renal medulla (19), the adrenal cortex (23), the gallbladder (27), and the joints (28). Descriptions of the pathology of the joints are scarce.

The glomerular changes in HSP have been studied extensively. They may show a wide spectrum, ranging from very mild changes to severe lesions. Most glomeruli may look normal by light microscopy with only a few showing mesangial proliferation. Other cases may show focal and segmental intracapillary and extracapillary proliferation with adhesions

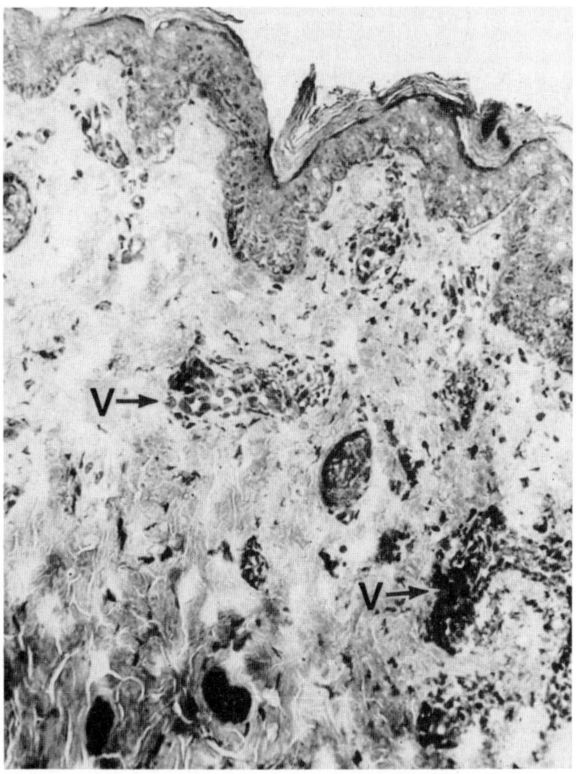

Figure 28A.1. Light micrograph of a skin biopsy from a child with HSP demonstrating a leukocytoclastic vasculitis. The boundary between many small capillaries and venules (**V**) within the dermis is obscured by an infiltrate consisting of primarily of polymorphonuclear leucocytes, both within and surrounding the vessel wall. (PAS stain X176.)

and small crescents. The most severe lesions consist of diffuse proliferation with infiltration of polymorphonuclear leukocytes and circumferential crescents in the majority of the glomeruli (Fig. 28A.2, *A*), as well as tubular atrophy and interstitial infiltration with mononuclear cells (7). Biopsies may sometimes show the typical picture of membranoproliferative glomerulonephritis. Probably the most consistent findings are the deposits of IgA in the mesangium (29) (Fig. 28A.2, *B*) and the walls of cutaneous capillaries (30). Deposits of IgA have also been described in the wall of mesenteric arteries (31). It should be stressed, however, that IgA deposits in cutaneous vessel walls are also found in various other forms of leukocytoclastic vasculitis.

The IgA deposited in the mesangium is mainly of the IgA1 subclass (32), although deposits of IgA2 have also been reported in HSP (33, 34). The detection of J-chain in the mesangial deposits correlates better with the presence of IgM than IgA (32). Secretory component could not be detected in the deposits (35). In addition to IgA, the deposits in mesangium and cutaneous capillaries frequently contain C3, IgG, and fibrin (36). The deposits of C3 are accompanied often by properdin, whereas C1q and C4 are commonly absent (37, 30). This indicates that the complement components in the deposits have been activated via the alternative pathway.

The site of the deposits within the glomeruli determines to a great extent the subsequent inflammatory reaction pattern and the renal histopathology in HSP. Mesangial deposits may stimulate the proliferation of mesangial cells. It is not known why some patients with heavy deposits of IgA have relatively little mesangial proliferation, whereas others show extensive mesangial proliferation. When the mesangial deposits extend to the subendothelial space of the peripheral capillary loops, focal and segmental changes may occur (38). Subepithelial deposits can also be found occasionally, but they are too scarce to lead to extensive spike formation (39).

DIFFERENTIAL DIAGNOSIS

The skin rash is an essential feature of the clinical presentation. Despite its variable character, the syndrome can be diagnosed easily when the purpura is accompanied by abdominal pain, arthralgia and renal involvement. A similar skin rash is occasionally seen in patients with acute poststreptococcal glomerulonephritis (40, 41) or in patients with systemic lupus erythematosus. Low complement levels and other serological evidence should help to differentiate these diseases from HSP. Other causes of purpura, such as septicemia, hemolytic uremic syndrome, thrombocytopenia, and coagulation abnormalities should be considered. When the gastrointestinal manifestations precede the skin rash other possible causes for an acute abdomen or gastrointestinal bleeding have to be excluded. The disease may also cause pancreatitis. A scrotal bleeding as a result of local vasculitis has to be differentiated from an incarcerated hernia, torsion of the testis, or traumatic orchitis (11). It is usually not difficult to discriminate the arthralgia in HSP from rheumatoid arthritis and acute rheumatic fever. The extrarenal manifestations are important clues to a systemic disorder.

Nephritis in HSP should be distinguished from other systemic forms of glomerulonephritis including bacterial endocarditis, systemic lupus erythematosus, and Goodpasture's syndrome. In adults it can be difficult to differentiate HSP from an overlap syndrome of polyarteritis combined with systemic small vessel vasculitis (42).

CLINICOPATHOLOGICAL CORRELATIONS AND PROGNOSIS

Aside from occasional abdominal complications, the morbidity and mortality of the disease are determined mainly by the severity of the renal complications. Although 10% to 15% of children were found to develop renal failure on long-term follow-up, the majority of children recover completely.

Between 50% to 70% of children have hematuria and mild or moderate proteinuria. Their renal biopsies usually show minor abnormalities or mesangial proliferation, which can either be diffuse or focal and segmental. These children usually have an excellent prognosis, although some have persistent symptomatic hematuria or mild proteinuria (<1 g/24 hours). There are however exceptions. Some children presenting with asymptomatic hematuria and proteinuria may develop later renal insufficiency. The prognostic index improves when both the clinical and the morphological manifestations of HSP are related to the long-term outcome of the disease. Patients who present with nephrotic syndrome and hematuria have a less favourable prognosis, particularly when these findings are accompanied by hypertension and a decreased glomerular filtration rate (7). Biopsies from these patients show focal

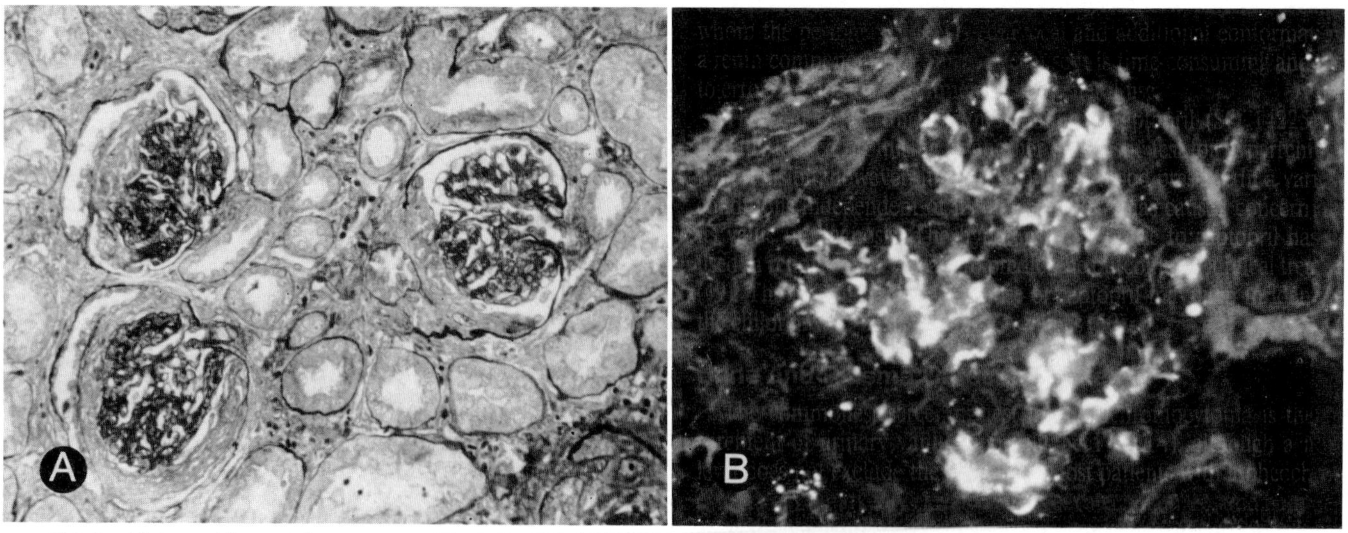

Figure 28A.2. Light and immunofluorescence (*IF*) micrographs of glomeruli from a kidney biopsy in a child with HSP. **A,** Demonstrating severe disease with crescents around most glomeruli and focal to diffuse mesangial proliferation. (PAS stain X221.) **B,** Distribution by IF of IgA, primarily within the mesangium, of a glomerulus from the above patient. (X400.)

proliferation involving segments of glomeruli, sometimes accompanied by necrosis of a tuft. These segmental lesions in capillary loops are frequently surrounded by small crescents, which are not only the result of proliferation of the visceral epithelium, but also may be a result of the influx of mononuclear phagocytes (43). When less than 50% of the glomeruli in the initial biopsy show small crescents, chronic renal disease may persist but relatively few patients develop renal failure. When patients present with nephrotic syndrome, hypertension, and a rapid deterioration of renal function, biopsies frequently show circumferential crescents in the majority of the glomeruli. A high proportion of these patients (about 60%) develop renal failure, either in the acute phase of the disease or after an interval of several years (5).

LABORATORY INVESTIGATIONS

Until now no laboratory test has been found to be diagnostic for HSP. In the first few days the peripheral blood count may show neutrophilic leukocytosis with a shift to the left. The erythrocyte sedimentation rate can be elevated. Platelet count, bleeding time, and clotting time are uniformly normal. Positive throat cultures and elevated ASO, anti-DNase, and anti-NADase titers have no diagnostic significance (44, 45). Tests for antinuclear antibodies and rheumatoid factor are negative.

Serum IgA levels can be transiently elevated, as was found in about 50% of children with HSP (46). About half of the children with HSP have cryoglobulins in their sera; IgA and properdin were found in several of these cryoglobulins (47). These findings suggest that cryoglobulins containing IgA can activate the alternative pathway. Although complement levels are consistently normal in HSP, C3d levels are significantly elevated in the acute phase of HSP (Fig. 28A.3) as an expression of a higher turn-over of C3, possibly by activation via the alternative pathway (4). The finding of deposits of IgA, C3, and C5 in cutaneous vessel walls in the absence of C1q and C4 supports this supposition (48).

Recently several groups of investigators have demonstrated independently that IgA-containing immune complexes (so called IgA-complexes) circulate in patients with HSP (4, 49, 50, 51). The methods used to detect IgA-complexes differed among these studies. Levinsky and coworkers (49) introduced an assay based on the principle that macromolecular IgA or IgA-complexes inhibit specifically the agglutination of IgA-coated latex beads by rabbit IgM antibodies directed against human IgA. A significant degree of inhibition was found in this study in 13 of 18 children (72%) with HSP. Kauffman and coworkers (4) used an assay based on a similar principle; radiolabeled goat IgM antibodies with a low avidity for IgA are inhibited by IgA-complexes from binding to IgA-coated Sepharose beads (a-IgAInhBA). The degree of inhibition is a measure of the amount of circulating IgA-complexes (52). With this assay IgA-complexes were found in 27 of 37 patients (73%). Hall and coworkers (50) used an assay based on the presence of C3-products in IgA-complexes. These complexes readily bind to C3b- and C3d-receptors of Raji cells, which are derived from a Burkitt's lymphoma and cultured continuously to serve as a detector reagent in immune complex assays (53). The class of the immunoglobulins in the complexes is then determined with the use of radiolabeled antibodies specific either for IgA or IgG (50). Four of the six patients with HSP were positive in this assay. Coppo and coworkers (51) used insolubilized bovine conglutinin to bind C3bi in IgA-complexes, which were then detected with enzyme-linked anti-IgA antibodies. With this assay 58% of patients with HSP had IgA-complexes. These findings all indicate that patients with HSP have macromolecular IgA or IgA-complexes in their circulation. After these complexes have deposited in the mesangium, arterioles, capillaries, and postcapillary venules, they may induce an inflammatory reaction and cause glomerulonephritis and leukocytoclastic vasculitis in HSP.

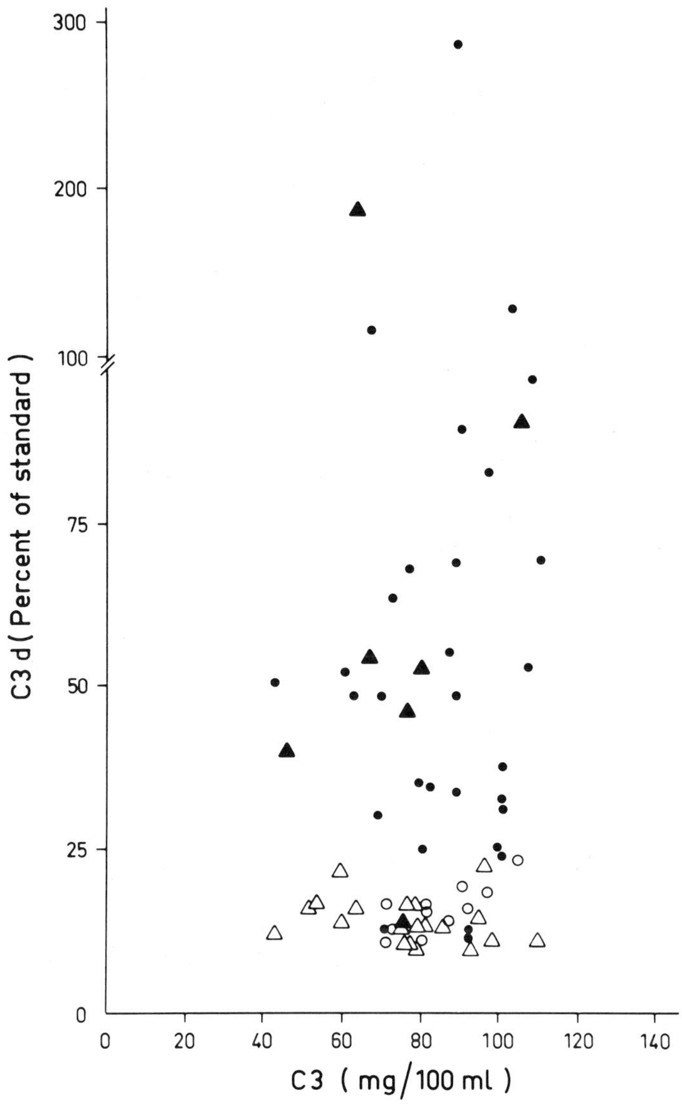

Figure 28A.3. C3 turn-over measured by C3d levels in children (●) and adults (▲) with HSP. Compared to the C3d levels in healthy children (○) and adults (△), the C3 turn-over is significantly higher in patients with HSP, although the serum C3 levels are not different between patients and controls. (From Kauffman RH, et al: Am J Med 69: 859, 1980.)

PATHOGENESIS

In 1914 Osler (54) alluded to the possibility that patients with urticaria and certain forms of purpura could be anaphylactic to certain proteins, as were patients with serum sickness. The term anaphylactoid purpura was introduced by Frank (55). Since then the idea that HSP is caused by a hypersensitivity reaction has developed into the concept that HSP is the result of an allergy to antigens derived from microorganisms, food, or drugs (56). Gairdner (8) reported on the high incidence of sore throat and positive cultures of hemolytic streptococci preceding the initial onset or relapses of HSP. His patients or their relatives did not have a higher incidence of allergies such as asthma, hay fever, or eczema than control patients. Others have reported a high incidence of upper respiratory tract infections preceding HSP (6, 14). However, Ayoub and Hoyer (45) were able to show by a carefully controlled study that patients with HSP do not have an increased frequency of positive cultures for hemolytic streptococci. In the majority of HSP cases an antecedent infection cannot be identified. Various microorganisms have been implicated in individual cases, including varicella (57), vaccinia (58), rubella (14), measles (14), influenza virus (59), and mycoplasma (60, 61).

Allergies to food and drugs have also been incriminated in the pathogenesis of HSP. The intake of dairy products, eggs, chocolate, wheat, and beans have been connected with the development of HSP (56). Only in a few cases was it shown that repeated intake of a particular kind of food provoked the disease.

A great variety of drugs have been implicated in the pathogenesis of HSP including penicillin, sulphonamides, tetracycline, erythromycin, quinidine, phenacetin, phenothiazines, and griseofulvin (10). However, several of these drugs were readministered after admission to the hospital without an exacerbation or recurrence of the disease (6). Although it cannot be excluded that drugs are involved in the pathogenesis of HSP, hard evidence fails to support this hypothesis.

HSP has been reported in adults with cancer of the gastrointestinal and respiratory tract (4, 62). It has also been described in a patient with monoclonal IgA gammopathy. Relapses of HSP could be prevented in this patient by cytotoxic treatment (63). This observation suggests that not only IgA-complexes, but also a monoclonal overproduction of IgA can cause HSP in the absence of antigen. Egido and coworkers (64) detected by sucrose density ultracentrifugation of sera from patients with HSP that these patients have an increase of IgA-oligomers in their circulation. It is of interest that others have found that B-lymphocytes from HSP patients produce more IgA and IgG in vitro than controls (65). This could be explained by a defective suppressor cell system in these patients (65). It is not known whether in HSP these B cells produce more polymeric IgA in vitro. Other studies indicate that the macromolecular IgA in sera of HSP patients is considerably larger than the size of IgA-oligomers (52). Oligomeric IgA can be distinguished from larger (>10^6 daltons) macromolecular IgA by precipitation in 3% polyethyleneglycol (PEG). When sera of patients with HSP are fractionated by sucrose density ultracentrifugation before and after PEG precipitation (Fig. 28A.4), the macromolecular IgA smaller than 19 S, detected in untreated serum, could no longer be detected in the PEG precipitate.

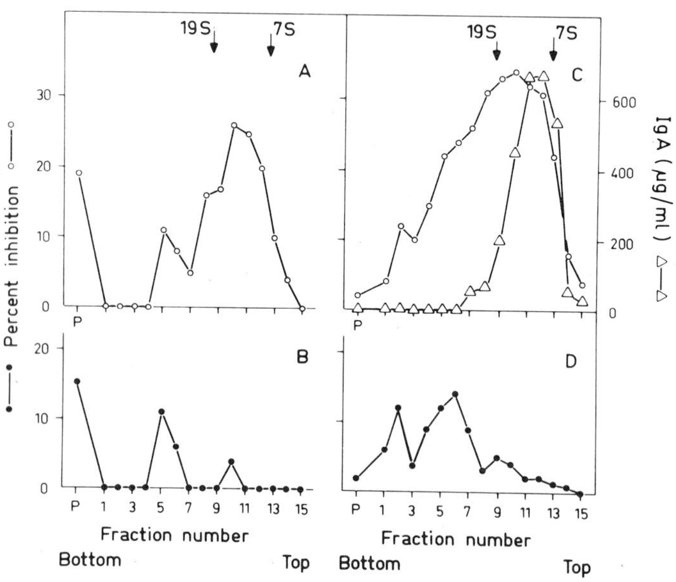

Figure 28A.4. Sucrose density ultracentrifugation of two sera from patients with HSP, showing the size distributions of the macromolecular IgA detected by the a-IgAInhBA, before (O——O) and after (●——●) precipitation with PEG. The PEG precipitate contains predominantly the large (>19 S) IgA-macromolecules or complexes. (From Kauffman RH, et al: J Immunol Meth 40: 117, 1981.)

Macromolecular IgA larger than 19 S could be detected in both serum and PEG precipitate. When sera from 20 patients with HSP were tested before and after PEG precipitation, only 50% of untreated sera were positive in the a-IgAInhBA, whereas all HSP patients were positive when their sera were first precipitated with PEG (52) (Fig. 28A.5). Because most of the macromolecular IgA in HSP patients is considerably larger than IgA-oligomers, it is more likely that this material represents antigen-antibody complexes. As long as antigens are not identified within these complexes, however, the use of the term IgA-complexes remains speculative. It has been suggested by several investigators that primary IgA nephropathy (Berger's disease) could be interpreted as a single expression of HSP. By precipitating sera with PEG, the size of the macromolecular IgA found in both diseases was found to be different (Table 28A.1). In HSP 34 of the 53 patients (64%) were positive in the a-IgAInhBA when PEG-precipitates of sera were tested, whereas only 6 of the 25 patients (24%) with primary IgA-nephropathy gave positive results when PEG precipitates of their sera were assayed. In contrast 16 patients with primary IgA nephropathy (64%) were positive in the a-IgAInhBA when their sera were tested without PEG precipitation. These data indicate that patients with HSP have larger macromolecular IgA or IgA-complexes

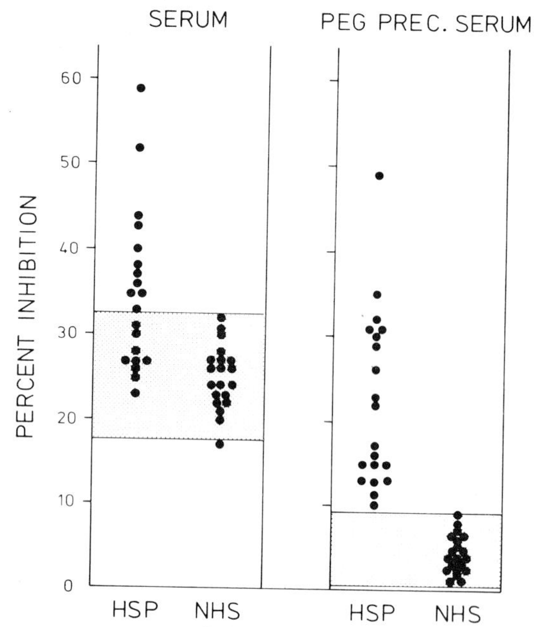

Figure 28A.5. By precipitating sera first with 3% PEG macromolecular IgA or IgA-complexes in sera of patients with HSP are distinguished better in the a-IgAInhBA from IgA in normal human sera (*NHS*). (From Kauffman RH, et al: J Immunol Meth 40: 117, 1981.)

Table 28A.1.
Sera from Patients with HSP and Primary IgA-Nephropathy (Berger's disease)[a]

Whole serum	3% PEG precipitate	HSP	IgA-N
+	+	14	5
+	−	1	11
−	+	20	1
−	−	18	8
TOTAL		53	25

[a] Patients were tested for the presence of larger (>10^6 daltons) and smaller (<10^6 daltons) IgA-macromolecules by testing sera before and after precipitation in 3% polyethyleneglycol in the a-IgAInhBA.

in their circulation than patients with primary IgA-nephropathy (66). It could also imply that the vasculitis in HSP is correlated with the presence of large (>10^6 daltons) IgA-complexes. Cryoglobulins can be detected in about half of the children with HSP (47). The finding of IgA deposits in the mesangium (38) and vessel walls (36) together with the detection of IgA-complexes in a high percent of the cases with HSP suggest that a humoral immune response is triggered by an antigen at the mucosal surfaces either of the respiratory or the gastrointestinal tract, which leads to the production of IgA antibodies that in turn form IgA-complexes with antigen in the circulation. A specific antigen is not required to trigger this reaction. Any material can cause IgA-complexes as long as it can induce the production and release into the circulation of IgA antibodies and can combine in the circulation with these antibodies.

To evaluate the pathogenicity of these IgA-complexes, it is relevant to correlate the presence of IgA-complexes with the clinical activity of the disease. Based on a limited number of patients, two studies were unable to show a correlation between the presence or levels of IgA-complexes and disease activity or organ manifestations (49, 50). However, Levinsky and coworkers found nephritis only in those patients who had not only IgA-complexes but also IgG-complexes (49). Based on the observation that IgA inhibits the phagocytosis of IgG-complexes by polymorphonuclear phagocytes (67), these authors have proposed that IgA-complexes play an indirect role in the pathogenesis of HSP by decreasing the clearance of IgG-complexes. Because of this decreased clearance and higher blood levels, these IgG-complexes will deposit in larger quantities in the mesangium and induce an inflammatory reaction in the glomeruli. A similar mechanism can be expected to occur in patients with C2 deficiency (61, 68). A deficiency in the classical complement pathway could be responsible for the ineffective clearance of immune complexes, leading to higher levels of circulating immune complexes.

A good correlation between the magnitude of microhematuria and the level of IgA-complexes, was found by Coppo and coworkers (51) using a solid phase conglutinin assay. No correlation was found between microhematuria and the level of IgG- or IgM-complexes (51). With the a-IgAInhBA, Kauffmann and coworkers (4) found a good correlation between both the presence and the levels of IgA-complexes and the clinical activity as measured by the appearance of new vasculitic lesions in the skin. The highest incidence (85%) of IgA-complexes was seen in the initial phase of the disease. These complexes could no longer be detected when the purpura and other signs of vasculitis disappeared. On the other hand when a solid phase conglutinin assay was used, IgA-, IgM-, and IgG-complexes were found until 3 weeks after the last signs of clinical activity were observed. The presence of IgA-complexes in the circulation correlated with the presence of IgA-complexes in the wall of cutaneous capillaries. The finding of IgA-complexes and IgA-deposits was concordant in 23 of the 25 cases (92%), when the a-IgAInhBA was used to detect complexes. When the IgA-complexes were detected with the conglutinin binding assay, circulating IgA-complexes and IgA-deposits were concordant in 16 of the 25 cases (64%). These findings suggest that the deposits of IgA in vessel walls probably represent IgA-complexes derived from the circulation. If IgA-complexes are capable of inducing an inflammatory response in vessel walls, this would also imply that the IgA-complexes detected in the circulation of patients with HSP represent the pathogenic factor responsible for the disease. The good correlation found between the clinical activity of the vasculitis and the presence and levels of circulating IgA-complexes suggests that such a causal relationship may exist. The hypothesis that HSP is an IgA-immune complex disease is attractive, since it would explain why it is so hard to identify a single etiological agent. If it were an immune-complex disease, then any antigen that can stimulate the secretory immune system and that can form complexes with circulating IgA antibodies would be potentially pathogenic and could cause HSP when the conditions are favourable for their deposition in glomeruli and vessel walls (69).

TREATMENT

The therapy of HSP has to be limited to general measures and treatment of the sequelae of the vasculitis, since specific intervention in the pathogenesis of the disease is presently not available. When a recent infection has preceded HSP, it should be treated. Vital signs, hemoglobin concentration and stools should be monitored to detect gastrointestinal hemorrhage. Severe hemorrhage, intussusception, and perforation should be treated by surgical intervention.

Fluid and electrolyte balance should be monitored in patients with nephrotic syndrome, nephritis or hypertension. Patients with renal insufficiency or renal failure should be seen by a pediatric nephrologist, who will have to decide on the need for a renal biopsy, the advisability of immunosuppressive therapy and the necessity of treatment by hemodialysis. Renal biopsies should be performed when the nephrotic syndrome persists even though other manifestations may have subsided and when renal function deteriorates. Treatment with corticosteroids alleviates the arthralgia and may sometimes influence the gastrointestinal manifestations (11). It does not influence the long-term outcome of renal disease. Although no controlled clinical trials have been performed with immunosuppressive drugs, no beneficial effects have been observed with azathioprine or cyclophosphamide (14, 7). The possible benefit of immunosuppressive therapy does not outweigh the potential hazards of its side-effects and complications. Although plasma exchange has given encouraging results in individual cases (70), this should be confirmed in a larger series of patients before this mode of therapy is recommended in children with HSP. Children who have demonstrated renal manifestations in the acute phase and continue to have hematuria or proteinuria should be seen every 3 to 6 months, since renal failure or hypertension can develop up to 10 years after the onset of the disease. When terminal renal failure develops, chronic hemodialysis should be instituted until a kidney is available for transplantation. Mesangial deposits of IgA are common in the graft, but they rarely lead to clinical manifestations of recurrent glomerulonephritis. Occasionally overt glomerulonephritis is seen in patients that have been on dialysis for a relatively short period before transplantation (5). The risk of recurrence, however, should not exclude a patient from transplantation.

References

1. Schönlein JL: Allgemeine und spezielle Pathologie, ed 3. Herisan, Literatur-Comptoir 1837, vol 2, p 48.
2. Henoch EH: Ueber eine eigenthümliche Form von Purpura. Berl Klin Wochnschr 11:641, 1874.
3. Henoch EH: Die hämorrhagische Diathese-Purpura. In Vorlesungen über Kinderkrankheiten, ed 9. Berlin, Hirschwald, 1895, p 847.
4. Kauffmann RH, Herrmann W, Meijer CJLM, et al: Circulating IgA-immune complexes in Henoch-Schönlein Purpura. A longitudinal study of their relationship to disease activity and vascular deposition of IgA. Am J Med 69:859, 1980.
5. Habib R, Cameron JS: Schönlein-Henoch Purpura In Bacon PA, Hadler NM (eds): The Kidney and Rheumatic Disease. London Butterworth Scientific, 1982, p 178.
6. Allen DM, Diamond LK, Howell DA: Anaphylactoid purpura in children (Schönlein-Henoch syndrome). Am J Dis Child 99:833, 1960.
7. Levy M, Broyer M, Assan A, et al: Anaphylactoid purpura nephritis in childhood: natural history and immunopathology. Adv Nephrol 6:183, 1976.
8. Gairdner D: The Schönlein-Henoch syndrome (Anaphylactoid purpura). Quart J Med 17:95, 1948.
9. Jones NF, Creamer B, Gimlette TMD: Hypoproteinemia in anaphylactoid purpura. Brit Med J 11:1166, 1966.
10. Cream JJ, Gampel JM, Peachy RDG: Schönlein-Henoch purpura in the adult. A study of 77 adults with anaphylactoid or Henoch-Schönlein purpura. Quart J Med 39:461–484, 1970.

11. Barratt TM, Drummond KN: The vasculitis syndromes: Henoch-Schönlein syndrome or anaphylactoid purpura. In Kelley VC (ed): Practice of Pediatrics. New York Ed. Harper & Row, 1979, vol 3.
12. Goldman LP, Lindenberg RL: Henoch-Schönlein Purpura. Gastrointestinal manifestations with endoscopic correlation. Am J Gastroenterol 75:357, 1981.
13. Rodriguez-Erdman F, Levitan R: Gastrointestinal and roentgenological manifestations of Henoch-Schönlein Purpura. Gastroenterology 54:260, 1968.
14. Meadow SR, Glasgow EF, White RHR, et al: Schönlein-Henoch nephritis. Quart J Med 41:243, 1972.
15. Feldt RH, Stickler GB: The gastrointestinal manifestations of anaphylactoid purpura in children. Mayo Clin Proc 37:465, 1962.
16. Hurley RM, Drummond KN: Anaphylactoid purpura nephritis: clinicopathological correlations. J Pediatr 81:904, 1972.
17. Imai T, Matsumoto S: Anaphylactoid purpura with cardiac involvement. Arch. Dis. Childh 45:727, 1970.
18. Kobayashi O, Wada H, Okawa K, et al: Henoch-Schönlein syndrome in children. Nephrology 4:48, 1977.
19. Norkin S, Weiner J: Involvement of other organs in Henoch-Schönlein syndrome. Am J Clin Path 33:55, 1960.
20. Modzelewska I, Korobowicz E: Goodpasture-syndrome in Verlauf einer anaphylactoiden Purpura Schönlein-Henoch. Acta Paed Acad Scien Hung 15:233, 1974.
21. Garner JAMcV: Acute pancreatitis as a complication of anaphylactoid (Henoch-Schönlein) purpura. Arch Dis Childh 52:971, 1977.
22. Puppala AR, Cheng JC, Steinheber FU: Pancreatitis—a rare complication of Schönlein-Henoch purpura. Am J Gastroenterol 69:101–104, 1978.
23. Levitt LM, Burbank B: Other organs involved in Henoch-Schönlein. N Engl J Med 248:530, 1953.
24. Lewis IC, Philpott: Neurological complications in the Schönlein-Henoch syndrome. Arch Dis Childh 31:369, 1956.
25. Meadow R: Schönlein-Henoch syndrome. In Edelman CM (ed): Paediatric Kidney Disease. Boston, Little, Brown, & Co., 1978, p 788.
26. Kaplan JM, Quintana P, Samson J: Facial nerve palsy with anaphylactoid purpura. Am J Dis Child 119:452, 1970.
27. Case 1980–14 Case records of the Massachusetts General Hospital: weekly clinicopathological exercises. N Engl J Med 302:853, 1980.
28. Krjukoff A, Agamaloff K: Problema semptom complexa Henocha vornutrennei patologii. Therap Arch 18:542, 1940.
29. Berger J, Neveu T, Morel-Maroger L, et al: Applications de l'immunofluorescence en nephrologie. Localisation des immunoglobulines et du fibrinogène dans les lésions glomérulaires. In Actuablités Nephrologiques de l'Hôpital Necker. Flammarion, 1967, p 161.
30. Baart de la Faille-Kuyper EH, Kater L, Kooyker CJ, et al: IgA-deposits in cutaneous blood vessel walls and mesangium in Henoch-Schönlein syndrome. Lancet 1:892, 1973.
31. Stevenson JA, Leong LA, Cohen AH, et al: Henoch-Schönlein purpura. Arch Pathol Lab Med 106:192, 1982.
32. Conley ME, Cooper MD, Michael AF: Selective deposition of immunoglobulin A in immunoglobulin A nephropathy, anaphylactoid purpura and systemic lupus erythematosus. J Clin Invest 66:1432, 1980.
33. André C, Berthoux FC, André F, et al: Prevalence of IgA_2 deposits in IgA nephropathies. N Engl J Med 303:1343, 1980.
34. Murakami T, Furuse A, Hattori S, et al: Glomerular IgA1 and IgA2 deposits in IgA nephropathies. Nephron 35:120, 1983.
35. Dobrin RS, Knudson FE, Michael AF: The secretory immune system and renal disease. Clin Exp Immunol 21:318–328, 1975.
36. Giangiacomo J, Tsai CC: Dermal and glomerular deposition of IgA in anaphylactoid purpura. Am J Dis Child 131:981, 1977.
37. Evans DJ, Gwyn Williams D, Peters DK, et al: Glomerular deposition of properdin in Henoch-Schönlein syndrome and idiopathic focal nephritis. Brit Med J 4:326, 1973.
38. Urizar RE, Michael A, Sisson S, et al: Anaphylactoid purpura II. Immunofluorescent and electron microscopic studies of the glomerular lesions. Lab Invest 19:437, 1968.
39. Zollinger HU, Mihatsch MJ, Gaboardi F, et al: Schönlein-Henoch glomerulonephritis. Characteristic ultrastructural changes in the glomerular basement membrane and localization of osmiophilic deposits. Virch Arch A Path Anat Histol 388:155, 1980.
40. Goodyer PR, de Chadarevian J-P, Kaplan BS: Acute poststreptococcal glomerulonephritis mimicking Henoch-Schönlein purpura. J Pediatr 93:412, 1978.
41. Ingelfinger JR, McCluskey RT, Schneeberger EE, et al: Necrotizing arteritis in acute postreptococcal glomerulonephritis—report of a recovered case. J Pediatr 91:228, 1977.
42. Fauci AS: The spectrum of vasculitis. Clinical, pathologic, immunologic and therapeutic considerations. Ann Int Med 89:660, 1978.
43. Atkins RC, Holdsworth SR, Glasgow EF, et al: The macrophage in human rapidly progressive glomerulonephritis. Lancet 1: 830, 1976.
44. Vernier RL, Worthen HG, Peterson RD, et al: Anaphylactoid purpura I. Pathology of the skin and kidney and frequency of streptococcal infection. Pediatrics 27:188–193, 1961.
45. Ayoub EM, Hoyer J: Anaphylactoid purpura: streptococcal antibody titers and β_1-globulin levels. J Pediatr 75:193, 1969.
46. Trygstad CW, Stiehm E: Elevated serum IgA globulin in anaphylactoid purpura. Pediatrics 47:1023, 1971.
47. Garcia-Fuentes M, Chantler C, Williams DG: Cryoglobulinemia in Henoch-Schönlein purpura. Brit Med J 2:163, 1977.
48. Baart de la Faille-Kuyper EH, van der Meer JB, Kater L, et al: Alternate-pathway complement activation by IgA in Schönlein-Henoch's syndrome. Neth J Med 17:5, 1974.
49. Levinsky RJ, Barratt TM: IgA immune complexes in Henoch-Schönlein purpura. Lancet 11:1100, 1979.
50. Hall RP, Lawley TJ, Heck JA, et al: IgA-containing circulating immune complexes in dermatitis herpetiformis, Henoch-Schönlein purpura, systemic lupus erythematosus and other diseases. Clin Exp Immunol 40:431, 1980.
51. Coppo R, Basolo B, Martina G, et al: Circulating immune complexes containing IgA, IgG and IgM in patients with primary IgA nephropathy and with Henoch-Schöenlein nephritis. Correlation with clinical and histologic signs of activity. Clin Nephrol 18:230, 1982.
52. Kauffmann RH, van Es LA, Daha MR: The specific detection of IgA immune complexes. J Immunol Meth 40:117, 1981.
53. Theofilopoulos AN, Dixon FJ: The biology and detection of immune complexes. In Dixon FJ, Kunkel HG (eds): Advances in Immunology. New York, Academic Press, 1979, vol 28, p 89.
54. Osler W: Visceral lesions of purpura and allied conditions. Brit Med J 1:517, 1914.
55. Frank E: Die essentielle Thrombopenie. Berl Klin Wochnschr 52:454, 1915.
56. Ackroyd JF: Allergic purpura, including purpura due to foods, drugs and infections. Am J Med 14:605, 1953.
57. Pedersen FK, Petersen EA: Varicella followed by glomerulonephritis. Acta Paediatr Scand 64:886, 1953.
58. Jiminez EL, Darrington HJ: Vaccination and Henoch-Schönlein purpura. N Engl J Med 279:1171, 1968.
59. Niederhoff H, Pernice W, Sedlacek H, et al: Purpura Schönlein-Henoch. Deutsche Medizin Wochnschr 104:1567, 1979.
60. Liew SW, Kessel I: Mycoplasmal pneumonia preceding Henoch-Schönlein purpura. Arch Dis Childh 49:912, 1974.
61. Sussman M, Jones JH, Almeida JD, et al: Deficiency of the second component of complement associated with anaphylactoid purpura and the presence of mycoplasma in the serum. Clin Exp Immunol 14:531, 1973.
62. Cairns SA, Mallick NP, Lawler W, et al: Squamous cell carcinoma of bronchus presenting with Henoch-Schönlein purpura. Brit Med J 474, 1978.
63. Dosa S, Cairns SA, Mallick NP, et al: Relapsing Henoch-Schönlein syndrome with renal involvement in a patient with an IgA monoclonal gammopathy. Nephron 26:145, 1980.
64. Egido J, Sancho J, Mampazo F, et al: A possible common pathogenesis of the mesangial IgA glomerulonephritis in patients with Berger's disease and Schönlein-Henoch syndrome. Proc EDTA 17:660, 1980.
65. Bannister KM, Drew PA, Clarkson AR, et al: Immunoregulation in glomerulonephritis, Henoch-Schönlein purpura and lupus nephritis. Clin Exp Immunol 53:384, 1983.
66. Valentijn RM, Kauffmann RH, Brutel de la Rivière G, et al: Presence of circulating macromolecular IgA in patients with hematuria due to primary IgA nephropathy. Am J Med 74:375–381, 1983.
67. Wilton JMA: Suppression by IgA of IgG-mediated phagocytosis by human polymorphonuclear phagocytes. Clin Exp Immunol 34:423, 1978.
68. Gelfand EW, Clarkson JE, Minta JO: Selective deficiency of the second component of complement in a patient with anaphylactoid purpura. Clin Immunol Immunopath 4:269, 1975.
69. Van Es LA: Factor affecting the deposition of immune complexes. Clin Immunol Allerg 1:281, 1981.
70. Kauffmann RH, Houwert DA: Plasmapheresis in rapidly progressive Henoch-Schönlein glomerulonephritis and the effect on circulating IgA immune complexes. Clin Nephrol 16:155, 1981.

28B Systemic lupus Erythematosus

JEFFREY L. PLATT
BARBARA A. BURKE
ALFRED J. FISH

Systemic lupus erythematosus (SLE) is a multisystem disease in which episodic or progressive injury to a number of organs results in an array of clinical findings, which may be pathognomonic or, more commonly, may resemble nearly any acquired syndrome (1–18). Indeed SLE can rarely be excluded from most differential diagnoses in the absence of compelling evidence suggesting another disease entity. While the pathogenesis of SLE is not completely understood, genetic, immunological, and hormonal factors have important roles in the onset and course (19–23).

The kidney is a frequent focus of tissue injury in SLE (1–16, 24–35). Renal pathological features may include proliferative glomerulonephritis, crescent formation, tuft necrosis, interstitial nephritis, and membranous nephropathy (10, 25–30, 32–37). These pathological changes are associated with a range of clinical syndromes including asymptomatic hematuria or proteinuria, acute and rapidly progressive nephritis, renal tubular acidosis, and hypertension.

CLINICAL MANIFESTATIONS

Since patients with renal disease resulting from SLE usually have signs and symptoms reflecting involvement of organs other than the kidney, the extrarenal manifestations will first be reviewed. Although any of the numerous manifestations of SLE may appear at onset, many patients experience fever, malaise, anorexia, weight loss, and arthralgia for weeks or months before a definitive diagnosis is made. The incidence of selected clinical features of SLE in children at the time of diagnosis are indicated in Table 28B.1. The diagnosis may be suggested by the presence of cutaneous lesions in association with systemic symptoms. Alternatively, during evaluation of major organ injury serological studies may point to SLE.

CUTANEOUS MANIFESTATIONS

Cutaneous lesions occur in most patients with SLE (38, 39). The butterfly rash usually first appears as erythema across the nasal bridge and cheeks (Fig. 28B.1). Papular, vesicular, or bullous lesions may occur in this region, and the rash may also involve the upper torso and anus. This characteristic rash of SLE is frequent in both children and adults and may arouse suspicion of SLE when other symptoms and findings are nondiagnostic. Discoid skin lesions are infrequent in childhood, but occur in approximately 20% of adults. They consist of raised well-delineated erythematous plaques or patches with central clearing, usually involving the cheeks and sometimes other portions of the head and neck. Other skin lesions seen include erythema, tender vasculitic papules with or without focal necrosis, livedo reticularis, petechiae, purpura, and urticaria. Tortuosity of nailbed capillaries (observed with a dissecting microscope) occurs in varying proportions of patients. Focal alopecia is another frequent manifestation of SLE. It may progress to involve the entire scalp and often remits with steroid therapy. Ulceration of the mucous membranes of the mouth, palate, and nasopharynx is a less common but prominant clinical feature of SLE. Cutaneous lesions may be brought about or exacerbated by exposure to sunlight; exacerbations of systemic involvement frequently follow sunburn.

Histopathological study of affected skin may reveal liquefactive degeneration of the basal layer, mononuclear inflammatory infiltrates in the dermis surrounding skin appendages and dermal vessels, hyperkeratosis, epidermal atrophy and acanthosis, dilatation of dermal vessels with edema of the papillary dermis, and thickening of the basement membrane (39). Immunofluorescence examination of skin reveals reactivity for IgG, IgM, and C3 at the dermal-epidermal junction (40, 41). This study, also called the "lupus band test," is positive in areas of apparently uninvolved skin in about 80% of patients with SLE (Fig. 28B.2) (40).

Although some of these cutaneous manifestations are rather uncommon, most patients with SLE exhibit one or another early in their course. Thus, the association of a skin lesion with a renal, hemopoietic, or other unexplained systemic disorder should arouse suspicion of SLE.

Cardiovascular and Pulmonary Involvement

The blood vessels, heart, and lungs are frequent foci of injury in SLE. Vascular involvement is occasionally manifest as Raynaud's phenomenon. Although this finding is considered a classic feature of SLE (42), its recognition should spur consideration of systemic sclerosis or mixed connective tissue disease with which it more frequently occurs (chapter 28E). Venous thrombosis associated with circulating lupus anticoagulant (vide infra) may appear as thrombophlebitis of the lower extremities,

Supported by NIH grants AI10704, AM25518, and AM26149, the Vikings Children's Fund, the Minnesota Medical Foundation, and the American Heart Association Minnesota Affiliate. Jeffrey L. Platt is under tenure of a Clinician Scientist Award from the American Heart Association.

Table 28B.1.
Initial Clinical Manifestations of SLE

	University of Minnesota (%)	Weighted mean of other surveys (%)	Range of other surveys (%)
Rash	77	64	36–76
Fever	63	70	59–74
Weight loss	29	39	38–43
Arthritis	61	70	48–84
Splenomegaly or lymphadenopathy	31	35	0–64
Leukopenia	33	41	20–60
PT/PTT prolongation	24	35	16–70
Thrombocytopenia	21	22	15–26
Coomb's Test positive	62	49	35–65
Hypocomplementemia	70	90	90
CNS findings	30	13	9–16
Renal involvement	71	63	40–84

From Platt JL, et al: Am J Kidney Dis II (suppl): 212, 1982 with permission.

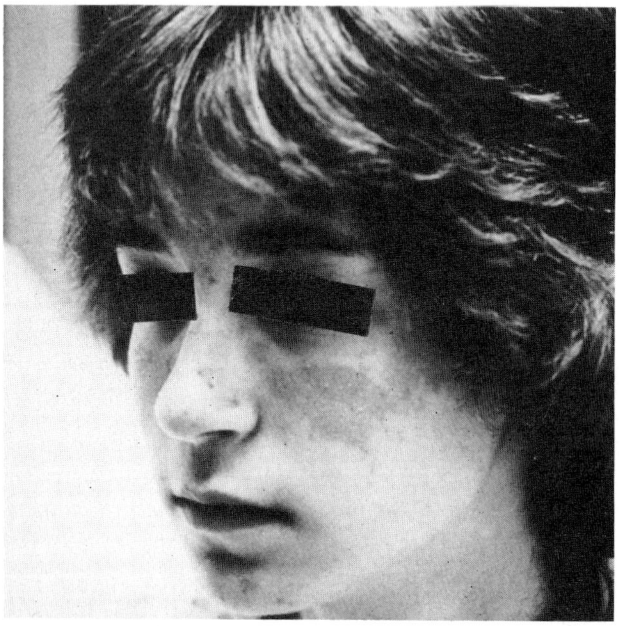

Figure 28B.1. Erythematous "butterfly rash" along cheeks and nasal bridge in young individual with SLE.

renal, or hepatic vein thrombosis and occasionally as recurrent pulmonary embolization. Nephrotic syndrome and corticosteroid administration may also increase the thrombotic diathesis in these patients.

Inflammation of the pericardium and pleura often occur in acute SLE, but are rarely life-threatening. Myocardial involvement because of coronary vasculitis or more commonly coronary emboli, thrombosis, and premature atherosclerosis are now recognized as important causes of morbidity and mortality from SLE, even in young patients (43, 44). Thus, chest pain, congestive heart failure, and arrhythmias must be fully evaluated regardless of the patient's age.

Verrucous lesions of the heart valves (Libman-Sacks endocarditis) and, less commonly, lesions on the mural endocardium and cordae tendineae are often noted at autopsy (45). Although these lesions may not result in clinical signs, they are potential sites for development of infectious endocarditis, which may be difficult to diagnose in the patient with acute SLE. Thus, the treatment of exacerbations of SLE should follow a careful physical examination to elicit findings (murmur, petechiae, or focal CNS signs) suggestive of endocarditis.

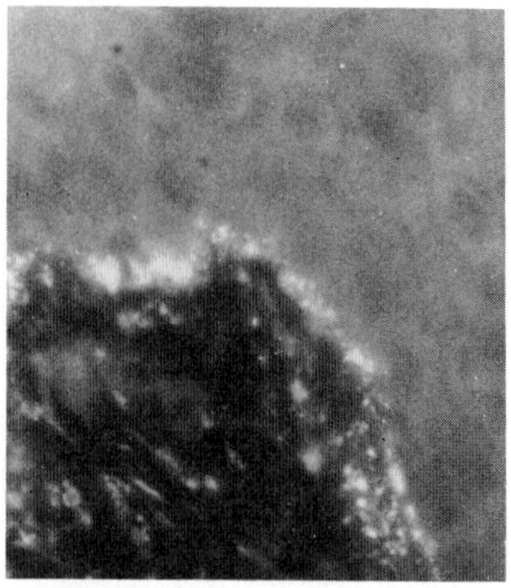

Figure 28B.2. Lupus band test: Granular immunofluorescence of C3 along dermal-epidermal junction of skin from patients with SLE. Fluorescence of IgG and IgM might have similar appearance. (X445.) (From Roy LP, et al., Prog Clin Immunol 1:1, 1972, with permission.)

Histopathologically, verrucous lesions consist of intermixed masses of fibrin, platelets, and eosinophilic staining material attached to a valve leaflet showing denudation of endothelium, foci of necrosis, fibrin deposition, granulation tissue, and mononuclear cell inflammation.

A few patients develop acute lupus pneumonitis characterized by interstitial edema and inflammation, alveolar exudation, and formation of hyaline membranes. However, pulmonary infection, embolus, or infarction are far more common. Diffuse intraalveolar hemorrhage can occur and when associated with renal involvement may resemble Goodpasture's syndrome (46).

Gastrointestinal Hepatic Involvement

Gastrointestinal (GI) tract symptoms, such as nausea, weight loss, and abdominal pain, are common in children with SLE and often abate as the disease is brought under control (10, 47). Rarely vasculitis of bowel may result in necrosis and perforation (necrotising enterocolitis) and may present as an acute surgical abdomen or a malabsorption syndrome. The potential development of peritonitis associated with nephrotic syndrome or of stress ulceration of the upper GI tract should be considered when patients with SLE develop acute abdominal pain. Pancreatitis associated with vasculitis or corticosteroid treatment is another potential cause of acute abdominal pain (48).

Hepatic involvement, suggested by hepatomegaly or modest increase of the SGOT or SGPT, is common in SLE, although in approximately one-half of such patients these findings result from secondary factors, such as drug toxicity and infection (49). Liver injury is rarely of clinical importance, however. Thus, notable abnormalities of liver function should prompt investigation of possible hepatic or portal vein thrombosis (Budd-Chiari syndrome or pyelophlebitis), hepatic abscess, or infectious hepatitis. Young women may develop granulomatous hepatitis associated with circulating antinuclear antibodies and mild rheumatic manifestations (47). There is little evidence, however, that this syndrome termed lupoid hepatitis is related to SLE.

Joint and Muscle Involvement

Arthralgia and nondeforming symmetrical polyarthritis occur in approximately 75% of patients. The proximal interphalangeal, metacarpophalangeal, wrist, and knee joints are most commonly involved. Joint destruction is rare, however, and symptoms generally respond well to corticosteroid therapy. Recrudescence of joint involvement is often the first indication of acute exacerbation of SLE.

Myalgia is a common symptom (50) and myositis clinically indistinguishable from that occuring in dermatomyositis or mixed connective tissue disease (MCTD) is occasionally observed. Since the distinction between MCTD and SLE are particularly important in estimating the prognosis of associated renal involvement, extensive serological analysis (vide infra) electromyography, and muscle biopsy may be needed.

Individuals with SLE are prone to develop aseptic necrosis of bone particularly involving the distal femoral condyl, femoral, humoral, or radial heads and bones of the feet and hands (51, 52). Although aseptic necrosis of bone occurs in the absence of corticosteroid therapy, the incidence is considerably greater in steroid-treated individuals. It may cause pain and limitation of joint motion, but is frequently not associated with symptoms (51). Therefore, radiological evaluation should be performed if joint symptoms or findings persist despite adequate therapy.

Neurological Manifestations

Overt neurological involvement occurs in at least one-third of patients with SLE (15, 53–55). Some of the more common manifestations are listed in the box below. CNS lupus in children may be subtle and consist only of minor personality or emotional changes, loss of handwriting skills, or minor seizure disorders (absence spells). Of special interest is the appearance of clinical findings typical of Sydenham's chorea, occurring months or years before the diagnosis of SLE can be established (15). In addition, headache and amenorrhea (a result of hypothalamic block) are quite common. Peripheral neuropathy sometimes in the form of mononeuritis multiplex may cause sensory or motor deficits. On the other hand CNS lupus may be mimicked by cerebrovascular disease, infection (meningitis and endocarditis), and drug-related phenomena, such as psychosis and pseudotumor cerebri.

Whereas CNS involvement is a major cause of morbidity and death, there is often notable disparity between the clinical and pathological findings (56). Multifocal microinfarcts may occur. These lesions are usually not associated with demonstrable occlusive disease or small vessel vasculitis. Cerebrovascular accidents involving thrombo-occlusive disease often occur in the absence of either vasculitis or atherosclerosis and are difficult to document. Hemorrhage into the subarachnoid space and diffuse petechial hemorrhage have also been described. Localization of immune complexes in the choroid plexus is a common feature of SLE in individuals with and without clinical evidence of CNS involvement (57). However, a defective blood-brain barrier and generation of antibrain autoantibodies may be more specifically related to CNS manifestations (58, 59).

Hematological Manifestations

Mild normochromic normocytic anemia occurs in more than one-half of patients with SLE (60). Hemolytic anemia is also common and may be associated with either a positive Coomb's test or with RBC fragmentation. Pure red cell aplasia and aplastic anemia resulting from SLE have also been described.

Leukopenia and especially lymphopenia are quite frequent and may be associated with circulating antibodies directed against white blood cells.

Thrombocytopenia occurs in about 20% of patients with SLE and may be associated with antiplatelet antibodies. Occasionally, patients thought to have idiopathic thrombocytopenic purpura will later develop manifestations of SLE. Further, the syndrome of thrombotic thrombocytopenic purpura has been described in a few patients with SLE. Although thrombocytopenia as a result of SLE may cause petechiae and purpura, the associations of these signs with sepsis and endocarditis should also be considered.

Coagulopathy in SLE may result in prolongation of the prothrombin time and partial thromboplastin time. Most commonly this coagulopathy is associated with the lupus anticoagulant, which is a circulating factor (probably an antibody) that inhibits the prothrombin-activator complex (61, 62). The lupus anticoagulant is recognized by persistence of abnormal prothrombin and partial thromboplastin times despite addition of normal plasma to the patient's plasma and is generally not of clinical significance. Rarely, circulating antibodies directed against factors VIII and IX are found, and these circulating anticoagulants can cause significant bleeding.

Renal Manifestations

Renal involvement in SLE may be signaled by nearly any recognized clinical syndrome (see box below). Of these, asymptomatic hematuria/proteinuria, nephrotic syndrome, and glomerulonephritis are most common. Up to three-fourths of patients have either decreased glomerular filtration rate (GFR), hematuria, or increased urinary protein excretion at some point in their course (1–18, 24–35). Since these findings may not be associated with specific symptoms (63) and occur episodically, the proportion of patients having evidence of renal disease in a given center will depend on the frequency that laboratory studies and renal biopsy are performed and on the duration of followup (30, 64, 65). Among 70 individuals followed at the University of Minnesota, more than 50% had a GFR <65 or urinary protein excretion >2.5 g/24 hours during the course of their disease (Fig. 28B.3) (15).

Among the most urgent (and fortunately uncommon) clinical renal syndromes of SLE is rapidly progressive glomerulonephritis (RPGN). RPGN as a result of SLE may be difficult to distinguish clinically from

Common Central Nervous System Manifestations of SLE

- Severe psychiatric disturbance—Psychosis or depression
- Chorea
- Cranial nerve lesion
- Ophthalmoplegia
- Seizures
- Clonus
- Acute hemiparesis/hemiplegia
- Cerebritis, coma

Renal Manifestations of SLE

- Asymptomatic proteinuria or hematuria
- Hypertension
- Acute nephritis
- Nephrotic syndrome
- Rapidly progressive glomerulonephritis
- Acute renal failure
- Renal tubular acidosis
- Cystitis
- Obstructive uropathy

Goodpasture's syndrome or anaphylactoid purpura nephritis if accompanied by pulmonary hemorrhage or lower extremity purpura, respectively. Since the management of these causes of RPGN differs, SLE must always be excluded. (chapter 26C).

Renal syndromes associated with extraglomerular urinary tract involvement have received little attention until recently. Renal acidosis of the classic distal type or associated with hyperkalemia because of impaired distal K+ excretion may be observed in SLE (66). These forms of RTA may have minimal impact on the immediate course of SLE; however, their recognition in children is important if optimal growth is to be achieved. Ureteral vasculitis and noninfectious cystitis are unusual manifestations of SLE (67). Either may result in obstructive uropathy leading to renal insufficiency (and could thus account for some instances of renal failure in patients with nearly normal glomerular morphology) or in lower urinary tract symptoms.

Renal Pathology

Extensive application of the renal biopsy technique has revealed a variety of pathological kidney lesions in SLE and has demonstrated the usefulness of pathological classification in the management of individual patients (68–70) (Fig. 28B.3). In this regard, correlation of light microscopic features with immunofluorescence and ultrastructural analysis is essential (68, 70, 71).

Most centers employ a modification of the World Health Organization classification that distinguishes glomerular lesions as normal, mesangial (or minimal), focal proliferative, diffuse proliferative, and membranous

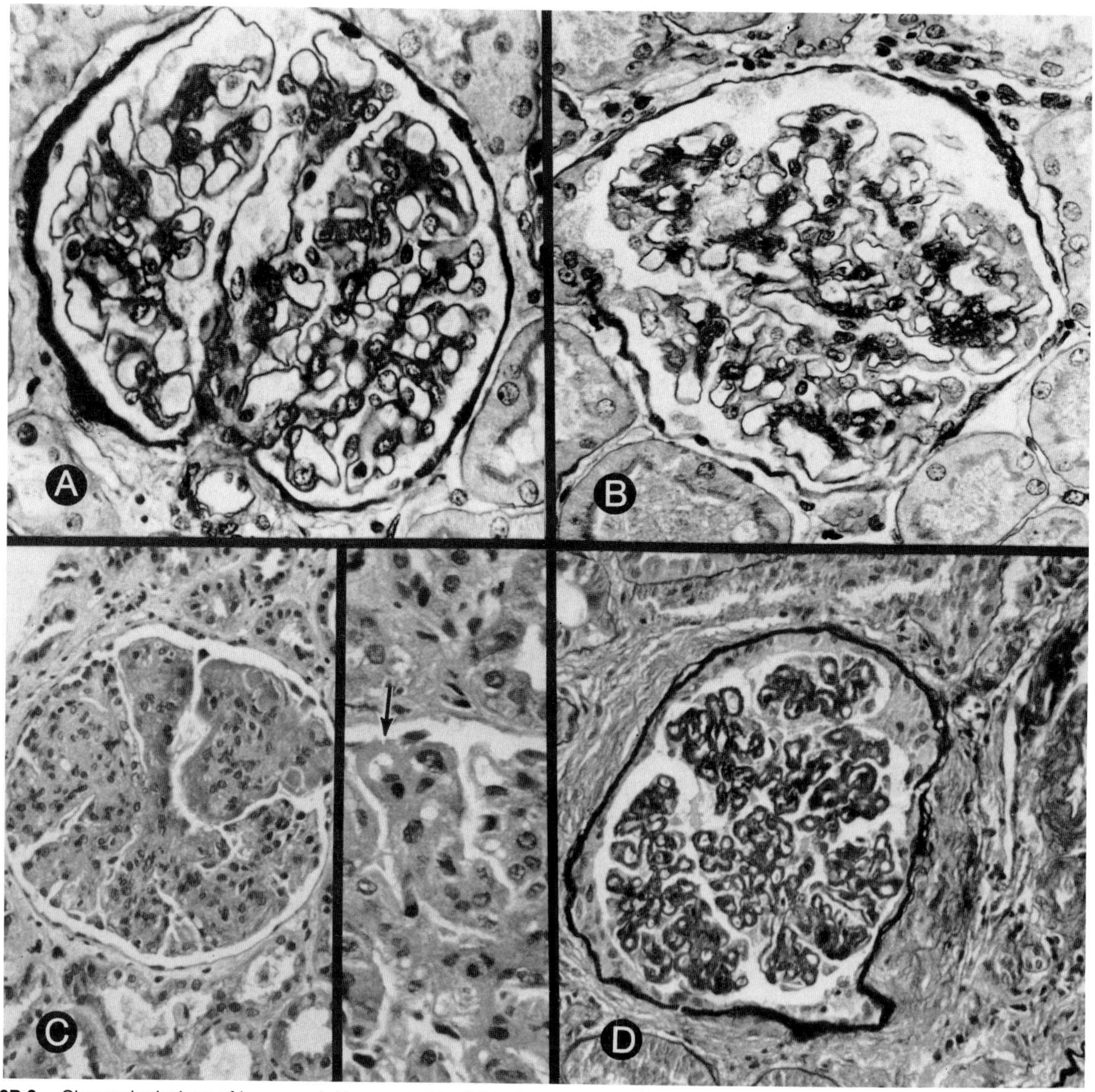

Figure 28B.3. Glomerular lesions of lupus nephritis revealed by light microscopy. **A,** Mesangial lupus nephritis characterized by segmental increase of mesangial matrix and hypercellularity. (X550.) *B,* Focal proliferative lupus nephritis characterized by focal and segmental increase in number of mesangial and endothelial cells. (X450.) **C,** Diffuse proliferative lupus nephritis with focal necrosis and characteristic wire-loop lesions (insert, *arrow*) (X250.) (Insert X1250.) **D,** Membranous lupus nephritis having diffuse thickening of glomerular capillary walls. (X300.) (**C** and **D** from Edelman CM (ed.): Pediatric Kidney Disease. Boston, Little, Brown & Co., 1978, with permission.)

lupus nephritis. Various modifications of this classification have been recommended (29–31, 35, 72, 73).

Normal glomeruli are not infrequently observed by light microscopy; however, immunofluorescence and electron microscopy often reveals lesions in such tissues suggestive of mesangial or membranous lupus nephritis (10, 68). Furthermore, individuals with normal glomeruli by light microscopy may have decreased renal function or proteinuria (15).

Mesangial lupus nephritis is characterized by mild mesangial hypercellularity with or without increase of mesangial matrix (Fig. 28B.3, *A*). Mesangial deposition of IgG and C3 by immunofluorescence and electron-dense mesangial deposits by electron microscopy, are usually observed. Minimal deposits in paramesangial and adjacent subendothelial regions may be seen. Patients with mesangial lupus nephropathy usually have evidence of mild renal functional impairment, proteinuria, or hematuria.

Focal proliferative lupus nephritis is characterized by focal-segmental proliferation of mesangial and endothelial cells usually involving fewer than 50% of glomeruli (Fig. 28B.3, *B*). Inflammatory cells may also be present. Some glomeruli may have foci of necrosis and fibrin deposition. Immunofluorescence microscopy reveals both mesangial and capillary wall (subendothelial) reactivity for IgG and C3 and frequently mesangial reactivity for IgA and IgM. Electron dense deposits in mesangial matrix, paramesangial areas, and subendothelial regions of the capillary wall may be observed by electron microscopy. Adjacent crescent formation and adhesions of proliferative or necrotizing tufts to these crescents may occur. Wire loops, hematoxyphil bodies, segmental and global sclerosis, and associated tubulointerstitial nephritis are occasionally seen. Since focal proliferative glomerulonephritis with mesangial deposition of IgA is also observed in IgA nephropathy and Henoch-Schönlein purpura nephritis, both must be excluded by clinical findings. Patients with focal proliferative lupus nephritis usually have proteinuria and hematuria, while renal functional impairment varies from mild to severe.

Diffuse (severe) proliferative lupus nephritis (DPLN) occurs in two distinct forms: an endocapillary proliferative lesion and a mesangiocapillary glomerulonephritis, the latter being similar to membranoproliferative glomerulonephritis, type I (Fig. 28B.3, *C*). This distinction, however, is questioned by some. In either form, crescents may be observed, and, when prolific, result in a diffuse crescentic pattern associated with a rapidly progressive clinical course as described above. Necrosis and crescent formation may be less common in the mesangiocapillary (membranoproliferative) form. Diffuse endocapillary proliferative glomerulonephritis is characterized by proliferation of mesangial and endothelial cells in more than 50% of glomeruli. Hyalin thrombi, which may be intraluminal extensions of subendothelial immune deposits, tuft necrosis, and glomerular infiltration by polymorphonuclear and mononuclear cells, are often seen and may correlate with prognosis.

Hematoxyphil bodies and wire-loop lesions are characteristic features of SLE nephritis most often seen in DPLN. Hematoxyphyl bodies are amorphous violaceous structures in hematoxylin & eosin stained sections located in areas of necrosis in glomeruli. They are thought to result from altered staining reactions of nuclear material and antinuclear antibodies analogous to the LE cell phenomenon. Although they are diagnostic of SLE, hematoxyphil bodies are rarely observed. Wire loops result from massive subendothelial deposition of immune complexes along the circumference of involved glomerular capillaries. The deposits are slightly refractile and brightly eosin positive. Wire loops are not diagnostic of SLE, but their presence is correlated with disease activity.

Mesangiocapillary glomerulonephritis is characterized by diffuse mesangial cell proliferation and interposition of mesangial cell cytoplasm between the endothelial cells and basement membrane along the circumference of the capillary walls. The presence of extended mesangial matrix forms a double contoured basement membrane appearance in affected capillary loops. Subendothelial immune deposits are also found in this form of lupus nephritis. Immunofluorescence microscopy reveals diffuse mesangial and irregular capillary wall fluorescence for IgG and C3 and often C1q, IgM, and IgA in subendothelial and sometimes subepithelial loci (Fig. 28B.4, *A*). Fibrin deposition is often observed in a subendothelial locus and in the mesangium, necrotic foci, and crescents. Both mesangial and capillary wall (subendothelial) deposits are demonstrated by electron microscopy in most glomeruli. Massive subendothelial de-

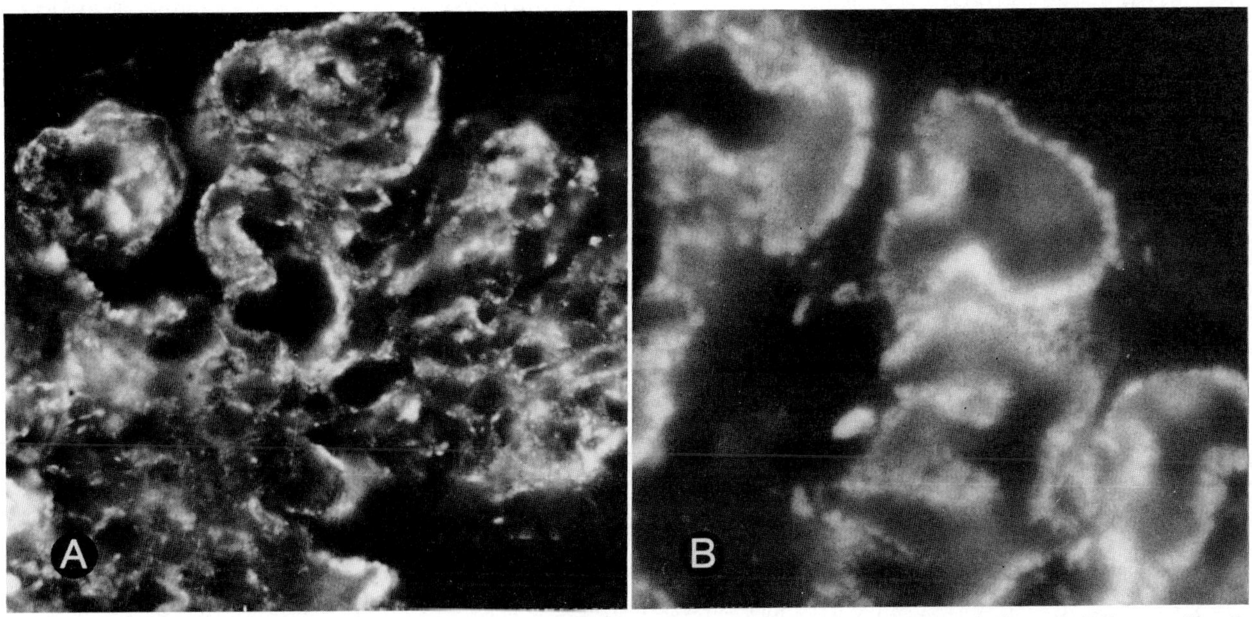

Figure 28B.4 Lesions of SLE nephritis demonstrated by immunofluorescence microscopy in frozen tissue sections. **A,** Diffuse proliferative lupus nephritis with fine granular fluorescence for IgG is present in subendothelial and mesangial loci. (X1050.) **B,** Membranous lupus nephritis with granular epimembranous fluorescence for IgG is observed. (X1400.) (From Edelman CM (ed.): Pediatric Kidney Disease. Boston, Little, Brown & Co., 1978, with permission.)

posits encircling capillary loops (wire-loops) may be found. The affected capillary lumena are narrowed and hyaline thrombi may be present. Occasionally, subendothelial deposits may extend into the GBM proper and become transmural. Both the quantity and persistence of subendothelial deposits have been implicated as prognostic factors in progressive glomerular disease. Subepithelial deposits are frequently noted, and a distinctive ultrastructural appearance of these deposits including irregular size and shape and the frequent presence of a finger print morphology and microtubular arrays have been described.

Patients with diffuse proliferative lupus nephritis have proteinuria, hematuria, and renal functional impairment. Nephrotic syndrome is present in 50% of patients.

Membranous lupus nephritis is characterized by diffuse thickening of capillary walls and is indistinguishable from idiopathic diffuse membranous glomerulonephritis by light microscopy. Mild mesangial hypercellularity with or without increased matrix material may be observed. Diffuse fine granular epimembranous deposits of IgG and C3 are characteristic immunofluorescence findings (Fig. 28B.4, *B*). IgA and IgM may be found in a similar location, but are generally not prominent. Fibrin deposits are uncommon. By electron microscopy, deposits are small and are uniformly distributed along the glomerular basement membrane in a subepithelial location. The same stages of progression of the capillary wall lesion in membranous lupus nephritis can be identified as are seen in idiopathic membranous glomerulopathy. In stage I, deposits are small and fewer than in later stages. By light microscopy the early lesions may be difficult to distinguish from normal. In stage II, the GBM appears thick and silver stains show typical basement membrane spikes extending between deposits. Ultrastructural studies confirm GBM thickening in stage II, and basement membranes appear to surround deposits. In stage III, spikes of basement membrane appear to have fused over deposits forming a layer of basement membrane between the deposits and the epithelium. Subsequently, in stage IV, deposits may become disorganized or resolved leaving a thickened, irregular basement membrane. Unlike idiopathic membranous glomerulonephritis, membranous lupus nephritis may be associated with mesangial deposits seen by electron microscopy or with focal proliferative lesions.

Patients with membranous lupus nephritis have proteinuria and many develop nephrotic syndrome. Hematuria is common, hypertension occurs occasionally, and renal functional impairment is usually mild. Because membranous lupus nephritis may be pathologically and clinically indistinguishable from idiopathic and secondary forms of membranous nephropathy these entities must be considered in the differential diagnosis. Hepatitis B, syphilis, drug toxicity, and other systemic illnesses associated with membranous lesions may falsely arouse suspicion of SLE on serological grounds. However, consideration of the patient's age and associated clinical manifestations will usually exclude most secondary forms of membranous nephropathy.

Glomerulosclerosis may be either segmental or global and in some cases represents the end result of a previous necrotizing process. It is most pronounced in patients with proliferative lupus nephritis, but can be seen in other forms of the disease as well.

Tubulointerstitial nephritis is a frequent concomitant of renal involvement in SLE and may rarely occur as a clinically significant lesion in the absence of glomerular abnormality by light microscopy (74, 75). The lesions are usually focal and consist of inflammatory cell infiltrates in the interstitium with degenerative changes in tubules associated with interstitial fibrosis and tubular atrophy. The cellular infiltrates are predominantly mononuclear. Tubular changes include thickening and splitting of tubular basement membranes and atrophy or degeneration of epithelial cells. Immunofluorescence microscopy may reveal granular or linear reactivity for IgG and C3 and less often IgA and IgM along tubular basement membranes. Tubulointerstitial nephritis is commonly associated with diffuse lupus nephritis and may contribute to the severity of renal functional abnormality.

Vasculitis involving arteries, arterioles, and venules is an uncommon manifestation of SLE. Necrotizing arteritis and arteriolitis resembling periarteritis nodosa has been described in the kidney, and disseminated vasculitis may occur in multiple organs including pancreas, bowel, pericardium, synovia, brain, skin, mesentery, and coronary arteries. Renal vascular lesions are most commonly associated with diffuse proliferative lupus nephritis, but may occur in other forms and rarely in the absence of glomerular involvement. These lesions are usually characterized by necrosis of vessel walls, with or without thrombosis, and by granular deposition of IgG and C3 within the vascular wall. The vasculitis of SLE may be associated with diastolic hypertension and accelerated renal failure.

Laboratory Findings

Some of the common laboratory findings of patients with SLE are listed in the box below. Most hematological abnormalities listed reflect production of autoantibodies that recognize RBC, WBC, or platelet antigens. Autoantibodies directed against the phospholipid cardiolipin are responsible for the false-positive VDRL reaction, as well as for prolongation of the PTT (lupus anticoagulant). These antibodies may also inhibit generation of prostacyclin resulting in a thrombotic diathesis (61, 62).

The most characteristic autoantibodies made by patients with SLE identify nuclear antigens, particularly native or double stranded-DNA (ds-DNA) (76, 79). Antinuclear antibodies are generally detected by the fluorescent antinuclear antibody (FANA) assay in which tissue sections (usually mouse liver) are overlayed with varying dilutions of the patient's serum and then with fluorescein labeled antisera specific for human Ig. If the patient's serum IgG has bound to nuclear antigens and in turn has been bound by the labeled antihuman antisera, then nuclear fluorescence will be observed with a fluorescence microscope. In this assay diffuse or peripheral (rim) patterns of antibody binding to hepatocyte nuclei suggest the presence of antideoxyribonucleoprotein and anti-DNA antibodies, respectively. A speckled pattern is generated by antibodies against "extractable," non-DNA, nuclear antigens (ENA), which may be present in SLE, other rheumatic, and nonrheumatic diseases, and in normal individuals. Nucleolar fluorescence reflects the presence of antibodies directed against ribonucleoprotein (RNP) and may be seen in SLE, systemic sclerosis, and dermatomyositis. Since a positive FANA may be obtained

Selected Serological and Hematological Abnormalities in SLE

- Positive FANA
- Circulating anti-DNA antibodies
- Circulating immune complexes present
- Cryoglobulins
- Hypocomplementemia
- Elevated ESR
- Hypergammaglobulinemia
- Positive VDRL
- Positive rheumatoid factor
- Positive Indirect Coomb's test
- Leukopenia
- Thrombocytopenia
- Anemia
- PTT prolongation

with serum from patients with other rheumatological diseases and occasionally in normal individuals, one should interpret the results in the context of the overall clinical picture. The rim pattern strongly favors the diagnosis of SLE, whereas a persistently negative FANA in an untreated patient opposes that diagnosis.

When the presence of circulating anti-DNA antibodies is suggested by the FANA, confirmation should be sought. A relatively simple immunofluorescence assay employs the kinetoplast of Crithida luciliae as a target to estimate the anti-DNA antibody titre. Because this test is not entirely specific, a positive result should be further confirmed by determination of DNA binding by radioassay or enzyme immunoassay (80).

In addition to anti-ds-DNA antibodies, patients with SLE may have autoantibodies directed against a variety of other identifiable nuclear components. Antibodies against single-stranded, denatured-DNA are common in SLE, but not specific as they are also observed in chronic liver disease, rheumatoid arthritis, and drug-induced lupus. Anti-RNA antibodies can often be detected; however, their significance is uncertain.

Autoantibodies directed against a variety of nonhistone nuclear proteins can be characterized in SLE sera (77, 81–83). Some, such as anti-SM antigen, are specific for SLE, whereas others are characteristically associated with other rheumatic diseases. Although not currently in general use, identification of autoantibody specificity may be useful in identifying subgroups of SLE patients or in distinguishing clinially similar diseases.

Decreases of the total hemolytic complement activity (CH_{50}), and serum levels of C1q, C3, and C4, are commonly observed in SLE and may correlate with activity of renal disease in some patients (84–86). Further, individuals with hereditary deficiency of complement components have an increased risk for development of SLE (84, 87). Decreased serum complement in part reflects consumption by classical and alternate pathways and may be associated with circulating immune complexes and cryoglobulins. In addition to SLE, hypocomplementemia occurs in acute glomerulonephritis (GN), membranoproliferative GN, dense deposit disease, serum sickness, and endocarditis. Still when the differential diagnosis of a multisystem illness is appropriately narrowed, hypocomplementemia may be rather specific for SLE (88).

Serological findings of SLE may be observed in the newborns as a result transplantal passage of autoantibodies. Associated manifestations that include skin rash, thrombocytopenia, and heart block (89) are temporary and renal disease is not observed. Serological abnormalities also occur in individuals treated with a variety of pharmacological agents (90, 91)); however, renal disease is rare in these drug-induced lupus syndromes.

Pathogenesis

The pathogenic mechanism underlying development of SLE remains obscure. Nevertheless, clinical and laboratory observations point to a number of factors that may have importance in mediating the onset of disease or conditioning the individual's response to factors that provoke the disease.

The primacy of inheritance as a pathogenic mechanism in SLE is suggested by association with female gender, with abnormalities of sex steroid metabolism, by familial clustering of manifest SLE and antinuclear antibody production, and by association of SLE with inherited syndromes of complement and IgA deficiency and autoimmunity (87, 92–96). These observations are supported by animal models, such as the NZB/NZW mouse in which autoimmunity per se and specific manifestations analogous to SLE in humans are closely associated with identifiable genotypes (97–99).

There is little evidence that SLE is caused by a specific infectious agent. However, clinical manifestations of SLE in humans and animals may resemble viral syndromes and some serological data have supported an association with viral infection. Nevertheless, attempts at viral isolation and ultrastructural identification have been unrewarding (100, 101).

Patients with SLE exhibit many abnormalities of humoral and cellular immunity and of complement metabolism (19–23, 84–86, 102–104). The disease is marked by production of antinuclear antibodies reflecting polyclonal B cell stimulation. While these antibodies do not appear to bind nuclear material of living cells, they may react with nuclear components released from disrupted and dying cells. The broad spectrum of renal lesions observed in SLE may reflect varying contributions of a number of pathogenic mechanisms which in turn reflect the physicochemical properties and site of formation of immune complexes, as well as defective Fc-mediated clearance of immune complexes (105, 106). Some of these complexes consist of DNA and anti-DNA antibodies and some of IgG and anti-IgG (103, 107, 108).

Formation of immune complexes in the circulation, particularly DNA-anti-DNA in SLE, may be responsible for immune deposit trapping in the mesangium. It is not certain, however, whether this mechanism is responsible for substantive renal injury (109). Furthermore, the association of circulating immune complexes with immune deposits in other glomerular loci is less certain. On the other hand subendothelial binding of circulating DNA to components of the glomerular basement membrane has been demonstrated and could presage in situ immune complex formation (108, 109). The source of subepithelial immune deposits may also reflect in situ complex formation or dissociation of subendothelial deposits and their subsequent reassociation at the subepithelial locus. The site of immune complex accumulation may be determined by properties such as immune complex size, charge, and antibody avidity (105, 106, 109), as discussed in Chapter 13.

Although accumulation of immune complexes might itself incite glomerular damage, recent investigations have pointed to the importance of complement activation and generation of the membrane attack complex (109–111). Further, recent studies suggest that cellular immunity and actions of phagocytic cells may underlie initiation and elaboration of immune complex glomerular disease (103, 109, 112, 113).

Autoantibodies directed against extranuclear antigens are frequently found in SLE sera (20, 23, 60, 104). These antibodies may incite tissue injury by immune complex formation as described. In addition, antibodies reactive with hemopoietic cells may be responsible for leukopenia, thrombocytopenia, anemia, or for selective depletion of immunoregulatory cells. Coagulopathies in SLE result from generation of antibodies against phospholipid (lupus anticoagulant) and occasionally against clotting factors VIII and IX (61). Further, autoantibodies, which bind to renal basement membranes, are occasionally detected.

Cellular immunity is notably abnormal in many patients with SLE. Impaired capacity to generate suppression and the autologous mixed lymphocyte reaction are among observations suggesting that defects in immunoregulation may be responsible for autoimmunity in SLE (19–23). These defects may in turn have a genetic basis or may reflect antibody mediated inactivation of some regulatory cells.

Although it is not possible to propose a unified mechanism of immune pathogenesis, one can identify distinct subsets of SLE in animals and humans based on genetic and immune parameters (19, 23, 114, 115). For example, stratification of patients according to peripheral blood T-cell subpopulations suggests that individuals having an increased ratio of helper to suppressor/cytotoxic T cells (recognized by monoclonal antibodies OKT4/Leu3 and OKT8/Leu 2, respectively) have manifestly different disease from those with normal or decreased ratios. Although it is not clear whether the relative proportions of T-cell subpopulations mediate disease or mark subgroups of SLE patients, these studies do point to increasing recognition of SLE as a syndrome rather than as a single disease.

Course and Prognosis

The course of SLE is generally characterized by exacerbations and remissions (1–18). Acute exacerbations may be precipitated by extrinsic factors such as infection and exposure to sunlight (47). Recurrence of systemic manifestations (flares), such as rash, arthralgia, fever, and weight loss, is often associated with changes in serological markers (hypocomplementemia or detectable anti-DNA antibodies) (85, 86). Worsening of renal disease may likewise be marked by changes in serological findings (28). However, in a given patient, renal injury may progress despite absence of clinical or serological abnormalities (63, 116, 117). Before the availability of corticosteroid and antimicrobial agents, SLE was considered an acute and almost uniformly fatal disease, most patients dying during acute flares or from infection. Currently, however, few patients die during the acute phase of the disease. Rather the most prevalent course is that of a chronic disease (punctuated by exacerbations) in which the ongoing manifestations reflect cumulative injury to the kidneys, brain, or cardiovascular system.

Clinical renal disease (see the box on p. 501), as detected by proteinuria or decreased GFR, is generally episodic over the course of the disease (Fig. 28B.5). Most patients including those with diffuse proliferative nephritis appear to respond clinically to corticosteroid or immunosuppressive therapy (118–120) (chapter 29). However, in some individuals, renal function inexorably deteriorates either because of ongoing autoimmune injury or because of progressive scarring and vascular injury. Curiously the emergence of renal failure may be associated with prolonged remission of systemic and serological manifestations, and spontaneous improvement in renal function has been documented in some patients thought to be permanently dependent on dialysis (121, 122). Allograft recipients with SLE often develop minimal disease in the allograft, with only mesangial deposition of immunoglobulin and complement. The long-term prognosis for renal allograft function is generally good although severe recurrent disease is reported (123).

Frequent histopathological transition distinguishes SLE from other forms of acute and chronic nephritis. Most transitions occur between mesangial, focal, and diffuse disease with worsening or improvement of pathological findings being paralleled by corresponding changes in renal function (15, 29, 31, 68, 69). Transitions to and from membranous lupus nephritis have also been observed.

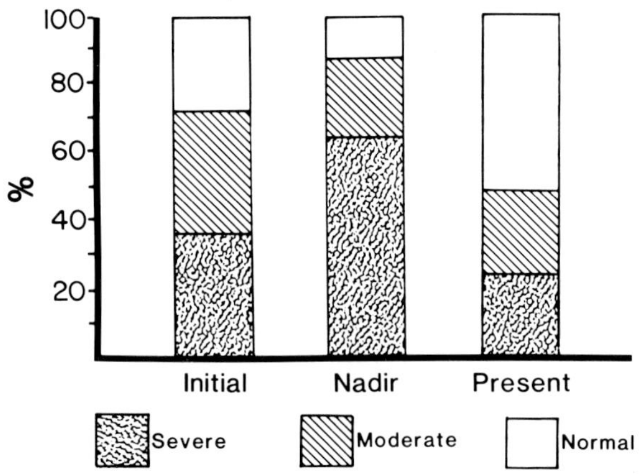

Figure 28B.5. Percentage of 70 patients with SLE in the first 2 decades of life having clinical evidence of severe, moderate, or absent renal disease at time of diagnosis, worst determination (nadir) and most recent determination. GFR <65 or proteinuria >2.5 g/24 hr is considered severe, GFR 66 to 90 or proteinuria 0.1 to 2.5 g is considered moderate, and GFR >90 and proteinuria <0.1 g is normal. (From Platt JL, et al: Am J Kidney Dis II(suppl):212, 1982, with permission.)

Pregnancy may influence the course of SLE and SLE nephritis. It is now clear that pregnancy can be safely undertaken by those with inactive disease and normal renal function. On the other hand, women with active SLE often experience worsening of renal function and fetal demise or prematurity (15, 124).

The past 30 years has witnessed a dramatic improvement of survival in patients with SLE (10, 13–16, 33, 125, 126). In our most recent analysis of 70 young patients with SLE, overall survival was 85% at 10 years and 77% at 15 years after diagnosis (15). Most deaths occurred early in the course of disease in patients with disseminated infection. Further, these data tend to underestimate prognosis, since most deaths occurred more than 15 years ago when less effective antibiotic agents were available and higher doses of immunosuppressive drugs were used.

On the other hand, a substantial incidence of coronary artery disease may be observed later in the course of SLE (43, 127). Thus, current survival data likely underestimate the risk of premature death from atherosclerosis or coronary vasculitis (127). It is hoped that application of newer criteria for diagnosis (128) and recognition of discrete subsets of the disease (77, 104, 115) will improve the accuracy of prognostic data and lead to more refined therapeutic strategies.

References

1. Zetterstrom R, Berglund G: Systemic lupus erythematosus in childhood. Acta Paed 45:189, 1956.
2. Gribetz D, Henley WL: Systemic lupus erythematosus in childhood. Mt Sinai Hosp J 26:289, 1959.
3. Cook CD, Wedgwood RJP, Craig JM, et al: Systemic lupus erythematosus. Pediatrics 26:570, 1960.
4. Jacobs JC: Systemic lupus erythematosus in childhood. Pediatrics 32:257, 1963.
5. Peterson RDA, Vernier RL, Good RA: Lupus erythematosus. Pediatr Clin N Am 10:941, 1963.
6. Hanson V, Kornreich H: Systemic rheumatic disorders ("collagen disease") in childhood. Bull Rheum Dis 17:435, 1967.
7. Robinson MJ, Williams AL: Systemic lupus erythematosus in childhood. Aust Paed J 3:36, 1967.
8. Meislin AG, Rothfield N: Systemic lupus erythematosus in childhood. Pediatrics 42:37, 1968.
9. Walravens PA, Chase HP: The prognosis of childhood systemic lupus erythematosus. Am J Dis Child 130:929, 1976.
10. Fish AJ, Blau EB, Westberg NG, et al: systemic lupus erythematosus within the first two decades of life. Am J Med 62:99, 1977.
11. King KK, Kornreich HK, Bernstein BH, et al: The clinical spectrum of systemic lupus erythematosus in childhood. Arthr Rheum 20(suppl):287, 1977.
12. Norris DG, Colon AR, Stickler GB: Systemic lupus erythematosus in children. Clin Pediatr 16:774, 1977.
13. Abeles M, Urman JD, Weinstein A, et al: Systemic lupus erythematosus in the younger patient. J Rheum 7:515, 1980.
14. Schaller J: Lupus in childhood. Clin Rheum Dis 8:219, 1982.
15. Platt JL, Burke BA, Fish AJ, et al: Systemic lupus erythematosus in the first two decades of life. Am J Kidney Dis II(suppl):212, 1982.
16. Glidden RS, Mantzouranis EC, Borel Y: Systemic lupus erythematosus in childhood. Clin Immunol Immunopathol 29:196, 1983.
17. Harvey AM, Shulman LE, Tumulty PA, et al: Systemic lupus erythematosus. Medicine 33:291, 1954.
18. Estes D, Christian CL: The natural history of systemic lupus erythematosus by prospective analysis. Medicine 50:85, 1971.
19. Decker JL, Steinberg AD, Reinertsen JL, et al: Systemic lupus erythematosus. Ann Intern Med 91:587, 1979.
20. Schwartz RS: Immunologic and genetic aspects of systemic lupus erythematosus. Kidney Intl 19:474, 1981.
21. Koffler D (editor): Current perspectives on the immunology of systemic lupus erythematosus. Arthr Rheum 25:721, 1981.
22. Hayslett JP, Hardin JA, editors: Advances in Systemic Lupus Erythematosus. New York, Grune and Stratton, 1983.

23. Steinberg AD: Recent advances on the mechanisms and genetic aspects of lupus erythematosus. Adv Nephrol 14:305, 1984.
24. Soffer LJ, Southren AL, Weiner HE, et al: Renal manifestations of systemic lupus erythematosus. Ann Intern Med 54: 215, 1961.
25. Rothfield NF, McCluskey RT, Baldwin DS: Renal disease in systemic lupus erythematosus. N Engl J Med 269:537, 1963.
26. Pollak VE, Pirani CL, Schwartz FD: The natural history of the renal manifestations of systemic lupus erythematosus. J Lab Clin Med 63:537, 1964.
27. Garin EH, Donnelly WH, Fennell III RS, et al: Nephritis in systemic lupus erythematosus in children. J Pediatr 89:366, 1976.
28. Hecht B, Siegel N, Adler M, et al: Prognostic indices in lupus nephritis. Medicine 55:163, 1976.
29. Baldwin DS, Gluck MC, Lowenstein J, et al: Lupus Nephritis. Am J Med 62:12, 1977.
30. Cameron JS, Turner DR, Ogg CS, et al: Systemic lupus with nephritis. Quart J Med XLVIII:1, 1979.
31. Ginzler EM, Bollet AJ, Friedman EA: The natural history and response to therapy of lupus nephritis. Ann Rev Med 31:463, 1980.
32. Morris MC, Cameron JS, Chantler C, et al: Systemic Lupus Erythematosus with Nephritis. Arch Dis Childh 56:779, 1981.
33. Glassock RJ, Goldstein DA, Findander P, et al: Glomerulonephritis in systemic lupus erythematosus. Am J Nephrol 1:53, 1981.
34. Wallace DJ, Podell TE, Weiner JM, et al: Lupus nephritis. Am J Med 72:209, 1982.
35. Austin HA, Muenz LR, Joyce KM, et al: Prognostic factors in lupus nephritis. Am J Med 75:382, 1983.
36. Baldwin DS, Lowenstein J, Rothfield NF, et al: The clinical course of the proliferative and membranous forms of lupus nephritis. Ann Intern Med 73:929, 1970.
37. Magil AB, Ballon HS, Chan V, et al: Diffuse proliferative lupus glomerulonephritis. Medicine 63:210, 1984.
38. Rowell NR: The natural history of lupus erythematosus. Clin Exp Dermatol 9:217, 1984.
39. Epstein JH, Tuffanelli DL: Discoid lupus erythematosus. In Dubois EL (ed): Lupus Erythematosus, ed 2. Los Angeles, University of Southern California Press, 1974.
40. Percy JS, Smyth CJ: The immunofluorescent skin test in systemic lupus erythematosus. JAMA 208:485, 1969.
41. Gilliam JN, Cheatum DE, Hurd ER, et al: Immunoglobulin in clinically uninvolved skin in systemic lupus erythematosus. J Clin Invest 53:1434, 1974.
42. Cohen AS, Reynolds WE, Franklin EC, et al: Preliminary criteria for the classification of systemic lupus erythematosus. Bull Rheum Dis 21:643, 1971.
43. Bulkley BH, Roberts WC: The heart in systemic lupus erythematosus and the changes induced in it by corticosteroid therapy. Am J Med 58:243, 1975.
44. Curry RC, Roberts WC: Status of the coronary arteries in the nephrotic syndrome. Am J Med 63:183, 1977.
45. Baehr G, Klemperer P, Schifrin A: A diffuse disease of the peripheral circulation (usually associated with lupus erythematosus and endocarditis). Trans Assoc Amer Phys 50:139, 1935.
46. Eagen JW, Memoli VA, Roberts JL, et al: Pulmonary hemorrhage in systemic lupus erythematosus. Medicine 57:545, 1978.
47. Dubois EL: The clinical picture of systemic lupus erythematosus. In Dubois EL (ed): Lupus Erythematosus, ed 2. Los Angeles, University of Southern California Press, 1974.
48. Baron M, Brisson M-L: Pancreatitis in systemic lupus erythematosus. Arthr Rheum 25:1006, 1982.
49. Runyon BA, LaBrecque DR, Anuras S: The spectrum of liver disease in systemic lupus erythematosus. Am J Med 69:187, 1980.
50. Oxenhandler R, Hart MN, Bickel J, et al: Pathologic features of muscle in systemic lupus erythematosus. Hum Pathol 13:745, 1982.
51. Bergstein JM, Wiens C, Fish AJ, et al: Avascular necrosis of bone in systemic lupus erythematosus. J Pediatr 85:31, 1974.
52. Klipper AR, Stevens MB, Zizic TM, et al: Ischemic necrosis of bone in systemic lupus erythematosus. Medicine 55:251, 1976.
53. Feinglass EJ, Arnett FC, Dorsch CA, et al: Neuropsychiatric manifestations of systemic lupus erythematosus. Medicine 55:323, 1976.
54. Cassidy JT, Sullivan DB, Petty RE, et al: Lupus nephritis and encephalopathy. Arthr Rheum 20(suppl):315, 1977.
55. Yancey CL, Doughty RA, Athreya BH: Central nervous system involvement in childhood systemic lupus erythematosus. Arthr Rheum 24:1389, 1981.
56. Ellis SG, Verity MA: Central nervous system involvement in systemic lupus erythematosus. Semin Arthr Rheum 8:212, 1979.
57. Boyer RS, Sun NCJ, Verity A, et al: Immunoperoxidase staining of the choroid Plexus in systemic lupus erythematosus. J Rheumatol 7:645, 1980.
58. Zvaifler NJ, Bluestein HG: The pathogenesis of central nervous system manifestations of systemic lupus erythematosus. Arthr Rheum 25:862, 1982.
59. Winfield JB, Shaw M, Silverman LM, et al: Intrathecal IgG synthesis and blood-brain barrier impairment in patients with systemic lupus erythematosus and central nervous system dysfunction. Am J Med 74:837, 1983.
60. Budman DR, Steinberg AD: Hematologic aspects of systemic lupus erythematosus. Ann Intern Med 86:220, 1977.
61. Thiagarajan P, Shapiro SS, De Marco L: Monoclonal immunoglobulin M coagulation inhibitor with phospholipid specificity. J Clin Invest 66:397, 1980.
62. Hughes GRV, Asherson RA: Atypical lupus with special reference to ANA negative lupus and lupus subsets. Adv Nephrol 14:333, 1985.
63. Mahajan SK, Ordonez NG, Feitelson PJ, et al: Lupus nephropathy without clinical renal involvement. Medicine 56:493, 1977.
64. Lee P, Urowitz MB, Bookman AAM, et al: Systemic lupus erythematosus. Quart J Med XLVI:1, 1977.
65. Grigor R, Edmonds J, Lewkonia R, et al: Systemic Lupus Erythematosus. Ann Rheum Dis 37:121, 1978.
66. DeFronzo RA, Cooke R, Goldberg M, et al: Impaired renal tubular potassium secretion in systemic lupus erythematosus. Ann Intern Med 86:268, 1977.
67. Orth RW, Weisman MH, Cohen AH, et al: Lupus cystitis. Ann Intern Med 98:323, 1983.
68. McCluskey RT: The value of renal biopsy in lupus nephritis. Arthr Rheum 25:867, 1982.
69. Baldwin DS: Clinical usefulness of the morphological classification of lupus nephritis. Am J Kidney Dis II(Suppl):142, 1982.
70. Grishman E, Gerber MA, Churg J: Patterns of Renal Injury in Systemic Lupus Erythematosus. Am J Kidney Dis II(Suppl):135, 1982.
71. Pirani CL, Olesnicky L: Role of electronmicroscopy in the classification of lupus nephritis. Am J Kidney Dis 2(Suppl):150, 1982.
72. Appel GB, Silva FG, Pirani CL, et al: Renal involvement in systemic lupus erythematosus (SLE). Medicine 57:371, 1978.
73. Hill GS: Systemic lupus erythematosus and mixed connective tissue disease. In Heptinstall RH (ed): Pathology of the Kidney, ed 3. Boston/Toronto, Little, Brown & Company, 1983.
74. Brentjens JR, Sepulveda M, Baliah T, et al: Interstitial immune complex nephritis in patients with systemic lupus erythematosus. Kidney Intl 7:342, 1975.
75. Schwartz MM, Fennell JS, Lewis EJ: Pathologic changes in the renal tubule in systemic lupus erythematosus. Hum Pathol 13:534, 1982.
76. Synkowski DR, Mogavero HS, Provost TT: Lupus erythematosus. Med Clin N Am 64:921, 1980.
77. Tan EM: Autoantibodies to nuclear antigens (ANA). Adv Immunol 33:167, 1982.
78. Hahn BH: Characteristics of pathogenic subpopulations of antibodies to DNA. Arthr Rheum 25:747, 1982.
79. Notman DD, Kurata N, Tan EM: Profiles of antinuclear antibodies in systemic rheumatic diseases. Ann Intern Med 83:464, 1975.
80. Eaton RB, Schnneider G, Schur PH: Enzyme immunoassay for antibodies to native DNA. Arthr Rheum 26:52, 1983.
81. Sharp GC: Subsets of SLE and mixed connective tissue disease. Am J Kidney Dis II(suppl):201, 1982.
82. Tan EM: Special antibodies for the study of systemic lupus Erythematosus. Arthr Rheum 25:753, 1982.
83. Beaufils M, Kouki F, Mignon F, et al: Clinical significance of Anti-SM antibodies in systemic lupus erythematosus. Am J Med 74:201, 1983.
84. Shur PH: Complement and lupus erythematosus. Arthr Rheum 25:793, 1982.
85. Morrow WJW, Isenberg DA, Todd-Pokropek A, et al: Useful laboratory measurements in the management of systemic lupus erythematosus. Quart J Med 51:125, 1982.
86. Lloyd W, Schur PH: Immune complexes, complement, and anti-DNA in exacerbations of systemic lupus erythematosus (SLE). Medicine 60:208, 1981.
87. Rynes RI: Inherited complement deficiency states and SLE. Clin Rheum Dis 8:29, 1982.
88. Weinstein A, Bordwell B, Stone B, et al: Antibodies to native DNA and serum complement (C3) levels. Am J Med 74:206, 1983.
89. Watson RM, Lane AT, Barnett NK, et al: Neonatal lupus erythematosus. Medicine 63:362, 1984.
90. Singsen BH, Fishman L, Hanson V: Antinuclear antibodies and lupus-like syndromes in children receiving anticonvulsants. Pediatrics 57:529, 1976.
91. Hess E: Introduction to drug related lupus. Arthr Rheum 24:6, 1981.
92. Lahita RG, Bradlow HL, Fishman J, et al: Abnormal estrogen and androgen metabolism in the human with systemic lupus erythematosus. Am J Kidney Dis II:206, 1982.
93. Miller MH, Urowitz MB, Gladman DD, et al: Systemic lupus erythematosus in males. Medicine 62:327, 1983.
94. DeHoratius RJ, Pillarisetty R, Messner RP, et al: Anti-nucleic acid antibodies in systemic lupus erythematosus patients and their families. J Clin Invest 56:1149, 1975.

95. Arnett FC, Shulman LE: Studies in familial systemic lupus erythematosus. Medicine 55:313, 1976.
96. Reveille JD, Bias WB, Winkelstein JA, et al: Familial systemic lupus erythematosus. Medicine 62:21, 1983.
97. Steinberg BJ, Smathers PA, Frederiksen K, et al: Ability of the xid gene to prevent autoimmunity in (NZB × NZW) F_1 mice during the course of their natural history, after polyclonal stimulation, or following immunization with DNA. J Clin Invest 70:587, 1982.
98. Dixon FJ: Murine lupus—an overview. Arthr Rheum 25:721, 1982.
99. Steinberg AD, Raveche ES, Laskin CA, et al: Systemic lupus erythematosus. Ann Intern Med 100:714, 1984.
100. Christian CL: Role of viruses in etiology of systemic lupus erythematosus. Am J Kidney Dis II(Suppl):114, 1982.
101. Pincus T: Studies regarding a possible function for viruses in the pathogenesis of systemic lupus erythematosus. Arth. Rheum 25:847, 1982.
102. Koffler D, Biesecker G, Katz SM: Immunopathogenesis of systemic lupus erythematosus. Arthr Rheum 25:858, 1982.
103. McCluskey RT: Evidence for an immune complex disorder in systemic lupus erythematosus (SLE). Am J Kidney Dis II(suppl):119, 1982.
104. Steinberg AD, Smith HR, Laskin CA, et al: Studies of immune abnormalities in systemic lupus erythematosus. Am J Kidney Dis II(suppl):101, 1982.
105. Mannix M: Pathophysiology of circulating immune complexes. Arthr Rheum 25:783, 1982.
106. Frank MM, Lawley TJ, Hamburger MI, et al: Immunoglobulin G Fc receptor-mediated clearance in autoimmune diseases. Ann Intern Med 98:206, 1983.
107. Izui S, Lambert P-H, Miescher PA: In vitro demonstration of a particular affinity of glomerular basement membrane and collagen for DNA. J Exp Med 114:428, 1976.
108. Yamada A, Miyakawa Y, Kosaka K: Entrapment of anti-DNA antibodies in the kidney of patients with systemic lupus erythematosus. Kidney Intl 22:671, 1982.
109. Couser WG, Salant DJ, Madaio MP, et al: Factors influencing glomerular and tubulointerstitial patterns of injury in SLE. Am J Kidney Dis II(suppl):126, 1982.
110. Biesecker G, Katz S, Koffler D: Renal localization of the membrane attack complex in systemic lupus erythematosus nephritis. J Exp Med 154:1779, 1982.
111. Falk RJ, Dalmasso AP, Kim Y, et al: Neoantigen of polymerized ninth component of complement. J Clin Invest 72:560, 1983.
112. Atkins RC, Holdsworth SR, Hancock WW, et al: Cellular immune mechanisms in human glomerulonephritis. Semin Immunopathol 5:269, 1982.
113. McCluskey RT, Bhan AK: Cell-mediated mechanisms in renal disease. Kidney Intl 21:S6, 1982.
114. Stobo JD: The influence of immune response genes on the expression of disease. J Lab Clin Med 100:822, 1982.
115. Smolen JS, Chused TM, Leiserson WM, et al: Heterogeneity of immunoregulatory T-cell subsets in systemic lupus erythematosus. Am J Med 72:783, 1982.
116. Lief PD, Barland P, Bank N: Diagnosis of lupus nephritis by skin immunofluorescence in the absence of extrarenal manifestations of systemic lupus erythematosus. Am J Med 63:411, 1977.
117. Morris RJ, Guggenheim SJ, McIntosh RM, et al: Simultaneous immunologic studies of skin and kidney in systemic lupus erythematosus. Arthr Rheum 22:864, 1979.
118. Donadio JV, Holley KE, Ferguson RH, et al: Treatment of diffuse proliferative lupus nephritis with prednisone and combined prednisone and cyclophosphamide. N Engl J Med 299:1151, 1978.
119. Pollak VE, Dosekun AK: Evaluation of treatment in lupus nephritis. Am J Kidney Dis II(Suppl):170, 1982.
120. Carette S, Klippel JH, Decker JL, et al: Controlled studies of oral immunosuppressive drugs in lupus nephritis. Ann Intern Med 99:1, 1983.
121. Coplon NS, Diskin CJ, Petersen J, et al: The long-term clinical course of systemic lupus erythematosus in end-stage renal disease. N Engl J Med 308:186, 1983.
122. Cheigh JS, Stenzel KH, Rubin AL, et al: Systemic lupus erythematosus in patients with chronic renal failure. Am J Med 75:602, 1983.
123. Amend WJC, Vincenti F, Feduska NJ, et al: Recurrent systemic lupus erythematosus involving renal allografts. Ann Intern Med 94:444, 1981.
124. Hayslett JP: Effect of pregnancy in patients with SLE. Am J Kidney Dis II(suppl):223, 1982.
125. Ginzler EM, Diamond HS, Weiner M, et al: A multicenter study of outcome in systemic lupus erythematosus I. Arthr Rheum 25:601, 1982.
126. Rosner S, Ginzler EM, Diamond HS, et al: A multicenter study of outcome in systemic lupus erythematosus II. Arthr Rheum 25:612, 1982.
127. Urowitz MB, Bookman AAM, Koehler BE, et al: The bimodal mortality pattern of systemic lupus erythematosus. Am J Med 60:221, 1976.
128. Tan EM, Cohen AS, Fries JF, et al: The 1982 revised criteria for the classification of systemic lupus erythematosus. Arthr Rheum 25:1271, 1982.

28C Vasculitis and Kawasaki Disease

BENJAMIN H. LANDING
ROSARIO NADORRA
EUNICE J. LARSON

Kawasaki disease or mucocutaneous lymph node syndrome (MCLS) is the most common disorder producing systemic arteritis in the pediatric age group. Although best studied and apparently more frequent in Japan and in children of Japanese descent in other countries, the disease appears to have a world-wide distribution.

Clinically, MCLS shows an acute febrile phase, followed by a subsidence or subacute phase and a convalescent phase (1, 2). Clinical features of the acute phase include fever with spikes to 40 °C or more, typically with sudden onset and duration greater than 5 days (average duration, 11 days) and without response to antibiotic therapy; conjunctival injection, generally without exudation, appearing usually 2 days after the onset of fever and lasting through the febrile period and for as long as 3 to 5 weeks; buccopharyngeal manifestations, including redness and fissuring of the lips, erythema of the pharynx, and strawberry appearance of the tongue, all with onset shortly after the beginning of the fever; indurative edema of the hands and feet, with erythema of the palms and soles, in the acute febrile phase, followed by desquamation of the skin of the fingers, palms, toes, and soles in the subsidence phase (usually beginning 2 to 3 weeks from onset of the fever); exanthematous rash, beginning with or shortly after the onset of fever, variably urticarial and pruritic, morbilliform or scarlatiniform, and usually lasting through the febrile phase; and unilateral cervical lymphadenomegaly, which regresses after the febrile period.

A variety of other manifestations can occur in patients with Kawasaki disease, including the following:

1. Urethritis, with leukocyturia, is relatively frequent (up to 70% of patients), but azotemia and elevation of serum creatinine are not features of MCLS.

2. Arthritis is seen in about 40% of patients with MCLS, with onset usually late in the febrile phase or in the subacute phase. Larger joints (knees, hips, and elbows) are most commonly affected.

3. Aseptic meningitis, with lymphocytic pleocytosis of cerebrospinal fluid to 25 to 100 white cells/mm^3, occurs in approximately one-fourth of patients. Irritability is regular in MCLS, lethargy is significant in about a third of patients, and semicoma or coma can occur.

4. Abdominal pain and diarrhea occur in a minority (about one-fourth) of patients.

5. Hydrops of the gallbladder, with right upper quadrant mass, is a more recently recognized feature of the acute or subsidence phases of MCLS; it typically regresses in 2 to 3 weeks. Elevation of serum bilirubin and of SGOT and SGPT levels is seen in about 10% of patients with MCLS.

The peak age of MCLS is approximately 1 year, although proven cases occur through childhood. Differentiation from toxic shock syndrome is necessary in older children and young adults. The cause of MCLS is not known, but its epidemiology suggests an infectious disease; much research directed to the possibility of a bacterial etiology is in progress.

RENAL INVOLVEMENT

Although pyuria resulting from urethritis is frequent in MCLS and renal artery involvement has been demonstrated in approximately 50% of autopsied patients with MCLS (3, 4), clinical features of parenchymal renal involvement are not a component of the disease. Melish (1) has stated that "true renal involvement in Kawasaki syndrome is so unusual that whenever it is encountered it should prompt serious reconsideration of the diagnosis."

The arterial lesion in Kawasaki disease is essentially limited to larger extraparenchymal or hilar renal arteries, including the main renal arteries, the primary anterior and posterior branches of the right and left main renal arteries and succeeding extraparenchymal branches of the anterior and posterior arteries, and to the arcuate arteries. In contrast, the vasculitis of classical adult polyarteritis (periarteritis) nodosa (APN) regularly affects also the smaller intrarenal interlobular and glomerular arteries, as well as the glomeruli proper which are rarely if ever affected in Kawasaki disease. Results of review of the patients in the study of Landing and Larson (3), with addition of some patients with MCLS seen more recently, are summarized in Table 28C.1, which demonstrates that MCLS is much more common, in pediatric autopsy series, than APN; that renal arterial lesions are not infrequent (56% in these data) in MCLS, but that true intrarenal disease occurs, statistically, only in APN; and that clinical manifestations of significant renal involvement are infrequent in MCLS. For example, hypertension was documented in only three of these 25 MCLS patients, and none developed renal insufficiency, although one did have a segmental renal infarct. Examples of the renal arterial lesions of MCLS are given in Figures 28C.2 to 4.

The general lack of glomerular or smaller intrarenal vascular disease in MCLS and the patchy distribution of the hilar arterial involvement imply that kidney biopsy will not generally be useful in diagnosis or confirmation of diagnosis of MCLS. The value of renal scans, flow studies, or angiography for these purposes may merit further study.

The data of Table 28C.1 show that pathologically early-stage and late-stage arterial lesions can be found in the same patient, as has been reported in other studies (3, 5). Figure 28C.1, based on autopsy studies

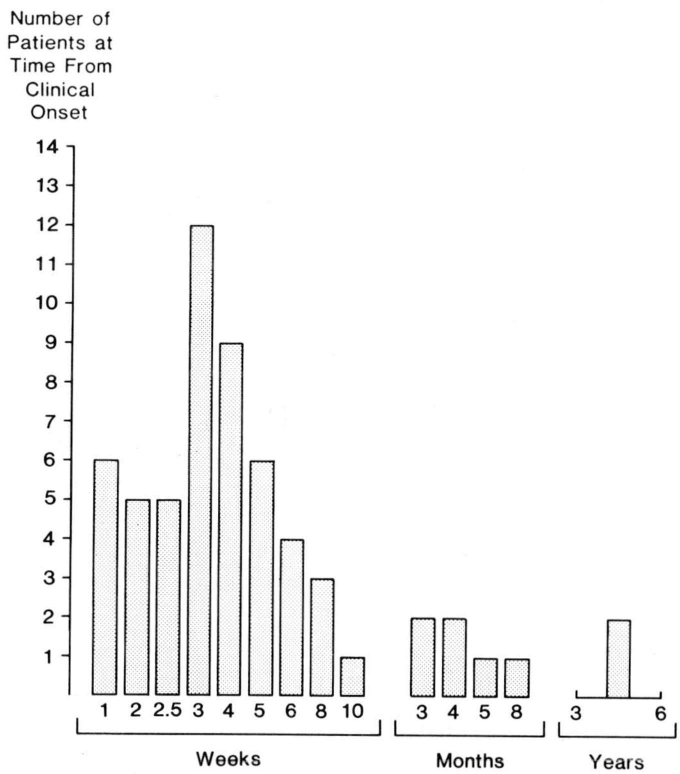

Figure 28C.1. Duration from onset of clinical disease to death, patients with MCLS from North America.

Table 28C.1.
Incidence and Type of Renal Arterial Lesions in MCLS and APN in Children

	Patients	Hilar/arcuate artery lesions: Early stage	Late stage	With thrombosis	No renal arterial lesion demonstrable	Glomerular artery and glomerular lesions	Clinical hypertension documented
MCLS	25	5	11	2	11	0	3
APN	3	1	2	1	0	3	3

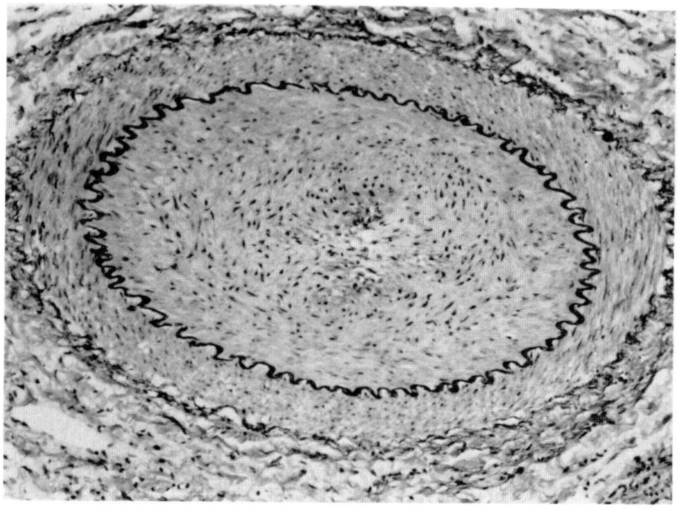

Figure 28C.2. Late-stage lesion of hilar branch of renal artery in 10-month-old female with Kawasaki disease, showing complete fibrous obliteration of arterial lumen, but good preservation of internal elastic layer and muscularis. (Verhoeff-van Gieson stain, X116.)

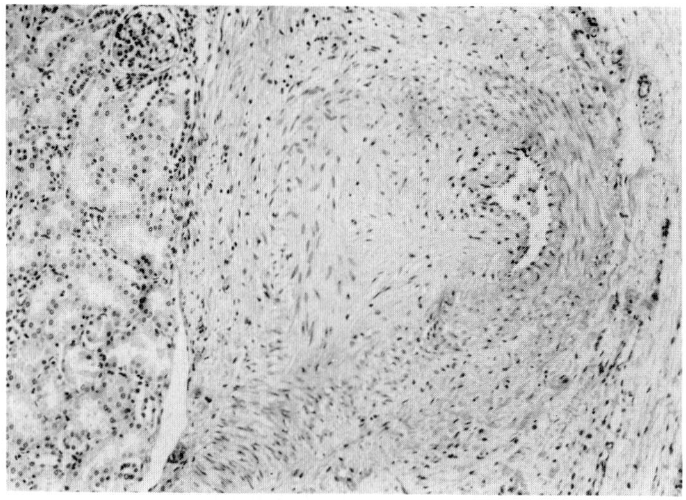

Figure 28C.4. Late-stage lesion of another hilar branch of renal artery in same patient as in Figure 28C.3, showing stenosis by intimal fibrosis, plus segmental destruction and fibrosis of elastic and muscular layers of the arterial wall. (H & E stain, X116.)

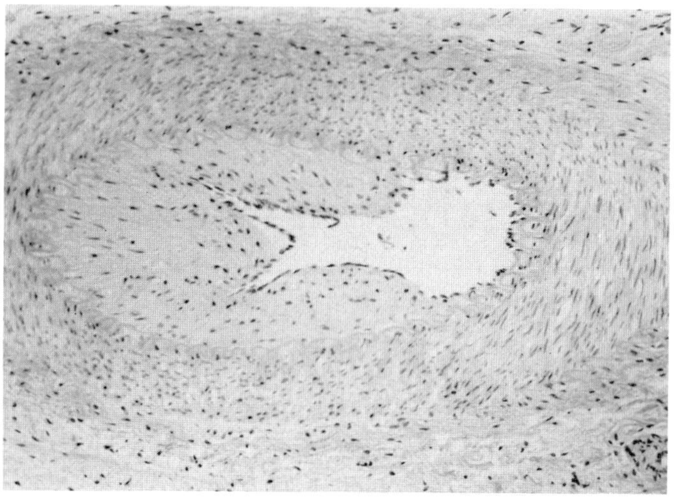

Figure 28C.3. Late-stage lesion of hilar branch of renal artery in MCLS (4-month-old male) showing stenosis by crescentic intimal fibrosis, but with preservation of internal elastic layer and muscularis. (H & E stain, X116.)

of patients with MCLS in North America, shows that the peak duration of disease in these patients, from onset to death, was 3 weeks, but that death could occur from within the first week of disease through the tenth week, as well as in the period 3 to 8 months from onset of disease, with rare patients dying from 3 to 6 years after the acute episode. Many studies have shown that the cause of death in MCLS is usually coronary artery disease, usually with occlusive thrombosis, and as far as we can determine, no patient with MCLS has been reported to have died of renal disease. Studies on the regression of the arterial aneurysms of MCLS (6) show that reformation of normal lumen contour is frequent over the first year after the acute disease, but that the "healing" process is usually the result of fibrous subintimal thickening, so that the involved vessels do not become truly normal. Late occlusive lesions of renal arteries perhaps can occur in MCLS, as has been well demonstrated for coronary arteries, but this event appears not to have been reported.

RENAL INVOLVEMENT IN POLYARTHERITIS NODOSA IN CHILDREN

As was mentioned, classical APN was a much less frequent disease in childhood than MCLS, its frequency in the autopsy material summarized in Table 28C.1 being only about one-tenth that of MCLS. (Since the death rate in MCLS is only about 0.5%, it is clear that APN is actually very rare in children.) APN variably affects arteries of skin, muscles, periarticular tissues, central nervous system, heart, gastrointestinal tract and mesentry, pancreas and retroperitoneum, and kidneys. The clinical features and prognosis depend on the organs and system involved. The most common presenting features are fever, myalgia, arthralgia, vasculitic skin lesions, hypertension, and abdominal pain (7–11). Testicular pain in males may occur early in the course of the disease and be mistaken for torsion of the testis (7). Myocarditis, pericarditis, coronary arteritis, and hypertension may lead to congestive heart failure. Neurological symptoms include transient ischemic attacks or stroke, paresthesias, and peripheral neuropathy (mononeuritis multiplex). Renal involvement may present as proteinuria, hematuria, and rapidly deteriorating renal function. Examples of the renal lesions of APN are given in Figures 28C.5 to 10. The arterial lesion of APN is typically necrotizing with definite "fibrinoid" necrosis and may or may not produce arterial aneurysms or ruptures. Pathological differential diagnosis of necrotizing renal arteritis in children includes Henoch-Schönlein disease, juvenile rheumatoid arthritis, systemic sclerosis (scleroderma), malignant hypertension, and allergic arteritis. Fibrinoid necrosis is not a significant feature of the arteritis of MCLS. The glomerular process of APN may be an acute diffuse glomerulonephritis, but is often crescentic glomerulonephritis (often now called "rapidly progressive glomerulonephritis") (12).

RENAL LESIONS OF WEGENER'S GRANULOMATOSIS IN CHILDHOOD

Wegener's granulomatosis is defined as a disorder with polyarteritis and a necrotizing granulomatous inflammatory process involving the nasal mucosa, the tracheobronchial tree and lungs, and the kidneys. There is male preponderance (2:1) as in adults (13). Most patients present with fever, malaise, vasculitic skin lesions, sinusitis, epistaxis, cough,

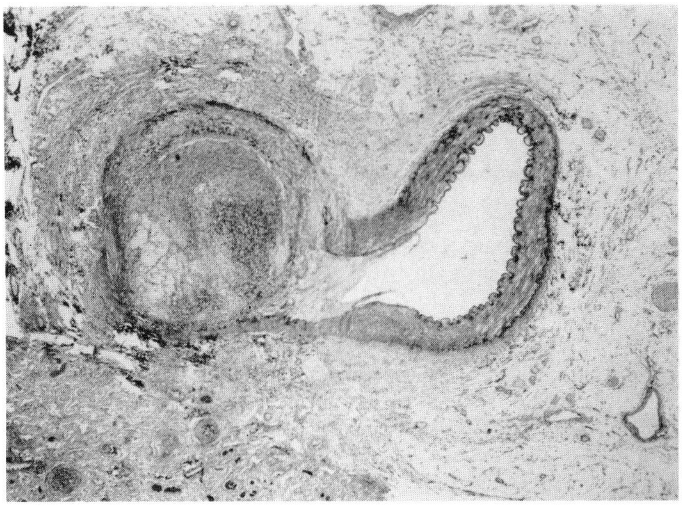

Figure 28C.5. Acute segmental destruction of wall of hilar renal artery in 18-year-old male with "adult" polyarteritis nodosa, showing aneurysm formation, with thrombosis of the aneurysm. (PAS stain, X46.)

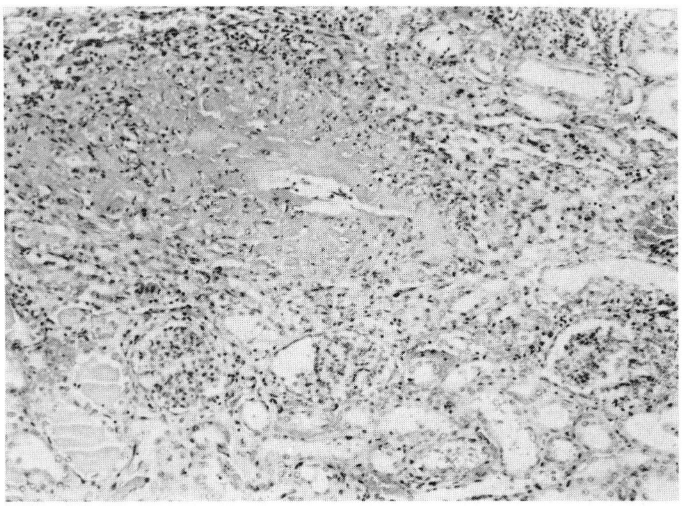

Figure 28C.6. Fibrinoid necrosis of intrarenal artery, with mural and perivascular inflammatory infiltration, in 8-year-old male with APN (H & E stain, X116.)

chest pain, and hematuria. Other not uncommon features are serous otitis media, eye lesions, polyarthralgia, and cardiac and neurological symptoms. Sinusitis may be accompanied by nasal mucosal ulceration and septal perforation. Eye lesions include granulomas of the optic nerve, conjunctiva, cornea and sclerae, and pseudotumors of the orbit. Pulmonary manifestations may be severe, with impairment of pulmonary function, but lesions sometimes are demonstrated radiographically in the absence of pulmonary symptoms. X-ray films of the lungs usually show bilateral nodular infiltrates or cavitating lesions. These wax and wane with disease activity; this feature aids differentiation of Wegener's granulomatosis from tumor or infectious granuloma (14). Cardiac involvement can be coronary arteritis, pancarditis, or conduction system granulomata (15). Neurological involvement in the pediatric age group, occurring in about 17% (14), is substantially less frequent than in adults, which occurs in about 54% (16). The most common neurological manifestation is mononeuritis multiplex (7), but cranial arteritis may also occur. Renal involvement is the leading cause of death in patients

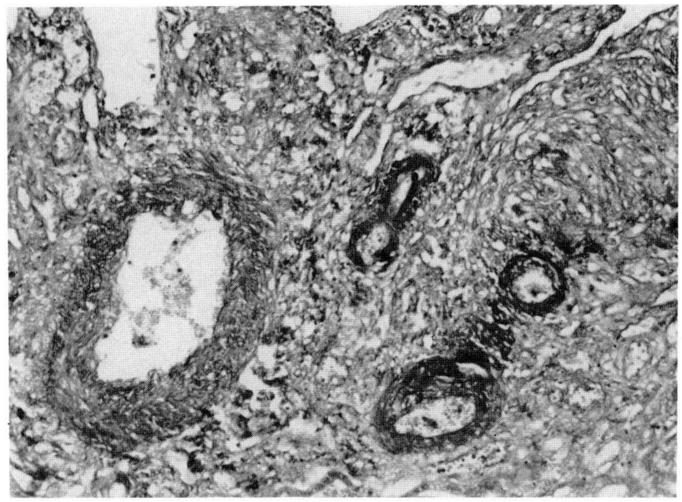

Figure 28C.7. Fibrinoid necrosis of smaller intrarenal arteries, in same patient with APN as in Figure 28C.5. (PAS stain, X116.)

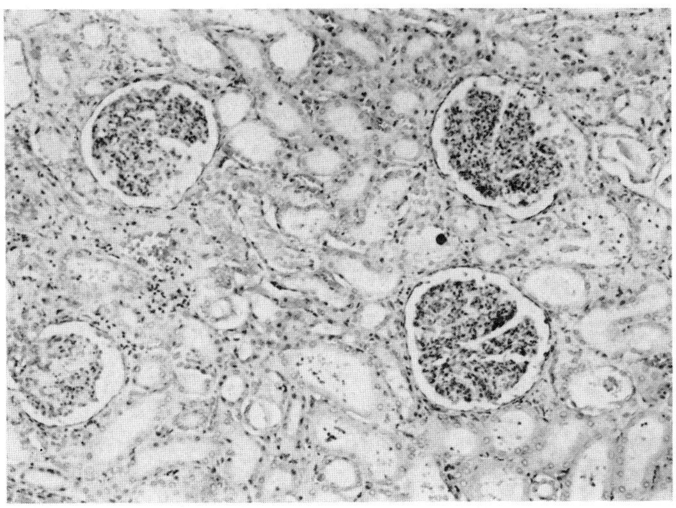

Figure 28C.8. Acute glomerulitis in APN (same patient as Figure 28C.6). (H & E stain, X116.)

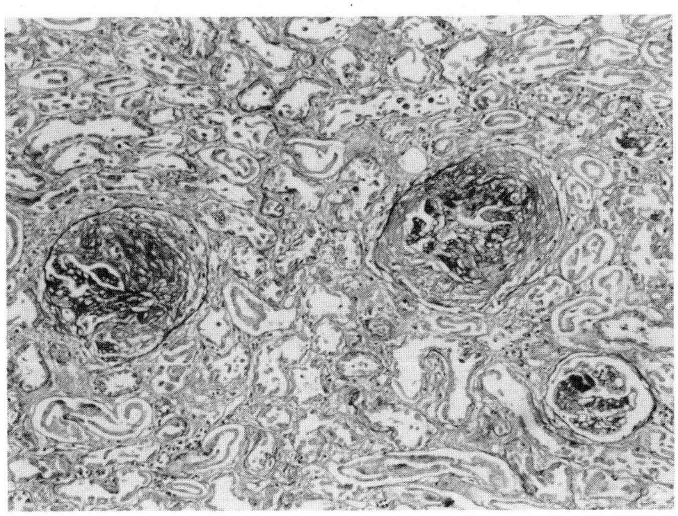

Figure 28C.9. Later stage of glomerular lesion of APN, with extensive crescent formation and glomerular scarring, in same patient as Figures 28C.5 and 7. (PAS stain, X116.)

with Wegener's granulomatosis. The urinary findings are typical of glomerulonephritis with proteinuria, hematuria, and red cell casts. The basic glomerular process is a segmental necrotizing glomerulonephritis, and crescentic glomerulonephritis resembling that which can occur in APN or SLE is frequent in Wegener's disease. Extraglomerular necrotizing granulomas, like those seen in the nasal and tracheobronchial mucosas, can occur in the kidneys. Pathological differential diagnosis of the renal lesions of Wegener's disease thus includes, not only APN and other causes of "rapidly progressive glomerulonephritis", but other causes of renal granulomas, including tuberculosis and sarcoid. A striking, but not pathognomonic, feature of the glomerular process of Wegener's disease is patchy destruction of the Bowman's capsular basement membrane. Excellent illustrations of the lesions of renal Wegener's disease are given by Brun and Olsen (12).

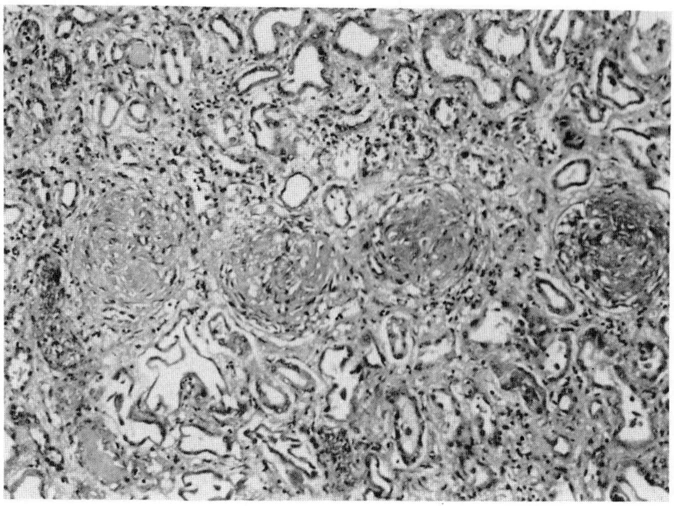

Figure 28C.10. Global glomerular sclerosis in late stage glomerular scarring of APN, in same patient as Figures 28C.5, 7, and 9. (H & E stain, X116.)

TAKAYASU'S DISEASE

The most detailed available data on patients with Takayasu's disease in North America are those of Lupi-Herrera and coworkers from the National Institute of Cardiology of Mexico (17). In their series of 107 patients, approximately 80% had onset of disease before age 20 years, the great majority between ages 10 and 20, but a few at younger ages with the youngest age of onset 3 years. Their series shows the typical female predominance (84% female). Hypertension was demonstrated in 72% of the patients, and renal vascular lesions were shown angiographically in 68 patients (62%), occurring on the right in 19, on the left in 17, and bilaterally in 31. Of 22 patients operated for unilateral renal vascular disease, only five benefited, suggesting that bilateral disease is more common than angiography indicates. Only about half the patients had characteristic sudden onset of fever, anorexia, weight loss, arthralgia, hypertension, and elevated sedimentation rate with partial or complete resolution of the acute features over about 3-months' time and subsequent development of "chronic phase" features of aortic and other vascular disease. The other half presented with features of arterial obstruction already present. The pathologic features of the late-stage renal arterial lesion are similar to those of late-stage Kawasaki disease (Fig. 28C.11), but the degree of aortic involvement in Takayasu's disease (present in 94% of the Mexico series) and the high frequency (45%) of severe pulmonary artery involvement in this condition should provide adequate distinction. Takayasu's arteritis should be suspected in adolescent girls or young women with hypertension, especially if features of reduced arterial blood flow or vascular bruits are present.

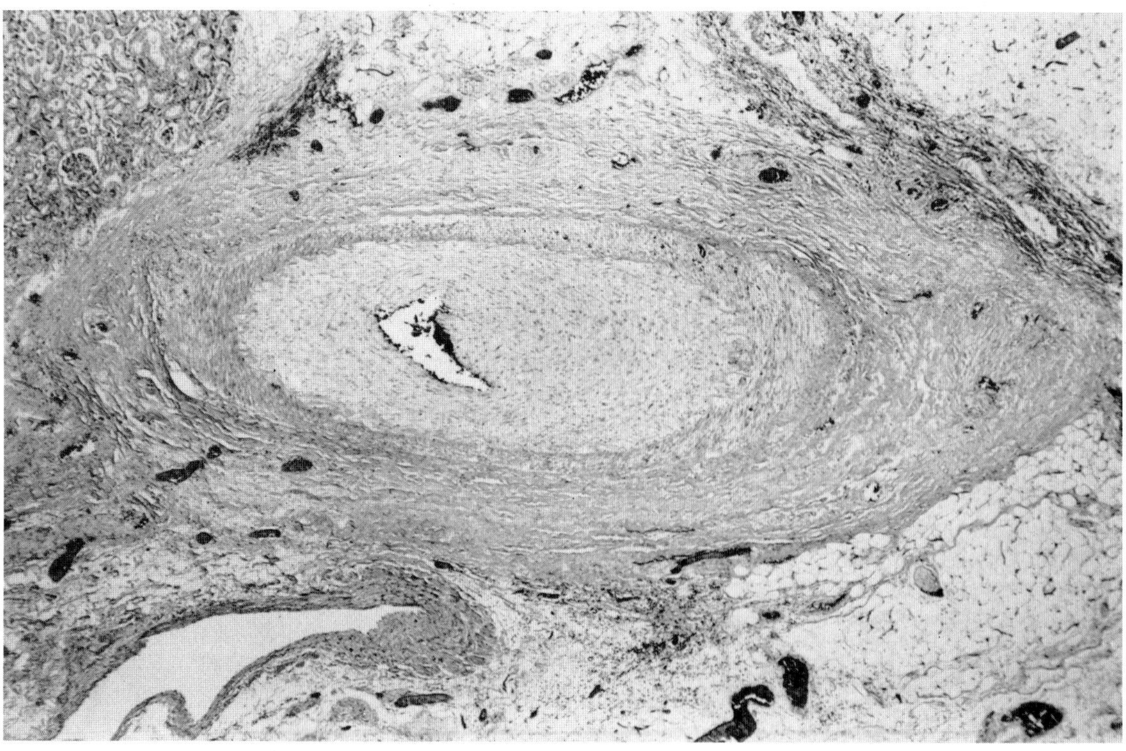

Figure 28C.11. Hilar renal artery of six-year-old black female with Takayasu disease, showing luminal obliteration of late-stage proliferative process. (H & E, X54). (Courtesy of Dr. Neva Gould, Chicago.)

References

1. Melish ME: Kawasaki syndrome (the mucocutaneous lymph node syndrome). Pediat Ann 11:251, 1982.
2. Japan MCLS Research Committee—Kawasaki Disease. Diagnosis, pathology, treatment and epidemiology. Tokyo, 1980.
3. Landing BH, Larson EJ: Are infantile periarteritis nodosa with coronary artery involvement and fatal mucocutaneous lymph node syndrome the same? Comparison of 20 patients from North America with patients with Hawaii and Japan. Pediatrics 59:651, 1977.
4. Amano S, Hazama F, Hamashima Y: Pathology of Kawasaki disease. 2. Distribution and incidence of the vascular lesions. Jap Circ J 43:741, 1979.
5. Amano S, Hazama F, Hamashima Y: Pathology of Kawasaki disease. 1. Pathology and morphogenesis of the vascular changes. Jap Circ J 43:633, 1979.
6. Sasaguri Y, Kato H: Regression of aneurysms in Kawasaki disease. A pathological study. J Pediatr 100:225, 1982.
7. Jacobs JC: Pediatric Rheumatology for the Practitioner. New York, Springer Verlag, Inc., 1982.
8. Blau EB, Morris RF, Yunis EJ: Polyarteritis nodosa in older children. Pediatrics 60:227, 1977.
9. Magilavy DB, Petty RE, Cassidy JT, et al: A syndrome of childhood polyarteritis. J Pediatr 91:25, 1977.
10. Reimold EW, Weinberg AG, Fink CW, et al: Polyarteritis in children. Am J Dis Child 130:534, 1976.
11. Ettlinger RE, Nelson AM, Burke EC, et al: Polyarteritis nodosa in childhood, a clinical pathologic study. Arthr Rheum 22:820, 1979.
12. Brun C, Olsen S: Atlas of Renal Biopsy. Philadelphia, W. B. Saunders Co., 1981.
13. Wolff SM, Fauci AS, Horn RG, et al: Wegener's granulomatosis. Ann Int Med 81:513, 1974.
14. Orlowski JP, Clough JD, Dyment PG: Wegener's granulomatosis in the pediatric age group. Pediatrics 61:83–90, 1978.
15. Forstot JZ, Overlie PA, Neufeld GK, et al: Cardiac complications of Wegener's granulomatosis: A case report of complete heart block and review of literature. Semin Arth Rheum 10:148, 1980.
16. Drachman DA: Neurological complications of Wegener's granulomatosis. Arch Neurol 8:145, 1963.
17. Lupi-Herrera E, Sánchez-Torres G, Marcushamer J, Mispireta J, Horwitz S, Espino Vela J: Takayasu's arteritis. Clinical study of 107 cases. Am Heart J 93:94, 1977.

28D Diabetes Mellitus

DAVID M. BROWN
S. MICHAEL MAUER

Diabetes mellitus constitutes one of the major causes of renal disease and renal failure. Approximately one of four patients developing uremia requiring hemodialysis are diabetic (1). Long-term follow-up of diabetic patients reveals an incidence of clinical proteinuria of approximately 35% (2, 3). Furthermore, patients with nephropathy often have other complications, such as neuropathy or retinopathy (4). In the natural course of progression of diabetic nephropathy, elevation of the serum creatinine to 2 mg/dl or greater is associated with rapid progression of renal failure (5). In fact, the presence of persistent proteinuria portends renal failure (6, 7). Close monitoring of insulin-dependent diabetics once proteinuria is detected, reveals progressive increments of proteinuria, decreasing glomerular filtration rate and increased blood pressure (8). Further refinement of techniques to measure urine albumin excretion has led to the observation that proteinuria detectable by standard screening techniques (Albustix positive) will eventually develop in a large proportion of patients who excrete 30 μg/min of albumin in their urine (9). Thus we can begin to appreciate that clinically significant nephropathy precedes by several years the gross proteinuria and decreased glomerular filtration rate (GFR), which accompanies the established glomerulosclerosis that probably is irreversible.

Although the pathological diagnosis of diabetic glomerulosclerosis in children is rare (10), it is important to recognize the factors that influence the onset and course of diabetic nephropathy, and that they probably represent a continuum beginning at the onset of disease. These make it imperative to define preventive and therapeutic measures and the nature of the population of diabetic patients who are at risk. This review will compare the current status of information of human diabetic nephropathy with the knowledge from experimental models, integrating the pathology, physiology, biochemistry, and clinical parameters. Since to the best of our present state of knowledge, diabetes mellitus and its renal complications are a continuum throughout the course of the disease, no attempt will be made to separate childhood from adult age groups, although the emphasis will be on insulin-dependent diabetes. The effects of diabetes mellitus on the kidney in both humans and experimental animals have been the subjects of recent reviews (11–13).

PATHOLOGY (Table 28D.1)

The most commonly occurring, although not unique, glomerular lesion found in diabetes is known as diffuse glomerulosclerosis. It consists of a generalized widening of the glomerular mesangium associated with the homogenous accumulation of glycoproteins, which by light microscopy stain uniformly with PAS (Fig. 28D.1) (11, 14). The accumulation within glomeruli of the nodular homogeneous staining acellular material in diabetic glomeruli, called the Kimmelstiel-Wilson lesion, is generally considered to be specific for diabetes and indicates an advanced stage of nephropathy (Fig. 28D.2). Although the origin of the nodular lesion is

Table 28D.1.
Pathology of Established Diabetic Nephropathy in Human Subjects

Always present[a]	Often present	Sometimes present
Glomerular basement membrane thickening, especially lamina densa	Kimmelsteil-Wilson[b] nodules (nodular glomerulosclerosis)	Hyaline "exudative" lesions, subendothelial
Mesangial widening with increased matrix material predominating (diffuse glomerulosclerosis)	Afferent and efferent[b] glomerular arteriolar hyalinization	Parietal Bowman's capsular surface[b] "capsular drop"
Intense glomerular basement membrane, tubular basement membrane, and Bowman's capsular immunofluorescent staining for albumin	Tubular basement membrane thickening	

From Mauer SM, et al: Am J Med 70:606, 1981.
[a] In combination, diagnostic of diabetic nephropathy.
[b] Highly characteristic of diabetic nephropathy.

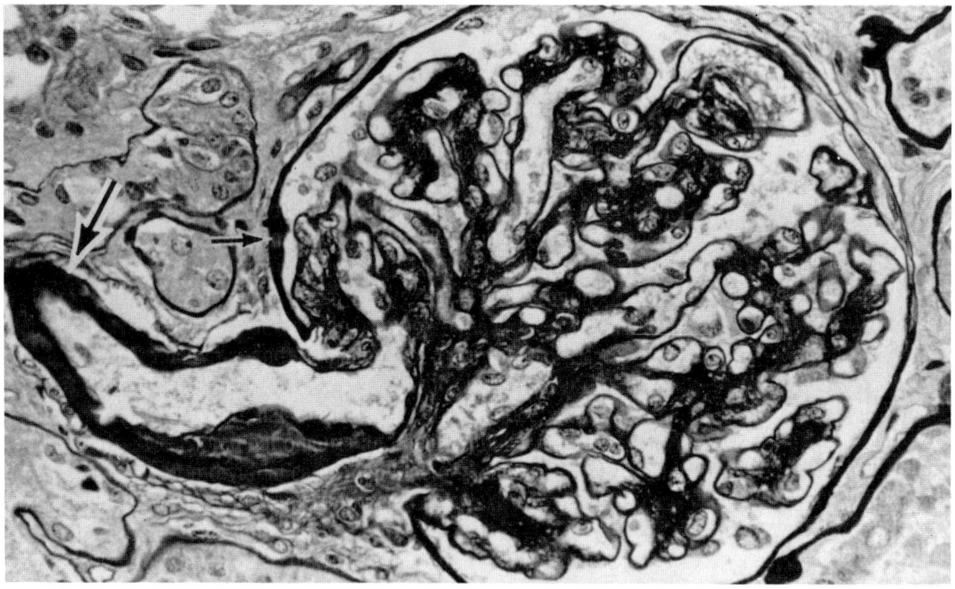

Figure 28D. 1. Moderate, diffuse increase in mesangial matrix in glomerulus from patient with diabetic nephropathy. The large arrow indicates the hyalinized arteriole and the small arrow points to a droplet within Bowman's capsule. (PAS X450.)

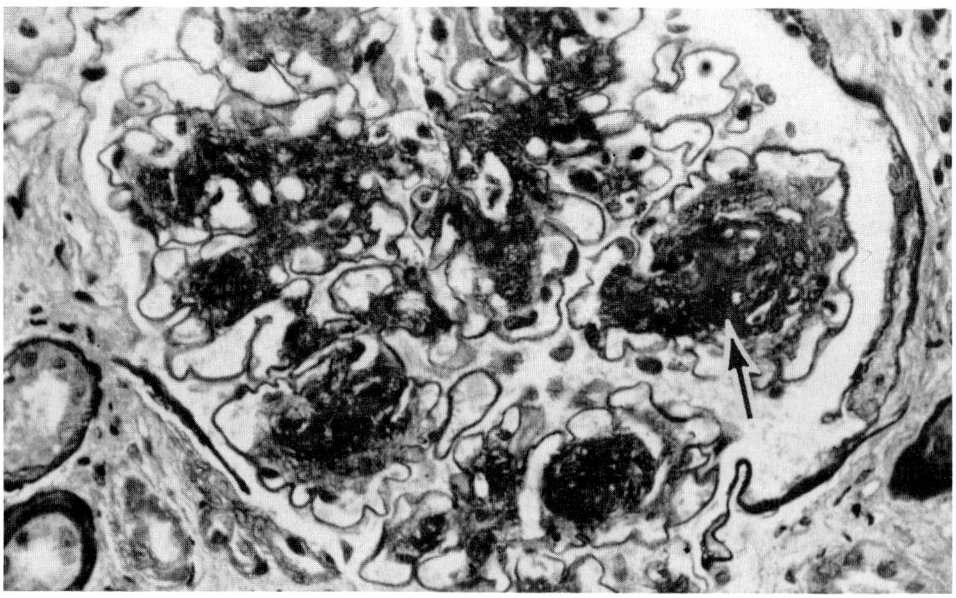

Figure 28D. 2. Typical advanced glomerular changes in diabetic nephropathy showing the nodular Kimmelstiel-Wilson lesions (*arrow*). (PAS X450.)

not well appreciated, it has generally been considered to be an extension of the diffuse glomerular lesion and is presumably derived from material that accumulates in the mesangial matrix. The third typical lesion is thickening of the glomerular basement membrane (GBM). Less common but highly characteristic of diabetic nephropathy are hyalinization of the afferent and efferent glomerular arterioles, thickening of the tubular basement membranes, subendothelial "exudative" hyaline lesions of the glomerulus, and "capsular drops" in the parietal Bowman's capsule. It has also been suggested that glomerular arteriolar and capillary dilatation in diabetes is comparable to the microaneurysms found in the diabetic retina (15). There is increased accumulation in the diabetic kidney of endogenous macromolecules, such as albumin within GBM (16) and tubular basement membrane (TBM) (17) as seen by immunohistochemistry; similar changes have been found in both vascular (18) and nonvascular (19) extrarenal tissues. Other studies have suggested that the quantity of albumin bound to GBM and TBM correlates with their total collagen content and shown that it is firmly bound, suggesting that the mechanisms of accumulation of albumin in diabetic membranes involves either a biochemical or electrostatic interaction (20).

The relationships between renal function and glomerular pathology have begun to provide clues to pathogenic factors in diabetic glomerulosclerosis and also help to define prognostic parameters. Quantitative assessments of glomerular components by morphometric analyses have revealed a direct relationship between the degree of widening of the glomerular mesangium and depression of the creatinine clearance, urinary albumin excretion, and hypertension (21). Thus, mesangial expansion encroaching on the subendothelial space eventually compromises the glomerular capillary lumen and blood flow, ultimately leading to constriction of the filtration surface or to glomerular capillary obliteration (22, 23). More recently we measured the total glomerular capillary filtration surface per glomerulus or per patient (24) and found a striking direct relationship between this structural parameter and glomerular filtration rate (GFR), across the entire range of GFR from hyperfiltration to moderate renal insufficiency. We further found that the structural parameters of total mesangial volume and glomerular volume together predict filtration surface with remarkable accuracy. These data contradict the conclusion that diffuse mesangial expansion represents a benign form of diabetic nephropathy (25). Although thickening of the GBM has been found to loosely correlate with urinary albumin exretion in a nonselected population of diabetic patients (21), there were patients in that study with either minimal or heavy albumin excretion who had either marked or minimal GBM thickness, respectively. No correlation was found in that study between GBM thickening and widening of the mesangium. These results suggest that the pathological expression of diabetic glomerulosclerosis represents varying pathophysiological mechanisms. Clearly, the GBM and mesangial changes can occur at different rates in the same patient.

In experimentally induced diabetes in rats, correction of the diabetic state by islet transplantation leads to reversal of albuminuria to normal and to reduction of the increased mesangial volume, while the thickened GBM remains unchanged (26, 27). Thus the concept of the distinctly differing functional implications of GBM and mesangial responses to diabetes is reinforced. One may speculate further that the thickening of the GBM observed microscopically represents a change in the scaffolding of the matrix as a result of diabetes, but as such is not the direct factor that regulates the glomerular filtration barrier impermeability. Thus specific biochemical matrix components of the barrier may change in diabetes leading to the architectural change, whereas other matrix components, not reflected in the thickening per se, also may change as a result of diabetes and may be the biochemical basis for altered impermeability. (This concept will be discussed further under Biochemistry).

The question of a metabolic vs a genetic influence to the occurrence of microvascular complications of diabetes has been long debated. It is important to emphasize that the pathology of the diabetic lesion has been found in conjunction with diabetes secondary to pancreatitis (29, 30). Furthermore, both in humans (31) and animals (32) the pathological lesions characteristic of diabetes recurs in the transplanted kidneys. Further, Osterby (33) has shown that kidney structure is normal at onset of diabetes in man. Finally we have noted that kidney structure is entirely normal in nondiabetic identical twins of diabetic subjects (unpublished observations). Thus it seems likely that the major, although perhaps not exclusive, factor influencing the development of microvascular complications of diabetes is the diabetic metabolic milieu. In this regard it is interesting that 6 to 14 years after kidney transplantation, only one third of diabetic patients develop severe diabetic lesions in the renal allograft (unpublished observations). These studies suggest that, at least in part, susceptibility to the renal complications of diabetes resides within the kidney itself.

PHYSIOLOGY

The early stages of insulin-dependent diabetes mellitus are marked by a generalized increase in the size of kidneys, as well as increased renal plasma flow (RPF) and GFR plus increase filtration fraction (34, 35). It has been suggested that the elevated RPF and GFR are related to hyperglycemia per se rather than insulin deficiency (36), although the elevated levels of plasma growth hormone and glucagon in poorly controlled diabetics have also been implicated in glomerular hyperfunction (35). Similar findings have been documented in experimental diabetes (37, 38). The extracellular volume in early diabetes in humans is normal (39) and may be increased in diabetic rats (38). Thus it has been postulated that diabetes results in renal vasodilatation accompanied by increased glomerular pressures and blood flows (40). The role of increased renal blood flow in the expression of diabetic glomerulopathy was first suggested by the observation in humans that constriction of blood flow to the diabetic kidney prevents full expression of the pathology of the diabetic state (41), which was confirmed subsequently by experimental reproduction of the same findings in the diabetic rat (42). Further uninephrectomy, presumably through adaptive glomerular hyperfiltration accelerates diabetic nephropathy in rats (43). However, increased renal plasma flow and glomerular filtration rate are not invariably associated with the appearance of diabetic glomerulopathy in experimental diabetes (43).

Several studies attribute renal dilatation and glomerular hyperfunction in diabetes to an alteration in vascular control mechanisms. Thus in experimental diabetes increased renal blood flow has been resistant to normal autoregulatory influences (44), while both afferent and efferent glomerular arteriolar resistances are decreased (37). It is possible that these physiological changes are a result of altered metabolism of vasoactive substances. Thus several studies in some human diabetics (45, 46) and in animals with experimental diabetes (47) have demonstrated decreased plasma renin activity. Increased glomerular synthesis of vasoactive arachidonic acid metabolites have been found in experimental diabetes (48) and may contribute to altered vascular tone and hence blood flow. Thus altered ratios of arachidonic acid metabolites, which control vasodilatation and vasoconstriction, may contribute to the abnormal vascular responsiveness of vascular structures in diabetes (48–52).

The vascular contractile mechanisms of the glomerulus, particularly the smooth muscle component of the mesangium are altered in diabetes. This postulate is reinforced by the finding of angiotensin II receptors (53) and nerve endings (54) in the mesangium. Furthermore, insulin is required for mesangial cell contractility (55). Recent studies suggest that angiotensin II receptors in the glomerulus of diabetic rats are decreased in number (56). Furthermore, there are increased quantities of actomyosin found in the mesangium in both the human (57) and rat (58) with diabetes.

Since, at the hilum, the mesangium extends outside the glomerulus (the extraglomerular mesangium), one may speculate that changes in the contractile mechanisms of the mesangium in diabetes are the basis for changes in blood flow regulatory mechanisms of the glomerulus. In addition to a possible role in regulating blood flow, the glomerular mesangium is responsible for processing circulating macromolecules (57). In diabetic rats the areas of the mesangium most thickened secondary to long-standing diabetes showed decreased capacity to clear injected macromolecules (60), whereas areas of the mesangium that appeared relatively normal had no such abnormality. Additional studies in diabetic mice have demonstrated that the juxtaglomerular apparatus and the distal tubule are involved in the processing of macromolecules apparently though the extraglomerular extension of the mesangium (61). Thus one may speculate that in diabetes there is an abnormality of the biochemistry of glomerular vascular contractile control mechanisms, which may involve both the end organ per se as well as the vasoactive substances that act on the end organ, in this case, the glomerular mesangium and the glomerular arterioles.

BIOCHEMISTRY

The major emphasis of studies on the biochemistry of the glomerulus in diabetes has been on the GBM (13). Until recently, it has been assumed that the major regulatory component of the macromolecular permeability barrier of the glomerular filter was the collagen component of the GBM. Although most of the studies of that component have demonstrated increased synthesis (62) and perhaps decreased degradation (63) of GBM collagen, they are all faulted by failure to appreciate that there are several distinct species of collagen in basement membranes (64). Furthermore it is currently not possible to isolate GBM per se without including mesangial matrix; therefore all published work actually represents GBM enriched fractions rather than "pure" GBM. A second technical problem that may add to the difficulty of interpreting the work in this field is the possibility that the procedures used to isolate the GBM fraction may result in selective but only questionably controllable losses of yet-to-be described chemical components of the filtration barrier.

A considerable amount of interest has been raised in the generalized phenomenon of nonenzymatic glucosylation of proteins to explain several of the microvascular and other complications of diabetes (65). Whereas it is possible to demonstrate that GBM, as is the case with other proteins, can readily be glucosylated by high concentrations of glucose (66) the pathological significance of this finding remains to be demonstrated. Although an early report suggested that the injection of glucosylated albumin led to glomerular damage in previously normal kidneys (67), recent studies have not demonstrated altered affinity of either glucosylated or nonglucosylated albumin for diabetic or normal renal basement membranes (68). Therefore it seems unlikely that glucosylation of endogenous macromolecules or of the tissues to which those macromolecules fix in diabetes are major factors in the pathogenesis of diabetic glomerulopathy.

Several noncollagen components of the GBM and filtration barrier have been discovered using both histochemical and biochemical techniques. These include such glycoproteins as laminin (69), fibronectin (70), entactin (71), proteoglycans (72–75), and sialoproteins (76). Although studies of the effects of diabetes on most of these substances is still incomplete, a great deal of emphasis is now being placed on the roles these glycoproteins may have in glomerular structural and functional relationships. For example, glomerular proteoglycans are known to be key determinants to glomerular filtration permeability (77). Recent studies with human (78) and rat (79) diabetic glomeruli suggest that the synthesis of glycosaminoglycans, the heteropolysaccharide of proteoglycans, is diminished. Additional studies in experimental diabetes have shown that the overall negative charge on glomerular proteoglycans is diminished (80). These findings suggest that alterations in the proteoglycans of glomeruli in diabetes may contribute to the altered permeability to endogenous macromolecules, which is characteristic of diabetes and may account for the concept of small pore changes early in diabetes (see Mechanisms of Proteinuria). In addition, the sialic acid content of GBM in diabetes is diminished (81), although the role of sialoproteins in glomerular function remains unknown.

Yet to be completely explained biochemically is the basis for the thickening of the GBM in diabetes (see Pathology) aside from the alterations in collagen metabolism. Recent studies have suggested that many matrix components of the GBM and mesangium, in addition to specific collagen moieties, are increased in diabetes (82). One may then speculate that the slow catabolism of many of these collagen and noncollagen components, once altered, retain a conformation change, which contributes to an altered "scaffold-like" structure of GBM that cannot reverse toward normal despite correction of the diabetic milieu (28, 83). However, it may be that other GBM components, such as proteoglycans, may respond more readily to an improvement in the diabetic environment thus accounting for reversibility of albuminuria despite the lack of an obvious morphological change of the GBM (27). It is likely that any of several changes in the biochemical relationships of the constituents of the GBM or the cell-coat substances, which control the binding of the glomerular endothelial and epithelial cells with each other and with the underlying GBM, will alter the permeability of the filtration barrier. How or whether those changes relate to the biochemical alterations of mesangial matrix and cellular constituents remains totally enigmatic.

Proteinuria in Diabetes

Increased urinary excretion of protein is a common finding in newly diagnosed diabetics of all ages (84–88). Proteinuria in diabetes has been recognized to consist of early microalbuminuria, which often progresses to overt clinically detectable proteinuria as glomerulosclerosis progresses. The early phase has been attributed to a loss of the electrostatic barrier of the glomerular filtration barrier during which there is slightly restrictive passage through the barrier of neutral dextran with small Einstein-Stokes radii associated with selective albuminuria but normal restriction of dextran particles with a larger radius (89); whereas in advanced nephropathy, when both urinary excretion of IgG and albumin are increased, large pore equivalents in the barrier are found with decreased passage of small dextran particles and increased passage of large radii dextran particles (90). Since the concept of pores in the glomerular filtration apparatus has yet to be proven by other than clearance techniques these conclusions must be considered as tentative. However, it remains useful in explaining the distinction between microalbuminuria and selective albuminuria vs the nonselective proteinuria accompanying advanced diabetic nephropathy.

Regardless of the specific etiology of proteinuria in diabetes, there is strong evidence that suggests an association of increased urinary albumin excretion with relatively poor metabolic control of the diabetic state (88, 91–94). However, in contrast with relatively early nephropathy, in advanced nephropathy no correlation has been found between the level of glycosylated hemoglobin ($HgBA_{1c}$) and proteinuria (94).

The question of the effects of intensive insulin management of diabetics on reversal of proteinuria remains controversial. Short-term correction of the metabolic derangement does correct increased microalbuminuria (93, 95–97). However, the results of long-term studies (6 months or longer) of intensive insulin therapy have yielded less optimistic and inconsistent results. Thus, in one study in which continuous subcutaneous insulin infusion for 6 months led to improvement in retinopathy, there was only minimal decrease in urinary albumin excretion, whereas the conventionally treated patients had marked increases in urinary albumin excretion (98). It has been suggested that precise glycemic control may not influence microalbuminuria when the patients are relatively well controlled at entry into the study, whereas patients with poor control may, with maximal glycemic managment, have a significant decrease in urinary albumin (99). Patients managed with tight control for 1 to 2 years, who already had diabetic nephropathy at the time of entry into the study, had ony a transient improvement in proteinuria that was not sustained (100).

What becomes obvious from the pathological studies cited earlier (21) and from the studies of the effects of insulin therapy on early vs established diabetic glomerulopathy is that once glomerular disease is well established, there may have occurred sufficient structural damage to prevent repair and that functional aberrations will persist. Whether or not institution of optimal insulin therapy at that time will prevent further deterioration is problematic, since it may be impossible to prevent progressive deterioration beyond some defined point. It has been suggested (71) that advanced mesangial expansion through the associated decrease in filtration surface, triggers adaptive physiological mechanisms that parallel those in the remnant kidney model of progressive nephron injury (37, 40, 100). This hypothesis suggests that once these adaptive changes are well established, the progression of glomerular injury is largely programmed and is independent of the diabetic state. Thus, as mentioned above, tight glycemic control may be ineffective once clinical nephropathy, overt proteinuria, hypertension, and decreased GFR are present. On the other hand careful treatment of hypertension at this stage of disease does slow (but does not stop) the progression to uremia (102).

Many difficult questions remain. How does one predict the risk of nephropathy? Although retrospective studies suggest that microalbuminuria predicts risk (103–105), this issue cannot be closed since we have failed to find any relationship between albuminuria and nephropathy (106). Thus there are patients with relatively advanced diabetic lesions and no albuminuria, as well as patients with microalbuminuria who despite 2 decades of diabetes have only minimal lesions. Will the prediction of risk allow prevention of progressive renal complications? Currently only glimpses of an answer can be perceived. Our preliminary findings (unpublished observations) suggest that early lesions can be reversed within 1 or 2 years following successful pancreatic transplantation in diabetic patients, whereas more advanced lesions show no such amelioration in the same time frame. This and the other studies described argue that early intervention may be important if the progression to

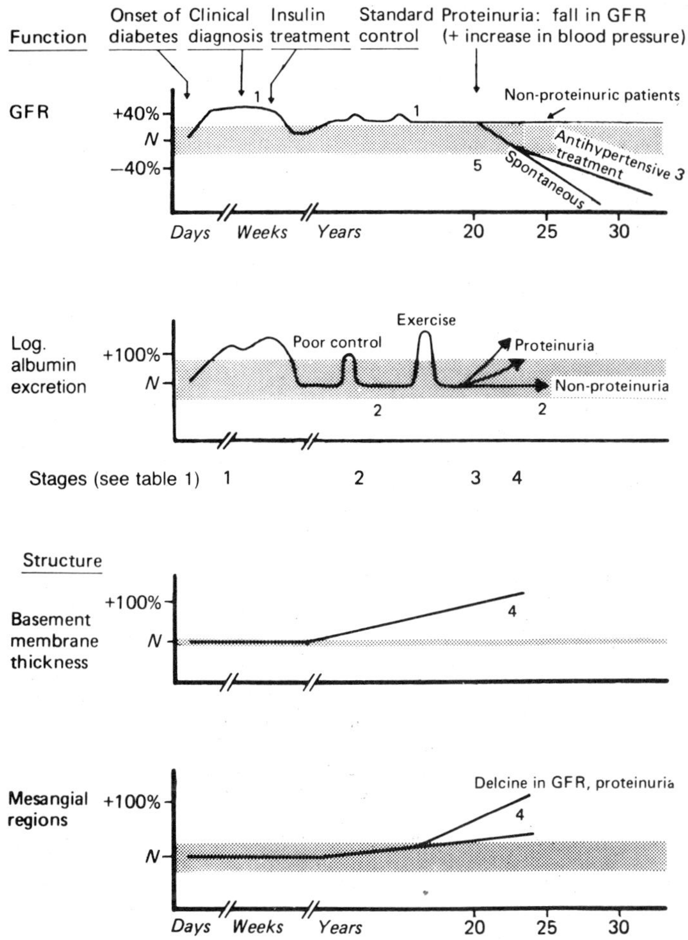

Figure 28D. 3. Chronology of renal changes in diabetes mellitus.

Table 28D.2.
The Kidney in Human Diabetes

Chronology or stages	Time to develop	Main features	Methods	Reversible or arrestable by strict glycemic control
Very early renal involvement Diabetic kidney lesions	Days or weeks, still present after many years when control imperfect >2 years, progression with time	Kidney hypertrophy—hyperfunction exercise—microalbuminuria[a]	Renal function test, morphometry and roentgenographic methods Renal biopsy	Reversible Stage I changes at least partially reverible; stage 2 probably not
Clinical incipient nephropathy	10 to 15 years (with great variation)	Slight or intermittent proteinuria and incipient blood pressure increase Aggravation during exercise[a]	Close clinical and laboratory observations; exercise provocation test	Studies in progress
Long-term diabetic nephropathy (a clinical diagnosis)	>10 to 20 years (with great variation)	Persistent proteinuria[b] and diabetes of long duration associated with a decline in GFR and hypertension	Close clinical and laboratory observation; renal function monitoring	Probably not arrestable, but studies are going on; ameliorated by antihypertensive treatment

[a] Different mechanisms likely to be operative in the early and in the late course.
[b] Exclude other causes in an atypical development.

uremia is to be avoided. Thus it seems prudent to continue to seek answers to those questions in carefully performed studies.

In the meantime, it is important to reemphasize that relatively conventional therapy, such as the treatment of hypertension, can effectively and beneficially influence the progression of nephropathy in long-term diabetics with proteinuria (102). Therefore, to prevent completion of the natural course of diabetic nephropathy in the potentially susceptible diabetic child (Table 28D.2) (Fig. 28D.3) (12), it seems reasonable to advise optimal diabetic and general clinical management of all diabetic patients with careful monitoring of the diabetic state per se, as well as of the function of the susceptible organs. In the case of the kidney, this includes annual creatinine clearance, quantitative urinary albumin testing by sensitive and accurate techniques, and regular monitoring of the blood pressure.

References

1. Rao TKKS, Hirsch S, Avram MM, et al: Prevalence of diabetic nephropathy in Brooklyn. In Friedman EA, L'Esperance FA Jr (eds): Diabetic Renal-Retinal Syndrome. New York, Grune and Stratton, 1980, p 205.
2. Knowles HC Jr, Guest GM, Lampe J, et al: The course of juvenile diabetes treated with unmeasured diet. Diabetes 14:239, 1965.
3. Deckert T, Poulsen JE, Larsen M: Prognosis of diabetes with diabetes onset before the age of thirty one. Diabetologia 14:363, 1978.
4. Pirart J: Diabetes mellitus and its degenerative complications: A prospective study of 4,400 patients observed between 1947 and 1973. Diabetes Care 1:168, 1978.
5. Jones RH, Mackay JD, Hayakawa H, et al: Progression of diabetic nephropathy. Lancet 1:1105, 1979.
6. Anderson AR, Anderson JK, Christiansen JS, et al: Prognosis for juvenile diabetics with nephropathy and failing renal function. Acta Med Scand 203:131, 1978.
7. Kussman MJ, Goldstein HH, Gleason RE: The clinical course of diabetic nephropathy. JAMA 236:1861, 1976.
8. Parving HH, Smidt VM, Friisberg B, et al: A prospective study of glomerular filtration rate and arterial blood pressure in insulin-dependent diabetics with diabetic nephropathy. Diabetologia 20:457, 1981.
9. Viberti GC, Jarrett RJ, Mahmud V, et al: Microalbuminuria as a predictor of clinical nephropathy in insulin-dependent diabetes mellitus. Lancet 1:1430, 1982.
10. Balodimos MC, Legg MA, Bradley RF: Diabetic glomerulosclerosis in children. Diabetes 20:622, 1971.
11. Mauer SM, Steffes MW, Brown DM: The kidney in diabetes. Am J Med 70:603, 1981.
12. Morgensen CE (editor): Diabetes mellitus and the kidney. Kidney Intl 21: 1982.
13. Brown DM, Andres GA, Hostetter TH, et al: Kidney complications. In Salans LB, Graham BJ (eds): Proceedings of a Task Force on Animals Appropriate for Studying Diabetes Mellitus and Its Complications. Diabetes 31(suppl 1):71, 1982.
14. Burkholder PM: Atlas of human glomerular pathology. Hagerstown, MD, Harper & Row, 1974, p 325.
15. Nakamoto Y, Takazakura E, Hayakawa H, et al: Intrarenal microaneurysms in diabetic nephropathy. Lab Invest 42:433, 1980.
16. Westberg NG, Michael AF: Immunohistopathology of diabetic glomerulosclerosis. Diabetes 21:163, 1972.
17. Miller K, Michael AF: Immunopathology of renal extracellular membranes in diabetes mellitus: specificity of tubular basement membrane immunofluorescence. Diabetes 25:701–708, 1976.
18. Chavers B, Etzwiler D, Michael AF: Albumin deposition in dermal capillary basement membrane in insulin-dependent diabetes mellitus. Diabetes 30:275, 1981.
19. Cohn RA, Mauer SM, Barbosa J, et al: Immunofluorescence studies of skeletal muscle extracellular membranes in diabetes mellitus. Lab Invest 39:13, 1978.
20. Michael AF, Brown DM: Increased concentration of albumin in kidney basement membranes in diabetes mellitus. Diabetes 30:843, 1981.
21. Mauer SM, Steffes MW, Sutherland DER, et al: Structuralfunctional relationships in diabetic nephropathy. J Clin Invest 74:1143, 1984.
22. Kimmelstiël P: Diabetic nephropathy. In Becker EL (ed): Structural Basis of Renal Disease. New York, Harper and Row, 1968, p 462.
23. Gundersen HJG, Osterby R: Glomerular size and structure in diabetes mellitus. II. Late abnormalities. Diabetologia 13:43, 1977.
24. Ellis EN, Steffes MW, Mauer SM: Relationship of glomerular structure to function in insulin dependent diabetes mellitus. Proc Am Soc Nephro 17:1112, 1984.
25. Bloodworth JMB Jr: Pathology of the diabetic kidney. In Friedman EA, L'Esperance FA Jr (eds): Diabetic Renal-Retinal Syndrome. New York, Grune and Stratton, 1980, p 159.
26. Mauer SM, Steffes MW, Sutherland DER, et al: Studies of the rate of regression of the glomerular lesions in diabetic rats treated with pancreatic islet transplantation. Diabetes 24:280, 1975.
27. Mauer SM, Brown DM, Matas AJ, et al: Effects of pancreatic islet transplantation on the increased urinary albumin excretion rates in intact and uninephrectomized rats with diabetes mellitus. Diabetes 27:959, 1978.
28. Steffes MW, Brown DM, Basgen JM, et al: Glomerular basement membrane thickness following islet transplantation in the diabetic rat. Lab Invest 41:116, 1979.
29. Verdonk CA, Palumbo PJ, Gharib H, et al: Diabetic microangiopathy in patients with pancreatic diabetes mellitus. Diabetologia 11:395, 1975.
30. Wellmann KR, Volk BW: Nodular intercapillary glomerulosclerosis in diabetes secondary to chronic calcific pancreatitis. Diabetes 25:713, 1976.
31. Mauer SM, Barbosa J, Vernier RL, et al: Immunopathology of renal extracellular membranes in kidneys transplanted into patients with diabetes mellitus. Diabetes 25:709, 1976.
32. Lee CS, Mauer SM, Brown DM, et al: Renal transplantation in diabetes mellitus in rats. J Exp Med 139:793, 1974.
33. Osterby R: Early phases in the development of diabetic glomerulosclerosis. Acta Med Scand 574(suppl):1, 1975.
34. Morgensen CE, Osterby R, Gunderson HJG: Early function and morphologic vascular renal consequences of the diabetic state. Diabetologia 17:71, 1979.
35. Christiansen JS, Gammelgaard J, Tronier B, et al: Kidney function and size in diabetics before and during initial insulin treatment. Kidney Intl 21:683, 1982.
36. Mogensen CE, Christensen NJ, Gunderson HJG: The acute effect of insulin on renal hemodynamics and protein excretion in diabetics. Diabetologia 15:153, 1978.
37. Hostetter TH, Troy JL, Brenner BM: Glomerular hemodynamics and experimental diabetes. Kidney Intl 19:410, 1981.
38. Michels LD, Davidman M, Keane WF: Determinants of glomerular filtration and plasma flow in experimental diabetic rats. J Lab Clin Med 98:869, 1981.
39. Brochner-Mortensen J, Ditzel J: Glomerular filtration rate and extracellular fluid volume in insulin dependent patients with diabetes mellitus. Kidney Intl 2:696, 1982.
40. Hostetter TH, Remke HG, Brenner BM: The case for intrarenal hypertension in the initiation and progression of diabetic and other glomerulopathies. Am J Med 72:375, 1982.
41. Berkman J, Rifkin H: Unilateral nodular diabetic glomerulosclerosis (Kimmelstiel-Wilson). Metabolism 22:715, 1973.
42. Mauer SM, Steffes MW, Azar S, et al: The effect of Goldblatt hypertension on the development of glomerular lesions of diabetes mellitus in the rat. Diabetes 27:738, 1978.
43. Brown DM, Steffes MW, Thibert P, et al: Glomerular manifestations of diabetes in the BB/Wistar rat. Metabolism 32:131, 1983.
44. Azar S, Weller D: Autoregulation of renal blood flow in the diabetic pancreatectomized rat. Eighth International Congress of Nephrology. Athens, 1981, p 18.
45. Christlieb AR, Kaldany A, D'Elia JA, et al: Aldosterone responsiveness in patients with diabetes mellitus. Diabetes 27:732, 1978.
46. Christlieb AR, Munichoodappa C, Braaten JT: Decreased response of plasma renin activity to orthostasis in diabetic patients with orthostatic hypotension. Diabetes 23:835, 1974.
47. Christlieb AR, Long R: Renin-angiotensin system in phlorozin compared with alloxan diabetes in the rat. Diabetes 28:106, 1979.
48. Brown DM, Gerrard JM, Peller J, et al: Glomerular prostaglandin metabolism in diabetic rats. Diabetes 29:219A, 1980.
49. Gerrard JM, Stuart MJ, Rao GHR, et al: Alteration in the balance of prostaglandin and thromboxane synthesis in diabetic rats. J Lab Clin Med 95:950, 1980.
50. Harrison HE, Reece AH, Johnson M: Decreased vascular prostacyclin in experimental diabetes. Life Sci 23:351, 1978.
51. Ziboh VA, Maruta H, Lord J, Cagle WD, et al: Increased biosynthesis of thromboxane A_2 by diabetic platelets. Eur J Clin Invest 9:223, 1979.
52. Johnson M, Harrison HE, Raftery AT, et al: Vascular prostacyclin may be reduced in diabetes in man. Lancet 1:325, 1979.
53. Osborne MJ, Droz B, Meyer P, et al: Angiotensin II: Renal localization in glomerular mesangial cells by autoradiography. Kidney Intl 8:245, 1975.
54. Barajas L, Mueller J: The innervation of the juxtaglomerular apparatus and the surrounding tubules: a quantitative analysis by serial section electron microscopy. J Ultrastruct Res 43:107, 1973.
55. Kreisberg JI: Insulin requirement for contraction of cultured rat glomerular mesangial cells in response to angiotensin II. Possible role for insulin in modulating glomerular hemodynamics. Proc Nat Acad Sci 70:4190, 1982.
56. Ballerman BJ, Dzau VJ, Skorecki KL, et al: Altered glomerular angiotensin II receptor modulation in untreated diabetic rats. Proc Amer Soc Nephrol 15:179A, 1982

57. Scheinman JI, Fish AJ, Matas AJ, et al: The immunohistopathology of glomerular antigens. The glomerular basement membrane, collagen and actomyosin antigens in normal and diseased kidneys. J Clin Invest 54:1144, 1974.
58. Scheinman JI, Steffes MW, Brown DM, et al: The immunhistopathology of glomerular antigens. III. Increased mesangial actomyosin in experimental diabetes in the rat. Diabetes 27:632, 1978.
59. Mauer SM, Fish AJ, Day NK, et al: The glomerular mesangium. II. Quantitative studies of mesangial function in nephrotoxic nephritis in rats. J Clin Invest 53:431, 1974.
60. Mauer SM, Steffes MW, Chern M, et al: Mesangial uptake and processing of macromolecules in rats with diabetes mellitus. Lab Invest 41:401, 1979.
61. Bower G, Brown DM, Steffes MW, et al: Studies of the glomerular mesangium and the juxtaglomerular apparatus in the genetically diabetic mouse. Lab Invest 43:333, 1980.
62. Spiro RG, Spiro MJ: Effect of diabetes on the biosynthesis of renal glomerular basement membrane. Studies on the glucosyltransferase. Diabetes 20:641, 1971.
63. Cohen MP, Surma ML, Wu V-Y: In vivo biosynthesis and turnover of glomerular basement membrane in diabetic rats. Am J Physiol 242:F385, 1982.
64. Houser MT, Scheinman JI, Basgen J, et al: Preservation of mesangium and immunohistochemically defined antigens in glomerular basement membrane isolated by detergent extraction. J Clin Invest 69:1169, 1982.
65. Cerami A, Stevens VJ, Monnier VW: Role of non-enzymatic glycosylation in the development of the sequelae of diabetes mellitus. Metabolism 28:431–437, 1979.
66. Cohen MP, Urdaniva E, Surma M, et al: Increased glycosylation of glomerular basement membrane collagen in diabetes. Biochem Biophys Res Commun 95:765, 1980.
67. McVerry BA, Hopp A, Fischer C, et al: Production of pseudodiabetic renal glomerular changes in mice after repeated injection of glycosylated proteins. Lancet 1:738, 1980.
68. Jeraj KP, Michael AF, Mauer SM, et al: Glucosylated and normal human or rat albumin do not bind to renal basement membranes of diabetic and control rats. Diabetes 32:380, 1983.
69. Scheinman JI, Foidart JM, Gehron-Robey P, et al: The immunohistology of glomerular antigens. IV. Laminin, a defined non-collagen basement membrane glycoprotein. Clin Immunol Immunopathol 15:175, 1980.
70. Scheinman JI, Fish AJ, Matas AJ, et al: The immunohistology of glomerular antigens. II. The glomerular basement membrane actomyosin and fibroblast surface antigens in normal, diseased and transplanted kidneys. Am J Pathol 90:71, 1978.
71. Chung AE, Jaffe R, Freeman IL, et al: Properties of a basement membrane-related glycoprotein synthesized in culture by a mouse embryonal carcinoma-derived cell line. Cell 16:277, 1979.
72. Kanwar YS, Farquhar MG: Heparan sulfate: presence in glomerular basement membrane. Proc Nat Acad Sci 76:1303, 1979.
73. Kanwar YS, Farquhar MG: Glycosaminoglycans (heparan sulfate): isolation from glomerular basement membranes. Proc Nat Acad Sci 76:4493, 1979.
74. Parthasarathy N, Spiro RG: Characterization of the glycosaminoglycan component of the renal glomerular basement membrane and its relationship to the peptide portion. J Biol Chem 256:507, 1981.
75. Vernier RL: Personal communication.
76. Nevins TE, Michael AF: Isolation of anionic sialoproteins from rat glomerulus. Kidney Intl 19:553, 1981.
77. Kanwar YS, Rosenzweig LJ, Kerjaschki DI: Glycosaminoglycans of the glomerular basement membrane in normal and nephrotic states. In Berlyne GM, Thomas S (eds): Renal Physiology. Basel, S. Karger Publishers, 1981, p 121.
78. Parthasarathy N, Spiro RG: Effects of diabetes on the glycosaminoglycan component of the human glomerular basement membrane. Diabetes 31:738, 1982.
79. Brown DM, Klein DJ, Michael AF, et al: ^{35}S-glycosaminoglycan and ^{35}S-glycopeptide metabolism by diabetic glomeruli and aorta. Diabetes 31:418, 1982.
80. Klein DJ: Personal communication.
81. Westberg NG, Michael AF: Human glomerular basement membrane: chemical composition in diabetes mellitus. Acta Med Scand 174:39, 1973.
82. Michael AF: Personal communication.
83. Gotzsche O, Gundersen HJG, Osterby R: Irreversibility of glomerular basement membrane accumulation despite reversibility of renal hypertrophy with islet transplantation in early experimental diabetes. Diabetes 30:481–485, 1981.
84. Brochner-Mortensen J, Ditzel J, Mogensen CE, et al: Microvascular permeability to albumin and glomerular filtration rate in diabetic and normal children. Diabetologia 16:307, 1979.
85. Mogensen CE: Urinary albumin excretion in early and long-term juvenile diabetics. Scand J Clin Lab Invest 28:183, 1971.
86. Morgensen CE, Vittinghus E: Urinary albumin excretion during exercise in juvenile diabetes. Scand J Clin Lab Invest 35:295, 1975.
87. Balodimos MC, Chlonverakis C, Gleason RE, et al: Urinary albumin excretion in the offspring of conjugal diabetics. Lancet 2:239, 1971.
88. Aronoff SL, Schnider S, Smeltzer J, et al: Urinary excretion and renal clearance of specific plasma proteins in diabetics of short and long duration. Diabetes 30:656, 1981.
89. Myers BD, Winetz JA, Chui F, et al: Mechanisms of proteinuria in diabetic nephropathy: A study of glomerular barrier function. Kidney Intl 21:633, 1982.
90. Winetz JA, Golbetz HV, Spencer RL, et al: Glomerular function in advanced human diabetic nephropathy. Kidney Intl 21:750, 1982.
91. Pettitt DJ, Lisse JR, Knowler WC, et al: Development of retinopathy and proteinuria in relation to plasma glucose concentrations in Pima Indians. Lancet 2:1050, 1980.
92. Parving H-H, Noer I, Deckert T, et al: The effect of metabolic regulation on microvascular permeability to small and large molecules in short-term juvenile diabetics. Diabetologia 12:161, 1976.
93. Viberti GC, Pickup JC, Jarrett RJ, et al: Effect of control of blood glucose on urinary excretion of albumin and 2-microglobulin in insulin-dependent diabetics. N Engl J Med 300:638, 1979.
94. Viberti GC, Macintosh D, Bilous RW, et al: Proteinuria in diabetes mellitus: Role of spontaneous and experimental variation of glycemia. Kidney Intl 21:714, 1982.
95. Christiansen JS, Frandsen M, Parving H-H: The effect of intravenous insulin infusion on kidney function in insulin-dependent diabetes mellitus. Diabetologia 20:199, 1981.
96. Viberti G, Pickup JC, Bilous RW, et al: Correction of exercise-induced microalbuminuria in insulin-dependent diabetics after 3 weeks of subcutaneous insulin infusion. Diabetes 30:818, 1981.
97. Vittinghus E, Mogensen CE: Graded exercise and protein excretion in diabetic man and the effect of insulin treatment. Kidney Intl 21:725, 1982.
98. Steno Study Group. Effect of 6 months of strict metabolic control of eye and kidney function in insulin-dependent diabetics with background retinopathy. Lancet 1:121, 1982.
99. Mogensen CE: Personal communication.
100. Tamborlane WV, Puklin JE, Bergman M, et al: Long-term improvement of metabolic control with the insulin pump does not reverse diabetic microangiography. Diabetes Care 5(suppl 1):58, 1982.
101. Hostetter TH, Olson JL, Rennke HG, et al: Hyperfiltration in remnant nephrons: A potentially adverse response to renal ablation. Am J Physiol 241:F85, 1981.
102. Mogensen CE: Progression of nephropathy in long-term diabetics with proteinuria and effect of initial anti-hypertensive treatment. Scand J Clin Lab Invest 36:383, 1976.
103. Parving H-H, Oxinbohl B, Svendsen PA, et al: Early detection of patients at risk of developing diabetic nephropathy. A longitudinal study of urinary albumin excretion. Acta Endocrinol (Copenhagen) 100:500, 1982.
104. Viberti GC, Jarrett RJ, Mahmud U, et al: Microalbuminuria as a predictor of clinical nephropathy in insulin dependent diabetes. Lancet 1:1430, 1982.
105. Mogensen CE, Christensen CK: Predicting diabetic nephropathy in insulin-dependent patients. N Engl J Med 311:89, 1984.
106. Chavers BC, Ellis E, Steffes MW, et al: Relationship of urinary albumin to glomerular structure in insulin dependent diabetes mellitus. Proc Am Soc Nephrol 17:37A, 1984.

28E Rheumatic Diseases

LAURIE C. MILLER
ROBERT L. VERNIER

With the exception of systemic lupus erythematosus (SLE) (chapter 28B), and systemic vasculitis (polyarteritis) (chapter 28C), rheumatic diseases do not prominently affect the kidney in childhood. However, renal disease may complicate juvenile rheumatoid arthritis (JRA), mixed connective tissue disease (MCTD), scleroderma, and dermatomyositis in childhood. Awareness of the renal manifestations of these diseases, as well as the potential nephrotoxicity of current drug treatments, is necessary when confronted with the child with a rheumatic disease complicated by hematuria, proteinuria, or renal insufficiency. In this circumstance it is also necessary to rule out evolution of the underlying rheumatic disease into SLE, vasculitis, or other overlap syndromes in which renal involvement may be life-threatening. Such transitions have been seen for all the rheumatic diseases of childhood. Children with rheumatic disease, especially if receiving nephrotoxic agents, should be regularly monitored for the development of hypertension, abnormal urinary sediment, renal insufficiency, and changing serology.

In this review we will discuss the major renal manifestations found in children with rheumatic diseases and the recognized renal complications occurring secondary to drug therapies commonly used in the management of these patients.

THE KIDNEY AND JUVENILE RHEUMATOID ARTHRITIS

Clinical renal abnormalities, including hematuria, proteinuria, abnormal urine sediment, decreased renal function, and hypertension are relatively common in children with juvenile rheumatoid arthritis (JRA). However, since virtually all patients with this chronic disease receive therapy with drugs that have potential nephrotoxicity, the incidence of primary renal disease in JRA is difficult to establish. Although primary renal disease is believed to be more common in patients with extraarticular manifestations, such as fever, rash, carditis, and vasculitis, these children usually receive more intensive drug treatment, making the distinction of primary from secondary renal involvement difficult. However, renal disease is especially important as it is the cause of death in as many as 40% to 50% of all children dying with JRA (1–4).

CLINICAL RENAL ABNORMALITIES

An early clinical study of 638 patients with JRA (5) noted persistent renal abnormalities in 47 children (7.4%). The majority had received drug therapy, including gold and corticosteroids. Proteinuria was the most frequent abnormality (43/47, including 9 with nephrotic syndrome); hematuria, leukocyturia, and casts were also seen. Diminished creatinine clearance was found in 23%; hypertension was found in 21% of the 47 children.

In a longitudinal study of 165 patients with JRA (6), urinalysis and renal function tests were done at presentation and at 2 to 3 month intervals (Table 28E.1). Proteinuria was found at some time during the course of 70 children, but was persistent in only 4. No patient became nephrotic. Proteinuria was noted in nine children before the institution of any drug therapy. Hematuria was found in 38 patients, but was persistent in only 7. Urinary tract infections were relatively common in girls in this study as described earlier (5). Reduced clearances were noted in 10% of patients; elevated clearance (>147 ml/min/1.73 M^2) were found in 30%, especially during periods of active disease. Hypertension was present early in the course of some children; 30% had hypertension at some time during the study. Although corticosteroids undoubtedly contribute to the hypertension described in JRA, only 20% of the patients with hypertension in this series received these drugs.

This study also found an association of renal manifestations with serological abnormalities and with therapy. Proteinuria was found more frequently in patients with antinuclear antibody ($p < .01$) or serum cryoprecipitates ($p < .001$). Treatment appeared to increase the fre-

Table 28E.1.
Common Renal Abnormalities Observed in 165 Children With Juvenile Rheumatoid Arthritis Followed Longitudinally

Abnormality	Percent
Proteinuria	
At sometime	42
Persistent	2
Prior to drug therapy	5
Hematuria	
At sometime	23
Persistent	4
Hypertension	
At sometime	30
Associated with steroid therapy	20
Renal function	
Reduced Ccr[a]: ≤80 ml/min/1.73 M^2	10
Increased Ccr: ≥147 ml/min/1.73 M^2	30
Urinary tract infection	
Females	21
Males	2

Adapted from Anttila R: Acta Paed Scand 227(suppl): 7, 1972.
[a] Ccr, Creatinine clearance.

quency of proteinuria, which was found in 29 of the 53 patients treated with gold and in about 25% of those treated with antimalarials, steroids, phenylbutazone, or salicylates.

Recent work has suggested that there may be an increased risk of hypercalciuria and hematuria in patients with JRA (7). Although most patients had systemic onset JRA, this complication is probably unrelated to the severity of the arthritis or drug therapies. The possible contributions of immobilization or periarticular bone resorption to the hypercalciuria has not been fully assessed.

KIDNEY PATHOLOGY

Few studies of the renal pathology in JRA are available, since biopsy specimens have been obtained primarily in those children with more significant clinical findings. Kidney tissue was examined in only 15 of the 638 patients with JRA (5), as discussed. Renal amyloid was the most common lesion found (10 patients), but glomerulonephritis, pyelonephritis, and nephrosclerosis were also seen. Renal biopsy or autopsy specimens were examined in 60 of the 165 children followed longitudinally (6), and significant pathology was noted in 23 patients (38%). Since only two patients had not received potentially nephrotoxic drugs, the difficulty of distinguishing primary from secondary renal injury is again raised. Glomerular abnormalities, consisting of focal mesangial proliferation, isolated glomerular basement membrane thickening, sclerosis, or capsular adhesions were noted in 17 biopsies. Tubulointerstitial disease, including tubular atrophy, interstitial fibrosis, and round cell infiltrates, were found in 16 biopsies. Vascular amyloid, without glomerular involvement, was seen in two specimens.

This report also confirms the association of abnormal serology with an increased incidence of renal disease as 50% of patients with histological abnormalities had hypergammaglobulinemia, and 34% had either antinuclear antibodies or cryoprecipitates. Since pathological lesions were less common in patients with extraarticular symptoms than in patients with only joint disease, this author did not feel that the histological abnormalities reflected unrecognized overlap syndromes. Other pathological abnormalities, including membranous, focal proliferative, or crescentic glomerulonephritis, glomerular sclerosis, and renal vascular disease (8–13), have been reported in adults with rheumatoid arthritis, presumably unrelated to drug therapy.

AMYLOIDOSIS

As indicated by the preceding general review of the renal pathology found in patients with JRA, amyloidosis is an uncommon but important lesion. With the eradication of tuberculosis and chronic osteomyelitis in the Western world, JRA has become the most common cause of secondary amyloidosis in children (14), although a curious disparity in geographical distribution exists (15). Anttila (6) summarized reports concerning 91 deaths occurring among 1664 JRA patients. Thirty-five of the deaths were a result of renal failure, and amyloidosis was the lesion in 24 patients (68%).

Amyloidosis usually occurs after many years of severe disease, although it has been reported as early as 18 months after onset of JRA (16, 17). A large English series reported an incidence of 4.3% after 10 years and 6.4% after 15 years of follow-up (18). All patients had proteinuria with normal renal function and half had hepatosplenomegaly; hypertension was uncommon. Seven of 21 deaths in this series were a result of amyloid. In a series of 230 JRA patients from Argentina (19) followed for 12 years, 5 patients developed renal amyloidosis and 4 had nephrotic syndrome. Renal vein thrombosis is another well-documented complication of renal amyloidosis (20). Confirmation of the diagnosis of renal amyloid usually requires thioflavin-T staining of biopsy material, however one report (21) suggests renal ultrasound may be helpful.

COMPLICATIONS OF THERAPY

Nonsteroidal Antiinflammatory Drugs

Increased use of nonsteroidal antiinflammatory drugs (NSAID) for adults with rheumatological disorders has been followed by widespread use of these agents in children. These agents inhibit the conversion of arachidonic acid to prostaglandins by inhibition of the enzyme cyclo-oxygenase, either by direct acetylation and permanent inactivation (aspirin compounds) or by interference with oxygen incorporation and reversible inhibition (other NSAID) (22). In neither case is the inhibition complete, as prostaglandin metabolites may still be measured in the urine. The adverse clinical reactions to cyclo-oxygenase inhibition may be broadly grouped into vascular, metabolic, and immunological categories.

The two major prostaglandins produced in the kidney are PGE_2 (cortex and medulla) and PGI_2 (cortex and endothelium) (23). Both act as vasodilators. Their synthesis is increased in states of relative or actual volume depletion, such as hypovolemia, diuretic therapy, or high circulating levels of catecholamines, angiotensin, bradykinin, or vasopressin. Although prostaglandins normally contribute little to renal blood flow regulation, they play a critical role in maintaining intrarenal blood flow in volume-compromised patients. Thus, patients with nephrotic syndrome, cirrhosis, congestive heart failure, and various other renal diseases are at risk for the development of reversible azotemia or acute oliguric renal failure when treated with NSAID (24–25). The rare occurrence of papillary necrosis may result from ischemia of the collecting system (26). Of all the NSAID, sulindac appears to have the least effect on renal blood flow (27, 28).

The metabolic effects of NSAID on the kidney include antagonism of prostaglandin-mediated natriuresis, diuresis, and kaliuresis. The salt and water effects may result from inhibition of prostaglandin-mediated vasodilation in the hypertonic medulla, thus decreasing passive sodium and water reabsorption. There may be additional direct tubular effects as well, and there is some evidence to suggest that prostaglandins partially antagonize antidiuretic hormone. The effects on potassium are mediated through the renin-aldosterone pathways thus explaining the utility of NSAID in Bartter's syndrome. A few case reports have described the occurrence of isolated edema or hyperkalemia (29–31); however, these effects are rare.

The more curious nephrotoxic reactions to NSAID may be immunological in nature. These include both glomerular and interstitial diseases that present as nephrotic syndrome, acute renal failure (ARF), interstitial nephritis, alone or in combination. These reactions have not yet been described in children. In a review of 36 adult patients (32) with these complications, 4 were nephrotic, 26 had ARF and nephrotic range proteinuria, and 6 had ARF without proteinuria. Renal biopsies or the presence of systemic signs of hypersensitivity appeared to rule out ischemic injury alone as a cause for the ARF. Eleven percent of these patients required dialysis, 34/36 recovered adequate renal function with and without steroid treatment. Other investigators have analyzed the prominent lymphocytic interstitial infiltrate in renal biopsy specimens from similar patients and have reported a preponderance of cytotoxic T cells (33, 34). The delayed onset of this syndrome after drug exposure and the lymphocytic interstitial infiltrate suggest that a delayed type hypersensitivity may play a role in the pathogenesis of this syndrome. Alternatively, increased synthesis of leukotrienes and other products of the lipoxygenase pathway may contribute to this syndrome.

Not to be confused with the proteinuria resulting from other drug treatment is the pseudoproteinuria described with tolmetin (35). When measured by acid precipitation methods, urinary protein measurements in the nephrotic range have been reported in patients receiving tolmetin. Recognition of this entity ("dipsticks tests" for albumin are negative) is important to spare the patient unnecessary investigation.

Salicylates

Salicylates (ASA) have been the mainstay of antiarthritis therapy since antiquity. Serious nephrotoxic effects are exceedingly rare considering the number of patients ingesting high-dose aspirin for years. Forty-six patients with arthritis followed 13 to 38 years developed no evidence of renal compromise despite ingestion of 12 to 28 kg of aspirin (36, 37).

However, like the other NSAID, salicylates reduce glomerular filtration rate and renal blood flow, probably by inhibiting intrarenal prostaglandin synthesis. This effect is more marked in the presence of sodium restriction or underlying renal disease (38, 39). This reduction in blood flow may predispose to the development of renal papillary necrosis that has been reported to occur in JRA (40). However, all of the described patients received other drugs concurrently. Analgesic nephropathy is exceedingly rare in patients given aspirin alone. Other studies have shown that long term ASA administration can be associated with diminished concentrating ability (41), without defects in glomerular or other tubular functions. The most frequently seen renal aspirin effect is the marked shedding of tubular cells into the urine when aspirin therapy is begun (42). Proteinuria has been described in association with salicylate therapy alone (43).

Gold

Intramuscular gold is a widely used and effective treatment for JRA. Nephrotoxic reactions are one of the most frequent side effects for which treatment is discontinued. Clinically, nephrotoxicity may be seen as transient proteinuria (0% to 26%) (44–46), microhematuria (0% to 10%) (47–49), nephrotic syndrome (.2% to 2.6%) (44–46), interstitial nephritis, or tubular dysfunction, including ATN (53–55). These abnormalities usually remit upon withdrawal of the gold and often gold can safely be restarted (56). Proteinuria has occurred with both parenteral and oral gold administration (50, 57) and is usually unrelated to the total dose received, serum gold levels, or level of urinary gold excretion (45, 49). In several large studies, proteinuria was more frequent with parenteral than oral gold. Generally, the prognosis is good, with resolution of the proteinuria in 80% of patients in 1 to 2 years (58). Renal biopsy specimens from patients receiving gold who develop nephrotic syndrome, usually show membranous nephropathy, sometimes recognizable only with immunofluorescent or electron microscopy. Other lesions, including nil lesion, mild mesangial proliferation, focal sclerosis, nonspecific immune complex deposition, and chronic interstitial nephritis have been described (59, 60).

The amount of injected gold excreted by the kidneys is 70% to 80%. Gold is found in the cells of the proximal tubule shortly after injection and later in distal tubule, glomerular epithelium, interstitial macrophages and glomerular mesangium, in the latter location for as long as 28 years after the last injection (61). Experimental models using rats or rabbits have shown that therapeutic doses of gold can result in proteinuria and membranous glomerulopathy (62, 63). One investigator has reported that antibody to renal tubular antigen (α-RTE) can be eluted from the kidneys of experimental animals with gold-induced membranous GN (64) and that α-RTE may be found in the serum of patients with gold-induced proteinuria (65). These observations support the theory that this complication results from an autoimmune response to RTE antigen released from gold-damaged renal tubular cells.

Other genetic and immunological factors may contribute to the development of gold toxicity. Several studies report correlations between the presence of HLA B8 and DR3 and increased risk for nephrotoxic reactions to gold (66–70). A recent report correlates the occurrence of an increased risk with development of subnormal levels of serum IgA during gold therapy (71).

Penicillamine

Similar renal complications have been reported with the use of penicillamine. The racemic form (DL-penicillamine) was initially used, but now D-penicillamine is used since it is less nephrotoxic. Proteinuria occurs in as many as 30% of patients (72) and the nephrotic syndrome occurs more often than in gold-treated patients (16% to 17%) (72, 73). Both are more frequent with higher doses and usually resolve when dosage is lowered or the drug discontinued. Again, renal biopsy specimens usually demonstrate membranous nephropathy (74–76). Several studies question whether there is an increased risk for the development of proteinuria with penicillamine when the patient has previously had such a reaction to gold (77). As with this complication in gold treated patients, a genetic predisposition may exist as HLA DR3 and B8 antigens are also reportedly increased (66–70). It is also possible that the chelating effect of penicillamine may enhance tissue release of previously administered gold in these patients. A similar mechanism may operate in penicillamine-treated patients also taking iron, who may develop nephropathy when the iron is discontinued and penicillamine absorption is increased (78).

Other nephrotoxic reactions to penicillamine have been reported. Microhematuria is a more worrisome sign, as penicillamine has been associated with the development of SLE (79), Goodpasture's syndrome (80), and necrotizing vasculitis with rapidly progressive glomerular nephritis (81). However, a more benign spectrum of abnormalities was seen in a study of 31 penicillamine-treated patients with hematuria (82). Of these patients, 11 had urinary tract infections, 1 each had bleeding from prostatic veins, trigonitis, mesangial IgA nephropathy, and 14 had unknown causes of hematuria. Three of 4 biopsies showed minimal glomerular changes.

The presumed pathogenesis of the membranous glomerulopathy induced by penicillamine may be somewhat different from that which occurs with gold therapy. Penicillamine may not be directly nephrotoxic, but may act as a hapten, modifying tissue proteins to induce neoantigens. Perhaps this occurs with RTE antigen, giving rise to the formation of RTE antigen-antibody complexes and the development of membranous nephropathy (83, 84).

MIXED CONNECTIVE TISSUE DISEASE

MCTD is a syndrome characterized by overlapping clinical features of SLE, dermatomyositis, scleroderma, rheumatoid arthritis, and the serological presence of antibody (often in extremely high titers) to an RNAse-sensitive saline extractable nuclear antigen, ribonucleoprotein (RNP). Renal disease was initially thought to be an unusual feature of this syndrome, in fact, early reports suggested the possibility of a protective effect of RNP antibodies against the development of renal disease (85). Most series suggested that the most frequent clinical findings were arthritis, arthralgias, sclerodactyly, Raynaud's syndrome, lymphadenopathy, anemia, and esophageal dysmotility (86–88).

However, sporadic reports (89–94) documented the occurrence of renal disease in MCTD, most often membranous nephropathy but also mesangial proliferative glomerulonephritis and sclerodermatous changes. A review (95) 8 years after Sharp's initial report of 25 patients with MCTD revealed that 2/8 deaths were related to renal disease and that an additional surviving patient had developed proteinuria.

Singsen's report (96) of 14 children with MCTD suggested that renal disease occurred even more frequently in young patients. Five children in this report had clinical renal disease, including proteinuria >1gr/24hrs, hematuria, and renal insufficiency. Histological findings in 4 of these patients showed mild interstitial nephritis, hypercellular glomeruli, and thickened glomerular basement membranes. Two patients had membranous nephropathy. Autopsy specimens from 2 patients without clinical renal disease showed mesangial proliferation, tubulointerstitial disease, and vascular sclerosis. A follow-up study (97) reported 7/15 children with clinical or histologic renal disease including two children with end-stage renal disease.

Baldassare and associates (98) reported the occurrence of proteinuria with normal renal function in 2/5 MCTD patients, one with mild mesangial proliferative and one with membranous nephropathy. Similarly, a Swedish group (99) described the development of glomerulonephritis in 2/6 children with MCTD. Both children had also developed hypocomplementemia and anti-DNA antibodies. Biopsy specimens showed diffuse proliferative or membranoproliferative glomerulonephritis and both patients eventually developed renal failure. Although these two patients may represent transition of MCTD to SLE, hypocomplementemia may occur with MCTD and may be associated with an increased risk of renal disease. Overall, a review of 50 reported cases of MCTD in children suggests that 28% have renal disease, compared to the 8% incidence in adults (100).

SCLERODERMA

Generalized and focal scleroderma are rare conditions in childhood. The renal disease of scleroderma in adults is well-known, however, renal disease is infrequently described in affected children. Kass and coworkers (101) reported that 4/16 children with scleroderma developed proteinuria. One also developed hematuria and renal failure. A report of autopsy findings in 6 children with progressive systemic sclerosis describes renal involvement in four patients (102). Other series do not report significant renal disease, in spite of lengthy follow-ups (103–106). Perhaps this observation relates to the low frequency in children of the "risk factors" for development of scleroderma renal disease. These factors were identified among 60 adults with scleroderma renal crisis as early onset and rapid progression of skin thickening, anemia, pericardial effusion, and congestive heart failure (107).

However, subclinical disease may exist in children as it does in adults. D'Angelo and coworkers (108) described a significantly low fractional sodium excretion in eight normotensive, normoreninemic scleroderma patients with normal PAH and inulin clearances. They postulate that this abnormal sodium retention may inhibit renin release in spite of renal hypoperfusion.

Histological abnormalities may also be subclinical, since 66% of adult patients with generalized scleroderma without clinical evidence of renal disease had arteriolar changes compatible with scleroderma on renal biopsy (109). Similarly, two children without clinical renal disease were found to have extensive renal vascular sclerosis and interstitial fibrosis by biopsy or at autopsy (101).

Children should be monitored for the evolution of diagnostic signs of other connective tissue diseases, such as SLE or MCTD or the development of antibodies to DNA. Anti-DNA antibodies are the only autoantibodies for which good evidence of renal pathogenicity exists (110, 111). Typical scleroderma may develop immunological and clinical features of SLE (112, 113).

DERMATOMYOSITIS

Although childhood dermatomyositis may be considered as a necrotizing vasculitis, there is little to suggest that endothelial injury occurs in the kidney. However, scattered reports of various renal findings and pathological lesions are available. Sheard (114) reported proteinuria in 18/25 patients with dermatomyositis. Bradley and coworkers (115) described a 7 year old with proteinuria and progressive renal insufficiency complicating dermatomyositis. In a careful autopsy study of eight patients, Banker and Victor (116) reported tubular and glomerular calcium deposits with arteriolar fibrosis in one patient who clinically had hematuria and pyuria. Bitnum and coworkers (117) also reported proteinuria, hematuria, or pyuria in 7/13 patients with dermatomyositis. Renal biopsy specimens in those patients showed mesangial hypercellularity, basement membrane thickening, capsular adhesions, hyperplastic vessels, and interstitial fibrosis. A nine-year-old male developed nephrotic syndrome with membranous glomerular changes by biopsy in association with dermatomyositis (118). Six adults have been reported with renal disease associated with polymyositis; five had proteinuria, hematuria, and focal mesangial proliferation, one had nephrotic syndrome, renal insufficiency, and focal sclerosis on renal biopsy (119, 120). These authors describe decreased proteinuria with steroid therapy. One 13 year old with typical dermatomyositis is reported to have developed glomerulonephritis, renal vasculitis, and polyarteritis, five years after presentation (121, 122). In another report of 21 children with dermatomyositis, one had persistent isolated microhematuria, whereas 19/21 had temporarily low creatinine clearances (70ml/min./1.73m^2) during active disease (123). However, no renal disease was recognized in large series of patients from Ann Arbor [n = 41] (122), Stanford [n = 13] (124), or Minnesota [n = 39] (125), although one of our patients presented with typical dermatomyositis 1 month after classic acute poststreptococcal glomerulonephritis. Of all the childhood rheumatic diseases, dermatomyositis has the least renal involvement.

References

1. Laakonsen AL: Acta Paed Scand (suppl):166, 1966.
2. Sury B, Vesterdal E: Extra-articular lesions in juvenile rheumatoid arthritis. Acta Rheum Scand 14:309, 1968.
3. Ansell BM, Wood PH: Prognosis in juvenile chronic polyarthritis. Clin Rheum Dis 2:397, 1976.
4. Baum J, Gutowska G: Death in juvenile rheumatoid arthritis. Arth Rheum 20:2 (suppl), 253, 1977.
5. Anttila R, Laaksonen AL: Renal disease in juvenile rheumatoid arthritis. Acta Rheum Scand 15:99, 1969.
6. Anttila R: Renal involvement in juvenile rheumatoid arthritis. Acta Paed Scand 227 (suppl):7, 1972.
7. Stapleton FB, Hanissian AS, Miller LA: Hypercalciuria in children with juvenile rhuematoid arthritis: association with hematuria. J Pediatr. 107:235, 1985.
8. Pollak VE, Pirani CL, Steck IE: The kidney in rheumatoid arthritis: studies by renal biopsy. Arth Rheum 5:1, 1962.
9. Brun C, Steenolsen T, Raaschon F, et al: Renal biopsy in rheumatoid arthritis. Nephron 2:65, 1965.
10. Sellars L, Siamopoulos K, Wilkinson R, et al: Renal biopsy appearances in rheumatoid disease. Clin Nephrol 20:114, 1983.
11. Friedman R, Gallo G, Buxbaum J: Renal disease in rheumatoid arthritis. Arth Rheum 23:781, 1980.
12. Davis JA, Cohen AH, Weisbart R, et al: Glomerulonephritis in rheumatoid arthritis. Arth Rheum 22:1018, 1979.
13. Meyers AM, Lewin J, Kraut P, et al: Rheumatoid arthritis and glomerulonephritis (abstract). Kidney Intl 16:89, 1979.
14. Straus RG, Schubert WK, McAdams AJ: Amyloidosis in childhood. J Pediatr 74:272, 1969.
15. Filipowicz-Sosnowska AM, Baum J: The amyloidosis of juvenile rheumatoid arthritis. Scand J Rheum 9:24, 1980.
16. Buts JP, Cornu G, Maes M, et al: Nephrotic syndrome with early renal amyloidosis in juvenile rheumatoid arthritis. Acta Paed Belg 29.51, 1976.
17. Trainer E, Greifer I, Spitzer A: Amyloidosis in juvenile rheumatoid arthritis. NY State J Med 78:72, 1978.

18. Smith ME, Ansell BM, Bywaters EGL: Mortality and prognosis related to the amyloidosis of Still's Disease. Ann Rheum Dis 27:137, 1968.
19. Garcia-Morteo O, Hubscher O, Gagliardi S: Amyloidosis in juvenile rheumatoid arthritis. Arth Rheum 21:867, 1978.
20. Barclay GPT, Cameron H, Longhridge LW: Amyloid disease of the kidney and renal vein thrombosis. Quart J Med 29:137, 1960.
21. Subramanyam BR: Renal amyloidosis in juvenile rheumatoid arthritis: sonographic features. Am J Roentgen 136:411, 1981.
22. Lifschitz MD: Renal effects of non steroid anti-inflammatory agents. J Lab Clin Med 102:313, 1983.
23. Dunn MJ: Clinical effects of prostaglandins in renal disease. Hosp Pract Mar: 99, 1984.
24. Boyer TD, Zia P, Reynolds TB: Effect of indomethacin and prostaglandin A on renal function and plasma renin activity in alcoholic liver disease. Gastroenterology 77:215, 1979.
25. Walshe JJ, Venuto RC: Acute oligenic renal failure induced by indomethacin. Ann Int Med 91:47, 1979.
26. Allen RC, Petty RE, Lirenman DS, et al: Renal papillary necrosis in children with chronic arthritis. Am J Dis Child 140:20, 1986.
27. Bunning RD, Barth WF: Sulindac: a potentially renal-sparing non-steroidal anti-inflammatory drug. JAMA 248:2864, 1982.
28. Calin A: In common clinical usage nonsteroidal anti-inflammatory drugs infrequently produce adverse effects on the kidney. Am J Kidney Dis 2:485, 1983.
29. Wilkinson EL, Brown H: The effect of phenylbutazone on water and electrolyte excretion. Am J Med Sci 225:153, 1953.
30. Tam SY, Shapiro R, Franco R: Indomethacin-induced prostaglandin inhibition with hyperkalemia. Ann Int Med 90:783, 1979.
31. Bennett WM: The adverse renal effects of nonsteroidal anti-inflammatory drugs. Am J Kidney Dis 2:477, 1983.
32. Abraham PA, Keane WF: Glomerular and interstitial disease induced by nonsteroidal anti-inflammatory drugs. Am J Nephrol 4:1, 1984.
33. Finkelstein A, Fraley D, Stachura I, et al: Fenoprofen nephropathy: lipoid nephrosis and interstitial nephritis, a possible T-lymphocyte disorder. Am J Med 72:81, 1982.
34. Bender WL, Whelton A, Beschorner WE, et al: Interstitial nephritis, proteinuria, and renal failure caused by nonsteroidal anti-inflammatory drugs. Am J Med 76:1006, 1984.
35. Wellborne FR, Claypool RG, Copley JB: Nephrotic range pseudoproteinuria in a tolmetin-treated patient. Clin Nephrol 19:211, 1983.
36. Emkey RD, Mills JA: Aspirin and analgesic nephropathy. JAMA 247:55, 1982.
37. Akyol SM, Thompson M, Kerr DNS: Renal function after prolonged consumption of aspirin. Brit Med J 284:631, 1982.
38. Kimberly RP, Plotz PH: Aspirin-induced depression of renal function. N Engl J Med 296:418, 1977.
39. Muther RS, Potter DM, Bennett WM: Aspirin-induced depression of glomerular filtration rate in normal humans: role of sodium balance. Ann Int Med 94:317, 1981.
40. Wortmann DW, Kelsch RC, Kuhns L, et al: Renal papillary necrosis in juvenile rheumatoid arthritis. J Pediatr 97:37, 1980.
41. Burry HC, Dieppe PA, Bresnihan FB, et al: Salicylates and renal function in rheumatoid arthritis. Brit Med J 1:613, 1976.
42. Prescott LF: Effects of acetylsalicylic acid, phenacetin, paracetamol and caffeine on renal tubular epithelium. Lancet 11:91, 1965.
43. Scott RH, Hanzlik RJ: The salicylates: III. Salicylate albuminuria. JAMA 67:1838, 1916.
44. Cooperative Clinics Committee of the ARA: A controlled trial of gold salt therapy in rheumatoid arthritis. Arth Rheum 16:353, 1973.
45. Furst D, Levine S, Scinivasan R, et al: A double-blind trial of high versus conventional dosages of gold salts for rheumatoid arthritis. Arth Rheum 20:1473, 1977.
46. Kean WF, Anastassiades TP: Long term chrysotherapy. Arth Rheum 22:495, 1979.
47. Empire Rheumatism Council: Gold therapy in rheumatoid arthritis. Ann Rheum Dis 19:95, 1960.
48. White EG, Smith DH, Zaphiropoulous GC: Haematuria occurring during anti rheumatoid therapy. Brit J Rheum 23:57, 1984.
49. Silverberg DS, Kidd EG, Shnitka TK: Gold nephropathy. Arth Rheum 13:812, 1970.
50. Katz WA, Blodgett RC, Pietrusko R: Proteinuria in gold-treated rheumatoid arthritis. Ann Int Med 101:176, 1984.
51. Vaamonde CA, Hunt FR: The nephrotic syndrome as a complication of gold therapy. Arth Rheum 13:826, 1970.
52. Blum M, Liron M, Aviram A: Nephrotic syndrome with reversible severe renal failure after gold therapy. Int J Clin Pharm 22:562, 1984.
53. Cramer CR, Hagler HK, Silva FG, et al: Chronic interstitial nephritis associated with gold therapy. Arch Pathol Lab Med 107:258, 1983.
54. Iesato K, Mori Y, Ueda S, et al: Renal tubular dysfunction as a complication of gold therapy in patients with rheumatoid arthritis. Clin Neph 17(1):46, 1982.
55. Derot M, Kahn J, Mazalton A, et al: Nephrite anurique aigue mortelle apres traitement aurique, chrysocyanose associee. Bull Soc Med Hop de Paris 70:234, 1954.
56. Watanabe I, Whithier FC, Moore J, et al: Gold nephropathy. Arch Path Lab Med 100:632, 1976.
57. Horton JR: Comparative safety and efficacy of auranofin and parenteral gold compounds. Scand J Rheum (suppl)51:100, 1983.
58. Newton P, Sunborn WR, Swanson DR: Proteinuria with gold therapy: when should gold be permanently stopped? Brit J Rheum 22:11, 1983.
59. Francis KL, Jenis EH, Jensen GE, et al: Gold-associated nephropathy. Arch Path Lab Med March, 1984.
60. Cramer CR, Hagler HK, Silva FG, et al: Chronic interstitial nephritis associated with gold therapy. Arch Path Lab Med 107:258, 1983.
61. Brun C, Olsen S, Raaschou F, et al: The localization of gold in the human kidney following chrysotherapy. Nephron 1:265, 1964.
62. Nagi AH, Alexander F, Barbas AZ: Gold nephropathy in rats. Exp Molec Pathol 15:354, 1971.
63. Yarom R, Stein H, Peters PD, et al: Nephrotic effects of parenteral and intra-articular gold. Arch Pathol 99:36, 1975.
64. Veda S, Wakashin Y: Gold nephropathy in guinea pigs (abstract). Seventh Int Cong Nephrol (K5), 1978.
65. Palosuo T, Provost T, Milgrom F: Gold nephropathy: serologic data suggesting an immune complex disease. Clin Exp Imm 25:311, 1976.
66. Panayi GS, Wooley P, Batchelor JR: Genetic basis of rheumatoid disease. Brit Med J 2:1326, 1978.
67. Wooley P, Griffin J, Panayi GS, et al: HLA-DR antigens and toxic reaction to sodium aurothiomalate and D-penicillamine in patients with rheumatoid arthritis. NEJM 303:300, 1980.
68. Bardin T, Dryll A, Debyre N, et al: HLA system and side effects of gold salt and D-penicillamine treatment of rheumatoid arthritis. Ann Rheum Dis 41:599, 1982.
69. Speerstra F, Reekers P, Putle LBA, et al: HLA-DR antigens and proteinuria induced by aurothiglucose and D-penicillamine in patients with rheumatoid arthritis. J Rheum 10:948, 1983.
70. Ford P: HLA antigens and drug toxicity in rheumatoid arthritis. J Rheum 11:259, 1984.
71. Van Riel PL, Putte LB, Gribnau FW, et al: Serum IgA and gold-induced toxic effects in patients with rheumatoid arthritis. Arch Int Med 144:1401, 1984.
72. Hill HF: Treatment of rheumatoid arthritis with penicillamine. Sem Arth Rheum 6:361, 1977.
73. Kirby JD, Dieppe PA, Huskisson EL, et al: D-Penicillamine and immune complex deposition. Ann Rheum Dis 38:344, 1979.
74. Stein HB, Chalmers A, Schroeder ML, et al: Selected adverse reactions of D-penicillamine. Clin Invest Med 7:73, 1984.
75. Bacon PA, Tribe CR, MacKenzie JC: Penicillamine nephropathy in rheumatoid arthritis. Quart J Med 45:661, 1976.
76. Neild GH, Gartner HV, Bohle A: Penicillamine induced membranous glomerulonephritis. Scand J Rheum (Suppl) 28:79, 1979.
77. Smith PJ, Swinburn WR, Swinson DR, et al: Influence of previous gold toxicity on subsequent development of penicillamine toxicity. Brit Med J 285:595, 1982.
78. Harkness JAL, Blake DR: Penicillamine nephropathy and iron. Lancet 8312:1368, 1982.
79. Chalmers A, Thompson D, Stein HE, et al: Systemic lupus erythematosus during penicillamine therapy for rheumatoid arthritis. Ann Int Med 97:659, 1982.
80. Hill HF: Penicillamine in rheumatoid arthritis: adverse effects. Scand J Rheum (suppl)28:94, 1979.
81. Banfi G, Imbasciati E, Guerra L, et al: Extracapillary glomerulonephritis with necrotizing vasculitis in D-penicillamine treated rheumatoid arthritis. Nephron 33:56, 1983.
82. Barraclough D, Cunningham TJ, Muirden KD: Microscopic hematuria in patients with rheumatoid arthritis on D-penicillamine. Aust NZ J Med 11:706, 1981.
83. Jaffe IA: Penicillamine in rheumatoid arthritis: clinical, pharmacological and biochemical properties. Scand J Rheum (suppl)28:58, 1979.
84. Hall CL: Gold and penicillamine induced renal disease. In Bacon PA, Hadler NM, (eds): The Kidney and Rheumatic Disease. London, Butterworth Scientific, 1982, p 246.
85. Reichlin M, Mattioli M: Correlation of a precipitin reaction to an RNA protein antigen and a low prevalence of nephritis in patients with SLE. N Engl J Med 286:908, 1972.
86. Sharp GC, Irvin WS, Tan EM, et al: Mixed connective tissue disease—an apparently distinct rheumatic disease associated with a specific antibody to an extractable nuclear antigen (ENA). Am J Med 52:148, 1972.
87. Bennett RM, O'Connell DJ: Mixed connective tissue disease: a clinicopathologic study of 20 cases. Sem Arth Rheum 10:25, 1980.
88. Farber SJ, Bole GG: Antibodies to components of extractable nuclear antigen. Arch Int Med 136:425, 1976.
89. Rao KV, Berkseth RO, Crosson JT, et al: Immune-complex nephritis in mixed connective tissue disease (letter). Ann Int Med 84:174, 1976.

90. Fuller TJ, Richman AV, Averbach D, et al: Immune-complex glomerulonephritis in a patient with mixed connective tissue disease. Am J Med 62:761, 1977.
91. Bennett RM, Spargo BH: Immune complex nephropathy in mixed connective tissue disease. Am J Med 63:534, 1977.
92. Cohen IM, Swerdlin AH, Steinberg SM, et al: Mesangial proliferative glomerulonephritis in mixed connective tissue disease. Clin Neph 13:93, 1980.
93. Palferman TG, McIntosh CS, Kershaw M: Mixed connective tissue disease with associated glomerulonephritis and hypocomplementaemia. Postgrad Med J 56:177, 1980.
94. Manthorpe R, Elling H, vander Meulen J, et al: Two fatal cases of MCTD. Scand J Rheum 9:7, 1981.
95. Nimelstein SH, Brody S, McShane D, et al: Mixed connective tissue disease: a subsequent evaluation of the original 25 patients. Medicine 59:239, 1980.
96. Singsen BH, Bernstein BH, Kornreich HK, et al: Mixed connective tissue disease in childhood. J Pediatr 90:893, 1977.
97. Singsen BH, Swanson VL, Bernstein B, et al: A histologic evaluation of mixed connective tissue disease in childhood. Am J Med 68:710, 1980.
98. Baldassare A, Weiss T, Auclair R, et al: Mixed connective tissue disease in children (abstract). Arth Rheum 19:788, 1976.
99. Eberhardt K, Svantesson H, Svensson B: Followup of 6 children presenting with a MCTD-like syndrome. Scand J Rheum 10:62, 1981.
100. Oetgen WJ, Boice JA, Lawless OJ: Mixed connective tissue disease in children and adolescents. Pediatrics 67:333, 1981.
101. Kass H, Hanson V, Patrick J: Scleroderma in childhood. J Pediatr 62:243, 1966.
102. Kornreich HK, King KK, Bernstein BH, et al: Scleroderma in childhood. Arth Rheum 20 (suppl):343, 1977.
103. Dabich L, Sullivan DB, Cassidy JT: Scleroderma in the child. J Pediatr 85:770, 1974.
104. Cassidy JT, Sullivan DB, Dabich L, et al: Scleroderma in children. Arth Rheum 20 (suppl):351, 1977.
105. Goel KM, Shanks RM: Scleroderma in childhood. Arch Dis Childh 49:861, 1974.
106. Diaz-Perez JL, Connolly SM, Winkelmann RK: Disabling pansclerotic morphea of children. Arch Dermatol 116:169, 1980.
107. Steen VD, Medsger TA, Osial TA, et al: Factors predicting the development of renal involvement in progressive systemic sclerosis. Am J Med 76:779, 1984.
108. D'Angelo A, Messa P, Fiocco U, et al: Functional renal involvement in normotensive patients with progressive systemic sclerosis. Arth Rheum 24:8, 1981.
109. Kovalchik MT, Guggenheim SJ, Silverman MH, et al: The kidney in progressive systemic sclerosis. A prospective study. Ann Int Med 89:881, 1978.
110. Leon SA, Green A, Ehrlich GE, et al: Avidity of antibodies in SLE: relations to severity of renal involvement. Arth Rheum 20:23, 1977.
111. Winfield JB, Faiterman I, Koffler D: Avidity of anti-DNA antibodies in serum and glomerular eluates from patients with SLE: association of high-avidity anti-native DNA antibody with glomerulonephritis. J Clin Invest 59:90, 1977.
112. Mitchell AJ, Rusin LJ, Diaz LA: Circumscribed scleroderma with immunologic evidence of SLE. Arch Dermatol 116:169, 1980.
113. Cassidy JT, Sullivan DB, Dabich L, et al: Scleroderma in children. Arth Rheum 20 (suppl):351, 1977.
114. Sheard C: Dermatomyositis. Arch Int Med 88:640, 1951.
115. Bradley JE, Drake ME, Mack HP: Dermatomyositis with nephritis in a negro girl. Am J Dis Child 81:403, 1951.
116. Banker BQ, Victor M: Dermatomyositis (systemic angiopathy) of childhood. Medicine 45:261–289, 1966.
117. Bitnum S, Daeschner CW, Travis LB, et al: Dermatomyositis. J Pediatr 64:101, 1964.
118. Debauchez C, Bessiere M, Etienne M: Syndrome nephrotique associe a une dermatomyosite. Ann Pediat 20:153, 1973.
119. Moutsopoulos H, Fye KH: Lipoid nephrosis and focal glomerulosclerosis in a patient with polymyositis. Lancet 1:1039, 1975.
120. Dyck RF, Katz A, Gordon DA, et al: Glomerulonephritis associated with polymyositis. J Rheum 6:336, 1979.
121. Sullivan DB, Cassidy JT, Petty RE, et al: Prognosis in childhood dermatomyositis. J Pediatr 80:555, 1972.
122. Sullivan DB, Cassidy JT, Petty RE: Dermatomyositis in the pediatric patient. Arth Rheum 20(suppl):327, 1977.
123. Pachman LM, Cooke N: Juvenile dermatomyositis: a clinical and immunologic study. J Pediatr 96:226, 1980.
124. Miller JJ: Late progression in dermatomyositis in childhood. J Pediatr 83:543, 1973.
125. Miller LC, Michael AF: Clinical features and long-term follow-up of 39 children with dermatomyositis. Unpublished observations.

28F Lymphoid Malignancies

ROBERT L. LYNCH

Lymphoid malignancies may lead to metabolic derangements as a consequence of direct tumor effects, secondary consequences of acute renal failure, or complications of either direct antitumor therapy or supportive measures. Serious disturbances of these types are unusual; however, when they do occur, they are often life threatening. Because these conditions are generally preventable or manageable, it is essential that these unusual complications be considered in patients at risk.

FINDINGS AT PRESENTATION

Initial work-up of the lymphoma or leukemia patient may demonstrate unilateral or bilateral kidney enlargement. This can be a result of infiltrative or nodular disease (1); however, its presence does not necessarily mean compromise of renal function. Such renomegaly may be demonstrated by IVP or ultrasound. These studies may also demonstrate mechanical obstruction of the urinary tract as a result of extrinsic tumor mass or, even more rarely, a result of uric acid stone. The most common cause of functional compromise at presentation in patients with lymphoid malignancies is uric acid nephropathy. The level of serum uric acid associated with renal compromise is quite variable, though renal function is frequently minimal if the uric acid is above 20 mg/dl. The source of the urate appears to be nucleic acid catabolism associated with the tumor mass, and levels are often highest in those patients with extensive disease.

Uric acid is largely filtered at the glomerulus and both reabsorbed and secreted by the renal tubule (2). As the tubular fluid becomes more concentrated and more acidic, solubility of uric acid decreases. These changes in the presence of a high serum uric acid level may result in generalized urate deposition within the collecting tubules causing intrarenal obstruction (3).

Some patients may also present with extreme elevations of serum phosphate, particularly when some renal compromise is present. Although many patients tolerate elevated phosphates without direct evidence of toxicity, some may be more sensitive, as evidence does exist suggesting nephrotoxicity as a result of phosphate occurring in some patients (4).

It must also be kept in mind that many of these patients present having been ill for some time with poor nutrition and hydration. Therefore, prerenal azotemia must frequently be distinguished from intrinsic renal disease.

In addition to acute renal failure, metabolic disturbances unrelated to renal function may be present (5). In particular, hypercalcemia, hypoglycemia, and metabolic acidosis appear to be occasional consequences of direct metabolic activity of tumor cells. Hypercalcemia may result from ectopic PTH-like activity, local affects on bone, and disturbances in other humoral systems. Elevated serum calciums may be complicated by conjunctivitis, gastrointestinal disturbance, hypertension, and renal failure, these later two occurring most frequently with serum total calciums above 15 mg/dl.

Hypoglycemia may occur particularly in patients with advanced tumors with quite variable onset, symptoms, and response to therapy. A variety of mechanisms probably contribute to hypoglycemia.

Patients with advanced disease may also develop the rare complication of severe lactic acidosis. This disturbance has been very difficult to manage and is likely a result of deranged metabolic pathways in the tumor cells leading to increased lactate production.

An additional renal manifestation of nonhodgkin's lymphoma at presentation may be nephrotic syndrome (6). The accompanying renal histology may be that of immune-complex disease or minimal-change disease. Successful treatment of the malignancy usually results in remission of the nephrotic syndrome.

TUMOR LYSIS COMPLICATIONS

Once specific antitumor therapy begins, patients with lymphoid malignancies are at risk of rapid metabolic deterioration as a result of the lysis of tumor cells with release of intracellular contents and metabolic products. In addition to providing an increased load of metabolic waste for excretion, these substances may be nephrotoxic, producing acute renal failure and blockade of normal excretory routes.

The patients at highest risk of complications of tumor lysis will be those with large tumor masses, rapidly growing tumors, tumors that are sensitive to cytotoxic therapeutic agents, and patients with some renal compromise before the initiation of specific therapy. Treatment protocols that produce a large cytolytic effect over a short time period are more likely to produce secondary complications. In general, one might expect regimens including large doses of prednisone, cyclophosphamide, or irradiation, to be cytolytic. One must be alert for the unusual, however, as illustrated by an acute lymphocytic leukemia (ALL) patient with dramatic splenomegaly who received 100 rads to the kidneys with partial inclusion of the spleen in the irradiated field. Within 6 hours, that patient's potassium was 8.4 mEq/L with moderate ECG changes. Emergency dialysis was required to prevent a fatal outcome.

As at presentation, urate nephropathy is a common consequence of rapid tumor lysis (7). The resulting acute renal failure magnifies the impact of the phosphate and hydrogen ion release occurring concurrently. Hyperphosphatemia may be nephrotoxic in itself and certainly may produce tetanic and convulsive complications as the result of inducing hypocalcemia. Metabolic acidosis may be pronounced and prolonged and may require such large amounts of bicarbonate that hypernatremia occurs as a secondary complication. It may, therefore, be necessary to dialyze such patients to control multiple electrolyte disturbances.

Of critical concern is control of serum potassium. It is quite possible for potassium to rise from a normal level to a life-threatening level within 8 hours following cytolytic therapy. The potassium elevation will be further exacerbated by any fall in serum pH. For example, a patient with a moderate potassium elevation of 7.0 mEq/L may develop asystole if respiratory acidosis occurring during a hypocalcemic convulsion pushes the serum potassium significantly higher.

In addition to biochemical disturbances, these patients may be threatened by fluid overload and hypertension. A small amount of pulmonary edema may be poorly tolerated in a patient who already has mediastinal tumor and pleural effusions, for example. Acute renal failure with fluid overload or hypercalcemia may contribute to elevations of blood pressure that are particularly dangerous in patients with severe thrombocytopenia. It is important, then, that physical findings, vital signs, and arterial oxygenation be considered in evaluating and monitoring these patients.

ADDITIONAL NEPHROTOXICITY

In addition to the cyclophosphamide sequelae of hemorrhagic cystitis and the inappropriate-ADH syndrome reported for vincristine and cyclophosphamide, nephrotoxicity is a well-described direct consequence of the anti-tumor agents methotrexate, cisplatin, and x-irradiation. Renal insufficiency has been associated with high-dose methotrexate therapy (8) and appears to be related to deposition of methotrexate in the tubular lumen in some patients and direct toxicity to tubular epithelial cells in others. This complication is minimized with substantial hydration, alkalinization, and metabolic "rescue" from methotrexate toxicity using agents such as citrovorum factor.

Cisplatin toxicity is complex in its relationship to total dose and dose delivered within a given time period. Renal failure may be profound and may occur after latent period of several days after dosage. Some patients may be at increased risk of acute renal failure if they receive other nephrotoxic drugs close to the time of administration of cisplatin. Nephrotoxicity from cisplatin is likewise best prevented with generous hydration, induced diuresis, and careful attention to dosage regimen and concurrent medications. A variety of effective regimens has been reviewed in detail (9).

Radiation nephritis may develop several months after the administered dosage and may lead to chronic renal failure (10). In general, this complication occurs when the dosage to a renal bed exceeds 2000 rads. Limitation of renal dosage to 1200 to 1500 rads seems a prudent measure.

These patients are at additional risk of renal insult because of infection and its treatment. Acute tubular necrosis may be associated with septic shock and prolonged poor renal perfusion, as well as aminoglycosides and other antibiotics with direct nephrotoxicity. Although the list of drugs that can be nephrotoxic is exceedingly long, one must particularly keep in mind gentamycin, tobramycin, amikacin, cephalosporins, and amphotericin B as culprits. It should be remembered that these drugs are unlikely to cause significant difficulty in the first few days of treatment and are therefore quite acceptable for initial therapy. Their appropriate management beyond that point requires careful clinical attention and adequate drug level monitoring (Table 28F.1).

EVALUATION AND PREVENTATIVE THERAPY

New or relapsing patients with nonhodgkins lymphoma may provide a history of ureteral colic and should be evaluated for fluid retention,

Table 28F.1.
Disturbances Associated With Malignancy

At presentation	Following therapy
Acute renal failure;	Tumor Lysis Syndrome
secondary to	↑ K^+, $PO_4^=$, urate, creatinine
Renal parenchymal encroachment	↓ Ca^{++}, pH
Obstructive uropathy—tumor mass or stone	Nephrotoxicity
Urate nephropathy	Methotrexate, cisplatin
Metabolic disturbances	X-irradiation
Hypoglycemia	Aminoglycosides, amphotericin B
Hypercalcemia	
Metabolic acidosis	

blood pressure, creatinine, electrolytes, calcium, phosphate, uric acid, LDH, and anatomical studies, such as a renal ultrasound and chest x-ray films.

In the absence of oliguric renal failure, high fluid intakes should be helpful in preventing many of the potential renal complications. In general, the range of 2.5 to 3 $l/m^2/24$ hours is appropriate; however, initial urinary output must be monitored closely to prevent overhydration of the patient already having renal compromise.

Further increases in tubular fluid flow can be achieved with mannitol. A test dose of 200 to 500 mg/kg should initially be administered, and the drug can be continued if appropriate urinary response occurs.

Induced diuresis is particularly important when using drugs such as extremely high dose methotrexate or cisplatin. Perhaps the safest diuretic to use at the present time is mannitol in combination with large fluid volume administration.

Since many renal complications in these patients involve urate nephropathy, alkalinization of the urine may be extremely important in minimizing risk. Sodium bicarbonate may be administered in patients at risk to increase the urinary pH to at least 7 to 8. More rapid alkalinization can be achieved with acetazolamide; however, this drug should not be continued for prolonged periods. Bicarbonate dosage can be begun at 100 $mEq/m^2/24$ hours. Acetazolamide dosage of 150 $mg/m^2/24$ hours is usually effective.

Urinary alkalinization is somewhat risky if a high calcium-phosphate product is present. In such patients one should probably not raise the urinary pH above 7. Alkaline urine favors calcium phosphate precipitation in the kidney, which may be more difficult to reverse than urate nephropathy.

Allopurinol is effective in decreasing uric acid production by inhibiting xanthine oxidase. It should be routine preventative therapy in patients at risk of urate nephropathy. Mercaptopurine and azathioprine metabolism are influenced by allopurinol and their dosage should be reduced.

Hyperphosphatemia can be somewhat alleviated with phosphate-binding antacids such as aluminum hydroxide.

Local irradiation of infiltrated kidneys may be of value in reducing the risk of renal insufficiency at the onset of cytolytic therapy. When appropriate, a dose of 400 rads given over 4 days may be initiated prior to systemic therapy.

In some patients conditions at presentation or developments during therapy may not be adequately managed conservatively. Dialysis may correct multiple problems simultaneously and may be called for on an emergency basis. Hemodialysis is certainly more rapid than peritoneal dialysis; however, either procedure has advantages and can be appropriately used to manage these patients. Aggressive use of dialysis, in general, makes overall management significantly easier.

References

1. Richmond J, Sherman RA, Diamond HD, et al: Renal lesions associated with malignant lymphomas. Am J Med 32:184, 1982.
2. Steel TH: Renal excretion of uric acid. Arthr Rheum 18(suppl):793, 1975.
3. Spencer HW, Yarger WE, Robinson RR: Alterations of renal function during dietary-induced hyperuricemia in the rat. Kidney Intl 9:489, 1976.
4. Kaplan BS, Hebert D, Morrell RE: Acute renal failure induced by hyperphosphatemia in acute lymphoblastic leukemia. Canad Med Assoc J 124(4):429, 1981.
5. Lynch RE, Kjellstrand CM, Coccia PF: Renal and metabolic complications of childhood non-hodgkin's lymphoma. Semin Oncol 4(3):325, 1977.
6. Gagliano RG, Costanzi JJ, Beathard GA, et al: The nephrotic syndrome associated with neoplasia: An unusual paraneoplastic syndrome. Am J Med 60:1026, 1976.
7. Arseneau JC, Canellos GP, Banks PM, et al: American Burkitt's lymphoma: A clinicopathologic study of 30 cases. I. Clinical factors relating to prolonged survival. Am J Med 58:314, 1975.
8. Pitman SW, Parker LM, Tattersall MHN, et al: Clinical trials of high dose methotrexate (NSC-740) with citrovorum factor (NSC-3590)—toxicologic and therapeutic observations. Cancer Chemother Rep (Part 3) 6:43, 1975.
9. Garnick MB, Mayer RJ, Abelson HT: Acute renal failure associated with cancer treatment. In Brenner BM, Lazarus JM (eds): Acute Renal Failure. Philadelphia, W.B. Saunders Co., 1983.
10. White DC: The histopathologic basis for functional decrements in late radiation injury in diverse organs. Cancer 37:1126, 1976.

CHAPTER 29

Therapy of Glomerular Disease

T. MARTIN BARRATT
D. F. GEARY
P. C. HOLLAND
M. LEVIN

INTRODUCTION

The management of glomerular disease can be considered under two headings: measures designed to ameliorate the consequences of glomerular dysfunction and specific treatment aimed at the reversal of glomerular pathology or at least the prevention of progressive glomerular damage.

Syndromes of Glomerular Disease

The glomeruli, being ultrafilters, have only a limited range of expression of disease. They may become leaky, blocked, or both. Leak has two manifestations: hematuria and proteinuria. Hematuria is a valuable sign of glomerular disease, but does not of itself need treatment. Proteinuria is an expression of the disturbed ultrafiltration characteristics of the glomeruli; if mild, it requires no therapy, but if heavy it leads to depletion of plasma proteins and edema, i.e., the nephrotic syndrome (NS). Block implies a reduction in glomerular filtration rate (GFR) and thus leads to renal failure. This may be sudden in onset—acute renal failure (ARF)—with various degrees of potential for recovery, or it may progress insidiously from an early phase of leak to irreversible chronic renal failure (CRF). Sudden onset of a partial block results in a limitation of the ability to excrete salt and water, leading to volume expansion, hypertension, and peripheral or pulmonary edema, i.e., the acute nephritic syndrome (ANS). The vascularity of the glomeruli focuses the effects of disordered endothelial-platelet interactions on the kidney in which renal failure is associated with erythrocyte fragmentation and thrombocytopenia, i.e., the microangiopathic syndrome.

Treatment of Glomerular Disease

Many glomerular diseases result from immunologically mediated injury, usually the deposition or formation in situ of immune complexes, but occasionally true autoantibody formation. In others, such as minimal-change nephrotic syndrome, as yet unidentified immunological mechanisms may be operative (chapter 13). Therefore, the rationale of specific therapy is usually based on attempts to modulate (suppress) the immune response or interfere with the recruitment of damaging mediator systems, such as platelets, polymorphs, complement, and coagulation. However, the tendency to immune complex formation might be the consequence of subtle forms of immunodeficiency rather than of overactivity of the immune response (1). Under those circumstances immunosuppression might aggravate rather than ameliorate the pathological process. For example, azathioprine therapy of malarial nephropathy increases the mortality from renal failure (2). Drug action is rarely specific, affecting one physiological system only. Thus, where beneficial effects have been observed, it is by no means certain by what mechanism the results have been achieved. Moreover, the wide range of immunopathological processes that may underlie apparently similar clinical syndromes, the unpredictable natural history of glomerular disease, the haphazard manner in which new forms of therapy have been introduced, and the relative paucity of adequately controlled clinical trials combine to make an objective assessment of current "specific therapy" a most difficult task.

Pathophysiology

The pathophysiology and management of ARF is described in Chapter 48 and of CRF in Chapter 49 and will not be considered here. Three syndromes of glomerular disease require further elaboration.

Nephrotic Syndrome

The term nephrotic syndrome is applied to any state in which there is heavy albuminuria leading to hypoalbuminemia and edema. Albumin accounts for most of the plasma oncotic pressure. A reduced concentration causes a disturbance of the Starling equilibrium with increased ultrafiltration of plasma into the interstitial compartment and results in hypovolemia and edema. Such hypoalbuminemic (flaccid) edema differs from the hypervolemic (turgid) edema of ANS or CRF, in that its distribution is more affected by gravity and tissue pressure.

Hypovolemia is the stimulus for sodium retention by the kidney. Sodium retention is a protective response, but it aggravates the edema. It is mediated by activation of renin release and consequent angiotension-stimulated aldosterone secretion, as well as by the factors that modulate proximal tubular sodium reabsorption. Since the plasma volume is contracted, there is hemoconcentration with a raised hematocrit. Significant hypovolemia is usually accompanied by abdominal pain and, if severe, by circulatory collapse. Arterial pressure occasionally may be raised, as a consequence of the intense vasoconstriction. The assumption that NS is invariably accompanied by hypovolemia is not always supported by direct measurement, but there are problems of artefact and interpretation in plasma volume determinations in the nephrotic state (3). Reduced renal perfusion leads to impaired water excretion and to the development of hyponatremia, reduction of GFR with uremia, and ultimately to acute tubular necrosis. The combination of hyponatremia and shock may resemble adrenal failure in a patient who has previously received corticosteroids.

Thrombotic episodes are common in NS. A variety of abnormalities of both platelets and the coagulation pathway have been documented. Platelets are hyperaggregable and frequently show spontaneous aggregation (4). Concentration of coagulation factors and fibrinogen are increased, and inhibitors of coagulation, particularly antithrombin III, are diminished. These abnormalities act in concert with the sluggish blood flow resulting from hypovolemia to cause thrombosis.

There is a generalised disturbance of plasma proteins in NS, with those of low molecular weight and particularly with slow plasma turnover times being reduced because of loss. On the other hand, concentrations of high molecular weight proteins, such as IgM, alpha 2-macroglobulin, fibrinogen, and beta-lipoprotein are increased for reasons that are not clear. Decreased concentrations of IgG and C3 proactivator predispose the nephrotic child to infection. Classically pneumococcal septicemia and primary peritonitis occur, but Hemophilus and gram-negative infections are also observed. In addition, edematous tissues are prone to cellulitis.

Hypercholesterolemia and hypertriglyceridemia are features of the nephrotic state. The latter may be associated with a deficiency of post-heparin lipoprotein lipase activity (5). Hyperlipidemia is, in part, responsible for the phenomenon of spontaneous platelet aggregation. Despite the hyperlipidemia and hypercoagulability, it has been surprisingly difficult to document an increased prevalence of arterial disease in patients with SRNS (6).

The nephrotic state thus is a complex biochemical and physiological disturbance that requires careful management and nonspecific treatment, in addition to that directed primarily at reversing the disorder of glomerular permeability.

Acute Nephritic Syndrome

ANS is characterized by the sudden onset of hematuria, proteinuria, hypertension, edema, and renal failure. The prototypic form is acute poststreptococcal glomerulonephritis, but the same syndrome can complicate other postinfectious or immunologically mediated vasculitic glomerulonephritides (chapter 26A). The characteristic functional disturbance is a moderate impairment of glomerular filtration with unusually severe salt and water retention (7). The cause of sodium retention is probably a reduced rate of delivery of filtrate into nephrons, which nevertheless have functioning tubular reabsorptive systems. The role of the renin-angiotensin system in this syndrome is not clear. While plasma renin activity and aldosterone concentration are not elevated, they are not as suppressed as would be expected in healthy individuals with a comparable degree of volume expansion (8).

Salt and water retention results in extracellular fluid (ECF) volume expansion affecting the intravascular, as well as the interstitial phases. Hypervolemia raises venous filling pressure. The cardiac response is characterized by bradycardia, increased stroke volume, gallop rhythm, and abolition of the reflex responses to the Valsalva maneuver (9). Hypertension (sometimes complicated by encephalopathy) and peripheral edema ensue, ultimately with left ventricular failure, cardiomegaly, and pulmonary edema.

It has been suggested that there is a diffuse disturbance of capillary permeability to account for the edema of the acute nephritic syndrome (10) or a direct myocardial effect responsible for the circulatory features (11); however, evidence for these additional mechanisms is insecure. From the point of view of therapy, inappropriate volume expansion should be considered the dominant feature of the syndrome.

A particularly complex disturbance is found in patients with a mixed nephritic-nephrotic pattern. This may be observed in patients with ANS and unusually heavy proteinuria, typical of those with the Henoch-Schönlein syndrome or lupus nephritis. In them it may be difficult to decide whether edema arises from hypervolemia or hypoproteinemia. Since the therapeutic strategies are diametrically opposed, it may be prudent to resolve the dilemma by direct measurements of central venous pressure (CVP).

Microangiopathic Syndrome

The association of renal failure with a hemolytic anemia characterized by erythrocyte fragmentation, thrombocytopenia, and hypertension is well established (12). There is a disturbance of the normal relationship between endothelium and platelets, with platelet deposition and secondary recruitment of the coagulation system. Hemolytic anemia is thought to be a consequence of the mechanical effect on the erythrocytes of the abnormal endothelial surface. This microangiopathy is characteristic of the hemolytic uremic syndrome (HUS) in which there sometimes appears to be defective endothelial production of prostacyclin (13). In mild cases, there is glomerular capillary thrombosis. In severe cases, there is arteriolar involvement with endothelial proliferation, severe hyperreninemia, and hypertension; in such circumstances, hypertension may be resistant to volume depletion (14).

A similar train of events can be initiated by hypertension itself; in the accelerated phase it can be associated with the complete microangiopathic syndrome. Whatever efforts are made at specific treatment of the underlying disorder, meticulous control of blood pressure is essential in the management of microangiopathy.

NONSPECIFIC TREATMENT

Hypovolemia

Symptomatic hypovolemia necessitates immediate volume expansion with plasma; with circulatory collapse, there is no question of the need for such therapy. However, it is prudent to avert such crises by recognizing the earlier signs of hypovolemia, particularly abdominal pain or a rise in hemoglobin concentration of 1 to 2 g/dl and by awareness of circumstances conducive to its development, particularly diarrhea, septicemia, diuretic therapy, and ascitic fluid drainage.

An initial infusion of plasma of 20 ml/kg is appropriate, though more may be required. When hypovolemia is complicated by infection, fresh frozen plasma may be an advantage; in general, purified plasma protein fraction, which is principally albumin, suffices. Salt-poor human serum albumin is not appropriate in this circumstance, for the correction of hypovolemia relies on withdrawal of interstitial fluid to the vascular compartment and is too slow.

The administration of plasma should be monitored by regular observation of the pulse, blood pressure, and jugular venous pulse. It is contraindicated if there is elevation of CVP, cardiomegaly, or pulmonary edema. Hypertension generally is a contraindication as well. Occasionally, elevation of blood pressure is not accompanied by other signs of circulatory overload, but is attributable to an excessive vasoconstrictor response; then further administration of plasma is appropriate. This conclusion can be reached only with considerable circumspection and usually with the assistance of direct CVP measurement.

Hypoalbuminemia

The use of human serum albumin to correct hypoalbuminemia is generally a fruitless and expensive undertaking, for the rates of urinary albumin loss are such that any advantage gained is transitory. Nevertheless, with a specific objective in mind, such as the preparation of a child for biopsy, albumin infusion may be helpful. Albumin infusions of 1 to 2 g/kg are appropriate, usually given as a 20% solution.

Edema

The use of diuretics to control hypoalbuminemic edema requires caution, because of the risk of precipitating hypovolemia. The presence of a mild degree of edema may be tolerated, but severe or increasing edema necessitates dietary sodium restriction and furosemide 0.5 to 2 mg/kg/24 hr, covered by plasma infusion if there is any suggestion of hypovolemia.

The control of long-standing severe edema, such as may afflict some children with focal segmental glomerulosclerosis (FSGS) or the congenital NS, is a difficult problem. It is appropriate to restrict dietary sodium intake, while at the same time maintaining a high protein intake, together with oral furosemide up to 5 mg/kg/24 hr. However, the prolonged administration of furosemide can be complicated by metabolic disturbances, particularly hypokalemic alkalosis, hyperglycemia, hyperuricemia, and hyperlipidemia (15), as well as occasionally by interstitial nephritis (an important possibility to consider when renal function declines in a chronically nephrotic child). To counteract hypokalemia, spironolactone, 0.5 to 5 mg/kg/24 hr, an aldosterone antagonist, is a useful additional diuretic agent provided renal function is good.

Hypervolemia

In contrast to the hypovolemia of NS, ANS is characterized by hypervolemia. Its treatment consists of dietary sodium restriction, diuretics, and dialysis if the first two measures do not suffice. The powerful loop diuretics are the most suitable, e.g., furosemide 1 to 2 mg/kg/24 hr orally or, if hypertension is severe or pulmonary edema imminent, by intravenous injection (up to 10 mg/kg/24 hr—at higher doses there is a risk of ototoxicity). The administration of furosemide reduces the duration of the hypertensive phase in acute nephritis (16). If pulmonary edema is actually present, then intravenous diuretics are indicated, but may be insufficient, and if hypoxemia is present as well, elective positive end-expiratory pressure ventilation should be considered. There is no place for digoxin in these circumstances.

Hypertension

The treatment of hypertension is considered in Chapter 47, which should be consulted for details of drug dosage and administration. The hypertension of ANS, being attributable essentially to hypervolemia, is best managed by the combination of a vasodilator and a diuretic, e.g., hydralazine and furosemide. Beta-adrenergic blockade carries some risk of exacerbation of cardiac decompensation and pulmonary edema and is best deferred until hypervolemia is corrected. Therefore, in acute severe hypertension with encephalopathy, parenteral hydralazine or nitroprusside are useful drugs: labetalol, a combined alpha-adrenergic and beta-adrenergic antagonist has also been used successfully. An anticonvulsant also may be necessary; diazepam is the most convenient.

In microangiopathic states hypertension, being renin driven, may be brittle or resistant to control by volume reduction and may coexist, with salt and water depletion, so that severe hypotension can follow the administration of an effective vasodilator. Great care must be exercised in the acute control of blood pressure of children with the microangiopathy of accelerated hypertension, for rapid reduction may cause cerebral damage, particularly infarction of the anterior visual pathways and blindness (chapter 46). Nevertheless, meticulous control of blood pressure is an essential aspect of the management of the microangiopathic state. Hypertension itself aggravates the disturbance, and, as the renin-angiotensin system is implicated, the converting enzyme inhibitor captopril is a suitable choice. Prostacyclin is also an effective antihypertensive agent in acute situations and has the additional merit of inhibiting platelet aggregation.

In children with chronic progressive glomerulonephritis, blood pressure surveillance and control is a most important aspect of follow-up, for this is one element of the factors leading to progressive renal destruction that is amenable to treatment. Therapy should be initiated if the diastolic blood pressure exceeds 2 SD above the mean for age. The combination of a vasodilator and beta-blocker, for example, hydralazine and propranolol, is suitable.

Coagulation

The tendency to thrombosis is a major risk to health in what is otherwise (in minimal-change cases) a benign disorder. There is a striking variation in the incidence of thrombotic episodes reported from different centers (17). The complication is avoidable by the early recognition and treatment of hypovolemic states and meticulous attention to venipuncture and intravenous infusion sites (particularly of radiological contrast media). Femoral venipuncture is to be avoided, for inadvertent arterial puncture may lead to thrombosis and loss of limb (18). Mobilization is recommended rather than bed rest wherever possible. This risk is a factor to be considered in the selection of patients for cyclophosphamide therapy to avert further relapses and periods of high-dose corticosteroid treatment.

Major thrombotic episodes should be treated by heparinization initially. A bolus dose of 100 u/kg followed by 25 u/kg/hr intravenously. Warfarin should be introduced after the initial heparin treatment at a dose adjusted to maintain the prothrombin time slightly less 2 to 3 times the control level for 2 months. Insofar as some of the thrombotic episodes are a consequence of platelet microthrombi resulting from spontaneous platelet aggregation, it may emerge that prostacyclin infusion is a useful way of managing these events (19). The prophylactic use of aspirin or other agents to prevent the thrombotic complications of NS has not yet been established.

Recently interest has been elicited by the possibility that FSGS is not a different and intrinsically more severe condition than minimal-change NS. The sclerotic lesions may represent the consequence of an uncontrolled nephrotic state, possibly platelet deposition in the glomerular capillary bed as a result of the tendency to spontaneous platelet aggregation compounded by the local effects of ultrafiltration (20). On this basis, aspirin and dipyridamole have been recommended as "antiplatelet therapy" in patients with FSGS to prevent the expected deterioration of renal function; a beneficial effect has been reported (21).

Hyperlipidemia

The disturbance of lipid metabolism is striking. In addition to a possible increase in arterial disease hyperlipidemia is associated with a tendency to spontaneous platelet aggregation and may play a role in the development of FSGS (22). However, as yet, no clear benefit has been demonstrated by the use of dietary or pharmacological measures to correct the lipid disturbance.

Infection

Eradication of an infection responsible for immune complex glomerulonephritis is an obvious principle of management, e.g., control of bacterial endocarditis, removal of an infected ventriculoatrial shunt, or treatment of congenital syphilis. However, control of infection does not guarantee cure of glomerulonephritis. Malarial nephropathy, for example, is unaffected by eradication of the parasite (23). A 2-week course of penicillin suffices for acute poststreptococcal glomerulonephritis; in contrast to rheumatic fever, continued penicillin prophylaxis is unnecessary as reinfection is very rare.

Nephrotic children are prone to infection. Septicemia should be considered in any sick nephrotic child; blood cultures should be taken and antibiotic therapy initiated. Penicillin and gentamicin are an appropriate combination, for the likely organism is either pneumococcus or a gram-negative organism, though the possibility of Hemophilus must not be overlooked. Abdominal pain and vomiting suggest primary peritonitis, though the differential diagnosis includes hypovolemia, acute pancreatitis, or a steroid-induced ulcer. The diagnosis may be confirmed by microscopy, counterimmunoelectrophoresis, and culture of a small sample of ascitic fluid obtained by fine-needle aspiration. Treatment should be initiated without delay, using high-dose ampicillin and gentamicin. Diagnostic laparatomy should be avoided, if possible, because the sudden release of ascitic fluid may precipitate hypovolemia. Edematous subcutaneous tissues are prone to cellulitis, which may spread at an alarming rate. Staphylococci and streptococci are often incriminated. Particular care is necessary at sites of venipuncture, intravenous infusion, and renal biopsy. The risk of infection, particularly pneumococcal, in a nephrotic child is such that it is prudent for them to be given prophylactic penicillin 20 mg/kg/24 hr for as long as hypoalbuminemia persists.

All children on immunosuppressive drugs are at risk of infection, particularly those with systemic lupus erythematosus who not only are intrinsically susceptible because of their primary disease and the associated NS, but are also the principal group of nephritic children currently being treated with long-term immunosuppressive therapy; in them, infection is now the principal cause of death (24).

Relapse of NS or episodes of hematuria in children with IgA nephropathy or convalescent acute poststreptococcal or Henoch-Schönlein nephritis is frequently precipitated by upper respiratory infections. Most are viral in origin and antibiotic prophylaxis is of no value. There is no indication for tonsillectomy, though there is a possibility that IgA nephropathy is less evident in individuals with tonsillectomies (25).

Although relapse of NS has been reported after immunization, there is no statistical basis for this association, and a full immunization program should be carried out. Measles infection can induce remission in a steroid-responsive nephrotic child. However, it can also cause a devastating illness in an immunosuppressed child, so it is well to ensure that measles immunization is achieved at an early phase of illness. Chicken pox is a serious illness in a nephrotic child on steroids. Exposure of such a child to the risk of infection should prompt the administration of zoster-immune globulin and development of a suitable vaccine will be of great help. A pneumococcal vaccine is available, but is not comprehensive so that penicillin prophylaxis cannot be omitted.

General Measures

Diet

The dietary management of acute and CRF is discussed in Chapters 48 and 49. Dietary sodium restriction is appropriate for both hypervolemic and hypoalbuminemic edema. It is difficult to reduce the dietary sodium intake <1 mmol/kg/24 hr without jeopardizing concurrent protein and energy intake. If further reduction in body sodium is necessary, diuretic therapy is preferable to more severe sodium restriction. Dietary sodium restriction is necessary only in a nephrotic child who is hypoalbuminemic. An occasional error occurs when persisting with a low sodium diet in a child who is in remission and in whom it is therefore no longer necessary.

Temporary protein restriction (about 1 to 2 g/kg/24 hr) may be necessary in ANS, whereas in NS a generous intake of 3 to 4 g/kg/24 hr is necessary to make up for urine protein losses. There is no evidence that hepatic albumin synthesis is augmented by higher protein intakes. Occasionally in congenital NS, where hypoalbuminemic edema appears intractable, some benefit may be obtained by nasogastric tube feeding of low sodium/high protein preparations that provide an additional 5 g protein/kg/24 hr.

Energy intake needs to be well maintained in ANS as in other forms of renal failure. In the nephrotic child on long-term corticosteroids, however, it may be necessary to reduce energy intake with a low carbohydrate diet to prevent obesity.

With advancing renal failure, phosphate intake should be reduced either by dietary means or by phosphate binding with calcium carbonate, not only to prevent the development of hyperparathyroidism, but also to retard the deterioration of renal function. The beneficial effect of dietary phosphate restriction on renal function in experimental glomerulonephritis is quite striking (26).

Bed Rest

There is no place for bed rest in the treatment of the child with glomerulonephritis, other than that desired by the child or necessary for the administration of other aspects of medical therapy. On the contrary, mobilization is desirable to maintain muscle tone, to preserve good skin condition, to minimize venous stasis thereby reducing the risk of thrombosis, and to maintain morale. In the past, severe restriction of physical exercise was advised in even quite mild cases of nephritis, perhaps because physical exercise can cause exacerbation of hematuria in patients with IgA nephropathy or healing poststreptococcal nephritis. There is no evidence, however, that this is harmful to renal function, and the lack of beneficial effect of bed rest in acute nephritis has been clearly demonstrated (27).

Psychosocial Factors

As with any chronic illness it is necessary to attend to the child's psychological, social, and educational development, as well as the needs of the family. With recurrent illness there is disruption of the child's educational program. The distortion of the child's body image by edema, corticosteroid obesity, or short stature is a psychological strain for both the patient and family. There is always anxiety about the long-term prospects of the illness. It is important to continue to express optimism about the outcome of a child with minimal-change NS and to reaffirm that the ultimate prognosis is good, that renal failure will not ensue, that dialysis and transplantation will not be necessary, and that the relapses will cease eventually.

CORTICOSTEROIDS

The introduction of adrenocorticotropic hormone (ACTH) in 1951 for the treatment of NS in children ushered in a new era in the specific treatment of glomerular disease (28). Since then new steroid drugs have been developed, and there is now no place for the use of ACTH in the treatment of renal disease. Corticosteroids have been used enthusiastically in almost all glomerular diseases, but there are few controlled trials demonstrating a beneficial effect. Their use in individual circumstances still remains a difficult and controversial decision. Furthermore, the possible beneficial effects have to be judged against numerous and severe side effects, which are responsible for a high morbidity in corticosteroid-treated patients.

Pharmacology

Mode of Action

Steroid therapy is usually initiated in the belief that the disease process will be ameliorated by modification of immunological factors. Steroids produce a variety of effects on the immune system, including a reduction in the numbers of circulating monocytes and lymphocytes, reduction in concentrations of immunoglobulin and complement components, suppression of leukocyte accumulation at the site of injury, and membrane stabilization (29, 30). Where a beneficial effect of corticosteroids has been observed it is not clear which mechanism of action is relevant.

Choice of Drug

Prednisone and its active metabolite, prednisolone, have greater antiinflammatory activity, cause less sodium retention than the natural hormone cortisol, and are the most widely used corticosteroid preparations in current nephrology practice. There is little to choose between them; conversion of prednisone to prednisolone is rapid and peak plasma levels are achieved in children within 2 hours of ingestion (31).

Methylprednisolone is available for intravenous administration. It has similar potency, but less salt-retaining properties than the oral preparation and is generally prescribed as a bolus of 10 to 30 mg/kg to be administered over approximately 30 minutes (28). It is used when a rapid effect is desired or when suppression of a flare-up of disease activity is required without increasing the daily maintenance steroid dosage. However, the advantage of such high doses of intravenous methylprednisolone over smaller doses given orally has not been proven, and its use has been questioned (32).

Pharmacokinetics

The half life of prednisolone in children is about 2 hours (31), but there appears to be some variation in the rates of clearance of the drug, with a few individuals being "fast inactivators" (33). Circulating prednisolone is protein-bound, and the proportion of free prednisolone is increased in nephrotic plasma (34).

At least a twice-daily dose is necessary for continuous action, but the suppressive effect on ACTH output by the pituitary is also greater than with a single daily dose. Administration of steroids on an alternate-day basis produces less pituitary suppression and is the recommended regimen provided adequate disease control is achieved (35). The total daily dose of steroids also affects the degree of pituitary suppression, which occurs only when the physiological cortisol output is exceeded (equivalent to a daily prednisolone dose of approximately 5 mg/m^2 SA). Suppression of the pituitary/adrenal axis persists for many months after steroid therapy and is a result of both failure of ACTH output by the pituitary and adrenal unresponsiveness (35).

Side Effects

Steroid side effects are numerous and some, particularly growth suppression, are more severe in younger children (in whom growth is fastest). Small stature, obesity, Cushingoid facies, and striae may distort the appearance of the child in a most distressing manner. Growth failure is probably a consequence of inhibition of growth hormone release, and low somatomedin levels are found in children on steroid therapy (31). A reduction in steroid toxicity and better growth is achieved by administration of steroids as a single dose in the morning on alternate days. Prolonged steroid therapy is associated with posterior lenticular opacities, but vision is rarely impaired (36). Gastrointestinal side effects (gastritis and ulceration) may be lessened by the use of enteric-coated prednisolone tablets.

Steroid metabolism is mostly hepatic with no dosage adjustment required in renal failure (37). However, patients with renal disease are at particular risk from some side effects, such as salt and water retention, hypertension, increased protein catabolism, and osteoporosis. Also, patients with renal disease are more prone to the infective complications associated with steroid therapy (38).

Withdrawal of steroids may expose suppression of the pituitary/adrenal axis. There is usually some anorexia; occasionally, benign intracranial hypertension may ensue, particularly in children with persistent hypoalbuminemia (39).

Indications

Minimal-change Nephrotic Syndrome

It is necessary to consider the natural history of minimal-change nephrotic syndrome (MCNS) before evaluating the role of steroids. The 5-year mortality rate in children with idiopathic NS, before the discovery of antimicrobial drugs, was 67%. This figure was halved following the introduction of sulfonamides and penicillin, but before the advent of steroids (40). It was first demonstrated in the early 1950s that ACTH was effective in inducing remission (28). Since then, following the introduction of cortisone and subsequently prednisone, increased expertise in their use, and improved diuretic and antibiotic therapy, the mortality rate has fallen to 4% (41). In earlier follow-up studies, renal histology was not ascertained; the diagnosis of MCNS being presumed on the basis of steroid response (41a). The presence of even a few patients with more serious forms of glomerular disease would have greatly influenced these figures, suggesting that the true mortality rate of MCNS might have been less. Such a favorable long-term prognosis demands that steroid use, with its attendant side effects, be carefully controlled.

Despite the introduction of steroids 20 years earlier and their subsequent widespread use, it was not until 1970 that the results of a controlled trial in patients with NS were published (42). A study by the British Medical Research Council confirmed the value of prednisolone in inducing remission in adults with MCNS, although a higher mortality rate was noted in the treated group as a whole than in the control patients. A relatively low dose of steroids (26 mg/24 hr prednisolone) was employed and continued for at least 6 months. With present-day regimens, using larger doses for shorter periods, a better response rate and fewer side effects would be expected. One regimen uses 60 mg/m2/24 hr prednisone for 4 weeks, followed by 40 mg/m2/24 hr for 3 days out of 7 (43), and another uses 2 mg/kg/24 hr prednisolone until the patient is protein-free for 3 days, followed by steroid withdrawal over 4 to 6 weeks (44).

Because patients with minimal histological lesions are the only cases of NS who consistently respond to steroid treatment, the diagnosis should be established with reasonable confidence before starting therapy. Although microscopic hematuria, hypertension, and impaired renal function may be found in more than 20% of children with MCNS (43), the diagnosis still may be predicted with sufficient accuracy (particularly in those <10 years) from clinical features alone because of the great preponderance of MCNS in this age group. Therefore, renal biopsy in nephrotic children may be deferred unless a pattern of steroid resistance emerges or unfavorable features are present at onset, particularly macroscopic hematuria, hypocomplementemia, or poorly selective proteinuria.

With steroid therapy, remission may be expected in more than 90% of patients with MCNS; 85% of responders becoming protein-free within 3 weeks (45). Despite initial response, relapses occur in as many as 80% of patients, especially in those who have developed adrenal suppression (46). About 40% of MCNS children have frequent relapses (47); and in them, the benefit of a prolonged course of maintenance alternate-day prednisone has been established as being superior to an intermittent regime (48). This study (48) used prednisone (35 mg/m SA/48 hr), but steroid toxicity necessitated withdrawal of 25% of patients from the trial. A 6-month course of maintenance prednisolone in frequently relapsing patients is appropriate, using the minimum dose necessary to prevent relapse (usually 10 to 20 mg/48 hr) as a single morning dose (44). Failure to maintain remission except at the expense of unacceptable corticosteroid toxicity is an indication for cyclophosphamide therapy.

Focal Segmental Glomerulosclerosis

Steroid therapy is not effective in most children with FSGS. This histology is often diagnosed by renal biopsy, which is undertaken because of steroid resistance (49). Nonetheless, a small number of patients with this lesion respond initially to steroids, although most of them ultimately become steroid-dependent or steroid-resistant (50). It is difficult to draw a rigorous distinction, on either clinical or histological grounds, between FSGS and MCNS.

Membranous Nephropathy

Membranous nephropathy (MN) is the most common underlying histology in adult patients with NS, and the clinical course is quite variable. Approximately 50% of patients maintain normal renal function, with complete or partial loss of proteinuria over an extended follow-up period (51). In 1970, the British Medical Research Council reported a possible effect of steroids in preventing deterioration of renal function in adults with MN, but the side effects of therapy appeared to outweigh the observed benefits (42). More recently a multicenter prospective controlled trial reevaluated steroid therapy in such patients and, using a higher steroid dose on an alternate-day basis for a period of only 8 weeks, confirmed the previously suggested beneficial effect (52). The mean follow-up period for patients in this study was <2 years, which is probably insufficient to evaluate a disease with a protracted course. In children the overall prognosis of MN is better than in adults; however, as the benefits of steroids are equivocal, their use is not generally indicated (53–55).

Membranoproliferative Glomerulonephritis

About half the patients with MPGN histopathology develop end-stage renal failure within 5 to 10 years from the time of diagnosis (56–59). Persistent NS, early onset of renal failure, and hypertension suggest a poor prognosis (58). Based on a retrospective analysis of their own data and a review of the literature, Habib and coworkers (56) concluded that steroids were not only ineffective, but also caused serious complications, particularly exacerbation of hypertension. However, prolonged use of prednisone (2 mg/kg/48 hr) has been associated with a survival of 89% at 15 years, the maximum benefit being noted in children with type 1 histology, but these results have not been confirmed and were not controlled studies (60). Surprisingly little steroid toxicity was noted and growth was affected only slightly. Preliminary results of a randomized controlled trial, using a slightly lower steroid dose in patients with type 1 MPGN, have not demonstrated any clear benefits attributable to steroids; drug toxicity necessitated withdrawal of 25% of treated patients from the study (61). Until this trial is complete, or more evidence accumulates in their favor, the use of steroids routinely in this disorder is not recommended.

Crescentic Glomerulonephritis

The presence of extensive epithelial crescents indicates a poor prognosis (rapidly progressive glomerulonephritis) with nearly all patients developing CRF within 2 years of diagnosis (62). The cases are heterogeneous, some being a result of antiglomerular basement membrane antibody, and other examples of type II MPGN or vasculitic disorders, such as Henoch-Schönlein syndrome, polyarteritis, or Wegener's granulomatosis.

Most reported results of treatment of crescentic glomerulonephritis are retrospective analyses, concern patients with a wide variety of underlying diseases of variable histological and clinical severity, and have used complex multiple drug regimes (63–65). Thus optimal treatment is not established, although (because of the grave prognosis) some attempt is usually made to arrest or reverse the disease process. Plasmapheresis (66), pulse methylprednisolone (67), and combinations of immunosuppressants, steroids, and anticoagulants (68) all have their advocates. It is difficult to make progress in this field unless a laboratory investigation closely related to the pathogenesis of the disorder (for example, antiglomerular basement membrane antibody in Goodpastures's syndrome) is available.

Systemic Lupus Erythematosus

Control of systemic lupus erythematosus (SLE) is generally achieved with prednisolone (1 to 2 mg/kg/24 hr) for 6 to 8 weeks, after which the dose is reduced to the lowest that maintains both serological and clinical remission. If the disease is not controlled with steroids or if the required dose is associated with the appearance of unacceptable side effects, azathioprine (2 mg/kg/24 hr) may be added. In an acutely ill patient, more rapid response may be obtained with intravenous doses of methylprednisolone (69) or plasmapheresis (70). There are no controlled trials of steroids in SLE nephritis in children, but it seems reasonable to ascribe the substantial improvement in prognosis in recent years to steroid and immunosuppressive drugs. The 5-year survival rate is currently about 80% (71).

As with other chronic illnesses, before starting steroids it is important to define the aims of treatment, but it is still uncertain whether the goal should be serological or clinical remission. On the one hand, lupus nephritis may be present without any overt urinary abnormality (72), while untreated patients may remain asymptomatic over extended periods, despite persistently abnormal serological tests (73). Prolonged control of serum complement levels within normal limits is associated with stabilization or improvement in renal function; this should probably be the objective (74).

In the allied disorder of mixed connective-tissue disease, renal involvement is more common in children than in adults, and a variety of histological abnormalities have been described (75). Steroids successfully control the disease in most patients, but long-term therapy may be required (76).

Henoch-Schönlein Syndrome

Approximately 25% of children with Henoch-Schönlein nephritis have persistent renal dysfunction 10 years after the onset of disease (77). Although steroids are helpful in the acute phase of the illness, particularly in controlling gastrointestinal manifestations of the disease, the general consensus is that they do not modify the natural history of renal involvement, except perhaps as part of a combined immunosuppressive and anticoagulant regimen in the rare case of crescentic nephritis. Similarly, there is no evidence that steroids affect the related disorder of IgA nephropathy.

Vasculitis Syndromes

Despite a lack of controlled trials, the available evidence suggests that steroids are beneficial in polyarteritis nodosa (78). Further improvement in outcome may be achieved with the addition of another cytotoxic agent, particularly cyclophosphamide. This combination may produce a remission when steroids alone have proved inadequate (79).

For Wegener's granulomatosis, which may be associated with a proliferative or crescentic glomerulonephritis, cyclophosphamide (1–2 mg/kg/day) is the treatment of choice. However, if it is associated with severe eye or serosal involvement, a short course of steroids also may be indicated (80). Intravenous methylprednisolone (30 mg/kg) may produce a rapid response in patients who are critically ill (81).

IMMUNOSUPPRESSIVE DRUGS

The use of nitrogen mustard to treat childhood NS was reported in 1958 (82), but alkylating agents were not further explored until the value of cyclophosphamide was demonstrated in 1963 (83). The gratifying results of cyclophosphamide in MCNS (84) led to its extensive use in the early 1970s, until concern about its toxicity engendered a more cautious approach (85). Meanwhile, experience with azathioprine in renal transplantation encouraged its use in the treatment of glomerular disease, but generally with rather disappointing results.

Alkylating Agents

Mode of Action

The major actions of alkylating agents, both cytotoxic and immunosuppressive, are related to their effect on DNA, interfering with cell division. Only metabolites with alkylating ability are effective in inducing immunosuppression (86). Both humoral and cell-mediated immunity are modified by cyclophosphamide, with a predominant effect on B cells.

Choice of Drug

Cyclophosphamide is an alkylating agent related to nitrogen mustard. It is well absorbed and peak levels are observed in plasma about 1 hour after oral administration (87). The native drug is activated by liver microsomal enzymes, and both active and inactive metabolites are excreted by the kidneys (87, 88). With impaired renal function, the elimination of these metabolites may be delayed and could result in their accumulation and possibly increased toxicity.

Chlorambucil is another alkylating agent whose precise mode of action is unknown, but is presumably similar to that of cyclophosphamide. Administration must be oral and absorption is reliable (87); metabolism takes place in the liver (88).

Side Effects

The side effects of alkylating agents are most evident in rapidly dividing cells. Thus, with both cyclophosphamide and chlorambucil, leukopenia is common, although reduction of the white cell count is not necessary for an immunosuppressive effect (89). Nausea and vomiting occur whether the drug is given orally or intravenously (87). Alopecia is a frequently noted side effect, which fortunately is reversible (87). Sterile hemorrhagic cystitis occurs in patients receiving high doses of cyclophosphamide; there are several reports of patients developing bladder neoplasia following its use (90, 91). Such effects probably result from prolonged exposure of the bladder wall to the metabolites of cyclophosphamide excreted in the urine and may be minimized by maintenance of a high urine flow rate.

The potential for gonadal toxicity is one of the more worrying features associated with the use of cyclophosphamide (85). Certain groups of patients have been identified who may be at particular risk. Those receiving the drug after the onset of puberty are more vulnerable than those exposed earlier in life (92–94). Ovarian function appears to be less affected than testicular (92, 94), although temporary amenorrhea may follow treatment with alkylating agents (87). Gonadal toxicity is dose related. Etteldorf and coworkers (95) found that a total dose of 210 mg/kg produced no histological abnormality of the testis. This dose represents more than the amount of cyclophosphamide known to produce a sustained effect in MCNS, which is about 3 mg/kg/24 hr for 8 weeks or a cumulative dose of 168 mg/kg. The safety of such a course, so far as spermatogenesis is concerned, has been confirmed (96). Prepubertal administration of twice this amount of cyclophosphamide also has been shown to produce only transient or minor abnormalities, suggesting that, if necessary, a second course could be considered.

As with cyclophosphamide, bone marrow suppression occurs with chlorambucil, but is rapidly reversible on withdrawal. Hemorrhagic cystitis, bladder neoplasia, and alopecia are less evident without chlorambucil; this lack of acute toxicity is one of the drug's attractive features. As with cyclophosphamide, however long-term toxicity of a more serious nature may follow its use. Thus, development of acute leukemia has been reported after immunosuppressive treatment of nonmalignant disease (97). Although several immunosuppressive agents may be implicated in such cases, this risk appears to be greatest with chlorambucil (98). Gonadal toxicity, which may be permanent, occurs in both pubertal and prepubertal patients treated with chlorambucil (99); ovarian function is affected less than the testis. This effect is dose related and may occur after a total dose of 8.2 mg/kg, equivalent to a 6-week course of 0.2 mg/kg/day (100).

Indications

Minimal-change Nephrotic Syndrome. A beneficial role of cyclophosphamide in the treatment of childhood NS was first described in 1963 (83), and support for this observation appeared over the next few years (101, 102). These reports were retrospective, concerned patients whose response to steroids was variable, and often did not provide histological confirmation of the underlying diagnosis.

In 1970 results were published of the first controlled trial of cyclophosphamide in steroid-responsive NS (84). This confirmed the value of cyclophosphamide in prolonging the period of remission in frequently relapsing patients; subsequent controlled studies supported this observation (103, 104). These later studies used different treatment protocols so that the question of appropriate dosage and duration of treatment remained unanswered. McCrory and coworkers (105) found that cyclophosphamide 2.5 mg/kg/24 hr for 90 days was just as effective and much less toxic than twice the dose given for half that time. Subsequently the efficacy of doses varying between 2.0 and 3.0 mg/kg/24 hr have been confirmed (106, 108); most authors now recommend an 8-week course of treatment at this dosage. The duration of remission, as well as the severity of side effects are less in those who remain on steroids for the duration of the course of cyclophosphamide (109).

Several attempts have been made to define the groups of patients who are most likely to respond to a course of cyclophosphamide. Siegel and coworkers (110) found that 38 of 40 children with a steroid-dependent frequently relapsing pattern of response to prednisone developed a complete remission after cyclophosphamide. The duration of remission and subsequent relapse rate were related only to the underlying histology. However, on the basis of both prospective (108) and retrospective studies (107), it is now apparent that the duration of response following a course of cyclophosphamide is much longer in frequently relapsing than in steroid-dependent patients. In steroid-resistant patients the response to cyclophosphamide is less predictable (104), although responders may again become steroid sensitive if they subsequently relapse (111).

The efficacy of chlorambucil in treating MCNS has also been clearly established. As with cyclophosphamide its chief benefit is noted in those who exhibit a frequently relapsing or dependent pattern of response to steroids, although some steroid-resistant patients may also respond (112). The minimum effective dose of chlorambucil has not been established, but a total dose of 11.2 mg/kg (equivalent to 0.2 mg/kg/24 hr for 8 weeks) is sufficient for induction of a sustained remission in most patients (113, 114). Following treatment with chlorambucil, the length of the ensuing remission appears to be greater than that achieved with cyclophosphamide (115). This factor, coupled with the relative lack of short-term side effects, has been the major argument in favor of its use; however, the specter of leukemia is a major concern (97, 98). The relative merits of one alkylating agent over another have not been proven, so that the choice of drug is often based on personal experience. Clearly, however, the use of both these drugs should be reserved for those who cannot be satisfactorily controlled with steroids alone.

Other Glomerular Disorders. Cyclophosphamide has been used to treat a variety of glomerular disorders other than MCNS in the hope of inducing a remission when management of the NS has been otherwise unsuccessful, when steroid toxicity is excessive, or in the face of a progressive deterioration of renal function. In these circumstances, its use may be justified, although proof of its efficacy has not been rigorously established.

In FSGS the response to cyclophosphamide is variable and patients who were initially steroid responsive are most likely to benefit (49, 50, 110). Some patients, however, while not responding completely to cyclophosphamide, may demonstrate a reduction in proteinuria, thus simplifying subsequent management and perhaps improving long-term prognosis (110). Similarly, in mesangial proliferative glomerulonephritis associated with NS, patients who are initially steroid resistant are unlikely to respond to cyclophosphamide later (116a, 117).

Cyclophosphamide also may be used in combination with steroids and anticoagulants to treat cresentic nephritis, but the benefit of such treatment has not been proven (63). It is also used as an immunosuppressive agent in conjunction with plasmapheresis in Goodpasture's syndrome (118).

Vasculitis Syndromes. Adequate control of the clinical and serological abnormalities of SLE is usually achieved with steroids, sometimes in combination with azathioprine. Cyclophosphamide further improves the outcome while permitting the use of less steroids (119, 120); however, with long-term therapy serious cyclophosphamide toxicity is almost inevitable. With a longer follow-up period, Decker and coworkers (121) were unable to demonstrate any clear advantage for patients receiving immunosuppressants beyond that attainable with steroids alone. The use of cyclophosphamide in SLE should probably be reserved for those who have proved unresponsive to less toxic therapy.

Vasculitis is associated with a wide variety of disorders including polyarteritis and many similar, but less well-defined conditions. While disease activity is sometimes controllable with steroids alone, this is often achieved only at the expense of severe toxicity. The use of cyclophosphamide, even in steroid-refractory patients, may produce a sustained remission and permit the discontinuance or reduction of steroids to tolerable levels (79). Cyclophosphamide is the drug of choice in Wegener's granulomatosis (80). In all these conditions, cyclophosphamide may have to be continued for a prolonged period, the usual dose being 1 to 2 mg/kg/day.

Purine Analogs

Pharmacokinetics

Azathioprine is a purine analog that undergoes transformation to 6-mercaptopurine in the tissues. It is available in both intravenous and oral forms, following which absorption is rapid. Metabolism occurs in the liver, and excretion of metabolites is via the kidneys; therefore, these may accumulate in renal failure unless the dosage is reduced (87).

Mode of Action

The precise mode of action of azathioprine is unknown, but probably includes effects on purine nucleotide synthesis and metabolism and alterations in the synthesis of RNA and DNA (87). Its immunosuppressive actions may result in a proportionate reduction of both B and T cells, although a greater sensitivity of B cells to the action of azathioprine has been noted (122, 123).

Side Effects

Bone marrow depression, usually manifest as leukopenia, is the most frequent side effect of azathioprine; the white cells may not return to normal for 7 to 10 days following cessation of the drug. Hepatitis, which may occur within 1 to 2 months of starting azathioprine, usually resolves on cessation of treatment. Macrocytosis, with or without anemia and unrelated to folate deficiency, has been described; it rarely antedates the development of red cell hypoplasia (124). As in patients receiving other immunosuppressants, an increased susceptability to infection is noted. Because the inactivation of 6-mercaptopurine is, in part, a result of the action of xanthine oxidase, there is an increased risk of toxic effects of azathioprine if it is prescribed in conjunction with allopurinol. In these circumstances, the dose of azathioprine should be reduced by approximately 75% (87).

Indications

Minimal-change Nephrotic Syndrome. The lesser toxicity of azathioprine when compared with cyclophosphamide has prompted its use in MCNS; unfortunately, comparable therapeutic benefits have not resulted. No difference between azathioprine and placebo was noted after 3 months of treatment in steroid-resistant patients (125). In this study, some benefit attributable to azathioprine was noted in frequently relapsing steroid-sensitive patients, although the results did not reach statistical significance. In a further controlled trial, no improvement in the stability of remissions after an 8-week course of azathioprine in frequently relapsing patients was observed (126). Hence, azathioprine is rarely used in the treatment of MCNS. Whether it might have a steroid-sparing effect and permit maintenance of remissions at a lower steroid dose in frequently relapsing or steroid-dependent patients has not been evaluated.

Systemic Lupus Erythematosus. The use of azathioprine in SLE should be aimed at achieving better disease control than that attainable with steroids alone or facilitating a reduction in maintenance steroid dosage below toxic levels. Conflicting results have been obtained from controlled clinical trials. There were no differences in mortality, disease control, renal function, or histological appearances when azathioprine and steroids were compared with steroids alone, whether evaluated at 6 (127) or 24 months (128). Hahn and coworkers (128) also evaluated the steroid-sparing effect of azathioprine, but found no difference in total steroid dosage or steroid toxicity between their two groups of patients (128). On the other hand, Cade and coworkers showed that, in patients with diffuse proliferative glomerulonephritis, the use of azathioprine in addition to steroids improved the prognosis for renal function above that achieved with steroids alone (129). Thus, although firm proof of its efficacy is lacking, azathioprine is used widely in SLE. It is therapeutically as effective as cyclophosphamide, although less toxic; for this reason, it is the drug of choice when steroids alone prove inadequate (130).

ANTICOAGULANT TREATMENT

Coagulation and Glomerular Disease

The role of coagulation mechanisms in glomerular disease and the evidence suggesting that activation of the coagulation pathways is involved in glomerular damage, has been discussed in detail in Chapter 14. In both experimental and human glomerulonephritis, fibrin is demonstrated in glomerular lesions either by immunofluorescence (131–132) or by electron microscopy (132–133). In animal experimental models, activation of coagulation is associated with glomerular damage (134). Anticoagulation with heparin is effective in reducing glomerular injury in experimental nephritis (135–136) as is defibrination with ancrod (137). However, there are other reports in which a beneficial effect has not been confirmed (138–139).

In human studies, further evidence for coagulation activation in glomerular disease has come from studies indicating increased fibrinogen turnover (21), elevated plasma and urinary fibrin degradation products (140–141), as well as evidence of persisting intravascular coagulation (142). This evidence, supporting involvement of the clotting system, has led to a number of therapeutic trials of anticoagulation. Despite numerous reports, the evidence that anticoagulation is beneficial is not completely clear. This may not be a result of treatment ineffectiveness, but rather to the heterogeneity of the patients studied, the lack of controlled trials, and the fact that anticoagulants were given in combination with antiplatelet agents, immunosuppression, and steroids, so that the contribution of each drug is difficult to assess.

Choice of Drug

Heparin

Heparin is a complex, highly anionic glycosaminoglycan that is extracted from animal sources. Its effect as an anticoagulant is immediate and depends on its ability to accelerate the action of the naturally occurring plasma coagulation inhibitor, antithrombin III, which neutralizes thrombin by forming a 1:1 enzyme inhibitor complex. Antithrombin III also inhibits factor IX and Xa activity. Heparin is not absorbed from the gastrointestinal tract and must be given parenterally. It is largely confined to the intravascular space and is strongly protein-bound. The half-life of heparin is about 90 minutes with average doses. There are contradictory data on heparin clearance in renal failure and it may be quite unpredictable. Other effects of heparin, not related to coagulation, are neutralization of cations such as platelet factor 4, release of lipoprotein lipase, as well as antikinin and anticomplement actions. Therefore, an effect of heparin therapy may not be solely a result of its anticoagulant activity.

Heparin can be given subcutaneously, by intermittent intravenous injection, or by continuous infusion. Absorption from depot sites is erratic, and hematomas are common. The needed dosages of heparin are extremely variable. In general, treatment regimens in children consist of an intravenous bolus of 100 U/kg, followed by 25 U/kg/hr by constant infusion.

There is considerable debate on the monitoring of heparin therapy. The most commonly recommended test is the activated partial thromboplastin time, which should be prolonged by 2 to 2.5 times. Minor bleeding can be treated by reducing or withdrawing the drug. If severe bleeding occurs, the anticoagulant effect can be reversed rapidly by protamine sulphate 1%, which should be given slowly, 1 mg/100 U heparin. Bleeding is the major complication, but occasionally thrombocytopenia and paradoxical thrombosis occur.

Oral Anticoagulants

The oral anticoagulants of the coumadin or indandione group act by inhibiting hepatic synthesis of the vitamin K-dependent clotting factors (prothrombin, VII, IX, and X), and the anticoagulant protein C. When a sufficient dose inhibits synthesis, these clotting factors disappear from the circulation at a rate dependent on their half-life.

Warfarin is generally the drug of choice. It is soluble and completely absorbed after oral administration. It is almost totally bound to plasma proteins, and only a small percentage of the drug is free. Biological half-life is between 35 and 45 hours. It is metabolized completely by hepatic microsomes, with which a variety of other drugs can interfere. The dose of warfarin should be adjusted to prolong the prothrombin time 1.5 to 2.5 times the control value.

The major side effect is bleeding, which is more likely when warfarin is used in conjunction with antiplatelet drugs or heparin. Bleeding is treated by administration of vitamin K1, and, if necessary, fresh frozen plasma may be given to produce rapid reversal.

Thrombolytic Agents

Both streptokinase and urokinase activate plasminogen to lyse fibrin thrombi. Streptokinase is a bacterial protein derived from filtrates of group C hemolytic streptococci. Urokinase is a plasminogen activator isolated from human urine. Streptokinase and urokinase are given systemically by intravenous infusion. If heparin is also used it should be discontinued as there is a considerable risk of bleeding. Urokinase is given with a loading dose of 4000 IU/kg body weight over 10 minutes, followed by a maintenance dose of 4000 U IV/kg/hr. With streptokinase, a loading dose is followed by 20 U/ml blood volume/hr. Alternatively, both drugs may be given as every 6-hour bolus injections. Treatment is continued for 3 to 5 days.

Allergic reactions to streptokinase include headache, fever, and anaphylaxis. Hydrocortisone may be given before treatment as a precaution. Bleeding is the major complication and is a particular risk in patients with recent surgery or invasive procedures, such as insertion of a peritoneal dialysis catheter or renal biopsy.

Indications

Anticoagulant therapy was introduced by Kincaid-Smith in 1968 in adults with crescentic nephritis (200). Beneficial effects of heparin treatment (usually combined with steroids, immunosuppression, or dipyridamol) were claimed later in a variety of conditions, including ARF, proliferative glomerulonephritis, malignant hypertension, and thrombotic thrombocytopenic purpura (132). Subsequent trials of heparin, warfarin, and antiplatelet agents in proliferative glomerulonephritis have given some encouraging results, but also conflicting ones.

Proliferative Glomerulonephritis

Cade and coworkers (143) studied 18 patients with chronic proliferative glomerulonephritis. Ten, including eight with crescents, were treated with daily subcutaneous depo-heparin for 1 year; eight (four with crescents) were untreated controls. Nine of the treated patients had stable or improving renal function, whereas 6/8 controls suffered a progressive decline in renal function. In five of the treated group, there was a rapid decline of renal function following discontinuation of treatment. The patients were not allocated randomly, and only a small number were treated.

Other studies in children on the use of anticoagulation for proliferative glomerulonephritis also produced encouraging results. Robson and coworkers treated six children with proliferative glomerulonephritis with necrosis or crescents, as well as evidence of active intravascular coagulation. Heparin was used initially in combination with azathioprine; phenindione and dipyridamol were commenced on discontinuation of heparin (142); anticoagulation was continued for 2 years and azathioprine for 1 year. All patients showed improved renal function, and several showed histological improvement. A heterogeneous group of children with various forms of nephritis were treated with heparin and some with warfarin by Herdman and coworkers (144); 5/13 showed improvement in renal function (144).

Combined anticoagulation and immunosuppression for MPGN were also reported to be of benefit in children with declining renal function in a nonrandomized or controlled trial, using the natural history of the disease or historical controls to assess benefit (145). Despite this uncontrolled report of a beneficial effect of combined therapy in MPGN, two recent controlled trials of warfarin, dipyridamol, and cyclophosphamide have shown no beneficial effect (146–147). These inconsistencies may be a result of differences in patient selection, stage of disease, or drug dosage and make definite conclusions and recommendations difficult.

Crescentic Nephritis

There have been no controlled trials of anticoagulation in crescentic nephritis because of the rarity of the disorder, poor prognosis, and heterogeneity of the patients studied.

Combinations of heparin followed by oral anticoagulants, antiplatelet drugs, and immunosuppression have been reported to improve renal function in both adults and children by several groups (63, 132, 148, 149). These reports, which suggest an improved prognosis in rapidly progressive nephritis treated with combination therapy, when compared with the untreated natural history of the disease, must be balanced against a high incidence of hemorrhagic complications (148, 150) and other studies showing no convincing beneficial effect (151–152). In particular, patients already anuric at the time of treatment are unlikely to improve, and treatment should perhaps be limited to those cases still passing urine (153). There are also reports that low dose heparin may be effective, but with diminished risk of hemorrhage (154).

Focal Segmental Glomerulosclerosis

Anticoagulation with heparin and dipyridamol was combined with steroids and cyclophosphamide in a controlled trial in nine patients with FSGS and compared with eight treated with steroids and cyclophosphamide alone. Significant improvement in renal function occurred in the anticoagulant group; 7/9 anticoagulant-treated patients had a complete remission, in contrast to only 3/8 of the untreated group (21).

Microangiopathy

The use of anticoagulants in the treatment of HUS and related disorders is considered in Chapter 27.

ANTIPLATELET THERAPY

Platelet Involvement in Glomerular Disease

The role of platelets in glomerular disease is now well established (155, 156). Platelets can be activated by a variety of stimuli, including immune complexes, exposed collagen, and vasoactive amines. In response to activation, they release several inflammatory substances that increase vascular permeability, degrade connective tissue, are chemotactic for neutrophils, and stimulate connective tissue proliferation (156). The importance of platelet activation in renal disease has been demonstrated in experimental animals. Intravascular platelet aggregation induces focal glomerular sclerosis and hypertension (157). In experimental immune complex disease, platelets are activated by immune complexes and release vasoactive substances that are important in the localization of immune complexes (158, 159).

In human studies, platelet turnover is increased in many glomerular diseases (21, 160, 161). Histologically platelets or platelet antigens have been demonstrated in glomeruli of patients with glomerular disease (162–165). In several forms of nephritis, platelet hyperaggregability has been shown in vitro (161, 166), as well as in vivo platelet aggregation (167), in the presence of platelet aggregating factors (168), and in the release of platelet granule contents (169).

The evidence that platelets are involved in glomerular disease has led to trials of antiplatelet agents in experimental glomerulonephritis. Blockade of platelet-released serotonin and histamine lessens tissue injury in experimental immune complex disease (159).

Induction of thrombocytopenia with antiplatelet serum inhibits proliferation in experimental proliferative glomerulonephritis (170). Both prostacyclin (PGI_2) and dipyridamol have lessened glomerular damage in Habu venom glomerulonephritis, whereas aspirin increased tissue damage (171), suggesting that aspirin may not only have inhibited thromboxane (TxA_2) production, but also blunted the protective effect of prostacyclin (PGI_2). In studies of Heymann nephritis, dipyridamol lessened proteinuria, but did not improve histological findings (172). In nehprotoxic serum nephritis, aspirin and ticlopidine diminished early inflammatory changes, but did not alter later glomerular damage (172).

While there are encouraging, but as yet inconclusive results of the use of antiplatelet agents in experimental nephritis, studies in human disease have been complicated by the following factors: (1) antiplatelet agents are often used in conjunction with immunosuppressants, anticoagulants, and plasma exchange, so that it is difficult to assess the contribution of any of these agents individually; (2) the patients are often heterogeneous, both in the nature and severity of the disease, so that it is difficult to compare the results obtained in the different studies; (3) drugs have been administered in varying doses and at different stages of the illness; (4) few of the reported studies have been randomized or adequately controlled; (5) a problem, particularly relevant to antiplatelet agents, such as aspirin and indomethacin, is the differing effect on vascular endothelium and platelets. Inhibition of platelet aggregation by blocking cyclo-oxygenase may be associated with simultaneous inhibition of endothelial PGI_2 production. The result, as shown in some animal studies (171), may actually be detrimental, without disproving the hypothesis that platelet inhibition may be of benefit in glomerulonephritis.

Choice of Drug

Dipyridamol

Dipyridamol acts to diminish platelet aggregation by inhibiting phosphodiesterase, and thus increasing intraplatelet cyclic AMP levels. Its effect is not easily demonstrated on in vitro aggregation studies, but has been shown in vivo. Dipyridamol is given orally in doses of 5 to 10 mg/kg/24 hr in three divided doses. Side effects include headache, gastrointestinal upset, bruising, and mild vasodilatation; however, in general, dipyridamol is a safe drug that is relatively free of major side effects.

Acetylsalicylic Acid

Aspirin causes irreversible inactivation of the enzyme cyclo-oxygenase. It blocks platelet TxA_2 production and is a powerful inhibitor of platelet aggregation induced by ADP, adrenalin, and arachidonic acid. As platelets are unable to synthesize cyclo-oxygenase, the effect persists for the life of the platelet. Therefore, aspirin's antiplatelet action lasts for a week to 10 days. Aspirin also inactivates endothelial cyclo-oxygenase and prevents PGI_2 production. This effect is less prolonged than that on the platelets and occurs only at higher doses. It follows that high dose aspirin inhibits both PGI_2 production and TxA_2 production, with an unpredictable final effect on platelet-endothelial interactions. In contrast, low dose aspirin inhibits TxA_2 production but leaves PGI_2 production intact, which should theoretically be more favorable for inhibition of platelet aggregation. Unfortunately, the dose and frequency of aspirin administration necessary for selective TxA_2 inhibition in the retention of PGI_2 production is not yet established in man. Most of the therapeutic trials of aspirin have been with doses high enough to block both TxA_2 and PGI_2 production and the results cannot be easily interpreted. Aspirin should be used as an antiplatelet agent in dosages much lower than those used previously, for example, 2 mg/kg on alternate days.

Indomethacin

Indomethacin inhibits cyclo-oxygenase of both platelets and vessel wall; therefore, it is similar to aspirin in its action. Major effects are diminution of GFR, headaches, and gastrointestinal irritation.

Clinical Experience

The results of trials in which antiplatelet agents are given in combination with immunosuppressive or anticoagulant therapy are difficult to interpret and will be discussed later. Specific antiplatelet therapy has been used infrequently.

Aspirin was used in a controlled prospective, double-blind study in 39 children (12 with idiopathic NS and 27 with proliferative glomerulonephritis) (173), who received 15 mg/kg/day aspirin or placebo for 16-week periods and were then crossed over. There were no significant changes in renal function or proteinuria, despite in vitro inhibition of platelet aggregation. The study is difficult to interpret because of the heterogeneity of patients (including seven with a family history of Alport's syndrome), the relatively short duration of treatment, and the fact that the aspirin dose used also could have inhibited endothelial PGI_2 production.

Dipyridamol has been used in combination with other drugs, including anticoagulants, other platelet inhibitors, or immunosuppressives. In a dosage of 300 to 450 mg/day, it has been reported to reduce proteinuria in NS (174) and proliferative glomerulonephritis (175).

In MPGN, a double-blind placebo-controlled study involving adults and children, showed that dipyridamol (225 mg/day) and aspirin (975 mg/day) caused a significant slowing of the rate of decline of renal function and improved platelet survival (176). A second controlled study, using dipyridamol and warfarin, also showed improved renal function in the treated group (177).

Combination of antiplatelet with anticoagulation and immunosuppressive drugs have been used frequently in uncontrolled studies of crescentic nephritis, MPGN, FSGS, and other forms of nephritis. Early enthusiastic reports of combination therapy (132) in a variety of glomerular diseases were followed by prospective randomized controlled trials of cyclophosphamide, dipyridamol, and warfarin in patients with MPGN (146–147). In both studies, no beneficial effect was demonstrated. These unsuccessful trials are in contrast to the previous uncontrolled studies that claimed a beneficial effect (142–145). Thus, no conclusion can be reached at this time on the efficacy of combined therapy.

Indomethacin is reported to reduce proteinuria in patients with glomerulonephritis, but the effect has not been confirmed (178–180).

PLASMA EXCHANGE

Plasmapheresis consists of the removal of plasma and return of red cells. It was introduced by Abel in 1914 as a means of obtaining large volumes of plasma (181) and was first used therapeutically in the hyperviscosity syndrome associated with macroglobulinemia (182). Apheresis is the general term for the removal of a blood component specified by the prefixes plasm-, leucocyt-, thrombocyt-, and so on. The therapeutic procedure discussed here is best termed plasma exchange, for the formed elements of the blood are returned with fresh plasma or other isoncotic fluid.

Technique

Equipment

Reliable plasma exchange is possible with the development of cell separators of two basic types: intermittent and continuous. Both have advantages, the former needs only one blood access line, but being slower and causing greater hemodynamic changes (particularly important in small children); the latter needs two access lines, but is generally faster and smoother in operation. Both involve separation of plasma from red cells by centrifugation and subsequent return of the red cells with the white cells and platelets suspended in replacement plasma. The development of plasma filters now also permits the extracorporeal separation of the formed elements of the blood from plasma without centrifugation.

Access

Good circulatory access is essential for successful plasma exchange, and, although flow rates as little as 10 ml/min can be used, the procedure then becomes prolonged and tedious (183). Arteriovenous shunts are the easiest to use; but, for short-term periods of treatment, central, or even peripheral venous lines suffice.

Replacement Fluid

The choice of replacement solution lies between plasma protein fraction (PPF), 5% albumin solution, or fresh frozen plasma (FFP). PPF is basically an albumin solution so that it leads to depletion of immunoglobulins, fibrinogen, and complement components, whereas FFP provides them (184). The choice between the two is confused because the relevant specific effect of plasma exchange is not well understood, and the consequences of depleting fibronogen and complement are not well defined.

Mode of Action

Some possible modes of action are the removal of antibody or immune complex, depletion of mediators of injury (fibrinogen and complement), anticoagulation, reversal of reticuloendothelial blockade, replacement of missing plasma component, and removal of inhibitor present in the plasma.

The relevant mode of action may be different in different diseases, for example, fibrinogen and complement depletion together with antibody removal, as in Goodpasture's syndrome (118), or the putative removal of an inhibitor of prostacyclin production in some cases of HUS (19). In an adult a 2-L exchange will remove 75% of an intravascular marker, a 4-L exchange 95%. However, the efficacy of depletion of a substance will also be affected by its distribution in body fluids, as well as by rates of synthesis and binding to tissues. With antibody removal, control of synthesis by immunosuppression is an essential adjunct to plasma exchange. The removal of immune complexes may be more related to reversal of endothelial blockade than to simple removal from plasma (185).

Complications

The complications associated with plasma exchange may be related to the type of replacement fluid or to the actual exchange procedure. An important consideration is in the type of replacement fluid, for there is a risk of severe anaphylactic reactions with FFP, which may also be responsible for the transmission of serum hepatitis.

The risk of infection, because of immunoglobulin depletion and other humoral factors, is uncertain and difficult to assess. Death has occurred following exchange, but the patients were usually receiving immunosuppressive therapy, as well as plasma exchange (38, 186, 187). Bleeding problems, a result of depletion of coagulation factors—especially fibrinogen, are rare, except when related to surgery or renal biopsy (188). The latter should not be performed within 48 hours of exchange, coagulation must be checked, and exchange should not be performed for at least 5 days after biopsy. Thrombocytopenia, if it occurs, could be a result of incorrect centrifuge settings in relation to flow rate. Thrombotic complications, such as cerebral thrombosis, pulmonary embolism, and vascular occlusion with gangrene, have been reported (189–190), perhaps related to depletion of antithrombin III. Prolonged apnea has been described when a general anesthetic was given, using suxamethonium within 72 hours of exchange, attributable to depletion of plasma cholinesterase activity (191).

Anticoagulation is effected with either acid-citrate-dextrose or heparin as a continuous infusion in the efferent line. With the former, citrate toxicity is well recognized, mediated principally by hypocalcemia (192). Parathesia, muscle twitching, tetany, and cardiac arrhythmias leading to death have been reported. Heparin, given as a bolus initially then as a slow infusion, has not proved troublesome and is partially removed with the plasma. Usually, reversal with protamine is not necessary.

Hemodynamic problems may occur with smaller children, particularly those <20 kg, but can be minimized with continuous separators and by priming with blood to the end of the return line. The edematous hypoalbuminemic patient is at particular risk of fluid overload, as correction of the hypoalbuminemia draws fluid into the intravascular compartment. The problem is more serious if the patient is also in renal failure. Recognition of the problems, ensuring that the patient is in a stable state before commencement of exchange, and close monitoring of blood pressure minimizes this risk. If necessary, the output and input flows can be adjusted to achieve a negative balance.

It is essential to give a careful explanation to the parents and child of the nature and purpose of the procedure and, with the older child, to show them the machine before it is used.

Indications

Plasma exchange is used in a wide variety of disorders with renal involvement with little substantiation of its efficacy by controlled trials. This situation has arisen, in part, because the individual conditions are rare and their prognosis is poor, so that there is a reluctance to have an untreated control population. Further, the technique has usually been combined with other treatments, which has complicated an analysis of the effect of the plasma exchange itself.

Goodpasture's Syndrome

Although rare in children, this condition has been described; the associated respiratory symptoms may be absent (193). It is caused by autoantibody production with specificity for the glomerular basement membrane (GBM). It is important to recognize it as a cause of rapidly progressive nephritis, since treatment initiated before anuria may prevent irreversible renal failure. An evaluation of the role of plasma exchange is helped by the ability to measure the antibody titer in plasma. It has been established with reasonable confidence that it is possible to arrest the deterioration of renal function (118). Control of lung hemorrhage is achieved by plasma exchange. The aim of treatment is the removal of antibody by intensive plasma exchange, together with long-term control of anti-GBM production by immunosuppression.

Prednisolone (2 mg/kg/24 hr) and immunosuppression with cyclophosphamide or azathioprine is essential to prevent rebound anti-GBM antibody production following removal by plasma exchange. Subsequent management is determined by renal function and the level of anti-GBM antibody. Compared with other forms of rapidly progressive nephritis the rate and volume of exchange should be more intensive because of the extravascular distribution and tissue fixation of the antibody. A minimum of 10 daily exchanges of 80 to 120 ml/kg is usually necessary. Relapses may occur, necessitating a further course of treatment.

Systemic Lupus Erythematosus

The implication of immune complexes in both the renal involvement and the systemic symptoms has led to the use of plasma exchange in an attempt to improve both aspects of SLE. Conventional therapy is aimed primarily at reducing the host antibody response and the initial inflammatory reaction elicited by the deposition of the immune complexes. Plasma exchange is aimed at reducing the level of immune complexes, as well as reduction of the steroid and cytotoxic dosage. In 1976, plasma exchange was used in eight cases as part of the treatment (194); four had circulating immune complexes that were reduced following exchange. Also, there was clinical improvement, with a reduction in proteinuria and a return to near normal in some cases of C3, C4, and DNA binding. In a follow-up study, 8/14 patients were considered to be improved following exchange, only 3 of whom had demonstrable circulating immune complexes (195).

Exchange with FFP rather than PPF may produce a more sustained improvement (196). It is not known whether it is the addition of complement or immunoglobulin in the FFP that might affect immune complex formation or clearance. Further work is required to ascertain whether the procedure of plasma exchange is necessary or whether the infusion of FFP alone will suffice (197).

Crescentic Nephritis

Patients with crescentic nephritis are characterized by rapid progression to renal failure. The condition may be associated with anti-GBM nephritis, MPGN postinfectious nephritis, or part of a multisystem disease, such as Henoch-Schönlein syndrome, polyarteritis, or SLE. On present data, assessment of the role of plasma exchange is difficult, because of small numbers of treated patients, variations of disease pattern, and the use of multiple therapy (199, 200). In 1977, nine cases of rapidly progressive nephritis were reported where plasma exchange was used in conjunction with prednisolone and cytotoxics; five of whom were thought to have improved as a result of plasma exchange (199). The disappearance of immune complexes or their return was temporally related to improvement of renal function. There have been isolated case reports, particularly in Henoch-Schönlein syndrome (201) and in MPGN type 2 (dense-deposit disease) suggesting improvement (202). In the Henoch-Schönlein syndrome, caution is necessary, as children with even a severe crescentic pattern may have a surprisingly good outcome. The situation is still rather unsatisfactory (203–204).

Hemolytic Uremic Syndrome

Plasmapheresis is beneficial in atypical cases of HUS associated with inhibition of prostacyclin production (19).

References

1. Soothill JF, Steward MW: The immuno-pathological significance of the heterogeneity of antibody affinity. Clin Exp Immunol 9:193, 1971.

2. Adeniyi A, Hendrickse RG, Soothill JF: A controlled trial of cyclophosphamide and azathioprine in Nigerian children with the nephrotic syndrome and poorly selective proteinuria. Arch Dis Childh 54:204, 1978.
3. Meltzer JI, Keim HJ, Laragh JL, et al: Nephrotic syndrome: vasoconstriction and hypervolemic types indicated by renin-sodium profiling. Ann Intern Med 91:688, 1979.
4. Levin M, Nokes TJC, Hardisty RM, et al: Spontaneous platelet aggregation in nephrotic syndrome. Int J Pediatr Nephrol 2:147, 1981 (abstract).
5. Yamada M, Matsuda I: Lipoprotein lipase in clinical and experimental nephrosis. Clin Chim Acta 30:787, 1970.
6. Wass VJ, Jarrett RJ, Chivers C, et al: Does nephrotic syndrome increase the risk of cardiovascular disease? Lancet 2:664, 1979.
7. Ichikawa I, Hoyer JR, Miele JF, et al: Mechanism of glomerulotubular balance in experimental glomerulonephritis. Kidney Intl 16:854, 1979, (abstract).
8. Birkenhager WH, Schalekamp MADH, Schalekamp-Kuyken MPA, et al: Interrelations between arterial pressure, fluid volumes, and plasma renin concentrations in the course of acute glomerulonephritis. Lancet 1:1086, 1970.
9. Sharpey-Schaffer EP: Venous Tone. Brit Med J 2:1589, 1961.
10. Warren JV, Stead EA: The protein content of edema fluid in patients with acute glomerulonephritis. Am J Med Sci 208:618, 1944.
11. Binak K, Sirmaci N, Ucak D, et al: Circulatory changes in acute glomerulonephritis at rest and during exercise. Brit Heart J 37:833, 1975.
12. Brain MC: The haemolytic uraemic syndrome. Semin Hematol 6:162, 1980.
13. Levin M, Barratt TM: Haemolytic uraemic syndrome. Arch Dis Childh 59:397, 1984.
14. Powell HR, Rotenberg E, Williams AL, et al: Plasma renin activity in acute poststreptococcal glomerulonephritis and the haemolytic-uraemic syndrome. Arch Dis Childh 49:802, 1974.
15. Mudge GH: Diuretics and other agents employed in the mobilisation of edema fluid. In AG Goodman, LS Goodman, A Gilman (eds): The Pharmacological Basis of Therapeutics, ed 6. New York, MacMillan, 1980, p 892.
16. Retan JW, Dillon HC: Furosemide in the treatment of acute post-streptococcal glomerulonephritis. South Med J 62:157, 1969.
17. Cameron JS, Ogg CS, Wass V: Complications of the nephrotic syndrome: hypercoagulability and thrombosis; infections; hyperlipoproteinaemia; loss of transport proteins in the urine; acute renal failure; tubular defects. In JS Cameron, RJ Glassock (eds): The Nephrotic Syndrome. New York, Marcel Dekker. (In press, 1984.)
18. Cameron JS, Ogg CS, Ellis FG, et al: Femoral artery thrombosis in nephrotic syndrome. Arch Dis Childh 46:215, 1971.
19. Mitchell JRA: Prostacyclin—powerful, yes: but is it useful? Brit Med J 287:1824, 1983.
20. George CRP, Clark WF, Cameron JS: The role of platelets in glomerulonephritis. Adv Nephrol 5:19, 1975.
21. Futrakul P, Postyachinda M, Mitrakul C: Focal sclerosing glomerulonephritis: a kinetic evaluation of hemostasis and the effect of anticoagulant therapy: controlled study. Clin Nephrol 10:180, 1978.
22. Moorhead JF, Chan MK, El-Nahas M, et al: Lipid nephrotoxicity in chronic progressive glomerular and tubulo-interstital disease. Lancet 2:1309, 1982.
23. Hendrickse RG, Glasgow EF, Adeniyi A, et al: Quartan malaria nephrotic syndrome. Lancet 2:1143, 1972.
24. Fish AJ, Blau EB, Westberg NG, et al: Systemic lupus erythematosus within the first two decades of life. Am J Med 62:99, 1972.
25. Bene MC, Favre B, Hurault de Ligny M, et al: Immunoglobulin A nephropathy. Quantitative immunohistomorphometry of the tonsillar plasma cells evidences an inversion of the immunoglobulin A versus immunoglobulin G secreting cell balance. J Clin Invest 71:1342, 1983.
26. Karlinsky ML, Haut L, Buddington B, et al: Preservation of renal function in experimental glomerulonephritis. Kidney Intl 17:293, 1980.
27. McCrory WW, Fleisher DS, Sohn WB: Effect of early ambulation in course of nephritis in children. Pediatrics 24:395, 1959.
28. Barnett HL, Farman CW, McNamara H, et al: The effect of adrenocorticotrophic hormone on children with the nephrotic syndrome. II. Physiologic observations on discrete kidney functions and plasma volume. J Clin Invest 30:227, 1951.
29. Fauci AS, Dale DC, Balow JE: Glucocorticosteroid therapy: mechanisms of action and clinical considerations. Ann Intern Med 84:304, 1976.
30. Baxter JD, Harris AW: Mechanism of glucocorticoid action: general features with reference to steroid mediated immunosuppression. Transplant Proc 7:55, 1975.
31. Green DC, Winter RJ, Kawahara RS, et al: Pharmokinetic studies of prednisolone in children. J Pediatr 93:299, 1978.
32. Anonymous: Prednisolone pulses in collagen disease; grammes or milligrammes? Lancet 1:280, 1983.
33. Nelson WF, Doherty CC, Douglas JF, et al: Plasma prednisolone concentration and kinetics in renal transplant patients. Proc Eur Dial Transplant Assoc 19:544, 1983.
34. Frey FJ, Frey BM: Altered prednisolone kinetics in patients with the nephrotic syndrome. Nephron 32:45, 1982.
35. Chamberlain P, Meyer WJ: Management of pituitary-adrenal suppression secondary to corticosteroid therapy. Pediatrics 67:245, 1981.
36. Brocklebank JT, Harcourt RB, Meadow SR: Corticosteroid induced cataracts in idiopathic nephrotic syndrome. Arch Dis Childh 53:30, 1982.
37. Bennett WM, Singer I, Golper T, et al: Guidelines for drug therapy in renal failure. Ann Intern Med 86:745, 1977.
38. Cohen J, Pinching AJ, Rees AJ, et al: Infection and immunosuppression. Quart J Med 51:1, 1982.
39. Nelville BGR, Wilson J: Benign intracranial hypertension following corticosteroid withdrawal in children. Brit Med J 3:554, 1976.
40. Arneil GC, Lam CN: Long term assessment of steroid therapy in childhood nephrosis. Lancet 2:819, 1966.
41. International Study of Kidney Disease in Children. Minimal change nephrotic syndrome in children: deaths during the first 5–15 years observation. Pediatrics 73:497, 1984.
41a. Siegel NJ, Goldberg B, Krassner LS, et al: Long term followup of children with steroid responsive nephrotic syndrome. J Pediatr 81:251, 1972.
42. Black DAK, Rose G, Brewer DB: Controlled trial of prednisone in adult patients with the nephrotic syndrome. Brit Med J 3:421, 1970.
43. International Study of Kidney Disease in Children. Nephrotic syndrome in children: prediction of histopathology from clinical and laboratory characteristics at time of diagnosis. Kidney Intl 13:159, 1978.
44. Barratt TM: Nephrotic syndrome. In Valman B (ed): Paediatric Therapeutics. Oxford, Blackwell, 1978, p 81.
45. Grupe WE: Primary nephrotic syndrome in childhood. Adv Pediatr 26:163, 1979.
46. Leisti S, Vilska J, Hallman N: Adrenocortical insufficiency and relapsing in the idiopathic nephrotic syndrome of childhood. Pediatrics 60:334, 1977.
47. Koskimies O, Vilska J, Rapola J, et al: Long term outcome of primary nephrotic syndrome. Arch Dis Childn 57:544, 1982.
48. Arbeitsgemeinschaft fur padiatrische nephrologie. Alternate day versus intermittent prednisone in frequently relapsing nephrotic syndrome. Lancet 1:401, 1979.
49. Gubler MC, Broyer M, Habib R: Signification des lesions de sclerose/hylinose segmentaire et focale dans la nephrose. Proc Seventh Intl Cong Nephrol 437, 1978.
50. Cameron JS, Turner DR, Ogg CS, et al: The long term prognosis of patients with focal segmental glomerulosclerosis. Clin Nephrol 10:213, 1978.
51. Glassock RJ, Cohen AH, Bennett CM, et al: Primary glomerular diseases. In Brenner B, Rector FC (eds): The Kidney, Ed 2. Philadelphia, W.B. Saunders, 1981, p 1351.
52. Collaborative Study of the Adult Idiopathic Nephrotic Syndrome. A controlled study of short term prednisone treatment in adults with membranous nephropathy. N Engl J Med 301:1301, 1979.
53. Habib R, Kleinknecht C, Gubler MC, et al: Membranous glomerulonephropathy in children. In Edelman C (ed): Pediatric Kidney Disease, Boston, Little, Brown & Co., 1978, p 646, vol 1.
54. Latham P, Poucell S, Konesaar A, et al: Idiopathic membranous glomerulopathy in Canadian children: a clinicopathologic study. J Pediatr 101:682, 1982.
55. Raminez F, Brouhard BH, Travis LB, et al: Idiopathic membranous nephropathy in children. J Pediatr 101:677, 1982.
56. Habib R, Kleinknecht C, Gubler MC, et al: Idiopathic membranoproliferative glomerulonephritis in children. Report of 105 cases. Clin Nephrol 1:194, 1973.
57. Davis AE, Schneeberger EE, Grupe WE, et al: Membranoproliferative glomerulonephritis (MPGN Type I) and dense deposit disease in children. Clin Nephrol 9:184, 1978.
58. Magil AB, Price JDE, Bower G, et al: Membranoproliferative glomerulonephritis Type 1: comparison of natural history in children and adults. Clin Nephrol 11:239, 1979.
59. Barbiano de Belgiojosa G, Tarantino A, Colasainti G, et al: The prognostic value of some clinical and histological parameters in membranoproliferative glomerulonephritis. Report of 112 cases. Nephron 19:250, 1977.
60. McEnery PT, McAdams AJ, West CD: Membranoproliferative glomerulonephritis: improved survival with alternate day prednisone therapy. Clin Nephrol 13:117, 1980.
61. International Study of Kidney Disease in Children. Alternate day steroid therapy in membranoproliferative glomerulonephritis: a randomized controlled clinical trial. Kidney Intl 21:150, 1982 (abstract).
62. Cameron JS. The natural history of glomerulonephritis. In Black DAK, Jones NF (eds): Renal Disease, Ed 4. Oxford, Blackwell Scientific, 1979, p 329.
63. Brown CB, Turner D, Ogg CS, et al: Combined immunosuppression and anticoagulation in rapidly progressive glomerulonephritis. Lancet 2:1166, 1974.
64. Cole BR, Brocklebank JT, Kienstra RA, et al: Pulse methylprednisolone therapy in the treatment of severe glomerulonephritis. J Pediatr 88:307, 1976.
65. Beirne GJ, Wagnild JP, Zimmerman SW, et al: Idiopathic crescentic glomerulonephritis. Medicine (Baltimore) 56:349, 1977.
66. Kincaid Smith P, D'Apice AJF: Plasmapheresis in rapidly progressive glomerulonephritis. Am J Med 65:564, 1978.

8

Metabolic And Tubular Disease

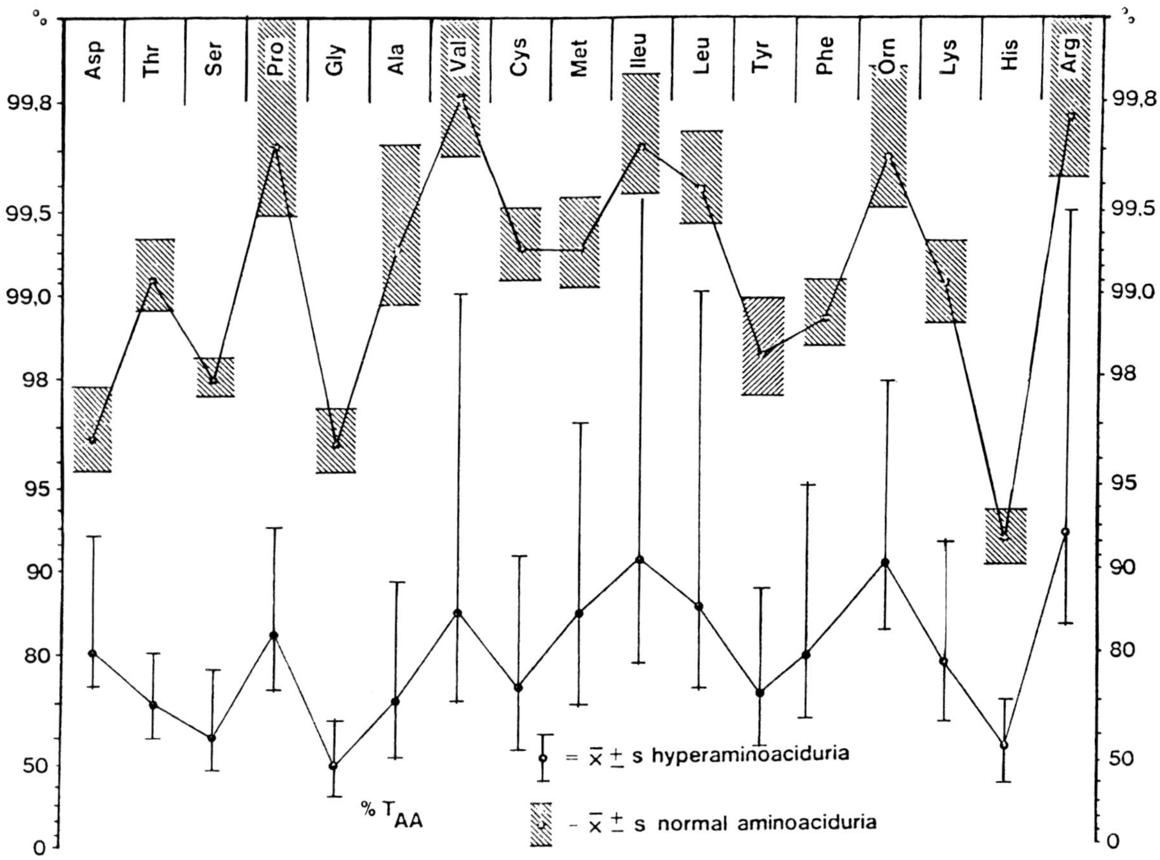

Figure 30.2. The mean values (x̄ ± SD) of percentage of tubular reabsorption in seven children with generalized hyperaminoaciduria in comparison with normal values of children. (From Brodehl J, Bickel H: Clin Nephrol 1:163, 1979)

the cell across the basolateral membrane also is carrier mediated. In the proximal convoluted tubule, where the bulk of AA reabsorption occurs, this movement is mediated predominantly by facilitated diffusion down the concentration gradient between the cell and peritubular fluid. In the proximal straight tubule, active transport across the basolateral membrane has been demonstrated, but its significance is not clear (17).

The urinary AA losses in the Fanconi syndrome do not cause any clinical difficulties because the losses are trivial in relation to intake and to dietary replacement of the losses. However, Paa levels tend to be lower than normal. In a few patients an impairment in intestinal AA transport contributes to the lower Paa levels.

Glucosuria

Glucosuria is another feature of the Fanconi syndrome and one of the originally recognized manifestations. The glucosuria is termed renal, because plasma glucose concentration is normal; often it is the first sign detected, since glucosuria is detected by routine urinalysis.

The presence of glucose in the urine with normal or even low plasma glucose concentrations indicates that the renal threshold, i.e., the plasma level of a solute when it first appears in the urine, is reduced. Tubular reabsorption rises with glucose loading, demonstrating that the tubule responds. Maximal tubular reabsorption of glucose (Tm_g) is normal in a few children with Fanconi syndrome. However, measuring Tm_g can be quite dangerous because of the risk of hypokalemia (18, 19). Adults with Fanconi syndrome have low renal threshold values and either normal or low Tm_g (20).

Glucosuria in the Fanconi syndrome may play a role in the disordered handling of phosphate and AA. Infusion of glucose, fructose, or galactose—but not xylose—in normal subjects results in phosphaturia and aminoaciduria (21). This response has been shown in isolated brush-border membrane vesicles as well (22).

Studies of glucose handling by the renal tubule have been reviewed (23). Glucose is nearly completely reabsorbed in early proximal tubule; little or none reaches the distal tubule when filtered loads are normal. The uptake of alpha-methylglucoside, a nonmetabolizable analogue of glucose, is active and is intimately linked to Na uptake (24). This process resides in the brush border of the proximal tubule (23, 25). Transport across the basolateral membrane is Na-independent, facilitated diffusion in both directions. Transport into the cell at this site may play an important role.

Hypophosphatemia

Hypophosphatemia and impairment in phosphate reabsorption is another important facet of the Fanconi syndrome. This defect is a result of depressed proximal tubular reabsorption of phosphate. In the normal state, approximately 60% to 70% of the filtered load of phosphate is reabsorbed in the pars convoluta and 10% in the pars recta of the proximal tubule (26). Phosphate is actively taken up by carriers in the brush border membrane in conjunction with Na^+ ions. Transport out of the cell across the basolateral membrane is also carrier mediated, but occurs passively down the electrochemical gradient (27). Brush-border membrane uptake is enhanced by dietary restriction (28, 29) and decreased by parathyroid hormone (30) and the generation of cyclic adenosine monophosphate (30).

The impaired phosphate reabsorption in the Fanconi syndrome is not usually reflected in hyperphosphaturia, except when the Fanconi syn-

Table 30.1.
Amino acid excretion in various types of the Fanconi syndrome

Type	24-Hr urinary amino acid excretion[a]			
	Normal	2 to 4×	5 to 10×	10×
Cystinosis ($N = 6$)[b]	SER, GLU MET, LYS HIS, TRY	ASP, THR ASN, GLN GLY, ALA CYS, ILE TYR, LEU PHE, DRN ARG	PRO, CIT VAL	
Lowe's syndrome ($N = 2$)[b]	ASP, THR SER, GLU MET, ILE LEU, TYR PHE, HIS	ASN, GLN GLY, ALA VAL, CYS ORN, LYS TRY, ARG	PRO CIT	
Lowe's syndrome ($N = 1$)[b]	HIS	GLU, CYS MET, ILE PHE	SER, GLY ALA, LEU TYR, ORN LYS, ARG	THR, ASN GLN,PRO CIT, VAL
Tyrosinemia ($N = 1$)	ASP, PRO VAL, ILE LEU, ORN ARG	GLN, GLU CIT, GLY CYS, LYS HIS	SER, ASN ALA, PHE	THR, MET TYR
Idiopathic ($N = 1$)	HIS		MET, TYR LYS	THR, SER GLU, PRO GLY, ALA CYS, VAL LEU, ILE ARG, PHE

[a] Headings denote the increase above normal. *N* denotes the number of patients studied. Abbreviations are defined as follows:

ASN—asparagine ASP—aspartic acid ARG—arginine
ALA—alanine CYS—cystine CIT—citrulline
GLN—glutamine GLU—glutamic acid GLY—glycine
HIS—histidine ILE—isoleucine LYS—lysine
LEU—leucine MET—methionine PHE—phenylalanine
PRO—proline SER—serine THR—threonine
TYR—tyrosine TRY—tryptophan VAL—valine

[b] Three patients with the same disease had two different patterns of amino acid excretion.

drome first develops. In a steady state, urinary phosphate excretion simply reflects dietary intake similar to that observed in X-linked hypophosphatemic rickets (31), vitamin D deficiency (32), and normals (33). Excessive phosphate excretion will be observed only when plasma phosphorus is above its steady state level.

Hypophosphatemia is the hallmark of depressed phosphate reabsorption in the Fanconi syndrome. Plasma phosphate concentration is governed by at least the following 3 factors: (1) renal phosphate threshold concentration, which is the theoretical plasma concentration of phosphate at which maximal tubular reabsorption would occur; (2) the net input of phosphate into ECF from the gastrointestinal tract, bone, and cells; and (3) the amount of ECF processed per unit time, i.e., GFR (34). The renal phosphate threshold concentration has the greatest effect. It, however, is influenced by the state of the ECF volume, the level of numerous hormones, e.g., growth hormone, estrogens, calcitonin, and especially parathyroid hormone. Vitamin D metabolites also play a role. The higher plasma phosphate level observed normally in children can be related to a higher renal phosphate threshold concentration (Tm_{PO_4}) and not to differences in various hormone levels (35). Dietary intake within a fairly wide range and GFR have only small influences until the GFR falls <25 ml/min/1.73m^2 (36), at which point dietary intake plays the central role in determining plasma phosphate.

Phosphate handling can be assessed by measuring the percent tubular reabsorption of phosphate (TRP), as described for AA. The TRP ranges from 80% to 95% in normal children (35). Much lower values are found in patients with Fanconi syndrome. A preferred way of estimating the renal handling of phosphate is to derive the Tm_{PO_4} related to GFR. This is determined from the fasting plasma phosphate, plasma creatinine, urinary phosphate, and urinary creatinine using the nomogram developed by Walton and Bijvoet (37). Normative data for children have been developed by Kruse and coworkers (35).

Phosphate handling by the kidney is altered by the level of parathyroid hormone (PTH). The rate of reabsorption decreases as the level of PTH is increased. However, the role of PTH in the Fanconi syndrome is not clear. Morris (38) found, in a patient with a parathyroidectomy and hereditary fructose intolerance, that both fructose and PTH were necessary to elicit the Fanconi syndrome , including the exaggerated phosphaturia. Kyle and coworkers (39) noted a normal phosphaturic effect with administered parathyroid extract, which indicated to them that excessive PTH was not causing the hypophosphatemia. Calcium infusions, which

192. Watson DK, Penny AF, Marshall RW, et al: Citrate induced hypocalcaemia during cell separation. Brit J Haematol 44:503, 1980.
193. Lockwood CM, Bolton-Jones JM, Lowenthal RM, et al: Recovery from Goodpasture's syndrome after immunosuppression treatment and plasmapheresis. Brit Med J 2:252, 1975.
194. Verrier-Jones J, Bucknell RC, Cumming RH, et al: Plasmapheresis in the management of acute systemic lupus erythematosis. Lancet 1:709, 1976.
195. Verrier-Jones J, Cumming RH, Bacon PA, et al: Evidence for a therapeutic effect of plasmapheresis in patients with systemic lupus erythematosis. Quart J Med 48:555, 1979.
196. Moran CJ, Parry HF, Mowbray J, et al: Plasmapheresis in systemic lupus erythematosis. Brit Med J 1:573, 1977.
197. Clark WF, Lindsay RM, Ulan RA, et al: Chronic plasma exchange therapy in SLE. Clin Nephrol 16:20, 1981.
198. Kincaid-Smith P, Saker BM, Fairley KF: Anticoagulants in irreversible acute renal failure. Lancet 2:1360, 1968.
199. Lockwood CM, Rees AJ, Pinching AJ, et al: Plasma exchange and immunosuppression in the treatment of fulminant immune complex mediated crescentic nephritis. Lancet 1:63, 1977.
200. Becker GJ, D'Apice AJF, Walker RG, et al: Plasmapheresis in the treatment of glomerulonephritis. Med J Aust 2:693, 1977.
201. Kauffmann RH, Houwert DA: Plasmapheresis in rapidly progressive Henoch-Schonlein glomerulonephritis and the effect on circulating IgA complexes. Clin Nephrol 16:155, 1981.
202. Montolin J, Bergada E, Arrizabalaga P, et al: Acute renal failure in dense deposit disease—recovery after plasmapheresis. Brit Med J 284:940, 1982.
203. Kincaid-Smith P, D'Apice AJF: Plasmapheresis in rapidly progressive nephritis. Am J Med 65:564, 1978.
204. Pinching AJ, Peters DK: Plasma exchange in nephritis (editorial). J Roy Soc Med 72:395, 1979.

suppresses PTH, lowered phosphate excretion in some (40–42), but not all, patients with the Fanconi syndrome (43–45). PTH levels were normal in one (46), but elevated in another (47) study. Bone histology of biopsy specimens from patients with the Fanconi syndrome did not show evidence of PTH effects (48).

Other influences on phosphate metabolism are vitamin D and its metabolites. Low levels of the activated form of vitamin D, 1,25-OH vitamin D have been noted in three patients with the Fanconi syndrome, two of whom had normal serum creatinine levels (49). Patients with the Fanconi syndrome have impaired conversion of [^{3}H]-25-vitamin D to [^{3}H]-1,25-vitamin D (50). In the experimental Fanconi syndrome caused by maleic acid administration, the activity of mitochondrial vitamin D hydroxylase was decreased, suggesting a cause for the low 1,25 dihydroxyvitamin D levels (51). Metabolic acidosis, a feature of the Fanconi syndrome, also impairs the conversion of 25-OH vitamin D to 1,25-OH vitamin D (52, 53), which may explain the observation that rickets in some patients with the Fanconi syndrome may heal with alkali alone (54).

Hypophosphatemia and low 1,25$(OH)_2$ vitamin D levels may explain the bone disease in patients with Fanconi syndrome. There is a wide spectrum of pathology—osteoporosis, osteomalacia, and, in children, rickets. However, hyperparathyroid changes are not common when GFR is normal or nearly so (48). Abnormalities in bone, if not treated, may lead to the growth retardation, fractures, and crippling deformities common in this syndrome. Most patients respond to large doses of vitamin D or 1,25$(OH)_2$ vitamin D and alkali; a few also require oral phosphate supplements.

Acidosis

Acidosis, another feature of the Fanconi syndrome, usually occurs in association with hyperchloremia and is a result of impaired bicarbonate reabsorption by the proximal tubule (55, 56). Normally, 80% to 90% of the filtered bicarbonate is reabsorbed proximally and from near zero to 5% is ultimately excreted. In the Fanconi syndrome, more than 30% of the normal filtered load may be excreted when plasma bicarbonate levels are normal, leading to low plasma bicarbonate levels and reduction in ECF volume. As the filtered load of bicarbonate and ECF volume contracts, a negligible fraction of the filtered bicarbonate is excreted. At this point, urine pH may be below 5.5 and H+ output balances input. Continuous retention of H+ does not occur. In this form of RTA, known as proximal RTA, retention of H+ is not sustained, as it is in distal RTA. Balance is obtained only when ECF volume and plasma bicarbonate level are depressed—the latter usually to between 12 to 18 mEq/l (chapter 22) (56).

Occasionally, there is a defect in distal acidification resulting from an inability to lower the urine pH <5.5 (55, 57–61). This probably is related to long-standing hypokalemia or nephrocalcinosis, either of which may affect the distal tubule. Ammoniagenesis is normal to increased, because of the hypokalemia and acidosis, unless glomerular impairment is significant (40, 62–64).

Sodium and Potassium Losses

Na and K losses may give rise to major problems in the Fanconi syndrome. Normally, 60% to 80% of the filtered load of Na is reabsorbed in the proximal tubule, but much less is reabsorbed in the Fanconi syndrome. Part of this loss is related to impaired bicarbonate reabsorption with the subsequent urinary excretion of $NaHCO_3$ and $KHCO_3$. In some cases, Na and K losses are so great that metabolic alkalosis and hyperaldosteronism result, simulating Bartter's syndrome in spite of the lowered bicarbonate threshold (62, 65). This occurs in part because of the delivery of Na distally, where Na for K exchange occurs, is excessive, leading to marked urinary K losses. The clearance of K may be twice that of the GFR (66). The hypokalemia and K deficiency may cause sudden death.

Dehydration

Polyuria, polydipsia, and frequent bouts of severe dehydration are common symptoms in patients with the Fanconi syndrome. Recurrent febrile episodes, as a consequence of the dehydration, are often the first sign of the Fanconi syndrome in infants with cystinosis. In some measure, the polyuria is related to an osmotic diuresis from the excessive urinary solute losses. In few patients, there also appears to be an impairment in distal tubule-concentrating ability, especially in those with prolonged hypokalemia, that aggravates the osmotic diuresis (57, 67, 68). The polyuria is commonly an hyposthenuria, as is often the case in K deficiency. Increased distal delivery of solute, particularly Na, increases free water clearance and the hyposthenuria.

Growth Retardation

A common feature of the Fanconi syndrome in children is growth retardation of varying severity. The cause probably is multifactorial in most patients. Hypophosphatemia, disordered vitamin D metabolism, or acidosis can impair growth. Chronic hypokalemia and extracellular volume contraction may be factors. Glucosuria and aminoaciduria probably are not. However, even with correction of all these metabolic abnormalities, most patients fail to grow, especially those with cystinosis.

Uricosuria

An impairment in renal handling of urate is present in the Fanconi syndrome, leading to hypouricemia, especially in adults (20, 44, 67, 69–72). The mechanism of renal tubular handling of uric acid in humans is not fully defined, but there is a large reabsorptive and simultaneous secretory flux in the proximal tubule (73). An alteration in either of these two fluxes could lead to the increased urinary excretion. However, a problem in a more distal secretory mechanism, which also appears to exist for urate, could underlie this loss. Urolithiasis from the uricosuria has not been reported. This probably is because the urine flow and pH are increased, inhibiting uric acid crystallization.

Proteinuria

Proteinuria, another feature of the Fanconi syndrome, was pointed out in the early descriptions of this syndrome and gave rise to the name, nephrotic-glucosuric dwarfism (4). Proteinuria usually is minimal, <40 $mg/m^2/hr$, except when the Fanconi syndrome develops in association with the nephrotic syndrome in its later stages, which is rare. The usual proteinuria consists of a low molecular weight species of protein in the range of 1900 to 30,000 daltons, e.g., enzymes, immunoglobulin light chains, and hormones (74–79); this pattern of proteinuria has been termed tubular. Proteinuria arises either from failure to reabsorb proteins filtered by the glomerulus or from proteins secreted by tubule cells, or both (79).

CAUSES

Patients with the Fanconi syndrome can be classified into two main categories: inherited and acquired (Table 30.2). In adults, the most common cause of the Fanconi syndrome is an exogenous toxin, such as a heavy metal; whereas in children, the most common cause is an inborn error of metabolism, such as cystinosis. Not considered in this classification are syndromes in which only two of the four cardinal signs of the Fanconi syndrome—glucosuria, hyperaminoaciduria, impaired phosphate reabsortion, and proximal tubular acidosis—are present, such as glucoglycinuria (80), glucoaminoaciduria (81), or glucophosphaturia (82).

Table 30.2.
Causes of the Fanconi Syndrome

Inherited	Acquired
Cystinosis	Heavy metal poisoning
Galactosemia	Glue sniffing
Hereditary fructose intolerance	Diachrome poisoning
Tyrosinemia	Azathiaprine
Wilson's disease	Gentamicin
Lowe's syndrome	Streptozotocin
Glycogenosis	Maleic acid
Cytochrome-c-oxidase deficiency	Multiple myeloma
Idiopathic	Sjogren's syndrome
	Hypergammaglobulinemia
	Light-chain proteinuria
	Amyloidosis
	Nephrotic syndrome
	Renal transplantation

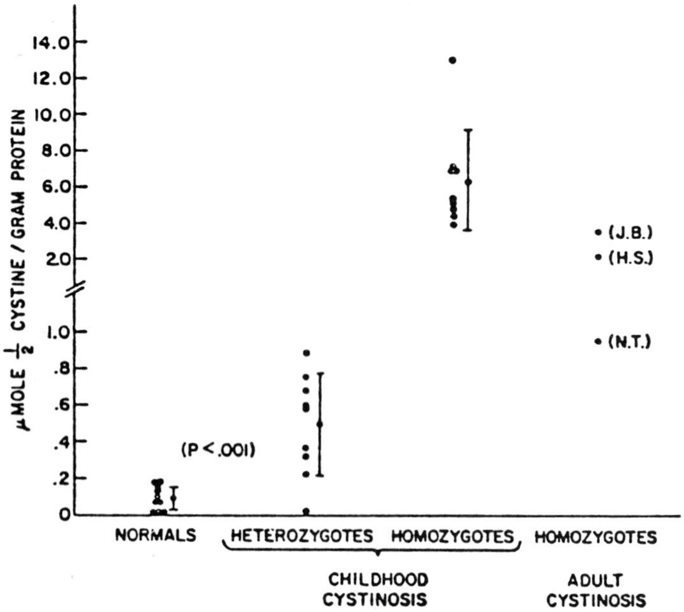

Figure 30.3. Free cystine content of leukocytes. Children are represented by open, and adult by closed circles. Note the scale change on the ordinate. The brackets indicate ±1 S.D. from the mean. (Reprinted by permission of The New England Journal of Medicine, vol. 279, p. 1255, 1968.)

Inherited Causes

Cystinosis

Cystinosis or cystine storage disease is an enigmatic disorder characterized biochemically by excessive storage of the AA, cystine, in numerous organs, including the kidney (83). Cystinosis, as is the case with most genetic disorders associated with the Fanconi syndrome, is transmitted as an autosomal recessive trait. The gene frequency, however, is unknown. This disorder is distinct from cystinuria in which cystine does not accumulate intracellularly and the Fanconi syndrome does not develop.

Three different types of cystinosis can be distinguished, based on the clinical course and the intracellular cystine content (84–86). Infantile or nephropathic cystinosis is the most common and is associated with the highest intracellular levels of cystine in leukocytes or cultured fibroblasts; it leads to severe renal injury and end-stage renal disease by late childhood (87–89). The benign or adult type has lower levels of intracellular cystine; crystals are observed only in the cornea and bone marrow. There is no renal involvement (2, 8–10). This form has been recognized only during routine ophthalmological examination. The adolescent form is intermediate, i.e., intracellular cystine levels are in between those of the infantile and adult forms. Renal involvement occurs but does not appear until later, usually in adolescence, is variable, and progresses slowly (86, 93, 94). Whether these represent allelic defects is not known but, if so, the intermediate form could be a double heterozygote of the other two.

The biochemical defect underlying cystinosis presently is unknown. Affected leukocytes contain 4 to 8 nMol/mg protein of ½ cystine, while normal cells contain virtually no cystine, but do contain small amounts of the reduced form, cysteine (84) (Fig. 30.3). The intracellular cystine appears to be stored in lysosomes (95, 96). Yet, unlike other lysosomal storage diseases, such as Gaucher's disease, there is not a progressive accumulation, since fetal tissue contains the same concentration as renal tissue removed at the time of renal transplantation (97, 98).

The source of this intracellular cystine pool and how it becomes entrapped in lysosomes is unclear. Several investigators have noted that cystinotic fibroblasts accumulate and store cystine much more avidly than normal fibroblasts, providing a convenient system for studying the biochemical basis of cystinosis (99, 100). Although cystinotic cells are marked by excessive cystine levels, there appears to be no defect in the capacity of these cells to reduce cystine to cysteine (101, 102).

Another important fate of cystine is incorporation into the tripeptide, glutathione. Whereas levels of the major intracellular form of this compound, reduced glutathione, are normal (103), levels of oxidized glutathione are, however, low. The activity of gamma-glutamyltranspeptidase, a glutathione cleavage enzyme, is high in fibroblasts from patients with cystinosis (104). Thus, the rapid turnover of oxidized glutathione back to its constituent amino acids could play a role in the high cystine levels.

Intralysosomal protein degradation has been proposed as the source of the intracellular cystine (105), but it may arise from extracellular protein or exogenous cystine as well. Recently, reports from two laboratories have described impaired cystine efflux from lysosomes of cystinotic cells (Fig. 30.4) (106–111). These investigators took advantage of the fact that lysozomes can be loaded with free AA when incubated with their methyl ester (112). Schneider's group also employed the mixed disulfide, cysteine-glutathione, to load lysosomes with cystine. With these techniques, they showed that cystine efflux, but not that of other AA, was slower from cystinotic lysosomes compared with normals; heterozygotes for cystinosis have intermediate values. Schneider's group also has raised the possibility that an ATP dependent proton pump in the lysosome is necessary for cystine efflux (110), although this was not confirmed by Schulman's group (106).

Remaining to be answered (if this is the biochemical defect in cystinosis) is how cystine enters the lysosome normally, since there is no uptake of free AA by the lysosome (112). The source of cystine in the cystinotic lysosome is also not known nor is the relationship of excessive intracellular cystine to the renal injury.

This high intracellular cystine level, the biochemical hallmark of this disease, is found in cells of the bone marrow, leukocytes, cornea, conjunctiva, retina, lymph nodes, and internal organs, including those of liver, spleen, intestine, thyroid, and kidney (83). The brain appears not to be affected. The usual tissues sampled to make the diagnosis are leukocytes (113), rectal mucosa (114), and bone marrow (115). Finding needle-shaped, tinsel-like refractile opacities in the cornea by slit lamp examination is usually diagnostic (Fig. 30.5) (116). Often, they are present early in the disease and they are invariably present after 2 years of age. A prenatal diagnosis can be made by measuring the cystine content of cells cultured from the amniotic fluid (114, 115).

The diagnosis of cystinosis usually is made in the latter half of the

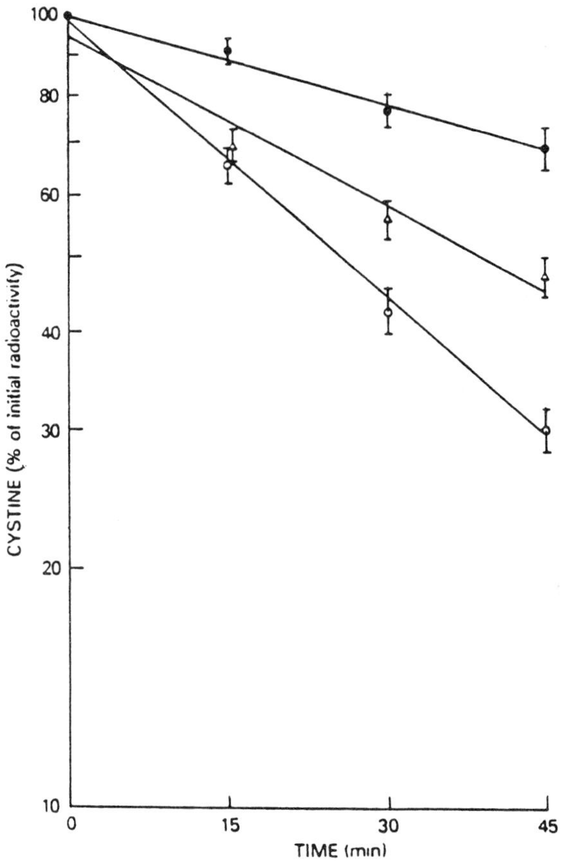

Figure 30.4. Cystine disposal from lysosome-rich granular fractions of normal, heterozygous and cystinotic leukocytes loaded with [^{35}S]-cystine dimethyl ester. Each point represents the mean ± S.E. for 13 cystinotic (●), 8 heterozygous (△), and 13 normal (○) preparations from 8 cystinotic, 8 heterozygous, and 11 normal subjects. (Reprinted from Gahl WA, et al: J Biol Chem 257:9572, 1982.)

first year of life (83, 88, 89, 117). The diagnosis can be made earlier in families with index cases, but there always is a delay between birth and the first symptoms. The early symptoms are polyuria, polydipsia, anorexia, failure to thrive, dehydration, and acidosis. Rickets usually does not occur in the first year. Assessment of renal tubular function before symptoms appear will show abnormalities, but there is a lag between birth and the appearance of abnormalities.

Children with cystinosis usually have fair complexions and blond hair, but dark hair has been observed in some. Cystinosis has been observed in blacks (118), but rarely. Affected children are not dysmorphic except for changes ascribed to rickets. Mental development is normal. Polyuria and polydipsia are invariable. The urine is dilute and contains 1 to 5 g/day of glucose, AA equal to 10 to 30 mg/day of alpha-amino nitrogen, and protein (0.2 to 1.5 g/day) before glomerular dysfunction is apparent (117). Tubular reabsorption of phosphate is <80% and the renal threshold for bicarbonate usually is between 12 to 15 mEq/l. Hypokalemia (K_s <3 mEq/l), hyperchloremic metabolic acidosis (bicarbonate level <18 mEq/l), hypophosphatemia (P_s <3 mg/dl), and hypouricemia (<3 mg/dl) are common (117). A few patients have hyponatremia; rarely, metabolic alkalosis is observed (65).

GFR always declines in infantile cystinosis. ESRD usually occurs between 7 to 10 years of age. Because GFR declines, the electrolyte supplements required initially may become harmful. Patients with cystinosis and ESRD tolerate chronic dialysis and transplantation with no greater difficulty than children with other forms of renal failure. Renal transplantation reverses the renal failure, but does not appear to improve the other symptoms of cystinosis (117, 119–121). Cystine accumulates in the monocytes and interstitial cells of transplanted kidneys, but symptoms because of proximal tubule dysfunction suggestive of cystinosis have not been noted.

Photophobia is common and usually appears between 3 and 6 years of age (116, 117). The severity of this symptom increases with age. In addition to the corneal and conjunctival crystal deposits, peripheral retinopathy occurs in which the appearance is quite variable, with either

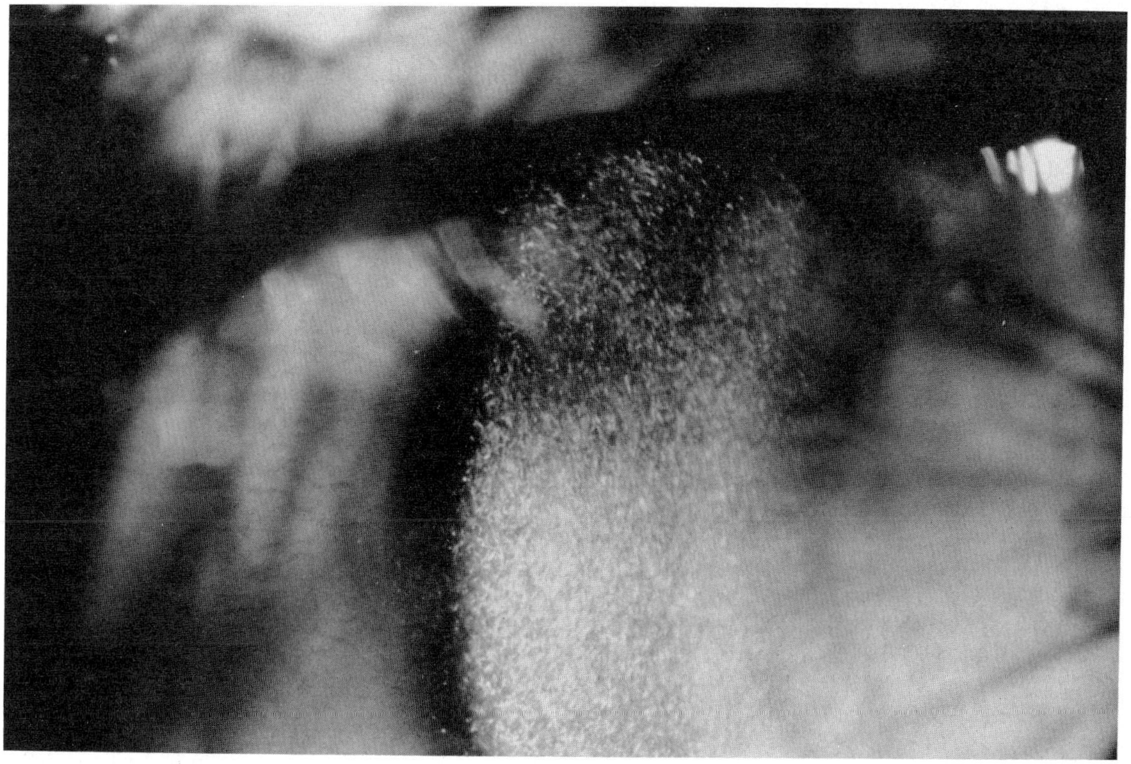

Figure 30.5. Tinsel-like refractile opacities in the cornea of a patient with cystinosis under slit lamp examination.

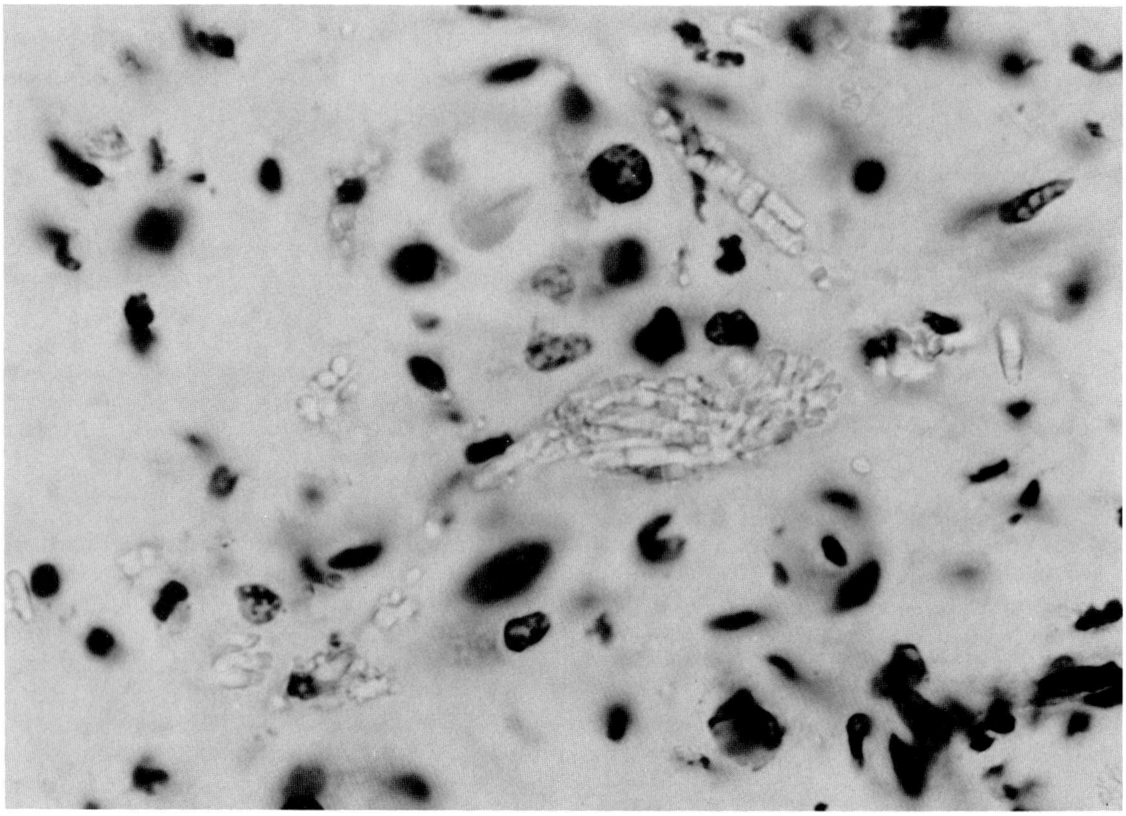

Figure 30.6. Cystine crystal deposition in the interstitial tissue of a cystinotic kidney.

hyperpigmented areas or the juxtaposition of hypopigmented and hyperpigmented areas as a salt and pepper pattern. It affects the temporal side more than the nasal, but occurs symmetrically in both eyes. Retinopathy tends to appear later in the course of the disease and to be progressive, although it has been observed before the first year of life. Visual impairment and blindness is severe in a few patients because of these eye abnormalities (117).

Growth failure is another major feature of cystinosis. Poor growth is usually evident before the first year of life and before the decline in the GFR. Growth failure occurs in spite of close attention to electrolyte imbalance. Renal failure as it develops adds to the poor growth. TSH levels may be elevated but normal T_3 and T_4 levels and no symptoms, characteristic of compensated hypothyroidism, often may be demonstrated in older children, presumably a result of cystine deposition (117, 122). The role this plays in growth failure is not clear; a few children have been frankly hypothyroid. Postrenal transplantation, growth improves in some. Adolescents with cystinosis are quite short in spite of well-functioning donor kidneys.

The morphological features of the kidney in cystinosis vary with the stage of the disease (123). Early in the disease, cystine crystals are present in tubular epithelial cells, interstitial cells and, rarely, in glomerular epithelial cells. A swan-neck deformity or thinning of the first part of the proximal tubule, originally thought to be pathognomonic of cystinosis, occurs in other forms of the Fanconi syndrome. Later in the course of the disease there is atrophy of many tubules, interstitial fibrosis, and abundant crystal deposition (Fig. 30.6). In the glomerulus, there is giant cell formation of the visceral epithelium, segmental sclerosis, and eventual obsolescence. Hyperplasia and hypertrophy of the juxtaglomerular apparatus have been noted and probably are related to abnormalities of the renin-angiotensin system. Electron microscopy studies have demonstrated crystalline inclusions surrounded by a single limiting membrane. Electron diffraction has shown the crystals to be L-cystine.

Until recently, treatment of infantile cystinosis has been symptomatic management of the Fanconi syndrome and, later, renal failure. These children almost invariably require supplemental K and alkali, which can be given as K citrate. Vitamin D supplementation, sometimes with neutral phosphate salts, is used to treat rickets (124). Careful attention to avoid dehydration, especially during gastroenteritis, is important. Agents that lower intracellular cystine in cultured fibroblasts have been given as treatment with limited success. Penicillamine (125, 126) and ascorbic acid (127) are not beneficial; in fact, ascorbic acid appears detrimental. Dithiothreitol has been used in two patients without a clear effect (128).

Cysteamine, given orally to 6 patients with cystinosis in a dose of 90 mg/kg/day, reduced the cystine content of their leukocytes (129). It also appeared to halt the progression of renal failure in two and, possibly, to improve the GFR in one of these two. No side effects were observed in these patients when the dose was slowly raised over three months. A serum-sickness reaction has been described in a few children treated with cysteamine who had a rapid increase in the dose (130). Cysteamine therapy did not improve either growth or the tubular dysfunction in these children. Of the two patients who responded, one was the youngest and the other had the least impairment in renal function when cysteamine was started, suggesting that beginning therapy early may be important. Restriction of methionine and cystine is not beneficial and can be dangerous if methionine is too severely limited (131).

Galactosemia

Galactosemia is an autosomal recessively inherited disorder of galactose metabolism (132). The most common type is the result of deficient activity of the enzyme galactose-1-phosphate uridyltransferase known as transferase deficiency galactosemia, with an incidence of 1/62,000 live births (132). This enzyme catalyzes the conversion of galactose-1-phosphate (Gal-1-PO_4) plus uridine diphosphate glucose to uridine diphosphate galactose (UDP-Gal) plus glucose-1-phosphate. UDP-Gal can then be further metabolized to either glucose or to CO_2 and H_2O via glycolysis. Deficiency of this enzyme leads to the accumulation of galactose-1-phosphate intracellularly, with damage to the liver, proximal renal tubule, brain, and lens.

A less frequent cause of galactosemia is a deficiency of galactose kinase, which forms galactose-1-phosphate from galactose. Cataracts are the only manifestation of this form, suggesting that galactose-1-phosphate and not galactose is the toxin in transferase deficiency galactosemia. How galactose-1-phosphate exerts its toxic effect is unknown.

The most common symptom of transferase deficiency galactosemia is failure to thrive (132–135). In part, this is a result of the vomiting and diarrhea that occur soon after ingesting milk containing lactose, the most common source of galactose in the diet. With the continued intake of galactose, jaundice and hepatomegaly soon appear; cataracts may appear within days after birth, although they often are detectable only with a slit lamp. Mental retardation may develop within a few months. Ascites occurs in some, especially in those infants who die. Neonatal death from fulminant *E. coli* sepsis occurs (136), which may be a result of inhibition of leukocyte bactericidal activity (137).

In addition to these clinical findings, galactose intake within days leads to the renal tubular dysfunction of the Fanconi syndrome, although not nearly as quickly as is the case when fructose is given to patients with hereditary fructose intolerance. The abnormalities are aminoaciduria, reduced phosphate reabsorption, proteinuria, metabolic acidosis, and mellituria. These dysfunctions appear after 1 to 2 weeks of galactose ingestion and take a similar period of time to resolve (133–135). The aminoaciduria is generalized and plasma AA are normal (138–141). Tubular reabsorption of phosphate decreases when galactose is given. Proteinuria of tubular origin also is evident, but resolves in time when galactose is discontinued (135). RTA with characteristics of proximal injury occurs (142). GFR may be reduced in the untreated state, which normalizes when galactose is withdrawn (19).

Mellituria, which is a cardinal feature of the Fanconi syndrome, is a result of galactosuria and not glucosuria (141). There seems to be little or no impairment in glucose handling by the renal tubule (19).

Galactosemia should be suspected whenever there is a urinary reducing substance that does not react in a glucose oxidase test. Identification of this reducing substance should be made, using either paper or gas-liquid chromatography, since lactose, pentose, and fructose may give similar results. Finding galactose in the urine does not establish the diagnosis, since it can be seen in severe liver disease, in the first week of life in normal newborns (143) and even for longer periods in premature infants (143, 144), and in some children with a high consumption of milk (145). Galactosuria will disappear in affected infants after the withdrawal of galactose, which can obscure the diagnosis. Confirmation should be made by demonstrating deficient transferase activity in either red blood cells, fibroblasts, leukocytes, or hepatocytes. Occasionally the characteristic liver pathology is helpful in establishing the diagnosis (146).

While the toxin responsible for the renal symptoms of galactosemia is not identified, Gal-1-PO_4, rather than galactose, is likely, because tubular dysfunction is found in transferase deficiency and not in kinase deficiency. The fall in Gal-1-PO_4 corresponds with the resolution of the symptoms. Aminoaciduria has been induced in normal rats fed a high galactose diet (147) and in normal human subjects given galactose intravenously (21). Incubation of slices of kidney cortex with galactose produces impairment of AA uptake (148).

Treatment of galactosemia is the elimination of galactose from the diet. Symptoms and signs resolve in a few days (20). Cataracts will also regress to some extent. With delay in treatment, recovery from brain damage may be incomplete. Intrauterine exposure of an affected fetus to galactose influences brain development. However, severe mental retardation as occurs in untreated phenylketonuria generally is not seen in transferase deficiency galactosemia (149).

Hereditary Fructose Intolerance

Hereditary fructose intolerance (HFI) is another disorder of carbohydrate metabolism associated with the Fanconi syndrome (150–153). Patients with this disorder experience nausea, vomiting, and symptoms of hypoglycemia shortly after ingesting fructose, sucrose, or sorbitol. These symptoms may progress to convulsions, coma, and even death, depending on the amount consumed. Concomitant serum biochemical findings after fructose ingestion are a fall in glucose, phosphate, and bicarbonate, with a rise in uric acid and lactic acid. Chronic exposure to fructose leads to failure to thrive, hepatomegaly, jaundice, hepatic cirrhosis, and nephrocalcinosis (58).

HFI is inherited as an autosomal recessive trait, with an unknown incidence, which, in Switzerland, is estimated to be 1/20,000 (154). It is caused by a deficiency of the enzyme fructose-1-phosphate aldolase B, which cleaves fructose-1-phosphate into D-glyceraldehyde and dihydroxyacetone phosphate for further conversion into glucose or CO_2 and H_2O (150).

The enzyme normally is present in liver, small intestine, and proximal renal tubule cells. Symptoms of HFI appear at weaning when fruit, vegetables, and sweetened cereals that contain fructose or sucrose are introduced (151). Symptoms will appear in the newborn period if the infant is fed a formula containing sucrose. The symptoms are more severe in infants than in older children and adults and are especially severe in newborns (150–152). Young infants with this disorder when exposed to fructose may have a catastrophic illness, with severe dehydration, shock, acute liver impairment, bleeding, or acute renal failure. Children with HFI learn to avoid sweets, with consequent lack of dental caries. The diagnosis should be suspected when symptoms develop following the ingestion of fructose. Confirmation can be made either by a carefully done fructose tolerance test or by assaying the activity of fructose-1-phosphate aldolase in a liver biopsy specimen (155).

Generalized aminoaciduria, glucosuria, proteinuria, and bicarbonaturia appears rapidly when these patients are given fructose (150–158). Changes in renal tubular phosphate handling are not clear because plasma phosphate falls with the accumulation of fructose-1-phosphate in cells following fructose ingestion, so that urinary phosphate excretion either remains unchanged or falls. The percent of tubular reabsorption of phosphate falls and metabolic acidosis will ensue (157, 158). Proximal bicarbonate reabsorption falls by 20% to 30%. The development of lactic acidosis adds significantly to the metabolic acidosis (159). As serum bicarbonate falls, bicarbonaturia diminishes, which is consistent with proximal RTA. In adults with HFI, chronic fructose ingestion may lead to nephrocalcinosis; distal RTA has been described (58). Although the onset of proximal tubule dysfunction is rapid after fructose loading, resolution of these symptoms may take days to weeks (153, 156).

Acute fructose loading in the rat has been used as a model for HFI (160–162). Fructose loading leads to depletion of intracellular phosphate as fructose-1-phosphate accumulates and adenine deaminase is activated. Adenine deaminase converts AMP to inosinic monophosphate (IMP) and ultimately to uric acid. A fall in AMP leads to a drop in ADP and ATP, since these levels are maintained at or near equilibrium by adenylate kinase. Therefore, a drop in intracellular phosphate may cause a massive depletion of ATP. Further, phosphate depletion impairs ATP regeneration by mitochondria. Fructose may induce a fall in tissue ATP in normal humans (162, 163), and to an even greater extent in patients with HFI. ATP depletion may impair substrate reabsorption in the kidney; although a direct correlation between ATP levels and solute reabsorption in vitro cannot be demonstrated (164).

Treatment of this disorder is strict avoidance of foods containing fructose and sucrose. Most patients develop a strong aversion to such foods, making this interdiction easy. The greatest risk to these patients is during infancy before they learn to avoid fructose. The inadvertent administration of fructose intravenously to affected individuals for unrelated medical reasons, e.g., after routine surgery also is a risk.

Glycogenosis

Fanconi syndrome has been described in patients with an enzymatically undefined glycogen storage disease (165–171). These patients do not belong to any of the ten known types of glycogenosis; yet, these patients accumulate large amounts of hepatic glycogen. This type of glycogen storage disease is inherited as an autosomal recessive trait; the majority of cases are in Europe. The syndrome is characterized by heavy glucosuria, which has led to the name renal glucose-losing syndrome (170). The glucose losses can amount to as much as 200 g/24 hr/1.73 m^2. The Fanconi syndrome may be present by the first few months of life and may precede the development of hepatomegaly. In these patients, the degree of tubular dysfunction—aminoaciduria, impaired phosphate reabsorption, or acidosis—in addition to the glucosuria is severe. Rickets, osteoporosis, and growth retardation develop. Glucose tolerance tests are diabetic in pattern, but glucagon stimulation only leads to a slight increase in blood sugar (166, 169, 171). Galactose tolerance also is impaired. Levels of galactose-1-phosphate uridyltransferase and galactokinase were normal in one patient (171) and erythrocyte galactose turnover was normal in another (169), excluding classical galactosemia. Ketonemia and ketonuria also are often features.

Treatment is frequent feeding and prevention of acute ketosis, which is prone to accompany intercurrent illnesses, by giving fluids and alkali. There appears to be no deterioration in GFR; the tubular dysfunction improves with time.

Tyrosinemia

Tyrosinemia was first described in 1956 in a patient with congenital cirrhosis of the liver and renal tubular defects, especially aminoaciduria and vitamin D-resistant rickets (172). Another patient had a similar picture and pronounced p-hydroxyphenyllactic aciduria (173). Since then, numerous cases have been described under several other names: tyrosyluria with hypermethioninemia, hypermethioninemia, and inborn hepatorenal dysfunction (174).

Tyrosinemia appears to have two distinct patterns, each of which is inherited as an autosomal recessive trait. Patients with the acute type develop symptoms and signs of liver dysfunction as early as the first month of life, characterized by jaundice, vomiting, failure to thrive, hepatomegaly, melena, ascites, and edema. Clotting difficulties develop early and are life threatening. Death from liver failure usually occurs within the first year of life despite attempts at dietary therapy.

Patients with the chronic form develop vitamin D-resistant rickets in late infancy and early childhood, with failure to thrive, nodular liver cirrhosis, hypoglycemia associated with hypertrophied islets of Langerhans, and, in some cases, mild to moderate mental retardation. Abdominal crises and polyneuropathy sometimes occur, which appear to be related to acute, intermittent porphyria-like abnormalities (175). Hepatoma is a late complication in 37% of patients (176). Death usually occurs by the end of the first decade. Renal failure does not occur, although a severe Fanconi syndrome is present in untreated cases.

Aminoaciduria is evident in patients with both forms of tyrosinemia. The aminoaciduria is generalized but tyrosine excretion is disproportionally increased. This is related, in part, to the elevated plasma tyrosine level that is a hallmark of this disorder and is present early (172, 176, 177). As the liver disease progresses, the aminoaciduria increases because plasma AA levels become elevated. Treatment with a diet low in phenylalanine and tyrosine may restore AA excretion to normal.

Glucosuria is intermittent and mild because plasma glucose levels are usually low (178, 179). Reabsorption of phosphate is severely impaired; plasma phosphate levels are correspondingly low. This leads to vitamin D-resistant rickets, one of the prominent clinical signs that develops after infancy (174, 178, 179). Metabolic acidosis is severe in both types of tyrosinemia and a result, at least in part, of renal tubular dysfunction. Proteinuria of tubular origin also is present (178, 179).

Tyrosinemia is associated with plasma tyrosine and methionine levels as much as 10 to 20 times normal. The hypermethioninemia imparts a cabbage-like odor to affected patients. In association with these changes, p-hydroxyphenolic compounds, especially p-hydroxyphenyllactic acid, are excreted in urine. These compounds are readily detected in urine from such patients by the formation of a red color when nitrosonaphthol is added.

These compounds arise from decreased activity of liver p-hydroxyphenylpyruvate dioxygenase, which converts p-hydroxyphenylpyruvic acid (PHPP), formed from tyrosine by tyrosine aminotransferase, to homogentisic acid (180, 181). Normally, homogentisic acid is oxidized to maleylacetoacetic acid (MAA) by homogentisic acid oxidase and MAA is converted to fumarylacetoacetic acid (FAA) by MAA isomerase. Finally, FAA is cleaved by FAA hydrolase to fumaric acid and acetoacetic acid, which are disposed of by the citric acid cycle.

It has been proposed that the primary defect in tyrosinemia is deficient activity of FAA hydrolase and MAA isomerase (182); the genetic basis for a decrease in both enzyme activities is speculative. Decreased activities of these enzymes have been documented in liver from affected patients (182–185), but not in other forms of liver failure. FAA hydrolase activity was 0–6% of control values in patients with the acute form of tyrosinemia and 20% in patients with the chronic form (185). PHPP dioxygenase, which has also been proposed as the enzymatic defect, is decreased in affected patients, but also has been described in other forms of hepatic disease, casting doubt on the primacy of this enzyme deficiency (186).

In the hypothesis proposed by Lindblad and coworkers (182), MAA and FAA accumulate in affected tissues and are converted to succinylacetoacetate (SAA) by PHPP dioxygenase. SAA and succinylacetone have been found in a number of patients (182, 187). Succinylacetone may arise by nonenzymatic decarboxylation of the alpha-keto acid SAA (182). Succinylacetone is structurally similar to maleic acid, known to induce the Fanconi syndrome. This may be the cause of the tubular dysfunction of tyrosinemia. Succinylacetone also inhibits porphobilinogen synthetase, which may explain the increased excretion of delta-aminolevulinic acid and the symptoms of acute porphyria sometimes observed in these patients (182, 188). MAA and FAA react with SH-containing compounds and may explain the decrease in reduced glutathione also noted in this order. A decrease in reduced glutathione may impair glutathione-dependent detoxification mechanisms (182).

The liver of these patients has nodular cirrhosis and marked regeneration of hepatic cells. Hepatoma develops in 37% of patients with the chronic form (189). The kidneys are enlarged from interstitial edema and marked tubular dilatation. The proximal tubule cells are swollen with degenerative changes. The pancreatic islets are often hyperplastic.

Treatment with a low phenylalanine and tyrosine diet dramatically improves the renal tubule dysfunction. In chronic cases, this diet leads to a rise in plasma phosphate, healing of rickets, a decrease in aminoaciduria and a disappearance of glucosuria and proteinuria (190–192). However, its efficacy in halting the liver disease is uncertain. There is a risk of inducing deficiency of phenylalanine or tyrosine (193). There is evidence for hepatic involvement prenatally before any elevations of tyrosine or methionine (194) that raises doubt that elevated levels of these AA are the cause of liver injury; therefore, therapy aimed at lowering these levels may not be beneficial. The low erythrocyte glutathione and plasma cystine levels have led some investigators to attempt treatment with cysteine supplementation or with penicillamine (183, 195). The long-term efficacy of such treatment remains to be determined. Liver transplantation offers a possible treatment for the patient with severe liver failure (196).

Several other disorders of tyrosine metabolism have been described, but are not associated with either liver or renal disease (174, 186). In 1932, Medes described an adult who excreted p-hydroxyphenylpyruvic acid and other p-hydroxyphenyl acids, but no particular symptoms could be ascribed to these phenolic acids; she named this condition tyrosinosis. Transient tyrosinemia is observed commonly in neonates, especially prematures. However, liver or renal dysfunction has not been noted in these infants and, as the name implies, this is only a transient disorder.

Tyrosinemia type II also is associated with elevated levels of tyrosine and p-hydroxyphenolic compounds. This form, caused by an absence of cytosolic tyrosine aminotransferase, is not associated with hepatic or renal disease, but rather mental retardation, skin, and corneal disorders.

Elevations of plasma tyrosine and methionine levels commonly occur with liver injury from any cause. Elevated levels of parahydroxyphenolic compounds also have been observed in liver disease and the Fanconi syndrome as a result of HFI and galactosemia.

Hereditary tyrosinemia occurs with a frequency of 1/120,000 in Sweden and 1/100,000 in Norway (197). The highest incidence is in the French-Canadian population of Quebec with an overall incidence of 1/12,500 (198). In the Chicoutimi-Lac St. Jean region of Quebec the heterozygote prevalence is 1/14 and 1/685 have the disease.

Wilson's Disease

In 1912, Wilson described a patient who died after a long illness characterized by muscular rigidity, tremor, and facial grimacing (199). At autopsy, there was cirrhosis of the liver and degeneration of the lenticular nuclei of the brain. Since then, numerous cases have been reported, with approximately 40% presenting with liver disease, 40% with extrapyramidal symptoms, and 20% with psychiatric or behavioral abnormalities (200). Although symptoms rarely occur before 6 years of age, the most common presentation in children is with chronic active hepatitis or cirrhosis with little or no neurological findings except those ascribable to hepatic failure. Greenish-brown rings at the limbus of the cornea, independently described by Kayser and Fleischer, are usually present and are pathognomonic of Wilson's disease, but may be visible only with a slit lamp; in young children with Wilson's disease, they may be absent.

The underlying problem in Wilson's disease is a severe impairment in biliary copper excretion, the major excretory route for copper, and in the incorporation of copper into ceruloplasmin, a plasma alpha$_2$-globulin. It is not clear whether ceruloplasmin functions as a copper transporting protein or is merely a copper-containing enzyme circulating in the plasma for iron oxidation and other functions. These abnormalities lead to the hallmark of Wilson's disease, which is excessive intracellular accumulation of copper in the liver with subsequent overflow into other tissues, such as brain, cornea, and renal proximal tubule.

Excessive storage of copper in the kidney leads to the Fanconi syndrome (61, 71, 200–203). Hematuria also has been noted. Renal plasma flow and GFR decrease as the disease progresses, but death from extrarenal causes will occur before the onset of renal failure. Tubular dysfunction overshadows the glomerular disease. Generalized aminoaciduria and normal plasma AA patterns are characteristic before the onset of hepatic failure (61, 71, 201–206). Renal glucosuria is usually intermittent and less severe than the aminoaciduria (61, 71, 201–203, 205, 206). A decrease in TmG has been described in 4 patients (71). Impaired phosphate resorption also has been noted, leading to hypophosphatemia, osteomalacia, and rickets, although hepatic dysfunction also plays a role (61, 71, 202, 205, 207, 208). RTA has been described and is consistent with a proximal tubular lesion in some (59, 71). Proteinuria is mild. Hypouricemia secondary to a marked uricosuria is common and can be a clue to the diagnosis (59, 61, 71, 202, 203, 206, 209, 210). The uric acid pool size is markedly diminished (210, 211). Hypercalciuria (61, 202, 203, 205, 207, 212, 213) with the development of renal stones (203) and nephrocalcinosis (59) also has been reported.

In addition to proximal tubular dysfunction, deranged distal tubular function also has been observed. Concentrating ability may be reduced (59, 61). A number of patients have distal RTA (59, 60). There is some evidence that the uricosuria may be a result in part of distal tubular dysfunction.

Histologically, the kidney in untreated Wilson's disease shows either no alterations on light microscopy or only some flattened proximal tubule cells without recognizable brush borders (202). Electron microscopy shows loss of the brush border, disruption of the apical tubular network, electron-dense bodies probably representing metalloproteins in the subapical region of tubule cell cytoplasm, and cavitation of the mitochondria with disruption of the normal cristae pattern. Rubeanic acid staining shows intracytoplasmic copper granules. The copper content of kidney tissue is markedly elevated (201).

The diagnosis of Wilson's disease should be suspected in children and young adults with unexplained neurological disease, chronic active hepatitis, acute hemolytic crisis, behavioral or psychiatric disturbances, or the appearance of the Fanconi syndrome. In such patients, the presence of Kayser-Fleischer rings would be an important clue in making the diagnosis; a slit-lamp examination may be necessary. Since serum ceruloplasmin levels are decreased in 96% of patients with Wilson's disease, this is a useful screening test. However, normal values in young children with severe liver disease are not uncommon. Two other laboratory tests useful in making the diagnosis are the serum and urine copper levels; serum copper usually is low and urinary copper is quite elevated and further increased after a dose of penicillamine in affected individuals. Copper levels in liver are increased in untreated patients, although in advanced cirrhosis this may not be the case. The ultimate test is negligible incorporation of radioactive copper into ceruloplasmin (214).

Treatment with D-penicillamine may lead to complete reversal of hepatic, renal, and neurological symptoms, depending on the degree of damage before the onset of therapy. Recovery, however, takes time; therapy may not benefit patients with hepatic failure. Liver transplantation has been used in a few patients (215). Patients treated before the onset of cirrhosis or neurological symptoms may lead a normal, healthy life. Penicillamine is recommended for asymptomatic but affected siblings.

Lowe's Syndrome

Lowe's syndrome (oculocerebrorenal syndrome) is characterized by congenital eye abnormalities, severe mental retardation, hypotonia with diminished to absent reflexes, and renal abnormalities (Fig. 30.7) (216). Initially, the renal abnormalities are those of the Fanconi syndrome, but later GFR is impaired. The disorder is transmitted as an X-linked recessive trait, although a few females have been reported (217, 218). This may be explicable by the Lyon hypothesis, or there are several

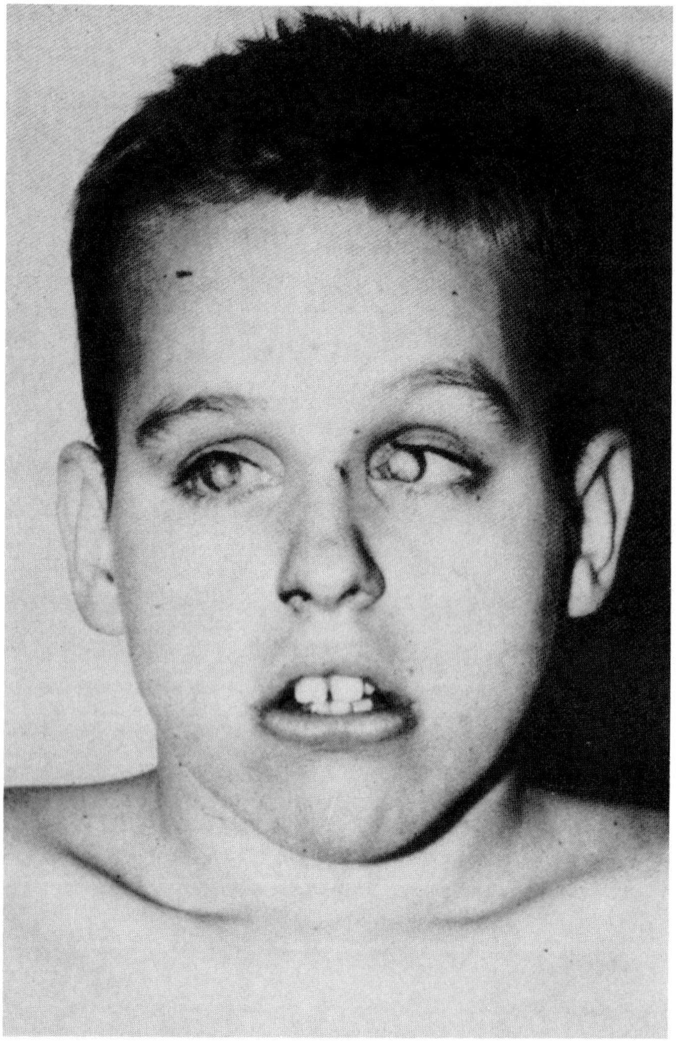

Figure 30.7. Patient with Lowe's syndrome demonstrating the cataracts and strabismus typical of this disorder. (From Wisniewski K, et al: Ann Neurol 16:42, 1984.)

modes of inheritance. Cataracts and punctate lens opacities have been noted in mothers of affected males (219–224). However, this has not proved to be a useful screening test for heterozygotes, because the incidence of such findings in the general population is high (225).

Aminoaciduria is a constant feature of Lowe's syndrome after the first several months of life. The aminoaciduria tends to decrease by 6 years of age (13, 223–227). The pattern is generalized, as in other disorders associated with the Fanconi syndrome. Several investigators have suggested that dibasic AA are relatively more affected than others (12, 13, 227), but this has not been a consistent finding (14). Decreased intestinal absorption of AA also has been inferred because AA in the stool are increased (228–230).

Defective ornithine metabolism has been proposed as a possible biochemical abnormality because ornithine loading produced aminoaciduria in one propositus and his mother (226). Ornithine loading in another family led to increased aminoaciduria in the propositus and his father, which is difficult to interpret in light of an X-linked inheritance pattern (231). Ornithine loading in a patient with Wilson's disease also led to aminoaciduria, casting doubt on the specificity of this finding in Lowe's syndrome (232).

Proteinuria is present from infancy and may become severe enough to lead to the nephrotic syndrome. They may also have evidence of reduced GFR. Glucosuria is minimal and only intermittently present. Phosphate reabsorption is variably impaired but may be severe (226). Proximal RTA is common (233).

The histology of the kidney by light microscopy is normal early in the disorder (218, 234–236). Swelling of endothelial cells with thickening and splitting of the glomerular basement membrane and fusion of the epithelial foot processes are observed by electron microscopy. In the proximal tubule cells, there is shortening of the brush border and enlargement of the mitochondria, with distortion and loss of the cristae. With progression, there is further thickening of the basement membrane, increased cellularity of the glomeruli, glomerular fibrosis, thickening of the tubular basement membrane, tubular atrophy, dilatation, and interstitial fibrosis.

Treatment of Lowe's syndrome is only symptomatic. During the neonatal period and infancy the major problems are related to the eyes. Later the symptoms resulting from the Fanconi syndrome, e.g., acidosis and rickets, become manifest. Renal insufficiency develops later and death from renal failure or intercurrent infection follows; the age of onset of renal failure is variable. Severe mental retardation is a major problem.

Cytochrome-c-oxidase Deficiency

In 1977, Biervliet described a family in which three infants died from a mitochondrial myopathy in association with lactic acidemia and the Fanconi syndrome (237). Subsequent to this report, two more infants with a similar clinical presentation were reported (238, 239). The infants were noted to have a weak cry and poor suck, with generalized hypotonia in the neonatal period. The hypotonia and weakness progressed in all 5 affected infants, leading to respiratory failure and death. In addition to the myopathy, all the infants had lactic acidosis and the Fanconi syndrome with a generalized aminoaciduria, glycosuria, mild proteinuria, and impaired phosphate reabsorption. Muscle from these babies showed lipid-filled vacuoles in type-I fibers, with swollen mitochondria containing disordered cristae. Biochemical evaluation of the muscle revealed a deficient activity of cytochrome-c-oxidase, an important enzyme in the electron-transport chain. This deficiency with its consequent impairment of oxidative phosphorylation appears to underlie the myopathy. Decreased activity of the enzyme was noted in the kidney of one of these infants, suggesting that impairment of the electron transport chain and energy generation in the cells of the renal tubule may be responsible for the observed Fanconi syndrome.

Acquired Causes

Exogenous Intoxications

Numerous substances have been described to cause tubular dysfunction; severe intoxications of a more general nature may lead to acute tubular necrosis and renal failure. The extent of the tubular dysfunction is quite variable and is dependent on the degree of intoxication and the host. Often the tubular dysfunction only results in an incomplete Fanconi syndrome, which usually is reversible after withdrawal of the intoxicant. A detailed history, therefore, is important in patients with tubular dysfunction to discover if a toxin is the cause.

A major cause of tubular dysfunctions is heavy metal intoxication. Lead poisoning induces Fanconi syndrome in both children and adults (240–243). In children, the tubular dysfunction usually is overshadowed by the involvement of other organs, especially the central nervous system. Generalized aminoaciduria is regularly present in children with moderate lead poisoning. Glycosuria and hypophosphatemia with impaired phosphate reabsorption also occur, but not as often. There is a rough correlation between the severity of the intoxication and the completeness of the Fanconi syndrome (241). In acute lead poisoning, the alterations in renal histology are mainly in the proximal tubule and include eosinophilic intranuclear inclusions with mitochondrial swelling (244).

Lead poisoning has been used as an experimental model of the Fanconi syndrome (245–246). Lead poisoning in animals causes both tubule dysfunction and morphological changes similar to those observed in humans. Isolated mitochondria from affected animals have a decreased rate of respiration with partially uncoupled oxidative phosphorylation. This may contribute to the tubular dysfunction.

Cadmium intoxication also leads to the Fanconi syndrome (242, 243, 248, 249). This poisoning was dramatized when a large number of cases appeared in the Jintsu River basin in Japan after World War II (248). It is characterized by severe bone pain, i.e., itai-itai (ouch-ouch) disease, aminoaciduria, glucosuria, hypophosphatemia with impaired phosphate reabsorption, hyposthenuria, and RTA. The cause was traced to industrial contamination of the soil and water with cadmium. Cadmium also has been used to induce an experimental Fanconi syndrome (250). In experimental cadmium poisoning, there is decreased activity of Na,K-ATPase, diminished ATP levels, and mitochondrial abnormalities. In addition to cadmium, several other heavy metals, e.g., uranium and mercury, may cause renal tubular dysfunction (57, 242, 251, 252).

Certain organic compounds may cause the Fanconi syndrome in man. Out-dated tetracycline causes a reversible Fanconi syndrome even in therapeutic doses (253–257). Affected patients experience dizziness, muscular weakness, acidosis and, occasionally, neurological symptoms. They have a generalized aminoaciduria, renal glucosuria, hypophosphatemia, RTA, hypokalemia, proteinuria, and hypouricemia; GFR is moderately reduced in some. Recovery is rapid when the degraded drug is stopped. The compound responsible for the tubular dysfunction is anhydro-4-epitetracycline formed from tetracycline by heat, moisture, and a low pH (258). This product also has been used experimentally to produce the Fanconi syndrome in dogs and rats (258–260). Tetracycline localizes in the mitochondria of hepatic and renal tubular cells, which may be a factor in causing the tubular dysfunction (261).

A number of other compounds also may give rise to the Fanconi syndrome, often in association with a reduced GFR; the renal injury usually is reversible. For example, methyl-3-chromone (diachrome) (262), 6-mercaptopurine (263), toluene (glue sniffing) (264), and Lysol (265) have each caused the Fanconi syndrome. Gentamicin and cephalothin in both children and adults have caused the Fanconi syndrome and renal failure (266, 267), as has streptozotocin, used to treat malignant insulinomas (268). Tubular dysfunction during recovery from acute renal failure from any cause occurs, diminishing the significance of some toxins as inducers of the Fanconi syndrome (269).

Maleic acid, the cis isomer of fumaric acid, has been used widely as an experimental model of the Fanconi syndrome (8, 9, 270–274). Intravenous or intraperitoneal injection leads to aminoaciduria, glucosuria, phosphaturia, proteinuria, and bicarbonaturia. Impaired sugar and amino acid transport occurs in renal cortical slices (8) or isolated tubules from mature and developing rats (275, 276) incubated with maleic acid. The major abnormality in vitro is accelerated loss of transported substrate (efflux) (8, 275). This corresponds to the data from double indicator and microperfusion studies in maleic acid treated animals, demonstrating an increased leakiness of the tubular cells (9, 275). Uptake in brush-border membrane vesicles isolated from proximal tubule cells is unaffected by maleic acid, indicating that the impaired solute reabsorption probably is not mediated by an effect on the luminal membrane (277). Maleic acid also had no effect on the physical state of the luminal and basolateral membranes (278).

Maleic acid appeared to inhibit the enzyme Na,K-ATPase, and it was postulated that inhibition of this enzyme leads to impaired substrate handling (279). However, these results were not confirmed by other investigators (276). Cellular depletion of the important cofactor, coenzyme A (CoA), leading to a decrease in ATP formation, has been suggested as the cause of the tubular dysfunction produced by maleic acid (280, 281). Maleic acid has been a useful experimental model of the Fanconi syndrome.

Other Acquired Disorders

Dysproteinemia associated with a number of diseases is a cause of the Fanconi syndrome. This is a cause mainly observed in adults, because the diseases are extremely rare in children. Dysproteinemia and the Fanconi syndrome are associated with multiple myeloma (4, 282–284), hypergammaglobulinemia (62), light chain proteinuria (285, 286), Sjogren's syndrome (287), and amyloidosis (288). The appearance of tubular dysfunction is correlated with Bence-Jones proteinuria, although some patients with Bence-Jones proteinuria do not have the Fanconi syndrome (289). Experimentally, incubation of renal cortical slices from both rabbits and rats with Bence-Jones proteins inhibits the uptake of para-aminohippurate, whereas incubation with urine proteins from patients with the nephrotic syndrome does not (290, 291).

The nephrotic syndrome rarely has been associated with the Fanconi syndrome (292–295). In those cases, the nephrotic syndrome began early in childhood and was resistant to steroid therapy. The Fanconi syndrome appeared 1 to 4 years later. These patients have hypokalemia, RTA, rickets, and growth retardation. Hypocalcemia and tetany are significant problems.

These patients have distal tubular dysfunction as well, e.g., polyuria and distal RTA. A similar combination of proximal and distal tubular abnormalities has been observed in the dysproteinemias. It is not known whether the excessive proteinuria causes tubular dysfunction. An alternative hypothesis is that the renal tubules are involved in the same process that affects the glomeruli (294).

The Fanconi syndrome has appeared rarely in postrenal transplant patients (119, 296, 297). The pathogenesis probably is multifactorial, e.g., sequelae of acute tubular necrosis, rejection, nephrotoxic drugs, ischemia from renal artery stenosis, and residual hyperparathyroidism (298). It occurs most commonly when these patients are uremic (299).

IDIOPATHIC FANCONI SYNDROME

A number of patients develop the complete Fanconi syndrome in the absence of any known cause. These cases have been called the idiopathic or primary Fanconi syndrome (44, 50, 67, 70, 300). Originally, only adults were thought to be affected; hence, it was called the adult Fanconi syndrome. However, it is now quite clear that the idiopathic Fanconi syndrome occurs in children as well (62, 63, 300–302). Indeed, some of the first patients described had initial symptoms in childhood. All of the features of the Fanconi syndrome may not be present when the patients are first studied; for example, 2 girls, described by Luder and Sheldon in 1955 (303), initially had only glucosuria and aminoaciduria. On reevaluation in 1961 they had hypophosphatemic rickets as well (300).

Several different modes of inheritance have been described in cases of idiopathic Fanconi syndrome, i.e., autosomal dominant (67, 300, 303, 304), autosomal recessive (63), and even an X-linked mode (302). However, most cases occur sporadically, without any evidence of genetic transmission (50, 62, 301). The possibility of an underlying enzymatic or other abnormality that has not yet been described as causing the Fanconi syndrome should always be remembered, especially in those in whom the syndrome is inherited. A number of patients, in whom the known causes of the Fanconi syndrome were excluded, still appeared to have an underlying metabolic abnormality (305–307). Chesney and coworkers (305) described two patients with the Fanconi syndrome who had galactose intolerance but normal levels of galactose-1-phosphate uridyltransferase and galactokinase activity; these patients also had glucose intolerance, insulinopenia, and ketonuria. The occurrence of the Fanconi syndrome and diabetes mellitus together has been noted by others (308, 309). Galactose intolerance in association with normal levels of galactose-1-phosphate uridyltransferase and galactokinase have been described in two other patients with idiopathic Fanconi syndrome (306, 307), one of whom had an elevated blood lactate level and an abnormal lactate to pyruvate ratio, suggesting an abnormal intracellular redox state (306).

Children with the idiopathic Fanconi syndrome usually have complaints related to growth failure, recurrent dehydration, and rickets, despite an adequate intake of vitamin D. They have polyuria, polydipsia, and recurrent episodes of vomiting. They also have hypokalemia, hypophosphatemia, RTA, aminoaciduria, glucosuria, and proteinuria. The GFR usually is normal. The prognosis in these children is variable. With careful management, death from dehydration and electrolyte imbalance can be avoided. However, some develop chronic renal failure 10 to 30 years after the onset (50, 119, 304, 305, 308–311).

Reports of the renal morphology of such cases are scanty. In one report, no abnormalities were found in tissue obtained by biopsy (62). In one autopsy specimen, zones of tubular atrophy with interstitial fibrosis were interspersed with areas of tubule dilatation (304); in another specimen, there was interstitial fibrosis and tubule dilatation, which was thought to be nonspecific (305). Brodehl reported markedly dilated tubules with swollen proximal tubular epithelium in a biopsy from a 7-year-old female; the rest of the renal structures were normal. Mitochondria were grossly swollen on electron microscopy, with displaced cristae (48).

Therapy for the idiopathic Fanconi syndrome is symptomatic. Careful follow-up of these patients is necessary because they are at risk for serious potentially fatal dehydration and electrolyte imbalance. In those with ESRD, renal transplantation has been done in a few (119, 305). In one patient, the Fanconi syndrome recurred in the allograft without evidence of rejection, suggesting in this case an extrarenal cause for the idiopathic Fanconi syndrome (119) (chapter 52).

THERAPY

Therapy, whenever possible, should be directed at an underlying cause, as in galactosemia, HFI, and hereditary tyrosinemia. Wilson's disease and heavy metal intoxication can be treated with chelation therapy. In these cases, resolution of the Fanconi syndrome usually is complete.

In other instances, therapy is directed to the biochemical abnormalities. Close attention to these problems is important. Bone pain, fractures, rickets, and growth failure that plague these patients can be ameliorated. Normal stature, however, is seldom attained in spite of careful management. Treatment of hypophosphatemia, RTA, and NaCl and K loss is important and prompt treatment of an electrolyte imbalance associated with an intercurrent illness is life-saving (chapters 7, 8, 32–34).

Hyperaminoaciduria, glucosuria, proteinuria, and hyperuricosuria usually do not lead to clinical difficulties and do not require specific treatment.

Proximal RTA associated with the Fanconi syndrome requires large doses of alkali for correction, i.e., 2 to 10 mEq/kg/day given in divided doses throughout the day. The amount of alkali needed may be so large that volume expansion ensues, with further bicarbonate wasting; in this situation, 1 to 3 mg/kg/day of hydrochlorthiazide prevents this (37, 296).

Electrolyte therapy may be given as Na bicarbonate or as the Na salts of metabolizable anions, such as citrate or lactate. A Na and K citrate mixture or K citrate solution corrects both acidosis and hypokalemia. Sometimes NaCl and other times KCl is necessary. Electrolyte therapy is important to restore body composition to normal and to improve growth and bone metabolism.

Treatment of rickets and osteomalacia commonly encountered in the Fanconi syndrome usually requires vitamin D; the preferred form is not known. The vitamin D resistance observed in this syndrome may be related to reduced synthesis of 1,25 $(OH)_2$ vitamin D (49, 50). Because levels of 1,25 vitamin D are low in spite of massive doses of vitamin D, some investigators advocate using the hydroxylated forms (47, 49, 54); others have proposed that these comounds offer no advantage over the usual forms (313). Further research in this area is necessary. Whatever form is employed, the dose should be enough to heal the rickets. With large doses of vitamin D, careful patient monitoring is necessary to prevent toxicity. Hypercalciuria may precede hypercalcemia and thus be a more subtle indicator of vitamin D toxicity.

Attention to the hypophosphatemia is also important for healing the bone disorders in the Fanconi syndrome. Increased vitamin D intake in some patients will normalize the serum phosphate concentration. In others, supplemental oral phosphate, usually in the range of 1 to 3 g as the neutral salt, is necessary (chapter 32) (124).

Adequate fluid intake must be assured, especially during infancy, early childhood, and with acute infections. Polyuria, and, in some patients, hyposthenuria, dehydration, and hypernatremia are a risk. A few children require supplemental NaCl in addition to a large free water intake because of renal NaCl wasting.

References

1. DeToni G: Remarks on the relations between renal rickets (renal dwarfism) and renal diabetes. Acta Paediatr 16:479, 1933.
2. Debré R, Marie J, Cléret F, et al: Rachitisme tardif coexistant avec une nephrite chronique et une glycosurie. Arch Med Enf 37:597, 1934.
3. Fanconi G: Die nicht diabetischen Glykosurien und Hyperglykamien des alteren Kindes. Jahrbuch Kinderheik 133:257, 1931.
4. Fanconi G: Der fruhinfantile nephrotisch-glykosurische Zwergwichs mit hypophosphatamischer Rachitis. Jahrbuch Kinderheik 147:299, 1936.
5. Segal S, Thier SO: Renal handling of amino acids. In Orloff J, Berliner RW (eds): The Handbook of Physiology: Renal Physiology. Washington DC, Am Physiol Soc, 1973, p 653.
6. Kinne R: Membrane-molecular aspects of tubular transport. In Thurauk (ed): International Review of Physiology. Kidney and Urinary Tract Physiology. Baltimore, University Park Press, 1976, p 169, Vol 2.
7. Cohen JJ, Kamm DE: Renal metabolism: Relation to renal function. In Brenner BM, Rector FC (eds): The Kidney, ed 2. Philadelphia, W. B. Saunders Co, 1981, p 144.
8. Rosenberg LE, Segal S: Maleic acid induced inhibition of amino acid transport in rat kidney. Biochem J 92:345, 1964.
9. Bergeron M, Dubord L, Hausser C: Membrane permeability as a cause of transport defects in experimental Fanconi syndrome. A new hypothesis. J Clin Invest 57:1181, 1976.
10. McCune DJ, Mason HH, Clarke HT: Intractable hypophosphatemic rickets with renal glycosuria and acidosis (the Fanconi syndrome). Am J Dis Child 65:81, 1943.
11. Brodehl J, Bickel H: Aminoaciduria and hyperaminoaciduria in childhood. Clin Nephrol 1:149, 1973.
12. Jagenburg OR: The urinary excretion of free amino acids and other amino compounds by the human. Scand J Clin Lab Invest (suppl 43) 11:5, 1959.
13. Manz F, Bremer HJ, Brodehl J: Renal transport of amino acids in children with oculocerebrorenal syndrome. Helv Paediatr Acta 33:37, 1978.
14. Roth KS, Foreman JW, Segal S: The Fanconi syndrome and mechanisms of tubular transport dysfunction. Kidney Intl 20:705, 1981.
15. Shih VE: Laboratory Techniques for the Detection of Hereditary Metabolic Disorders. Cleveland, CRC Press, 1973, p 11.
16. Ullrich KJ: Sugar, amino acid and sodium cotransport in the proximal tubule. Ann Rev Physiol 41:181, 1979.
17. Schafer JA, Barfuss DW: Membrane mechanisms for transepithelial amino acid absorption and secretion. Am J Physiol 238:F335, 1980.

18. Bradley SE: Disorders of renal tubular function. Am J Med 20:457, 1956.
19. Brodehl J: The Fanconi syndrome. In Edelmann CM (ed): Pediatric Kidney Disease. Boston, Little, Brown, and Co, 1978, p 955.
20. Reem GH, Isaacs M, Vanamee P: Renal transport of urate, phosphate and glucose in the Fanconi syndrome. J Clin Endocrinol Metab 27:1141, 1967.
21. Fox M, Thier S, Rosenberg L, et al: Impaired renal tubular function induced by sugar infusion in man. J Clin Endocrinol Metab 24:1318, 1964.
22. Thierry J, Poujeol P, Ripoche P: Interactions between Na^+-dependent uptake of D-glucose, phosphate and L-alanine in rat renal brushborder membrane vesicles. Biochim Biophys Acta 647:203, 1981.
23. Silverman M: Glucose transport in the kidney. Biochim Biophys Acta 457:303, 1976.
24. Segal S, Genel M, Holtzapple P, et al: Transport of alpha methyl-D-glucoside by human kidney cortex. Metabolism 22:67, 1973.
25. Turner RJ, Silverman M: Sugar uptake into brushborder vesicles from normal human kidney. Proc Natl Acad Sci (USA) 74:2825, 1977.
26. Goldberg M, Agus ZS, Goldfarb S: Renal handling of phosphate, calcium and magnesium. In Brenner BM, Rector FC (eds): The Kidney. Philadelphia, W. B. Saunders Co, 1976, p 344.
27. Dousa TP, Kempson SA: Regulation of renal brushborder membrane transport of phosphate. Min Elect Metab 7:113, 1982.
28. Kempson SA, Dousa TP: Phosphate transport across renal cortical brushborder membrane vesicles from rats stabilized on a normal, high or low phosphate diet. Life Sci 24:881, 1979.
29. Stoll R, Kinne R, Murer H, et al: Phosphate transport by rat renal brushborder membrane vesicles. Influence of dietary phosphate, thyroparathyroidectomy, and 1,25 dihydroxy-vitamin D_3. Pfleuger Arch Euro J Physiol 380:47, 1979.
30. Evers H, Murer H, Kinne R: Effects of parathyrin on the transport properties of isolated renal brushborder vesicles. Biochem J 172:49, 1978.
31. Krohn H-P, Brandis M, Brodehl J, et al: Tubulärer Phosphattransport bei der vitamin D resistenten Rachitis. Monatschr Kinderheilk 122:583, 1974.
32. Krohn H-P, Brodehl J, Offner G, et al: Über die Veränderungder Nierenfunktion bei der Vitamin D Mangel-Rachitis. Monatschr Kinderheilk 121:327, 1973.
33. Robertson WG: Urinary excretion. In Nordin BEG (ed): Calcium, Phosphate and Magnesium Metabolism. London, Churchill-Livingstone, 1976, p 113.
34. Bijvoet OLM: Indices for the measurement of the renal handling of phosphate. In Massry SG, Fleisch H (eds): Renal Handling of Phosphate. New York, Plenum Medical Book Co, 1980, p 1.
35. Kruse K, Kracht U, Gopfert G: Renal threshold phosphate concentration. Arch Dis Childh 57:217, 1982.
36. Friis T, Hahnemann S, Weeke E: Serum calcium and serum phosphorus in uremia during administration of sodium phytate and aluminum hydroxide. Acta Med Scand 183:497, 1968.
37. Walton RJ, Bijvoet OLM: A simple slide-rule method for the assessment of renal tubular reabsorption of phosphate in man. Clin Chim Acta 81:273, 1977.
38. Morris RC Jr, McSherry E, Sebastian A: Modulation of experimental renal dysfunction of hereditary fructose intolerance by circulating parathyroid hormone. Proc Natl Acad Sci (USA) 68:132, 1971.
39. Kyle LH, Meroney WH, Freeman ME: Study of the mechanism of bone disease in hypophosphatemic glycosuric osteomalacia. J Clin Endocrinol Metab 14:365, 1954.
40. Callis L, Castello F, Fortuny G, et al: Effect of hydrochlorothiazide on rickets and on renal tubular acidosis in two patients with cystinosis. Helv Paediatr Acta 25:602, 1970.
41. Fellers FX, Ko KW, Nicolaidou M: A defect of tubular secretory function in the deToni-Fanconi syndrome. Am J Dis Child 100:558, 1960.
42. Haquani AH, Ram MM: Renal tubular insufficiency. J Pediatr 61:242, 1962.
43. Fraser D, Leeming JM, Cerwenka EA: Über die Handhabung von Phosphat durch die Nieren bei hypophosphatamischer vitamin D-resistent Rachitis der einfachen Art und bein Cystinspeicherkrankheit:Reaktion auf verlängerte Calciuminfusion. Helv Paediatr Acta 14:497, 1959.
44. Wilson DR, Yendt ER: Treatment of adult Fanconi syndrome with oral phosphate supplement and alkali. Am J Med 35:487, 1963.
45. Rodriquez-Soriano J, Houston IB, Boichis H, et al: Calcium and phosphorus metabolism in the Fanconi syndrome. J Clin Endocrinol Metab 28:1555, 1968.
46. Fanconi A, Fischer JA, Prader A: Serum parathyroid hormone concentrations in hypophosphatemic vitamin D resistent rickets. Helv Paediatr Acta 29:187, 1974.
47. Chesney RW, Harrison HE: Fanconi syndrome after bowel surgery and hepatitis reversed by 25-hydroxycholecalciferol. J Pediatr 86:857, 1975.
48. Brodehl J: Tubular Fanconi syndrome with bone involvement. In Bickel H, Stern J (eds): Inborn Errors of Calcium and Bone Metabolism. Lancaster, England, MTP Press, 1976, p 191.
49. Chesney RW, Rosen JF, Hamstra AJ, et al: Serum 1,25-dihydroxy-vitamin D levels in normal children and in vitamin D disorders. Am J Dis Child 134:135, 1980.
50. Brewer ED, Tsai HC, Morris RC: Evidence for impairment of metabolism of 25-hydroxyvitamin D_3 in children with Fanconi syndrome. Clin Res 24:154A, 1976.
51. Brewer ED, Tsai HC, Szeto KS, et al: Maleic acid-induced impaired conversion of $25(OH)D_3$: implications for Fanconi syndrome. Kidney Intl 12:244, 1977.
52. Lee SW, Russell J, Avioli LV: 25-Hydroxycholecalciferol: conversion impaired by systemic acidosis. Science 195:944, 1977.
53. Booth BE, Tsai HC, Morris RC Jr: Metabolic acidosis in the vitamin-D deficient chick. Metabolism 26:1099, 1977.
54. Chesney RW: 1,25-dihydroxyvitamin D_3 in childhood bone disease. In DeLuca HF, Anast CS (eds): Pediatric Diseases Related to Calcium. New York, Elsevier, 1981, p 387.
55. Rodriquez-Soriano J, Edelmann CM: Renal tubular acidosis. Ann Rev Med 20:363, 1969.
56. Morris RC Jr: Renal tubular acidosis: Mechanisms, classification and implications. N Engl J Med 281:1405, 1969.
57. Lee DNB, Drinkard JP, Rosen VJ, et al: The adult Fanconi syndrome. Medicine 51:107, 1972.
58. Mass RF, Smith WR, Walshe JR: The association of hereditary fructose intolerance and renal tubular acidosis. Am J Med Sci 251:516, 1966.
59. Fulop M, Sternlieb I, Scheinberg IM: Defective urinary acidification in Wilson's disease. Ann Int Med 68:770, 1968.
60. Walshe JM: Effect of penicillamine on failure of renal acidification in Wilson's disease. Lancet 1:775, 1968.
61. Leu ML, Strickland GT, Gutman RA: The renal lesion on Wilson's disease: Response to penicillamine therapy. Am J Med Sci 260:381, 1970.
62. Houston IB, Boichis H, Edelmann CM: Fanconi syndrome with renal sodium wasting and metabolic alkalosis. Am J Med 44:638, 1968.
63. Illig R, Prader A: Primäre tubulopathien:II. Ein Fall von idiopathischem Gluko-Amino-Phosphat-Diabetes (De Toni-Debre-Fanconi syndrome). Helv Paediatr Acta 16:622, 1961.
64. Kamm DE, Fischer MS: Proximal renal tubular acidosis and the Fanconi syndrome in a patient with hypergammaglobulinemia. Nephron 9:208, 1972.
65. O'Regan S, Mongeau J-G, Robitaille PO: A patient with cystinosis presenting with features of Bartter's syndrome. Acta Paediatr Belg 33:51, 1980.
66. Brodehl J, Hagge W, Gellissen K: Die Veränderungen der Nierenfunktion bei der Cystinose. Teil 1:Die Inulin-, PAH-und Elektrolyte-Clearance in verschiedenen Stadien der Erkrankung. Ann Paediatr (Basel) 205:131, 1965.
67. Ben-Ishay D, Dreyfuss F, Ullmann TD: Fanconi syndrome with hypouricemia in an adult. Am J Med 31:793, 1961.
68. Bloomer HA, Canary JJ, Kyle LH, et al: The Fanconi syndrome with renal hyperchloremic acidosis. Am J Med 33:141, 1962.
69. Sirota JH, Hamerman D: Renal function studies in an adult subject with Fanconi syndrome. Am J Med 16:138, 1954.
70. Wallis LA, Engle RL Jr: The adult Fanconi syndrome:II. Review of eighteen cases. Am J Med 22:13, 1957.
71. Bearn AG, Yu TF, Gutman AB: Renal function in Wilson's disease. J Clin Invest 36:1107, 1957.
72. Wilson DM, Goldstein NP: Renal urate excretion in patients with Wilson's disease. Kidney Intl 4:331, 1973.
73. Chonko AM, Grantham JJ: Disorders of urate metabolism and excretion. In Brenner BM, Rector FC (eds): The Kidney, ed 2, Philadelphia, W. B. Saunders Co, 1981, p 1023.
74. Butler EA, Flynn FV: The proteinuria of renal tubular disorders. Lancet 2:978, 1958.
75. Harrison JF, Blainey JD: Low molecular weight proteinuria in chronic renal disease. Clin Sci 33:381, 1967.
76. Harrison JF, Lunt GS, Scott P, et al: Urinary lyzozyme, ribonuclease and low-molecular-weight protein in renal disease. Lancet 1:371, 1968.
77. Barratt TM, Crawford R: Lyzozyme excretion as a measure of renal tubular dysfunction in children. Clin Sci 39:457, 1970.
78. Dillard MG, Pesce AJ, Pollark VE, et al: Proteinuria and renal protein clearance in patients with renal tubular disorders. J Lab Clin Med 78:203, 1971.
79. Waldmann TA, Strober W, Mogielnicki RP: The renal handling of low molecular weight proteins:II. Disorders of serum protein. Catabolism in patients with tubular proteinuria, the nephrotic syndrome or uremia. J Clin Invest 51:2162, 1972.
80. Käser H, Cottier P, Antener I: Glucoglycinuria, a new familial syndrome. J Pediatr 61:386, 1962.
81. Oetliker O, Käser H, Donath A, et al: Beitrag zur Familiaritat der idiopathischen Gluko-Hyperaminoacidurie. Helv Paediatr Acta 19:556, 1964.
82. Dent CE: Rickets and osteomalacia from renal tubule defects. J Bone Joint Surg 34B:266, 1952.
83. Schneider JA, Schulman JD: Cystinosis. In Stanbury JB, et al (eds): The Metabolic Basis of Inherited Disease, ed 5. New York, McGraw-Hill Book Co, 1982, p 1844.

84. Schneider JA, Wong V, Bradley KH, et al: Biochemical comparisons of the adult and childhood forms of cystinosis. N Engl J Med 279:1253, 1968.
85. Aaron K, Goldman H, Scriver CR: Adolescent cystinosis. A "new" phenotype. A possible role for dithiothreitol (DTT) in treatment. In Hereditary Disorders of Sulphur Metabolism. Eighth annual conference of the Society for the Study of Inborn Errors of Metabolism, Belfast, 1970.
86. VanHooft C, Carton D, DeSchrijver F: Juvenile cystinosis in two siblings. In Hereditary Disorders of Sulphur Metabolism. Eighth annual conference of the Society for the Study of Inborn Errors of Metabolism, Belfast, 1970.
87. Bickel H: Entwicklung der biochemischen Lasion bei Lignac-Fanconi scher Krankheit. Helv Paediatr Acta 10:259, 1955.
88. Bickel H, Baar HS, Astley R, et al: Cystine storage disease with amino-aciduria and dwarfism (Lignac-Fanconi disease). Acta Paediatr (suppl 90) 42:1, 1952.
89. Worthen HG, Good RA: The deToni-Fanconi syndrome with cystinosis. Am J Dis Child 95:653, 1958.
90. Brubaker RF, Wong VG, Schulman JD, et al: Benign cystinosis: The clinical biochemical and morphological findings in a family with two affected siblings. Am J Med 49:546, 1970.
91. Cogan DG, Kuwabara T, Kineshita J, et al: Cystinosis in an adult. JAMA 164:394, 1957.
92. Lietman PS, Frazier PD, Wong VG, et al: Adult cystinosis-a benign disorder. Am J Med 40:511, 1966.
93. Goldman H, Scriver CR, Aaron K, et al: Adolescent cystinosis: Comparisons with infantile and adult forms. Pediatrics 47:900, 1971.
94. Hooft C, Carton D, DeSchrijver F, et al: Juvenile cystinosis in two siblings. In Carson NA, Raine DN (eds): Inherited Disorders of Sulphur Metabolism. London, Churchill-Livingstone, 1971, p 141.
95. Hummeler K, Zajal BA, Genel M, et al: Human cystinosis: Intracellular deposition of cystine. Science 166:859, 1970.
96. Patrick AD, Lake BD: Cystinosis: Electron microscopic evidence of lysosomal storage of cystine in a lymph node. J Clin Path 21:571, 1968.
97. Schneider JA, Verroust FM, Kroll WA, et al: Prenatal diagnosis of cystinosis. N Engl J Med 279:1253, 1968.
98. States B, Blazer B, Harris D, et al: Prenatal diagnosis of cystinosis. J Pediatr 87:558, 1975.
99. Schneider JA, Rosenbloom FM, Bradley KH, et al: Increased free-cystine content of fibroblasts cultured from patients with cystinosis. Biochem Biophys Res Commun 29:527, 1967.
100. States B, Harris D, Segal S: Uptake and utilization of exogenous cystine by cystinotic and normal fibroblasts. J Clin Invest 53:1003, 1974.
101. Tietze F, Bradley KH, Schulman JD: Enzymatic reduction of cystine by subcellular fractions of cultured and peripheral leukocytes from normal and cystinotic individuals. Pediatr Res 6:649, 1972.
102. Kaye IC, Nadler HL: Enzymatic reduction of cystine and glutathione in cultivated human fibroblasts from normal subjects and patients with cystinosis. J Lab Clin Med 86:422, 1975.
103. States B, Scardigli K, Segal S: Glutathione in fibroblasts from normal and cystinotic children. Life Sci 22:31, 1978.
104. States B, Segal S: Levels of gamma-glutamyl-transpeptidase in cultured skin fibroblasts from cystinotics and normals. Life Sci 27:1985, 1980.
105. Thoene JG, Oshima RG, Ritchie DG, et al: Cystinotic fibroblasts accumulate cystine from intracellular protein degradation. Proc Natl Acad Sci (USA) 74:4505, 1977.
106. Steinberg R, Tietz F, Raiford D, et al: Patterns of amino acid efflux from isolated normal and cystinotic human leucocyte lysosomes. J Biol Chem 257:6041, 1982.
107. Gahl WA, Tietz F, Bashan N, et al: Defective cystine exodus from isolated lysosome rich fractions of cytinotic leucocytes. J Biol Chem 257:9570, 1982.
108. Gahl WA, Bashan N, Tietz F, et al: Cystine transport is defective in isolated leukocyte lysosomes from patients with cystinosis. Science 217:1263, 1982.
109. Steinberg R, Tietz F, Triche T, et al: Heterozygote detection in cystinosis using leukocytes exposed to cystine dimethyl ester. N Engl J Med 306:1468, 1982.
110. Jonas AJ, Smith ML, Schneider JA: ATP dependent lysosomal cystine efflux is defective in cystinosis. J Biol Chem 257:13185, 1982.
111. Jonas AJ, Green AA, Smith ML, et al: Cystine accumulation and loss in normal, heterozygous, and cystinotic fibroblasts. Proc. Natl Acad Sci (USA) 79:4442, 1982.
112. Reeves JP: Accumulation of amino acids by lysosomes incubated with amino acid methyl esters. J Biol Chem 254:8914, 1979.
113. Schneider JA, Bradley K, Seegmiller JE: Increased cystine in leukocytes from individuals homozygous and heterozygous for cystinosis. Science 157:1321, 1967.
114. Holtzapple PG, Genel M, Yakovac WC, et al: Diagnosis of cystinosis by rectal biopsy. N Engl J Med 218:143, 1969.
115. Esser M: Zur diagnose der Cystinkrankheit. Ann Paediat 156:344, 1940.
116. Wong VG: The eye and cystinosis. In Schulman JD (ed): Cystinosis. Washington, DC, US Government Printing Office, 1973, p 23.
117. Broyer M, Guillot M, Guber MC, et al: Infantile cystinosis: a re-appraisal of early and late symptoms. Adv Nephrol 11:137, 1981.
118. Jonas AJ, Schneider JA: Cystinosis in a black child. J Pediatr 100:934, 1982.
119. Briggs WA, Kominami N, Wilson RE, et al: Kidney transplantation in Fanconi syndrome. N Engl J Med 286:25, 1972.
120. Hembridge KM, Goodman SI, Walravens PA, et al: Accumulation of cystine following renal hemotransplantation for cystinosis. Pediatr Res 3:364, 1969.
121. Mahoney CP, Striker GE, Hickman RO, et al: Renal transplantation for childhood cystinosis. N Engl J Med 283:397, 1970.
122. Chen AM, Lynch MJG, Bailey JD, et al: Hypothyroidism in cystinosis. A clinical, endocrinologic and histologic study involving 16 patients with cystinosis. Am J Med 48:678, 1970.
123. Spear GS: The pathology of the kidney. In Schulman JD (ed): Cystinosis. Washington, DC, US Government Printing Office, 1973, p 37.
124. Rasmussen H, Pechet M, Anast C, et al: Long-term treatment of familial hypophosphatemic rickets with oral phosphate and 1 α-hydroxyvitamin D_3. J Pediatr 99:16, 1981.
125. Crawhall JC, Leitman PS, Schneider JA, et al: Cystinosis: plasma cystine and cysteine concentrations and the effect of D-penicillamine and dietary treatment. Am J Med 44:330, 1968.
126. Clayton BE, Patrick AD: Use of dimercaprol or penicillamine in the treatment of cystinosis. Lancet 2:909, 1961.
127. Schneider JA, Schlesselman JJ, Mendoza SA, et al: Ineffectiveness of ascorbic acid therapy in nephropathic cystinosis. N Engl J Med 330:756, 1979.
128. Depape-Brigger D, Goldman H, Scriver CR: The in vivo use of dithiothreitol in cystinosis. Pediatr Res 11:124, 1977.
129. Yudkoff M, Foreman JW, Segal S: Effects of cysteamine therapy in nephropathic cystinosis. N Engl J Med 304:141, 1981.
130. Corden BJ, Schulman JD, Schneider JA, et al: Adverse reactions to oral cysteamine use in nephropathic cystinosis. Dev Pharmacol Ther 3:25, 1981.
131. Bickel H, Lutz P, Schmidt H: The treatment of cystinosis with diet and drugs. In Schulman JD (ed): Cystinosis. Washington, DC, US Government Printing Office, 1973, p 199.
132. Segal S: Galactosemia. In Stanbury JB, et al (eds): The Metabolic Basis of Inherited Disease, ed 5. New York, McGraw-Hill Book Co, 1982, p 167.
133. Hsia DYY, Walker FA: Variability in the clinical manifestations of galactosemia. J Pediatr 59:872, 1961.
134. Nadler HL, Inouye T, Hsia DYY: Clinical galactosemia: A study of 55 cases. In Hsia DYY (ed): Galactosemia. Springfield, Ill, Charles C Thomas, 1969, p 127.
135. Komrower GM, Schwartz V, Holzel, et al: A clinical and biochemical study of galactosemia. A possible explanation of the nature of the biochemical lesion. Arch Dis Childh 31:254, 1956.
136. Levy HL, Sepe SJ, Shih VE, et al: Sepsis due to *Escherichia coli* in neonates with galactosemia. N Engl J Med 297:823, 1977.
137. Litchfield WJ, Wells WW: Effect of galactose on free radical reactions of polymorphonuclear leukocytes. Arch Biochem Biophys 188:26, 1978.
138. Cusworth DC, Dent CE, Flynn FV: The aminoaciduria in galactosemia. Arch Dis Childh 30:150, 1955.
139. Holzel A, Komrower GM, Wilson VK: Aminoaciduria in galactosemia. Brit Med J 1:194, 1952.
140. VanGeffel R, Devriendt A, Dustin I-P, et al: La maladie du galactose, considerations genetiques, etude de l'amino-acidemie et de l'amino-aciduric. Arch Fr Pediatr 16:158, 1959.
141. Darling S, Mortensen O: Aminoaciduria in galactosemia. Acta Paediat 43:337, 1954.
142. Arthurton MW, Meade BW: Congenital galactosemia: Report of a case. Brit Med J 2:618, 1954.
143. Dahlquist A, Svenningsen NW: Galactose in the urine of newborn infants. J Pediatr 75:454, 1969.
144. Haworth JC, MacDonald MS: Reducing sugars in urine and blood of premature babies. Arch Dis Childh 32:417, 1952.
145. Hall WK, Cravey CE, Chen PT, et al: An evaluation of galactosuria. J Pediatr 77:625, 1970.
146. Smetana HF, Olen F: Hereditary galactose disease. Am J Clin Path 38:3, 1962.
147. Rosenberg L, Weinberg A, Segal S: The effect of high galactose diets on urinary excretion of amino acids in the rat. Biochim Biophys Acta 48:500, 1961.
148. Thier S, Fox M, Rosenberg L, et al: Hexose inhibition of amino acid uptake in the rat-kidney-cortex slice. Biochim Biophys Acta 93:106, 1964.
149. Donnell GN, Koch R, Bergren WR: Observations on results of management of galactosemic patients. In Hsia DYY (ed): Galactosemia. Springfield, IL, Charles C Thomas, 1969, p 247.
150. Gitzelmann R, Steinmann B, VanDen Berghc G: Essential fructosuria, hereditary fructose intolerance and fructose-1,6-diphosphatase deficiency. In Stanbury JB, et al (eds): The Metabolic Basis of Inherited Diseases, ed 5. New York, McGraw-Hill Book Co, 1982, p 118.

151. Baerlocher K, Gitzelmann R, Steinmann B, et al: Hereditary fructose intolerance: A major diagnostic challange. Helv Paediatr Acta 33:465, 1978.
152. Odièvre M, Gentil C, Gautier M, et al: Hereditary fructose in-tolerance in childhood. Am J Dis Child 132:605, 1978.
153. Levin B, Snodgrass GJAI, Oberholzer VG, et al: Fructosemia. Observations in seven cases. Am J Med 45:826, 1968.
154. Cornblath M, Schwartz R: Disorders of carbohydrate metabolism in infancy. In Major Problems in Clinical Pediatrics, ed 2. Philadelphia, WB Saunders Co, 1976, p 322, vol 3.
155. Steinmann B, Gitzelmann R: The diagnosis of hereditary fructose intolerance. Helv Paediatr Acta 36:297, 1981.
156. Levin B, Oberholzer VG, Snodgrass GJAI, et al: Fructosemia: An inborn error of fructose metabolism. Arch Dis Childh 38:220, 1963.
157. Morris RC Jr: An experimental renal acidification defect in patients with hereditary fructose intolerance: I. Its resemblance to renal tubular acidosis. J Clin Invest 47:1389, 1968.
158. Morris RC Jr: An experimental renal acidification defect in patients with hereditary fructose intolerance: II. Its distinction from classic renal tubular acidosis and its resemblance to the renal acidification defect associated with the Fanconi syndrome of children with cystinosis. J Clin Invest 47:1648, 1968.
159. Richardson RMA, Little JA, Patten RL, et al: Pathogenesis of acidosis in hereditary fructose intolerance. Metabolism 28:1133, 1979.
160. Burch HB, Lowry OH, Meinhardt L, et al: Effect of fructose, dihydroxyacetone, glycerol and glucose on metabolites and related compounds in liver and kidney. J Biol Chem 245:2092, 1970.
161. Morris RC Jr, Nigon K, Reed EB: Evidence that depletion of inorganic phosphate determines the severity of the disturbance of adenine nucleotide metabolism in the liver and renal cortex of the fructose-loaded rat. J Clin Invest 61:209, 1978.
162. Bade JC, Zelder O, Rumpelt HF, et al: Depletion of liver adenine phosphates and metabolic effects of intravenous infusion of fructose or sorbitol in man and in the rat. Europ J Clin Invest 3:436, 1973.
163. Hultman E, Nilsson LH, Sahlin K: Adenine nucleotide content of human liver: Normal values and fructose induced depletion. Scand J Clin Lab Invest 35:245, 1975.
164. Rea C, Segal S: ATP content of rat kidney cortex slices: Relations to α-aminoisobutyric acid uptake. Kidney Intl 2:101, 1972.
165. Fanconi G, Bickel H: Die chronische Amino-acidurie (Aminosaurendiabetes oder nephrotisch-glukosurischer Zwergwuchs) bei der Glykogenose und der Cystinkrankheit. Helv Paediatr Acta 4:359, 1949.
166. Rotthauwe HW, Finchsel H, Heldt HW, et al: Glykogenose der Leber mit Aminoacidurie und Glokusurie. Klin Wchnschr 41:818, 1963.
167. Odiève M: Glycogénose hepato-rénale avec tubulopathy pathie complex. Rev Int Hepatol 26:1, 1966.
168. Lampert F, Mayer H: Glykogenose der Leber mit Galaktoseverwertungsstorung und schwerem. Fanconi-Syndrom. Ztschr Kinderheilk 98:133, 1967.
169. Bauer B: Debré-De-Toni-Fanconi Syndrom mit Glykogenose der Leber. Klin Wchnschr 46:317, 1968.
170. Brodehl J, Gellissen K, Hagge W: The Fanconi Syndrome in hepato-renal glycogen syndrome disease. In Peters G, Roch-Ramel F (eds): Progress in Nephrology. Berlin, Springer, 1969, p 241.
171. Garty R, Cooper M, Tabachnik E: The Fanconi Syndrome associated with hepatic glycogenosis and abnormal metabolism of galactose. J Pediatr 85:821, 1974.
172. Barber MD: A case of congenital cirrhosis of the liver with renal tubular defects akin to those in the Fanconi Syndrome. Arch Dis Childh 31:335, 1956.
173. Sakai K, Kitagawa T: An atypical case of tyrosinosis (1-parahydroxyphenyllactic aciduria). 1. Clinical and laboratory findings. Jikeikai Med J 4:1, 1957.
174. La Du BN, Gjessing LR: Tyrosinosis and tyrosinemia. In Stanbury JB, et al (eds): Metabolic Basis of Inherited Disease, ed 5. New York, McGraw-Hill Book Co, 1978, p 256.
175. Strife CF, Zuroweste EL, Emmett EA, et al: Tyrosinemia with acute inter-mittant porphyria: amino-levulinic acid dehydratase deficiency related to elevated urinary aminolevulinic acid levels. J Pediatr 90:400, 1977.
176. Larochelle J, Mortezai A, Belanger M, et al: Experience with 37 infants of tyrosinemia. Canad Med Assoc J 97:105, 1967.
177. Gaull GE, Rassin DK, Solomon GE, et al: Biochemical observations on so-called hereditary tyrosinemia. Pediatr Res 4:337, 1970.
178. Lelong M, Alagille D, Gentil C, et al: Cirrhose congénitale et familiale avec diabete phospho-gluco-amine, rachitisme vitamino-resistant et tyrosinurie massive. Rev Fr Etud Clin Biol 8:37, 1963.
179. Gentz J, Jagenburg R, Zetterström R: Tyrosinemia: An inborn error of tyrosine metabolism with cirrhosis of the liver and multiple renal tubule defects (de Toni-Debre-Fanconi-syndrome) J Pediatr 66:670, 1965
180. Taniguchi K, Gjessing LR: Studies on tyrinosis. Activity of the trans-aminase, paralydroxyphenylpyruvate oxidase and homogentisic oxidase. Brit Med J 1:968, 1965.
181. LaDu BA: The enzymatic deficiency in tyrosinemia. Am J Dis Child 113:54, 1967.
182. Lindblad B, Lindstedt S, Steen G: On the enzymatic defects in hereditary tyrosinemia. Proc Natl Acad Sci (USA) 74:4641, 1977.
183. Fällstrom SP, Lindblad B, Lindstedt S, et al: Hereditary tyrosinemia-fumarylacetoacetase deficiency. Pediatr Res 13:78, 1979.
184. Kirttingen EA, Jellum E, Stokke O: Assay of fumarylacetoacetate fumarylhydrolase in human liver-deficient activity in a case of hereditary tyrosinemia. Clin Chem Acta 115:311, 1981.
185. Lescault A, Laberge C, Grenier A, et al: Deficiency of liver fumarylacetoacetate hydrolase in acute and chronic hereditary tyrosinemia. (In Press.)
186. Goldsmith L: Tyrosinemia and related disorders. In Stanbury JB, et al (eds): The Metabolic Basis of Inherited Disease, ed 5. New York, McGraw-Hill Book Co, 1982, p 287.
187. Grenier A, Lescault A, Laberge, et al: Detection of succinylacetone and the use of its measurement in mass screening for hereditary tyrosinemia. Clin Chim Acta 123:93, 1982.
188. Ebert PA, Hess RA, Frykholm BC, et al: Succinylacetone, a potent inhibitor of heme biosynthesis: Effects on cell growth, heme content and delta-aminolevulinic acid dehydratase activity of malignant murine erythroleukemia cells. Biochem Biophys Res Commun 88:1382, 1979.
189. Weinberg AG, Mize CE, Worthen HG: The occurrence of hepatoma in the chronic form of hereditary tyrosinemia. J Pediatr 88:434, 1976.
190. Aronsson S, Engelson G, Jagenburg R, et al: Long-term dietary treatment of tyrosinosis. J Pediatr 72:620, 1968.
191. Fairney A, Francis D, Ersser RS, et al: Diagnosis and treatment of tyrosinosis. Arch Dis Childh 43:540, 1968.
192. Halvorsen S, Gjessing LR: Studies on tyrosinosis: 1. Effect of a low tyrosine and low phenylalanine diet. Brit Med J 2:1171, 1964.
193. Cohn RM, Yudkoff M, Yost B, et al: Phenylalanine-tyrosine deficiency syndrome as a complication of the management of hereditary tyrosinemia. Am J Clin Nutr 30:209, 1977.
194. Hostetter MK, Levy HL, Winter HS, et al: Evidence for liver disease preceding amino acid abnormalities in hereditary tyrosinemia. N Engl J Med 308:1265, 1983.
195. Slordahl S, Lie SO, Jellum E, et al: Increased need for L-cysteine in hereditary tyrosinemia. Pediatr Res 13:74, 1979.
196. Frisch RO, McCabe ERB, Doeden D, et al: Homotransplantation of the liver in a patient with hepatoma and hereditary tyrosinemia. J Pediatr 93:592, 1978.
197. Halvorsen S: Screening for disorders of tyrosine metabolism. In Bickel H, et al (eds): Neonatal Screening for Inborn Errors of Metabolism. New York, Springer-Verlag, 1980, p 45.
198. Bergeron P, Laberge C, Grenier A: Hereditary tyrosinemia in the province of Quebec: Prevalence at birth and geographic distribution. Clin Genet 5:156, 1974.
199. Wilson SAK: Progressive lenticular degeneration. A familial nervous disease associated with cirrhosis of the liver. Brain 34:295, 1912.
200. Sass-Kortsak A, Bearn A: Hereditary disorders of copper metabolism. In Stanbury JB, et al (eds): The Metabolic Basis of Inherited Disease, ed 4. New York, McGraw-Hill Book Co, 1978, p 1098.
201. Bickel H, Neale FC, Hall G: A clinical and biochemical study of hepatolenticular degeneration (Wilson's disease). Quart J Med 26:527, 1957.
202. Reynolds ES, Tannen RL, Tyler HR: The renal lesion in Wilson's disease. Am J Med 40:518, 1966.
203. Monro P: Effect of treatment on renal function in severe osteomalacia due to Wilson's disease. J Clin Path 23:487, 1970.
204. Uzman L, Denny-Brown, D: Amino-aciduria in hepato-lenticular degeneration (Wilson's disease). Am J Med Sci 215:599, 1948.
205. Cooper AM, Eckhardt RO, Faloon WW, et al: Investigation of the aminoaciduria in Wilson's disease (hepatolenticular degeneration), demonstration of a defect in renal function. J Clin Invest 29:265, 1950.
206. Schonheider F, Gregerson G, Hansen HE, et al: Renal clearances of different amino acids in Wilson's disease before and after treatment with penicillamine. Acta Med Scand 190:395, 1971.
207. Cavallino R, Grossman H: Wilson's disease presenting with rickets. Radiology 90:493, 1968.
208. Joshua GE: Hepatolenticular degeneration (Wilson's disease) and rickets in children. Indian J Med Res 61:1876, 1973.
209. Bishop C, Zimdahl WT, Talbott JH: Uric acid in two patients with Wilson's disease (hepatolenticular degeneration). Proc Soc Exp Biol Med 86:440, 1954.
210. Mahoney JP, Sandberg AA, Gabler CJ, et al: Uric acid metabolism in heptolenticular degeneration. Proc Soc Exp Biol Med 88:427, 1955.
211. Sorenson LB, Kappas A: The effects of penicillamine on uric acid metabolism in Wilson's disease. Trans Assoc Am Phys 79:157, 1966.

212. Finby N, Bearn AG: Roentgenographic abnormalities of the skeletal system in Wilson's disease (hepatolenticular degeneration). AJR 79:603, 1958.
213. Litin RB, Randall RV, Goldstein NP, et al: Hypercalciuria in hepatolenticular degeneration (Wilson's disease). Am J Med Sci 238:614, 1959.
214. Sternlieb I, Scheinberg IH: Role of radioactive copper in the diagnosis of Wilson's disease. Gastroenterology 77:138, 1979.
215. DuBois RS, Rodgerson DO, Martineau G, et al: Orthotopic liver transplantations for Wilson's disease. Lancet 1:505, 1971.
216. Lowe CU, Terrey M, McLachlan EA: Organic-aciduria, decreased renal ammonia production, hydrophthalmus, and mental retardation. Am J Dis Child 83:164, 1952.
217. Svorc I, Masopust I, Komarkowa A, et al: Oculo-cerebro-renal syndrome in a female child. Am J Dis Child 114:186, 1967.
218. Sagel I, Ores RO, Yuceoglu AM: Renal function and morphology in a girl with oculo-cerebro-renal syndrome. J Pediatr 77:124, 1970.
219. Seedorff HH: Ocular changes in certain forms of aminoaciduria. Acta Ophthal 37:125, 1959.
220. Illig R, Dummaruth G, Prader A: Das oculo-cerebro-renal syndrom (Lowe): Klinische, metabolishe und elektroencephalographische Befunde bei 3 Fallen. Helv Paediatr Acta 18:173, 1963.
221. Wilson WA, Richards W, Donnell GN: Oculo-cerebro-renal syndrome of Lowe: A review of eight cases noting the genetic inheritance. Arch Ophthalmol 70:5, 1963.
222. Richards W, Donnell GN, Wilson W, et al: The oculo-cerebro-renal syndrome of Lowe. Am J Dis Child 109:185, 1965.
223. Abassi V, Lowe CU, Calcagno PL: Oculo-cerebro-renal syndrome: A review. Am J Dis Child 115:145, 1968.
224. Holmes LB, McGowan BL, Efron ML: Lowe's syndrome: A search for the carrier state. Pediatrics 44:358, 1969.
225. Hambraeus L, Pallisgaard G, Kildeberg P: The Lowe's syndrome: Observations on the amino acid metabolism in a 2-year-old affected boy. Acta Paediatr Scand 59:631, 1970.
226. Texier JL, Jully G, Bach C: Syndrome de Lowe. Ann Pediatr (Paris) 18:825, 1971.
227. Schwartz R, Hall PW, Gabuzda GJ: Metabolism of ornithine and other amino acids in the cerebro-oculo-renal syndrome. Am J Med 36:778, 1964.
228. Bartsocas CS, Levy HL, Crawford JD, et al: A defect in intestinal amino acid transport in Lowe's syndrome. Am J Dis Child 117:93, 1969.
229. Colombo JP: Hinweis auf eine tubuläre und intestinale Malabsorption der Aminosauren beim Lowe-Syndrom. Schweiz Med Wchnschr 101:968, 1971.
230. Antener I, Nordio S, Kaeser M, et al: Etude Clinique de l'absorption intestinale des acides amines: Determination des acides amines dans les selles. Ann Nestle 62:18, 1972.
231. Matsuda I, Sugai M, Kajii T: Ornithine loading test in Lowe's syndrome. J Pediatr 77:127, 1970.
232. Chutorian A, Rowland LP: Lowe's syndrome. Neurology 16:115, 1966.
233. Oetliker O, Rossi E: The influence of extracellular fluid volume on the renal bicarbonate threshold: A study of two children with Lowe's syndrome. Pediatr Res 3:140, 1969.
234. Van Acker KJ, Roels H, Beelaerts W, et al: The histologic lesions of the kidney in the oculo-cerebro-renal syndrome of Lowe. Nephron 4:193, 1967.
235. Witzleben CL, Schoen EJ, Tu WE, et al: Progressive morphologic renal changes in the oculo-cerebro-renal syndrome of Lowe. Am J Med 44:319, 1968.
236. Ores RO: Renal changes in oculo-cerebro-renal syndrome of Lowe. Arch Path 89:221, 1970.
237. Biervliet JPAM, Bruinvis L, Ketting D, et al: Hereditary mitochondrial myopathy with lactic acidemia, a DeToni-Fanconi-Debre syndrome, and a defective respiratory chain in voluntary striated muscle. Pediatr Res 11:1088, 1977.
238. DiMauro S, Mendell JR, Sahenk Z, et al: Fatal infantile mitochondrial myopathy and renal dysfunction due to cytochrome-c-oxidase deficiency. Neurology 30:795, 1980.
239. Heiman-Patterson TD, Bonilla E, DiMauro S, et al: Cytochrome-c-oxidase deficiency in a floppy infant. Neurology 32:898, 1982.
240. Chisolm JJ, Harrison HC, Eberlein WR, et al: Aminoaciduria, hypophosphatemia and rickets in lead poisoning. Am J Dis Child 89:159, 1955.
241. Chisolm JJ: Aminoaciduria as a manifestation of renal tubular injury in lead intoxication and a comparison with patterns of aminoaciduria seen in other diseases. J Pediatr 60:1, 1962.
242. Clarkson TW, Kench JE: Urinary excretion of amino acids by men absorbing heavy metals. Biochem J 62:361, 1956.
243. Goyer RA, Tsuchuja K, Leonard DL, et al: Aminoaciduria in Japanese workers in the lead and cadmium industries. Am J Clin Path 57:635, 1972.
244. Galle P, Morel-Maroger L: Les lésions rénales du saturnisme humain et experimental. Nephron 2:273, 1945.
245. vonStudnitz W, Haeger-Aronsen B: Urinary excretion of amino acids in lead-poisoned rabbits. Acta Pharmacol Toxicol 19:36, 1962.
246. Goyer RA: The renal tubule in lead poisoning: I. Mitochondrial swelling and aminoaciduria. Lab Invest 19:71, 1968.
247. Goyer RA, Krall A, Kimball JP: The renal tubule in lead poisoning: II. In vitro studies of mitochondrial structure and function. Lab Invest 19:78, 1968.
248. Emmersen BT: "Ouch-ouch" disease: The osteomalacia of cadmium nephropathy. Ann Intern Med 73:854, 1970.
249. Kazantzis G, Flynn FV, Spowage JS, et al: Renal tubular malfunction and pulmonary emphysema in cadmium pigment workers. Quart J Med 32:165, 1963.
250. Gonick HC, Indraprasit S, Rosen VJ, et al: Experimental Fanconi syndrome: III. Effect of cadmium on renal tubular function, the ATP-Na-K-ATPase transport and renal tubular ultrastructure. Min Electro Metab 3:21, 1980.
251. Rothstein A, Berke HJ: Aminoaciduria in uranium poisoning: The use of amino-acid nitrogen to creatinine ratio in "spot" samples of urine. J Pharmacol Exp Ther 96:179, 1049.
252. Rützler L: Passageres tubuläres Syndrome durch Vergiftung mit einer organischen Quecksilberverbindung (Glyceromerfen) bei einem 1] jährigen Madchen. Schweiz Med Wchnschr 103:678, 1973.
253. Gross JM: Fanconi syndrome (adult type) developing secondary to ingestion of outdated tetracycline. Ann Intern Med 56:523, 1963.
254. Frimpter GW, Timpanelli AE, Eisenmenger WJ, et al: Reversible Fanconi syndrome caused by degraded tetracycline. JAMA 184:111, 1963.
255. Ehrlich LI, Stein WJ: Abnormal urinary findings following administration of Achromycin V. Pediatrics 31:339, 1963.
256. Cleveland WW, Adams WC, Mann JB, et al: Acquired Fanconi syndrome following degraded tetracycline. J Pediatr 66:333, 1965.
257. Brodehl J, Gellisson K, Hagge W, et al: Reversibles renales Fanconi-Syndrom durch toxisches Abbauprodukt des tetrazyklins. Helv Paediatr Acta 23:373, 1968.
258. Benitz KF, Diermeir HF: Renal toxicity of tetracycline degradation products. Proc Soc Exp Biol Med 115:930, 1964.
259. Lindqvist RR, Fellers FX: Degraded tetracycline nephropathy: Functions, morphologic and histochemical observations. Lab Invest 15:864, 1966.
260. Lowe MB, Tapp E: Renal damage caused by anhydro-4-EPI-tetracycline. Arch Pathol 81:362, 1966.
261. DuBuy HG, Showacre JL: Selective localization of tetracycline in mitochondria of living cells. Science 133:196, 1961.
262. Otten J, Vis HL: Acute reversible renal tubular dysfunction following intoxication with methyl-3-chromone. J Pediatr 73:422, 1968.
263. Butler HE, Morgan JM, Smythe CM: Mercaptopurine and acquired tubular dysfunction in adult nephrosis. Arch Int Med 116:853, 1965.
264. Moss AH, Gabow PA, Kaehny WD, et al: Fanconi syndrome and distal renal tubular acidosis after glue sniffing. Ann Int Med 92:69, 1980.
265. Spencer AG, Franglen GT: Gross aminoaciduria following a lysol burn. Lancet 1:190, 1952.
266. Schwartz JH, Schein P: Fanconi syndrome associated with cephalothin and gentamicin therapy. Cancer 41:769, 1978.
267. Russo JC, Adelman RD: Gentamicin-induced Fanconi syndrome. J Pediatr 96:151, 1980.
268. Schein P, Kahn R, Gordon P, et al: Streptozotocin for malignant insulinomas and carcinoid tumor. Arch Int Med 132:555, 1973.
269. Emslie-Smith D, Johnstone JH, Thomson MB, et al: Aminoaciduria in acute tubular necrosis. Clin Sci 15:171, 1976.
270. Berliner RW, Kennedy TJ, Hilton JG: The effect of maleic acid on renal function. Proc Soc Exp Biol Med 75:791, 1950.
271. Harrison HE, Harrison HC: The experimental production of renal glucosuria, phosphaturia, and aminoaciduria by injection of maleic acid. Science 120:606, 1954.
272. Angielski S, Niemiro R, Makarewicz W, et al: Aminoaciduria caused by maleic acid. Acta Biochim Polon 5:431, 1958.
273. Silverman M, Huang L: Mechanism of maleic acid-induced glycosuria in dog kidney. Am J Physiol 231:1024, 1976.
274. Maesaka JK, McCaffery M: Evidence for renal tubular leakage in maleic acid-induced Fanconi syndrome. Am J Physiol 239:F507, 1980.
275. Roth KS, Hwang SM, Segal S: Effect of maleic acid on the kinetics of α-methyl-D-glucoside uptake by isolated rat renal tubules. Biochim Biophys Acta 426:675, 1976.
276. Roth KS, Goldmann DR, Segal S: Developmental aspects of maleic acid-induced inhibition of sugar and amino acid transport in the rat renal tubule. Pediatr Res 12:1121, 1978.
277. Reynolds RA, McNamara PD, Segal S: On the maleic acid induced Fanconi syndrome: Effects on transport by isolated rat kidney brushborder membrane vesicles. Life Sci 22:39, 1978.
278. LeGrimellac C, Carrière S, Cardinal J, et al: Effect of maleate on membrane physical state of brushborder and basolateral membranes of the dog kidney. Life Sci 30:1107, 1982.
279. Kramer HJ, Gonick HC: Experimental Fanconi. 1. Effect of maleic acid on renal cortical Na-K-ATPase activity and ATP level. J Lab Clin Med 76:799, 1970.

280. Rogulski J, Pacanis A, Adamonicz W, et al: On the mechanism of maleate action on rat kidney mitochondria. Effect on oxidative metabolism. Acta Biochim Polon 21:403, 1974.
281. Pacanis A, Rogulski J, Ledochowski H, et al: On the mechanism of maleate action on rat kidney mitochondria. Effect on substrate-level phosphorylation. Acta Biochim Polon 22:1, 1975.
282. Engle RL, Wallis LA: Multiple myeloma and the adult Fanconi syndrome. 1. Report of a case with crystal-like deposits in the tumor cells and the epithelial cells of the kidney. Am J Med 22:5, 1957.
283. Constanza DJ, Smoller M: Multiple myeloma with Fanconi syndrome. Am J Med 34:125, 1963.
284. Headley RN, King JS, Cooper MR, et al: Multiple myeloma presenting as adult Fanconi syndrome. Clin Chem 18:293, 1972.
285. Harrison JF, Blainey JD: Adult Fanconi syndrome with monoclonal abnormality of immunoglobulin light chain. J Clin Path 20:42, 1967.
286. Smithline N, Kassirer JP, Cohen JJ: Light-chain nephropathy: Renal tubular dysfunction associated with light-chain proteinuria. N Engl J Med 294:71, 1976.
287. Shearn MA, Tu WH: Nephrogenic diabetes insipidus and other defects in renal tubular function in Sjögren syndrome. Am J Med 39:312, 1965.
288. Finkel PN, Kronenberg K, Pesce AJ, et al: Adult Fanconi syndrome, amyloidosis and marked X-light chain proteinuria. Nephron 10:1, 1973.
289. Kyle RA, Maldonado JE, Bayrd ED: Idiopathic Bence-Jones proteinuria—a distinct entity? Am J Med 55:222, 1973.
290. Preuss HG, Hammack WJ, Murdaugh HV: The effect of Bence-Jones proteins on the in vitro function of rabbit renal cortex. Nephron 5:210, 1967.
291. Preuss HG, Weib FR, Iammarino RM, et al: Effects on rat kidney slice function in vitro of proteins from the urines of patients with myelomatosis and nephrosis. Clin Sci Mol Med 46:283, 1974.
292. Hooft C, Vermassen A: Syndrome de DeToni-Debré-Fanconi chez un efant atteint de nephrose lipoidique. Ann Pediatr (Basel) 190:1, 1958.
293. Stickler GB, Hayles AB, Power MH, et al: Nephrotic syndrome complicated by renal tubular dysfunction. Am J Dis Child 98:647, 1959.
294. Doolan PD, Morris MD, Harper HA: Amino aciduria in an elderly man with the nephrotic syndrome and a young man with a variant of the Fanconi syndrome. Ann Intern Med 56:448, 1962.
295. Royer P, Delaitre R, Mathieu H, et al: Le syndrome nephrotique avec insuffisance tubulaire globale et tetanic recidivante. Ann Pediatr (Paris) 10:583, 1963.
296. Massry SG, Preuss HG, Maher JF, et al: Renal tubular acidosis after cadaver kidney homotransplantation. Am J Med 42:284, 1967.
297. Vertuno LL, Preuss HG, Argy WP, et al: Fanconi syndrome following homotransplantation. Arch Intern Med 133:302, 1974.
298. Better OS: Tubular dysfunction following kidney transplantation. Nephron 25:209, 1980.
299. Standbury SW, Lumb GA: Metabolic studies of renal osteodystrophy: 1. Calcium, phosphorus and nitrogen metabolism in rickets, osteomalacia and hyperparathyroidism complicating chronic uremia and in the osteomalacia of the adult Fanconi syndrome. Medicine 41:1, 1963.
300. Sheldon W, Luder J, Webb BA: A familial tubular absorption defect of glucose and amino acids. Arch Dis Childh 36:90, 1961.
301. Christiaens L, Biserte G, Farriaux J, Fontaine G, et al: La forme idiopathique du syndrome de deToni-Debré-Fanconi. Sem Hôp Paris Ann Pediatr 41:49, 1965.
302. Neimann N, Pierson M, Marchal C, et al: Nephropathie familial glomerulo-tubulaire avec syndrome de deToni-Debré-Fanconi. Arch Fr Pediatr 25:43, 1968.
303. Luder J, Sheldon WA: Familial tubular absorption defect of glucose and amino acids. Arch Dis Childh 30:160, 1955.
304. Hunt DD, Stearns G, McKinley JB, et al: Long-term study of a family with the Fanconi syndrome without cystinosis (deToni-Debré-Fanconi syndrome). Am J Med 40:492, 1966.
305. Chesney RW, Kaplan BS, Teitel D, et al: Metabolic abnormalities in the idiopathic Fanconi syndrome: Studies of carbohydrate metabolism in two patients. Pediatrics 67:113, 1981.
306. Chesney RW, Kaplan BS, Colle E, et al: Abnormalities of carbohydrate metabolism in idiopathic Fanconi syndrome. Pediat Res 14:209, 1980.
307. Aperia A, Bergqvist G, Linne T, et al: Familial Fanconi syndrome with malabsorption and galactose intolerance, normal kinase and transferase activity. Acta Paediatr Scand 70:527, 1981.
308. McCune DJ, Mason HH, Clarke HT: Intractable hypophosphatemic rickets with renal glycosuria and acidosis (The Fanconi syndrome). Am J Dis Child 65:81, 1943.
309. Smith R, Linderbaum RH, Walton RJ: Hypophosphatemic osteomalacia and Fanconi syndrome of adult onset with dominant inheritance. Possible relationship with diabetes mellitus. Quart J Med 69:387, 1976.
310. Patrick A, Cameron JS, Ogg CS: A family with a dominant form of idiopathic Fanconi syndrome leading to renal failure in adult life. Clin Nephrol 16:289, 1981.
311. Friedman AL, Trygstad CW, Chesney RW: Autosomal dominant Fanconi syndrome with early renal failure. Am J Clin Genet 2:225, 1978.
312. Rampini S, Fanconi A, Illig R, et al: Effect of hydrochlorothiazide on proximal renal tubular acidosis in a patient with idiopathic deToni-Debre-Fanconi syndrome. Helv Paediatr Acta 23:13, 1968.
313. Balsan S, Garabedian M, Sorgniard R, et al: 1,25-dihydroxyvitamin D_3 and 1,α-hydroxyvitamin D_3 in children: Biologic and therapeutic effects in nutritional rickets and different types of vitamin D resistance. Pediatr Res 9:586, 1975.

CHAPTER 31

Aminoaciduria

CHARLES R. SCRIVER
MICHEL BERGERON

INTRODUCTION

In this chapter we will discuss the hereditary hyperaminoacidurias of humans. The prefix hyper implies that aminoaciduria is a natural phenomenon, whereas too much aminoaciduria is a deviant phenotype. Whether the aberrant phenotype is indicative of disease requires knowledge of its biological significance.

The first task is to define normal amino acid excretion in urine. Since the amount excreted is determined both by the amount filtered and the ability of the nephron to reabsorb amino acids from filtrate, measurement of urinary amino acids is a useful indicator of abnormal prerenal amino acid metabolism and of abnormal renal reabsorption. If the disturbance of amino acid homeostasis compromises adaptation to the experiences of life, it is a disease; if it does not, it is a benign variation in phenotype.

The process of amino acid reabsorption by the nephron is complex. It is relevant to know something about the process because it determines how much amino acid will be excreted into bladder urine from filtrate. Mutations that impair net tubular reabsorption in humans are markers of components in the process. They reflect the evolutionary process that endows our species with mechanisms dedicated to the metabolic homeostasis that underlies our health.

This chapter begins with an overview of the normal phenotype and its heritability. A description of the mechanism of amino acid transport follows, which leads to a description of the origin of deviant phenotypes (cause); a classification of the latter is given. Selected inborn errors of amino acid transport are examined, translating theory into an analysis of the disadaptive processes that cause disease (pathogenesis). Then we look at ontogeny, a process that further delineates transport functions in the nephron; awareness of ontogeny averts misclassification of a developmental phenotype as a potential disease. Finally, in an appendix, we provide capsule summaries of eight Mendelian disorders of amino acid transport expressed in the kidney.

NORMAL VARIATION (HOMEOSTASIS) ILLUSTRATED BY AMINOACIDURIA

In this section the normal variation in renal handling of amino acids is described.

Only a small fraction (≈3%) of total urinary nitrogen (N) in humans is excreted in the form of free amino acids (AA) (largely as the L-stereoisomers). The excreted fraction is less than 5% of the filtered AA load. The excretion pattern is informative about the reabsorption process. Fractional reabsorption is lower for short-chain aliphatic α-amino acids than for long-chain analogues (Fig. 31.1). Net reabsorption under endogenous conditions is more efficient for α-amino acids relative to non-α-amino analogues. L-isomers are reabsorbed more efficiently than D-isomers. Renal clearance is influenced by filtered load, and disorders of prerenal homeostasis influence fractional excretion through saturation of the reabsorption process. If catabolism of the AA by the tubular epithelium is important to the process of reabsorption, its impairment, as occurs in some states of inborn errors of metabolism, may contribute to impaired reabsorption and hyperaminoaciduria. Fractional excretion is also influenced by the age of the individual and other physiological factors. Clearance rates of some AA are elevated in the human infant, e.g., for proline and glycine, a circumstance that reflects renal ontogeny. The available but rather inadequate data on normal variation in renal clearance of amino acids in man, expressed as range or mean and standard deviation (SD) are summarized in Table 31.1.

Renal clearance of an amino acid (C_{AA}) (equation 1) requires a timed urine volume and usually is adjusted to rate per unit surface area (SA).

$$C_{AA}\ (\text{ml/min}) = \frac{U_{AA}\ (\mu\text{mole/ml}) \cdot \text{volume (ml/min)}}{P_{AA}\ (\mu\text{mole/ml})} \qquad (1)$$

The fractional excretion of amino acid (FE_{AA}) can be derived from an untimed specimen using the clearance of creatinine (C_{Cr}) as the reference (equations 2 and 3):

$$FE_{AA} = C_{AA}/C_{Cr} \qquad (2)$$

$$FE_{AA} = \frac{U_{AA} \cdot P_{Cr}}{P_{AA} \cdot U_{Cr}} \qquad (3)$$

C_{AA} and FE_{AA} are metrical parameters of net renal reabsorption of amino acids. As such, they have central tendencies and dispersion, which reflect intraindividual and interindividual variation. A third variation in Fe_{AA} (or C_{AA}) is a result of the crudeness of the measurement itself; it is dependent on an imprecise "black box" technique whose contribution to the observed variance is considerable if not precisely known (2).

Of the biological variation consider FE_{AA} (or C_{AA}) as a phenotype (P), which is the product of genotype (G) and environmental events (E)

$$P = G + E \qquad (4)$$

Since there is variability (V) in these biological entities, it follows that

$$V_p = V_G + V_E \qquad (5)$$

It is of interest to know how much of the phenotypic variance (V_p) is derived from genotype and how much from environment. A measure of this is called heritability (h^2). The broad definition of heritability (3) is

$$h^2 = V_G/V_p \qquad (6)$$

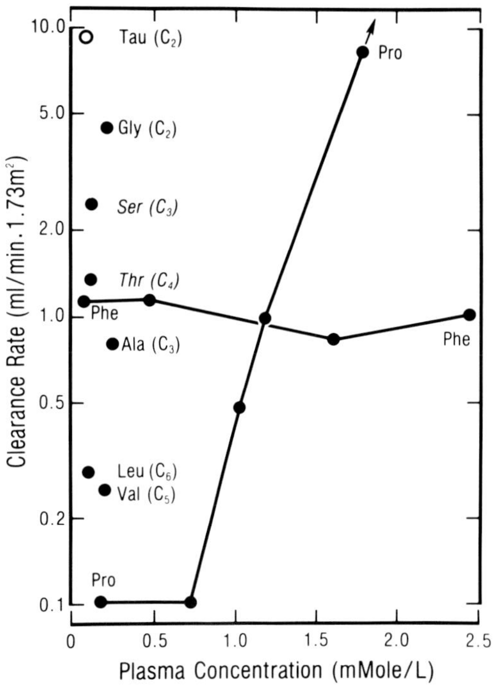

Figure 31.1. Endogenous renal clearance is an indirect measure of the net tubular absorption of amino acids under endogenous conditions. α-Amino acids (●) with long, apolar side chains have low (leucine, isoleucine, and valine) renal clearance rates (high tubular reabsorption) relative to those with short carbon chains (alanine, threonine, serine, and glycine). Renal clearance rate for β-amino acid (○) is greater than for α-amino analog. Clearance rates for proline (*pro*) show saturation of tubular transport process (transport or metabolic runout); the proline system saturates at relatively low plasma concentrations. Phenylalanine does not easily saturate its transcellular reabsorption process; it is absorbed with equal efficiency at high and at normal concentrations of phenylalanine in the plasma. Source of data is a patient with phenylketonuria, off and on treatment. (Modified from Scriver CR: Pediatrics 44:348, 1969.)

Mendelian forms of deviant or mutant phenotype have high heritability, e.g., cystinuria. By contrast, hyperaminoaciduria, associated with intravenous alimentation, has low heritability. Two quite different studies indicate that there is heritability in the normal aminoaciduria phenotype.

First, the variability of aminoaciduria is smaller in human monozygotic (MZ) twin pairs than in nontwin pairs examined under equivalent environmental conditions (1).

Second, rats of the same strain have 30-fold less intraindividual variation relative to the observed interindividual variation in FE_{AA} (4) (Fig. 31.2). For example, a constant weight-corrected infusion of α-aminoisobutyrate (AIB), which is neither metabolized nor incorporated into protein, minimizes V_E; accordingly, any difference in FE_{AIB} between animals (V_p) must reflect variability in genotype (V_G). By this analysis, Fe_{AIB} has heritability.

The steady-state plasma AIB level is inversely related to FE_{AIB} (Fig. 31.2), which implies that renal handling influences homeostasis of the free AA pool. This relationship is less evident for most natural AA, because other metabolic components contribute to homeostasis in extracellular fluid (ECF). However, renal handling is an important determinant of taurine homeostasis.

To state the argument another way, mutation (V_G) will modify the AA excretion phenotype (FE_{AA}) either by an effect on the renal reabsorption process or on amino acid catabolism, which indirectly influences reabsorption.

Extreme deviation from the optimal metabolic steady-state can be disadaptive to health. In this context, health is a state of adaptive homeostasis; disease is disadaptive dishomeostasis (5). It is not surprising that many inborn errors affecting AA transport are identified early in life, because the disadaptation or disease induces symptoms shortly after birth. Problems arise when screening procedures identify deviant phenotypes in the form of abnormal urinary amino acid excretion without symptoms. The significance of the finding depends on whether it is indicative of an incipient disease or is a normal variant, i.e., is not disadaptive. We will classify aminoaciduria phenotypes into those that are not usually disadaptive from those that are.

THE PROCESS OF TRANSEPITHELIAL REABSORPTION

This section addresses matters relevant to understanding the pathogenesis of hyperaminoaciduria, in abbreviated fashion, as an appropriate background to an understanding of the pathogenesis of disease and the taxonomy of aminoaciduria, without which classification will be soon forgotten.

With evolution, differentiation of function and chemical content of cells developed (6). Cells partition extracellular from intracellular aqueous environments by means of a hydrophobic lipid bilayer; subcellular compartmentation is achieved by other boundary membranes, which affect the ability to transfer hydrophilic substances, e.g., AA, across a hydrophobic boundary. Some transport processes have catalytic specificity as a result of membrane-bound protein. The specificity of transport proteins is genetically controlled, i.e., renal transport of L-amino acids can be modified by mutation; mutation can be used to probe the process.

Renal Transport of Amino Acids General Features

Renal transport encompasses net reabsorption from filtrate and uptake from extracellular fluid (ECF). The former is a transcellular process; the latter supports cell nutrition.

The process of reabsorption has several general characteristics (7). At endogenous filtered loads, over 80% of reabsorption of most AA occurs within the early portion of the proximal nephron. Glycine and taurine are exceptions that share a greater portion of their reabsorption in the S_3 (pars recta) segment of proximal nephron. When filtered loads increase, reabsorption of other AA extends to late portions of proximal nephron. The distal nephron does not participate in net reabsorption of AA (2).

The principal driving force for reabsorption is the inward transport of Na^+ across the luminal membrane; reabsorption of AA is secondary to active transport or cotransport (8). Energy is invested at the basolateral membrane to pump Na from the cell to maintain the gradient for Na at the brush-border membrane. The transport process for substrate can operate against an electrochemical gradient.

The carrier in brush-border membrane interacting with the amino acid and Na^+ is saturable and follows Michaelis-Menten kinetics. Passive, Na^+-independent, diffusion of most AA plays a lesser role in their net reabsorption (7). The transport sites have higher affinity for L-isomers of the AA and specificity for substrate. The latter can be divided into sites that have group specificity (7, 9) with high capacity and low affinity relative and more selective systems for single AA, which have higher affinity and lower capacity. Oligopeptides and dipeptides are transported at sites independent of those serving free AA.

The "carrier" mechanism is not the γ-glutamyl cycle as proposed by some (10); but its actual nature is not known.

Transport at the basolateral membrane shares most of the features described for the reactive sites in brush-border membrane. Uptake is Na^+-dependent for some AA and probably Na^+-independent for others.

Table 31.1.
Endogenous Renal Clearance of Amino Acids (ml/min/1.73M²)[a]

Amino Acid	Infants		Children			Adults
	Range	Mean ± SD	Mean ± SD	Mean	Range	Range
Taurine	0.1–3.8	—	—	13.7	9.9–26.2	1.7–14
Hydroxyproline	tr–34	—	—	—	0–tr	
Aspartic Acid	tr–16	—	3.6 ± 0.9	2.8	tr–8.8	0–2.4
Threonine	3.0–8.2	2.0 ± 1.4	1.0 ± 0.2	1.4	0.5–2.5	0.8–1.5
Serine	4.5–13	4.1 ± 1.9	2.4 ± 0.5	2.4	1.2–3.4	1.9–3.0
Asn + Gln[b]	1.2–3.6	—	—	1.3	0.1–2.3	0.7–1.8
Proline	1.7–14	1.0 ± 0.7	0.3 ± 0.2	—	0–0.3	
Glutamic Acid	0.1–3	—	—	0.8	0.1–2.4	0.3–1.7
Glycine	12–44	7.4 ± 3.2	4.2 ± 1.4	4.4	1.2–8.3	2.7–5.8
Alanine	1.5–4.2	1.6 ± 0.7	0.8 ± 0.4	0.8	0.2–1.3	0.3–0.9
Valine	0.2–0.6	0.3 ± 0.1	0.2 ± 0.1	0.2	0.18–0.3	0.1–0.3
Half Cystine	2.5–8.8	1.1 ± 0.3	0.8 ± 0.2	—	1.0–1.4	0.7–2.9
Methionine	2.3–5.8	0.8 ± 0.5	0.8 ± 0.3	1.9	1.0–3.4	1.1
Isoleucine	0.4–1.7	0.3 ± 0.2	0.3 ± 0.1	0.5	0.2–1.0	0.2–1.0
Leucine	0.4–1.3	0.8 ± 0.5	0.5 ± 0.1	0.5	0.2–0.9	0.2–0.9
Tyrosine	0.5–2.6	1.8 ± 0.4	2.0 ± 0.8	2.0	0.8–3.3	1.0–1.7
Phenylalanine	1.0–2.2	1.7 ± 0.9	1.5 ± 0.3	1.2	0.3–2.3	0.7–1.4
Ornithine	0.6–1.1	0.4 ± 0.1	0.4 ± 0.1	0.5	0.2–0.8	tr
Lysine	1.6–6.3	1.3 ± 0.4	1.2 ± 0.4	1.1	0.3–2.4	0.2–1.9
Histidine	12–29	8.5 ± 4.4	9.5 ± 2.6	9.2	1.9–21.8	4.7–9.1
Arginine	tr–1.0	0.4 ± 0.1	0.3 ± 0.1	0.5	0.15–1.2	0.2–0.8

Adapted from Scriver CR, Rosenberg LE: Distribution of amino acids in body fluids. In Amino Acid Metabolism and Its Disorders. Philadelphia, W. B. Saunders, 1973.
[a] Clearance rates were obtained from overnight fasted subjects (children and adults) or before feeding (infants).
[b] Asparagine and glutamine combined.

Saturability, stereospecificity, substrate specificity, and energy dependence for uptake into the cell also operate at the basolateral membrane. Whether specificity for cell influx mirrors specificity for efflux is not settled (11, 12). These are cell uptake systems at the basolateral membrane along the whole length of the nephron, whereas reabsorption sites in brush-border membrane are confined to proximal nephron (7). Events at the brush-border membrane are the major determinants of net reabsorption and these plus filtered load determine AA composition of urine.

The Transepithelial Transport Process

Renal epithelium is a permeability barrier to AA in filtrate by virtue of tight junctions at the luminal pole of the tubular cells (13). Amino acid enters proximal tubular cells at the luminal surface (Fig. 31.3). Because the luminal surface faces an environment topologically "outside" the organism and the antiluminal surface faces a milieu topologically "inside", i.e., the membranes have different functions, inborn errors of transport are either disorders of the brush-border membrane or the basolateral membrane or occasionally of both membranes (11). Since most of the substrate-specific inborn errors are primarily disorders of only one membrane, we can appreciate why they appear to have little impact on the general health of renal tubular cells; substrate necessary for cell metabolism may be derived from either surface and cell nutrition is sustained despite a mutant phenotype on one surface. Impact of mutation is thus more on homeostasis in the "milieu interieur" and less on these intervening cellular interfaces between internal and external environments.

Because renal epithelium functions as an interface between two different environments, we need to summarize the mechanisms that underlie flux asymmetry, which sustains net reabsorption (11, 12), for these are relevant to interpretation of mutant phenotypes.

During net reabsorption of a specific AA, the trans-transepithelial inward flux (J_1 in Fig. 31.3) must exceed the outward flux (J_2). Each flux conforms to the general equation

$$J = K \cdot [A] \tag{7}$$

where K is the rate coefficient, [A] is the AA chemical activity.† Net reabsorption from the lumen of the nephron requires only that flux J_3, the influx component at the brush-border membrane, exceed flux J_4, the efflux component at the same membrane (Fig. 31.3). If we assume that passive diffusion by cellular and paracellular routes is not its principal determinant then net reabsorption is determined by events at the brush-border membrane.

The transport of amino acid at brush-border membrane fits Michaelis and diffusional equations

$$J_3 = J_{in} = \frac{Jmax_{in} \cdot A_l + Kd \cdot \overset{*}{A_l}}{Km_{in} + A_l} \tag{8}$$

where the subscripts *in* and *l* refer to influx and lumen, respectively. The corresponding equation for efflux at the brush-border membrane is

$$J_4 = J_{eff} = \frac{Jmax_{eff} \cdot A_c + Kd \cdot \overset{*}{A_c}}{Km_{eff} + A_c} \tag{9}$$

where subscripts *eff* and *c* refer to efflux and cell, respectively. The influx of L-amino acid uses the energy of the Na^+ electrochemical gradient ($\Delta\bar{\mu}Na$) as described by the equation

$$\Delta\bar{\mu}Na = \frac{-RTln\ (Na^+)_c}{(Na^+)_l} - F \cdot V_{BBM} \tag{10}$$

† Chemical activity indicated by asterisk and concentration are not necessarily synonymous. There is little difference for neutral AA, but activity and concentration may be different with taurine, for example.

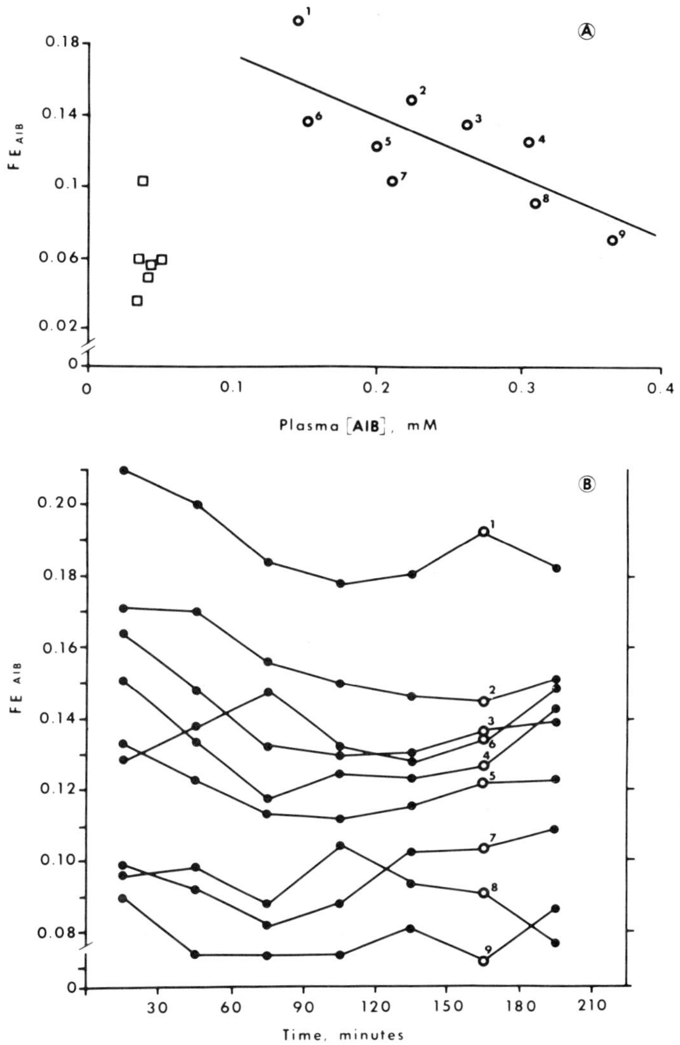

Figure 31.2. **Top,** Relation of FE_{AIB} to plasma [AIB] at steady state in the sixth clearance period (150 to 180 min), in rats preinjected with AIB 16 hours before zero time. Two amounts of AIB were injected; 6 rats received 0.115 mmole/kg (*open squares*); 9 rats received 1.22 mmole/kg (*open circles*). The regression of FE_{AIB} on plasma AIB in the high-dose group is significant ($r = 0.734$; $p < 0.05$). **Bottom,** Interindividual variation of FE_{AIB} is 30-fold greater than the intraindividual variation ($n = 9$ rats; 63 clearance periods). Threefold interindividual variation in FE_{AIB} (0.07 to 0.21) is observed; the intraindividual variation is less than 10% around the mean per single animal. (From McInnes RR, Scriver CR: Am J Physiol 240: F1, 1981, with permission.)

where R is the gas constant, T the absolute temperature, F the Faraday constant, and V_{BBM} the brush-border membrane potential. Tubular reabsorption of AA proceeds against an electrochemical gradient (14, 15).

Given flux asymmetry at the brush-border membrane and the ability of proximal epithelium to concentrate substrate, we must consider how the moment-to-moment in vivo steady state, compatible with net reabsorption, is kept far from the situation where J_4 equals J_3. To put it another way, the circumstance that tolerates net reabsorption is a local condition in a far-from-equilibrium open system.

Two possibilities exist to explain this situation: either the effective intracellular concentration of amino acid ($[A]_c$) is kept below the equilibrium concentration or Km_{eff} is higher than Km_{in}. At present, we have no data on the latter possibility; however, there are two mechanisms that could achieve the former. First, amino acids in the cytoplasmic pool are reduced by amino acid metabolism (degradation), and second, efflux at

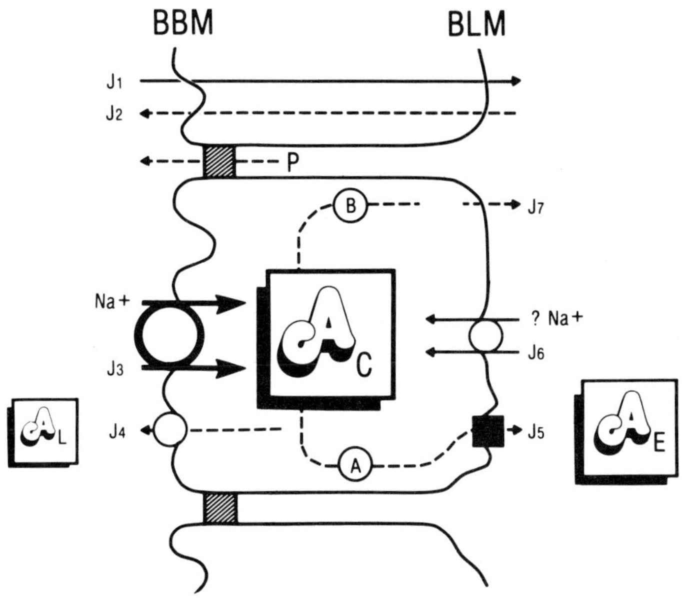

Figure 31.3. A scheme to describe transepithelial transport of amino acids applicable to nephron (and small intestine). *A*, amino acid; *BBM*, brush-border membrane; *BLM*, basal-lateral membrane; *Na^+*, sodium ion; *A_L*, luminal substrate; *A_C*, cellular substrate; *A_E*, extracellular (antiluminal) substrate (size of boxes indicates relative concentrations); *J*, flux; *J_1*, transcellular absorptive flux; *J_2*, transcellular outward flux; *J_3*, absorptive flux at BBM; *J_4*, backflux at BBM; *J_5*, outward flux at BLM; *J_6*, uptake flux at BLM; *J_7*, metabolic runout flux; *A*, permeability runout of A_c at steady-state; *P*→, diffusional flux from intercellular space to lumen via tight junction; ⇄ and ⇄, carrier mediated transport of A.

the basolateral membrane (J_5) exceeds influx (J_6) (Fig. 31.3). Mediation of the permeability mechanism for amino acids in the renal basolateral membrane differs from that in the brush-border membrane (17, 18), so that transepithelial fluxes in situ at the two membranes accommodate net reabsorption as required. From this reasoning one can anticipate that specific abnormalities of either brush-border or basolateral membrane permeability or of metabolism of AA or a combination of these can impair net reabsorption of amino acid (11) (Fig. 31.4).

Heterogeneity (Specificity) of the Transport Process

Mutations that alter the function of specific transport proteins identify these transport proteins. Homozygotes or genetic compounds with two mutant alleles at the same locus synthesise only abnormal gene product. The resulting hyperaminoaciduria reflects the altered carrier, channel, or reactive site in the membrane.

Carriers in human renal membranes that have been defined by mutation affect the following groups of AA (9): (1) the cationic group or dibasic AA—lysine, arginine and ornithine; (2) the cationic group plus cystine; (3) a large neutral group excluding glycine and the iminoacids—proline and hydroxyproline; (4) a neutral group comprising secondary AA—glycine, sarcosine, and the imino acids; (5) the anionic group—glutamate and aspartate; and (6) the β-amino group—taurine, β-alanine, and β-aminoisobutyrate. This classification (summarized in Fig. 31.5) was defined first by human geneticists; it has been largely confirmed by physiologists (7, 19). Physiological studies employ laboratory animals, using in vitro or in situ techniques impossible to apply to human subjects, for example, microperfusion, micropuncture, and perfusion of isolated nephron segment perfusions. Any discrepancy between the genetic and physiological classifications of sites probably reflects either methodological refinements or species differences.

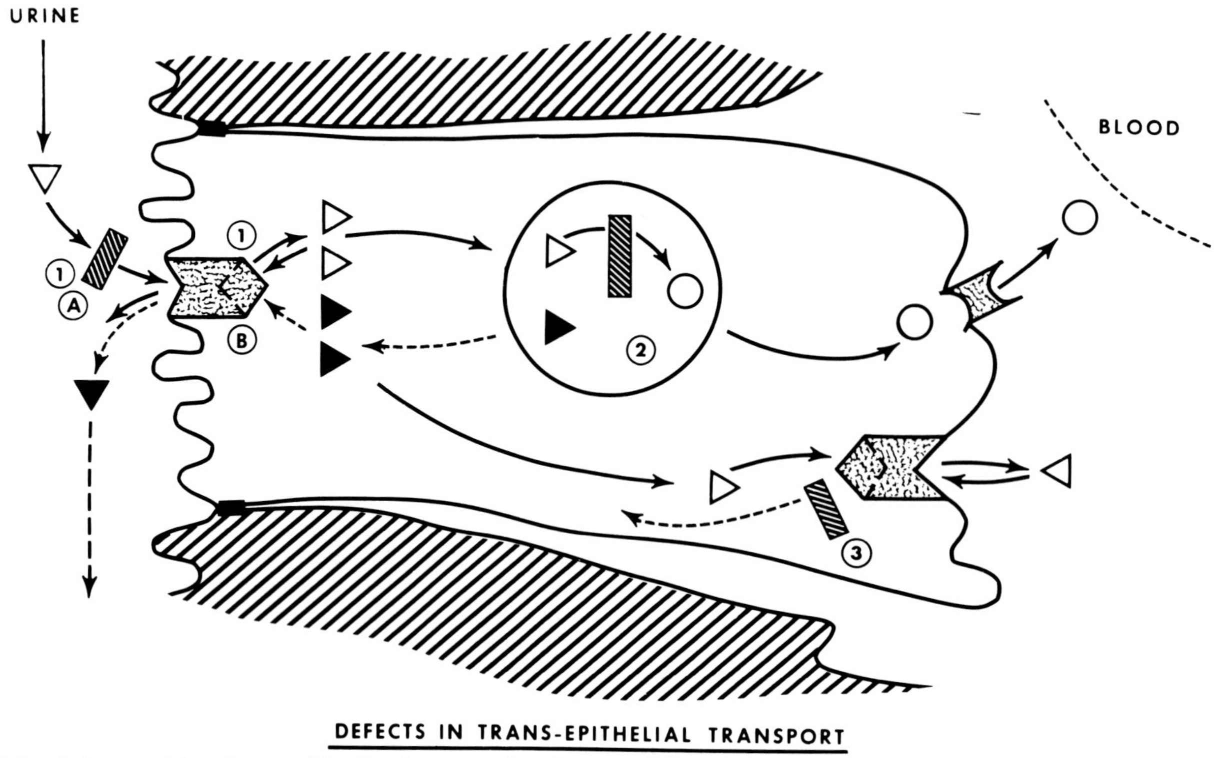

Figure 31.4. A diagram delineating possible sites for expression of mutant allele causing hereditary disorders of tubular reabsorption. Appropriate recognition of the vectorial flux in secretory transport allows the model to be adapted also to disorders of secretion. Defect 1A, mutant site (carrier) blocks entry; defect 1B, mutant carrier permits excessive exodus (backflux) from internal pool (Δ); defect 2, blocked catabolic mutant state prevents metabolic "runout" to alternate form (○) leading to accumulation of original solute in the internal pool (Δ) and exaggerated exodus (backflux) on normal carrier; and defect 3, defect in exodus at basolateral membrane leads to intracellular accumulation as in defect 2. All lead to reduction of net transepithelial flux. From Scriver CR, Chesney RW, McInnes RR: Kidney Intl 9:149, 1976.)

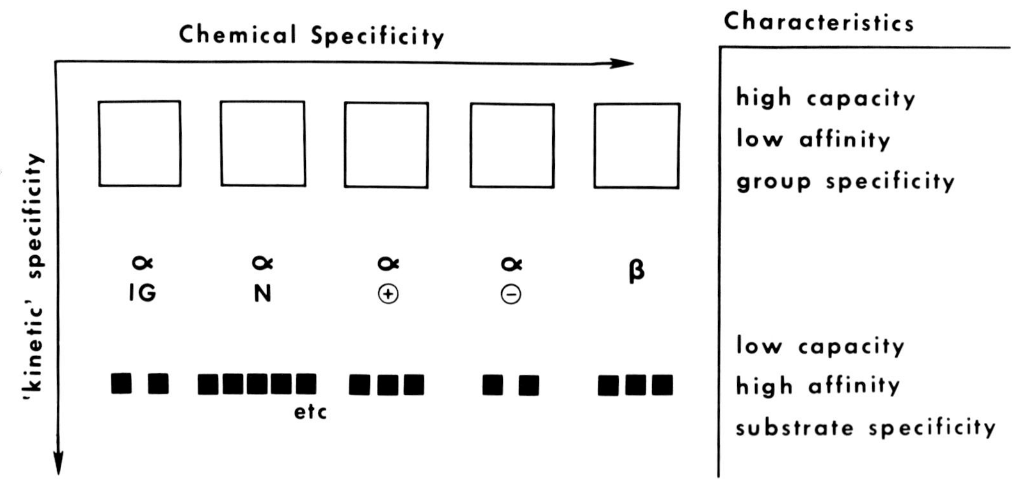

Figure 31.5. Apparent array of transport (recognition) sites in renal brush-border and basolateral (plasma) membranes for amino acid uptake. Sites have at least two types of specificity, one for the chemical nature of solute, another with respect to the concentration of substrate. Specificity is broad, capacity is great, and affinity for substrate is low when the substrates are at "high" concentration (i.e., above the usual plasma concentration range); sites for uptake at low substrate concentration have the opposite characteristics (From Scriver CR, Hechtman P: Adv Hum Gen 1:211, 1970, with permission.)

The group-specific sites are shared by several substrates and, in general, have higher maximal transport rates and lower affinities for member AA in the group. It is apparent that they are not the only available transport mediations operating in the nephron (7, 20). We know this because the homozygote with an inborn error of renal AA transport generally does not lose all reabsorptive function for the affected AA. Additional mechanisms serving transport of AA apparently exist. Thus we have evidence for specific sites serving cystine, histidine, glycine, tyrosine, and so on. Sites of this nature tend to have higher affinity and greater specificity while transporting substrate at lower maximal rates. This heterogeneity of function confers an adaptive advantage, since mutation in single-copy DNA would not ablate all renal transport activity for a particular amino acid.

Axial Heterogeneity of Amino Acid Transport in the Nephron

Whereas, the heterogeneous reactive sites just described are confined to the proximal nephron, their topological distribution in that portion is lagely unknown. However, there is evidence that sites for glycine, for example, observe axial heterogeneity (17). Glycine transport at brush-border membrane in S_1 and S_2 segments has high capacity and low affinity; transport also occurs in pars recta (S_3 segment), but the latter process has lower capacity and higher affinity. This evidence was obtained by perfusion experiments with isolated rat nephron segments. Failure to delineate more than one system with the brush-border membrane vesicle preparation may reflect only a failure to obtain a mixture of membranes from the appropriate segments of the nephron (21).

Axial differentiation of sites with different kinetic properties is a useful mechanism to "tune" the reabsorption process. While physiological and biochemical studies attempting to delineate this form of functional heterogeneity are sparse or often negative in their evidence, genetic and ontogenetic phenotypes still imply that kinetic (and topological) heterogeneity of amino acid transport mechanisms in proximal nephron does exist.

PATHOGENESIS OF ABNORMAL AMINOACIDURIA

In the preceding section, we described the normal process of AA transport in proximal nephron and thus the components of net reabsorption. A harmonious relationship between the demand placed on the process and the operation of its components determines the normal phenotype of aminoaciduria. Any deviation from the normal demand or any change (acquired or inherited) in the components and the way they function must alter the process (reabsorption). If the demand exceeds or the change impairs the capacity of the process, tolerance of the system will be exceeded and dishomeostasis will result, with consequences for phenotype. This consequence is recognized as hyperaminoaciduria.†† In this section we will describe pathogenesis of the hyperaminoacidurias and offer a systematic classification of deviant phenotypes.

General Model

The normal steady state of AA excretion reflects the balance between the filtered load of each AA and the ability to reabsorb each from filtrate; the latter reflects the balance of events occurring at brush-border and basolateral membranes (permeability) and in cell metabolism of the AA. The overall relationship represents a steady state in an open system operating at far-from-equilibrium (22).

To describe the vectorial process in simple terms, let the normal steady state be either

$$A_F \overset{K_1}{\rightleftharpoons} Ac_{BB} \overset{K_2}{\rightleftharpoons} Ac_{BL} \overset{K_3}{\rightleftharpoons} A_p \qquad (11)$$

or

$$A_F \overset{K_1}{\rightleftharpoons} Ac_{BB} \overset{K_2}{\rightharpoonup} Bc \overset{K_3}{\rightharpoonup} Bc_{BL} \overset{K_4}{\rightleftharpoons} B_p \qquad (12)$$

In equation 11, A_F is AA in filtrate, Ac_{BB} is AA inside the cell at the luminal (brush-border pole), Ac_{BL} is AA at the antiluminal (basolateral) pole, and A_p is AA in peritubular fluid or plasma; K_1 and so on are equilibrium constants for each step. In equation 12, Bc is the intracellular metabolic conversion product of Ac; Bc_{BL} and B_p are terms analogous to those in equation 11.

Since A_F is constantly added to the system and A_p or B_p are constantly removed, chemical equilibrium is never attained in vivo in this open system. When the rate of input of A_F equals the rate of removal of A_p (or B_p), a steady state exists, which is a local equilibrium condition in a far-from-equilibrium system. All of this is simply a shorthand description of the process of net reabsorption. It follows that the final concentration of A_F at the end of proximal nephron is the principal determinant of AA concentration in bladder urine. Thus, hyperaminoaciduria will occur if A_F exceeds the capacity for reabsorption by the system, for example

$$100\ A_F \vdots \dashrightarrow 10\ A_p \qquad (13)$$

Hyperaminoaciduria will also occur if operation of any single component in the system is impaired, for example

$$10A_F \rightarrow | \text{------}\ Ac_{BB} \dashrightarrow \qquad \text{(brush-border membrane defect)} \quad (14)$$

or

$$10A_F \rightleftharpoons 10Ac_{BB} \rightarrow | \text{—} Bc \dashrightarrow \qquad \text{(metabolic runout defect)} \quad (15)$$

or

$$10A^F \rightleftharpoons 10Ac_{BL} \rightarrow | \text{—} Ac_{BL} \dashrightarrow A_p$$

$$\text{(basolateral membrane defect)} \quad (16)$$

Since transport across the membrane (brush-border or basolateral) requires a carrier and its capacity is finite, saturation of the carrier leads to hyperaminoaciduria. Since carriers have selective preference for the AA, excess of one substrate may displace others they share. Finally, change in the carrier (affinity for its substrate or rate at which it can operate) can also impede transport (reabsorption), thus altering the steady state and causing hyperaminoaciduria.

With these relationships explained it is a simple matter to delineate the specific mechanisms of hyperaminoaciduria in clinical terms and to offer a logical classification (Table 31.2).

Specific Mechanisms of Hyperaminoaciduria

Four primary mechanisms explain all hyperaminoacidurias.

Saturation. AA appears at elevated concentration in filtrate and approaches far exceeds the capacity of the reabsorption process (equation 7). Excessive excretion of phenylalanine in phenylketonuria or branched-chain AA (leucine, isoleucine, and valine) in maple-syrup urine disease illustrate this mechanism. "Overflow" and "prerenal" are descriptive terms.

Competition and Saturation. One AA at an elevated concentration in filtrate displaces others present at normal concentration from a carrier shared by the set of substrates. Excessive excretion of glycine and hydroxyproline occurs in hyperprolinemia (Table 31.2), because all three substrates share a common carrier to which proline has preferential access. The hyperiminoglycinuria could thus be the result of competition for the carrier or a defect in the carrier itself (Table 31.2).

Modifications of Carrier or Net Flux. If the carrier is impaired in its capacity (rate of transport activity, equivalent to Tm) or in its ability to take on substrate (affinity for substrate, equivalent to "splay"), the net rate at which the vectorial process functions will be impaired even though the concentration of AA in filtrate is not elevated. This mechanism reflects a primary disorder of membrane transport (equations 14 and

†† Hypoaminoaciduria is not discussed, although it can occur as the consequence of a reduced filtered load, as in glomerular insufficiency. The phenotypes (either hypo or hyperaminoacidurias), while variant, are not necessarily disorders with medical significance (Table 31.2).

Table 31.2.
The Hyperaminoacidurias: Pathogenetic Classification[a]

GROUP 1A

The primary disorder is one of AA catabolism. The specific AA normally has low renal clearance. Hyperaminoaciduria occurs by saturation of the reabsorption process. Assignment to this group indicates that screening (and diagnosis) is performed preferentially by analysis of blood (plasma or serum).

Condition or disease	Amino acid affected	Enzyme affected (synonym) (Enzyme commission No.)	Inheritance	Remarks
		Common Perinatal (Adaptive) Traits[b]		
Neonatal hyperphenylalaninemia	Phenylalanine	Phenylalanine 4-monooxygenase (phenylalanine-hydroxylating system [1.14.16.1]	—	Benign; may respond to folic acid; often occurs with tyrosinemia
Neonatal tyrosinemia	Tyrosine	4-Hydroxyphenylpyruvate dioxygenase (ρ-hydroxyphenylpyruvic acid hydroxylase) [1.13.11.27]	—	Benign; responds to ascorbic acid and reduced protein intake
Hypermethioninemia	Methionine	Methionine adenosyltransferase (ATP:L-methionine S-adenosyltransferase [2.5.1.6]	—	Benign; usually found with high protein intake
Hyperhistidinemia	Histidine	L-Histidine ammonia-lyase [4.3.1.3]	—	Benign; related to high protein intake
		Inherited Traits		
Hyperphenylalaninemias				
Phenylketonuria and other hydroxylase variants, e.g.:	Phenylalanine	Phenylalanine 4-monooxygenase (L-phenylalanine, tetrahydrobiopterin:oxygen oxidoreductase [4-hydroxylating) [1.14.16.1]	AR	Plasma phenylalanine >1 mM causes mental retardation when untreated. L-phenylalanine tolerance in diet is 250–500 mg/day
Atypical phenylketonuria	Ibid	Same as above		Dietary tolerance for L-phenylketonuria is >500 mg/day
Transient phenylketonuria	Ibid	Same as above	(AR)	Change in status, several months or years after birth
Benign hyperphenylalaninemia	Ibid	Same as above	AR	Plasma phenylalanine <1 mM on normal diet; benign trait
Tetrahydrobiopterin deficient forms of hyperphenylalaninemia	Phenylalanine	Dihydropterin reductase [1.6.9.7] or deficient biosynthesis of tetrahydrobiopterin	AR	Requires specific diagnosis of tetrahydrobiopterin status
Hypertyrosinemias				
Tyrosinosis (Medes)	Tyrosine	? Tyrosine aminotransferase (L-tyrosine: α-ketoglutarate aminotransferase) [2.6.1.5]	AR	One case known; myasthenia gravis probably incidental finding
Hypertyrosinemia	Tyrosine	Soluble (cytosol) tyrosine aminotransferase [2.6.1.5]	AR	Associated with developmental retardation; Richner-Hanhart syndrome in some patients
Hereditary tyrosinemia	Tyrosine (and methionine in acute stage)	Fumarylacetoacetate hydrolase [3.7.1.2]	AR	Hepatic cirrhosis and renal tubular failure with Fanconi syndrome
Hyperhistidinemias[c]				
Classic form	Histidine (alanine elevated in some cases)	L-Histidine ammonia-lyase [4.3.1.3]; liver, epidermis	(AR)	Benign disorder
Variant form	Histidine	L-Histidine ammonia-lyase [4.3.1.3]; liver only	(AR)	Same as above
Hypertryptophanemia	Tryptophan	? Tryptophan pyrrolase	(AR)	Mental retardation; motor disorders; behavioural disorders; dermatitis
Branched-chain hyperaminoacidemia[d]				
Classic "maple-syrup urine disease	Leucine, isoleucine, valine, alloisoleucine	Branched-chain α-ketoacid lipoate oxidureductase (probably decarboxylase component) [1.2.4.3(4)]	AR	Postnatal collapse; mental retardation in survivors; diet therapy effective
Intermittent form	Leucine, isoleucine, valine, alloisoleucine	Branched-chain	(AR)	Intermittent symptoms; development may be otherwise normal

Table 31.2. *Continued*

Condition or disease	Amino acid affected	Enzyme affected (synonym) (Enzyme commission no.)	Inheritance	Remarks
Mild form	Same as above	Same as above	(AR)	Intermittent
Thiamin-response form	Same as above	Same as above	(AR)	Mild form; responsive to thiamin (vitamin B_1)
Multiple dehydrogenase form	Same as above (plus pyruvate and α-ketoglutarate)	Dihydrolipoyl dehydrogenase (E_3) [1.8.1.4]	(AR)	Congenital lactic acidosis plus branched-chain amino-keto acid disorder
Hypervalinemia	Valine	Branched-chain amino-acid aminotransferase (valine aminotransferase) [2.6.1.66]	AR	Retarded development and vomiting; responds to diet
Hyperleucinemia	Leucine, isoleucine	Branched-chain amino-acid amino-transferase (leucine/isoleucine aminotransferase) [2.6.1.42]	(AR)	Retarded development
Sulfur aminoacidemias				
Homocyst(e)inuria[c] (cystathionine β-synthase deficiency)	Methionine and homocyst(e)ine	Cystathionine β-synthase (L-serine hydroxylase [adding homocysteine]) [4.2.1.22]	AR	Usually associated with thromboembolic disease, mental retardation, and Marfan-like phenotype; pyridoxine responsive & unresponsive forms
Homocyst(e)inuria (methylene THF reductase deficiency)	Homocyst(e)ine (high), methionine (low); plus methylmalonate	Defective cobalamin coenzyme biosynthesis or deficiency of 5,10-methyltetrahydrofolate reductase [1.7.99.5]	AR	Defective remethylation of homocysteine and methylmalonyl-CoA mutase (MMA mutase) activity; neurologic signs and acidosis
Cystathioninuria[c]	Cystathionine	Cystathionine γ-lyase [4.4.1.1]	AR	Probably benign trait; vitamin B_6 corrects biochemical trait in most patients
Hyperglycinemias				
Ketotic form	Glycine and other gluconeogenic amino acids	Propionyl-CoA carboxylase (ATP-hydrolyzing) (propionyl-CoA:carbon-dioxide ligase [ADP-forming]) [6.4.1.3]	AR	Ketosis, neutropenia, mental retardation; often fatal; detectable in skin fibroblasts
Ibid.		Methylmalonyl-CoA mutase [5.4.99.2]	(AR)	Symptoms are those of methylmalonic aciduria with acidosis (some mutase affected patients are responsive to vitamin B_{12})
Ibid.		Acetyl-CoA acyltransferase (β-ketothiolase) [2.3.1.16] deficiency	(AR)	Symptoms are those of α-methyl-β-hydroxybutyric aciduria (with or without tiglic aciduria) and acidosis
Nonketotic form	Glycine	Glycine cleavage reaction (CO_2, NH_3, and hydroxymethyltetrahydrofolate formed) [1.4.4.2, 2.1.2.10]	AR	Severe CNS depression soon after birth; high CSF/plasma glycine ratio; benzoate decreases plasma glycine; no effect on CNS prognosis; strychnine improves seizures
Sarcosinemia[c]	Sarcosine	Sarcosine oxidase (sarcosine oxygen oxidoreductase [demethylating]) [1.5.3.1]	AR	Benign (probably)
"Sarcosinemia" (glutaric aciduria, type II)	Sarcosine (glutaric acid and multiple fatty acids)	Electron transfer flavoprotein (affecting multiple aryl-CoA dehydrogenases) [1.3.99.2–3]	AR	Postnatal lethargy, vomiting, coma, and acidosis; odor; multiple abnormalities of fatty acid oxidation
Hyperprolinemias				
Type I	Proline	L-Proline dehydrogenase (oxidase) [1.5.99.8]	AR	Benign trait
Type II	Proline	1-Pyrroline dehydrogenase (Δ'-pyrroline-5-carboxylate: NAD^+ oxidoreductase) [1.5.1.12]	AR	Benign trait; Δ'-pyrroline-5-carboxylate and 3-hydroxy-1-pyrroline-5-carboxylate excreted in urine; proline concentration >type I.

Table 31.2. *Continued*

Condition or disease	Amino acid affected	Enzyme affected (synonym) (Enzyme commission no.)	Inheritance	Remarks
Hydroxyprolinemia	Hydroxyproline	4-Hydroxy-L-proline dehydrogenase (oxidase) [1.1.1.104]	AR	Benign trait
Hyperlysinemias				
Type I	Lysine (and glutamine)	Saccharopine dehydrogenase (NADP$^+$, lysine-forming) [1.5.1.8]	AR	Associated with mental retardation and hypotonia
Saccharopinuria[c]	Lysine, saccharopine, citrulline	? Saccharopine dehydrogenase (NADP$^+$, L-glutamate-forming) (saccharopine dehydrogenase) [1.5.1.10]	AR	Associated with mental retardation
Hydroxylysinemia	Free hydroxylysine	? Hydroxylysine kinase [2.7.1.81]	(AR)	Mental retardation
α-Aminoadipic acidemia	α-Aminoadipic acid (and α-ketoadipic acid)	? "α-Ketoadipate dehydrogenase"	(AR)	Mental retardation
Pipecolic acidemia[c]	Pipecolic acid	L-Pipecolate dehydrogenase (pipecolate oxidase) [1.5.99.3]	AR	Hepatomegaly and mental retardation [Peroxisomal disease]
Hyperammonemias				
Carbamyl phosphate synthetase (CPS) deficiency	Glycine, glutamate	Carbamate kinase (ATP: carbamate phosphotransferase) [2.7.2.2]	AR	This group of diseases has ammonia intoxication, protein intolerance, hepatomegaly, vomiting, etc.; argininosuccinic aciduria also has trichorrhexis nodosa
Ornithine transcarbamylase (OTC) deficiency	Glutamine	Ornithine carbamoyltransferase (carbamoylphosphate: L-ornithine carbamoyltransferase) [2.1.3.3]	XL	
Citrullinemia	Citrulline	Argininosuccinate synthase (L-citrulline:L-aspartate ligase [AMP-forming]) [6.3.4.5]	AR	
Argininosuccinic-aciduria	Argininosuccinic acid	Argininosuccinate lyase (L-succinic arginine-lyase) [4.3.2.1]	AR	
Hyperargininemia	Arginine	Arginase (L-arginine amidinohydrolase) [3.5.3.1]	AR	
Hyperornithinemias	Ornithine	a. L-Ornithine; 2-oxoacid aminotransferase [2.6.1.13]	AR	a. Associated with gyrate atrophy of choroid and retina but no hyperammonemia
		b. Unknown (mitochondrial ornithine transport system ?)	AR	b. Associated with hyperammonemia and homocitrullinemia (HHH syndrome)
Hyperalaninemias	Alanine	Pyruvate dehydrogenase (lipoate) (pyruvate dehydrogenase) [1.2.4.1]; pyruvate carboxylase [6.4.1.1]; other enzymes	AR	Lactic acidosis, intermittent ataxia, mental retardation
Miscellaneous				
Aspartylglucosaminuria	Glycoasparagines	Aspartylglucosylaminase (2-acetaminido-1-[β^1-L-aspartamido]-1-2-dideoxyglucose amidohydrolase) [3.5.1.26]	AR	Lysosomal disease; mental retardation
"Glutathionemia"	Glutathione or related peptide	γ-Glutamyltransferase (γ-glutamyl-transpeptidase) [2.3.22]	(AR)	Mental retardation associated with finding
		Acquired conditions that may affect amino acids in plasma		
Protein-calorie malnutrition	Tryptophan, leucine, isoleucine, valine decreased; tyrosine, glycine, proline increased	—	—	Degree of dishomeostasis related to severity of malnutrition
Prolonged fasting	Decreased alanine; threonine and glycine increased	—	—	Early fasting does not cause same pattern

Table 31.2. *Continued*

Condition or disease	Amino acid affected	Enzyme affected (synonym) (Enzyme commission no.)	Inheritance	Remarks
Obesity	Leucine, isoleucine, valine, phenylalanine and tyrosine all increased; glycine decreased	—	—	Reflects insulin insensitivity
Hepatitis	Methionine, tyrosine both increased			Reflects severity of liver disease

GROUP 1B[a]

The primary defect is in catabolism. There is a high renal clearance of amino acid and hyperaminoaciduria occurs by saturation of transepithelial transport. Detection in the urine is preferable.

Condition or disease	Amino acid affected (synonym)	Enzyme affected (synonym) (Enzyme commission no.)	Inheritance	Remarks
Hypophosphatasia	Phosphoethanolamine	? Deficiency of ethanolamine-phosphate phospho-lyase (Q-phosphorylethanolamine phospho-lyase) [4.2.99.7]	AR	Defective bone mineralization unresponsive to Vitamin D; craniosynostosis; hypercalcemia
Pseudohypophosphatasia	Phosphoethanolamine	"Alkaline phosphatase" activity present but altered (Km mutant)	AR	Same as above
β-Aminoisobutyric-aciduria	β-Aminoisobutyric acid	?	AD/AR	Benign polymorphic trait
Hyper-β-alaninemia	β-Alanine	? β-Alanine-pyruvate aminotransferase (β-alanine transaminase) [2.6.2.18]	(AR)	Seizures; somnolence; mental retardation
Carnosinemia	Carnosine	Aminoacyl-histidine dipeptidase (carnosinase) [3.4.13.3]	AR	Seizure and mental retardation; or benign possibly
Pyroglutamic aciduria	L-pyroglutamic acid (5-oxo-L-proline; pyrrolidone-2-carboxylic acid)	Glutathione synthetase [6.3.2.3]	AR	L-pyroglutamic acid (5-oxo-L-proline) results from overproduction via modified γ-glutamyl cycle

[a] Urine screening is as efficient as, or even more reliable, than blood screening in these conditions.

GROUP 2

There is a primary defect in catabolism and a secondary defect in transport. Hyperaminoaciduria is of combined origin—saturation and competition. Detection is possible in both plasma and urine.

Disease	Amino acids		Remarks
	Affected in Plasma	Present in Urine	
Hyperprolinemia, types I and II	Proline	Proline, + hydroxyproline and glycine	See entries in Group IA; competition occurs on iminoglycine transport system (see Group III)
Hyper-β-alaninemia	β-Alanine	β-Alanine, + β-aminoisobutyric acid and taurine	See entry in Group IB; competition occurs on β-amino transport system
Hyperlysinemia	Arginine	Ornithine and lysine, and sometimes generalized hyperaminoaciduria	See entry in Group IA; competition occurs on "dibasic" transport system (see Group III); pathogenesis of generalized aminoaciduria unknown.

GROUP 3

The primary defect is in the renal transport process. There is a high renal clearance of amino acid, and detection is possible only in the urine. Hetz, heterozygote; homoz, homozygote.

Trait	Substance Affected	Activity Affected Common Perinatal (Adaptive) Trait	Remarks
Neonatal iminoglycinuria	Proline, hydroxyproline, glycine	Specific proline and specific glycine transport (probably)	Benign adaptive trait; prolinuria subsides at ≈100 days, glycinuria at ≈200 days after full term birth
Noonatal cystinuria	Cystine and dibasic amino acids (lysine, ornithine, and arginine)	Specific dibasic transport system	Transient; evident in newborn period in some but not all infants

Group 3 *Continued*

Table 31.2. *Continued*
Mendelian Disorders of Renal Transport of Amino Acids

Substrate and cellular membrane affected	Condition (and McKusick catalogue no.)	Inheritance	Other tissues affected
Amino acids (groups)			
Lysine, Ornithine, Arginine	Hyperdibasic-aminoaciduria(s)		
(at BBM in 12600)?	(12600)	AD[a]	Intestine and Liver (in 22270)
(at BLM in 22270)	(22270)	AR[a]	
Lysine, Ornithine, Arginine & Cystine (at BBM)	Cystinuria (22010)	AR[a] (>1 allele)	Intestine (Types I & II)
Neutral Amino Acids (excl. Gly, Pro, Hypro) (at BBM)	Hartnup (23450)	AR[a]	Intestine (in some types)
Proline (Hydroxyproline), Glycine, (Sarcosine) (?)	Iminoglycinuria (24260)	AR[a] (>1 allele)	Intestine (in some types)
Aspartate, Glutamate (?)	Dicarboxylicaminoaciduria (22293, 23165)	AR[a]	?
Amino acids (single)[b]			
Histidine	Hyperhistidinuria (23583)	AR	Intestine
Cystine (at BBM probably)	Hypercystinuria (23450)	AR	?
Lysine	Lysine malabsorption (24795)	(AR)	intestine

[a] *How to use the classification.* The classification is based on the physiological process by which renal filtration and renal reabsorption of amino acids influence urinary composition (aminoaciduria). The pathogenesis of hyperaminoaciduria primarily involves either a disorder in substrate catabolism with increased filtered load (Group 1, the "prerenal" aminoacidurias) or a disorder of transport with decreased net reabsorption (Group 3, the "renal" aminoacidurias). The primary mechanism, in general, determine which fluid (plasma or urine) is preferred for analysis to obtain a diagnosis; there is a further subdivision of catabolic defects (Groups I and II) into those involving either low renal clearance amino acids (Group 1A) or high renal clearance substrates (group 1B) plasma being preferred for the former, urine for the latter to obtain a diagnosis. Conditions characterized by "combined" aminoaciduria (prerenal and renal) are found in Group 2.

[b] These conditions have been detected by screening methods applied in the newborn period of life. They should not be misdiagnosed as permanent disorders of amino acid metabolism also identifiable by screening.

[c] Urine screening is as efficient as, or even more reliable than, blood screening in these conditions.

[d] A number of disorders of branched-chain amino acid catabolism cause accumulation of substances which are ninhydrin-negative. These compounds can usually be detected by gas-liquid chromatographic methods. (Goodman SI: Am J Hum Genet 32:781, 1980.)

[e] Inheritance pattern confirmed.

[f] Two other inborn errors of single amino acid transport are known: methionine malabsorption (25090); tryptophan malabsorption (Blue-diaper syndrome) (21100); neither involves kidney, both involve intestine.

16); it may occur at either the brush-border or basolateral membrane. Some so-called "renal" aminoacidurias reflect this mechanism.

Should the metabolic runout of an AA (equation 12) be a significant determinant of the steady state, impairment of substrate metabolism in the renal cell will also alter the steady state. Substrate concentration in the cell (Ac) will rise, the normal steady state at the brush-border membrane will change, back flux into filtrate will occur, and since the latter is moving down the nephron, substrate will be removed distally into bladder urine. A portion of the hyperprolinuria in hyperprolinemia is attributable to this mechanism, since renal oxidation of proline is a significant determinant of its net reabsorption (23, 24).

The rate at which the carrier operates is apparently determined by its coupling to cellular energy metabolism. Since coupling is common to all carriers, the predictable effect of disrupted energy metabolism is a generalized impairment of permeability. This is the domain of the Fanconi syndrome (chapter 30).

General Classification of Hyperaminoacidurias

The hyperaminoacidurias are classified according to the primary mechanism (pathogenesis) that alters phenotype (Table 31.2). Groups 1A and 1B in the classification recognize the "saturation" mechanism. The subdivisions are offered to give clinical guidance. Group 1A includes AA with low renal clearance; these disorders are best recognized (screened) by measurement of plasma (prerenal) concentration of the affected AA. Group 1B includes AA with high renal clearance; these disorders are best detected by measurement (screening) of urine amino acid content. Group II contains hyperaminoacidurias explained by the "combined" mechanism (saturation + competition). Group III is concerned with "renal" aminoaciduria—the primary inborn errors of AA transport. They are discussed further in the next section and classified in more detail in Table 31.2.

The classification in Table 31.2 delineates the specific component of the hyperaminoaciduria or hyperaminoacidemia, the mutant gene product (in the Mendelian disorders), and the major associated disease (clinical phenotype). When the aminoaciduria phenotype is the result of immature development (ontogeny) rather than mutation, the "disorder" is designated as an adaptive trait.

CLASSIFICATION OF INBORN ERRORS OF AMINO ACID TRANSPORT IN HUMANS

The purpose of classifying inborn errors of AA transport (IET) (Table 31.2, Group III) is to satisfy categorical needs and to illustrate the obvious: that mutation is a powerful probe of renal membrane functions. Classification has practical value in diagnosis, prognosis, treatment, and prediction of recurrence in relatives of the proband. Our classification implies the following:

1. Mutation can be expressed in one tissue, such as the kidney, and not in another, such as, intestine or erythrocyte, even though the AA is transported in each. This implies that the carrier protein in each tissue is controlled by different gene loci. Such diversity is the basis of adaptive homeostasis and reflects the process of natural selection.

2. Mutation can be expressed in one membrane brush-border or basolateral and not in the other, which affirms the difference between brush-border and basolateral function, as well as morphology.

3. The derangements of renal transport are Mendelian. Therefore, specific gene loci are associated with each IET, which will eventually be mapped to specific chromosomes and bands in the human chromosome map. The message that flows from the segregation analysis of Mendelian disorders of renal transport of AA is that they observe a separatist hierarchy; any federalism in their transport lies not in the domains of their carriers as in their coupling to Na^+ transport through the process of secondary active transport (25).

4. Mutations inherited as homozygous (recessive), compound (codominant), or dominant (autosomal or X-linked) phenotypes do not necessarily ablate all transport activity for the specific substrate controlled by the normal allele. One explanation for "residual" activity is a mutation causing a qualitative change in the gene product that retains some quantity of normal activity. Another postulates a mutation that impairs quantitative translation of the gene and yields a diminished amount of cellular gene product. Yet another, and it is apparently the more usual explanation, is the presence of more than one type of carrier accessible to the substrate; mutation at one locus affects only one carrier leaving the other with normal functional integrity. The latter phenomenon is relevant to the larger view of adaptive homeostasis. A function as vital to the organism as membrane transport of essential L-amino acids is well served if there is diversity of carriers.

THE INBORN ERRORS OF AMINO ACID TRANSPORT AS EXPERIMENTS OF NATURE

The specific systems that constitute the normal process are open systems and they experience a continuous flux of AA through their compartments. Any change (mutation) in the genetic instructions of the components will modify the output of the process; accordingly, phenotype changes. The change can be measured either as an altered rate in transport of specific AA or as deviation from the optimal steady state defined by the AA concentration in urine or plasma. Thus, these disorders generate phenotypes characterized by specific hyperaminoacidurias, which in some, cause the plasma concentration of amino acids also to be deviant. When the changes are disadaptive, disease occurs; otherwise, the finding is part of normal variation. Some of the entries from Table 31.2 illustrate this.

Cystinuria

In his lectures on the inborn errors of metabolism (26), Garrod considered cystinuria to be a disorder of AA catabolism; only later was it appreciated that the functional target of mutation in this phenotype was not catabolism but transport. Dent and colleagues (27, 28) proposed that cystinuria is an inborn error of transport to explain the mutant phenotype that involved not one but four AA (cystine plus lysine, ornithine, and arginine).

Cystinuria is the homozygous phenotype that is inherited as an autosomal recessive (29). There are at least two mutant alleles at the relevant locus in man. These alleles are variably expressed in kidney and intestine. The phenotype is significant because of the low solubility of L-cystine in urine. Because urinary cystine levels in these patients usually exceeds the solubility limit, calculi form.

Lysine is an essential AA and its impaired intestinal absorption might affect nutrition in cystinuria patients, but this does not appear to be the case.

Because cystinuria is the classical prototype for an hereditary renal aminoaciduria, it has fascinated investigators. The principal question posed during the past quarter century was which AA transport system of intestinal and renal epithelium is involved in cystinuria? The initial answer was direct and simple (27, 28): it was a "carrier" in the nephron selective for the four AA. Trouble came when the putative carrier (for cystine and dibasic AA) could not be demonstrated in the renal cortex slice preparation in mammalian kidney (30, 31). This was a puzzling finding since there was convincing evidence for a carrier, both in vivo and in situ, that transported the four AA back from filtrate in man (28, 32). Even more frustrating was the evidence that cystine uptake was normal in renal cortex slices obtained at nephrectomy from patients with cystinuria (33).

The resolution of this paradox came when it was realized that transport of the amino acid tetrad at brush-border and basolateral membranes is achieved by independent carriers in the two membranes. The slice preparation exposes the basolateral membrane (34), whereas cystinuria is a disorder of brush-border membrane (29) in the intestine (35) and apparently in the kidney.

Transport of these four AA is served by different carriers at brush-border and basolateral membranes of kidney and intestine (36, 37). Transport at the basolateral membrane employs one for the dibasic amino acids, another for cyst(e)ine; at the brush-border membrane, transport is affected by multiple carriers, among which is one shared by all four AA (29, 37), another for dibasic amino acids only, and a third system for cystine only. Cystinuria is a specific disorder of brush-border membrane transport of both kidney and intestine. Direct evidence to support this hypothesis has been obtained from intestinal biopsy material (35) and these findings are presumably applicable to the kidney also. Because plasma membranes of parenchymal cells are more analogous to the basolateral membrane, it is not surprising that transport appears to be normal in leukocytes and fibroblasts of cystinuria patients (29).

The unfolding of knowledge about cystinuria has occupied almost 2 centuries. It began in 1812 with Woolaston's discovery of cystine in bladder calculi; it advanced significantly with Garrod's proof of Mendelian inheritance in cystinuria; it has now settled into a somewhat comfortable framework of cellular biology. In the meantime, we have learned something more about dibasic AA transport from another Mendelian disorder called lysinuria-protein intolerance.

Lysinuria-Protein Intolerance (Hyperdibasic Aminoaciduria, Type II)

Lysinuria-protein intolerance (LPI) is an autosomal "ethnic" disease. It is most prevalent among Finns (38) and rare in other populations. The homozygous phenotype is disadaptive conferring failure to thrive and intolerance to a protein-rich diet. Hyperammonemia with low blood urea reflects a disorder of the urea cycle.

Intestinal biopsy material from patients with LPI indicates that dibasic AA transport is deficient only at the basolateral membrane (39). Studies of renal reabsorption in vivo (40), noting the obligatory conversion of citrulline to arginine in renal tubular cells, indicate a basolateral membrane defect in kidney. This lesion causes hyperammonemia, because ornithine levels are low. Dietary supplementation with L-citrulline (41) enhances tolerance for dietary protein. This finding suggests that the transport defect is present also in hepatocytes, making them "auxotrophic" for ornithine and arginine in the mutant phenotype. Citrulline is beneficial because it is a metabolic precursor of arginine and ornithine; it can readily enter the hepatocyte on the neutral AA carrier(s) restoring homeostasis of ammonia disposal and urea synthesis. LPI illustrates a practical rationale for seeking the identity and topology of membrane transport systems; it also has a logic satisfying to the embryologist who perceives the developmental homology of basal-lateral membranes in nephron and intestine and the plasma membrane of hepatocytes.

Dibasic Aminoaciduria Type 1

Dibasic aminoaciduria type 1 is different from the LPI phenotype. It has no protein intolerance and its geographic/ethnic distribution is different. Obligate heterozygotes have modest dibasic aminoaciduria in contrast to LPI heterozygotes who have no findings (42, 43).

One can speculate that dibasic aminoaciduria type I is a disorder of brush-border membrane transport with deficient activity of the dibasic AA carrier that excludes cystine. The equally prominent dibasic aminoaciduria in cystinuria and in type I dibasic aminoaciduria, each representing loss of only one type of brush-border membrane carrier, implies that both carriers have nearly equivalent roles to play in renal reabsorption of their substrates. How can one explain hyperaminoaciduria in the heterozygote with type-I dibasic aminoaciduria, and hyperaminoaciduria in the incompletely recessive cystinuria heterozygote, if each is deficient in only one quarter of the total number of available carriers? Clearly, there is more to be learned about transport of dibasic amino acids in the nephron.

Hartnup Disorder

Hartnup disorder is a variant of hyperaminoaciduria in which transport in the kidney and intestine of a large group of neutral α-amino acids is involved. Dibasic AA, anionic AA (glutamate and aspartate), the imino acids (proline and hydroxyproline) glycine, and the β-amino acids (taurine, β-alanine, and β-AIB) are not involved. The phenotype is inherited as an autosomal recessive and is expressed in homozygotes, but not in heterozygotes under endogenous conditions, implying that half the normal membrane transport activity is adequate for normal homeostasis (44, 45).

Three features of the condition are of special clinical interst. First, the original patients (46) were discovered during investigation of a pellagra-like condition; but symptomatic (disadaptive) Hartnup disorder is the exception rather than the rule. Disadaptation in Hartnup disorder is not fully understood. It may reflect a relationship that involves six essential AA—tryptophan, phenylalanine, valine, leucine, isoleucine, and threonine—in relation to their intestinal absorption and renal conservation. Nicotinamide homeostasis is impaired (45). Marginal nicotinamide intake, which in normal subjects is compensated by dietary tryptophan, is compromised in these patients, because of tryptophan depletion. Interindividual variation measured by this difference in plasma AA and nicotinamide in the population with Hartnup disorder have not been correlated with symptomatology. We would anticipate that the occasional symptomatic patients are outliers in the distribution of essential AA and nicotinamide levels in plasma of all the patients with Hartnup's disorder which develops under marginal dietary conditions. We speculate to illustrate how an inborn error of transport might compromise health only when an external stress develops.

Second, we should ask why plasma levels of the six essential AA are not always low in the Hartnup phenotype. Evidence for supplementary cell mechanisms that prevent severe decompensation of nutrition and metabolic homeostasis in the homozygote is of interest because it provides evidence of adaptive flexibility. Other processes, not controlled by the Hartnup gene, sustain transport of the "Hartnup" AA. These cell processes include oligopeptide carriers and intracellular peptidases (47) and specific carriers for single AA (identified in some cases, surmised in others (2)) (Fig. 31.5). Accordingly, loss of the shared "Hartnup" carrier does not ablate all transport activity for the neutral AA. Nonetheless, existence of the Hartnup phenotype implies that its particular group-specific, neutral AA preferring carrier is an important determinant of the normal phenotype. As a corollary, we can anticipate mutant phenotypes that are inborn errors of AA transport, which involve only single AA in the Hartnup mosaic. Three such disorders have been identified: methionine malabsorption (48); tryptophan malabsorption (blue diaper syndrome) (49); and the renal and intestinal transport of histidine (50). It is unclear how disadaptive these phenotypes are, although each came to attention through patients with rare disease.

The third feature concerns topology of the Hartnup gene product. Which membrane—brush-border or basolateral—is involved in the Hartnup disorder? While the evidence is oblique, it implicates the brush-border membrane of intestine and presumably of proximal nephron as well (2, 45). The data came from studies of the plasma AA response to ingestion of a dipeptide or one of its constituent free AA (51). The plasma response is normal in individuals with Hartnup disorder following dietary challenge with dipeptide, and it is attenuated only following a challenge with the constituent free AA. This observation implies that transport of dipeptide at the brush border can deliver the AA, after intracellular hydrolysis, at a normal rate to plasma because flux at the basolateral membrane is not impaired by the mutation. The free AA from dipeptide gains access to the basolateral membrane carrier only after entering the cell on the dipeptide-preferring brush-border membrane carrier and following intracellular hydrolysis. Since appearance in plasma is attenuated, after challenge with free AA, it follows that entry of free AA at the brush-border membrane is deficient. Therefore, the Hartnup gene product is apparently located in the brush-border membrane. Hartnup disorder is of historical significance because it was among the first of the inborn errors of transport to be interpreted from this viewpoint.

ONTOGENY AND ADAPTATION

Homeostatic systems are hierarchical. They have controlled and controlling components and limbs. They adjust the disturbing signals and restore the controlled components toward the normal central tendency, provided the displacement does not overwhelm the capacity to restore homeostasis. The capacity for adjustment is the process of health; displacement that overwhelms it with biological consequence constitutes disease. Renal adaptation during the transition from intrauterine to extrauterine life (perinatal ontogeny) is the response to a disturbing signal; so is renal adaptation to nutrient (AA) deprivation. Accordingly, both processes are homeostatic in response to change that is disturbing. In this section we describe examples of renal response to disturbing signals.

Postnatal Ontogeny Affecting Aminoaciduria

Renal clearance of AA is higher in the postnatal period than in later life (Table 31.1 and Fig. 31.6), and the pattern of aminoaciduria is correspondingly different in infants and mature subjects (52–54). This phenomenon is particularly evident with the iminoglycine group (proline, hydroxyproline, and glycine) of neutral AA and with the dibasic-cystine group (lysine, ornithine, arginine, and cystine). To recognize ontogeny has clinical relevance; misclassification of the normal postnatal phenotype as hyperaminoaciduria is avoided, and one need not consider neonatal iminoglycinuria, for example, as an indication of hyperprolinemia with combined hyperaminoaciduria (Table 31.2) or of renal iminoglycinuria (Table 31.2).

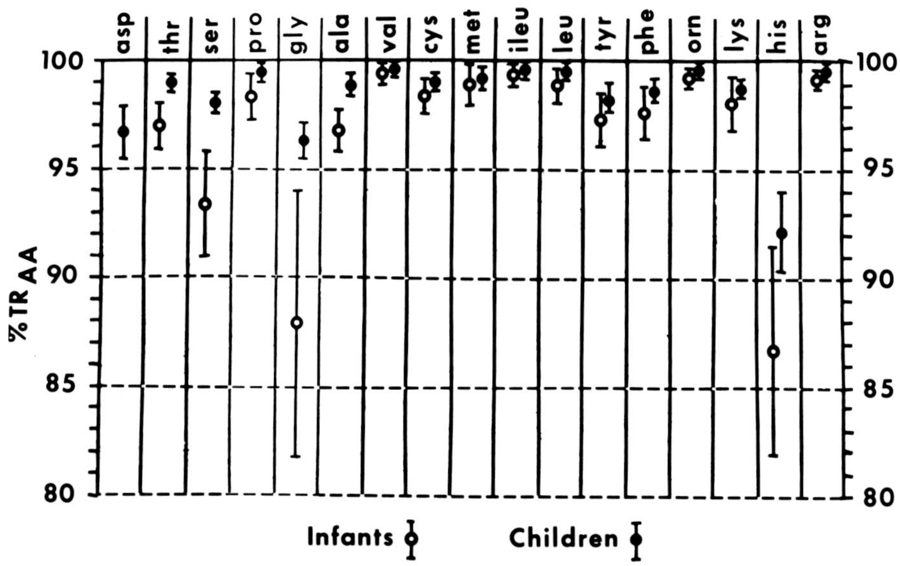

Figure 31.6. Tubular reabsorption of amino acids (expressed as percent of filtered load) in the infant with immature tubular function (○) compared with the child (●) with mature function. Ontogeny involves decreased net reabsorption; certain amino acids, particularly short-chain neutral aliphatics (Fig. 31.1), proline, and histidine, are more influenced by ontogeny than others (Adapted from Brodehl J, Gellissen K: Pediatrics 42:395, 1968.)

In the case of neonatal "cystinuria," we and others have noted that asymptomatic heterozygotes for the cystinuria mutation(s) have prominent selective hyperaminoaciduria involving the cystine-dibasic AA group in the first month or two after birth. Since heterozygotes have only half the population of transport sites controlled by the normal gene, the specific neonatal hyperaminoaciduria apparently reflects a relative overload (saturation) at a filtered load normal for age; in other words—a renal mechanism of hyperaminoaciduria. Since mature heterozygotes do not have the degree of hyperaminoaciduria evident in the infant heterozygote, ontogeny must affect either the remainder of the sites controlled by the normal allele or sites sharing the load that are controlled by other loci (e.g., the dibasic AA selective system and the cystine-selective system) (Table 31.2) or both together. The practical point at issue is this: newborn "cystinuria" should be monitored through the period of ontogeny before concluding that the phenotype is homozygous (or compound). Heterozygotes for cystinuria are approximately 200 times more frequent than homozygotes in the population and "neonatal cystinuria" is far more likely to be the phenotype for one or other form of heterozygous cystinuria modified by ontogeny.

The mechanism of human neonatal iminoglycinuria has been clarified by comparing iminoglycinuria of the normal newborn with that found in infants, at comparable age, who are homozygous for the inborn error of AA transport, renal iminoglycinuria (55). The mutant homozygous newborn has normal concentrations of proline and glycine in plasma, normal maturation of glomerular filtration, and greatly elevated renal clearance of proline, hydroxyproline, and glycine. Fractional excretion of iminoacids and glycine in these infants is far in excess of that expected for the normal infant and on occasion it approachs 100% of the filtered load. A schedule of postnatal maturation is observed in homozygotes that parallels that of normal infants; proline reabsorption matures before glycine reabsorption. These findings suggest an explanation for renal ontogeny of iminoglycine transport. There are three (or more) membrane gene products (carriers) serving tubular reabsorption of iminoacids and glycine in human kidney (Fig. 31.7). One system, affected by the renal iminoglycinuria mutation, is responsible for a transport activity shared by iminoacids, glycine, and other secondary amino acids; the second, with preference for proline and not affected by the mutation, has an early schedule of postnatal maturation; the third, with preference for glycine and also not affected by the mutation, has a late schedule of maturation. This interpretation is supported by two independent sets of evidence. First, human renal cortical brush-border membrane have two carriers for proline uptake (56). Second, mammalian nephron has two sites for glycine reabsorption, one in the proximal convolution, the other in pars recta (17).

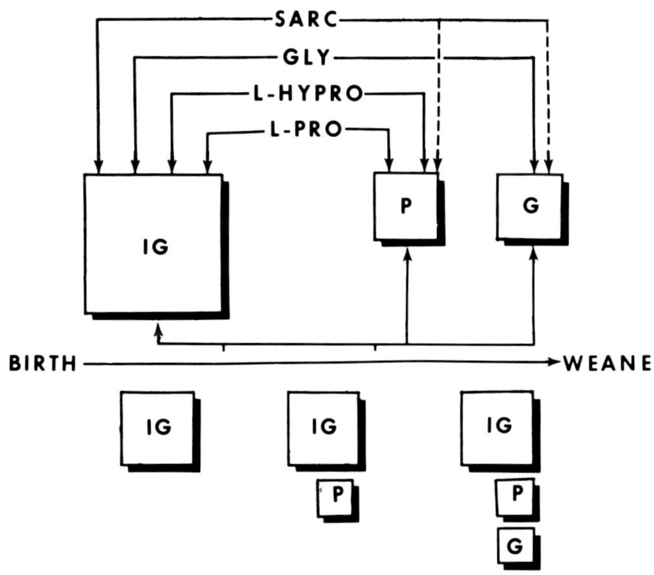

Figure 31.7. Scheme depicting array of transport sites selective for the secondary amino acids (L-proline, L-hydroxyproline, and sarcosine) and glycine. Sarcosine interacts with the shared high-capacity, low-affinity carrier (*IG*) and also with the low capacity, high affinity. More selective carriers (*P* for proline preferring and *G* for glycine preferring). Ontogeny influences activity of the carriers (lower half); the IG system operates alone at birth; the proline system appears before the glycine system during postnatal ontogeny. This schedule of sites and of ontogeny explains the process of neonatal iminoglycinuria in normal subjects and in mutant homozygotes with renal iminoglycinuria.

Additional conclusions can be drawn from the evidence. Ontogeny of iminoglycine transport appears to involve two mechanisms. First, there is enhancement of specific activity of sites in proximal nephron; second, enhancement of total available activity. The first implies appearance of carriers to increase specific activity in the membrane; the second, implies multiplication of carriers to increase total activity. Yet other studies indicate adaptation at the basolateral membrane as well (14). Indeed, a mosaic of events is implicated during development of mature function, encompassing proliferation of brush border and basolateral membranes, heterogeneity of sequential activities, changes in permeability, and oscillations of intracellular metabolism. Each of these events contributes to the schedule of ontogeny. The signals for postnatal adaptation of transport activity in proximal nephron have not been identified nor has the cellular mechanism whereby specific activity of transport sites is altered. One expects adaptation to the challenge of extrauterine life to be complex, and indeed it is in the nephron.

Adaptive Response to Disturbing (Metabolic) Signals in Kidney

Endowment of the nephron with substrate-specific AA transport systems that operate with high affinity and low capacity and shared systems with lower affinity and higher capacity for constituent amino acids has adaptive advantages. The former capture AA in conditions of "famine;" the latter still operate efficiently when "feasted" (2, 58). But what would happen to renal excretion of a particular AA under conditions of deprivation or abundance if there were only one carrier in the luminal membrane?

Taurine (2-aminoethane sulfonic acid) is an AA for which there appears to be only one carrier in renal brush-border membrane (59). This β-amino compound is prominent in human body fluids (plasma, urine, milk, and bile) and tissues (myocardium, skeletal muscle, platelet, retina, and brain) (60). It has been implicated as a modulator of intracellular calcium activity and ion fluxes. Renal transport of taurine is achieved by a β-amino acid preferring system. Human infants are relatively deficient in taurine and respond to dietary deprivation of the substance by conservation of filtered taurine so that fractional excretion is drastically reduced (61). This finding suggests that taurine is a conserved (quasiessential) metabolite in humans and that kidney is an important arbiter of taurine homeostasis. As yet there are no studies in humans to confirm that renal adaptation in response to taurine deprivation actually occurs or that there is a renal mechanism responsive to signals that perturb taurine homeostasis; but there are studies in the mouse that indicate an adaptive renal system.

Mouse kidney responds to taurine deprivation or supplementation (62). Fractional renal excretion decreases or increases respectively, beyond the normal range in response to changes in taurine homeostasis. The response to deprivation is not directed solely at taurine transport; brush-border membranes show enhanced transport of both taurine and alanine (the only other AA measured so far). Maximal adaptation occurs with selective taurine deprivation; but the essential amino acid phenylalanine can also act as a signal for a modest adaptive response in taurine transport. Change in brush-border membrane transport of taurine correlates best with change in plasma taurine suggesting that taurine homeostasis itself is, in some manner, the initial signal for adaptation. How the signal is translated and by what mechanism the membrane transporter responds is still unknown. The purpose in mentioning these intriguing findings is to enlarge the picture of AA reabsorption and to encourage our readers to consider the phenomenon of renal adaptation when interpreting variation in amino aciduria.

Acknowledgment

We are grateful to our colleagues for their contributions to this chapter through their work and discussion. Lynne Prevost typed the manuscript. Our work was supported in part by grants from the Medical Research Council of Canada, the Kidney Foundation of Canada, and the Quebec Network of Genetic Medicine.

APPENDIX
Clinical Phenotypes of the Mendelian Renal Hyperamino Aciduria

This section provides resumés of the major diagnostic criteria, the clinical phenotype and complications, the presumed etiology, the apparent pathogenesis, and other facts pertaining to the Mendelian disorders of renal amino acid transport of greatest clinical interest. The Fanconi syndrome is discussed in Chapter 30. The disorders are described in alphabetical order by their usual designations: (1) cystinuria; (2) dicarboxylic amino aciduria; (3) Hartnup disorder; (4) hypercystinuria; (5) hyperdibasic aminoaciduria(s); (6) hyperhistidinuria; and (7) iminoglycinuria. (The material is adapted from relevant sections written by the authors for the Birth Defects Compendium.)

CYSTINURIA: (Cystine-lysine-arginine-ornithinuria (29); Excludes: Cystinosis; lysine-protein intolerance (LPI) (hyperdibasic-aminoaciduria type II); hyperdibasic-aminoaciduria type I; hypercystinuria.

Major diagnostic criteria: Urinary cyanide-nitroprusside test produces magenta red color; specific cystine-lysine-arginine-ornithinuria identifiable by paper chromatography, paper electrophoresis, or column chromatography; normal or slightly decreased plasma concentrations of cystine and dibasic amino acids.

Major clinical findings: Formation of radiopaque cystine calculi in renal pelvis, ureter, or bladder and cystine crystalluria occur when cystine content of urine exceeds 250 mg/L at neutral pH. Renal clearance and excretion of cystine, lysine, arginine, and ornithine are markedly increased. Defective intestinal absorption of cystine, lysine, arginine, and ornithine also occurs in some (allelic?) forms of cystinuria (type I, II). Distribution of height values is said to be toward the low side of normal.

Complications: Renal or ureteral colic, hematuria, dysuria, and urinary tract infection are secondary to cystine stone formation; renal insufficiency and uremia secondary to infection and chronic obstruction of ureteral tract. Incidence of mental retardation or psychiatric disturbance is possibly increased in homozygotes (and genetic compounds).

Etiology: Autosomal recessive transmission with genetic heterogeneity. There are at least 3 mutant alleles (types I, II, III) with homozygous or "compound" expression (McKusick catalogue entry 22010).

Pathogenesis: The mutation(s) affect(s) the carrier protein in brush-border membrane serving shared transport of cystine, lysine, arginine, and ornithine in proximal renal tubule. Defective renal tubular reabsorption of cystine produces excessive urinary excretion and crystalluria; lithiasis is due to limited solubility of cystine in urine (maximum solubility about 300 mEq/L) in urine. The renal phenotype is similar in homozygotes/compounds for any combination of alleles. Dibasic aminoaciduria component has no known clinical significance. Impaired intestinal absorption of lysine (an essential amino acid) in phenotypes with intestinal transport defect (types I and II) may explain the moderate shortness of stature.

Genetics sex ratio: M1:F1, prevalence, about 1 in 10,000 live births. Risk of recurrence for patient's siblings: 1 in 4 (25%) for each; for patient's child: 1 in 100. Phenotype detectable at birth.

Detection of heterozygote: Type I heterozygotes have normal aminoaciduria but intestinal absorption of cystine and dibasic amino acids is impaired. This allele occurs in $\frac{1}{2}$ to $\frac{2}{3}$ of cystinuria heterozygotes. Type II and type III heterozygotes excrete increased amounts of cystine and dibasic amino acids in urine.

Treatment: Primary prevention: genetic counseling. Secondary prevention: high fluid intake, alkalinization of the urine to increase cystine solubility; oral administration of D-penicillamine (1–2 gm/24 hr in divided doses) if necessary to dissolve calculi. Surgical removal of renal, ureteral, or vesical calculi may be necessary. There is no evidence that the different genotypes responsible for cystinuria lead to clinically different syndromes. Cystine calculi may be formed occasionally by type II or type III heterozygotes, suggesting that such individuals should also be encouraged to maintain high free water clearance. Patients with cystinuria may form stones of mixed composition and even noncystine stones; any patient with renal tract calculi should have a nitroprusside test to exclude this disorder. D-penicillamine is effective in prevention and dissolution of stones but also produces a variety of deleterious effects including serum sickness, leukopenia, thrombocytopenia, and a reversible nephrotic syndrome.

Prognosis: In the absence of symptomatic treatment, in patients with calculi, life span apparently shortened by more than 10 years in affected males and by less than 10 years in affected females; death a result of renal failure.

DICARBOXYLIC AMINOACIDURIA (Glutamic-aspartic aciduria) (63, 64); Excludes: Dicarboxylic aciduria

Major diagnostic criteria: Selectively increased fractional excretion of L-glutamate and L-aspartate in urine (dicarboxylicmonoamino aciduria); identifiable by partition chromatography, electrophoresis, or elution chromatography on ion exchange resin columns. The corresponding plasma concentrations are normal or slightly depressed. Endogenous renal clearances of both dicarboxylic amino acids can exceed endogenous creatinine clearance.

Clinical findings: Probably a benign condition (Melancon, S. pers. comm. 1982). Fasting hypoglycemia, increased serum ketone bodies, and low plasma bicarbonate without a defect in ammoniagenesis, and modest hyperprolinemia were observed in only one of the known patients. Significance lies with evidence for a transport process selective for the anionic dicarboxylic amino acids.

Etiology: Presumed to be homozygous phenotype with autosomal recessive transmission involving either a defect in selective membrane transport of dicarboxylicmonoamino acids, or in their intracellular metabolic runout (McKusick catalogue entries 22273, 23165).

Pathogenesis: Simple defect in uptake at brush-border membrane will not explain why C_{glu} and C_{asp} are greater than C_{Cr}. Impaired intracellular conversion of L-amino acids to keto acids (metabolic runout) with intracellular accumulation and backflux as a possible alternative. Intestinal uptake defect also suspected; pathogenesis (and etiology) of intestinal defect presumably similar to renal defect.

Related facts: Sex ratio: presumably 1:1. Incidence: 1:50,000 births (Melancon, S. Pers. Comm., 1982). Risk of recurrence for patient's siblings: presumed 1 in 4 (25%) for each; for patient's child: not increased unless mate is carrier or homozygote. Phenotype detectable in newborn period. Heterozygotes have normal urine and plasma amino acid concentrations and normal renal clearance of glutamate and aspartate.

Treatment: Frequent feeding of L-glutamate prevented hypoglycemia in the single symptomatic proband (63). Most subjects do not need treatment.

Prognosis: Apparently benign condition.

HARTNUP DISORDER Selective neutral amino aciduria (45, 46). Excludes: Pellagra and hypertryptophanemia.

Major diagnostic criteria: Probands are usually asymptomatic; some have episodic behavioural disturbances and about 10% may experience attenuated development (neuromotor and somatic) in infancy. The specific hyper-(alpha)-aminoaciduria, involves neutral aliphatic and ring-structured amino acids. Excluded are dicarboxylic and dibasic amino acids, the imino acids and glycine, and β-amino acids. The same group of neutral amino acids is also found in excess in the feces of most patients; a variant of the disorder without the intestinal defect (presumably a different allele), has been reported.

Clinical findings: The phenotype is usually asymptomatic. It is frequently discovered by urine screening of healthy newborns; occasionally, in patients with intermittent psychiatric disorder, or mild delay in mental development. Photosensitivity of the exposed skin may occur after sufficient UV exposure. Behavioral manifestations (when present) are intermittent. Threshold factors, if they exist, have not been fully clarified, but marginal essential amino acid nutrition is suspected as a precipitating event along with impaired nicotinic acid nutrition.

Plasma levels of tryptophan are slightly depressed as are the levels of the other essential amino acids involved in the transport disorder (i.e., lysine is not affected).

Complications: Pellagra-like symptoms under marginal nutritional intake.

Etiology: Autosomal recessive inheritance (with genetic heterogeneity probably) (McKusick catalogue entry 23450).

Pathogenesis: Deficiency of a group-specific membrane transport system selective for several free aliphatic and ring-structured neutral (alpha)-amino acids. Transport of the same amino acids in (oligo)peptide linkage is normal.

Phenotype is expressed in kidney and intestine; a variant without intestinal phenotype may exist. Urine may contain excessive amounts of tryptophan derivatives, such as indoxyl sulfate, indole-3-acetic acid, and indolylacetyl glutamine; all are of intestinal origin, secondary to impaired intestinal absorption of tryptophan; the latter findings can be suppressed with neomycin.

Genetics: sex ratio: M1:F1 (approximate). Incidence: 1 in 15,000 to 1 in 100,000 live births depending on geographic region (and ethnic population). Risk of recurrence for patient's siblings: 1 in 4 (25%) for each. For patient's child: not increased unless mate is carrier or homozygote. Phenotype detectable in newborn. There are no identifying characteristics in the heterozygote under endogenous conditions.

Treatment: augmented protein nutrition particularly in patients with low plasma concentrations of essential amino acids; nicotinic acid supplements to offset proposed deficiency in endogenous synthesis of coenzyme to prevent pellagra-like symptoms.

Prognosis: good with normal life span, benign with appropriate treatment.

HYPERCYSTINURIA (isolated) (65).
Excludes: Cystinuria; cystinosis; homocystinuria.

Minimal diagnostic criteria: Positive urinary cyanide-nitroprusside test; increased renal clearance of cystine alone; (clearance of lysine, arginine, or ornithine must be normal).

Clinical findings: Disorder has been described in only 1 family to date; proband did not have urolithiasis but the risk is presumably present.

Complications (associated): Hypocalcemia and tetany reported in 1 of 2 affected sibs.

Etiology: Presumed to be autosomal recessive disorder (McKusick catalogue entry 23820).

Pathogenesis: Transport defect involves cystine-specific carrier in renal tubule (probably in brush-border membrane). It leads to increased renal clearance and excretion of cystine. Urinary tract calculi are a potential complication.

Genetics: sex ratio: M:F 1:1 presumably; risk of occurrence: unknown (apparently rare); risk of recurrence for patient's siblings: presumed 1 in 4 (25%) for each; for patient's child: not increased unless mate is carrier of homozygote. Phenotype detectable at birth, presumably.

Treatment: Prevention of calculi (see entry for cystinuria).

Prognosis: Normal life span, presumably.

Detection of carrier: Parents of the only reported patients excrete normal amounts of cystine in the urine.

Special considerations: Phenotype is significant because it provides evidence for a tubular transport system specific for cystine (in brush-border membrane?) unshared with the dibasic amino acids. No data are available concerning intestinal transport of cystine.

HYPERDIBASIC-AMINOACIDURIAS (Type I) (42, 43) and type II (lysinuria-protein intolerance) (38)
Excludes: Cystinuria.

Major diagnostic criteria: Lysinuria-protein intolerance (LPI), also called type II dibasic aminoaciduria, has failure to thrive (after weaning from breast milk), protein aversion, growth failure, hepatomegaly and splenomegaly, vomiting and episodes of stupor or coma after excessive protein feeding, normal or slightly elevated blood ammonia during fasting, and hyperammonemia with orotic aciduria after protein feeding. There is a selective increase in renal excretion of lysine, arginine and ornithine and normal urinary cystine concentration. Intestinal absorption of dibasic amino acids is also impaired. Concentration of dibasic amino acids in plasma are lower than normal. Symptomatic patients are homozygous; heterozygotes are symptom free and do not have hyperdibasic aminoaciduria.

A second form of dibasic aminoaciduria (type I) does not have LPI. Asymptomatic heterozygotes manifest the aminoaciduria phenotype. Symptomatic (homozygous?) patients have impaired mental development. Dibasic aminoaciduria pattern is similar in the type I and type II phenotypes.

Clinical findings: Type I aminoaciduria phenotype is dominantly inherited. Heterozygotes are apparently asymptomatic. Reported homozygotes (rare) have mental retardation. Type II clinical phenotype (LPI) is found predominantly in the Finnish population. Only homozygotes are symptomatic and have hyperdibasic aminoaciduria.

Hyperammonemia is provoked in LPI by high protein intake or loading with alanine; symptoms can be prevented by reduction of protein in the diet, and by citrulline supplementation. Heterozygotes are symptom-free. Twelve patients with apparent LPI from outside Finland and of various genetic backgrounds have been reported.

Patients with LPI also fail to absorb dibasic amino acids from dietary oligopeptides implying that the transport defect is in the basolateral membrane of epithelial cells.

Complications: Type II (LPI) impaired growth, osteoporosis, and muscular hypotonia. Increased protein intake causes periods of stupor and, if recurrent, can result in mental retardation through hyperammonemia. If mental retardation is a genuine consequence of the type I mutation, its pathogenesis is obscure.

Etiology: Autosomal recessive inheritance of the symptomatic type II phenotype (LPI); heterozygotes for LPI have no obvious expression of the mutant allele in vivo. Type I hyperdibasicaminoaciduria is expressed dominantly; homozygotes are rare and probably symptomatic (mental retardation). Two different genes proposed [McKusick catalogue entries 12600 (for type I) and 22270 (for type II)]; (the phenotypic descriptions in the catalogues are confusing).

Pathogenesis: All patients have selective deficiency of one or other of the membrane transport systems that are shared by "dibasic" amino acids and exclude cystine. Two Mendelian types of hyperdibasic aminoacidurias exist; therefore two different systems are involved. In the Type I phenotype, transport is clearly defective in the renal tubule (and perhaps in the intestine); the defect is likely to be located in the luminal (brush-border) membrane of the epithelial cell. In the Type-II phenotype (with LPI) the defect is almost certainly located in the basolateral antiluminal membrane of both renal and intestinal epithelial cells. Dibasic amino acids taken up by epithelial cells, either in the free form or as oligopeptides, do not permeate the basolateral surface normally. The liver probably shares the transport defect in the Type II phenotype. A functional deficiency of urea cycle intermediates (arginine and ornithine) impairs urea synthesis, causing hyperammonemia; orotic aciduria appears as a consequence after excessive amino nitrogen loading.

Genetics: Sex ratio: M1:F1. Incidence: Unknown but rare for Type I phenotype. Type II (LPI): approximately 1 in 60,000 live births in Finland; rarer elsewhere. Risk of recurrence for patient's siblings: as for autosomal recessive or autosomal dominant inheritance in type II and type I aminoaciduria phenotypes respectively; clinical phenotypes are apparently recessive for both mutations. Patient's child: as for autosomal recessive or autosomal dominant phenotypes. Phenotypes detectable in newborn.

Detection of heterozygote: Type I: modest hyperdibasicaminoaciduria in heterozygotes. Normal dibasic amino excretion in type II (LPI) heterozygote.

Treatment: No treatment advised for type I heterozygotes. None attempted for type I homozygotes with MR. For type II (LPI), protein intake should be restricted (to less than 1.5 q/kg/day). L-citrulline supplement (0.5 mmol/g of dietary protein) is beneficial; measurement of daily urinary orotic acid excretion is a useful monitor.

Prognosis: Normal life span in Type I heterozygotes: prognosis for mental development may be poor in homozygotes. Development and prognosis of Type II (LPI) phenotype is improved with treatment.

Special considerations: In the Type II (LPI) phenotype the transport defect is located in the basolateral plasma membrane; it may be shared by the plasma membrane of liver. Impairment of the urea cycle, hyperammonemia, and protein intolerance are part of the phenotype, because the liver is apparently deprived of urea cycle intermediates. Citrulline feeding bypasses the transport defect and primes the urea cycle in LPI.

HYPERHISTIDURIA (Renal histidinuria) (66–68).
Excludes: Histidinemia; Hartnup disorder.

Major diagnostic criteria: All patients reported had CNS signs (mental retardation or myoclonic seizures). A selective hyperaminoaciduria comprising histidine alone occurs in the presence of a normal plasma histidine level. Intestinal absorption of histidine may also be impaired.

Clinical findings: In the four reported patients (including 2 siblings), renal histidinuria was identified during investigation of mental retardation or myoclonic seizures. Whether renal histidinuria is ever asymptomatic is not known. The phenotype seems not to have been reported in newborn urine screening programs.

Etiology: Autosomal recessive (tentative) (McKusick catalogue entry 23583)

Pathogenesis: Deficient activity of a specific membrane transport system for L-histidine in renal (and intestinal?) epithelium would explain the following: 1) high renal clearance of histidine (reabsorption less than the normal 90% of filtered load) at normal plasma histidine level; 2) impaired plasma response to oral histidine load in some but not all patients. CSF histidine is normal (in cases examined). Urine histidine metabolites are normal.

Genetics: Sex ratio: should be M1:F1 if autosomal recessive. Incidence: probably very rare. Risk of recurrence: as for AR conditions. Age of detectability: presumably in newborn; (but no cases reported yet by newborn urine screening programs). Some obligate carriers are said to show attenuated intestinal absorption of histidine but there was no apparent increase of renal histidine clearance under endogenous conditions in these subjects.

Significance: Isolated Mendelian hyperhistidinuria is evidence for a histidine-specific membrane carrier. In this context, the phenotype is analogous to hypercystinuria (section 7.4), methionine malabsorption (ref. 48) and tryptophan malabsorption (ref. 49).

IMINOGLYCINURIA (69).
Excludes: Hyperprolinemia; Iminoglycinuria of normal newborn.

Major diagnostic criteria: Homozygotes have normal plasma concentration of proline and hydroxyproline, (both are imino acids), and glycine. Large amounts of imino acids and glycine persist in urine after 6 months of age. Heterozygotes (one allelic type) have glycinuria exceeding 160 mmoles/g total urinary nitrogen, or renal clearance exceeding 8.6 $ml/min/1.73M^2$; other (silent) heterozygotes have normal glycine excretion.

Clinical findings: No proven disease associated with the trait. Its occasional association with seizures or mental retardation, is probably fortuitous (bias of ascertainment). Numerous healthy children and adults have been recognized with selective impairment of cellular transport of proline, hydroxyproline and glycine. Plasma levels of affected amino acids are normal. In homozygotes, net renal tubular reabsorption of proline, hydroxyproline and glycine is about 80, 80 and 60% of normal respectively. An intestinal transport defect restricted to the iminoglycine group of amino acids has also been identified in some, but not in all pedigrees. Most heterozygotes have abnormal endogenous glycine reabsorption. There is evidence of a "silent" heterozygous phenotype. (see Special considerations). From this and other evidence, it is assumed that more than one allele determines the renal iminoglycinuria trait.

Etiology: Autosomal recessive transmission (McKusick catalogue entry 24260).

Pathogenesis: Presumed deficiency of high-capacity, low-affinity, group-specific membrane transport system in brush-border membrane shared by proline, hydroxyproline, and glycine.

Genetics: Sex ratio: M1:F1 (approximate). Incidence: about 1 in 17,000 live births for mutant homozygous phenotype. Risk of recurrence for patient's siblings: 1 in 4 (25%) for each; for patient's child: not increased unless mate is carrier or homozygote. Age of detectability: at birth. Detection of heterozygote: hyperglycinuria associated with one allelic form.

Treatment: None indicated (benign condition).

Prognosis: Normal life span.

Special considerations: Evidence for more than one mutant genotype rests on: (1) different form of heterozygosity; (2) demonstration of an intestinal transport defect in some homozygotes and failure to identify this feature in others; (3) Mendelian evidence for genetic compounds.

References

1. Scriver CR, Rosenberg LE: Distributions of amino acids in body fluids. In Amino Acid Metabolism and Its Disorders. Philadelphia, W.B. Saunders, 1973.
2. Scriver CR, Bergeron M: Amino acid transport in kidney. The use of mutation to dissect membrane and transepithelial transport. In Nyhan WL (ed): Heritable Disorders of Amino Acid Metabolism. New York, John Wiley & Son, 1974, p 515.
3. Vogel F, Motulsky AG: Human Genetics: Problems and Approaches. New York, Springer-Verlag, 1979, p 152–154.
4. McInnes RR, Scriver CR: Net reabsorption of α-amino-isobutyric acid by rat kidney in vivo. Am J Physiol 237:F274, 1979.
5. Scriver CR: Window panes of eternity. Health, disease, and inherited risk. Yale J Biol Med 55:487, 1983.
6. Tanford C: The hydrophobic effect and the organization of living matter. Science 200:1012, 1978.
7. Silbernagel S: Renal transport of amino acids. Klin Wchnschr 57:1009, 1979.
8. Aronson PS: Identifying secondary active solute transport in epithelia. Am J Physiol 240:F1, 1981.
9. Scriver CR, Hechtman P: Human genetics of membrane transport with emphasis on amino acids. Adv Hum Gen 1:211, 1970.
10. Silbernagl S, Pfaller W, Heinle H, et al: Topology and function of renal γ-glutamyl transpeptidase. In Sies H, Wendel A (eds): Functions of Glutathione in Liver and Kidney. Berlin, Springer-Verlag, 1978, p 60.
11. Scriver CR, Chesney RW, McInnes RR: Genetic aspects of renal tubular transport: diversity and topology of carriers. Kidney Intl 9:149, 1976.
12. Schafer JA, Barfuss DW: Membrane mechanisms for transepithelial amino acid absorption and secretion. Am J Physiol 238:F335, 1980.
13. Diamond JM: Tight and leaky junctions of epithelia: a perspective on kisses in the dark. Fed Proc 33:2220, 1974.
14. Baerlocher KE, Scriver CR, Mohyuddin F: The ontogeny of amino acid transport in rat kidney. I. Effect on distribution ratios and intracellular metabolism of proline and glycine. Biochim Biophys Acta 249:353, 1971.
15. Holtzapple P, Genel M, Rea C, et al: Metabolism and uptake of L-proline by human kidney cortex. Pediatr Res 7:818, 1973.
16. Barfuss DW, Mays JM, Schafer JA: Peritubular uptake and transepithelial transport of glycine in isolated proximal tubules. Am J Physiol 238:F324, 1980.
17. Barfuss DW, Schafer JA: Active amino acid absorption by proximal convoluted and proximal straight tubules. Am J Physiol 236:F149, 1979.
18. Slack EN, Liang C-CT, Sacktor B: Transport of L-proline and D-glucose in luminal (brush-border) and contraluminal (basal-lateral) membrane vesicles from the renal cortex. Biochem Biophys Res Commun 77:891, 1977.
19. Ullrich KJ: Sugar, amino acid, and Na^+ cotransport in the proximal tubule. Ann Rev Physiol 41:181, 1979.
20. Scriver CR, Wilson OH: Amino acid transport: Evidence for genetic control of two types of human kidney. Science 155:1428, 1967.
21. Hammerman MR, Sacktor B: Na^+-dependent transport of glycine in renal brush border membrane vesicles. Evidence for a single specific transport system. Biochim Biophys Acta 686:189, 1982.
22. Herman RH: The principles of metabolic control. In Herman RH, et al (eds): Principles of Metabolic Control in Mammalian Systems. New York, Plenum Press, 1980.
23. Scriver CR, McInnes RR, Mohyuddin F: Role of epithelial architecture and intracellular metabolism in proline uptake and transtubular reclamation in PRO/Re mouse kidney. Proc Nat Acad Sci (USA) 72:1431, 1975.
24. Scriver CR, Smith RJ, Phang JM: Disorders of proline and hydroxyproline metabolism. In Stanbury JB, et al (eds): The Metabolic Basis of Inherited Disease, ed 5. New York, McGraw-Hill Book Co, 1983, p 360.
25. Alvarado F: Intestinal transport of sugars and amino acids: Independence or Federalism? Am J Clin Nutr 23:824, 1970.
26. Garrod AE: The Croonian Lectures. Lancet 2:1, 73, 142, 204, 1908.
27. Dent CE, Rose GA: Amino acid metabolism in cystinuria. Quart J Med 20:205, 1951.
28. Robson EB, Rose GA: The effect of intravenous lysine on the renal clearances of cystine, arginine and ornithine in normal subjects, in patients with cystinuria and Fanconi syndrome and in their relatives. Clin Sci 16:75, 1957.
29. Segal S, Thier SO: Cystinuria. In Stanbury JB, et al (eds): The Metabolic Basis of Inherited Disease, ed 5. New York, McGraw-Hill Book Co, 1983, p 1774.
30. Rosenberg LE, Downing SJ, Segal S: Competitive inhibition of dibasic amino acid transport in rat kidney. J Biol Chem 237:2265, 1962.
31. Schwartzman L, Blair A, Segal S: A common renal transport system for lysine, ornithine, arginine and cysteine. Biochem Biophys Res Comm 23:220, 1966.
32. Kato T: Renal handling of dibasic amino acids and cystine in cystinuria. Clin Sci Molec Med 53:9, 1977.
33. Fox M, Thier S, Rosenberg I, et al: Evidence against a single renal transport defect in cystinuria. N Engl J Med 270:556, 1964.
34. Arthus MF, Bergeron M, Scriver CR: Topology of membrane exposure in the renal cortex slice. Studies of glutathinone and maltose cleavage. Biochim Biophys Acta 692:371, 1982.
35. Coicadan L, Heyman M, Grasset E, et al: Cystinuria: reduced lysine permeability at the brush border membrane of intestinal cells. Pediatr Res 14:109, 1980.
36. Craan AG, Bergeron M: Experimental cystinuria: the cycloleucine model. II. Amino acid efflux from intestinal and renal tissues. Metabolism 27:1613, 1978.
37. Foreman JW, McNamara PD, Segal S: Renal transport of cystine by isolated renal tubules and brush-border membrane vesicles. In Belton MR, Toothill C (eds): Transport and Inherited Disease. Baltimore, University Park Press, 1981, p 263.
38. Norio R, Perheentupa J, Kekomaki M, et al: Lysinuric protein intolerance, an autosomal recessive disease. A genetic study of 10 Finnish families. Clin Genet 2:214, 1971.
39. Desjeux JF, Simell RO, Dumontier AM, et al: Lysine fluxes across the jejunal epithelium in lysinuric protein intolerance. J Clin Invest 65:1382, 1980.
40. Rajantie J, Simell O, Perheentupa J: Lysinuric protein intolerance. Basolateral transport defect in renal tubuli. J Clin Invest 67:1078, 1981.
41. Rajantie J, Simell O, Perheentupa J: Intestinal absorption in lysinuric protein intolerance: impaired for diamino acids, normal for citrulline. Gut 21:519, 1980.
42. Whelan DT, Scriver CR: Hyperdibasicaminoaciduria: an inherited disorder of amino acid transport. Pediatr Res 2:525, 1968.
43. Oyanagi K, Miura R, Yamanoucki T: Congenital lysinuria: a new inherited transport disorder of dibasic amino acid. J Pediatr 77:259, 1970.
44. Scriver CR: Hartnup disease a genetic modification of intestinal and renal transport of certain neutral alpha-amino acids. N Engl J Med 273:530, 1965.
45. Jepson B: Hartnup Disease. In Stanbury JB, et al (eds): The Metabolic Basis of Inherited Disease, ed 4. New York, McGraw-Hill Book Co, 1978, p 1563.
46. Baron DN, Dent CE, Harris H, et al: Hereditary pellagra-like skin rash with temporary cerebellar ataxia, constant renal aminoaciduria and other bizarre biochemical features. Lancet 2:421, 1956.
47. Silk DB, Dawson AM: Intestinal absorption of carbohydrate and protein in man. Int Rev Physiol 19:151, 1979.
48. Hooft C, Timmermans J, Snoeck J, et al: Methionine malabsorption syndrome. Ann Paediat 205:73, 1965.
49. Drummond KN, Michael AF, Ulstrom RA, et al: The Blue Diaper Syndrome: familial hypercalcemia with nephrocalcinosis and indicanuria. Am J Med 37:928, 1964.
50. Holmgren G, Hambreus L, de Chateau P: Histidinemia and "Normo-histidinemic histidinuria". Acta Paediat Scand 63:220, 1974.
51. Navab F, Asatoor AM: Studies on intestinal absorption of amino acids and a dipeptide in a case of Hartnup disease. Gut 11:373, 1970.
52. Brodehl J, Gellissen K: Endogenous renal transport of free amino acids in infancy and childhood. Pediatrics 42:395, 1968.
53. Brodehl J: Postnatal development of tubular amino acid reabsorption. In Silbernagl S, et al (eds): Amino Acid Transport and Uric Acid Transport. Stuttgart, Georg Thieme, 1976.
54. Woolf LI, Norman AP: The urinary excretion of amino acids and sugars in early infancy. J Pediatr 50:271, 1957.
55. Lasley L, Scriver CR: Ontogeny of amino acid reabsorption in human kidney. Evidence from the homozygous infant with familial renal iminoglycinuria for multiple proline and glycine systems. Pediatr Res 13:65, 1979.
56. McNamara PD, Ozegovic B, Pepe LM, Segal S. Proline and glycine uptake by renal brush border membrane vesicles. Proc. Natl. Acad. Sci. (USA) 73:4521, 1976.

57. Scriver CR, Arthus MF, Bergeron M: Neonatal iminoglycinuria: Evidence that the prolinuria originates in selective deficiency of transport activity in the proximal nephron. Pediatr Res 16:684, 1982.
58. Scriver CR: The human biochemical genetics of amino acid transport. Pediatrics 44:348, 1969.
59. Rozen R, Tenenehouse HS, Scriver CR: Taurine transport in renal brush-border membrane vesicles. Biochem J 180:245, 1979.
60. Rozen R, Goodyer PR, Scriver CR: Metabolism of GABA and taurine in mammals. What are metabolites like this doing in places like that? Contemp Metab 2:189, 1982.
61. Gaull GE, Rassin DK, Raihi NCR, et al: Milk protein quantity: quality in low-birth-weight infants. III. Effects on sulfur amino acids in plasma and urine. J Pediatr 90:348, 1977.
62. Rozen R, Scriver CR: Renal transport of taurine adapts to perturbed taurine homeostasis. Proc Natl Acad Sci (USA) 79: 2101, 1982.
63. Teijema HL, van Gelderin HH, Giesberts MAH, et al: Dicarboxylic aminoaciduria: An inborn error of glutamate and aspartate transport with metabolic implications in contribution with hyperprolinemia. Metabolism 23:115, 1974.
64. Melançon SB, Dallaire L, Lemieux B, et al: Dicarboxylic aminoaciduria: An inborn error of amino acid conservation. J Pediatr 91:422, 1977.
65. Brodehl J, Gellissen K, Kowalewski S: Isolierter defect der tubularen cystin-ruck resorption in einer familie mit idiopathischem hypoparathyroidisms. Klin Wschr 45:38, 1967.
66. Holmgren G, Hambraeus L, de Chateau P: Histidinemia and "Normohistidinemic Histidinuria". Acta Paediat Scand 63:220, 1974.
67. Sabater J, Ferre C, Puliol M, et al: Histidinemia: A renal and intestinal histidine transport deficiency found in two mentally retarded children. Clin Gen 9:117, 1976.
68. Kamoun PP, Parvy P, Cathelineau L, et al: Renal histidinuria. J Inher Metab Dis 4:217, 1981.
69. Scriver CR: Familial Iminoglycinuria. In Stanbury JB, et al (eds): The Metabolic Basis of Inherited Disease, ed 5. New York, McGraw-Hill Book Co, 1983, p 1792.

CHAPTER 32

Disorders of Tubular Transport of Calcium and Phosphorus

RUSSELL W. CHESNEY
SHERMINE DABBAGH

Disorders of renal tubular transport reflect an alteration in the physiological process responsible for the net tubular reaccumulation of a given ion or organic solute (1–3). The disorders that alter calcium (Ca) and phosphorus (P) handling by the kidney appear to have the following features: (1) these defects often are inherited; (2) a renal tubular transport protein or site may be altered or may function in an atypical fashion; (3) the usual response of the tubule to a hormonal signal—particularly parathyroid hormone (PTH)—is altered; and (4) the function of a regulatory protein within the tubular epithelium may be defective. An understanding of the pathophysiology and the clinical expression of these syndromes has been improved by the ability to measure ionic Ca, PTH, vitamin D metabolites, and cyclic nucleotides (cAMP) in plasma and urine. The information derived from renal clearance and fractional excretion of Ca and P have assisted in defining differences in the clinical presentations of these syndromes. Three syndromes are described: primary hypophosphatemic rickets, pseudohypoparathyroidism, and hypercalcemia-hypercalciuria syndromes.

PRIMARY HYPOPHOSPHATEMIC RICKETS

Primary hypophosphatemic rickets describes a group of disorders in which the following are found: (1) osteomalacia or rickets caused by a deficiency of phosphorus (P) in the extracellular fluid (ECF) of bone such that normal mineralization of osteoid does not occur; (2) an increased urinary P excretion despite hypophosphatemia, and (3) a genetic pattern of inheritance in some instances (3). Hyperphosphaturic hypophosphatemia secondary to hyperparathyroidism resulting from vitamin D-deficiency rickets, and vitamin D-dependency rickets not responsive to calcitriol (1,25$(OH)_2$-vitamin D) (vitamin D-dependency type II) are excluded. Five types of primary hypophosphatemic rickets have been defined (Table 32.1), the first type is the most common and will be discussed in detail.

The common type is the X-linked form (Table 32.1) (4) in which patients present with growth retardation and bowing of the lower limbs on weight-bearing. They have hypophosphatemia, normocalcemia, and an elevated serum alkaline phosphatase activity. Clinical features include coxa vara, genu valgum, and pelvic deformities (5) (Figs. 32.1*A* and *B*). The corresponding radiological findings are rickets in the epiphysis and metaphysis with a widening of the bone shaft and a loose reticular pattern of bone trabeculae. Premature craniostenosis occurs and leads to a bulging forehead and an enlarged bridge of the nose. Enamel formation of the teeth is normal, but dentin formation (intraglobular dentin) is defective (6). The patients have a waddling gait, but myopathy is not a feature. Neither aminoaciduria nor glucosuria are present.

In the X-linked type, males are hemizygotes and females are heterozygotes (4). As a result, males are more severely affected, whereas females generally have only mild disease—fasting hypophosphatemia and minimal bowing. Untreated males are short in stature, reaching an adult height of 140 to 155 cm. Degenerative joint disease commonly develops in adult life so that prevention of joint disease is reason for treating asymptomatic adults (3).

Dr. Chesney is recipient of a Research Career Development Award KO4-AM00421. Dr. Dabbagh is supported by the Stetler Research Fund for Women Physicians. Supported in part by USPHS Grant AM 31682.

Table 32.1.
Types of Primary Hypophosphatemic Rickets

Condition	Inheritance pattern	Associated finding	Salient clinical features	Age detected	Therapy
X-linked hypophosphatemic rickets (also called vitamin D-dependent rickets or familial hypophosphatemic rickets)	X-linked dominant, rarely autosomal dominant or autosomal recessive	Occasional patient has parathyroid adenomas or hyperplasia	Bowing of lower segment, short stature, no myopathy; usually affects males more severely	9 to 13 months	Oral phosphate, 1–4 gm/24 hr given 4 to 5 times each day; 1,25$(OH)_2D$ at 65–75 ng/kg/24 hr
Hypophosphatemic nonrachitic bone disease	Autosomal dominant or sporadic		No radiological evidence of rickets; disease is milder and short stature may appear in late adolescence	3 years to adult	Oral phosphate and vitamin D; may be healed by 1,25$(OH)_2D$
Hereditary hypophosphatemic rickets with hypercalcuria	Autosomal recessive; consanguinity	High calcitriol level; increased intestinal Ca absorption; hypercalcuria low urinary cAMP	Rickets, short stature, osteomalacia, sexes equally affected	Early childhood	Oral phosphate reverses biochemical features
Oncogenous rickets with phosphaturia	Sporadic or autosomal dominant, autosomal recessive	Sometimes, neurofibromatosis, polyostotic fibrous dysplasia, and epidermal nevus syndrome	Rickets is healed by removal of tumor; where measured serum 1,25$(OH)_2D$ values are low	Birth onwards	Oral phosphate and 1,25$(OH)_2D$ will reverse hypophosphatemia; surgery may be curative if tumor is totally removed
Adult sporadic hypophosphatemic osteomalacia	Sporadic	Glycinuria	Severe bone pain, vertebral flattening, Looser's zones, severe myopathy, and weakness	Adult	Oral phosphate, plus vitamin D in any form

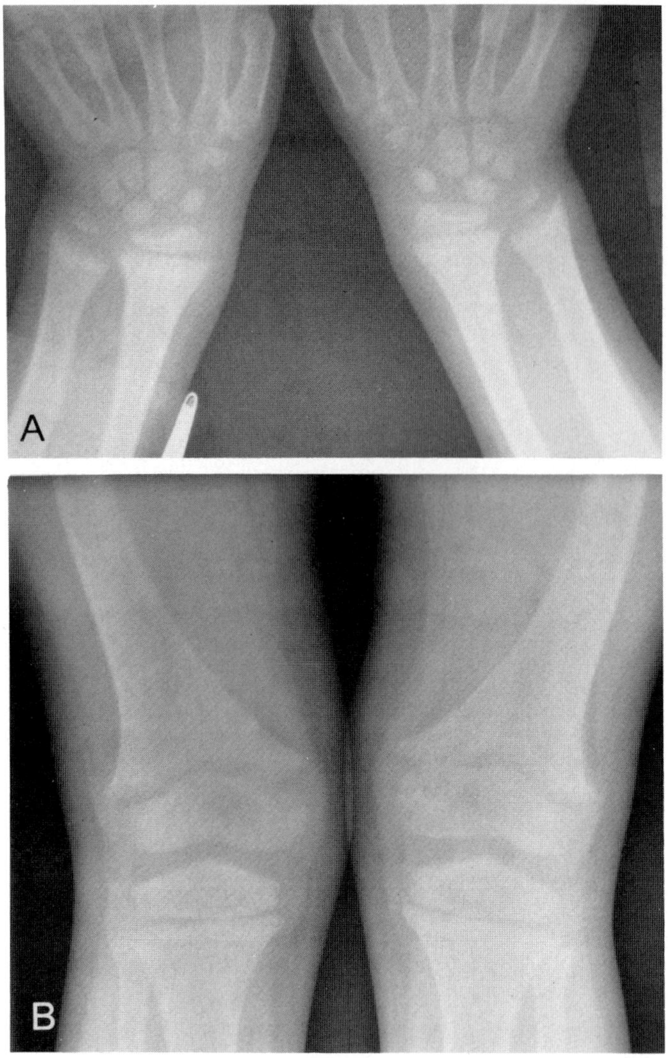

Figure 32.1. **A**, Radiographs of hands and wrists and, **B**, knees of an 8-year-old girl with untreated X-linked hypophosphatemic rickets. Note the smooth bowing of the femur, as well as the cupping and fraying at the metaphysis of the radius, ulna, femur, tibia, and fibula.

Hypophosphatemia serum phosphorus between 1.0 and 2.5 mg/dl (0.32–.81 mM/L) is the biochemical characteristic; in neonates and infants with this disease, serum phosphorus may be as high as 4.0 mg/dl (4, 5). Serum Ca usually is in the low normal range averaging 9.0 mg/dl (2.3 mM/L). Urinary Ca excretion is low, urinary P excretion is high (3–6). Despite hypophosphatemia, the reabsorption of P in relation to glomerular filtration rate (GFR) is low, as reflected by a $TmPO_4$: GFR ration of <1.8 mg/100 ml in comparison to normal childhood values of 4.5 to 8.0 (7). The fecal concentration of both Ca and P is elevated (8). Yet, despite a reduction in intestinal calcium absorption, the circulating values of iPTH are normal and rise only after oral phosphate therapy (9). A subgroup of patients has been described with both a renal P "leak" and secondary parathyroid hyperplasia that may necessitate surgical removal of the parathyroid glands (10).

The pathogenesis of the hyperphosphaturia is uncertain. At least two hypotheses have been proposed (11, 12): (1) a renal tubular transport protein is missing that normally affects the reabsorption of P and (2) a defect in vitamin D metabolism results in decreased intestinal Ca absorption, secondary hyperparathyroidism, and renal P wasting. The finding that iPTH values are normal has caused the second hypothesis to be modified, i.e. the renal tubule is overly sensitive to the phosphaturic action of PTH (11, 12). The fact that there is no evidence for excess PTH action, e.g., hypercalcemia, aminoaciduria, and elevated urinary cAMP, favors the first hypothesis. The report of a patient in whom hypophosphatemic rickets and hypoparathyroidism occurred together also favors this hypothesis (13). In this patient raising serum calcium (Ca_s) by giving 1,25(OH)-vitamin D (calcitriol) orally, caused phosphaturia despite the absence of PTH (8). A block in intestinal P absorption suggested in some but not all studies also support the first hypothesis (8).

The second hypothesis, that the nephron in patients with X-linked hypophosphatemia is overly sensitive to the phosphaturic action of PTH, is examined by studies of response to PTH and Ca infusion. PTH evokes a rise in urinary (nephrogenous) cAMP in 2 studies (11, 14) but not in a third (12). The intravenous infusion of calcium, which suppresses PTH secretion, reduces P and cAMP excretion. The question is whether these actions operate only at the level of the parathyroid glands. Scriver (15) has argued that while Ca infusion blocks these PTH-induced effects (11, 14), Ca may be acting directly at the level of the renal tubule to reduce urinary P excretion, because Ca_s levels of 13 to 15 mg/dl must be achieved before urinary cAMP and P excretion decrease.

At least two conclusions are possible from these findings. This condition may be heterogeneous, i.e., patients from certain families have primary hypophosphatemia and patients from other families are supersensitive to the phosphaturic effect of PTH. Alternatively, the pathogenic sequence may be more complex than is explained by either the hypothesis of deficiency of transport protein or that of hyperresponsiveness to PTH, e.g., the latter may be a result of a defect in vitamin D metabolism.

In his original description of X-linked hypophosphatemic rickets, Fuller Albright theorized that abnormalities of vitamin D metabolism play an important role in the pathogenesis of this disorder (16). Recent studies indicate that vitamin D metabolism is abnormal. Serum calcidiol (25(OH)D) values are normal (17) and increase appropriately when patients are treated with high doses of vitamin D_2 or D_3 (18). Serum levels of $24,25(OH)_2D$ are slightly reduced, but rise into the normal range with vitamin D therapy (19) (Fig. 32.2). There is an inverse correlation between calcidiol and calcitriol ($1,25(OH)_2D$) levels (Fig. 32.3) (18, 19). Calcitriol levels are low despite hypophosphatemia, and the infusion of

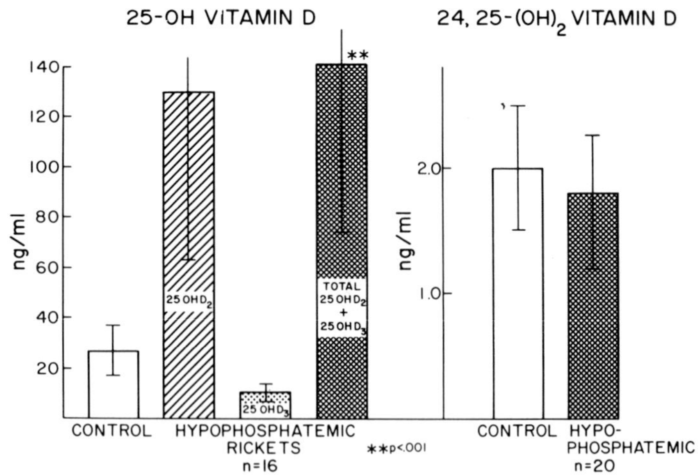

Figure 32.2. Effects of vitamin D_2 on circulating values of 25(OH)D and $24,25(OH)_2D$ in 16 patients with X-linked hypophosphatemic rickets. Note the finding that the $25(OH)D_2$ fraction is increased and that the $25(OH)D_3$ fraction is normal. A slight reduction in $24,25(OH)_2D$ values is evident (Unpublished data of Chesney, Rose, Hamstra, Mazess, and DeLuca).

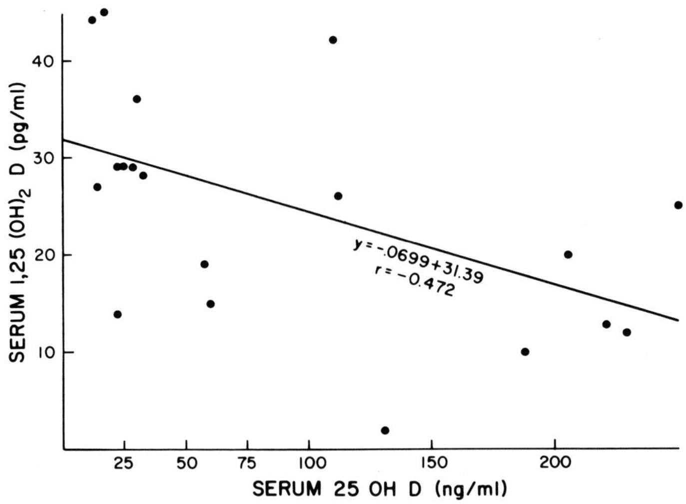

Figure 32.3. Relationship between serum 1,25(OH)$_2$D and 25(OH)D in 12 patients with X-linked hypophosphatemic rickets. This indicates that the lowest values of 1,25(OH)$_2$D are found in association with high circulating values of 25(OH)D related to treatment with vitamin D_2. (From Chesney RW, et al: Pediatrics 71:559, 1983.)

PTH does not lead to the expected increase (20). In a preliminary study in which these patients were deprived of P, the calcitriol levels fell, whereas in normal subjects calcitriol levels rise (12). Because high doses of calcitriol used in conjunction with oral phosphate heals rickets in these patients, the healing may be related to a rise in calcitriol levels (19, 22, 23).

In summary, the abnormality in vitamin D metabolism is a low or low normal calcitriol level despite hypophosphatemia. Higher doses of calcitriol appear to be required to heal rickets in these patients than is required to heal the rickets caused by renal osteodystrophy.

A model of X-linked hypophosphatemic rickets has been described in (Hyp/Y) mice, which is characterized by rickets, hypophosphatemia, short stature, decreased intestinal Ca and P absorption, and osteopenia (24–26). Sodium-dependent, arsenate-inhibitable phosphate transport by brush-border membrane vesicles is impaired in the Hyp/Y (male) mouse and, to a lesser extent, in the female heterozygote. When the female heterozygote is fed a low P diet, the uptake of P by brush-border vesicle increases by 200%, indicating that the renal epithelium in these mice adapts to an altered dietary intake. The Hyp/Y mouse does not show the same response (27). As in the human disease, serum PTH values in the mice are normal and PTH infusion does not alter renal tubular P handling. Moreover, after acute thyroparathyroidectomy and P loading, a renal tubular phosphate leak is still evident (8). These results strongly suggest that a renal P leak is important in this animal model.

The absolute levels of vitamin D metabolites in these mice are normal, but are low in view of the hypophosphatemia. After phosphate deprivation, the serum levels of 1,25(OH)$_2$D rise in normal mice, but they either do not change or actually fall in Hyp/Y mice, as is the case in humans (21). One explanation is that phosphate pools in the renal cortex are not lower in Hyp/Y mice despite hypophosphatemia (28). Therapy with oral phosphate improves bone mineralization. Therapy with 1,25(OH)$_2$D improves intestinal Ca transport, but does not influence transport of P. Although either 1α-(OH)D (a synthetic analogue) or calcitriol increases urinary P conservation and improves rachitic bone, only the synthetic analogue will improve P homeostasis by raising plasma values. However, others have noted improvement in bone histology after oral P and 1,25(OH)$_2$D therapy (29).

At present, a simple unified theory of the pathogenesis of primary hypophosphatemic rickets in man is not possible. At least six major questions remain:

1. Does the human disease have a defect in brush-border membrane vesicle transport analogous to that in the mouse?
2. Is the renal handling of P altered by changing plasma PTH levels without changing any of its other actions?
3. Do the normal or subnormal circulating values for 1,25(OH)$_2$D found in patients represent relative deficiency considering the presence of hypophosphatemia?
4. Does Ca infusion result in an appreciable alteration of phosphate handling in this condition so that studies using this approach to suppress endogenous PTH secretion should be viewed with caution?
5. Is Ca homeostasis important in setting the $TmPO_4$/GFR as suggested in the patient described by Lyles and coworkers (13)?
6. Does the paradoxical fall in serum 1,25(OH)$_2$D values after dietary phosphate deprivation indicate an important defect in vitamin D metabolism? Or does this occur because renal cortical P content is actually normal despite plasma hypophosphatemia (8, 29)? Until these questions are answered, a unified hypothesis is speculative.

Therapy

Treatment of hypophosphatemic rickets with large daily doses of vitamin D will improve the radiological appearance of the epiphyseal lesion. This form of therapy, often requiring doses of 150,000 units (3,333 μg) of vitamin D per day, does not prevent the continuing deformity of the lower limbs nor prevent recurrence of the deformity after surgical correction or restore growth to normal (30, 31). The risk-benefit ratio of vitamin D alone is high; toxicity: hypercalcemia, hypercalcuria, nephrocalcinosis, and renal damage, as evidence by a fall in creatinine clearance, is frequent (30, 31).

Although early studies indicated disappointing results using P supplements, when more frequent and larger doses were given that were sufficient to lead to P retention, rickets healed (32, 33). In long-term studies in which 1 to 4 gm of inorganic P are given every 4 to 5 hours, rickets has healed and growth velocity has increased (34). If oral P is started early in life, near normal height can be achieved. These doses of oral phosphate can lead to hyperparathyroidism and bone disease.

Ninety to 120 minutes after an oral phosphate dose, P_s peaks and returns to baseline values in 4 hours (34). Vitamin D_2 therapy in moderately high doses and oral Ca will prevent this effect of high dose oral phosphate therapy.

Therapy with calcidiol and supplemental P have not led to correction of the bone lesion and does not appear to offer any advantage over vitamin D_2 therapy (35).

Patients given short-term trials of calcitriol therapy have had improved intestinal Ca absorption and a transient rise in P_s values. In these trials, which lasted only 2 weeks, no healing of the bone disease was noted (36); this mode of therapy does not correct the renal tubular P leak.

Long-term P and calcitriol (65 ng/kg/day) therapy improved Ca and P retention, increased bone mineralization and linear growth rate (Fig. 32.4) (37). The rachitic lesion at the growth plate and the mineralization defect at the endosteal surface were corrected; this has not been shown for any other form of treatment. The renal tubular phosphate leak is unchanged and $TmPO_4$/GFR is either unchanged or falls. Where vitamin D_2 and P treatment fail, therapy with calcitriol and phosphate is effective (37), although complete healing does not occur always (38, 39). We do not know whether calcitriol and phosphate given over decades will prevent the degenerative joint disease so prevalent in adult patients.

Four other primary phosphaturic conditions have been described

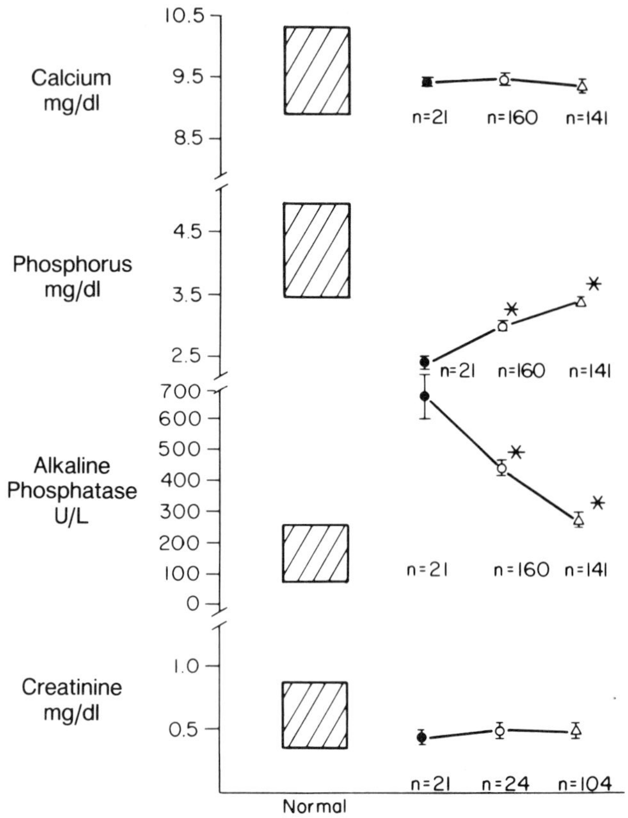

Figure 32.4. The effect of different treatment regimens on serum chemical determinations in X-linked hypophosphatemic rickets. *O*, vitamin D_2 (same dose) plus phosphate (1 to 4 gm by mouth per day, given every 4 hours); Δ, 1,25$(OH)_2$D (65 ng/kg/day in two divided doses) plus phosphate (1 to 4 gm by mouth per day, given every 4 hours); and *, $p < .01$ from preceding value. The last treatment regimen results in normalization of serum phosphorus and alkaline phosphatase values without changing calcium and creatinine values. (From Chesney RW, et al: Pediatrics 71:559, 1983.)

(Table 32.1). Hypophosphatemic nonrachitic bone disease is an autosomal dominant or sporadic condition in which hypophosphatemia occurs without the radiological appearance of rickets. In contradistinction to the X-linked form, the $TmPO_4$/GFR is normal when the patient is hypophosphatemic. The values of 1,25$(OH)_2$D are normal. Vitamin D and oral phosphate are recommended (30).

Hereditary hypophosphatemic rickets with hypercalcuria (HHRH) is a familial condition with rickets, short stature, increased renal phosphate clearance, hypercalciuria (a level of 8.6 ± 0.1 mg/kg/24 hr), normocalcemia, and increased intestinal Ca and P absorption (64). In contrast to X-linked hypophosphatemic rickets where serum calcitriol level is low or low normal and to HMB where the value is normal, the circulating values of calcitriol are 2 to 5 times normal. The pathogenesis of this disorder is felt to be a renal phosphate leak resulting in hypophosphatemia, which stimulates increased synthesis of calcitriol with higher calcitriol levels, intestinal Ca absorption increases, PTH secretion is suppressed, and hypercalcuria develops. In support of this pathogenic sequence, fasting reduces and an oral Ca load increases urinary Ca excretion. Long term oral phosphate supplementation appears to reverse all of the biochemical defects except the reduced $TmPO_4$/GFR.

Oncogenous rickets with phosphaturia is a disorder in which a mesenchymal tumor of soft tissue or bone appears to elicit a substance causing phosphaturia with hypophosphatemic osteomalacia (1, 3, 8). The circulating values for 1,25$(OH)_2$D are low. Removal of the tumor results in a cure. This condition is also rarely found in polyostotic fibrous dysplasia, neurofibromatosis, and the epidermal naevus syndrome. Adult sporadic hypophosphatemic osteomalacia occurs in adolescents as well as adults. Glycinuria occurs in conjunction with the hyperphosphaturia. Oral phosphate therapy is indicated (1, 3, 8).

PSEUDOHYPOPARATHYROIDISM

Pseudohypoparathyroidism (PHP) is a pleitropic hereditary disorder characterized by signs and symptoms of hypoparathyroidism in association with distinctive skeletal and developmental stigmata. It is the first disease in humans to be attributed to end-organ resistance to the action of a hormone. In contradistinction to hypoparathyroidism, there is hyperplasia of the parathyroid glands and excess secretion of PTH. Since the original description of the disease in 1942, it has become apparent that PHP is a heterogeneous condition and the basic pathophysiology is not clear.

Historical Perspective

The syndrome was first reported by Albright and coworkers (40), who described three patients with tetany, seizures, hypocalcemia and hyperphosphatemia. Unlike patients with hypoparathyroidism, these patients failed to show either a hypercalcemic or a phosphaturic response to PTH, i.e., the target organs, kidney and bone, were resistant to the action of PTH. These patients, in addition to these biochemical abnormalities, have other abnormalities (Table 32.2). These findings are collectively known as Albright's hereditary osteodystrophy (AHO). Later, Albright (41) described a patient with the phenotypic features of AHO but with normal Ca_s and P_s. This syndrome is termed "pseudopseudohypoparathyroidism" (PPHP) and may represent a variant in the expressivity of PHP. The presence of hyperplastic parathyroid glands and elevated iPTH levels in PHP patients have confirmed the state of secondary hyperparathyroidism, as originally suggested.

Chase and coworkers (43) noted that patients with PHP failed to increase the urinary (nephrogenous) excretion of cAMP in response to the intravenous PTH. This lack of response characterizes PHP, type I. A different form of PHP, type II, is characterized by the failure of exogenous PTH to elicit a hyperphosphaturic or hypercalcemic effect, but causes a normal increase in urinary cAMP (44). The cAMP response of patients with PPHP is variable.

Patients with the biochemical abnormalities of PHP, but without the

Table 32.2.
Clinical Features of Pseudohypoparathyroidism and Albright's Hereditary Osteodystrophy

Abnormality	Feature
Developmental	Round facies, short neck
	Obesity
	Thick stocky body build
	Short stature
Skeletal	Brachydactyly (short metacarpals, metatarsals or phalanges)
	Increased bone density
	Hyperostosis fontralis interna
	Thickened calvaria
	Abnormal dentition
Soft-tissue calcification	Subcutaneous
	Cataracts
	Basal ganglia

osteodystrophic features of AHO have also been reported (45). Furthermore, patients with and without the phenotypic features have been reported to have radiological and clinical evidence of bone-responsive, but renal nonresponsive, disease (46). Some of these patients have appeared to have rickets, but actually have osteitis fibrosa (46, 47).

Clinical Features

The symptoms of PHP reflect increased neuromuscular irritability secondary to hypocalcemia (45). These include: tetany, convulsions, muscle cramps, seizures, and episodes of laryngeal spasm. Poor vision may result from cataracts.

The defect in the cAMP response is present at birth, yet Ca_s and P_s remain normal for years. PTH levels may be elevated. The average age of onset of the symptoms is about 8 years (45).

The phenotype of AHO–short stature, round facies, short neck, thick, stocky body build—sometimes include other skeletal abnormalities, e.g., shortness of metacarpal and metatarsal bones and of the phalanges. The most common finding is shortening of the fourth and fifth metacarpal or metatarsal; the defect may be unilateral. When only one digit is involved, it is the fourth. These abnormalities seem to be secondary to premature closure of the epiphyses (Table 32.2).

These patients may manifest normal or increased bone density by x-ray, particularly in the skull where thick calvarium, widened spongy diploe, hyperostosis frontalis interna, and abnormal dentition is sometimes present. Changes compatible with osteitis fibrosa cystica and hyperparathyroid bone disease, including subperiosteal bone resorption (Figs. 32.5, *A* and *B*), are present in a few patients (46). Brown tumors, cysts, slipping of the femoral capital epiphyses, fractures, and osteopenia have been noted. Histologically, evidence of hyperparathyroid bone disease is common.

Cutaneous and subcutaneous placques of Ca may be present near joints (Figs. 32.6, *A* and *B*), on the abdomen and elsewhere. These placques may include elements of true bone. Basal ganglia calcifications are common, occurring in as many as 50% of the patients with PHP and AHO (45). The intellect is usually, but not always, diminished.

The degree of osteodystrophy varies. In some, the features are quite characteristic; in others, they are not definite enough to establish the diagnosis. Many patients who lack the phenotypic changes are classified as having idiopathic hypoparathyroidism. The correct diagnosis is established only when PTH levels and the renal responses to exogenous PTH are characteristic.

Most, but not all, of the patients have hypocalcemia and hyperphosphatemia (48). PTH levels are increased. Alkaline phosphatase levels are normal except when osteitis fibrosa cystica is present. Vitamin D levels are low in most patients with PHP and hypocalcemia (49) (infra vide).

Pathogenesis

The underlying biochemical abnormality in PHP type I is impaired cAMP response to PTH (43). The normal cAMP response is dependent on three components: hormone receptors; a catalytic unit which converts ATP to cAMP; and the N or G protein, which couples the receptors and catalytic unit (50). Patients with PHP have a reduction of about 50% of the N or G protein in erythrocytes, platelets, transformed lymphoblasts, and fibroblasts and have both the somatic and biochemical features of PHP type I with AHO. None of the patients with normal phenotype had the defect. However, the reverse was consistently the case, i.e., patients with PHP and AHO have had normal N- or G-protein activity. Thus, those patients with the reduction in the coupling protein activity are now characterized as having PHP type Ia to distinguish them from those who have normal G-protein activity, now known as PHP type Ib (51, 52).

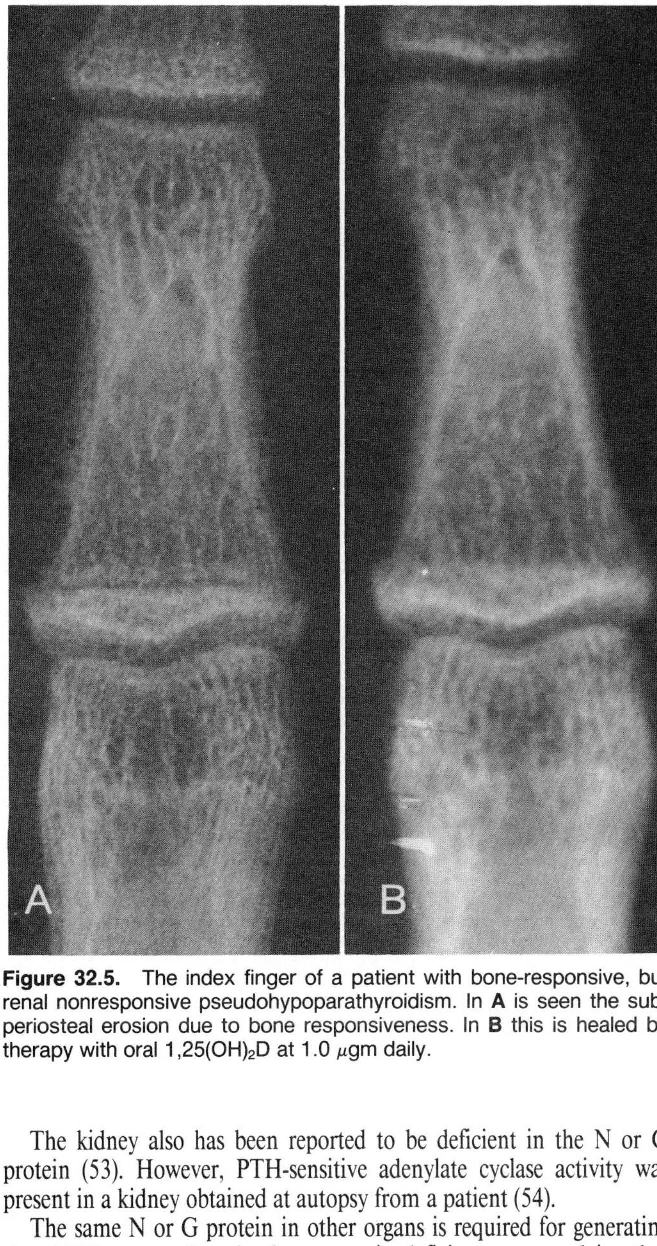

Figure 32.5. The index finger of a patient with bone-responsive, but renal nonresponsive pseudohypoparathyroidism. In **A** is seen the subperiosteal erosion due to bone responsiveness. In **B** this is healed by therapy with oral $1,25(OH)_2D$ at 1.0 μgm daily.

The kidney also has been reported to be deficient in the N or G protein (53). However, PTH-sensitive adenylate cyclase activity was present in a kidney obtained at autopsy from a patient (54).

The same N or G protein in other organs is required for generating the cAMP response by other hormones; its deficiency may explain other hormone resistance. Thyroid function is abnormal in most patients with PHP, type Ia (51). Basal thyroid hormone levels are slightly low and thyrotropin (TSH) is elevated. The release of TSH and prolactin following the administration of thyrotropin-releasing hormone (TRH) is abnormal. Although these patients do not have clinical signs of nephrogenic diabetes insipidus, they have a reduced ability to concentrate urine in response to water deprivation (51). Gonadal hypofunction and a blunted cAMP response to glucagon was noted, although the glycemic response was normal in one report (55). In PHP type II, the abnormality is presumed to be a defect beyond the PTH stimulated cAMP generation.

Genetics

The variability of PHP (Table 32.3) indicates considerable genetic heterogeneity. Although the familial nature has long been recognized, the mode of inheritance has not been established (56). There are twice as many females as males with AHO, which suggests X-lined dominant inheritance. There are no documented examples of male-to-male trans-

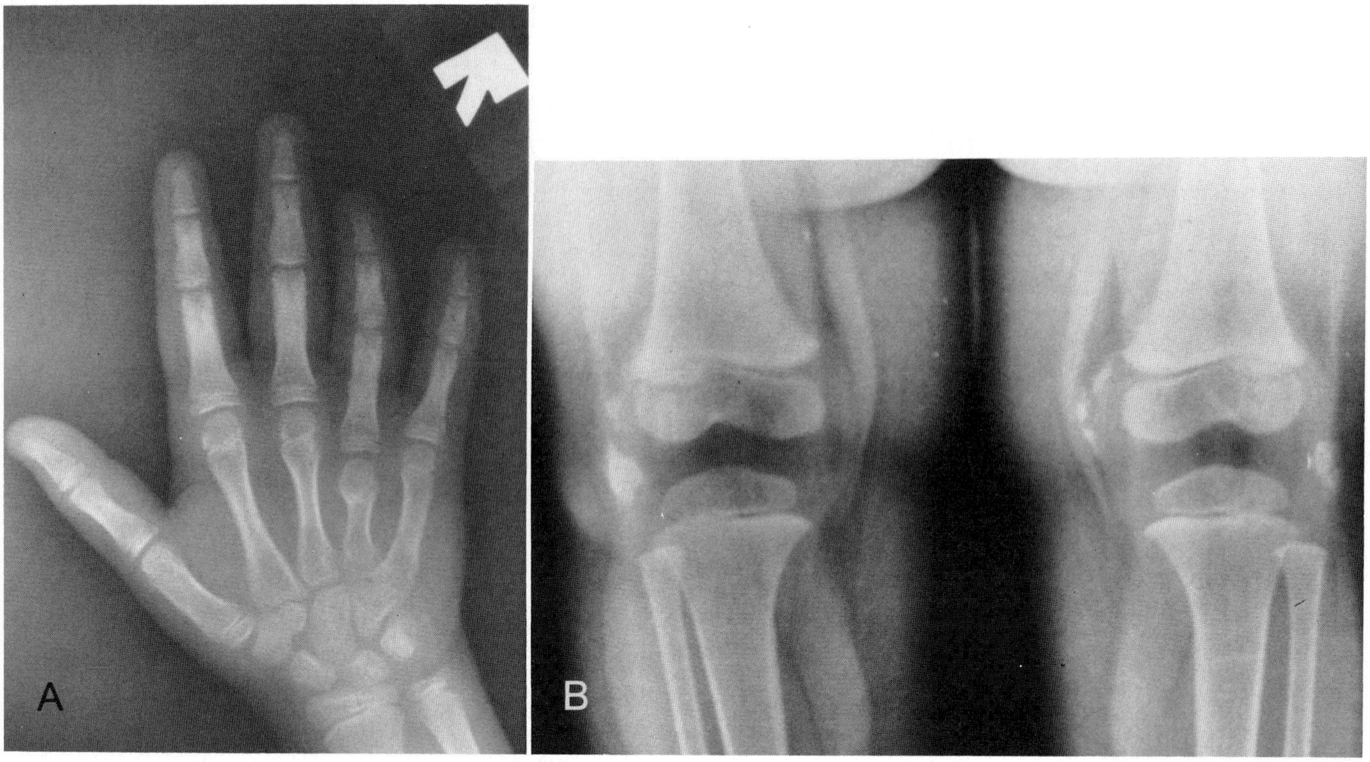

Figure 32.6. **A** and **B**, Hand and knee radiographs of a patient with type I (classical) pseudohypoparathyroidism. This patient had an absent response to infused parathyroid extract. Note the brachydactaly of the fourth metacarpal and the subcutaneous calcifications about the knees.

Table 32.3.
Biochemical and Clinical Aspects of Pseudohypoparathyroidism

Diagnosis	AHO	Serum PTH	Serum ca	Serum 25(OH)D_3	Serum 1,25$(OH)_2D_3$	N-protein activity	Generalized hormone resistance	Urine cAMP/PO_4 response to PTH
PHP Ia	+	↑	Usually ↓	N	↓	↓	+/−	↓/↓
PHP 1b	+/−	↑	↓ or N	N	↓ or N	N	+/−	↓/↓
PHP II	+/−	↑	↓	N	↓	N	−	N/↓
PPHP	+	↑	N	?	?	N or	−	N or ↓/N or ↓

AHO, Albright's hereditary osteodystrophy; *PHP*, Pseudohypoparathyroidism; *PPHP*, Pseudopseudoparathyroidism.

mission. The possibility of autosomal dominant inheritance with sex modification has been reported recently (58).

Measurement of the N or G protein activity should be useful in studying the inheritance pattern. However, when different variants, e.g., PPHP, bone-responsive PHP, or biochemical PHP with a normal phenotype, appear within the same family genetic, analysis will be difficult.

Treatment

Patients with PHP and hypocalcemia are treated with vitamin D. The choice of the vitamin D preparation is controversial. The level of 1,25$(OH)_2D_3$ is low in most patients with PHP and hypocalcemia (50) and the reduced levels may result from decreased renal 1α-hydroxylation of 25(OH)D_3, secondary to resistance to PTH and to the inhibitory effects of hyperphosphatemia. The absence of hypercalcemic response to PTH in patients with PHP is similar to that observed in patients with vitamin D deficiency and chronic renal failure (CRF).

In view of the postulated impairment in renal 1α-hydroxylation, calcitriol or its analogue dihydrotachysterol is recommended (59). The recommended dose of calcitriol is 14 to 21 ng/kg/day. Treatment restores the Ca_s to normal and restores the hypercalcemic response to PTH (50). However, treatment does not restore the cAMP response to PTH. The hyperphosphaturic response to PTH was restored with treatment. Treatment with vitamin D_2, 50,000 to 100,000 units per day and additional calcium as lactate or gluconate also is successful. The aim of therapy is to achieve a normal Ca_s (Fig. 32.7).

Patients with PPHP do not require treatment. Patients with PPHP and other hormonal imbalances, e.g., hypothyroidism, should receive appropriate replacement therapy.

HYPERCALCEMIA-HYPERCALCURIA-NEPHROPATHY SYNDROMES

Renal stones secondary to hypercalcuria are discussed elsewhere (chapter 42). Hypercalcuria—defined as urinary Ca excretion >4–6 mg/kg/24 hr or a urinary Ca/creatinine ratio >0.2 (61)—is associated with a number of familial hypercalcemic states, which are described in this section. Hypercalcemia secondary to sarcoidosis, malignancies, the milk alkali syndrome, and vitamin D intoxication are not discussed, since these are seldom pediatric conditions.

Some children with familial hypercalcuria have abnormal responses

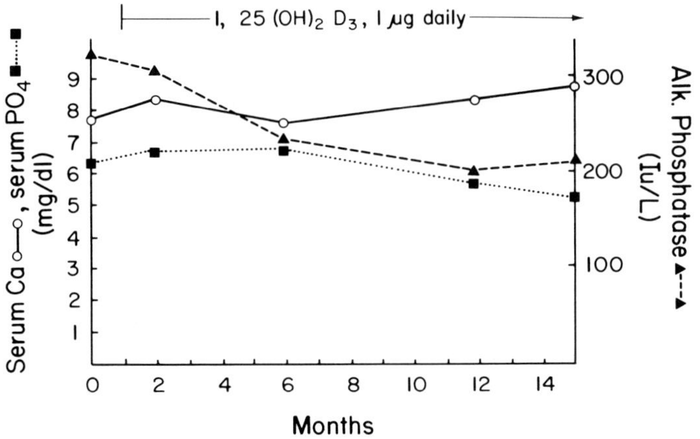

Figure 32.7. The clinical course of the patient in Figure 32.6 before and after therapy with $1{,}25(OH)_2D$.

Table 32.4.
Etiology of Neonatal Hypercalcemia

Uncertain Pathophysiological Sequence
- Idiopathic infantile hypercalcemia (mild)
- Severe idiopathic infantile hypercalcemia (William's syndrome with elfin facies)
- Fat necrosis
- Infantile hypophosphatasia
- Familial hypocalcuric hypercalcemia (benign familial hypercalcemia)

Increased Vitamin D
- Maternal vitamin D toxicity
- Maternal high-dose vitamin D for a disorder of vitamin D metabolism
- High-dose $1{,}25(OH)_2$-vitamin D therapy to mother with vitamin D target organ abnormalities

Increased Parathyroid Hormone
- Neonatal hyperparathyroidism (familial)
- Maternal hypoparathyroidism with fetal parathyroid gland hyperplasia

to conventional maintenance doses of vitamin D (400 U/day) have absorptive hypercalcuria; others have renal hypercalcuria (62). Hypercalcemic-hypercalcuria syndromes in neonates are more serious and have many causes (Table 32.4).

Hypercalcemia can lead to renal damage by altering glomerular hemodynamics or by causing Ca depositions in the renal medulla (nephrocalcinosis) or in the renal parenchyma and microvasculature (renal calcification). Ca may affect the ultrafiltration permeability coefficient (Kf) of glomerular capillaries. PTH dependent hypercalcemia is associated with a fall in Kf, which is reversed by thyroparathyroidectomy (63). Ca appears to affect the tubuloglomerular feedback control of GFR, e.g., hypercalcemia reduces single nephron GFR (64). Either filtered or intracellular Ca in the renal medulla influences the release of arachidonic acid and prostaglandin, which may influence the concentrating mechanism of the kidney (65). Nephrocalcinosis is associated with a defect in the concentrating mechanism (66). Vascular calcifications are associated with patchy areas of necrosis and tubular atrophy.

At least five clinical syndromes of hereditary hypercalciuria are delineated: (1) idiopathic infantile hypercalcemia, (2) severe idiopathic infantile hypercalcemia (Williams syndrome), (3) fat necrosis, (4) severe infantile hypophosphatasia, and (5) familial hypocalcuric hypercalcemia.

Idiopathic Infantile Hypercalcemia

Many authors include all infants with hypercalcemia in the neonatal period whose serum PTH and/or parathyroid gland appearance are

Table 32.5.
Forms of Idiopathic Infantile Hypercalcemia Syndrome

Form	Mild	Severe[a]
Hypercalcemia	11–15 mg/dl	11–20 mg/dl
Facial appearance	Normal	Elfin facies with cupid bow upper lip and flat, upturned nose
Teeth	Normal	Peg-like with numerous caries
Cardiac	10% murmurs	Supravalvular aortic stenosis, pulmonic stenosis, and other abnormalities
Intelligence	Normal	Mild to moderate retardation, IQ of 40-80
Behavior	Normal, except irritable when hypercalcemic	Cocktail party patter; outgoing and friendly; 15% have severe behavioral difficulties
Prognosis	Excellent	Long-term chronic medical problems
Frequency	Rare	Not infrequent
Birth weight	Normal	Small for gestational age

[a] Also known as Williams elfin facies syndrome.

normal as idiopathic infantile hypercalcemia (IIH) (67, 68). Fanconi and coworkers (69) used the terms "mild variant" and "severe variant" of IIH. The syndrome was reported by Lightwood in 1952 (70), and more than 200 cases were described in England by 1956. This disorder has been rare in North America and it is no longer common in Europe (67, 68, 71).

The clinical signs of the mild variant are thirst, dehydration, and fever (67, 68, 71). Mild azotemia, leukocyturia, and cylinduria are common. The prognosis of mild IIH is good. The clinical signs of the severe form include cardiac abnormalities, mental retardation, elfin features, and poor growth (Table 32.5).

The large number of cases reported in England in the 1950s was associated with a policy introduced after World War II to supplement milk and other staples with vitamin D. Intakes from these sources frequently exceeded 2000 U daily. Lowering the supplement to levels where intakes seldom exceed 400 U daily has been associated with the incidence decreasing to the occasional case. Several affected children with IIH had levels of vitamin D activity in plasma that were distinctly elevated (68, 71). The experience in England appear to represent an example of an environmental change—an increase in vitamin D intake—eliciting an adverse response in a genetically sensitive subpopulation. Their experience and the various hereditable forms of vitamin D resistance point to a genetic divergence in sensitivity to vitamin D action over a broad spectrum. The infants who developed IIH are an example of the very sensitive (67, 68).

The cases appearing since then are examples of more extreme hereditable disorder with hypercalcemia and hypercalciuria resulting.

In one report of a 9-month-old patient with IIH, 25(OH)D levels were normal and $1{,}25(OH)_2D$ synthesis and urinary cAMP were decreased, as would be anticipated in response to hypercalcemia. In an infant with IIH and hypercalcuria, we observed a low $1{,}25(OH)_2D$ level (44 pg/ml vs 85 $\pm$ 15 pg/ml in 1- to 12-month-old controls) and normal 25(OH)D values (26.2 ng/ml vs 30.4 $\pm$ 5 ng/ml in controls). Thus, as stated by Fraser and coworkers "a direct causal relationship between vitamin D and infantile hypercalcemia has not yet been proven" (67).

Therapy of this disorder is aimed at reducing the intake of both vitamin D and calcium. A meat-based formula has been used successfully; the recipe for this special formula is available (67, 68). Glucocorticoids, which impair intestinal calcium absorption, have been used on a short-term basis (67, 68, 72).

Severe Idiopathic Infantile Hypercalcemia

A peculiar elfin facial appearance is characteristic of the severe form of IIH (69, 73). Williams and coworkers (74) pointed out the association between the peculiar facies and supravalvular aortic stenosis, others recognized that hypercalcemia was also present (75). The term "Williams syndrome" now describes children with a medial eyebrow flare, ocular hyperteliorism, depressed nasal bridge, short palpebral fissures, strabismus, pale blue eyes with a star-like pattern to the iris, full prominent lips with an open mouth, malar hypoplasia, and antiverted nares (76, 77). Although this condition is considered to be sporadic, it has been found in siblings and in twins.

Low birth weight is common. Growth failure and mental deficiency are more common than either hypercalcemia or supravalvular aorta stenosis. The facies are apparent at birth, a variety of other cardiac and vascular lesions, e.g., atrial septal defect and mesenteric, celiac, and renal artery stenosis, are associated. These children have an unusual personality and exhibit a "cocktail party patter."

The association of hypercalcemia, hypercalcuria, and nephrocalcinosis has led to the hypothesis that these patients are similar to individuals with vitamin D toxicity. Fellers and Schwartz (73) reported vitamin D-like material in plasma to be 30 to 40 times normal in three patients. Massive doses of vitamin D given to pregnant rabbits led to offspring that had a high incidence of arterial stenosis (78). However, the cardiac lesions in the rabbits differed in histology from those seen in patients with typical Williams syndrome. From Germany, hypercalcemia, typical facies, and supravalvular aortic stenosis were reported in infants whose mothers had taken 500,000 IU of vitamin D during pregnancy (79). Weisman and coworkers (80) have theorized that hypercalcemia could be the result of a defect in esterification of $1,25(OH)_2D$, a step found in the transfer of radiolabelled vitamin D from mother to fetus across the rat placenta. Taylor and coworkers (77) examined the handling of vitamin D in six normocalcemic children with Williams syndrome and in age-matched controls given vitamin D 1500 IU/kg for 4 days. Plasma 25(OH)D levels increased to supranormal values in patients with Wiliam's syndrome, but not in controls (Fig. 32.8). Plasma $1,25(OH)_2D$ and Ca were unchanged in both groups. The higher 25(OH)D is not related to higher vitamin D binding-protein levels (81). Whether this increase in circulating 25(OH)D value seen in children with Williams syndrome is causally related to hypercalcemia in more severe cases is not clear, but it gives some support to the idea that vitamin D metabolites are affected in William's syndrome. Mothers of infants with William's syndrome seldom have histories of excessive intakes of vitamin D during pregnancy. This has led to skepticism over the role vitamin D might play in the pathogenesis of this syndrome (67, 68, 82).

Forbes and coworkers (82) demonstrated a prolonged half-life to Ca_s elevated by giving an infusion of Ca in eight children with this syndrome. Because the decrease in the increment in Ca_s following Ca infusion was unrelated to the action of vitamin D on intestinal absorption, these authors theorized that the bone resorption rate did not fall in these patients and that a deficiency of calcitonin could account for these changes. However, they did not measure immunoreactive calcitonin.

At present, evidence that abnormalities of vitamin D metabolism are central to the hypercalcemia of William's syndrome is inconclusive. The recent observations of Taylor and coworkers (77) need to be corroborated by additional studies, and more patients need to be examined during the hypercalcemic phase. Hypercalcemia is transient in this condition, and

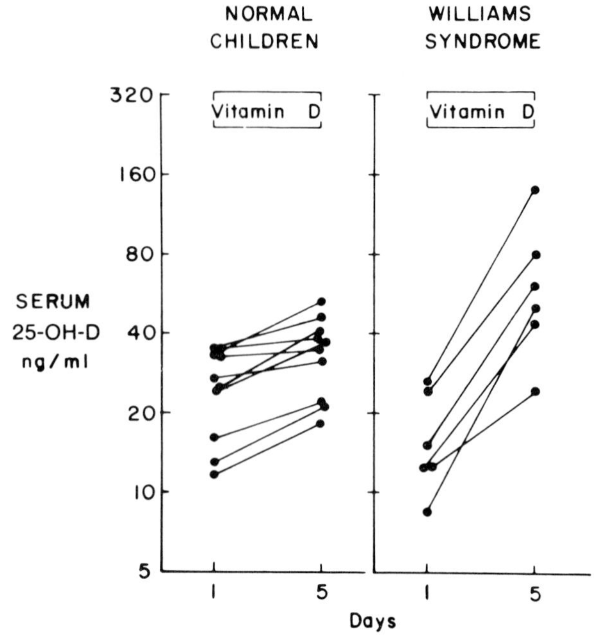

Figure 32.8. Effects of vitamin D_2 (1500 IU/kg/day) given for 4 days to normal children and six patients with Williams syndrome. Note that the scale of the ordinate is logarithmic. The increase in normal children was 41% and in Williams syndrome 298% (From Taylor AB, et al: N Engl J Med 306:972, 1982, with permission.)

a low-calcium, low-vitamin D diet is rarely indicated (73). If hypercalcuria and nephrocalcinosis persist, these should be treated accordingly. The prognosis for survival of the disorder is good, but most patients are seriously retarded (IQ between 40 and 80). An occasional patient may display bizarre or antisocial behavior.

Fat Necrosis

An association between infantile hypercalcemia and subcutaneous fat necrosis has long been appreciated (83). By history, these infants are either premature or small for gestational age or have evidence of neonatal stress—hypothermia, hypoxia, birth trauma, or were delivered by cesarean section. The antecedent factors resemble those associated with hypocalcemia. These infants develop high serum calcium values, 16 and 22 mg/dl, coincident with the appearance of tender, bluish-red discolored areas of induration in the subcutaneous fat, particularly in pressure sites (67, 74, 84). By histological examination, the necrotic adipose tissue shows fatty acid crystals, presumably a calcium salt, plus giant cells and mononuclear infiltrates (83). These patients exhibit all the consequences of hypercalcemia, e.g. azotemia, nephrocalcinosis, radiological evidence of subcutaneous dystrophic calcification, and growth retardation. The levels of 25(OH)D are normal and those of $1,25(OH)_2D$ are suppressed appropriate to the degree of hypercalcemia (84). A low Ca, low vitamin D diet, and glucocorticoids are recommended to reverse the hypercalcemia when present (67, 68, 83). Urinary prostaglandin E_2 was elevated in one affected patient (84). The elevation of urinary prostaglandin E_2 may be the cause or consequence of hypercalcemia or fat necrosis in as much as renal prostaglandin excretion is related to urine volume, which, in hypercalcuria, is high (65).

Severe Infantile Hypophosphatasia

Severe infantile hypophosphatasia is a rare autosomal recessive disorder associated with hypercalcemia. It is characterized by severe bone demineralization at the growth plate, a low serum alkaline phosphatase activity, elevated urinary concentrations of phosphoethanolamine, and premature loss of teeth (85). Hypophosphatasia is usually divided into an infantile, a childhood, and an adult form. The infantile type is most common and may be diagnosed in utero (86). Another subset of patients die in utero or shortly after birth, because bony support of the thorax and skull is inadequate (87). The histological picture of bone is identical to rickets with marked osteodosis and disruption of the normal columnar arrangement of cartilage cells. Wormian bones are present in the skull. The isoenzymes of alkaline phosphatase activity are present in the bone, kidney, liver, and intestine (85, 88).

Hypercalcemia, hypercalcuria, and nephrocalcinosis probably occur as a result of the failure of Ca deposition in the bone with a resultant increase in Ca_s. Abnormalities in vitamin D metabolism do not appear to contribute to the hypercalcemia (89, 90); the values of $1,25(OH)_2D$ are reduced appropriate to the hypercalcemia. iPTH levels are elevated in some patients (91), but in most patients they are reduced when the patients are hypercalcemic (89, 90). Restriction of dietary Ca and vitamin D result in hypocalcemia and an increase in iPTH and $1,25(OH)_2D$ levels. One patient on the low Ca and vitamin D diet developed rickets, which caused serum alkaline phosphatase activity to increase. Other factors that normally stimulate bone turnover, e.g., phenobarbital, glucocorticoids, and vitamin A did not increase alkaline phosphatase activity in one patient (89). In a 6-month-old patient, hypercalcemia and hypercalcuria were controlled by the intravenous infusion of alkaline phosphate-rich plasma (92). This finding supports the hypothesis of Rasmussen and Bartter (85) that alkaline phosphatase is important for bone mineralization, because it stimulates Ca uptake in bone matrix vesicles.

Familial Hypocalcuric Hypercalcemia

Foley and coworkers (93) described a kindred of 12 members with hypercalcemia who had no symptoms associated with hypercalcemia, i.e., fatigue, weakness, mental disturbances, polydipsia and polyuria, arthralgia, or headache. The inheritance was autosomal dominant. In subsequent cases urinary Ca excretion was low, and nephrocalcinosis, stone formation, and azotemia were infrequent (94, 95). Since urinary Ca/creatinine ratio is usually under 0.01, the term familial hypocalcuric hypercalcemia (FHH) has been used. Two consequences of prolonged hypercalcemia in FHH appear to be chondrocalcinosis and pancreatitis (94, 96).

The pathogenesis of the hypercalcemia is not clear; both iPTH and vitamin D levels are normal (95). The normal iPTH values are associated with mild parathyroid hyperplasia (97). Not only is Ca elevated in the face of hypocalcuria, but serum magnesium also is elevated with relative hypomagnesuria (94). Marx (95) has theorized that the kidney and parathyroid are insensitive to Ca_s; the kidney fails to excrete excess Ca and parathyroid gland hyperplasia with increased hormone secretion results. Following parathyroidectomy, Ca_s becomes normal only transiently; hypercalcemia rapidly recurs. This condition may involve an alteration of one of the Ca binding proteins, e.g., calmodulin or vitamin D-dependent calcium-binding protein.

In three kindred with FHH, severe hyperparathyroidism has been reported in at least four infants in the neonatal period (98). These infants had life-threatening hypercalcemia, muscular hypotonia, and skeletal undermineralization. The cause of the extreme parathyroid hyperplasia and hypercalcemia in these infants is not known; it may represent a relative insensitivity of the fetal parathyroid gland to the high concentration of calcium found in the intrauterine environment. On the other hand, most hypercalcemic infants born into kindreds of FHH are asymptomatic.

References

1. Scriver CR, Chesney RW, McInnes RI: Genetic aspects of renal tubular transport diversity and topology of carriers. Kidney Intl 9:149, 1976.
2. Chesney RW: Defects of renal tubular transport. In Massry SG, Glassock R (eds): Textbook of Nephrology. North Holland, Elsevier, 1983, p 3.178.
3. Chesney, R. W. Tubular defects in phosphate reabsorption in clinical medicine. In Massry SG, Fleish H (eds): The Renal Handling of Phosphorus. New York, Plenum Press, 1980, p 321.
4. Fraser, D, Scriver CR: Familial forms of vitamin D-resistant rickets revisited: X-linked hypophosphatemia and autosomal recessive vitamin D dependency. Am J Clin Nutr 29:1315, 1976.
5. Harrison HE, Harrison HC: Disorders of Calcium and Phosphate Metabolism in Childhood and Adolescence. Philadelphia, W. B. Saunders, 1979, p 53.
6. Gorlin R: Thoma's Oral Pathology. St. Louis, C. V. Mosby, 1970.
7. Kruse K, Kracht U, Gopfert G: Renal threshold phosphate concentration ($TmPO_4$/GFR). Arch Dis Child 57:217, 1982.
8. Chesney RW: Phosphaturic syndromes. In Gonick H (ed): Renal Tubular Disorders. Marcel Dekker, Inc., 1985, pp 201–238.
9. Arnaud C, Glorieux F, Scriver CR: Serum parathyroid hormone in X-linked hypophosphatemia. Science 173:845, 1971.
10. Kleerekoper M, Coffey R, Greco T, et al: Hypercalcemic hyperparathyroidism in hypophosphatemic rickets. J Clin Endocrinol Metab 45:86, 1977.
11. Hahn TJ, Scharp CR, Halstead LR, et al: Parathyroid hormone status and renal responsiveness in familial hypophosphatemic rickets. J Clin Endocrinol Metab 41:926, 1975.
12. Glorieux F, Scriver CR: Loss of a parathyroid hormone-sensitive component of phosphate transport in X-linked hypophosphatemia. Science 175:997, 1972.
13. Lyles KW, McNamara CR, Drezner MK: Coincidence of hypoparathyroidism and X-linked hypophosphatemic rickets: An experiment of nature illuminating the physiological factors which regulate the renal tubular defect. Calcif Tissue Int 33:309A, 1981.
14. Short E, Morris RC Jr, Spencer M: Exaggerated phosphaturic response to circulating parathyroid hormone in patients with familial X-linked hypophosphatemic rickets. J Clin Invest 58:152, 1976.
15. Scriver CR: Rickets and the pathogenesis of impaired tubular transport of phosphate and other solutes. Am J Med 57:43, 1974.
16. Albright F, Butler AM, Bloomberg E: Rickets resistant to vitamin D therapy. Am J Dis Child 54:529, 1937.
17. Haddad JG, Chyu KJ, Hahn TJ, et al: Serum concentrations of 25-hydroxyvitamin D in sex-linked hypophosphatemic vitamin D-resistant rickets. J Lab Clin Med 81:22, 1973.
18. Chesney RW, Mazess RB, Rose P, et al: Supranormal 25-hydroxyvitamin D and subnormal 1,25-dihydroxyvitamin D: Their role in X-linked hypophosphatemic rickets. Am J Dis Child 134:140, 1980.
19. Drezner MK, Lyles KW, Harrelson JM: Vitamin D-resistant osteomalacia: Evaluation of vitamin D metabolism and response to therapy. In Cohn DV, et al (eds): Hormonal Control of Calcium Metabolism. New York, Excerpta Media, 1981, p 243.
20. Lyles KW, Drezner MD: Parathyroid hormone effects on serum 1,25-dihydroxyvitamin D levels in patients with X-linked hypophosphatemic rickets: Evidence for abnormal 25-hydroxyvitamin D-1-hydroxylase activity. J Clin Endocrinol Metab 54:638, 1982.
21. Insogna K, Stewart A, Gertner J: Impaired phosphorus conservation and 1,25 dihydroxyvitamin D generation during phosphorus deprivation in familial hypophosphatemic rickets. J Clin Invest 71:1562, 1983.
22. Drezner MK, Lyles KW, Haussler MR, et al: Evaluation of a role for 1,25-dihydroxyvitamin D_3 in the pathogenesis and treatment of X-linked hypophosphatemic rickets and osteomalacia. J Clin Invest 66:1020, 1980.
23. Glorieux FH, Marie PJ, Pettifor JM, et al: Bone response to phosphate salts, ergocalciferol and calcitriol in hypophosphatemic vitamin D-resistant rickets. N Engl J Med 303:1023, 1980.
24. Eicher EM, Southard JL, Scriver CR, et al: Hypophosphatemia: Mouse model for human familial hypophosphatemic (vitamin D-resistant) rickets. Proc Natl Acad Sci (USA) 73:4667, 1976.
25. O'Doherty PJA, DeLuca HF, Eicher EM: Intestinal calcium and phosphate transport in genetic hypophosphatemic mice. Biochem Biophys Res Commun 71:617, 1976.
26. Giasson SD, Brunetti MG, Danan G, et al: Micropuncture study of renal phosphorus transport in hypophosphatemic vitamin D-resistant rickets mice. Pfluegers Arch 371:33, 1977.
27. Muhlbauer RC, Bonjour J-P, Fleisch H: Abnormal tubular adaptation to dietary P_i restriction in X-linked hypophosphatemic mice. Am J Physiol 242:F353, 1982.
28. Sabina RL, Drezner MK, Holmes EW: Reduced renal cortical ribonucleoside tri-

phosphate pools in three different hypophosphatemic animal models. Biochem Biophys Res Commun 109:649, 1982.
29. Marie PJ, Travers R, Glorieux FH: Bone response to phosphate and vitamin D metabolites in the hypophosphatemic male mouse. Calcif Tissue Int 34:158, 1982.
30. Scriver CR: On phosphate transport and genetic screening, "Understanding Backward—Living Forward" in human genetics: William Allen Memorial Award Address. Am J Hum Genet 31:243, 1979.
31. Harrison HE, Harrison HC, Lifshitz F, et al: Growth disturbance in hereditary hypophosphatemia. Am J Dis Child 112:290, 1966.
32. Gerbeaux-Balsan S: L'absorption intestinale du phosphore dans le rachitisme vitamine-resistant hypophosphatemique hereditaire. Effets de fortes surcharges de phosphore et des regimes tres pauvres en calcium. Rev Fr Etud Clin Biol 10:65, 1965.
33. West CD, Blanton JD, Silverman FN, et al: Use of phosphate salts as an adjunct to vitamin D in the treatment of hypophosphatemic vitamin D-refractory rickets. J Pediatr 64:469, 1964.
34. Glorieux FH, Scriver CR, Reade TM, et al: Use of phosphate and vitamin D to prevent dwarfism and rickets in X-linked hypophosphatemia. N Engl J Med 287:481, 1972.
35. Puschett JB, Genel M, Rastegar A, et al: Long-term therapy of vitamin D-resistant rickets with 25-hydroxycholecalciferol. Clin Pharmacol Ther 17:202, 1975.
36. Glorieux FH, Scriver CR, Holick MF, et al: X-linked hypophosphatemic rickets: Inadequate therapeutic response to 1,25-dihydroxycholecalciferol. Lancet 2:287, 1973.
37. Chesney RW, Mazess RB, Rose P, et al: Long-term influence of calcitriol (1,25$(OH)_2$ vitamin D) and supplemental phosphate in X-linked hypophosphatemic rickets. Pediatrics 71:559, 1983.
38. Marie PJ, Glorieux FH: Stimulation of cortical bone mineralization and remodeling by phosphate and 1,25-dihydroxyvitamin D in vitamin D-resistant rickets. Metab Bone Dis Rel Res 3:159, 1981.
39. Marie PJ, Glorieux FH: Histomorphometric study of bone remodeling in hypophosphatemic vitamin D-resistant rickets. Metab Bone Dis Rel Res 3:31, 1981.
39a. Teider M, Modai D, Samuel R, et al: Hereditary hypophosphatemic rickets with hypercalcuria. N Engl J Med 312:611, 1985.
40. Albright F, Burnett CH, Smith PH, et al: Pseudohypoparathyroidism—an example of the "Seabright-Bantam syndrome." Endocrinology 30:922, 1942.
41. Albright F, Forbes AP, Henneman PH: Pseudopseudohypoparathyroidism. Trans Assoc Am Phys 65:337, 1952.
42. Tashjian AH Jr, Frantz AG, Lee JB: Pseudohypoparathyroidism: Assays of parathyroid hormone and thyrocalcitonin. Proc Natl Acad Sci 56:1138, 1966.
43. Chase LR, Melson GL, Aurbach GD: Pseudohypoparathyroidism: Defective excretion of 3′,5′-AMP in response to parathyroid hormone. J Clin Invest 48:1832, 1969.
44. Drezner M, Nelson FA, Lebovitz HE: Pseudohypoparathyroidism type II: A possible defect in the reception of the cyclic-AMP signal. N Engl J Med 289:1056, 1973.
45. Bronsky D, Kushner DA, Dubin A, et al: Idiopathic hypoparathyroidism and pseudohypoparathyroidism. Case reports and review of the literature. Medicine (Baltimore) 37:317, 1958.
46. Kidd GS, Schaff M, Adler RA, et al: Skeletal responsiveness in pseudohypoparathyroidism. A spectrum of clinical disease. Am J Med 68:722, 1980.
47. Dabbagh S, Chesney RW, Langer L, et al: Normal vitamin D metabolism in renal non-responsive, bone-responsive pseudohypoparathyroidism (PHP) manifesting with rickets. Am J Dis Child 138:1030, 1984.
48. Drezner MD, Haussler MR: Normocalcemic pseudohypoparathyroidism. Association with normal vitamin D_3 metabolism. Am J Med 66:503, 1979.
49. Drezner MK, Neelon FA, Haussler M, et al: 1,25-Dihydroxycholecalciferol deficiency: The probable cause of hypocalcemia and metabolic bone disease in pseudohypoparathyroidism. J Clin Endocrinol Metab 46:621, 1976.
50. Ross EM, Gilman AG: Biochemical properties of hormone-sensitive adenylate cyclase. Ann Rev Biochem 49:533, 1980.
51. Farfel Z, Brickman AS, Kaslow HR, et al: Defect of receptor-cyclase coupling protein in pseudohypoparathyroidism. N Engl J Med 303:237, 1980.
52. Farfel Z, Bourne HR: Pseudohypoparathyroidism: Mutation affecting adenylate cyclase. Min Elec Metab 8:227, 1982.
53. Downs RW Jr, Levine MA, Drezner MK, et al: Deficient adenylate cyclase regulatory protein in renal membranes from a patient with pseudohypoparathyroidism. J Clin Invest 71:231, 1983.
54. Markus R, Wilber JF, Aurbach GD: Parathyroid hormone-sensitive adenyl cyclase from the renal cortex of a patient with pseudohypoparathyroidism. J Clin Endocrinol Metab 33:537, 1981.
55. Levine MA, Downs RW, Lasker RD, et al: Resistance to multiple hormones in pseudohypoparathyroidism and deficient guanine nucleotide regulatory protein (abstract). Clin Res 29:412A, 1981.
56. Monn E, Osnes JB, Oye I, et al: Pseudohypoparathyroidism. Acta Pediatr Scand 65:487, 1976.
57. Mann JB, Alderman S, Hills AG: Albright's hereditary osteodystrophy and pseudohypoparathyroidism. Ann Intern Med 50:315, 1962.
58. Fitch N: Albright's hereditary osteodystrophy: A review. Am J Med Genet 11:11, 1982.
59. Kooh SW, Fraser D, DeLuca HF, et al: Treatment of hypoparathyroidism and pseudohypoparathyroidism with metabolites of vitamin D: Evidence for impaired conversion of 25-hydroxyvitamin D to 1α,25-dihydroxyvitamin D. N Engl J Med 293:840, 1975.
60. Stogmann, W, Fischer JA: Pseudohypoparathyroidism: Disappearance of the resistance to parathyroid extract during treatment with vitamin D. Am J Med 59:140, 1975.
61. Roy S III, Stapleton FB, Noe NH, et al: Hematuria preceding renal calculus formation in children with hypercalciuria. J Pediatr 99:712, 1981.
62. Greer F, Chesney RW: Calcium disorders in the neonate. In Kurtzman NA, Moore ES (eds): Seminars in Nephrology—Pediatric Nephrology: Rose of the Kidney in Mineral Homeostasis in Early Life. New York, Grune & Stratton, 1983, p 100.
63. Humes HD, Ichikawa I, Troy JL, et al: Evidence for a parathyroid hormone-dependent influence of calcium on the glomerular ultrafiltration coefficient. J Clin Invest 61:32, 1978.
64. Bell PD, Navar LG: Intrarenal feedback control of glomerular filtration rate. Semin Nephrol 2:289, 1982.
65. DeRubertis FR, Craven PA: Prostaglandin metabolism in the kidney: Physiologic implications. Semin Nephrol 2:302, 1982.
66. Chesney RW, Friedman AL: Chapters on hypertensive emergencies, maintenance fluid needs, dehydration fluid needs, disorders of sodium and potassium metabolism, disorders of calcium metabolism and acute renal failure. In Cohen S (ed): Handbook of Emergency Pediatrics. New York, Prentice-Hall, 1982, p 147, 178.
67. Harrison HE, Harrison HC: Disorders of calcium and phosphate metabolism in childhood and adolescence. Philadelphia, W. B. Saunders, 1979, p 100.
68. Fraser D, Kidd BSL, Kooh SW, et al: A new look at infantile hypercalcemia. Pediatr Clin N Am 13:503, 1966.
69. Fanconi G, Giradet P, Schlesinger B, et al: Chronische hypercalcamie, lobiniert mit osteosklerose, hyperazotamie, minderwuchs und kongenitalen missbildungen. Helv Paediatr Acta 4:314, 1952.
70. Lightwood R: Idiopathic hypercalcaemia with failure to thrive. Arch Dis Child 27:302, 1952.
71. Smith DW, Blizzard RM, Harrison HE: Idiopathic hypercalcemia: A case report with assays of vitamin D in the serum. Pediatrics 24:258, 1959.
72. Aarskog D, Asknes L, Markestad T: Vitamin D metabolism in idiopathic infantile hypercalcemia. Am J Dis Child 135:1021, 1981.
73. Fellers FX, Schwartz R: Etiology of the severe form of idiopathic hypercalcemia of infancy. N Engl J Med 259:1050, 1958.
74. Williams JCP, Barratt-Boyes BG, Lowe JB: Supravalvular aortic stenosis. Circulation 24:1311, 1961.
75. Black JA, Bonham Carter RE: Association between aortic stenosis and facies of severe infantile hypercalcemia. Lancet 2:745, 1963.
76. Jones KL, Smith DW: The Williams elfin facies syndrome: A new perspective. J Pediatr 86:718, 1975.
77. Taylor AB, Stern PH, Bell NH: Abnormal regulation of circulating 25-hydroxyvitamin D in the William's syndrome. N Engl J Med 306:972, 1982.
78. Friedman WF, Roberts WC: Vitamin D and the supravalvular aortic stenosis syndrome: The transplacental effects of vitamin D on the aorta of the rabbit. Circulation 34:77, 1966.
79. Beuren AJ, Schulze C, Eberle P, Harmjanz D: Syndrome of supravalvular aortic stenosis, peripheral pulmonary stenosis, mental retardation and similar facial appearance. Am J Cardiol 13:471, 1964.
80. Weisman Y, Harell A, Edelstein S: Infantile hypercalcemia: A defect in the esterification of 1,25-dihydroxyvitamin D? Med Hypoth 5:379, 1979.
81. Diager SP, Miller M, Romeo G, et al: Vitamin D binding protein in the William's syndrome and idiopathic hypercalcemia. N Engl J Med 298:687, 1978.
82. Forbes GB, Bryson MF, Manning J, et al: Impaired calcium homeostasis in the infantile hypercalcemic syndrome. Acta Paediatr Scand 61:305, 1972.
83. Michael AF, Hong R, West CD: Hypercalcemia in infancy. Am J Dis Child 104:235, 1962.
84. Veldhuis JD, Kulin HE, Demers LM, et al: Infantile hypercalcemia with subcutaneous fat necrosis: Endocrine studies. J Pediatr 95:460, 1979.
85. Rasmussen H, Bartter FC: Hypophosphatasia. In Stanbury JB, et al (eds): The Metabolic Basis of Inherited Disease, ed 4. New York, McGraw-Hill, 1978, p 1340.
86. Mulivor RA, Mennuti M, Zackai EH, et al: Prenatal diagnosis of hypophosphatasia: Genetic, biochemical and clinical studies. Am J Hum Genet 30:271, 1978.
87. Fraser D: Hypophosphatasia. Am J Med 22:730, 1957.
88. Vanneuville FJ, Leroy JG: Enzymatic diagnosis of congenital lethal hypophosphatasia in tissues, plasma and diploid skin fibroblasts. J Inher Metab Dis 4:129, 1981.
89. Opshaug O, Maurseth K, Howlid H, et al: Vitamin D metabolism in hypophosphatasia: Case report. Acta Paediatr Scand 71:517, 1982.
90. Whyte MP, Seino Y: Circulating vitamin D metabolite levels in hypophosphatasia. J Clin Endocrinol Metab 55:178, 1982.

91. Wolfish NM, Heick H: Hyperparathyroidism and infantile hypophosphatasia: Effect of prednisone and vitamin K therapy. J Pediatr 95:1079, 1979.
92. Whyte MP, Valdes R, Ryan LM, et al: Infantile hypophosphatasia: Enzyme replacement therapy by intravenous infusion of alkaline phosphatase-rich plasma from patients with Paget bone disease. J Pediatr 101:379, 1982.
93. Foley TP, Harrison HC, Arnaud CD, et al: Familial benign hypercalcemia. J Pediatr 31:1060, 1972.
94. Marx SJ, Spiegel AM, Levine MA, et al: Familial hypocalciuric hypercalcemia: The relation to primary parathyroid hyperplasia. N Engl J Med 307:416, 1982.
95. Marx SJ, Attie MF, Levine MA, et al: The hypocalciuric or benign variant of familial hypercalcemia: Clinical and biochemical features in fifteen kindreds. Medicine 60:397, 1981.
96. Davies M, Klimiuk PS, Adams PH, et al: Familial hypocalciuric hypercalcaemia and acute pancreatitis. Brit Med J 282:1023, 1981.
97. Thorgeirsson U, Costa J, Marx SJ: The parathyroid glands in familial hypocalciuric hypercalcemia. Human Pathol 12:229, 1981.
98. Marx SJ, Attie MF, Spiege AM, et al: An association between neonatal severe primary hyperparathyroidism and familial hypocalciuric hypercalcemia in three kindreds. N Engl J Med 306:257, 1982.

CHAPTER 33

Disorders of Renal Tubular Handling of Sodium and Potassium

MICHAEL J. DILLON

INTRODUCTION

The pathological states associated with hypokalemia and hyperkalemia are inseparably linked to disturbances of sodium (Na) and hydrogen ion balance. It is therefore difficult to consider them in isolation, even though, at times, the biochemical changes may predominantly involve one cation. The primary object of this chapter is to discuss disorders in renal tubular handling of Na and potassium (K) in which hypokalemia and hyperkalemia are striking manifestations. Among the hypokalemic states, Bartter's syndrome and similar disorders will be emphasized and the hyperkalemic conditions will encompass those associated with mineralocorticoid deficiency or unresponsiveness.

HYPOKALEMIC STATES

If inadequate dietary intake, gastrointestinal and skin loss, and certain conditions associated with redistribution of K from extracellular fluid (ECF) to intracellular fluid (ICF) are excluded, hypokalemia may be considered under intrinsic and extrinsic defects of renal K conservation. The intrinsic category includes Bartter's and related syndromes, the Fanconi syndrome, renal tubular acidosis (RTA), and certain other renal parenchymal disorders. Within the extrinsic category are primary mineralocorticoid excess as a result of Conn's syndrome, Cushing's syndrome, cortisol IIβ hydroxysteroid dehydrogenase deficiency, and secondary mineralocorticoid excess associated with increased renin production. Pharmacological and osmotic diuretics, nonreabsorbable anion administration, e.g., penicillin, and ketoacidosis are often extrinsic causes of kaliuresis and hypokalemia (chapter 7).

Intrinsic Defects of K Conservation

Intrinsic defects of K conservation implies primary defects in renal tubular function resulting in, among other things, K deficiency but excluding conditions classified as extrinsic. For descriptions of Fanconi syndrome and distal renal tubular acidosis, see Chapters 30 and 34, respectively.

Bartter's Syndrome

In 1962, Bartter and coworkers (1) described a new syndrome of growth and mental retardation, hypokalemic alkalosis, increased aldosterone secretion rate, and increased plasma angiotensin II concentration in the presence of normal blood pressure. Juxtaglomerular cell hyperplasia was seen on renal biopsy, a pitressin-resistant hyposthenuria was demonstrated, and there was decreased pressor responsiveness to infused angiotensin II. Since that time, many reports have appeared in the literature describing a wide spectrum of clinical and biochemical features that are considered to be manifestations of this condition. This diversity has raised some doubt as to whether the term "Bartter's syndrome" is applicable to all the patients reported, which in turn has created difficulties in identifying criteria for diagnosis. For the diagnosis of Bartter's syndrome to be seriously considered the following must be present: hypokalemia, hypochloremia, alkalosis, hyperreninemia in the presence of a normal blood pressure, and elevated urinary K and Cl excretion in the absence of other conditions that might cause similar features. The diagnosis is therefore still one of exclusion even though a degree of specificity has been applied to certain biochemical investigations in recent years.

In addition to the basic components of the syndrome, a number of other clinical and biochemical findings have been described. Some of these are probably essential aspects of Bartter's syndrome and help in understanding the pathophysiology of the condition; others may serve to distinguish between the "classic" syndrome and "Bartter-like" disorders; still others are just epiphenomena. The basic components are evidence of defective proximal and/or distal renal tubular handling of Na and K (2–11), abnormal chloride (Cl) reabsorption in the ascending limb of the loop of Henle (8, 11, 12), and abnormal intracellular electrolyte concentrations in red cells (13–16) and muscle cells (18, 19). In addition, the following are reported: abnormal red cell Na and K transport (13, 15, 16, 19–21); hypercalcemia (22); hypophosphatemia (22–26); hypercalciuria; nephrocalcinosis and progressive impairment of renal function (14, 22); rickets (22–24); magnesium (Mg) deficiency (27); defective renal tubular acidification (28, 29); excess renal prostaglandin production with response to prostaglandin synthetase inhibitors (9, 20, 22, 30–40); abnormalities of skin fibroblast prostaglandin production (41); defects in platelet aggregation (20, 42, 43); abnormalities of the kallikrein-kinin system (34, 44–46); renal biopsy abnormalities (1, 2, 25, 47); a circulating inhibitor of phytohemagglutinin-induced lymphocyte proliferation (48); a familial incidence (9, 20, 22, 49–52); a characteristic facial appearance (49); and several odd clinical features including chondrocalcinosis (22, 53).

Clinical Features. The majority of patients present with failure to thrive, vomiting, and constipation during the first 2 years of life. The most common age of onset of symptoms is between 6 to 12 months of age (22); there may be a preceding history of hydramnios during the pregnancy. There may be evidence of clinical ECF volume depletion with complaints of fatigue, muscle cramps, polydipsia, and polyuria. Developmental delay, although initially reported by Bartter (1) is variable. The majority of these features are explained by the renal tubular dysfunction cited above and the effects of K deficiency and hypokalemia. Rickets may be present (22–24); occasionally there is a history of carpopedal spasm (9). Some patients have a distinctive facial appearance characterised by prominence of the forehead, triangular facies, drooping mouth, large eyes, and pinnae (49).

The patients are normotensive; an increased blood pressure casts considerable doubt on the diagnosis. Occasionally a child who is asymptomatic might be identified by a routine investigation revealing hypokalaemic alkalosis (22). Most affected sibships are symptomatic (9, 20, 49–51), although in one family neither affected child had obvious symptoms (22).

Biochemical and Laboratory Findings. The characteristic laboratory abnormality is hypokalemia accompanied by alkalosis and increased fractional urinary excretion of K and Cl. Evidence of urinary Na wasting may be present, although some patients conserve Na appropriately when they are placed on a low Na diet. Hypercalciuria, seen in up to 50% of cases (14, 22, 29), may be linked to the association between Na and Ca excretion secondary to the effect natriuresis has on Ca reabsorption in the proximal tubule. Pitressin-resistant hyposthenuria is often present and may be severe enough to cause polyuria. It is, however, interesting that maximal free-water clearance also may be reduced and patients may have difficulty in producing extremely dilute urine under conditions of hypotonic saline loading (4, 8). Several patients have been reported with hypercalcemia. The etiology of this is not clear, but it has been proposed that alkalosis may modify protein binding of Ca (54) and in at least one case ionized Ca was normal (22). An alternative explanation for the hypercalcemia is excess bone release under the influence of prostaglandins (55). Hypophosphatemia, phosphaturia and florid rickets have been reported (22, 23). Mg depletion with or without evidence of excessive urinary Mg loss is well recognized in Bartter's syndrome (20, 27, 56). It is still unclear whether this is related to hyperaldosteronism (55) or a primary abnormality of tubular magnesium handling. It may contribute to hypokalemia; magnesium supplementation in affected patients has led to an increase in plasma potassium (27, 56). Hypomagnesemia in patients with Bartter's syndrome needs to be distinguished from primary disorders of renal Mg wasting in which hypokalemia also occurs (vide infra) (57–60).

Some patients with Bartter's syndrome have presented with a defect of urinary acidification or have been shown to have such a defect on ammonium-chloride loading (20, 22, 28, 29, 61). The significance of these observations is controversial, and it has been considered that patients with acidification defects may not be examples of Bartter's syndrome but of incomplete distal renal tubular acidosis (RTA) (62–64). However, there are those patients who in spite of the similarity to incomplete distal renal tubular acidosis, fulfill in other respects the criteria for the diagnosis of Bartter's syndrome (20, 22, 28, 61). In these it is possible that the minimal inadequacy of urine acidification under conditions of acid loading is related to a decrease in ammonium excretion or a decrease in the rate of distal hydrogen ion secretion rather than an inability to generate a steep pH gradient across the distal nephron (65). This defect may be identified by demonstrating an inability of urine to blood P_{CO_2} gradient to increase appropriately with bicarbonate loading (66). There are reports of patients with evidence of other renal tubular disturbances, e.g., mild glycosuria or aminoaciduria, which need to be distinguished from that resulting from the Fanconi syndrome (22, 23).

Hyperreninemia is consistently present and this is accompanied in some children by high plasma aldosterone levels. However, in others, possibly a result of the low plasma K, plasma aldosterone is suppressed yet increases subsequently when hypokalemia is corrected (22). An infusion of angiotensin II is associated with a blunted increase in blood pressure in patients with Bartter's syndrome, but this lack of response is not diagnostic; it may reflect sodium depletion (2).

Urine prostaglandins PGE_2 and PGF_2 alpha, which are principally derived from renal synthesis, are increased in most patients with Bartter's syndrome (32, 33, 40). Urine 6-keto-PGF_1 alpha, the metabolite of prostacyclin, may be increased (39) but plasma levels are normal (20, 67). The therapeutic use of prostaglandin synthetase inhibitors has been associated with significant decreases in urine prostaglandin values, but controversy still exists concerning the role of prostaglandins in the etiology of the syndrome. Basal release of PGE_2 from cultured skin fibroblasts is reduced in patients compared to controls, but bradykinin-stimulated release of prostacyclin is higher. The reasons for these differences are not clear, although the permeability of cell membranes to potassium may play a part (41). A defect in the first and second phase of platelet aggregation response to ADP, epinephrine, collagen, and thrombin has been reported (20, 42). This effect may be related to Na depletion, for it improves when supplementary salt is given (42).

The renal handling of water and electrolytes in response to hypotonic saline loading have demonstrated characteristic abnormalities in Bartter's syndrome (4, 68); the fractional excretion of NaCl and K and the osmolar clearance (Cosm) is increased. Maximal free-water clearance (CH_2O) is decreased (8, 11, 20). Fractional reabsorption of electrolytes from the proximal tubule is normal in most patients, but reabsorption of Na, K, and Cl from the ascending limb of the loop of Henle is decreased (8, 9, 11). The administration of indomethacin to these patients increases proximal tubule reabsorption of Na, Cl and K during hypotonic saline loading (11) although the distal tubular reabsorptive defect is not corrected. However, in some patients reabsorption of electrolytes from the proximal tubule is decreased and this finding appears to be associated with a blunted response to indomethacin treatment.

Abnormalities in cation content and in cation transport properties of red blood cells (RBC) have been described in patients with Bartter's syndrome. The RBC level of Na is increased or the level of K is decreased for most but not all patients (16, 19, 20, 21, 30, 38); muscle cell cations are similarly affected (18).

The permeability of the RBC membrane to Na measured in a number of ways is increased (13, 16, 19–21, 69). Active Na and K transport of RBC is decreased (13, 20), and the number of ouabain-sensitive Na pump sites is reduced (20, 69).

Response to therapy has varied. K supplementation has increased muscle K (18); sodium supplementation did not affect RBC Na or K (20). Indomethacin corrects the intracellular cation abnormalities (20, 30, 38), but has little effect on membrane cation transport properties (16, 20).

Renal biopsy findings are variable. Juxtaglomerular cell (1) and renomedullary cell hyperplasia (30) are present with varying degrees of glomerular hyalinization and atrophy (1, 2) and tubular atrophy and vacuolization (2, 25).

Diagnosis. The diagnosis in Bartter's syndrome is made when the following criteria are met: hypokalemia; hypochloremic alkalosis, with elevated urinary potassium and chloride; and hyperreninemia in the presence of normal blood pressure. The differential diagnosis includes the Fanconi syndrome, incomplete distal RTA (29, 61), use of diuretics (70), laxative abuse (71), cyclical vomiting (72), chloride deficient diets (73), cystic fibrosis (74), alkalosis associated with administration of impermeable anions (75), mineralocorticoid excess (76), and primary Mg-losing kidney disease, i.e., Gitelman's syndrome (57).

Aminoaciduria and glycosuria point to the Fanconi syndrome; hyperchloremic acidosis points to distal RTA. A low urine chloride would be suggestive of laxative abuse, cyclical vomiting, dietary chloride deficiency, or cystic fibrosis. The history of administration of an anion, such as sulphate or carbenicillin, may be available, and hypertension may point to a mineralocorticoid excess state.

The most difficult entity to distinguish from Bartter's syndrome is Gitelman's syndrome associated with renal Mg wasting with excessive urinary losses of Mg (57–60). These patients are often hypocalcemic and may present with tetany. Hypokalemia usually is present; plasma-renin activity (PRA) and aldosterone concentration are increased, but less so when compared with the values characteristic of Bartter's syndrome. A moderate defect in distal tubular electrolyte reabsorption is demonstrable during hypotonic saline loading, similar to but less than that reported in patients with Bartter's syndrome (67). Nephrocalcinosis, interstitial nephropathy, and impaired renal function are present in some patients. Oligospermia and osteochondrosis have been reported (60). The condition is characterized by a primary defect in renal tubular reabsorption of magnesium, but the site of the defect is not known. The disorder is familial and apparently genetically transmitted. Management consists of magnesium supplementation.

Treatment. Treatment of Bartter's syndrome, although not fully satisfactory, has improved over the last 8 years. K and NaCl supplementation and K-sparing diuretics, e.g., spironolactone and triamterine, improve the clinical state (1, 50, 78). K supplementation is required in the majority of patients; NaCl supplementation is required in some. Renin-suppressing agents, e.g., methyldopa (79) and propranolol (78), do not appear to help.

Indomethacin, the prostaglandin synthetase inhibitor (30, 31), has improved results considerably. Hypokalemia has been corrected and catch-up weight gain and growth in stature has occurred. The patients have thrived (22). In some patients, notably those with reduced glomerular filtration rate (GFR), function decreased. Indomethacin appears to act by redistributing renal tubular blood flow and by improving proximal renal tubular reabsorption. The distal tubular defect in Cl reabsorption (8, 11) and the RBC membrane transport defect (69) persist, whereas intracellular Na decreases (69) toward normal. In some patients clinical and biochemical relapse (80) occurs even though prostaglandin levels remain suppressed; in others, clinical improvement occurs but prostaglandins are not suppressed (22). Other drugs that inhibit prostaglandin synthesis, e.g., aspirin, ketoprofen, and ibuprofen (32, 34, 37) have not been more effective than indomethacin.

Indomethacin is given in a daily dose of 2 to 5 mg/kg/day in 4 to 6 doses daily. Patients tolerate indomethacin well with few side effects. Occasionally gastrointestinal intolerance occurs, but resolves with reduction of dose. Decreases in GFR that occur with treatment usually improve with reduction or discontinuation of therapy. There is as yet no satisfactory evidence that treatment has modified mental development or improved renal function in those patients in whom mental development or renal function were impaired. Some patients require Mg, phosphate, or vitamin D supplementation when signs of deficiencies of any of these develop.

Causal Theories. There is yet no unifying hypothesis that explains the range of abnormalities seen in Bartter's syndrome. Initially, Bartter (1) considered the disorder to be one in which there was a defect in pressor response to angiotensin II, which resulted in hypotension leading to secondary hyperreninemia and aldosteronism. The latter, it was felt, caused the hypokalemia and potassium deficiency, which, in turn, resulted in the defect in urine concentration. Later, some form of primary hyperreninemia was considered to be the proximal cause (78), but this seemed unlikely when treatment of affected patients with renin suppressant agents failed to modify the abnormalities (78).

The increase in urinary prostaglandin and the effect of indomethacin have led to the proposal that a disturbance in prostaglandin synthesis at some site is the primary cause of the syndrome (9, 20, 22, 28, 30–41). However, several findings mitigate against this hypothesis: (i) the inconsistent prostaglandin levels (36), (ii) the clinical and biochemical escape that occurs when patients are on chronic indomethacin therapy, although urinary prostaglandins remain low (80), and (iii) the lack of improvement when urinary prostaglandins are suppressed with mepacrine (9). Furthermore, prostaglandin synthetase inhibition does not correct the tubular defect in chloride reabsorption (8, 11) or the changes in RBC Na flux even though it does improve intracellular Na concentration (69). The observations on skin fibroblast showing basal PGE_2 to be reduced and stimulated PGI_2 release to be increased in Bartter patients, however, need to be carefully considered, since these might point to a primary defect in prostaglandin synthesis (41).

The abnormalities of renal tubular function have been considered to be the prime defect (2–11), although there is controversy as to which of these tubular dysfunctions is the critical abnormality. The defect in Cl reabsorption in the ascending limb of the loop of Henle associated with passive loss of sodium and potassium is a current hypothesis. Indomethacin does not affect the defect. This defect, demonstrated by hypotonic saline loading, has been reported in two studies (8, 11). It has been proposed that all the other pathophysiological features could be secondary to this abnormality. However, some doubt has been cast on this finding because it is much less evident when fractional electrolyte reabsorption is measured during water rather than hypotonic saline diuresis (20). The findings can be explained by a defect in cell wall electrolyte transport affecting muscle, RBC, and renal tubule cells. This explanation currently fits the clinical and biochemical features of the condition most accurately.

Prognosis. Before the use of indomethacin many patients with Bartter's syndrome were chronically ill throughout childhood and were at risk of dying from episodes of electrolyte imbalance. Those that survived these episodes failed to thrive and some were mentally retarded. Since PG synthetase–inhibiting drugs have been used, the outlook for patients is better. Most children whose electrolyte imbalance is controlled have the potential to attain normal stature and to maintain normal kidney function. Some gradually develop chronic renal failure usually associated with nephrocalcinosis (14, 18, 22). Currently we recommend that patients remain on indomethacin until growth is complete. Asymptomatic adults of normal height appear to require no form of therapy (22).

HYPERKALEMIC STATES

Hyperkalemia may be caused by renal failure, either acute or chronic, because GFR has diminished to such an extent that the potential for K secretion to balance intake is insufficient; the need for dialysis is imminent unless K intake can be reduced. However, hyperkalemia in chronic renal insufficiency may develop before this occurs because the tubule becomes unresponsive to aldosterone, a form of acquired pseudohypoaldosteronism, or because hyporeninemic hypoaldosteronism develops (81, 82). The majority of children with persistent hyperkalemia in the absence of chronic renal failure or iatrogenic potassium oversupplementation have adrenal disease or some form of tubular unresponsiveness to aldosterone's action.

Mineralocorticoid Deficiency

Several adrenal disorders are associated with inadequate production of aldosterone. They are nearly always associated with salt-wasting and can be considered under the headings of congenital adrenal hypoplasia, congenital adrenal hyperplasia, Addison's disease, and isolated defects of aldosterone biosynthesis.

Congenital Adrenal Hypoplasia

Affected children present in early infancy with a hyperkalemic, salt-wasting state, but without evidence of virilization (83). Both mineralocorticoid and glucocorticoid synthesis are impaired, and investigations demonstrate that PRA is increased but plasma aldosterone (PA) is inappropriately low (84). There is evidence of glucocorticoid failure as well. Urinary values of glucocorticoid and mineralocorticoid metabolites are low and precursors are not present in excess.

Treatment with NaCl, hydrocortisone and mineralocorticoid replacement therapy—either DOCA or 9 alpha-fludrocortisone—is successful in reversing the clinical abnormalities. The condition may be sporadic or familial. There are three anatomical variants: (i) the "anencephalic" pattern resembling the adrenals seen in anencephaly, (ii) the "cytomegalic" pattern only seen in males, and (iii) the "miniature" pattern. Of these the "anencephalic" pattern seems to be inherited on a recessive basis, and the "cytomegalic" and "miniature" forms on an X-linked basis, although all three can occur sporadically. See Forest (85) for a review of this subject.

Congenital Adrenal Hyperplasia

Most cases of congenital adrenal hyperplasia associated with hyperkalemia are a result of 21-hydroxylase deficiency. Patients with 21-hydroxylase deficiency have been divided into those who are overt salt wasters and those who are not. A majority of patients have a tendency for salt wasting, but the tendency varies in severity (86, 87). In some patients, salt wasting is suspected by the clinical signs of ECF volume contraction, i.e., loss of skin turgor and hypotension. Hyponatremia and hyperkalemia are present and urinary sodium chloride excretion is inappropriately high. In other patients salt wasting is less obvious. In some, PA may be normal, but the PRA is high, i.e., although the PA value is within the normal range it is inappropriately low in relation to the simultaneously measured PRA and the degree of salt wasting (84). Those classified as salt wasters have a marked defect in aldosterone synthesis. In these patients ECF volume contraction often becomes apparent toward the end of the first week of life and is associated with an increase in precursors of cortisol such as 17-hydroxyprogesterone (88, 89). These precursors have natriuretic effects in their own right. In the infant, Na reabsorption under aldosterone control in the distal nephron is proportionally greater than normal so that the natriuresis is exaggerated; hyperkalemia develops, PRA increases, and PA is inappropriately low (84, 87). PA may not be absolutely low—it is low in comparison with the elevated PRA. In patients who do not show clinical signs of ECF volume contraction, an increased PRA indicates that Na homeostasis is impaired (87).

Children with 21-hydroxylase deficiency should be treated with NaCl supplementation, physiological doses of hydrocortisone, and either DOCA, aldosterone or 9 alpha-fludrocortisone. NaCl should replace urinary salt losses. In the neonatal period infusion of NaCl may be necessary. Pharmacological doses of cortisone are not required unless the infant is stressed. Glucorcorticoid administration should suppress the corticotropin-releasing factor sufficiently to normalize ACTH levels. The dose may be adjusted by the plasma levels of ACTH and androgens or urinary steroid levels and should be such that it does not suppress growth. The dose of glucocorticoid is adjusted as the individual grows (90). It is customary to express the dose as a function of surface area.

The question of how long mineralocorticoid therapy should be used is controversial. There is no doubt that it is indicated in patients with salt depletion and hyperkalemia who become symptomatic in the first week of life. There is disagreement about its use in the child with less obvious salt depletion. We recommend that when patients are treated the dose of mineralocorticoid be adjusted by following PRA values. The appropriate dose is associated with normal PRA values; an overdose by its suppression to low values.

Mineralocorticoid treatment has in the past been withdrawn as the child reaches 3 to 4 years of age (91). This practice was based on the ability of these children to remain in sodium balance at this age under normal conditions. This is a mistake. The maturation of the proximal nephron and the tendency for dietary salt to increase may sustain salt balance in the absence of stress, but most of these patients retain their tendency for salt wasting (92). All patients who have 21-hydroxylase deficiency should be treated with mineralocorticoids (86). Treatment safeguards these children against sudden salt-wasting crises associated with an intercurrent illness at a time when their cortisol requirements may increase and natriuretic steroids reappear in the circulation (93). The requirement for hydrocortisone is reduced and the adverse effect this drug has on growth is lessened (87). Hyperreninemia stimulates ACTH production and directly affects the production of steroid precursors of cortisol (94). This leads to a loss of glucocorticoid control. Therefore mineralocorticoid therapy should be given always and supplemental salt adjusted to a point where PRA is within the normal range.

Isolated Defects of Aldosterone Biosynthesis

Isolated defects of aldosterone biosynthesis other than 21-hydroxylase deficiency also cause hyperkalemia. The defects occur towards the end of the aldosterone biosynthetic pathway (chapter 7). In 1964, Visser and Cost (95) reported an 18-oxidation defect in infants with a salt-wasting syndrome, which subsequently was shown to be a defect in 18-hydroxylation (96). A 5-month-old infant with identical clinical findings had a defect in 18-dehydrogenation of corticosterone (97), i.e., there were at least two sites where the 18-oxidation step was blocked that could result in inadequate aldosterone synthesis.

Several subsequent reports have confirmed the 18-dehydrogenation defects (98–101). Recently Ulick (102) suggested that the mechanism involves a defect in corticosterone methyloxidase. Type I (CMOI) converts corticosterone to a transient, oxygenated steroid-metallo enzyme complex, which is substrate for a second oxidase (CMOII). A second hydroxylation here precedes spontaneous dehydration to aldehyde. A defect in CMOII leads to decomposition to the labile intermediate, and with the formation of 18-hydroxycorticosterone.

Children with these disorders usually present in early infancy with severe hyperkalemia and salt wasting. Occasionally they have a less dramatic course, presenting at a few months of age with unexplained failure to thrive (100). There is no evidence of virilization. Glucocorticoid patterns and renal function are normal. PRA is high and PA levels are low (100). Urinary levels of aldosterone and aldosterone metabolites (tetrahydro aldosterone) are low; the urinary levels of aldosterone precursors are high depending on the site of the enzymatic block (103). Analyses of urine for steroids by gas chromatographic and mass spectrometric techniques are at the limit of methodological sensitivity. Interpretation is made more difficult by the fact that urinary steroid excretion patterns vary with age. In the newborn and young infant, a knowledge of the normal patterns of excretion is essential before attempting to define the abnormality (104, 105). These values are influenced when extraneous steroids are administered.

Affected children sometimes present with febrile episodes unassociated with infection and not a result of dehydration (95, 100). These febrile attacks may be precipitated by pyrogenic metabolites of precursors of aldosterone with similar structure to etiocholanolone (106). Aldosterone deficiency is treated with NaCl supplements—often large quantities, e.g., 20 mmol/kg/day in infants—and mineralocorticoid replacement also in large amounts (100), e.g., up to 0.5 mg of 9 alpha-fludrocortisone per day is sometimes needed initially to sustain normal ECF volume. The need for the high dose is a result of the competitive effect of aldosterone precursors on mineralocorticoid given as replacement therapy. After some months, 9 alpha-fludrocortisone can be reduced to maintenance requirements, 0.05 mg/day. The defect is lifelong. While it has been shown that children can stop mineralocorticoid therapy, at 12 to 18 months of age they retain the tendency to lose salt (101). This is analogous to the situation described in 21-hydroxylase deficiency; the proximal tubule matures and salt intake increases. Withdrawal of mineralocorticoid is not advisable; we recommend continuing mineralocorticoid therapy for life (100). It appears that 18-oxidation defects are inherited on an autosomal recessive basis (95, 98).

Addison's Disease. This form of primary chronic adrenocorticoid insufficiency is rare but important to recognize. In the past the main cause was tuberculosis; now "autoimmune adrenalitis" is the more common cause (85). This may be isolated or associated with other endocrine diseases, such as hypoparathyroidism, hypothyroidism, or diabetes mellitus (85). Antiadrenal antibodies are found in the circulation, but do not correlate with the severity of the adrenal disease (107). Familial occurrence is frequent (108) and the inheritance of the abnormality of immune response is probably autosomal recessive although females are more affected (109).

Clinical features are related to deficiency of glucocorticoid and mineralocorticoid hormones—hyperpigmentation, hypoglycemia, gastrointestinal disturbances, and progressive weakness (85). Characteristic laboratory findings include hyponatremia, hyperkalemia, and hypoglycemia. Plasma ACTH is increased, and there is no rise of plasma cortisol to ACTH stimulation; PRA is high and PA is low. Precursors to glucocorticoid or mineralocorticoid biosynthesis will be low or absent. Treatment consists of cortisol replacement, 12–15 $mg/m^2/day$ or its equivalent and 9 alpha-fludrocortisone 0.05 to 0.2 mg/day. Adrenal crises because of salt wasting or hypoglycemia occur and require intravenous isotonic saline, glucose, and additional glucocorticoid. Patients with Addison's disease given correct treatment live a normal life.

Adrenal leukodystrophy (Addison-Schilder's disease) (110) is an important condition to be differentiated from isolated Addison's disease. It is characterised by progressive neurological disease associated with primary adrenal insufficiency. A sex-linked inheritance occurs affecting male children. At present no therapy is effective in arresting the progressive neurological disease.

Mineralocorticoid Unresponsiveness

Pseudohypoaldosteronism

Pseudohypoaldosteronism (PHA) presents in a fashion identical to that described for 18-oxidation defect, i.e., failure to thrive, hyperkalemia, and a salt-wasting state. It was first reported by Cheek and Perry in 1958 (111), who noted that mineralocorticoid therapy seemed to be ineffective and did not modify the urine $Na+/K+$ ratio. Since that time, many cases have been reported (112–135). Although plasma electrolyte findings are similar to those seen in 18-oxidation defects, there are certain distinguishing features. First, both PRA and PA levels are markedly increased, and, second, urinary steroid analysis reveals increased amounts of aldosterone metabolites in a characteristic pattern (117, 131, 135).

The condition is a result of renal tubular unresponsiveness to aldosterone. There is some doubt about where in the nephron the NaCl losses take place; initially the distal tubule was considered the likely site (111); more recent observations implicate a more proximal site (127, 129, 136). The nature of the defect is not defined, but it is thought to be the result of a decrease in Na,K-ATPase in the renal tubule (114).

There is overlap between PHA and childhood type 4 RTA (137, 138) (chapter 34). The latter characteristically is not associated with overt salt wasting, but there is reduced tubular responsiveness to aldosterone. PRA and urinary aldosterone excretion are increased even though superficially there is only a defect of distal tubular $H+$ and $K+$ secretion (139). Children with type 4 RTA also are growth retarded and have frequent bouts of vomiting (138). Hyperchloremic and hyperkalemic acidosis with aciduria are the laboratory features of this disorder. Although salt wasting is not obvious, there is sufficient evidence from the PRA and PA levels to suggest that there is some salt depletion as well. In view of this it seems likely that PHA and early childhood type 4 RTA are similar disorders with differing degrees of salt wasting.

PHA is treated with NaCl supplementation, which expands ECF volume. Tubular flow and delivery of solute to the distal nephron increases creating a favourable gradient for K secretion (140, 141). This occurs in spite of the fact that there is little or no mineralocorticoid stimulation of K secretion. The amount of NaCl required often is large; the correct dose is deduced from the decrease in K and PRA, and from the clinical improvement of the patients who gain weight and thrive (117). By the age of 18 to 24 months, these patients may be able to manage without NaCl supplementation (111, 115, 117, 126). However, as with 18-oxidation defects, the disorder persists for life (124, 129, 142), and the apparent recovery is probably related to proximal tubular maturation and the tendency of the child to ingest more salt. Administering aldosterone or other mineralocorticoid is without effect.

Prostaglandins may play a part in the NaCl wasting that occurs in this condition. In one child with PHA, treatment with indomethacin was successful (127). The drug appears to act by decreasing proximal renal tubular perfusion and improving sodium reabsorption at this site, compensating for more distal losses (77).

Since 1976 several children have been described with PHA in whom there is mineralocorticoid unresponsiveness affecting various target organs including the colon, sweat and salivary glands (123, 135, 143).

It seems likely that the condition is most commonly inherited on an autosomal recessive basis (114, 128), although there are reports by Roy

(129) and Lauras and coworkers (120) that suggest there may be a form transmitted by dominant inheritance as well. PHA may be more common than thought. It can masquerade as congenital adrenal hyperplasia, especially in boys. This may result in unnecessary use of glucocorticoids that may increase the risk of growth retardation. The only appropriate treatment is salt supplementation.

References

1. Bartter FC, Pronove P, Gee JR, et al: Hyperplasia of the juxtaglomerular complex with hyperaldosteronism and hypokalemic alkalosis. Am J Med 33:811, 1962.
2. Cannon PJ, Leeming JM, Sommers SC, et al: Juxtaglomerular cell hyperplasia and secondary hyperaldosteronism (Bartter's syndrome): a reevaluation of the pathophysiology. Medicine (Baltimore) 47:107, 1968.
3. White MG: Bartter's syndrome. A manifestation of renal tubular defects. Arch Int Med 129:41, 1972.
4. Chaimovitz C, Levi J, Better OS, et al: Studies on the site of renal salt loss in a patient with Bartter's syndrome. Pediatr Res 7:89, 1973.
5. Chan JCM, Malakzedah MH, Anand SK: Defect in renal tubular sodium reabsorption in a patient with Bartter's syndrome. Clin Proc Child Hosp Nat Med Cen 31:67, 1975.
6. Bartter FC, Delen CS, Kawasaki T, et al: The adrenal cortex and the kidney. Kidney Int 6:272, 1974.
7. Tomko DJ, Yeh BPY, Falls WF: Bartter's syndrome. Study of a 52-year-old man with evidence of a defect in proximal sodium reabsorption and comments on therapy. Am J Med 61:111, 1976.
8. Gill JR, Bartter FC: Evidence of a prostaglandin independent defect in chloride reabsorption in the loop of Henle as a proximal cause of Bartter's syndrome. Am J Med 65:766, 1978.
9. Delaney VB, Oliver JF, Simms M, et al: Bartter's syndrome: physiological and pharmacological studies. Quart J Med 50:213, 1981.
10. Vribarri J, Alveranga D, Man S, et al: Bartter's syndrome due to a defect in salt reabsorption in the distal convoluted tubule. Nephron 40:52, 1985.
11. Rosa FC, Shah V, Dillon MJ: Effects of indomethacin on GFR, fractional distal delivery and reabsorption in Bartter's syndrome. Int J Ped Nephrol 2:129, 1981.
12. Kurtzman NA, Gutierrez LF: The pathophysiology of Bartter's syndrome. JAMA 234:753, 1975.
13. Gall G, Vaitukaitis J, Haddow JE, et al: Erythrocyte Na flux in a patient with Bartter's syndrome. J Clin Endocrinol Metab 32:562, 1971.
14. McCredie DA, Rotenberg E, Williams AL: Hypercalciuria in potassium-losing nephropathy: a varient of Bartter's syndrome. Aust Paediatr J 10:286, 1974.
15. Oliver JF, Delaney VB, Bourke E: Increased erythrocyte sodium permeability in patients with Bartter's syndrome. Min Elect Metab 1:225, 1978.
16. Cole CH, O'Regan S: Effect of treatment with prostaglandin synthetase inhibitors on the erythrocyte sodium transport abnormality of Bartter's syndrome. Pediatr Res 15:926, 1981.
17. Haljamae H, Enger E, Sigstrom L: Cellular potassium transport and ATPase activity in Bartter's syndrome. Scand J Clin Lab Invest 35:53, 1975.
18. Delaporte C, Stulzaft J, Loirat C, et al: Muscle electrolytes and fluid compartments in six children with Bartter's syndrome. Clin Sci Molecular Med 54:223, 1978.
19. Gardner JD, Simopoulis AP, Lapey A, et al: Altered membrane sodium transport in Bartter's syndrome. J Clin Invest 51:1565, 1972.
20. Solomon LR, Bobinski H, Astley P, et al: Bartter's syndrome—observations on the pathophysiology. Quart J Med 51:251, 1982.
21. Mongeau JG, Garay R, de Mondonca M, et al: Erythrocyte Na+ and K+ transport systems in children with Bartter's syndrome: increase in passive sodium permeability. Kidney Intl 23:530, 1983.
22. Dillon MJ, Shah V, Mitchell MD: Bartter's syndrome: 10 cases in childhood. Results of long term indomethacin therapy. Quart J Med 48:429, 1979.
23. Fricker H, Frey K, Vallotton MB, et al: Bartter-syndrome und tubulare funktionsstorungen. Helv Paediatr Acta 30:61, 1975.
24. Sann L, David L, Bernheim J, et al: Hypophosphatemia and hyperparathyroidism in a case of Bartter's syndrome. Helv Paediatr Acta 33:299, 1978.
25. Arant BS, Brackett NC, Young RB, et al: Case studies of siblings with juxtaglomerular hyperplasia and secondary aldosteronism associated with severe azotemia and renal rickets—Bartter's syndrome or disease? Pediatr 46:344, 1970.
26. Godard C, Vallotton MB, Broyer M, et al: A study of the inhibition of the renin-angiotensin system in renal potassium wasting syndromes, including Bartter's syndrome. Helv Pediatr Acta 27:495, 1972.
27. Mace JW, Hambidge KM, Gotlin RW, et al: Magnesium supplementation in Bartter's syndrome. Arch Dis Childh 48:485, 1973.
28. Donker AJM, de Jong PE, Statins van Eps LW, et al: Indomethacin in Bartter's syndrome. Does the syndrome represent a state of hyperprostaglandinism? Nephron 19:200, 1977.
29. Rodriguez-Soriano J, Vallo A, Oliveros R: Bartter's syndrome presenting with features resembling renal tubular acidosis. Improvement of renal tubular defects by indomethacin. Helv Paediatr Acta 33:141, 1978.
30. Verberckmoes R, Van Damme B, Clement J, et al: Bartter's syndrome with hyperplasia of renomedullary cells: successful treatment with indomethacin. Kidney Intl 9:302, 1976.
31. Fichman MP, Telfer N, Zia P, et al: Role of prostaglandins in the pathogenesis of Bartter's syndrome. Am J Med 60:785, 1976.
32. Gill JR, Frolich JC, Bowden RE, et al: Bartter's syndrome: a disorder characterized by high urinary prostaglandins and a dependence of hyper-reninemia on prostaglandin synthesis. Am J Med 61:43, 1976.
33. Norby L, Lentz R, Flamenbaum W, et al: Prostaglandins and aspirin therapy in Bartter's syndrome. Lancet 2:604, 1976.
34. Halushka PV, Wohltmann H, Privitera PJ, et al: Bartter's syndrome: urinary prostaglandin E-like material and kallikrein; indomethacin effects. Ann Intern Med 87:281, 1977.
35. Bowden RE, Gill JR, Radfar N, et al: Prostaglandin synthetase inhibitors in Bartter's syndrome. JAMA 239:117, 1978.
36. Dray F: Bartter's syndrome: contrasting patterns of prostaglandin excretion in children and adults. Clin Sci Molecular Med 54:115, 1978.
37. Littlewood JM, Lee MR, Meadow SR: Treatment of Bartter's syndrome in early childhood with prostaglandin synthetase inhibitors. Arch Dis Childh 53:43, 1978.
38. Proesmans W, Muaka BK, Monnens L: Indomethacin therapy in Bartter's syndrome. Acta Paediatr Belg 30:31, 1977.
39. Gullner HG, Cerletti C, Bartter FC, et al: Prostaglandin overproduction in Bartter's syndrome. Lancet 2 :767, 1979.
40. Rosa FC, Shah V, Dillon MJ: Urine prostaglandins in healthy children and in patients with Bartter's syndrome. Int J Ped Nephrol 3:112, 1982.
41. Mullner G, Gahwiler T, Luthy C, et al: Comparison of prostaglandin production of skin fibroblasts grown from patients with Bartter's syndrome and from age and sex matched controls. Prost Leuko Med 11:83, 1983.
42. Stoff JS, Stemerman M, Steer M, et al: A defect in platelet aggregation in Bartter's syndrome. Am J Med 68:171, 1980.
43. MacIntyre DE, Smith M, Levine L, et al: Is the platelet defect in Bartter's syndrome associated with a plasma prostaglandin? In Samuelsson B, et al (eds): Advances of Prostaglandin and Thromboxane Research, vol 7. New York, Raven Press, 1980, p 1185.
44. McGiff JC: Bartter's syndrome results from an imbalance of vasoactive hormones. Ann Intern Med 87:369, 1977.
45. Lechi A, Covi G, Lechi C, et al: Urinary kallikrein excretion in Bartter's syndrome. J Clin Endo Metab 43:1175, 1976.
46. Vinci JM, Gill JR, Bowden RE, et al: The kallikrein-kinin system in Bartter's syndrome and its response to prostaglandin synthetase inhibition. J Clin Invest 61:1671, 1978.
47. Salomon MI, Tchertkoff V: Bartter's syndrome: an overview. Angiology 28:806, 1977.
48. Garin EH, Sausville PJ, Richard GA: Serum inhibitor of phytohemagglutinin-induced lymphocyte proliferation in Bartter's syndrome. J Pediatr 102:569, 1983.
49. James T, Holland NH, Preston D: Bartter's syndrome. Typical facies and normal plasma volume. Am J Dis Child 129:1205, 1975.
50. Trygstad CW, Mangos JA, Bloodworth JMB, et al: A sibship with Bartter's syndrome: failure of total adrenalectomy to correct the potassium wasting. Pediatrics 44:234, 1969.
51. Sutherland LE, Hartcroft P, Balis JU, et al: Bartter's syndrome: a report of four cases, including three in one sibship, with comparative histological evaluation of the juxtaglomerular apparatuses and glomeruli. Acta Paediatr Scand 201(suppl):1, 1970.
52. Ogihara T, Maroyama A, Nugent CA, et al: Familial Bartter's syndrome. Arch Intern Med 142:906, 1972.
53. Goulon M, Raphael JC, Rohan P: Syndrome de Bartter et chondrocalcinose. Une association non fortuite. Nouv Presse Med 9:1291, 1980.
54. Robertson WG: Measurement of ionised calcium in body fluids—a review. Ann Clin Biochem 13:540, 1976.
55. Seyberth HW, Segre GV, Morgan JL, et al: Prostaglandins as mediators of hypercalcemia associated with certain types of cancer. N Engl J Med 293:1278, 1975.
56. Baehler RW, Work J, Kitchen TA, et al: Studies on the pathogenesis of Bartter's syndrome. Am J Med 69:933, 1980.
57. Gitelman HJ, Graham JB, Welt LG: A new familial disorder characterised by hypokalemia and hypomagnesemia. Trans Assoc Am Phys 79:221, 1966.
58. McCredie DA, Blair-West JR, Scroggins BA, et al: Potassium losing nephropathy of childhood. Med J Aust 1:129, 1971.
59. Paunier L, Sizonenko PC: A symptomatic chronic hypomagnesemia and hypokalemia in a child: cell membrane disease? J Pediatr 88:51, 1976.

60. Evans RA, Carter JN, George CRP, et al: The congenital magnesium-losing kidney. Report of two patients. Quart J Med 50:197, 1981.
61. Takeda R, Mortimoto S, Kuroda M, et al: Renal tubular acidosis, presenting as a syndrome resembling Bartter's syndrome, in a patient with arachnodactyly. Acta Endocrinol (Copenh) 73:531, 1973.
62. Buckalew VM, McCurdy DK, Ludwig GD, et al: Incomplete renal tubular acidosis. Am J Med 45:32, 1968.
63. Sebastian A, Morris RC Jr: Renal tubular acidosis. Clin Nephrol 7:216, 1977.
64. Wrong O, Davies HE: The excretion of acid in renal disease. Quart J Med 23:259, 1959.
65. Battle D, Grupp M, Gavira M, et al: Distal renal tubular acidosis with intact capacity to lower urinary pH. Am J Med 72:751, 1982.
66. Halperin ML, Goldstein MB, Haig A, et al: Studies on the pathogenesis of type I (distal) renal tubular acidosis as revealed by the urinary pCO_2 tensions. J Clin Invest 53:669, 1974.
67. Stoff JS, MacIntyre DI, Brown RS, et al: Prostacyclin overproduction in Bartter's syndrome. Lancet 2:1196, 1979.
68. Rodriguez-Soriano J, Vallo A, Castillo G, et al: Renal handling of water and sodium in infancy and childhood: a study using clearance methods during hypotonic saline diuresis. Kidney Intl 20:700, 1981.
69. Rosa FC, Bobinski H, Shah V, et al: A plasma factor's role in the red blood cell sodium pump abnormality in Bartter's syndrome. Europ J Pediatr 140:153, 1983.
70. Ben-Ishay D, Levy M, Birnbaum D: Self-induced secondary hyperaldosteronism simulating Bartter's syndrome. Isr J Med Sci 8:1835, 1972.
71. Schwartz WB, Relman AS: Metabolic and renal studies in chronic potassium depletion resulting from overuse of laxatives. J Clin Invest 32:258, 1953.
72. Demers LM, Valdhuis JD, Ramos E: The clinical entity of pseudo-Bartter's syndrome. In Samuelsson B, et al (eds): Advances in Prostaglandins and Thromboxane Research, vol 7. New York, Raven Press, 1980, p 1203.
73. Roy S, Arant BS: Hypokalemic metabolic alkalosis in normotensive infants with elevated plasma renin activity and hyperaldosteronism: role of dietary chloride deficiency. Pediatrics 67:423, 1981.
74. Gottleib RP: Metabolis alkalosis in cystic fibrosis. J Pediatr 79:930, 1971.
75. Lipmer HI, Ruzany F, Dasgupta M, et al: The behaviour of carbenicillin as a non reabsorbable anion. J Lab Clin Med 86:183, 1975.
76. Schambelan M, Slaton PE, Biglieri EG: Mineralocorticoid production in hyperadrenocorticism: role in pathogenesis of hypokalemic alkalosis. Am J Med 51:299, 1971.
77. Kinuthia DMW, Rosa FC, Dillon MJ: Fractional electrolyte delivery and reabsorption during hypotonic saline diuresis in familial hypokalemia/hypomagnesemia (Gitelman's syndrome), and pseudohypoaldosteronism compared with observations in Bartter's syndrome. Int J Pediatr Nephrol 3:126, 1982.
78. Modlinger RS, Nicholis GL, Krakkoff LR, et al: Some observations on the pathogenesis of Bartter's syndrome. N Engl J Med 289:1022, 1973.
79. Straus RG, Mohammed S, Loggie JMH, et al: The effect of methyl dopa on plasma renin activity in a child with Bartter's syndrome. J Pediatr 77:1071, 1970.
80. Guesry P, Dray F, Broyer M: Abstracts of the 4th International Symposium of Paediatric Nephrology, Helsinki, 1977.
81. Hoey H, Grant DB, Dillon MJ, et al: Male pseudohermaphroditism associated with salt wasting and hyporeninaemia. Pediatr Res 16:898, 1982.
82. Monnens L, Fiselier T, Bos B, et al: Hypo-reninemic hypoaldosteronism in infancy. Nephron 35:140, 1983.
83. Pakravan P, Kenny FM, Depp R et al: Familial congenital absence of adrenal glands: evaluation of glucocorticoid, mineralocorticoid and estrogen metabolism in the perinatal period. J Pediatr 84:74, 1974.
84. Dillon MJ, Ryness JM: Plasma renin activity and aldosterone concentration in children. Brit Med J 4:314, 1975.
85. Forest MG: Adrenal steroid deficiency states. In Brook CGD (ed): Clinical Paediatric Endocrinology. Oxford, Blackwell Scientific, p 396, 1981.
86. Gillet P, Francois R: L'hyperplasia surrenale congenitale. In Journees Parisiennes de Pediatrie. 1974, p 71.
87. Grant DB, Dillon MJ, Atherton SM, et al: Congenital adrenal hyperplasia: renin and steroid values during treatment. Europ J Pediatr 126:89, 1977.
88. Jacobs DR, Van der Poll J, Gabrilove JL, et al: 17 alpha-hydroxyprogesterone—a salt-losing steroid: relation to congenital adrenal hyperplasia. J Clin Endocrinol Metab 21:909, 1961.
89. Landau RL, Lugibihl K: Inhibition of sodium-retaining influence of aldosterone by progesterone. J Clin Endocrinol Metab 18:1237, 1958.
90. Brook CGD: Congenital adrenal hyperplasia. In Brook CGD (ed): Clinical Paediatric Endocrinology. Oxford Blackwell Scientific, 1981, p 453.
91. Newns GH: Congenital adrenal hyperplasia. Arch Dis Childh 49:2, 1974.
92. Hughes IA, Walton A, Lole CA, et al: Continuing need for mineralocorticoid therapy in salt-losing congenital adrenal hyperplasia. Arch Dis Child 54:350, 1979.
93. Loras B, Haour F, Bertrand J: Exchangeable sodium and aldosterone secretion in children with congenital adrenal hyperplasia due to 21-hydroxylase deficiency. Pediatr Res 4:145, 2970.
94. Rosler A, Levine LS, Schneider B, et al: The interrelationships of sodium balance, plasma renin activity and ACTH in congenital adrenal hyperplasia. J Clin Endocrinol Metab 45:500, 1977.
95. Visser HKA, Cost WS: A new hereditary defect in the biosynthesis of aldosterone: urinary C21-corticosteroid pattern in three related patients with a salt-losing syndrome, suggesting an 18-oxidation defect. Acta Endocrinol 47:589, 1964.
96. Degenhart HJ, Frankena L, Visser HKA, et al: Further investigation of a new hereditary defect in the biosynthesis of aldosterone: evidence for a defect in 18-hydroxylation of corticosterone. Acta Physiol Pharmacol Neerlandica 14:88, 1966.
97. Ulick S, Gautier E, Vetter KK, et al: An aldosterone biosynthetic defect in a salt-losing disorder. J Clin Endocrinol Metab 24:669, 1964.
98. David R, Golan S, Drucker W: Familial aldosterone deficiency: enzyme defect, diagnosis and clinical course. Pediatrics 41:403, 1968.
99. Hamilton W, McCandless AE, Ireland JT, et al: Hypoaldosteronism in three sibs due to 18-dehydrogenase deficiency. Arch Dis Childh 51:576, 1976.
100. Milla PJ, Trompeter R, Dillon MJ, et al: Salt-losing syndrome in 2 infants with defective 18-dehydrogenation in aldosterone biosynthesis. Arch Dis Childh 52:580, 1977.
101. Rappaport R, Dray F, Legrand JC, et al: Hypoaldosteronisme congenital familial par defaut de la 18-OH-dehydrogenase. Etude hormonale avant et apres guerison du syndrome de parte de sel. Pediatr Res 2:456, 1968.
102. Ulich S: Diagnosis and nomenclature of the disorders of the terminal portion of the aldosterone biosynthetic pathway. J Clin Endocrinol Metab 43:92, 1976.
103. Shackleton CHL, Honour JW, Dillon M, et al: Multi-component gas chromatographic analysis of urinary steroids excreted by an infant with a defect in aldosterone biosynthesis. Acta Endocrinol 81:762, 1976.
104. Shackleton CHL, Taylor NF: Identification of the androstenetriolones and androstenetetrols present in the urine of infants. J Steroid Biochem 6:1393, 1975.
105. Taylor NF, Curnow DH, Shackleton CHL: Analysis of glucocorticoid metabolites in the neonatal period: catabolism of cortisone acetate by an infant with 21-hydroxylase deficiency. Clin Chim Acta 85:219, 1978.
106. Cara J, Beas F, Soach C, Lic SC, et al: Increased urinary and plasma etiocholanolone and related steroids in a boy with virilizing adrenal hyperplasia and periodic fever. J Pediatr 62:521, 1963.
107. Nerup J: Addison's disease: clinical studies; seriological studies. Acta Endocrinol (Copenh) 76:127, 1974.
108. Bamatter F, Koegel R, Haller J de, et al: Maladie d'Addisons familiale. Insuffisance corticosurrenale chez quatre freres et plusiers cas probables dans deux generations de la meme famille. Helv Pediatr Acta 21:109, 1966.
109. Perheentupa J, Tiilikainen A, Lokki ML: Autoimmune poly-endocrinopathy-candidosis syndrome (APECS): clinical variation, inheritance and HLA association in 40 Finnish patients. Pediatr Res 12:1087, 1978.
110. Forsyth GC, Forbes M, Cummings JN: Adrenocortical atrophy and diffuse cerebral sclerosis. Arch Dis Childh 46:273, 1971.
111. Cheek DB, Perry JW: A salt-wasting syndrome in infancy. Arch Dis Childh 33:252, 1958.
112. Barakat AY, Papadopoulou ZL, August GP: A hyperkalaemic salt-wasting syndrome in infancy. Pediatr Res 6:394, 1972.
113. Barthe P, Thai VK, Bouisou F, et al: A propos d'un cas de pseudohypoaldosteronisme (Etude du taux de secretion d'aldosterone). Arch Fr Pediatr 31:973, 1974.
114. Bierich JR, Schmidt U: Tubular Na K-ATPase deficiency, the cause of the congenital renal salt-losing syndrome. Europ J Pediatr 121:81, 1976.
115. Blacher Y, Kaplan BS, Griffel B, et al: Pseudohypoaldosteronism. Clin Nephrol 11:281, 1979.
116. Corbel L: Diabete salin du nourrisson sans insuffisance surrenalienne. Pediatrie 18:557, 1963.
117. Dillon MJ, Leonard JV, Buckler JM, et al: Pseudohypoaldosteronism. Arch Dis Childh 55:427, 1980.
118. Donnell GN, Litman N, Roldan M: Pseudohypoadrenalcorticism. Renal sodium loss, hyponatremia and hyperkalemia due to renal tubular insensitivity to mineralocorticoids. Am J Dis Child 97:813, 1959.
119. Kaufman E, Hayek A, Greenberg R: Pseudohypoaldosteronism in triplets. Pediatr Res 11:426, 1977.
120. Lauras B, Ravussin J-J, David M, et al: Pseudohypoaldosteronism chez l'enfant. A propos de quatre observations dont deux concernant des freres. Pediatrie 33:119, 1978.
121. Lelong M, Alagille D, Philippe A, et al: Diabete salin par insensibilite congenitale du tubule a l'aldosterone: pseudohypoadrenocorticisme. Rev Fr d'Etudes Clinique et Biologiques 5:558, 1960.
122. Limal JM, Rappaport R, Dechaux M, et al: Familial dominant pseudohypoaldosteronism. Lancet 1:51, 1978.
123. Oberfield SE, Levine LS, Carey RM, et al: Pseudohypoaldosteronism: multiple

target organ unresponsiveness to mineralocorticoid hormones. J Clin Endocrinol Metab 48:228, 1979.
124. Petersen S, Giese J, Kappelgaard AM, et al: Pseudohypoaldosteronism. Clinical, biochemical and morphological studies in a long term follow-up. Acta Pediatr Scand 67:255, 1978.
125. Proesmans W, Guessens H, Corbel L, et al: Pseudohypoaldosteronism. Am J Dis Child 126:510, 1973.
126. Raine DN, Roy J: A salt-losing syndrome in infancy. Pseudohypoadrenocorticalism. Arch Dis Childh 37:548, 1962.
127. Rampini S, Furrer J, Keller HP, et al: Congenital pseudohypoaldosteronism: a case report and review. Effect of indomethacin during sodium chloride depletion. Helv Paediatr Acta 33:153, 1978.
128. Rosler A, Theodor R, Boichis H, et al: Metabolic responses to the administration of angiotensin II, K and ACTH in two salt-wasting syndromes. J Clin Endocrinol 44:292, 1977.
129. Roy C: Pseudohypoaldosteronisme familial (a propos de 5 cas). Arch Fr Pediatr 34:37, 1977.
130. Royer P, Bonnette J, Mathieu H, et al: Pseudohypoaldosteronisme. Ann Pediatr 39:596, 1963.
131. Shackleton CHL, Snodgrass GHAI: Steroid excretion by an infant with an unusual salt-losing syndrome: a gas chromatographic-mass spectrometric study. Ann Clin Biochem 11:91, 1974.
132. Honour JW, Dillon MJ, Shackleton CHL: Analysis of steroids in urine for differentiation of pseudohypoaldosteronism and aldosterone biosynthetic defect. J Clin Endocrinol Metab 54:325, 1982.
133. Stubbe P, Manouguina G: Der pseudohypoaldosteronisme. Bericht eines weiteren falles. Monatsschr Kinderheilk 125:234, 1977.
134. Trung PH, Piussan C, Rodary C, et al: Etude du taux de secretion de l'aldosterone et de l'activite de la renine plasmatique d'un cas de pseudohypoaldosteronism. Arch Fr Pediatr 27:603, 1970.
135. Savage MO, Jefferson IG, Dillon MJ, et al: Pseudohypoaldosteronism; severe salt wasting in infancy caused by generalised mineralocorticoid unresponsiveness. J Pediatr 101:239, 1982.
136. Proesmans W, Muaka BK, Eeckel R: Pseudohypoaldosteronism: a proximal tubular sodium wasting disease. Proceedings of Fourth International Symposium of Pediatric Nephrology, Helsinki, 1977, p 86.
137. McSherry E: Renal tubular acidosis in childhood. Kidney Intl 20:799, 1981.
138. Sebastian A, Hulter HN, Kurtz I, et al: Disorders of distal nephron function. Am J Med 72:289, 1982.
139. McSherry E: Current issues in hydrogen ion transport. In Gruskin AB, Norman ME (eds): Developments in Nephrology 3—Pediatric Nephrology. The Hague, Martinus Nijhoff, 1981, p 403.
140. Good DW, Wright FS: Luminal influence on potassium secretion: sodium concentration and fluid flow rate. Am J Physiol 236:F192, 1979.
141. Wright FS: Sites and mechanisms of potassium transport along the renal tubules. Kidney Intl 11:415, 1977.
142. Postel-Vinay MC, Alberti GM, Ricour C, et al: Pseudohypoaldosteronism: persistence of hyperaldosteronism and evidence for renal tubular and intestinal responsiveness to endogenous aldosterone. J Clin Endocrinol Metab 39:1038, 1974.
143. Anand SK, Frobeg L, Northway JD, et al: Pseudohypoaldosteronism due to sweat gland dysfunction. Pediatr Res 10:677, 1976.

CHAPTER 34

Renal Tubular Acidosis

ANTHONY A. PORTALE
BEVERLEY E. BOOTH
R. CURTIS MORRIS, JR.

INTRODUCTION

This review of renal tubular acidosis (RTA) begins with a presentation of selected aspects of the normal renal acidification process, which establishes the context for a pathophysiological classification of the various types of renal tubular acidosis. Clinical aspects of diagnosis and treatment of the disorder are emphasized.

A more detailed discussion of normal renal acidification and acid-base metabolism is given in Chapters 5 and 8.

RENAL ACIDIFICATION

Under normal physiological conditions, the kidneys participate in the regulation of the acid-base composition of extracellular fluid (ECF) by regulating the plasma concentration of bicarbonate at normal levels (1). The kidneys perform this function by reabsorbing nearly all of the bicarbonate filtered at the glomerulus and by excreting acid as titratable acid and ammonium. Urinary excretion of acid results in the generation of new bicarbonate in an amount equal to that lost in buffering the endogenous load of noncarbonic acid i.e., sulfuric, phosphoric, and organic acids. Net endogenous production of noncarbonic acid averages approximately 1 mEq/kg/day (range 0.4 to 1.6) in normal adults ingesting typical diets (2) and approximately 1 to 3 mEq/kg/day in healthy infants and young children (3, 3a). Current evidence suggests that both the reabsorption of bicarbonate and the excretion of acid are mediated by renal tubular secretion of hydrogen ion (H^+) (1, 4–7). For each mole of H^+ secreted by renal tubular cells into the tubular lumen, one mole of bicarbonate ion is generated in intracellular fluid and returned to the blood.

In the proximal tubule, H^+ secretion results in the reabsorption of approximately 80% to 90% of the filtered load of bicarbonate at normal plasma bicarbonate concentrations (1, 6, 8–10). Filtered bicarbonate is not reabsorbed directly, but combines in the lumen with secreted H^+ to form carbonic acid (H_2CO_3), which in turn rapidly dissociates to H_2O and CO_2; luminal CO_2 rapidly equilibrates with peritubular CO_2 (Fig. 34.1, upper panel). The dissociation of H_2CO_3 is catalyzed by the enzyme, carbonic anhydrase, located at the brush-border membrane of the proximal tubule. By reducing the steady state concentration of luminal H_2CO_3 and, hence, of luminal H^+, carbonic anhydrase greatly facilitates tubular secretion of H^+ (4, 5, 7). Carbonic anhydrase located in the cytoplasm catalyzes the reaction between cytoplasmic CO_2 and H_2O to yield HCO_3^-, which then diffuses into the blood. When the activity of carbonic anhydrase is inhibited, as with acetazolamide, H_2CO_3 accumulates in the tubular lumen, inducing an increase in the cytoplasm-to-lumen H^+ concentration gradient and thereby a decrease in the rate of H^+ secretion and in bicarbonate reabsorption (4, 5, 7). The acidification process of the proximal tubule has a high capacity for H^+ secretion, but a relatively low capacity to generate steep pH gradients between blood and urine.

In the distal nephron, H^+ secretion results in reabsorption of the 10% to 20% of filtered bicarbonate not reabsorbed in the proximal tubule, thereby decreasing the pH of tubular fluid to less than about 6.4. As luminal pH decreases, secreted H^+ continues to combine with the major nonbicarbonate urinary buffers, Na_2HPO_4 and NH_3, forming NaH_2PO_4 and NH_4^+, measured in the urine as titratable acid and as ammonium ion, respectively (Fig. 34.1, lower panel).

The amount of H^+ excreted as titratable acid and ammonium, minus the normally negligible excretion of bicarbonate, is referred to as net acid excretion. Net acid excretion is a quantitative measure of the net renal input of bicarbonate into body fluid, which under steady state conditions equals the net endogenous production of noncarbonic acid (11); net acid balance is zero (Chapter 8). Net acid excretion normally accounts for no more than 3% of renal H^+ secretion at normal plasma bicarbonate concentrations; bicarbonate reabsorption accounts for more than 97%.

Although the distal nephron has the ability to generate and maintain a large pH gradient between blood and urine, its capacity to secrete H^+ is small relative to that of the proximal tubule. A relatively small increase in distal delivery of bicarbonate increases urinary pH, as a result of increased buffering of secreted H^+ by bicarbonate. This decreases the amount of H^+ excreted as titratable acid and ammonium. Thus, for a given distal H^+ secretory capacity, the rates of excretion of titratable acid and ammonium vary inversely with the rate of distal delivery of bicarbonate and with urinary pH. Since distal delivery of bicarbonate is determined by the amount of bicarbonate not reabsorbed in the proximal tubule, the rate of H^+ secretion (bicarbonate reabsorption) by the proximal tubule and the plasma concentration (filtered load) of bicarbonate are critical and complementary modulators of urinary pH and net acid or net base excretion.

A number of factors influences the rates at which the proximal and distal nephrons secrete H^+ (1). In the proximal tubule, H^+ secretion

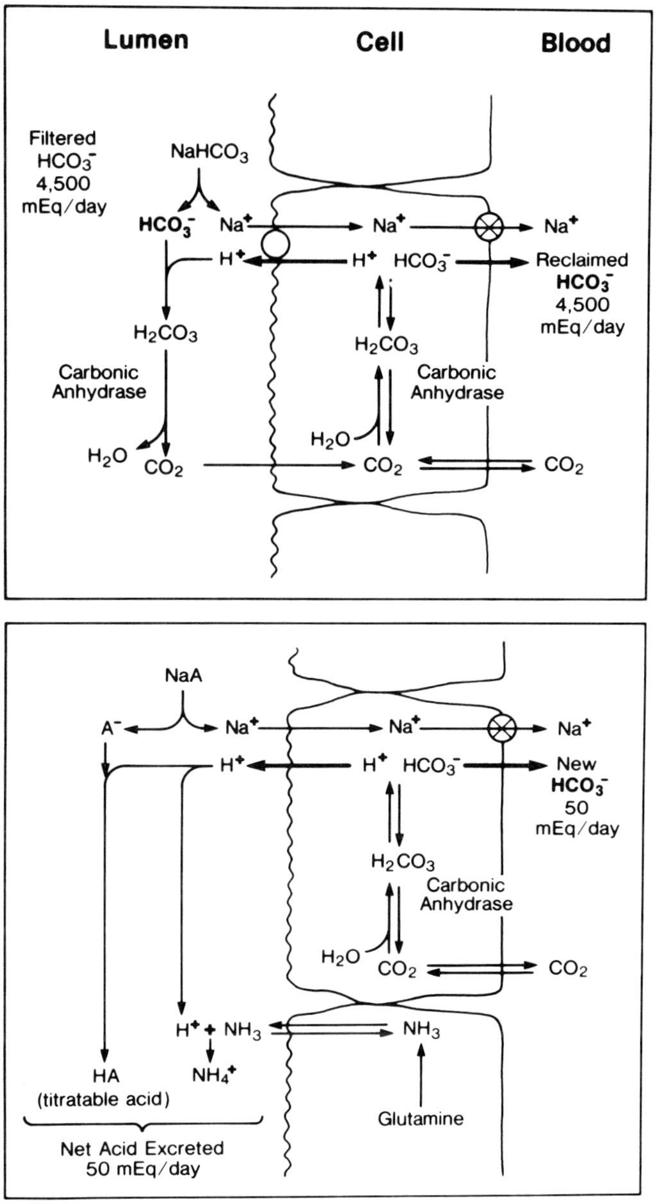

Figure 34.1. Schematic diagram of the normal mammalian renal acidification process. Upper panel, Bicarbonate reabsorption in the proximal and distal tubule. Lower panel, Excretion of titratable acid and ammonium in the distal tubule.

varies directly with luminal bicarbonate concentration and pH (12–14), luminal flow rate (15–16), and peritubular P_{CO_2} (14, 17–20) and varies inversely with peritubular bicarbonate concentration and pH (14, 18, 21–23), and with the state of potassium balance (22, 24).

In the distal tubule, H^+ secretion appears to vary directly with luminal bicarbonate concentration and pH (1). The rate of distal H^+ secretion is principally modulated by the kind and quantity of nonbicarbonate sodium salts delivered to the distal nephron and by its resorptive avidity for sodium (Na). Resorptive avidity for Na is determined by many factors including the level of circulating aldosterone (Chapter 6). When distal avidity for Na is high, as occurs with volume depletion or administration of mineralocorticoid hormone, increased distal delivery of Na will increase the lumen-negative electrical potential difference in the distal nephron, thus stimulating H^+ secretion (25, 26). When the Na delivered to the distal nephron is largely accompanied by chloride, which is usually the case, the stimulus for H^+ secretion is less because chloride is passively reabsorbed, thus dissipating the electrical gradient to some extent. Aldosterone appears to stimulate H^+ secretion directly in the absence of an effect on Na transport, in both the turtle bladder (27) and mammalian medullary collecting tubule (28, 29).

Expansion of the ECF volume reduces the overall net rate of H^+ secretion (30–32). Acute administration of parathyroid hormone (PTH) to rats and dogs inhibits proximal bicarbonate reabsorption and increases urinary pH (33–37); chronic administration of PTH to rats and dogs (38–40) and to humans (41) induces metabolic alkalosis and an increase in net acid excretion.

Secretion of H^+ by the renal tubule is thought to occur by two general mechanisms: (1) electroneutral Na^+-H^+ exchange across the luminal membrane (42–44) and (2) electrogenic H^+ secretion by the luminal membrane (28, 29, 45). Electroneutral Na^+-H^+ exchange is driven by the downhill lumen-to-cytoplasm Na^+ concentration gradient that is generated and maintained by extrusion of Na across the basolateral membrane by the Na, K-ATPase system located there (46). Current evidence suggests that H^+ secretion in the proximal tubule is mediated principally by electroneutral Na^+-H^+ exchange.

Electrogenic H^+ secretion is mediated by a proton-translocating ATPase located in the luminal membrane. In the turtle bladder, the epithelium of which resembles that of the mammalian collecting tubule, H^+ secretion is electrogenic; that is, it is capable of transporting a net positive charge into the lumen and is not dependent on Na reabsorption. On the other hand, the rate of H^+ secretion may be influenced by the lumen-negative electrical potential difference generated by Na reabsorption (47–50). Hydrogen secretion can occur in the absence of a favorable transepithelial electrical potential difference and against a transepithelial H^+ concentration gradient, until the H^+ concentration in mucosal fluid exceeds that in serosal fluid by about 1000, i.e., 3.0 pH units. At this gradient, H^+ secretion stops. There is direct evidence for a reversible proton-translocating ATPase in the luminal membrane of the turtle bladder (51). Studies of isolated perfused cortical and medullary collecting tubules of the rabbit suggest that H^+ secretion in the mammalian distal nephron is mediated by electrogenic H^+ secretion (28–29).

RENAL TUBULAR ACIDOSIS

RTA is a clinical syndrome of disordered renal acidification characterized by hyperchloremic metabolic acidosis, inappropriately high urinary pH, and reduced urinary excretion of titratable acid and ammonium (52–72). The disorder of renal acidification can occur with little or no reduction of renal mass, which distinguishes RTA from the acidosis that accompanies renal insufficiency.

Type 1 or Distal Renal Tubular Acidosis

Physiological Characteristics

In untreated patients with type 1 or distal RTA, urinary pH is inappropriately high, usually greater than 6.0, during all degrees of acidosis, severe as well as mild (Fig. 34.2) (52, 53, 55–60, 63–67). As a consequence, bicarbonate delivered to the distal nephron is incompletely reabsorbed resulting in persisting urinary excretion of bicarbonate, and urinary excretion of titratable acid and ammonium is reduced (52, 53, 55–60, 63–67). Renal reabsorption of glucose, amino acids, and phosphorus is not impaired.

Adults. In adult patients with type 1 RTA, the amount of bicarbonate excreted in the urine at normal plasma bicarbonate concentrations usually is less than 5% of the filtered load of bicarbonate (55, 56, 73). Because the magnitude of bicarbonaturia is relatively constant over a

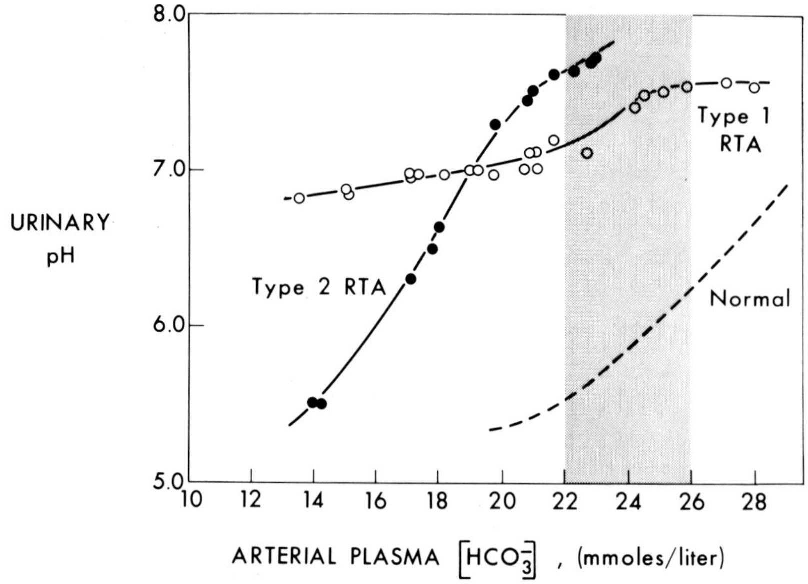

Figure 34.2. The relationship between urinary pH and plasma bicarbonate concentration in patients with type 1 or distal and type 2 or proximal RTA. In patients with type 1 RTA, urinary pH is high during severe, as well as mild, degrees of acidosis. In patients with type 2 RTA, the urinary pH may be inappropriately high or appropriately low, depending on the severity of systemic acidosis. (Shaded area represents the range of normal plasma bicarbonate concentration). (From Sebastian A: Calif Med 116: 34, 1972.)

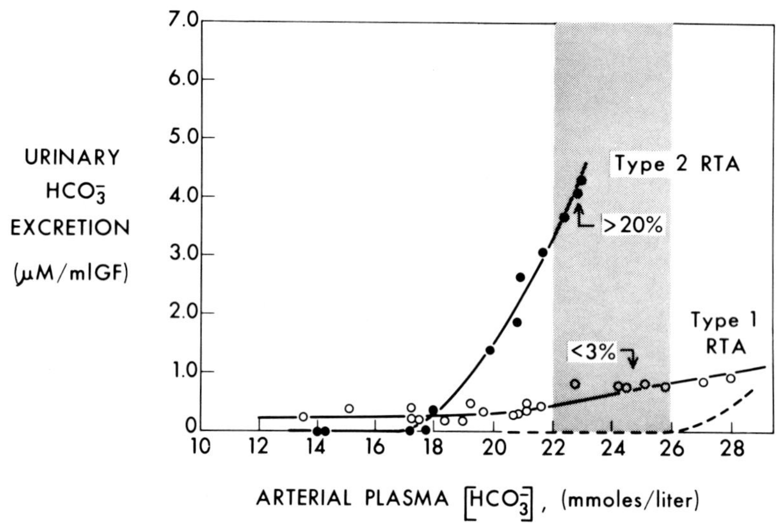

Figure 34.3. The relationship between urinary bicarbonate excretion and plasma bicarbonate concentration in patients with type 1 or distal and type 2 or proximal RTA. In patients with type 1 RTA, bicarbonaturia occurs during all degrees of acidosis, severe as well as mild. In adult patients the magnitude of bicarbonaturia is relatively modest, usually less than 5% of the filtered bicarbonate load, and is relatively constant over a broad range of normal and reduced plasma bicarbonate concentrations. In patients with type 2 RTA, bicarbonaturia is absent during severe acidosis, but is of large magnitude at normal plasma bicarbonate concentrations, often being greater than 15% of the filtered bicarbonate load. (Shaded area represents range of normal plasma bicarbonate concentrations). (From Sebastian A: Calif Med 116: 34, 1972.)

broad range of normal and reduced plasma bicarbonate concentrations (Fig. 34.3), it has been inferred that reabsorption of bicarbonate by the proximal tubule is not substantially impaired.

In some adult patients with type 1 RTA, the rate of excretion of bicarbonate at normal plasma bicarbonate concentrations exceeds the combined rate of excretion of titratable acid and ammonium, i.e., there is urinary excretion of net base (65). Hence, the acidosis of those patients results not only from their reduced urinary excretion of titratable acid and ammonium, but also from their moderate urinary excretion of net base. In a group of 11 adult patients with type 1 RTA studied at normal plasma bicarbonate concentrations, the amount of alkali required to sustain correction of acidosis averages 1.5 mEq/kg/day, i.e., an amount that neutralizes endogenous production of noncarbonic acid (approximately 1 mEq/kg/day) and replaces the urinary excretion of net base (approximately 0.5 mEq/kg/day) (65).

Infants and Children. By contrast, in many infants and children with type 1 RTA, the amount of bicarbonate excreted in the urine and hence the urinary excretion of net base is considerably greater than that in affected adults (65, 67, 68, 72, 74). The fractional excretion of bicarbonate ($FEHCO_3$) at normal plasma bicarbonate concentrations ranges from 5% to 15% of the filtered load (65, 67, 74). Such children are said to have severe "renal bicarbonate wasting." The substantial urinary excretion of net base accounts for the progressive and life-threatening acidosis that occurs in untreated infants with type 1 RTA. The magnitude of urinary bicarbonate excretion at normal plasma bicarbonate concentrations is the major determinant of the amount of alkali required to sustain correction of the acidosis, an amount that ranges from 5 to 14 mEq/kg/day (67, 68, 72, 74).

Renal bicarbonate wasting is common in infants and young children with type 1 RTA. It may be present from the outset of the disorder (65, 67, 68, 72), and it may increase in severity several weeks to months after initiation of alkali therapy when growth velocity has greatly increased (68). It may decrease in magnitude after the age of 4 to 6 years, reaching values of bicarbonate excretion similar to or slightly greater than those observed in affected adult patients (72). It has been proposed that renal bicarbonate wasting in children with type 1 RTA reflects, in part, functional immaturity of the proximal nephron that results in increased delivery of bicarbonate to an already impaired distal nephron (67). But, if bicarbonate wasting were to reflect only an impairment in proximal reabsorption of bicarbonate, one would expect the magnitude of the leak from the proximal nephron to vary directly with the filtered load of bicarbonate and this is not the case. In the majority of infants with type 1 RTA and renal bicarbonate wasting, the magnitude of bicarbonaturia is relatively fixed over a broad range of normal and subnormal plasma bicarbonate concentrations (Fig. 34.4) (65, 67, 68, 74). Renal bicarbonate wasting in children with type 1 RTA could result from a more severe impairment in the acidification process of the distal nephron such that its inability to lower urinary pH below 7.0 even during severe acidosis would result in a greater impairment in distal bicarbonate reabsorption (65). Infants with type 1 RTA and bicarbonate wasting were formerly designated as having type 3 RTA. Since renal bicarbonate wasting is now recognized to be a characteristic feature of type 1 RTA in infancy, the designation type 3 RTA has been dropped.

Pathogenesis

The pathophysiological characteristics of type 1 RTA are a consequence of a reduced net rate of H^+ secretion by the distal nephron. Such a reduction might result from either of two general mechanisms (Table 34.1): (1) a reduced rate of active H^+ secretion from cell to lumen, (2) increased cell membrane permeability that permits passive backleak of secreted H^+ from lumen to cell or backleak of HCO_3^- from cell to lumen. Active H^+ secretion might be reduced because the distal nephron is unable to secrete H^+ against a large plasma-to-lumen pH gradient, a result of a primary disorder of the H^+ secretory pump or to a decrease

Table 34.1.
Hypothetical Mechanisms Of Impaired Collecting Duct Function Resulting In Renal Tubular Acidosis

Reduced cell-to-lumen unidirectional active H^+ secretion
Disorder of H^+ secretory pumps
Reduced strength (protonmotive force) of pumps
Reduced proton "conductance"
Decreased number of pumps
Defect in active transport pathway
Defect in metabolic energy production
Defect in metabolic energy utilization
Structural defect of pump
Reduction in electrochemical gradient that ordinarily promotes H^+ secretion
Reduced lumen-negative transtubular electrical potential
Reduced sodium reabsorption
Enhanced potassium secretion
Enhanced chloride reabsorption
Reduced availability of cellular H^+
Impaired exit of cellular bicarbonate or OH^- to peritubular fluid
Carbonic anhydrase defect
Increased luminal H^+ secondary to reduced concentration of luminal proton acceptors
Impaired ammoniagenesis
Impaired medullary ammonia delivery
Hypophosphaturia
Impaired luminal acidification despite normal or increased cell-to-lumen unidirectional active H^+ secretion
Permeability defect
Backleak of luminal H^+ through cell membrane or between cells
Increased luminal entry of HCO_3^-, $CO_3^=$, or OH^-
Abnormal stimulation of active HCO_3^- secretion or HCO_3^-/Cl^- exchange

From Morris RC Jr, Sebastian A: Renal tubular acidosis and Fanconi syndrome. In The Metabolic Basis of Inherited Disease, ed 5. New York, McGraw-Hill, 1983.

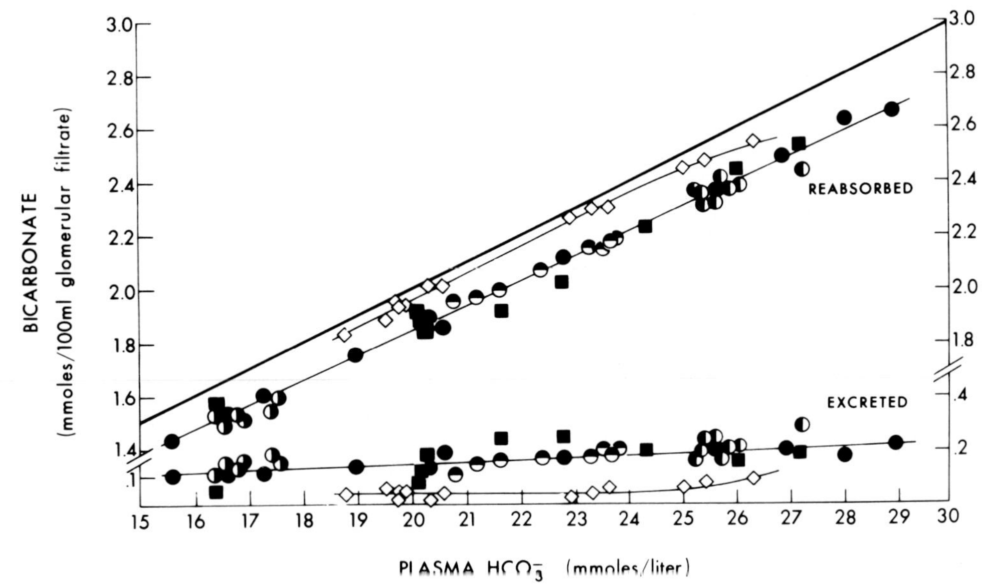

Figure 34.4. The relationship between plasma concentration, renal tubular reabsorption, and urinary excretion of bicarbonate in three infants with type 1 RTA studied during the first year of life. Two infants had renal bicarbonate wasting (*circles* and *squares*), and one did not (diamonds). (From McSherry E, et al: J Clin Invest 51: 499, 1972.)

in the lumen-negative electrical potential difference that normally augments H^+ secretion. An abnormality that allowed passive backleak of secreted H^+ or increased luminal entry of HCO_3^- would prevent an appropriately large plasma-to-lumen pH gradient from being maintained.

Evidence that function of the distal nephron is impaired in patients with type 1 RTA is the finding that urinary carbon dioxide tension (PCO_2) does not increase to normally high values during loading with $NaHCO_3$ (75, 76). Under normal circumstances, when urinary pH and bicarbonate concentration are greatly increased by administration of $NaHCO_3$, urinary PCO_2 increases to values considerably higher—usually >20 mm Hg—than those of blood; the difference in PCO_2 between urine and blood varies directly with the urinary bicarbonate concentration (69, 76–78). The increase in PCO_2 in alkaline urine is thought to reflect principally an increase in H^+ secretion in the distal tubule and collecting duct, augmented by the high luminal bicarbonate concentration. Secreted H^+ and luminal HCO_3^- combine to form H_2CO_3, which dissociates to H_2O and CO_2 at an uncatalyzed rate, since luminal fluid is not in functional contact with carbonic anhydrase in the distal nephron. Because the CO_2 is generated in distal segments of the collecting duct, where medullary trapping of CO_2 can occur, and in the renal pelvis and bladder, where conditions are unfavorable for absorption of CO_2 into blood, CO_2 appears in the urine in increased amounts. In bicarbonate-loaded patients with type 1 RTA, the finding that urine-blood PCO_2 is considerably less than that of normal subjects with comparable urine bicarbonate concentrations (77) has been interpreted as evidence that the total amount of H_2CO_3 generated in the lumen of the distal nephron is greatly reduced because of a greatly reduced net rate of H^+ secretion. Since bicarbonate loading causes urinary pH to be higher than that of blood, any reduction in the rate of H^+ secretion would reflect decreased cell-to-lumen H^+ secretion rather than backleak of H^+ from lumen-to-cell.

In patients with type 1 RTA, a reduction in urinary PCO_2 during bicarbonate loading might reflect not only reduced generation of H_2CO_3 but also a permeability abnormality of the distal nephron that permits backleak of that H_2CO_3 generated in the lumen (73). Such a permeability abnormality might also permit passive backleak of secreted H^+ from lumen to cell during acidosis, when urinary pH is lower than that of blood. Accordingly, an abnormally reduced urinary PCO_2 during bicarbonate loading provides evidence for reduced H^+ secretion by the distal nephron and is consistent with either of the two major mechanisms proposed as causal of type 1 RTA; i.e., decreased cell-to-lumen H^+ secretion and increased backleak of luminal H^+.

Type 1 RTA develops de novo in patients with amphotericin B nephrotoxicity (79, 80), providing evidence that a permeability abnormality of the distal nephron underlies the impairment of urinary acidification in some patients with type 1 RTA. In the turtle bladder, amphotericin B impairs acidification by increasing the permeability of the luminal membrane to H^+, thus permitting increased passive backleak of H^+ from lumen to cell (81, 82). In the rat with amphotericin-induced type 1 RTA, urinary PCO_2 increases normally during bicarbonate loading, suggesting that amphotericin does not increase luminal membrane permeability to H_2CO_3.

In adult patients, type 1 RTA occurs in a number of diseases characterized by hypergammaglobulinemia, e.g., Sjogren's syndrome (83–86) and chronic active hepatitis (87–89), suggesting that immunological disease impairs distal renal acidification. In such patients, the RTA seems not to be caused by the hypergammaglobulinemia per se, but rather to be the functional renal expression of a general autoimmune disorder. Both humoral and cell-mediated immunological mechanisms may play a role (90).

Pathophysiology

Sodium and Potassium.—Renal wasting of Na and K are characteristic of untreated type 1 RTA (56–58, 65, 91–94). Na reabsorption by the distal nephron is reduced (91, 94), presumably a result of reduced H^+ secretion and reduced Na^+-H^+ exchange. Na reabsorption by the proximal nephron is reduced during metabolic acidosis per se (95). Contraction of the ECF volume stimulates secretion of renin and aldosterone, leading to renal K wasting (91). When the acidosis of patients with type 1 RTA is corrected with alkali therapy, urinary pH increases and the gradient restriction on H^+ secretion no longer operates to limit H^+ secretion. Both H^+ secretion and distal Na^+-H^+ exchange increase, resulting in correction of Na depletion, reversal of hyperaldosteronism, retention of potassium, and correction of hypokalemia (Fig. 34.5). However, in some patients with type 1 RTA, a persistent impairment in renal conservation of Na (94) and frank renal K wasting (93) occur, despite sustained correction of acidosis with alkali therapy. The persisting renal K wasting is thought to reflect, at least in part, persisting hyperaldosteronism (93).

Calcium, Phosphorus, and Citrate. The urinary excretion of (Ca) and renal clearance of phosphorus (P) are predictably increased during metabolic acidosis (52, 96, 97). It is not clear whether the increases seen in untreated patients with type 1 RTA are greater than would occur in normal individuals made acidotic. Urinary excretion of citrate also is reduced (57, 98–104). Medullary nephrocalcinosis and recurrent nephrolithiasis, formed as calcium phosphate or oxalate, commonly occur in

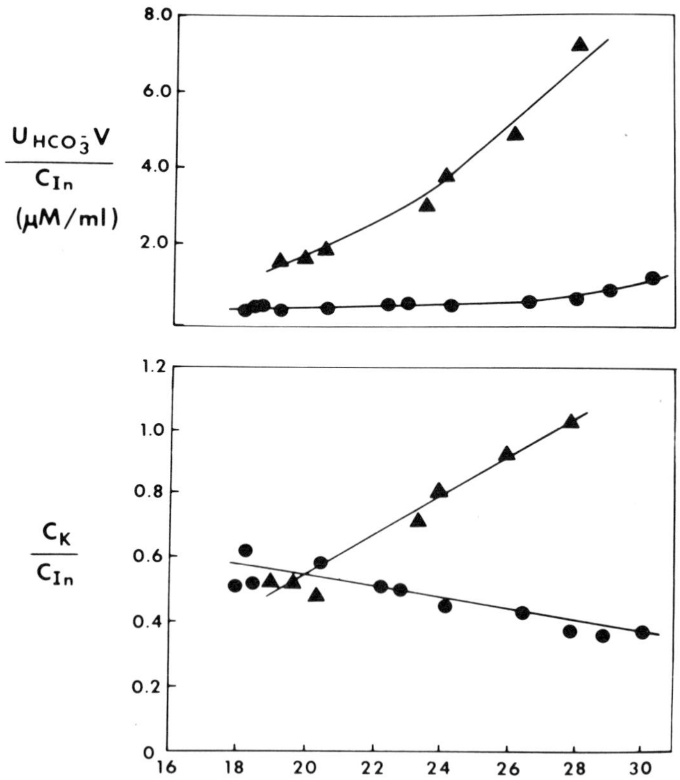

Figure 34.5. Effect of an acute progressive increase in plasma bicarbonate concentration (intravenous administration of sodium bicarbonate) on the fraction of the filtered load of potassium excreted in the urine (C_K/C_{in}) and on the urinary excretion of bicarbonate ($U_{HCO3}V/C_{in}$) in a patient with type 1 RTA (*circles*) and in a patient with type 2 RTA (*triangles*). (From Morris RC Jr, et al: Kidney Intl 1: 322, 1972.)

these patients (52–55, 57, 60, 66, 67, 72) and are presumed to be a result of persistent hypercalcuria (52, 72) and reduced urinary citrate excretion (57, 98–104a) in the presence of alkaline urine. Urinary citrate forms a soluble complex with Ca and prevents the precipitation of Ca as phosphate or oxalate. With reduced urinary citrate excretion, such chelation does not occur. The hypocitraturia of patients with type 1 RTA could be a consequence of metabolic acidosis per se, since acute ammonium chloride-induced metabolic acidosis decreases urinary citrate excretion (105). In some patients with type 1 RTA, impaired gut absorption, as well as increased renal excretion of Ca (52, 106), can give rise to hypocalcemia, hyperparathyroidism (107, 108), and hypophosphatemia, which are a basis for the rickets and osteomalacia that can occur (53, 109–111).

With sustained correction of acidosis, urinary excretion of Ca (52, 68, 72) and renal clearance of P decrease, urinary excretion of citrate can increase (98, 101–104a), gut absorption of Ca increases (52), and the serum concentrations of Ca and P become normal (52). Although nephrocalcinosis and nephrolithiasis persist, stones may be passed less frequently (112). Rickets and osteomalacia can heal with alkali therapy alone (109–111).

The possibility has been considered that metabolic acidosis induces an impairment in the metabolism of vitamin D that contributes to the intestinal malabsorption of Ca and metabolic bone disease of patients with RTA. In vitamin D-deficient animals, ammonium chloride-induced metabolic acidosis is associated with a decrease in the activity of renal 25-hydroxyvitamin D-1-hydroxylase and in the conversion of 25-hydroxyvitamin D (25-OHD) to 1,25-dihydroxyvitamin (1,25-$(OH)_2D$), the biologically active metabolite of vitamin D (112a–112d). But chronic ammonium chloride-induced acidosis in normal adults neither reduced the basal serum level of 1,25-$(OH)_2D$ nor attenuated the increment in serum 1,25-$(OH)_2D$ induced by administration of parathyroid extract (113). On the other hand, in rats made continuously acidotic with ammonium chloride (NH_4Cl), dietary Ca restriction failed to cause the otherwise predictable increase in serum level of 1,25-$(OH)_2D$ (113a). In children with proximal and distal RTA, the serum concentrations 25-OHD and 1,25-$(OH)_2D$ were found to be normal during acidosis and to remain unchanged after acidosis was corrected with alkali therapy (114).

Clinical Spectrum

Complete Syndrome of Renal Tubular Acidosis. Type 1 RTA may occur either alone or in association with a number of acquired or genetically transmitted systemic diseases (Table 34.2). In children, type 1 RTA most commonly occurs alone as either a sporadic or familial disorder. Different genotypes can give rise to different clinical expressions of the disorder. Type 1 RTA can occur as an autosomal dominant trait in which the genetic defect is fully expressed in early childhood (68, 110, 115–117). In one kindred of patients with type 1 RTA, 12 members over 4 successive generations were affected; acidosis was present as early as the first few months of life, and nephrocalcinosis was radiographically demonstrable as early as 5 years of age (68, 110, 116, 117). The genetic defect in this kindred did not, however, compel the occurrence of nephrocalcinosis. In four children from this kindred and in three children from a second kindred in whom high-dose alkali therapy (4 to 12 mEq/kg/day) was initiated before 4 years of age, neither radiographically demonstrable nephrocalcinosis nor nephrolithiasis has developed with treatment ranging from 10 to 20 years in duration. Furthermore, the glomerular filtration rate (GFR) of these patients has remained normal (104). In these patients, the hypercalciuria and hypocitraturia were corrected by high-dose alkali therapy (104). Thus, in some children with type 1 RTA, nephrocalcinosis and loss of renal function could be prevented.

Table 34.2.
Clinical Spectrum of Type 1 or Distal RTA

Primary (without associated systemic disease)
Genetically transmitted (68, 110 115–117)
Sporadic (52–57, 60, 65–68, 72)
Genetically transmitted systemic diseases
Ehlers-Danlos syndrome (118)
Hereditary elliptocytosis (119)
Sickle-cell anemia (120, 121)
Osteopetrosis (122)
Carbonic-anhydrase deficiency (122, 124, 125)
Marfan syndrome (126)
Sensorineural deafness (127, 128)
Autoimmune diseases
Hypergammaglobulinemia
Hyperglobulinemic purpura (129)
Cryoglobulinemia (83)
Sjogren's syndrome (84–86, 130)
Chronic active hepatitis (87–89)
Primary biliary cirrhosis (89, 131, 132)
Thyroiditis (133)
Fibrosing alveolitis (134)
Systemic lupus erythematosus (135, 136)
Disorders causing nephrocalcinosis
Hypercalciuria
Familial (137, 138)
Idiopathic (139, 140)
Primary hyperparathyroidism (141, 142)
Vitamin D intoxication (143)
Hyperthyroidism (144)
Medullary sponge kidney (145, 146)
Hereditary fructose intolerance (after chronic fructose ingestion) (147)
Wilson's disease (148)
Fabry's disease (149)
Drug-or-toxin-induced nephropathy
Amphotericin B (79, 80)
Toluene (150)
Analgesics (151, 152)
Lithium (153)
Cyclamate (154)
Other renal diseases
Obstructive uropathy (155, 159)
Pyelonephritis (associated with urolithiasis) (160)
Renal transplantation (161, 162)
Leprosy (163)
Miscellaneous disorders
Hepatic cirrhosis (164–165a)

Adapted from Morris RC Jr, Sebastian A: Renal tubular acidosis and Fanconi syndrome. In The Metabolic Basis of Inherited Disease, ed 5. New York, McGraw-Hill, 1983.

Incomplete Syndrome of Renal Tubular Acidosis. The term incomplete RTA has been used to describe patients in whom systemic acidosis does not occur spontaneously, but in whom urinary acidification is impaired. Urinary pH is abnormally high and urinary excretion of titratable acid abnormally low when acidosis is induced by administration of NH_4Cl (57, 103, 166, 167); urinary excretion of ammonium can be normal or increased (57, 166). Incomplete RTA commonly is associated with nephrocalcinosis and nephrolithiasis, hypercalciuria, and reduced urinary excretion of citrate (57, 103, 166, 167).

It should be pointed out that the evidence that patients with incomplete RTA do not have acidosis is not convincing. We now know that measured values of blood pH and plasma bicarbonate concentration must be assessed in relation to the prevailing rate of endogenous acid production (167a) and the set-point at which plasma P_{CO_2} is regulated by the respiratory system (167b), before the values can be said to be normal. Incomplete RTA may reflect only "incomplete" evaluation of the acid-base status of blood.

In some kindreds in which an autosomal dominant disorder of renal acidification is present, the genetic defect is expressed as incomplete RTA, hypercalciuria, and hypocitraturia (103, 112, 166). Progression to frank acidosis occurs in association with the development of nephrocalcinosis or nephrolithiasis. Accordingly, in some genotypes of type 1 RTA, hypercalciuria and hypocitraturia may be not only the primary metabolic manifestations of the genetic defect, but also critical events in the pathogenesis of nephrocalcinosis and nephrolithiasis, and in the progression of incomplete to complete RTA.

In some kindreds in which hypercalciuria appears to occur as an autosomal dominant trait, both complete and incomplete RTA have been found in the hypercalciuric members, usually in association with nephrocalcinosis (137, 138). It has been proposed that over time, hypercalciuria gives rise to nephrocalcinosis, which damages the renal tubule, impairs acidification, and thereby furthers the pathogenesis of the nephrocalcinosis.

Type 2 or Proximal Renal Tubular Acidosis

Physiological Characteristics

Patients with type 2 or proximal RTA have severe renal bicarbonate wasting when plasma bicarbonate concentration is normal, but during severe acidosis their bicarbonaturia ceases, urinary pH decreases to less than 5.5, and net acid excretion approximates net acid production, suggesting that the acidification process in the distal nephron is intact (Fig. 34.2) (1, 60, 62–65). In these patients, greater than 15% of the filtered load of bicarbonate may be excreted in the urine when plasma bicarbonate concentration is normal. This suggests that bicarbonate reabsorption by the proximal tubule is impaired, because this nephron segment in the normal monkey and rat reabsorbs greater than 85% of the filtered load of bicarbonate (6, 8, 10, 168).

The physiological characteristics of type 2 RTA can be explained in the following manner: at normal plasma bicarbonate concentrations in normal subjects, approximately 15% of the filtered load of bicarbonate escapes reabsorption by the proximal tubule and is reabsorbed in the distal nephron; urinary excretion of bicarbonate is negligible, urinary pH is appropriately low, and net acid excretion is normal. In patients with type 2 RTA, the capacity of the proximal tubule to reabsorb bicarbonate is reduced. At normal plasma bicarbonate concentrations, more than 15% of the filtered load of bicarbonate escapes reabsorption and supernormal amounts of bicarbonate are delivered to the distal nephron. This load overwhelms its limited capacity to reabsorb bicarbonate, and substantial bicarbonaturia occurs, net acid excretion ceases, and metabolic acidosis ensues (Fig. 34.3). As metabolic acidosis develops and the plasma bicarbonate concentration decreases, the filtered load of bicarbonate decreases to a point at which the amount of bicarbonate that escapes reabsorption by the impaired proximal tubule is sufficiently small so that it can be completely reabsorbed by the distal nephron. Bicarbonaturia ceases, urinary pH is appropriately low, and net acid excretion is normal.

Pathogenesis

Type 2 RTA occurs in a variety of diseases (73), usually as part of Fanconi syndrome, a generalized dysfunction of the proximal tubule characterized by impaired reabsorption of amino acids, phosphate, glucose, and usually bicarbonate and sometimes uric acid (chapter 30). This chapter focuses primarily on those conditions in which the type 2 RTA defect is isolated (Table 34.3).

Table 34.3.
Clinical Spectrum of Type 2 RTA Not Associated with Fanconi Syndrome

Carbonic anhydrase inhibition, alteration, or deficiency
Drugs
Acetazolamide (169–171)
Sulfonamide (172)
Mafenide acetate (173)
Sporadic (174)
Familial
With nerve deafness (124)
With osteopetrosis (122)
Primary
Sporadic
Transient (61, 66)
Adult onset (175)
With cyanotic congenital heart disease (176)
Renal vascular accidents (176a)
Familial (177)

The mechanisms of transport impairment in type 2 RTA have not been defined; inhibition, deficiency, or alteration of carbonic anhydrase activity has been implicated in certain cases. Normal renal acidification depends on two forms of renal carbonic anhydrase; carbonic anhydrase II (also known as carbonic anhydrase C) present in the cytoplasm of renal tubular cells, and an isoenzyme present in the brush-border membrane of the proximal tubule with different amino acid composition and immunoreactivity (178). Drugs that inhibit carbonic anhydrase activity cause type 2 RTA presumably through inhibition of one or both of these carbonic anhydrases (169–173, 179). In one patient with type 2 RTA, administration of acetazolamide did not increase the severity of renal bicarbonate wasting, which was interpreted as evidence that deficiency of renal carbonic anhydrase was the cause of the type 2 RTA (174). In recent studies of patients with familial type 2 RTA associated with osteopetrosis, carbonic anhydrase II activity was low in red blood cells of affected family members, suggesting that the RTA in these patients was caused by deficiency of carbonic anhydrase II (122, 123). In such patients, the renal acidification defect has characteristics of type 1 and type 2 RTA, in that urinary pH remains inappropriately high during moderately severe acidosis, but fractional excretion of bicarbonate is substantial at normal plasma bicarbonate concentrations (180–183). However, when severe acidosis was induced in some of these patients by giving NH_4Cl, urinary pH decreased to less than 5.5 (180, 184), suggesting either that the capacity of the distal nephron to acidify the urine is not totally dependent on carbonic anhydrase or that renal carbonic anhydrase was partially active.

In affected members of another pedigree in which RTA was associated with nerve deafness (124), red blood cell carbonic anhydrase I activity (also known as B) was reduced; the enzyme present had electrophoretic and immunological identity with carbonic anhydrase I from normal subjects. In two patients with RTA associated with Fanconi syndrome, carbonic anhydrase I activity was normal (124). Because carbonic anhydrase I has not been demonstrated in either cytoplasm or brush border of renal tubule cells, the relationship between inactive red blood cell carbonic anhydrase I and the occurrence of RTA is unclear.

There is a transient form of RTA with onset during the first 2 years of life, which disappears as early as 3 years of age. It has physiological characteristics that are consistent with type 2 RTA (61, 66). Patients with this disorder have renal bicarbonate wasting at normal plasma bicarbonate concentrations (61, 66), and at least 10–15 mEq/kg/24 hr of alkali are required to maintain normal plasma bicarbonate concentrations (66).

These patients could acidify their urine (61) and had no evidence of Fanconi syndrome. Adult-onset RTA, persisting isolated type 2 RTA (175), isolated type 2 RTA in association with cyanotic congenital heart disease (176) or renal vascular accidents (176a), and a familial form of isolated type 2 RTA present in early childhood (177) also have been reported.

Pathophysiology

Calcium, Phosphorus, and Bone Metabolism. Children with transient or familial isolated type 2 RTA have normal serum concentrations and urinary excretions of calcium and phosphorus despite the presence of metabolic acidosis (61, 66, 177, 185); bone age may be retarded (177). Rickets or osteomalacia has been reported to occur in patients with isolated type 2 RTA, but only in those in whom vitamin D or calcium intake appears to have been marginal (175, 186). The infrequency of bone disease in untreated patients may be explained by the capacity of these children to excrete normal amounts of net acid, i.e., to excrete H^+ in an amount equal to their endogenous production of noncarbonic acid, as reflected by a net external H^+ balance that is approximately zero (185). When bone disease occurs, supplemental calcium or vitamin D usually is needed to effect healing. By contrast, in patients with untreated, apparently type 1 RTA, metabolic bone disease can occur in the absence of dietary deficiency of vitamin D or calcium and can be healed with alkali therapy alone (53, 109, 111). Patients with untreated type 1 RTA, like those with chronic renal insufficiency, have long-standing, positive net H^+ balance (11, 187–189). It has been postulated that the retained H^+ is titrated by alkaline bone salts and that this loss is the basis for the metabolic bone disease that occurs with chronic metabolic acidosis (187, 190–192). In some patients with RTA and osteopetrosis, radiographic evidence of rickets has been observed (180, 193). The renal acidification defect in these patients has characteristics of both type 1 and type 2 RTA; rickets may occur because net acid balance is positive and bone mineral salts are titrated as occurs in type 1 RTA.

Type 4 or Hyperkalemic Renal Tubular Acidosis

Physiological Characteristics

Hyperkalemia and decreased renal clearance of K occurs in some patients with RTA, most commonly in adults with chronic tubulointerstitial renal disease in whom the GFR is moderately reduced (i.e., GFR about 25 ml/min/1.72m^2 or greater) (194–198). The severity of the acidosis and hyperkalemia is disproportionately great for the degree of renal insufficiency. In these patients, reabsorption of bicarbonate is reduced at normal plasma bicarbonate concentrations (sustained by alkali therapy), but the magnitude of the reduction ($FEHCO_3$ less than 15%) is not so great as to implicate impaired bicarbonate reabsorption by the proximal tubule (196, 197). Urinary pH in these patients can be less than 5.5 during acidosis (194, 197). Despite the low urinary pH, urinary excretion of ammonium and hence of net acid is low. Renal production of ammonia appears to be reversibly suppressed by the hyperkalemia of these patients (1977). Renal clearance of K is greatly reduced, and the serum concentration of K (K_s) increases greatly when dietary K is increased (198). Proximal tubule function is unimpaired as judged by the absence of hyperaminoaciduria, glycosuria, or increased renal clearance of P. The syndrome of hyperkalemia and RTA, as characterized, has been designated type 4 RTA (197–200).

Pathogenesis and Pathophysiology

The physiological characteristics of type 4 RTA are those predicted to occur in patients with aldosterone deficiency or impairment in its renal physiological effect. When aldosterone deficiency is induced experimentally in dogs, hyperkalemia and hyperchloremic acidosis occur and net acid excretion is decreased (200). The decrease in net acid excretion is a result principally of a decrease in renal excretion of ammonium secondary to diminished renal production of ammonia. The reduced ammonia production in the dog appears to be a result in part of hyperkalemia, because the rate of ammonia excretion varies inversely with the plasma potassium concentration, and ammonia excretion is suppressed to a lesser extent when hyperkalemia is prevented by restricting potassium intake when mineralocorticoid is discontinued (200). In the rabbit, mineralocorticoid hormone stimulates H^+ secretion in both the cortical and outer medullary collecting tubules (28, 29). Adrenalectomy reduces the rate of H^+ secretion in the medullary collecting tubule, and aldosterone replacement restores the rate, providing evidence that normal levels of aldosterone maintain the normal rate of H^+ secretion in this segment (29). Since the outer medullary collecting tubule is a quantitatively major site of distal nephron acidification in the rabbit (201), mineralocorticoid hormone-stimulated H^+ secretion may be the major determinant of H^+ secretion in the mammalian distal nephron. The results of studies of aldosterone deficiency in the dog and rabbit are consistent with the results of in vitro studies in turtle bladders, which indicate that aldosterone deficiency decreases the maximal rate of active H^+ secretion in the absence of an opposing transepithelial electrical gradient, but does not impair the ability of the H^+ secretory pump to establish steep H^+ concentration gradients between serosa and mucosa (27).

In humans with adrenalectomy receiving adequate glucocorticoid replacement, plasma bicarbonate concentration and net acid excretion decrease when mineralocorticoid is discontinued and increase when mineralocorticoid is initiated (202). The changes in net acid excretion vary directly with the changes in plasma total CO_2 and in sodium balance and inversely with the changes in potassium balance. These findings provide strong evidence that in humans, renal acidification is under tonic stimulation by physiological levels of mineralocorticoid hormone.

Clinical Variants

The designation type 4 RTA can be applied to all patients with hyperkalemia and RTA in whom the ability to lower urinary pH is intact, whether aldosterone deficiency is present or absent, or whether the status of aldosterone activity and renal responsiveness is known (203). Type 4 RTA occurs in a wide variety of clinical disorders with and without associated renal parenchymal disease (Table 34.4). In the initial group of patients in whom the syndrome was characterized, chronic tubulointerstitial renal disease and reduced GFR were associated with hypoaldosteronism, but normal secretion of glucocorticoid hormone (195, 197). In the majority of such patients, the decrease in secretion of aldosterone appears to be causally related to a decrease in renal secretion of renin (197, 198), so called hyporeninemic hypoaldosteronism (196–198, 213–217). Possible causes of decreased secretion of renin are primary destruction of cells of the juxtaglomerular apparatus, decreased neurally mediated renin release in patients with diabetic nephropathy and neuropathy, and defective renal conversion of the inactive renin precursor, big renin, to its normally active form (216). In patients with tubulointerstitial renal disease in whom type 4 RTA is associated with aldosterone deficiency, administration of physiological amounts of mineralocorticoid hormone can decrease urinary pH, increase net acid excretion, and substantially correct metabolic acidosis and hyperkalemia (Fig. 34.6). Administration of superphysiological doses of mineralocorticoid is required for correction of the acidosis in some of these patients, suggesting that some degree of renal tubular unresponsiveness to mineralocorticoid occurs (Fig. 34.7) (197).

The syndrome of type 4 RTA and aldosterone deficiency can occur

Table 34.4.
Clinical Spectrum Of Type 4 RTA

Aldosterone deficiency
- Combined deficiency of aldosterone and adrenal glucocorticoid hormones
  - Inherited impairment of steroidogenesis: 21-hydroxylase deficiency—congenital adrenal hyperplasia (204–206)
  - Addison's disease
  - Bilateral adrenalectomy
- Isolated deficiency of aldosterone
  - Inherited impairment of aldosterone biosynthesis: corticosterone methyl oxidase deficiency (207–212)
  - Secondary to deficient renin secretion
    - Chronic tubulointerstitial disease with renal insufficiency-"hyporeninemic hypoaldosteronism" (196–198, 213–217)
    - Indomethacin administration (218)
  - Chronic idiopathic hypoaldosteronism in children (219–221) and adults (222–224)

Attenuated renal response to aldosterone with secondary hyperreninemia and hyperaldosteronism—pseudohypoaldosteronism
- Pseudohypoaldosteronism of infancy (209, 225–234)
- Chronic tubulointerstitial disease with renal insufficiency-"saltwasting nephritis" (235, 236)
- Obstructive uropathy in infancy (237)
- Drugs
  - Spironolactone
  - Amiloride
  - Triamterene

Attenuated renal response to aldosterone with aldosterone deficiency
- Selective tubule dysfunction with impaired renin secretion (238–246)
- Chronic tubulointerstitial disease with renal insufficiency
  - Associated deficient renin secretion (196, 197, 213–217)
  - Renin status uncertain
- Obstructive uropathy with deficient renin secretion (217)
- Renal transplantation with deficient renin secretion (247, 248)
- Lupus nephritis with deficient renin secretion (249)

Uncertain pathophysiology
- Chronic pyelonephritis (194, 250)
- Lupus nephritis (251)
- Renal transplantation (252)
- Acute glomerulonephritis (253)
- Renal amyloidosis (254)

Adapted from Morris RC Jr, Sebastian A: Renal tubular acidosis and Fanconi syndrome. In The Metabolic Basis of Inherited Disease, ed 5. New York, McGraw-Hill, 1983.

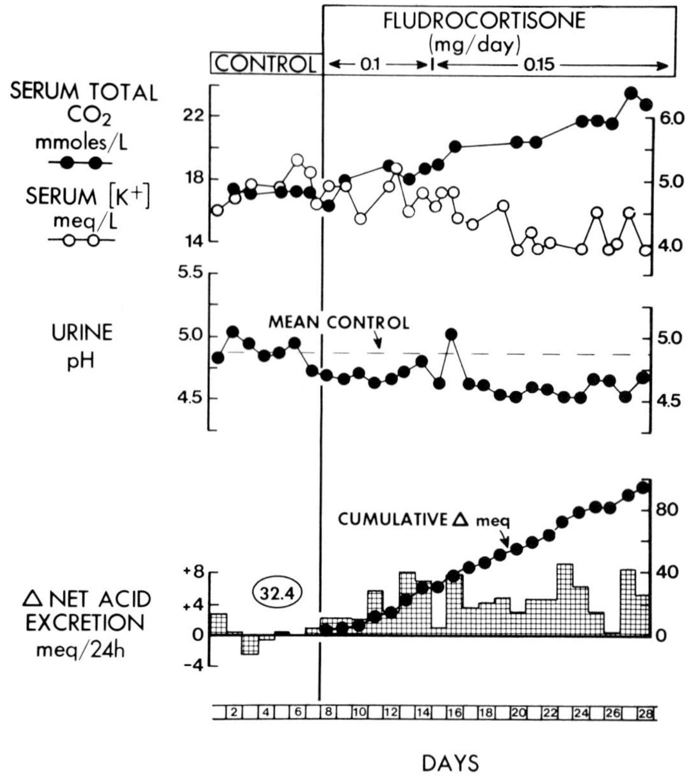

Figure 34.6. Effect of orally administered fludrocortisone on serum total CO_2 and potassium concentration, urinary pH, urinary titratable acid, ammonium, and net acid excretion in a patient with hyporeninemic hypoaldosteronism and chronic renal insufficiency (creatinine clearance, 13 ml/min/1.73 m^2). Systemic acidosis had not previously been treated. The severity of hyperkalemia had been mitigated before the study was initiated by provision of a low-normal dietary intake of potassium. The hatched bars represent the difference between the measured value of acid excretion and the mean value before therapy; the magnitude of the difference is indicated by the scale on the left-hand side of the panel. The mean control value is designated by the numerals within the elipse. The accumulated values of the daily differences are shown by the solid circles and are indicated by the scale on the right-hand side of the panel. (Adapted from Sebastian A, et al: N Engl J Med 297: 576, 1977.)

in a number of clinical conditions in which diffuse renal parenchymal damage is not present (Table 34.4). Deficiency of aldosterone may be associated with deficiency of glucocorticoid hormone, as in infants with the salt-wasting form of congenital adrenal hyperplasia, 21-hydroxylase deficiency (204–206) or in patients with bilateral adrenal insufficiency. An isolated deficiency of aldosterone that can give rise to sodium depletion, failure to thrive, hyperkalemia, and metabolic acidosis can occur in children because of an inborn error of aldosterone biosynthesis, corticosterone methyl oxidase deficiency (207–212). Isolated deficiency of aldosterone can be secondary to congenital deficiency of renin (219–221). In these disorders, mineralocorticoid replacement therapy and sodium supplements correct the hyponatremia, hyperkalemia, and metabolic acidosis and improve the growth rate (Chapter 33).

In some patients with type 4 RTA, there is evidence for end-organ resistance to the renal action of aldosterone. In infants with pseudohypoaldosteronism, failure to thrive, dehydration, hyponatremia, hyperkalemia, and hyperchloremic acidosis occur as an apparently congenital disorder that is sometimes familial (209, 225–234). Plasma-renin activity and urinary and plasma aldosterone levels are increased, whereas plasma levels of glucocorticoid hormones are normal. Prolonged administration of superphysiological amounts of mineralocorticoid hormone fails to correct renal Na wasting and decreased renal clearance of K, whereas large supplements of NaCl reverses the hyponatremia and hyperkalemia, relieves symptoms, and permits normal or improved growth. Renal Na wasting and K retention spontaneously remit after infancy, and supplemental NaCl is no longer necessary, although plasma levels of renin and aldosterone remain supernormal (Chapter 33). The renal dysfunction persists, because hyponatremia and hyperkalemia reappear when dietary sodium chloride is restricted (229). The pathophysiological manifestations of the disorder are consistent with depressed cellular response to aldosterone in those segments of the renal tubule normally responsive to aldosterone, i.e., the collecting tubules and ducts.

A rare syndrome of hyperkalemia, hyperchloremic acidosis, and hypertension has been reported in a few children and adults without evidence of renal parenchymal disease (238–246). Plasma levels of renin are low or undetectable and aldosterone secretion is low or normal. It

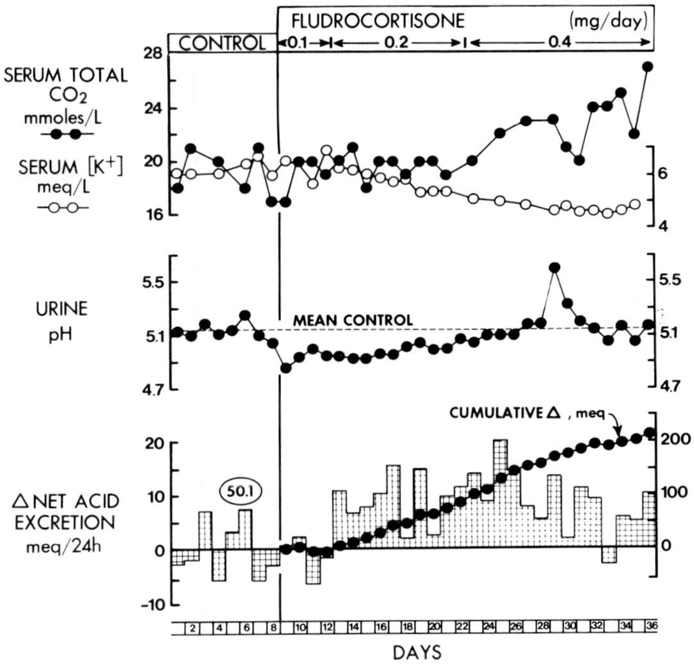

Figure 34.7. Effect of orally administered fludrocortisone on serum total CO_2 and potassium concentration, urinary pH, urinary titratable acid, ammonium, and net acid excretion in a patient with hyporeninemic hypoaldosteronism and chronic renal insufficiency (creatinine clearance 35 ml/min/1.73 m^2). Systemic acidosis had not been previously treated. See legend Figure 34.6 for explanation of symbols. (Adapted from Sebastian A, et al: N Engl J Med 297: 576, 1977.)

Table 34.5.
Prototypic Characteristics of the Various Types of RTA

	Type 1	Type 1 with HCO_3^- wasting	Type 2	Type 4
At subnormal $[HCO_3^-]_p$[a]				
Urine pH	>6.0	>6.0	<5.5	<5.5
TA and NH_4 excretion	↓	↓	nl or ↓	↓
Urinary citrate excretion	↓	↓	↑	?
Serum K^+	nl or ↓	nl or ↓	usually ↓	↑
Renal K^+ clearance	>20%	>20%	>20%	<20%
At normal $[HCO_3^-]_p$				
TA and NH_4 excretion	↓	↓	↓	↓
$FEHCO_3$[b]	3–5%	5–10%	>15%	1–15%
Urinary citrate excretion	nl	nl	↑	?
Serum K^+	nl	nl	nl or ↓	nl or ↑
(U-B) Pco_2[c] (mmHg)	<20	<20	>20	?
Therapeutic alkali requirement (mEq/kg/day)	1–3	5–10	5–20	1–5
Osteomalacia	rare	rare	frequent	absent
Nephrocalcinosis/nephrolithiasis	common	common	rare	absent

[a] Plasma bicarbonate concentration.
[b] Fractional excretion of HCO_3^-.
[c] When urinary pH is greater than blood pH.

has been suggested that in such patients, a primary abnormality of the distal nephron that increases its reabsorptive avidity for chloride gives rise to a decrease in the lumen-negative, sodium and mineralocorticoid dependent electrical driving force for potassium and H^+ secretion, resulting in hyperkalemia and acidosis; and an increase in distal sodium reabsorption resulting in ECF volume expansion, hypertension, and suppression of the renin-aldosterone system (246). Restriction of dietary sodium chloride or administration of diuretics corrects the hyperkalemia and acidosis in these patients.

DIAGNOSIS OF RENAL TUBULAR ACIDOSIS

Clinical Findings

The untreated child with RTA has nonspecific symptoms, such as failure to thrive, polydypsia and polyuria, constipation, anorexia, vomiting, and listlessness. The presence of certain signs and symptoms suggests a particular type of RTA (Table 34.5). Children with type 1 RTA usually are diagnosed before rickets has become clinically apparent. Rickets and osteomalacia are uncommon in patients with isolated type 2 RTA, whereas in those with type 2 RTA associated with Fanconi syndrome, metabolic bone disease may be a prominent presenting feature, often in association with hypophosphatemia and mild hypocalcemia (255). Nephrocalcinosis is common in patients with type 1 RTA, but occurs only rarely in patients with type 2 RTA and has not been reported in patients with type 4 RTA (255). Muscle weakness may be a prominent feature in untreated patients with osteomalacia or hypokalemia who have type 1 RTA or type 2 RTA associated with Fanconi syndrome.

Determination of Acid-Base Status

In healthy infants and young children, the normal values for blood Pco_2 and plasma bicarbonate and total CO_2 concentrations are lower than those in healthy adults; the values increase with age (Table 34.6) (256–262). In healthy adults, the plasma pH and bicarbonate concentration are determined to a large extent by the set point at which Pco_2 is regulated by the respiratory system (167a) and by the rate of endogenous acid production (167b); the latter being largely determined by diet composition (2). Although the normal range of values of plasma bicar-

Table 34.6.
Normal Values for Plasma Acid-Base Composition in Infants and Children[a]

Age		pH	Arterialized venous[b]		
			pCO_2	$[HCO_3^-]$[c]	$[TCO_2]$[d]
			mmHg	mEq/L	mEq/L
1–24 mos	mean	7.40	34	19	20
	range	7.34–7.46	26–41	16–22	17–23
2–12 yrs	mean	7.40	38	22	23
	range	7.36–7.44	33–43	19–25	20–26
12–18 yrs	mean	7.40	40	24	25
	range	7.36–7.44	36–44	21–27	22–28

From references 256–262.
[a] The ranges depicted are calculated as mean ± 1 S.D.
[b] In venous blood, pH is approximately 0.02 units lower, Pco_2 approximately 4 mm Hg higher, and $[HCO_3^-]$ and $[TCO_2]$ 1 mEq higher than in arterialized blood.
[c] Bicarbonate concentration $[HCO_3^-]$ is a calculated value derived from the pH and Pco_2 values using the Henderson-Hasselbach equation.
[d] Most clinical laboratories measure the total CO_2 content (TCO_2) and not the bicarbonate concentration, even though the value obtained may be reported as plasma bicarbonate concentration, HCO_3^-. Total CO_2 content is equal to the sum of HCO_3^- + dissolved CO_2 + H_2CO_3. The H_2CO_3 is negligible and the dissolved CO_2 content is equal to 0.03 × Pco_2. Thus the true HCO_3^- = TCO_2 − 0.03 × Pco_2 or approximately 1 mEq less than TCO_2.

bonate concentration is broad, the concentration in a given individual varies little from day-to-day under steady state conditions (167a, 167b). In normal infants, the plasma bicarbonate concentration varies directly with P_{CO_2} (258) and inversely with the amount of protein and presumably potential net acid in the diet (263, 264). Metabolic acidosis may be present in a child even though the values of plasma pH and bicarbonate concentration fall within the broad range of published values observed in healthy children consuming diets of unknown composition (256–262).

The metabolic acidosis of patients with RTA is associated with a normal "anion gap." Other disorders that can cause metabolic acidosis with a normal anion gap are those that result in a loss of bicarbonate from the gastrointestinal tract, e.g., diarrhea, gastrointestinal fistulas, or nasojejunal suctioning; ingestion of chloride-containing acid salts such as NH_4Cl, arginine hydrochloride, or chloride-containing amino acid mixtures as found in some intravenous or oral alimentation preparations; and dilutional acidosis induced by intravenous administration of large amounts of NaCl. When metabolic acidosis is associated with retention in plasma of anions of endogenously produced or exogenously administered (nonchloride-containing) acids, the anion gap is increased; this may occur with ingestion of toxins, in uremic acidosis, with ketoacidosis, lactic acidosis, and with certain inborn errors of metabolism usually seen in infants.

The diagnosis of RTA should be considered in patients with persisting hyperchloremic metabolic acidosis in whom extrarenal causes of the acidosis have been excluded, especially when the urinary pH seems inappropriately high for the severity of the acidosis. To evaluate the latter, one should obtain an arterial or arterialized venous blood sample for measurement of blood pH, P_{CO_2}, and total CO_2 concentration, near simultaneously with obtaining a urine sample for measurement of pH. Arterialized venous blood can be obtained by warming the extremity with a heating pad for 20 minutes before blood is drawn; blood should be drawn without a tourniquet. The values for pH and bicarbonate concentration determined in arterialized venous blood are virtually the same as those determined in arterial blood (265). The urine sample for measurement of pH should be promptly covered with a thin layer of mineral oil or taken up in a syringe to prevent loss of CO_2 and an increase in pH; pH should be measured using a pH meter. The child not toilet trained fitted with a urine collection bag often voids while the blood is being drawn.

The relationship in normal infants and children between urinary pH and plasma total CO_2 has been evaluated only in subjects made acutely acidotic by administration of ammonium chloride (257–260). In normal infants 2 to $11\frac{1}{2}$ months of age, urinary pH is less than 6.0 and usually less than 5.5 when plasma (arterialized capillary) total CO_2 concentration decreases to less than 21 mEq/l (257). In normal children 4 to 13 years of age, urinary pH is less than 6.0 when plasma total CO_2 concentration is below 23.5 mEq/l; urinary pH is less than 5.5 when plasma total CO_2 concentration is 19.5 mEq/l (260).

Characterization of the Type of Renal Tubular Acidosis

In patients with suspected RTA in whom the severity of the acidosis is only moderate (plasma total CO_2 concentration of about 18 mEq/l), and in whom urinary pH is greater than 6.0, it is recommended that NH_4Cl be given to increase the severity of the acidosis to distinguish type 1 RTA from type 2 or type 4 RTA (Fig. 34.2).

The NH_4Cl loading test is performed as follows. First, obtain a urine sample for determination of pH and an arterialized venous blood sample for determination of acid-base status. Then give NH_4Cl 0.15 g/kg, by mouth over 30 to 45 minutes (tablets may be crushed and given in food or liquid or placed in gelatin capsules). The patient may eat and should be encouraged to drink during the study. Urine is collected hourly in older children or as voided in younger children, for 4 hours, at which time a second blood specimen is obtained. In most subjects, the induced acidosis is maximal 4 hours after giving NH_4Cl, but in some children the nadir of plasma total CO_2 concentration may not occur until 6 or 8 hours. If after 4 hours urinary pH remains above 5.5 and plasma total CO_2 concentration is only minimally depressed, it may be prudent to continue to collect urine samples and to obtain another blood sample 6 or 8 hours after giving NH_4Cl.

If urinary pH decreases to less than 5.5, the diagnosis of type 1 RTA can be ruled out. If urinary pH remains greater than 5.5 despite a severe degree of acidosis (plasma total CO_2 concentration less than 15 mEq/l), it is likely that the patient has type 1 RTA. However, in some patients with type 2 RTA, urinary pH may not fall below 5.5 until the plasma total CO_2 concentration falls below 12 mEq/l (174).

In patients with type 2 or type 4 RTA in whom acidosis is severe, urinary pH may be appropriately acidic, i.e., less than 5.5. Their urinary pH will become greater than 6.0 when acidosis is partially corrected with oral alkali, which distinguishes them from patients with an extrarenal cause of acidosis in whom urine pH remains less than 6.0 until plasma bicarbonate concentration is normalized by alkali therapy. Renal handling of bicarbonate can be estimated by calculating the fraction of filtered bicarbonate excreted in the urine at normal plasma bicarbonate levels. In patients with type 2 RTA, fractional excretion of bicarbonate is often greater than 15%.

Renal acidification may also be evaluated by determining the difference in P_{CO_2} between urine-blood (U-B) P_{CO_2} when urinary pH is rendered greater than blood pH by administration of alkali. In adult patients with type 1 RTA, values of (U-B) P_{CO_2} are less than 20, whereas in normal adults, (U-B) P_{CO_2} increases to values above 25 to 30 mgHg when urine bicarbonate concentration is greater than about 80 mEq/l (69, 71, 77). Values of (U-B) P_{CO_2} in patients should be compared with those of controls at comparable urine bicarbonate concentrations.

Additional Characteristics

In patients with type 1 RTA, the urinary calcium and citrate excretion are reduced during acidosis, but increase to normal values when acidosis is corrected with alkali therapy (52, 57, 68, 72, 98–104). By contrast, in patients with type 2 RTA associated with Fanconi syndrome, urinary citrate excretion is increased during acidosis and after its correction, the fractional renal clearance of phosphate, amino acids, glucose, and potassium are increased, and hypophosphatemia and hypokalemia occur. In patients with type 1 RTA, hypokalemia is usually attenuated when the acidosis is corrected, whereas in patients with type 2 RTA and Fanconi syndrome, hypokalemia may increase in severity when alkali is administered (Fig. 34.5). (92). In patients with type 4 RTA, evaluation of the status of renin-aldosterone activity may help distinguish aldosterone deficiency from aldosterone-resistant states.

TREATMENT AND PROGNOSIS OF PATIENTS WITH RENAL TUBULAR ACIDOSIS

Type 1 or Distal Renal Tubular Acidosis

In patients with previously untreated type 1 RTA or in children with type 1 RTA and bicarbonate wasting in whom alkali therapy is omitted, severe acidosis, hypokalemia, and hypocalcemia may occur. Hypokalemia can be severe enough to cause respiratory depression in some patients; when severe, hypokalemia should be corrected with intravenously administered K, 1 to 3 mEq/kg, 6 to 12 hours before acidosis is corrected. Sustained correction of acidosis can be achieved by oral administration of $NaHCO_3$ or Na citrate (Shohl's solution). K intake should at least equal maintenance levels (3 mEq/100 kcal/day) (Chapter 11). In infants and young children, alkali can be initiated at a dose of about 3 mEq/kg/day and increased at 2 to 4 day intervals until the plasma bicarbonate concentration is normal. In the first weeks to months after initiation of alkali therapy when growth velocity increases strikingly, the dose of alkali per kilogram body weight often increases (68). The amount of alkali required to sustain correction of acidosis may range from 5 to 14 mEq/kg/day, the amount being determined principally by the magnitude of renal bicarbonate wasting. Such large amounts of alkali are preferably administered to children in four divided doses or to infants with each feeding of formula. After the age of 4 to 6 years, alkali requirements become less, although some children continue to require amounts in excess of 3 mEq/kg/day (58, 62). In adult patients with type 1 RTA, the amount of alkali required to correct acidosis is 1 to 2 mEq/kg/day, administered in three divided doses.

With sustained correction of acidosis with $NaHCO_3$ alone, renal wasting of potassium diminishes and hypokalemia is corrected in the majority of patients (Fig. 34.5). However, in some patients, potassium supplements may be required to sustain normokalemia; 20% to 50% of the alkali requirement can be given as $KHCO_3$ or K citrate.

In growth retarded infants with type 1 RTA, growth velocity increases within weeks of initiating alkali therapy and within 3 to 6 months, normal stature can be attained (68). Older children may take several years to attain normal height (68). In infants and children with type 1 RTA in whom acidosis is corrected over years with alkali therapy, normal growth is usually attained and maintained (68). Bone disease does not occur in treated patients.

Nephrocalcinosis may be present radiographically as early as the first few months of life (67, 72, 74) and appears to be invariably present by 4 years of age in untreated children with type 1 RTA or in those receiving alkali in amounts of 3 mEq/kg/day or less. However, nephrocalcinosis may be prevented. In a group of infants and children with type 1 RTA in whom alkali therapy was initiated before the age of 4 years and in amounts greater than 4 mEq/kg/day, neither radiographically demonstrable nephrocalcinosis nor nephrolithiasis have developed with treatment ranging from 10 to 20 years in duration (104). With correction of acidosis, urinary calcium excretion decreases (52, 68, 72) and citrate excretion increases (98, 101–104a). It has been suggested that urinary calcium excretion is a sensitive guide to therapy and that an attempt should be made to keep the excretion rate within the range of normal (72).

Type 2 or Proximal Renal Tubular Acidosis

Correction of acidosis in patients with type 2 RTA requires administration of alkali in amounts sufficient both to titrate the endogenous production of noncarbonic acid and to offset the urinary excretion of net base that occurs when plasma bicarbonate is normal. At normal plasma bicarbonate concentrations, urinary excretion of net base can vary from as little as 2 to 3 mEq/kg/day in patients with minimal impairment of proximal bicarbonate reabsorption or with greatly reduced GFR, to values greater than 20 mEq/kg/day in patients with more marked dysfunction or more normal GFR. Thus, alkali requirements must be determined empirically for each patient.

Hypokalemia and renal potassium wasting are not characteristic of patients with isolated type 2 RTA (61, 66, 175), and the acidosis can be corrected by giving $NaHCO_3$ alone. In patients with type 2 RTA and Fanconi syndrome, correction of hypokalemia can be achieved by giving a substantial fraction, often 50% or more, of the alkali requirement as $KHCO_3$ or K citrate. When the amount of alkali required to correct acidosis is prohibitively large, restriction of dietary NaCl or coadministration of hydrochlorothiazide at an initial dosage of 1.5 to 2 mg/kg/day may be helpful. This agent may increase proximal bicarbonate reabsorption by inducing contraction of extracellular fluid volume or may stimulate H^+ secretion directly and thus may permit correction of acidosis with lesser amounts of alkali. Hydrochlorothiazide may, however, exacerbate renal potassium wasting. When type 2 RTA is associated with Fanconi syndrome, treatment is directed where possible towards removal of those substances critical to its causation, as in the case of hereditary fructose intolerance, galactosemia, Wilson's disease, and tyrosinemia (type 2) (Chapter 30).

Short stature is characteristic of children with isolated type 2 RTA. Indeed, in children with transient (61, 66) or familial isolated type 2 RTA (177), impaired growth usually is the presenting complaint. Metabolic acidosis per se may be a critical pathogenetic determinant of impaired somatic growth. In growth retarded infants and children with transient isolated type 2 RTA, growth velocity increases dramatically with alkali therapy sufficient to correct the acidosis (61, 66).

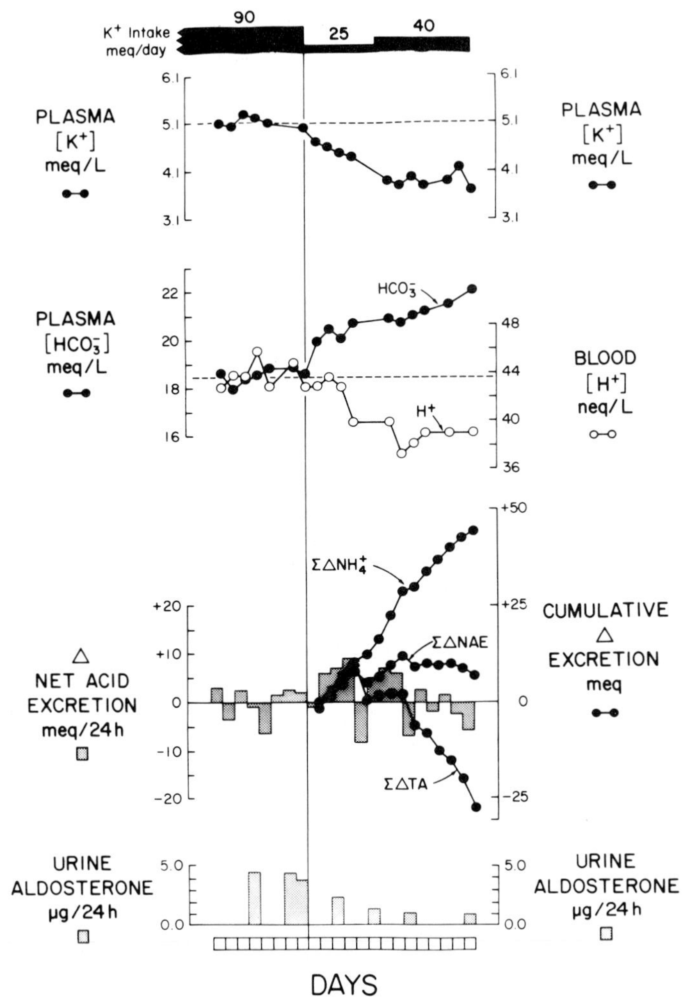

Figure 34.8. Effect of restriction and partial replenishment of dietary potassium on plasma potassium concentration, bicarbonate and blood hydrogen ion concentrations, and urinary excretion of ammonium, titratable acid, net acid, and aldosterone in a patient with hyperkalemia, metabolic acidosis, and chronic renal insufficiency (creatinine clearance 36 ml/min/1.73 m²). See Figure 34.6 for explanations of symbols. (Adapted from Maher T, et al: J Lab Clin Med 103: 432, 1984.)

Type 4 or Hyperkalemic Renal Tubular Acidosis

In adult patients with type 4 RTA who have tubulointerstitial renal disease and reduced GFR, administration of mineralocorticoid in either physiological replacement doses (fludrocortisone, 0.10 to 0.15 mg/day) or superphysiological amounts is associated with a reduction in urinary pH, an increase in net acid excretion, and a substantial amelioration of metabolic acidosis and hyperkalemia (Figs. 34.6 and 7) (197). However, in patients with hypertension or evidence of increased ECF volume, treatment with mineralocorticoid may not be indicated because of its effect to increase renal reabsorption of sodium chloride, which may exacerbate hypertension or lead to other adverse effects of an increased ECF volume.

Restriction of dietary K in patients with type 4 RTA and moderate renal insufficiency has resulted in correction of hyperkalemia and amelioration of metabolic acidosis (Fig. 34.8) (266). Administration of furosemide has also been shown to ameliorate acidosis and hyperkalemia in these patients (267). Administration of $NaHCO_3$, 1 to 2 mEq/kg/day, may be sufficient to correct acidosis and partially correct the hyperkalemia.

In patients without intrinsic renal parenchymal disease in whom type 4 RTA is a result of deficiency of aldosterone, either isolated or combined with deficiency of glucocorticoid hormone, administration of physiological amounts of synthetic mineralocorticoid hormone can correct hyponatremia, hyperkalemia, and metabolic acidosis and improve the growth rate (204–212, 219–221). In patients with pseudohypoaldosteronism, administration of supplemental NaCl often suffices (Chapter 34).

References

1. Alpern RJ, Warnock DG, Rector FC Jr: Renal acidification mechanisms. In Brenner BM, Rector FC Jr (eds): The Kidney, ed 3. Philadelphia, W. B. Saunders, 1986, Chapter 7.
2. Lennon EJ, Lemann J Jr, Litzow JR: The effects of diet and stool composition on the net external acid balance of normal subjects. J Clin Invest 45:1601, 1966.
3. Kildeberg P: Disturbances of hydrogen ion balance occurring in premature infants. II. Late Metabolic Acidosis. Acta Pediat 53:517, 1964.
3a. Chan JCM: Calcium and hydrogen ion metabolism in children with classic (Type 1/Distal) renal tubular acidosis. Ann Nutr Metab 25:65, 1981.
4. Rector FC Jr, Carter NW, Seldin DW: The mechanism of bicarbonate reabsorption in the proximal and distal tubules of the kidney. J Clin Invest 44:278, 1965.
5. Vieira FL, Malnic G: Hydrogen ion secretion by rat renal cortical tubules as studied by an antimony microelectrode. Am J Physiol 214:710, 1968.
6. Bennett CM, Brenner BM, Berliner RW: Micropuncture study of nephron function in the rhesus monkey. J Clin Invest 47:203, 1968.
7. DuBose TD Jr, Pucacco LR, Carter NW: Determination of disequilibrium pH in the rat kidney in vivo: evidence for hydrogen secretion. Am J Physiol 240:F138, 1981.
8. Gottschalk CW, Lassiter WE, Mylle M: Localization of urine acidification in the mammalian kidney. Am J Physiol 198:581, 1960.
9. DuBose TD Jr, Pucacco LR, Lucci MS, et al: Micropuncture determination of pH, PCO_2 and total CO_2 concentration in accessible structures of the rat renal cortex. J Clin Invest 64:476, 1979.
10. Cogan MG, Maddox DA, Lucci MS, et al: Control of proximal bicarbonate reabsorption in normal and acidotic rats. J Clin Invest 64:1168, 1979.
11. Relman AS: Renal acidosis and renal excretion of acid in health and disease. Adv Intern Med 12:295, 1964.
12. Malnic G, de Mello-Aires M: Kinetic study of bicarbonate reabsorption in proximal tubule of the rat. Am J Physiol 220:1759, 1971.
13. Alpern RJ, Cogan MG, Rector FC Jr: Effect of luminal bicarbonate concentration on proximal acidification in the rat. Am J Physiol 243:F53, 1982.
14. Sasaki S, Berry CA, Rector FC Jr: Effect of luminal and peritubular HCO_3^- reabsorption in rabbit proximal convoluted tubules perfused in vitro. J Clin Invest 70:639, 1982.
15. Pitts RF, Lotspeich WD: Bicarbonate and the renal regulation of acid-base balance. Am J Physiol 147:138, 1946.
16. Lemieux G, Methot AL, Gagnon-Burnette M, et al: The effect of renal artery constriction on tubular reabsorption of bicarbonate. Nephron 5:362, 1968.
17. Levine DZ: Effect of acute hypercapnia on proximal tubular water and bicarbonate absorption. Am J Physiol 221:1164, 1971.
18. de Mello Aires M, Malnic G: Peritubular pH and PCO_2 in renal tubular acidification. Am J Physiol 228:1766, 1975.
19. Jacobson HR: Effects of CO_2 and acetazolamide on bicarbonate and fluid transport in rabbit proximal tubules. Am J Physiol 9:F54, 1981.
20. Cogan MG: Effects of acute alterations in PCO_2 on proximal bicarbonate, chloride and water reabsorption in the rat. Am J Physiol 246:F21, 1984.
21. Giebisch G, Malnic G, de Mello GB, et al: Kinetics of luminal acidification in cortical tubules of the rat kidney. J Physiol 267:571, 1977.
22. Chan YL, Biagi B, Giebisch G: Control mechanisms of bicarbonate transport across the rat proximal convoluted tubule. Am J Physiol 242:F532, 1982.
23. Alpern RJ, Cogan MG, Rector FC Jr: Effects of extracellular fluid volume and plasma bicarbonate concentration on proximal acidification in the rat. J Clin Invest 71:736, 1983.
24. Kunau RT Jr, Frick A, Rector FC Jr, et al: Micropuncture study of the proximal tubular factors responsible for the maintenance of alkalosis during potassium deficiency in the rat. Clin Sci 34:223, 1968.
25. Schwartz WB, Jenson RL, Relman AS: Acidification of the urine and increased ammonium excretion without change in acid-base equilibrium: Sodium reabsorption as a stimulus to the acidifying process. J Clin Invest 34:673, 1955.
26. Clapp JR, Rector FC Jr, Seldin DW: Effect of unreabsorbed anions on proximal and distal transtubular potentials in rats. Am J Physiol 202:781, 1962.
27. Al-Awqati Q, Norby LH, Mueller A, et al: Characteristics of stimulation of H^+ transport by aldosterone in turtle urinary bladder. J Clin Invest 58:351, 1976.
28. Koeppen BM, Helman SI: Acidification of luminal fluid by the rabbit cortical collecting tubule perfused in vitro. Am J Physiol 242:F521, 1982.
29. Stone DK, Seldin DW, Kokko JP, et al: Mineralocorticoid modulation of rabbit medullary collecting duct acidification: a sodium-independent effect. J Clin Invest 72:77, 1983.
30. Purkerson ML, Lubowitz H, White RW, et al: On the influence of extracellular fluid volume expansion on bicarbonate reabsorption in the rat. J Clin Invest 48:1754, 1969.
31. Kurtzman NA: Regulation of renal bicarbonate reabsorption by extracellular volume. J Clin Invest 49:586, 1970.
32. Cogan MG: Volume expansion predominantly inhibits NaCl rather than $NaHCO_3$. Am J Physiol 245:F272, 1983.
33. Bank N, Aynedjian HS: A micropuncture study of the effect of parathyroid hormone on renal bicarbonate reabsorption. J Clin Invest 58:336, 1976.
34. Puschett JB, Zurbach P: Acute effects of parathyroid hormone on proximal bicarbonate transport in the dog. Kidney Intl 9:501, 1976.
35. Iino Y, Burg MB: Effect of parathyroid hormone on bicarbonate absorption by proximal tubules in vitro. Am J Physiol 236:F387, 1979.
36. McKinney TD, Myers P: Bicarbonate transport by proximal tubules: Effect of parathyroid hormone and dibutyryl cyclic AMP. Am J Physiol 238:F166, 1980.
37. McKinney TD, Myers P: PTH inhibition of bicarbonate transport by proximal convoluted tubules. Am J Physiol 239:F127, 1980.
38. Mitnick PA, Greenberg A, Coffman T, et al: Effects of two models of hypercalcemia on renal acid-base metabolism. Kidney Intl 21:613, 1982.
39. Hulter HN, Sebastian A, Toto RD, et al: Renal and systemic acid-base effects of the chronic administration of hypercalcemia-producing agents: Calcitriol, PTH, and intravenous calcium. Kidney Intl 21:445, 1982.
40. Toto RD, Hulter HN, Sebastian A, et al: Chronic renal metabolic alkalosis in models of primary and secondary hyperparathyroidism. Clinical Res 29:478A, 1981.
41. Hulter HN, Peterson JC: Acid-base homeostasis during chronic PTH excess in humans. Kidney Intl 28:187, 1985.
42. Murer H, Hopfer U, Kinne R: Sodium/proton antiport in brushborder membrane vesicles isolated from rat small intestine and kidney. Biochem J 154:597, 1976.
43. Kinsella JL, Aronson PS: Properties of the Na^+-H^+ exchanger in renal microvillus membrane vesicles. Am J Physiol 238:F461, 1980.
44. Warnock DG, Reenstra WW, Yee VJ: Na^+/H^+ antiporter of brush border vesicles: Studies with acridine orange uptake. Am J Physiol 242:F733, 1982.
45. Kinne-Saffran E, Kinne R: Further evidence for the existence of an intrinsic bicarbonate-stimulated Mg^{++}-ATPase in brush border membranes isolated from rat kidney cortex. J Membr Biol 49:235, 1979.
46. Glynn IM, Karlish SJD: The sodium pump. Ann Rev Physiol 37:13, 1975.
47. Steinmetz PR: Characteristics of hydrogen ion transport in urinary bladder of water turtle. J Clin Invest 46:1531, 1967.
48. Ziegler TW, Fanestil DD, Ludens JH: Influence of transepithelial potential difference on acidification in the toad urinary bladder. Kidney Intl 10:279, 1976.
49. Al-Awqati Q, Mueller A, Steinmetz PR: Transport of H^+ against electrochemical gradients in turtle urinary bladder. Am J Physiol 233:F502, 1977.
50. Steinmetz PR: Cellular defects in urinary acidification and renal tubular acidosis.

In Andreoli TE, Hoffman JF, Fanestil DD (eds): Physiology of Membrane Disorders. New York, Plenum Press, 1978, p 987.
51. Dixon TE, Al-Awqati Q: Urinary acidification in turtle bladder is due to a reversible proton-translocating ATPase. Proc Natl Acad Sci (USA) 76:3135, 1979.
52. Albright F, Burnett CH, Parson W, et al: Osteomalacia and late rickets. Medicine 25:399, 1946.
53. Pines KL, Mudge GH: Renal tubular acidosis with osteomalacia: Report of three cases. Am J Med 11:302, 1951.
54. Lightwood R, Payne WW, Black JA: Infantile renal acidosis. Pediatrician 12:628, 1953.
55. Smith LH Jr, Schreiner GE: Studies on renal hyperchloremic acidosis. J Lab Clin Med 43:347, 1954.
56. Reynolds TB: Observations on the pathogenesis of renal tubular acidosis. Am J Med 25:503, 1958.
57. Wrong O, Davies HEF: The excretion of acid in renal disease. Quart J Med 28:259, 1959.
58. Elkinton JR, Huth EJ, Webster GD Jr, et al: The renal excretion of hydrogen ion in renal tubular acidosis. Am J Med 29:554, 1960.
59. Relman AS: Renal acidosis and renal excretion of acid in health and disease. Adv Intern Med 12:295, 1964.
60. Rodriquez-Soriano J, Boichis H, Edelman CM Jr: Bicarbonate reabsorption and hydrogen ion excretion in children with renal tubular acidosis. J Pediatr 71:802, 1967.
61. Rodriguez-Soriano J, Boichis H, Stark H, et al: Proximal renal tubular acidosis. A defect in bicarbonate reabsorption with normal urinary acidification. Pediatr Res 1:81, 1967.
62. Morris RC Jr: An experimental renal acidification defect in patients with hereditary fructose intolerance. J Clin Invest 47:1648, 1968.
63. Rodriquez-Soriano J, Edelmann CM Jr: Renal tubular acidosis. Ann Rev Med 20:363, 1969.
64. Morris RC Jr: Renal tubular acidosis: Mechanisms, classification and implications. N Engl J Med 281:1405, 1969.
64a. Morris RC Jr, Sebastian A, McSherry E: Renal acidosis. Kidney Intl 1:322, 1972.
65. McSherry E, Sebastian A, Morris RC Jr: Renal tubular acidosis in infants: The several kinds, including bicarbonate-wasting, classic renal tubular acidosis. J Clin Invest 51:499, 1972.
65a. Sebastian A: Renal tubular acidosis. Calif Med 116:34, 1972.
66. Nash MA, Torrado AD, Greifer I, et al: Renal tubular acidosis in infants and children. J Pediatr 80:738, 1972.
67. Rodriquez-Soriano J, Vallo A, Garcia-Fuentes M: Distal renal tubular acidosis in infancy: A bicarbonate wasting state. J Pediatr 86:524, 1975.
68. McSherry E, Morris RC Jr: Attainment and maintenance of normal stature with alkali therapy in infants and children with classic renal tubular acidosis. J Clin Invest 61:509, 1978.
69. Stinebaugh BJ, Schloeder FX, Tam SC, et al: Pathogenesis of distal renal tubular acidosis. Kidney Intl 19:1, 1981.
70. Rodriguez-Soriano J: Renal Tubular Acidosis. In Pediatric Kidney Disease. Little, Brown, Boston, 1978, Chapter 83.
71. Batlle D, Kurtzman NA: Distal renal tubular acidosis: Pathogenesis and classification. Am J Kidney Dis 6:328, 1982.
72. Rodriguez-Soriano J, Vallo A, Castillo G, et al: Natural history of primary distal renal tubular acidosis treated since infancy. J Pediatr 101:669, 1982.
73. Morris RC Jr, Sebastian A: Renal tubular acidosis and Fanconi syndrome. In The Metabolic Basis of Inherited Disease, ed 5. New York, McGraw-Hill, 1983.
74. Leumann EP, Steinmann B: Persistent and transient distal renal tubular acidosis with bicarbonate wasting. Pediatr Res 9:767, 1975.
75. Pak Poy RK, Wrong O: The urinary PCO_2 in renal disease. Clin Sci 19:631, 1960.
76. Halperin ML, Goldstein MB, Haig A, et al: Studies on the pathogenesis of type 1 (distal) renal tubular acidosis as revealed by the urinary PCO_2 tensions. J Clin Invest 53:669, 1974.
77. Stinebaugh BJ: Distal renal tubular acidosis: A review of current concepts and pathogenesis. In Barcelo R, Bergeron M, Carriere S, Dirks JH, Drummond K, Guttman RD, Lemieux G, Mongeau JG, Seely JF (eds): Proc Seventh Int Cong Nephrol Karger AG, Basel, 1978, p 337.
78. Stinebaugh BJ, Esquenazi R, Schloeder FX, et al: Control of the urine-blood Pco_2 gradient in alkaline urine. Kidney Intl 17:31, 1980.
79. McCurdy DK, Frederic M, Elkinton JR: Renal tubular acidosis due to amphotericin B. N Engl J Med 278:124, 1968.
80. Patterson RM, Ackerman GL: Renal tubular acidosis due to amphotericin B nephrotoxicity. Arch Intern Med 127:241, 1971.
81. Steinmetz PR, Lawson LR: Defect in urinary acidification induced in vitro by amphotericin B. J Clin Invest 49:596, 1970.
82. Finn JT, Cohen LH, Steinmetz PR: Acidifying defect induced by amphotericin B: Comparison of bicarbonate and hydrogen ion permeabilities. Kidney Intl 11:261, 1977.
83. LoSpalluto J, Dorward B, Miller W, et al: Cryoglobulinemia based on interaction between a gamma macroglobulin and 7S gamma globulin. Am J Med 32:142, 1962.
84. Morris RC Jr, Fundenberg HH: Impaired renal acidification in patients with hypergammaglobulinemia. Medicine 46:57, 1967.
85. Talal N, Zisman E, Schur PH: Renal tubular acidosis, glomerulonephritis and immunologic factors in Sjogren's syndrome. Arthritis Rheum II:774, 1968.
86. Shioji R, Furuyama T, Onodera S, Saito H, Ito H, Sasaki Y: Sjogren's syndrome and renal tubular acidosis. Am J Med 48:456, 1970.
87. Seedat YK, Rain ER: Active chronic hepatitis associated with renal tubular acidosis and successful pregnancy. S Afr Med J 39:595, 1965.
88. Bridi GS, Falcon PW, Brackett NC Jr, Still WJS, Sporn IN: Glomerulonephritis and renal tubular acidosis in a case of chronic active hepatitis with hyperimmunoglobulinemia. Am J Med 52:267, 1972.
89. Tsantoulas DC, McFarlane JG, Portmann B, et al: Cell-mediated immunity to human Tamm-Horsfall glycoprotein in autoimmune liver disease with renal tubular acidosis. Brit Med J 4:491, 1974.
90. Andres GA, McCluskey RT: Tubular and interstitial renal disease due to immunologic mechanisms. Kidney Intl 7:271, 1975.
91. Gill JR Jr, Bell NH, Bartter FC: Impaired conservation of sodium and potassium in renal tubular acidosis and its correction by buffer anions. Clin Sci 33:577, 1967.
92. Sebastian A, McSherry E, Morris RC Jr: On the mechanism of renal potassium wasting in renal tubular acidosis associated with the Fanconi syndrome (type 2 RTA). J Clin Invest 50:231, 1971.
93. Sebastian A, McSherry E, Morris RC Jr: Renal potassium wasting in renal tubular acidosis (RTA): Its occurrence in types 1 and 2 RTA despite sustained correction of systemic acidosis. J Clin Invest 50:667, 1971.
94. Sebastian A, McSherry E, Morris RC Jr: Impaired renal conservation of sodium and chloride during sustained correction of systemic acidosis in patients with type 1, classic renal tubular acidosis. J Clin Invest 58:454, 1976.
95. Glassman VP, Safirstein R, DiScala VA: Effects of metabolic acidosis on proximal tubule ion reabsorption in dog kidney. Am J Physiol 227:759, 1974.
96. Lemann J Jr, Litzow JR, Lennon EJ: Studies on the mechanisms by which chronic metabolic acidosis augments urinary calcium excretion in man. J Clin Invest 46:1318, 1967.
97. Lemann J Jr, Litzow JR, Lennon EJ: The effects of chronic acid loads in normal man: Further evidence for participation of bone mineral in the defense against chronic metabolic acidosis. J Clin Invest 45:1608, 1966.
98. Gyory AZ, Edwards KDG: Renal tubular acidosis: A family with an autosomal dominant genetic defect in renal hydrogen ion transport, with proximal tubular and collecting duct dysfunction and increased metabolism of citrate and ammonia. Am J Med 45:32, 1968.
99. Harrison HE: Mechanisms of action of vitamin D. Pediatr 14:285, 1954.
100. Dedmon RE, Wrong O: The excretion of organic anion in renal tubular acidosis with particular reference to citrate. Clin Sci 22:19, 1962.
101. Morrissey JF, Ochoa M Jr, Lotspeich WD, et al: Citrate excretion in renal tubule acidosis. Ann Intern Med 58:159, 1963.
102. Brodwall EK, Westlie L, Myhre E: The renal excretion and tubular reabsorption of citric acid in renal tubular acidosis. Acta Med Scand 192:137, 1972.
103. Norman ME, Feldman NI, Cohn RM, et al: Urinary citrate excretion in the diagnosis of distal renal tubular acidosis. J Pediatr 92:394, 1978.
104. McSherry EM, Pokroy MV: The absence of nephrocalcinosis in children with type 1 RTA on high dose alkali therapy since infancy. Clin Res 26:470, 1978.
104a. Harrington TM, Bunch TW, Van Den Berg CJ: Renal tubular acidosis: A new look at treatment of musculoskeletal and renal disease. Mayo Clin Proc 58:354, 1983.
105. Simpson DP: Citrate excretion: A window on renal metabolism. Am J Physiol 244:F223, 1983.
106. Greenberg AJ, McNamara H, McCrory WW: Metabolic balance studies in primary renal tubular acidosis: Effects of acidosis on external calcium and phosphorus balances. J Pediatr 69:610, 1966.
107. Coe FL, Firpo JJ: Evidence for mild reversible hyperparathyroidism in distal renal tubular acidosis. Arch Intern Med 135:1485, 1975.
108. Coe FL, Firpo JJ, Hollandsworth DL, et al: Effect of acute and chronic metabolic acidosis on serum immunoreactive parathyroid hormone in man. Kidney Intl 8:262, 1975.
109. Foss GL, Perry CB, Wood FJY: Renal tubular acidosis. Quart J Med 25:185, 1956.
110. Randall RE Jr, Targgart WH: Familial renal tubular acidosis. Ann Intern Med 54:1108, 1961.
111. Richards P, Chamberlain MJ, Wrong OM: Treatment of osteomalacia of renal tubular acidosis by sodium bicarbonate alone. Lancet 11:994, 1972.
112. Coe FL, Parks JH: Stone disease in hereditary distal renal tubular acidosis. Ann Intern Med 93:60, 1980.
112a. Lee SW, Russell J, Avioli LV: 25-Hydroxycholecalciferol to 1,25-dihydroxychole-

calciferol: Conversion impaired by systemic metabolic acidosis. Science 195:994, 1977.
112b. Weber HP, Gray RW, Dominguez JH, et al: The lack of effect of chronic metabolic acidosis on 25-OH-vitamin D metabolism and serum parathyroid hormone in humans. J Clin Endocrinol Metab 43:1047, 1976.
112c. Kraut JA, Gordon E, Horst RL, et al: The effect of chronic metabolic acidosis in man on basal and stimulated plasma levels of 1-25(OH)$_2$D$_3$. Proc Fifth Workshop on Vitamin D 193, 1982.
112d. Bushinsky DA, Favus MJ, Sen PK, et al: Effects of chronic metabolic acidosis (CMA) on serum 1,25-dihydroxyvitamin D$_3$ (1,25d$_3$) levels in the rat. Kidney Intl 21:130A, 1982.
113. Kraut JA, Gordon EM, Ransom JC, et al: Effect of chronic metabolic acidosis on vitamin D metabolism in humans. Kidney Intl 24:644, 1983.
113a. Bushinsky DA, Favus MJ, Sen PK, et al: Effects of chronic metabolic acidosis on serum 1,25-dihydroxyvitamin D$_3$ levels in the rat. Am J Physiol 243:F570, 1982.
114. Chesney RW, Kaplan BS, Phelps M, et al: Renal tubular acidosis does not alter circulating values of calcitriol. J Pediatr 104:51, 1984.
115. Schreiner GE, Smith LH Jr, Kyle LH: Renal hyperchloremic acidosis. Am J Med 15:122, 1953.
116. Pitts HH, Schulte JW, Smith DR: Nephrocalcinosis in a father and three children. J Urol 73:208, 1955.
117. Randall RE Jr: Familial renal tubular acidosis revisited. Ann Intern Med 66:1024, 1967.
118. Levine AS, Michael AF Jr.: Ehlers-Danlos syndrome with renal tubular acidosis and medullary sponge kidneys. J Pediatr 71:107, 1967.
119. Baehner RI, Gilchrist GS, Anderson FJ: Hereditary elliptocytosis and primary renal tubular acidosis in a single family. Am J Dis Child 115:414, 1968.
120. Goosens JP, Van Eps LWS, Schouten H, et al: Incomplete renal tubular acidosis in sickle cell disease. Clin Chim Acta 41:149, 1972.
121. Kong H H-P, Alleyne GAO: Defect in urinary acidification in adults with sickle cell anemia. Lancet 2:954, 1968.
122. Sly WS, Hewett-Emmett D, Whyte MP, Yu Y-S L, et al: Carbonic anhydrase II deficiency identified as the primary defect in the autosomal recessive syndrome of osteopetrosis with renal tubular acidosis and cerebral calcification. Proc Natl Acad Sci (USA) 80:2752, 1983.
123. Sly WS: Personal Communication.
124. Shapira E, Ben-Yoseph Y, Eyal FG, et al: Enzymatically inactive red cell carbonic anhydrase B in a family with renal tubular acidosis. J Clin Invest 53:59, 1974.
125. Kondo T, Taniguchi N, Taniguchi K, et al: Inactive form of erythrocyte carbonic anhydrase B in patients with primary renal tubular acidosis. J Clin Invest 62:610, 1978.
126. Takeda R, Morimoto S, Kuroda M, et al: Renal tubular acidosis, presenting as a syndrome resembling Bartter's syndrome, in a patient with arachnodatcyly. Acta Endocrinol 73:531, 1973.
127. Donckerwolke RA, Van Biervliet JP, Koorvaar G, et al: The syndrome of renal tubular acidosis with nerve deafness. Acta Paediatr Scand 65:100, 1976.
128. Dunger DB, Brenton DP, Cain AR: Renal tubular acidosis and nerve deafness. Arch Dis Childh 55:221, 1980.
129. Cohen A, Way BJ: The association of renal tubular acidosis with hyperglobulinaemic purpura. Aust Ann Med 11:189, 1962.
130. Mason AMS, Golding PL: Hyperglobulinaemic renal tubular acidosis: A report of nine cases. Brit Med J 3:143, 1970.
131. Golding PL: Renal tubular acidosis in chronic liver disease. Postgrad Med J 51:550, 1975.
132. Cochrane AMG, Tsantoulos DC, Moussouros A, et al: Lymphocyte cytotoxicity for kidney cells in renal tubular acidosis of autoimmune liver disease. Brit Med J 2:276, 1976.
133. Mason AMS, Golding PL: Renal tubular acidosis and autoimmune thyroid disease. Lancet 2:1104, 1970.
134. Mason AMS, McIllmurray MB, Golding PL, et al: Fibrosing alveoitis associated with renal tubular acidosis. Brit Med J 4:596, 1970.
135. Tu WH, Shearn MA: Systemic lupus erythematosus and latent renal tubular dysfunction. Ann Int Med 67:100, 1967.
136. Jessop S, Rabkin R, Mumford G, et al: Renal tubular function in systemic lupus erythematosus. S Afr Med J 47:132, 1973.
137. Buckalew VM Jr, Purvis ML, Shulman MG, et al: Hereditary renal tubular acidosis. Medicine 53:229, 1974.
138. Hamed JA, Czerwinski AW, Coats B, et al: Familial absorptive hypercalcuria and renal tubular acidosis. Am J Med 67:385, 1979.
139. Dent CE, Harper CM, Parfitt AM: The effect of cellulose phosphate on calcium metabolism in patients with hypercalciuria. Clin Sci 27:417, 1964.
140. Parfitt AM, Higgins BA, Nassim JR, et al: Metabolic studies in patients with hypercalciuria. Clin Sci 27:463, 1964.
141. Cohen SI, Fitzgerald MG, Fourman P, et al: Polyuria in hyperparathyroidism. Quart J Med 26:423, 1957.
142. Reynolds TB, Bethune JE: Renal tubular acidosis secondary to hyperparathyroidism. Clin Res 17:169, 1969.
143. Ferris T, Kashgarian M, Levitin H, et al: Renal tubular acidosis and renal potassium wasting required as a result of hypercalcemic neuropathy. N Engl J Med 265:924, 1961.
144. Zisman E, Buccino RA, Gorden P, et al: Hyperthyroidism and renal tubular acidosis. Arch Int Med 121:118, 1968.
145. Deck MDF: Medullary sponge kidney with renal tubular acidosis: A report of 3 cases. J Urol 94:330, 1965.
146. Morris RC Jr, Yamauchi H, Palubinskas AJ, et al: Medullary sponge kidney. Am J Med 38:883, 1965.
147. Mass RE, Smith WR, Walsh JR: The association of hereditary fructose intolerance and renal tubular acidosis. Am J Med Sci 251:516, 1966.
148. Fulop M, Sternlieb J, Scheinberg IH: Defective urinary acidification in Wilson's disease. Ann Intern Med 68:770, 1968.
149. Yeoh SA, Asan P: Fabry's disease with renal tubular acidosis. Singapore Med J 8:275, 1967.
150. Taher SM, Anderson RJ, McCartney R, et al: Renal tubular acidosis associated with toluene "sniffing". N Engl J Med 290:765, 1974.
151. Steele TW, Edwards KDG: Analgesic nephropathy. Changes in various parameters of renal function following cessation of analgesic abuse. Med J Aust 1:181, 1971.
152. Steele TW, Gyory AZ, Edwards KDG: Renal function in analgesic nephropathy. Brit Med J 2:213, 1969.
153. Perez GO, Oster JR, Vaamonde CA: Incomplete syndrome of renal tubular acidosis induced by lithium carbonate. J Lab Clin Med 86:386, 1975.
154. Yong JM, Sanderson KV: Photosensitive dermatitis and renal tubular acidosis after ingestion of calcium cyclamate. Lancet 2:1273, 1969.
155. Berlyne GM: Distal tubular function in chronic hydronephrosis. Quart J Med 30:339, 1961.
156. Better OS, Arieff AI, Massry SG, et al: Studies on renal function after relief of complete unilateral ureteral obstruction of three months' duration in man. Am J Med 54:234, 1973.
157. Hutcheon RA, Kaplan BS, Drummond KN: Distal renal tubular acidosis in children with chronic hydronephrosis. J Pediatr 89:372, 1976.
158. Wilson DR: Renal function during and following obstruction. Ann Rev Med 28:329, 1977.
159. Thirakomen K, Kozlov N, Arruda JAL, et al: Renal hydrogen ion secretion after release of unilateral ureteral obstruction. Am J Physiol 231:1233, 1976.
160. Cochran M, Peacock M, Smith DA, et al: Renal tubular acidosis of pyelonephritis with renal stone disease. Brit Med J 2:721, 1968.
161. Gyory AZ, Steward H, George CRP, et al: Renal tubular acidosis, acidosis due to hyperkalaemia, hypercalcemia, disordered citrate metabolism and other tubular dysfunctions following human renal transplantation. Quart J Med 38:231, 1969.
162. Wilson DR, Siddigui AA: Renal tubular acidosis after kidney transplantation. Ann Intern Med 79:352, 1973.
163. Drutz DJ, Gutman RA: Renal tubular acidosis in leprosy. Ann Intern Med 75:475, 1971.
164. Shear L, Bonkowsky HL, Gabuzda GJ: Renal tubular acidosis in cirrhosis. N Engl J Med 280:1, 1969.
165. Better OS, Goldschmid Z, Chaimowitz C, et al: Defect in urinary acidification in cirrhosis. Arch Intern Med 130:77, 1972.
165a. Oster JR, Hotchkiss JL, Carbon M, et al: Abnormal renal acidification in alcoholic liver disease. J Lab Clin Med 85:987, 1975.
166. Buckalew VM Jr, McCurdy DK, Ludwig GD, et al: Incomplete renal tubular acidosis: Physiologic studies in three patients with a defect in lowering urine pH. Am J Med 45:32, 1968.
167. Konnak JW, Kogan BA, Lau K: Renal calculi associated with incomplete distal renal tubular acidosis. J Urol 128:900, 1982.
167a. Madias NE, Adrogue HJ, Horowitz GL, et al: A redefinition of normal acid-base equilibrium in man: carbon dioxide tension as a key determinant of normal plasma bicarbonate concentration. Kidney Intl 16:612, 1979.
167b. Kurtz I, Maher T, Hulter HN, et al: Effect of diet on plasma acid-base composition in normal humans. Kidney Intl 24:670, 1983.
168. Sebastian A, McSherry E, Ueki I, et al: Renal amyloidosis, nephrotic syndrome, and impaired renal tubular reabsorption of bicarbonate. Ann Int Med 69:541, 1968.
169. Nadell J: The effects of the carbonic anhydrase inhibitor "6063" on electrolytes and acid-base balance in two normal subjects and two patients with respiratory acidosis. J Clin Invest 32:622, 1953.
170. Leaf A, Schwartz WB, Relman AS: Oral administration of a potent carbonic anhydrase inhibitor ("Diamox"). N Engl J Med 250:759, 1954.
171. Seldin DW, Portwood RM, Rector FC Jr, et al: Characteristics of renal bicarbonate reabsorption in man. J Clin Invest 38:1663, 1959.

172. Beckman WW, Rossmeisl EC, Pettingill RB, Bauer W: Study of the effects of sulfanilamide on acid-base metabolism. J Clin Invest 19:635, 1940.
173. White MG, Asch MJ: Acid-base effects of topical mafenide acetate in the burned patient. N Engl J Med 284:1281, 1971.
174. Donckerwolcke RA, Van Stekelenburg GJ, Tiddens HA: A case of bicarbonate-losing renal tubular acidosis with defective carboanhydrase activity. Arch Dis Childh 45:769, 1970.
175. York SE, Yendt ER: Osteomalacia associated with renal bicarbonate loss. Canad Med Assoc J 94:1329, 1966.
176. Rodriquez-Soriano J, Vallo A, Chouza M, et al: Proximal renal tubular acidosis in tetralogy of fallot. Acta Ped Scand 64:671, 1975.
176a. Stark H, Geiger R: Renal tubular dysfunction following vascular accidents of the kidneys in the newborn period. J Pediatr 83:933, 1973.
177. Brenes LG, Brenes JN, Hernandez MM: Familial proximal renal tubular acidosis. Am J Med 63:244, 1977.
178. Wistrand PJ: Renal membrane-bound carbonic anhydrase: Purification and properties. Upsala J Med Sci 26(suppl):75, 1979.
179. Cogan MG, Maddox DA, Warnock DG, et al: Effect of acetazolamide on bicarbonate reabsorption in the proximal tubule of the rat. Am J Physiol 237:F447, 1979.
180. Guibaud P, Larbre F, Freycon M-T, et al: Osteopetrose et acidose renale tubulaire deux cas de cette association dans une fratrie. Arch Franc Pediat 29:269, 1972.
181. Vainsel M, Fondu P, Cadranel S, et al: Osteopetrosis associated with proximal and distal tubular acidosis. Acta Paediat Scand 61:429, 1972.
182. Bregman H, Brown J, Rogers A, et al: Osteopetrosis with combined proximal and distal renal tubular acidosis. Am J Kid Dis 2:357, 1982.
183. Bourke E, Delaney VB, Mosawi M, Reavey P, Weston M: Renal tubular acidosis and osteopetrosis in siblings. Nephron 28:268, 1981.
184. Whyte MP, Murphy WA, Fallon MD, et al: Osteopetrosis, renal tubular acidosis and basal ganglia calcification in three sisters. Am J Med 69:64, 1980.
185. Lemann J Jr, Wilz DR, Brenes LG: Acid, calcium and phosphorous balances in proximal renal tubular acidosis. Kidney Intl 10:561, 1976.
186. Ishitsu T, Matsuda I, Seino Y, et al: Anticonvulsant-induced rickets associated with renal tubular acidosis and normal level of serum 1,25-dihydroxyvitamin D. Am J Dis Child 135:1140, 1981.
187. Goodman AD, Lemann J Jr, Lennon EJ, et al: Production, excretion and net balance of fixed acid in patients with renal acidosis. J Clin Invest 44:495, 1965.
188. Litzow JR, Lemann J Jr, Lennon EJ: The effect of treatment of acidosis on calcium balance in patients with chronic azotemic renal disease. J Clin Invest 46:280, 1967.
189. Chan JCM: Calcium and hydrogen ion metabolism in children with classic (type 1/distal) renal tubular acidosis. Ann Nutr Metab 25:65, 1981.
190. Albright F, Drake TG, Sulkowitch HW: Renal osteitis fibrosa cystica. Bull Johns Hop Hosp 60:377, 1937.
191. Liu SH, Chu HI: Studies of calcium and phosphorus metabolism with special reference to pathogenesis and effects of dihydrotachysterol and iron. Medicine 22:103, 1943.
192. Schwartz WB, Relman AS: Acidosis in renal disease. N Engl J Med 256:1184, 1957.
193. Ohlsson A, Stark G, Sakati N: Marble brain disease: Recessive osteopetrosis, renal tubular acidosis and cerebral calcification in three Saudi Arabian families. Develop Med Child Neurol 22:72, 1980.
194. Carroll HJ, Farber SJ: Hyperkalemia and hyperchloremic acidosis in chronic pyelonephritis. Metabolism 13:808, 1964.
195. Sebastian A, McSherry E, Schambelan M, et al: Renal tubular acidosis (RTA) in patients with hypoaldosteronism caused by renin deficiency. Clin Res 21:706, 1973.
196. Perez GO, Oster JR, Vaamonde CA: Renal acidosis and renal potassium handling in selective hypoaldosteronism. Am J Med 57:809, 1974.
197. Sebastian A, Schambelan M, Lindenfeld S, et al: Amelioration of metabolic acidosis with fludrocortisone therapy in hyporeninemic hypoaldosteronism. N Engl J Med 297:576, 1977.
198. Schambelan M, Sebastian A, Biglieri EG: Prevalence, pathogenesis, and functional significance of aldosterone deficiency in hyperkalemic patients with chronic renal insufficiency. Kidney Intl 17:89, 1980.
199. Phelps KR, Lieberman RL, Oh MS: Pathophysiology of the syndrome of hyporeninemic hypoaldosteronism. Metabolism 29:186, 1980.
200. Hulter HN, Ilnicki LP, Harbottle JA, et al: Impaired renal H^+ secretion and NH_3 production in mineralocorticoid-deficient glucocorticoid-replete dogs. Am J Physiol 232:F136, 1977.
201. Lombard WE, Jacobson HR, Kokko JP: Collecting duct bicarbonate transport: Comparison of cortical and medullary segments. Kidney Intl 16:827, 1979.
202. Sebastian A, Sutton JM, Hulter HN, et al: Effect of mineralocorticoid replacement therapy on renal acid-base homeostasis in adrenalectomized patients. Kidney Intl 18:762, 1980.
203. Sebastian A, Schambelan M, Hulter HN, et al: Hyperkalemic renal tubular acidosis. In Buckalew VM Jr., Gonick HC (eds): Renal Tubular Disorders, New York, Marcel Dekker, Chapter 10, 1985.
204. Imai M, Igarashi Y, Sokabe H: Plasma renin activity in congenital virilizing adrenal hyperplasia. Pediatrics 41:897, 1968.
205. Oetliker OH, Zurbrugg RP: Renal tubular acidosis in salt-losing syndrome of congenital adrenal hyperplasia (CAH). J Clin Endocrinol Metab 31:447, 1970.
206. Oetliker OH, Zurbrugg RP: Renal regulation of fluid, electrolyte and acid-base homeostasis in the salt-losing syndrome of congenital adrenal hyperplasia (SL-CAH). ECF volume: A compensating factor in aldosterone deficiency. J Clin Endocrinol Metab 46:543, 1978.
207. David R, Goland S, Drucker W: Familial aldosterone deficiency: Enzyme defect, diagnosis and clinical course. Pediatrics 41:403, 1968.
208. Ulick S: Diagnosis and nomenclature of the disorders of the terminal portion of the aldosterone biosynthetic pathway. J Clin Endocrinol Metab 43:92, 1976.
209. Rosler A, Rabinowitz D, Theodor R, et al: The nature of the defect in a salt-wasting disorder in Jews of Iran. J Clin Endocrinol Metab 44:279, 1977.
210. Rosler A, Theodor R, Boichis H, et al: Metabolic responses to the administration of angiotensin II, K and ACTH in two salt-wasting syndromes. J Clin Endocrinol Metab 44:292, 1977.
211. Veldhuis JD, Kulin HE, Santen RJ, et al: Inborn error in the terminal step of aldosterone biosynthesis: Corticosterone methyl oxidate type II deficiency in a North American pedigree. N Engl J Med 303:117, 1980.
212. Curtis JA, Monaghan HP, New MI, et al: Selective hypoaldosteronism in infancy. Am J Dis Child 137:633, 1983.
213. Schambelan M, Stockigt JR, Biglieri EG: Isolated hypoaldosteronism in adults, a renin deficiency syndrome. N Engl J Med 287:573, 1972.
214. Perez G, Siegel L, Schreiner GE: Selective hypoaldosteronism with hyperkalemia. Ann Intern Med 76:757, 1972.
215. Weidmann P, Reinhert R, Maxwell MH, et al: Syndrome of hyporeninemic hypoaldosteronism and hyperkalemia in renal disease. J Clin Endocrinol Metab 36:965, 1973.
216. DeFronzo RA: Hyperkalemia and hyporeninemic hypoaldosteronism. Kidney Intl 17:118, 1980.
217. Batlle DC, Arruda JAL, Kurtzman NA: Hyperkalemic distal renal tubular acidosis associated with obstructive uropathy. N Engl J Med 304:373, 1981.
218. Tan SY, Shapiro R, Franco R, et al: Indomethacin-induced prostaglandin inhibition with hyperkalemia. Ann Intern Med 90:783, 1979.
219. Russell A, Levin B, Sinclair L, et al: A reversible salt-wasting syndrome of the newborn and infant. Arch Dis Childh 38:313, 1963.
220. Shuper A, Eisenstein B, Stark H, et al: Hyporeninemic hypoaldosteronism in a child with lactic acidosis, deafness, and mental retardation. J Pediatr 100:769, 1982.
221. Landier F, Guyene TT, Boutignon H, Nahoul K, Corvol P, Job J-C: Hyporeninemic hypoaldosteronism in infancy: A familial disease. J Clin Endocrinol Metab 58:143, 1984.
222. Marieb NJ, Melby JC, Lyall SS: Isolated hypoaldosteronism associated with idiopathic hypoparathyroidism. Arch Intern Med 134:424, 1974.
223. McGiff JC, Muzzarelli RE, Duffy PA, et al: Interrelationships of renin and alosterone in a patient with hypoaldosteronism. Am J Med 48:247, 1970.
224. Mellinger RC, Petermann FL, Jurgenson JC: Hyponatremia with low urinary aldosterone occurring in an old woman. J Clin Endocrinol Metab 34:85, 1972.
225. Cheek DB, Perry JW: A salt-wasting syndrome in infancy. Arch Dis Childh 33:252, 1958.
226. Donnell GN, Litman N, Roldan M: Pseudohypo-adrenalocorticism. Am J Dis Child 97:813, 1959.
227. Raine DN, Roy J: A salt-losing syndrome in infancy. Pseudohypoadrenocorticalism. Arch Dis Childh 37:548, 1962.
228. Alvarez MN, Barnes ND, Stickler GB: Salt wasting nephropathy or "pseudohypoaldosteronism" in twins. Pediatr Res 8:453, 1974.
229. Postel-Vinay M-C, Alberti GM, Ricour C, et al: Pseudohypoaldosteronism: Persistence of hyperaldosteronism and evidence for renal tubular and intestinal responsiveness to endogenous aldosterone. J Clin Endocrinol Metab 39:1038, 1974.
230. Petersen S, Giese J, Kappelgaard AM, et al: Pseudohypoaldosteronism: Clinical, biochemical and morphological studies in a long-term follow-up. Acta Paediatr Scand 67:255, 1978.
231. Blacher Y, Kaplan BS, Griffel B, et al: Pseudohypoaldosteronism. Clin Nephr 11:281, 1979.
232. Oberfield SE, Levine LS, Carey RM, et al: Pseudohypoaldosteronism: Multiple target organ unresponsiveness to mineralocorticoid hormones. J Clin Endocrinol Metab 48:228, 1979.
233. Rosenberg S, Franks RC, Ulick S: Mineralocorticoid unresponsiveness with severe neonatal hyponatremia and hyperkalemia. J Clin Endocrinol Metab 50:401, 1980.
234. Dillon MJ, Leonard JV, Buckler JM, et al: Pseudohypoaldosteronism. Arch Dis Childh 55:427, 1980.
235. Popovitzer MM, Katz FH, Pinggera WF, et al: Hyperkalemia in salt-wasting nephropathy: Study of the mechanism. Arch Intern Med 132:203, 1973.
236. Cogan MG, Arieff AI: Sodium wasting, acidosis, and hyperkalemia induced by

methicillin interstitial nephritis: Evidence for selective distal tubular dysfunction. Am J Med 64:500, 1978.
237. Rodriguez-Soriano J, Vallo A, Oliveros R, et al: Transient pseudohypoaldosteronism secondary to obstructive uropathy in infancy. J Pediatr 103:375, 1983.
238. Stokes GS, Gentle JL, Edwards KDG, et al: Syndrome of idiopathic hyperkalemia and hypertension with decreased plasma renin activity: Effects on plasma renin and aldosterone of reducing the serum potassium level. Med J Aust 2:1050, 1968.
239. Arnold JE, Healy JK: Hyperkalemia, hypertension and systemic acidosis without renal failure associated with a tubular defect in potassium excretion. Am J Med 47:461, 1969.
240. Gordon RD, Geddes RA, Pawsey GK, et al: Hypertension and severe hyperkalaemia associated with suppression of renin and aldosterone and completely reversed by dietary sodium restriction. Aust Ann Med 4:287, 1970.
241. Spitzer A, Edelmann CM Jr, Goldberg LD, et al: Short stature, hyperkalemia and acidosis: A defect in renal transport of potassium. Kidney Intl 3:251, 1973.
242. Weinstein SF, Allan DME, Mendoza SA: Hyperkalemia, acidosis, and short stature associated with a defect in renal potassium excretion. J Pediatr 85:355, 1974.
243. Brautbar N, Levi J, Rosler A, et al: Familial hyperkalemia, hypertension and hyporeninemia with normal aldosterone levels: A tubular defect in potassium handling. Arch Intern Med 138:607, 1978.
244. Farfel Z, Iaina A, Rosenthal T, et al: Familial hyperpotassemia and hypertension accompanied by normal plasma aldosterone levels. Possible hereditary cell membrane defect. Arch Intern Med 138:1828, 1978.
245. Lee MR, Ball SG, Thomas TH, et al: Hypertension and hyperkalaemia responding to bendrofluazide. Quart J Med 48:245, 1979.
246. Schambelan M, Sebastian A, Rector FC Jr: Mineralocorticoid-resistant renal hyperkalemia without salt-wasting (type II pseudohypoaldosteronism): Role of increased renal chloride reabsorption. Kidney Intl 19:716, 1981.
247. DeFronzo RA, Goldberg M, Cooke CR, et al: Investigations into the mechanisms of hyperkalemia following renal transplantation. Kidney Intl 11:357, 1977.
248. Batlle DC, Mozes MF, Manaligod J, et al: The pathogenesis of hyperchloremic metabolic acidosis associated with kidney transplantation. Am J Med 70:786, 1981.
249. DeFronzo RA, Cooke R, Goldberg M, et al: Impaired renal tubular potassium secretion in systemic lupus erythematosus. Ann Intern Med 86:268, 1977.
250. Lathem W: Hyperchloremic acidosis in chronic pyelonephritis. N Engl J Med 258:1031, 1958.
251. Handler NM, Gill JR Jr, Gardner JD: Impaired renal tubular secretion of potassium, elevated sweat sodium chloride concentration and plasma inhibition of erythrocyte sodium outflux as complications of systemic lupus erythematosus. Arthritis Rheum 15:515, 1972.
252. Gyory AZ, Steward JH, George CRP, et al: Renal tubular acidosis, acidosis due to hyperkalemia, hypercalcemia, disordered citrate metabolism and other tubular dysfunctions following human renal transplantation. Quart J Med 38:231, 1969.
253. Rubini ME, Sanford JP, Meroney WH: Studies of potassium secretion in glomerulonephritis. Am J Med 42:790, 1957.
254. Luke RG, Allison MEM, Davidson JF, et al: Hyperkalemia and renal tubular acidosis due to renal amyloidosis. Ann Intern Med 70:1211, 1969.
255. Brenner RJ, Spring DB, Sebastian A, et al: Incidence of radiographically evident bone disease, nephrocalcinosis, and nephrolithiasis in various types of renal tubular acidosis. N Engl J Med 307:217, 1982.
256. Cassels DE, Morse M: Arterial blood gases and acid-base balance in normal children. J Clin Invest 32:824, 1953.
257. Peonides A, Levin B, Young WF: The renal excretion of hydrogen ions in infants and children. Arch Dis Childh 40:33, 1965.
258. Bartels O, Wenner J: Standardbicarbonat, pH und CO_2-Druck im "arterialisierten" Blut gesunder Sauglinge nach der Neugeborenenperiode bis zum Ende des ersten Lebensjahres. Klin Wchnschr 43:30, 1965.
259. Morris SA, Winters RW: Acid-base equilibrium of blood in normal infants. Pediatrics 37:728, 1966.
260. Edelmann CM Jr, Boichis H, Rodriguez-Soriano J, et al: The renal response of children to acute ammonium chloride acidosis. Pediatr Res 1:452, 1967.
261. Edelmann CM Jr, Rodriguez-Soriano J, Boichis H, et al: Renal bicarbonate reabsorption and hydrogen ion excretion in normal infants. J Clin Invest 46:1309, 1967.
262. Vavrova V, Mrzena B, Vokac Z: pH, PCO_2 et composante non respiratoire de L'equilibre acido-basique du sang cutane arterialise chez 97 enfants sains ages de 3 mois a 15 ans. Le Poumon et le Coeur 25:1121, 1969.
263. Kerpel-Fronius E, Heim T, Sulyok E: The development of the renal acidifying processes and their relation to acidosis in low birth-weight infants. Biol Neonate 15:156, 1970.
264. Raiha NCR, Heinonen K, Rassin DK, et al: Milk protein quantity and quality in low birth-weight infants: I. Metabolic responses and effects on growth. Pediatrics 57:659, 1976.
265. Forster HV, Dempsey JA, Thomson J, et al: Estimation of arterial PO_2, PCO_2, pH, and lactate from arterialized venous blood. J Appl Physiol 32:134, 1972.
266. Maher T, Schambelan M, Kurtz I, et al: Amelioration of metabolic acidosis by dietary potassium restriction in hyperkalemic patients with chronic renal insufficiency. J Lab Clin Med 103:432, 1984.
267. Sebastian A, Schambelan M, Sutton JM: Amelioration of hyperchloremic acidosis with furosemide therapy in patients with chronic renal insufficiency and type 4 renal tubular acidosis. Am J Nephrol 4:287, 1984.

CHAPTER 35

Nephrogenic Diabetes Insipidus

SOLOMON A. KAPLAN

Vasopressin-resistant (nephrogenic) diabetes insipidus is an inherited disorder in which the kidneys are unable to respond to the antidiuretic hormone, vasopressin. The production of large volumes of hypotonic urine, even in the dehydrated state, may lead to severe dehydration and hypertonicity. No anatomic abnormality of the kidneys has been found to account for the disorder, and it is not associated with parenchymatous or obstructive diseases of the kidneys that could lead to impairment of their response to vasopressin.

The term nephrogenic was introduced by Williams and Henry in 1947 to describe a form of diabetes insipidus in patients whose symptoms were not relieved by administration of vasopressin (1). The disease had been recognized previously by Waring and coworkers (2) and was included as a separate form of diabetes insipidus by Forssman in his report in 1945 (3). In the next 15 years over 100 additional cases were reported (4). The prevalence of the disorder remains unknown, but it is assumed to be quite rare, since it is observed infrequently in large pediatric endocrinology and nephrology clinics.

PATHOPHYSIOLOGY

In normal individuals, the kidneys respond to vasopressin administration or endogenous production by reducing urine flow and increasing the solute concentration of the urine. In vasopressin-resistant diabetes insipidus, administration of large doses of vasopressin has little or no effect on urine flow or urine osmolality. In the 12-year-old male studied by Orloff and Burg (5), infusion of as much as 50 mU vasopressin per minute for 40 minutes effected no change in urine flow, urine osmolality, plasma osmolality, or glomerular filtration rate (GFR). In the same individual, dehydration led only to a slight decrease of urine volume from about 10 to about 7 ml per minute. Urine osmolality remained below 90 mOsm/L and plasma osmolality rose from 282 to 296 mOsm/L. GFR remained virtually unchanged at about 80 ml/min. The fact that neither exogenous nor endogenous vasopressin enhances renal concentrating ability rules out the possibility that the defect is caused by synthesis of an abnormal form of vasopressin.

From time to time reports have appeared that an abnormality in the structure of the nephrons of patients with nephrogenic diabetes insipidus can be revealed by microdissection. The abnormality described is a shortening of the proximal segments of the nephrons (6, 7). It has been suggested that this abnormality could lead to a reduction in proximal reabsorption and increased delivery of hypotonic fluid from the ascending limb of Henle to the distal portion of the nephron. It is unlikely that such a mechanism could lead to vasopressin-resistance, however. It would be more likely to lead to isosthenuria and solute diuresis (such as occurs in renal insufficiency) than to persistent excretion of hypotonic urine.

The nature of the renal resistance to vasopressin is not established. Vasopressin action is dependent on its ability to stimulate activity of adenylate cyclase after attaching to its receptor in its target tissues (8). In other endocrine disorders resulting from end-organ resistance, such as type I pseudohypoparathyroidism, the defect is apparently an inability of the hormone to generate cyclic AMP in its target organs (9). The defect of pseudohypoparathyroidism type I, may be a deficiency of the protein responsible for coupling the occupied receptor to the adenylate cyclase system (10). In nephrogenic diabetes insipidus, however, urinary excretion of cyclic AMP is normal and individuals with pseudohypoparathyroidism do not evidence signs of vasopressin resistance (11).

GENETICS

In most family pedigrees, vasopressin-resistant diabetes insipidus occurs in males. It has been deduced therefore that the mode of transmission is through a defect on the X chromosome. While this is the most likely explanation, the issue is complicated by the fact that symptoms have been observed in females and that male-to-male transmission has been reported (12). The fact that symptoms may occur in females is not inconsistent with an X-chromosome defect, but regular male-to-male transmission is. That Cannon's information may have been incomplete or incorrect has been assumed by McKusick (13). In any case, significant symptoms in females sufficient to require treatment may occur (4, 12).

SYMPTOMS AND SIGNS

A remarkable feature of the disorder is the extraordinary variability in intensity of symptoms and signs (4). The disorder is congenital and characteristically, manifestations of the disorder occur shortly after birth. The most typical symptoms are polydipsia and polyuria, but because they appear early in infancy, they may not be recognized promptly. Instead, irritability, poor feeding, and poor weight gain are often the initial symptoms. They suck eagerly, but may vomit during or shortly after the feeding. Such infants may have fever and not infrequently their symptoms are first considered to be caused by an infection. It is not unusual therefore for such infants to be studied extensively for signs of bacterial, viral, or parasitic disease. From time to time the true nature of the disorder is first revealed when the parent tells the physician that the irritability disappears whenever the infant ingests fluids.

While these severe symptoms may develop early in life, some affected children (even males) suffer very little. They progress through infancy and childhood with very little evidence of the consequences of dehydration. They consider their polydipsia and polyuria little more than an inconvenience and may never feel the need to consult a physician.

PHYSICAL FINDINGS

Physical examination may show impairment of normal growth. The infant may be irritable and, as indicated previously, may have an increased temperature. Dehydration may be evidenced by dryness of the skin, loss of normal skin turgor, recession of the eyeballs, increased periorbital fold depth, recession of the anterior fontanelle and scaphoid abdomen. Adequate hydration of the infant may be accomplished by the oral route following which a remarkable change in behavior may be seen. In spite of the dehydration the diapers are constantly wet.

LABORATORY TESTING

The most useful initial laboratory test is the serum sodium, which usually is in excess of the normal range and may be higher than 180 mEq/L. There is also an increase in concentration of serum chloride and, during the episodes of dehydration, retention of urea and creatinine. Metabolic acidosis occurs because of the dehydration and hypovolemia. Urine is increased in quantity, and, despite the dehydration, is hypotonic. Once adequate quantities of fluid are administered, however, serum sodium, chloride, bicarbonate, pH, urea, and creatinine return to normal. Diminished GFR, renal blood flow, hydrogen ion secretion, and ammonia production all return to normal when adequate quantities of fluid are administered.

COMPLICATIONS

The most serious complication, encephalopathy, may occur because of repeated damage from dehydration and hypernatremia. Psychomotor retardation may develop, associated with a short attention span and learning disorder. If the disease goes untreated, dilation of the renal pelvis, ureters, and bladder may be demonstrated by urography or ultrasonography. Urinary tract obstruction and infection are not a part of the disorder, however.

DIAGNOSIS

There are two steps in the diagnosis of this disorder. The first is to establish that a renal-concentrating defect exists, and the second is to establish the etiology of the defect. The first is accomplished by careful history taking, family history, observation of polyuria in a dehydrated infant, and the finding of a high serum sodium concentration.

Once the presence of polyuria is established, a differential diagnosis must be made between chronic renal disease, diabetes mellitus, vasopressin-responsive diabetes insipidus, and vasopressin-resistant diabetes insipidus. Pitressin-resistant hyposthenuria because of disease of the kidney other than vasopressin-resistant diabetes insipidus is described elsewhere (chapter 50) and will not be discussed here. Diabetes mellitus is characterized by glucosuria and hyperglycemia. During episodes of dehydration in diabetes mellitus, the serum sodium tends to be normal or diminished in concentration and the acidosis is associated with the presence of acetone, acetoacetic acid and beta-hydroxybutyric acid in plasma and urine.

Vasopressin responsive or central diabetes insipidus may be caused by tumors involving the hypothalamic area or posterior pituitary and other organic lesions of this area (14). In perhaps one-third to one-half, the disturbance is primary (idiopathic). In a small proportion the disease is genetically transmitted as an autosomal dominant or X-linked dominant disorder. A history of polyuria or polydipsia in relatives, therefore, may suggest either vasopressin-resistant or vasopressin-deficient diabetes insipidus. In both disorders, dehydration is associated with persistent polyuria, hypotonic urine, and hypernatremia. Generally the vasopressin resistant form is present from birth, whereas the vasopressin sensitive form occurs later in the first decade of life. The vasopressin sensitive form may occur during infancy, however, especially the inherited form.

To confirm the presence of polyuria and to distinguish the vasopressin-sensitive form from the vasopressin-resistant form, the following test is carried out. In children (3 years of age or older), a water deprivation test is performed as follows (15): after breakfast, access to water is removed and the child is kept under constant supervision up to a maximum of seven hours. This part of the test is to determine if polyuria is indeed present. Children with normal concentrating powers will soon develop oliguria. On the other hand, if diabetes insipidus is present, urine volumes will continue to be excessive and the child will experience significant weight loss. The test should be done during the day, not overnight, to permit careful observation of the child and to permit a decision to be made when to terminate the test. Older children or adolescents may be able to urinate at regular intervals. Each urine sample should be checked for volume and osmolality. If progressive dehydration occurs, the test should be terminated and samples of blood and urine should be obtained for measurement of osmolality. If dehydration does not occur to a significant degree, the test should be terminated after 7 hours of water deprivation, at which time the samples of blood and urine are taken. If the ratio of urine to plasma osmolality is greater than 1.5, the patient may be judged to have normal concentrating powers (16).

Once the blood and urine samples are obtained, if polyuria persists, DDAVP (1-desamino-8-D-arginine vasopressin) should be administered intranasally in a dosage of 10 μg in infants or 20 μg in older children. If the polyuria is a result of the lack of vasopressin, antidiuresis will promptly develop and a further sample of blood and urine should be obtained within the first hour for measurement of osmolality. In vasopressin-sensitive individuals, the ratio of urine to plasma osmolality will exceed 1.5. If antidiuresis does not develop, the child is given fluids orally every hour in amounts equivalent to the urinary output of the previous hour. The test continues for a maximum of four hours at the end of which time blood and urine samples are again collected for measurement of plasma osmolality (15).

In infants the total period of water deprivation should not exceed 4 hours and the period of observation after vasopressin administration should not be prolonged in excess of 2 hours. The water deprivation test (7 hours) and intranasal installation of DDAVP are easily the best and safest tests for the differential diagnosis of polyuria. Tests based on infusion of hypertonic saline are more hazardous and often yield little useful information. If a diagnosis of vasopressin-sensitive diabetes insipidus is made, a careful search must be made for a lesion involving the hypothalamic or posterior pituitary. The best available treatment for vasopressin-sensitive diabetes insipidus is the intranasal instillation of DDAVP (17).

TREATMENT

Because nephrogenic diabetes insipidus is resistant to treatment with vasopressin, other means have to be used. While treatment of vasopressin-sensitive diabetes insipidus is fairly simple and straightforward, the treatment of the vasopressin-resistant form is difficult and often only partially effective. Large volume feedings are necessary throughout the day and night. During infancy protein intake should be reduced to equal that of human milk—approximately 6% of calories as protein, c.a.p. (chapter 10) and sodium intake to less than 0.7 mEq/kg/day. After infancy dietary protein should remain <8% c.a.p. and Na intake <0.7 mEq/kg/day. This is done to minimize renal solute excretion, which requires obligatory water excretion. The protein must not be reduced to a level where anabolism and growth are impaired nor should the Na be reduced to a degree that leads to hyponatremia (14). Breast milk is preferable to most formula feedings because of its lower solute content. If calorie intake is inadequate, it is preferable to make up the deficit by adding glucose to the water intake.

A dramatic improvement in the treatment of vasopressin-resistant diabetes insipidus occurred in 1959 with the introduction by Crawford and Kennedy of chlorothiazide for the treatment of this disorder (18). These investigators reasoned that administration of these diuretic agents would decrease sodium reabsorption in the cortical diluting segment and increase urinary sodium loss. Contraction of the plasma volume would ensue, leading to enhanced absorption of fluid in the proximal tubule. The dosage used was 30 mg/kg of chlorthiazide or 3 mg/kg hydrochlorthiazide per day in three divided doses. If this treatment is used the serum sodium must not be permitted to fall below the range of 133–137 mEq/L by dietary sodium restriction or the treatment will be unsuccessful. The plasma concentration of potassium must also be carefully monitored and if hypokalemia occurs, oral intake of K salts must be increased. Na intake should not exceed 1.5 mg/kg/da.

This form of treatment represents a substantial advance over what was available previously and often permits progression of normal growth and psychomotor development. Nevertheless, in many subjects, this treatment is not sufficient to achieve these goals. Recently attention has been focussed on other agents that might be used separately or in conjunction with chlorothiazides to enhance the efficacy of therapy. One group of agents that appears to show promise is the prostaglandin synthetase inhibitors. The actions of prostaglandins on renal function are quite complex and their effects on renal NaCl and water excretion may vary with the prostaglandin used and the conditions of the experiment (19) (chapters 5, 6, and 16). In conscious humans, however, it appears that prostaglandin synthetase inhibitors usually inhibit water excretion. In 1976, Fichman and coworkers (20) showed that administration of the prostaglandin synthetase inhibitor, indomethacin, to two adults with nephrogenic diabetes insipidus led to a significant decrease in water excretion. Recently Monn (21) reported improvement in two children with nephrogenic diabetes insipidus in whom either indomethacin or acetylsalicylic acid was added to the diuretic and low salt diet regimen. In the seven-year-old child, eneuresis abated. In the infant, oral feedings replaced tube feedings; growth and development improved. These results are encouraging but more experience is necessary before the effectiveness of these combinations can be ascertained.

References

1. Williams RH, Henry C: Nephrogenic diabetes insipidus transmitted by females and appearing during infancy in males. Ann Intern Med 27:84, 1947.
2. Waring AJ, Kajdi L, Tappan V: A congenital defect of water metabolism. Am J Dis Child 69:323, 1945.
3. Forssman H: On hereditary diabetes insipidus with special regard to a sex-linked form. Acta Med Scand 159 (suppl):1, 1945.
4. Kaplan SA, Yuceoglu AM, Strauss J: Vasopressin-resistant diabetes insipidus. Am J Dis Child 97:309, 1959.
5. Orloff JJ, Burg MB: Vasopressin-resistant diabetes insipidus. In Stanbury JB, et al (eds): The Metabolic Basis of Inherited Disease, ed 13. New York, McGraw-Hill, 1972.
6. MacDonald WB: Congenital pitressin resistant diabetes insipidus of renal origin. Pediatrics 15:298, 1955.
7. Darmady E, Prince J, Stranack F: The proximal convoluted tubule in the renal handling of water. Lancet 2:1254, 1964.
8. Orloff J, Handler JS: The role of adenosine 3′-5 phosphate in the action of antidiuretic hormone. Am J Med 42:757, 1967.
9. Chase LR, Melson GL, Aurbach GD: Pseudohypoparathyroidism: defective excretion of 3′5′-AMP in response to parathyroid hormone. J Clin Invest 48:1832, 1969.
10. Farfel Z, Brickman AS, Kaslow HR, et al: Defect in receptor-cyclase coupling protein in pseudohypoparathyroidism. N Engl J Med 303:237, 1980.
11. Moses AM, Coulson BB: Absence of overlapping resistance to vasopressin and parathyroid hormone in patients with nephrogenic diabetes insipidus and pseudohypoparathyroidism. J Clin Endocrinol Metab 55:699, 1983.
12. Cannon JF: Diabetes insipidus. Clinical and experimental studies with consideration of genetic relationships. Arch Int Med 96:215, 1955.
13. McKusick VA: Mendelian Inheritance in Man. Catalogs of Autosomal Dominant, Autosomal Recessive, and X-Linked Phenotypes, ed 3. Baltimore, Johns Hopkins Press, 1971.
14. Bode HH: Disorders of the posterior pituitary. In Kaplan SA (ed): Clinical Pediatric and Adolescent Endocrinology. Philadelphia, W. B. Saunders Co, 1982.
15. Hendricks SA, Lippe BM, Kaplan SA, et al: Differential diagnosis of diabetes insipidus: Use of DDAVP to terminate the seven hour water deprivation test. J Pediatr 98:244, 1981.
16. Frasier SD, Kutnick LA, Schmidt RT, et al: A water deprivation test for the diagnosis of diabetes insipidus in children. Am J Dis Child 114:157, 1967.
17. Lee W-NP, Lippe BM, La Franchi SH, et al: Vasopressin analog DDAVP in the treatment of diabetes insipidus. Am J Dis Child 130:166, 1976.
18. Crawford JD, Kennedy GC: Chlorothiazide in diabetes insipidus. Nature 183:891, 1959.
19. Friedman WF, Molony DA, Kirkpatrick SE: Prostaglandins. Physiological and clinical correlations. In Barnes LA (ed): Advances in Pediatrics, Chicago, Year Book Medical Publishers, 1978, vol 25.
20. Fichman MP, Speckart P, Zia P, et al: Antidiuretic response to prostaglandin inhibition by indomethacin in nephrogenic diabetes insipidus. Clin Res 24:(2)161, 1976.
21. Monn E: Prostaglandin synthetase inhibitors in the treatment of nephrogenic diabetes insipidus. Acta Pediatr Scand 70:39, 1981.

9

Genitourinary Tract Disease

CHAPTER 36

Clinical Aspects of Urinary Tract Infection

J. WINBERG

Urinary tract infection (UTI) is one of the major bacterial diseases of children. The cumulative risk of a girl falling ill during childhood with a symptomatic UTI is at least 3%, and of a boy about 1% (1, 2). The prevalence of asymptomatic bacteriuria (ABU) in girls of preschool and school age is approximately 1% (3, 4). About half the children with symptomatic UTI and 80% or more of those with ABU will have one or several recurrences. Some girls of late preschool or school age have an almost endless sequence of UTI.

About 5% to 10% of children with asymptomatic UTI acquire a renal scar; a proportion of these develop renal stones, hypertension, end stage renal disease, or complications of pregnancy. These severe complications probably can be prevented by adequate care. Both quantitatively and qualitatively, UTI is a disease of major concern. Proper management of UTI usually calls for expensive microbiological, nephrological, and radiological examinations, with several follow-up visits after the first diagnosis. The majority of patients take antibiotics for short or long periods. UTI causes morbidity and inconvenience to many patients and is a large financial burden for the family and society.

DEFINITIONS AND CLASSIFICIATIONS

UTI is the term applied to all conditions that have one feature in common: the presence of significant numbers of bacteria in the urine. It is used in this chapter to encompass all such conditions irrespective of the localization of the infection in the urinary tract. Several mechanisms may lead to the establishment of UTI, and consequently the course and the prognosis are diverse. UTI can be classified with regard to pathogenesis, localization, and the circumstances of its occurrence.

Pathogenesis

It is helpful to classify children with UTI into subgroups for clincal as well as for scientific purposes, and Table 36.1 provides a tentative pathogenetic classification. UTI may be primary (uncomplicated) or secondary to an anatomical abnormality of the urinary tract (complicated). Obstructed infections make up only a minority of cases of UTI in childhood (1% to 2% in girls, 5% to 10% in boys) but are qualitatively important, since irreversible renal damage may occur rapidly. Vesicoureteric reflux (VUR) is not considered to be an obstructive anomaly as significant as urethral valves, ureterocele, or others; however, it has the potential to transport bacteria to the upper urinary tract and, when associated with intrarenal reflux, into the renal parenchyma, which probably accounts for the great impact of VUR on the prognosis of UTI.

Uncomplicated UTI may be symptomatic or asymptomatic. Screening bacteriuria (asymptomatic; symptomless; covert; latent; or other terms) is revealed by examination of healthy populations and occurs mainly in girls. A special host-parasite relationship in many of these patients in this group may warrant placing it in a separate classification, although the pathogenetic mechanisms are probably the same as in uncomplicated symptomatic infections.

Localization

Cystitis and Pyelonephritis

Cystitis and pyelonephritis are self-explanatory terms. Localizing measures are described on pp 630–1.

Pyelitis

Pyelitis is an inflammation of the renal pelvis and the term is used, especially in Europe, to denote febrile UTI. It may be the forerunner of pyelonephritis. Since it is difficult to show that an infection involves the pelvis but not the renal tissue, there is little reason to use the term pyelitis any longer.

Chronic Pyelonephritis

Chronic pyelonephritis is a confusing term, since it is used in different ways to describe: (a) certain characteristic histological lesions of the renal parenchyma; (b) focal renal parenchymal defects visible on roentgenograms and usually consisting of papillary shrinking with a defect of the corresponding part of the renal outline (focal scarring); and (c) a clinical condition characterized by continuous excretion of bacteria or by frequent recurrences of infection. Thus, the term "chronic pyelonephritis" may be misleading. True chronic infections of the renal parenchyma are probably rare but may occur in association with staghorn calculi and in such specific infections as tuberculosis.

Table 36.1.
Classification of Urinary Tract Infection (UTI)[a]

Uncomplicated
Symptomatic nonobstructed with and without gross reflux
Neonates
Girls
Boys
"Screening bacteriuria"
Complicated
Obstructed[b]
Associated with a neurogenic bladder

[a] UTI is used in this chapter as a common designation for conditions with significant bacteriuria.
[b] Valves, ureterocele, foreign bodies, stones, diverticula, and others.

Cystourethral Syndrome

Cystourethral syndrome (cystourethritis, abacterial cystitis, urethritis, uninhibited bladder, detrusor-sphincter instability) is a vague term often used to describe patients with the classic symptoms of cystitis, such as urgency, frequency, or pain, who lack the laboratory criteria for UTI. The condition is not uncommon in prepubertal girls and is often associated with uninhibited contractions of the detrusor and instability of the sphincter function. Squatting and pant-wetting are common symptoms. Pyuria, suggesting inflammation, may be present. Vulvitis and balanitis should be ruled out by inspection. The cause is unknown, and its association with UTI is complex and far from understood. It remains to be proven that true bacterial urethritis exists (except for gonococcal infection).

Circumstance

There is a need for an operational classification of UTI, in order to determine the clinical aspects of management. Stamey suggested four simple categories: (a) first infection; (b) unresolved bacteriuria during therapy (failure to sterilize the urine); (c) bacterial persistance (in a locus not amenable to antibiotics); and (d) reinfection (5). A distinction is made between failure to sterilize (a) the urine (unresolved bacteriuria) and (b) a localised site within the urinary tract (bacterial persistence), in which case voided urine may be sterile temporarily.

First Infection

Bacteria causing the initial (onset) infection in infants and children are, with few exceptions, sensitive to most antimicrobial agents. Sulfonamides will cure almost all these patients. In infants and toddlers, the first infection usually is associated with fever and probably involves the renal parenchyma. Demonstration of the presence or absence of gross reflux is essential in follow-up and prophylaxis.

Unresolved Bacteriuria during Therapy

The clinician often fails to recognize unresolved bacteriuria during therapy, either because urine cultures are not obtained during treatment or, if they are obtained, bacterial counts of $<10^5$/ml are misinterpreted as contaminants. Clearly, if any bacteria of the infecting strain are present in a midstream specimen of urine during therapy, one cannot be certain that the bacteriuria has been eradicated. According to Stamey (5), the causes of the unresolved bacteriuria, in descending order of importance, are as follows.

1. Bacterial resistance to the drug selected for therapy. If a patient has received therapy in the recent past, there is a considerable chance that resistant organisms from the fecal flora may be responsible for the current bacteriuria (see Chapter 14). Resistant mutants also may be selected from an initially sensitive bacterial population in the urinary tract.
2. Occurrence of two different bacterial species simultaneously in the bladder that have mutually exclusive antimicrobial sensitivities; initial therapy unmasks the presence of a second species.
3. Renal failure. Unresolved bacteriuria may continue with sensitive bacteria if renal failure prevents the attainment of the urinary concentration of antibiotic required to kill the organism.
4. Staghorn calculi associated with a "critical mass" of sensitive bacteria too great for antimicrobial inhibition. The role of stagnant urine in therapeutic failure has been emphasized (6).

The first two of these causes for failure to sterilize the urine can be resolved by in vitro antimicrobial sensitivity testing.

Bacterial Persistence

Once the urine is sterile, the same organism may reappear from a site within the urinary tract. This may occur in two circumstances: (a) in the presence of infected stones (struvite) and (b) with chronic bacterial prostatitis. The existence of prostatitis in children is unlikely. A structural abnormality, such as a nonfunctioning duplication, a urachal cyst, or a nonrefluxing ureteral stump, may represent other causes of bacterial persistence.

Reinfection

Reinfection may be inferred when a new species or serotype of an infectious organism is found.

DIAGNOSTIC PROCEDURES

Demonstration of a "significant" number of bacteria in the urine is the only valid criterion for the diagnosis of UTI. Other commonly accepted diagnostic signs, such as pyuria, decreased concentrating capacity, elevated antibody titers, are only secondary phenomena and therefore give only supportive evidence. Some patients with obvious infections have only a few bacteria in the urine (7, 8). The reason for this is obscure.

Bacterial Culture

Bacterial culture is described in Chapter 14.

Secondary Phenomena

Pyuria

White blood cells (WBC) in the urine are a sign of inflammation—bacterial or nonbacterial—of the genital region or urinary tract; demonstrating their presence cannot replace bacterial culture in the diagnosis of UTI. A normal WBC count does not exclude UTI. In consecutive urine specimens from patients with UTI the number of WBC may vary between normal and gross pyuria (9). It is more common to find a normal WBC with recurrent infections than with apparent first-time infections (Fig. 36.1).

Quantifying urinary WBC is best done on uncentrifuged urine in a counting chamber, e.g., the Fuchs-Rosenthal (10). Healthy boys should have <10 WBC/mm^3 in voided specimens; girls usually also have few WBC and counts as high as 50 and 100 WBC/mm^3 may be found without demonstrable disease. Microscopic investigation of the urinary sediment is valuable in demonstrating WBC casts. Presence or absence of WBC esterase in the urine can be demonstrated by means of paper strips (Cytur), but WBC counting is helpful in four situations: (a) in making a tentative diagnosis in acutely ill patients before the results of culture are available; (b) in suggesting renal involvement by appearance of WBC casts; (c) in supporting the diagnosis in patients with low level bacteriuria, with symptoms of doubtful significance, or with asymptomatic bacteriuria; and (d) in all boys <4 yr in whom preputial bacteria may contaminate the urine sample heavily.

Testing for proteinuria is of no help in the diagnosis of UTI. Hematuria is not uncommon.

Antibody Response

Agglutinating and hemagglutinating antibodies to the O-antigen of the infecting *Escherichia coli* can be demonstrated regularly in the serum of patients with pyelonephritis but not in those with cystitis (11, 12). The antibodies are highly specific and can be used diagnostically to verify that the isolated bacteria are causing the infection. This may be clinically useful, for example, in patients with low-count bacteriuria.

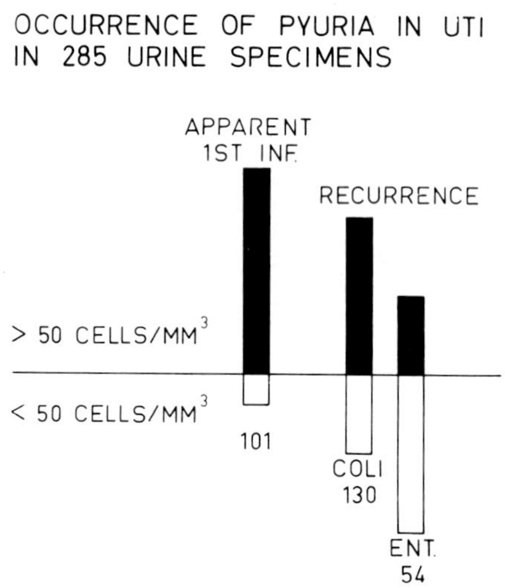

Figure 36.1. Occurrence of pyuria in girls with urinary tract infections. A count of <50 cells/mm³ in the uncentrifuged urine is common, especially in recurrent infection. ENT-enterococci.

Renal Function

In acute infection of a previously healthy kidney, renal concentrating capacity is reduced temporarily. In uncomplicated UTI, it improves rapidly but is not restored completely until after 8 to 12 weeks (Fig. 36.2) (13). If it does not return to normal, obstruction of urine flow, renal scarring, or persistent infection should be considered.

An increase in plasma urea or creatinine concentration is uncommon in uncomplicated acute pyelonephritis. If present, it suggests obstruction with bilateral hydronephrosis or marked parenchymal destruction. During the newborn period, however, plasma urea concentration may increase even in the absence of obstruction (14).

In scarred kidneys, all types of functional defects may be seen, including reduced ability to excrete a sodium load (15) and lowering of the renal threshold for bicarbonate (16), which may be the earliest functional defect to become manifest.

Inulin and para-aminohippurate clearances performed three to five days after onset of treatment for febrile infections have demonstrated increased glomerular filtration rate (GFR) and effective renal plasma flow (ERPF) (17). However, gamma camera studies with ^{131}I-hippuran in the acute phase of untreated pyelonephritis in monkeys have shown a considerable increase in renal transit time, possibly due to edema, and later a decrease in ERPF (18). The studies in monkeys may show the true effect of infection, whereas the clinical study may reflect the effect of early treatment on renal function.

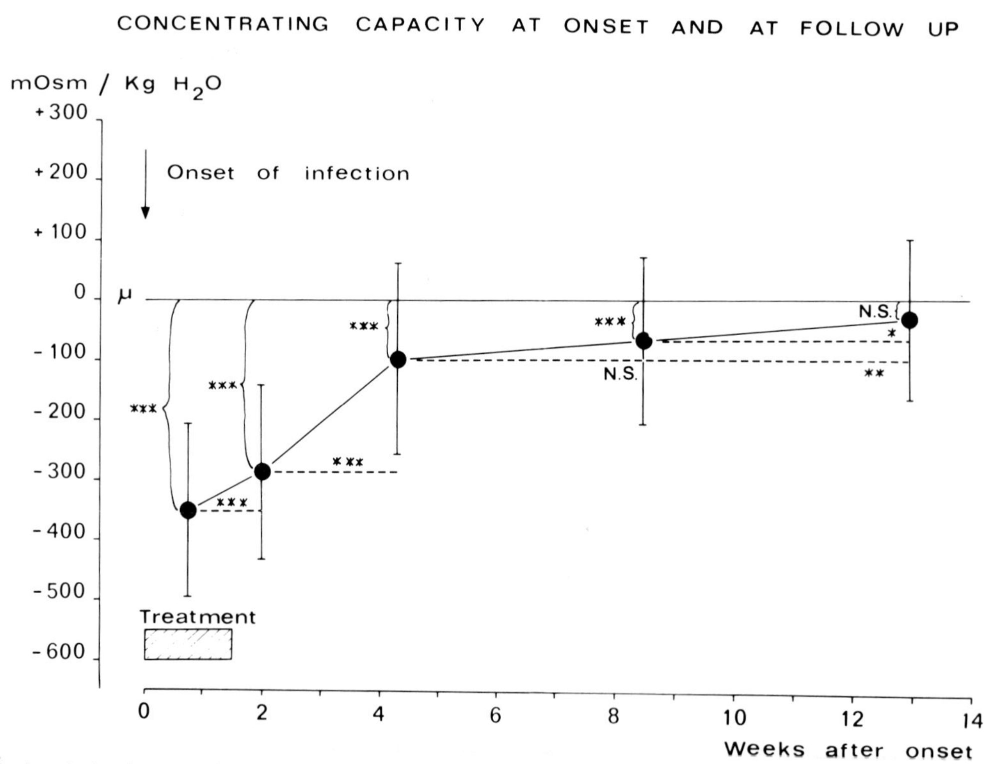

Figure 36.2. Statistical analysis of repeated concentration tests in 95 girls, selected on the basis of a rectal temperature of ≥38° C, a sedimentation rate of ≥20 mm/h, and significant bacteriuria and pyuria. 0 = normal mean for age [13]. The vertical axis gives deviation from normal mean. * $p < 0.05$; ** $p < 0.01$; *** $p < 0.001$.

Diagnostic Radiology

Aims

The appropriate modalities of renal imaging are discussed in Chapter 20. There are three main aims of intravenous urography (IVU) and micturating cystourethrography (MCU):

1. To detect factors predisposing to infection and to kidney damage, principally congenital or acquired obstructions of the urinary flow, calculi, vesicoureteric reflux, and intrarenal reflux.

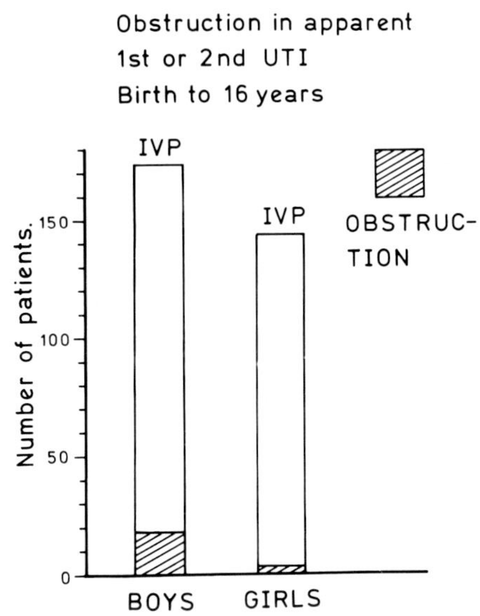

Figure 36.3. Occurrence of obstruction in 174 apparent first-time infections in boys and in 144 first or second infections in girls. Onset between birth and 16 yr. Obstructions in boys: Urethral valves proven in 3 patients and suspected in 2 patients; bladder stone and diverticula in 2 patients; ureteral obstruction in 11 patients. (From Winberg J, Anderson HJ, Bergström T, et al: Epidemiology of symptomatic urinary tract infection in childhood. Acta Paediatr Scand (suppl 252) 63: 1, 1974.)

2. To detect and outline narrowing of renal parenchyma and calyceal dilatation, which may be an early sign of progressive renal scarring.

3. To determine the rate of growth of the kidney, which may be a valuable aid in assessing the effect of treatment (19–21).

Referral centers have reported that 25% to 50% of their children with UTI have anatomical malformations. In general practice, however, the frequency of obstruction is much less: 5% to 10% in boys and 1% to 2% in girls (Fig. 36.3) (1, 2).

Methods

Intravenous Urography. When evaluating renal size and form it is important to visualize the nephrographic phase approximately one min after the injection of contrast medium. Symmetry in the excretion of contrast as well as the time for appearance should be noted. Morphological changes of the parenchyma (scars, necroses, cysts), of the renal pelvices (hydronephrosis, calyceal deformities, stones) and of the ureters (obstruction, dilatation, abnormal course) should be noted. The width of the ureters should be measured, with scars classified according to Smellie (Fig. 36.4) (22).

Each examination should include a measurement of the kidneys. Diagrams of the normal parenchymal thickness, renal length, and area at different ages and in relation to the L1 to L3 distance are available (19–21). Area measurements are most suitable to follow the growth of the kidney, but the length measurement is simple and may be used instead. To demonstrate focal scarring, measurement of parenchymal thickness is superior. It should be noted that in little children the kidney poles are relatively much thicker than in older children or adults, so that retarded renal growth in the poles is easily overlooked.

Micturating and Cystourethrography. Micturating cystourethrography (MCU) should include at least one frontal and one side projection during micturition. The frontal picture should be large enough to visualize urethra, bladder, and the whole kidneys. Morphological changes as well as the ability of the bladder to empty and the appearance of the urethra should be noted. One film should be taken after the end of the micturition to evaluate the ability to empty.

If there is VUR it should be graded. There are three-, four-, and five-

Vesico-ureteric reflux and renal scarring

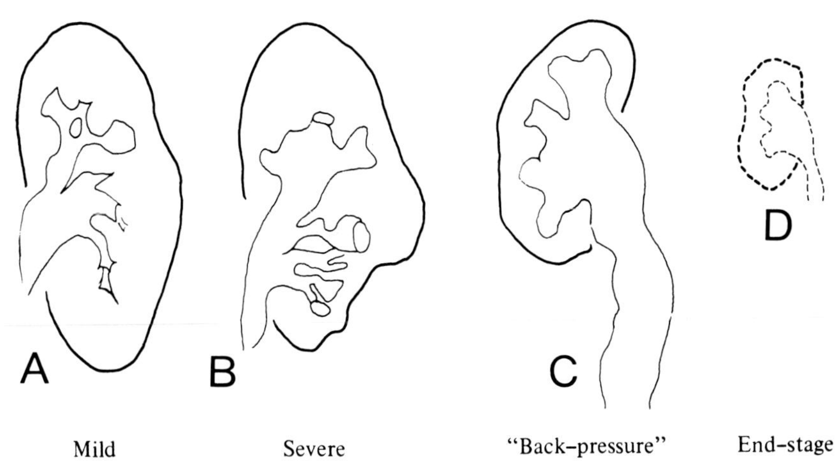

Figure 36.4. Classification of focal renal scarring. **A**, Mild form—not more than two focal scars. **B**, Severe form—more than two scars; some areas with normal tissue thickness remain. **C**, "Back pressure" type—in addition to a generalized deformity of the calyces (as in obstructive uropathy) the thin mantle of parenchyma shows irregular, thin areas, possibly representing scars caused by infections. **D**, Totally shrunken kidney with no or poor function. (From Smellie JM, Edwards D, Hunter N, et al; Vesico-ureteric reflux and renal scarring. Kidney Int 8: 65, 1975.

Grades of Reflux

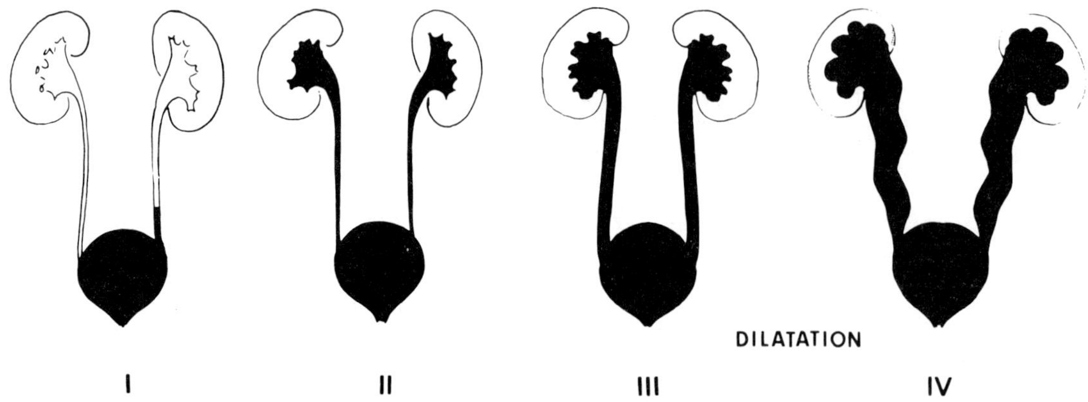

Figure 36.5. Grades of reflux in a four-graded scale, not taking into account whether reflux is free or not. (From Winberg J, Larson H, Bergström T. Comparison of the natural history of urinary infection in children with and without vesico-ureteric reflux. In Kincaid-Smith P, Fairley K (eds): *Renal Infection and Renal Scarring*, Melbourne, Mercedes, 1971).

grade systems (Fig. 36.5). In all systems, VUR without dilatation is probably of no clinical importance. There is some disagreement as to whether VUR occurs in healthy children during the first and second year of life, but gross reflux that dilates the upper urinary tract is always abnormal. In such cases, it should be noted whether intrarenal reflux (usually pyelotubular backflow) is present or not.

Indications

Apparent First Infection. Suggested indications include (a) a mass seen or palpated over the symphysis after micturition, indicating incomplete bladder emptying; (b) a mass palpated in the upper part of the abdomen, indicating hydronephrosis; (c) increased plasma urea or creatinine concentration, or persistently lowered concentrating capacity, or UTI associated with acidosis; (d) increased blood pressure; (e) an infection that fails to resolve in spite of an adequate antibiotic; (f) infants with symptomatic infections; (g) all boys with symptomatic infections, irrespective of age; (h) all girls with febrile infections (a roentgenogram may be unnecessary in a girl if a first infection is associated with lower tract symptoms only and she is afebrile and otherwise healthy).

Many clinics do not have the capacity for radiological investigation of all children with UTI; selecting suitable patients for roentgenography is then a question of the patient's age and sex, personal experience and the referral pattern.

Recurrent Infections. Patients of all ages and either sex with a history of recurrent infections that have not been previously examined roengenographically should have an IVU and an MCU.

Follow-up. Only tentative suggestions for radiological follow-up can be made. It is appropriate to check patients with persistently recurrent UTI in order to monitor renal growth and calyceal appearance, at intervals of six months during the first year of life, an interval of 12 months during the second year of life, and later on at intervals of two to three yr. Since preserving renal tissue is the therapeutic goal, documentation of growth of the kidneys by IVU is the most relevant observation and repeated MCU in conservatively treated patients with VUR (Fig. 36.5) should be avoided. For follow-up after reflux surgery see Chapter 37.

Localization

Localization of the infection site is mainly a research objective in studies in which it is essential to know whether an infection involves the renal parenchyma. Demonstration of persistent unilateral infection, however, may also guide elective surgery. The washout techniques, such as the Stamey type (23) with ureteral catheterization and the Fairley type (24) using only bladder catheterization, are useful but have their pitfalls. The discharge of bacteria may be intermittent, so results may indicate bladder infection when in fact there is renal parenchymal involvement. A reverse misinterpretation is also possible if bacteria are carried up from the bladder, either by the catheter or by reflux. Even minimal amounts of the bladder disinfectant left behind after saline irrigation in the Fairley technique inhibit bacterial growth and may erroneously suggest infection confined to the bladder. Although these methods are often referred to as direct, the only truly direct technique for demonstrating renal infection is biopsy, which can be performed only in selected cases.

A transitory decrease in renal concentrating capacity or an increase in serum antibody titer against the O-antigen of infecting bacteria, as determined by hemagglutination or direct agglutination, indicates renal involvement. Although these tests seem valuable in defining groups of patients with renal infection, they have limitations in any individual patient (25, 26). A low concentrating capacity and a high antibody titer may have explanations other than a renal infection.

There is a good correlation between concentrating capacity, antibody titer, and sedimentation rate in patients with apparent first symptomatic infection, but it is less good in patients with frequent recurrences or ABU. In these instances, the infection is often caused by bacteria with a deficient cell wall. When such bacteria are used as antigen sources, measured antibody titer is lower than when a laboratory strain with a more complete antigenic structure is used (26). Unfortunately, it is mainly in patients with frequent recurrences or asymptomatic bacteriuria that localization studies may be needed.

Demonstration of antibody-coated bacteria in the urine has been suggested to distinguish renal from bladder infection (27). This elegant and simple method seems less reliable in children. Determination of C-reactive protein discriminates rather well between renal and nonrenal infections in patients with symptomatic (25) but not in asymptomatic infections (26, 28).

At present, it is difficult to say which method is most reliable. All have their drawbacks. Antibody determination involves a number of technical problems and pitfalls. Washout methods are inconvenient for the patient. Easiest to evaluate is the concentrating capacity, especially when a low value is demonstrated in two consecutive tests. Administration of des-D-amino-arginine vasopressin (DDAVP) has made this test more convenient (29). Determination of C-reactive protein is easy to perform but is not reliable when most needed. With these difficulties, it is unlikely that localization studies will have much impact on the clinical management of symptomatic UTI.

EPIDEMIOLOGY

Symptomatic Infections

The age and sex distribution of 523 consecutive cases (excluding neonates) with presumed first (onset) infections appearing within a defined population during a defined period of time are shown in Figure 36.6 (1, 2). From these data, the risk of a child falling ill with a symptomatic UTI before the age of 11 yr has been calculated as 1.1% for boys and 3.0% for girls. Such figures may be subject to local variations, e.g., epidemic outbreaks of UTI caused by especially virulent "clones" of *E. coli* (see Chapter 14). Most infants and small children with acute symptomatic infections seem to grow out of their susceptibility to UTI, boys usually during the second year of life, girls later. A proportion of girls continue to have repeated infections for many years. This explains why, even though onset infections have a peak incidence during the first year of life, girls of school age with UTI predominate among the pediatrician's patients.

Screening Bacteriuria

Screening bacteriuria (asymptomatic bacteriuria [ABU] or covert, latent, symptomless bacteriuria) is defined here as UTI diagnosed during surveys of apparently healthy populations. The designation "asymptomatic" may not be adequate, since some of these patients feel more comfortable after eradication of bacteriuria than they did before. In apparently healthy girls between 4 and 16 yr of age, the incidence is between 0.7% and 2.0% with no definite increase with age, although a yearly acquisition rate of 0.32% has been observed (4). In males, the frequency is very low (4, 30).

In neonates, "asymptomatic" bacteriuria associated with heavy pyuria may be seen in 1% to 3% of males (31, 32). A randomized population-based survey during the first year of life reveals a frequency of UTI of about 2.7% and 0.7% in males and females, respectively (33). The significance of neonatal and early infantile asymptomatic bacteriuria is unknown.

BACTERIAL ETIOLOGY AND RESISTANCE PATTERN

E. coli causes most UTI in patients without a complicating disorder of the urinary system, such as calculus, obstruction, or neuropathic bladder (Table 36.2). *E. coli* isolates in the urine are usually of the same serotype as those dominating the fecal flora (34). *Proteus* is a common invader in older boys, and *Staphylococcus saprophyticus* in girls at puberty. *Klebsiella* is often seen in newborns (Table 36.2).

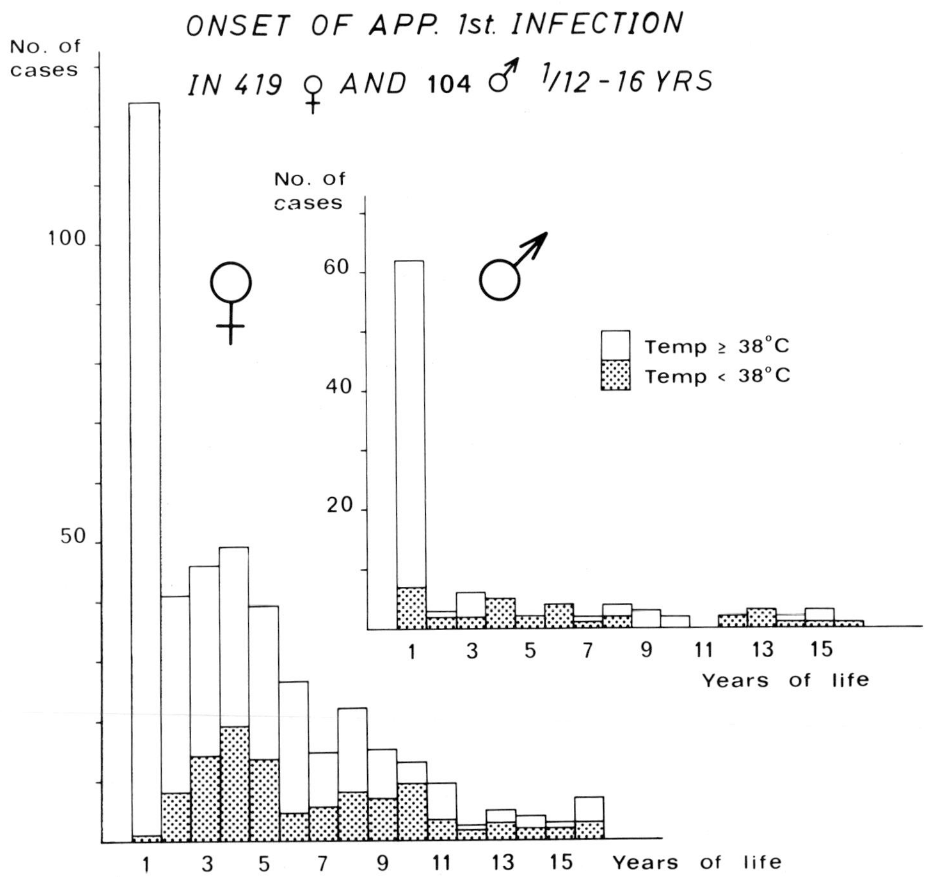

Figure 36.6. Apparently primary onset of symptomatic UTI in 419 girls and 104 boys between second month and 16 yr. The proportion of nonfebrile infections was very small during the first year of life, but increased with age. Not included are 54 boys and 21 girls with neonatal infections (0 to 30 days). (From Winberg J, Andersen HJ, Bergström T, et al: Epidemiology of symptomatic urinary tract infection in childhood. Acta Paediatr Scand (suppl 252) 63:1, 1974).

Table 36.2.
Bacterial Etiology in 596 Apparent First Nonobstructed Urinary Tract Infections in Relation to Sex and Age

Bacteria	Percent of neonates of both sexes (N = 73)	Percent of girls		Percent of boys	
		1 mo–10 yr[a] (N = 389)	10–16 yr (N = 30)	1 mo–1 yr (N = 62)	1–16 yr[a] (N = 42)
E. coli	75[b]	83	60	85	33
Klebsiella	11	<1	0	2	2
Proteus	0	3	0	5	33
Enterococci	3	2	0	0	2
Staphylococcus albus	1	<1	30	0	12[c]
Other bacteria	4	<1	0	3	2
Mixed etiology	4	1	3	2	5
Unknown	1	9	7	3	10

[a] No differences between girls 1 month to 1 yr and 1 to 10 yr. No differences between boys 1 to 10 and 10 to 16 yr except for *S. albus*; see footnote c.

[b] In girls, 57%; in boys, 83%; χ^2: $p = 0.016$.

[c] Four of the five patients were >11 years of age. (From Winberg J, Andersen HJ, Bergström T, et al: Epidemiology of symptomatic urinary tract infection in childhood. Acta Paediatr Scand (suppl 252) 63:1, 1974.)

The majority of infecting bacteria are sensitive to most commonly used antimicrobials, including sulfonamides. There are exceptions. It is especially noteworthy that antibiotics often induce a multiple resistance of the gram-negative fecal flora, which may determine the resistance pattern of recurrent urinary infections (35). The microbiology of UTI is discussed in Chapter 14.

PATHOGENESIS AND PREDISPOSING FACTORS

Bacteria seem to enter the urinary tract by the ascending route. It is generally assumed, but not proven, that infections appearing during the newborn period are blood-borne. Presumed ascending infection seems to affect 3% to 5% of all girls. The risk of reinfection increases with the number of previous infections (Fig. 36.7) and may be up to 50 times the risk in a previously healthy girl (1, 2).

Obstructive Malformation, Hematogenous Versus Ascending Infection, Fecal Soiling, Urethral Length, and "Maturation"

The typical age and sex distribution of onset infection (Fig. 36.6) helps to define possible pathogenetic mechanisms. The average number of new cases per month of life at different ages was calculated from this population (Fig. 36.8). More than 50 males fell ill in the first month of life; during the next five months, there were about 10 new cases per month; in the next six months there were 1 or 2 per month. Thus, UTI in boys is largely a disease of early infancy. The decline in the morbidity rate for females was similar but slower.

Several possibilities must be considered to explain the slope of the curves in Figure 36.8: (a) Obstructive malformations do not account for the age distribution, since these patients were excluded in the studies. (b) The pathogenetic factors operating in the early infections may be different from those occurring later e.g., gram-negative septicemia may explain the early peak incidence. This can, however, hardly be valid beyond the first month of life. Furthermore, ABU, which probably is ascending rather than hematogenous, appears in 1% to 3% of newborn boys (31–33) and is not infrequent during the following first six months of life (33). This suggests a decreased local defense at this age. (c) Fecal soiling, proposed as a predisposing factor, can hardly be important since the rapid decrease in frequency of UTI starts during the first few months of life.

Female preponderance in UTI is usually explained with reference to

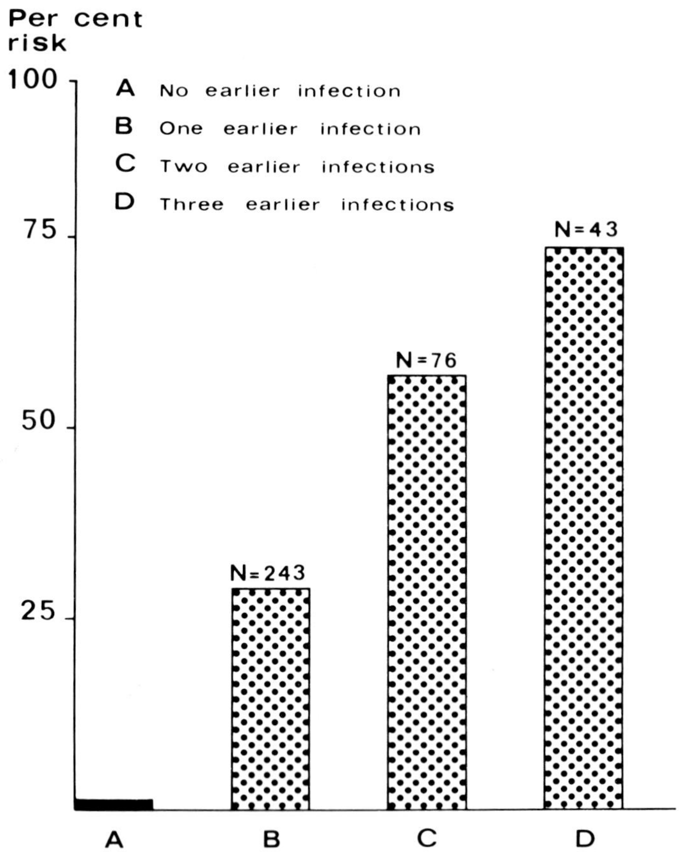

Figure 36.7. Recurrence rate within 1 yr of a preceding infection, related to the number of earlier infections. **A**, Approximate risk of a 30-day-old healthy girl having a symptomatic infection <11 yr of age. **B**, Observed risk in 243 girls with one earlier infection. **C**, Observed risk in 76 patients with two earlier infections. **D**, Observed risk in 43 patients with three earlier infections. (From Winberg J, Andersen HJ, Bergström T, et al: Epidemiology of symptomatic urinary tract infection in childhood. Acta Paediatr Scand (suppl 252) 63:1, 1974.

the short female urethra. The successive change of the sex ratio with age demonstrated in Table 36.3 is hardly compatible with this view; it is more suggestive of a successive functional maturation of a defense

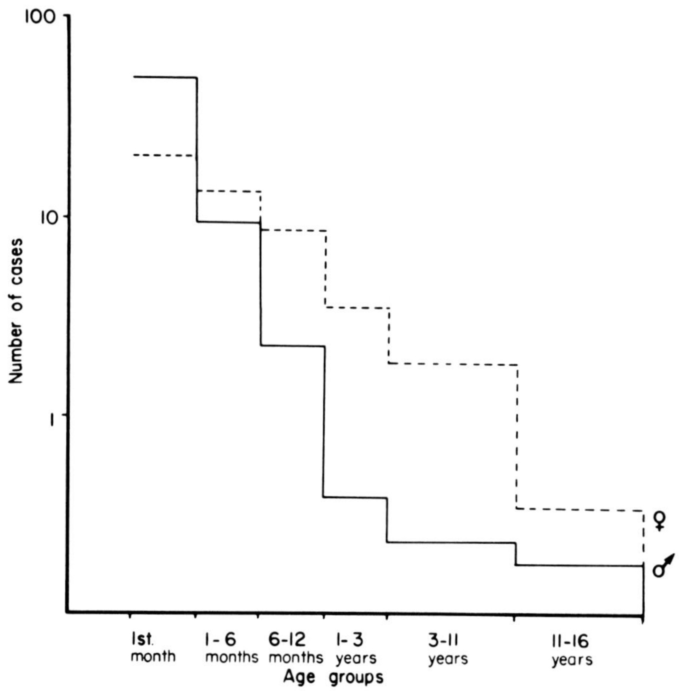

Figure 36.8. Mean number of new cases per month in different age groups in males and females. (From Winberg J, Anderson JH, Bergström T, et al: Epidemiology of symptomatic urinary tract infection in childhood. Acta Paediatr Scand (suppl 252) 63:1, 1974. Modified by Asscher AW [137].

Table 36.3.
Sex Ratio at Time of First Nonobstructed Urinary Tract Infection in Different Age Groups

Age group	Female-male ratio
First month	0.4
2–6 months	1.5
7–12 months	4
2–3 yr	10
4–11 yr	9

mechanism or the disappearance of a predisposing factor that progresses at different speeds in the two sexes.

Meatal Stenosis, Bladder Neck Obstruction, Incomplete Bladder Emptying, Vesicoureteral Reflux

So-called bladder neck obstruction and urethral meatal stenosis often have been mentioned as causes of recurrent infections. Critical evaluation suggests that these conditions play little, if any, role (36). Incomplete emptying of the urinary system (6, 37) may encourage infection in some patients, especially in those with posterior urethral valves, ureterocele, bladder diverticula, neuropathic disorders, or calculus. This group is very small.

VUR also has been incriminated as a factor facilitating infection of the bladder. Evidence seems to be more against than for this hypothesis (36, 38), with the possible exception of gross reflux. The role of reflux in the pathogenesis of pyelonephritis is discussed in Chapter 37. The micturition disturbances associated with daytime wetting may in some instances predispose to UTI (39, 40).

Cooling, Hygiene, Social Conditions, and Genetic Factors

Although it is commonly observed that cooling may provoke urgency, there is so far no rigorous proof that it predisposes to infection, nor is there evidence in regard to swimming, hygiene, or social conditions (41). Acute respiratory infections were reported to precede UTI in 13% of cases (41). With regard to genetic factors, black girls may be more resistant to infection than white (42).

Immune Response, Periurethral Flora, and Bacterial Adhesion to the Epithelial Surface of the Urogenital Region

Since simple anatomical and hygienic explanations for repeated reinfections have been largely abandoned, other factors of possible pathogenetic importance, like those mentioned, have been sought. This is discussed in Chapter 14.

CLINICAL FEATURES

Symptomatology and Findings

Depending on the clinical situation in which UTI appears, the following points merit special attention.

1. The clinical features may be influenced by the age and sex of the patient, presence of anatomical disorders of the urinary tract, localization of the infection, number of earlier infections, and the time interval since the last infection.
2. An infection associated with high fever is presumed to be pyelonephritis, although the evidence for this is only indirect. On the other hand, a renal infection may be unaccompanied by any symptoms.
3. The more infections a patient has had, or the closer a recurrence follows an earlier infection, the less serious the symptoms seem to be. Endotoxin tolerance or the effect of antibodies to lipid-A have been suggested as explanations (43–45). Other suggestions are that recurrent infections are often caused by bacteria with a deficient cell wall (46) and, therefore, reduced virulence (47).
4. Bacteria, such as enterococci, *Proteus*, *Pseudomonas*, and *Staphylococcus epidermidis*, often cause fewer symptoms than *E. coli.*
5. Increased plasma urea concentration and/or severe acidosis in patients >2 months of age or arterial hypertension almost always indicate the existence of bilateral hydronephrosis or advanced renal parenchymal destruction.
6. Children experiencing frequency, urgency, burning, micturition pains, and often diurnal enuresis may have sterile urine or insignificant bacteriuria. The condition may or may not be associated with pyuria; however, bladder puncture studies suggest that the number of bacteria sometimes may be very small, i.e., a few thousand per milliliter even in true infections (7, 8). Also, infections caused by bacteria not grown on traditional culture media may escape attention (48). Renal tuberculosis should not be forgotten in countries where this disease still occurs.
7. Most commonly, children with urgency, diurnal enuresis, and other above-mentioned symptoms but normal urinary findings have a detrusor-sphincter imbalance or other urodynamic disturbances.

Sex and Age in Unobstructed Infections

Neonatal Infections

It is generally thought, but not proven, that symptomatic neonatal UTI is a manifestation of a generalized septicemia. The symptoms are varied (14) (Table 36.5) and may precede positive urinary findings by several days. Classic symptoms of infantile UTI are sluggishness, feeding difficulties, irritability, and tenderness to touch. A change in an initially normal weight curve often may be noted before any other symptoms and should focus early attention on the possibility of UTI.

An abnormally slow weight gain also may be noted for several weeks after successful treatment. The central nervous system symptoms in neonatal UTI (Table 36.5) consist of generalized convulsions with loss of consciousness, marked hypotonicity or irritability, respiratory inadequacy, and absent or difficult-to-elicit primitive reflexes. Pleocytosis without demonstrable bacterial meningitis is found in one third of those who have a spinal tap. In this series, bacteremia was found in 50% of those examined; plasma urea concentration was increased in 20% of cases (14). There may be marked oliguria and a temporary increase in renal size.

Girls and Boys from One Month to Three Years

Symptomatic infections of acute onset, especially if it is the first infection, are usually accompanied by fever. Meningism, irritability, and abnormal sensitivity to touch are common symptoms, as are distended abdomen, abdominal pain, vomiting, a pale or even gray skin color, and "smelly" diapers. A few patients have macroscopic hematuria. Otherwise, symptoms pointing to the urinary tract are usually lacking.

"Failure to thrive" (feeding difficulties, sluggishness, poor weight gain, abdominal discomfort) is a leading feature of UTI during the first few years of life. Although some infections may start with such symptoms, they are more usually the features of long-standing infections that were overlooked during the acute febrile stage, which later assume a "low-grade" character.

Diagnosis during the initial stage of febrile UTI requires liberal use of urine culture and sediment examinations in patients with an acute febrile illness not readily explained by other symptoms.

Table 36.4.
Characteristics of *E. coli* Strains Isolated from Patients with Pyelonephritis and Asymptomatic Bacteriuria

Characteristics of urinary *E. coli*	Pyelonephritis (N = 119) (percent)	Asymptomatic bacteriuria (N = 115) (percent)
O serogroups: O_1, O_2, O_4, O_6, O_7, O_{16}, O_{18}, O_{75}	80	31
Spontaneous agglutination	2	45
Serum bactericidal sensitivity:		
Strains highly[a] resistant	69	12
Strains highly[b] sensitive	4	70

[a] <50% of bacteria killed.

[b] >99% of bacteria killed. (From Lindberg U, Hanson LA, Jodal U, et al: Asymptomatic bacteriuria in schoolgirls. II. Differences in *Escherichia coli* causing asymptomatic and symptomatic bacteriuria. Acta Paediatr Scand 64:432, 1975.)

Table 36.5.
Prominent Symptoms in Neonatal (0–30 days) Nonobstructed Urinary Tract Infection

Symptom	Percent (N = 75)
Weight loss[a]	76
Fever	49
Cyanosis or gray color	40
Distended abdomen	16
Central nervous system symptoms (purulent meningitis not included)	23
History of generalized convulsions	7
Purulent meningitis	8
Jaundice (conjugated bilirubin increased)	7
Other	16

[a] Registered only for 46 patients falling ill on days 0–10. Weight loss was not explained by vomiting, diarrhea, or refusal to eat.

Older Girls

With increasing age, lower urinary tract symptoms, including enuresis, appear more frequently, as does abdominal discomfort. Pain in the loin appears later during childhood, but tenderness on palpation may be noted in younger children.

Older Boys

In boys over two years of age, generalized symptoms are not prominent. Fever occurs occasionally and is usually moderate. Macroscopic or microscopic hematuria is common (49). Pain on micturition or urgency may be present. Coliform bacteria do not dominate to the same extent as in girls. *Proteus* and other "atypical" bacteria are relatively frequent invaders. In late-onset infection in boys, the kidneys often show focal scarring at the time of the first infection. Such patients may have had earlier undiagnosed infections (49).

Infections With Underlying Obstruction

If complicated by congenital lower urinary tract obstruction (urethral valves, ureterocele, prune belly syndrome, neuropathic bladder) causing bilateral hydronephrosis, infection usually starts during the first few months of life. In children with obstruction of the upper urinary tract, the onset of infection may be at any age.

The presenting features of these complicated infections are the same as those of infantile infections. On physical examination, a palpable bladder or a mass in the loin may be found. When an acute UTI is associated with arterial hypertension, dehydration, a high BUN, electrolyte disturbances—including acidosis, or all these conditions it should raise the suspicion of an obstructive complication until the reverse is shown (50, 51). Straining at micturition, dribbling, or a poor urinary stream usually characterizes urethral obstruction; however, such symptoms may be absent even if the obstruction is marked.

ASYMPTOMATIC BACTERIURIA

Girls of Preschool and School Age

Clinical Examination

About one third of children found to have ABU have a past history of symptoms referable to the urinary tract. Pyuria is often absent. Reflux is seen in 20% to 35% and focal renal scars in 10% to 25% (4, 30, 52–55).

Bacteriology

There are marked differences between *E. coli* isolates from patients with symptomatic pyelonephritis or cystitis and those from individuals with ABU (Table 36.4). Some differences may be caused by selection of polysaccharide-deficient mutants (46, 57), which may be of low virulence (47). This process may be due to "antigenic drift," i.e., the bacteria have changed to survive the pressure from the immune response in the urinary tract. Bacteria isolated from patients with ABU also have a low adherence capacity (58).

Localization

Localization of the infection in ABU is difficult (26, 28). There is a poor correlation between washout tests, concentrating capacity, C-reactive protein, antibody titers, and sedimentation rate. It is possible that the changed *E. coli* strains do not evoke the usual inflammatory response. It is still uncertain how often the infection involves the renal parenchyma.

Therapy

A short course of antibiotics eliminates infection in >90% of patients, but only 20% to 25% remain uninfected one to two years later (4, 59–61). Spontaneous "cures" lasting one year appear in about 10% (3, 61). Recent follow-up studies suggest that renal function and renal growth of scarred and unscarred kidneys is equal in medically treated as well as untreated patients. This appears to be true even in the presence of reflux (62). Progress of scarring is uncommon after the age of five years.

Sometimes patients feel better after treatment even though they have not complained of symptoms. On the other hand, restriction of chemotherapy may be advisable in ABU. Thus, elimination of cell wall-deficient bacteria by therapy is sometimes followed by symptomatic recurrence (59, 63) caused by bacteria with intact cell wall arising from the fecal reservoir (59). Restriction of antibiotics is also motivated by the large increase in the side effects reported after antibiotic treatment. It would seem reasonable to limit treatment to patients with symptoms (even if slight) or with foul-smelling urine.

Course and Prognosis

ABU is often a phase in the natural history of symptomatic infections, although in some instances infections seem to begin as asymptomatic ones, as in neonates or during the first year of life, and possibly later. There is no evidence that ABU itself causes renal growth retardation, focal renal scarring, or renal functional impairment (54, 61). For example, renal scarring in patients with ABU was observed with the same frequency at four years and at 12 years of age (54). A frequency of scarring of up to 25% has been reported in some studies (30, 54, 55) but was considerably lower in others (4, 53). This incidence of scarring is higher than in patients with symptomatic UTI (Table 36.6). A possible interpretation is that patients with symptomatic infection have often been diagnosed, treated, and checked, whereas the initial symptomatic infection of many patients with ABU may not have been diagnosed and treated. School screening programs, including radiological examinations, seem to register events that happened some time previously. If resources are limited, it seems more urgent to screen a different group, namely, infants and small children with fever, for UTI, rather than to spend money on school screening programs.

Table 36.6.
Radiological Scarring in Girls with Symptomatic and Asymptomatic Bacteriuria

	Percent with scarring	
	England	Sweden
Symptomatic	13[a,b] (N = 281)	4.5[c,d] (N = 440)
Asymptomatic	26[e] (N = 296)	10[f] (N = 119)

[a] Referred with a history of recurrent infection.
[b] Recalculated from Smellie and Normand (134).
[c] Followed prospectively from first symptomatic infection.
[d] From Winberg J, Andersen HJ, Bergström T, et al (1).
[e] From Savage DCL, Wilson MI, McHardy M, et al (55).
[f] From Lindberg U, Claësson I, Hanson LA, et al (53).

Neonatal and Early Infantile Bacteriuria

Asymptomatic urinary excretion of bacteria occurs in 1% to 3% of newborns, mainly boys (32). The significance of this finding is unknown. Neonatal ABU as well as symptomatic UTI rarely occur within four or five days of delivery, which may explain why some studies have revealed few if any neonatal infections (64). So far, there is no clinical reason for screening healthy neonates, except possibly premature infants (64).

In a population-based study of children <1 yr, cases of ABU has been examined by repeated cultures during the first year. At the same time, from symptomatic infections in the same population, two important observations have been reported. Asymptomatic infections did not develop into symptomatic ones. Conversely, patients in the group with symptomatic infections had not had a preceding asymptomatic infection (33, 65).

VESICOURETERIC REFLUX AND INTRARENAL REFLUX

Pioneering and comprehensive work by Hodson, Ransley, and Risdon, Smellie and Normand, and by others (73–76, 88–89) has shown beyond any doubt that gross VUR, when associated with intrarenal reflux (IRR) and UTI, may lead to extensive renal damage. However, the generally held view of reflux as the absolutely dominating factor in initiation of renal infection and renal scarring (vigorously expressed in the term reflux nephropathy) seems less well founded.

The reflux phenomenon and its importance are discussed in full in Chapter 37. Presented here are selected data that show an epidemiological approach based on studies of patients in primary care, which give a more complete picture of the overall importance of reflux. Only the uncomplicated situation is considered here, i.e., VUR in children without bladder outlet obstruction, neuropathic bladder dysfunction, true ectopia of the ureteral orifices or previous bladder surgery.

Developmental Physiology

Basic knowledge of normal, developmental physiology is the appropriate foundation for evaluating supposed pathological states and their management. This knowledge is deficient with regard to the ureterovesical junction. Although the morphology and the successive elongation of the intramural course of the ureter is well described, the developmental aspects of valvular function, especially the competence in different ages, are but little explored. Most studies are based on children beyond the first and second year of life and suggest that VUR does not occur normally. There is, however, only one planned systematic study of healthy children at different ages (66): it suggests a high frequency of VUR during the first year of life, with a rapid decrease thereafter (Fig. 36.9) (66–68). Köllermann's methodology in performing MCU has been criticized, but the results suggest that the morphologic maturation of the ureterovesical junction has a functional correlate (66).

Genesis of Reflux

Obstruction is now ruled out as a major cause of VUR (69, 70), nor does infection seem to have any causal role in the development of reflux. The analysis of a large volume of material suggests "that reflux and UTI are independent variables that often coexist" (69). This view concurs with the comparison of girls with and without UTI shown in Figure 36.9. The findings in girls also correspond strikingly well to the age-adjusted frequency of VUR in monkeys.

A genetic predisposition seems, however, to play a role in the genesis of reflux (71, 72). Since reflux disappears with growth (22, 73), a maturation process seems to take place. It may be the rate of this functional maturation that is genetically controlled.

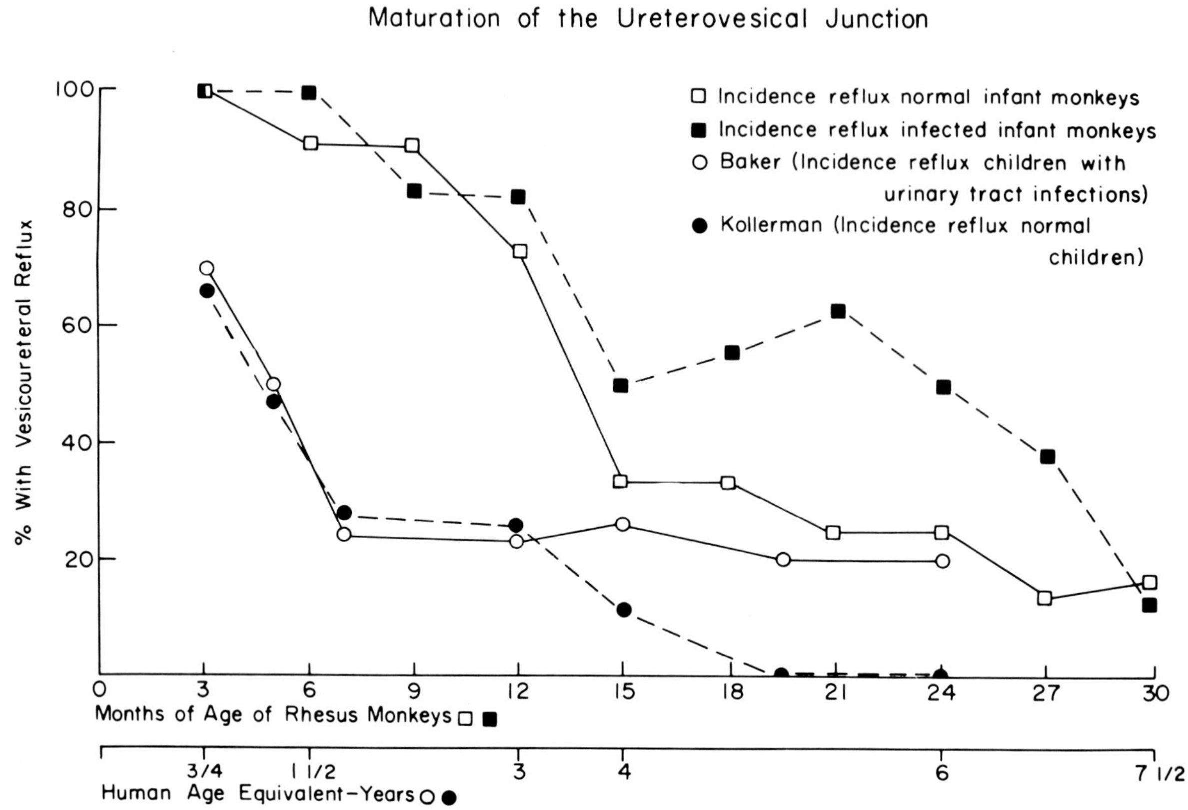

Figure 36.9. A comparison of normal infant humans and monkeys versus those with recurrent UTI. Notice that, over time, the incidence of reflux declines (thus, maturation of the ureterovesical junction occurs) despite infection. (From Roberts JA: Studies of vesicoureteral reflux: a review of work in a primate model. South Med J 71:28, 1978.)

Even if infection does not cause VUR, it may interfere with the rate of maturation and lead to a delay in disappearance of reflux in humans and monkeys, as suggested by the gap in reflux frequency between infected and noninfected cases (Fig. 36.9). This process could account for the often demonstrated coexistence of infection and reflux.

Reflux and Initiation of Renal Infection and Damage: Bacterial Adherence

How bacteria reach the renal tissue in patients with acute, clinical pyelonephritis has long remained an enigma. VUR provides a mechanism for the ascent of bacteria from the bladder to the pelvis and IRR for the spread into the renal parenchyma. Gross VUR with IRR into conglomerate papillae has been identified as a major risk factor for progressive renal damage (74–76); however, among infants and children appearing in a primary care center with an acute attack of presumed clinical pyelonephritis (high fever, CRP, sedimentation rate, *E. coli* IgM antibodies, and prolonged lowering of concentrating capacity as shown in Fig. 36.2), only a minority had VUR demonstrable by MCU—40% and 25%, respectively (1). IRR is found in an even smaller number; nor is progressive scarring always associated with demonstrable VUR. During a prospective study based on material from primary care, 23 kidneys developed focal scarring, yet VUR with dilatation was demonstrated in only one third of patients at the time of the first infection (Table 36.7) (77). Furthermore, in some children with VUR the infection still seems to be limited to the bladder. Obviously, the mechanistic concept of pathogenesis of pyelonephritis and renal scarring (expressed in the term "reflux nephropathy") needs amendment and expansion.

The discrepancies may be reconciled by some studies in the monkey suggesting a different mechanism for pyelorenal backflow. In a series of experiments, Roberts and coworkers (18, 79–82) showed that some, but not all, *E. coli* strains caused ureteral paralysis, which could be associated with an increase in ureteral perfusion pressure, flattening of a highly compliant papilla, and pyelorenal backflow. This was invariably followed by progressive renal damage. It was later shown that bacteria highly adherent to monkey ureteral and renal epithelial cells, i.e., P-fimbriated (see Chapter 14), were a prerequisite for these effects (83, 84). These experimental studies, combined with the adherence concept, might explain the obvious fact that renal infection and renal scarring are found even in the absence of gross VUR. Interestingly, the damaging effect may occur through the same final pathway as in gross VUR-pyelorenal backflow. In this context it is also interesting that, in the absence of gross reflux, about 95% of episodes of acute pyelonephritis are caused by P-fimbriated *E. coli* (85) (highly pyelonephritogenic strains) (Chapter 14), but in the presence of gross VUR P-fimbriated *E. coli* are less common (86). A cornerstone in this reasoning is the recent demonstration that inoculation of P-fimbriated *E. coli* into the bladder of adult nonrefluxing monkeys results in acute and chronic pyelonephritis (83). In conclusion,

Table 36.7.
Demonstration of VUR at Time of First Infection in 23 Kidneys Developing Focal Scarring

Grade	%
0–1	39
2	26
3	35
4	0

Data from Winberg J, Bollgren I, Källenius G, et al (77).

bacterial adhesion in association with induced ureteral malfunction may lead to renal damage in the absence of VUR.

Treatment of VUR

Obviously VUR, when gross and especially when associated with IRR, enhances the risk for renal scarring, at least in association with infection (22, 76, 87–89). Gross or minor VUR as shown by MCU, is not, however, a prerequisite for renal infection and renal damage, and reflux correction does not necessarily improve the situation of the patient. Although operative correction of VUR has been practiced for three decades, its value is still unproven. The only controlled studies (90) and the preliminary data from the Birmingham reflux study group (91) suggest that surgery does not influence the prognosis. Uncontrolled data (19, 62, 92, 93) point in the same direction, i.e., that renal growth can take place even in the presence of reflux. Further data are, however, needed.

Sterile Reflux and Renal Lesion

Hodson and coworkers (74) have shown in the pig that sterile reflux can lead to renal scars in the areas of IRR; however, this model requires bladder neck obstruction, which creates increased voiding pressure. This model thus mimics only the clinical situation of patients with obstruction or with neuropathic bladder dysfunction, as originally studied by Hutch (94). Experimental work (75, 95, 96) suggests that there is no renal damage from reflux unless associated with persistently raised pressure or infection. Studies in humans show that sterile reflux does not prevent renal growth or even compensatory hypertrophy.

FOCAL RENAL SCAR

Diagnostic Criteria

Infections may cause renal growth retardation, focal scars, or both; such changes also may have causes other than infection. A scar is wedge-shaped, with the tip in the papilla, and has a distinct demarcation from healthy renal tissue (97). The cause of the characteristic demarcation is uncertain; the distribution of IRR has been suggested, as have vascular and immunological barriers. In any case, the distribution clearly suggests the ascending nature of the infection.

Radiological criteria have been defined by Hodson and Wilson (98); these consist of a papillary lesion, in the most advanced cases with "clubbing," and a corresponding defect in the renal outline. It may take up to 24 months before a scar becomes visible on roentgenogram (87). Differentiation from congenital renal dysplasia sometimes may be difficult. The diagnosis of dysplasia should rest exclusively on strictly defined histological criteria (99). It is striking how silently even extensive renal destruction may develop (54, 100).

Determinants of Renal Scarring

The ultimate goal of the care of children with UTI is to prevent progressive renal damage with its consequences, such as hypertension, complications of pregnancy, and renal failure. Prevention will become more successful if the main causes are recognized. The association of huge reflux and of obstruction with scarring is well established, but there are also other determinants of renal damage following infection (77). The role of obstruction, especially when associated with infection, in severe renal damage, is well established and will not be dealt with here.

Age

The growing kidney of the young child seems to be much more vulnerable than that of the adult to focal scarring and growth retardation. This also has been shown in the experimental animal (101). The kidneys of small children with gross reflux are particularly vulnerable (22, 87).

Scars may be present at the first roentgenographic examination. Smellie and Normand (89) rightly point out that, in such instances, the damage is congenital or that the first infection, went unrecognized. The second possibility is strongly favored, since scarring and renal growth retardation are less commonly seen at the first roentgenographic examination in infantile infections than when the first recognized infection occurs at an older age (2). Table 36.8 shows that among boys with a first infection during the first year of life, only 1 of 116 had a scar at the first intravenous pyelogram, whereas 6 of 116 (about 5%) developed a scar later. Among those >1 yr of age at the so-called "first infection," a focal scar was already present at the first intravenous pyelogram in one fourth. Table 36.8 indicates, firstly, that when infections are diagnosed during the first year and treated immediately and checked after treatment, the infection carries a rather low risk for scar formation. Secondly, when UTI is diagnosed after the first year of life, the patient often may have had at least one earlier (probably unrecognized and untreated) infection that caused scarring in a high percentage of cases. As a group, girls seem to have their debut infection later than the boys, and scars develop usually up to about the age of three to four years, sometimes later. The findings of McLachlan and coworkers emphasize that attempts to prevent renal damage should be directed toward very young children (54).

Postmortem examinations of adults show that focal renal scars are as common in males as in females. Since urinary infections are about 10 times more common in females, it has been questioned whether infections have much to do with such scars (102, 103); however, a 1/1 (18/20) male/female ratio of scarring also was seen at follow-up of children with proven UTI (1, 2). If the kidneys are most vulnerable before one year of age, this sex ratio for pyelonephritic scarring would be expected, since the male/female ratio for UTI among 0- to 12-month old infants was 0.8, and among 0- to 6-month-old infants, 1.1 (Table 36.9).

Increased attention to the possibility of pyelonephritis in infants and children with unexplained fever is necessary to prevent renal damage.

Therapeutic Delay

One important determinant of renal damage is the duration of infection before treatment begins. A few days of persistent infection may be enough to cause severe renal and ureteral damage. In 41 girls in whom the first known infection was inadequately treated, the incidence of renal

Table 36.8.
Renal Scarring in Males at "First" Infection and at Follow-up

Age at 'first' UTI	n	% with scars	
		At 'first' infection	At follow-up[a]
<1 yr	116	1	5
>1 yr	44	25	0

[a] In earlier undamaged kidneys. (Data from Winberg J, Andersen HJ, Bergström T, et al [1].)

Table 36.9.
Sex Distribution Among 258 Consecutive "First" Symptomatic UTI During Infancy

Age (months) at first infection	Male/female ratio	
	Absolute N	Relative
0–12	113/145	0.8
0–6	102/91	1.1

(Data from Winberg J, Andersen HJ, Bergström T, et al [1].)

damage was four times as high as in 440 girls in whom diagnosis and treatment were prompt and adequate (Table 36.10).

The impact of therapeutic delay is demonstrated in two experimetnal studies (104, 105). Pyelonephritis was induced in rats and therapy delayed for varying periods. With each prolongation of the interval, from hours to seven days, the renal damage became more and more severe (Table 36.11). These findings correspond well with the clinical observations.

In an analysis of causes of ureteral and renal damage, attention should be given to the duration of the first febrile infection before treatment began.

Inflammatory Response

The importance of the inflammatory response for tissue damage in general has been explored during the last decade. Its relevance for initiation of parenchymal damage in renal infections has been analyzed (106, 107). The damaging effect of the inflammatory response seems to be caused by the release of large amounts of free oxygen and hydroxyl radicals, which are highly toxic to bacteria, but also to parenchymal cells. If the release of these agents exceeds the capacity of the host to metabolize them, tissue damage will occur.

The results of the studies in experimental infections can be briefly summarized. In a rat experimental model, suppuration after inoculation of bacteria was maximal at three days. This was followed by scarring, which was extensive if the suppuration had persisted more than three days. Scarring was less severe if suppuration was aborted through early treatment of the infection. Scarring also was reduced if suppuration was aborted, but infection persisted through "partial treatment" with antibiotics. Similarly and most interestingly, scarring became limited when suppuration was aborted in the presence of an augmented number of bacteria, a situation caused by colchicine-induced depression of leukocyte migration. The in vivo significance of these findings has been shown by Roberts and coworkers (108). Administration of superoxide dismutase, a scavenger of free radicals, prevented acute and chronic renal damage in experimental infections in monkeys.

These studies suggest that tissue damage may be caused not so much by bacteria but by the inflammatory response through free radicals liberated from leukocytes. The studies emphasize that the elapsed time between initiation of infection and onset of treatment is critical in determining the extent of the renal damage. One possibility, emerging from these studies, is that renal bacteriuria not associated with pyuria may be of minor importance.

Table 36.10.
Care and Prognosis in Symptomatic UTI

Care at first infection	Total N	Scarring N	Scarring %
Adequate	440	20	4.5
Delayed	41	7	17

(Data from Winberg J, Bollgren I, Källenius G, et al [77].)

Table 36.11.
Delayed Antimicrobial Therapy Versus Gross Renal Lesions

Nontreated controls: Renal surface involved (percent)	Treated animals: Start of therapy after challenge	Treated animals: Renal surface involved (percent)
	8 hr	2.5
	1 day	6
27	2 days	9
	3 days	13
	4 days	14
	7 days	21

(Data from Miller T, Phillips S [104].)

Individual Susceptibility

Some individuals are more prone to infections than others. This feature is associated with abnormal gram-negative colonization of the introitus (109) and periurethral area (110) preceding infection. Also the anaerobic flora is abnormal (111); however, the mere presence of abundant *E. coli* in the periurethral area is insufficient to induce infection. An additional factor must be postulated. Studies of bacterial adherence have demonstrated that uroepithelial cells from infection-prone women bind *E. coli* more avidly than cells from nonsusceptible women (112, 113). Whether such females run a greater risk for renal damage is so far open to discussion (Chapter 14).

Bacterial Virulence

A number of bacterial factors have been proposed to be associated with uropathogenicity (114). The ability to bind to epithelial cells by specific adhesions may be the most relevant (Chapter 14).

Other Factors

Other factors that induce renal damage have been suggested: (a) persistence of bacterial antigen; (b) formation of immune complexes with complement fixation; (c) cross-reactions between kidney and certain *E. coli* antigens with formation of autoantibodies; (d) a direct toxic effect of lipid A (115); and (e) infection with atypical bacteria (48). The possible role of such mechanisms in the pathogenesis of renal scar formation has been reviewed by Hanson and coworkers (57) and Holmgren and Smith (45).

DIAGNOSIS, THERAPY, AND FOLLOW-UP

The goal of care is to prevent progressive renal damage. Chemotherapy and close follow-up, including radiological and urological exploration and, if needed, surgical treatment, are complementary aspects of management.

Obstruction

The physician's first concern should be to look for evidence of obstruction of the urinary flow. He or she should examine thoroughly the genital organs and the abdomen, especially the suprapubic area. A palpable bladder, a mass in the loin, arterial hypertension, clinical signs of dehydration, a high BUN, or an electrolyte disturbance, including acidosis, should evoke suspicion of an obstruction.

The main key to differentiation between obstructed and nonobstructed infections is the response to treatment. If the temperature has not become normal after two to three days of therapy and if sediment has not cleared after four to five days, it is likely that the bacteria are resistant to the antibiotic given or that there is an obstruction. The same is true if the renal concentrating capacity does not approach normality within three weeks. Such patients should have a full radiological investigation as soon as possible.

If urethral obstruction is suspected on physical examination, the patient should have bladder drainage until an expert evaluation can be performed. If the radiological examination confirms obstruction, the catheter should be left in place until a free urinary flow is established surgically. Direct drainage of a unilaterally obstructed pelvis may sometimes be necessary. It should be remembered that infection in itself may cause moderate dilatation of ureters and pelves, owing to muscle damage or interference with transmission of nerve impulses (79, 116). If the infant is severely ill or dehydrated, an intravenous drip and parenteral administration of antimicrobials are necessary.

Follow-Up

Table 36.12 gives guidelines for follow-up during and after treatment of pyelonephritis and cystitis.[117] The program might be less ambitious in girls over 5–6 years.

Antibiotics

A 10-day course of a suitable antibiotic will eradicate infection in almost all patients, provided the bacteria are sensitive to it (Fig. 36.10). The high rate of recurrence after a short course of antibiotic treatment was formerly interpreted as being due to recrudescence of incompletely eradicated infections. This was the original basis for the "long-term treatment," the idea being that bacteria in the renal tissue could be eliminated only after therapy lasting weeks and months. This reason for long-term treatment is rarely, if ever, relevant, since most recurrences are reinfections, i.e., therapy of the foregoing infection has been effective but new bacteria have invaded (118). This is true even when recurrences appear within two to three days after discontinuation of therapy. The current approach, therefore, is to attempt to eradicate infection by a short course of an antimicrobial agent and, in selected cases, to continue with a small prophylactic dose of antibiotic to prevent reinfection. Some physicians prefer to put all patients on long-term prophylaxis (119); others select such a regimen only for those who have had repeated infections at very short intervals (35, 42). Because of the high risk for renal scarring in infants and toddlers with grade IV reflux, these patients should be given prophylaxis even before they have demonstrated susceptibility to recurrence.

Although most recurrences are reinfections, a few are not. The latter are caused by unresolved bacteriuria or persistence of bacteria in a situation not amenable to antibiotic treatment. A change in drug or dosage is usually helpful in unresolved bacteriuria, whereas surgery is the answer in most instances for persistence of bacteria.

Table 36.12.
Program of Follow-up During and After Treatment of Pyelonephritis and Cystitis

Time after onset of treatment	Pyelonephritis (temperature ≥38 °C, CRP-positive[a])	Cystitis (temperature <38 °C, CRP-negative)
3 days	Dipslide culture[b] WBC[c] in urine Possibly IVU[d]	Dipslide culture[e] WBC
2–3 weeks	Dipslide culture[b] WBC CRP ESR Possible referral for radiological examination[d]	Dipslide culture WBC
2 months	Dipslide culture WBC	Dipslide culture Possibly IVU[d,e]
3–4 months	Dipslide culture WBC	Dipslide culture WBC
12 months	Dipslide culture WBC	Dipslide culture[e] WBC
Later	If possible, a checkup should be performed at 24 months and 36 months after onset	

[a] C-reactive protein.
[b] A dipslide culture is performed and extra urine stored at 4 °C for 24 hr. If the dipslide is positive, the urine is sent to a microbiologist for quantitative culture and resistance pattern.
[c] White blood cell count.
[d] See text.
[e] Can be omitted.

Initial Treatment of Acute Infections

Choice of antimicrobial drugs and duration of treatment should be considered in relation to the situation of the patient; whether there have been single episodes at long intervals or frequently repeated infections; whether the patient is severely dehydrated and vomiting; whether he/she has a neurogenic bladder or renal insufficiency; or whether the patient is a newborn. With all drugs, 10 days of therapy will eradicate infection, even in febrile pyelonephritis. Night time doses are not needed. Shorter courses may work as well. In afebrile infections 5 days are probably sufficient. Some studies suggest that one single dose of a suitable drug is enough for eradication of infection (120, 121). Single dose therapy should pend further evaluation.

Single episodes of symptomatic infections separated by long intervals. Sulfonamide still holds its position as a good first choice in these patients, whether they have pyelonephritis or "cystitis". In vivo sulfonamide resistance has usually remained uncommon in these patients, as contrasted to those with frequently recurring infecions, but local differences may exist. Cure of the infection will follow a 10-day course in almost 100 per cent of treated cases (see Figure 36.10).

In addition to efficacy, solubility, frequency of side reactions and cost should guide the choice of sulfonamide compound. Preparations with a short excretion time, such as sulfafurazole (Gantrisin) and sulfasomidine (Elkosin) have a high solubility in urine, and allergic reactions are infrequent. Sulfonamide preparations with a "long" or "half-long" excretion time do not seem to hold any advantages. Even with "rapidly excreted" drugs, the antibacterial activity of urine remains high 12 to 24 hours, sometimes even 48 hours, following a single dose (120, 122).

Urine concentrations may be more essential than blood concentrations in treatment of UTI (23, 123). Considering this, it is possible that intervals between doses can be prolonged. Studies to prove this are lacking, however.

In addition to sulfonamide, other suitable first choice drugs are nitrofurantoin, amoxicillin and related penicillin substances, trimethoprim-sulfamethoxazole, trimethoprim, nalidixic acid, and third generation cephalosporins. Indications, doses, and complications are listed in Table 36.13.

Nitrofurantoin is, in view of its limited ecologic effects (see page 641), a very suitable drug. There are, however, no controlled studies of its efficiency in treating acute febrile pyelonephritis. Gastointestinal side effects will be few with a dosage of 3 mg/kg/24 hours. Allergic pulmonary reactions and pulmonary fibrosis have been reported with increasing frequency in the elderly. Such reactions are rare in children. Nitrofurantoin is ineffective when glomerular filtration rate is reduced to about 50 per cent of normal or less.

The previously reported rapid development of primary chromosomal resistance to nalidixic acid in a formerly sensitive bacterial population during therapy (124) seems to occur mainly with underdosage (125).

The combination of trimethoprim with a sulfonamide (Septrin, Bactrim, Eusaprim) are widely used. Both compounds interfere with bacterial folate metabolism, but on different levels, and both have a synergistic effect at least in vitro. Dosages of 5 to 7 mg/kg body weight of trimethoprim and 25 to 35 mg/kg body weight of sulfamethoxazole twice daily for 10 days are used in small children as well as in adults.

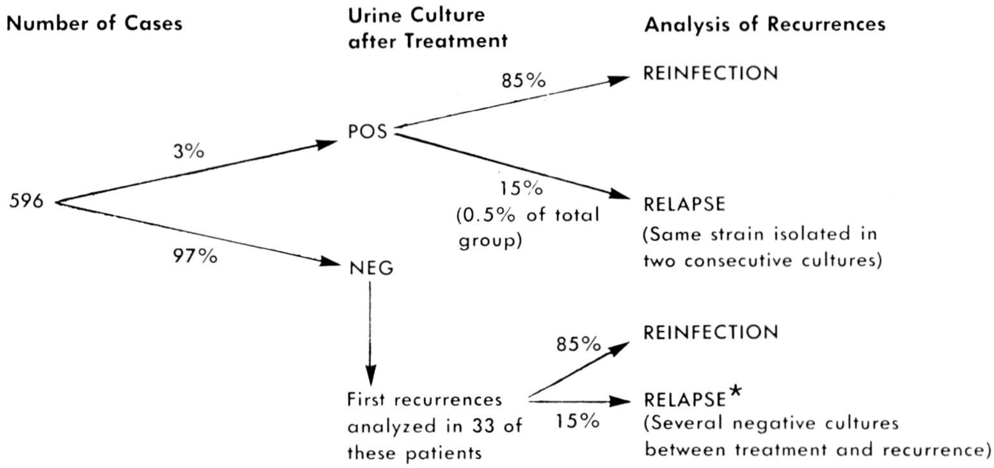

Figure 36.10. Approximate figures for immediate cure rate after treatment with sulfonamide (10 to 60 days—no difference). Only 0.5% of the total group of patients had a relapse without a preceding negative culture. * Same strain isolated in onset infection and first recurrence, but several negative cultures in between these two infections. (From Winberg J, Berström T, Jacobsson B: Morbidity, age and sex distribution, recurrences and renal scarring in symptomatic urinary tract infection in children. Kidney Int 8:101, 1975.)

Table 36.13.
First-Choice Drugs in Treatment of UTI

Compound	Dosage mg/kg body weight/24 hr[a]	No. of doses per day	Duration of therapy (days)[b]	Remarks
Short-acting sulfonamide:				
Sulfafurazole	100–200	4	7–10	Not to be used so long as neonatal jaundice persists.
Sulphasomidine	100	4	7–10	
Nitrofurantoin	3	4	7–10	Not to be used the first month of life. Not effective when GFR is about 50% of normal or less. Pulmonary side reactions reported with increasing frequency; seem so far to be rare in children. Limited ecologic side effects.
Nalidixic acid	60	3–4	7–10	Not to be used in newborns. Dosage at 1 to 4 months of age, 30 mg/kg/24 hr. Rise in intracranial pressure described in infants and children.
Trimethoprim-	6	3–4	7–10	Not to be used before 6 weeks of life.
Sulfamethoxazole	30			Diffuses into prostate and vagina.
Trimethoprim	6	3–4	7–10	
Amoxicillin	25–50	3–4	7–10	Neonatal infections often caused by *Klebsiella* resistant to ampicillin. Gastrointestinal complications common with ampicillin.
Pivampicillin	25–50			

[a] First dose at waking up, the last at bedtime, one or two in between. Nighttime doses not necessary.
[b] Duration of therapy, especially single-dose treatment, is discussed on p 639.

Trimethoprim, unlike other antimicrobial substances, seems to concentrate by nonionic diffusion across vaginal as well as prostatic epithelium. This may play a major role in the treatment, and especially in the prevention, of certain urinary infections (126, 127).

Checkup after therapy. First checkup should preferably be done after therapy has been discontinued for 2 to 3 days, and then again 2 to 3 weeks later. The next three checkups are spread out over the first year after the infection. If possible, the patients should be followed a few more years. If check-up cultures are done during therapy or within 1–2 days after the last dose evaluation of negative or doubtfully positive cultures will be difficult.

This schedule is used for all infants and small children with acute onset, symptomatic infections. Older children with mainly lower urinary tract symptoms and no renal scarring are checked with longer intervals. Infants and small children with grade IV reflux (see Figure 36.5) are checked each week during the first 1 to 2 months after an acute pyelonephritis. Home culture with dip slide or similar devices may be used after thorough instruction of the parents.

Management of recurrent infections. The bacterial etiology and resistance pattern of recurrent infections are more variable than in single infections. If the patient's condition allows, therapy should be postponed until the resistance of the bacteria has been examined. If this is impracticable, a drug of a type different from that used in the preceding infection should be given. Dosage and duration of therapy are as described previously.

Prophylaxis is carried through after treatment in patients with frequent reinfections. Nitrofurantoin is the drug of choice because of its insignificant effect on the gut flora (35). Dosage is 1 mg/kg/24 hours, as a night-dose. If this does not work the dose may be divided into one morning and one evening dose. Trimethoprim with sulfamethoxazole is a good alternative. This combination may keep the vestibular area clean (127). Trimethoprim without sulfonamide has also been used as a prophylactic in a single night dose of about 2 mg/kg body weight. It is effective, but there is some concern about increased risk for selection of resistant strains. Nalidixic acid, 20 mg/kg/24 hours may be another alternative for prophylaxis.

With regard to duration of prophylaxis, a trial-and-error approach is suggested. Let the initial period of prophylaxis last for 2 to 4 months. If a recurrence occurs shortly after prophylactic therapy is stopped, a new therapeutic course should be given, followed by prophylaxis for half a year and so on. Some patients need prophylactic treatment for several years. Elo (128) suggests a more rigid schedule in patients with recurrent infections. If there have been three infectious episodes within a year, treatment of the third one should be followed by a prophylactic course. The length of the prophylaxis depends on the interval between the second and the third episodes. If this is shorter than three weeks, prophylaxis is administered for one year; if it is between three weeks and three months prophylaxis is given for three months; if the interval between the second and third infection is more than three months no prophylaxis is prescribed.

Check-up is done 2 to 3 days after each therapeutic course and at every second or third month during prophylaxis, depending on the susceptibility of the patient to recurrence. In patients more than 4–5 years without scarring and without gross (grade IV) reflux, the intervals between check-up examinations might be considerably prolonged. With co-operative and understanding families we see such patients once or twice a year if there are no problems. The use of dip-slide (or "dip-stream") cultures (129) facilitates check-up for both patient and doctor (see Chapter 14).

Management of infections in patients with neurogenic bladders, specifically with myelomeningocele—a pediatrician's view. Therapy has three main goals: to protect the kidneys from damage, to make the patient socially continent and to decrease the number of infections. Intermittent catheterization—clean but not sterile—has improved the situation for many of these patients (130). It should be started before dilatation of the upper urinary tract has occurred. Children over 6–7 years can often learn to do it themselves. Catheterization will diminish the pressure in the upper urinary tract and in the kidneys. Infections seem to occur less frequently and to run a more benign course. During continence training pharmacologic agents which increase bladder volume, relax the external sphincter, and stimulate detrusor contraction, are often helpful.

A true obstruction of the outflow region of the bladder may complicate these cases. The patients should be cared for by urologist and pediatrician in cooperation. The etiology and resistance pattern of the infecting bacteria are unpredictable. In nonacute infections, therapy is best postponed until the results of culture and sensitivity tests are available. Antimicrobial therapy should be given to patients who have either urinary symptoms or a high sedimentation rate, or unspecific symptoms such as tiredness or anorexia that have no other obvious explanation. Antimicrobial treatment of asymptomatic infections in these patients is probably of little value. Recurrences, which usually are reinfections, are almost impossible to prevent by prophylaxis.

Management of infections in newborns. Infections in this age group are often caused by *E. coli* with a K1 antigen that seems to be a virulence factor (131). These infections are sometimes part of a generalized septicemia. A combination of gentamicin and ampicillin is a good choice. Glomerular filtration rate is often severely reduced by infection; therefore, the serum concentration of any potentially toxic drug should be monitored. If renal infection is the only manifestation, ampicillin, 100 to 200 mg/kg body weight, may be sufficient. If response is not quick, therapy should be changed, since *Klebsiella* or *Enterobacter* are common pathogens in this age group. When diagnosed early, neonatal *E. coli* pyelonephritis has a good prognosis (14). For dosage of gentamicin, see Nelson and McCracken (132).

Management of patients with renal insufficiency and urinary infection. The ideal qualities of an antimicrobial agent for patients with both urinary infection and renal insufficiency can be summarized as follows: (1) Rapid renal excretion; (2) low toxicity, even in high serum concentrations; (3) slow metabolism by the liver; and (4) no alternative pathways of excretion. Ampicillin is a suitable drug before antibiotic sensitivity results are obtained. Sulfonamides with a short half-life are more useful than those with a long half-life. Nitrofurantoin should not be used. Gentamicin can be used, but with great caution, if the dosage is guided by determination of serum concentrations.

Management of patients with screening bacteriuria. (See page 635)

Chemotherapy, Fecal Flora, and Transmissible Chemoresistance (R Factors)

The management of UTI is seriously hampered by the increasing frequency of infections caused by organisms with R factor mediated multiresistance. Urinary infections caused by such strains are often *preceded* by their appearance in feces and in the periurethral flora (35) usually favored by a selective antibiotic pressure.

The problem of resistant urinary infections should therefore be considered in the light of the influence of therapy on the intestinal and periurethral flora. The evaluation of any drug used for treatment of UTI should be done with regard to its effect on these physiologic bacterial reservoirs. These questions are dealt with in Chapter 14.

COURSE AND PROGNOSIS

This can be evaluated at different levels: the risk of recurrence, the risk of scarring and renal growth retardation, and the risk of development of hypertension or end-stage renal disease or complications of pregnancy. Some of the figures given below are from a prospective study in which the patients were diagnosed, treated and checked at an apparent first infection (1, 2). If one can bring a child up to puberty without renal damage, the future risk for scarring is very small if existing at all.

Main Determinants of Renal Damage

These are summarized in Table 36.14.

Infections Complicated by Obstruction

The nature of the obstruction, the success of the surgical intervention, and the time lapse between onset of infection and establishment of adequate drainage are the main factors determining the degree of postnatal renal damage. Clinically, such damage—if bilateral—may manifest itself as failure to thrive, growth retardation, water-losing nephropathy, generalized acidosis necessitating sodium bicarbonate replacement, uremia, or a combination of these disorders.

Repeated infections will occur in some patients even though the obstruction has been removed. In these patients, as in others with frequent recurrences, absence of symptoms or pyuria never excludes infection. Check-up of these patients only by history or examination of urinary sediment is inadequate. For a detailed discussion, the reader is referred to Chapter 38.

Girls Without Obstruction Falling Ill Beyond the Newborn Period

Recurrence rate. The most characteristic feature of this group of patients is their susceptibility to recurrences, which often continue to appear for many years, sometimes for decades (133). In such cases, it is not the infection but the inclination to acquire repeated infections that is "chronic". This distinction is essential with regard to selection of therapy.

Table 36.14.
Main Determinants of Renal Damage

Anatomical obstruction
Gross VUR with IRR
Age
Therapeutic delay
Inflammatory response
Individual susceptibility
Bacterial virulence

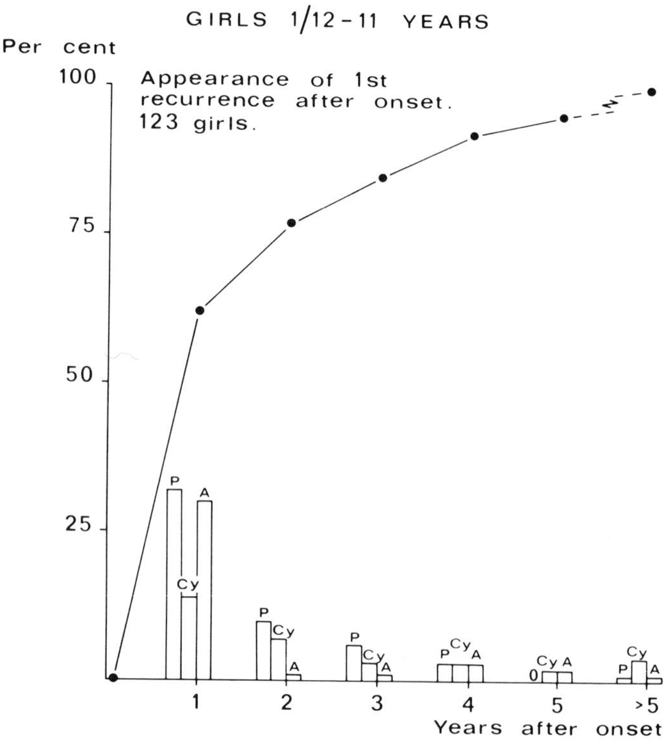

Figure 36.11. Appearance of a first recurrence after the primary infection, studied in a sample of 123 girls (aged ½ to 11 yr) with at least one recurrence. Bars denote main symptom: P, febrile infection; Cy, afebrile, symptomatic infection; A, asymptomatic infection. (From Winberg J, Andersen HJ, Bergström T, et al: Epidemiology of symptomatic urinary tract infection in childhood. Acta Paediatr Scand (suppl 252) 63:1, 1974.)

The risk of recurrence is about 30 per cent the first year after an onset infection and probably around 50 per cent for the next five years. An unexplained phenomenon is that reinfections tend to occur soon after the preceding infection (Fig. 36.11). The risk of recurrence seems to increase with the number of preceding infections (Fig. 36.7), which suggests that the postulated defect of the defense mechanisms vary in severity. There seems to be no obvious correlation between susceptibility to recurrence and age, localization of infection, and presence or absence of reflux. There may be a positive correlation between residual urine volume, even if small, and susceptibility to recurrence (56).

From a practical point of view, in the majority of schoolgirls with frequent nonfebrile infections, scarring of a previously intact kidney rarely if ever occurs, and renal growth continues at a normal rate (Fig. 36.12). It can be questioned whether the rigorous follow-up so often practiced in these patients is necessary.

Prognosis

Scarring and Renal Growth Retardation

A young girl falling ill with her first acute symptomatic UTI may run a risk of some 5% of developing a scar; the risk for a boy may range from 10% to 15%. These figures are for children in whom the infection is diagnosed early, treated, and checked (1). With inadequate or delayed care, these figures are higher (Tables 36.10, 36.11). In fact, scars already are often present at the first examination, especially in boys (Table 36.8) and, in patients not seen during their apparent first infection, the frequency of scarring is considerably greater (133, 134). A 25% frequency of scarring in asymptomatic bacteriuric girls, probably representing a selection with an early and unrecognized symptomatic infection, may estimate the approximate risk in untreated patients (Table 36.6). Scarring is often accompanied by renal growth retardation. If scarring is unilateral, there is a compensatory hypertrophy of the undamaged kidney. Even a

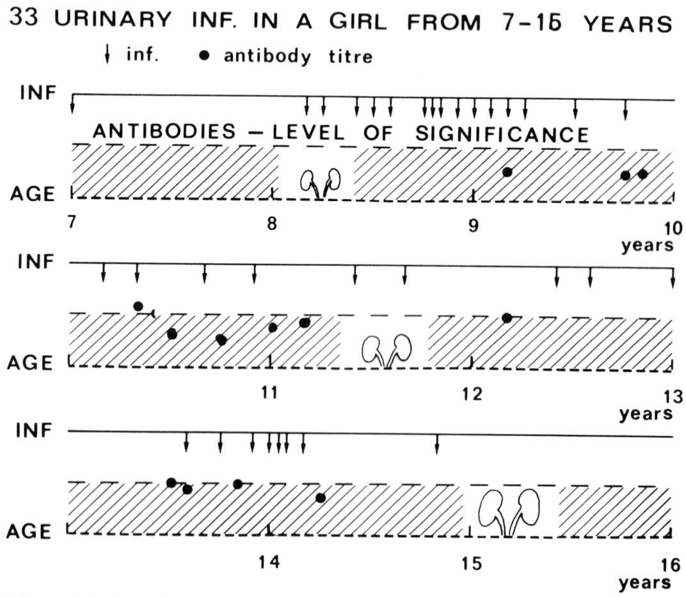

Figure 36.12. Radiographic follow-up of a girl with 33 recorded infections which, with one or two exceptions, were not accompanied by fever, observed from age 7 to 16 yr. In this kind of patient renal growth retardation and renal scarring rarely occur. Infections (↓) and specific *E. coli* antibody titers (●) are indicated. Dashed line at the level of significance for antibody titer.

damaged kidney shows a remarkable catchup growth at puberty (Fig. 36.13).

Clinically Severe Long-Term Effects

It is unknown how often patients with recurrent infections develop hypertension, uremia, distal tubular insufficiency, obstructing stones, or complications of pregnancy. In patients with "reflux nephropathy" severe clinical manifestations may appear much more often during adulthood than during childhood. In the absence of obstruction, the risk of such severe disease seems to be remote. Since UTI is common, however, the total number of patients with severe long-term complications may be considerable. Chantler and coworkers (135) reported that so-called "reflux nephropathy" made up 21% of 75 children with end stage renal failure; Holland (136) found that among children with hypertension, many had suspected focal renal damage. Complications of pregnancy, such as intrauterine fetal death, prematurity, and intrauterine growth retardation, are other possible consequences of childhood infections with renal damage.

Neonatal Infections

These early infections seem to be part of a generalized bacteremia, the course of which determines the early prognosis. Early recurrences during the months following the first infection appear in about one fourth of patients (14). Recurrences after more than one year seem to be rare. This feature clearly distinguishes the infections appearing during the newborn period from those of older girls. The frequency of scarring following neonatal infection is unknown.

Boys

Boys falling ill during the first year of life (neonates excluded) have early recurrences, as do girls; however, infant boys, like neonates, seem to grow out of their susceptibility to infection. Thus, it is rare to see a recurrence more than one year after the onset of infection (2). Scarring may be more common than in girls.

There seems to be no systematic observation of UTI without obstruction in boys aged 1 to 16 years. Early recurrences do occur after onset infection, as in girls; late recurrences, however, are less common (49). Focal renal scarring, sometimes extensive, is a common finding, even at the so-called first infection (49). They are probably consequences of early unrecognized infections (Table 36.8).

CONCLUSIONS

The pathogenesis of the kind of UTI seen in girls and women without obstruction is unknown; however, more and more clearly the picture unfolds as a disease (a) that begins during the first years of life; (b) in which the tendency to acquire UTI often remains for many years, perhaps for life, and (c) in which the prognosis is to a great extent determined by the way the patient is cared for during infancy or early childhood. Against this background, both increased knowledge of the clinical manifestations of the disease in infancy and improved inexpensive diagnostic methods that are practical and usable by practitioners are important. The reader is also referred to recent surveys and position papers (77, 82, 121, 137–141).

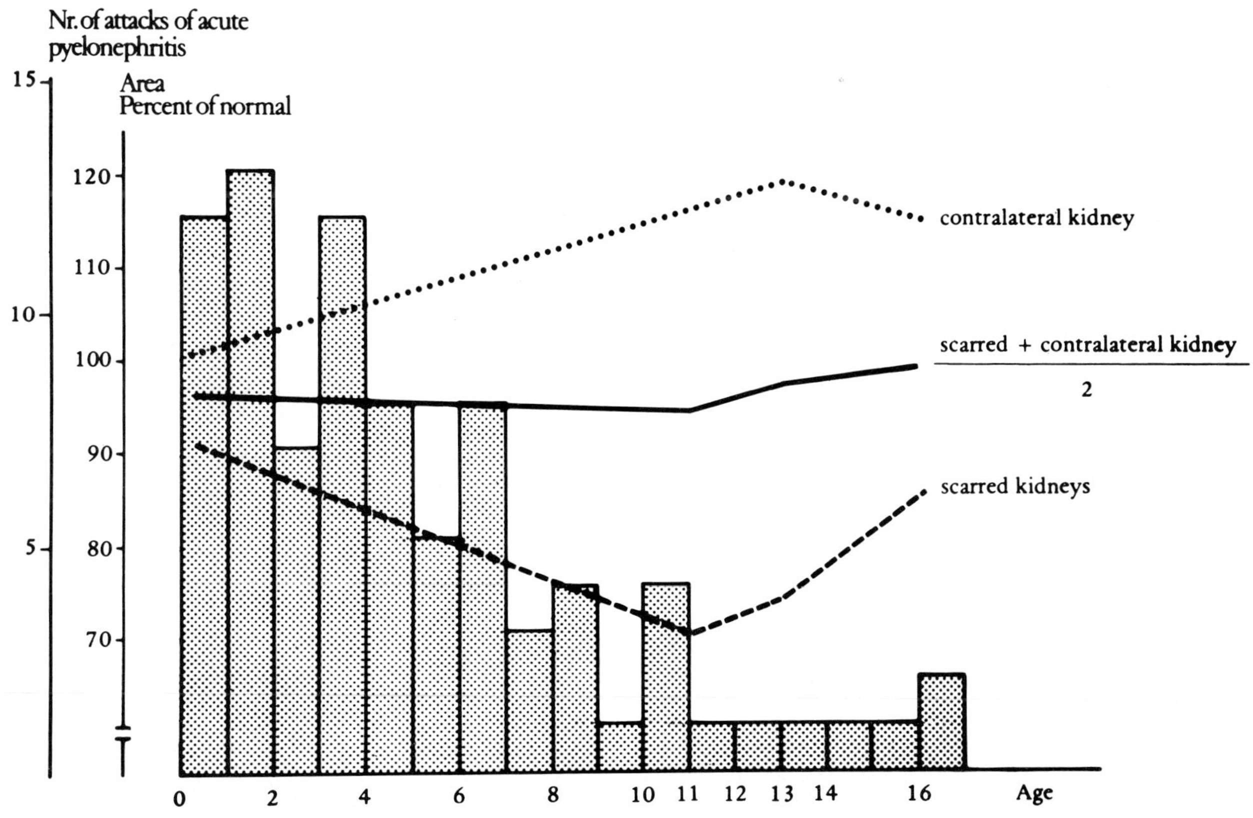

Figure 36.13. Renal parenchymal area in percent of normal in 16 girls with unilateral scarring. The areas of the scarred and the contralateral kidneys and the mean total renal area are given as function of age. The bars indicate the total number of attacks of pyelonephritis for each year of age. There is a catchup growth of the scarred kidneys at puberty. (From Cläesson I, Jacobsson B, Jodal U, et al: Compensatory kidney growth in children with urinary tract infection and unilateral renal scarring: a epidemiologic study. Kidney Int 40:759, 1981.)

References

1. Winberg J, Andersen HJ, Bergström T, et al: Epidemiology of symptomatic urinary tract infection in childhood. Acta Paediatr Scand (suppl 252) 63:1, 1974.
2. Winberg J, Bergström T, Jacobsson B: Morbidity, age and sex distribution, recurrences and renal scarring in symptomatic urinary tract infection in childhood. Kidney Intl 8:101, 1975.
3. Asscher AW, McLachlan MSF, Verrier-Jones R, et al: Screening for asymptomatic urinary-tract infection in schoolgirls. Lancet 2:1, 1973.
4. Kunin CM, Deutscher R, Paquin A: Urinary tract infection in school children: a epidemiologic, clinical and laboratory study. Medicine 43:91, 1964.
5. Stamey TA: A clinical classification of urinary tract infections based upon origin. South Med J 68:934, 1975.
6. O'Grady F, Mackintosh IP, Greenwood D, et al: Treatment of "bacterial cystitis" in fully automatic mechanical models simulating conditions of bacterial growth in the urinary bladder. Br J Exp Pathol 54:283, 1973.
7. Stamm WE, Counts GW, Running KR, et al: Diagnosis of coliform infection in acutely dysuric women. N Engl J Med 307:463, 1982.
8. Bollgren I, Engström CF, Hammarlind M, et al: Low urinary counts of P-fimbriated *Escherichia coli* in presumed acute pyelonephritis. Arch Dis Child 59:102, 1984.
9. Geisinger JF: Intermittency of pyuria at the level of the renal papillae. J Urol 25:649, 1931.
10. Houston IB: Pus cell and bacterial counts in the diagnosis of urinary tract infections in childhood. Arch Dis Child 38:600, 1963.
11. Percival A, Brumfitt W, de Louvois J: Serum-antibody levels as an indication of clinically inapparent pyelonephritis. Lancet 2:1027, 1964.
12. Winberg J, Andersen HJ, Hanson LA, et al: Studies of urinary tract infections in infancy and childhood. Br Med J 2:524, 1963.
13. Winberg J: Determination of the renal concentration capacity in infants and children without renal disease. Acta Paediatr Scand 48:318, 1959.
14. Bergström T, Larson H, Lincoln K, et al: Studies of urinary tract infections in infancy and childhood: XII. Eighty consecutive patients with neonatal infection. J Pediatr 80:858, 1972.
15. Aperia A, Berg U, Broberger O: Control of sodium homeostasis in children with recurrent infections and reduced glomerular filtration rates. Acta Paediatr Scand 60:695, 1971.
16. Berg U, Aperia A, Broberger O: Subclinical defects in renal regulation of acid base balance in children with recurrent urinary tract infections. Acta Paediatr Scand 60:521, 1971.
17. Berg U: Renal function in acute febrile urinary tract infection in children: pathophysiologic aspects on the reduced concentrating capacity. Kidney Intl 30:753, 1981.
18. Janson L, Roberts JA: Experimental pyelonephritis. V. Functional characteristics of pyelonephritis. Invest Urol 15:397, 1978.
19. Claësson I, Jacobsson B, Jodal U, et al: Compensatory kidney growth in children with urinary tract infection and unilateral renal scarring: an epidemiologic study. Kidney Intl 40:759, 1981.
20. Claësson I, Jacobsson B, Jodal U, et al: Early detection of nephropathy in childhood urinary tract infection. Acta Radiol (Diagn) (Stockh) 22:315, 1981.
21. Claësson I, Jacobsson B, Olsson T, et al: Assessment of renal parenchymal thickness in normal children. Acta Radiol 32:305, 1981.
22. Smellie JM, Edwards D, Hunter N, et al: Vesico-ureteric reflux and renal scarring. Kidney Intl 8:65, 1975.
23. Stamey TA, Govan DE, Palmer JM: The localization and treatment of urinary tract infections: The role of bacterial urine levels as opposed to serum levels. Medicine (Baltimore) 44:1, 1965.
24. Fairley KF, Carson NE, Gutch RC, et al: Site of infection in acute urinary tract infection in general practice. Lancet 2:615, 1971.
25. Jodal U, Lindberg U, Lincoln K: Level diagnosis of symptomatic urinary tract infections in childhood. Acta Paediatr Scand 64:201, 1975.
26. Lindberg U, Jodal U, Hanson LA, et al: Asymptomatic bacteriuria in schoolgirls: IV. Difficulties of level diagnosis and the possible relation to the character of infecting bacteria. Acta Paediatr Scand 64:574, 1975.
27. Thomas V, Shelokov A, Forland M: Antibody-coated bacteria in the urine and the site of urinary tract infection. N Engl J Med 290:588, 1974.
28. Hellerstein S, Duggan E, Welchert E, et al: Serum C-reactive protein and the site of urianry tract infections. J Pediatr 100:21, 1982.
29. Abyholm G, Monn E: Intranasal DDAVP-test in the study of renal concentrating capacity in children with recurrent urinary tract infections. Eur J Pediatr 130:149, 1979.
30. Meadow WR, White RHR, Johnston NM: Prevalence of symptomless urinary tract disease in Birmingham school children: I. Pyuria and bacteriuria. Br Med J 3:81, 1969.
31. Lincoln K, Winberg J: Studies of urinary tract infection in infancy and childhood: II. Quantitative estimation of bacteriuria in unselected neonates with special reference to the occurrence of asymptomatic infections. Acta Paediatr Scand 53:307, 1964.
32. Winberg J: Screening in the newborn period. In Colloquium on Pyelonephritis, Proceedings of 14th International Congress of Pediatrics, Buenos Aires, 1974.
33. Wettergren B, Jodal U, Jonasson G: Epidemiology of bacteriuria during the first year of life. Acta Pediat Scand 74:925, 1985.
34. Gruneberg RN, Leight DA, Brumfitt W: *Escherichia coli* serotypes in urinary tract infection: studies in domiciliary, antenatal and hospital practice. In O'Grady F, Brumfitt W (eds): Urinary Tract Infection. London: Oxford University Press, 1968, p 68.
35. Winberg J, Bergström T, Lidin-Janson G, Treatment trials in urinary tract infection (UTI) with special reference to the effect of antimicrobials on the fecal and periurethral flora. Clin Nephrol 1:142, 1973.
36. Kendall AR, Karafin L: Urinary tract infection in children: Fact and fantasy. J Urol 107:1068, 1972.
37. O'Grady F, Cattell WR: Kinetics of urinary tract infection: II. The bladder. Br J Urol 38:156, 1966.
38. Govan DE, Fair WR, Friedland GW, et al: Urinary tract infections in children: III. Treatment of ureterovesical reflux. Western Med J 121:382, 1974.
39. Berg I, Fielding D, Meadow R: Psychiatric disturbance, urgency, and bacteriuria in children with day and night wetting. Arch Dis Child 52:651, 1977.
40. van Gool JD, Kuijten RH, Donckerwolcke RA, et al: Bladder-sphincter dysfunction, urinary function and vesico-ureteral reflux with special reference to cognitive bladder training. In Hodson CJ, Heptinstall RH, Winberg J (eds): Contribution to Nephrology: Reflux Nephropathy Update. Basle: Karger, 1984, p 190.
41. Stansfeld JM: Clinical observations relating to incidence and aetiology of urinary tract infections in children. Br Med J 1:631, 1966.
42. Kunin CM: Pattern of recurrent urinary tract infections in girls. In Symposium on Pyelonephritis. Edinburgh: Livingstone, 1966, p 1.
43. McCabe WR, Anderson V: Endotoxin tolerance: I. Its induction by experimental pyelonephritis. J Clin Invest 42:610, 1963.
44. McCabe WR: Endotoxin tolerance: II. Its occurrence in patients with pyelonephritis. J Clin Invest 42:618, 1963.
45. Holmgren J, Smith JW: Immunological aspects of urinary tract infections. Progr Allergy 18:289, 1975.
46. Lindberg U, Hanson LA, Jodal U, et al: Asymptomatic bacteriuria in schoolgirls. II. Differences in *Escherichia coli* causing asymptomatic and symptomatic bacteria. Acta Paediatr Scand 64:432, 1975.
47. Roantree RJ: The relationship of lipopolysaccharide structure to bacterial virulence. In Kadis S, Weinbaus G, Ajl S (eds): Microbial Toxins. V. Bacterial endotoxins. New York: Academic Press, 1971, p 1.
48. Fairley KF, Birch DF: Unconventional bacteria in urinary tract disease: Gardnerella vaginalis. Kidney Intl 23:862, 1983.
49. Bergström T: Sex differences in childhood: Urinary tract infection. Arch Dis Child 47:227, 1972.
50. Ericsson NO, Winberg J, Zetterström R: Renal function in infantile obstructive uropathy. Acta Paediatr 44:444, 1955.
51. McCrory WW, Shibuya M, Leuman E, et al: Studies of renal function in children with chronic hydronephrosis. Pediatr Clin North Am 18:445, 1971.
52. Anders D, Anders I, Sitzmann FC: Feldstudie zur Epidemiologie inapparenter Harnweginfektionen bei Mädchen im Vorschulalter. Med Klin 69:1850, 1974.
53. Lindberg U, Claësson I, Hanson LA, et al:. Asymptomatic bacteriuria in schoolgirls: I. Clinical and laboratory findings. Acta Paediatr Scand 64:425, 1975.
54. McLachlan MSF, Meller ST, Verrier-Jones ER, et al: Urinary tract infections in schoolgirls with covert bacteriuria. Arch Dis Child 50:253, 1975.
55. Savage DCL, Wilson MJ, McHardy M, et al: Covert bacteriuria of childhood, a clinical and epidemiological study. Arch Dis Child 48:8, 1973.
56. Lindberg U, Bjure J, Haugstvedt S, et al: Asymptomatic bacteriuria in schoolgirls: III. Relation between residual urine volume and recurrence. Acta Paediatr Scand 64:437, 1975.
57. Hanson LA, Ahlstedt S, Jodal U, et al: The host-parasite relationship in urinary tract infections. Kidney Intl 8:28, 1975.
58. Svanborg-Edén C, Hanson LÅ, Jodal U, et al: Variable adherence to normal human urinary tract epithelial cells of *Escherichia coli* strains associated with various forms of urinary tract infections. Lancet 2:490, 1976.
59. Lindberg U: Asymptomatic bacteriuria in schoolgirls: V. The clinical course and response to treatment. Acta Paediatr Scand 64:718, 1975.
60. Savage DCL: Natural history of covert bacteriuria in schoolgirls. Kidney Intl 8:90, 1975.
61. Verrier-Jones ER, Meller ST, McLachlan MSF, et al: Treatment of bacteriuria in schoolgirls. Kidncy Intl 8:85, 1975.
62. Verrier Jones K, Asscher AW, Verrier-Jones ER, et al: Glomerular filtration rate in schoolgirls with covert bacteriuria. Br Med J 285:1307, 1982.

63. Asscher AW, Sussman M, Waters, WE, et al: Asymptomatic bacteria in the non-pregnant woman: II. Response to treatment and follow-up. Br Med J 1:804, 1969.
64. Edelmann CM, Ogwo JE, Fine BP, et al: The prevalence of bacteriuria in full-term and premature newborn infants. J Pediatr 82:125, 1973.
65. Märild S, Hellström M, Jodal U, et al: UTI during the first year of life in a Göteborg area 1977–79: II. Symptomatic infections. Pediatr Res 14:981, 1980.
66. Köllermann MW, Ludwig H: Ueber den vesico-ureteralen Reflux beim normalen Kind im Saüglings- und Kleinkindalter. Z Kinderheilk 100:185, 1967.
67. Baker R, Maxted W, Maylath J, et al: Relation of age, sex, and infection to reflux: Data indicating high spontaneous cure rate in pediatric patients. J Urol 95:27, 1966.
68. Roberts JA: Studies of vesicoureteral reflux: a review of work in a primate model. South Med J 71:28, 1978.
69. Gross GW, Lebowitz RL: Infection does not cause reflux. Am J Roentgenol 137:929, 1981.
70. Ehrlich RM: Vesicoureteral reflux: A surgeon's perspective. Pediatr Clin North Am 29:827, 1982.
71. De Vargas A, Evans K, Ransley P, et al: A family study of vesicoureteric reflux. J Med Genet 15:85, 1978.
72. Jerkins GR, Noe HN: Familial vesicoureteral reflux: a prospective study. J Urol 128:774, 1982.
73. Edwards D, Normand ICS, Prescod N, et al: Disappearance of vesicoureteric reflux during long-term prophylaxis of urinary tract infection in children. Br Med J 2:285, 1977.
74. Hodson CJ, Maling TMJ, McManamon PJ, et al: The pathogenesis of reflux nephropathy (chronic atrophic pyelonephritis). Br J Radiol (suppl. 13) 48:1, 1975.
75. Ransley PG, Risdon RA: Reflux and renal scarring. Br J Radiol (suppl 14):1, 78.
76. Rolleston GL, Maling TMJ, Hodson CJ: Intrarenal reflux and the scarred kidney. Arch Dis Child 49:531, 1974.
77. Winberg J, Bollgren I, Källenius G, et al: Clinical pyelonephritis and focal renal scarring. A selected review of pathogenesis, prevention, and prognosis. Pediatr Clin North Am 29:801, 1982.
78. Winter AL, Hardy BE, Alton DJ, et al: Acquired renal scars in children. J Urol 129:1190, 1983.
79. Roberts JA: Experimental pyelonephritis in the monkey. III. Pathophysiology of ureteral malfunction induced by bacteria. Invest Urol 13:117, 1975.
80. Roberts JA, Angel JR, Roth JK: The hydrodynamics of pyelorenal reflux: II. The effect of chronic obstructive changes on papillary shape. Invest Urol 18:296, 1981.
81. Angel JR, Smith TW, Roberts JA: The hydrodynamics of pyelorenal reflux. J Urol 122:20, 1979.
82. Roberts JA: Vesicoureteral reflux in the monkey. A review. J Urol (in press).
83. Svenson SB, Källenius G, Korhonen TK, et al: Initiation of clinical pyelonephritis. The role of P-fimbriae-mediated bacterial adhesion. In Hodson CJ, Heptinstall RH, Winberg J (eds): Contributions to Nephrology: Reflux Nephropathy Update, Basle, Karger, 1984, p 252.
84. Roberts JA, Kaack B, Källenius G, et al: Receptors for pyelonephritogenic *Escherichia coli* in primates. J Urol 131:163, 1984.
85. Källenius G, Möllby R, Svenson SB, et al: Occurrence of P-fimbriated *Escherichia coli* in urinary tract infections. Lancet 2:1369, 1982.
86. Lomberg H, Hanson LÅ, Jacobsson B, et al: Correlation of P blood group, vesicoureteral reflux, and bacterial attachment in patients with recurrent pyelonephritis. N Engl J Med 308:1189, 1983.
87. Filly R, Friedland GW, Govan DE, et al: Development and progression of clubbing and scarring in children with recurrent urinary tract infections. Radiology 113:145, 1974.
88. Hodson CJ, Edwards D: Chronic pyelonephritis and vesicoureteric reflux. Clin Radiol 11:219, 1960.
89. Smellie JM, Normand ICS: Bacteriuria, reflux and renal scarring. Arch Dis Child 50:581, 1975.
90. Elo J, Tallgren LG, Alfthan O, et al: Character of urinary tract infections and pyelonephritic renal scarring after antireflux surgery. J Urol 129:343, 1982.
91. Birmingham Reflux Study Group: Prospective trial of operative versus non-operative treatment of severe vesicoureteric reflux: Two years' observation in 96 children. Br Med J 287:171, 1983.
92. Smellie JM, Edwards D, Normand ICS, et al: Effect of vesicoureteric reflux on renal growth in children with urinary tract infection. Arch Dis Child 56:593, 1981.
93. Govan DE, Fair WR, Filly RA, et al: Management of children with urinary tract infections. The Stanford experience. Urology 6:273, 1975.
94. Hutch JA: Vesico-ureteral reflux in the paraplegic: Cause and correction. J Urol 68:457, 1952.
95. Lenaghan D, Cass AS, Cussen LJ, et al: Long-term effect of vesicoureteral reflux on the upper urinary tract of dogs. J Urol 107:758, 1972.
96. Mendoza JM, Roberts JA: Effects of sterile high pressure vesicoureteral reflux on the monkey. J Urol 130:602, 1983.
97. Heptinstall RH: Pathology of the Kidney. Little, Brown, Boston, 1966, p 421.
98. Hodson CJ, Wilson S: Natural history of chronic pyelonephritic scarring. Br Med J 2:191, 1965.
99. Bernstein J: Developmental abnormalities of the renal parenchyma: Renal hypoplasia and dysplasia. In Sommers SC (ed): Pathology Annual 1968, New York, Appleton-Century-Crofts, 1969.
100. Andersen HJ, Jacobsson B, Larson H, et al: Hypertension, asymmetric renal parenchymal defect, sterile urine and high *E. coli* antibody titre. Br Med J 3:14, 1973.
101. Asscher AW, Chick S: Increased susceptibility of the kidney to ascending *Escherichia coli* infection following unilateral nephrotomy. Br J Urol 44:202, 1972.
102. Freedman LR: Chronic pyelonephritis at autopsy. Ann Intern Med 66:697, 1967.
103. Kleeman SET, Freedman LR: The finding of chronic pyelonephritis in males and females at autopsy. N Engl J Med 263:988, 1960.
104. Miller T, Phillips S: Pyelonephritis: The relation between infection, renal scarring and antimicrobial therapy. Kidney Intl 19:654, 1981.
105. Slotki IN, Asscher AW: Prevention of scarring in experimental pyelonephritis in the rat by early antibiotic therapy. Nephron 30:262, 1982.
106. Bille J, Glauser MP: Protection against chronic pyelonephritis in rats by suppression of acute suppuration: Effect of colchicine and neutropenia. J Infect Dis 146:220, 1982.
107. Glauser MP, Lyons JM, Braude AI: Prevention of chronic experimental pyelonephritis by suppression of acute suppuration. J Clin Invest 61:403, 1978.
108. Roberts JA, Roth JK, Domingue G, et al: Immunology of pyelonephritis in the primate model: V. Effect of superoxide dismutase. J Urol 128:1394, 1982.
109. Stamey TA, Timothy M, Millar M, et al: Recurrent urinary infections in adult women: the role of introital enterobacteria. Calif Med 115:1, 1971.
110. Bollgren I, Winberg J: The periurethral aerobic flora in girls highly susceptible to urinary infections. Acta Paediatr Scand 65:81, 1976.
111. Bollgren I, Nord CE, Pettersson L, et al: Periurethral anaerobic microflora in girls highly susceptible to urinary infections. J Urol 125:715, 1981.
112. Fowler JE, Stamey TS: Studies of introital colonization in women with recurrent urinary infections: VII. The role of bacterial adherence. J Urol 117:472, 1977.
113. Källenius G, Winberg J: Bacterial adherence to periurethral epithelial cells in girls prone to urinary-tract infections. Lancet 2:540, 1978.
114. Winberg J, Bollgren I, Källenius G, et al: Bacterial virulence and host defence in pathogenesis of renal infection and renal scarring. In François B and Perrin P (eds); Urinary Infection, Insights and Prospects, London, Butterworth and Co., 1983, p 19.
115. Westenfelder M, Galanos C, Madsen PO: Experimental lipid A induced nephritis in the dog. Invest Urol 12:337, 1975.
116. Teague W, Boyarksy S: The effect of coliform bacteria upon ureteral peristalsis. Invest Urol 5:423, 1968.
117. Winberg J, Bollgren I: Care of children with urinary tract infection. In Asscher AW (ed): The Management of Urinary Tract Infection, 1980. Oxford, The Medicine Publishing Foundation.
118. Bergström T, Lincoln K, Ørskov F, et al: Studies of urinary tract infections in infancy and childhood: VIII. Reinfection vs relapse. J Pediatr 71:13, 1967.
119. Normand ICS, Smellie JM: Prolonged maintenance chemotherapy in the management of urinary infection in childhood. Br Med J 1:1023, 1965.
120. Källenius G, Kallings L-O, Winberg J: Single dose treatment of children using Sulphafurazole. In Bailey RR (ed): Single Dose Therapy of Urinary Tract Infection. Sidney and Bristol, Adis Health Science Press, 1983, p 63.
121. Bailey RR (ed): Single Dose Therapy of Urinary Tract Infection. Sidney and Bristol, Adis Health Science Press, 1983.
122. Tschudi Madsen S: Antibacterial effect of urine after single oral doses of sulphonamide. Chemotherapia 13:16, 1968.
123. Stamey TA, Fair WR, Timothy MM, et al: Serum versus urinary antimicrobial concentrations in cure of urinary tract infections. N Engl J Med 291:1159, 1974.
124. Ronald AR, Turck M, Petersdorf RA: A critical evaluation of nalidixic acid in urinary tract infections. N Engl J Med 275:1081, 1966.
125. Stamey TA, Bragonje J: Resistance to nalidixic acid: a misconception due to underdosage. JAMA 236:1857, 1976.
126. Stamey TA, Bushby SRM, Bragonje J: The concentration of trimethoprim in prostatic fluid: Nonionic diffusion or active transport? J Infect Dis (suppl) 128:S686, 1973.
127. Stamey TA, Condy M: The diffusion and concentration of trimethoprim in human vaginal fluid. J Infect Dis 131:261, 1975.
128. Elo J: Treatment and prophylaxis of urinary tract infection in children. A retrospective study. Drugs Exp Clin Res 9:357, 1983.
129. Arneil GC, McAllister TA, Kay, P: Measurement of bacteriuria by plane dipslide culture. Lancet 1:94, 1973.
130. Scott JES, Deegan S: Management of neuropathic urinary incontinence in children by intermittent catheterisation. Arch Dis Child 57:253, 1982.

131. Robbins JB, McCracken GH, Gotschlich EC, et al: *Escherichia coli* K_1 capsular polysaccharide associated with neonatal meningitis. N Engl J Med 290:1216, 1974.
132. Nelson JD, McCracken GH: The current status of gentamicin for the neonate and young infant. Am J Dis Child 124:13, 1972.
133. Lindblad BS, Ekengren K: The long-term prognosis of nonobstructive urinary tract infection in infancy and childhood after the advent of sulphonamide. Acta Paediatr Scand 58:25, 1969.
134. Smellie JM, Normand ICS: Experience of follow-up of children with urinary tract infection. In O'Grady F, Brumfitt W (eds); Urinary Tract Infection. London, Oxford University Press, 1968, p 123.
135. Chantler C, Carter JE, Bewick M, et al: 10 years' experience with regular haemodialysis and renal transplantation. Arch Dis Child 55:435, 1980.
136. Holland NH: Reflux nephropathy and hypertension. In Hodson J, Kincaid-Smith P (eds): Reflux Nephropathy. New York, Masson 1979, p 257.
137. Asscher AW: The Challenge of Urinary Tract Infections, London, Academic Press; New York, Grune & Stratton; 1980.
138. McCurdy FA, Vernier RL: Unique consequences of kidney infections in infants and children: pathogenesis, early recognition, and prevention of scarring. Am J Nephrol 1:184, 1981.
139. Hellerstein S: Recurrent urinary tract infections in children. Pediatr Infect Dis 1:271, 1982.
140. Winberg J: P-fimbriae, bacterial adhesion, and pyelonephritis. Arch Dis Child 59:180, 1984.
141. Winberg J, Larson H, Bergström T: Comparison of the natural history of urinary infection in children with and without vesico-ureteric reflux. In Kincaid-Smith P, Fairley K (eds): Renal Infection and Renal Scarring, Melbourne, Mercedes, 1971, p 293.

CHAPTER 37

Vesicoureteric Reflux and Renal Scarring

N. P. GOLDRAICH
T. M. BARRATT

The term vesicoureteric reflux (VUR) denotes the retrograde passage of urine from the bladder into the ureter. The phenomenon occurs rarely enough in healthy children to be considered abnormal. It is a consequence of dysfunction of the ureterovesical junction. VUR is associated with urinary tract infection (UTI) and the coarse renal scarring designated chronic pyelonephritis or reflux nephropathy. This nephropathy is the commonest cause of end-stage renal failure and severe hypertension in children and young adults (1, 2)

VUR is a controversial subject, in part because of the variation in its severity and in associated bladder pathology is insufficiently recognized, and in part because the pathogenetic mechanisms of scarring, particularly the relative contributions of dysplasia and postnatally acquired pyelonephritic damage, have not been defined.

VESICOURETERIC REFLUX

Historical Background

The valvular nature of the ureterovesical junction was known to Galen and is attested by the fact that when the pig's bladder was used as a football in medieval times it was not considered necessary to ligate the ureters.

VUR was demonstrated in vivo in dogs and rabbits by Sampson in 1903 (3). In these species it occurs more frequently in apparently healthy animals than it does in pigs or humans. Clinically, Kretschmer (4) demonstrated VUR in four children in 1916, and in 1924 Bumpus (5) reported VUR in 8.6% of 1036 cystograms in patients with a variety of urological disorders, establishing the condition as a nosological entity. The late 1950s witnessed a rapidly expanding phase of clinical activity with the description by Politano and Leadbetter (6) of a surgical technique for the correction of VUR, the clinical-radiological studies of Hodson and Edwards (7), and the contributions of Stephens and Lenaghan (8), Tanagho (9), and Williams (10).

Recently there has been a swing away from the surgical enthusiasm of earlier years (11), with a better understanding of the pathogenesis of scarring (12) and a recognition of the particular vulnerability of young children to pyelonephritic damage (13). Even so, the controlled clinical trials necessary to formulate a rational management policy are only now beginning to be undertaken (14, 15).

Definition and Detection

Concepts of VUR have been defined and limited by the techniques used for its detection, all of which have their shortcomings. The extent to which contrast medium or radioisotope ascends the urinary tract during micturition gives an incomplete picture of the movement of unopacified urine or pressure transients.

Micturating Cystourethrogram

The micturating cystourethrogram (MCU) is the definitive means of diagnosing VUR (Fig. 37.1) (see Chapter 20). There are, however, a number of technical details that affect the examination (16): the infusion technique; the contrast agent used; the amount given; the rate of infusion and the pressure applied; the state of hydration and urine flow in the patient; the position of the patient; the use of sedation or general anesthesia; the radiographic technique; the temporal relationship to UTI; the preparation of the patient; and the experience of the observer.

Radionuclide Cystogram

The radionuclide cystogram (RNC) was introduced by Winter in 1959 (17) and has since undergone many modifications. The three principal methods are the indirect (intravenous) (18, 19, 20, 21), the direct (22, 23), and the suprapubic (24, 25); they differ in the route of administration of the radiopharmaceutical. Using a gamma camera, regions of interest are defined over the kidney and bladder areas. Following micturition there is normally an abrupt drop in bladder activity without any increase in the renal areas, but with VUR activity in the renal areas rises and then falls again as refluxed urine is returned to the bladder (Fig. 37.2).

RNC permits detection of VUR and quantitation of the postvoiding bladder residue but does not provide anatomical information about the bladder or urethra. It therefore cannot replace the MCU as an initial investigation in boys, especially newborns and infants, but is ideal for older children and for follow-up. Results are better in toilet-trained children (26, 27). The technique can be linked to urodynamic evaluation

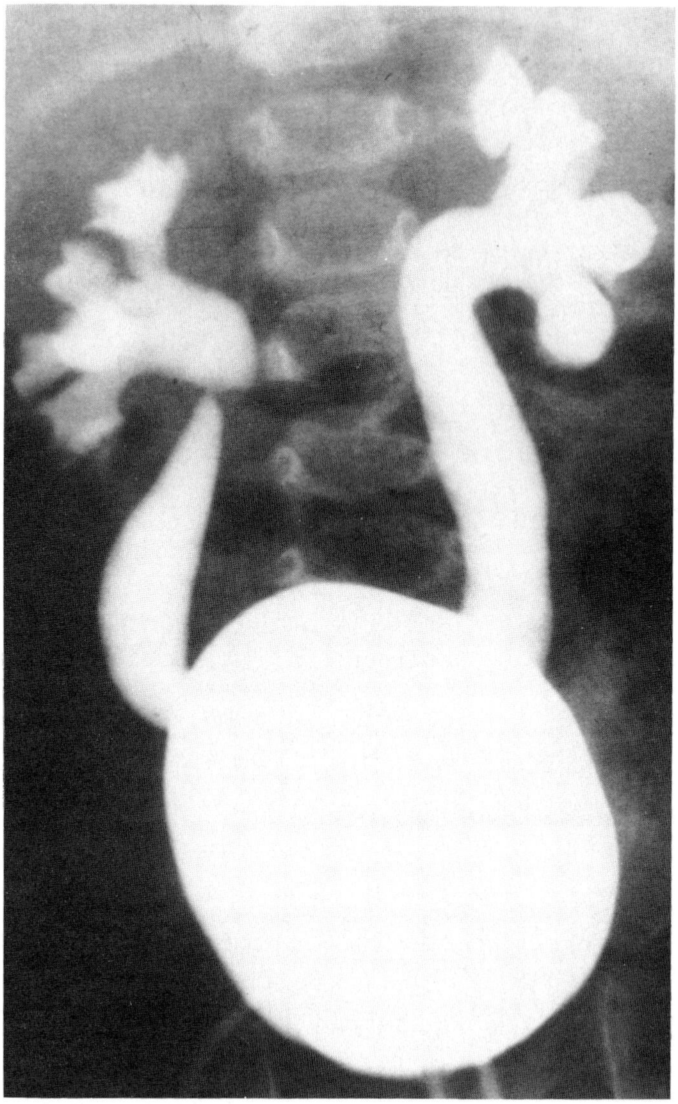

Figure 37.1. Micturating cystogram showing bilateral vesicoureteric reflux.

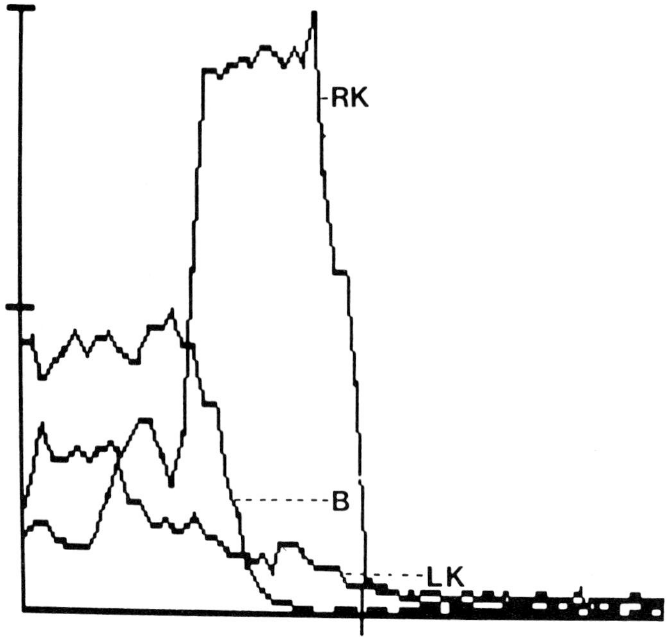

Figure 37.2. Quantitative data from a suprapubic radionuclide cystogram illustrating right VUR. RK = right kidney, LK = left kidney, B = bladder.

(28). The principal advantages of RNC over the MCU lie in the lower radiation dosage (23), the opportunity for continuous recording and, with the indirect and suprapubic techniques, the avoidance of urethral catheterization.

Indirect Cystography. 99m-Technetium diaminotetraethylpentacetic acid (^{99m}Tc-DTPA) is injected intravenously, rapidly cleared from the circulation, and excreted by glomerular filtration. Counts are obtained from renal and bladder areas before and after micturition as previously described. The technique's advantage is that bladder filling takes place by physiological means and that the voiding posture is normal. It is, however, difficult to ensure that the bladder is completely full before micturition, and VUR during the early phase of bladder filling may be missed. Nevertheless, the indirect RNC compares favorably with the MCU in detecting VUR (18, 20, 26).

Direct Cystography. The bladder is catheterized, and 1 mCi of ^{99m}Tc-pertechnetate is introduced, followed by warmed saline solution until the bladder is full. Images are obtained before and after micturition. The advantages over the indirect method are that it depends less on the cooperation of the child, is not influenced by renal function, permits evaluation of VUR during the filling phase, avoids uncertainty about the origin of radioactivity in the upper tract, and involves a lower radiation dosage. On the other hand, the bladder is not filled in a physiological manner, and there is a risk of introducing UTI. The direct RNC involves less radiation (23) and is superior to the MCU in detecting VUR (22, 29); Conway (22) estimated that it detected 30% more cases of VUR than the MCU and 25% more than indirect RNC.

Suprapubic Cystography. ^{99m}Tc-DTPA is injected by suprapubic puncture of a full bladder. The child is asked to hold urine for as long as possible and then void in front of the gamma camera. The technique does not require bladder catheterization, does not depend on renal function, and permits normal physiological bladder filling and emptying; it has proved very satisfactory in demonstrating VUR (24, 25) (Fig. 37.3).

Causes and Classification

Reflux is a consequence of dysfunction of the ureterovesical junction (UVJ), whose competence depends on an adequate length of intravesical ureter being compressed during voiding. It is considered primary if unassociated with any other structural abnormality, secondary if combined with other major urological malformations. In its primary form, which is the principal concern of this chapter, VUR can be considered as a congenital abnormality of the UVJ, presumably present since embryonic life. In practice, a clear-cut distinction between primary and secondary VUR is not always possible, for VUR cannot be considered in isolation from concomitant bladder function. There are cases in which the UVJ is obviously abnormal with a short intramural segment of ureter and a gaping orifice, others in which bladder function is clearly abnormal due to neuropathy or outflow obstruction; there are also intermediate cases with a marginally incompetent UVJ and subtle disorders of bladder function characterized by detrusor instability and high voiding pressures. The intravesical segment of ureter increases in length with age so that an incompetent junction may mature into a competent one (30). Thus VUR is not necessarily a permanent phenomenon, which raises problems for the epidemiologist and the geneticist. Furthermore, the competence of the UVJ may be transiently affected by UTI caused by edema around the intramural segment of ureter and the paralyzing effect of bacterial

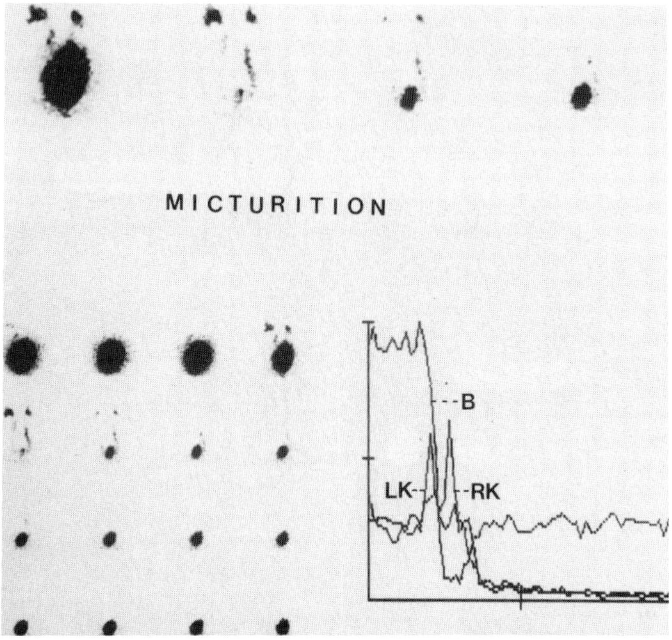

Figure 37.3. Direct suprapubic radionuclide cystogram showing bilateral VUR on filling with a postvoiding residue.

toxins on ureteric musculature. VUR occurring only in association with UTI is generally thought to be of less significance, but this view may lead to a false sense of security, for it is during infected episodes that the kidney is most at risk of pyelonephritic damage.

There are also special anatomical circumstances to consider, for example, VUR associated with an ectopic ureter or a duplex system (see Chapter 39); with other pathology at the UVJ such as obstruction, a diverticulum or previous surgery; or with widespread uropathology as in the prune belly syndrome (see Chapter 38), neuropathic bladder (see Chapter 40), or urethral valves (see Chapter 38).

Severity and Grading

In addition to heterogeneous anatomical causes and associations, VUR varies in degree or grade. This is conventionally judged by the level to which contrast medium is perceived to ascend during the MCU and by the degree of dilatation of the upper urinary tract. The commonly used classifications of VUR according to intensity are the three grades proposed by Rolleston and coworkers (31), the four grades proposed by Smellie and coworkers (32) and by Dwoskin and Perlmutter (33), and the five grades proposed by Heikel and Parkkulainen (34), which was adopted by the International Reflux Study Committee (14). These classifications are illustrated in Figure 37.4. There are several caveats to these systems of grading, for the apparent degree of VUR may vary considerably in the same individual on different occasions, depending on the degree of bladder filling, the recent occurrence of UTI, and the practical details of the cystographic technique (see section on technique) (16, 35, 36, 37). For these reasons, elaborate systems of grading are inappropriate, and a simple classification such as that presented by Rolleston and coworkers (31) is preferred.

In some cases VUR is observed during the filling phase of the MCU, in others only during or after micturition, leading to a distinction between low-pressure and high-pressure reflux, it being implied that the latter is less significant. This terminology is, however, confusing, for recently the term high-pressure reflux has come to be used for those troublesome cases in which VUR is associated with bladder dysfunction and high resting bladder pressures.

Intrarenal reflux is an associated phenomenon, defined for practical purposes by the detection of contrast medium in the renal parenchyma during cystography. It is found with severe VUR in young children and outlines segments of the kidney at particular risk of scarring with UTI (see below).

Prevalence and Incidence

There has been considerable debate about whether VUR is a "normal" finding, perhaps a reflection of immaturity of the UVJ. The evidence is against this view. Kjellberg and coworkers (38) investigated 101 children (aged 2 days to 13 yr) without evidence of urological disorder and could not demonstrate VUR in any of them; Jones and Headstream (39) studied 100 children (mean age 3.5 yr) without any suggestion of urinary tract disease and found bilateral VUR in only one 4-year-old boy in whom subsequent investigations showed a trabeculated bladder with a significant postvoiding residue; Gibson (40) investigated 43 children up to 12 yr of age without any history of urinary problems and found unilateral VUR in two of them. Lich and coworkers (41) studied 26

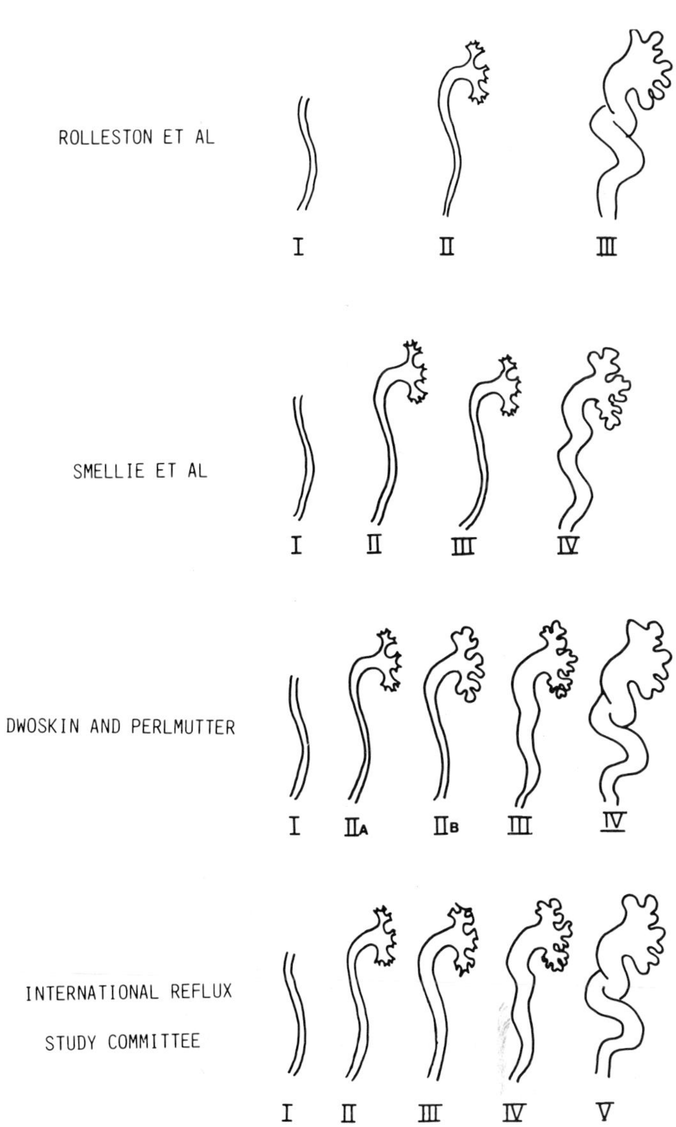

Figure 37.4. Grading of VUR: classifications of Rolleston and coworkers (31), Smellie and coworkers (in grade II VUR occurs only during micturition; in grade III it occurs at rest) (32), Dwoskin and Perlmutter (33), and the International Reflux Study Committee (14).

neonates (less than 48 hr of life) with normal physical examination findings and negative urine cultures and were not able to demonstrate VUR in any of them. Peters and coworkers (42) examined 66 premature infants weighing 1970 to 2465 g and did not find VUR; however, this group included a high proportion of black children, who are known to have a significantly lower incidence of VUR than whites (43, 44). Finally, Booth and coworkers (45) collected 28 cases of fetal cystograms accidentally performed during intrauterine red blood cell transfusion in fetuses affected by erythroblastosis fetalis. Bilateral VUR was detected in only one case. This child, a girl, had an MCU at 1 year of age that demonstrated persistent VUR.

Bailey (46) reviewed the literature in an attempt to establish the incidence of VUR in the population as a whole. He encountered several difficulties: different age groups were included in the various reports; inadequate information was presented on the radiological techniques used; the indications for undertaking x-ray studies were not always clear; and insufficient information concerning the severity of VUR was given. He concluded that VUR was present in 0.4% to 1.8% of unselected children, with the lower figure probably being more correct. In neonates the data of Abbott (47) and Drew and Acton (48) suggest an incidence of VUR of 0.21 to 0.55%. The incidence is significantly lower in black children (43, 44, 49).

VUR is reported with greater frequency in females (50, 51, 52). In children who present with UTI, VUR is found with a similar frequency in the two sexes (38, 53, 54, 55). As UTI is much commoner in females except in the neonatal period and is the usual event leading to the diagnosis of VUR, it may be that the greater reported prevalence of VUR in females is a result of bias in ascertainment.

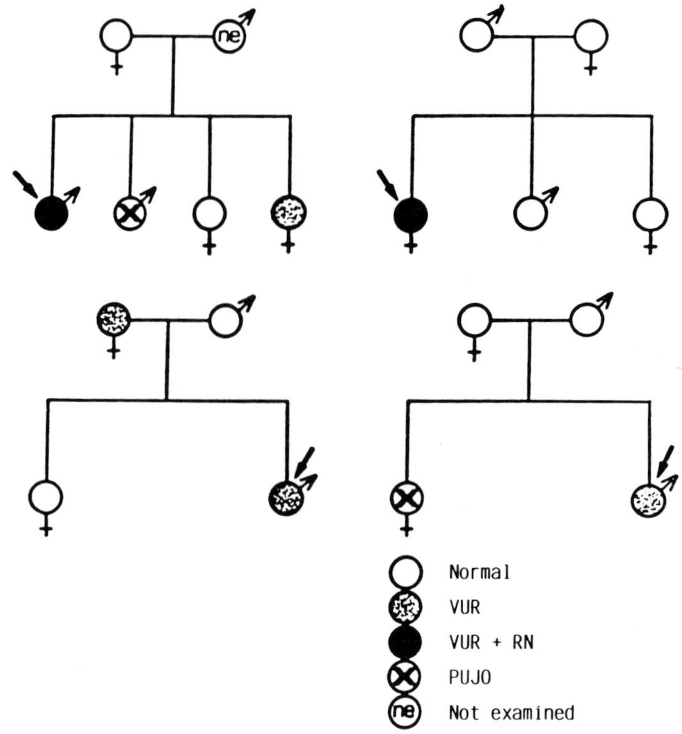

Figure 37.5. Familial VUR showing different patterns of inheritance (VUR = vesicoureteric reflux, RN = reflux nephropathy, PUJO = pelvi-ureteric junction obstruction).

Genetic Aspects

There are strong hereditary factors in the genesis of VUR. Stephens and coworkers (56) described VUR in identical twins in 1955, and since then there have been several other reports of its occurrence in twins (57, 58), in sibships (49, 59–66), and in different generations of the same family (49, 61, 63–67) (Fig. 37.5). The mode of inheritance has not been established, but analysis of pedigrees in the literature suggests autosomal dominance with incomplete penetrance (62, 66, 68). This hypothesis is compatible with the observed familial incidence, the racial differences, the variable severity within families, and the unilateral or bilateral occurrence (68). Alternatively, as with other congenital malformations such as cleft palate, polygenic mechanisms may be operative (61). This pattern of inheritance might explain the apparent difference in incidence of VUR in the two sexes, for it is possible that males have a higher threshold of manifestation requiring a greater number of predisposing genes for clinical expression of the abnormality (68). Sex-linked inheritance has also been suggested (67).

In reviewing reports on the familial incidence of VUR it is necessary to take account of the severity of VUR and scarring in the index case and any bias toward symptomatic individuals in the selection of family members studied. The method of investigating family members presents some problems, for an MCU will only detect those individuals with continuing VUR but not those in whom VUR existed previously but ceased when the UVJ matured. An intravenous urogram (IVU) will reveal scarring in some of these, but even combining these two investigations will underestimate the true familial incidence of VUR.

In prospective studies the prevalence of VUR in siblings of index cases ranges between 15% and 32% (60, 61, 63–65, 69). The highest incidence of VUR is found in siblings of index patients with radiological evidence of reflux nephropathy (62, 65, 66). VUR, reflux nephropathy, or both may be found in completely asymptomatic siblings, and in one study the presence of symptoms referable to the urinary tract was of no value in identifying affected individuals (64). Other urological abnormalities such as duplex systems and pelviureteric obstruction are also more common in these families (62–64, 69).

Studies on histocompatability antigens in patients with VUR and end-stage renal failure have suggested a linkage with HL-A antigen (70–73), but is unclear from the data of the literature if HL-A can be used as a marker in affected families.

Screening family members provides the opportunity to identify VUR before UTI occurs in those at risk of developing scarring. It may also permit detection of asymptomatic individuals with severe scarring liable to hypertension or end-stage renal failure. We therefore advise that newborns with a first-degree relative with VUR, reflux nephropathy, or both be investigated by MCU in the first two months of life. Older siblings of newly diagnosed cases should be screened for reflux nephropathy by IVU, ^{99m}Tc-DMSA scan, or with ultrasound, which is convenient but less accurate.

Clinical Presentation

VUR itself is asymptomatic. The most common event leading to its detection is UTI—85% of children with VUR reported by Goldraich (74). Lenaghan and coworkers (75) reported that VUR presented with UTI in 93% of girls and 71% of boys. Cussen (76) observed that, in a series of 747 autopsies, VUR was three times more common in males than females and concluded that, as a consequence of UTI being less common in boys, VUR was more often occult in them during life. Smellie and coworkers (77) reviewed the records of children with UTI and were not able to identify any symptom that suggested the presence of VUR. Fever was more common in the children with VUR, but the difference from children with UTI but without VUR was not statistically significant.

VUR may be discovered during the investigation of children with chronic renal failure (CRF) or hypertension. It is not infrequently revealed during the evaluation of children with other urological disorders or with multiple congenital abnormalities, particularly malformation of the gastrointestinal or biliary tracts, when the incidence may be as high as 50% (78, 79, 80, 81). Its detection by family studies is described in the previous section.

Consequences

VUR has three major consequences: (a) it maintains a residual volume of urine in the bladder, predisposing to UTI; (b) in the presence of UTI it transmits bacteria to the upper urinary tract; and (c) it permits the transmission of bladder pressure to the kidney.

VUR is the most common abnormality found in children with UTI, being reported in 30% to 50% of affected children (31, 43, 48, 55, 82), whether or not the infection is symptomatic (83, 84) or asymptomatic (85–87). In newborns with UTI, VUR is found in 42% to 57% of cases (47, 48); however, VUR is not the only factor in the genesis of UTI in these children, for recurrent infections may continue in spite of spontaneous cessation or surgical correction of the reflux (15).

The association of VUR and UTI in the genesis of pyelonephritic scarring is considered in the following section. Whether VUR itself can cause renal damage by transmitting bladder pressure remains a moot point, both clinically and experimentally (13, 88).

Natural History

VUR is an unusual congenital abnormality in that it often disappears spontaneously. Hutch (30), observing that the intramural ureter grows from 0.5 cm in the newborn to 1.3 cm in the adult, proposed that the cessation of VUR was attributable to maturation of the UVJ. Baker and coworkers (51) demonstrated progressive disappearance of VUR starting at 2 yr of age. Edwards and coworkers (89) reported the disappearance of VUR in 71% of children and in 79% of ureters of 75 children observed for periods up to 15 yr under conservative treatment. Spontaneous cessation occurred in 85% of the ureters of normal caliber and in 41% of the dilated ureters. Lenaghan and coworkers (75) observed 167 ureters with VUR in 102 patients up to 18 yr and recorded spontaneous disappearance of VUR in 50% of the ureters and in 42% of the patients. Sixty-six percent of the normal-caliber ureters and 26% of the dilated ureters ceased refluxing. Goldraich and coworkers (90) observed cessation of VUR in 65% of 210 ureters in 142 children observed up to 4.5 yr. VUR disappeared spontaneously in 78% of the ureters with slight VUR and in 49% of the ureters with severe VUR. Heale (91) observed that VUR ceased spontaneously in 75% of 268 infants observed into early adult life, ranging from 98% cessation rate in patients with moderate or slight VUR, which largely ceased within 3 yr, to a 25% rate with gross VUR that ceased 3 to 18 yr after birth. Rolleston and coworkers (31) reported disappearance of VUR in 66% of the infants with moderate VUR followed for up to five yr. The spontaneous cessation of VUR is thus well documented.

RENAL SCARRING

The association between coarse renal scarring and VUR is sufficiently well established for it to have earned the designation "reflux nephropathy" (RN) (92); parenchymal bacterial infection is taken to be the primary cause of the renal damage. VUR, however, is also associated with renal dysplasia, which may be difficult on morphological grounds to distinguish from chronic pyelonephritis.

Pathology

Wagner (93), in 1882, studying 150 specimens of small scarred kidneys, identified five cases associated with conditions such as stricture of the urethra, chronic cystitis, or chronic pyelitis that had certain features in common. It is the report of Löhlein (94), however, in 1917, which describes the clinical and pathological findings in three young women who died of uremia, that the modern era of study of chronic pyelonephritis begins. In 1933, Longcope and Winkenwerder (95), based on their experience of nine fatal cases in young women, pointed out the absence of major urological abnormalities, the progression to CRF, and the high prevalence of severe hypertension in the terminal phase. In 1939 and 1940 Weiss and Parker (96, 97) described the histopathological characteristics and the variability of the clinical evolution of chronic pyelonephritis, emphasizing the importance of the vascular lesions induced by infection and their relationship to hypertension. The term reflux nephropathy was used for the first time by Heale and coworkers (98) in 1972, but it was the report of Bailey (92) in 1973 that marked the separation of this entity from the rest of chronic pyelonephritis. The name reflux nephropathy emphasizes that VUR is the important factor in the pathogenesis of the renal lesions, and although there are criticisms of the term (99), it is now being used with increasing frequency. It encompasses all renal lesions associated with VUR, which are similar to those previously described as nonobstructive chronic pyelonephritis. Reflux nephropathy is a focal disease; a scar related to one or more dilated calyces, with a chronic inflammatory reaction, is the specific lesion. The gross examination of the kidney is as important as microscopy in identifying reflux nephropathy, since the microscopic findings themselves are nonspecific (Fig. 37.6). Heptinstall (100) does not believe that it is possible to diagnose chronic pyelonephritis without radiological findings on the caliceal system and the clinician's report concerning the presence of UTI.

VUR and Renal Scarring

In 1960 Hodson and Edwards (7), in a report that is still the most important contribution to the study of VUR, established the relationship between the presence of VUR and the occurrence of chronic pyelonephritis. They demonstrated the association of these findings in 20 patients, 8 of whom did not have a history of UTI. They concluded that VUR was the principal cause of chronic pyelonephritis and observed that the disease could progress to CRF without any urinary symptoms or even UTI. These findings were confirmed by Hutch and coworkers (101) in 14 adults and by McGovern and Marshall (102) in 23 women and 11 men.

Reflux was demonstrated by Rosenheim (103) in 64% of 36 patients with chronic pyelonephritis aged 7 to 46 yr and in 85% of 125 patients studied by Weber and Weylman (104). Servadio and Schachner (105) found VUR in 23% of 60 adults investigated, but in those in whom there was a history of urinary symptoms from childhood, VUR was found in 50%.

In children, Smellie and coworkers (82) observed VUR in 27 of 33 kidneys with chronic pyelonephritis. Scott and Stansfeld (106) observed that renal scars were eight times more frequent in children with UTI if VUR was present: they found VUR in 85% of 114 scarred kidneys. Rolleston and coworkers (31) investigated the relationship between the degree of VUR and the renal lesions and concluded that scars were to be found only in the presence of severe VUR. Additional evidence was obtained from patients with duplex systems in whom scars were found only in the refluxing segments (107).

Vermillion and Heale (108) established a relationship between the position and the configuration of the ureteric orifice and the presence of renal scars in adults, from which they concluded that 89% of 97 kidneys with scars resulted from VUR in childhood and that in 46% of them VUR was still present in adult life.

Several authors (13, 82, 103, 109) observed that the development of

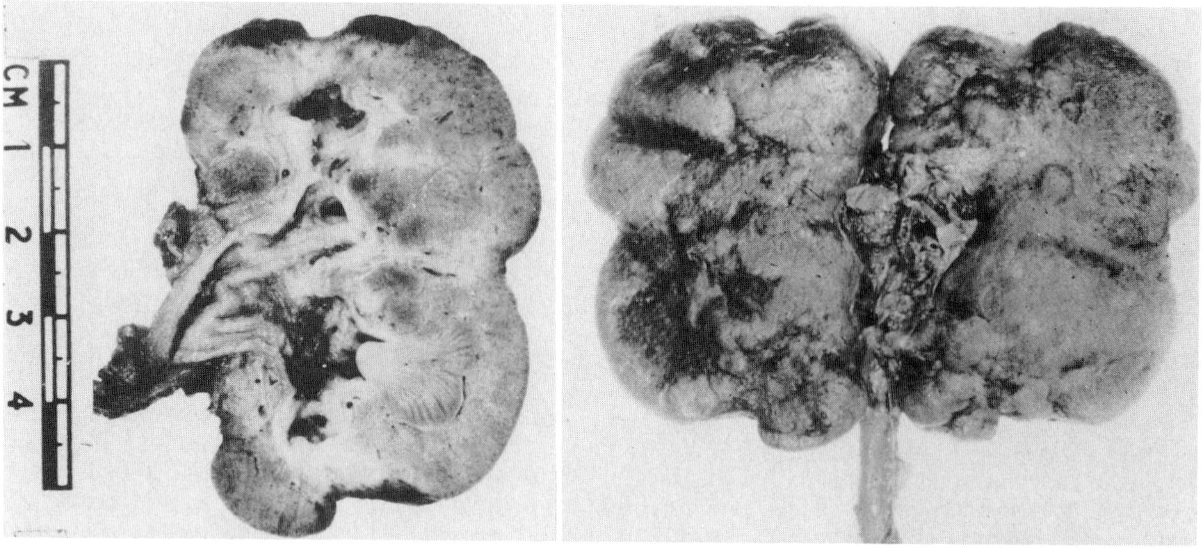

Figure 37.6. Reflux nephropathy in an 18-year-old girl with chronic renal failure and hypertension (courtesy Dr. J. Hodson).

the coarse scars of reflux nephropathy is a phenomenon that is characteristic of the period of rapid growth of the kidney, when it appears to be more susceptible to the effects of VUR. Hodson (109) pointed out that this form of nephropathy is characteristic of children and young adults.

Intrarenal Reflux

Intrarenal reflux is defined in the clinical context by the presence of radiological contrast medium in the renal parenchyma during cystography (Fig. 37.7). It is reported with frequency that varies from 4% to 15% in children with VUR aged less than 16 yr (Table 37.1). Rolleston and coworkers (110, 114) listed the important technical factors that affect the detection of intrarenal reflux; (a) definition of the renal areas; (b) degree of bladder filling; (c) comparison between the films taken before injection of contrast medium and during the peak of VUR; (d) presence of feces in the colon.

Intrarenal reflux was observed for the first time in 1965 by Brodeur (115) in five children with VUR. Amar (116), in 1970, reported the occurrence of intrarenal reflux in 8 patients who were between 2 and 59 yr of age. He suggested that it was a route by which bacteria could enter the renal tubules and parenchyma. Rolleston and coworkers (13, 110) observed that intrarenal reflux occurred only in children younger than 4 yr of age with moderate or severe VUR and demonstrated that scars developed in these areas previously outlined by intrarenal reflux. Bourne and coworkers (111) discussed the possibility of a process of maturation of the renal papillae to explain the infrequency of intrarenal reflux in patients older than 6 yr of age. Scars in areas exposed to intrarenal reflux are observed with a frequency that varies between 27% and 88% (110–113). During follow-up, new scars can be visualized in more than 20% (110). Experimental studies in the minipig, an animal with multipapillary kidneys like humans, confirmed the occurrence of intrarenal reflux and the relationship between it and the development of scars (12, 117). Intrarenal reflux in young minipigs depends on the architecture of the renal papilla and is an all-or-none phenomenon, requiring a critical minimum level of intrapelvic pressure to occur but not increasing in distribution with higher pressure (12, 88, 118, 119, 120). Ransley and Risdon (118, 119, 120) provided an explanation for the confinement of intrarenal reflux to certain papillae. They described two types of renal papillae: simple and compound. The former are conical structures in which the papillary ducts open obliquely on the surface through small slitlike orifices in such a way that increased pressure closes them, preventing intrarenal reflux (Fig. 37.8). Eighty-eight percent of the renal papillae in children and 46% in the minipig are of the simple variety. Compound papillae result from the fusion of two or three adjacent ones with the result that the area cribosa is flattened or even concave. In this circumstance, the papillary ducts open at right angles to the surface, which permits intrarenal reflux to occur. In the minipig as well as in children these compound papillae are found in the polar regions, where the scars of reflux nephropathy are also most prone to occur. Studies in humans indicate that one third of the kidneys contain only simple papillae and are therefore not predisposed to intrarenal reflux, but other combinations of papillary architecture can be found with consequences ranging from complete immunity to bilateral susceptibility to intrarenal reflux.

Intravesical Pressure

Intravesical pressure is another factor that may affect renal scarring in children with VUR. For a long time it has been known that some affected children have bladder sphincter dysfunction expressed clinically by urgency, frequency, and daytime wetting (121, 122). Urodynamic assessment suggests that obstructive uropathy, UTI, and VUR may be consequences of a functional disorder of the bladder in which the activities of the external urethral sphincter and the detrusor are not properly coordinated (121, 123).

When VUR is present, abnormally high bladder pressures may be transmitted to the renal pelvis and papillae where, under normal circumstances, the pressure does not exceed 10 cm of water (124). These abnormal pressures facilitate intrarenal reflux and can last for long periods of time during the phase of bladder filling, though only briefly during voiding.

Two different functional conditions precipitated by UTI can be identified in children with VUR who are otherwise neurologically normal (Fig. 37.9):

1. *Sphincter overactivity or voiding dysfunction.* The children void against an abnormally high pressure resulting from incoordination of detrusor contraction and relaxation of the external sphincter. They have an increased bladder capacity, a postvoiding urine residue, and various degrees of bladder trabeculation with upper tract dilatation (121, 123, 125, 126).

2. *Detrusor overactivity or filling dysfunction.* This is the more com-

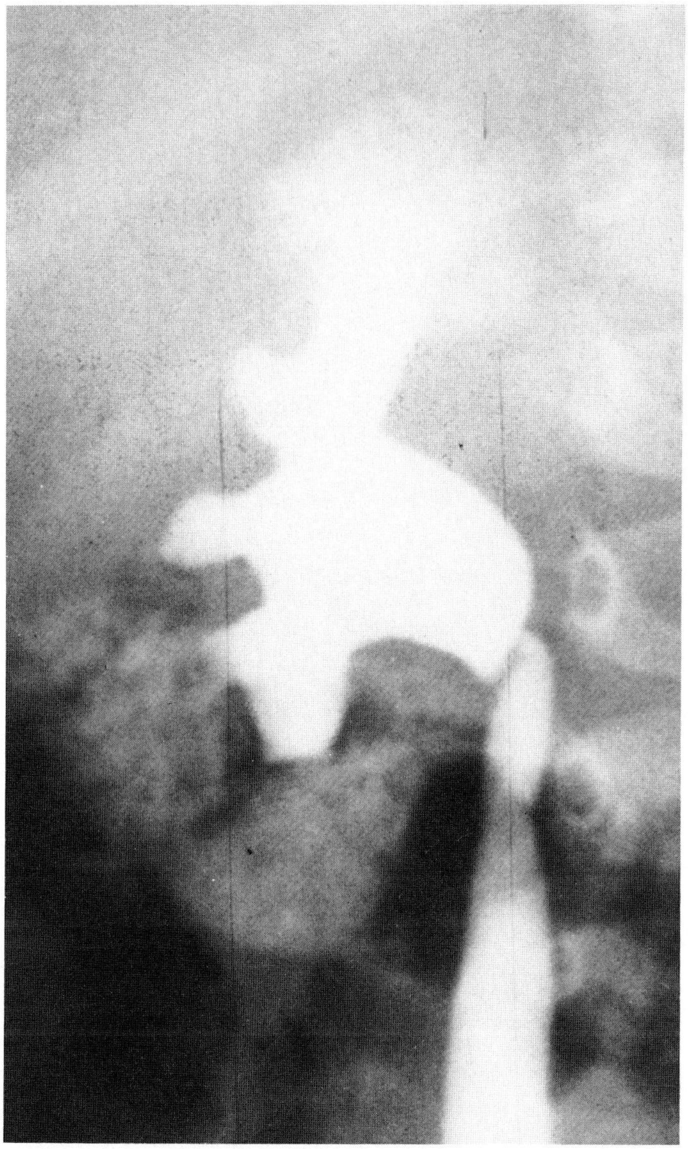

Figure 37.7. Intrarenal reflux demonstrated by cystography in the upper and lower poles.

Table 37.1.
Prevalence of Intrarenal Reflux in Children with Vesicoureteral Reflux

Source	Group studied (age in years)	Number with VUR	IRR n	IRR %
Rolleston (110)	0–4	241	16	6.7
Goldraich (74)	0–5	47	2	4.3
Bourne (111)	<6	47	7	14.9
Rolleston (110)	0–12	344	16	4.6
Uldall (112)	0–13	76	7	9.2
Bourne (111)	0–14	119	8	6.7
Rose (113)	0–16	150	15	10.0

mon urodynamic abnormality found among children with VUR (127). It occurs in children who have uninhibited detrusor contractions; to achieve continence, these children voluntarily increase the tone of their external sphincter. This functions as obstruction to the normal emptying mechanism of the bladder. Pressures exceeding 150 cm of water have been recorded (128). This type of obstruction occurs only during the phase of bladder filling, when the uninhibited detrusor contractions develop, and not during voiding. The signs and symptoms in each patient depend on the relationship between the frequency and intensity of uninhibited detrusor contractions and the effectiveness of sphincter contraction. One feature considered almost pathognomic of uninhibited detrusor contractions is Vincent's curtsey, a maneuver in which the child squats down and compresses the perineum and urethra with a heel to prevent urinary incontinence (129). In this group, the bladder capacity is small, as is residual volume (122, 125, 126, 128, 130).

In children with VUR, sphincter overactivity is significantly associated with renal scarring (131, 132), but this association is not found in children with detrusor overactivity, suggesting that factors other than bladder pressure are involved. The period of toilet training is critical because of alterations occurring in the lower urinary tract with the transition from infantile to adult patterns of urinary control; an increased prevalence of UTI; a greater vulnerability of the kidney to the combined effects of UTI and VUR, and the possibility of persistence of functional disturbances acquired during this period (110, 123, 124, 128, 131, 133).

Urinary Tract Infection

The evidence that both VUR and UTI are necessary for the development of renal scarring is derived from clinical and experimental studies. Patients with VUR but without UTI have been observed for periods up to 23 yr without showing any deterioration of renal function or development of apparent abnormalities on roentgenograms (134, 135). The kidneys of children with VUR and UTI grow normally after the control of infection (136, 137). A convincing argument for the role of UTI was provided by Smellie (137), who compared her experience in the long-term follow-up of children with VUR with that of Lenaghan and coworkers (75) and was able to demonstrate that whereas fresh scarring occurred in 21% of 102 patients observed by Lenaghan and coworkers for 5 to 18 yr on intermittent antibacterial treatment, it was only seen in 1% of her 75 children kept on continuous low-dose prophylaxis for periods of 7 to 15 yr. In addition, all reports on new scars (133, 138–142), with the exception of that from Rolleston and coworkers (110), emphasize a close relationship with UTI.

Hodson and coworkers (88, 117) developed an experimental model in the pig in which they were able to produce different degrees of VUR by section of the ureteral orifice and partial obstruction of the urethra. They demonstrated the occurrence of intrarenal reflux and the development of lesions that were indistinguishable from those of chronic pyelonephritis in those areas with intrarenal reflux. The urine was sterile, and they did not find a polymorph infiltrate or microscopic or immunological evidence of bacterial invasion of the renal parenchyma. They concluded that UTI was not an essential factor in scarring, but they did show that when UTI was superimposed on VUR the time necessary for scars to develop was shorter and the renal damage more severe.

Ransley and Risdon (12, 143) also studied the pig model of VUR, though they used a different sex and strain and a slightly different surgical technique from that of Hodson and coworkers (in which the urethra was partially obstructed) and were able to produce renal scars only in the presence of UTI and not if the urine remained sterile. They showed that when the urine was infected, renal damage occurred rapidly in the course of one to three weeks and were also able to demonstrate that if antimicrobial therapy was started early (in the first week), it was possible to prevent the histological alterations and the development of scarring. More recently, they (144) also produced scars in the sterile condition, but only when high voiding pressures were caused by partial urethral obstruction.

Roberts (145, 146), in studies on the monkey, which has unipapillary

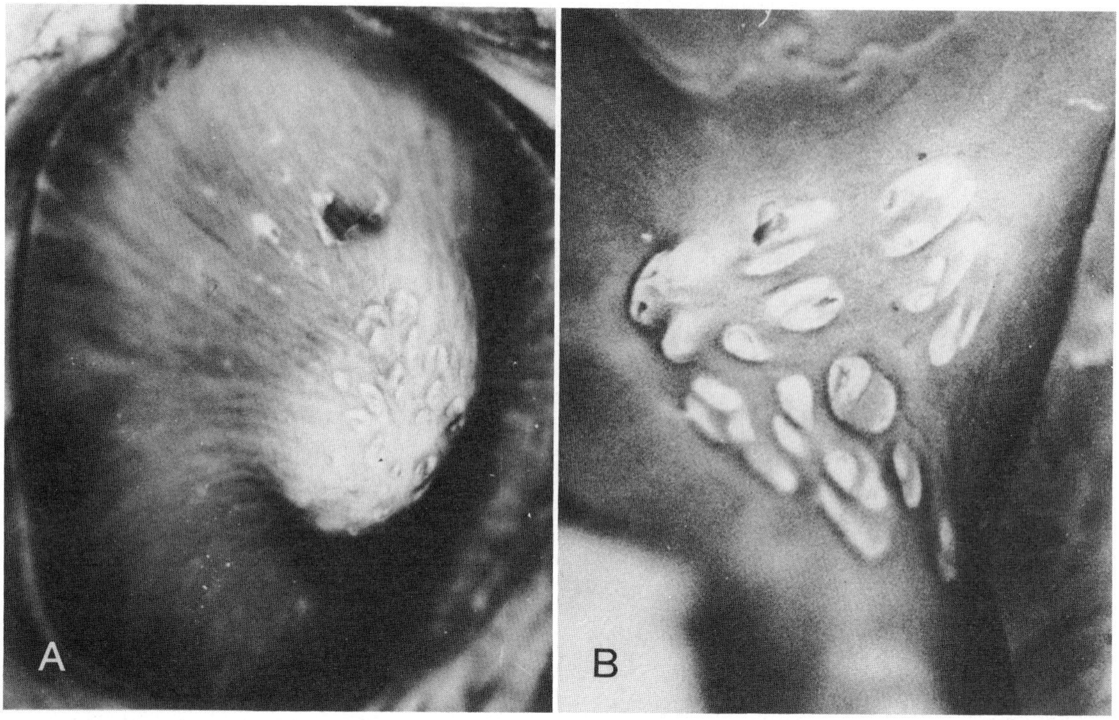

Figure 37.8. Renal papillae in the pig. **A**, Simple papilla. **B**, Compound papilla (courtesy Mr. P. G. Ransley.)

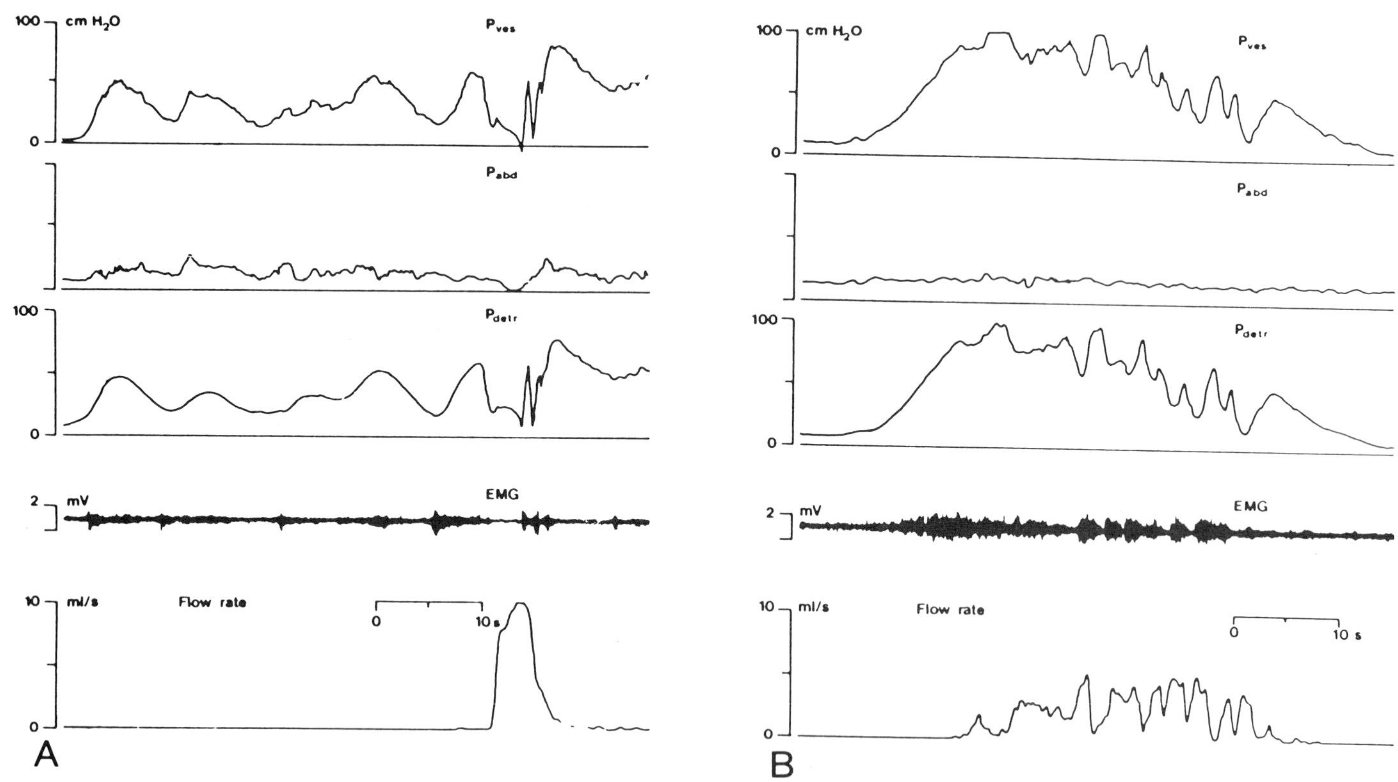

Figure 37.9. Bladder pressure (P ves), rectal pressure (P abd), and calculated detrusor pressure (P detr); pelvic floor electromyogram and urine flow rate in **A**, child with VUR with detrusor overactivity (filling dysfunction) and **B**, child with VUR and sphincter overactivity (emptying dysfunction). (Courtesy Dr. J. D. van Gool (126), reproduced with permission.)

kidneys but shows an age-related maturation of the competence of the UVJ, demonstrated that some strains of *Escherichia coli* produced ureteritis, which altered ureteral mobility and led to functional obstruction. There was an increase in the pressure in the renal pelvis, acute pyelonephritis, and progressive renal damage. Studies on bacterial adhesion (14) have identified *E. coli* containing P-fimbriae as most likely to cause acute pyelonephritis (see Chapter 14). In subsequent studies in the monkey (147), it was shown that the *E. coli* poducing these abnormalities are those that have P-fimbriae and that the monkey has P-fimbriae receptors; this suggests an interplay of host and bacterial factors in the pathogenesis of scarring.

Renal Dysplasia

Renal dysplasia is defined as an abnormal differentiation of the renal parenchyma characterized histologically by the presence of primitive collecting ducts and cartilaginous metaplasia (148–150). It is well established that renal dysplasia results from abnormal development of the ureteral bud (150–153). Beck (154), Potter (155), and Bernstein (149) have shown that retrograde pressure starting early in intrauterine life produces renal dysplasia.

In 1953, Marshall (156) found fetal structures in pyelonephritic kidneys and concluded that in children, renal dysplasia was the cause of coarse scarring associated with VUR. Ericsson and Ivemark (152, 153) confirmed the findings of Marshall. Persky (157, 158) identified focal areas of dysplasia in pyelonephritic kidneys without obstruction and postulated that in childhood shrunken kidneys might be the result of dysplasia and not of infection. Stephens and Lenaghan (8) suggested that the congenital abnormalities that occur in patients with VUR (megaureter, bladder diverticula, multiple ureters, and renal dysplasia) are frequently associated with generalized maldevelopment of the ureteral bud. This maldevelopment may have a genetic origin (159) or may result from retrograde transmission of pressure by VUR to the ureteral bud (151, 152, 160). Bialestock (161) found that severe dysplasia was more frequent in patients with VUR and obstruction than in cases with VUR alone. Cussen (76) found a significant association between VUR and renal dysplasia in 21 children with primary VUR identified in the course of 747 consecutive autopsies. Stecker and coworkers (160) also found dysplastic kidneys in six children with VUR. During a study of double ureters, Mackie and Stephens (162) demonstrated a significant association between the position of the ureteral orifice and the presence or absence of renal dysplasia: the more ectopic the ureteral orifice, the more abnormal the kidney. According to these authors, UTI in childhood merely leads to the diagnosis of this abnormal situation and is not involved in the pathogenesis of scarring.

Summary

With the knowledge derived from experimental studies and clinical observations it is apparent that the term reflux nephropathy subsumes three different situations:

1. Maldevelopment of the ureteric bud, resulting in renal dysplasia associated with VUR.
2. High-pressure VUR, usually sterile (but when infected, the renal damage is accelerated), resulting in generalized thinning of the renal parenchyma and dilatation of the pelvis and all the calyces.
3. A combination of UTI and VUR leading to the focal form of scarring in areas at risk because of intrarenal reflux.

Diagnosis

Intravenous Urogram (IVU)

Reflux nephropathy is normally assessed in vivo by its radiological features (92). Hodson (109, 163) established the criteria for the diagnosis of reflux nephropathy on the intravenous urogram (IVU); they consist of localized contraction of the renal parenchyma (scar) with clubbing of the adjacent calyx, resulting from focal destruction of kidney parenchyma with blunting and retraction of the renal papilla. This association is characteristic but not specific for reflux nephropathy (Fig. 37.10).

Analysis of a large number of IVUs from apparently healthy children of different ages demonstrates that (a) the growth of the normal kidney is related to the increase in body height of the child; (b) the renal parenchyma compared to kidney length is proportionally thicker in the child than in the adult; (c) it is not until the end of the second decade that the adult kidney size is reached; (d) the size of both kidneys is similar unless a duplex system or other anomaly is present; (e) the thickness of the renal parenchyma is similar in the four polar regions (163–165).

In patients with VUR, the earliest sign of renal damage is asymmetry of the two kidneys resulting from growth arrest of the diseased kidney and accentuated by the compensatory hypertrophy of the other one. It is important to observe that when there is severe unilateral disease and the contralateral kidney remains within normal size limits, it cannot be regarded as healthy. When the disease is bilateral, growth of both kidneys decreases, but even in this situation kidney size is usually not symmetrical (109, 165–167).

Several reports (99, 110, 166) suggest the possibility of two forms of reflux nephropathy defined according to the radiological features:

1. Focal features. Coarse scars in a distribution characteristic of reflux nephropathy. They are usually polar, and their localization depends on the lobar composition of the kidney and the presence of the compound papillae described by Ransley and Risdon (120).
2. Diffuse features. Calyceal dilatation with thinning of the parenchyma that is indistinguishable from obstructive nephropathy. This form is often first diagnosed in an advanced state and is usually not identified in its early stages, when the papillary changes are subtle and the damage can only be assessed by measuring parenchyma thickness (166).

Hodson and Wilson (168) point out that the pattern of scarring is the best way of grading the severity of renal damage. In 1970 Rolleston and coworkers (31) proposed three degrees of scarring, and in 1975, Lindberg and coworkers (169) also quantified the renal damage in three grades. It is, however, Smellie's and coworkers' (11) four-grade classification of renal scarring that has become best established and is the classification adopted by the International Reflux Study Committee (14) (Fig. 37.11):

Grade A. Mild scarring: not more than two scarred areas.

Grade B. Severe scarring: more generalized scars but with areas of normal tissue between them.

Grade C. "Back-pressure" type: contraction of the whole kidney without or with very few scars in the outline, similar to obstructive nephropathy.

Grade D. End-stage shrunken kidney with little or no function, indistinguishable radiologically from a hypoplastic or dysplastic kidney.

The different types of reflux nephropathy do not represent different phases of disease progression. New scars are occasionally formed, but progression from the focal (grades A and B) to a generalized form (grade C) has not been reported.

The contraction produced by the scar, accentuated by the hypertrophy of the normal surrounding renal tissues, is not immediately visualized on the IVU after the causative UTI. Hodson and Wilson (168) observed in one patient that severe bipolar scars took 15 months to develop. Filly and coworkers (139) found, during the follow-up of children with VUR, that the scar and the papillary abnormalities were fully developed only after two years. This is also the experience of Smellie and Normand (133), although Smellie and coworkers reported that the minimum period for a scar to become apparent in a previously normal kidney was nine months (11). Hugosson et al (141) documented in infants and preschool children an interval of eight months as the shortest period for a scar to be evident on the IVU.

There are some difficulties with the use of the IVU to diagnose reflux nephropathy in children: (a) inadequate visualization of the renal outlines, especially in infants and preschool children, due to excessive amounts of gas in the bowel combined with the poor ability of the renal tubules to concentrate the radiological contrast medium; (b) latency period necessary for complete development of the scar; (c) interference of several factors (respiratory movements, position of the patient, distortion) on sequential measurements of renal size; (d) dose of radiation, especially when repeated IVUs are required in the follow-up of the patient.

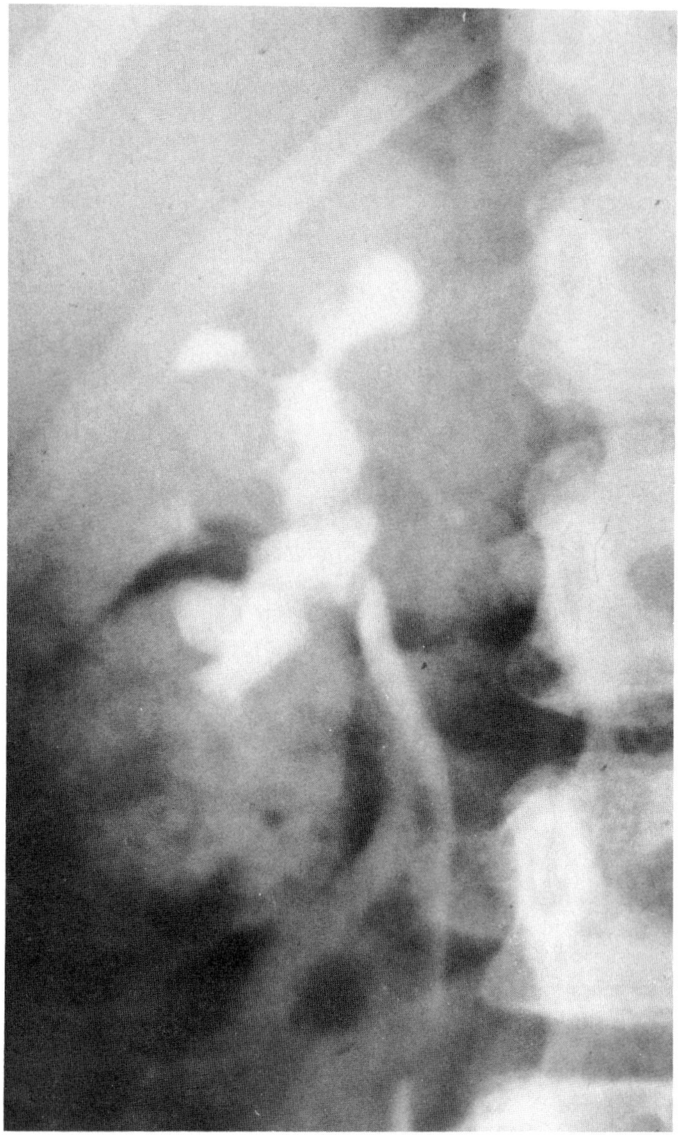

Figure 37.10. IVU demonstrating reflux nephropathy.

^{99m}Tc-DMSA Scan

^{99m}Tc-DMSA, a radiopharmaceutical introduced in 1974 by Lin and coworkers (170), is a cortical marker that provides both functional (absolute individual and total renal function) and anatomical data (presence of scars, contraction of the whole kidney, or both) (171–175). This is particularly useful in a disease such as reflux nephropathy, in which even when bilateral, the renal damage is always asymmetrical. A scar is defined as a defect in the kidney outline with reduced ^{99m}Tc-DMSA uptake. Reflux nephropathy is identified by the presence of scars or by contraction of the whole kidney (Fig. 37.12).

The ^{99m}Tc-DMSA renal scan is now the most suitable method for the initial assessment and follow-up observation of kidneys of children with VUR. It does not require patient preparation and is not affected by bowel gas. It avoids risks inherent with contrast material; it gives better visualization of the renal parenchyma (especially with combined posterior and oblique views) than the IVU; and the radiation dose is less than with conventional radiography, permitting more frequent follow-up. The absolute uptake of the injected dose of ^{99m}Tc-DMSA in each kidney of healthy children is $33 \pm 3.3\%$ (175).

Smellie's four-grade radiological classification of renal scarring (see section on IVU) can be adapted to the findings of the ^{99m}Tc-DMSA scan to grade the intensity of chronic pyelonephritis (90, 176):

Type 1: no more than two scarred areas.

Type 2: more than two scars with some areas of normal parenchyma in between.

Type 3: generalized damage to the whole kidney, similar to obstructive nephropathy, i.e., contraction of the whole kidney with or without scars in the outline.

Type 4: end-stage, shrunken kidney with little or no uptake of ^{99m}Tc-DMSA, i.e., less than 10% of the overall renal function.

The ^{99m}Tc-DMSA scan is superior to the IVU in demonstrating the alterations characteristic of reflux nephropathy. It is now not sufficient to define a kidney as normal in a child with VUR on the basis of the IVU findings alone (177–179).

Goldraich and coworkers (179, 180) undertook a prospective comparison of the IVU and the ^{99m}Tc-DMSA scan in the initial assessment of children with VUR. Two hundred and ninety-nine kidneys in 202 patients were evaluated by both methods. All the children had sterile urine for at least four weeks before the tests were performed and between the two investigations, which were usually done with an interval of one week or less. The results of this study are shown in Table 37.2. Discrepancies were observed in 37 kidneys of 31 patients. Thirty-four kidneys in 28 children were normal on the IVU but had reflux nephropathy on the ^{99m}Tc-DMSA scan (type 1 in 24, type 2 in 6, and type 3 in 4). Three

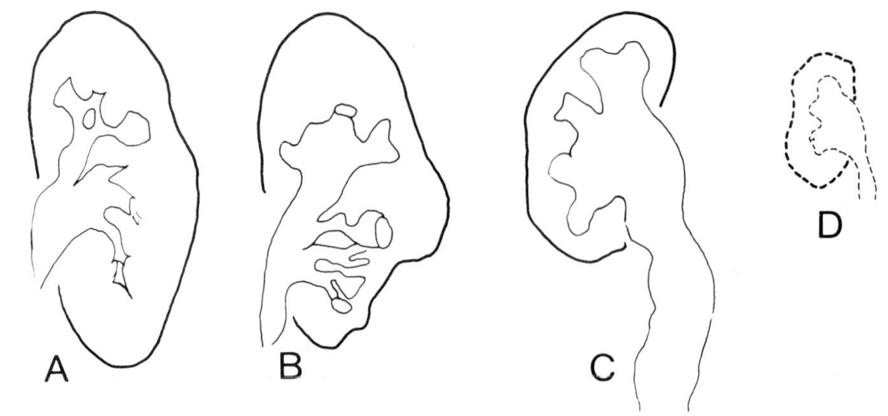

Figure 37.11. Grading of renal scarring adopted by International Reflux Study Committee (14).

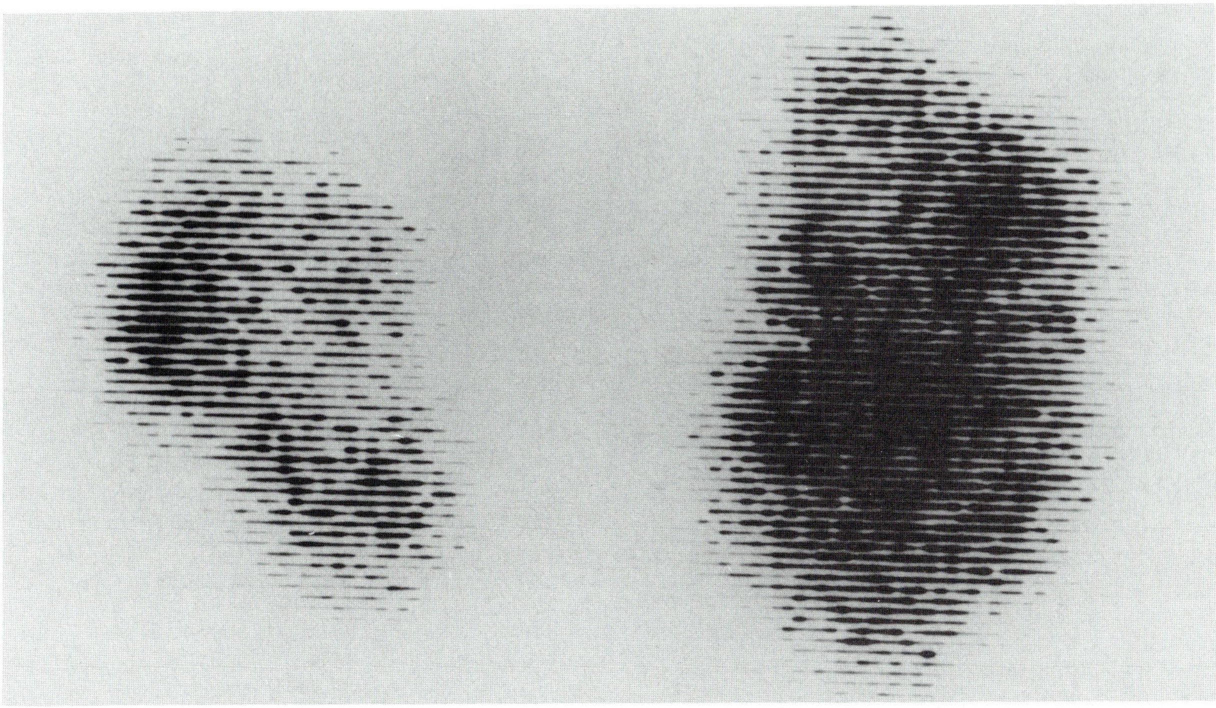

Figure 37.12. Right oblique view of ^{99m}Tc-DMSA scan showing bilateral reflux nephropathy more severe (type III) in right side.

kidneys from three patients with VUR were diagnosed as scarred on the IVU but appeared normal on the ^{99m}Tc-DMSA scan. The abnormalities identified on the ^{99m}Tc-DMSA scan may precede the radiological findings. New scars that are seen in sequential IVU can be visualized significantly earlier by the ^{99m}Tc-DMSA scan and shortly after the UTI. Focal defects in the static images and a decrease in ^{99m}Tc-DMSA uptake may be transiently and reversibly associated with acute UTI. To avoid misleading results, the ^{99m}Tc-DMSA renal scan should only be performed after four weeks of sterile urine.

Differential Diagnosis

The differential diagnosis of reflux nephropathy in childhood includes persistent fetal lobulation, postobstructive atrophy, renal dysplasia, and renovascular accidents (papillary necrosis, medullary necrosis, cortical necrosis, and renal vein thrombosis) (11, 92, 109, 181, 182).

In persistent fetal lobulation, the deformities in the renal outline are situated between the calyces and not immediately adjacent to them (109). In postobstructive atrophy there is a symmetrical involvement of the calyces and reduction of the thickness of renal parenchyma (181); however, when there is a generalized form of reflux nephropathy (grade C of Smellie's radiological classification or type 3 of the ^{99m}Tc-DMSA renal scan classification), it may be impossible to differentiate the two entities. Also, renal dysplasia can be indistinguishable from reflux nephropathy grade D of Smellie's classification or type 4 of the radionuclide classification. Renovascular accidents, especially if partial or unilateral, may escape recognition. They result later in a shrunken kidney with scars and papillary abnormalities. These patients can also develop hypertension and renal impairment and are more prone to develop UTI (182).

Prevalence

Prevalence Detected by IVU

Wide variation in the prevalence of scarring in children with VUR has been reported in the literature. The factors that should be considered when comparing the results from different series are (a) age of patients

Table 37.2.
Comparative Study Between Intravenous Urogram and ^{99m}Tc-DMSA Scan for Diagnosis of Reflux Nephropathy[a]

IVU	^{99m}Tc-DMSA	Infants n	Infants %	Preschool n	Preschool %	School-age n	School-age %	Total n	Total %
0	+	9	10	22	17	3	4	34	11
0	0	66	73	75	56	41	55	182	61
+	0	2	2	1	1	0	0	3	1
+	+	14	15	35	26	31	41	80	27
Total		91	100	133	100	75	100	299	100

[a] (+ = present, 0 = absent)

included; (b) severity of VUR; (c) source of referral; (d) quality of the radiology employed. Tables 37.3 and 37.4 list different reports on the prevalence of reflux nephropathy at diagnosis of VUR.

Smellie and Normand (188) compared the prevalence of scarring between children with symptomatic UTI and those with asymptomatic bacteruria identified during screening and did not find any significant difference. They also showed that scarring was present in a higher proportion in children with recurrent rather than with presumed first UTI.

Prevalence Detected by ^{99m}Tc-DMSA Scan

Goldraich (179) studied 300 kidneys with VUR but without other major abnormalities on the MCU in 203 children. The criteria for including patients in this prospective study were (a) plasma creatinine concentration less than 2 mg/dl; (b) proteinuria less than 200 mg/24 hr; (c) no previous radiological, endoscopic, or surgical procedure on the urinary tract. The prevalence of reflux nephropathy using the static images of the ^{99m}Tc-DMSA scan is given in Table 37.5. There was a significant association between the age of the patients when VUR was diagnosed, the grade of VUR and the presence of reflux nephropathy. Table 37.6 shows the distribution of types of reflux nephropathy in the 115 affected kidneys. The data presented in Table 37.6 confirm the

Table 37.3.
Prevalence of Reflux Nephropathy on Intravenous Urogram at Diagnosis of Vesicoureteral Reflux According to Number of Patients

Source	Group studied	Patients with VUR	RN n	RN %
Woodard (183)	Children	118	23	20
Williams (184)	Children	276	88	32
Newcastle (86)	School-age girls	54	18	33
Dwoskin (33)	Children (0–15 yr)	281	98	35
Smellie (11)	Children (0–12 yr)	56	22	39
Goldraich (185)	Children (0–14 yr)	59	25	42

Table 37.4.
Prevalence of Reflux Nephropathy on Intravenous Urogram at Diagnosis of Vesicoureteral Reflux According to Number of Kidneys with Vesicoureteral Reflux

Source	Group studied	Kidneys with VUR	RN n	RN %
Rolleston (110)	Children <5 yr	365	58	16
Rolleston (13)	Infants (0–1 yr)	130	29	22
Goldraich (179)	Children (0–12 yr)	299	83	28
Lenaghan (75)	Children	120	44	37
Savage (186)	School-age children	45	25	55
Filly (139)	Girls <10 yr	77	48	62
Kern (187)	Men <50 yr	12	10	83

findings previously reported by others (11, 13) based on the IVU that the generalized form (type 3) is the most common type of reflux nephropathy in infants.

New Scars

A consistent finding in the long-term follow-up of children with VUR is that the renal scars are already present in the first examination and that new scars are rarely seen to develop in previously normal kidneys. Children with VUR included in prospective studies are not an appropriate population in which to study the natural history of scarring since they are kept under careful medical observation, with the majority of them on prophylactic chemotherapy, so recurrence of UTI is not a usual event. There is now an almost general agreement that if the kidneys are normal on the first examination of a child over 5 yr of age it is not necessary to repeat the imaging of the kidneys even if the child has several recurrences of UTI.

There are many reports showing that new scars can develop in previously normal kidneys (11, 110, 138–142, 168, 189). In all, except in the patients reported by Rolleston and coworkers (110), a relationship between UTI and scarring was present. It has also been shown that new scars usually develop during the first five years of life when the kidney is more vulnerable to the combined effects of UTI and VUR (49, 139–141).

Functional Assessment

For an adequate assessment of the effects of VUR on the kidney it is necessary to combine anatomical evaluation with functional information. Aperia and coworkers (190) used inulin clearance and measurement of tubular reabsorption of glucose in children with unilateral external ureteric compression and observed that when VUR was slight or moderate the renal function was not affected, but that when severe VUR was present there was a functional impairment that was already present at the beginning of the study and that became more accentuated with increasing age of the children. They did not relate their findings to the presence or absence of scarring.

Verrier-Jones and coworkers (191) studied individual glomerular filtration in schoolgirls with asymptomatic bacteriuria using ^{99m}Tc-DTPA. They demonstrated that there was no significant difference in mean glomerular filtration rate between kidneys with and without VUR. When the kidneys were normal on the IVU, mean glomerular filtration rate was significantly greater than the mean or scarred kidneys. They concluded that the difference in the glomerular filtration rate depended on the presence of reflux nephropathy rather than from the effects of VUR itself.

Goldraich and coworkers (90, 192) assessed individual renal function using the absolute uptake of ^{99m}Tc-DMSA. They showed that 25% of 210 refluxing kidneys had functional impairment when VUR was diagnosed. No significant differences were found in the functional index of different age groups in spite of different prevalence of reflux nephropathy, indicating that compensatory hypertrophy of undamaged parenchyma can mask the effects of reflux nephropathy on kidney function. In a further study (179), in which 300 kidneys with VUR in 203 children were assessed, they demonstrated that when the kidneys were classified as anatomically normal on the ^{99m}Tc-DMSA scan image, the functional index was normal or increased. When there was scarring, however, the functional index could be normal, increased, or reduced (Fig. 37.13). It is important to consider the interaction between the two kidneys in these patients with VUR. To compensate for the effects of loss of normal renal parenchyma, there is hypertrophy of the rest of the normal parenchyma in the affected kidney and in the contralateral kidney. The long-term consequences of this situation are unknown but may lead to hyperfiltration injury and late deterioration of renal function (193).

Consequences

The consequences of renal scarring are hypertension, CRF, glomerulopathy, and complications during pregnancy.

Hypertension

Hypertension is a late complication of reflux nephropathy. It may be

Table 37.5.
Prevalence of Reflux Nephropathy on ^{99m}Tc-DMSA Scan in Children with Vesicoureteral Reflux

	Infants	Preschool	School-age	Total
n kidneys	92	133	75	300
n RN	24	57	34	115
% RN	26	43	45	38

Table 37.6.
Distribution of Kidneys with Reflux Nephropathy According to Degree of Scarring on ^{99m}Tc-DMSA Scan

RN	Infants n	Infants %	Preschool n	Preschool %	School-age n	School-age %
Type 1	4	17	18	32	11	32
Type 2	7	29	22	39	8	24
Type 3	13	54	17	30	13	38
Type 4	0	0	0	0	2	6
Total	24	100	57	100	34	100

benign and relatively easy to control or may, less frequently, present as malignant hypertension (104). Hypertension occurs in both unilateral and bilateral reflux nephropathy. Ischemic vascular lesions and the renin-angiotensin system have been implicated in its pathogenesis (96, 194), but the role of the latter is still controversial (195, 196).

Reflux nephropathy was reported as a cause of severe and persistent hypertension in childhood in 33% of the 55 children studied by Still and Cottom (197), in 30% of the 32 patients reported by Goldraich and coworkers (198), in 19% of the 100 children in the series of Gill and coworkers (199), and 18% of the 326 patients reported by Dillon (200) (see Chapter 47).

Several authors (201–203) have described a syndrome characterized by the occurrence of severe hypertension, bilateral VUR, and bilateral scarred kidney. Holland (204) reviewed the literature of this subject and analyzed 177 reports on children and young adults. The renal abnormality was described as "chronic pyelonephritis" in 99, "segmental hypoplasia" in 49, "primary interstitial nephritis" in 15, "reflux nephropathy" in 8, and "Ask-Upmark kidney" in 6. The ages of the patients varied between 3 and 40 yr, but the majority were adolescent. The ratio of females to males was 5:1.

Various prevalences of hypertension among children with VUR (see Table 37.7) and patients with scarred kidneys (see Table 37.8) have been reported in the literature.

Chronic Renal Failure

Reflux nephropathy is an important cause of CRF in children and young adults. In a series of children with end-stage CRF, reflux nephropathy was responsible for 9.6% of the 270 patients reported by Habib and coworkers (210), for 21.3% of the 75 patients reported by Chantler and coworkers (211); for 15% of the 63 cases reported by Goldraich and coworkers (212); and for 50% of the 12 patients reported by Bailey and

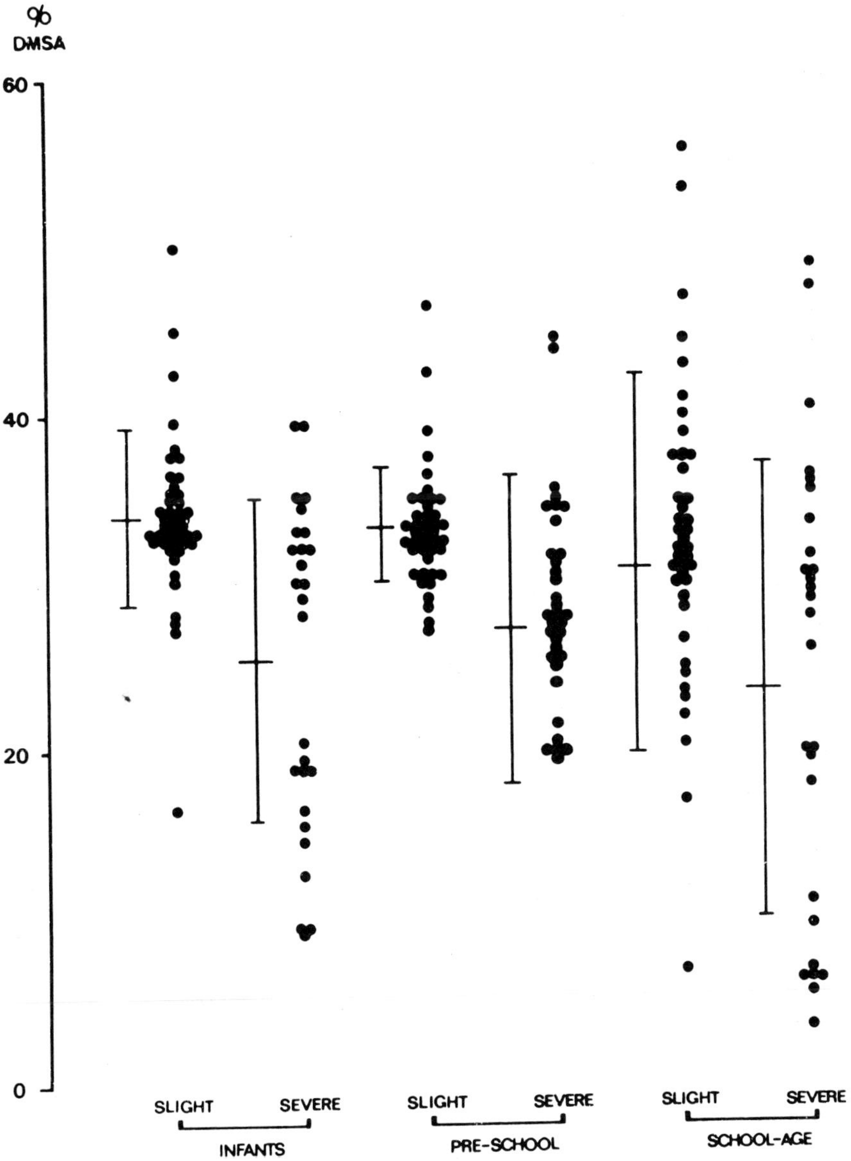

Figure 37.13. Absolute renal uptake of ^{99m}Tc-DMSA, expressed as a percentage of the administered dose, in children with slight (Rolleston grade I and II) or severe (Rolleston grade III) VUR (179).

Table 37.7.
Prevalence of Hypertension among Children with Vesicoureteral Reflex

Source	Number of children with VUR	Hypertension n	Hypertension %
Savage (186)	36	0	0
MacGregor (52)	92	2	2.2
Still[a] (197)	276	8	3.0
Lenaghan (75)	102	10	9.8
Smellie (82)	56	7	12.5
Goldraich (205)	58	9	15.5

[a] Included only children with diastolic pressure >95 mm Hg.

Table 37.8.
Prevalence of Hypertension in Patients with Reflux Nephropathy

Source	Group studied	Number with RN	Hypertension n	Hypertension %
Savage (186)	Children	24	0	0.0
Ambrose (206)	Adults	45	7	15.6
Hutch (207)	Adults	22	4	18.0
Smellie (11)	Children	83	17	20.5
Servadio (105)	Adults	60	15	25.0
Goldraich (205)	Children	47	3	27.6
McGovern (102)	Adults	35	10	28.6
Rosenheim (208)	Children + adults	36	11	30.6
Hinman (209)	Adults	9	3	33.3

Lynn (2). In the Combined Report on Regular Dialysis and Transplantation in Children in Europe, 1980 (1), reflux nephropathy was responsible for 21.9% of the 2778 cases included. Data from the Australasian Renal Replacement Programmes for the period 1971–1980 show that when patients under the age of 16 yr were considered, 34% of 158 in Australia and 19% of 32 in New Zealand that entered the program had end-stage CRF secondary to reflux nephropathy (2).

In adults, reflux nephropathy was found in 8.4% of the 403 patients on regular hemodialysis in New South Wales (213) and in 10% of the 667 patients with end-stage CRF included in the Australia and New Zealand Combined Dialysis and Transplant Registry from November 1980 to October 1981 (2).

Based on the data of the European Dialysis and Transplant Association Registry from 1977, Bailey and Lynn (2) calculated that 0.3 to 0.4 children/million of the population/year under the age of 15 yr will present with CRF due to reflux nephropathy. In the adult population, Kincaid-Smith (214) estimated that 5 to 10 women/million population/year go into end-stage CRF secondary to reflux nephropathy. These figures may be an underestimate, for sometimes it is difficult to identify the association between end-stage renal failure in the adult and VUR in childhood.

MacGregor (215) studied the outcome of children with scarred kidneys and VUR and suggested that there was among them a small subgroup with a malignant course who died in adolescence or in early adult life with CRF, associated or not with hypertension; he called the condition "pyelonephritis lenta." The patients usually remained asymptomatic until they went into end-stage CRF.

The rate of progression of CRF with reflux nephropathy is variable. Lewy and Sorrenti (203) followed the renal function of 18 patients aged 7 to 16 yr. At the beginning of the study 8 of them had a plasma creatinine concentration less than 1.6 mg/100 ml. During a period of four to six yr, 6 of them remained with stable renal function but other 2 required dialysis treatment. The remaining 10 patients initially had a plasma creatinine concentration above 2 mg/100 ml, and 8 of them entered a dialysis program in periods that ranged from one to seven yr. Salvatierra and coworkers (216) observed during the follow-up of 18 patients with end-stage CRF secondary to reflux nephropathy that the mean age at which CRF was identified as 19.1 yr, but that the range was 5 to 36 yr. Kincaid-Smith and coworkers (217) reported that males with CRF due to reflux nephropathy required dialysis earlier (mean age: 22 yr) than females (mean age: 33 yr). They also observed that CRF secondary to reflux nephropathy developed at an earlier age compared with other categories of CRF (mean age: 33 yr for men and 39 yr for women).

Reflux Glomerulopathy

According to Kincaid-Smith (214, 217), proteinuria is the most important feature heralding a poor outcome in patients with reflux nephropathy. Once proteinuria has developed, the course of progression to renal failure is normally gradual but inexorable over 5 to 10 yr and may be accelerated by malignant hypertension or pregnancy. She also pointed out the association of proteinuria with atypical and fastidious microorganisms in the urinary tract (214).

Zimmerman and coworkers (218), Kincaid-Smith (219), Bhathena and coworkers (220), Torres and coworkers (221), Goldraich and coworkers (222), and Bailey and coworkers (223), among others, described the glomerular lesions in patients with reflux nephropathy now known as reflux glomerulopathy. There is a general agreement that this glomerulopathy is responsible for the deterioration of the renal function in patients with reflux nephropathy. In all the 23 cases reported by Bhathena and coworkers (220) and in 78% of the 122 patients of the series of Kincaid-Smith (219), the histological findings were categorized as focal glomerulosclerosis. Kincaid-Smith (219) pointed out that the more advanced and widespread lesions were found in patients with severely impaired renal function. Reflux glomerulopathy has even been found in the contralateral nonscarred normal-sized or hypertrophied kidney (217, 223).

Cotran (224) listed four mechanisms that might be involved in the genesis of this glomerulopathy: (a) immunological injury; (b) macromolecular trapping and mesangial dysfunction; (c) vascular changes and hypertension; (d) glomerular hyperfiltration. The hypothesis now considered most plausible is that the glomerular lesions are secondary to the hemodynamic alterations (hyperfiltration) resulting from a reduction in renal mass. The focal lesions of reflux nephropathy are similar to those observed after subtotal nephrectomy and in other situations leading to glomerular hyperperfusion (193, 221, 224).

Pregnancy

Complications during pregnancy are a prominent feature in women with reflux nephropathy. Pregnancy also accelerates the deterioration of renal function in women with reflux nephropathy and impaired renal function.

Kincaid-Smith and Becker (225) reviewed the data on 48 women aged 16 yr or more with reflux nephropathy and VUR and found that 13 (27%) of them developed their first symptom in relation to pregnancy (10 presented with UTI, 1 with hypertension, and 2 with postpartum edema and proteinuria). Thirty-seven women had 85 pregnancies, and complications occurred in 59 of them, principally hypertension, edema, and UTI.

Verrier-Jones (226) analyzed the data on 52 pregnancies occurring in nine women with scarred kidneys and in 27 with normal kidneys with or without VUR who had been identified during a bacteriuria survey of children in Oxford and Cardiff in 1972, and compared the findings with those in healthy control subjects. Women with reflux nephropathy had significantly higher blood pressure and heavier proteinuria during the third trimester than the controls and the women with normal kidneys. They were also more likely to require obstetric intervention with induction of labor and operative delivery.

Natural History

The natural history of reflux nephropathy can be divided into three phases. The first begins in childhood and is characterized by UTI, usually recurrent; it is during this period that the irreversible lesions of reflux nephropathy develop. The second phase is asymptomatic and follows the cessation of VUR. A few patients reach the third phase in adolescence or early adult life, which is again symptomatic as a consequence of hypertension, impairment of renal function, or both.

It is remarkable that there is a period that is absolutely asymptomatic and that lasts for years before hypertension or CRF develop. Although there is a considerable body of information in the literature on the two symptomatic phases, little is known about the intermediate one. It is not known what proportion of patients with VUR have a poor outcome since only those that enter the third symptomatic phase are identified. In contrast to VUR, which is characterized by a high rate of spontaneous resolution, reflux nephropathy is a progressive disease that may lead to hypertension, CRF, glomerulopathy, and complications during pregnancy.

MANAGEMENT

Clinical Observations

The demonstration of a high rate of spontaneous resolution of VUR (11, 51) and the realization that new scars are not formed if UTI is adequately controlled (90, 133) have changed the approach to children with VUR that previously had been essentially surgical. Also, reports showing that successful reimplantation of the ureters did not prevent the development of hypertension in children with scarring (227), nor alter or delay the progression to end-stage CRF in patients who already had impaired renal function (228), reinforced the conservative approach.

Following the careful but uncontrolled studies of Smellie and coworkers (11, 89), the first reports of controlled studies of conservative versus operative management of VUR have now been published. In 1983, the Birmingham Reflux Study Group (15, 229) presented the two-year follow-up results on 96 children with severe primary VUR (grade III of Rolleston's classification), with or without reflux nephropathy. The patients were stratified in three age groups and then allocated randomly to conservative or surgical treatment. At the end of two yr of follow-up, there was no significant difference between the groups in the incidence of breakthrough UTI (25% in each group), ^{51}Cr-edetic acid glomerular filtration rate, renal length, new scar formation, or progression of existing scars on IVU. Surgery was successful in correcting VUR in 97% of the cases, and 74% of the ureters treated conservatively still refluxed at the end of two yr. The five-yr follow-up data on these patients are now available and do not show any significant difference between treatment groups (230).

The preliminary results of the International Collaborative Study on Reflux in Children (231), which included 116 children up to 10 yr of age with primary VUR (grades IV and V of the International classification) allocated randomly to medical and surgical treatment, did not show any significant differences in the results of the two treatments after five yr; however, it is important to emphasize that this is still a short period in which to draw conclusions on the natural history of VUR treated conservatively or surgically.

Vesicoureteric Reflux

Conservative Treatment

The principle of conservative treatment is to prevent UTI while VUR persists in order to avoid progression of renal damage. One of the difficulties with conservative treatment is that there is no guide to predict if or when VUR is going to disappear. All the parameters suggested (cystoscopic appearance of the ureteral orifices, age at diagnosis of VUR, degree of ureteral dilatation, presence of reflux nephropathy, occurrence of UTI during conservative treatment) have proved unsuccessful.

Simple Measures. Children with VUR who are susceptible to recurrent UTI should be guided in simple measures that reduce the risks of bacterial infection: regular and complete voiding and control of constipation. Maintenance of high fluid intake should be advised provided uninhibited detrusor contractions have been excluded (128).

Chemoprophylaxis. Antimicrobial therapy in most instances prevents recurrence of UTI. Retrospective comparison of results from different centers suggests that renal damage is less when infections are carefully controlled by prophylaxis (11) than when care is less rigorous (75). Nevertheless it is important to emphasize that there is no prospective controlled study to support the use of regular antibiotic prophylaxis. In the Cardiff-Oxford survey (232), control of asymptomatic bacteriuria in schoolgirls did not offer any advantages over the treatment of symptomatic infections alone. Further, the development of a new scar in an apparently normal kidney in a child over 5 yr of age is uncommon, even if VUR is persistent and UTI recurrent.

With these considerations in mind, continuous chemoprophylaxis is recommended in all children under 5 yr of age with VUR and in older children with scarring who continue to have VUR and recurrent UTI. Chemoprophylaxis in children over 5 yr of age with VUR but without renal scarring is not necessary unless infections are troublesomely symptomatic. Opinions differ on the necessity for continued chemoprophylaxis in children over 5 yr of age with renal scarring who are not prone to UTI—usual practice is to continue antibiotics until about 12 yr of age if VUR persists. Many different antibiotics schedules have been used. It is important to avoid the selection of resistant strains of *E. coli* in bowel flora. In this respect, nitrofurantoin (1 to 3 mg/kg body weight) or trimethoprim (4 mg/kg body weight), alone or in combination with a sulfonamide, as a single dose at night usually suffices. In special situations cephalexin (125 mg or 250 mg—daily single dose) may be used. It is rarely necessary to increase the dose to adjust to the growth of the child.

Follow-up. Children with VUR in the categories deemed appropriate for chemoprophylaxis should have regular urinalysis—when symptomatic and monthly during the first six months and subsequently every two or three months—without stopping the chemoprophylaxis. All patients should have urine tested every time they present with fever even if a respiratory infection is present. Dip slide cultures are ideal for this purpose.

When there is a breaktrough UTI, compliance with chemoprophylaxis has to be checked. Resistance to nitrofurantoin occurs rarely.

The presence of VUR in most cases is initially established by conventional MCU. Follow-up studies of VUR are best undertaken by radionuclide cystography and since there is less radiation involved, the test can be repeated every two years or so to review the need for prophylactic chemotherapy.

When the history suggests dysfunctional voiding (126) or there are difficulties in controlling UTI despite adequate treatment and compliance, a thorough evaluation of lower urinary tract function should be undertaken (see Chapter 36).

Surgical Treatment

The surgical treatment of VUR consists of reimplantation of the ureter or nephroureteretomy.

Antireflux Surgery. In spite of a quarter of a century of vigorous clinical activity, the place of surgical correction of VUR is still uncertain. There is, however, general agreement that there is no need for ureteric reimplantation in children with slight or moderate VUR or in cases in which chemoprophylaxis can maintain sterile urine. Surgery should be considered for those children with severe VUR in whom UTI persists in spite of adequate medical management, especially those under the age of 5 yr. Factors affecting the success rate of an antireflux surgery are a kidney with impaired function, a dilated and atonic ureter, a trabeculated bladder, and dysfunctional voiding (126, 128).

The Politano-Leadbetter ureteroneocystostomy (6) has now largely given way to the ureteric advancement technique of Cohen (233), which has a low complication rate and is very effective in preventing VUR. The experience of the surgeon is a factor that has to be considered. Even in the best units the success rate of antireflux surgery is around 95%, but it is important to observe that the majority of the published series includes both moderate and severe VUR (14, 213, 234). Among the complications of surgery are persistence of VUR and postoperative obstructions of the new VUJ. Even with effective surgery, however, the incidence of UTI remains high, about 25% (15), and the decision about surgery should take into account the well-established tendency for VUR to cease spontaneously (51). Some studies have claimed increased growth of the kidney after reimplantation (235, 236), but prospective studies have not so far shown any difference in renal function between medically and surgically managed cases (229, 231). There are, however, many difficulties: the asymmetry of the disease, the long-time course of the natural history, and the existence of many subsets within the whole group of children with VUR.

In ideal circumstances children about to undergo antireflux surgery should have a urodynamic assessment to evaluate bladder function, a radionuclide cystography before surgery and after three months to spout assess VUR, and a ^{99m}Tc-DTPA renal scan one month after surgery to exclude the complication of obstruction. The urine should be regularly tested for UTI and prophylactic chemotherapy contined for three to six months after surgery.

Ureteronephrectomy. Ureteronephrectomy is indicated in those cases in which there is extreme dilatation of the ureter and severe scarring (grade D on the IVU or type 4 on the ^{99m}Tc-DMSA scan), with the kidney contributing less than 10% of the overall renal function.

Reflux Nephropathy

Renal scarring is irreversible; management consists of anticipation, early detection, and treatment of complications.

Follow-up

Observation of patients with renal scarring should emphasize blood pressure, UTI, proteinuria, renal function, and progressive renal scarring. Renal scarring is best detected by the ^{99m}Tc-DMSA scan, which should be repeated every year or so with patients under the age of 5 yr, every two to three yr until age 12, and thereafter every three to four yr if VUR persists.

Hypertension

More than 10% of children with renal scarring become hypertensive within 10 yr at follow-up (227). All patients should therefore have their blood pressure measured yearly throughout life. If untreated, the hypertension can evolve into a malignant phase with cerebral and ocular damage as well as further deterioration of renal function (see Chapter 48). These complications can be prevented by early detection and treatment.

Chronic Renal Failure

The late deterioration of renal function that occurs in reflux nephropathy and other forms of extensive renal damage has been attributed to two factors: phosphate nephrotoxicity (237) and hyperfiltration of residual functioning nephrons (193). The former is amenable to dietary phosphate restriction, the latter to protein restriction, which should be considered if GFR is less than 30 ml/min/1.73 m^2SA (see Chapter 49).

Pregnancy and Contraception

Pregnant women with renal scarring require especially close supervision of blood pressure, proteinuria, and UTI. The newborn infant should be screened for VUR. Contraceptive pills are better avoided in patients with scarred kidneys, as they increase the risk of hypertension. If no other contraceptive measure seems adequate for the individual patient, a low estrogen dose should be used and blood pressure should be carefully monitored.

References

1. Broyer M, Donckerwolcke RA, Brunner FP, et al: Combined report on regular dialysis and transplantation in children in Europe, 1980. Proc Eur Dial Transplant Assoc 18:60, 1981.
2. Bailey RR, Lynn KL: End-stage reflux nephropathy. Contrib Nephrol 39:102, 1984.
3. Sampson JA: Ascending renal infection with special reference to the reflux of the urine from the bladder into the ureters as an etiologic factor in its causation and maintenance. Bull John Hopkins Hosp 14:334, 1903.
4. Kretschmer HL: Cystography, its value and limitations in surgery of the bladder. Surg Gynecol Obstet 23:709, 1916.
5. Bumpus HC: Urinary reflux. J Urol 12:341, 1924.
6. Politano VA, Leadbetter WF: An operative technique for the correction of vesicoureteral reflux. J Urol 79:932, 1958.
7. Hodson CJ, Edwards D: Chronic pyelonephritis and vesicoureteric reflux. Clin Radiol 11:219, 1960.
8. Stephens FD, Lenaghan D: The anatomical basis and dynamics of vesicoureteral reflux. J Urol 87:669, 1962.
9. Tanagho EA, Pugh RCB: The anatomy and function of the ureterovesical junction. Br J Urol 35:151, 1963.
10. Williams DI: The ureter, the urologist and the paediatrician. Proc R Soc Med 63:595, 1970.
11. Smellie JM, Edwards D, Hunter N, et al: Vesico-ureteric reflux and renal scarring. Kidney Int (suppl 4):S-65, 1975.
12. Ransley PG, Risdon RA: Reflux and renal scarring. Br J Radiol (suppl 14):1, 1978.
13. Rolleston GL, Shannon FT, Uttley WLF: Follow-up of vesico-ureteric reflux in the newborn. Kidney Int (suppl 4):S-59, 1975.
14. International Reflux Study Committee: Medical versus surgical treatment of primary vesicoureteral reflux: a prospective international reflux study in children. J Urol 125:277, 1981.
15. The Birmingham Reflux Study Group: A prospective trial of operative versus non-operative treatment of severe vesico-ureteric reflux: 2 years' observation in 96 children. Contrib Nephrol 39:169, 1984.
16. Friedland GW: The voiding cystourethrogram: an unreliable examination. In Hodson J, Kincaid-Smith P (eds): Reflux Nephropathy. New York, Masson, 1979, p 91.
17. Winter CC: A new test for vesicoureteral reflux: an external technique using radioisotopes. J Urol 81:105, 1959.

18. Merrick MV, Uttley WS, Wild R: A comparison of two techniques of detecting vesico-ureteric reflux. Br J Radiol 50:792, 1977.
19. Rothwell DL, Constable AR, Albrecht M: Radionuclide cystography in the investigation of vesicoureteric reflux in children. Lancet 1:1072, 1977.
20. Pollett JE, Sharp PF, Smith FW, et al: Intravenous radionuclide cystography for the detection of vesicorenal reflux. J Urol 125:75, 1981.
21. Anselmi OE, Goldraich IH, Goldraich NP, et al: Cistografia indireta con ^{99m}Tc-DTPA. In Temas-livres 2a: Jornada Brasileira de Nefrologia Pediátrica, Sao Paulo, Brazil, 1983, p 35.
22. Conway JJ, Belman B, King LR: Direct and indirect radionuclide cystography. Semin Nucl Med 4:197, 1974.
23. Conway JJ: Radionuclide cystography. Contrib Nephrol 39:1, 1984.
24. Silva N, Goldraich NP, Goldraich IH, et al: Cistografia radioisotópica direta por punção suprapúbica. In Temas-Livres 4: Congresso de Sociedade Brasileira de Biologia e Medicina Nuclear, Pôrto Alegre, Brazil, 1984, p 46.
25. Goldraich NP, Silva N, Goldraich IH, et al: Emprego da cistografia radioisotópica suprapúbica na avaliação do refluxo vesicoureteral. In Temas-Livres 3a: Jornada Brasileira de Nefrologia Pediátrica, Belo Horizonte, Brazil, 1985, p 113.
26. Merrick MV, Wild SR, Uttley W: Radionuclide cystography vs micturating cystourethography for diagnosing vesico-ureteric reflux in children. Br J Radiol 53:263, 1980.
27. Mellor ST, Ward BCH, Eckstein HB: Radionuclide cystography vs micturating cystourethrography for diagnosing vesico-ureteric reflux in children. Br J Radiol 53:262, 1980.
28. Maizels M, Weiss S, Conway JJ, et al: The cystometric nuclear cystogram. J Urol 121:203, 1979.
29. Nasrallah PF, Nara S, Crawford J: Clinical applications of nuclear cystography. J Urol 128:550, 1982.
30. Hutch JA: Theory of maturation of the intravesical ureter. J Urol 88:169, 1962.
31. Rolleston GL, Shannon FT, Uttley WLF: Relationship of infantile vesicoureteric reflux to renal damage. Br Med J 1:430, 1970.
32. Smellie JM, Pursell R, Prescod N, et al: Relationship between serum antibody titre and radiological findings in children with urinary tract infection. In Brumfitt W, Asscher AW (eds): Urinary Tract Infection: Proceedings of the Second National Symposium Held in London, March 1972. London, Oxford University Press, 1973, p 31.
33. Dwoskin JY, Perlmutter AD: Vesicoureteral reflux in children: a computerised review. J Urol 109:888, 1970.
34. Heikel PE, Parkkulainen KV: Vesico-ureteric reflux in children: a classification and results of conservative treatment. Ann Radiol 9:37, 1966.
35. Fairley KF: The effect of a diuresis on vesicoureteral reflux. In Hodson J, Kincaid-Smith P (eds): Reflux Nephropathy. New York, Masson, 1979, p 102.
36. Thompson RM, Reilly RJ, Gleason DM: Does the conventional cystogram exaggerate reflux? J Urol 121:206, 1979.
37. Hodson CJ: Micturating cystography—an unassessed method of examination. Int J Pediatr Nephrol 1:2, 1980.
38. Kjellberg SR, Ericsson NO, Rudhe U: Selected aspects of urinary tract infection. In The Lower Urinary Tract in Childhood: Some Correlated Clinical and Roengtenologic Observations. Stockholm, Almqvist & Wiksell, 1957, p 182.
39. Jones BW, Headstream JM: Vesicoureteral reflux in children. J Urol 80:114, 1968.
40. Gibson HM: Ureteral reflux in the normal child. J Urol 62:40, 1949.
41. Lich R Jr, Howerton LW Jr, Davis LA: Ureteral reflux and the vesical neck of the normal newborn. In Kass EH (ed): Progress in Pyelonephritis. Philadelphia, FA Davis, 1965, p 645.
42. Peters PC, Johnson DE, Jackson JH: The incidence of vesicoureteral in the premature child. J Urol 97:259, 1967.
43. Kunin CM, Zacha E, Paquin AJ: Urinary tract infections in school children. I. Prevalence of bacteriuria and associated urologic findings. New Engl J Med 266:1287, 1962.
44. Askari A, Belman AB: Vesicoureteral reflux in black girls. J Urol 127:747, 1982.
45. Booth EJ, Bell TE, McLain C, et al: Fetal vesicoureteral reflux. J Urol 113:258, 1975.
46. Bailey RR: Vesicoureteric reflux in healthy infants and children. In Hodson J, Kincaid-Smith P (eds): Reflux Nephropathy. New York, Masson, 1979, p 59.
47. Abbott GD: Neonatal bacteriuria: a prospective study in 1,460 infants. Br Med J 1:267, 1972.
48. Drew JH, Acton CM: Radiological findings in newborn infants with urinary infection. Arch Dis Child 51:628, 1976.
49. Schmidt JD, Hawtrey CE, Flocks RH, et al: Vesicoureteral reflux. An inherited lesion. JAMA 220:821, 1972.
50. King LR, Surian MA, Wendel RM, et al: Vesico-ureteral reflux; a classification based on cause and the results of treatment. JAMA 203:169, 1968.
51. Baker R, Maxted DW, Maylath J, et al: Relation to age, sex and infection to reflux: data indicating high spontaneous cure rate in pediatric patients. J Urol 95:27, 1966.
52. MacGregor ME, Freeman P: Childhood urinary infection associated with vesicoureteric reflux. Q J Med 44:481, 1975.
53. Kelalis PP: Proper perspective on vesicoureteral reflux. Mayo Clin Proc 46:807, 1971.
54. Kincaid-Smith P, Becker GJ: Reflux nephropathy and chronic atrophic pyelonephritis: a review. J Infect Dis 138:774, 1978.
55. Baker R, Barbaris HT: Comparative results of urological evaluation of children with initial and recurrent urinary tract infection. J Urol 116:503, 1976.
56. Stephens FD, Joske RA, Simmons RT: Megaureter with vesicoureteric reflux in twins. Aust NZ J Surg 24:192, 1955.
57. Mebust WK, Foret JD: Vesicoureteral reflux in identical twins. J Urol 108:635, 1972.
58. Hampel N, Levin DR, Gersh I: Bilateral vesico-ureteral reflux with pyelonephritis in identical twins. Br J Urol 47:535, 1975.
59. Amar AD: Familial vesicoureteral reflux. J Urol 108:969, 1972.
60. Bredin HC, Winchester P, McGovern JH, et al: Family study of vesicoureteral reflux. J Urol 113:623, 1975.
61. De Vargas A, Evans K, Ransley P, et al: A family study of vesicoureteric reflux. J Med Genet 15:85, 1978.
62. Heale WF, Shannon FT, Uttley WL, et al: Familial and hereditary reflux nephropathy. In Hodson J, Kincaid-Smith P (eds): Reflux Nephropathy. New York, Masson, 1979, p 48.
63. Goldraich IH, Cunha L, Goldraich NP: Anormalidades no trato urinário identificadas durante a investigação sistemática de familiares de portadores de refluxo vesicoureteral primário. J Bras Nefrol 3:4, 1981.
64. Goldraich NP: Discussion on chapters 4–12. In Hodson CJ, Heptinstall RH, Winberg J (eds): Reflux Nephropathy Update: 1983. Basel, Karger, 1984, p 132.
65. Jerkins GR, Noe HN: Familial vesicoureteral reflux: a prospective study. J Urol 128:774, 1982.
66. Bailey RR, Janus E, McLoughlin K, et al: Familial and genetic data in reflux nephropathy. Contrib Nephrol 39:40, 1984.
67. Middleton GW, Howards SS, Gillenwater JY: Sex-linked familial reflux. J Urol 114:36, 1975.
68. Burger RH: Theory on the nature of transmission of congenital vesicoureteral reflux. J Urol 108:249, 1972.
69. Dwoskin JY: Sibling uropathology. J Urol 115:726, 1976.
70. Bailey RR, Wallace M: HLA-B12 as a genetic marker for vesicoureteric reflux? Br Med J 1:47, 1978.
71. Sengar DPS, McLeish WA, Rashid A, et al: Histocompatibility antigens in urinary tract infection and vesicoureteral reflux: a preliminary communication. Clin Nephrol 10:166, 1978.
72. Sengar DPS, Rashid A, Wolfish NM: Familial urinary tract anomalies: association with the major histocompatibility complex in man. J Urol 121:194, 1979.
73. Torres VE, Moore SB, Kurtz SB, et al: In search of a marker for genetic susceptibility to reflux nephropathy. Clin Nephrol 14:217, 1980.
74. Goldraich NP: Refluxo vesicoureteral primário: reprecussões renais. MSc thesis in nephrology, Universidade Federal do Rio Grande do Sul. Pporto Alegre, Brazil, 1977.
75. Lenaghan D, Whitaker JG, Jensen F, et al: The natural history of reflux and long-term effects of reflux on the kidney. J Urol 115:728, 1976.
76. Cussen LJ: Vesicoureteral reflux in children; frequency and associated urologic abnormalities. Invest Urol 8:640, 1971.
77. Smellie JM, Normand ICS, Katz G: Children with urinary infection: a comparison of those with and those without vesicoureteral reflux. Kidney Int 20:717, 1981.
78. Atwell JD, Beard RC: Congenital anomalies of the upper urinary tract associated with esophageal atresia and tracheoesophageal fistula. J Pediatr Surg 9:825, 1974.
79. Goldraich NP, Kilpp JC, Koff WJ, et al: Diseases of the genito-urinary tract associated to malformations of the upper digestive tract and extra-hepatic biliary tract. In Abstracts of the International Forum for Paediatric Gastroenterology and Nutrition, Sao Paulo, Brazil, 1977, p 27.
80. Rickwood AMK, Spitz L: Primary vesicoureteric reflux in neonates with imperforate anus. Arch Dis Child 55:149, 1980.
81. Narasimharao KL, Prasad GR, Mukhopadhyay B, et al: Vesicoureteric reflux in neonates with anorectal anomalies. Br J Urol 55:268, 1983.
82. Smellie JM, Hodson CJ, Edwards D, et al: Clinical and radiological features of urinary infection in childhood. Br Med J 2:1222, 1964.
83. Stansfeld JM: Clinical observations relating to incidence and aetiology of urinary-tract infection in children. Br Med J 1:631, 1966.
84. Winberg J, Anderson HJ, Bergström T, et al: Epidemiology of symptomatic urinary tract infection in childhood. Acta Paediatr Scand (Suppl 252):3, 1974.
85. Savage DCL, Wilson MI, McHardy M, et al: Covert bacteriuria of childhood: a clinical and epidemiologic study. Arch Dis Child 48:8, 1973.
86. Newcastle Asymptomatic Bacteriuria Research Group: Asymptomatic bacteriuria in school children in Newcastle upon Tyne. Arch Dis Child 50:90, 1975.

87. McLachlan MSF, Mellor ST, Verrier-Jones ER, et al: Urinary tract in schoolgirls with covert bacteriuria. Arch Dis Child 50:253, 1975.
88. Hodson CJ, Maling TMJ, McManamon PJ, et al: Reflux nephropathy. Kidney Int 8 (suppl 4):S-50, 1975.
89. Edwards D, Normand ICS, Prescod N, et al: Disappearance of vesicoureteric reflux during long-term prophylaxis of urinary tract infection in children. Br Med J 2:285, 1977.
90. Goldraich NP, Goldraich IH, Anselmi OE, et al: Reflux nephropathy: the clinical picture in South Brazilian children. Contrib Nephrol 39:52, 1984.
91. Heale WF: Prolonged follow-up of infants with reflux and reflux nephropathy. Eur J Pediatr 140:160, 1983.
92. Bailey RR: The relationship of vesico-ureteric reflux to urinary tract infection and chronic pyelonephritis—reflux nephropathy. Clin Nephrol 1:132, 1973.
93. Wagner EL: Handbuch der Krankherten des Harnapparates: I Hälfte der Morbus Brightii. In von Ziemssen HW (ed): Handbuch der Speciellen Pathologie und Therapei, ed 3. Leipzig, Vogel, 1882, vol. 9, pt. 1, p. 309. Quoted by Heptinstall RH: Pyelonephritis: pathologic features. In Pathology of the Kidney. ed 3, Boston, Little, Brown, 1983, vol 3, p 1323.
94. Löhlein M.: Über Schrumpfnieren. Beitr. Pathol. Anat. 63:570, 1917. Quoted by Heptinstall RH: Pyelonephritis: pathologic features. In Pathology of the Kidney, ed 3, Boston, Little, Brown, 1983, vol 3, p 1323.
95. Longcope WT, Winkenwerder WL: Clinical features of the contracted kidney due to pyelonephritis. Bull Johns Hopkins Hosp 53:255, 1933.
96. Weiss S, Parker F: Pyelonephritis: its relation to vascular lesions and to arterial hypertension. Medicine 18:221, 1939.
97. Weiss S, Parker F: Relation of pyelonephritis and other urinary-tract infections to arterial hypertension. N Engl J Med 223:959, 1940.
98. Heale WF, Rolleston GL, Shannon FT, et al: Chronic pyelonephritis in infants, children and adults. In Abstracts of the 5th International Congress of Nephrology, Mexico City, 1972, p 576.
99. Heptinstall RH: Urinary tract infection, reflux and pyelonephritis. In Heptinstall RH (ed): Pathology of the Kidney, ed 3. Boston, Little, Brown, 1983, vol 3, p 1257.
100. Heptinstall RH: The limitations of the pathological diagnosis of chronic pyelonephritis. In Black DAK (ed): Renal Disease, ed 2. Oxford, Blackwell, 1967, p 350.
101. Hutch JA, Hinman F Jr, Miller ER: Reflux as a cause of hydronephrosis and chronic pyelonephritis. J Urol 88:169, 1962.
102. McGovern JH, Marshall VF: Reflux and pyelonephritis in 35 adults. J Urol 101:668, 1969.
103. Rosenheim ML: Vesico-ureteric reflux. In Kass EH (ed): Progress in Pyelonephritis. Philadelphia, FA Davis, 1965, p 599.
104. Weber AL, Weylman WT: Evaluation of vesicoureteral reflux by intravenous pyelography and cine cystography. Radiology 87:489, 1966.
105. Servadio C, Schachner A: Observations on vesicoureteral reflux and chronic pyelonephritis in adults. J Urol 103:722, 1970.
106. Scott JES, Stansfeld JM: Ureteric reflux and kidney scarring in children. Arch Dis Child 43:468, 1968.
107. Johnston JH, Heal MR: Reflux in complete duplicated ureters in children: management and techniques. J Urol 105:881, 1971.
108. Vermillion DC, Heale WF: Position and configuration of the ureteral orifice and its relationship to renal scarring in adults. J Urol 109:579, 1973.
109. Hodson CJ: The radiological contribution toward the diagnosis of chronic pyelonephritis. Radiology 88:857, 1967.
110. Rolleston GL, Maling TMJ, Hodson CJ: Intrarenal reflux and the scarred kidney. Arch Dis Child 49:531, 1974.
111. Bourne HH, Condon VR, Hoyt TS, et al: Intrarenal reflux and renal damage. J Urol 115:304, 1976.
112. Uldall P, Frøkjaer O, Ibsen KK: Intrarenal reflux. Acta Paediatr Scand 65:711, 1976.
113. Rose JS, Glassberg KI, Waterhouse K: Intra-renal reflux and its relationship to renal scarring. J Urol 37:531, 1965.
114. Maling TMJ, Rolleston GL: Intra-renal reflux in children demonstrated by micturating cystography. Clin Radiol 25:81, 1974.
115. Brodeur AE, Goyer RA, Melick W: A potential hazard of barium cystography. Radiology 85:1080, 1965.
116. Amar AD: Calicotubular backflow with vesicoureteral reflux: relation to pyelonephritis. JAMA 213:293, 1970.
117. Hodson CJ, Maling TMJ, McManamon PJ, et al: The pathogenesis of reflux nephropathy (chronic atrophic pyelonephritis). Br J Radiol (suppl 13):1, 1975.
118. Ransley PG, Risdon RA: Renal papillary morphology in infants and young children. Urol Res 3:111, 1975.
119. Ransley PG: Intrarenal reflux: anatomical, dynamic and radiological studies. Part I. Urol Res 5:61, 1977.
120. Ransley PG, Risdon RA: The renal papilla, intrarenal reflux, and chronic pyelonephritis. In Hodson J, Kincaid-Smith P (eds): Reflux Nephropathy. New York, Masson, 1979, p 126.
121. Allen TD: The non-neurogenic neurogenic bladder. J Urol 117:232, 1977.
122. Koff SA, Lapides J, Piazza DH: Association of urinary tract infection and reflux with uninhibited bladder contractions and voluntary sphincteric obstruction. J Urol 122:373, 1979.
123. Allen TD: Vesicoureteral reflux as a manifestation of dysfunctional voiding. In Hodson J, Kincaid-Smith P (eds): Reflux Nephropathy. New York, Masson, 1979, p 171.
124. von Gool JD: Bladder infection and pressure. In Hodson J, Kincaid-Smith P (eds): Reflux Nephropathy. New York, Masson, 1979, p 181.
125. Koff SA: Bladder-sphincter dysfunction in childhood. Urology 29:457, 1982.
126. von Gool JD, Kuitjen RH, Donckerwolcke RA, et al: Bladder-sphincter dysfunction urinary infection and vesico-ureteral reflux with special reference to cognitive bladder training. Contrib Nephrol 39:190, 1984.
127. Taylor CM: Unstable bladder activity and the rate of resolution of vesico-ureteric reflux. Contrib Nephrol 39:238, 1984.
128. Koff SA, Lapides J, Piazza DH: The uninhibited bladder in children: a cause for urinary obstruction, infection and reflux. In: Hodson J, Kincaid-Smith P (eds): Reflux Nephropathy. New York, Masson, 1979, p 161.
129. Koff SA, Murtagh D: The uninhibited bladder in children: effect of treatment on vesicoureteral reflux resolution. Contrib Nephrol 39:211, 1984.
130. Taylor CM, Corkery JJ, White RHR: Micturition symptoms and unstable bladder activity in girls with primary vesicoureteric reflux. Br J Urol 54:494, 1982.
131. Anders D, Bolter D, Reither M: Dysfunctional voiding and psychodynamic patterns maintaining chronic recurrent urinary tract infections (UTI) in girls. Int J Pediatr Nephrol 3:107, 1982.
132. Whiteside CG, Arnold EP: Persistent primary enuresis: a urodynamic assessment. Br Med J 1:364, 1975.
133. Smellie JM, Normand ICS: Bacteriuria, reflux and renal scarring. Arch Dis Child 50:581, 1975.
134. Sargent JW: Bilateral ureteral reflux observed in a patient over a 23-year period: case report. J Urol 91:650, 1964.
135. Stephens FD: Clinical features and prognosis of vesico-ureteral reflux. J Coll Radiol Australas 7:17, 1963.
136. Shopfner CE: Vesicoureteral reflux; five year reevaluation. Radiology 95:637, 1970.
137. Smellie J: Childhood urinary infections and their significance. In Asscher AW (ed): The Management of Urinary Infection: An International Symposium. Oxford, Medicine Publishing Foundation, 1980, p 29.
138. Berström T, Larson H, Lincoln K, et al: Studies of urinary tract infection in infancy and childhood. XII. Eighty consecutive patients with neonatal infection. J Pediatr 80:858, 1972.
139. Filly RA, Friedland GW, Govan DE, et al: Development and progression of clubbing and scarring in children with recurrent urinary tract infections. Radiology 113:145, 1974.
140. Randolph MF, Morris KF, Gould EB: The first urinary tract infection in the female infant; prevalence, recurrence, and prognosis: a 10-year study in private practice. J Pediatr 86:342, 1975.
141. Hugosson CO, Chrispin AR, Wolverson MK: The advent of the pyelonephritic scar. Ann Radiol 19:1, 1976.
142. Smellie JM, Ransley PG, Normand ICS, et al: The development of new renal scars. A collaborative study. Br Med J 290:1957, 1985.
143. Ransley PG, Risdon RA: Reflux nephropathy: effects of antimicrobial therapy on the evolution of the early pyelonephritis scar. Kidney Int 20:733, 1981.
144. Ransley PG, Risdon RA, Godley ML: High pressure sterile vesicoureteral reflux and renal scarring: an experimental study in the pig and minipig. Contrib Nephrol 39:320, 1984.
145. Roberts JA: Experimental pyelonephritis in the monkey. III. Pathophysiology of ureteral malfunction induced by bacteria. J Urol 13:117, 1975.
146. Roberts JA: Pathogenesis of pyelonephritis. J Urol 129:1102, 1983.
147. Svenson SB, Kallenius G, Korhonen TK, et al: Initiation of clinical pyelonephritis—the role of P-fimbriae-mediated bacterial adhesion. Contrib Nephrol 39:252, 1984.
148. Habib R: Renal dysplasia, hypoplasia and cysts. In Strauss J (ed): Pediatric Nephrology. New York, Stratton Intercontinental Medical Books, 1974, vol 1, p 209.
149. Bernstein J: A classification on renal cysts. In Gardner Jr KD (ed): Cystic Diseases of the Kidney. New York, John Wiley, 1976, p 3.
150. Kissane JM: Congenital malformations. In Heptinstall RH (ed): Pathology of the Kidney, ed 3. Boston, Little, Brown, 1983, vol 1, p 83.
151. Ashley DJB, Mostofi FK: Renal agenesis and dysgenesis. J Urol 83:211, 1960.
152. Ericsson NO, Ivemark BI: Renal dysplasia and pyelonephritis in infants and children. Part I. Arch Pathol 66:255, 1958.
153. Ericsson NO, Ivemark BI: Renal dysplasia and pyelonephritis in infants and children. II. Primitive ductules and abnormal glomeruli. Arch Pathol 66:264, 1958.
154. Beck AD: The effect of intra-uterine urinary obstruction upon the development of the fetal kidney. J Urol 105:784, 1971.
155. Potter EL: Normal and Abnormal Development of the Kidney. Chicago, Year Book Medical Publishers, 1972, p 209.

156. Marshall AG: The persistence of foetal structures in pyelonephritic kidneys. Br J Surg 41:38, 1953.
157. Persky L: Pyelonephritis in children. J Urol 94:20, 1965.
158. Persky L, Izant R, Bolande R: Renal dysplasia. J Urol 98:431, 1967.
159. Lewy PR, Belman AB: Familial occurrence of nonobstructive, non-infectious vesicoureteral reflux with renal scarring. J Pediatr 86:851, 1975.
160. Stecker JF, Rose JG, Gillenwater JY: Dysplastic kidneys associated with vesicoureteral reflux. J Urol 110:341, 1973.
161. Bialestock D: Studies of renal malformations and pyelonephritis in children with and without associated vesico-ureteral reflux and obstruction. Aust NZ J Surg 35:120, 1965.
162. Mackie GG, Stephens FD: Duplex kidneys: a correlation of renal dysplasia with position of the ureteral orifice. J Urol 114:274, 1975.
163. Hodson CJ: The radiological diagnosis of pyelonephritis. Proc R Soc Med 52:669, 1975.
164. Hodson CJ, Drewe JA, Karn MN, et al: Renal size in normal children; a radiographic study during life. Arch Dis Child 37:616, 1962.
165. Hodson CJ: Radiological diagnosis of renal involvement. In O'Grady F, Brumfitt W (eds): Urinary Tract Infection: Proceedings of the First National Symposium held in London, April 1968. London, Oxford University Press, 1968, p 108.
166. Hodson CJ: Reflux nephropathy: scoring the damage. In Hodson J, Kincaid-Smith P (eds): Reflux Nephropathy. New York, Masson, 1979, p 29.
167. Hodson CJ: Pyelonephritis in children. Ann Radiol 7:355, 1964.
168. Hodson CJ, Wilson S: Natural history of chronic pyelonephritic scarring. Br Med J 2:191, 1965.
169. Lindberg V, Claësson I, Hanson LÅ, et al: Asymptomatic bacteriuria in schoolgirls. 1. Clinical and laboratory findings. Acta Paediatr Scand 64:425, 1975.
170. Lin TH, Khentigan A, Winchell HS: A ^{99m}Tc-chelate substitute for organo-radiomercurial renal agents. J Nucl Med 15:34, 1974.
171. Kawamura J, Hosokawa S, Yoshida O, et al: Validity of ^{99m}Tc dimercaptosuccinic acid renal uptake for an assessment of individual kidney function. J Urol 119:305, 1978.
172. Merrick MV, Uttley WS, Wild SR: The detection of pyelonephritic scarring in children by radioisotope imaging. Br J Radiol 53:544, 1980.
173. Abbou CC, Moretti JL, Chopin D, et al: La scintigraphie au dimercaptosuccinate de technetium: DMSA ^{99m}Tc; apport dans l'évaluation de la fonction rénale séparée. Nouv Presse Med 10:1475, 1981.
174. Daly MJ, Henry RE: Defining renal anatomy and function with 99m-technetium dimercaptosuccinic acid: clinical and renographic correlation. J Urol 126:5, 1981.
175. Goldraich NP, Goldraich IH: Reflux nephropathy: assessment using DMSA renal uptake. Int J Pediatr Nephrol 3:120, 1982.
176. Goldraich IH, Goldraich NP, Ramos OL: Classification of reflux nephropathy according to findings at DMSA renal scan. Eur J Pediatr 140:212, 1983.
177. Goldraich IH, Goldraich NP, Anselmi OE, et al: Comparative study between intravenous urography and DMSA renal scan in the diagnosis of reflux nephropathy in infants and preschool children. Eur J Pediatr 140:177, 1983.
178. Shulman CC: Guest editor's notes. Dial Pediatr Urol 7:2, 1984.
179. Goldraich NP: Nefropatia do refluxo: avaliação com a cintilografia renal com ^{99m}Tc-DMSA. PhD thesis in nephrology. Sao Paulo, Brazil, Escola Paulista de Medicina, 1984.
180. Goldraich NP, Goldraich IH, Ramos OL: Comparative study between intravenous urography and ^{99m}Tc-DMSA: a prospective study in 202 children with vesicoureteral reflux (in preparation).
181. Hodson CJ, Craven JD: The radiology of obstructive atrophy of the kidney. Clin Radiol 17:305, 1966.
182. Barratt TM: Renal failure in the first year of life. Br Med Bull 27:115, 1971.
183. Woodard JR, Holden S: The prognostic significance of fever in childhood urinary infections. Observations in 350 consecutive patients. Clin Pediatr 15:1051, 1976.
184. Williams DI, Eckstein HB: Surgical treatment of reflux in children. Br J Urol 37:13, 1965.
185. Goldraich NP, Goldraich IH, Cunha L, et al: Nefropatia do refluxo: prevalência. Clín Ger 12:39, 1978.
186. Savage DCL: Natural history of covert bacteriuria in schoolgirls. Kidney Int 8 (suppl 4):S-90, 1975.
187. Kern HB, Malament M: Vesico-ureteral reflux and the adult male. Br J Urol 41:295, 1969.
188. Smellie J, Normand C: Reflux nephropathy in childhood. In Hodson J, Kincaid-Smith P (eds): Reflux Nephropathy. New York, Masson, 1979, p 14.
189. Winter AL, Hardy BE, Alton DJ, et al: Acquired renal scars in children. J Urol 129:1190, 1983.
190. Aperia A, Broberger O, Ericsson NO, et al: Effect of vesicoureteral reflux on renal function in children with recurrent urinary tract infections. Kidney Int 9:418, 1976.
191. Verrier-Jones K, Asscher AW, Verrier-Jones E, et al: Glomerular filtration rate in schoolgirls with covert bacteriuria. Br Med J 285:1307, 1982.
192. Goldraich NP, Goldraich IH, Anselmi OE, et al: Assessment of individual renal function with DMSA renal scan in children with primary vesico-ureteric reflux. Eur J Pediatr 140:212, 1983.
193. Brenner BM, Meyer TW, Hostetter TH: Dietary protein intake and the progressive nature of the kidney disease: the role of hemodynamically mediated glomerular injury in the pathogenesis of progressive glomerular sclerosis in aging, renal ablation, and intrinsic renal disease. New Engl J Med 307:652, 1982.
194. Heptinstall RH: Pyelonephritis: pathologic features. In Heptinstall RH (ed): Pathology of the Kidney, ed 3. Boston, Little, Brown, 1983, vol 3, p 1323.
195. Bailey RR, Lynn KL, McRae CV: Unilateral reflux nephropathy. Contrib Nephrol 39:116, 1984.
196. Dillon MJ, Smellie JM: Peripheral plasma renin activity, hypertension and renal scarring in children. Contrib Nephrol 39:68, 1984.
197. Still JL, Cottom D: Severe hypertension in childhood. Arch Dis Child 42:34, 1967.
198. Goldraich NP, Goldraich IH, Pranke ML: Como eu trato: hypertensão arterial em pediatria. Atual Méd 1:53, 1979.
199. Gill DG, Mendes da Costa, Cameron JS, et al: Analysis of 100 children with severe and persistent hypertension. Arch Dis Child 51:951, 1976.
200. Dillon MJ: Modern management of hypertension. In Meadow R (ed): Recent Advances in Pediatrics, No 7. Edinburgh, Churchill Livingstone, 1984, p 35.
201. Andersen HJ, Jacobsson B, Larsson H, et al: Hypertension, asymmetrical renal parenchymal defect, sterile urine and high E coli antibody titre. Br Med J 3:14, 1973.
202. Holland NH, Kotchen T, Bhathena D: Hypertension in children with chronic pyelonephritis. Kidney Int 8 (suppl 5):S-243, 1975.
203. Lewy PR, Sorrenti R: Severe hypertension (HT) in children with renal scarring and/or atrophy (RSA). Kidney Int 10:502, 1976.
204. Holland NH: Reflux nephropathy and hypertension. In Hodson J, Kincaid-Smith P (eds): Reflux Nephropathy. New York, Masson, 1979, p 257.
205. Goldraich NP, Goldraich IH, Pranke ML: Associação entre hipertensão e refluxo vesicoureteral primário na infância. In Temas-Livres. 9º Congresso Brasileiro de Nefrologia. Rio de Janeiro, 1978, p 57.
206. Ambrose SS: Reflux pyelonephritis in adults secondary to congenital lesions of the ureteral orifice. J Urol 102:302, 1969.
207. Hutch JA, Miller ER, Hinman F: Vesicoureteral reflux; role in pyelonephritis. Am J Med 34:338, 1963.
208. Rosenheim ML: Problems of chronic pyelonephritis. Br Med J 2:1433, 1963.
209. Hinman F Jr, Hutch JA: Atrophic pyelonephritis from ureteral reflux without obstructive signs ("reflux pyelonephritis"). J Urol 87:230, 1962.
210. Habib R, Broyer M, Benmaiz H: Chronic renal failure in children; causes, rate of deterioration and survival data. Nephron 11:209, 1973.
211. Chantler C, Carter JE, Bewick M, et al: 10 years' experience with regular haemodialysis and renal transplantation. Arch Dis Child 55:435, 1980.
212. Goldraich IH, Goldani JC, Goldraich NP, et al: Insuficiência renal crônica na infância: etiologia. J Bras Nefrol 3:15, 1981.
213. Stewart JH, McCarthy SW, Storey BG, et al: Diseases causing end-stage renal failure in New South Wales. Br Med J 1:440, 1975.
214. Kincaid-Smith P: Reflux nephropathy. Br Med J 286:2002, 1983.
215. MacGregor ME: Pyelonephritis lenta; consideration of childhood urinary infection as a forerunner of renal insufficiency in later life. Arch Dis Child 45:159, 1970.
216. Salvatierra O Jr, Kounts SL, Belzer FO: Primary vesicoureteral reflux and end-stage renal disease. JAMA 226:1454, 1973.
217. Kincaid-Smith PS, Bastos MG, Becker GJ: Reflux nephropathy in the adult. Contrib Nephrol 39:94, 1984.
218. Zimmerman SW, Uehling DT, Burkholder PM: Vesicoureteral reflux nephropathy. Evidence for immunologically mediated glomerular injury. Urology 2:534, 1973.
219. Kincaid-Smith P: Glomerular lesions in atrophic pyelonephritis (RN). In Hodson J, Kincaid-Smith P (eds): Reflux Nephropathy. New York, Masson, 1979, p 268.
220. Bhathena DB, Weiss JH, Holland NH, et al: Focal and segmental glomerular sclerosis in reflux nephropathy. Am J Med 68:886, 1980.
221. Torres VE, Velosa JA, Holley KE, et al: The progression of vesicoureteral reflux nephropathy. Ann Int Med 92:776, 1980.
222. Goldraich NP, Goldraich IH, Saad FA: Glomerulonefrite em pacientes com refluxo vesico-ureteral. J Bras Nefrol 3:4, 1981.
223. Bailey RR, Swainson CP, Lynn KL, et al: Glomerular lesions in the "normal" kidney in patients with unilateral reflux nephropathy. Contrib Nephrol 39:126, 1984.
224. Cotran RS: Glomerulosclerosis in reflux nephropathy. Kidney Int 21:528, 1982.
225. Kincaid-Smith, P, Becker GJ: Reflux nephropathy in the adult. In Hodson J, Kincaid-Smith P (eds): Reflux Nephropathy. New York, Masson, 1979, p 21.
226. Verrier-Jones K: Personal communication, 1985.
227. Wallace DMA, Rothwell DL, Williams DI: The long-term follow-up of surgically treated vesicoureteric reflux. Br J Urol 50:479, 1978.
228. Senekjian HO, Stinebaugh BJ, Mattioli CA, et al: Irreversible renal failure following vesicoureteral reflux. JAMA 241:160, 1979.
229. Birmingham Reflux Study Group: Prospective trial of operative versus non-operative

treatment of severe vesicoureteric reflux: two years' observation in 96 children. Br Med J 287:171, 1983.
230. Taylor CM: Personal communication, 1985.
231. International Collaborative Study of Reflux in Children: Clinical trial of medical vs surgical treatment of vesicoureteral reflux (VUR). Pediatr Res 18:373A, 1984.
232. Cardiff-Oxford Bacteriuria Study Group: Sequelae of covert bacteriuria in schoolgirls. A four-year follow-up study. Lancet 1:889, 1978.
233. Cohen SJ: The Cohen technique of ureteroneocytostomy. In Eckstein HB, Hohenfellner R, Williams DI (eds): Surgical Pediatric Urology. Stuttgart, Georg Thieme, 1977, p 269.
234. Coleman JW, McGovern JH: A 20-year experience with pediatric ureteral reimplantation: surgical results in 701. In Hodson J, Kincaid-Smith P (eds): Reflux Nephropathy. New York, Masson, 1979, p 299.
235. Scott JES, Stansfeld JM: Treatment of vesico-ureteric reflux in children. Arch Dis Child 43:323, 1968.
236. McRae CV, Shannon FT, Utley WLF: Effect on renal growth of reimplantation of refluxing ureters. Lancet 1:1310, 1974.
237. Ibels LS, Alfrey AC, Haut L, et al: Preservation of function in experimental renal disease by dietary restriction of phosphate. N Engl J Med 298:122, 1978.

CHAPTER 38

The Dilated Urinary Tract

T. M. BARRATT
G. A. MANZONI

INTRODUCTION

Obstructive lesions of the urinary tract are a most important group of disorders, for they constitute a major preventable cause of chronic renal failure. At first sight, they may seem straightforward mechanical problems, but such simplicity is illusory, for the range of anatomical variants is wide, the nature of the obstruction is poorly defined in urodynamic terms, and the consequences for renal function are ill understood.

Dilatation of the urinary tract is the most characteristic result of obstruction, but that cannot be assumed to be always the cause, for other factors may be operative: maldevelopment, infection, polyuria, or reflux. For example, the ureteric dilatation associated with the prune belly syndrome is as much caused by disordered development of the whole urinary tract as by a specific obstructive lesion. Urinary tract infection (UTI), especially in young infants, may result in considerable dilatation that is completely reversible with medical treatment alone (1); experimentally it has been shown that bacterial toxins are capable of paralyzing ureteric muscle (2). Continued polyuria may also cause ureteric dilatation, typically seen in hereditary nephrogenic diabetes insipidus (3). The ureteric dilatation associated with vesicoureteric reflux (VUR) varies considerably from time to time, being much more evident during cystography than during urography because of bladder pressure. Further, ureteric dilatation may persist even though satisfactory surgical correction of the obstruction has been achieved. From these examples it is clear that demonstrating ureteric dilatation alone cannot be accepted as unequivocal evidence of obstruction.

NORMAL AND ABNORMAL FUNCTION

Upper Tract

Transport of urine from the kidney to the bladder is effected by a coordinated system of ureteric peristalsis. The contractions are initiated by pacemaker sites in the renal pelvis (4), and excitation is propagated from cell to cell across tight cellular junctions (5). Intraureteric pressures as high as 50 mm Hg are generated by peristaltic contractions, but apposition of the ureteric walls generates a stripping wave that propels a bolus of urine forward in addition to protecting the kidney from the retrograde transmission of pressure (6).

Acute ureteric obstruction leads to an increased frequency and amplitude of peristaltic contractions with an elevation of resting intraureteric pressure. With time, however, resting pressure falls and the ureter dilates. The Laplace relationship indicates that the pressure in the ureter is directly proportional to the stress in the wall and inversely proportional to the radius. Thus, with increasing dilatation, muscular contraction is less effective in generating intraureteric pressure, and once apposition of the ureteric walls fails, the contractions lose their efficiency for urine transport—the obstruction is said to be decompensated.

Lower Tract

As urine accumulates in the bladder, there is initially little rise in pressure. Eventually, pressure increases, and the desire to micturate is stimulated. Micturition is initiated and maintained by a complex series of neural reflexes, resulting in detrusor contraction and relaxation of the internal and external sphincter mechanisms.

Obstruction to the flow of urine during micturition may be the consequence of incoordinated detrusor-sphincter activity or of urethral abnormality. Peak urine flow rates during micturition are decreased and intravesical voiding pressure increased. There is hypertrophy of bladder musculature. Voiding is incomplete, and the residue of urine predisposes to UTI. With raised bladder pressure there is difficulty in ureteric emptying, this increased pressure is transmitted to the upper urinary tract, and hydronephrosis ensues.

The rate of urine flow during micturition is determined by voiding pressure and urethral resistance, but the relationship is not simple because of the effects of turbulence in the urinary stream (7).

Definition of Obstruction

It has proved surprisingly difficult to define urinary tract obstruction rigorously. Ultimately it must be seen as a disturbance of the normal pressure-flow relationships in the urinary tract, and it is only by an increase in pressure that the effects of obstruction are transmitted back to the kidney.

In the upper tract, obstruction is best demonstrated by antegrade perfusion (8). The normal ureter can accommodate flows up to 10 ml/min without the pressure rising above 15 mm Hg, and a pressure above 20 mm Hg strongly suggests obstruction. In dilated capacious systems it is important to continue perfusion long enough to ensure that a steady state is obtained. The state of bladder filling should be defined, for it may influence the function of the ureterovesical junction (UVJ).

The lower urinary tract is more accessible to direct measurement of pressure and flow (see Chapter 40), but urodynamic studies may be difficult in young children because of lack of cooperation. It has, however, proved possible to define urethral obstruction in terms of abnormal resistance to flow (7).

CONSEQUENCES OF URINARY TRACT OBSTRUCTION

Embryological Consequences

Complete or severe degrees of urinary obstruction in fetal life result in oligohydramnios with resultant compression disorders: Potter facies, crumpled ears, talipes, dislocated hips, and skin dimples on pressure points. Pulmonary hypoplasia is a common accompaniment, frequently presenting as pneumothorax in the neonatal period.

Gross abdominal distention in early pregnancy results in disordered development of the abdominal wall. The pathogenesis of the prune belly syndrome is believed to be a transient period of complete urethral obstruction resulting in bladder distension; later the urethra recanalizes, but the consequences of maldevelopment of kidney, ureters, and abdominal wall remain (9, 10).

Morphological Consequences

Kidney

Dysplasia. There is a strong association between congenital obstructive uropathy and renal dysplasia. Bernstein defined renal dysplasia as the presence of microscopic abnormalities variously attributed to developmental arrest, to failure of differentiation, and to the persistence of fetal structures or mesonephric tissues; he considered the most characteristic features to be primitive ducts lined by columnar epithelium and surrounded by fibromuscular collars, and nests of metaplastic cartilage (11). There may also be primitive fetal glomeruli and cyst formation. There are two possible explanations for this association: either dysplasia and obstruction may be regarded as parallel manifestations of the same teratogenic process, or the dysplasia may be the consequence of intrauterine urinary tract obstruction.

Some insight into this problem has been provided by experimental fetal surgery. Beck reported that ureteric ligation in the fetal lamb in the second half of pregnancy causes simple hydronephrosis but earlier in pregnancy resulted in renal dysplasia and, if the contralateral kidney was removed, in an appearance resembling polycystic disease (12). Tanagho confirmed that dysplasia was not a feature of experimental fetal urinary tract obstruction in the lamb during the second half of gestation (13–15). Glick and coworkers showed that early midtrimester ureteric ligation in fetal lambs caused renal dysplasia that could be ameliorated by cutaneous end-ureterostomy in utero after 20 to 60 days (16, 17).

Hydronephrosis and Postobstructive Atrophy. The gross changes of hydronephrosis are well known: the renal calyces become clubbed with flattening of the papillae. At first the changes are reversible, but later there is parenchymal atrophy. Experimentally the sequence of events after ureteric obstruction has been described by Hodson (18, 19) in the multipapillate kidney of the minipig. The atrophy is most evident after the obstruction has been relieved and the kidney has contracted, but clearly the process of nephron destruction is continuous throughout the period of obstruction, and the potential for recovery depends on the extent of this loss.

Urinary Tract

Ureter. The characteristics of obstructive dilatation depend on age at onset. With fetal obstruction the ureter is very wide, whereas the renal pelvis remains relatively small; the later in life that obstruction occurs, the less the consequent ureteric dilatation. This effect is possibly a result of the increase of the population of ureteric elastic fibers and smooth muscle cells that occurs with growth (20). On the other hand, surgical relief of urinary obstruction in the neonate results in a rapid return of ureteric caliber to normal, whereas later in life recovery is slower and less complete, perhaps raising difficult diagnostic considerations, for significant residual obstruction may be suspected.

Bladder. The bladder responds to outflow obstruction by muscular hypertrophy, evident as trabeculation.

Physiological Consequences

Consequences during Obstruction

Experimental Data. A large body of experimental work on obstructive uropathy has illuminated some of the physiological problems involved, but its clinical relevance must always be critically examined. In the first place, there are important anatomical differences between the kidneys of humans, the dog, and the rat, particularly in papillary structure. Secondly, most of the experimental models are not precisely comparable to the situation in which a partially obstructive lesion has been present from early fetal life.

There are three basic experimental models for the study of the physiology of urinary obstruction. In the first, ureteric ligation causes complete obstruction; the model is amenable to short-term and long-term studies, but as no urine is secreted, classic clearance methods are inapplicable. The second method involves ureteric catheterization and the imposition of external pressures; it is suitable for experiments on acute conditions only. Finally, chronic partial obstruction simulating congenital lesions can be created surgically.

With experimental complete ureteric obstruction there is at first a rise in renal blood flow (RBF) (21, 22); however, with prolonged obstruction, RBF falls to 70% of control values at 24 hr and 30% at one week (23). The initial rise is attributed to vasodilator prostaglandins and can be inhibited by indomethacin (24); the later fall can be attributed to the vasoconstrictive effect of thromboxane A2 (25).

As the tubular pressure rises, the glomerular filtration pressure gradient and hence filtration rate fall. Even with complete obstruction, however, it is probable that glomerular filtration does not cease completely, for there is continued reabsorption of salt and water by the tubules. Water and solutes are to some extent reabsorbed from the renal pelvis also; for example ^{131}I-labeled albumin injected into an obstructed renal pelvis can be detected in venous blood (26). The exact route of this reabsorption is still a matter of debate, and four different mechanisms have been discussed: pyelovenous, pyelotubular, pyelointerstitial, and pyelolymphatic back-flow (27). Renal lymphatic flow increases threefold in dogs with acute ureteric obstruction, but its composition is unchanged, suggesting that the effect is due to increased lymph formation rather than pyelolymphatic back-flow of urine (28).

Even small increments in ureteric pressure cause a fall in glomerular filtration rate (GFR). Tubular function is characterized by a reduced ability to concentrate the urine, associated with a decline in papillary sodium and urea content (29). Permeability characteristics of the tubular epithelium are altered, for the urinary recovery of inulin injected into the proximal tubule is not complete (30). The fractional excretion of filtered sodium is reduced (31). During water diuresis, increased ureteric pressure on one side causes a decrease in urine flow rate and sodium concentration, with an increase in urea concentration and osmolality compared to the urine of the control kidney (32). During hypotonic saline infusion there is a reduction in fractional excretion of filtered water compared to the control kidney; the finding is similar in renal artery stenosis and implies increased sodium reabsorption by the proximal tubule (33).

With chronic partial ureteric obstruction, functional characteristics are different. Both GFR and RBF are substantially reduced, and during hypotonic saline expansion there is an increased fractional excretion of filtered water; the data suggest that many nephrons have ceased to function and that the remaining functional nephrons are carrying an increased excretory load, as in other forms of chronic renal failure (33).

Clinical Data. There are formidable problems inherent in studying the functional aspects of obstructive uropathy in children. In the first place, the clinical cases are heterogeneous and, as indicated previously, the diagnosis of significant urinary obstruction is not susceptible to rigorous confirmation. The two kidneys are frequently unequally affected, and the observed data may be influenced by concomitant urinary tract infection, renal dysplasia, or salt and water depletion. The dilatation of the ureter and pelvis proximal to the site of obstruction creates a large reservoir of varying volume that makes short-term timed urine collections inaccurate and that may mask changes in concentrations of solutes in the urine secreted by the kidney. For this reason, if the investigation involves the imposition of an acute stimulus on the kidney, it is necessary to demonstrate that the urinary response achieves a plateau before it can be concluded that the urine passed externally is representative of that secreted by the kidney. Passage of catheters above the site of obstruction does not resolve this problem, for the urodynamics are altered in the process. Finally it must be remembered that sick infants tolerate investigational procedures poorly, and that there is often some urgency to proceed to definitive surgical treatment. Under these circumstances it is hardly surprising that data on renal function in infants with obstructive uropathy are limited.

The principal aspects of renal function whose derangement in obstructive uropathy may be clinically important are glomerular filtration, sodium conservation, hydrogen ion excretion, and urinary concentration and dilution. The degree of suppression of GFR is quite variable, usually being more marked with lower urinary tract than with upper tract lesions, even if the latter are bilateral, and it is possible for the measured GFR to be within the normal range in spite of unequivocal radiological evidence of urinary obstruction.

Perhaps the most striking effect of urinary tract obstruction is on the urinary concentrating mechanisms (34). Obligatory hyposthenuria is common (35) and may mimic nephrogenic diabetes insipidus (36); in infants the defect may be so extreme that there is difficulty in maintaining water balance, particularly if high solute diets are offered.

The capacity of the child with obstructive uropathy to dilute the urine in response to a water load is interesting in relation to the observation of Suki and coworkers (33) on the differences between acute and chronic experimental obstructive uropathy previously described. Acute obstruction, in which the impairment of renal function is potentially reversible, is characterized by a decreased fractional excretion of filtered water, and Barratt and Chantler reported an inverse relationship between the minimum urine osmolality during preoperative water diuresis and the immediate increase in GFR after release of obstruction (37).

Defective hydrogen ion excretion is common: Berlyne (36) documented failure of maximal urinary acidification after administration of ammonium chloride in six of seven patients with hydronephrosis, and a low gradient between urine and plasma P_{CO_2} during bicarbonate infusion suggests that distal tubular hydrogen ion secretion is at fault (38).

After Relief

Postobstructive Natriuresis. Following the relief of urinary obstruction there may be an exaggerated urinary loss of sodium, which can sometimes achieve massive proportions (39). Osmotic diuresis due to the excretion of retained urea and other solutes plays a role (40) but seems an inadequate explanation for the more extreme cases. In a minor degree the phenomenon is common: in infants with obstructive uropathy the urine sodium excretion on the first postoperative day is 59% above preoperative levels, in contrast to the usual antinatriuretic response to surgery (41). Excessive postoperative urine sodium losses are typically seen in the child who has a good nephrogram preoperatively and in whom renal function recovers well; there is a correlation between the increase in urine sodium excretion immediately after operation and the increment in GFR (41).

Postoperative natriuresis in the rat has been extensively studied as an experimental model. Following 24-h bilateral ureteric ligation, relief of the obstruction in one ureter results in considerable diuresis; this does not happen if only one ureter is occluded (42) unless contralateral nephrectomy is undertaken or urine from the unobstructed kidney is reinfused, suggesting that urea retention and volume expansion are important determinants of the diuresis in these experiments (43).

Recovery of Function. There is anecdotal evidence that some recovery of renal function may occur in humans after a period of complete ureteric obstruction of as much as three months (44). In dogs the degree of recovery is a function of the duration of obstruction and the time elapsed following its relief; the full potential for recovery may not be realized for three months. After relief following one week of complete ureteric obstruction the GFR reaches 68% of the control kidney value, but if the obstruction is prolonged for four weeks, recovery to only 22% is seen (45). These data are, however, of questionable relevance to the child with a partially obstructive congenital lesion, and there is unfortunately little intelligible data on the long-term recovery of function of these children, principally due to the heterogeneity of their clinical course.

The factors affecting recoverability of renal function after relief of obstruction may be summarized as follows: it is possible to recognize two polar types of urinary obstruction, which may be designated "acute" and "chronic" though it must be admitted that it is not clear whether the duration of the obstruction is in fact the principal determinant of the physiological characteristics. In acute obstruction the intrapelvic pressure is high, renal blood flow is well maintained, and glomerular filtration continues, but there is avid proximal reabsorption of filtrate so that the nephrogram is prominent, the secretory phase of the renogram persists, and there is limitation of the ability of the kidney to dilute the urine; the GFR rises after relief of obstruction, which is often accompanied by a significant postoperative natriuresis. On the other hand, in the chronically obstructed kidney the intrapelvic pressure may only be raised under diuretic conditions, there is a reduction in RBF with a poor secretory phase in the renogram, and an inconspicuous nephrogram; fractional sodium reabsorption in the proximal tubule is diminished, as in other forms of chronic renal failure: these kidneys do not improve after relief of obstruction.

Radiological Consequences

Urography

The hallmark of acute urinary tract obstruction is a delayed but increasingly dense prolonged nephrogram on the intravenous urogram (IVU) (46) (Fig. 38.1, *A*). This may be juxtaposed with dilated calyces that fill sluggishly with contrast medium so that in early films the effect is of a "negative pyelogram." The physiological basis of this type of nephrogram is continuing glomerular filtration with concentration of the dye within the tubular lumen caused by the salt and water reabsorption previously described; its presence suggests there will be a good return of renal function when the obstruction is relieved. A good nephrogram may

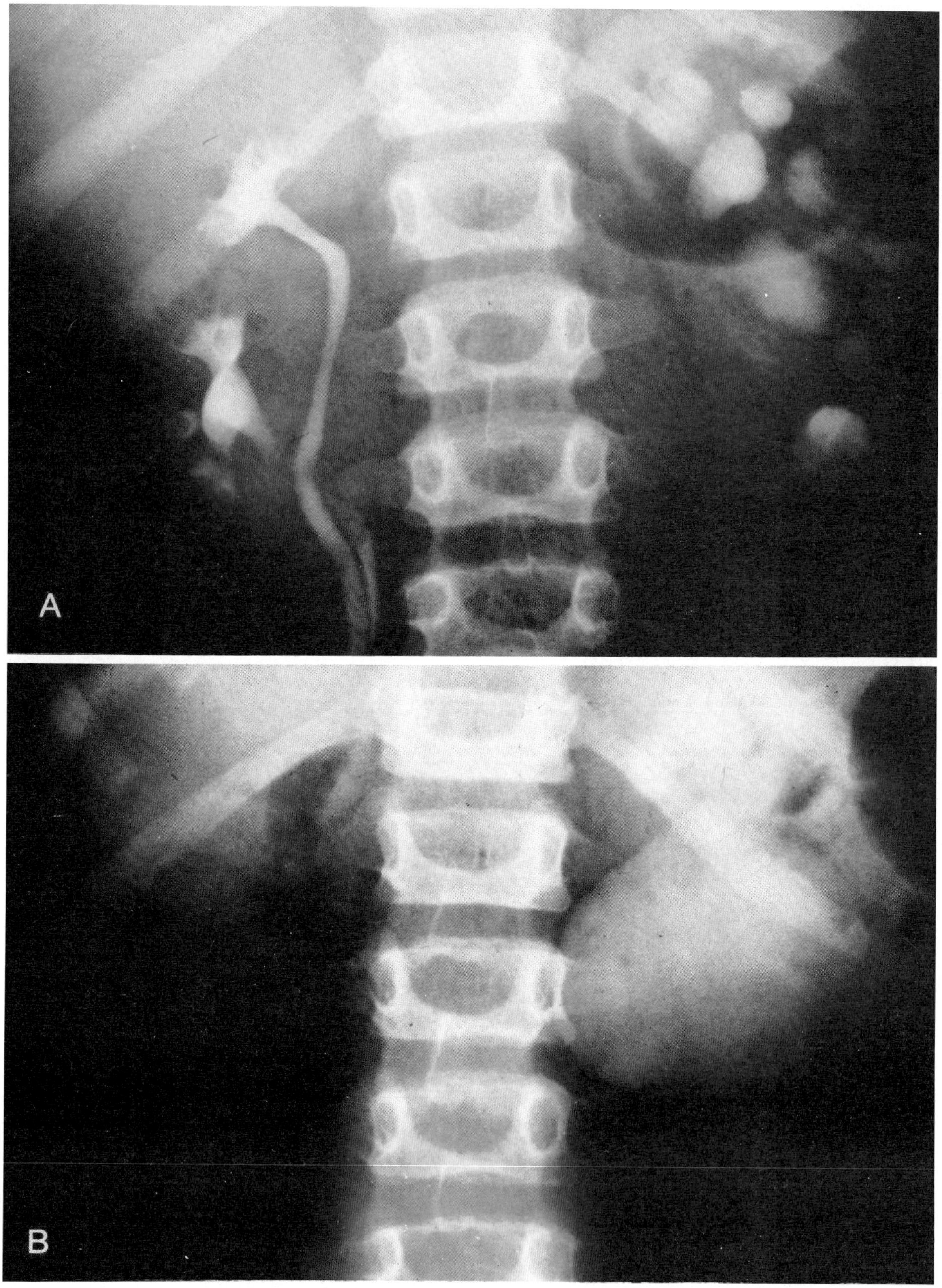

Figure 38.1. **A,** Pelviureteric junction obstruction on left side with dense nephrogram and pooling of contrast medium in hydronephrotic calyces. Duplex system on right side. **B,** Later film showing the dilated renal pelvis.

be seen with congenital lesions in spite of the fact they are by definition long standing, suggesting that the duration of obstruction is not necessarily the principal determinant of the radiological appearances.

There is a variant of the obstructive nephrogram in which a particularly dense rim of contrast medium surrounds the calyx; presumably the contrast medium is within the collecting ducts stretched over the hydronephrotic sac. Such a "shell nephrogram" indicates good potential for recovery.

Isotope Scanning

The effect of obstruction is best displayed by gamma camera quantitation of the renal excretion of 99m-technetium diethylenetriamine-pentacetic acid (^{99m}Tc-DTPA) (see Chapter 20). Following intravenous injection there is, with obstruction, decreased uptake of the chelate by the kidney, prolonged renal transit time and delayed removal of activity from the renal pelvis. The decreased uptake is due to reduced GFR. The prolonged parenchymal transit time is the isotopic equivalent of the obstructive nephrogram and reflects decreased tubular flow caused by enhanced salt and water reabsorption. Transit time has been elegantly evaluated by deconvolutional analysis in adult patients with hydronephrosis, and a distinction has been drawn between obstructive uropathy, in which renal function is normal, and obstructive nephropathy, in which transit time is prolonged (47). In children, however, it has not proved possible to define areas of renal parenchyma with sufficient reliability for this type of analysis, and the whole kidney transit time is dominated by the rate of turnover in the renal pelvis (48).

Delayed clearance of isotope from the renal pelvis is difficult to analyze quantitatively; however, the response to diuretics has been found useful, and a good clearance of isotope following furosemide suggests that there is no significant obstruction (49), but the test is not reliable if underlying renal function is poor.

Bacteriological Consequences

The association between urinary tract infection and obstruction is well known; infection is often the event that draws attention to an obstructive lesion and is one of the major factors that causes loss of renal function in such cases. Lower urinary tract obstruction increases the residual volume in the bladder and thereby facilitates ascending infection. The effects of ureteric ligation in the rat have been studied by Guze and Beeson; complete obstruction increases the susceptibility to hematogenous infection, but the effects of partial ureteric obstruction are less marked (50, 51). The obstructed kidney receives the same inoculum as the control kidney after intravenous injection of *Escherichia coli*, for the viable bacterial counts are the same during the first few hours in the two kidneys, but the numbers decline on the control side and multiply rapidly on the obstructed side.

ETIOLOGY OF CONGENITAL URINARY TRACT OBSTRUCTION

There is surprisingly little information on the etiology of congenital obstructive uropathy, but both genetic and environmental factors probably operate.

Genetic Aspects

Several families with hydronephrosis caused by pelviureteric junction (PUJ) or ureterovesical junction (UVJ) obstruction have been described, and McKusick lists familial hydronephrosis as a possible autosomal dominant, though in some pedigrees males seem particularly affected and the generally rather low familial incidence suggests polygenic inheritance (51a). Hydronephrosis is occasionally found in the dominantly inherited syndromes of Ehlers-Danlos, Marfan, multiple lentigines, and Apert's acrocephalosyndactyly. Recessively inherited syndromes that may include hydronephrosis are Laurence-Moon-Biedl, Fanconi's anemia, and ectromelia-icthyosis (see Chapter 25).

Of the chromosomal anomalies, trisomies 13 and 18 are complicated by obstructive uropathy in about 20% and trisomy 21 (mongolism) and Turner's syndrome in 4% of cases (52).

A number of inbred mice strains have developed hydronephrosis in association with various congenital malformations (53). Lozzio described an interesting syndrome in the rat in which inherited midureteric strictures are variably associated with hydronephrosis or renal dysplasia, and this in some ways seems the most appropriate experimental model for studies of congenital obstructive uropathy (54).

Teratogenesis

The critical stage in the development of the human kidney is at the 5.5 to 7 mm stage (28–30 days), when the ureteric bud arises from the posteromedial wall of the wolffian duct. If the congenital anomaly results from an isolated teratogenic episode, it is likely to have occurred at this early stage of pregnancy, but no such factors have been identified in humans, except with maternal thalidomide ingestion, which occasionally resulted in hydronephrosis in the fetus. There are, however, numerous experimental models, reviewed by Warkany (53): maternal vitamin A deficiency or excess, pantothenic acid deficiency, pteroylglutamic acid deficiency, and irradiation have all been reported to cause the development of hydronephrosis in the rat.

Obstructive lesions of the urinary tract are frequently associated with other congenital malformations, particularly congenital heart disease (55) and anorectal malformations (56). Constellations of congenital malformations, including obstructive uropathy, which constitute recognized syndromes occur: the prune belly syndrome; Russell-Silver dwarfism (hemihypertrophy, dwarfism, craniofacial dysostosis and sometimes PUJ obstruction); and the Rubenstein-Taybi syndrome (broad thumbs, hypoplastic maxillae, and megaureter).

LEVELS OF URINARY TRACT OBSTRUCTION

Pelviureteric Junction

Pathology

The PUJ is the commonest site of obstruction in the upper urinary tract in childhood. The condition is usually congenital and may have a mechanical basis with intrinsic stenosis or external compression. Several lesions have been described: pelviureteral angulation with high insertion of the ureter (57), adhesions, aberrant lower pole vessels (58), and persisting fetal folds (59, 60). The obstruction may also be functional, resulting from ureteropelvic incoordination or secondary to an overdistensible renal pelvis (61). There may be a structural abnormality of which the consequence is disordered peristalsis (62–65). PUJ obstruction may be associated with fused or ectopic kidneys or affect one part (usually the lower pole) of a duplex system.

Presentation

Antenatal Presentation. In recent years the use of prenatal ultrasonography has led to the diagnosis of hydronephrosis in utero and therefore to an awareness of its presence in asymptomatic neonates (66–69) (see Chapter 57).

Neonatal Presentation. The most common presenting feature in the neonatal period is an abdominal mass (70–74). Infants with bilateral PUJ obstruction may have a significant degree of renal failure, which is unusual in cases presenting in later childhood. Vomiting and failure to thrive may be a consequence of pain or superimposed UTI.

Older Children. In older children the clinical presentation is intermittent loin pain, colicky in nature, accompanied by vomiting and nausea, and lasting a few hours but followed by complete relief of symptoms (75–80). Equally common is a presentation with UTI. Hematuria may be the first sign, sometimes precipitated by slight abdominal trauma—perhaps the result of increased intrapelvic pressure leading to sudden distention of the pelvis and rupture of a dilated vessel.

Diagnosis

In the classic case, the diagnosis can be easily confirmed by ultrasound and ^{99m}Tc-DTPA scan (66). In the neonate a micturating cystourethrogram (MCU) should also be undertaken to exclude VUR. A poorly functioning kidney with PUJ obstruction has to be differentiated from a multicystic kidney. Ultrasound may do this, but in doubtful cases an antegrade pyelogram is helpful and has eliminated the need for retrograde pyelography.

In older children an IVU is useful, particularly if there is doubt about the anatomical abnormality at the PUJ itself, for example, the possibility of papillomata (81, 82). In the classic PUJ obstruction, the IVU shows a prolonged nephrogram with negative pyelogram and subsequently a dilated renal pelvis with nonvisualization of the ureter below (Fig. 38.1, *A*). Delayed films are important to determine the true level of obstruction (Fig. 38.1, *B*).

In equivocal cases several techniques have been proposed: antegrade pressure-flow studies (83, 84), diuretic urography (85), and diuretic radionuclide renography (49, 86, 87), but none have proved absolutely reliable.

Management

The surgical relief of obstruction can be performed in a variety of ways, the most frequently chosen being the Anderson-Hynes operation in which the pelviureteric junction is excised and a new pelviureteric anastomosis created (88). If the function of the kidney is very poor and the opposite kidney is apparently normal, nephroureterectomy should be considered. The choice between pyeloplasty and nephrectomy may be difficult, and a conservative approach should be adopted because potential for recovery of the kidney is greater in children than in adults. A preliminary temporary urinary diversion with percutaneous insertion of a nephrostomy catheter may be helpful in functional assessment and prediction of outcome.

The management of infants with hydronephrosis diagnosed in utero remains controversial (see Chapter 57). A few authors have stressed the need for early surgery (72, 73, 89). A group of 26 cases (3 with bilateral obstruction) have been observed for two years at the Hospital for Sick Children, London. Renal function was assessed by ^{99m}Tc-DTPA scan and assessed as poor in 4 kidneys, moderate in 9, and good in 12. The kidneys with poor function were drained by percutaneous nephrostomy and recovered sufficient function to merit subsequent pyeloplasty. Kidneys in the moderate group were managed by pyeloplasty, and half showed improvement in function. The kidneys classified as having good function were managed conservatively, and function was well maintained in them with only one case undergoing subsequent pyeloplasty because of UTI. There is thus no need for emergency surgery in the neonate diagnosed as having PUJ obstruction with good renal function.

Ureterovesical Junction

Pathology

Obstruction at the UVJ results in ureteric dilatation. In its primary form the condition is often referred to as obstructive megaureter. The term megaureter of itself merely indicates ureteric dilatation without any implication of pathogenesis. Four categories of megaureter are recognized: (a) refluxing, (b) obstructive, (c) nonrefluxing and nonobstructive, and (d) refluxing and obstructive (90, 91).

Primary obstructive megaureter is associated with a segment of the lower ureter, which though of normal caliber, fails to propel the bolus of urine adequately, thereby effectively causing obstruction. The precise pathogenesis is disputed. Abnormal muscular arrangements with an excess of circular in proportional to longitudinal fibers (92–95) and segmental defects (96, 97) have been described. Ultrastructural studies have shown an excess of collagen and muscular hypertropy and hyperplasia in the dilated segment (98–101). There may be two different pathogenetic groups, with the primary muscular abnormality residing at the UVJ in one and in the dilated segment in the other (102–104).

Presentation

In most series there is a male preponderance (106, 107). The left ureter is affected more often than the right, but the condition may be bilateral albeit asymmetrical. The presentation may be in early childhood with fever and loin pain due to urinary tract infection. The obstruction may be complicated by stone formation. Hematuria may occur, even in absence of stones.

Diagnosis

The diagnosis can ordinarily be made on IVU, if necessary with diuresis or late films, to delineate the bulbous lower part of the dilated ureter (Fig. 38.2). An MCU is required to exclude VUR or bladder outflow obstruction. VUR does not exclude obstruction, which may be suggested by dilution of the refluxed contrast medium in the pool of urine in the dilated obstructed ureter. It is not always clear whether a dilated ureter is significantly obstructed, in which case an antegrade study with pressure-flow measurements and a ^{99m}Tc-DTPA scan are helpful (108).

Management

Obstructive megaureter is best treated by excising the lower stenotic segment and ureteric reimplantation with an antireflux technique (108–110). In many cases a narrowing of the dilated ureter is required, either with tailoring or plication, both to improve ureteric function and to allow the submucosal tunnel in the bladder to be effectively valvular (111–114). The results of surgery are very satisfactory, with both the megaureter and the related kidney having considerable capacity for recovery; only rarely is nephroureterectomy appropriate.

Posterior Urethral Valve

Pathology

A congenital posterior urethral valve (PUV) is the most common and severe obstructive lesion in male infants. The typical valve, described by Young and coworkers as type I (115), consists of a fold of mucosa hanging down from the verumontanum with a small sagittal slit posteriorly. The impression of two valve leaflets is an artifact of the technique of displaying the postmortem pathology by incision of the anterior wall of the urethra. Young's type III valve consists of a diaphragmatic structure with a central orifice (115, 116), which may occasionally be dragged downstream in the manner of a wind sock (117). Type II valves are a doubtful entity. The term type IV valve is sometimes applied to the conical urethral abnormality associated with prostatic hypoplasia in the prune belly syndrome.

The valve obstructs the flow of urine and therefore leads to bladder hypertrophy and trabeculation, which may be marked. The ureters are dilated and tortuous with bilateral hydronephrosis. Because obstruction is present in utero there may be severe renal dysplasia, particularly in kidneys exposed to VUR (118, 119).

Urinary extravasation may occur in the perinatal period with a perirenal urinoma or urinary ascites (120, 121). Extravasation is usually associated with a reasonably good kidney, as though the leak protected it from the deleterious effects of back pressure.

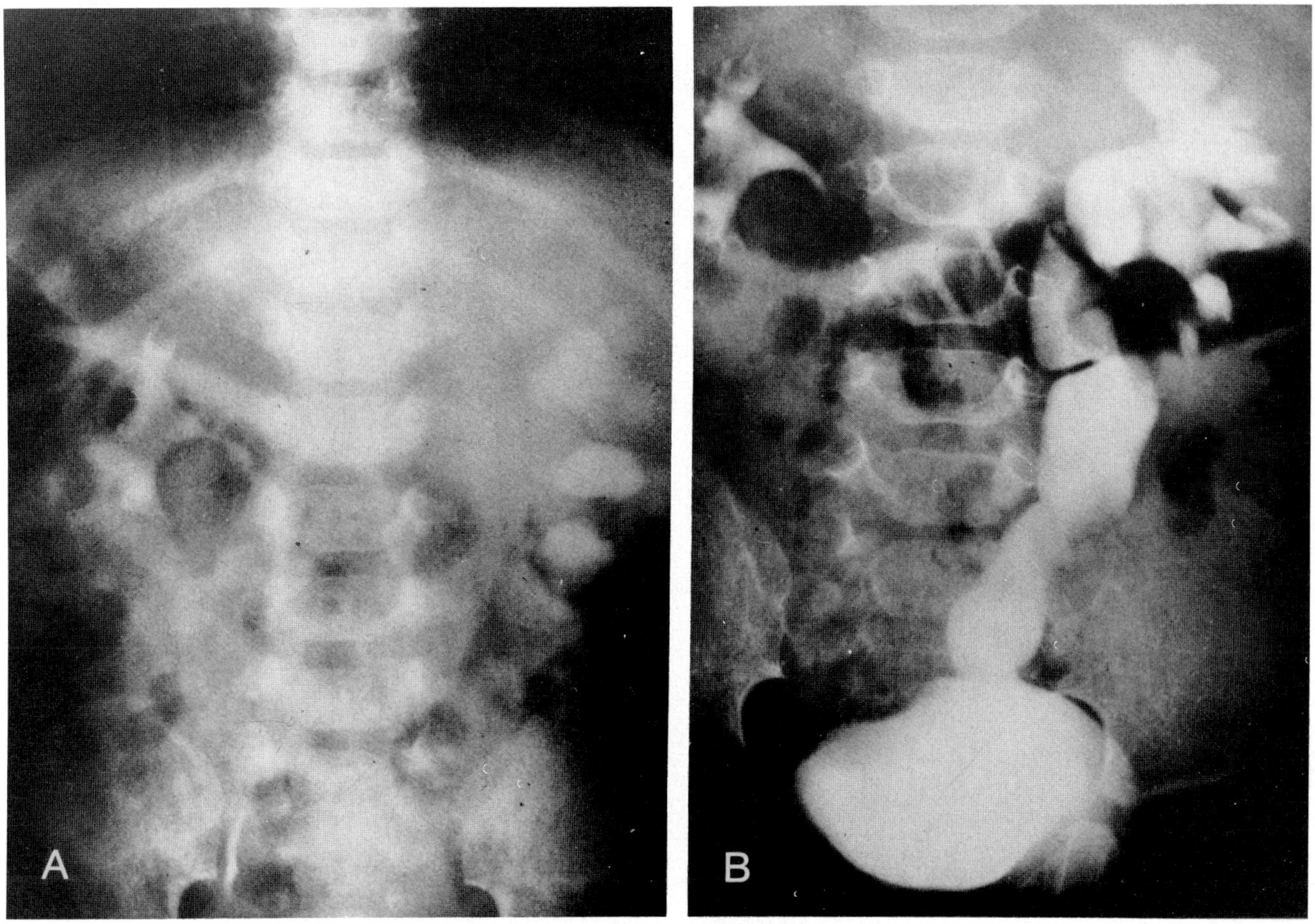

Figure 38.2. Obstructive megaureter on left side: **A,** Hydronephrosis. **B,** Later film showing dilated ureter.

Presentation

Antenatal Presentation. Hydronephrosis as a consequence of PUV is now frequently detected by routine ultrasonography in pregnancy (122, 123) (see Chapter 58).

Neonatal Presentation. The typical presentation is urinary retention or dribbling with a poor urinary stream (124–127). Sometimes the abnormality is first discovered by the detection of a palpable kidney or bladder on routine neonatal examination. However, the condition can be overlooked as detrusor hypertrophy may enable a moderately good urinary stream to be achieved, and a palpable bladder may be missed in a neonate in whom the umbilical cord has not separated. Abdominal distention and vomiting may lead to an initial suspicion of a bowel disorder. Hematuria may occur. The renal failure may cause vomiting, dehydration, and failure to thrive. If dysplasia has caused poor renal function, other problems may result from the oligohydramnios, particularly pulmonary hypoplasia and pneumothorax. Later, when UTI supervenes, the infant may present acutely ill with renal failure and possibly septicemia and meningitis (128).

Older Children. The pattern of presentation of PUV is changing. In earlier series some cases were diagnosed in boys who were investigated for UTI or incontinence in the first few years of life (129, 130). There is a concentrating defect secondary to the obstructive nephropathy, and renal failure may be responsible for poor growth and osteodystrophy, so cases were found among children investigated for polyuria, rickets, or growth failure. With increasing standards of neonatal care more cases are being detected in early life, and late presentation is now unusual.

Diagnosis

In the sick neonate, ultrasound examination is by far the best initial investigation. The following features can be assessed: the degree of hydronephrosis, the thickness of the renal parenchyma, the presence of extravasated urine, the degree of ureteric dilatation, residual bladder urine, bladder wall thickening, and posterior urethral dilatation (Fig. 38.3, *A*) (131). An MCU is necessary to demonstrate the valve itself, with oblique views taken during micturition after removal of the catheter to demonstrate the anatomy clearly (Fig. 38.3, *B*).

Later, a ^{99m}Tc-DTPA scan is necessary to assess individual kidney function, which may be surprisingly asymmetrical, even though the obstruction is intravesical because of the association of renal dysplasia with VUR. There is now little place for an IVU in the evaluation of these infants.

Management

A rapid initial assessment of the state of hydration, electrolyte disturbance, uremia, and sepsis is necessary. Rehydration, antibiotic therapy, and treatment of acute renal failure as outlined in Chapter 48 are appropriate (132).

The bladder should be drained by an indwelling catheter and upper tract deflation checked by ultrasound. Endoscopic resection should be undertaken as soon as the child's general condition permits (133–135). Previously, temporary upper tract diversion by nephrostomy or ureterostomy was frequently undertaken but is now less necessary as techniques of endoscopic valve resection have improved (136, 137). Diversion tends

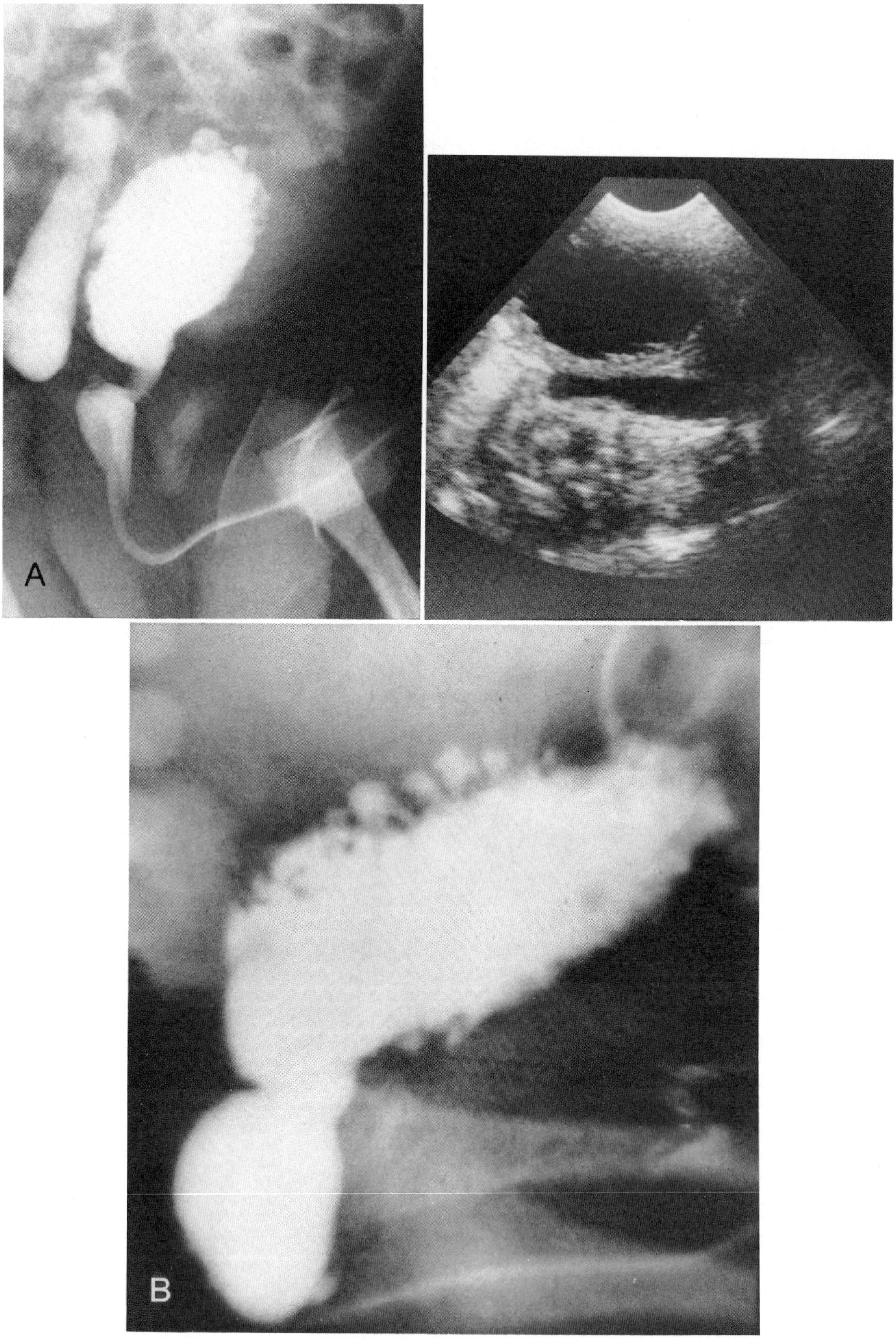

Figure 38.3. **A,** Micturating cystourethrogram (*left*) and ultrasound examination (*right*) of infant with posterior urethral valve showing bladder hypertrophy, dilated refluxing right ureter, and enlarged posterior urethra. **B,** Posterior urethral valve demonstrated by micturating cystourethrogram.

to generate further problems because of contraction of the defunctioned bladder and the need for a complex program of reconstructive ureteric surgery; however, there is still a place for vesicostomy in the management of small premature infants (138).

Following valve resection, another MCU and cystourethroscopy are necessary to ensure that valve ablation is complete. Vesicoureteric reflux is frequently associated but should be managed conservatively with chemoprophylaxis. A ^{99m}Tc-DTPA scan indicates the adequacy of urinary drainage and provides a baseline for further follow-up. It may also identify a nonfunctioning kidney, which if associated with VUR is best removed. These children require indefinite urological follow-up to ensure that urinary drainage remains adequate and that late sequelae such as urethral stricture are not overlooked.

Renal function should be monitored carefully in the postoperative period. There may be natriuresis, which is usually appropriately replaced as $NaHCO_3$, about 2 mmol/kg/24 hr. Subsequently the babies should have a calorie intake of at least 100 cal/kg/24 hr, and if renal function is impaired, modest protein restriction is appropriate. Extra fluid may be required because of the urinary concentrating defect.

Outcome

Nearly all affected infants now survive the initial phase of diagnosis and surgery. In a few, however, renal dysplasia is severe, with end-stage renal failure ensuing in a few months. The majority have much better renal function, but long-term follow-up studies indicate a high incidence of hypertension and renal failure in teenage boys (139). Growth is often poor but has been alleged to be better with early diversion (140). Urinary continence is impaired but improves at puberty (141).

Other Causes

Ureter

The ureter may be obstructed by stricture (142), valves (143), polyps (81), or stone. In retrocaval and retroiliac ureters, external compression by vascular structure may be obstructive (144, 145). Extrinsic compression by abcess or tumor may result in acquired obstruction.

Bladder

Ureteroceles may obstruct the ureterovesical junction of bladder outflow (see Chapter 39). A dysfunctional bladder due to overt or occult nephropathy may be responsible (see Chapter 40). Bladder neck obstruction in other circumstances is now considered a rare abnormality in children (146).

Urethra

The urethra may be obstructed by a polyp at any position (147). The so-called anterior urethral valve is really a wide-mouthed diverticulum with an obstructive anterior lip (148). Urethral stricture may follow catheterization. There is a tendancy during MCU to concentrate on the posterior urethra and UVJ, so that anterior urethral lesions are often overlooked.

PRUNE BELLY SYNDROME

The association of deficiency of abdominal musculature, urological abnormality, and cryptorchidism has been called the prune belly syndrome (PBS) (149), the Eagle-Barrett syndrome (150), or triad syndrome (151). The prune-like appearance of the abdominal wall is so striking that the term prune belly syndrome is now preferred (Fig. 38.4) (152, 153). The condition is estimated to occur about once in 35,000 to 50,000 live births (154) but is more common in twin pregnancies (155). By the previously given definition, it is confined to male patients but occasionally similarly affected girls are seen (156). Familial cases have been recorded (157), but most appear sporadically.

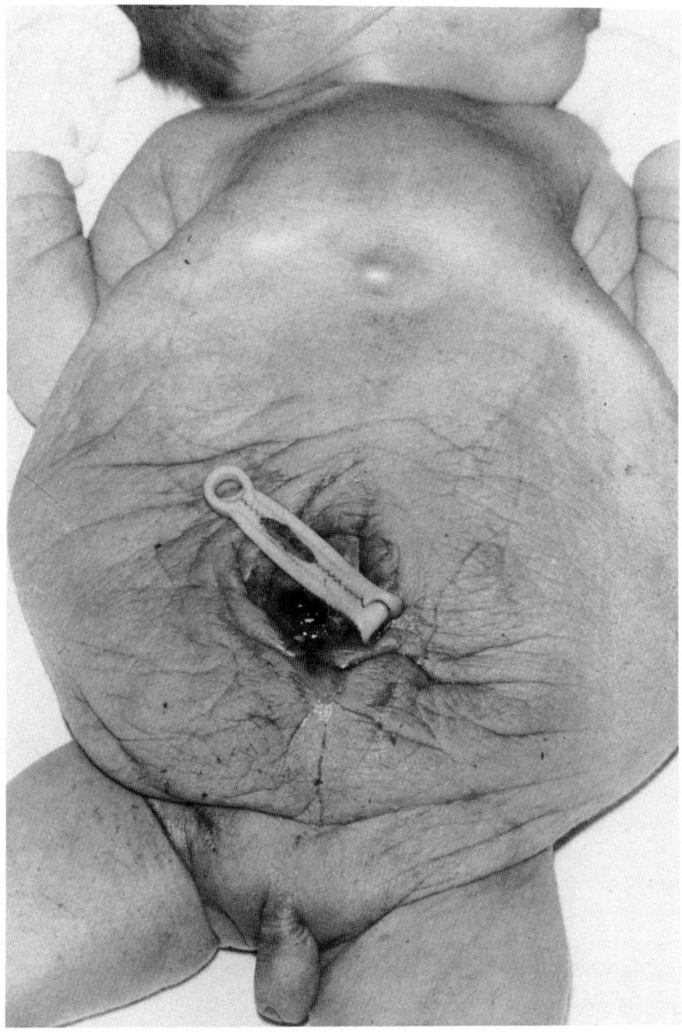

Figure 38.4. Prune belly syndrome.

Pathology

Abdominal Wall

Abdominal wall musculature is absent or sparse (158, 159). The extent of the defect is variable, but typically the lower abdomen is most severely involved. There are cases in which the urological and testicular abnormalities are typical of the prune belly syndrome, yet the abdominal wall musculature appears normal ("pseudoprunes") (160).

Urological Abnormalities

Renal dysplasia is usually found in prune belly syndrome. It may be asymmetrical and vary from extreme cystic dysplasia to a mild dysmorphic abnormality. Renal function may be surprisingly well preserved, even with gross urological abnormality. The ureters are usually severely dilated and tortuous, and typically there is a disparity, with the lower part being more markedly affected than the upper (161, 162) (Fig. 38.5, *A*). The bladder is enlarged and functions abnormally (163). The apex is frequently tethered to the umbilicus: in more severe cases associated with complete urethral obstruction the urachus may be patent, draining urine.

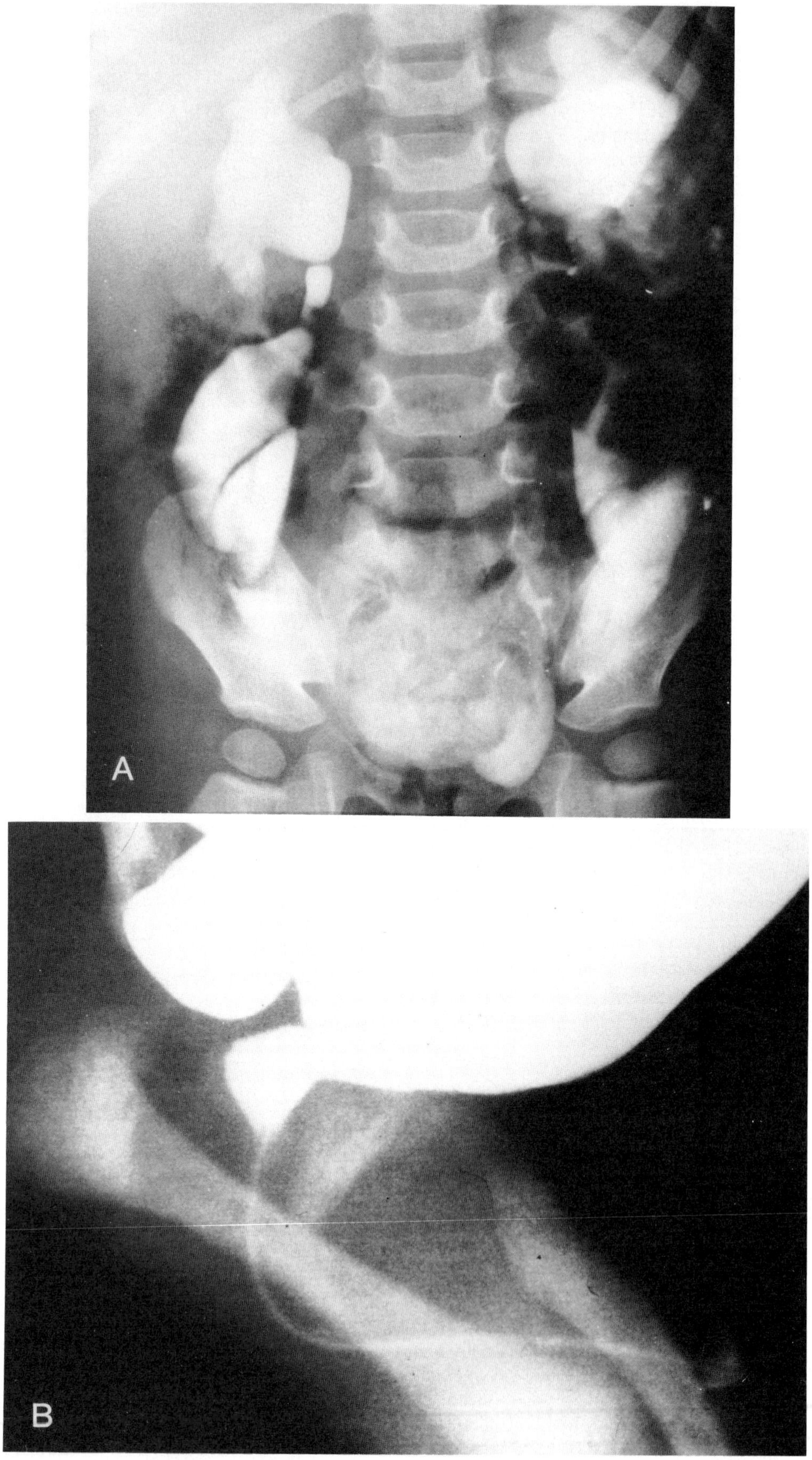

Figure 38.5. Prune belly syndrome: **A,** Dilated ureters shown by intravenous urography. **B,** Conical posterior urethra shown by micturating cystourethrogram.

The posterior urethra is wide, tapering in a conical fashion to a point in the membranous urethra (Fig. 38.5, *B*). The degree of obstruction at this point differs in individual cases. The prostate is hypoplastic (164). Occasionally there is dilatation of the anterior urethra, or megalourethra (165).

Testes

Cryptorchidism is the rule, spermatogenesis is poor, and there is a risk of neoplasia (166).

Other Systems

There is an association with major anomalies of the gastrointestinal tract (167). Cases of prune belly syndrome usually have a short universal mesentery so that malrotation may occur. Cardiac anomalies have been reported.

Some of the abnormalities in prune belly syndrome are the consequence of oligohydramnios with Potter facies, talipes, and dislocated hips. A rather characteristic abnormality is skin dimpling over pressure sites on the lateral aspects of elbows and knees (153). Pulmonary hypoplasia may be associated with the oligohydramnios, and the deficient abdominal musculature is a handicap to ventilation, predisposing these children to postoperative respiratory complications (152, 168).

Pathogenesis

The pathogenesis of prune belly syndrome has recently been the subject of an interesting debate. Pagon and coworkers proposed that the abdominal wall defect was the consequence of abdominal distention by a full bladder secondary to transient urethral obstruction (9), which Moerman and coworkers attributed to prostatic hypoplasia (10). Woodhouse and coworkers do not accept this thesis, however, for it fails to explain the abdominal wall defect in cases in which bladder drainage has been maintained during pregnancy by a patent urachus (160).

Presentation

The urological abnormality associated with prune belly syndrome has been detected by antenatal ultrasound (169, 170). The condition is obvious at birth. Woodhouse and coworkers (161) presented a clinical classification of 47 cases of prune belly syndrome: Group 1: Perinatal death, often with hypoplastic or atretic urethra (5 cases). Group 2: Neonatal emergency presentation with infection and gross urinary tract dilation (13 cases). Group 3: Well in the neonatal period. Good renal function despite very abnormal radiological findings (29 cases).

Management

Medical Management

Neonates with prune belly syndrome may present as medical emergencies with acute renal failure due to renal dysplasia complicated by the effects of sepsis, obstruction, and perinatal asphyxia. The renal failure should be managed in a spirit of optimism according to the principles outlined in Chapter 48: the 13 cases in group 2 of Woodhouse and coworkers survived the neonatal period, and half of them grew up normally with good health and renal function.

The large volume of stagnant urine presents a major risk of urinary tract infection, which if established, may be serious. Instrumentation of the urinary tract or catheterization (e.g., for MCU) should therefore be avoided unless absolutely essential; conversely, an infected urinary tract should be properly drained. Infection with a urea-splitting organism such as *Proteus* has been reported to cause hyperammonemic encephalopathy due to absorption of ammonia from the urinary tract (171).

Surgical Management

With the realization of the generally good outcome of children with prune belly syndrome, the aggressive surgical approach of the 1970s, with extensive use of urinary diversion and ureteric remodeling (172, 173), has given way to more conservative management with minimal surgical intervention (152, 153) and an acceptance of upper tract dilatation, the emphasis being on the maintenance of bladder drainage by urethral surgery if necessary. A vesicostomy, though, is a helpful temporary diversion in the infant with urinary tract infections (175).

Current practice is to correct the cryptorchidism surgically. In the first months of life, it may prove possible to move the testis into the scrotum without diversion of the spermatic vessels (176), but in older children it may be necessary to rely on a strip of peritoneum for vascularization (177); even in the second instance the success rate of operation is 75% (178). Redundant abdominal wall is sometimes removed by plication, principally for cosmetic reasons.

References

1. Pais VM, Retik AB: Reversible hydronephrosis in the neonate with urinary sepsis. N Engl J Med 292:465, 1975.
2. Teague N, Boyarsky S: Further effects of coliform bacilli on ureteral peristalsis. J Urol 99:702, 1968.
3. Ten Bensel RW, Peters ER: Progressive hydronephrosis, hydroureter and dilatation of the bladder in siblings with congenital nephrogenic diabetes insipidus. J Pediatr 77:439, 1970.
4. Weiss RM, Wagner ML, Hoffman BF: Localisation of pacemaker for peristalsis in intact canine ureter. Invest Urol 5:42, 1967.
5. Notley RG: Electron microscopy of the upper ureter and pelviureteric junction. Br J Urol 40:37, 1968.
6. Boyarsky S, Gottschalk CW, Tanagho EA, et al (eds): Urodynamics; Hydrodynamics of the Ureter and Renal Pelvis. New York, Academic Press, 1971.
7. Gierup J, Ericsson NO: Micturition studies in infants and children. Urodynamics in boys with disorders of the lower urinary tract. Scand J Urol Nephrol 5:1, 1971.
8. Whitaker RH: Methods of assessing obstruction on dilated ureters. Br J Urol 45:15, 1973.
9. Pagon RA, Smith DW, Shepherd TM: Urethral obstruction malformation complex: a cause of abdominal muscle deficiency and the "prune-belly". J Pediatr 94:900, 1979.
10. Moerman P, Fryns J-P, Goddeeris P, et al: Pathogenesis of prune-belly syndrome: a functional urethral obstruction caused by prostatic hypoplasia. Pediatrics 73:470, 1984.
11. Bernstein J: Developmental abnormalities of the renal parenchyma—renal hypoplasia and dysplasia. Pathol Ann 3:213, 1968.
12. Beck AD: The effect of intrauterine urinary obstruction upon the development of the fetal kidney. J Urol 105:784, 1971.
13. Tanagho EA: Surgically induced partial urinary obstruction in the fetal lamb. I. Technique. Invest Urol 10:19, 1972.
14. Tanagho EA: Surgically induced partial urinary tract obstruction in the fetal lamb. II. Urethral obstruction. Invest Urol 10:25, 1972.
15. Tanagho EA: Surgically induced partial urinary obstruction in the fetal lamb. III. Ureteral obstruction. Invest Urol 10:35, 1972.
16. Glick PL, Harrison MR, Noall RA, et al: Correction of congenital hydronephrosis in utero. III. Early mid-trimester ureteral obstruction produces renal dysplasia. J Pediatr Surg 18:681, 1983.
17. Glick PL, Harrison MR, Adzick NS: Correction of congenital hydronephrosis in utero IV: in utero decompression prevents renal dysplasia. J Pediatr Surg 19:649, 1984.
18. Matz LR, Craven VD, Hodson CJ: Experimental obstructive uropathy in the pig. Br J Urol (suppl)51:21, 1969.
19. Hodson CJ: Post-obstructive renal atrophy (nephropathy). Br Med Bull 28:237, 1972.
20. Cussen LJ: The structure of the normal human ureter in infancy and childhood. Invest Urol 5:179, 1967.
21. Selkurt EE: Effect of ureteral blockade on renal blood flow and urinary concentrating ability. Am J Physiol 205:286, 1963.
22. Murphy GP, Scott WW: The renal haemodynamic response to acute and chronic ureteral obstruction. J Urol 95:636, 1966.
23. Vaughan ED, Sorenson EJ, Gillenwater JW: The renal hemodynamic response to chronic unilateral complete ureteral occlusion. Invest Urol 8:78, 1970.

24. Allen JT, Vaughan ED, Gillenwater JY: The effect of indomethacin on renal blood flow and ureteral pressure in unilateral ureteral obstruction in awake dogs. Invest Urol 15:324, 1978.
25. Vaughan ED, Albanese CT, Marion DN, et al: Thromboxane A2 inhibition partially reverses the increased renal vascular resistance found at 24 hours of complete unilateral ureteral occlusion in the dog. Kidney Int 21:266, 1982.
26. Persky L, Bonte FJ, Austen G: Mechanism of hydronephrosis: radioautographic backflow patterns. J Urol 75:190, 1956.
27. Chisholm CG, Osborn DE: Pathophysiology of obstructive uropathy. In Williams DI, Chisholm GD (eds): Scientific Foundations of Urology, ed 1. London, Heinemann, 1976, p 64.
28. Henry NM, O'Morchoe PJ, O'Morchoe CC: The renal lymphatic system during obstructed urine flow. J Urol 106:455, 1971.
29. Jaenike JR, Bray GA: Effects of acute transitory urinary obstruction in the dog. Am J Physiol 199:1219, 1960.
30. Lorentz WW, Lassiter WE, Gottschalk CW: Renal tubular permeability during increased intrarenal pressure. J Clin Invest 51:484, 1972.
31. Fulop M, Brazeau P: Increased ureteral back pressure enhances renal tubular sodium reabsorption. J Clin Invest 49:2315, 1970.
32. Kiil F, Aukland K: Effect of high ureteral pressure on urine concentration during water diuresis. Scand J Clin Lab Invest 13:268, 1961.
33. Suki W, Eknoyan G, Rector FC, et al: Patterns of nephron perfusion in acute and chronic hydronephrosis. J Clin Invest 45:122, 1966.
34. Ericsson NO, Winberg J, Zetterstrom R: Renal function in infantile obstructive uropathy. Acta Paediatr Scand 44:444, 1955.
35. Winberg J: Renal function in water-losing syndrome due to lower urinary tract obstruction before and after treatment. Acta Paediatr Scand 48:149, 1959.
36. Berlyne GM: Distal tubular function in chronic hydronephrosis. Q J Med 30:339, 1961.
37. Barratt TM, Chantler C: Obstructive uropathy in infants. Proc R Soc Med 63:1248, 1970.
38. Hutcheon RA, Drummond KN, Kaplan BS: Distal renal tubular acidosis (DRTA) in children with chronic hydronephrosis. Pediatr Res 9:375, 1975.
39. Bricker NS, Shwayri EI, Reardan JB, et al: An abnormality in renal function resulting from urinary tract obstruction. Am J Med 23:554, 1957.
40. Maher JF, Schreiner GE, Waters TS: Osmotic diuresis due to retained urea after release of obstructive uropathy. N Engl J Med 268:1099, 1963.
41. Ghazali S, Barratt TM: Sodium excretion after relief of urinary tract obstruction in children. Br J Urol 46:163, 1974.
42. Yarger WE, Aynediian HS, Bank N: A micropuncture study of postobstructive diuresis in the rat. J Clin Invest 51:625, 1972.
43. Harris RH, Yarger WE: The pathogenesis of postobstructive diuresis. The role of circulating natriuretic and diuretic factors, including urea. J Clin Invest 56:880, 1975.
44. Better OS, Arieff AI, Massry SG, et al: Studies on renal function after relief of complete ureteral obstruction of three months duration in man. Am J Med 54:234, 1973.
45. Kerr WS: Effects of complete ureteral obstruction in dogs on kidney function. Am J Physiol 184:521, 1956.
46. Kelsey-Fry I, Catell WR: Nephrographic patterns during excretion urography. Br Med Bull 28:227, 1972.
47. Whitfield HN, Britton KE, Hendry WF, et al: The distinction between obstructive uropathy and nephropathy by radioisotope transit times. Br J Urol 50:433, 1978.
48. Vivian GC, Barratt TM, Todd-Pokropek A, et al: Renal parenchymal determination and analysis during dynamic ^{99m}Tc-DTPA scans in children. Nuclear Med Comm 5:35, 1984.
49. O'Reilly PH, Testa HJ, Lawson RS, et al: Diuresis renography in equivocal urinary tract obstruction. Br J Urol 50:76, 1978.
50. Guze LB, Beeson PB: Experimental pyelonephritis. I. Effect of ureteral ligation on the course of bacterial infection in the kidney of the rat. J Exp Med 104:803, 1956.
51. Guze LB, Beeson PB: Experimental pyelonephritis. II. Effect of partial ureteral obstruction on the course of bacterial infection in the kidney of the rat and rabbit. Yale J Biol Med 30:315, 1958.
51a. McKusick VA: Mendelian inheritance in man. Catalogs of Autosomal Dominant, Autosomal Recessive and X-linked Phenotypes. 6th Edition, Johns Hopkins University Press, Baltimore, 1983.
52. Egli F, Stadler G: Malformations of kidney and urinary tract in common chromosomal aberrations. I. Clinical Studies. Humangenetik 18:1,1973.
53. Warkany J: Congenital Malformations. Chicago Year Book Medical Publishers Inc, 1971, p 1053.
54. Lozzio BB: Hereditary renal disease in a mutant strain of rats. Science 156:1792, 1967.
55. Chrispin AR, Lillie JG: The pyelogram following angiocardiography in children with congenital heart disease. Proc R Soc Med 59:419, 1966.
56. Williams DI, Grant J: Urological complications of imperforate anus. Br J Urol 41:288, 1969.
57. Hanley HG: The pelvi-ureteric junction: a cine-pyelography study. Br J Urol 31:377, 1959.
58. Stephens FD: Ureterovascular hydronephrosis and the "aberrant" renal vessels. J Urol 128:984, 1982.
59. Östling K: Genesis of hydronephrosis. Acta Chir Scand (suppl)86:5, 1942.
60. Johnston JH: The pathogenesis of hydronephrosis in childhood. Br J Urol 41:724, 1969.
61. Whitaker RH: Some observations and theories on the wide ureter and hydronephrosis. Br J Urol 47:377, 1975.
62. Notley RG: Electron microscopy of the upper ureter and pelvi-ureteric junction. Br J Urol 40:37, 1968.
63. Hanna MK, Jeffs RD, Sturgess JM, et al: Ureteral structure and ultrastructure. II. Congenital UPJ obstruction and primary obstructive megaureter. J Urol 116:725, 1976.
64. Puigvert A: L'hydronephrose chez l-enfant. Facteurs pathogeniques. Acta Urol Belg 31:304, 1964.
65. Ruano-Gil D, Coca-Payeras A, Tejedo-Maten A: Obstruction and normal recanalisation of the ureter in the human embryo. Its relation to congenital ureteric obstruction. Eur Urol 1:287, 1975.
66. Pope TL, Alford BA, Buschi AJ, et al: Nuclear scintigraphy and ultrasound in the diagnosis of congenital ureteropelvic junction obstruction. J Urol 124:917, 1980.
67. Martin JJ, Taylor ES: Diagnosis of bilateral hydronephrosis in utero by ultrasonography. Urology 17:272, 1981.
68. Cass A, Veeraraghavan K, Smith S, et al: Prenatal diagnosis of fetal urinary tract abnormalities by ultrasound. Urology 18:197, 1981.
69. Fourcroy JL, Blei CL, Glassman LM, et al: Prenatal diagnosis by ultrasonography of genitourinary abnormalities. Urology 22:223, 1983.
70. Williams DI, Karlaftis CM: Hydronephrosis due to pelvi-ureteric obstruction in the newborn. Br J Urol 38:138, 1966.
71. Perlmutter AD, Kroovand RL, Lai Y-W: Management of ureteropelvic obstruction in the first year of life. J Urol 123:535, 1980.
72. Bejjani B, Belman BA: Ureteropelvic junction obstruction in newborns and infants. J Urol 128:770, 1982.
73. Roth DR, Gonzales ET: Management of ureteropelvic junction obstruction in infants. J Urol 129:108, 1983.
74. Robson WJ, Rudy SM, Johnston JH: Pelviureteric obstruction in infancy. J Pediatr Surg 11:57, 1976.
75. Williams DI, Kenawi MM: The prognosis of pelviureteric obstruction in childhood. Eur Urol 2:57, 1976.
76. Johnston JH, Evans JP, Glassberg KI, et al: Pelvic hydronephrosis in children: a review of 14 years of experience. J Urol 119:649, 1978.
77. Drake DP, Stevens PS, Eckstein HB: Hydronephrosis secondary to ureteropelvic obstruction in children: a review of 14 years of experience. J Urol 119:649, 1978.
78. Kelalis PP, Culp OS, Stickler GB, et al: Ureteropelvic obstruction in children: experience with 109 cases. J Urol 106:418, 1971.
79. Hendren WH, Radhakrishan J, Middleton AW: Pediatric pyeloplasty. J Pediatr Surg 15:133, 1980.
80. Thomas DFM, Agrawal M, Laidin AZ, et al: Pelviureteric obstruction in infancy and childhood. A review of 117 patients. Br J Urol 54:204, 1982.
81. Mirandi D, De Assis AS: Transitional cell papilloma of ureter in a young boy. Urology 5:559, 1975.
82. Johnston JH: Upper urinary tract obstruction. In Williams DI, Johnston JH (eds): Paediatric Urology. London, Butterworths, 1982, p 194.
83. Man D, Ransley PG: Antegrade pyelogram in children. Br J Urol 56:237, 1984.
84. Whitaker RH: Clinical assessment of pelvic and ureteral function. Urology 12:146, 1978.
85. Whitfield HN, Britton WF, Hendry WF, et al: Furosemide intravenous urography in the diagnosis of PUJ obstruction in childhood. Br J Urol 51:445, 1979.
86. Koff SA, Thrall JH, Keyes JW: Diuretic radionuclide uropathy: a non-invasive method for evaluating nephro-ureteral dilatation. J Urol 122:451, 1979.
87. O'Reilly PH, Lawson RS, Shields RA, et al: Idiopathic hydronephrosis—the diuresis renogram: a new non-invasive method of assessing equivocal PUJ obstruction. J Urol 121:153, 1979.
88. Anderson JC, Hynes W: Retrocaval ureter: cause diagnosed preoperatively and treated successfully by plastic operation. Br J Urol 21:209, 1949.
89. King LR, Coughlin PWF, Bloch EC, et al: The case for immediate pyeloplasty in the neonate with ureteropelvic obstruction. J Urol 132:725, 1984.
90. Stephens FD: The ABC of megaureters. Birth Defects 13:1, 1977.
91. King LR: Megaloureter: definition, diagnosis and management. J Urol 123:222, 1980.
92. Murnaghan GF: Experimental investigation of the dynamics of the normal and dilated ureter. Br J Urol 29:403, 1957.

93. Tanagho EA, Smith DR, Guthrie TH: Pathophysiology of functional obstruction. J Urol 104:73, 1970.
94. Tanagho EA: The pathogenesis and management of megaloureter. Johnston JH, Goodwin WE (eds): Reviews in Pediatric Urology. Amsterdam, Excerpta Medica, 1974, p 85.
95. McLaughlin P, Pfister RC, Leadbetter WF, et al: The pathophysiology of primary megaloureter. J Urol 109:805, 1973.
96. MacKinnon KJ, Foote JW, Wigleswoth FW, et al: The pathology of the adynamic distal ureteral segment. J Urol 103:134, 1970.
97. Gregoir W, Debled G: L'etiologie due reflux congenital et du megauretere primaire. Urol Int 24:119, 1969.
98. Notley RG: Electron microscopy of primary obstructive megaloureter. Br J Urol 44:229, 1972.
99. Hanna MK, Jeffs RD, Sturgess JM: Ureteral structure and ultrastructure. II. Congenital ureteropelvic junction obstruction and primary obstructive megaureter. J Urol 116:725, 1976.
100. Cussen LJ: The morphology of congenital dilatation of the ureter: intrinsic ureteral lesions. Austr N Z J Surg 41:185, 1971.
101. Stephens FD: Idiopathic dilatations of the urinary tract. J Urol 112:819, 1974.
102. Tokunaka S, Koyanagi T, Tsuji I, et al: Histopathology of the non-refluxing megaureter: a clue to its pathogenesis. J Urol 127:238, 1982.
103. Tokunaka S, Koyanagi J: Morphologic study of primary nonreflux megaureters with particular emphasis on the role of ureteral sheath and ureteral dysplasia. J Urol 128:399, 1982.
104. Tokunaka S, Gotoh T, Koyanagi I, et al: Muscle dysplasia in megaureters. J Urol 131:383, 1984.
105. Williams DI, Hulme-Moir I: Primary obstructive megaureter. Br J Urol 42:140, 1970.
106. Hanna MK, Jeffs RD: Primary obstructive megaureter in children. Urology 6:419, 1975.
107. Pfister RC, Newhouse JH, Hendren WH: Percutaneous pyeloureteral urodynamics. Urol Clin North Am 9:41–49, 1982.
108. Politano VA, Leadbetter WF: An operative technique for the correction of ureteric reflux. J Urol 79:932, 1958.
109. Bischoff P: Operative treatment of megaureter. J Urol 85:268, 1961.
110. Ahmed S: Transverse advancement ureteral reimplantation: pull-through alternative in megaureter. J Urol 123:218, 1980.
111. Tanagho EA: Ureteral tailoring. J Urol 106:194, 1971.
112. Hendren WH: Operative repair of megaureter in children. J Urol 101:491, 1969.
113. Kalcinsky Z, Kansy J, Kotabinska B, et al: Surgery of megaureters. Modification of Hendren's operation. J Pediatr Surg 12:183, 1977.
114. Weiss RM, Biancani P: Rationale for ureteral tapering. Urology 20:482, 1982.
115. Young HH, Frontz WA, Baldwin JC: Congenital obstruction of the posterior urethra. J Urol 3:289, 1919.
116. Robertson WB, Hayes JA: Congenital diaphragmatic obstruction of the male posterior urethra. Br J Urol 41:592, 1969.
117. Field PL, Stephens FD: Congenital urethral membranes causing urethral obstruction. J Urol 111:250, 1974.
118. Henneberry MD, Stephens FD: Renal hypoplasia and dysplasia in infants with posterior urethral valves. J Urol 123:912, 1980.
119. Milliken LD, Hodgson NB: Renal dysplasia and urethral valves. J Urol 108:960, 1972.
120. Cass AS, Khan AU, Smith S, et al: Neonatal perirenal urinary extravasation with posterior urethral valves. Urology 18:258, 1981.
121. Greenfield SP, Hensle TW, Bordon WE, et al: Urinary extravasation in the newborn male with posterior urethral valves. J Pediatr Surg 17:751, 1982.
122. Harrison MR, Filly RA, Parer JT, et al: Management of the fetus with a urinary tract malformation. JAMA 246:635, 1981.
123. Harrison MR, Golbus MS, Filly RA: Management of the fetus with a correctable congenital defect. JAMA 246:774, 1981.
124. Cass AS, Stephens FD: Posterior urethral valves; diagnosis and management. J Urol 112:519, 1974.
125. Williams DI: Male urethral obstruction. In Williams DI, Johnston JH (eds): Paediatric Urology, ed 2. London, Butterworths, 1982, p 254.
126. Evins SC, Lorenzo RL: Posterior urethral valves: current concepts in diagnosis and treatment. J Urol 121:76, 1979.
127. Atwell JD: Posterior urethral valves in the British Isles: a multicenter BAPS review. J Pediatr Surg 18:70, 1983.
128. Gonzales R, Sheldon CA: Septic obstruction and uremia in the newborn. Urol Clin North Am 9:297, 1982.
129. Campbell MF: Obstruction of the posterior urethral valve in infancy and childhood: a study of 18 cases. JAMA 96:592, 1931.
130. Williams DI, Whitaker RH, Barratt TM, et al: Urethral valves. Br J Urol 45:200, 1973.
131. Cremin BJ, Aaronson IA: Ultrasonic diagnosis of posterior urethral valves in neonates. Br J Radiol 56:435, 1983.
132. Sheldon CA, Gonzalez R, Mauer SM et al: Obstructive uropathy, renal failure and sepsis in the neonate—a surgical emergency. Urology 16:457, 1980.
133. Hendren H: A new approach to infants with severe obstructive uropathy: early complete reconstruction. J Pediatr Surg 5:184, 1970.
134. Hendren H: Posterior urethral valves: management. J Urol 110:682, 1973.
135. Parkkulainen KV: Posterior urethral obstruction: valvular or diaphragmatic? Endoscopic diagnosis and treatment. Birth Defects 13:63, 1977.
136. Garg SK, Lawrie JH: the perineal urethrotomy approach to posterior urethral valves. J Urol 130:1146, 1983.
137. Williams DI, Cromie WJ: Ring ureterostomy. Br J Urol 47:789, 1976.
138. Lome LG, Williams DI: Urinary reconstruction following temporary cutaneous diversion in children. J Urol 108:162, 1972.
139. Duckett JW: Current management of posterior urethral valves. Urol Clin North Am 1:471, 1974.
140. Williams DI: Urethral valves: a 100 cases with hydronephrosis. In Bergsma D, Duckett JW (eds): Urinary System Malformations in Children. New York, Alan R Liss, 1977.
141. Krueger RP, Hardy BE, Churchill BM: Growth in boys and posterior urethral valves. Primary valve resection vs upper tract diversion. Urol Clin North Am 7:265, 1980.
142. Whitaker RH, Keeton JE, Williams DI: Posterior urethral valves: a study of urinary control after operation. J Urol 108:167, 1972.
143. Allen TD: Congenital ureteral strictures. J Urol 104:196, 1970.
144. Gosalbez R, Garat JM, Piro C, et al: Congenital ureteral valves in children. Urology 21:237, 1983.
145. Kenawi MM, Williams DI: Circumcaval ureter: a report of 4 cases in children with a reveiw of the literature and a new classification. Br J Urol 48:183, 1976.
146. Hanna MK: Bilateral retroiliac artery ureters. Br J Urol 44:339, 1972.
147. Johnston JH: Bladder disorders. In Williams DI, Johnston JH (eds): Paediatric Urology, ed 2. London, Butterworth, 1982, p 225.
148. Williams DI, Abbassian A: Solitary pedunculated polyp of the posterior urethras in children. J Urol 96:483, 1966.
149. Williams DI, Retik AB: Congenital valves and diverticula of the anterior urethra. Br J Urol 41:228, 1969.
150. Burke EC, Smith MH, Kelalis PP: Prune belly syndrome: clinical findings and survival. Am J Dis Child 117:668, 1969.
151. Eagle JF, Barrett GS: Congenital deficiency of abdominal musculature with associated genitourinary abnormalities, a syndrome; reports of 9 cases. Pediatrics 6:721, 1950.
152. Nunn IN, Stephens FD: The triad syndrome: a composite anomaly of the abdominal wall, urinary system and testes. J Urol 86:782, 1961.
153. Williams DI: Prune belly syndrome. In Williams DI, Johnston JH (eds): Paediatric Urology. London, Butterworths, 1982, p 289.
154. Woodard JR: Prune-belly syndrome. In Kelalis PP, King LR, Belman AB (eds): Clinical Pediatric Urology, ed 2. Philadelphia, Saunders, 1981, vol 2, p 805.
155. Garlinger P, Ott J: Prune belly syndrome—possible genetic implications. Birth Defects 10:173, 1974.
156. Ives EJ: The abdominal muscle deficiency triad syndrome—experience with 10 cases. Birth Defects 10:127, 1974.
157. Rabinowitz R, Schillinger JF: Prune belly syndrome in the female subject. J Urol 118:454, 1974.
158. Adeyokunnu AA, Familusi JB: Prune belly syndrome in two siblings and a first cousin. Am J Dis Child 136:23, 1982.
159. Afifi AK, Rebeiz JM, Andonian SJ, et al: The myopathy of the prune belly syndrome. J Neurol Sci 15:153, 1972.
160. Mininberg DT, Montoya F, Okada K, et al: Subcellular muscle studies in the prune belly syndrome. J Urol 109:524, 1973.
161. Woodhouse CRJ, Ransley PG, Williams DI: Prune belly syndrome—report of 47 cases. Arch Dis Child 57:856, 1982.
162. Erlich RM, Brown WJ: Ultrastructural anatomic observations of the ureter in the prune belly syndrome. Birth Defects 13:101, 1977.
163. Palmer JM, Tesluk H: Ureteral pathology in the prune belly syndrome. J Urol 111:701, 1974.
164. Snyder HM, Harrison NW, Whitfield HN, Williams DI: Urodynamics in the prune belly syndrome. Br J Urol 48:663, 1976.
165. Delklerk DP, Scott WW: Prostatic maldevelopment in prune belly syndrome. A defect in prostatic stroma-epithelial interaction. J Urol 120:241, 1978.
166. Sellers BB, McNeil R, Smith RV, et al: Congenital megalourethra associated with prune belly syndrome. J Urol 116:814, 1976.
167. Woodhouse CRJ, Ransley PG: Teratoma of the testis in the prune belly syndrome. Br J Urol 56:580, 1983.
168. Silverman FM, Huang N: Congenital absence of abdominal muscle associated with

malformation of the genitourinary and alimentary tracts: Report of cases and review of literature. Am J Dis Child 80:9, 1950.
169. Karamanian K, Kravath B, Nagashima H, et al: Anaesthetic management of "prune belly" syndrome: case report. Br J Anaesth 46:897, 1974.
170. Smythe AR: Ultrasonic detection of fetal ascites and bladder dilatation with resulting prune belly. J Pediatr 98:978, 1981.
171. Christopher CR, Spinelli A, Severt D: Ultrasonic diagnosis of prune belly syndrome. Obstet Gynecol 59:391, 1982.
172. Samtoy B, de Beukelaer MM: Ammonia encephalopathy secondary to urinary tract infection with Proteus mirabilis. Pediatrics 65:294, 1980.
173. Hendren WH: Restoration of function in the severely decompensated ureter. In Johnston JH, Scholtmeijer RJ (eds): Problems in Pediatric Urology. Amsterdam, Excerpta Medica, 1972, p 1.
174. Jeffs R, Comisarow RH, Hanna MK: The early assessment for individualized treatment in prune belly syndrome. Birth Defects 13:97, 1977.
175. Woodhouse CRJ, Kellett MJ, Williams DI: Minimal surgical interference in prune belly syndrome. Br J Urol 51:475, 1979.
176. Duckett JW: The prune belly syndrome. In Kelalis PP, King LR, Belman AB (eds): Clinical Pediatric Urology, ed 2. Philadelphia, Saunders, 1980, p 802.
177. Woodard JR, Parrott TS: Orchidopexy in prune belly syndrome. Br J Urol 50:348, 1978.
178. Fowler R, Stephens FD: The role of testicular vascular anatomy in the salvage of high undescended testes. In Stephens FD (ed): Congenital Malformations of the Rectum, Anus and Genitourinary Tract. Endinburgh, Livingstone, 1963, p 306.
179. Gibbons MD, Cromie WJ, Duckett JW: Management of the abdominal undescended testis. J Urol 122:76, 1979.

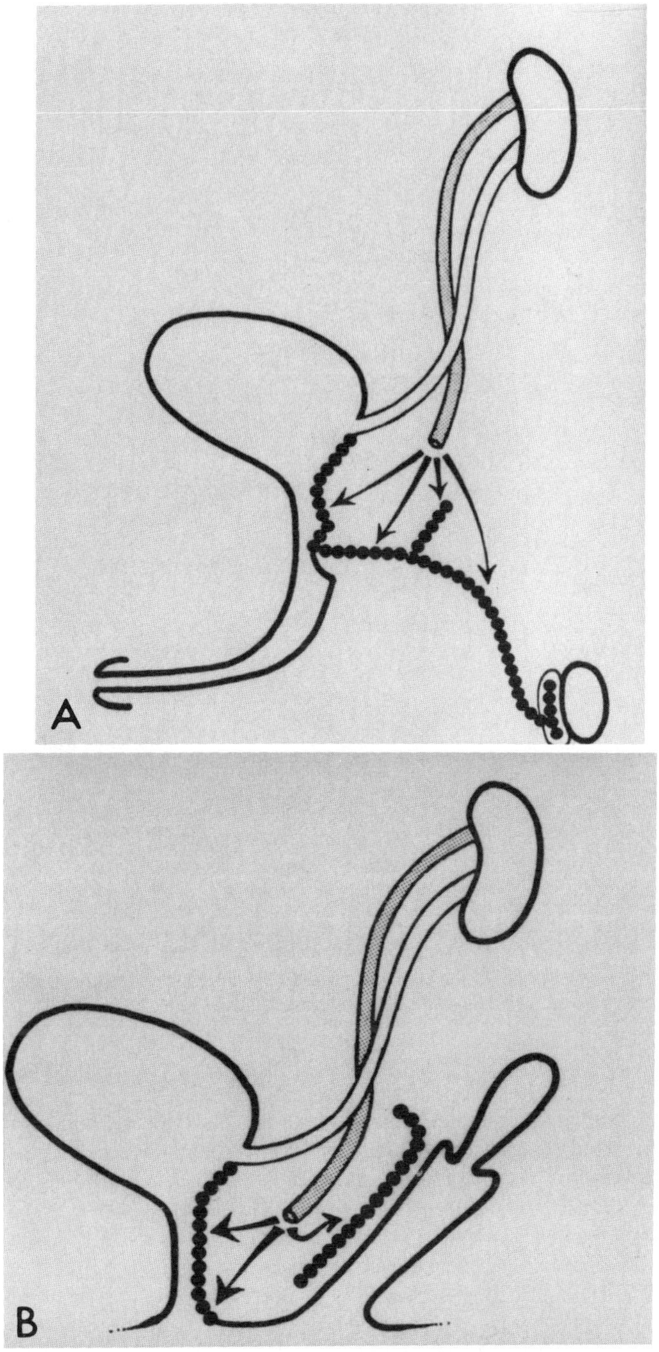

Figure 39.3. **A,** Ectopic ureters in male: possible sites of ectopic ureter are all above external sphincter. **B,** Ectopic ureter in female: ectopic ureter may be located beyond sphincters and lead to incontinence. From Johnston JH: Problems in the diagnosis and management of ectopic ureters and ureteroceles. In Johnston JH, Scholtmeijer RJ (eds): Problems in Pediatric Urology. Amsterdam, Excerpta Medica, 1972, p 57.

not removed and only rarely is later excision required because of VUR into the stump during voiding, leading to infection or dribbling incontinence after voiding.

Males

In the male, an ectopic ureteric orifice may lie anywhere along the ectopic pathway that extends to the verumontanum and encompasses the mesonephric duct derivatives (vas deferens, epididymis, and seminal vesicle). In about half the cases, the ectopic orifice is in the posterior urethra (Fig. 39.5). Drainage of an ectopic ureter into the male genital tract may produce epididymitis. For this reason, the prepubertal male with epididymitis should be evaluated for an ectopic ureter. Ectopic ureters entering the posterior urethra do not produce incontinence because they are above the external sphincter but may occasionally lead to urgency and frequency from the constant drip of urine into the posterior urethra.

The diagnosis of an ectopic ureter in the male requires considerable suggestive evidence. An ectopic ureter entering the genital tract is often single and draining a nonfunctioning renal element (14). Ultrasound may be useful in establishing the diagnosis. When the ectopic ureter is from the upper pole of a duplicated system, the indirect lower pole signs of hydroureteronephrosis that have been described previously may be found. The most difficult diagnostic problems arise in duplicated systems with a tiny upper pole draining into a minimally obstructed ectopic ureter. The diagnosis may be suggested by finding contralateral duplication. Only about 15% of ectopic ureters in males reflux. As in the female, ectopic ureters at the level of the sphincters may exhibit the paradox of both obstruction and reflux. Treatment generally requires removing the associated poorly functioning renal tissue. When the ectopic ureter enters the male genital ducts, they are usually rendered unfit for the passage of sperm; to avoid recurrent epididymitis, it is wise to ligate the vas.

Bilateral Single Ectopic Ureters

Bilateral single ectopic ureters are a rare entity; fewer than 50 cases have been reported in the literature (15). When no ureteric orifice embryologically joins the bladder, the bladder neck and trigonal musculature are deficient. Incontinence and a small bladder are the result. This situation is seen only when bilateral single ectopic ureters are very distal in their location. Cases with bilateral single ectopic ureters ending at the bladder neck level may present with infection and upper urinary tract dilatation from obstruction or reflux but have a better prognosis with respect to continence and bladder function.

Diagnosis may be possible by IVU and MCU. Often, however, the kidneys exhibit poor function, and although the MCU may demonstrate a small bladder with no evidence of a bladder neck, it may not show the ureters if they are farther down the ectopic pathway than the urethra. Ultrasound can be most useful.

Treatment of the incontinent child with bilateral single ectopic ureters constitutes one of the major surgical challenges of pediatric urology. Reimplantation of the ureters into the bladder with surgical augmentation of the bladder neck and possibly an intestinal cystoplasty may be required. The artificial urinary sphincter may have merit in these cases. If a continent reservoir can be created, clean intermittent catheterization may be required for emptying, but this would appear to be a small price to pay to effectively deal with this difficult clinical problem.

URETEROCELE

A ureterocele is defined as a cystic dilatation of the intravesical submucosal ureter. Most often, they are associated with the upper pole ureter of a kidney with complete ureteral duplication. Ureteroceles are much more common in girls than in boys. The ureterocele may vary in size from one so small that it is difficult to visualize to ones large enough to fill the entire bladder. The orifice of the ureterocele may be intravesical or extravesical and it may be stenotic, normal in size, or even patulous in a minority of cases. The wall of the ureterocele typically demonstrates attenuated muscle and excessive collagen.

Understanding of ureteroceles was advanced by Ericsson's classification in 1954 (16). He defined simple ureteroceles as ones contained

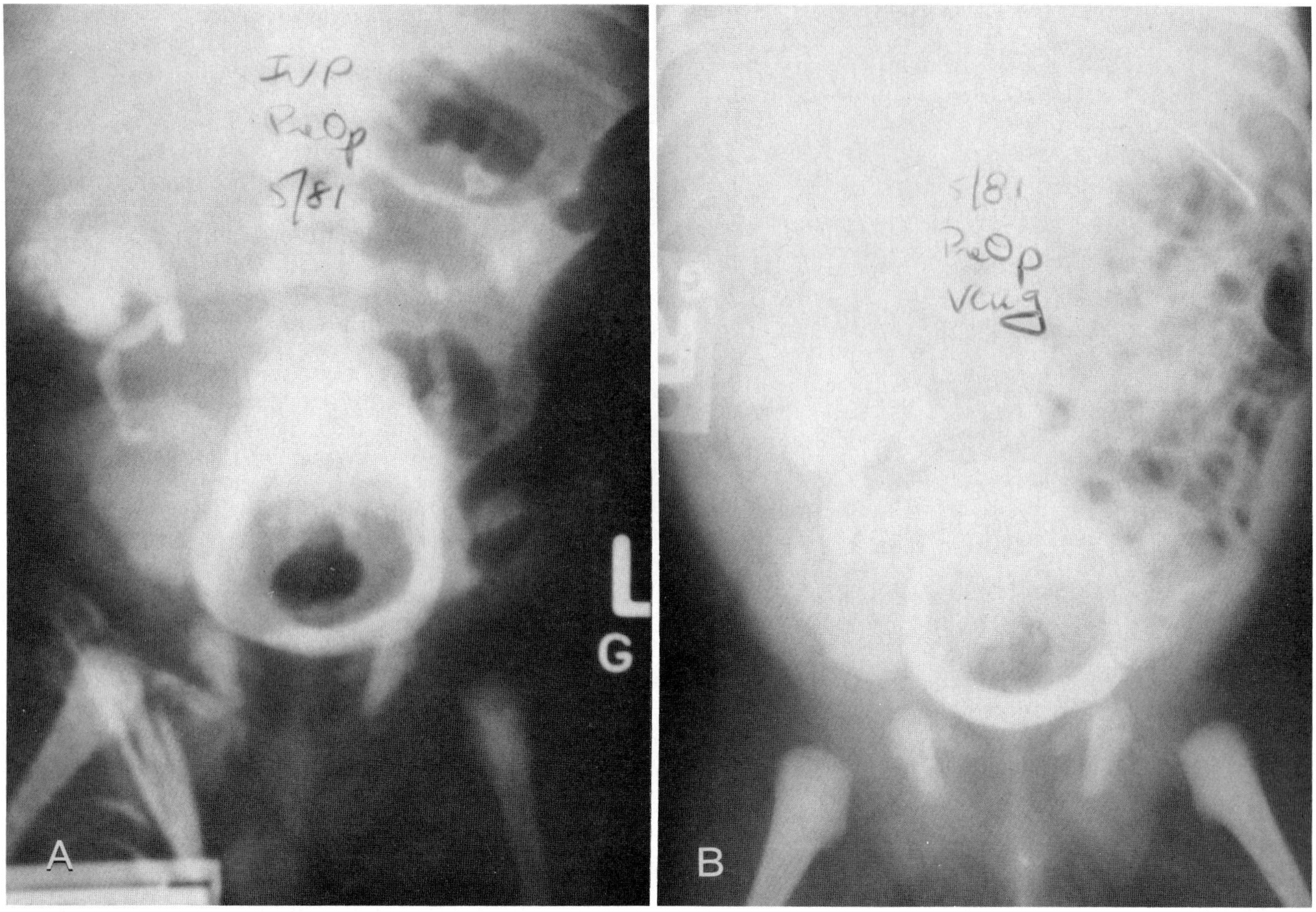

Figure 39.4. Right ureteral duplication with ureterocele in infant who presented with sepsis. **A,** Intravenous pyelogram showing large ureterocele associated with nonfunctioning upper pole of right kidney. Lower pole collecting system is displaced downward and laterally—"drooping lily sign." Right lower pole ureter is displaced laterally and is tortuous as it wraps around the dilated upper pole ureter. **B,** Voiding cystourethrogram shows ipsilateral lower pole vesicoureteral reflux.

entirely within the bladder. These are most common with single ureters. Ectopic ureteroceles were defined as ones that extended to the bladder neck or urethra. Although there are more complex classifications (17), Ericsson's continues to be the most widely used today.

The incidence of ureteroceles has been reported from 1/500 autopsies in children (18) to 1/4000 (19). Ureteroceles are common in whites and rare in blacks. Four to seven times as many ureteroceles are seen in females as males. Some series have demonstrated a left-sided predominence; 10% to 15% are bilateral. Duplication of the ureter is present in 75% of children with ureteroceles. Ectopic ureteroceles, as opposed to simple ones, make up 60% to 80% of most series (20, 21, 22). Single-system ectopic ureteroceles are rare and are usually seen in males. There are frequent associated urological anomalies. When the ureterocele is associated with ipsilateral ureteral duplication, there is a 30% to 50% chance of contralateral duplication. Renal anomalies, especially fusions and ectopia, are common. Dysplasia or hypoplasia of the renal moiety associated with the ureterocele is frequent.

The most common presentation of a child with a ureterocele is infection. Often this occurs in the first few months of life with full gram-negative sepsis. Infants may also exhibit failure to thrive or gastrointestinal symptomatology as is common with obstructive uropathies in early life. Occasionally, an infant will be found to have a palpable abdominal mass. Prolapse of the ureterocele may lead to bladder outlet obstruction. This is the most common cause of urethral obstruction in young girls; however, most ureteroceles do not produce obstruction because they are compressible during voiding. Trauma to an associated dilated drainage system or from the presence of a stone secondary to stasis may lead to hematuria. Flank or abdominal pain is more common with simple than ectopic ureteroceles. Incontinence may be a presenting symptom as well. Most commonly, this is caused by bladder infection; however, if the ureterocele is large with an intraurethral extension, an abnormal internal sphincter occasionally may permit incontinence even after the surgical treatment of the ureterocele (23).

The diagnosis of a ureterocele is usually possible from examination of the IVU (24). When the function of the associated kidney is adequate, there is a typical "cobra head" deformity produced by opacified urine in the ureterocele surrounded by a radiolucent halo produced by the wall of the ureterocele (Fig. 39.6). This is seen most commonly with simple ureteroceles. Most ectopic ureteroceles are associated with a poor or nonfunctioning renal unit, and the degree of associated hydroureteronephrosis is greater. Because of poor function, the radiographic signs are the indirect changes in the lower pole unit that have been described previously for ectopic ureters with duplication (Fig. 39.4). In the bladder, there is typically a negative shadow reflecting the ureterocele. This may vary from a large, tense, rounded shadow filling much of the bladder to a poorly defined irregularity along the floor of the bladder. It is wise to

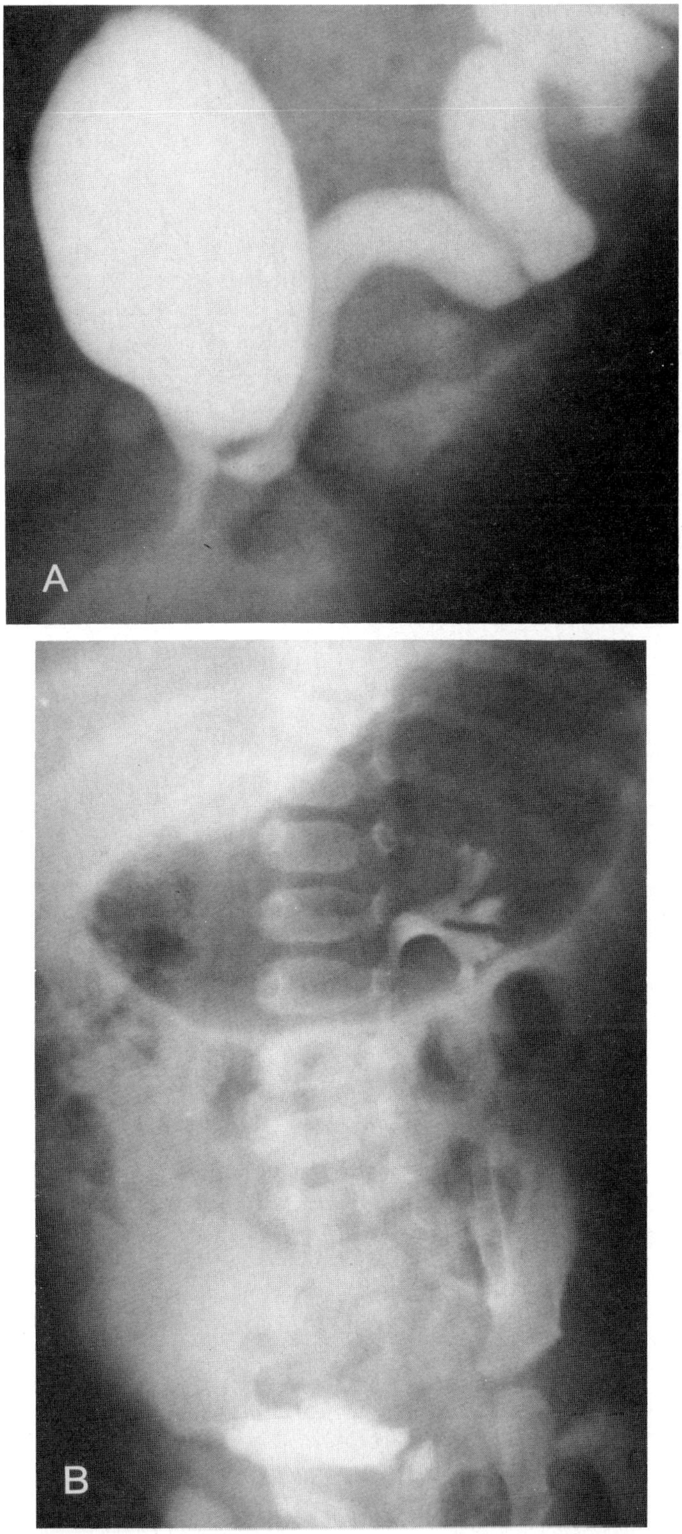

Figure 39.5. Ectopic ureter to posterior urethra in male infant who presented with sepsis. **A,** Voiding cystourethrogram showing vesicoureteral reflux into single ectopic ureter to posterior urethra from solitary left kidney. **B,** Intravenous pyelogram following reimplant of ectopic ureter into bladder.

examine early films from the pyelogram because once the bladder is filled with opaque dye, the ureterocele may be obscured.

An MCU is an essential part of ureterocele evaluation. When the ureterocele is associated with the upper pole of a duplication, reflux to the lower pole occurs in about one half of cases (Fig. 39.4). In 10% to 15%, there is reflux into the ureterocele itself. The typical radiographic sign of a ruptured ureterocele is the filling of an irregular cavity beyond the bladder outline with an edge that forms a filling defect within the bladder shadow. If detrusor backing for the ureterocele is poor, the ureterocele may prolapse through the detrusor during voiding and the radiographic picture may mimic that of a bladder diverticulum. Interestingly, after decompression of the ureterocele, the detrusor backing may appear to substantially improve. Tense ureteroceles may obstruct the ipsilateral lower pole ureter or contralateral ureter and may prolapse into the bladder neck, producing bladder outlet obstruction. Ultrasonography has been useful in helping to sort out these diagnositc dilemmas (25). Cystoscopic examination may prove to be diagnostically useful but requires an observer experienced with this type of pathology. Retrograde injection of the ureterocele may help to sort out which unit is involved when the ureterocele is large and both upper tracts exhibit pathological findings.

For the simple ureterocele associated with a single ureter, excision of the ureterocele and reimplantation of the ureter by an antirefluxing technique is the most successful approach (26). Endoscopic unroofing of a ureterocele is rarely needed to decompress a septic system in the era of modern antibiotics and is usually followed by reflux requiring a secondary operation. Occasionally, a simple ureterocele is small, minimally obstructive, and requires no surgical intervention (Fig. 39.6).

When a simple ureterocele is associated with the upper pole of a duplicated system, rarely there may be adequate function and a small enough ureter to permit a common sheath reimplantation of the two ureters following ureterocele excision. Usually, however, the ureter is too dilated for reimplantation without tapering, and if function justifies salvage, a ureteropyelostomy or ureteroureterostomy is performed (Fig. 39.7). This form of treatment is the exception rather than the rule. Usually the upper pole demonstrates such poor function that an upper pole partial nephrectomy and partial ureterectomy is carried out.

In the treatment of ectopic ureteroceles, there are a number of surgical options (Fig. 39.8). In recent years, the approach to ectopic ureteroceles has changed considerably, and some issues continue to be debated. The traditional approach to an ectopic ureterocele associated with a ureteral duplication was to excise the ureterocele, reconstruct the bladder wall, and reimplant the ipsilateral lower pole ureter and contralateral ureter if necessary (27). Through a separate flank incision, an upper pole partial nephroureterectomy was then performed. Whether done in a single stage or as a two-staged procedure, this operative undertaking was of considerable technical challenge and led a number of centers to examine alternative methods of treatment (28, 29). As the upper pole renal unit with ectopic ureteroceles with duplication rarely warrants salvage, an approach based on a primary upper pole partial nephrectomy with decompression of the ureterocele and a staged approach to surgery at the bladder level was tried in some centers. Decompression of the ureterocele would let it shrink down. It was felt that if a secondary bladder operation were necessary, it would be a simpler procedure. With this approach, it was noted that frequently ipsilateral and contralateral reflux or obstruction would subside. Even cases where the ureterocele appeared to be associated with a weakness in the bladder wall were observed on occasion after ureterocele decompression to lose this bladder wall weakness. Usually the ureterocele collapsed so well that it was hard to see subsequently by radiography. Persistence of ipsilateral lower pole reflux was the most common indication for a secondary procedure. Some series have now reported as low as a 25% to 30% need for secondary operations at the bladder level. It is becoming increasingly evident that the staged approach to the treatment of ectopic ureteroceles will eliminate the need

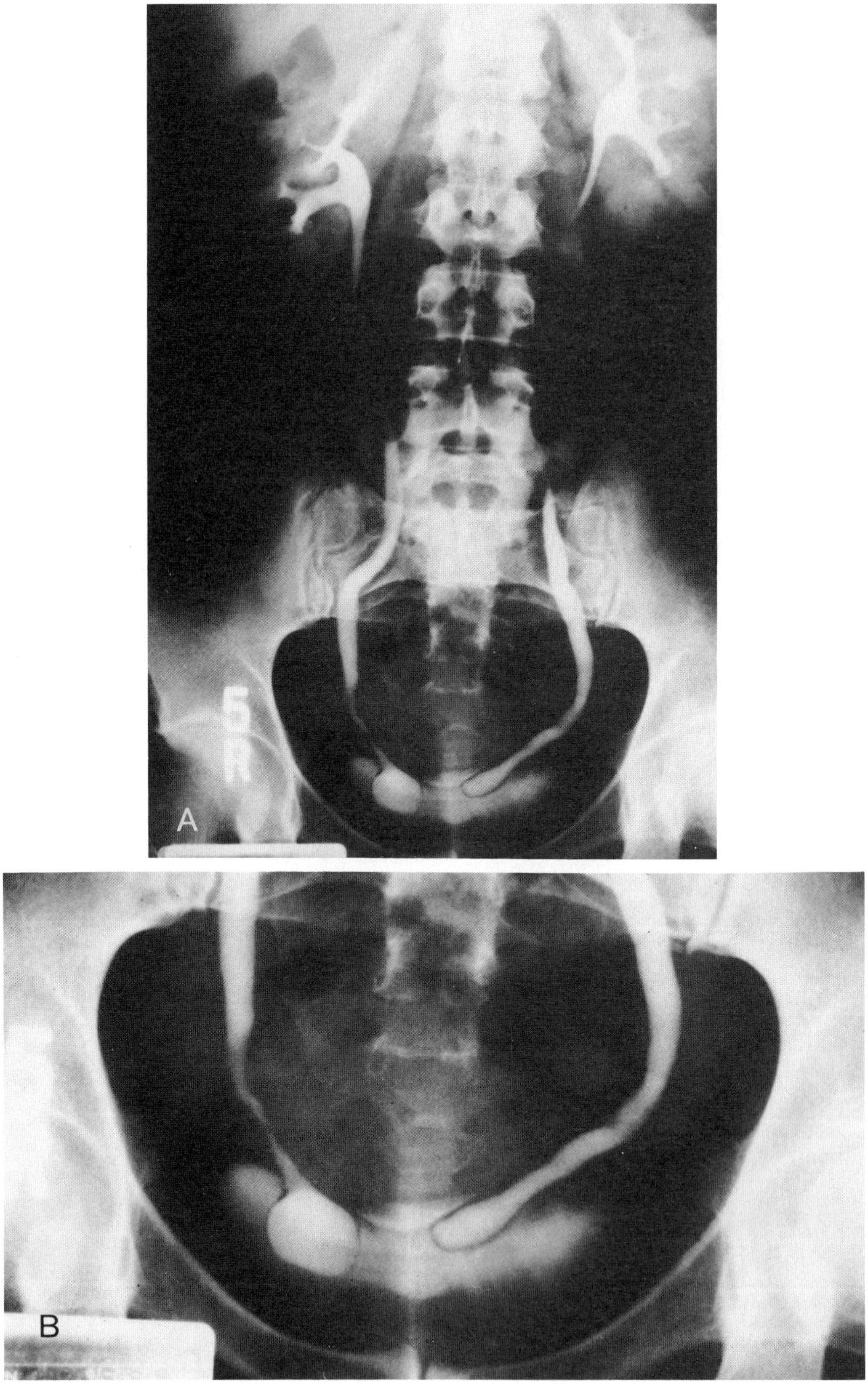

Figure 39.6. Bilateral single system simple ureteroceles. **A,** Intravenous pyelogram showing normal kidneys and minimal obstruction. **B,** Bladder showing "cobra head" deformity of ureterocele with good renal function.

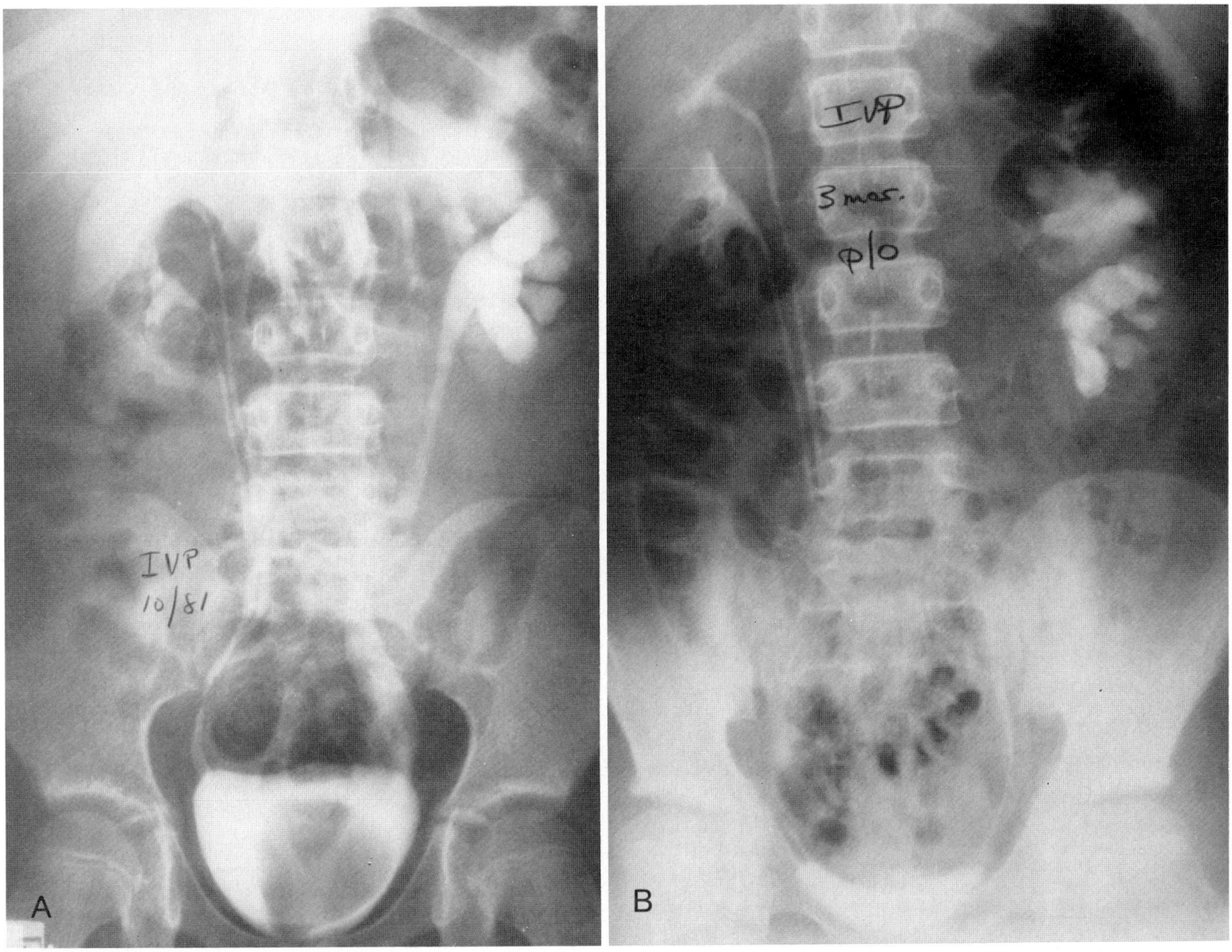

Figure 39.7. Ureterocele with left ureteral duplication and good function of upper pole treated by ureteroureterostomy. **A,** Preoperative intravenous pyelogram shows bilateral duplication and ureterocele associated with left upper pole with good function. **B,** Postoperative intravenous pyelogram shows decompression of left upper pole. The ureterocele is collapsed and no longer can be seen in bladder.

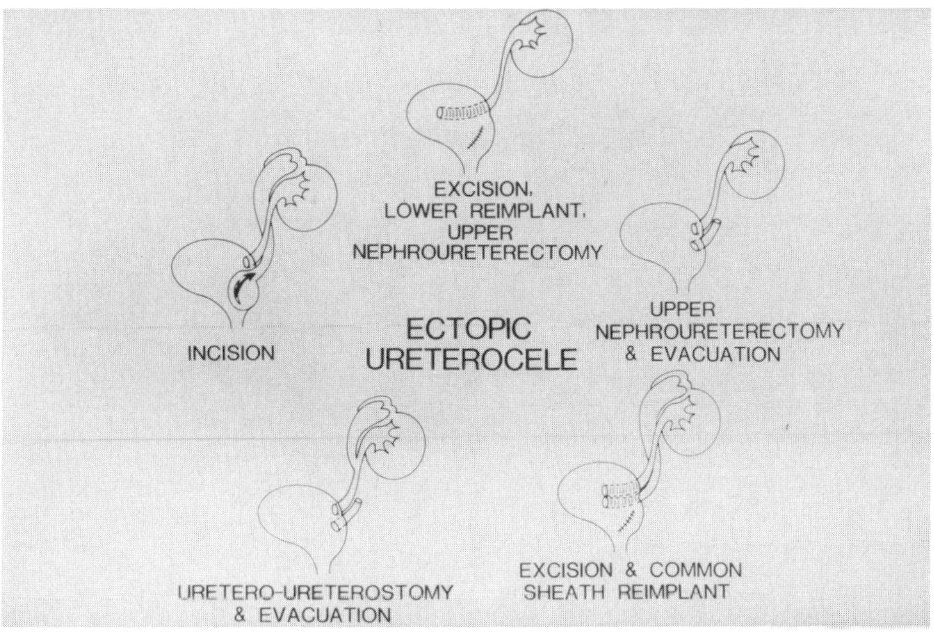

Figure 39.8. Ectopic ureterocele: surgical options. Primary upper pole partial nephroureterectomy and evacuation of ureterocele without ureterocele excision is current "simplified approach." (Courtesy of Dr. A. Colodny.)

for secondary bladder procedures in many children. This simplified approach is most widely accepted among pediatric urologists today.

When the upper pole renal unit associated with an ectopic ureterocele exhibits function warranting salvage (fewer than 10% of cases), a high ureteroureterostomy or ureteropyelostomy is appropriate. The decompressed ureterocele can be managed as mentioned previously. Occasionally, an ectopic ureterocele is associated with such a severe degree of ipsilateral lower pole obstruction or reflux that the lower pole is virtually destroyed. In this situation, a primary nephroureterectomy may be justified.

References

1. Chwalla R: The process of formation of cystic dilatations of the vesical end of the ureter and of diverticula at the ureteral ostium. Urol Cutan Rev 31:499, 1927.
2. Stephens FD: Caecoureterocele and concepts on the embryology and aetiology of ureteroceles. Aust NZ J Surg 40:239, 1971.
3. Tanagho EA: Embryologic basis for lower ureteral anomalies: a hypothesis. Urology 7:451, 1976.
4. Mackie GG, Stephens FD: Duplex kidneys: a correlation of renal dysplasia with position of the ureteral orifice. J Urol 114:274, 1975.
5. Campbell MF: Anomalies of the ureter. In Campbell MF, Harrison JH (eds): Urology, ed 3. Philadelphia, Saunders, 1970.
6. Cohen N, Berant M: Duplications of the renal collecting system in the hereditary osteo-onychodysplasia syndrome. J Pediatr 89: 261, 1976.
7. Atwell JD, Cook PL, Howell CJ, et al: Familial incidence of bifid and double ureters. Arch Dis Child 49:390, 1974.
8. Privett JTJ, Jeans WD, Roylance J: The incidence and importance of renal duplication. Clin Radiol 27:521, 1976.
9. Schulman CC: The single ectopic ureter. Eur Urol 2:64, 1976.
10. Malek RS, Kelalis PP, Stickler GB, et al: Observations on ureteral ectopy in children. J Urol 107:308, 1972.
11. Williams DI: The ectopic ureter: diagnostic problems. Br J Urol 26: 253, 1954.
12. Johnston JH, Davenport TJ: The single ectopic ureter. Br J Urol 41:428, 1969.
13. Gill B: Ureteric ectopy in children. Br J Urol 52:257, 1980.
14. Cendron J, Bonhomme C: Uretere a terminaison ectopique extra-vesicale chez des sujets de sexe masculin (a propos de 10 cas). J Urol Nephrol (Paris) 74:31, 1968.
15. Williams DI, Lightwood RG: Bilateral single ectopic ureters. J Urol 44:267, 1972.
16. Ericsson NO: Ectopic ureterocele in infants and children. Acta Chir Scand (suppl) 197:8, 1954.
17. Stephens FD: Congenital malformations of the rectum, anus and genitourinary tracts. London, Livingstone, 1963.
18. Uson AC, Lattimer JK, Melicow MM: Ureteroceles in infants and children: a report based on 44 cases. Pediatrics 27:971, 1961.
19. Campbell M: Ureterocele: a study of 94 instances in 80 infants and children. Surg Gynecol Obstet 93:705, 1951.
20. Mandell J, Colodny AH, Lebowitz R, et al: Ureteroceles in infants and children. J Urol 123:921, 1980.
21. Caldamone A, Snyder HM, Duckett JW: Ureteroceles in children: Follow-up of management with upper tract approach. J Urol 131:1130, 1984.
22. Brock WA, Kaplan GW: Ectopic ureteroceles in children. J Urol 119:800, 1978.
23. Gomez F, Stephens FD: Cecoureterocele: morphology and clinical correlation. J Urol 129:1017, 1983.
24. Sherwood T, Stevenson JJ: Ureteroceles in disguise. Br J Radiol 42:899, 1969.
25. Athey PA, Carpenter RJ, Hadlock FP, Hedrick TD: Ultrasonic demonstration of ectopic ureterocele. Pediatrics 71:568, 1983.
26. Snyder HM, Johnston JH: Orthotopic ureteroceles in children. J Urol 119:543, 1978.
27. Hendren WH, Mitchell MF: Surgical correction of ureteroceles. J Urol 121:590, 1979.
28. Cendron J, Melin Y, Valayer J: Simplified treatment of ectopic ureteroceles in 35 children. Eur Urol 7:321, 1981.
29. King LR, Kozlowski JM, Schacht MJ: Ureteroceles in children: a simplified and successful approach to management. JAMA 249:1461, 1983.

CHAPTER 40

Dysfunctional Voiding and Neurogenic Bladder

W. R. TURNER JR.

ANATOMY AND PHYSIOLOGY

The anatomy and physiology of the lower urinary tract is a subject of great complexity and controversy that cannot be described fully in the space available. The view presented here, however, serves satisfactorily as a basis for the clinical evaluation of dysfunctional voiding.

From an anatomical and functional standpoint, the lower urinary tract may be divided into the bladder body, or detrusor, and the internal and external continence mechanisms. The structure and functional significance of each of these entities tends to be described differently by different authors, but the concepts of Goslin concerning the functioning of the lower tract are particularly useful in understanding clinical voiding problems (1). The detrusor (Fig. 40.1) refers to that portion of the bladder above the bladder neck, extending to the trigone, composed of interlacing bundles of smooth muscle, which contrary to common belief, have no clearly delineated layers. The detrusor muscle cells are supplied primarily with parasympathetic innervation; thus, the primary bladder contractile stimulation is cholinergic. There is little sympathetic innervation to the body of the bladder. Goslin noted that sympathetic influence on the detrusor probably results from a modulating effect on the parasympathetic system (1). The trigone consists of a thin layer of smooth muscle lying between the ureteral orifices, extending through the bladder neck to the verumontanum in the male and the proximal urethra in the female. The trigone has negligible sympathetic innervation and little functional impact on the bladder, other than influencing the ureteral orifices.

The configuration of the bladder neck musculature differs widely in the male and female. In the male preprostatic area, the smooth muscle bundles form a concentric collar at the base of the bladder, the fibers shading distally to fuse and become indistinguishable from the prostatic capsule. Not only does this bladder neck form a separate unit morphologically from the detrusor, but it is heavily innervated by α-adrenergic fibers, in contrast to the β-innervation of the detrusor. The female bladder neck does not have well-developed circularly oriented smooth muscle but has oblique and longitudinally oriented fibers that fade out into the proximal urethra. The sympathetic innervation to these fibers is also adrenergic but much less than in the male bladder neck.

In the male, Goslin describes a striated muscle sphincter in the region of the membranous urethra composed of "slow twitch" striated muscle fibers (1). These muscle fibers are able to sustain contraction over long periods of time without fatigue, thus creating a basic urethral tone that aids continence. Also in the area of the membranous urethra are the fibers of the pelvic diaphragm, made up of fast and slow twitch fibers. The fast twitch fibers contract rapidly and forcefully but fatigue rapidly; they are useful in stopping voiding or increasing the urethral tone for short periods of time when bladder continence is challenged, e.g., by coughing or sneezing.

In the female, there is not only a mass of "slow twitch" fibers around the midportion of the urethra but also "fast twitch" and "slow twitch" fibers that arise from the pelvic diaphragm to invest the urethra. There are fewer fibers in the female than in the male. The "slow twitch" fibers are innervated by the pelvic nerve and the pelvic diaphragm by the pudendal nerve. This innervation pattern explains the fact that pudendal nerve block does not affect the "slow twitch" component of continence, and patients may remain continent after a bilateral pudendal neurectomy.

ETIOLOGY

The term dysfunctional voiding implies abnormal bladder function that may be congenital or acquired in onset and functional or anatomical in etiology. A neuropathic or neurogenic bladder is one in which there is an overt neuroanatomical explanation for the disorder. By common usage the term simple dysfunctional voiding is restricted to those cases in which there is no overt anatomical or neurological lesion.

The most common type of true neurogenic bladder in childhood is that associated with myelomeningocele. Although the numbers of such patients are decreasing due to antenatal diagnosis and the early delinea-

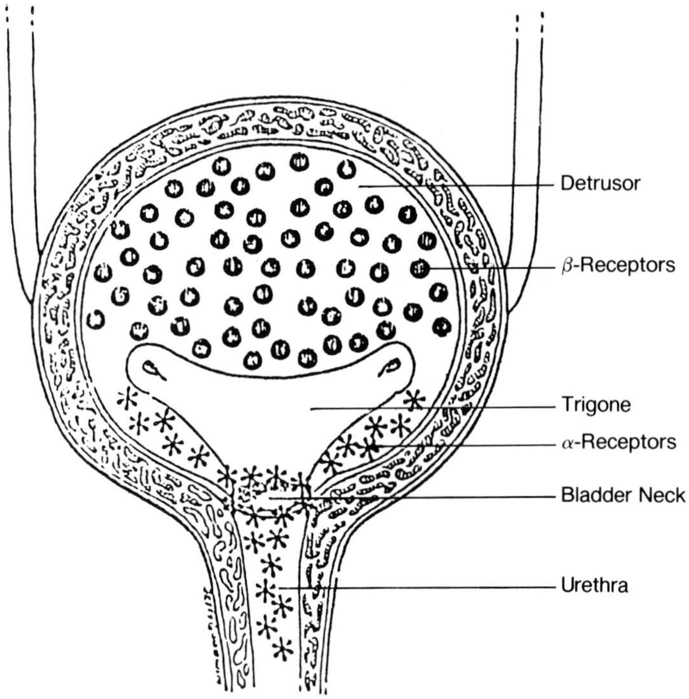

Figure 40.1. Receptor innervation of the bladder.

tion of risk factors, Eckstein and Williams point out that the skin-covered lesions may not be diagnosed antenatally because α-fetoprotein is not elevated (2). Thus, some cases of neurogenic bladder will "be always with us."

The type of bladder dysfunction with a myelomeningocele varies widely, and no distinct correlation can be made between the level of the lesion and the cystometric findings (3). Of those patients with absent reflexes or no voluntary activity below the first sacral segment, however, 92% have areflexia or flaccid bladder. Duckett has proposed a useful classification of meningomyelocele: those patients whose bladder fails to store and those in whom the bladder fails to empty (4). This simple concept has much to recommend it when considering types of treatment for the neurogenic bladder.

Other vertebral or bony anomalies associated with neurogenic bladder are diastematomyelia, sacral agenesis, and trauma. Spinal arachnoiditis and tumors of the conus medullaris and cauda equina also may lead to bladder dysfunction, usually resulting in a flaccid or hyporeflexic bladder. The most clandestine neurological lesion to cause bladder dysfunction is the tethered cord; since there are no specific symptoms, the syndrome is difficult to diagnose. A tethered cord should be considered in a child more than 3 yr of age who develops incontinence or bladder dysfunction that worsens with increasing age (2).

Some abnormal voiding appears to be caused by neurological disease, because of failure of coordination of voiding with the resultant bladder and renal injury patterns, yet careful evaluation demonstrates no neurological lesion. These children have what is termed dysfunctional voiding of nonneurogenic etiology, sometimes called dyssynergic, nonneurogenic neurogenic bladder, or occult neuropathic bladder. In them, the basic problem is failure of the voiding cycle to be coordinated, i.e., proper contraction of the detrusor with relaxation of the continence mechanisms. Although several other dysfunctional voiding syndromes have been described (2, 3), the concept that voiding dysfunction with bladder and renal damage could be related to failure of the bladder to function in a coordinated manner was proposed by Hinman and Bauman (5) and subsequently by Allen (6). Hinman and Bauman proposed that failure to relax the continence mechanisms could lead to a syndrome of damage similar to that caused by obstruction (5). Allen termed the syndrome the nonneurogenic neurogenic bladder, a functional and anatomical finding, which suggested a neurogenic bladder but without neurological abnormality (6). Williams and coworkers also noted this unusual combination and called it an occult neuropathic bladder (7).

SYMPTOMATOLOGY

The patient history should provide insight into the problem of a child with dysfunctional voiding, but the questioning must be purposeful, bearing in mind the information sought.

Frequency is a difficult term to define accurately. As a solitary complaint, it indicates that the bladder is unable to accommodate the volume of urine presented to it in a given period of time. The cause may be a high urine output caused by diabetes mellitus or insipidus, failure to concentrate urine because of renal damage, or excess fluid intake. A decrease in bladder capacity also may produce frequency; however, other symptoms usually are present that result from the causative condition. Psychosomatic frequency usually affects the patient only during the day, without any complaint of nocturia.

If the patient complains of *urgency* and frequency, conditions that increase bladder contractility should be considered. If dysuria is present, an irritative cause should be suspected, most commonly infection, but possibly a foreign body such as a stone. Urgency without dysuria usually points to a bladder that contracts inappropriately or without central control. This is called a hyperreflexic or unstable bladder, particularly if the symptom is precipitated by change of position, coughing, sneezing, and so on.

Enuresis without other urological symptoms indicates a maturational delay in the control of micturition; genitourinary pathology is rarely present. When nocturnal enuresis is coupled with daytime wetting, a more complex problem may be present and a urological evaluation is usually indicated. A child with a urinary tract infection should always be evaluated urologically, even with the first infection and especially if associated with daytime wetting. Daytime incontinence is the key symptom suggesting a neurogenic bladder, but consistent encopresis or squatting maneuver, in which the child squats or crosses the legs to remain continent, should also cause concern.

Hesitancy, although a common complaint in adults, is unusual in children, since they may not understand or have experienced normal voiding. Hesitancy denotes the inability of the patient to initiate voiding at will, so the bladder gradually increases the pressure until enough is generated to result in voiding. It may be caused by a defect in muscle contractility, as in a flaccid neuropathic bladder; be psychogenic, as in an individual who cannot void in public; or be caused by obstructive uropathy.

Incontinence may indicate several types of bladder dysfunction. In the distended bladder that cannot empty, chronic overflow dribbling can occur. This is termed paradoxical incontinence since the patient is not incontinent but is in retention. If the continence mechanism is damaged, the child dribbles because he or she is unable to retain urine. Anomalies such as an ectopic ureter opening below the bladder neck may lead to continuous incontinence. Incontinence associated with squatting, complaints of urgency, or leg-crossing indicate a hyperactive bladder and should cause concern that the patient is a dysfunctional voider generating high bladder pressures and thus having a high risk of renal damage—particularly if there is vesicoureteric reflux.

EVALUATION

Physical examination may reveal a lower midline abdominal mass indicating a distended bladder; flank masses may be hydronephroses.

The most helpful physical findings in the child with dysfunctional voiding are those that point to neurological diseases. The presence of a tuft of hair, a dimple, or other lesion over the sacroiliac area may indicate the presence of a vertebral column or spinal cord anomaly with associated neurological deficit. The lack of a gluteal fold can suggest sacral agenesis; palpation of the sacrococcygeal region will substantiate this. Rectal examination will provide information about rectal sphincter tone. Eliciting the bulbocavernous reflex by squeezing the penis or the clitoris and feeling the rectal sphincter contract determines that the sacral nerves (S2, 3, 4) are intact. An absent ankle jerk or asymmetry of leg length may point to spinal dysraphism. Neurological deficits must be carefully sought, but as emphasized by Eckstein and Williams, the neurological lesions in these children tend to be incomplete and result in a confusing clinical picture (2).

Accurate information about the dysfunctional lower urinary tract can be obtained from the proper use of various tests and radiological examinations, which must be carried out in logical sequence to answer specific questions. One of the simplest tests is measurement of the urine flow rate or the amount of urine voided per unit time (usually milliliters per second). Flow rate may be evaluated by elaborate electronic devices, simple mechanical measures, or by measuring the amount voided per second with a stopwatch, as suggested by Bloom (8). Torrens and Abrams stated that peak flow rates in a child under 10 yr of age should be 15 ml/sec, in those 10 yr or older, about 20 ml/sec (9). Although measurement of flow rate is an excellent screening procedure, a normal flow rate does not necessarily mean that no lower tract anomaly exists; however, it does show that the lower tract is functionally normal and that, if an abnormality is present, there has been compensation.

Radiological studies are an integral part of the urological evaluation of patients with dysfunctional voiding, and much information can be derived from the excretory urogram and voiding cystourethrogram. A proper flat x-ray film of the abdomen may demonstrate many useful findings, including bony anomalies, often associated with neurogenic bladder; a distended bladder; and such renal masses as hydronephrosis. The excretory pyelogram may demonstrate renal scarring, hydronephrosis, hydroureters and provide gross informaion about the bladder, such as the "Christmas tree" configuration associated with neurogenic bladder. A postvoiding film provides an estimate of voiding function by indicating the volume of urine left in the bladder. In children whose problem does not necessitate complete information, micturition views may be obtained by using the contrast left in the bladder after pyelography and following the procedure for a voiding cystogram. No information concerning reflux will be obtained. Abnormalities of the excretory urogram, coupled with symptoms of dysfunctional voiding, suggest the need for urological consultation. The voiding cystogram is one of the most helpful tests if performed and interpreted properly. A static cystogram is of little aid, and the voiding cystogram with random static pictures may be less than optimal. The cine-voiding cystourethrogram is perhaps the most useful radiological test in the evaluation of bladder function. Since the fluoroscopic examination is recorded on videotape, the films can be played over and over, and the phases of voiding can be stopped or slowed to compare the dynamic voiding process with the pressure measurements obtained with urodynamic studies. The cine-voiding films permit observation of the coordination of voiding, such as the opening and closing of the bladder neck, the urethral configuration, and so on. The information obtained from the cine-voiding films more than justifies the increased cost over the simple voiding cystourethrogram, and the radiation exposure can be rigidly controlled by the radiologist using fluoroscopy. This is not to say cine-cystograms are indicated in all cases or even routinely. When the administration of contrast media or catheterization is not advisable, ultrasound is helpful in locating kidneys, delineating hydronephrosis, demonstrating distended bladder, assessing residual urine, and is very useful in following the progress of urological conditions.

URODYNAMICS

Urodynamics are invasive studies and at times overused, but when indicated, they provide a valuable amount of information about bladder function. The evaluation usually consists of recording bladder filling and voiding pressures concurrent with urinary flow rate, intra-abdominal pressure, and the electrical activity of the external sphincter (Fig. 40.2). Urethral pressure profiles, i.e., the measurement of pressures throughout the urethra, require more cooperation than can usually be obtained from children.

As the bladder fills, it expands for a period without an increase in intravesical pressure (Fig. 40.2). This phenomenon is known as accommodation and is grossly related to how well the bladder can accommodate the fluid load. As the bladder pressure rises during voiding, the electrical activity in the area of the pelvic sphincter decreases, indicating relaxation of the pelvic floor and the continence mechanism, which results in unimpeded voiding. Figure 40.2 does not indicate specific volumes or pressures, as these vary with each child; intra-abdominal pressures are not indicated to avoid confusion; however, intra-abdominal pressure is an important measurement because it reveals how much of the pressure within the bladder is generated by bladder contraction and how much by abdominal straining. An example of the importance of the second factor is that many adult females void by abdominal pressure alone and not by generating bladder contractions.

The methods for urodynamic studies vary considerably. One approach is as follows. Under general anesthesia the child is cystoscoped in routine fashion, then two 8FG Silastic tubes are passed percutaneously through the skin into the bladder and positioned under direct vision. These are sutured to the abdominal skin, and the child is sent back to the ward with catheters in place. The child resumes normal activities in the afternoon and by the next day is almost oblivious of these catheters.

The procedures are explained carefully to the child, who is then taken to the urodynamic laboratory. There, one of the previously placed tubes is attached to a bottle of saline and the other to a pressure transducer. A catheter is passed into the rectum to record intra-abdominal pressures, and pediatric electrocardiographic electrodes are pasted to the skin around the anus to record the electrical activity of the pelvic floor. Saline is dripped into the bladder while bladder pressures are measured. When the child is ready to void into a flow meter, the flow rate, the pressure within the bladder, and the electromyogram are recorded at the time of

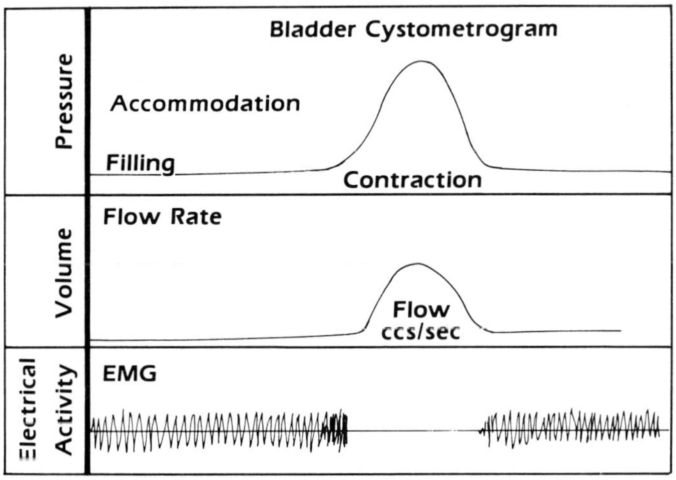

Figure 40.2. Example of a urodynamic study demonstrating coordination of detrusor and sphincteric action and resultant urine flow rate.

voiding (Fig. 40.2). This procedure is repeated until a pattern can be consistently duplicated. Often, a picture suggestive of dysfunction turns out to be nothing more than an indication of the child's fear and inability to relax and void normally; this disappears as the child becomes adjusted. If the child is voiding abnormally, the study may be repeated several times to show the child how to correct this problem. After several trials, the child understands these functions and how it feels to control them. This may provide the basis for biofeedback training of bladder dysfunction.

Voiding should be considered from the standpoint of force and efficiency of the detrusor, the capacity of the bladder, and the action of the continence mechanisms. From a urodynamic standpoint these functional abnormalities show similar patterns regardless of cause, so they carry similar therapeutical implications. Obviously, although the child with dysfunctional voiding may respond to treatment and be cured, and the child with a true neurological deficit may continue to require therapy, their management may be similar. Once the history or workup suggests functional bladder abnormality, the dysfunction should be categorized in terms of bladder capacity, bladder contractility, and sphincter activity. Bladder capacity may be large, normal, or small; with these capacities, the muscle may be hyporeflexic, normal, or hyperreflexic. The sphincter activity with each of these configurations may be hyperactive, hypoactive, uncoordinated, or normal and coordinated.

The large-capacity bladder may be associated with several combinations of factors. One of the more common combinations is the "lazy bladder syndrome," in which a large-capacity hyporeflexic bladder has a sphincter mechanism that relaxes appropriately and contracts with the voiding cycle; in this example, the capacity and contractility are abnormal but the sphincter functions normally (10). These children with a "lazy bladder" usually present with encopresis as well and have similar rectal function difficulties, with a large and relatively atonic bowel full of feces.

Large-capacity hyporeflexic bladders also occur with meningomyelocele, cord lesions, or other abnormalities of the sacral area. The sphincter activity in these lesions varies according to the neural damage and may range from hypoactive in the meningomyelocele to hyperactive in the true dyssynergic patient. The child with dyssynergic or nonneurogenic bladder have a large-capacity bladder but also have hyporeflexia or hyperreflexia, the latter usually associated with high bladder pressures. In these cases the sphincter classically shows an inability to relax during voiding and thus presents a functional obstruction; many of these children have bladder and upper tract damage. The colon is full of feces, and the child presents with encopresis caused by failure of the perineal sphincter mechanism to relax when a bowel movement is attempted. The dyssynergic patient is at great risk for renal damage, and the diagnosis should be pursued vigorously.

A small-capacity bladder may be associated with hyperreflexic contractions and is seen most commonly with suprasacral cord lesions. Sphincter mechanism in these patients depends on the anatomical lesion. It may be hyperactive and present obstruction, with a likelihood of damage to the upper tracts or, at the other extreme, hypoactivity and resulting incontinence. A bladder with hyporeflexia may result from total lack of sphincter control because the bladder cannot store urine, resulting in an incontinent patient with little bladder capacity.

Bladders of normal capacity may demonstrate muscular contractions that the patient cannot control; these are termed unstable contractions. Although the sphincter mechanism will show activity during these unstable contractions, it will relax normally during purposeful voiding. This is an appropriate action for the sphincter in that the patient is trying to suppress incontinence from the unstable contractions but can allow the sphincter to relax during normal micturition. Some children with normal-capacity bladders may show transient lack of sphincter coordination, but often this is spurious and induced by the child's failure to relax the sphincter during test conditions. Dyssynergia, or lack of coordination of the pelvic sphincter, is an overdiagnosed problem.

TREATMENT

Several methods have been devised to treat the dysfunctional bladder: pharmacological, mechanical, and surgical.

Pharmacological Treatment

Drug therapy depends on a selective action on specific areas of the urinary system. The primary focus is on drugs that affect three areas of reference: capacity, contractile force, and the sphincter or continence mechanisms. Several drugs have actions that affect more than one area of the voiding cycle; in others, controversy exists as to the exact site of drug function.

Drugs that alter the contractility of the bladder musculature are of several types: (a) cholinergic, which stimulate bladder contraction; (b) anticholinergic, i.e., those blocking cholinergic function; (c) antispasmodic, i.e., those that directly suppress activity of the bladder musculature.

The most commonly used cholinergic drug, bethanechol chloride, acts by releasing acetylcholine at the terminals of postganglionic parasympathetic fibers in smooth muscle, thus increasing the tone of the detrusor and producing a voiding contraction (11, 12). It is useful when faced with a problem of decreased detrusor tone, such as the flaccid bladder of a cord lesion. The drug is usually effective only in large doses. Lapides and coworkers took advantage of this effect and proposed a test for neurogenic bladder in which a pressure rise of more than 15 ml of water after subcutaneous injection of bethanechol indicated denervation sensitivity (13). The effectiveness of oral bethanechol has been questioned, but from clinical standpoint it still appears useful (14).

Several drugs decrease the contractile force of the bladder; each has its own peculiar effect, and it is important to understand the pharmaceutical differences. Anticholinergic drugs, such as propantheline bromide, atropine, or dicyclomine hydrochloride, produce a competitive blockade of acetylcholine at the postganglionic receptors, thus decreasing bladder contractility (15). Even though this type of drug would seem useful in hyperreflexic and hypertonic bladders, no orally administered drug can stabilize a truly unstable bladder (15).

Another class of drug that affects bladder contractility is the antispasmodic group, or what Benson terms musculotropic drugs, which function distal to cholinergic receptors, thus blocking at the muscular level (16). Oxybutynin, a musculotropic drug, also seems to have some anticholinergic effects and produces local anesthesia, thus proving useful in the treatment of enuretics and in patients with hyperreflexic or hypertonic bladders (16).

Imipramine is a controversial drug in that its mode of action is not clear. Some report it to be musculotropic and anticholinergic, whereas others think it exerts its effect by antihistaminic action and local anesthesia (17). Creed reports that its action is on the central nervous system (18), but Milroy has suggested that it increases urethral tone by potentiating the effect of norepinephrine and thus increasing the α-adrenergic effect on the urethra (19). Whatever the action of this drug, it is useful in the treatment of enuretics and in some children with hyperreflexic bladders.

The use of these drugs allows manipulation of bladder function to a certain degree; subsequently, the sphincter mechanisms may be approached. As noted previously, the bladder neck in the male is heavily populated with α-adrenergic receptors, though to a lesser degree in the female. α-adrenergic stimulation, therefore, tends to increase the voiding resistance and improve continence; conversely, blockade of the α-receptors decreases resistance to voiding. Ephedrine is the most commonly used of the α-stimulators; other drugs with similar stimulatory action are pseudoephedrine hydrochloride and phenylpropanolamine hydrochloride. In adult males, the use of such drugs for the relief of symptoms of the "common cold" sometimes cause urinary retention. Ephedrine is the most useful of these drugs and, because of the density of bladder neck α-receptors, its effect is more pronounced in males than females. Dibenzyline causes α-blockade and decreases smooth muscle tone in the bladder neck and urethra, again with an effect more noticeable in the male. Because the external sphincter is not a single entity but a "continence complex," the striated components that permit volitional control over voiding are not directly affected by the α-receptors. The most effective striated muscle relaxant is diazepam, which is useful in cases of external or striated muscle hyperactivity and hypertonicity such as dyssynergia.

The therapy should be aimed at a specific functional abnormality. For example, in a child with meningomyelocele, use of ephedrine may tighten the bladder neck and result in complete retention, thus allowing the use of intermittent catheterization with the child continent between catheterizations. In similar patients, the addition of oxybutynin or an anticholinergic drug may render the bladder flaccid and increase capacity. The child with dyssynergia or nonneurogenic bladder has a high risk of renal damage. The bladder may be hyporeflexic and require bethanechol to increase contractions; however, the continence mechanism must first be relaxed. Diazepam has been effective in patients who lack striated muscle coordination, whereas a dibenzyline-like drug is more appropriate in treating those patients with internal sphincter dyssynergia. Thus, the outflow resistance can be decreased with diazepam or a dibenzyline like drug and the contractility increased with bethanechol.

The volume of small-capacity bladders may be increased by the muscle-relaxing effect of anticholinergic or musculotropic drugs or by imipramine, which also seems to affect accommodation.

Mechanical Treatment

The most commonly used mechanical therapy for dysfunctional voiding in the child with a large residual volume or retention is intermittent catheterization; artificial sphincters or bladder-tightening procedures are used with incontinent children. Lapides' and coworkers suggestion that clean intermittent catheterization could be used in bladders that did not empty properly is one of the major advances in the treatment of children with dysfunctional voiding (20). Sterile catheterization is not necessary, so almost any child with chronic retention can be treated without surgical intervention.

Credé has been a mechanical method for managing bladders that did not empty properly; Eckstein and Williams have noted its usefulness in infants (2). However, this mechanical method must be used cautiously and is rarely applicable. Before selecting this method, it must be clear that no obstruction or sphincter hypertonicity exists, otherwise extremely high intravesical pressures would be created. Particular care should be exercised when using this method in patients with reflux. Raz noted that abdominal straining with the intermittent catheterization maneuvers in patients with suprasacral lesions elicited a reflex contraction of the pelvic floor, with consequent increase in obstruction (12).

Other Treatments

Hinman has suggested the use of hypnotism to change the pattern of voiding (5); several authors have demonstrated good results with biofeedback in the dysfunctional voiding pattern for children (19).

Surgical Treatment

Cutaneous vesicostomy may be useful for the poorly functioning bladder, especially with myelodysplasia. As popularized by Duckett, the dome of the bladder is brought to the skin and thus temporarily diverted until the time is right for the definitive continence procedure (21). Vesicostomy is one of the most useful surgical procedures in the infant or small child with a bladder that does not empty well. Implantation of electrical stimulation has not been helpful, and the Young-Dees-Leadbetter procedure, which creates a new bladder neck, has been disappointing in a child with neurogenic bladder. Supravesical indwelling catheters are to be condemned except for short periods of time, and supravesical diversion is to be avoided because of the high incidence of renal damage associated with ileal conduits. Ileocecocystoplasty and ileocystoplasty may be used to increase bladder capacity, but these must be chosen with care. External sphincterotomy seems to have a place in children with spastic external sphincters, but sacral blocks and pudendal nerve blocks have shown too high an incidence of impotence to be used routinely (22). Artificial sphincters are beginning to be used with increasing success in the incontinent child and seem to be the hope of the future.

References

1. Goslin J: The structure of the bladder and urethra in relation to function. Urol Clin North Am 6:31, 1979.
2. Eckstein HB, Williams DI: Neuropathic bladder. In Williams DI, Johnston JH (eds): Paediatric Urology, ed. 2. London, Butterworth Scientific, 1982, p 326.
3. Blaivas JG, Labib KB, Bauer SB, et al: Changing concepts in the urodynamic evaluation of children. J Urol 117:778, 1977.
4. Raezer DM, Benson GS, Weir AJ, et al: The functional approach to the management of the pediatric neuropathic bladder: a clinical study. J Urol 117:649, 1977.
5. Hinman F Jr, Bauman FW: Vesical and ureteral damage from voiding dysfunction in boys without neurologic or obstructive disease. J Urol 109:727, 1973.
6. Allen TD: The nonneurogenic neurogenic bladder. J Urol 117:232, 1977.
7. Williams DI, Hirst G, Doyle D: The occult neuropathic bladder. J Pediatr Surg 9:35, 1974.
8. Bloom DA: Personal communication, 1982.
9. Torrens M, Abrams P: Urine flow studies. Urol Clin North Am 6:1979.
10. Bauer SB, Retik AB, Colodny AH, et al: The unstable bladder of childhood. Urol Clin North Am 7:1980.
11. Koelle G: Parasympathetic agents. In Goodman LS, Gilman A (eds): The Pharmacological Basis of Therapeutics, ed 4. New York, MacMillan, 1975, p 672.
12. Raz S, Bradley WE: Neuromuscular dysfunction of the lower urinary tract. In Harrison J (ed): Campbell's Urology, ed 4. Philadelphia, WB Saunders, 1979, Vol 2, p 1250.
13. Lapides J, Friend CR, Ajemian EP, et al: Denervation supersensitivity as a test for neurogenic bladder. Surg Gynaecol Obstet 114:241, 1962.
14. Innes IR, Nickerson M: Atropine, scopolamine and related antimuscarinic drugs. In Goodman LS, Gilman A (eds): The Pharmacological Basis of Therapeutics, ed 4. New York, MacMillan, 1975, p 516.
15. Milroy E: Pharmacological management of common urodynamic problems. Urol Clin North Am 6:265, 1979.
16. Benson GS, Sharshik SA, Raezel DM et al: Bladder muscle contractility. Urology 9:34, 1977.
17. Labay P, Boyarsky S: The action of imipramine on the bladder musculature. J Urol 109:385, 1973.
18. Creed AG: Drugs and the treatment of psychiatric disorders. In Goodman LS, Gilman A (eds): The Pharmacological Basis of Therapeutics, ed 5. New York, MacMillan, 1980, p 418.
19. Milroy E: Treatment of detrusor instability. Urol Clin North Am 6:265, 1979.
20. Lapides J, Dickens AC, Sibler JJ, et al: Clear intermittent cath in the treatment of urinary tract disease. J Urol 127:458, 1972.
21. Duckett JW: Cutaneous vesicostomy in childhood. Urol Clin North Am 1:485, 1974.
22. Missak SJ, Bunts RC, Ulmer JL, et al: Nerve interruption procedures in the urological management of paraplegic patients. J Urol 88:397, 1962.

CHAPTER 41 Enuresis

S. R. MEADOW

Enuresis is the lack of bladder control in a person who has reached an age at which control is to be expected. Nocturnal enuresis means nighttime wetting, i.e., bed-wetting, and diurnal enuresis means daytime wetting.

NOCTURNAL ENURESIS

Most children become able to remain dry at night between the ages of 3 and 3½ yr, but there is a wide variation in the time at which the skill is acquired. Some children become reliably dry at night as early as 6 months and others not until 5 yr. By the age of 3½ yr, 75% of children are reliably dry at night. This may be the result of a sudden acquisition of dryness, having been previously wet all the time or, more commonly, gradual acquisition of dryness. Although this may be influenced by the attitudes and regimes that parents impose, evidence suggests that it is an inborn skill the emerges regardless of "training" (1–3). Quite simply, it is a rule of nature that healthy animals do not foul their sleeping quarters.

Characteristics

Most children who present to the physician with bed-wetting have never had a prolonged period when they were reliably dry; however, they will almost always have had one or two nights during which they have been dry. True primary enuresis—never having had a single dry night—is exceedingly rare over the age of 5 yr. In my experience, it accounts for 1% to 2% of school children. The usual pattern is one of intermittent nocturnal enuresis in which the child, at least on occasions, has a day or two or a period of days of being dry. A small proportion of children, about 20%, will have had more than a year of being reliably dry. For them, it is reasonable to apply the term "secondary" or "onset" enuresis. For that subgroup, it is customary to look more carefully for a specific cause for the wetting (though rarely is one found).

It is usual for the parent to say that their child "always" wets the bed and is a "deep sleeper." Close questioning will reveal that the first is not true, and the evidence from electroencephalography (EEG) and other studies does not suggest that children who wet the bed sleep particularly deeply. Bed-wetting is more common in boys, in first-born children, in the lower socioeconomic classes, and in children who have experienced severe stress, e.g., prolonged separation or loss of a parent between the ages of 1 and 4 yr (4–6).

There is a definite association between enuresis and psychiatric disorders, particularly the common neurotic and conduct disorders. But it is important to recognize that most children with the problem of bed-wetting are well adjusted and normal. Moreover, for that minority who are disturbed, it is by no means clear whether the disturbance is the cause or the result of bed-wetting (7, 8). Most children who wet the bed are not awakened by the wetting and awaken in the morning in a wet bed. The minority wake up soon after wetting and climb into the bed of their parents or siblings.

The prevalence of bed-wetting decreases with age. In Western Europe, 10% to 15% of 5-year-olds wet the bed at least once a week, 7% of 10-year-olds, and 1% of 15-year-olds (9). The prevalence in North America and Australia seems to be slightly higher. In some cultures, it is very much lower (10, 11).

Bed-wetting can occur at most stages of sleep but not during REM (rapid eye movement) sleep. There is a suggestion that the EEG, particularly the EEG response to hyperventilation, is different in children who wet the bed (12). The significance is uncertain.

There is a strong genetic factor associated with bed-wetting. Nearly three quarters of children who wet the bed have at least one parent who also wet the bed after the age of 5. On measuring, they have a functionally small bladder capacity, but the bladder itself is healthy, and it is usual for the pattern of micturition by day to be normal. Up to 10% may have a small amount of daytime wetting (9).

Children who wet the bed are slow in acquiring the skill of bladder control. Although they have immature bladder function at night, it is rare for disease or a structural disorder to be responsible.

Conditions that predispose to bed-wetting are those that cause polyuria or bladder irritation.

Polyuria

Commonly, children presenting with diabetes mellitus or chronic renal failure have recently developed bed-wetting after previously being dry, i.e., they have secondary nocturnal enuresis. It is, however, extremely rare to find anything to suggest an organic disorder in a child whose main complaint is nocturnal enuresis. The rare serious organic disorders that may cause nocturnal enuresis nearly always present in other ways.

Bladder Irritation

Urinary tract infection is the most common factor that "irritates" the bladder, increases bladder detrusor activity, and reduces functional bladder capacity. Bed-wetting is the presenting symptom in a small proportion of children with urine infection. Infected urine is found in between 5% and 10% of girls with bed-wetting and about 1% of boys (13). Eradication of the infection cures the bed-wetting in fewer than half of those children.

Assessment and Investigation

A careful history of the conditions should be taken, which should banish the need for any investigation apart from careful urine examination. The history will reveal that the child has had at least an occasional dry night. That tells the physician, child, and parents that dryness is possible and that there is no permanent leak. The history should reveal a child with normal drinking and voiding habits, apart from bed-wetting. A small degree of frequency or urgency may be apparent by day, but there will be no difficulty in passing urine or an interrupted stream of urine. The bed-wetting child usually provides a healthy and unexceptional history, apart from being unhappy and perhaps a bit disturbed by the problem. The presence of another first-degree relative who had suffered from bed-wetting is further confirmation that the child has inherited a familial tendency for lateness in acquiring bladder control at night.

Physical examination is an important part of therapy; it impresses on the child and parents that there is no organic disorder. The results of an examination will be normal. Examination of the urine and a check for urine infection is obligatory, and any infection should be treated. Few people would consider further investigation in an otherwise healthy school child, though some request a roentgenogram of the urinary tract for the child over the age of 12 yr of age or for those with secondary enuresis. However, if the child is assessed carefully and competently, radiological examination of an otherwise healthy bed-wetting child is not warranted. Urodynamic investigations, cystoscopy, and other urosurgical procedures are not helpful.

Management

The details of management vary from culture to culture and among therapists. Most physicians rely on a combination of general and specific measures. There is agreement that the therapist's attitude is critical, in order to make full use of simple and effective psychotherapy. The parent and child need to know that there is no permanent structural disorder or disease and that cure will occur. A daily record of the wetting events can be kept as a star chart or diary for the child to fill in. This is an important record for the physician, as well as an encouragement for the child. Most parents will have tried to restrict fluid and will have tried rewards and punishment and found that they do not work. Although it is important for the child to want to be dry and to know that the wetting is a nuisance for everyone, too much tension in the form of excessive rewards and punishments does not help the child acquire a natural skill. Many parents have found that going to their child's room last thing at night, to lift the child out of bed to empty his bladder, results in less volume of wetting (and less dirty laundry). My practice is to let them continue this until management is well advanced and cure is in sight.

The two main measures for the treatment of bed-wetting are drugs and behavioral and conditioning therapy.

Drugs

A host of drugs has been used to manage bed-wetting. Few have been shown to be effective in satisfactorily conducted controlled trials (14, 15).

Two groups of drugs are of proven value:

1. Tricyclic antidepressant drugs, e.g., imipramine. Fifty percent of children become dry while taking these drugs, but their effect is not long-lasting and most children relapse when the drug is stopped. Tricyclic antidepressants have many undesirable side effects and are dangerous for young children if taken in excess. Their place in the treatment of bed-wetting is limited.

2. Antidiuretic drugs. Desmopressin (DDAVP) is the drug of choice in this group. It is administered in the evening in a dose of 10 to 40 μg. The antidiuretic effect of a single dose lasts for 7 to 10 hr and allows many children to be dry that night. The number of children remaining dry after conclusion of a one-month course of DDAVP is higher than after imipramine. Nevertheless, an unsatisfactorily high proportion of children relapse once the drug is stopped (16).

Drugs therefore have a limited role. A short course of drug therapy can be useful in showing a desperately unhappy child with persistent bed-wetting that dryness is possible. A short course of drug therapy also can be useful to cover a period in which the child is away from home, on holiday, or at camp. Drugs can also be useful for that group of children for whom behavior conditioning therapy cannot be used, but there is a danger of carrying on with the drugs for too long a period. Drugs should not be used for children under the age of 5. The parental complaints and anxieties should be diverted away from such specific therapy in a compassionate and acceptable way.

Behavioral and Conditioning Therapy

Many forms of behavior therapy have been tried, and many have been successful. Impressive results have been obtained by intensive behavioral therapy for a short period of a few nights (17). These "dry-bed" techniques require a dedicated and skilled therapist, as well as parents and child who will cooperate (18, 19). For many pediatricians, the techniques involved seem too punitive and impractical.

Conditioning therapy in the form of a buzzer alarm is much more popular, but one should not underestimate some of the practical difficulties in using the alarms and the dedication required by the therapist and family. A variety of enuresis alarms are available. All depend on the principle that a sensor pad will become wet when the child wets the bed, and then sound an alarm. The child is instructed to wake up, turn off the alarm, go to the toilet, and empty his or her bladder. As treatment continues with the buzzer alarm, the child wakes up earlier and earlier, so that the size of the wet patch decreases and, in addition, the number of wetting occasions decreases. Thus, at the end of treatment the child is either tolerating a full bladder during the night and not needing to empty it at all, or is awakening to the stimulus of a full bladder and going to the toilet. The time to dryness with the use of the buzzer is usually about eight weeks. The average child requires about 18 buzzes and wet nights before being reliably dry, but the range is wide and some children need to use the buzzer for up to six months. If improvement does not occur after four months of use, it is probably kinder to abandon treatment.

Many buzzer alarms are available in different countries, but even in one country several alarms may be available that differ significantly in sensitivity, ease of use, and benefit to the child (20). Some children may cooperate well with a minialarm, which is attached to the child's pajama jacket, but others are only able to cooperate with an alarm that is out of reach of the bed so that when the alarm rings they have to get up to turn it off. The buzzer alarm requires a dedicated therapist who is willing to spend time with the parents and child, see them regularly, and help them with the problems that arise. It is helpful to give printed instructions or a booklet to the family to help them to understand the problem of enuresis and to use the alarm effectively (21). Many problems arise with the use of buzzer alarms, but there is a wealth of guidance available in the literature on how to overcome them (22–24).

To cooperate with the alarm, most children need to be of an emotional or mental age of 7 yr or more, though intelligent and emotionally mature children of 6 may be able to cope with it. The family should be relatively settled and able to devote time to the procedure for the next few months. Results with the use of the alarm are less good in the presence of adverse housing conditions or where several children sleep in the same bed. However, gratifying success can be achieved even for this group of children (22).

Those with more severe behavior disturbance are also less easy to treat, and the results with alarm therapy are not so good (22, 25–27). Nevertheless, most of these children will still fall within the care of a pediatrician. In my experience with 157 children referred because of bed-wetting, only 4 had a degree of behavior disturbance that made referral to a child psychiatrist seem appropriate.

Without any treatment, the spontaneous remission rate for children with nocturnal enuresis under the age of 10 is 14%/year; over the age of 10 it is 16%/year (28). With energetic therapy, more than 70% should be cured within a year.

DIURNAL ENURESIS

Much less has been written about diurnal (daytime) enuresis than nocturnal. Moreover, it is difficult to compare the few available published studies because of differences in definition. Most healthy children are reliably dry during the day by the age of 3 yr; however, few parents would be worried by a 3½- or 4-year-old who occasionally had some dribbling and damp pants when busy playing outside. Even when the child first attends school it is likely that a small degree of daytime wetting will be tolerated by the teachers and not noticed by the children. But by the time the child is 6, others are less tolerant and wetting becomes a problem. Stains appear on the clothing, the child is smelly, teased, and embarrassed.

Daytime wetting can be classified into three grades:

Grade 1 is dampening of the pants that does not soak through the outer clothing.

Grade 2 is a degree of dampening that does soak through the outer clothing so that, for instance, a girl will always be wearing dark-colored jeans rather than light ones that would show the wet patch.

Grade 3 is a degree of wetting that leaves a puddle on the seat or floor. It must be stressed that most daytime wetting is grade 1 or grade 2; for the child to be taken to the physician, it is likely that grade 1 or grade 2 wetting occurs at least two or three times a week.

Incidence

Accurate figures are difficult to obtain because of poor definition of daytime wetting. From the large survey of 7-year-old Swedish school children (5) and the National Child Development study of British 6-year-old children born in 1958, about 3% were reported to have daytime wetting (9). Of these, approximately two-thirds also had nighttime wetting. For older children, the prevalence is less; approximately 1% was found in Dutch children at the age of 10 (29). Most surveys suggest that daytime wetting is more common in girls.

Characteristics

Most children will not have had a prolonged period, e.g., one year, of being reliably dry by day. Secondary, or onset, diurnal enuresis is uncommon and accounts for <20% of the wetting children. Untreated, it is likely that the spontaneous remission rate is about 15%/year (28).

Day-wetting is strongly associated with urgency: an urge to micturate at the first signal and an inability to delay for more than a minute or two. Many of the children press their perineum with their hands, heels, the side of a chair, or by squeezing the thighs together to hold on better. Frequency of micturition is associated with urgency more than with daytime wetting itself (10). The detrusor instability, or hyperreflexia, has been well studied. In contrast to children with nocturnal enuresis, those with daytime enuresis nearly always show this bladder instability (30).

The most common story is that the wetting is worse after school, when the child is playing out or busy with friends; however, there are some important variations. A few children have an adult type of stress incontinence in that the wetting occurs only on the most vigorous physical exertion. For others, it is more common at the time of coughing or laughing (the rare group who have true giggle micturition are considered separately).

Children with daytime wetting are likely to show more behavior disturbance than those with night-wetting alone or in the general population; soiling appears to be common, particularly in boys (10). This behavior disturbance should not be overstressed. Many children who wet by day show no abnormality on psychological assessment; even for those that do, it is difficult to sort out whether the behavior disturbance is a cause of, or a result of, the troublesome symptom.

Causes

The reason for the unstable bladder is uncertain. Adequate family studies are lacking, so the genetic influence is uncertain, though likely to be as strong as it is for nocturnal enuresis.

Urinary tract infection is an important association in girls with daytime wetting but much less important in boys. Forty percent to 50% of school girls who present with daytime wetting have significant bacteriuria (10). Eliminating that bacteriuria allows many of them to become reliably dry. Bacteriuria predisposes to daytime wetting. Daytime wetting predisposes to bacteriuria, presumably because of the soggy perineum and clothing that attract bacteria and predispose to ascending infection.

Other organic causes are not worth considering at length. Theoretically, any condition associated with polyuria might predispose to daytime wetting, but in practice they do not present in that way. Although it is common to cite an ectopic ureter as a possible reason for daytime wetting, I have not encountered one presenting in that way. It is important to remember that in nearly all children with a wetting problem one can quickly establish that there are days or periods of days when the child is reliably dry; therefore, there can be no "leak in the plumbing." A small and unfortunate minority are boys who have had previous operations for urethral valves and are left with impaired control of micturition and, quite often, some daytime wetting.

Management

The initial history and physical examination of the child are important parts of the therapy, for they are reassuring to the parents and the child. If, as is usual, the child is otherwise healthy, further investigations have a limited place. Examination and culture of the urine for infection is essential because of the high prevalence of urinary tract infection. Moreover, if the day-wetting child is a girl, she should have regular checks, monthly or bimonthly, during the period of management, as acquisition of infection is likely and will interfere with cure.

Compared with children with nocturnal enuresis, there is a high incidence of abnormality on roentgenogram, but the findings rarely influence management. Therefore, such investigation is not generally warranted. An intravenous urogram is likely to be normal, but voiding cystourethrography will show an appreciable incidence of vesicoureteral reflux. This is not surprising in view of the association between daytime wetting and urinary tract infection.

As with nocturnal enuresis, general as well as specific measures are important in measurement. The general measures include several supportive and encouraging measures mentioned in the section on bed-wetting. In addition to the positive, optimistic, and yet sympathetic approach, it is important to remember some of the practical problems. Apart from regular and thorough washing of body and pants, the unpleasant smell is alleviated by dusting the clothes and affected skin with a bacteriostatic and fungicidal powder. For children who have the symptoms of stress incontinence, an intensive spell of bladder training—holding onto the urine for increasing periods—may help. Dissuade the child who wants to go to the toilet until after a count of about 10 sec. The following day, the child is asked to wait 30 sec, and so on until a 10- or 15-min delay can be achieved satisfactorily.

For most children, a trial period of positive warning to empty the bladder at regular intervals is helpful. The child can be given a kitchen cooking alarm timer or a small minielectronic alarm that goes off every hour or two and reminds the child to go to the toilet.

No specific measures for the treatment of daytime wetting have been shown to be effective in satisfactorily conducted controlled trials.

Anticholinergic and tricyclic antidepressant drugs that might be expected to reduce detrusor tone have not been found superior to placebo (31). Trials with a small portable daytime alarm, sounding when the child wets, have yet to be concluded.

Throughout any period of management it is essential to determine that the urine is free from infection. If recurrent bacteriuria is a problem, as it is so often in girls, then long-term low-dose chemotherapy may be needed. My own practice is to use nitrofurantoin in a dose of 25 mg each night. Once the child has become dry, it is worthwhile to continue the check for bacteriuria for several months because its recurrence may soon cause daytime wetting again and set back the final cure by many months.

Hypnotherapy has been shown to be effective for women with detrusor instability (32). There are anecdotal reports of its success for children with daytime wetting. In view of the lack of proven effective methods for children with daytime wetting, it would seem reasonable to try hypnotherapy on selected children if it is easily and inexpensively available.

GIGGLE MICTURITION

As originally described, the term giggle micturition was applied to children who, on giggling as opposed to laughing, had complete emptying of the bladder that they were unable to stop (33). In this form, it is a rare condition; however, it has become clear that many variations exist.

Leaving aside the many children who have a small degree of stress incontinence when giggling or laughing vigorously, there is a group who have giggle micturition in a variety of forms. For some, wetting occurs only if they are standing when they giggle; others only when in the company of friends and when having an embarrassed giggle. Some have complete bladder voiding both on giggling and on laughing. As with all forms of daytime wetting, it is more common in girls. The natural history is uncertain. There are a few children who continue with the distressing problem into adulthood but, more recently, cures have been reported (34).

My own practice is to inquire carefully about the circumstances in which the giggle micturition occurs, then try to find ways of minimizing the risk. For instance, if it only occurs when standing, then the child should watch the TV comedy program sitting down. For all children, it is worth stressing the importance of regular voiding and keeping the bladder relatively empty to minimize the chance of a large and embarrassing wetting event. I have also used the anticholinergic drug, propantheline, with apparent success (34).

References

1. MacKeith RC, Meadow SR, Turner RK: How children become dry. In Kolvin I, MacKeith RC, Meadow SR (eds); Bladder Control and Enuresis (Clinics in Developmental Medicine Nos. 48/49). Philadelphia, Lippincott, 1973, p 3.
2. Oppel WC, Weiner G, Harper PA, Rider RV: The age of attaining bladder control. Pediatrics 42:614, 1968.
3. Roberts KE, Shoellkopf JA: Eating, sleeping, and elimination practices of two- and two-and-one-half-year-old children. Am J Dis Child 82:121, 1951.
4. Douglas JWB: Early disturbing events and later enuresis. In Kolvin I, MacKeith RC, Meadow SR (eds): Bladder Control and Enuresis, London, William Heinemann, 1973.
5. Hallgren B: Enuresis. A clinical and genetic study. Acta Psychiatr Neurol Scand (suppl 114) 32:1, 1957.
6. MacKeith R: A frequent factor in the origins of primary nocturnal enuresis: anxiety in the third year of life. Dev Med Child Neurol 10:465, 1968.
7. Rutter M, Yule W, Graham P: Enuresis and behavioural deviance: some epidemiological considerations. In Kolvin I, MacKeith RC, Meadow SR, (eds): Bladder Control and Enuresis (Clinics in Developmental Medicine Nos. 48/49). Philadelphia, Lippincott, 1973, p 137.
8. Shaffer D: Enuresis. In Kolvin I, MacKeith RC, Meadow SR (eds): Bladder Control and Enuresis. London, William Heinemann, 1973.
9. Essen J, Peckham C: Nocturnal enuresis in childhood. Dev Med Child Neurol 18:577, 1976.
10. Berg I, Fielding D, Meadow R: Psychiatric disturbance, urgency, and bacteriuria in children with day and night wetting. Arch Dis Child 52:65, 1977.
11. DeVries MW, DeVries MR: Cultural relativity of toilet training readiness: a perspective from East Africa. Pedatrics 60:170, 1977.
12. Kaoda B, Retvedt A: Enuresis and hyperventilation response in the EEG. Dev Med Child Neurol 23:591, 1981.
13. Stansfeld JM: Enuresis and urinary tract infection. In Kolvin I, MacKeith RC, Meadow SR (eds): Bladder Control and Enuresis (Clinics in Developmental Medicine Nos. 48/49). Philadelphia, Lippincott, 1973, p 102.
14. Blackwell B, Currah J: The psychopharmacology of nocturnal enuresis. Enuresis (Clinics in Developmental Medicine Nos. 48/49). Philadelphia, Lippincott, 1973, p 231.
15. Meadow SR: Drugs for bed-wetting, Arch Dis Child 49:257, 1974.
16. Birkasova M, Birkas O, Flynn MJ, Cort JH: Desmopressin in the management of nocturnal enuresis in children: a double-blind study. Pediatrics 62:970, 1978.
17. Azrin NH, Thienes PM: Rapid elimination of enursis by intensive learning without a conditioning apparatus. Behav Ther 9:342, 1978.
18. Azrin NH, Besabel-Azrin V: Bedwetting Eliminated Through Training. New York, Simon and Schuster, 1979.
19. Griffiths P, Meldrum C, McWilliam R: Dry bed training in the treatment of nocturnal enuresis in childhood: a research report: J Child Psychol Psychiatr 23:485, 1982.
20. Finley WW, Wansley RA: Auditory intensity as a variable in the conditioning treatment of enuresis nocturna. Behav Res Ther 15:181, 1977.
21. Meadow R: Help for Bed Wetting. London, Churchill Livingstone, 1980.
22. Dische S: In Kolvin I, Mackeith RC, Meadow SR (eds): Bladder Control and Enuresis (Clinics in Developmental Medicine Nos. 48/49). Philadelphia, Lippincott, 1973, Chapter 24.
23. Meadow R: How to use buzzer alarms to cure bed-wetting. Br Med J 2:1073, 1977.
24. Morgan R: The management and treatment of nocturnal enuresis in children. J Behav Social Work Abstracts 2:1, 1982.
25. Berg I, Forsythe I, McGuire R: Response of bedwetting to the enuresis alarm. Arch Dis Child 57:394, 1982.
26. Dische S, Yule W, Corbett J, Hand D: Childhood nocturnal enuresis: factors associated with outcome of treatment with an enuresis alarm. Dev Med Child Neurol 18:577, 1983.
27. Wagner W, Bennett Johnson S, Walker D, et al: A controlled comparison of two treatments for nocturnal enuresis. Pediatrics 101:302, 1982.
28. Forsythe WI, Redmond A: Enuresis and spontaneous cure rate. Arch Dis Child 49:259, 1974.
29. DeJonge GA: Epidemiology of enuresis: a survey of the literature. In Kolvin I, MacKeith RC, Meadow SR (eds): Bladder Control and Enuresis (Clinics in Developmental Medicine Nos. 48/49). Philadelphia, Lippincott, 1973, p 66.
30. Whiteside CG, Arnold EP: Persistent primary enuresis: a urodynamic assessment. Br Med J 1:364, 1975.
31. Meadow R, Berg I: Controlled trial of imipramine in diurnal enuresis. Arch Dis Child 57:714, 1982.
32. Freeman RM, Baxby K: Hypnotherapy for incontinence caused by the unstable detrusor. Br Med J 284:1831, 1982.
33. MacKeith RC: Micturition induced by giggling. Guys Hosp Rep 113:250, 1964.
34. Brocklebank JT, Meadow SR: Cure of giggle micturition. Arch Dis Child 56:232, 1981.

CHAPTER 42

Urolithiasis and Nephrocalcinosis

T. M. BARRATT

INTRODUCTION

The presence of crystalline material within the kidney or urinary passages characterizes a wide range of renal, urological, endocrine, and metabolic disorders (1–6). A distinction is drawn between urolithiasis, i.e., stone in the urinary tract, and nephrocalcinosis, which refers to an increase in calcium content of the kidney, though the two conditions may coexist. Many different crystal species may be identified in urinary calculi in children (Table 42.1), and their relative frequency has striking epidemiological features. Radiologically evident nephrocalcinosis is much less common and may be focal, occurring in an area of previously damaged renal parenchyma; or generalized, usually a consequence of an underlying metabolic disorder.

STONE COMPOSITION AND FORMATION

Chemical composition

The principal varieties of urinary calculi are shown in Table 42.1. Some calculi have many constituents, and most struvite (magnesium ammonium phosphate) stones contain apatites (basic calcium phosphates) as well. The presence of calcium atoms renders the stone radiopaque; cystine stones are also radiopaque due to the presence of sulfur. Nonopaque stones are almost certainly composed of purines.

Activity Products

In spite of considerable research, the physicochemical principles underlying the formation of renal calculi remain incompletely understood (7). The precipitation of a salt occurs when the product of the activity of its ionic constituents exceeds a certain critical level, but there are several complexities in such an analysis. In the first place, it may be difficult to ascertain what proportion of a solute is present in ionized form. For example, only 30% to 60% of urinary calcium is ionized: the remainder is complexed to polyvalent anions such as sulfate, phosphate, oxalate, and citrate. This proportion may be deduced from a knowledge of urinary composition, but many different complexes have to be considered and the calculations are elaborate.

Secondly, it may not be clear which species of salt is first precipitated and which ion product is therefore relevant: with calcium phosphate it is probably octocalcium phosphate, which converts spontaneously into the less soluble hydroxyapatite. Finally, there are two critical activity products to be considered: the solubility product, below which is the undersaturated region where added crystals would dissolve, and the formation product, above which is the labile region in which spontaneous precipitation occurs. Between the solubility product and the formation product lies the metastable region in which existing crystals grow, but precipitation does not occur unless the system is perturbed.

With these considerations, it is not surprising that there is substantial overlap of the urinary octocalcium phosphate and calcium oxalate ion products between stone-formers and healthy individuals. Because of these complex interactions between ions, unexpected factors may be important; for example, within the physiological range, the activity product of octocalcium phosphate is more influenced by increase in urine pH than by increase in calcium concentration.

Inhibitors of Crystallization

Because the activity products of octocalcium phosphate and calcium oxalate lie in the metastable region in many healthy individuals, a search has been made for the factors that inhibit precipitation. Thus, an inhibitor of the growth of calcium oxalate crystals, found in normal urine, is absent in the urine of many stone-forming individuals (7), and calcium oxalate microcrystals form spontaneously if the urine of stone-formers is allowed to stand. Low excretion rates of pyrophosphate and citrate and low urinary magnesium/calcium and sodium/calcium ratios have all been reported to characterize patients with urinary calculi.

Organic Matrix

In addition to crystalline constituents, all urinary stones contain a glycoprotein matrix, which is particularly prominent in infective calculi (8, 9). The chemistry of these substances is complex. Boyce and coworkers described matrix substance A, a glycoprotein of molecular weight 30,000 to 40,000 daltons (10). Tamm-Horsfall glycoprotein and the closely related uromucoid are often present. The subject requires reinvestigation with modern techniques of glycoprotein chemistry.

EPIDEMIOLOGY

The incidence, composition, and clinical characteristics of urinary calculi in children vary greatly from one part of the world to another and from one historical period to the next. It is, however, possible to discern four major epidemiological patterns.

In some areas of the world, such as Turkey (12) and the Far East (particularly Thailand (13)), childhood urolithiasis is endemic; in boys

Table 42.1.
Urinary Calculi

Chemical composition	Crystalline structure
Calcium phosphates	Hydroxyapatite
	Carbonate-apatite
	Brushite
	Whitlockite
	Octocalcium phosphate
Magnesium ammonium phosphate	Struvite
Calcium oxalates	Whewellite
	Wedellite
Purines	Ammonium acid urate
	Uric acid
	2,8-dihydroxyadenine
	Xanthine
Cystine	

especially it accounts for a significant proportion of children admitted to hospital. In these cases the stones usually are found in the bladder and are composed of ammonium acid urate and oxalate. Evidence implicates dietary factors in their pathogenesis, particularly dependence on a cereal or rice diet (14). Such stones used to be common in England, particularly in rural areas like East Anglia, but declined in incidence in this century, possibly as a consequence of improved standards of nutrition (15).

Secondly, in the United Kingdom and certain other European countries, urolithiasis is somewhat less common, with a frequency of one or two children per million total population per annum (16, 17). There is an impression in the United Kingdom that during the last decade stones in children have become less common. Approximately 90% of these children have upper tract calculi composed of organic matrix and struvite (magnesium ammonium phosphate), and in the majority of these there is evidence of *Proteus* urinary tract infection (3).

For reasons that are not understood, the incidence of such infective calculi varies considerably and is low in, for example, Scandinavia and the United States of America. These areas have a third epidemiological pattern, in which urolithiasis in children is rare, and cases can generally be attributed to metabolic disorders (hypercalciuric states, particularly distal renal tubular acidosis [RTA]; hyperoxaluria; cystinuria; and disorders of purine metabolism) (5, 6). Fourthly, in areas where the incidence of calcium stones is high in adults, such as the stone belt of the American South, a few older children may be found to be similarly affected, often with a background of idiopathic hypercalciuria (18).

The incidence of radiologically evident nephrocalcinosis in children is much less than that of urinary calculi: for example, only 31 cases were reported from Hospital Necker-Enfants Malades, Paris, in a 15-yr period (19)

CLINICAL FEATURES

The presence of urolithiasis may be declared by the passage of stone or gravel but is more commonly revealed during the investigation of a child for urinary tract infection (UTI) or hematuria, or with obstructive phenomena such as renal colic or renal failure in bilateral cases or with a solitary functioning kidney.

All children with UTI, particularly those with *Proteus* infection, should have a plain abdominal roentgenogram to exclude a calculus. An ultrasound scan is insufficient for this purpose, for although the typical acoustic shadow may be present, small stones may pass undetected. On the other hand, ultrasound is more sensitive than conventional radiology in detecting nephrocalcinosis (Fig. 42.1), and may point to the presence of radiotranslucent purine stones.

Likewise, all children with hematuria should be investigated for calculi, even if there is another obvious cause for the bleeding. Renal colic or loin pain also suggests stone, though the association of loin pain with hematuria may also occur with hydronephrosis or some cases of IgA nephropathy. Occasionally, a patient with cystinuria may present with colic and hematuria, having passed the stone unnoticed. There is an association between recurrent hematuria and hypercalciuria even in the absence of stone formation (20, 21), but the relationship of this syndrome to calculus disease is not clear (22).

Urinary obstruction from stone may cause renal damage with postobstructive atrophy or, if infection is present, pyonephrosis may ensue, causing severe destruction of kidney tissue and constitutional symptoms. Nephrocalcinosis is itself asymptomatic, but there may be clinical features of the underlying illness such as polyuria.

INVESTIGATION

Children in whom a renal calculus is detected should have a full radiological investigation of the urinary tract in a search for other stones, for an underlying urological abnormality, and to assess the degree of urinary obstruction and renal damage. Crystalline elements observed on urine microscopy may suggest the nature of the stone.

Chemical analysis of urinary calculi is important but often inadequately performed in routine hospital laboratories: the wet stone should be solubilized and quantitatively analyzed for the main ingredients (i.e., calcium, phosphorus, magnesium, ammonium, oxalate, and urate) and should in addition be tested for cystine (23). X-ray diffraction analysis is helpful as a research tool (24).

The extent to which a child with urolithiasis should be screened for metabolic abnormality varies in different clinical circumstances: thus sterile urine, nephrocalcinosis, recurrence, and calculi in older children should lead to close metabolic scrutiny; on the other hand the yield of metabolic diagnoses from screening children with renal calculi and *Proteus* infection is small. All children with stone must be screened for cystinuria, as the diagnosis may modify the surgical program and the condition may be amenable to medical treatment. The 24-hr urinary calcium and oxalate excretion and plasma calcium and uric acid concen-

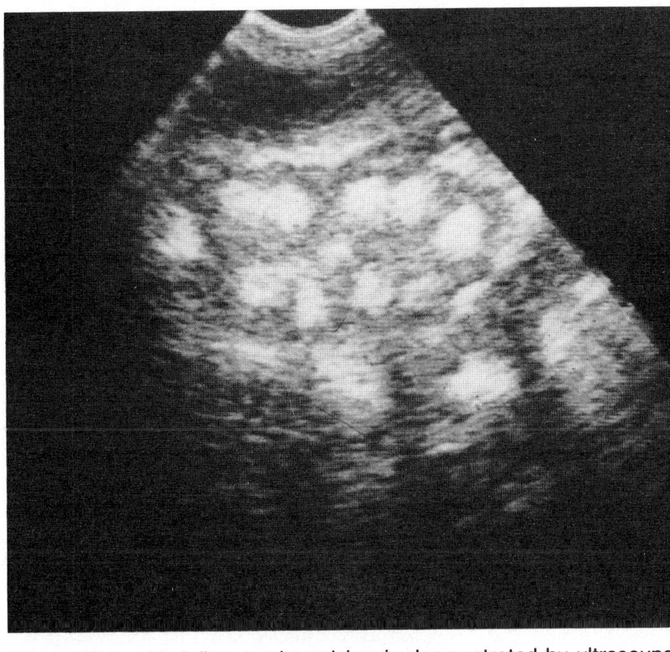

Figure 42.1. Medullary nephrocalcinosis demonstrated by ultrasound in a 3-year-old girl. No underlying metabolic abnormality was detected.

trations should be estimated preoperatively. An observation of urine pH of 5.3 or less under any circumstances, either spontaneous or following ammonium chloride loading, excludes the diagnosis of distal RTA, but if the urine is infected, particularly with *Proteus*, it may prove difficult to exclude this diagnosis, and formal examination of the capacity to acidify the urine should be deferred until the stone has been removed and the urine sterilized. Nonopaque stones are probably purine and require careful analysis by an experienced laboratory.

INFECTIVE STONES

Presentation

Seventy-five percent of children with infective calculi are aged less than 5 yr at the time of diagnosis; peak incidence occurs at 2 yr of age. Of these young children, 80% are male and 93% have infected urine (5). The presentation is with the usual features of a urinary tract infection but one that is often resistant to antibiotic therapy; there may also be loin pain and hematuria. Sometimes fragments may be passed in the urine; these stones are often very soft and may be described as toothpaste or a discharge. In some children, particularly those with a pyonephrosis, the constitutional symptoms of malaise and failure to thrive may be prominent.

The stone is in the upper urinary tract in 85% of cases, usually in the kidney. The left side is involved twice as often as the right, and in 15% the calculi are bilateral.

Diagnosis

The cardinal feature of urolithiasis in younger children is the association with *Proteus* urinary tract infection; the organism can be isolated from the urine at diagnosis in 75% of all patients under 5 yr of age. In some cases with sterile urine or *Escherichia coli* infection, *Proteus* may be isolated from the interior of the stone or from the cut surface of the kidney at surgery; in others, review of the child's medical history may reveal that the initial infection was with *Proteus*, even though other organisms were subsequently isolated.

The diagnosis of stone should be carefully considered in all children with *Proteus* urinary tract infection (Fig. 42.2). The stones are usually evident on the plain x-ray film taken before intravenous urography, but they may not be very radiopaque and therefore not well visualized, particularly if there is gaseous abdominal distention, in which case tomography, screening, or ultrasound may be helpful. Ultrasound alone is not a satisfactory technique to exclude stone.

Stone Composition

There is a large matrix component in these calculi, of which the Tamm-Horsfall glycoprotein is a prominent component. The inorganic constituents are struvite (magnesium ammonium phosphate) and apatite (basic calcium phosphate). The significance of the *Proteus* organism lies in its urease activity, for the formation of ammonia from urea raises the urine pH, which favors the precipitation of calcium phosphate and also leads directly to an increase in ammonium ion concentration, thereby raising the magnesium ammonium phosphate ion product.

Associated Urological Abnormalities

In one third of the cases there is an underlying urological malformation other than vesicoureteric reflux. Thirty-five percent of the remainder have reflux preoperatively, but it ceases spontaneously in two thirds of these soon after removal of the calculi so ureteric reimplantation is only rarely necessary. In many there is dilatation of the lumbar ureter, which may at first suggest obstructive megaureter, but this is a consequence of the calculus or the associated infection, for it recedes rapidly after surgery (Fig. 42.3).

Calcium Excretion

In 15% of apparently straightforward infective calculi the urine calcium excretion exceeds 0.15 mmol/kg/24 hr and in another 15% it is

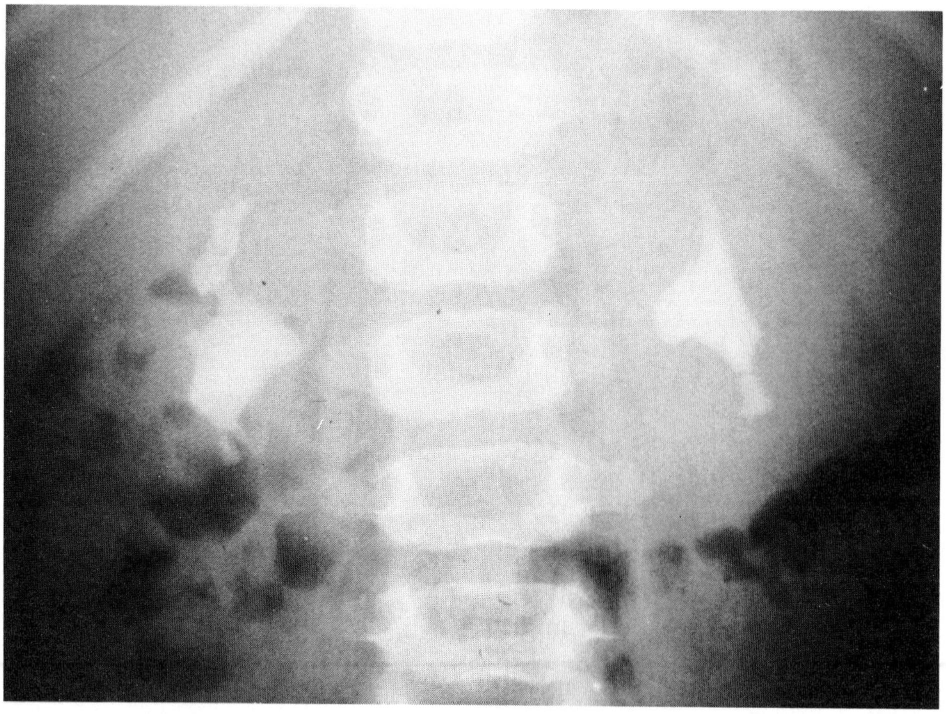

Figure 42.2. Bilateral staghorn calculi associated with *Proteus* infection.

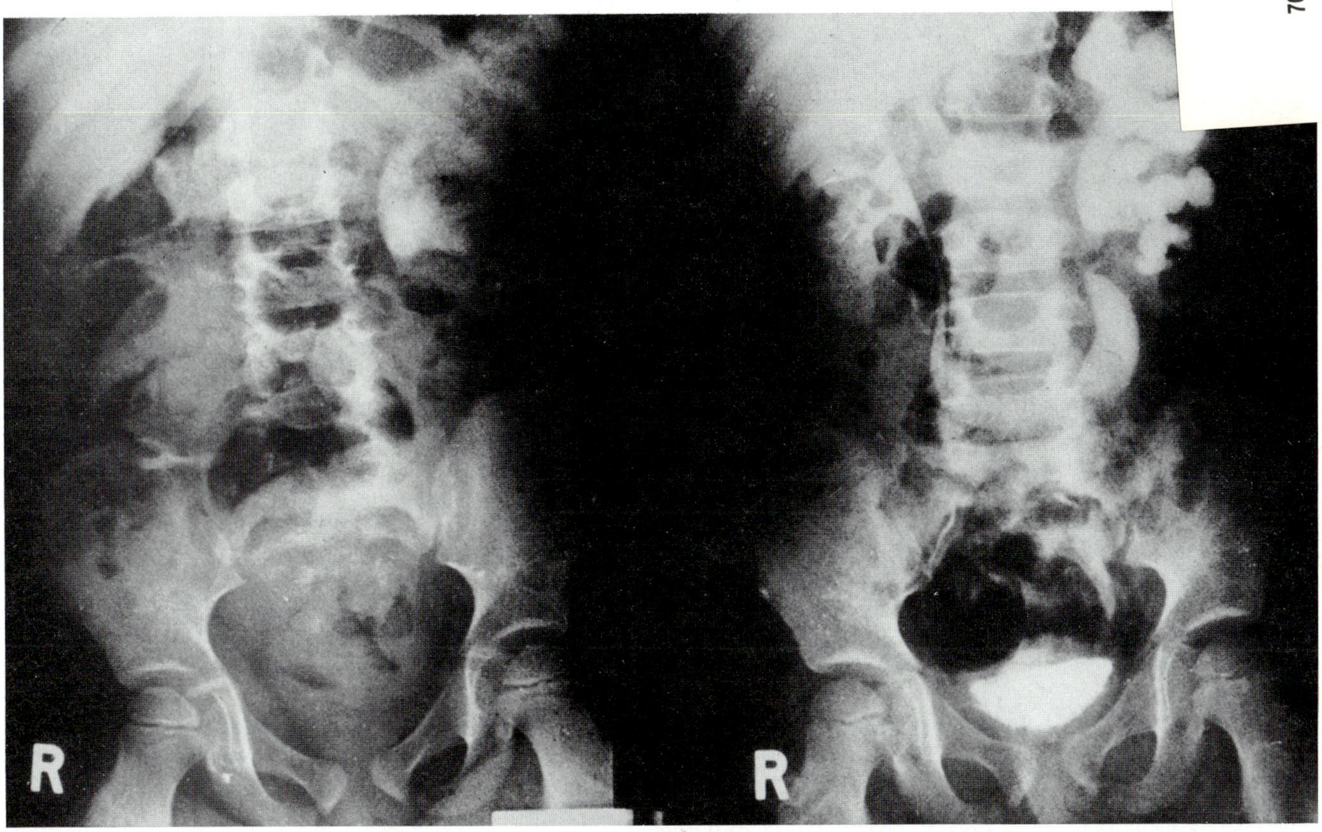

Figure 42.3. Left: Plain abdominal roentgenogram in a 6-year-old girl presenting with *Proteus* urinary tract infection; a left-sided staghorn calculus is shown. Right: The intravenous urogram shows the typical dilatation of the lumbar ureter associated with the stone.

between 0.10 and 0.15 mmol/kg/24 hr (5). However, the hypercalciuria is of the same order as observed in other children with urinary tract infection but without stone, and it subsides after the calculus is removed, which suggests that the hypercalciuria is an epiphenomenon reflecting immobilization and ill health rather than an underlying metabolic disorder predisposing to stone formation.

Treatment

The stones must be removed surgically; there is almost no place in children for conservative management of such infective calculi, for if left untreated pyonephrosis may supervene, leading to complete destruction of the kidney. Nephrectomy is necessary on this account in about 10% of cases. Under such circumstances the kidney will be found to be full of caseous material, and some cases described as xanthogranulomatous pyelonephritis are really examples of this disease (25).

The recurrence rate is low, less than 10%, and can usually be attributed to failure to remove all the fragments or to persistent *Proteus* infection (26). There is no evidence that these infective calculi herald a problem of urolithiasis in adult life, though of course the associated pyelonephritic scarring may be responsible for hypertension and occasionally chronic renal failure.

Pathogenesis

Any hypothesis of the pathogenesis of such infective calculi must recognize the close association with *Proteus* yet explain why children with neurogenic bladder, who frequently have *Proteus* infection, are only occasionally afflicted with stone. It must also account for the curious epidemiological characteristics of the disease and its predilection for young male children. At present there is not a satisfactory hypothesis that accounts for all these features.

CALCIUM STONES

Calcium-containing stones are frequently the expression of an underlying metabolic abnormality, especially if nephrocalcinosis is present.

Generalized Nephrocalcinosis

An increase in calcium content of the kidney without histological or radiological evidence of calcification can be produced in several experimental models. Calcium phosphate crystals can be demonstrated by von Kossa's stain and are a not infrequent finding in a wide variety of renal conditions. There must be a substantial increase in the calcium content of the kidney before nephrocalcinosis becomes radiologically evident.

Nephrocalcinosis associated with metabolic disease is most prominent in the medulla, especially at the corticomedullary junction. It must be distinguished from the punctate nephrolithiasis complicating medullary sponge kidney and renal tubular ectasia.

The three most frequent causes are hypercalcemic states, defects of urinary acidification, and the hyperoxalurias (27). In adult patients hyperparathyroidism accounts for one third of cases of nephrocalcinosis, but it is much rarer in childhood (28). The nephrocalcinosis associated with hyperoxaluria is of a coarser pattern than the other varieties, involving the cortex as well as the medulla; in infants it may cause renal failure without stone formation. Nephrocalcinosis may complicate diuretic therapy, especially with the carbonic anhydrase inhibitor acetazolamide. It is seen in some cases with features of Bartter's syndrome (29), in association with hypomagnesemia (30), and in other cases no cause is found (Fig. 42.1).

Cortical nephrocalcinosis may be a consequence of cortical necrosis, as in severe cases of the hemolytic-uremic syndrome, or following venous thrombosis in the neonatal period. In the latter instance there may be adrenal calcification as well, as a consequence of adrenal hemorrhage.

Hypercalcemia

The hypercalcemic syndromes of childhood are more frequently complicated by nephrocalcinosis than by urolithiasis. Causes of hypercalcemia and nephrocalcinosis or stone in this age group include hyperparathyroidism, vitamin D intoxication, immobilization, idiopathic hypercalcemia in its mild or severe form, hypothyroidism (32–34), alkaptonuria (35), indicanuria (36), hypophosphatasia, and tumors.

Hyperparathyroidism has only rarely been recognized in children (37–40) and usually presents with bone lesions; it may on occasion cause renal calculi. It may be part of the endocrine adenomatosis syndrome, and there is a rare neonatal variant related to familial hypocalciuric hyperparathyroidism (41). Hypothyroidism is easily overlooked as a cause of hypercalcemia, but with earlier diagnosis this complication is now rare. It may be difficult to establish retrospectively the diagnosis of vitamin D intoxication when the plasma calcium returned to the normal range; the possibility should be considered in a child with a renal calculus who comes from a country where the administration of vitamin D is haphazard. The risks of nephrocalcinosis complicating the treatment of hypophosphatemic rickets is much less now that vitamin D therapy has been superceded by the use of the shorter-acting 1,25-dihydroxycholecalciferol (42).

Hypercalciuria

There has been difficulty in establishing standards for urinary calcium excretion in healthy children, for there may be considerable variation between different nationalities or decades as a consequence of diet or habits of vitamin D prescription. In the older literature there is as well some uncertainty about the technical adequacy of the methods used to measure urinary calcium concentration. Royer (43) reported the upper limit of calcium excretion to be 0.15 mmol/kg/24 hr (6 mg/kg/24 hr), but in 52 British children aged 1 to 14 yr, Ghazali and Barratt found the upper limit was 0.10 mmol/kg/24 hr (4 mg/kg/24 hr) (44). There is considerable diurnal variation in calcium excretion, but a calcium/creatinine concentration ratio greater than 0.7 mmol/mmol (0.25 mg/mg) in the second urine specimen voided in the morning strongly suggests hypercalciuria; this simple screening test avoids the problems inherent in 24-hr urine collections in children. Stapleton and coworkers reported similar results (45, 46). It should be recalled that even straightforward surgical operations result in sufficient immobilization to cause hypercalciuria, so studies of calcium excretion in stone-forming patients should be undertaken either preoperatively or after convalescence.

Urinary calcium excretion is increased in the hypercalcemic syndromes previously described. Hypercalciuria with normal plasma calcium concentration may be caused by increased gastrointestinal absorption (vitamin D excess and idiopathic hypercalciuria [(47]); to increased bone mobilization of calcium (immobilization, Cushing's syndrome, and neoplastic deposits including leukemia in bone); and to renal tubular disorders such as distal renal tubular acidosis (RTA), Bartter's syndrome, and Wilson's disease. Royer and coworkers have also described idiopathic hypercalciuria apparently caused by a tubular leak associated with dwarfism but not with urolithiasis (48).

During immobilization, calcium is lost from the skeleton. Children undergoing orthopedic surgery or with extensive burns are particularly at risk. Even slight activity reduces the negative calcium balance, and a high fluid intake helps to prevent stone formation. Many children with apparently straightforward infective stones also have hypercalciuria, but as discussed previously, this is probably just an epiphenomenon of a severe infective illness.

Acidification Defects

Of the hypercalciuric states previously described, distal RTA is the most important, since recurrence of calculi is typical but may be prevented by adequate treatment (49). Distal RTA is characterized by the failure to establish a significant hydrogen ion gradient between tubular fluid and plasma (see Chapter 34). A metabolic acidosis ensues; as renal failure with divalent anion retention is not present, the anion gap is normal, and thus the acidosis is associated with hyperchloremia. There is renal wastage of sodium, potassium, and calcium and defective urinary concentration. Citrate excretion is low, particularly when assessed in relation to urine pH. The combination of hypercalciuria, alkaline urine, and low citrate excretion favors precipitation of calcium salts; a similar situation is observed with acetazolamide therapy. Osteomalacia or rickets may occur, and growth may be poor. The disease may be associated with autoimmune phenomena, and in some cases there is a familial pattern suggestive of dominant inheritence, but there is also an autosomal recessive variant associated with nerve deafness.

The combination of nephocalcinosis and calculi is characteristic of this condition (Fig. 42.4), although a similar pattern may be seen in primary hyperoxaluria. Sometimes the stones may drop into the ureter and obstruct the flow of urine, in which case surgery is necessary, but in general the surgical approach should be conservative because the condition tends to recur. The diagnosis may be evident from a review of plasma bicarbonate and urine pH data, and the observation of a urine pH less than 5.3 (often observed in health in the morning urine specimen) excludes the condition. In borderline cases it may be necessary to stress urinary acidification by the administration of ammonium chloride (50). If there is urinary tract infection, particularly with a urea-splitting organism such as *Proteus*, urinary acidification tests cannot be carried out, and sometimes it is necessary to defer formal study until the stones have been removed and the infection eradicated.

Treatment consists of the administration of sufficient alkali to neutralize endogenous acid production: about 2 mmol/kg/24 hr of sodium or potassium bicarbonate, depending on diet. Sufficient alkali must be given to ensure a normal plasma bicarbonate concentration throughout the 24-hr day. Urine calcium excretion decreases, and there may be catchup growth and healing of rickets without any additional vitamin D therapy. Unfortunately, however, stone formation sometimes continues in spite of seemingly adequate alkali therapy.

OXALATE STONES

Primary Hyperoxaluria

Oxalic acid is an end-product of metabolism: approximately 15% of urinary oxalate originates from dietary sources and the remainder is derived in more or less equal amounts from the metabolism of glyoxalate and ascorbic acid. Ethylene glycol (antifreeze) and the anesthetic agent methoxyflurane are also converted to oxalic acid in vivo. Oxalate excretion (expressed in terms of anhydrous oxalic acid) in health is 0.2 to 0.5 mmol (20–50 mg)/24 hr/1.73 m^2SA. Measurement of urinary oxalate concentration has some problems, and critical analyses should be reconfirmed by experienced laboratories.

The primary hyperoxalurias are genetically determined conditions characterized by increased urinary oxalate excretion, typically above 1 mmol/24 hr/1.73 m^2SA, recurrent calcium oxalate nephrolithiasis that usually presents in childhood, nephrocalcinosis, and frequently death from end-stage renal failure in early adult life (51, 52). Small spiky stones form in sterile urine and are often associated with hematuria or renal colic. There may be episodes of urinary obstruction, but the principal cause of renal damage is the precipitation of calcium oxalate within the renal parenchyma. In later stages of the illness there may be oxalate deposition (oxalosis) in other organs as well—particularly the cardiac conducting system—which causes arrhythmias.

Type I hyperoxaluria, the commoner variety, is characterized in addition by increased excretion of glyoxylate and glycolate; there is a

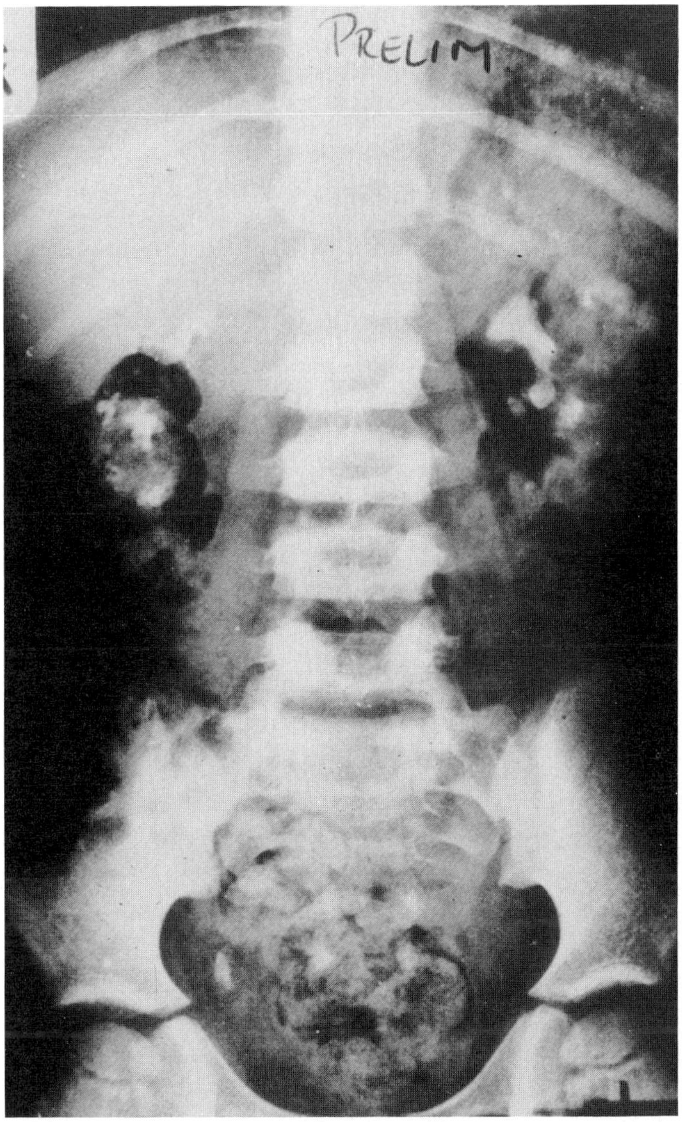

Figure 42.4. Intravenous urogram in a 10-year-old boy with distal renal tubular acidosis. There is medullary nephrocalcinosis, renal calculi, and a calculus at the lower end of the right ureter.

deficiency of the enzyme 2-oxo-glutarate:glyoxylate carboligase, which converts glyoxylate and 2-oxo-glutarate to 2-hydroxy-3-oxo-adipate, and thus there is a buildup of glyoxylate and glycolate with increased conversion of glyoxylate to oxalate. In type II hyperoxaluria there is increased excretion of L-glycerate as well; a deficiency of the enzyme D-glycerate dehydrogenase has been described, but the pathogenesis of the hyperoxaluria remains uncertain.

There is no satisfactory treatment for either type of hyperoxaluria at present. A few type I patients respond to large doses of pyridoxine, but other drugs have not been effective in reducing oxalate excretion. It is obviously appropriate to try to diminish calcium excretion by reducing dietary calcium in order to reduce the calcium oxalate ion product. It has also been suggested that increased magnesium concentration in the urine tends to inhibit calcium oxalate precipitation, but it is difficult to influence urinary magnesium excretion by dietary supplementation.

Surgical treatment should be confined to the removal of obviously obstructing calculi and should if anything err on the conservative side, as recurrence is inevitable. Transplantation has in general been accompanied by the rapid recurrence of oxalate calculi, and dialysis by the progression of oxalosis, so these patients have poor prospects on renal replacement programs.

The majority of adult patients who form calcium oxalate stones, even those with a family history of urolithiasis, do not have primary hyperoxaluria; many of these have idiopathic hypercalciuria, and this type of calcium oxalate stone is occasionally seen in older children (53). Oxalate stones have also been described in association with hyperglycinuria (54).

Bowel Disease

Hyperoxaluria, occasionally complicated by renal stones, occurs in some patients with bowel disease, particularly that affecting the terminal ileum such as ileal resection of Crohn's disease (55, 56). The mechanism is not certain, but it has been observed that bile salts and unsaturated fatty acids promote the absorption of oxalate by the colon. Increased oxalate excretion is seen in some children with celiac disease but has not yet been reported to be associated with urolithiasis.

CYSTINURIA

In cystinuria there is defective tubular reabsorption of the dibasic amino acids cystine, ornithine, arginine, and lysine from the glomerular filtrate (57) (see Chapter 31); the transport defect is also present in the gut in some individuals. There is more than one mode of inheritance,

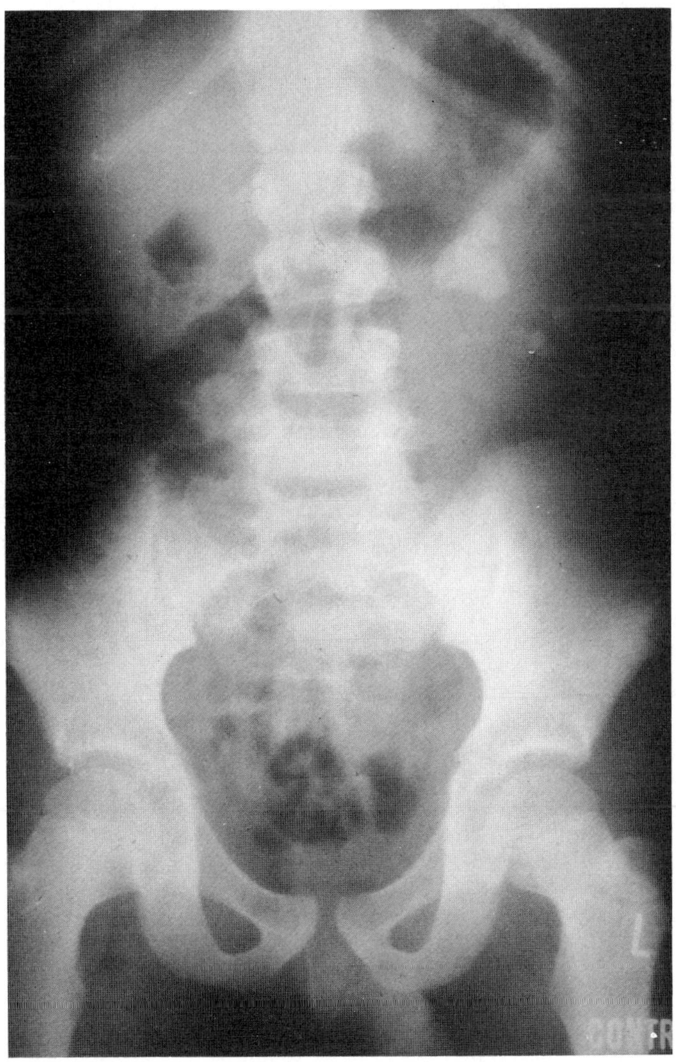

Figure 42.5. Cystinuria.

and three variants are recognized. The only clinical abnormality in these children is recurrent formation of urinary calculi. A presumptive diagnosis may be made on the basis of the purple color that develops when the urine is mixed with cyanide-nitroprusside, and it should be confirmed with further studies of urinary amino acids by chromatography or high-voltage electrophoresis.

Cystine stones may occur in children at all ages. In the very young, bladder calculi are not uncommon; later in childhood renal calculi are predominant, often large rounded stones or branched stones in the renal pelvis with multiple calculi in the dilated calices (Fig. 42.5). Some cystine stones may be passed spontaneously, and in cases of renal colic where no explanation is evident, the urine should be tested for cystine. All cystine calculi are opaque to x-rays, though they are not as dense as many calcium-containing stones and often not as dense as the opaque medium during intravenous urography. If the calculus lies over a transverse process, the bone may be visible on x-ray film behind the stone.

The attractive simplicity of the view that cystinuria represents a genetic deficiency of the transport system of the dibasic amino acids is threatened by the genetic heterogeneity alluded to previously, by the observation that the cystine clearance frequently exceeds the inulin clearance, and by the recognition of phenotypes in which there is an isolated failure of reabsorption of cystine or of the other members of the group without involvement of cystine.

The solubility of cystine in urine of pH less than 7.5 is about 1 mmol/liter. Above this pH there is a substantial increase in solubility, but it is difficult to maintain the urinary pH consistently in this region with alkali therapy. A knowledge of the quantitative cystine excretion enables the minimum safe urine volume to be calculated: in adult patients who excrete about 4 mmol/24 hr this is approximately 4 liters daily.

A high fluid intake, sustained throughout the day and night, prevents the formation of cystine stones and may result in their dissolution. The treatment is inconvenient and difficult to follow but has the merit of being cheap and effective if the cooperation of the patient can be maintained. This is sometimes lost with the rebellious attitudes of adolescence, particularly if it is many years since an episode of renal colic. An alternative treatment with D-penicillamine results in the excretion of the mixed cysteine-penicillamine disulfide, which is more soluble than cystine. The drug is expensive and has many side effects and should be reserved for patients in whom continuous hydration fails. Surgery is occasionally required for the removal of bladder stones and of obstructing renal and ureteric stones, particularly if complicated by infection.

DISORDERS OF PURINE METABOLISM

Uric Acid

Uric acid is a weak acid with a pK of 5.6; below this pH it exists predominantly in the un-ionized form, which is considerably less soluble than the urate ion; in contrast to calcium phosphate, acid urine favors its precipitation. These stones may develop in situations of uric acid overproduction such as leukemia or lymphoma, especially after cytotoxic chemotherapy, but occasionally as the presenting feature of leukemia. Uric acid gravel in both kidneys may lead to acute renal failure without radiological evidence of calculus: allopurinol and sodium bicarbonate are valuable in preventing this complication of leukemia therapy.

Primary gout with uric acid calculi occasionally occurs in older children. Another variant is the Lesch-Nyhan syndrome (58)—a disorder characterized by progressive choreoathetosis, self-multilation, and hyperuricemia with uric acid calculi. The deficient enzyme is guanine-

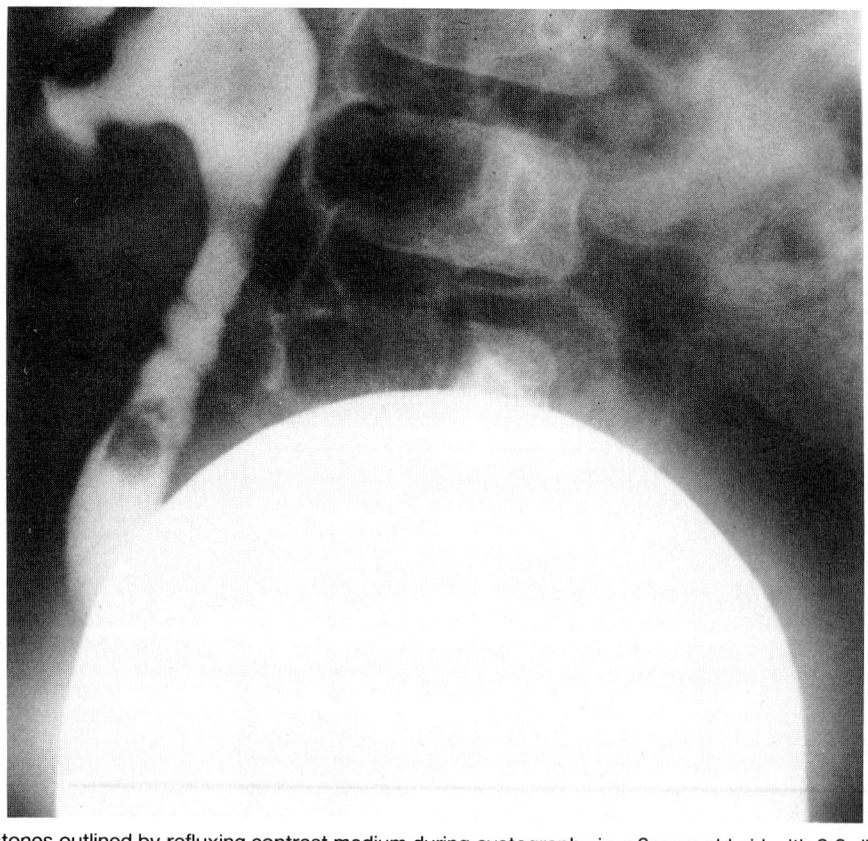

Figure 42.6. Nonopaque stones outlined by refluxing contrast medium during cystography in a 3-year-old girl with 2,8-dihydroxyadenine urolithiasis.

hypoxanthine phosphoribosyltransferase (59). Infants may present with renal failure (59), and calculi may precede neurological manifestations. Hyperuricosuria with calculus formation may also occur in type 1 glycogen storage disease; the mechanism is not clear.

In some patients, particularly males of Mediterranean stock, there is a tendency to uric acid stone formation without hyperuricemia or uricosuria; the syndrome is sometimes familial and is occasionally seen in childhood, but some of these patients may in fact have had dihydroxyadenine calculi, which are not distinguished from uric acid calculi by routine laboratory techniques.

Dihydroxyadenine

A new inborn error of purine metabolism has recently been recognized with a deficiency of the enzyme adenine phosphoribosyl-transferase resulting in the diversion of adenine metabolism to 2,8-dihydroxyadenine, which is relatively insoluble and forms nonopaque stones (Fig. 42.6) (61–63). These stones require specialized chemical analysis to distinguish them from uric acid stones, but the diagnosis is important as alkalinization of the urine decreases the solubility of 2,8-dihydroxyadenine, but the condition responds satisfactorily to allopurinol therapy. Parenchymal deposits, however, may lead to renal failure (64).

Xanthinuria

Xanthinuria is a rare condition in which there is a deficiency of xanthine oxidase and hence a failure of conversion of xanthine to uric acid (65). The plasma uric acid concentration is therefore low, and as xanthine is relatively insoluble in acid urine, radiolucent calculi develop. A xanthine nephropathy may also be precipitated by the use of allopurinol in patients with high uric acid excretion rates.

DYSTROPHIC CALCIFICATION

Irregular patches of calcification may occur in damaged renal parenchyma. This may be the consequence of cortical necrosis, venous infarction, or papillary necrosis. The calcification may be sited in abnormal vasculature, as in angiomata, aneurysms, and familial calcific arterial stenosis. Infections, particularly tuberculosis, may be responsible, and patchy calcification may be seen in tumors, particularly nephroblastoma. An end-stage kidney from almost any cause may have calcification in it.

References

1. Barratt TM, Ghazali S: The aetiology of renal stones in children. Postgrad Med J 53:35, 1977.
2. Broyer M, Gagnadoux MF, Beurton D: Urinary lithiasis in children. Review of 100 cases. Adv Nephrol 10:389, 1981.
3. Ghazali S, Barratt TM, Williams DI: Childhood urolithiasis in Britain. Arch Dis Child 48:291, 1973.
4. Malek RS: Urolithiasis: In Kelalis PP, King LR, Belman AB (eds): Clinical Pediatric Urology, cd 2. Philadelphia, WB Saunders, 1985, vol 2, p 1093.
5. Malek RS, Kelalis PP: Pediatric urolithiasis. J Urol 113:545, 1975.
6. Wenzel JE, Burke EC, Stickler GB, et al: Nephrolithiasis and nephrocalcinosis in children. Pediatrics 41:57, 1968.
7. Robertson WG, Nordin BEC: Physicochemical factors governing stone formation. In Williams DI, Chisholm GD (eds): Scientific Foundations of Urology. London, Heinemann, 1976, vol 1, p 254.
8. Williams DI: Matrix calculi. Br J Urol 35:411, 1963.
9. Wickham JEA: The matrix of renal calculi. In Williams DI, Chisholm GD (eds): Scientific Foundations of Urology. London, Heinemann, 1976, vol 1, p 323.
10. Boyce WH, Stanton-King J, Fielden ML: Total non-dialysable solids in human urine. XIII. Immunological detection of a component peculiar to renal calculus matrix and to urine of calculous patients. J Clin Invest 41:1180, 1962.
11. Blacklock NJ: Epidemiology of urolithiasis. In Williams DI, Chisholm GD (eds): Scientific Foundations of Urology. London, Heinemann, 1976, vol 1, p 235.
12. Eckstein HB: Endemic urinary lithiasis in Turkish children (a clinical study of 119 cases). Arch Dis Child 36:137, 1961.
13. Chutikorn C, Valyaseri H, Halstead SB: Studies of bladder stone disease in Thailand. II. Hospital experience: urolithiasis at Ubol Provincial Hospital, 1956–62. Am J Clin Nutr 26:1027, 1973.
14. Anderson DA: Historical and geographical differences in the pattern of urinary stones considered in relation to possible aetiological factors. In Hodgkinson A, Nordin BEC (eds): Renal Stone Research Symposium. London, Churchill, 1969, p 7.
15. Lett H: On urinary calculus with special reference to stone in the bladder. Br J Urol 8:205, 1936.
16. Ghazali S: Childhood urolithiasis in the United Kingdom and Eire. Br J Urol 47:739, 1975.
17. Gaches CGC, Gordon IRS, Shore DF, et al: Urinary lithiasis in childhood in the Bristol clinical area. Br J Urol 47:109, 1975.
18. Moore ES, Coe FL, McMann BJ, et al: Idiopathic hypercalciuria: prevalence and metabolic characteristics. J Pediatr 92:906, 1978.
19. Mathieu H, Cuisinier-Gleizes P: Nephrocalcinoses et rein des hypercalcemies. In Royer P, Habib R, Mathieu H, Broyer M (eds): Nephrologie Pediatrique, ed 3. Paris, Flammarion, 1983, p 200.
20. Kalia A, Travis LB, Brouhard BH: The association of idiopathic hypercalciuria and asymptomatic gross hematuria in children. J Pediatr 99:716, 1981.
21. Stapleton FB, Roy S, Noe N, et al: Hypercalciuria in children with hematuria. N Engl J Med 310:1345, 1984.
22. Roy S, Stapleton FB, Noe HN, et al: Hematuria preceding renal calculus formation in children with hypercalciuria. J Pediatr 99:712, 1981.
23. Westbury EJ, Omenogor P: A quantitative approach to the analysis of renal calculi. J Med Lab Technol 27:462, 1970.
24. Sutor DJ: Crystallographic analysis of urinary calculi. In Williams DI, Chisholm GD (eds): Scientific Foundations of Urology. London, Heinemann, 1976, vol 1, p 244.
25. Habib R, Levy M, Royer P: La pyelonephrite chronique xanthogranulomateuse. Arch Franc Pediatr 25:489, 1968.
26. Androulakakis PA, Barratt TM, Ransley PG, et al: Urinary calculi in children: a 5- to 15-year follow-up with particular reference to recurrent and residual stones. Br J Urol 54:176, 1982.
27. Cremin B, Wiggelinkhuisen J, Bonnici F: Nephrocalcinosis in children. Br J Radiol 55:413, 1982.
28. Wrong OM, Feest TG: Nephrocalcinosis. In Peters DAK (ed): Advanced Medicine 12. Tunbridge Wells, England, Pitman, 1976, p 394.
29. McCredie DA, Rottenberg E, Williams AL: Hypercalciuria in potassium losing nephropathy. Austr J Pediatr 10:286, 1974.
30. Manz F, Scharer K, Janka P, et al: Renal magnesium wasting, incomplete tubular acidosis, hypercalciuria and nephrocalcinosis in siblings. Eur J Pediatr 128:67, 1978.
31. Lightwood R: Idiopathic hypercalcemia with failure to thrive: nephrocalcinosis. Proc R Soc Med 45:401, 1952.
32. Bateson EM, Chandler S: Nephrocalcinosis in cretinism. Br J Radiol 38:581, 1965.
33. Naylor JM: A case of hypothyroidism with nephrocalcinosis. Arch Dis Child 30:165, 1955.
34. Royer P, Matthieu H, Balsan S: Troubles de metabolisme calcique dans l'insuffisance thyroidienne de l'enfant. Acta Endocrinol 29:610, 1982.
35. Goldberg BH, Penson JS, Stern LM, et al: Alcaptonuria with nephrocalcinosis. J Pediatr 88:518, 1976.
36. Drummond KN, Michael AF, Ulstrom RA, et al: The blue diaper syndrome—familial hypercalcemia with nephrocalcinosis and indicanuria: a new familial disease with definition of the metabolic abnormality. Am J Med 37:928, 1964.
37. Klein R, Hadow J: Hyperparathyroidism. In Gardner LI (ed): Endocrine and Genetic Disorders of Childhood and Adolescence, ed 2. Philadelphia, Saunders, 1975, p 400.
38. Malek RS, Kelalis PP: Urologic manifestations of hyperparathyroidism in childhood. J Urol 115:717, 1976.
39. Matsuo M, Okita K, Takemine H, et al: Neonatal primary hyperparathyroidism in familial hypocalciuric hypercalcemia. Am J Dis Child 136:728, 1982.
40. Vasquez AM: Nephrocalcinosis and hypertension in juvenile hyperparathyroidism. Am J Dis Child 125:104, 1973.
41. Marx SJ, Attie MF, Spiegel AM, et al: An association between neonatal severe primary hyperparathyroidism and familial hypocalciuric hypercalcemia in three kindreds. N Engl J Med 306:257, 1982.
42. Moncrieff MV, Chance GM: Nephrotoxic effect of vitamin D therapy in vitamin D refractory rickets. Arch Dis Child 44:571, 1969.
43. Royer P: Explorations biologique du metabolism calcique chez l'enfant. Helv Paed Acta 16:320, 1961.
44. Ghazali S, Barratt TM: Urinary excretion of calcium and magnesium in children. Arch Dis Child 48:291, 1974.
45. Stapleton FB, Noe NH, Jerkins GL: Urinary excretion of calcium following an oral calcium load. Pediatrics 69:594, 1982.
46. Stapleton FB, Noe NH, Roy C, et al: Hypercalciuria in children with urolithiasis. Am J Dis Child 136:675, 1982.
47. Coe FL, Parks JH, Moore ES: Familial idiopathic hypercalciuria. N Engl J Med

300:357, 1979.
48. Royer P, Mathieu H, Gerbeaux S, et al: Hypercalciurie idiopathique avec nanisme et atteinte renale chez l'enfant. Sem Hop Paris 38:147, 1962.
49. McSherry E: Renal tubular acidosis in childhood. Kidney Int 20:799, 1981.
50. Wrong O, Davies HEF: The excretion of acid in renal disease. Q J Med 28:259, 1959.
51. Hodgkinson A: Oxalate metabolism and hyperoxaluria. In Williams DI, Chisholm GD (eds): Scientific Foundations of Urology. London, Heinemann, 1976, vol 1, p 289.
52. Williams HE, Smith LH: Primary hyperoxaluria. In Stanbury JB, Wyngaarden JB, Frederickson DS, et al (eds): Metabolic Basis of Inherited Disease. ed 5. New York, McGraw-Hill, 1983, p 2021.
53. Resnick M, Prigden DB, Goodman HO: Genetic predisposition to formation of calcium oxalate renal calculi. N Engl J Med 278:1313, 1968.
54. De Vries A, Kochwa S, Lazebrik J, et al: Glycinuria, a hereditary disorder associated with nephrolithiasis. Am J Med 23:408, 1957.
55. Smith LH, Fromm H, Hoffman AF: Acquired hyperoxaluria, nephrolithiasis, and intestinal disease. N Engl J Med 286:1371, 1972.
56. Harrison AR: Urinary calculi in bowel disorders. In Williams DI, Chisholm GD (eds): Scientific Foundations of Urology. London, Heinemann, 1976, vol 1, p 315.
57. Segal S, Thier SO: Cystinuria. In Stanbury JB, Wyngaarden JB, Fredericksen DS, et al (eds): The Metabolic Basis of Inherited Disease, ed 5. New York, McGraw-Hill, 1983, p 1774.
58. Lesch M, Nyhan WL: A familial disorder of uric acid metabolism and central nervous system function. Am J Med 36:351, 1964.
59. Seegmiller JE, Rosenbloom FM, Kelley WN: An enzyme defect associated with a sex-linked human neurological disorder and excessive purine synthesis. Science 155:1682, 1967.
60. Holland PC, Dillon MJ, Pincott J, et al: Hypoxanthine guanine phosphoribosyl transferase deficiency presenting with gout and renal failure in infancy. Arch Dis Child 58:831, 1983.
61. Van Acker KJ, Simmonds HA, Potter CE, et al: Complete deficiency of adenine phosphoribosyltransferase. Report of a family. New Engl J Med 297:127, 1977.
62. Barratt TM, Simmonds HA, Cameron JS, et al: Complete deficiency of adenine phosphoribosyltransferase: a third case presenting as renal stones in a young child. Arch Dis Child 54:25, 1979.
63. Simmonds HA, Van Acker KJ: Adenine phosphoribosyltransferase deficiency: 2,8-dihydroxyadenine lithiasis. In Stanbury JB, Wyngaarden JP, Frederickson DS, et al (eds). The Metabolic Basis of Inherited Disease, ed 5. New York, McGraw-Hill, 1983, p 1144.
64. Greenwood MC, Dillon MJ, Simmonds HA, et al: Renal failure due to 2,8-dihydroxyadenine urolithiasis. Eur J Pediatr 138:346, 1982.
65. Dent CE, Philpot GR: Xanthinuria, an inborn error (or deviation) of metabolism. Lancet 1:172, 1954.

CHAPTER 43

Miscellaneous Urological Diseases

BARRY A. KOGAN

HEMATURIA FROM A UROLOGICAL VIEWPOINT

Hematuria is a common presenting complaint in childhood. A major consideration for the urologist is whether bleeding is caused by a surgically correctable abnormality; thus, attention is first directed toward differentiating glomerular from nonglomerular cases.

Clinical Evaluation

The initial evaluation consists of a careful history, physical examination, and urinalysis, any of which can significantly affect the further workup. For instance, age is one important consideration, since gross hematuria in neonates is associated with significant nonglomerular renal pathology, including renal vein thrombosis, infantile polycystic kidney disease, and obstructive uropathy (1) (see Chapter 57). Voiding symptoms (initial or terminal hematuria or dysuria) point to a lower urinary tract abnormality; an upper abdominal mass suggests an upper tract, though nonglomerular, cause. Examination of the urine is essential. Significant proteinuria or red blood cell casts indicate a glomerular cause for the bleeding but do not necessarily exclude other disease processes. Careful evaluation of red blood cells by phase contrast microscopy, or even light microscopy with minimal light, can differentiate glomerular from nonglomerular bleeding, based on the morphology of the individual cells (2, 3) (Fig. 43.1).

Excretory Urography

Whether the clinical evaluation permits the exclusion of the excretory urogram (IVP) from the workup of the child with hematuria is still unclear. Large screening studies suggest that the IVP is not cost-effective and is associated with needless radiation exposure, (4, 5), particularly if a glomerular source is suspected. However, a large percentage of children with upper urinary tract tumors, calculi, or obstruction present with hematuria, and their diagnosis and appropriate management would be delayed if screening IVPs were not performed (Fig. 43.2). Furthermore, medicolegal concerns in the United States induce most pediatric urologists to obtain an IVP in these children. A current alternative would be ultrasonography of the kidney and bladder, which would pick up most lesions with minimal radiation exposure.

Cystoscopy

Although the utility of the IVP is still controversial, it is well accepted that endoscopy is not indicated in children with isolated hematuria (6, 7). In adults, endoscopy must rule out transitional cell carcinoma, but this lesion is extremely rare in childhood. The more common rhabdomyosarcoma generally presents with obstructive symptoms, not hematuria.

GENITOURINARY TRAUMA

Accidental injuries are a significant source of morbidity and the leading cause of death in children. Genitourinary trauma accounts for 5% to 10% of such injuries, and its frequency seems to be increasing. At least 50% of the genitourinary injuries are renal, most of the others being bladder and urethral. Ureteral trauma is seen with less frequency.

Renal Trauma

The kidney of the child is more prone to traumatic injury than that of the adult because it is relatively larger and has less protection from the rib cage and paravertebral musculature. Further, perirenal and Gerota's fascia are incompletely developed before age 10. Most childhood renal injuries are caused by blunt trauma. Preexisting disease (e.g., hydronephrosis, renal ectopy, or neoplasia) predisposes to these injuries and is seen in up to 23% of cases (8), but this incidence is disputed by others who have found abnormalities in as few as 2% (9). This discrepancy is most likely related to the severity of the trauma. Relatively minor trauma is likely to yield significant injury to a distended hydronephrotic kidney, whereas a normal kidney would be unaffected. On the other hand, renal trauma caused by a rapid deceleration injury will occur with equal frequency in the normal and abnormal kidney. This explanation is supported by the low incidence of motor vehicle accidents in the former (29%) as opposed to the latter (77%).

Diagnosis

The diagnosis of renal injury is made from a history of trauma, flank pain and tenderness, and hematuria. The symptoms and signs can be extremely subtle, or the patient may present in profound shock. Hematuria is nearly always present, although there are reports of major renal

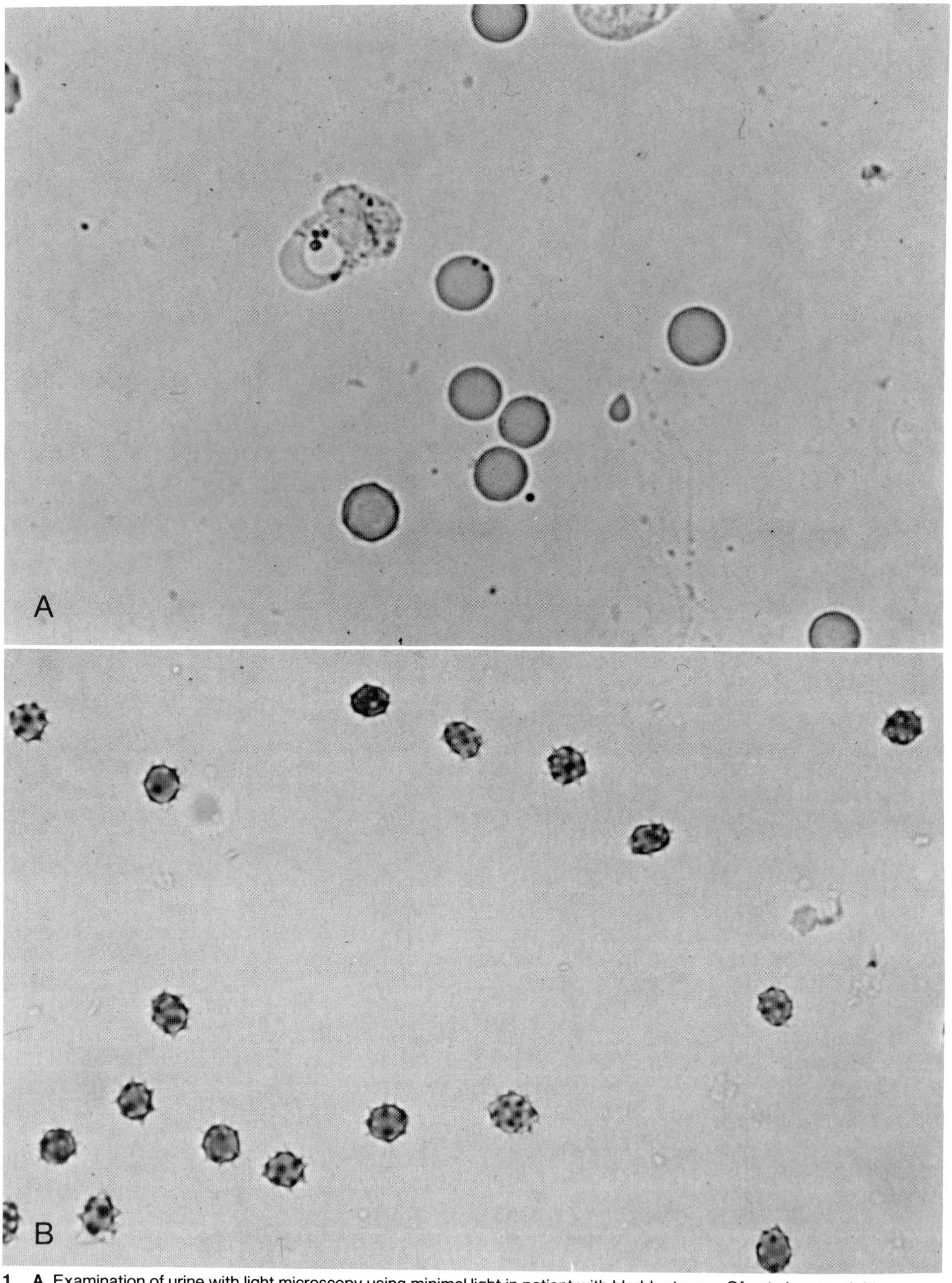

Figure 43.1. **A,** Examination of urine with light microscopy using minimal light in patient with bladder tumor. Of note is smooth biconcave appearance of red blood cells. **B,** Comparable examination in patient with glomerulonephritis. Red cells are obviously irregular. (Courtesy T. Stamey and R. Kindrachuk.)

artery lesions or complete avulsion of the ureteropelvic junction in which the urine is totally clear (9). Although sonography and renal nuclear medicine studies can be helpful, the evaluation should most commonly proceed with a high-dose IVP (e.g., 2 to 4 ml/kg 60% Hypaque). The quality of the study may be less than optimal in an acutely ill patient, but it is important to rule out a significant renal pedicle injury (which

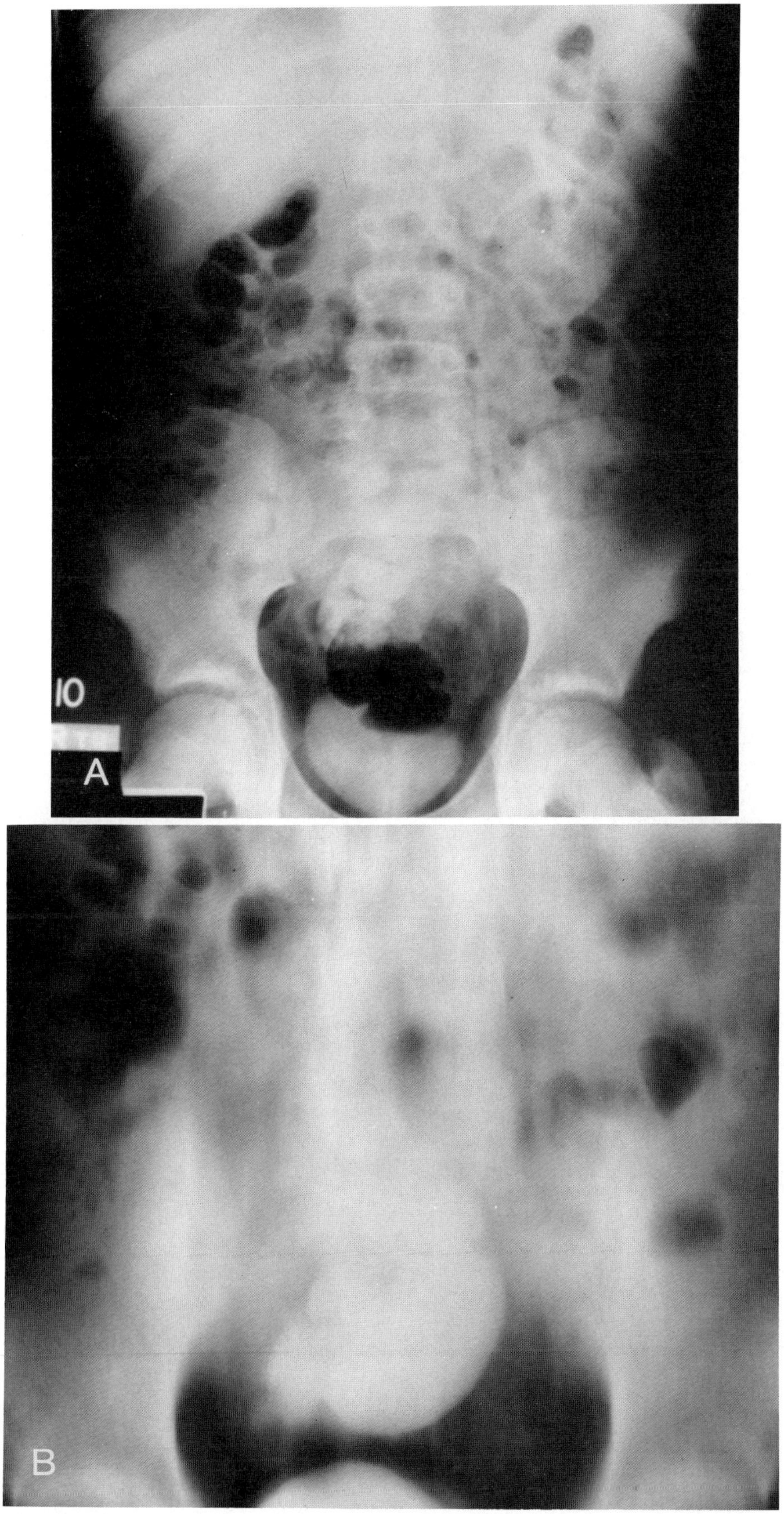

Figure 43.2. **A,** Excretory urogram from a 12-year-old boy with hematuria, red blood cell casts, and mild abdominal pain. **B,** An ectopic right pelvic kidney with ureteropelvic junction obstruction is seen on tomography.

would present as nonvisualization) and absolutely essential to document the presence and normality of the opposite kidney. Next, whenever possible, tomograms should be obtained to define the renal margins, calyceal architecture, and any extravasation.

Although the IVP is presently the most widely available study, recent experience with computed tomography suggests that it may become the study of choice (10). In many trauma centers, it can be performed on short notice at any time of the day. It provides superior images of renal cortex, hematoma, and contrast extravasation, and it clearly delineates major associated intraperitoneal injuries (Fig. 43.3). Arteriography can also be helpful in delineating the anatomy; however, at present it should be reserved for those cases in which a pedicle injury is suspected.

Management

Appropriate management depends on the exact nature of the injury. In general, the findings will permit classification into one of the categories shown in Figure 43.4. Contusions and minor lacerations are the most common abnormalities and are appropriately managed expectantly. Major lacerations with extravasation, shattered kidneys, and pedicle injuries require early surgical intervention to maximize renal salvage. Inevitably, there is a "gray zone" between the minor and major injuries. In these instances, therapy is most controversial. Some authors propose immediate surgery; others, delayed exploration; still others prefer nonoperative management (9, 11–14).

Proponents of different approaches report widely differing results, as the degree of renal trauma, the associated injuries, and the surgeon's experience vary widely. There is general concensus, however, that the most important principle of operative intervention is early transperitoneal control of the renal pedicle (15). It is critical to accomplish this before opening Gerota's fascia; otherwise, the ensuing hemorrhage often results in renal loss. With this technique, the operative nephrectomy rate has dropped dramatically (16). Ultimately, the management of each patient must be individualized, based on the exact anatomy and clinical condition.

Complications

Long-term sequelae are uncommon but evidence of them should nonetheless be sought. Hypertension is seen periodically and is related

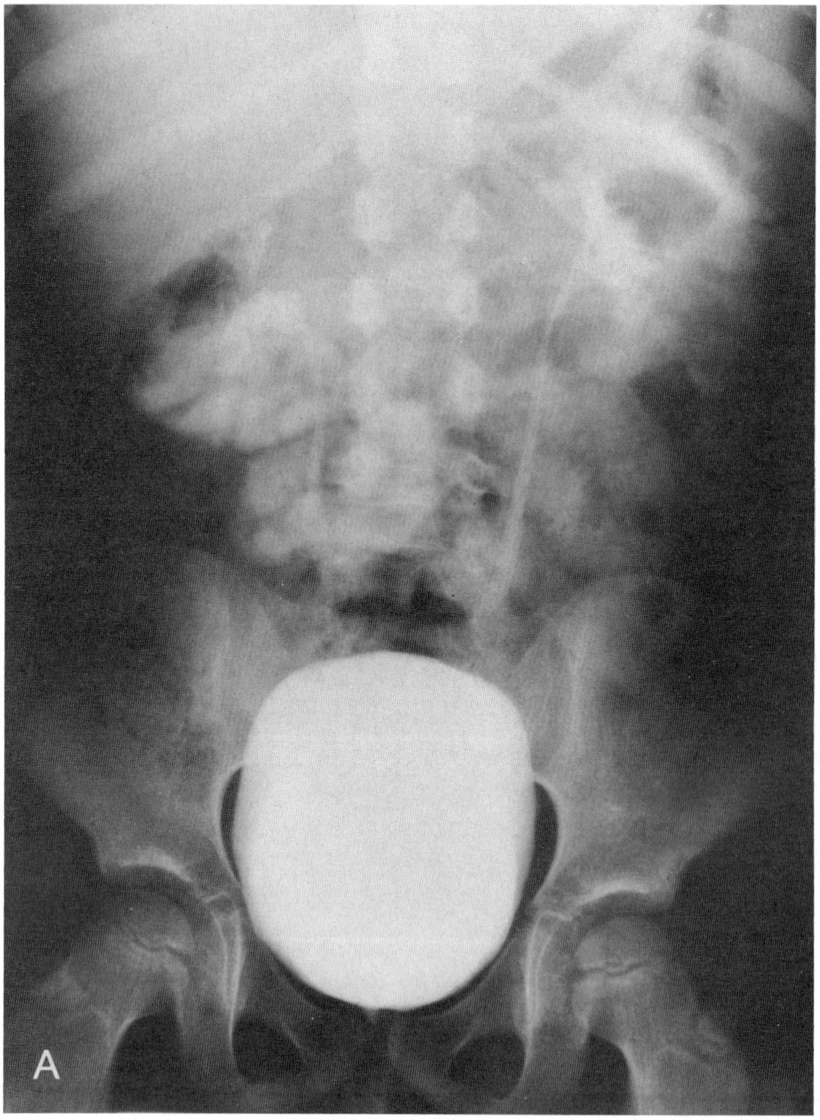

Figure 43.3. A 6-year-old boy hit by an automobile in the left flank. **A,** Plain film of the abdomen following high-dose intravenous and oral contrast administration. Kidneys look normal, although there is questionable extravasation of contrast above the left kidney.

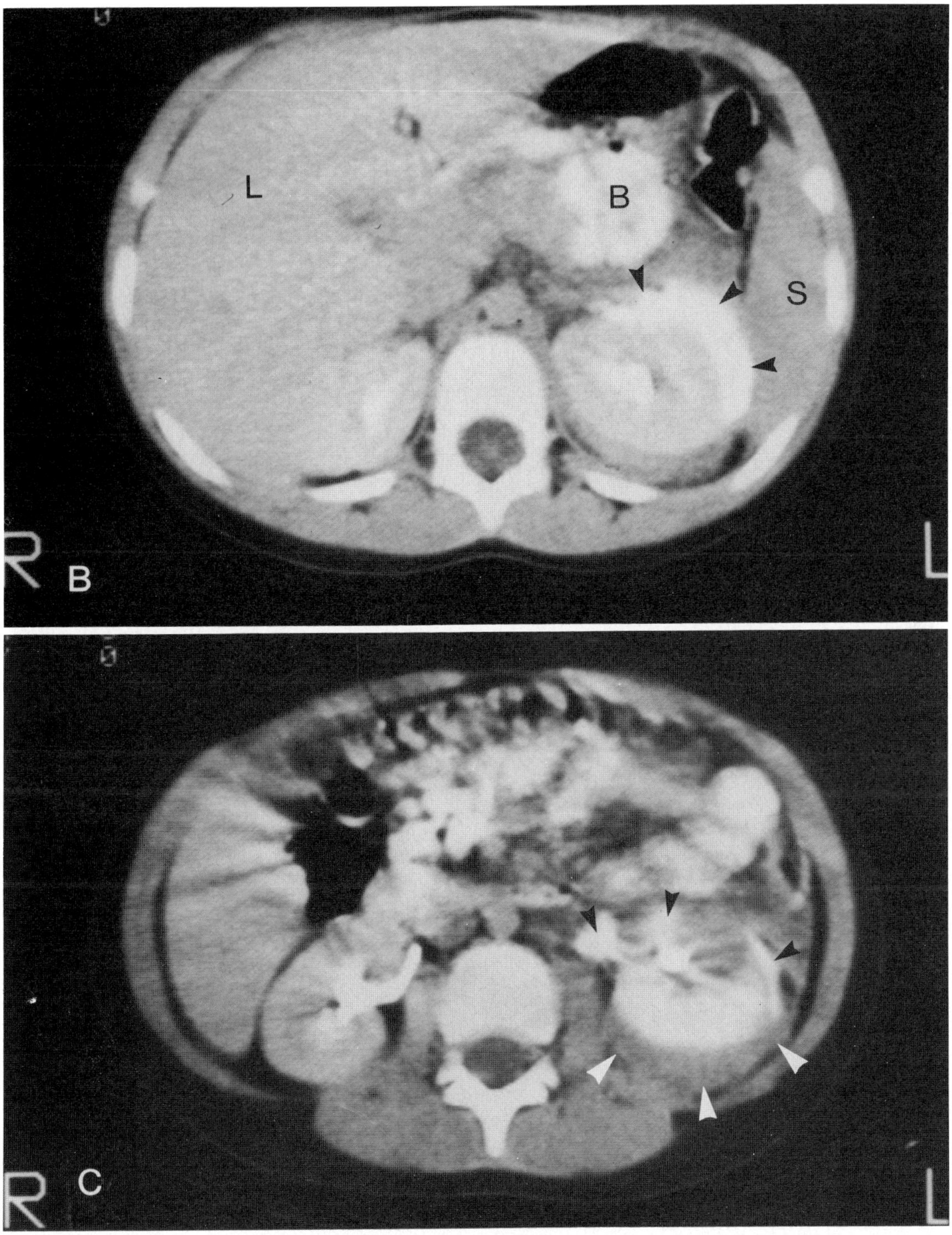

B, Simultaneous computed tomographic image of upper poles demonstrating obvious extravasation of contrast (*black arrows*). Both liver (L) and spleen (S) are normal. There is oral contrast in the bowel (B). **C,** Computed tomographic image through hilum of kidneys demonstrates large retroperitoneal hematoma displacing left kidney (*white arrows*). The extravasation is again clearly seen laterally and around the renal pelvis and proximal ureter (*black arrows*). (Courtesy J. W. McAninch.)

either to renal ischemia following a vascular injury or to perinephric fibrosis following resolution of a perirenal hematoma (11, 17, 18). Other posssible complications are segmental hydronephrosis due to scarring as a calyceal laceration heals and perirenal pseudohydronephrosis in which a well-loculated urinoma persists (11). These findings are obvious on follow-up IVP or ultrasonography.

Bladder Trauma

Bladder ruptures account for virtually all significant bladder injuries and are classified as intraperitoneal or extraperitoneal. The former occur most commonly with blunt trauma to a distended bladder, whereas the latter are nearly always associated with a pelvic fracture. When such ruptures are suspected, a cystogram should be performed before the IVP.

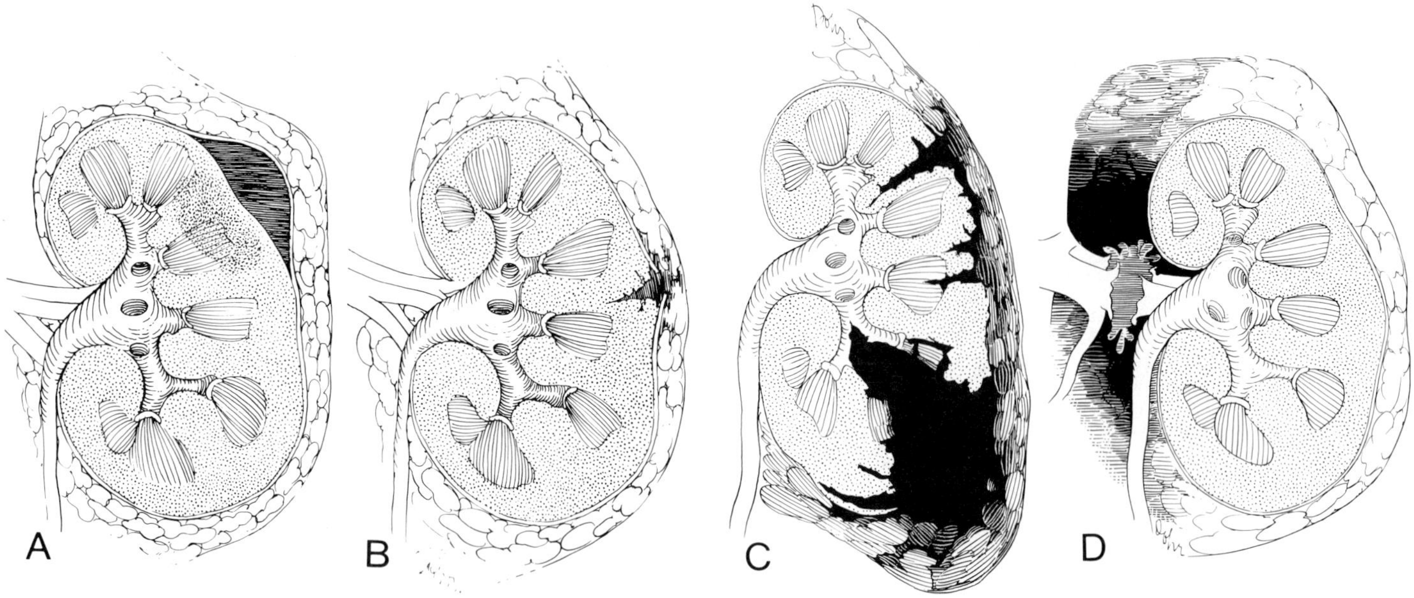

Figure 43.4. Renal contusion **(A)** and minor parenchymal laceration **(B)** are generally best managed expectantly. Major parenchymal lacerations **(C)** and injuries to the renal vascular pedicle **(D)** are best managed with early operative intervention. (Reprinted with permission from McAninch JW: Injuries to the urinary system. In Blaisdell WF and Trunkey DD (eds): Trauma Management. New York, Thieme Stratton, 1985.)

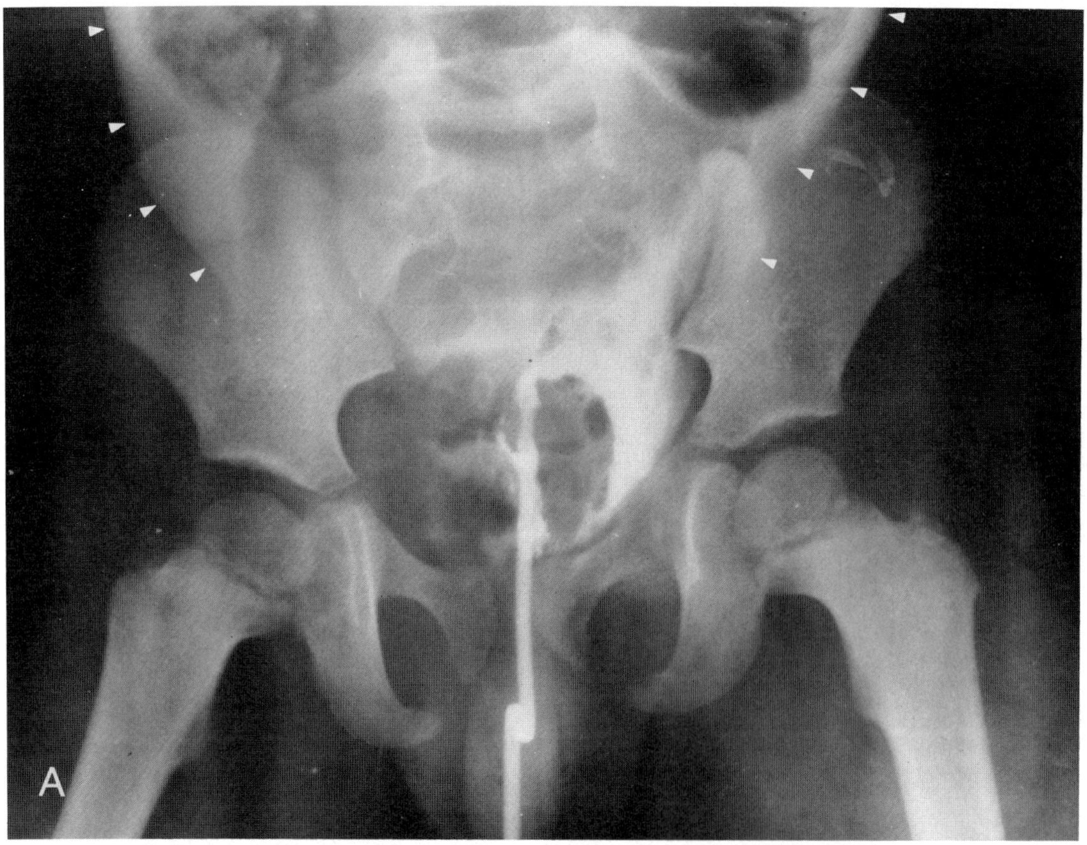

Figure 43.5. A, Intraperitoneal bladder rupture in a 3-year-old male following a motor vehicle accident. There is a large filling defect in the bladder (hematoma) and marked extravasation of contrast that surrounds the bowel (*arrows*). **B,** Extraperitoneal bladder rupture in 18-year-old male following a motor vehicle accident. There is a pelvic fracture. Bladder has been catheterized and filled with contrast. There is extravasation in at least two places (*arrows*), but it is limited to pelvis. **C,** On postemptying film, it is clear contrast is outside the bladder. This film is crucial as the extravasation may be missed on routine anterior-posterior images.

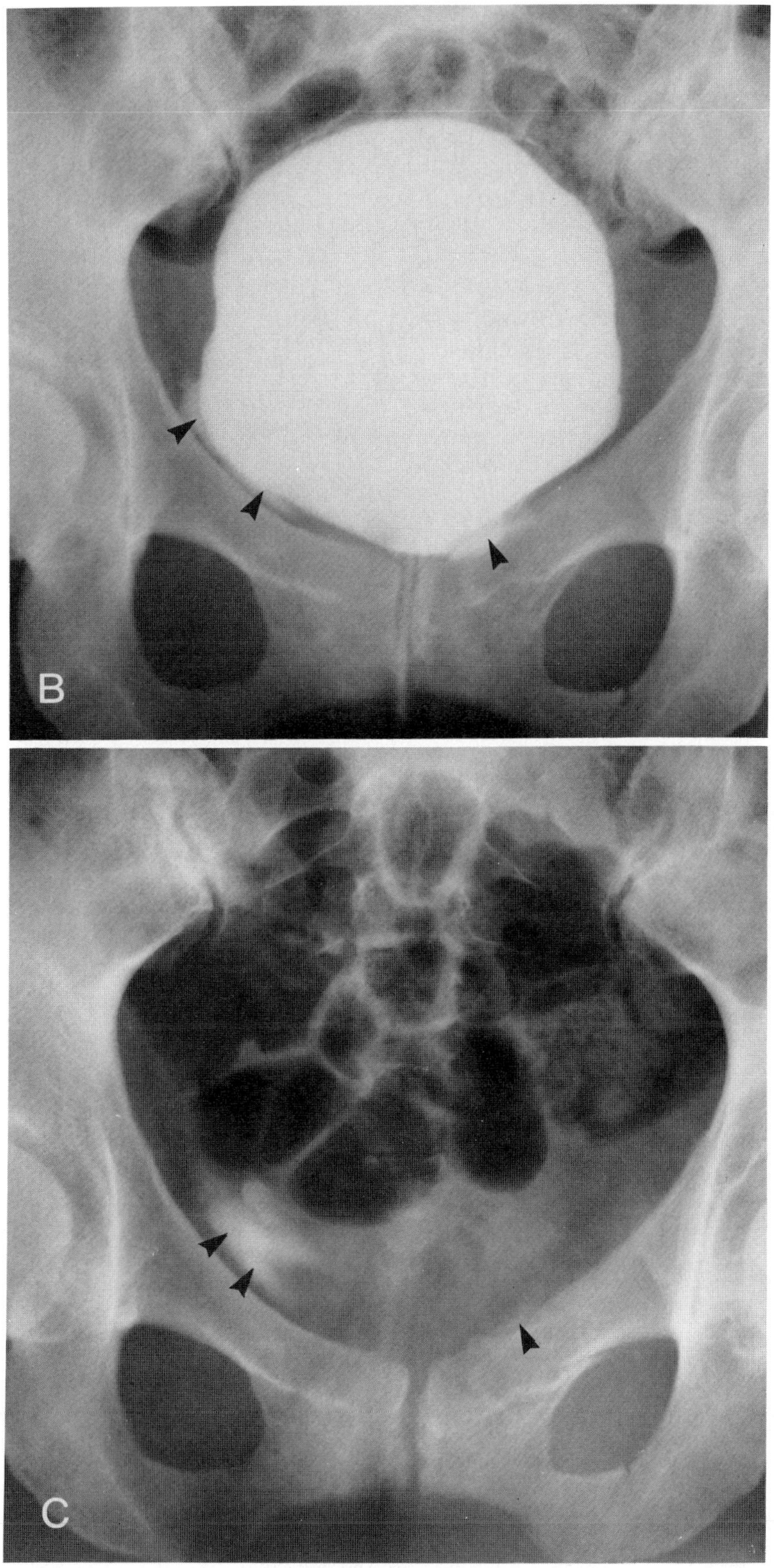

Figure 43.5. B and C

A large volume of contrast along with oblique and postemptying views are necessary for accurate diagnosis (19). A rupture is present when contrast medium is seen outside the bladder, either surrounding loops of bowel (intraperitoneal rupture) or within the pelvis (extraperitoneal rupture) (Fig. 43.5).

Although recent studies suggest that some of these cases can be managed by urethral catheter drainage alone (20, 21), surgical management must still be considered standard for all except the small extraperitoneal perforation. At operation, the laceration is easily closed and the bladder drained with suprapubic cystostomy. Complications are rare.

Urethral Trauma

Two types of urethral injuries are commonly seen. These are different in their etiology, position, repair, and sequelae.

Prostatomembranous Urethra

The prostatomembranous urethral rupture occurs in conjunction with a major pelvic fracture, most often caused by motor vehicle trauma. The patient usually has blood coming from the urethral meatus and is unable to void. The most appropriate initial study is a gentle retrograde urethrogram, which generally delineates a complete rupture and demonstrates elevation of the bladder out of the pelvis by a large hematoma. After initial resuscitation, operative intervention is mandatory. At a minimum, a suprapubic cystostomy should be performed. In infants, a cutaneous vesicostomy is a good alternative. Some surgeons advocate this as the only procedure necessary during the acute phase (22). As the hematoma resolves, the anatomy returns to normal; in some cases, the urethra heals appropriately. In the majority, however, a short stricture remains to be dealt with when the acute inflammation has resolved.

Others have advocated primary realignment of the urethra (23–25). This can be accomplished by antegrade placement of a urethral catheter or operative exposure of the rupture and primary repair. When attempted in children, the catheter can be brought out through a perineal urethrostomy, thereby allowing placement of a larger catheter and eliminating trauma to the distal urethra (26). Regardless of the approach, stricture formation is a frequent complication; others include incontinence and impotence. In general, there appear to be fewer complications when minimal surgery is done at presentation (22). Nonetheless, excellent long-term results have been reported with both techniques (22, 23).

Bulbous Urethra

Injury to the bulbous urethra in the male is generally the result of a straddle type of trauma in which the urethra is crushed against the inferior margin of the pubis. The trauma can be severe enough to cause complete rupture but more commonly results in mild injury heralded by initial hematuria. Undoubtedly, a number of these injuries have minimal symptoms and go unrecognized. They are significant in that the patient can present, years later, with a short, posttraumatic, bulbous urethral stricture. This type of stricture is amenable to excision and end-to-end anastomosis, with excellent results (27).

GENITOURINARY TUMORS

Malignant disease in childhood is uncommon, although in developed countries, it is the second leading cause of death. The tumors most often seen are acute leukemia, lymphomas, and central nervous system neoplasms. Approximately 15% of childhood tumors are abdominal neoplasms, primarily nephroblastoma and neuroblastoma. Other genitourinary neoplasms include rhabdomyosarcoma of the bladder, prostate, vagina, or paratesticular tissues, and testicular neoplasms. All are rare, and only referral centers see more than occasional cases.

Nephroblastoma (Wilms' Tumor)

Nephroblastoma occurs in approximately 1/200,000 children each year. It is a tumor of undifferentiated renal blastema. Primitive tubules are seen, along with variable amounts of connective tissue, cartilage, osteoid, and even muscle. There is some suggestion that the disease results from two gene mutations. This is particularly true for bilateral tumors, where a high incidence of genetic abnormalities is seen, and there is association with a number of congenital anomalies (e.g., aniridia and hemihypertrophy) (28, 29).

Diagnosis

An abdominal mass is the most common presenting sign. Because these are relatively asymptomatic, they can reach huge proportions before being discovered. Abdominal pain occurs rarely; hematuria is noted in about one third of patients at the time of presentation. Fever, anemia and weight loss may be seen but are less common. Hypertension occurs frequently, although its incidence is uncertain because not every child has an accurate blood pressure determination preoperatively.

Classically, the diagnosis has been made by IVP. There is generally no calcification on the scout film; after administration of contrast, an intrarenal mass is seen. The lesion distorts the collecting system and occasionally causes segmental hydronephrosis. Computed tomography, when available, seems far superior (30–32), since the mass is delineated more clearly and its relations are visualized; the liver, great vessels, and opposite kidney are also well seen (Fig. 43.6).

The most common sites of metastases are lymph nodes, liver, and lung. Hence, computed tomography (including the chest) is also valuable for staging. Spread to bone occurs only rarely; hence, marrow biopsy is part of the preoperative evaluation in some centers. A positive result suggests the diagnosis of neuroblastoma rather than nephroblastoma.

Treatment

Treatment has changed considerably in recent decades. Although surgical excision remains the cornerstone of therapy, the combination of radiation and chemotherapy has led to a markedly improved survival rate.

Present therapy is multimodal, with surgical excision of bulk disease the initial step. The tumor is radiosensitive, but in young children there is considerable musculoskeletal, renal, and hepatic toxicity (33), and recent studies have attempted to limit radiotherapy. The National Wilms' Tumor Studies I and II showed that radiotherapy is not necessary when disease is localized to the kidney and is entirely removed surgically (34, 35); however, it remains a useful adjunct in more advanced disease.

Chemotherapy is used in nearly every case. There are four known active agents (actinomycin D, vincristine, doxorubicin, and cyclophosphamide), and combination therapy is more effective than treatment with a single agent. In cases of incompletely resected, widespread, or bilateral disease, second-look surgery (after radiation and chemotherapy) helps to allow complete excision or to evaluate the amount of further therapy needed.

Preoperative therapy is no longer in vogue in the United States. Its benefits have not been conclusively demonstrated; indeed, a number of cases were misdiagnosed and, therefore, inappropriately treated (36). Increased use of computed tomography should lessen this problem, but sometimes it is still possible to misdiagnose a renal or retroperitoneal tumor preoperatively.

Prognosis

Prognosis is related to stage and grade at the time of presentation. Recent studies have distinguished favorable from unfavorable histological findings, which appear to be the major determinant of survival (37). Although unfavorable histological findings (marked cytologic atypia or sarcomatous pattern) occurred in only 12% of patients in the National Wilms' Tumor Study I, these conditions accounted for 52% of deaths. This effect appears to be independent of stage. Nonetheless, the presence of metastasis in lymph nodes or in distant organs does have a negative effect on prognosis (38).

National Wilms' Tumor Study II staging and survival rates are shown in Figure 43.7 and Table 43.1. As survival rates have improved, increasing attention has been given to late effects of therapy, including the incidence

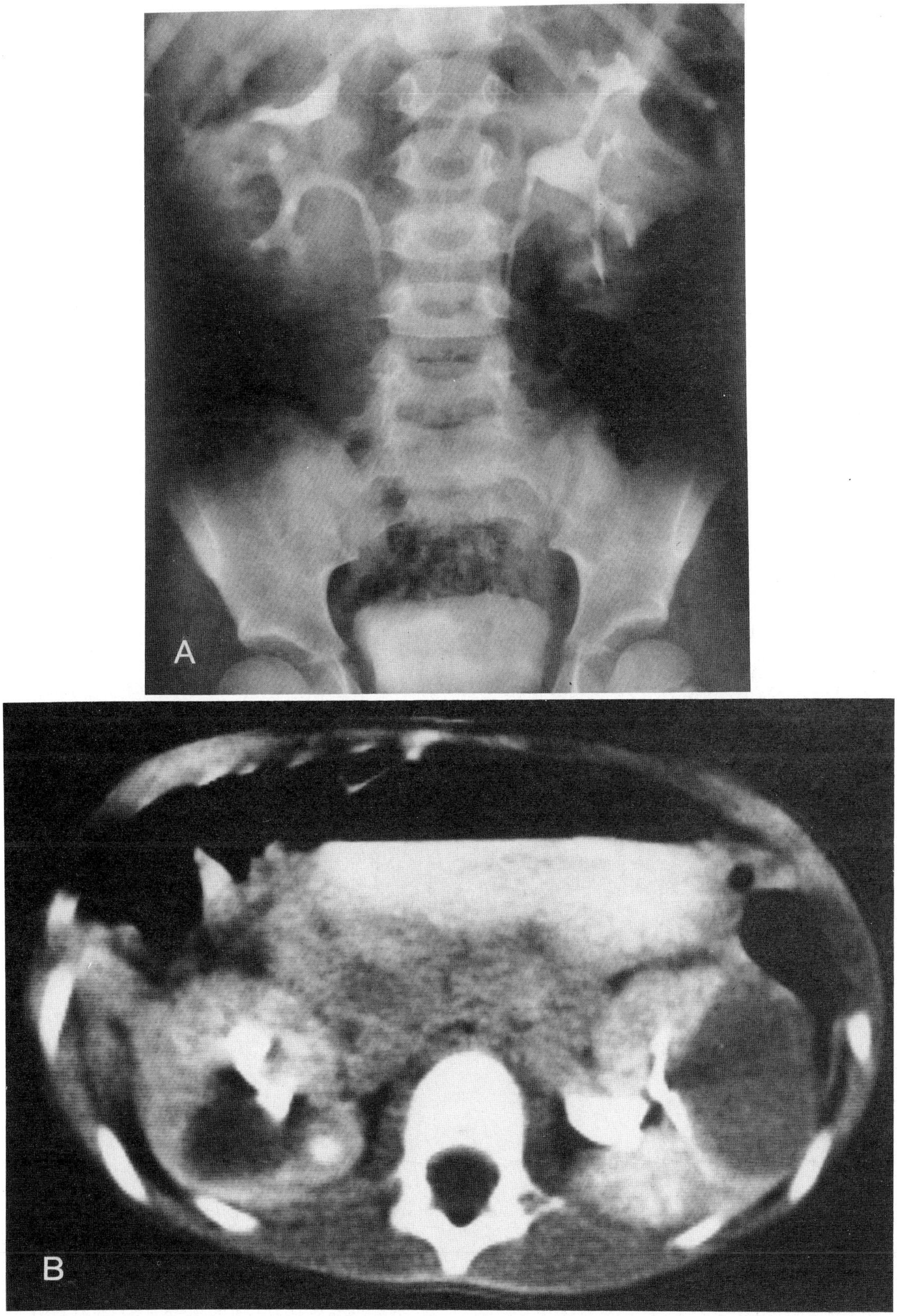

Figure 43.6. **A,** Excretory urography in a 6-year-old girl with bilateral Wilms' tumor. There is stretching of calyces on left and perhaps involvement of right upper pole. **B,** Bilateral involvement is obvious on this contrast computed tomogram taken at level of left renal pelvis. Extent of disease is well delineated, and radiographs at other levels show liver and retroperitoneum to be free of gross disease.

of second neoplasms. As a result, further trials are underway to reduce therapy.

Rhabdomyosarcoma, angiomyolipoma, renal cell carcinoma, leukemia, and lymphoma may all occur in the child's kidney, however, the most important diseases that can be confused with nephroblastoma are the mesoblastic nephroma and the neuroblastoma.

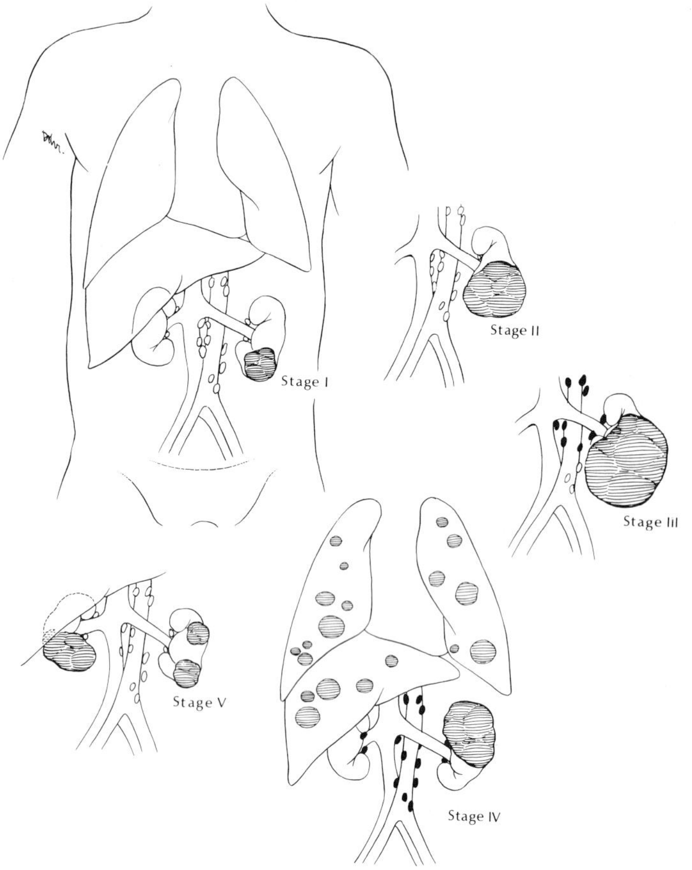

Figure 43.7. Current staging of Wilms' tumor.

Table 43.1.
Summary of Statistical Analysis for National Wilms' Tumor Study II

	Actuarial rates	
	Relapse-free survival 1-2 yr (%)	Survival at 2 yr (%)
Stage I: favorable histology (treatment with actinomycin D for 6 months)	98	100
Stage I: unfavorable histology (initial treatment as for favorable histology)	51	75
Stage II: favorable histology (treatment with actinomycin D, vincristine, doxorubicin, and radiation)	91	91
Stage III: favorable histology (same treatment as stage II)	95	92
Stage II/III: unfavorable histology (same initial treatment)	46	77
Stage IV: favorable and unfavorable histology (same treatment as stages II/III)	53	62

(Courtesy Arthur Ablin, M.D.)

Mesoblastic Nephroma

Mesoblastic nephroma is a congenital neoplasm only seen early in life, at which time it is more common than nephroblastoma. It is a benign-acting lesion and has in the past been misdiagnosed as nephroblastoma, accounting for the excellent prognosis that neonatal Wilms' tumors were thought to have (39). The mesoblastic nephroma can be locally invasive, but metastases are extremely rare. Treatment consists of surgical excision, often a nephrectomy, as these lesions are not well encapsulated. In general, radiotherapy or chemotherapy is contraindicated (40).

Neuroblastoma

Neuroblastoma is a tumor of the sympathochromaffin tissue. It most commonly originates in the adrenal medulla or intra-abdominal sympathetic ganglia; however, the neoplasm can occur anywhere the precursor cells migrate. Computed tomography is the best diagnostic tool (demonstrating an abdominal mass that displaces the kidney), and the diagnosis is often confirmed by finding metabolites of catecholamines in the urine (vanillylmandelic acid or homovanillic acid is excreted in 80% of cases). Bone marrow and liver metastases should always be sought. Surgical excision is the cornerstone of therapy. When gross total excision is possible, survival is approximately 75% (41). Unfortunately, 66% of children present with widespread metastatic disease. Except for one group (stage IV-S), survival in children with metastatic disease is only 5% to 10% despite modern multimodal therapy (42). In stage IV-S (the young child with a small primary tumor and metastasis limited to liver, skin, and/or bone marrow), there is a remarkably high incidence of spontaneous regression, apparently dependent on the child's host defenses. Thus, immunosuppressive therapy is contraindicated. About 80% of this select group will survive. Modern chemotherapeutic regimens have not been shown to significantly benefit children with neuroblastoma, as they have those with nephroblastoma, and many new therapies are being suggested, including the use of monoclonal antibodies or retinoic acid (43). Total body irradiation followed by toxic doses of chemotherapy, with later rescue using bone marrow transplantation, appears to be more promising. Preliminary results have been encouraging (44).

Rhabdomyosarcoma

Tumors of the lower urinary tract are considerably less common than renal tumors in childhood. Although transitional cell neoplasms do occur rarely, the most frequently seen neoplasm is the rhabdomyosarcoma, usually arising in the bladder base, although prostatic and vaginal tumors are seen. Occasionally, the growth may be so extensive that the site of origin cannot be determined.

These children generally present with stranguria and obstructive voiding symptoms, often urinary retention. Urinary infection and renal failure are frequently associated conditions. Unlike adults, children rarely present because of hematuria. A mass may be palpable on rectal examination. IVP or voiding cystourethrography is usually diagnostic, although computed tomography provides much more information. Histological confirmation is obtained by endoscopic or perineal needle biopsy.

Although initial salvage rates were poor (45), the combination of radical cystectomy, chemotherapy (vincristine, actinomycin D, and cyclophosphamide) and high-dose radiation has effected an overall relapse-free survival rate of 70% (46). As this regimen produces considerable morbidity, recent studies have attempted to minimize the side effects, especially those related to exonerative surgery and radiation therapy (47); however, survival rates, while good, have not been optimal. At the present time, initial treatment should be aggressive chemotherapy. Residual disease should be monitored endoscopically. If the response is not complete, a decision must be made for radical surgery or radiotherapy. It should be borne in mind that although radical surgery and permanent urinary diversion are significant deterrents, high-dose pelvic irradiation in young children also has numerous side effects, including not only cystitis and proctitis but poor growth of the bony pelvis as well. Overall, survival rates have improved tremendously, but the quality of life remains less than optimal for such children.

CRYPTORCHIDISM

Although cryptorchidism has been recognized for thousands of years, it remains an enigma. Not only are the etiology, complications, and treatment of the undescended testis debatable, but in many cases the diagnosis is even in dispute.

Incidence

The condition is best diagnosed in the newborn in whom there is no cremasteric reflex. Approximately 3% of newborn males have an undescended testis (48). Because the testes descend during the third trimester, premature infants have a much higher incidence (as high as 21% in those weighing <2500 g). Of these, most testes descend spontaneously during the first months of life, leaving an incidence of 0.8% by 9 months. It is doubtful that these testes will descend without treatment after 9 months of age, as the incidence in adults is almost identical (49).

Unfortunately, many cases of "undescended testis" are not seen until the child is several years old, at which time the active cremasteric reflex makes it difficult to distinguish between the undescended and the retractile testis. Not only does this affect individual patient care, but it casts doubt on the validity of studies on this subject that have not been controlled and double-blinded. Since retractile testes are not thought to be associated with an increased incidence of malignancy or infertility (50), inclusion of even a few of these patients in a cryptorchid series may falsely suggest beneficial effects of therapy.

Etiology

Cryptorchidism is not really a single disease; rather it is a symptom that can be seen in a number of different circumstances. Hence, the etiology may not be the same in each instance. For example, a child with prune belly syndrome may have undescended gonads due to mechanical abnormality, whereas in Kallmann's syndrome the problem may be strictly endocrinological. The majority of cryptorchid patients are grossly normal. It is not known whether there is a subtle endocrinological abnormality, a mechanical or gubernacular problem, or even a primary, inherently abnormal testis, although preliminary data suggest diminished luteinizing hormone and testosterone levels in cryptorchid newborns (51). Epididymal abnormalities, however, are common (52) and suggest a mechanical problem. Further, experimental data suggest that abnormalities of the vas or epididymis can lead to testicular abnormalities (53). Finally, the failure of orchiopexy, as previously performed to prevent the complications of cryptorchidism (i.e., infertility and testicular malignancy), has led many clinicians to conclude that these testes are inherently dysgenetic, which may prevent normal descent. Unfortunately, there are not enough data to draw conclusions about any of these theories.

Complications

The undescended testis does seem more prone to both trauma and torsion and is frequently associated with a patent processus vaginalis, hence an indirect inguinal hernia. However, the most serious potential complications (infertility and testicular neoplasia) take 20 to 30 yr to present, and most studies are of necessity retrospective. What is noteworthy is that the fertility rate is abnormal, not only in 50% of those treated for bilateral cryptorchidism (54), but also in 25% of patients with untreated unilateral undescent (55), suggesting the possibility of an autoimmune basis for the infertility. Unfortunately, there are limited data on this subject. It is known that testicular biopsies performed on children at the time of orchiopexy show a progressive decrease in the number of spermatogonia starting at age 2 (56). Therefore, it is not surprising that orchiopexy performed at puberty and even at age 5 or 6 yr may be ineffective in preserving fertility. Whether earlier orchiopexy can improve these results remains to be seen. These testes may be inherently abnormal and thus not amenable to treatment.

Retrospective studies of patients with testicular neoplasms show that from 6% to 14% of the tumors occur in an undescended gonad (57). Since only 4/1000 testes are undescended, this is a startlingly high rate. A number of these neoplasms develop in testes that have previously been operated on (58), suggesting that orchiopexy has no influence on the development of neoplasia. Unfortunately, in most of these studies the patients were operated on in a different era, with most not undergoing orchiopexy until after 6 yr of age (59). The effects of earlier treatment are as yet unknown. It may be that these gonads are inherently abnormal, a theory also supported by the higher than normal incidence of testicular neoplasms in the scrotal testis of patients with unilateral undescent (60).

Treatment

Therapy consists of hormonal manipulation or surgical repair. Shortly after it was discovered that urine from pregnant monkeys could cause testicular descent in other monkeys (61), human chorionic gonadotropin (HCG) was used to stimulate testicular descent. The dosage depends on the size of the child. In a 15-kg boy, a regimen of 500 IU (intramuscularly) twice a week for five weeks has been suggested (62). Initial reports were very enthusiastic (>50% success) (63), but inclusion of retractile testes could easily skew the results. A very careful study has shown descent in 38% of bilateral and 16% of unilateral cases (64).

Unfortunately, to this day there have been no controlled double-blind studies with HCG. In light of its questionable efficacy, especially in young children, and the fact that HCG must be given in repeated intramuscular injections, it is rapidly losing popularity. An alternative available in Europe but not in the United States is luteinizing hormone-releasing hormone (LHRH). This can be given as an intranasal spray, with minimal toxicity, and was shown in two double-blind controlled studies to be superior to placebo (65, 66). Even so, only a third of cases responded; the remainder required operative intervention.

Numerous techniques of testicular fixation have been proposed, but the one caveat for all methods is adequate mobilization of the cord structures to achieve placement of the testis in the scrotum without undue tension. If this is achieved, the method of fixation is probably not important; if there is tension on the spermatic cord, no degree of fixation will be effective. In instances where adequate length cannot be achieved, mobilization may be easier at a second-stage procedure six months later (67). An alternative is the Fowler-Stephens method, in which the artery and vein are divided and testicular viability is maintained by collaterals from vasal vessels (68). Some difficult cases are being treated by dividing the testicular vessels and performing a microsurgical anastomosis between the testicular and inferior epigastric vessels (69).

As it has become clear that late orchiopexy is ineffective in preventing infertility and neoplasia, the recommended age of treatment has dropped. At the present time, most pediatric urologists in the United States suggest intervention before 18 months. Nevertheless, it is essential to recognize that even this may be ineffective if the testes are inherently abnormal.

HYPOSPADIAS

Appearance

It is critical that the diagnosis of hypospadias be made at birth, as children with this condition should not be circumcised, so that the prepuce remains for future surgical reconstruction. Hypospadias is recognized by the pediatrician as an abnormal-appearing phallus with a meatus opening on the ventral aspect, proximal to its usual position on

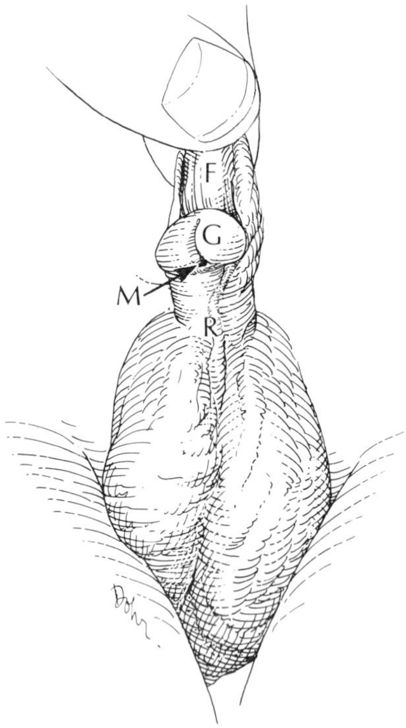

Figure 43.8. Diagrammatic sketch of child with coronal hypospadias. There is redundant "hooded" foreskin (F) on the dorsum. Ventral foreskin has not developed. Glans (G) is somewhat splayed and flattened, as opposed to being conical. The median raphe (R) is displaced laterally, leading to penile torsion. The meatus (M) is at the level of the corona. The chordee commonly seen in children with proximal hypospadias is not illustrated.

the glans (Fig. 43.8). The foreskin is present only on the dorsal aspect and its "hooded" nature accounts for the abnormal appearance. A contributing factor is that the glans is usually splayed open ventrally. Although less important cosmetically, virtually all the children with a meatus proximal to the glans have an associated ventral chordee. This curvature may be apparent only during erection, but is of major consequence with regard to sexual function and hence requires surgical repair.

Etiology

Penile morphogenesis is completed late in the first trimester and depends on androgenic stimulation (70). The exact etiology of hypospadias is unknown, but it probably results from interference with normal endocrinological stimulation (71): exogenous progesterone given to the mother; diminished testosterone secretion by the fetal testes; mild deficiencies in the conversion of testosterone to dihydrotestosterone; or a lack of androgenic receptors in the phallic tissues. Regardless of the precise cause, hypospadias should be considered a mild form of intersex. When there is any other indication of intersexuality, e.g., undescended testes, a complete endocrinological evaluation is indicated. In uncomplicated cases, no workup seems necessary.

Upper Urinary Tract Evaluation

The need for routine excretory urography in these patients has been debated for many years. If the defect is primarily endocrinological, there is no reason to suspect a high incidence of renal lesions. Nonetheless, the data are conflicting. One study has demonstrated no statistical difference in the incidence of urinary tract anomalies between patients with hypospadias and the general population (72); another group has reported a 5% incidence of significant lesions (73). These anomalies seem to occur primarily in patients with very proximal hypospadias and in those with other anomalies (74). Perhaps the high-risk cases can be screened with ultrasound.

Treatment

From a therapeutic standpoint, hypospadias can be classified, based on the position of the meatus, as distal (glandular or coronal) or proximal (penile, penoscrotal, or perineal). The distal form predominates and often causes minimal disability. There may be little or no chordee. The only significant functional abnormality is a downward spraying of the urinary stream caused by a small skin flap just distal to the meatus. When the major disability is cosmetic, it is difficult to justify any surgical procedure that carries with it a significant risk of complication (75). Hence, some recommend only a dorsal or "anterior" meatotomy and excision of the hooded dorsal prepuce (76). Recently, MAGPI (meatal advancement and glanduloplasty) has been proposed (77). This technique has minimal complications, can be performed with little or no hospital stay, and gives an excellent cosmetic result. A number of surgeons have documented its effectiveness (78, 79), and it is becoming increasingly popular.

A vast number of different repairs have been recommended for more proximal hypospadias. This, in part, represents the diversity of the disorder but, more importantly, reflects the fact that no repair is ideal. In any case, the chordee must be corrected first, followed by the urethroplasty. The urethra is reconstructed using local skin, free grafts, or, more recently, vascularized pedicles. There has been a trend from two- and three-stage to one-stage repairs, particularly those in which the neourethra is based on a vascularized pedicle (77, 80). Complications, particularly stenosis and fistulae, occur regardless of the technique and a further procedure is necessary in 10% to 30% of cases.

There is general agreement that repair should be completed before school age. Two years of age was formerly the most common time for the initial procedure; however, optical magnification has allowed the surgery to begin as early as 6 months of age without compromising the repair (81–83). There may be psychological reasons for performing the repair before 1 yr (84, 85), but long-term follow-up data addressing this are limited.

EXSTROPHIC ANOMALIES

Exstrophic abnormalities occur in approximately 1/10,000 births. There are many related anomalies varying considerably in severity, but bladder exstrophy and epispadias are the most common. All the anomalies result from a premature breakdown of the infraumbilical membrane. If this occurs before the formation of the urorectal septum, cloacal exstrophy results, with both bladder and bowel exposed; if it occurs later and only the caudal portion of the membrane is involved, epispadias alone is seen. In bladder exstrophy, the timing of the defect is intermediate.

Cloacal Exstrophy

Clocacal exstrophy occurs rarely but when present it poses difficult ethical problems. The defect itself is severe, and other anomalies often coexist. Exomphalos is nearly always present, and the intestine is congenitally short, with an imperforate anus. Urinary tract abnormalities are present in half the cases (multicystic kidney, renal dysplasia, or even bilateral renal agenesis), and various degrees of spina bifida are frequent as well. The external genitalia are always malformed, with duplication being common; in males, the phallus is not only duplicated but generally rudimentary.

Fluid and electrolyte imbalance results from the renal and alimentary tract abnormalities and is likely to be fatal without urgent therapy. Even

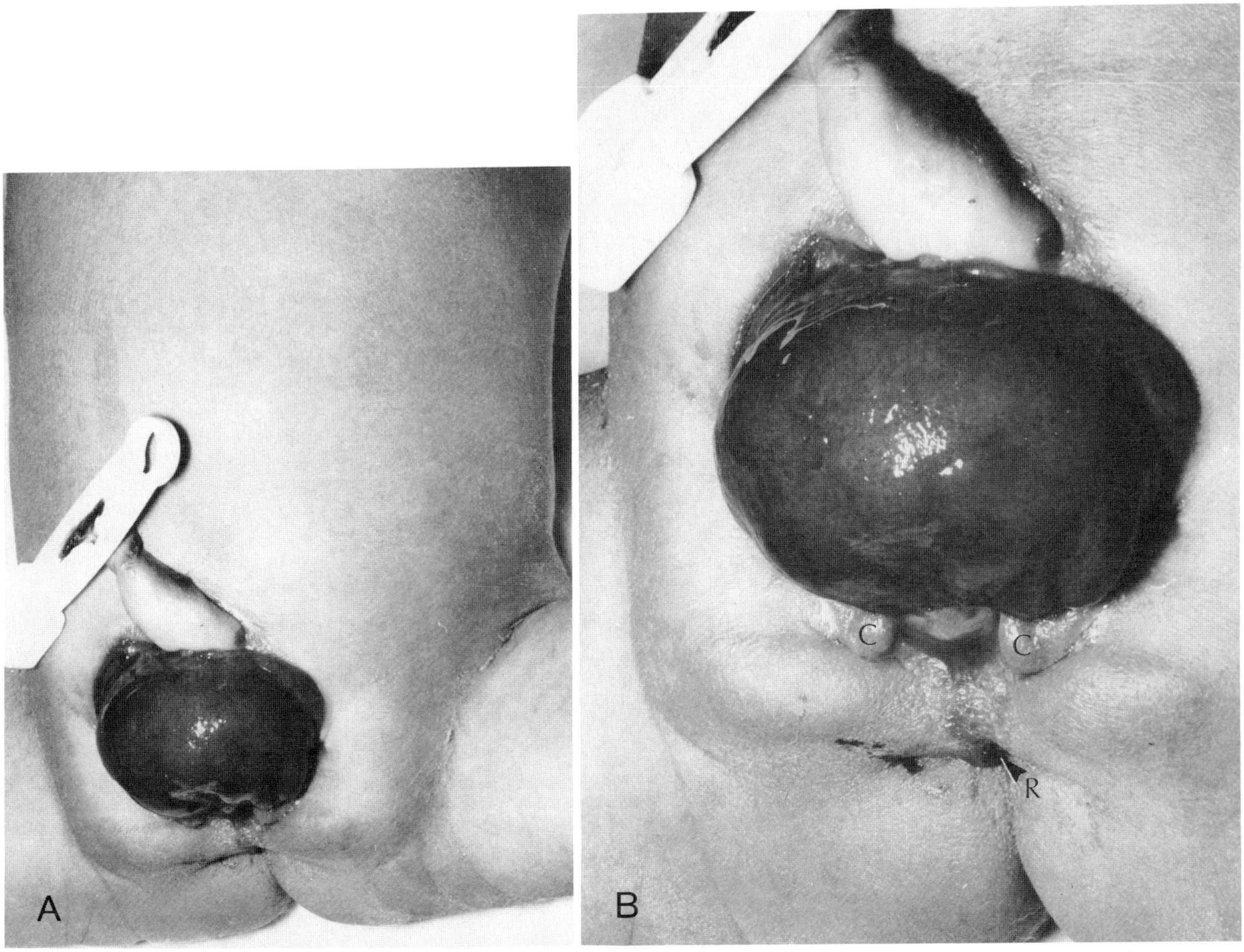

Figure 43.9. **A,** Newborn girl with bladder exstrophy. **B,** Closeup photo showing prolapsed bladder, bifid clitoris (C), and the anterior rectum (R). Although not seen, this infant had two vaginal orifices.

with optimal treatment, the child will likely have both fecal and urinary stomas. Genital reconstruction will be necessary, and many males may need to be sex-reversed. Further, the problems of spina bifida require considerable attention. Aside from the surgical aspects, the quality of life for the patient and the emotional and financial stress on the family must be considered. Although acceptable results can be obtained (86), not every case is amenable to an aggressive approach. The moral questions regarding care of these children are wide-ranging and require hard choices soon after birth.

Bladder Exstrophy

Bladder exstrophy is always associated with epispadias and a widened pubic symphysis, but only rarely are other congenital anomalies present (Fig. 43.9). Hence, attention is directed to appropriate surgical management of the bladder and external genitalia.

Treatment

Early attempts at reconstruction were invariably unsuccessful (87), with urinary diversion the treatment of choice in the first half of this century. The most common procedure was the ureterosigmoidostomy. Although a continent internal diversion was usually achieved, long-term follow-up revealed a high incidence of upper urinary tract deterioration (88). Other methods of treatment were therefore developed, including improved techniques for ureterosigmoidostomy, external diversion with bowel conduits, and surgical reconstruction. At the present time, it is appropriate to explore all options with the parents, but attempts at reconstruction seem the most reasonable course, provided the bladder is pliable and of adequate size (89). This is a staged procedure, the initial step being closure of the bladder and repair of the lower abdominal fascial defect with musculofascial and skin flaps (90, 91) or, with the aid of simultaneous iliac osteotomies, by bringing the bladder, fascia, and skin together in the midline (91, 92). If the repair is done within the first 72 hr of life, the effects of maternal relaxin may be enough to allow a midline closure without osteotomies (93). Regardless of the technique, no attempt is made to make the child continent, the goal of initial surgery being to convert the patient to complete epispadias. At 3 to 4 yr of age, a bladder neck reconstruction is performed, based on a posterior or an anterior bladder flap (94, 95). Since reflux is nearly always present, bilateral ureteral reimplantation is performed at the same time. In males, reconstruction of the epispadiac penis is performed as a later procedure (96).

Results

Results vary considerably from one report to another (91–93, 97–99), reflecting both the selection of patients for closure and the varying definitions of continence. One consideration is that a number of patients who are only partially continent during childhood develop much better control at puberty, perhaps due to prostatic growth (100). The effects of newer methods of therapy for incontinence, including pharmacotherapy and the artificial sphincter, have yet to be fully explored. On average, results are disappointing, with only 10% to 30% of patients obtaining an acceptable result (defined as normal urinary control and no upper tract deterioration). Several groups, however, have recently reported significantly better results (70% to 80% success) (98, 99). The exact reasons for their improved results are unclear, but their data have further encouraged attempts at reconstruction.

Follow-up

The bladder epithelium is invariably abnormal in these cases and is prone to neoplasia, most commonly adenocarcinoma (101). It is thought that the neoplasms are caused by chronic inflammatory changes; however, at least one tumor has been reported in a patient after successful neonatal bladder closure (102). They generally do not develop until adult life and, albeit malignant, are slow-growing. Although the risk is not so great as to obviate reconstruction, life-long follow-up, with urine cytology and cystoscopy, is advisable. If the patient requires permanent diversion, cystectomy is recommended.

Epispadias

Epispadias, without exstrophy, occurs most commonly in boys (Fig. 43.10). It varies in degree, depending on the location of the urethral meatus. The penis is short, often with an associated dorsal chordee. The glans is splayed open dorsally, with the prepuce on the ventral aspect only. In severe forms, the bladder neck and posterior urethra are affected and the patient has severe, virtually total, stress incontinence—the major disability.

Incontinence

Urodynamic evaluation of these patients reveals minimal resistance in the posterior urethra (103). Further, there is almost no change with electrical stimulation of the pelvic floor, implying that the abnormality affects the anatomy of the pelvic floor as well as the smooth muscle. The bladder is often small and thin-walled as well; perhaps because the incontinence is so severe, it has never been used for voiding.

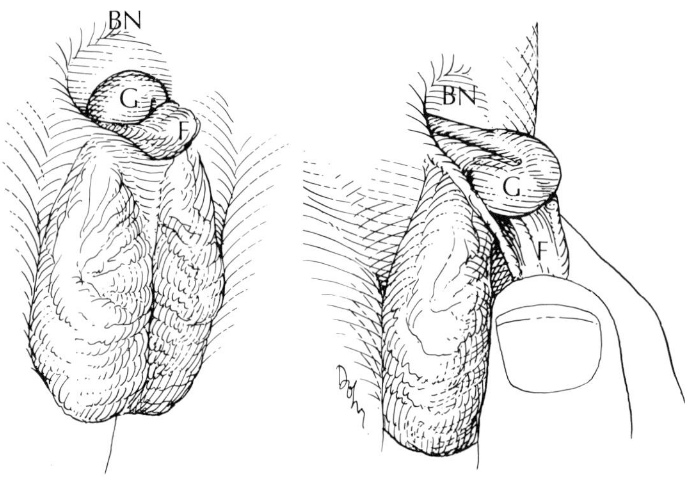

Figure 43.10. Diagram of boy with epispadias. The bladder neck (BN) is wide open and the boy is totally incontinent. Penis is short and upturned, with only the glans (G) visible. The foreskin (F) is only developed on the ventrum.

Reconstruction of the bladder neck is most often accomplished by creating a long tube of healthy smooth muscle which, based on its intrinsic tone and elastic properties, will provide adequate urethral resistance to maintain continence. This can be achieved with an anterior or a posterior bladder flap (94–95). As in the patient with a reconstructed bladder exstrophy, a marked improvement in continence is frequently achieved at the time of puberty (100). Similarly, pharmacological therapy or the artificial sphincter may be useful in treating these patients.

Penile Deformity

After bladder neck reconstruction, attention is turned to the penile deformity. The phallus may need to be lengthened; partially detaching the crus of the corpora cavernosa from the pubic symphysis that is widely separated will allow the phallus to project further and will release the chordee (104). As in hypospadias, many approaches for urethral reconstruction have been proposed (100). In general, they involve local skin flaps or free grafts. They are fraught with the same problems as those for hypospadias, i.e., fistulae and strictures, but an acceptable result can ultimately be achieved in nearly every case. The splayed open glans should be closed at the same time. Even when urinary diversion is necessary for incontinence or upper tract deterioration, the genitalia in most patients with exstrophy or epispadias can be corrected to enable reasonably normal appearance and function (105, 106).

CIRCUMCISION

Neonatal circumcision is one of the most controversial subjects in medicine. Although there are some objective data upon which to base decisions, there are many social and religious considerations as well. For the parents, the decision is often emotional; despite attempts at parental education, it is frequently based on considerations that are medically insignificant. Even among medical professionals, the issue is argued passionately, recent writings being entitled "The Rape of the Phallus" (107) and "Whither the Foreskin?" (108).

Social Considerations

Various societies have placed different values on circumcision. In the United States, 80% to 90% of newborn males are circumcised. In other countries, the rates are lower, with circumcision being distinctly uncommon in Northern Europe, Central and South America, and Asia (109). Clearly, one society's idea of a "normal" phallic appearance differs from another's, and it is likely that this is the major determinant in the decision to circumcise.

Medical Considerations

There is no question that carcinoma of the penis can be almost totally prevented by routine neonatal circumcision, with only nine cases reported in adults circumcised at birth (110). In studies of African tribes in Kenya and Uganda, the rate of penile cancer is significantly higher in those tribes where circumcision is not practiced routinely (111). It can be argued, however, that penile cancer is so rare (cumulative lifetime risk $166/10^5$) (112) that routine neonatal circumcision is unjustified. Further, it has been suggested that good penile hygiene is also protective and that patient education is a more appropriate use of medical resources (113). Undoubtedly, environment also plays a significant role: one might expect a higher rate of penile cancer in Africa, where warmer temperatures and relatively poor hygiene are likely to lead to chronic penile inflammation.

The low rate of carcinoma of the cervix in Jewish women in Israel led to suggestions that circumcision protected against this disease (114). However, there are many genetic and social considerations. A careful study of husbands of women with cervical cancer revealed no significant difference in their circumcision status compared with controls (115).

Similarly, it is doubtful that circumcision in any way prevents prostatic carcinoma or venereal disease.

It has been argued that circumcision eliminates phimosis and posthitis (inflammation of the foreskin) and reduces the incidence of balanitis (inflammation of the glans), thereby obviating the need for later childhood circumcision with the attendant risks of general anesthesia and psychological trauma related to genital surgery. The rate of nonneonatal circumcision is not well established, but is most likely between 2% and 10% (109). On the other hand, true meatal stenosis, although rare, occurs exclusively in circumcised males. The foreskin undoubtedly plays a role in preventing meatal irritation.

Aesthetic appearance and sexual function in circumcised men have been the subject of numerous debates, but there is little objective information. Nonetheless, it is not infrequent for the clinician in the United States to be presented with the uncircumcised child or adolescent who objects to being different and ultimately insists on a circumcision. Conversely, a patient who requests reconstruction of the foreskin is exceedingly rare.

Other than the expense of routine neonatal circumcision, the major objection is the morbidity and mortality associated with the procedure. Although a number of horrendous complications have been reported (116), a recent series of over 5000 consecutive circumcisions performed during a 20-yr period at a teaching hospital revealed only 14 significant complications (117). There was no bleeding significant enough to require transfusion and there were no deaths. Eight of the complications, the inadvertent circumcision of children with hypospadias, could probably have been prevented had a more experienced person performed the procedure. Severe complications, such as loss of the glans or even death, should be rare in experienced hands. A number of delayed complications are seen; most are minor, but some require operative revision. The exact percentage is impossible to determine.

Overall, there remains considerable dispute over the most appropriate approach. The American Academy of Pediatrics has recently concluded: "There is no absolute medical indication for routine circumcision of the newborn" (113). Nonetheless, attempts to present this information to American parents, even before delivery, have had no discernible effect on the rate of circumcision (118, 119).

Recommendations

Should parents elect to proceed with neonatal circumcision, a penile nerve block is easy to perform and has been shown to reduce stress significantly in these infants (120, 121). Should the parents elect not to have their child circumcised, clear instruction regarding proper hygiene should be given. This has not been done in the past, probably because the best course remains controversial (122). In general, good external penile hygiene should be recommended until the foreskin is easily retractable; thereafter, cleansing beneath the foreskin would seem appropriate. It should be emphasized that phimosis is normal in newborns and there appears to be no need for forcible release of the adhesions between the prepuce and glans; most of these adhesions will resolve spontaneously in the first years of life (123).

The choice of whether to circumcise a child is based primarily on social considerations. Perhaps this is appropriate, since objective data are so conflicting. The physician's role remains advisory, but caution should be exercised since parents generally have strong feelings and often regret being forced into the decision one way or the other.

References

1. Emanuel B, Aronson N: Neonatal hematuria. Am J Dis Child 128:204, 1974.
2. Fairley KF, Birch DF: Hematuria: A simple method for identifying glomerular bleeding. Kidney Int 21:105, 1982.
3. Rizzoni G, Braggion F, Zacchello G: Evaluation of glomerular and nonglomerular hematuria by phase-contrast microscopy. J Pediatr 103:370, 1983.
4. Northway JD: Hematuria in children. J Pediatr 78:381, 1971.
5. Dodge WF, West EF, Smith EH, Bunce H III: Proteinuria and hematuria in schoolchildren: epidemiology and early natural history. J Pediatr 88:327, 1976.
6. Wyatt RJ, McRoberts JW, Holland NH: Hematuria in childhood: significance and management. J Urol 117:366, 1977.
7. Walther PC, Kaplan GW: Cystoscopy in children: indications for its use in common urologic problems. J Urol 122:717, 1979.
8. Persky L, Forsythe WE: Renal trauma in childhood. JAMA 182:709, 1962.
9. Cass AS: Blunt renal trauma in children. J Trauma 23:123, 1983.
10. McAninch JW, Federle MP: Evaluation of renal injuries with computerized tomography. J Urol 128:456, 1982.
11. Ahmed S, Morris LL: Renal parenchymal injuries secondary to blunt abdominal trauma in childhood: a 10-year review. Br J Urol 54:470, 1982.
12. Mandour WA; Lai MK, Linke CA, Frank IN: Blunt renal trauma in the pediatric patient. J Pediatr Surg 16:669, 1981.
13. Kuzmarov IW, Morehouse DD, Gibson S: Blunt renal trauma in the pediatric population: a retrospective study. J Urol 126:648, 1981.
14. Carlton CE Jr: Editorial comment to Kuzmarov et al. (ref. 13). J Urol. 126:649, 1981.
15. Scott R Jr: Transperitoneal approach to renal pedicle. Urology 4:223, 1974.
16. McAninch JW, Carroll PR: Renal trauma: kidney preservation through improved vascular control—a refined approach. J Trauma 22:285, 1982.
17. Sobel IP: So-called essential hypertension in childhood. Am J Dis Child 61:280, 1941.
18. Page IH: The production of persistent arterial hypertension by cellophane perinephritis. JAMA 113:2046, 1939.
19. Carroll PR, McAninch JW: Major bladder trauma: the accuracy of cystography. J Urol 130:887, 1983.
20. Mulkey AP Jr, Witherington R: Conservative management of vesical rupture. Urology 4:426, 1974.
21. Hayes EE, Sandler CM, Corriere JN Jr: Management of the ruptured bladder secondary to blunt abdominal trauma. J Urol 129:946, 1983.
22. Morehouse DD, MacKinnon KJ: Management of prostatomembranous urethral disruption: 13-year experience. J Urol 123:173, 1980.
23. Malek RS, O'Dea MJ, Kelalis PP: Management of ruptured posterior urethra in childhood. J Urol 117:105, 1977.
24. Glass RE, Flynn JT, King JB, Blandy JP: Urethral injury and fractured pelvis. Br J Urol 50:578, 1978.
25. Pierce JM Jr: Management of dismemberment of the prostatic membranous urethra and ensuing stricture disease. J Urol 107:259, 1972.
26. Johnston JH: Urinary tract injuries. In Williams DI, Johnston JH, (eds): Paediatric Urology. London, Butterworths, 1982, p 376.
27. Turner-Warwick R: Observations on the treatment of traumatic urethral injuries and the value of the fenestrated urethral catheter. Br J Surg 60:775, 1973.
28. Bond JV: Bilateral Wilms' tumour: age at diagnosis, associated congenital anomalies, and possible pattern of inheritance. Lancet 2:482, 1975.
29. Strong LC, Riccardi VM: Genetics of Wilms tumor. In Ehrlich RM (ed): Dialogues in Pediatric Urology. Pearl River, NY, William J. Miller Associates, 1983, p 6.
30. Stephenson TF, Iyengar S, Rashid HA: Comparison of computerized tomography and excretory urography in detection and evaluation of renal masses. J Urol 131:11, 1984.
31. Cohen MD, Siddiqui A, Weetman R, et al: A rational approach to the radiologic evaluation of children with Wilms' tumor. Cancer 50:887, 1982.
32. Cohen MD, Weber T, Smith JA, Reider JI: The role of computerized tomography in the diagnosis and management of patients with bilateral Wilms' tumor. J Urol 130:1160, 1983.
33. Thomas PRM, Griffith KD, Fineberg BB, et al: Late effects of treatment for Wilms' tumor. Am J Radiat Oncol Biol Phys 9:651, 1983.
34. D'Angio GJ, Evans AE, Breslow N, et al: The treatment of Wilms' tumor. Results of the National Wilms' Tumor Study. Cancer 38:633, 1976.
35. D'Angio GJ, Evans A, Breslow N, et al: The treatment of Wilms' tumor. Results of the Second National Wilms' Tumor Study. Cancer 47:2302, 1981.
36. Ehrlich RM, Bloomberg SD, Gyepes MT, et al: Wilms tumor, misdiagnosed preoperatively: a review of 19 National Wilms Tumor Study I cases. J Urol 122:790, 1979.
37. Beckwith JB, Palmer NF: Histopathology and prognosis of Wilms' tumor. Results from the first National Wilms' Tumor Study. Cancer 41:1937, 1978.
38. Breslow NE, Palmer NF, Hill LR, et al: Wilms' tumor: prognostic factors for patients without metastases at diagnosis. Cancer 41:1577, 1978.
39. Bolande RP, Brough AJ, Izant RJ Jr: Congenital mesoblastic nephroma in infancy. A report of either cases and the relationship to Wilms' tumor. Pediatrics 40:272, 1967.

40. Howell CG, Othersen HB, Kiviat NE, et al: Therapy and outcome in 51 children with mesoblastic nephroma: a report of the National Wilms' Tumor Study. J Pediatr Surg 17:826, 1982.
41. Evans AE, D'Angio GJ, Koop CE: The role of multimodal therapy in patients with local and regional neuroblastoma. J Pediatr Surg 19:77, 1984.
42. Evans AE: Staging and treatment of neuroblastoma. Cancer 45:1799, 1980.
43. Seeger RC, Siegel SE, Sidell N: Neuroblastoma: clinical perspectives, monoclonal antibodies, and retinoic acid. Ann Intern Med 97:873, 1982.
44. Pritchard J, McElwain TJ, Graham-Pole J: High-dose melphalan with autologous marrow for treatment of advanced neuroblastoma. Cancer 45: 86, 1982.
45. MacKenzie AR, Whitmore WF Jr, Melamed MR: Myosarcomas of the bladder and prostate. Cancer 22:833, 1968.
46. Hays DM, Raney RB Jr, Lawrence W Jr, et al: Bladder and prostatic tumors in the intergroup rhabdomyosarcoma study (IRS-I). Results of therapy. Cancer 50:1472, 1982.
47. Hays DM, Raney RB Jr, Lawrence W Jr, et al: Primary chemotherapy in the treatment of children with bladder-prostate tumors in the intergroup rhabdomyosarcoma study (IRS-II). J Pediatr Surg 17:812, 1982.
48. Scorer CG: The descent of the testis. Arch Dis Child 39:605, 1964.
49. Baumrucker GO: Incidence of testicular pathology. Bull U.S. Army Med Dept. 5:312, 1946.
50. Puri P, Nixon HH: Bilateral retractile testes—subsequent effects on fertility. J Pediatr Surg 12:563, 1977.
51. Gendrel D, Roger M, Job J-C: Plasma gonadotropin and testosterone values in infants with cryptorchidism J Pediatr 97:217, 1980.
52. Heath AL, Man DWK, Eckstein HB: Epididymal abnormalities associated with maldescent of the testis. J Pediatr Surg 19:47, 1984.
53. Marshall FF, Ewing LL, Zirkin BR, Cochran RC: Testicular atrophy associated with agenesis of the epididymis in the ACI rat. J Urol 127:155, 1982.
54. Bramble FJ, Houghton AL, Eccles S, et al: Reproductive and endocrine function after surgical treatment of bilateral cryptorchidism. Lancet 2:311, 1974.
55. Lipshultz LI, Caminos-Torres R, Greenspan CS, Snyder PJ: Testicular function after orchipexy for unilateral undescended testis. N Engl J Med 295:15, 1976.
56. Mengel W, Hienz HA, Sippe WG II, Hecker W Ch: Studies on cryptorchidism: a comparison of histological findings in the germinative epithelium before and after the second year of life. J Pediatr Surg 9:445, 1974.
57. Campbell HE: The incidence of malignant growth of the undescended testicle: a reply and re-evaluation. J Urol 81:663, 1959.
58. Batata MA, Whitmore WF Jr, Chu FCH, et al: Cryptorchidism and testicular cancer. J Urol 124:382, 1980.
59. Martin DC: Germinal cell tumors of the testis after orchiopexy. J Urol 121:422, 1979.
60. Kuber W: Testicular tumor and cryptorchidism. Eur Urol 8:280, 1982.
61. Engle ET: Experimentally induced descent of the testis in the Macacus monkey by hormones from the anterior pituitary and pregnancy urine. Endocrinology 16:513, 1932.
62. Bierich JR: Gonadotropin therapy for the undescended testis. In Kogan SJ, Hafez ESE (eds): Pediatric Andrology. The Hague, Martinus Nijhoff Publishers, 1981, p 163.
63. Brunet J, Mowbray RR de, Bishop PMF: Management of the undescended testes. Br Med J 1:1367, 1958.
64. Ehrlich RM, Dougherty LJ, Tomashefsky P, Lattimer JK: Effect of gonadotropin in cryptorchidism. J Urol 102:793, 1969.
65. Illig R, Exner GU, Kollmann F, et al: Treatment of cryptorchidism by intranasal synthetic luteinising-hormone releasing hormone. Lancet 2:518, 1977.
66. Westphal O: Current treatment of cryptorchidism. In Ehrlich RM, (ed): Dialogues in Pediatric Urology. Pearl River, NY: William J. Miller Associates, 1983, p 4.
67. Firor HV: Two-stage orchiopexy. Arch Surg 102:598, 1971.
68. Fowler R Jr, Stephens FD: The role of testicular vascular anatomy in the salvage of high undescended testes. Aust NZ J Surg 29:92, 1959.
69. Silber SJ, Kelly J: Successful autotransplantation of an intra-abdominal testis to the scrotum by microvascular technique. J Urol 115:452, 1976.
70. Bellinger MF: Embryology of the male external genitalia. Urol Clin North Am 8:375, 1981.
71. Allen TD, Griffin JE: Endocrine studies in patients with advanced hypospadias. J Urol 131:310, 1984.
72. McArdle R, Lebowitz R: Uncomplicated hypospadias and anomalies of upper urinary tract. Need for screening? Urology 5:712, 1975.
73. Fallon B, Devine CJ Jr, Horton CE: Congenital anomalies associated with hypospadias. J Urol 116:585, 1976.
74. Khuri FJ, Hardy BE, Churchill BM: Urologic anomalies associated with hypospadias. Urol Clin North Am 8:565, 1981.
75. Mills C, McGovern J, Mininberg D, et al: An analysis of different techniques for distal hypospadias repair: the price of perfection. J Urol 125:701, 1981.
76. Johnston JH: Abnormalities of the penis. In Williams DI, Johnston JH (eds): Paediatric Urology. London, Butterworths, 1982.
77. Duckett JW: Hypospadias. Clin Plast Surg 7:149, 1980.
78. Livne PM, Gibbons MD, Gonzales ET Jr: Meatal advancement and glanuloplasty: an operation for distal hypospadias. J Urol 131:95, 1984.
79. Shapiro SR: Complications of hypospadias repair. J Urol 131: 518, 1984.
80. Hodgson NB: A one-stage hypospadias repair. J Urol 104:281, 1970.
81. Manley CB, Epstein ES: Early hypospadias repair. J Urol 125:698, 1981.
82. Belman AB, Kass EJ: Hypospadias repair in children less than 1 year old. J Urol 128:1273, 1982.
83. Wacksman J: Results of early hypospadias surgery using optical magnification. J Urol 131:516, 1984.
84. Lepore AG, Kesler RW: Behavior of children undergoing hypospadias repair. J Urol 122:68, 1979.
85. Schultz JR, Klykylo WM, Wacksman J: Timing of elective hypospadias repair in children. Pediatrics 71:342, 1983.
86. Howell C, Caldamone A, Snyder H, et al: Optimal management of cloacal exstrophy. J Pediatr Surg 18:365, 1983.
87. Trendelenburg F: The treatment of ectopia vesicae. Ann Surg 44:281, 1906.
88. Harvard BM, Thompson GJ: Congenital exstrophy of the urinary bladder: late results of treatment by the Coffey-Mayo method of uretero-intestinal anastomosis. J Urol 65:223, 1951.
89. Lattimer JK, Beck L, Yeaw S, et al: Long-term followup after exstrophy closure: late improvement and good quality of life. J Urol 119:664, 1978.
90. Marshall VF, Muecke EC: Functional closure of typical exstrophy of the bladder. J Urol 104:205, 1970.
91. Williams DI, Keeton JE: Further progress with reconstruction of the exstrophied bladder. Br J Surg 60:203, 1973.
92. Johnston JH, Kogan SJ: The exstrophic anomalies and their surgical reconstruction. Curr Probl Surg Aug. 1974.
93. Ansell JS: Surgical treatment of exstrophy of the bladder with emphasis on neonatal primary closure: personal experience with 28 consecutive cases treated at the University of Washington hospitals from 1962 to 1977: techniques and results. J Urol 121:650, 1979.
94. Leadbetter GW Jr: Surgical correction of total urinary incontinence. J Urol 91:261, 1964.
95. Tanagho EA, Smith DR: Clinical evaluation of a surgical technique for the correction of complete urinary incontinence. J Urol 107:402, 1972.
96. Lepor H, Shapiro E, Jeffs RD: Urethral reconstruction in boys with classical bladder exstrophy. J Urol 131:512, 1984.
97. Megalli M, Lattimer JK: Review of the management of 140 cases of exstrophy of the bladder. J Urol 109:246, 1973.
98. Mollard P: Bladder reconstruction in exstrophy. J Urol 124:525, 1980.
99. Lepor H, Jeffs RD: Primary bladder closure and bladder neck reconstruction in classical bladder exstrophy. J Urol 130:1142, 1983.
100. Culp OS: Treatment of epispadias with and without urinary incontinence: Experience with 46 patients. J Urol 109:120, 1973.
101. Jakobsen BE, Olesen S: Bladder exstrophy complicated by adenocarcinoma. Danish Med Bull 15:253, 1968.
102. Engel RME: Bladder exstrophy: vesicoplasty or urinary diversion? Urology 2:20, 1973.
103. Johnston JH: The exstrophic anomalies. In Williams DI, Johnston JH, (eds): Paediatric Urology. London, Butterworths, 1982.
104. Johnston JH: Lengthening of the congenital or acquired short penis. Br J Urol 46:685, 1974.
105. Johnston JH: The genital aspects of exstrophy. J Urol 113:701, 1975.
106. Hendren WH: Penile lengthening after previous repair of epispadias. J Urol 121:527, 1979.
107. Morgan WKC: The rape of the phallus. JAMA 193:123, 1965.
108. Preston EN: Whither the foreskin? A consideration of routine neonatal circumcision. JAMA 213:1853, 1970.
109. Kaplan GW: Circumcision: an overview. Curr Probl Pediatr 7:3, 1977.
110. Leiter E, Lefkovits AM: Circumcision and penile carcinoma. NY State J Med 75:1520, 1975.
111. Dodge OG, Linsell CA, Davies JNP: Circumcision and the incidence of carcinoma of the penis and the cervix. A study in Kenya and Uganda Africans. East Afr Med J 40:440, 1963.
112. Kochen M, McCurdy S: Circumcision and the risk of cancer of the penis. A life-table analysis. Am J Dis Child 134:484, 1980.
113. Thompson HC, King LR, Knox E, Korones SB: Report of the Ad Hoc Task Force on Circumcision. Pediatrics 56:610, 1975.
114. Hochman A, Ratzkowski R, Schreiber H: Incidence of carcinoma of the cervix in Jewish women in Israel. Br J Cancer 9:358, 1955.

115. Terris M, Wilson F, Nelson JH Jr: Relation of circumcision to cancer of the cervix. Am J Obstet Gynecol 117:1056, 1973.
116. Editorial. The case against neonatal circumcision. Br Med J 1:1163, 1979.
117. Gee WF, Ansell JS: Neonatal circumcision: a ten-year overview. With comparison of the Gomco clamp and Plastibell device. Pediatrics 58:824, 1976.
118. Herrera AJ, Cochran B, Herrera A, Wallace B: Parental information in highly motivated couples with higher education. Pediatrics 71:233, 1983.
119. Maisels MJ: Circumcision: the effect of information on parental decision making. Pediatrics 71:453, 1983.
120. Kirya C, Werthmann MW Jr: Neonatal circumcision and penile dorsal nerve block—a painless procedure. J Pediatr 92:998, 1978.
121. Williamson PS, Williamson ML: Physiologic stress reduction by a local anesthetic during newborn circumcision. Pediatrics 71:36, 1983.
122. Osborn LM, Metcalf TJ, Mariani EM: Hygienic care in uncircumcised infants. Pediatrics 67:365, 1981.
123. Gairdner D: The fate of the foreskin. A study of circumcision. Br Med J 2:1433, 1949.

10

Hypertension

CHAPTER 44

The Kidney in Blood Pressure Control and Hypertension

ARTHUR C. GUYTON

INTRODUCTION

It is almost impossible to develop chronic hypertension without the kidneys being pathologically or functionally part of the cause. This concept, however, is not widely held and probably would not be supported by more than a small percentage of those who work in the field of hypertension. Therefore, we will develop briefly some of the historical highlights in the evolution of hypertensive theory and then return to our thesis.

Studies on "Bright's disease" in the mid-1800s convinced many physicians that diseased kidneys could cause hypertension, which at that time could be diagnosed only by a hard pulse and thrusting heart because of lack of adequate pressure-measuring apparatus. It was natural to assume that since the kidneys were responsible for removing fluid and salt from the body, one possible mechanism for hypertension might be simply too much fluid volume in the body. Yet even from the beginning, Bright's own description of the disease also emphasized the possibility of a vasoconstrictor substance in the genesis of the disease (1).

Over the years, many separate observations have deprecated the "obvious" fluid volume hypothesis while at the same time fortifying the vasoconstrictor hypothesis. Most important of all, in the late 1800s and early 1900s, when it became possible to measure blood volume, extracellular fluid (ECF) volume, and cardiac output, it became clear that all of these were normal or nearly normal in most patients with hypertension. Yet in all these patients the total peripheral resistance was high. Therefore, the natural assumption was that the initiating cause of hypertension was some factor that increased total peripheral resistance.

With the discovery of the renin-angiotensin system, and especially following the extensive study of this system in the 1930s and 1940s by Page (2) and Braun-Menendez and his coworkers (3), a general belief ensued that at last the mythical vasoconstrictor substance of hypertension had been found. With better measuring techniques, however, it was soon learned that most patients with essential hypertension have a normal or low circulating renin.

During this time, many investigators were convinced that the nervous system was the basis for hypertension. Studies on the sympathetic nervous system, especially in the 1920s and 1930s, furthered this concept because many experiments demonstrated the powerful capability of the sympathetic nervous system to drive the heart to greatly increased activity while constricting the peripheral vessels. This led to the great epoch in the 1940s of performing sympathectomies for the treatment of hypertension. The acute results of these operations were astounding: blood pressure returned to normal within seconds after section of the last greater splanchnic nerve. Yet again the enthusiasm was short-lived. Much of the belief in the nervous system as the main progenitor of hypertension became greatly dampened because statistical analysis of blood pressures in those patients showed that within a few months pressure usually returned to their original elevated levels.

Therefore, most concepts of chronic hypertension genesis have met major roadblocks. The "mosaic theory" of hypertension, coined by Page (4) avoids this dilemma by stating that hypertension can be caused by multiple factors. This chapter also advocates a multiple-factor theory of hypertension, with one major addition: every factor that causes hypertension must in some way operate directly or indirectly through the kidneys to elevate the pressure.

BLOOD PRESSURE CONTROL

Renal Mechanisms

The kidneys control blood pressure by two primary mechanisms and by multiple secondary mechanisms. A primary kidney mechanism is one in which some function of the kidney itself responds directly to changes in arterial blood pressure and in turn causes some feedback effect on the circulatory system to return the blood pressure toward its previous level.

One of the primary mechanisms, the renin-angiotensin system, causes angiotensin to form in response to falling blood pressure; the multiple effects of angiotensin then return the pressure toward normal. Another primary mechanism, one that is much more fundamental but unfortunately far less well understood, is the renal-blood volume-pressure control mechanism. Multiple experiments in the past few years have shown it to be crucial in the long-term control of blood pressure, as opposed to short-term pressure control over a period of minutes or hours in which this renal-blood volume-pressure control mechanism plays almost no role.

The secondary renal mechanisms for pressure control include the effects of multiple extrinsic factors acting on the two primary kidney pressure control mechanisms to alter their control characteristics. For instance, aldosterone affects the kidney by causing water and salt retention and is an important secondary renal pressure control mechanism. Likewise, antidiuretic hormone (ADH) mildly affects renal pressure control. The nervous system, acting primarily through the sympathetic nervous system may have long-term effects on kidney function that could alter its pressure control capability. In addition, such factors as diet composition, effect of hormones other than aldosterone and ADH, and even the effect of such physical factors as exercise might have effects on renal function that would secondarily affect pressure control.

Nonrenal Mechanisms

Even in patients who do not have kidneys and who regularly go two to three days between dialysis sessions, arterial pressure is controlled during the intervening time. If the kidneys are so important in pressure control, how can this be true? The answer is that the renal-blood volume-pressure control mechanism functions for long-term control over weeks and months. Actually, the dialysis sessions themselves substitute for the kidney mechanisms and provide a long-term background control base from which short-term pressure control systems can function.

The minute-to-minute and hour-to-hour control of pressure between dialysis sessions is effected mainly through several different nervous mechanisms. The most widely known is the baroreceptor-sympathetic feedback system, in which stretch receptors in the carotid sinuses and aortic arch elicit nerve reflexes that feed back mainly through the sympathetics to the heart, peripheral arterioles, and veins to alter circulatory dynamics, thereby controlling arterial pressure.

Less well known are two other major nervous feedback control mechanisms. One is the chemoreceptor mechanism, which is initiated by depressed oxygen or excessive carbon dioxide concentration in the blood acting on chemoreceptors in the carotid and aortic bodies, then eliciting sympathetic feedback effects similar to those elicited by the baroreceptor mechanism. The other is the central nervous system ischemic mechanism, which is excited by diminished blood flow to the vasomotor center in the medullar oblongata and also leading to sympathetic feedback effects.

In addition, several hormonal mechanisms can control blood pressure entirely independently of the kidneys. The best known of these is the sympathetic activation of the epinephrine-norepinephrine system that then participates along with the baroreceptor, chemoreceptor, and central nervous system (CNS) ischemic feedback mechanisms. Less well known is the fact that vasopressin (or ADH) release from the posterior pituitary gland in response to hypotension is also an important short-term pressure controller. Studies by Cowley and coworkers (5) convincingly demonstrate that the amount of ADH released during hypotensive episodes can sometimes correct as much as two-thirds to three-quarters of the fall in pressure. This correction occurs within a few minutes, as the concentration of ADH builds up in the circulating blood.

Dominance of the Renal-Blood Volume-Pressure Control Mechanism Over All Other Mechanisms

Compared with almost all of the other pressure-controlling systems, the renal-blood volume-pressure control mechanism is slow to act; however, it has a special feature not shared by any of the others. It is an *integrating control mechanism* that continues to cause progressively more feedback until the arterial pressure returns all the way to the target pressure level dictated by this control mechanism alone (6). Therefore, over long periods of time, the renal-blood volume-pressure control mechanism becomes extremely powerful, a characteristic that it exhibits hardly at all during the first few hours of control. As a consequence, it almost certainly is the basis for long-term pressure control.

RENAL-BLOOD VOLUME AND PRESSURE CONTROL

Basic Mechanism

The basic mechanism of the renal-blood volume-pressure control system is the following. An increase in renal arterial pressure directly increases renal output of both water and salt, which is illustrated by the curve in Figure 44.1 called a *renal function curve.* This curve is a composite drawn from studies by many different research investigators, including Selkurt (7), Thompson (8), Shipley (9), and Narvar (10). Note that at 100 mm Hg mean arterial pressure, the output of water and salt is exactly equal to the net intake of water and salt (when net intake is defined as the total intake minus the water and salt leaving the body by nonrenal routes). Thus, normally, there is a state of exact fluid and salt balance; however, when the renal perfusion pressure decreases to 60 mm Hg, the output of both water and salt essentially ceases. At the other extreme of 200 mm Hg, the output of water and salt increases to about

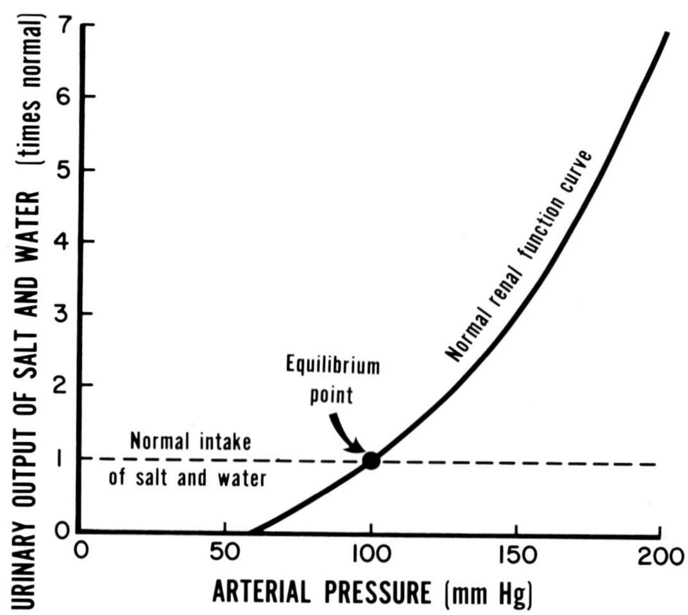

Figure 44.1. The "pressure-analysis diagram," showing normal renal function curve equated with normal level of intake of salt and water. Equilibrium point defines operating level of system. (Modified from Guyton AC: Arterial Pressure and Hypertension. Philadelphia, W. B. Saunders Co., 1980.)

seven times normal. Therefore, so long as the salt intake remains constant and the kidneys also remain normal, any pressure above this "equilibrium point" of 100 mm Hg will cause a decreasing body fluid volume that will continue decreasing indefinitely until the pressure falls back to the control value of 100 mm Hg. Conversely, if the arterial pressure falls below 100 mm Hg, the renal output of water and salt will become less than the intake, progressively increasing body fluid volume until the pressure again returns to the equilibrium point of 100 mm Hg.

Thus, the renal-blood volume-pressure control mechanism is a simple one. Whenever the pressure falls too low, the body fluid volume increases until the pressure returns to the control value; conversely, whenever the pressure rises too high, the volume decreases until the pressure again returns to the control value. The complexities of this system are not so easy to understand, however.

"Infinite Gain" Principle

The infinite gain principle, as it applies to the renal-blood volume-pressure control system, can best be understood by referring to Figure 44.1. Note that at any pressure greater than the "equilibrium point," even if the pressure is only a fraction of a millimeter of mercury greater, there will be negative water and salt balance. Therefore, net loss of water and salt from the body will never stop until the pressure decreases *all the way back to the equilibrium point.* This is what is meant by the inifinite gain principle. That is, the effects of the mechanism keep accumulating (which is the principle of integration and is the reason that this mechanism is called an integrating control system) until eventually any pressure different from the equilibrium point pressure will be corrected. To state this still another way, if given time to become fully operative, the feedback gain of this system for control of arterial pressure is infinite.

In view of the infinite gain principle, one can readily see that it would be impossible for the arterial pressure ever to stabilize at any level except at the equilibrium point, where the line in Figure 44.1 depicting net intake of water and salt intersects with the renal function curve. The infinite gain principle thus underlies two physiological laws that help in understanding long-term arterial pressure control (11). These are:

Law 1. The long-term pressure level at which the arterial pressure is controlled cannot change to a new level without changing the pressure level of the equilibrium point, where the renal function curve for salt and water output intersects the net salt and water intake level.

Law 2. If the pressure level of the equilibrium point changes to a new pressure level, the arterial pressure will after a few days also be controlled to this new level. From this law, one can also deduce that there are two separate determinants of the long-term arterial pressure level. These are the degree of shift of the renal function curve along the pressure axis and the net level of salt and water intake.

Finally, the diagram in Figure 44.1 has been called the pressure-analysis diagram because, if each of the two curves is known, one can predict from the diagram the eventual long-term arterial pressure level.

NonCauses of Chronic Hypertension

A sudden increase in heart strength or total peripheral resistance or a decrease in vascular capacitance increases arterial pressure. In fact, these three factors are the principal controllers of arterial pressure in the short run; however, the infinite gain principle, in effect, states that not any one of these three factors can play a role in determining the long-term arterial pressure level unless it in some way affects the net intake of salt and water or the degree of shift of the renal function curve along the pressure axis. The reason for this is that the renal-blood volume-pressure control system uses still a fourth pressure-controlling factor not normally used by the acute pressure control mechanisms: changes in blood volume. Furthermore, because of the infinite gain principle, blood volume changes caused by the renal-blood volume-pressure control system can compensate fully for abnormalities of any one of the three factors previously mentioned. In fact, that is what is meant by the infinite gain principle. How does the blood volume factor compensate for each of these?

Capacitance

Assume that the vascular capacitance suddenly decreases and remains decreased thereafter. This causes an acute rise in arterial pressure because of increased return of blood to the heart; however, it also increases the renal arterial pressure. The pressure-analysis diagram in Figure 44.1 shows that negative fluid balance immediately develops and continues until the blood volume decreases enough to bring the pressure exactly back to its original value. In other words, for each decrease in volume holding capacity of the circulation, the renal-blood volume-pressure control system eventually decreases the blood volume in same amount exactly, which fully compensates the effect of the capacitance change.

Heart Strength

Assume that heart strength suddenly increases and remains increased thereafter. The sudden increase in heart strength causes a small or, in some instances, a great increase in arterial pressure. If, however, the intake of water and salt remains constant and the renal function curve does not shift along the pressure axis, negative fluid balance again ensues and continues until the pressure returns to its normal level. There are numerous examples of this effect in the clinical literature. Perhaps the most striking occurs following surgical operations on the heart; these occasionally increase the pumping capability of the heart as much as two- to three-fold, but nevertheless do not cause hypertension.

Total Peripheral Resistance

Almost all persons with hypertension have greatly increased total peripheral resistance. Yet strangely enough, the infinite gain principle states that a primary increase in total peripheral resistance will not cause hypertension so long as the increase in resistance does not change the intake of water and salt or shift the renal function curve toward higher pressure levels. For instance, assume that the total peripheral resistance increases suddenly to a very high level but without affecting the degree of shift of the renal function curve along the pressure axis. That is, let us constrict all of the arterioles in the body except those in the kidneys so that the kidneys will continue to function normally. The increase in total peripheral resistance will obviously increase the arterial pressure acutely; yet even though the total peripheral resistance remains elevated indefinitely, the pressure will still return to normal because any pressure greater than that of the equilibrium point will cause a negative fluid balance until the pressure returns to the original equilibrium point as defined by the pressure-analysis diagram of Figure 44.1.

Does this lack of an effect of total peripheral resistance on the long-term arterial pressure level fit with clinical experience? Figure 44.2 illustrates that it does. This figure shows average arterial pressures and cardiac outputs in different clinical abnormalities in which the total peripheral resistance is too low or too high but in which renal function remains unaffected. Note that the arterial pressures are all in the normal range but also that the different levels of total peripheral resistance are all associated with exact inverse changes in cardiac output. Therefore, total peripheral resistance is a long-term controller of cardiac output, not of arterial pressure.

Why is hypertension so often associated with increased total peripheral resistance? There are several reasons for this: First, an increase in renal resistance, especially if the increase is preglomerular, has an especially

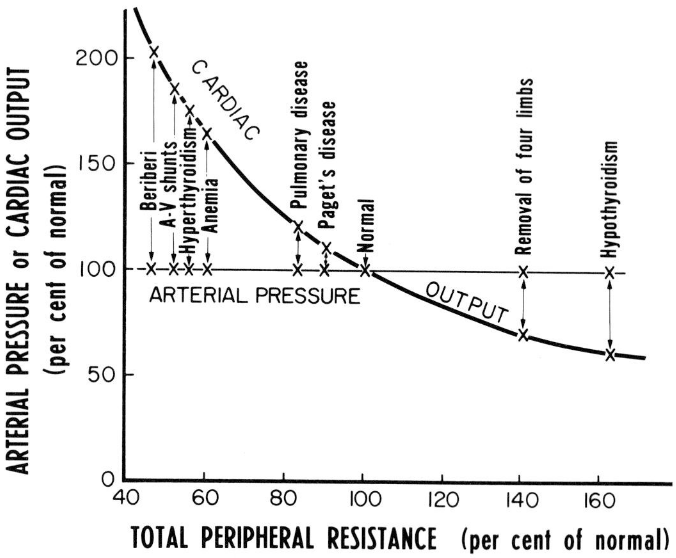

Figure 44.2. Effect of total peripheral resistance on arterial pressure and cardiac output in a number of different clinical conditions causing abnormal total peripheral resistances but not affecting renal function. (From Guyton AC: Arterial Pressure and Hypertension. Philadelphia, W. B. Saunders Co., 1980.)

powerful effect to shift the renal function curve toward higher pressure levels. Therefore, when the renal resistance increases along with the increase in total peripheral resistance, which usually occurs when there is a generalized vasoconstrictor factor, hypertension also occurs. It should be recognized, however, that it is not the increase in total peripheral resistance that is the cause of the hypertension but the increase in renal resistance. Though this may appear to be a subtle point, it is critical in understanding causative factors in hypertension development, because it states that increased resistance in all parts of the body besides the kidneys will not lead to chronic hypertension. Secondly, in many instances of hypertension, if not most, the increase in total peripheral resistance occurs secondarily to the hypertension rather than as the cause of it. This will be discussed in relation to the role of autoregulation in pressure control.

The Autoregulation Effect

Role of Autoregulation in the Pressure Control System

Autoregulation of blood flow means the ability of each local tissue to control its own blood flow in relation to its local need. Most often, the need for oxygen is the most powerful of the local autoregulating factors (12). That is, when the tissues are inadequately supplied with oxygen, the local arterioles dilate and blood flow increases. On the other hand, when the tissues are more than adequately supplied with oxygen, exactly opposite effects occur: the arterioles constrict and blood flow decreases. Other local tissue factors that affect local blood flow include carbon dioxide concentration, pH, potassium ion concentration, glucose concentration, and organic substances released from the tissues, the most important of which is adenosine.

But what role does autoregulation play in hypertension? Though the answer to this depends upon the circumstances, the following are the principal ingredients of the answer.

First, autoregulation never *causes* hypertension. Some investigators have coined the term "autoregulation theory of hypertension"; however, autoregulation does not autoregulate pressure; it autoregulates blood flow. Therefore, there is no such thing as an autoregulation theory of hypertension, although this does not mean that autoregulation does not have significant effects in hypertension.

Second, when hypertension is caused by some vasoconstrictor factor that constricts the renal arterioles at the same time that it constricts the arterioles in all other tissues of the body, the autoregulation mechanism might not be operative at all. That is, the renal arteriolar constriction causes the hypertension, but the increase in arterial pressure does not increase the blood flow in the peripheral tissues because of arteriolar constriction in these tissues as well as in the kidneys. Therefore, since the tissue blood flow is already normal, the autoregulation mechanism is not activated.

Third, whenever the cardiac output becomes abnormal, local blood flow in the peripheral tissues must also become abnormal. Under these conditions, local blood flow autoregulation becomes highly operative, attempting to return the blood flow back to its required level. In doing so, it often markedly affects circulatory dynamics. One instance where these effects are exceedingly important is in volume-loading hypertension.

Role of Autoregulation in Volume-Loading Hypertension

The basic mechanism of volume-loading hypertension is the following. Increased blood volume increases venous return, which then causes the heart to pump extra blood, resulting in increased cardiac output. The increase in cardiac output increases local tissue blood flow throughout the body. The increase in cardiac output also increases the arterial pressure; however, the increased tissue blood flow also activates the autoregulation mechanism, which increases the resistance throughout the body. This returns the tissue blood flow toward normal, thus decreasing the venous return and returning cardiac output back toward normal as well. Pressure remains high, however, because of the increasing resistance.

These principles are illustrated in Figure 44.3, which shows approximate composite quantitative results recorded in a series of volume-loading hypertension experiments in dogs spanning a period of 20 years (13–17). In each experiment, about 70% of the renal mass was removed several weeks before volume-loading by removing the two poles of one kidney and later removing the entire second kidney, leaving only the central portion of a single kidney. On the average, this removal of renal tissue increased the arterial pressure about 6 mm Hg. After several weeks of adjustment, the dogs were given large amounts of salt and water, either as saline solution in place of drinking water or by intravenous infusion of saline. Since the remaining kidney mass could not excrete the large saline load, fluid accumulated in the body and hypertension ensued. The curves of Figure 44.3 illustrate the experimental results during the first 2 weeks of the salt and water loading. Note the immediate increases in extracellular fluid volume, blood volume, and cardiac output, which are the usual effects associated with increased body fluid volume. However, note also that the early effect on total peripheral resistance was to decrease it, not to increase it. Even so, as illustrated by the lowermost curve of the figure, the arterial pressure rose despite the negative effect of decreased total peripheral resistance on the pressure. During the next few days, the decrease in total peripheral resistance reversed, and the resistance then increased to 30% to 35% above normal during the ensuing 10 days. Simultaneously, the ECF volume, blood volume, and cardiac output returned so nearly to normal that the remaining abnormality in each was not statistically significant.

How does autoregulation affect volume-loading hypertension? Measurement of cardiac output provides the answer. After an initial large rise, cardiac output returned almost to normal within a week or two. This is exactly the effect one would expect as a consequence of autoreg-

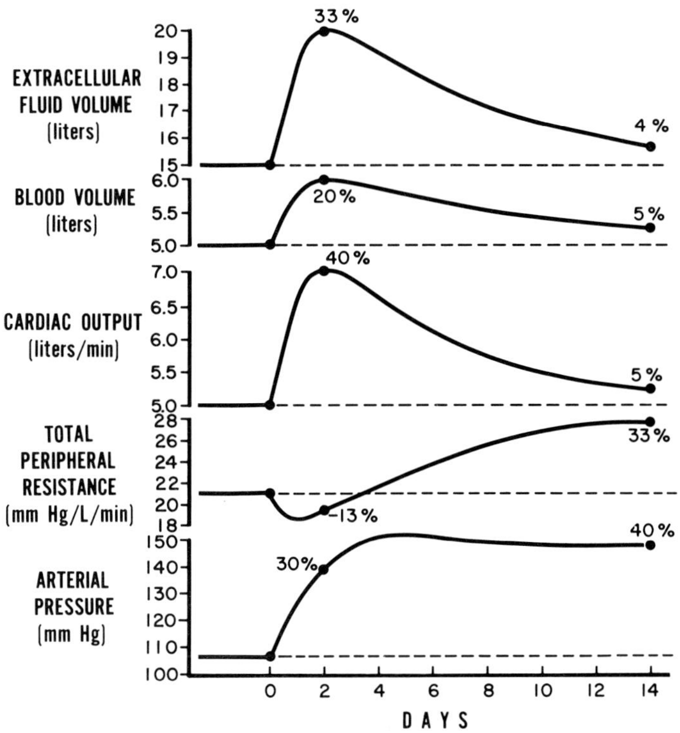

Figure 44.3. Approximate composite quantitative results from series of volume-loading hypertension experiments, showing that hypertension is initially a high cardiac output and high volume hypertension but that this converts to a high total peripheral resistance hypertension within a week or so. (Modified from Guyton AC: Arterial Pressure and Hypertension. Philadelphia, W. B. Saunders Co., 1980.)

ulation, because the initial elevation of cardiac output caused abnormally high tissue blood flow, which is the activating stimulus for autoregulation. The autoregulation in turn reduced both tissue blood flow and cardiac output to the normal level.

One problem, however, with this thesis is whether the autoregulatory mechanism has a high enough feedback gain to bring the blood flow so nearly back to normal as observed in the experiments. This problem has probably been solved by studies on local blood flow in patients with coarctation of the aorta, in which the autoregulatory mechanism also appears to operate strongly (18, 19). In several such studies, it has been shown that the local tissue blood flow in the upper part of the body, where the pressure is high, and blood flow in the lower part of the body, where the pressure is low, are both normal compared with flows in persons without coarctation of the aorta. Since both the upper and lower body tissues are exposed to the same circulating vasoconstrictor factors and, presumably, to the same nervous vasoconstrictor factors, it appears that the local tissues themselves are capable of a degree of blood flow autoregulation that is almost perfect. Therefore, it is reasonable to believe that the return of the cardiac output almost to normal (Fig. 44.3) was caused by autoregulation.

Some investigators have attempted to limit the term autoregulation to immediate blood flow autoregulation that occurs in a matter of minutes and not to include the long-term effects that occur in coarctation of the aorta. The origin of the term, however, allows one to speak of both "immediate autoregulation," which is usually rather weak, and "long-term autoregulation," which appears from coarctation studies to have a very high feedback gain. Long-term autoregulation has been shown to results from structural changes in the vessels (20), which is not true in immediate autoregulation.

Role of Autoregulation in Total Peripheral Resistance

Note in Figure 44.3 that as cardiac output returned toward normal, total peripheral resistance rose far above normal. This is exactly what would be expected, because the way in which autoregulation decreases the cardiac output is to increase the resistances in the local tissues throughout the body.

Even more important is the relative timing of the increase in arterial pressure in relation to the increase in total peripheral resistance. Note that the arterial pressure rose several days ahead of the rise in total peripheral resistance. Therefore, the conclusion must be that the increase in total peripheral resistance had nothing to do with the initial development of the hypertension. Instead, the increased total peripheral resistance was a secondary phenomenon.

Effect of Autoregulation on ECF and Blood Volume

Note also in Figure 44.3 that both the ECF volume and blood volume returned to normal at the same time that the cardiac output decreased. These decreases in volume can be explained by two effects. The autoregulatory mechanism constricts principally the arterioles, which would be expected to reduce the capillary pressure; this in turn would favor osmotic absorption of fluid from the interstitial spaces into the circulation. The rise in arterial pressure as the hypertension develops has a direct effect on the kidneys to cause greatly increased output of water and salt, in accordance with the renal function curve (Fig. 44.1). Consequently, the kidneys would be expected to excrete greatly increased quantities of fluid until both the ECF volume and blood volume are returned nearly to normal.

The main conclusion of the studies illustrated in Figure 44.3, therefore, is that volume-loading hypertension in the chronic stage is not a high volume nor high cardiac output hypertension but instead a high total peripheral resistance hypertension.

Long-Term Effect on ECF and Blood Volume. After a few weeks of volume loading the net increases in ECF volume and blood volume were extremely small (Fig. 44.3), even though the arterial pressure had increased as much as 40%. Yet it was certain that the cause of the hypertension was the volume loading itself, because when the volume loading was stopped, the arterial pressure returned to the original control values in two to three days. From this it can be concluded that increases in ECF volume or blood volume of as little as 4% to 5%, which is a body weight change of about 1%, can cause significant hypertension.

Do these data fit with clinical observations? Bits of evidence from the literature suggest that they do. In hypertensive patients successfully treated with diuretics, there is usually an initial significant decrease in plasma volume; however, after a week or so the plasma volume returns almost to normal even though the blood pressure remains reduced (21). These effects are almost opposite to those in the volume-loading hypertension illustrated in Figure 44.3. Patients with acute glomerular nephritis go through a sequence of fluid volume and arterial pressure changes similar to those illustrated in Figure 44.3; therefore, the hypertension of acute glomerular nephritis is likely to be mainly a volume-loading type.

Three conclusions appear from this line of reasoning 1. Prolonged body fluid volume changes equivalent to no more than a few percent of the body weight appear to be capable of causing marked changes in arterial pressure. This is true even though the same fluid volume changes that occur immediately have almost no effect on arterial pressure, mainly because the nervous pressure control systems can block the immediate effects.

2. The real importance of the autoregulation mechanism is not to cause hypertension but to reduce the fluid volumes and cardiac output to normal or nearly normal after the hypertension has developed or

while it is developing. In this manner, the hypertension is converted from a high cardiac output type to a high resistance type. Consequently, when a physician sees a hypertensive patient with high total peripheral resistance, this does not mean that the high total peripheral resistance results from some primary vascular cause. It is likely to be the result of autoregulation, occurring secondarily or parallel to the hypertension, not as the cause.

3. The fact that one cannot demonstrate elevated fluid volumes nor elevated cardiac output in hypertension does not eliminate volume-loading as the initiating cause of the hypertension.

"SALT-LOADING" AND BLOOD PRESSURE CONTROL

Because salt plays an important role in blood pressure control, especially in renal disease, it is important to know the effect of chronic salt-loading on the renal function curve. Figure 44.4 illustrates, for comparitive purposes, the normal acute renal function curve, which is the same curve as that illustrated in Figure 44.1, and a "salt-loading renal function curve" recorded in a series of dogs in the following manner (22).

A salt solution was infused intravenously at four different rates, each rate for three or more days, beginning at about one-fifth the normal salt intake and increasing to about eight times the normal intake, a total increase of about 40-fold. After several days at each salt infusion level, the rate of salt output was essentially equal to the intake. Therefore, the salt output was determined from the measurement levels of intake and plotted in relation to the arterial pressure, thus producing what we have called the "salt-loading renal function curve" or the "chronic renal function curve."

Note that the salt-loading renal function curve is far steeper (about 25 times) than the acute renal function curve. The obvious reason for this is that many more factors affect urinary output than pressure alone. Therefore, the acute renal function curve shifts to different levels as the salt intake changes, as illustrated in Figure 44.5 (23).

At the lowest salt intake level, excess formation of angiotensin, excess secretion of aldosterone, and probably a number of other factors reduce the acute renal function curve to the lowest curve illustrated in this figure. Conversely, at high salt intakes, opposite hormonal effects shift the curve to the highest level.

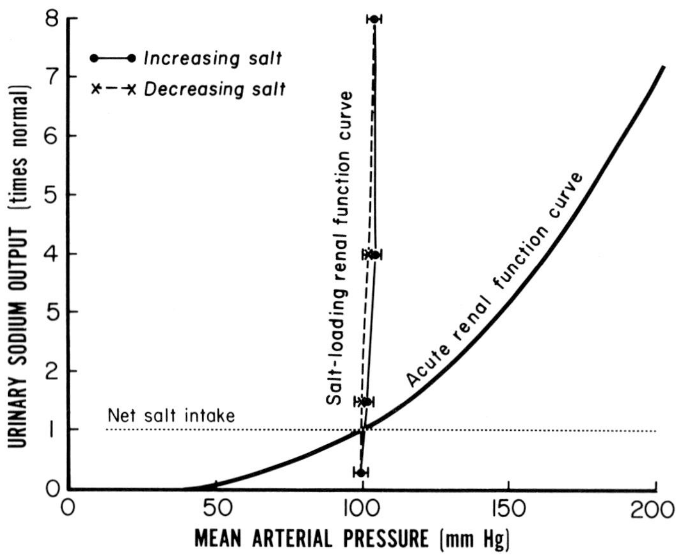

Figure 44.4. Comparison of "salt-loading renal function curve" (measured in intact animals over a period of weeks) with the acute renal function curve (measured acutely in isolated kidneys). (Modified from Guyton AC: Arterial Pressure and Hypertension. Philadelphia, W. B. Saunders Co., 1980.)

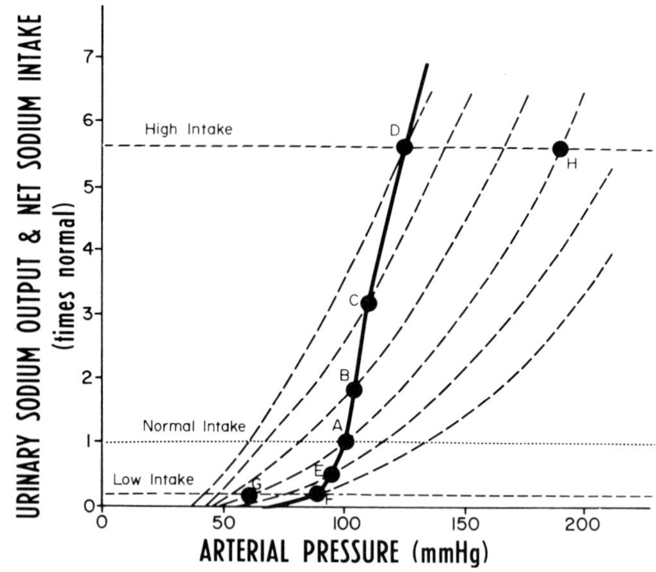

Figure 44.5. Effect of progressive increase in sodium intake to cause upward and leftward shift of acute renal function curve, thus explaining steepness of salt-loading renal function curve. (Modified from Guyton AC, Coleman TG, Cowley AW, et al.: Arterial pressure regulation: overriding dominance of the kidney in long-term regulation and in hypertension. Am J Med 52:584, 1972.)

The very dark curve (Figure 44.5) shows the measured changes in arterial pressure and urinary output at the different salt intake levels—the salt-loading renal function curve. This curve is important in analyzing different types of hypertensive states because it factors into the equation not only the effect of arterial pressure on urinary output, as represented by the acute renal function curve, but also the effect of salt-loading to shift this curve from one level to another. Furthermore, the salt-loading curve is easily measured in normal unanesthetized animals or human beings by changing the salt intake level, whereas the acute curve is virtually impossible to measure in the intact animal.

Arterial Pressure Analysis

Figure 44.6 illustrates a normal salt-loading renal function curve and five abnormal curves, four of which are associated with hypertension: reduced renal mass, continuous infusion of aldosterone or angiotensin, Goldblatt hypertension or spontaneously hypertensive rats, and hypertension caused by reduced glomerular filtration coefficient. The first three of these curves have been measured in animals, and the fourth has been approximated from anecdotal data in the literature (11). Some hypertensive factors cause the function curve to shift parallel to the normal curve, for example, in Goldblatt hypertension and spontaneous hypertension of the rat. Others cause the slope of the curve to decrease, for example, aldosterone or angiotensin infusion and reduced glomerular filtration coefficient. Finally, the "reduced renal mass" curve is shifted far to the right at the higher salt intake but not at low salt intake.

Remembering that the arterial pressure is determined by the equilibrium point where the renal function curve intersects the salt intake level in the pressure-analysis diagram, one can use the curves of Figure 44.6 to predict the arterial pressure level for any specific curve at any specific salt intake level. For instance, when considering the normal curve at normal salt intake, the arterial pressure is 100 mm Hg, and at high salt intake it is 102 mm Hg, hardly any change. For the Goldblatt or

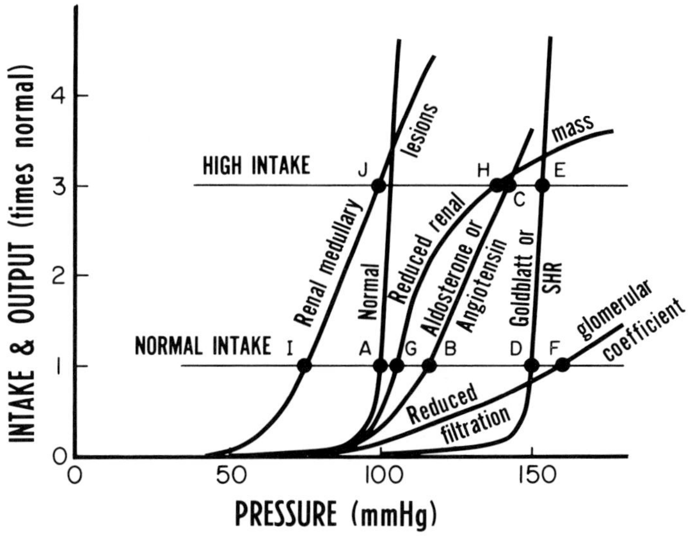

Figure 44.6. A pressure-analysis diagram showing salt-loading renal function curves for a number of different abnormal functional states of the kidneys. Points of intersection with normal and high intake lines are predictions of average long-term arterial pressure levels for respective renal conditions at two salt intake levels. (From Guyton AC: Arterial Pressure and Hypertension. Philadelphia, W. B. Saunders Co., 1980.)

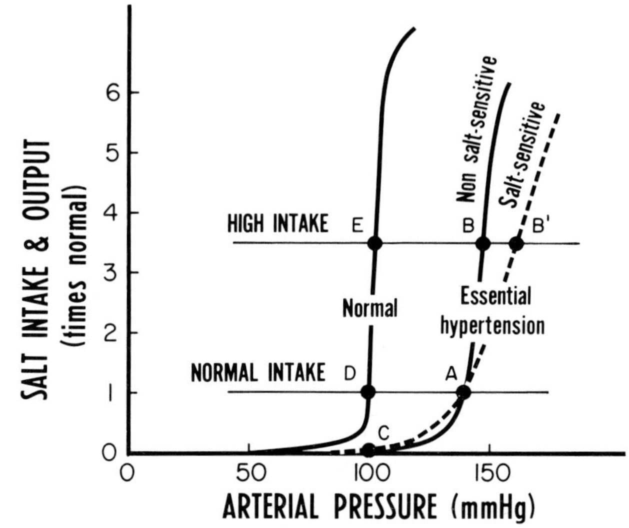

Figure 44.7. Analysis of long-term arterial pressure control in non-salt-sensitive and salt-sensitive essential hypertension. (From Guyton AC: Arterial Pressure and Hypertension. Philadelphia, W. B. Saunders Co., 1980.)

spontaneously hypertensive rat curve, the arterial pressure is 150 mm Hg at normal salt intake or 152 mm Hg at high salt intake, again hardly a change related to salt intake. Thus, these two types of hypertension are said to be "salt-insensitive."

With aldosterone or angiotensin infusion at normal salt intake, the arterial pressure is approximately 115 mm Hg; at high salt intake, it is approximately 135 mm Hg (Fig. 44.6). Thus, both types of hypertension are "salt-sensitive." Likewise, reduced renal mass hypertension and reduced glomerular filtration coefficient hypertension are salt-sensitive types.

Figure 44.6 (left) is a salt-loading renal function curve labeled "renal medullary lesions," which is drawn only approximately from different measurements of renal function in dogs with medullary lesions (Balfe, Hall, and Guyton, unpublished observations). It illustrates that these animals must have a high salt intake to maintain normal pressure. Elimination of their high salt intake causes arterial pressure to fall rapidly from normal to about 75 mm Hg. Clinical conditions that might have a similar effect would be Bartter syndrome and salt-losing syndromes caused by interstitial nephritis; however appropriate measurements have not yet been made.

Essential Hypertension

What is the cause of essential hypertension? Certainly, no vasoconstrictor factor has yet been found that can explain essential hypertension. Also, almost all measurements of cardiac output in severe essential hypertension show the output to be normal or slightly below normal in most patients, whereas the total peripheral resistance is greatly elevated. Patients with severe essential hypertension usually also have renal blood flows less than half normal (24), which alone would account for a 10% reduction in cardiac output; therefore, blood flow through the nonrenal portions of the body might be slightly elevated on the average. Thus essential hypertension has many characteristics similar to those of the volume-loading hypertension, namely, very high total peripheral resistance but cardiac output, ECF volume, and blood volume all within normal limits.

Whether or not essential hypertension is strictly a volume-loading type, it can still be analyzed using the pressure-analysis diagram (Fig. 44.7). This figure shows a normal salt-loading renal function curve for reference and two other salt-loading curves that approximate the equivalent measurements made by Bartter and his colleagues in essential hypertensive patients (25). One of these two curves is for salt-insensitive essential hypertension, and the other for the salt-sensitive type. In both instances, the renal function curve is shifted far to the right on the arterial pressure axis, so it must be presumed that this shift explains the essential hypertension. Consequently, the question is; what is the factor that shifts the curve? Possible answers include pathologically constricted renal arterioles that reduce blood flow into the glomerulus, excess nervous stimulation of the arterioles that cause secondary renal vascular constriction, hormonal factors that cause secondary renal vascular constriction, pathologically reduced glomerular filtration coefficient, or hormonal factors or renal disease that increase tubular reabsorption of salt and water.

Recent studies by Folkow and his colleagues have demonstrated increased preglomerular vascular resistance in the spontaneously hypertensive rat (26). Electron microscope studies in this same rat by Evan and his colleagues showed that the porosity of the glomerular membrane is decreased (27). Therefore, two abnormalities in this genetic type of hypertension can shift the renal function curve to a higher pressure level that is similar to the shift illustrated in Figure 44.7 for essential hypertension.

Tubular Absorption Versus Glomerular Filtration Capability

The study of different disorders that *decrease* the kidney's glomerular filtration capability reveals that *all* have the potential for causing hypertension. These disorders include increased preglomerular vascular resistance caused by intrinsic pathology in the kidney or extrinsic factors that constrict the preglomerular vessels (sympathetic stimulation, infused norepinephrine, or perhaps other hormonal factors that cause constriction) and decreased glomerular filtration coefficient resulting from decreased glomerular surface area or decreased permeability.

Abnormalities of tubular reabsorption also affect pressure control but in exactly the opposite manner; i.e., *increased* tubular reabsorption of water and electrolytes causes increased arterial pressure. The classic example of this is aldosterone acting to increase tubular reabsorption as well as arterial pressure.

Thus, the opposing effects of tubular reabsorption and glomerular filtration lead to the concept that the final long-term arterial pressure level can be represented approximately by the following equation (11):

$$\text{Arterial Pressure} \propto \frac{\text{Tubular reabsorptive capability}}{\text{Glomerular filtration capability}}$$

This equation is important because it explains most of the conditions that cause uremia but not hypertension. When large portions of the renal mass are removed, there is little increase in pressure. For instance, in experimental dogs, we removed progressively greater portions of the renal mass, attempting to cause hypertension (Baer, Navar, and Guyton, unpublished observations). The greatest rise in pressure observed before the animals developed uremia was about 8 mm Hg. We concluded that removing renal mass fails to increase arterial pressure significantly because both tubular reabsorption and glomerular filtration capabilities are reduced about equally by this procedure. In accordance with the above equation, this would not lead to a significant change in pressure.

In fact, mathematical analyses of renal function have suggeted that body fluid balance could probably be maintained satisfactorily by as little as 5% to 10% of the normal kidney mass, so long as the appropriate ratio between tubular reabsorption capability and glomerular filtration capabilities are maintained. The reason for this is that the kidneys normally reabsorb over 99% of the water and electrolytes so that only a moderate decrease in this reabsorption percentage could easily control body fluid volume, even in a person with very little renal mass. On the other hand, elimination of many of the urinary waste products is directly proportional to the effective renal mass, so that uremia would be expected to occur long before hypertension if the only abnormality were reduced numbers of functional nephrons. This is what we found in our experiment.

RENIN-ANGIOTENSIN SYSTEM

The renin-angiotensin system plays an important role in hypertension because it increases total peripheral resistance. However, the vasoconstrictor effect of angiotensin on blood vessels can elevate pressure only temporarily; therefore, it is necessary to look at other functions of angiotensin to explain its chronic hypertensive effect.

Angiotensin is known to have significant effects on the kidneys themselves in addition to its extrarenal effects. These renal effects, some of which are mediated through aldosterone but the more potent of which act directly on the kidneys, can shift the renal function curve along the pressure axis (Fig. 44.8). The middle curve of this figure is the salt-loading curve for the normal dog, which is the same curve as that in Figure 44.4. The left-hand curve is for dogs whose renin-angiotensin system was blocked entirely by the converting enzyme inhibitor captopril (11). The right-hand curve is for dogs that were infused continuously for several weeks with angiotensin II at a low rate of infusion (22). The values in parentheses represent measured or calculated circulating levels of angiotensin II as compared to a normal level of 1 for the normal dog with normal salt intake. The significant shift between the left- and right-hand curves of this figure, caused by a relatively small amount of circulating angiotensin, explains the chronic hypertension caused by long-term continuous infusion of angiotensin II.

Study of the relationship of the "normal" renal function curve in Figure 44.8 to the other two curves can lead to still another important concept, i.e., that the renin-angiotensin system is capable of "buffering"

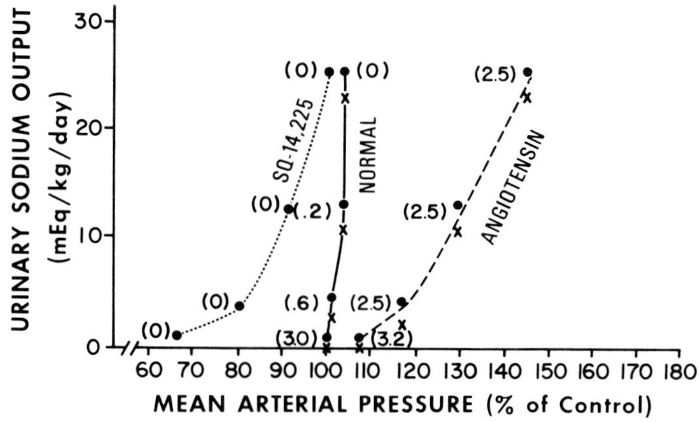

Figure 44.8. Salt-loading renal function curves measured in dogs under three different conditions: (1) when renin-angiotensin system was blocked by converting enzyme inhibitor Captopril (SQ-14,225), (2) under normal conditions, and (3) when angiotensin was infused continuously at a low rate (5 ng/kg/min). Note shift of renal function curve by approximately +40 to +50 mm Hg between zero angiotensin state and elevated angiotensin state. Note also that top of "normal" curve fits approximately on zero angiotensin curve while bottom of normal curve fits approximately on bottom of angiotensin curve. (From Guyton AC: Arterial Pressure and Hypertension. Philadelphia, W. B. Saunders Co., 1980.)

arterial pressure changes caused by greatly differing levels of salt intake. Note that circulating angiotensin in the normal animal was about three times normal on a very low salt intake, but at very high salt intake it was zero. Furthermore, the top of the "normal" function curve fits almost exactly at the top of the curve in which there was zero circulating angiotensin-II because of the converting enzyme inhibitor; the bottom of the "normal" curve fits almost exactly at the bottom of the angiotensin infusion curve. Thus, salt-loading, because of changes in the angiotensin system, shifts the top of the "normal" curve to the left, whereas salt deprivation shifts the bottom of the curve to the right. The importance of this is that the control capability of the renin-angiotensin system makes it possible for us to eat either extremely small amounts or extremely large amounts of salt, with almost insignificant effects on the arterial pressure level. On the other hand, when the renin-angiotensin system becomes nonresponsive to the level of salt intake, the person's arterial pressure then becomes highly sensitive to the intake level, i.e., arterial pressure becomes "salt-sensitive."

References

1. Bright R: Tabular view of the morbid appearances in 100 cases connected with albuminous urine. With observations. Guy's Hosp Reports 1:380, 1936.
2. Page IH: Some regulatory mechanisms of renovascular and essential arterial hypertension. In Hypertension, Genest J, Koiw E, Kuchel O, (eds): New York, McGraw-Hill, 1977, p 576.
3. Braun-Menendez E, Fasciolo JC, Leloir LF, Muñoz JM: La sustancia hipertensora de la sangre del riñón isquemiado. Rev Soc Argent Biol 15:420, 1939.
4. Page IH: On the nature of the pressor action of renin. J Exp Med 70:521, 1939.
5. Cowley AW, Jr, Switzer SJ, Guinn M: Evidence and quantification of the vasopressin arterial pressure control system in the dog. Circ Res 46:58, 1980.
6. Guyton AC, Coleman TG, Cowley AW Jr, Manning RD Jr, et al: A systems analysis approach to understanding long-range arterial blood pressure control and hypertension. Circ Res 35:159, 1974.
7. Selkurt EE, Hall PW, Spencer MP: Influence of graded arterial pressure decrement on renal clearance of creatinine, ρ-amino hippurate and sodium. Am J Physiol 159:369, 1949.
8. Thompson DD, Pitts RF: Effects of alterations of renal arterial pressure on sodium and water excretion. Am J Physiol 168:490, 1952.
9. Shipley RE, Study RS: Changes in renal blood flow, extraction of inulin, glomerular

filtration rate, tissue pressure, and urine flow with acute alterations of renal artery blood pressure. Am J Physiol 167:676, 1951.
10. Navar LG, Guyton AC: Intrarenal mechanisms for regulating body fluid volume, In Guyton AC, Taylor AE, Granger HJ (eds): Circulatory Physiology II: Dynamics and Control of the Body Fluids, Philadelphia, W. B. Saunders Co., 1975, p 243.
11. Guyton AC: Arterial Pressure and Hypertension. Philadelphia, W. B. Saunders Co., 1980.
12. Jones RD, Berne RM: Local regulation of blood flow in skeletal muscle. Circ Res 15(Suppl. I), 30, 1964.
13. Langston JB, Guyton AC, Douglas BH, Dorsett PE: Effect of changes in salt intake on arterial pressure and renal function in nephrectomized dogs. Circ Res 12:508, 1963.
14. Douglas BH, Guyton AC, Langston JB, Bishop VS: Hypertension caused by salt loading. II. Fluid volume and tissue pressure changes. Am J Physiol 207:669, 1964.
15. Coleman TG, Guyton AC: Hypertension caused by salt loading in the dog. III. Onset transients of cardiac output and other circulatory variables. Circ Res 25:152, 1969.
16. Cowley AW JR, Guyton AC: Baroreceptor reflex effects on transient and steady-state hemodynamics of salt-loading hypertension in dogs. Circ Res 36:536, 1975.
17. Manning RD Jr, Coleman TG, Guyton AC, et al: Essential role of mean circulatory filling pressure in salt-induced hypertension. Am J Physiol 236:R40, 1979.
18. Wakim KG, Slaughter O, Clagett OT: Studies on the blood flow in the extremities in cases of coarctation of the aorta: determination before and after excision of the coarctate region. Proc Mayo Clin 23:347, 1948.
19. Patterson GC, Shepherd JT, Whelan RF: The resistance to blood flow in the upper and lower limb vessels in patients with coarctation of the aorta. Clin Sci 16:627, 1957.
20. Folkow B, Hallbäck M, Lundgren Y, Weiss L: Structurally based increase of flow resistance in spontaneously hypertensive rats. Acta Physiol Scand 79:737, 1970b.
21. Gifford RW, Jr, Mattox VR, Orivs AL, et al: Effect of thiazide diuretics on plasma volume, body electrolytes, and excretion of aldosterone in hypertension. Circulation 24:1197, 1961.
22. DeClue JW, Guyton AC, Cowley AW Jr, et al: Subpressor angiotensin infusion, renal sodium handling, and salt-induced hypertension in the dog. Circ Res 43:503, 1978.
23. Guyton AC, Coleman TG, Cowley AW, et al: Arterial pressure regulation: overriding dominance of the kidney in long-term regulation and in hypertension. Am J Med 52:584, 1972.
24. Kolsters G, Schalekamp MADH, Birkenhager WH, Lever AF: Renin and renal function in benign essential hypertension: evidence for a renal abnormality. In Berglund G, Hansson L, Werko L, et al (eds): Pathophysiology and Management of Arterial Hypertension, Mölndal, Sweden, 1975, p 54.
25. Kawasaki T, Delea CS, Bartter FC, Smith H: The effect of high-sodium and low-sodium intakes on blood pressure and other related variables in human subjects with idiopathic hypertension. Am J Med 64:193, 1978.
26. Göthberg G, Lundin S, Ricksten SE, Folkow B: Apparent and true vascular resistances to flow in SHR and NCR kidneys as related to the pre/post-glomerular resistance ratio. Acta Physiol Scand 105:282, 1979.
27. Evan AP, Luft FC, Gattone V, et al: The glomerular filtration barrier in the spontaneously hypertensive rat. Hypertension 3:I-154, 1981.

CHAPTER **45**

Normal Blood Pressure

M. DE SWIET

An elevation in systemic arterial blood pressure is a common and well-recognized manifestation of renal disease; hypertension, therefore must be considered in any text on clinical nephrology. There is, however, a problem in the field of pediatric nephrology. The use of the term hypertension implies that normal tension has been satisfactorily defined. Although the normal range of blood pressure is well described in adults, only recently have normal standards for blood pressure been reported for infants and young children. This is largely because of difficulties in measurement but also because for many years hypertension was considered to be a disease of adults and was neglected in children.

This chapter considers various techniques available for measuring blood pressure; the normal range of blood pressure in children; the relationship of blood pressure to weight, age, and other variables; and, finally, "tracking" for blood pressure: at what age do children develop pressures that are representative of those they will have in adult life? Is essential hypertension in childhood a valid concept?

BLOOD PRESSURE MEASUREMENT

Techniques for measuring blood pressure may be divided into direct methods using intra-arterial catheters and indirect noninvasive techniques, which at present rely on sphygmomanometry. Although direct measurements from umbilical artery catheters have been used to establish normal blood pressures in neonates (1), such techniques are too invasive for general use outside the intensive care ward and cannot be applied to healthy children. All epidemiological studies, therefore, rely on indirect estimates of arterial blood pressure.

There are two sources of variation in the indirect technique: the system for detecting the pulse (conventional sphygmomanometry with auscultation, Doppler ultrasound, infrasound) and the system for pressure measurement in the sphygmomanometer cuff (mercury, aneroid, pressure transducer).

Detection of Pulse

It is difficult to use auscultation (as in conventional sphygmomanometry) to detect the pulse in the small arms of infants and children younger than about 5 yr, presumably because the blood vessels do not transmit sufficient energy for the Korotkoff sounds to be audible with an ordinary stethoscope. An alternative has been to use the "flush technique," which relies on a visual assessment of blood flow into a previously blanched limb. Elseed and coworkers studied the flush technique and conventional sphygmomanometry and compared them with the Doppler method (2). They found that blood pressure varied much more with conventional sphygmomanometry and the flush technique than with the Doppler method. The flush technique gives a blood pressure nearer to mean than to systolic or diastolic pressure, and both the older techniques have now been superseded by the Doppler method or one of its variants.

We use the Parks' Doppler ultrasound system (2); its advantages over other ultrasound systems are that it is relatively inexpensive and the sensor is small and separate from the sphygmomanometer cuff. The system detects red cell and blood vessel wall movement by the frequency shift that they induce in the reflected ultrasound waves. To measure the blood pressure, the brachial artery is located first at the elbow with the sensor. Then a sphygmomanometer cuff is inflated in the usual way above systolic pressure, when red cell and blood vessel wall movements cease in the arm distal to the cuff. As the cuff is deflated, blood flow resumes when the systolic pressure is reached and is detected by hearing the rhythmical Doppler tones.

The Parks' Doppler system measures only systolic blood pressure, but this is more valuable than diastolic blood pressure for epidemiological purposes (3) and perfectly adequate for most clinical uses. Other instruments measure diastolic blood pressure as well, but the correlation between observed diastolic blood pressure and intra-arterial measurement is not as good as for systolic blood pressure (4). For epidemiological purposes, we also use a random zero sphygmomanometer to reduce observer bias (5).

It is tempting to use an instrument such as the Physiometrics Infrasonde recorder, which relies on electronic detection of the Korotkoff sounds, or one in which the Doppler signal is automatically detected and compared with a cuff pressure measured by a transducer, thus permitting a digital printout of the blood pressure. These instruments are not reliable in measuring diastolic blood pressure in children (6). The inherent problem is that the calibration of the transducer may drift as it ages (also a difficulty with aneroid sphygmomanometers) so these instruments are therefore not recommended (7). Digital readout of blood pressure, though easy to read, gives a spurious sense of accuracy. We still favor an ultrasound system and sphygmomanometer in children up to the age of 5 yrs and conventional sphygmomanometry in older children.

Cuff Pressure

An inherent problem of indirect sphygmomanometry is the possibility that the pressure in the sphygmomanometer cuff is not that "seen" by the artery being compressed. Cuff size is crucial if the pressure is to be accurately transmitted to the artery. We employ cuffs with inflation bags 4 by 13.5 cm and 7.6 by 15.5 cm, using the larger cuff wherever possible. We have found that these accurately measure blood pressure in children up to the age of 8 yrs with arm circumferences up to 22 cm (8). Disposable cuffs are also available, and these too appear to give satisfactory results if the correct size is chosen (9).

NORMAL BLOOD PRESSURE

American Task Force Study

Normal values for blood pressure are available in older children and have been reviewed and published in percentile form from age 2 yrs by the American Task Force for Blood Pressure Control (Fig. 45.1) (10). For the age group from 2 to 5 yrs, however, data were drawn from a group of only 100 children; until recently, there were no data for blood pressure in a large group of younger healthy children.

Brompton Study

We selected a group of 2000 children born consecutively in one hospital and observed their blood pressures from age 4 days (8, 11). The percentile distribution of systolic blood pressure from this study up to 5 yrs is also given in Figure 45.1. The data show that blood pressure rises rapidly between the ages of 4 days and 6 weeks. Further studies, measuring blood pressure during the first 6 weeks, have shown that systolic blood pressure rises from a mean of 70 mm Hg at the age of 2 days to 84 mm Hg at 2 weeks in awake babies (12). There is a further rise to 93 mm Hg by the age of 6 weeks. Most of the 14 mm Hg increase therefore takes place in the first 2 weeks of life. The mean blood pressure of infants who are asleep when their blood pressure is measured is lower at all ages but rises in a similar manner.

Figure 45.1 shows that after the initial rise of blood pressure in infancy, pressure remains stable from age 1 to 5 yrs and then starts to rise again. The mechanism of this physiological rise in blood pressure during the neonatal period has not been determined in humans; however, studies in sheep have demonstrated that cardiac output falls at the time of the rise in systolic pressure, implying a marked rise in peripheral resistance during the neonatal period (13). If this were also the case in humans, it would indicate that, in addition to the sudden increase in peripheral vascular resistance that occurs at delivery with cord clamping and lung expansion, there is a further rise in total peripheral vascular resistance during the first 6 weeks of life. A noninvasive method of measuring cardiac output would be necessary to confirm this.

It is not clear why blood pressure should be stable from 1 to 5 yrs and then start to rise again. Although the stability of blood pressure from ages 1 to 5 in the Task Force data is confirmed by the Brompton Study, the precise age at which blood pressure begins to rise is at present unresolved. The Task Force data are based on different study groups which change between ages 5 and 6 yrs, and this may account for the apparent rise at this age; however, there is no doubt that at some age between 5 and 10 yrs, blood pressure starts rising again. The 50th and 95th percentiles for blood pressure, based on the Brompton and Task Force data, are given in Table 45.1.

Other Studies

There are few other large population studies of blood pressure in the first year of life. The Task Force for Blood Pressure Control in Children did not present data in children younger than 2 yrs. Other studies of blood pressure measured by indirect techniques in the neonatal period usually have been made in small groups of selected infants. Kirkland and Kirkland, using the Parks' Doppler ultrasound system, reported a range of systolic blood pressures of 67 to 79 mm Hg in 42 neonates who were both "resting and sucking" (14). The data are similar to those of the Brompton Study at these ages (68 to 92 mm Hg), even though in the Brompton Study measurements were not made while the infants were

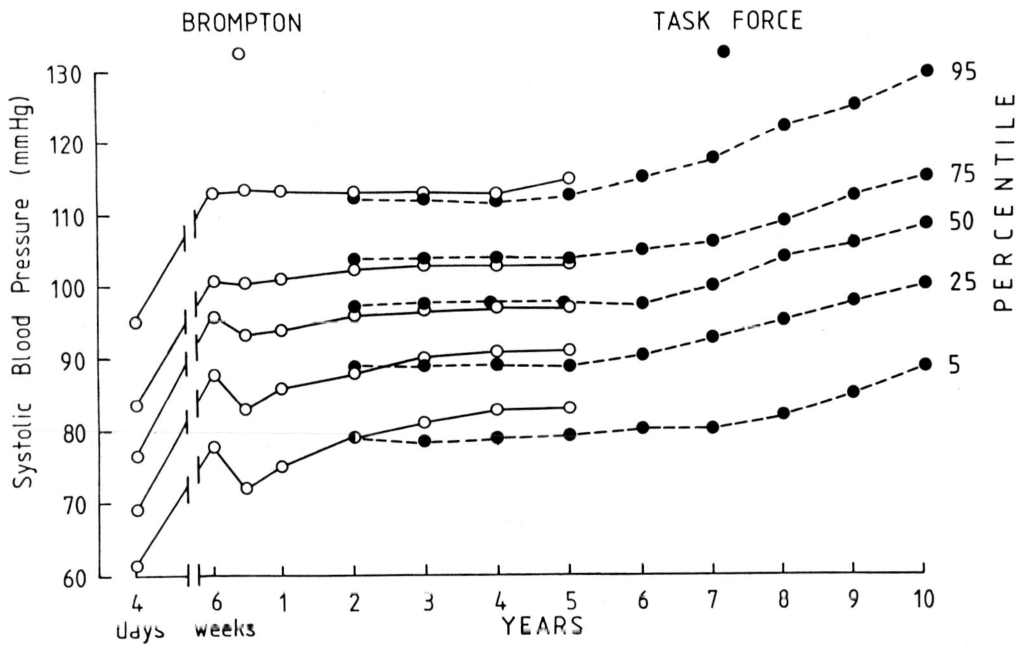

Figure 45.1. Blood pressure in children. ○ (age 4 days to 5 yrs) from the Brompton Study (8); ● (age 2 to 10 yrs) from the Task Force for Blood Pressure Control in Children (10).

Table 45.1.
Systolic Blood Pressure (mm Hg) in Children Age 4 Days to 5 Yrs (Brompton Study) and 9 Yrs to 18 Yrs (Task Force Data) (8, 10)

	50th systolic BP awake	95th percentile awake
4 days	76	95
6 weeks	96	113
6 months	93	113
1 yr	94	113
5 yrs	95	115
9 yrs	108	125
13 yrs	119	138
18 yrs[a]	128	152

[a] Boys only; girls about 5 mm Hg lower.

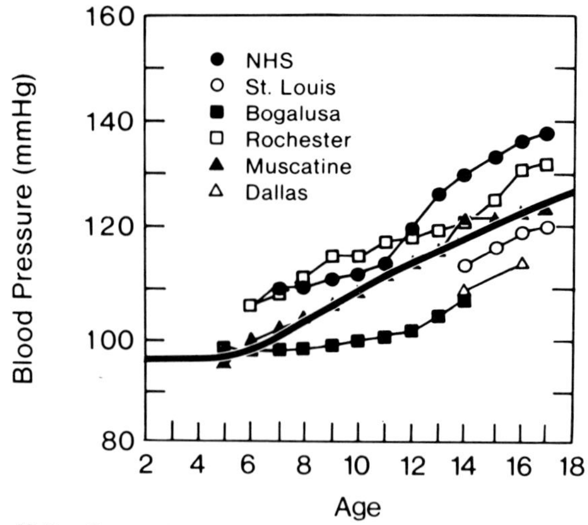

Figure 45.2. Comparisons of mean systolic blood pressure for boys of different ages in selected studies: National Health Survey (31, 32), St. Louis (33), Bogalusa (34), Rochester (34), Muscatine (34) and Dallas (35) as reviewed by Fixler (19). The heavy line represents the mean systolic blood pressure values reported by the Task Force on Blood Pressure Control in Children (10). Reproduced with permission from Hypertension, volume 2, supplement 1, 1980.

sucking, because it had previously been found that blood pressure was more variable under these circumstances (15).

Zinner and coworkers studied 837 infants of varied ethnic origins aged 1 to 6 days and found a systolic blood pressure between 69 and 83 mm Hg, depending on the age and level of consciousness (16), values that are about 5 mm Hg higher than those of the Brompton Study (8). They used the Arteriosonde, a different Doppler system, in which the cuff is more rigid and also contains the transducer. Hennekens and coworkers studied 43 infants from black families (17), also using the Arteriosonde, and found substantially higher mean systolic pressures of 78 mm Hg at 2 days and 103 mm Hg at 1 month: they did not specify the level of consciousness and made measurements exclusively in a hospital environment, which could well account for the higher values observed. Previous studies have not shown any difference in blood pressure between black and white infants (16, 18).

Fixler and coworkers reviewed six population studies of blood pressure in the young; Figures 45.2 and 45.3 show the results for mean and 95th percentile pressures (19). There is a fairly wide range of values between the different studies. The Task Force data are well placed in the middle range for both mean and 95th percentile for blood pressure. The factors accounting for this variability are likely to include genuine differences between populations, race (in older children), body mass, different cuff sizes, environmental differences at the time of measurement (including previous venipuncture), and in the case of the 95th percentile, the taking of multiple blood pressure measurements with subsequent regression toward the mean.

For clinical purposes, the 20 mm Hg difference at age 18 yrs between the lowest (140 mm Hg) and the highest 95th percentile value (160 mm Hg) is unlikely to be important. Most children with renovascular hypertension have blood pressures considerably in excess of these limits; however, occasionally there are borderline cases, so it is important to be aware of the differences between populations. Ideally, each center should have its own set of normal data obtained under precisely defined circumstances.

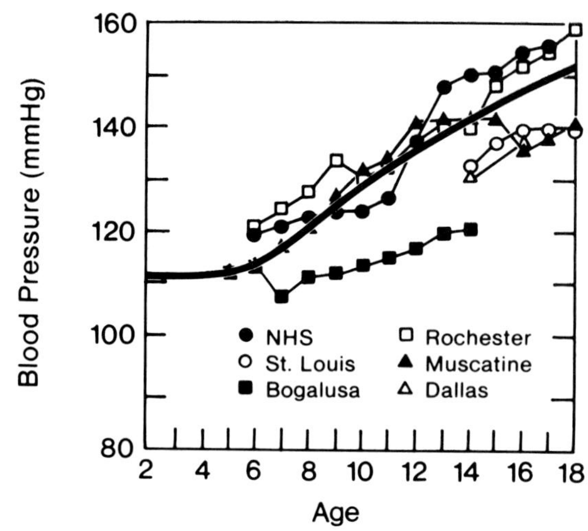

Figure 45.3. Comparisons of mean diastolic blood pressure for boys as in Figure 2. Reproduced with permission from Hypertension, volume 2, supplement 1, 1980.

In the first year of life, boys have slightly higher blood pressures than girls. The difference is less than 1.5 mm Hg (8); however, boys are heavier at birth than girls and, after adjusting for weight, the difference in pressure due to gender is largely eliminated (8). The Task Force data indicate that when blood pressure starts rising at age 6 to 7 yrs, it does so more rapidly in boys than in girls until the age of 18, when the 50th percentile for systolic pressure in boys is about 5 mm Hg higher than for girls (10). Although differences in body mass are likely to be the major determinants of this relatively small difference in blood pressure, the different hormonal environment may also contribute (21).

FACTORS AFFECTING BLOOD PRESSURE

Weight and Sex

Although the correlation coefficients are low, there is a statistically significant correlation between infant blood pressures and weights at all ages studied from 4 days to 4 yrs (8, 11). At age 1, each kilogram increase in body weight is associated with a 1 mm Hg increase in systolic pressure (8). At age 7, there is a difference of 15 mm Hg in systolic pressure between children in the 5th percentile for weight and those in the 95th percentile (20).

Wakefulness

At the age of 4 days, the mean blood pressure is about 5 mm Hg greater in awake than in asleep infants, and at age 6 weeks the difference is about 7 mm Hg (8). The effect of wakefulness can be demonstrated even in the youngest neonates and is independent of age. In the Brompton Study, infants were categorized as awake if their eyes were open and asleep if their eyes were closed at the onset of blood pressure measurement; on this basis, higher pressures were found in awake babies (15). Indeed, whenever the effect of wakefulness has been examined, the blood pressure always has been found to be higher in awake than in sleeping babies. In older children the effect of wakefulness has not been studied. For comparison with other studies, blood pressure should be measured in children sitting quietly after 5 min of rest whenever possible.

Environment

In children in the Brompton study the possible influences of place of blood pressure measurements (home versus school), time of day (10.00 to 15.00 hrs), time since previous meal (up to 5 hrs), and ambient temperature (14° to 25° C) were investigated. None of these factors significantly affected pressure. Mild intercurrent illness that required medication from a physician, but permitting blood pressure measurement at home or school, did not systematically affect pressure. It is probable that the variability of blood pressure and its measurement is so large that minor differences due to environmental factors are obscured.

Familial Aggregation

Familial aggregation of blood pressure in adults is well recognized. In children, some studies have shown significant correlations between mother and infants for both systolic and diastolic blood pressure (16, 17, 21–23). It is not clear to what extent these correlations reflect a shared environment in addition to genetic factors. Biron and Mongeau examined about 400 French Canadian families, each containing at least one adopted child (24). They found that correlations between the blood pressures of natural relatives were all significant, whereas correlations between the pressures of adopted children and their new families were not. This implies that environment is not important, or that the adopted children had not been relocated long enough for the effect of environment to be observed. Alternatively, if there was an effect of environment, it might be that it was most significant in the first few months and years of life.

Twin data also show significant correlations for blood pressure at age 7 yrs (25) and throughout childhood (26). Interestingly, the McIlhany study also showed a significant correlation in the degree of blood pressure elevation caused by the stress of a cold pressor test, as well as the absolute pressure (26).

BLOOD PRESSURE TRACKING

The tendency for individuals to maintain their position within the percentile distribution of blood pressure for chronological age has been described as "tracking." This is a phenomenon that is well established for adults. Once an individual is found to be hypertensive, he or she appears to remain hypertensive for the rest of life unless treated. However, the blood pressures of adults show regression toward the mean; i.e., those with extreme blood pressures on one occasion tend to have pressures nearer the mean when they are next studied.

Tracking of blood pressure has been demonstrated in children by examining the correlation in pressures measured on one occasion with those on subsequent occasions. A matrix of correlation coefficients for the children of the Brompton Study is shown in Table 45.2. After the age of 1 yr, the year-to-year correlation coefficient of pressure rises with age. Between the ages of 3 and 4 it is 0.47. The Brompton Study originally reported a significant correlation in pressure between 4 days and 6 weeks and this was taken to be evidence of tracking (27); however, there is only a weak correlation between blood pressures measured at 4 days and later pressures, and it is now believed that the original 4 day to 6 week correlation was more likely due to confounding circumstances, such as method of delivery.

Table 45.2.
Serial Correlations in Children's Blood Pressure, Corrected for Weight and Level of Consciousness, Between the Ages of 4 Days and 4 Yrs

	6 Weeks	6 M	1 Yr	2 Yr	3 Yr	4 Yr
4 days	0.17[a]	0.09[b]	−0.01	−0.05	−0.04	0.10[c]
6 weeks		0.04	0.05	0.02	0.10[b]	0.18[a]
6 months			0.12	0.12[c]	0.18[a]	−0.03
1 yr				.26[a]	0.27[a]	0.23[a]
2 yr					0.35[a]	0.32[a]
3 yr						0.47[a]

[a] $p < 0.001$. [b] $p < 0.01$. [c] $p < 0.05$.

Rosner and coworkers demonstrated tracking from the age of 5 yrs (28). They showed that the correlation coefficient of blood pressure measurements repeated at 4-yr intervals between the ages of 5 and 75 yr rises with age from 0.25 to about 0.65. The "Thousand Aviator" study also showed that those young adult Air Force recruits with relatively high blood pressures at age 18 tended to maintain their positions in the blood pressure distribution when observed 24 yrs later (29). Thus there is evidence that blood pressure tracking starts at age 1 yr and continues into adult life when measured at different ages, even though a longitudinal study of measurements made in the same individuals is not available. Nevertheless, the correlation coefficients of blood pressure in childhood are still relatively low, and tracking will only account for a small proportion (no more than 25%) of the blood pressure variance.

It is inappropriate to label a child as hypertensive because of a single blood pressure reading above the 95th percentile. Even if children have pressures persistently in excess of the 95th percentile, there is no evidence to support intervention with drug therapy. Under these circumstances, weight reduction, avoiding excessive sodium intake (30), and, later, caution against smoking and the contraceptive pill are the principal measures to be recommended.

If, however, the hypertension is due to renal disease, if there is evidence of end-organ damage, or if the patient is symptomatic, specific antihypertensive therapy is indicated.

References

1. Kitterman JA, Phibbs PH, Tooley WH: Aortic blood pressure in normal newborn infants during the first 12 hours of life. Pediatrics 44:959, 1969.
2. Elseed AM, Shinebourne EA, Joseph MC: Assessment of techniques for measurement of blood pressure in infants and children. Arch Dis Child 48:932, 1973.
3. Kannel WB, Gordon T, Schwartz MJ. Systolic versus diastolic blood pressure and risk of coronary heart disease. The Framingham study. Am J Cardiol 27:335, 1971.
4. Whyte RK, Elseed AM, Fraser CB, et al: Assessment of Doppler ultrasound to measure systolic blood pressures in infants and young children. Arch Dis Child 50:542, 1975.
5. Wright BM, Dore CF: A random zero sphygmomanometer. Lancet 1:337, 1970.
6. Van Den Berg BJ: Comparisons of blood pressure measurements by auscultation and Physiometrics Infrasonde recording techniques. Hypertension (Supplement 1):8, 1980.
7. Perlman LV, Chiang BH, Keller J, et al: Accuracy of sphygmomanometers in hospital practice. Arch Intern Med 125:1000, 1970.
8. de Swiet M, Fayers P, Shindbourne EA: Systolic blood pressure in a population of infants in the first year of life: The Brompton Study. Pediatrics 65:1028, 1980.
9. Steinfeld L, Dimich I, Reder R, et al: Sphygmomanometry in the pediatric patient. J Pediatr 92:934, 1978.
10. Report of the Task Force on Blood Pressure Control in Children: Pediatrics 59 (Supplement):707, 1977.

11. de Swiet M, Fayers P, Shinebourne EA: Value of repeated blood pressure measurements in children: The Brompton study. Br Med J 280:1567, 1980.
12. Earley A, Fayers P, Ng S, et al: Blood pressure in the first six weeks of life. Arch Dis Child 55:755, 1980.
13. Klopfenstein HS, Rudolph AM: Post natal changes in the circulation and responses to volume loading in sheep. Circ Res 42:839, 1978.
14. Kirkland RT, Kirkland JC: Systolic blood pressure measurement in the newborn infant with the transcutaneous Doppler method. J Pediatr 80:52, 1972.
15. de Swiet M, Fancourt R, Peto J: Systolic blood pressure variation during the first 6 days of life. Clin Sci Molec Med 49:557–61, 1975.
16. Zinner SH, Lee YH, Rosner B, et al: Factors affecting blood pressure in new born infants. Hypertension 2 (Supplement 1):101, 1980.
17. Hennekens CH, Jesse MJ, Klein BE, et al: Aggregation of blood pressure in infants and their siblings. Am J Epidemiol 103:457, 1976.
18. McDonough JR, Garrison GE, Hames CG: Blood pressure in hypertensive disease among negroes and whites: A study of Evans County, Georgia. Ann Intern Med 61:208, 1964.
19. Fixler DE, Kautz JA, Dana K: Systolic blood pressure differences among pediatric epidemiological studies. Hypertension 2 (Supplement 1):7, 1980.
20. Katz SH, Hediger ML, Schall JI, et al: Growth and blood pressure. In: Kotchen TA, Kotchen JM (eds): High Blood Pressure in the Young. Boston, Wright PSG, 1983.
21. Katz SH, Hediger ML, Schall JI, et al: Blood pressure, growth and maturation from childhood through adolescence. Mixed longitudinal analysis of the Philadelphia Blood Pressure Project. Hypertension 2 (Supplement 1):55, 1980.
22. Lee Y, Rosner B, Gould JB, et al: Familial aggregation of blood pressures of newborn infants and their mothers. Pediatrics 58:722, 1976.
23. Gupta JM, Scopes JW: Observations on blood pressure in newborn infants. Arch Dis Child 40:637, 1965.
24. Biron P, Mongeau JG: Familial aggregation of blood pressure and its components. Pediatr Clin North Am 25:29, 1978.
25. Havlik RJ, Garrison RJ, Katz SH, et al: Detection of genetic variance in blood pressure of seven-year-old twins. Am J Epidemiol 109:512, 1979.
26. McIlhany ML, Shaffer JW, Hines EA: The heritability of blood pressure: An investigation of 200 pairs of twins using the cold pressor test. John Hopkins Med J 136:57, 1975.
27. de Swiet M, Fayers P, Shinebourne EA: Blood pressure survey in a population of newborn infants. Br Med J 2:9–11, 1976.
28. Rosner B, Hennekens CH, Kass EH, et al: Age-specific correlation analysis of longitudinal blood pressure data. Am J Epidemiol 106:306, 1977.
29. Oberman A, Lane NE, Harlan W, et al: Trends in systolic blood pressure in the thousand aviator cohort over a twenty four year period. Circulation 36:812, 1967.
30. de Swiet M: Blood pressure, sodium, and take away food. Arch Dis Child 9. 57:645, 1982.
31. Blood Pressure Levels of Youths 6–11 Years: United States Vital and Health Statistics: Series 11, Data from the National Health Survey, No. 135, DHEW Publication No. (HRA) 74-1617. Washington, DC, U.S. Government Printing Office, 1973.
32. Blood Pressure of Youths 12–17 Years: United States Vital and Health Statistics: Series 11, Data from the National Health Survey, No. 163 DHEW Publication No. (HRA) 77-1645. Washington, DC, U.S. Government Printing Office, 1977.
33. Goldring D, Londe S, Sivakoff M, et al: Blood pressure in a high school population. J Pediatr 91:884, 1977.
34. Cardiovascular Profile of 15000 Children of School Age in Three Communities 1971–1975: DHEW Publication No. (NIH) 78-1472, Washington, DC, U.S. Government Printing Office, 1978.
25. Fixler DE, Laird WP, Fitzferald V, et al: Hypertension screening in schools: Results of the Dallas Study. Pediatrics 63:32, 1979.

CHAPTER 46

Clinical Aspects of Hypertension

M. J. DILLON

The overall incidence of high blood pressure in children is estimated at between 1% and 3% (1), though the definition of hypertension is necessarily somewhat arbitrary. Most of these children have only a mild increase in blood pressure, which is classified as primary or essential hypertension; however, there is a smaller number of children with much higher blood pressure who, in most cases, suffer from secondary hypertension and often require specific treatment (2–4). The prevalence of secondary hypertension in children is about 0.1% (1, 5)—similar to that of childhood diabetes mellitus. Hypertension also should be differentiated between transient and sustained.

The sequelae of untreated hypertension depend on its severity, duration, and cause. The mild increases in blood pressure seen in childhood essential hypertension may have little adverse effect until adult life. Moderate hypertension, however, has been shown to be a major factor in the genesis of arterial disease in adults. No long-term data on the natural history of moderately hypertensive children are available. However, severe hypertension in children, if untreated, is known to carry a high risk of morbidity and mortality. The most frequent complications of severe hypertension involve the central nervous system: hypertensive encephalopathy, facial palsy, visual impairment, cerebral infarction, and hemorrhage. Cardiac decompensation and renal failure are also well-recognized sequelae of uncontrolled severe hypertension.

A reduction in renal function that results from severe hypertension may be reversible, especially if there is no glomerular disease; however, severe hypertension usually is secondary to renal disease and even a short period of uncontrolled hypertension may cause severe and irreversible loss of renal function if control of blood pressure is delayed. There is good evidence of a link between the onset of hypertension and the deterioration of renal function in patients with reflux nephropathy (7).

PRESENTING FEATURES

Symptoms of hypertension vary considerably in affected children; often there are none, even in severe hypertension. Physical signs, similarly, frequently are minimal and may be overlooked or misinterpreted unless hypertension is considered and the blood pressure recorded. On the other hand, the symptoms of loss of consciousness, convulsions, and hemiplegia may develop dramatically in children who have had no symptoms or only minor symptoms that might have drawn attention to their hypertension earlier (8).

Presenting features differ according to age. During infancy, congestive cardiac failure, respiratory distress, vomiting and irritability, or failure to thrive are the most common features; whereas in older children headache, nausea, vomiting, polydipsia, polyuria, visual symptoms, tiredness, irritability, cardiac failure, facial weakness, epistaxis, and growth retardation are characteristic (1, 9, 10) (Tables 46.1 and 46.2). Palpitations, sweating, and pallor at any age may suggest an underlying pheochromocytoma, but these symptoms occur sometimes with other causes of hypertension, such as renovascular disease.

Physical examination may reveal signs of cardiomegaly or hypertensive retinopathy. There may be signs associated with the specific underlying cause of the hypertension, e.g., delayed pulses and blood pressure differences between the upper and lower limbs in coarctation of the aorta; a bruit in the abdomen or flank associated with renovascular disease or collateral vessels secondary to it; cafe-au-lait skin patches or other features of neurofibromatosis with renal artery disease; skeletal, perianal, or abdominal wall abnormalities that may point to a neuropathic bladder or an obstructive uropathy; abdominal masses in nephroblastoma and neuroblastoma; and cushingoid features or evidence of virilization in disturbances of adrenocortical function.

Of these signs and symptoms, several neurological features are particularly important. Headache is a common presenting symptom in children beyond infancy (1) and may precede the detection of hypertension by months or years. Not infrequently it is considered to be caused by migraine, which it resembles, especially if there are associated vomiting and visual symptoms. Another common mistake is to attribute the headache to a refractive error. Occasionally, in very young children, behavior disorders, including head-banging, appear to be linked to hypertension possibly caused by headache; these improve with antihypertensive therapy.

Another important sign of hypertension in childhood is facial palsy, a well-recognized presenting feature (1, 11, 12) that may be recurrent. At the Hospital for Sick Children, Great Ormond Street, 16 children with severe hypertension have presented during the past 10 yr with facial palsy (7 of these had chronic pyelonephritic scarring and 6 had renovascular disease), an incidence of 7% among children treated for severe hypertension. The facial palsy of hypertension is thought to be caused by hypertensive vascular damage to the vasa nervorum serving the facial nerve in its canal and is a reflection of severe long-standing hypertension rather than a short-lived episode. It usually is reversible once the hypertension is controlled.

Visual disturbances in malignant hypertension deserve special men-

Table 46.1.
Incidence of Major Clinical Features of Hypertension in Infants

Clinical feature	Percentage
Congestive cardiac failure	56
Respiratory distress	36
Failure to thrive, vomiting	29
Irritability	20
Convulsions	11

From Leumann EP: Blood pressure and hypertension in childhood and adolescence. Ergebnisse der Inneren Medizin und Kinderheilkunde 43:109, 1979.

Table 46.2.
Major Clinical Features of Hypertension in Older Children

	Percentage
Headache	30.0
Nausea, vomiting	13.0
Hypertensive encephalopathy	10.6
Polydipsia, polyuria	7.4
Visual problems	5.2
Tiredness, irritability	4.5
Cardiac failure	4.5
Facial palsy	3.4
Epistaxis	3.0
Growth retardation, weight loss	2.7
Cardiac murmur	2.7
Abdominal pain	1.8
Enuresis	1.2

From Leumann EP: Blood pressure and hypertension in childhood and adolescence. Ergebnisse der Inneren Medizin und Kinderheilkunde 43:109, 1979.

tion: they may be caused by direct retinal disruption associated with retinal infarcts, hemorrhages, papilledema, cortical blindness (9, 13); vitreous hemorrhage; or infarction of the anterior visual pathways (12, 14, 15). The last is particularly important since it may result in permanent visual loss; it should be borne in mind when treatment strategies are being planned, as it may be precipitated by sudden hypotension when long-standing high blood pressure is being reduced and autoregulatory forces fail to ensure adequate perfusions of the optic nerve. The cause is damage to the microvasculature in the ciliary artery bed that supplies the anterior part of the optic nerve, coupled with effects on perfusion of optic disc swelling (15).

Children may complain of transient mild disturbances such as blurred vision, "flashing lights," or more serious episodes of visual loss. Physical examination may reveal the obvious retinal changes of arterial narrowing, arteriovenous nicking, exudates, hemorrhages, papilledema, or vitreous hemorrhage. An important additional observation is the pupillary reaction to light. In cortical blindness and in most patients with retinal blindness, the light reflex is retained; in anterior ischemic optic neuropathy it is lost, yet the accommodation reflux remains normal.

Children may present with encephalopathy that develops into devastating neurological complications due to cerebral infarction or hemorrhage. Major neurological complications have been reported by several authors (2, 3); at the Hospital for Sick Children, 23% of 326 children admitted with severe hypertension experienced these complications. Recognizing the presenting features of the neurological complications of hypertension is thus critical.

STRATEGY OF INVESTIGATION

The extent to which investigation is warranted depends on the severity of the hypertension and the circumstances in which it was detected. There are clearly important differences between mild hypertension identified incidentally in an asymptomatic child and severe hypertension observed in a patient with clinical symptoms related to it. Symptomatic hypertension, in general, is moderate to severe and secondary in nature; however, severe hypertension may be detected in an asymptomatic form. All children with hypertension should undergo some evaluation, but the question arises as to how intensive it should be. The degree of investigative zeal might be defined by the level and consistency of blood pressure recorded and the age of the patient.

Leumann (1) defined borderline hypertension as systolic or diastolic pressures repeatedly above the 90th and occasionally above the 95th percentile; mild-to-moderate hypertension as blood pressure repeatedly exceeding the 95th percentile but not as high as in severe hypertension and without target organ involvement; and severe hypertension as blood pressures repeatedly exceeding the 95th percentile by more than 15 mm Hg or any elevation of blood pressure with signs of target organ involvement.

On this basis, borderline hypertension requires a history with special reference to family members affected by hypertension or cardiovascular disease and, in girls, questions concerning the use of the contraceptive pill. Clinical examination should include repeated blood pressure recordings to establish the consistency of the blood pressure readings and physical examination that includes careful fundoscopy and examination for bruits and pulse deficits. Laboratory tests should include routine urinalysis and measurement of plasma creatinine, urea, electrolytes, calcium, cholesterol, and urate.

Mild-to-moderate hypertension requires more extensive evaluation and should include some form of renal imaging. This may consist of an abdominal ultrasound study and a technetium 99m-DMSA scan or a rapid sequence intravenous urogram. The measurement of plasma renin activity, aldosterone level, and a 24-hour urine VMA or plasma catecholamine measurement are also recommended. An electrocardiogram (ECG) and chest roentgenogram would complete this preliminary investigative protocol (Table 46.3).

Severe hypertension justifies all these investigations and, depending on initial findings, more complex or invasive procedures as well. These may include angiography, renal vein renin sampling, vena caval catecholamine measurements, urine steroid estimations, computerized tomography (CT) studies, voiding cystourethrogram (VCU), bone marrow examination, echocardiography, cardiac catheterization, and steroid suppression tests.

INVESTIGATIONS

The investigation of a hypertensive child depends not only on the severity of the hypertension but also on whether the child is symptomatic and hypertension is the suspected cause. Possible investigative procedures range from routine tests available in most hospitals to more refined invasive procedures available in specialized units.

Routine Investigations

All children with moderate-to-severe hypertension should have a complete blood count, plasma (or serum) electrolytes, urea nitrogen (BUN), creatinine, and calcium; urinalysis including estimation of proteinuria; a chest roentgenogram, an electrocardiogram; and some form of renal imaging. This protocol will identify the presence of significant anemia with or without fragmentation of red cells or iron deficiency

Table 46.3.
Investigation of Children with Hypertension

A	Complete blood count Plasma electrolytes, calcium, urate, cholesterol, urea, creatinine Urinalysis
B	Abdominal ultrasound ^{99}Tc-DMSA scan or rapid sequence IVU +/− Micturating cystourethrogram Peripheral plasma renin and aldosterone 24-hr urine VMA or plasma catecholamine Chest roentgenogram and ECG
C	Angiography, digital vascular imaging Main and segmental renal vein renin sampling Vena caval catecholamine sampling Computerized tomography Urine steroid analysis 2D echocardiogram, cardiac catheterization ^{99}Tc-DTPA scan ^{131}I MIBG scan ^{131}I 19-iodo cholesterol scan Pharmacological blockade or renin angiotensin system Pharmacological catecholamine blockade Bone marrow Steroid suppression tests, adrenal venous steroid

Strategy of Investigation (see text for details)
Borderline hypertension: A (at least)
Mild-to-moderate sustained hypertension: A and B (at least)
Moderate-to-severe sustained hypertension: A and B + items from C

changes; hypokalemia (which may be due to primary or secondary hyperaldosteronism); impaired renal function; hypercalcemia; urinary tract infection or hematuria with or without proteinuria; evidence of left ventricular hypertrophy implying significant hypertension; and obvious structural and functional anomalies of the kidneys.

Renal Imaging

The value of the intravenous urogram (IVU) in the investigation of hypertension is beginning to be questioned. Undoubtedly an IVU may reveal obvious asymmetry of kidney size and function, kidney displacement, and the presence of parenchymal loss or other structural anomaly such as hydronephrosis, tumor, or cystic disease. It may also demonstrate, by rapid sequence technique, a delayed nephrogram appearance and a dense prolonged pyelogram on the side of a unilateral main renal artery stenosis. However, it has its disadvantages: the solute load may be unacceptable in a child with poorly controlled hypertension; it may not reveal the kidneys at all if renal function is seriously impaired; it may fail to demonstrate parenchymal loss, especially if renal scars are situated anteriorly or posteriorly; and its reliability in detecting renal artery stenosis in children is limited by the incidence of bilateral and intrarenal arterial lesions.

Recent advances in ultrasound (US) have resulted in high-quality images with a resolution of 2 to 3 mm. No specific pediatric ultrasound unit is required, although appropriate transducers to examine neonates and infants are necessary. US is valuable in assessing abdominal masses, differentiating between solid and cystic lesions, and identifying the origin of a mass, for example, intrarenal or extrarenal. US may be used to determine renal size and to demonstrate renal scarring or the presence of calculi. Dilatation of the collecting systems, the presence of a duplex system, ureterocele, thickened bladder wall, and dilatation of the posterior uretha can be demonstrated. There are, however, shortcomings to its use in hypertension. It does not indicate a level of renal function and therefore must be coupled with some other form of imaging for this; it can often miss pathological conditions in the region of the upper renal poles because the rib acoustic shadows may obscure these, and its value is very much operator-dependent.

The VCU obviously is indicated when vesicoureteric reflux or obstructive uropathy is considered. Its use poses no problem in hypertension since there is no solute load; when renal function is impaired it may provide considerable information about pelvicalyceal appearance and, of course, the presence or absence of urethral valves or other lower urinary tract anomalies.

Special Investigations

Special investigations include specific imaging techniques such as radionuclide imaging, angiography, digital vascular imaging, computerized tomography; measurements of active hormones in urine and peripheral, vena caval, renal, and adrenal venous blood; tests dependent on pharmacological blockade of active hormones; and steroid suppression tests.

Radionuclide Imaging

Images obtained by the gamma camera after injection of radiopharmaceuticals containing gamma-emitting nuclides have revolutionized diagnostic investigation during the last decade. Although this will have already been dealt with in some detail in Chapter 20, specific mention is made here of the techniques and its value in childhood hypertension.

Technetium 99m-Dimercaptosuccinic Acid (DMSA) Scan. The ^{99m}Tc-DMSA scan is an example of a "static" renal scan and is a useful means of evaluating the renal parenchyma. In healthy children approximately 50% of the administered dose is localized in the kidneys in one hour; the cortical to medullary ratio is high. The bound isotope appears to reflect the functioning proximal tubular mass and has been especially valuable in childhood hypertension in detecting areas of pyelonephritic scarring (17, 18) and ischemic areas of kidney due to renovascular disease (19). The DMSA scan also has an important role in identifying small, poorly functioning kidneys and renal tumors and for obtaining information about differential renal function (20). Radiation is much less than in the standard IVU examination; the gonadal radiation dose is very low. Although these advantages are offset slightly by the persistence of the DMSA within the kidney after injection, the half-life of ^{99m}Tc is very short, so that total kidney irradiation remains low; i.e., a 1 mCi dose of ^{99m}-Tc-DMSA gives only 730 mrads to the kidneys; the majority of children receive less than this because of size-related dose reduction. The correlations between regions of scarring and ischemia identified by ^{99m}Tc-DMSA and renal artery anomalies identified by arteriography or regions of high renin release by segmental renal vein renin sampling (18, 19) are good. DMSA demonstrates pathological tissue within kidneys that the IVU and US fail to detect and therefore makes a valuable contribution in hypertensive investigation (Fig. 46.1). Combined with the US it provides a useful initial imaging of the kidneys without a solute load or excess radiation.

^{99m}Tc-Diethylene Triamine Pentacetic Acid (DTPA) Scan. ^{99m}Tc-DTPA is filtered by the glomeruli of the kidney and is neither reabsorbed nor excreted by the tubules. It is a dynamic scan that gives information on renal perfusion, glomerular filtration rate (GFR), and renal transit time. The collecting systems also are visualized. The scan may be used to measure relative GFR in each kidney; with adaptation, GFR may be quantified. Obstructive uropathy can be demonstrated using the washout of isotope from the renal tract with furosemide; vesicoureteric reflux

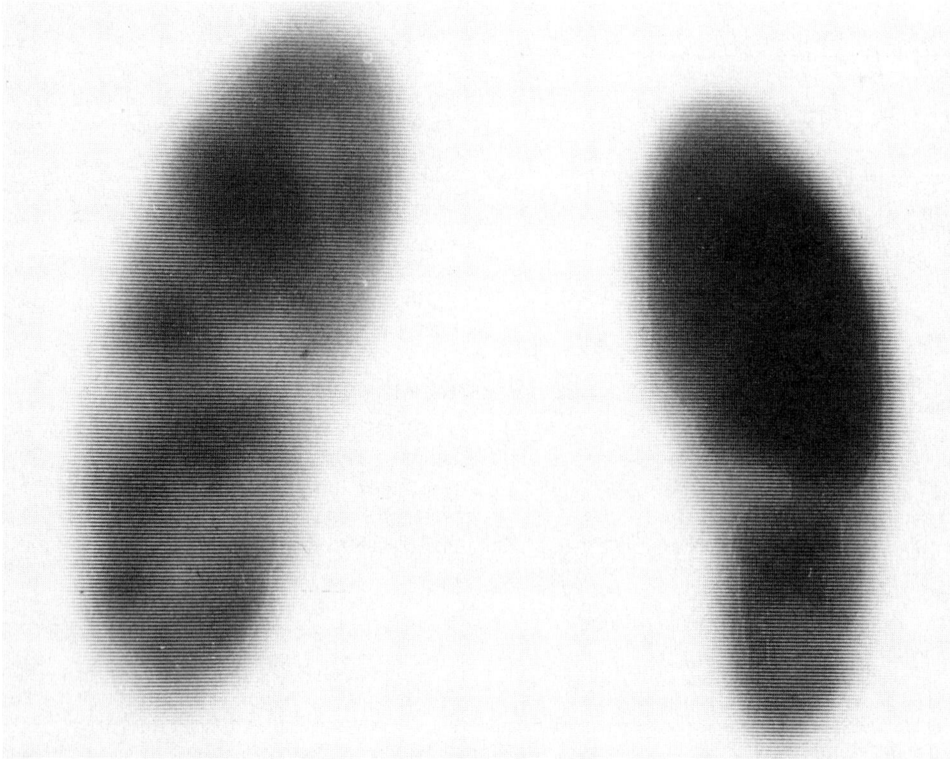

Figure 46.1. ^{99m}Tc DMSA scan undertaken in a hypertensive child with widespread intrarenal vascular disease demonstrating multiple regions of decreased isotope uptake in renal parenchyma. IVU and US were normal.

can be identified by means of the indirect technique. Finally, the inferior vena cava can be outlined by injecting isotope into a foot or leg vein (20–23); however, in spite of initial promise, DTPA has not proved as valuable in hypertension as anticipated. It can demonstrate decreased renal perfusion in unilateral main renal artery stenosis but is not particularly helpful when bilateral or intrarenal arterial disease is present (19). When renal function is seriously impaired, $Na^{123}I$ is more useful.

^{131}I-19-Iodocholesterol Scintigraphy. This technique may be used to localize adrenal lesions in Cushing syndrome and in primary hyperaldosteronism (24). It is rarely used in children. The thyroid gland needs protection by prior administration of potassium perchlorate or iodide.

^{131}I Meta-iodobenzylguanidine scintigraphy (^{131}I MIBG). ^{131}I MIBG resembles norepinephrine in molecular structure and concentrates in adrenergic tissue through a pathway related to function. It has localized pheochromocytomas when other methods have failed (25). The test is quicker than iodocholesterol scans—two days as opposed to seven or eight days for iodocholesterol. Experience is limited, but so far the method offers hope of a safe diagnostic tool. Its value is still undefined.

Angiography

Angiography is invasive. Its use is indicated in childhood hypertension under certain circumstances: (a) when coarctation of the aorta is suspected, it would be part of an angiocardiographic examination; (b) when renovascular disease is suspected, in which case a flush aortogram and selective renal arteriograms would be necessary; (c) when a renal tumor is suspected and not identified by other investigative modalities; (d) in the investigative procedures for pheochromocytoma; and (e) occasionally in the presence of an adrenocortical tumor. It is most commonly undertaken in children with renin-dependent hypertension in whom no obvious cause, such as pyelonephritic scarring, is present and in whom the prospect of a surgical cure for the hypertension exists. The study is usually combined with and preceded by renal vein renin sampling. It must not be performed in the presence of poorly controlled hypertension, and blood pressure monitoring must be undertaken throughout, especially at times of contrast medium injection. In the presence of a possible pheochromocytoma, angiography is even more prone to complications unless the child is given α- and β-sympathetic blocking drugs beforehand. In suspected pheochromocytoma the study usually is combined with and preceded by caval venous sampling for catecholamine. It is important that oblique as well as anteroposterior views are obtained when attempting to identify small intrarenal vessel abnormalities or tumor vasculature serving a small adrenal tumor. See Chapter 20 for more detail concerning technique and interpretation.

Digital Vascular Imaging (DVI)

Digital vascular imaging (DVI) is a new method of demonstrating renal and other vasculature by intra-arterial or intravenous injection of relatively small quantities of contrast medium; it is still being evaluated (26, 27). The noninvasiveness of the intravenous route makes it attractive for use with children; however, our limited experience so far suggests that although major vessels are demonstrated clearly by IV injection, the technique is not particularly effective in outlining the intrarenal vasculature, which is so often abnormal in childhood renovascular disease. Using DVI with standard angiography, superb definition is obtained with minute amounts of injected contrast medium. Khoury and coworkers (28) have shown that DVI also is useful in evaluating the vascular anatomy in renal transplant recipients.

Computerized Tomography

Computerized tomographic (CT) scanning can identify the presence and position of intra-abdominal masses when other investigative procedures have failed. Although its usefulness has been demonstrated in, for

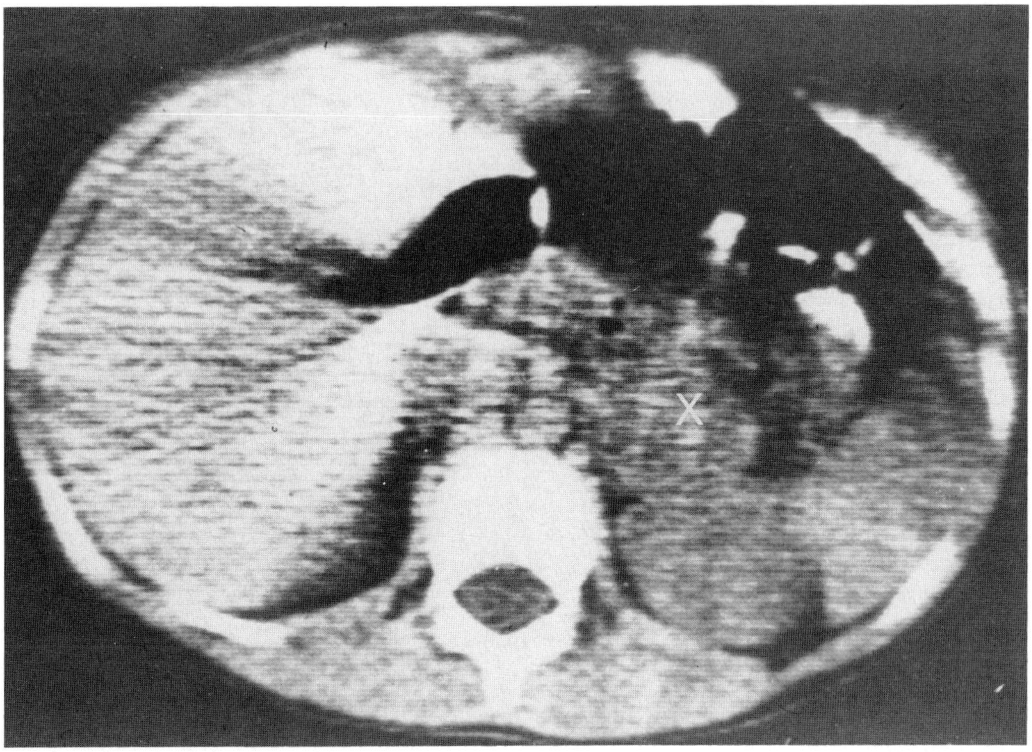

Figure 46.2. Computerized tomogram of abdomen of child with left-sided pheochromocytoma situated above and anterior to left kidney.

example, the investigation of adrenal tumors such as pheochromocytomas (Fig. 46.2), it can fail to demonstrate fairly obvious lesions (29). CT scans of the head have been valuable in assessing the child with neurological complications of hypertension in which brain swelling, cerebral infarct, or hemorrhage may be suspected.

Peripheral Venous Renin Measurements

The ischemic kidney secretes renin and, through the vasopressor effects of angiotensin II, causes hypertension. There is some controversy over whether the measurement of peripheral renin levels, such as plasma renin activity (PRA), can demonstrate that the renin-angiotensin aldosterone system (RAAS) is stimulated in childhood hypertension (30, 31); however, most children with hypertension secondary to renovascular disease or pyelonephritic scarring have raised peripheral PRA values (Fig. 46.3) (31, 32). Hypertensive children may have an increased PRA without underlying renal disease (30), but the converse rarely occurs. A very low PRA in an hypertensive child may be due to salt and water overload or be the clue to an underlying mineralocorticoid excess state (33–35).

Measurement of peripheral PRA may eventually have a role in predicting which children with pyelonephritic scarring will subsequently develop hypertension. Approximately 10% of children with renal scarring become hypertensive (36), and it is important to identify those at risk for this complication. If overproduction of renin in this situation is the cause of the hypertension, early measurement of PRA may have predictive value. In a study by Savage and coworkers (32), 8 of 100 normotensive children with renal scarring had peripheral PRA values above the normal range for age and the negative correlation between PRA and age was much weaker for the children with renal scarring than in normal children. During a five-year follow-up period the negative correlation between renin and age in this group of children was obliterated, yet in individual subjects there is no clear relationship between initial PRA and subsequent development of hypertension. Patients with renal scarring require long-term longitudinal follow-up because hypertension may develop later than the five-year follow-up now reported.

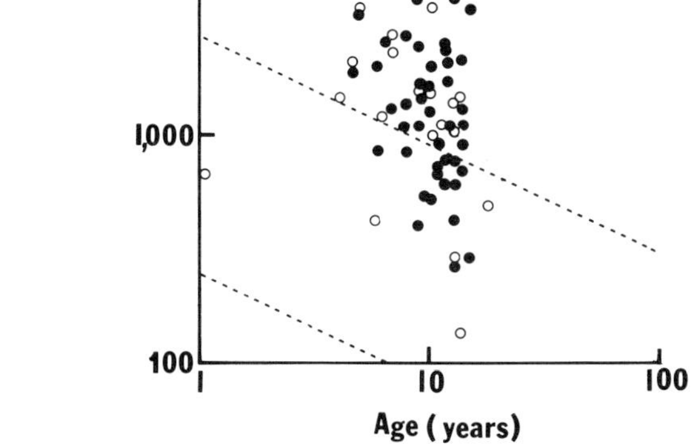

Figure 46.3. Peripheral plasma renin activity of hypertensive children. Dotted lines indicate upper and lower limits of normal range. Open circles represent patients with renovascular disease and closed circles patients with coarse renal scarring due to reflux nephropathy.

In practical terms an untreated, elevated PRA in a moderately hypertensive child strongly suggests renin-dependent hypertension. Conversely, a low or normal PRA is a strong indication that renin-dependent hypertension is not present. If PRA is very low, a mineralocorticoid excess state is likely.

Renal Venous Renin Measurements

Bilateral renal venous renin levels have been established as important in diagnosing surgically curable forms of renal hypertension in adults (37); this technique has also been successfully applied to the investigation of hypertensive children (30, 38, 39). Gerdts and coworkers (40) have established a reference range for renal venous PRA values in normotensive children free from renal disease. This study supported a ratio of 1.5 as an acceptable upper limit of normality for the interpretation of renal venous PRA ratios in the investigation of children with suspected renal hypertension.

In hypertensive children in whom renal venous renin measurements have been taken, the ratio of 1.5 or above between the main renal veins has been shown to be a good predictor of surgical success in patients with renal lesions amenable to surgical treatment (Fig. 46.4) (39). The value of this method may be limited however, because ratios less than 1.5:1 occur when a lesion exists and only the main renal venous blood is sampled (38). This problem is diminished when segmental renal venous sampling is used (Fig. 46.5) (19, 41, 42). Current practice at the Hospital for Sick Children is to undertake main vein, inferior vena caval, and segmental sampling from the upper, middle, and lower zones of each kidney in every child undergoing renal vein sampling. Results from segmental renal vein renin studies, DMSA scan and angiography usually agree in children with renovascular disease (19, 43). Results from segmental renal vein renin studies and DMSA scans in children with reflex nephropathy also agree (18). Appropriate surgical interventions have been possible as a result.

Plasma Renin-Aldosterone Profile

Parallel measurements of peripheral PRA and plasma aldosterone concentration (PA) may be helpful in identifying mineralocorticoid excess states (44). A suppressed PRA with inappropriately raised PA is characteristic in hyperaldosteronism, whereas a low or normal PA is characteristic in the hypertensive forms of congenital adrenal hyperplasia, e.g., 11-hydroxylase deficiency and the low renin hypertension of cortisol-11β-hydroxysteroid dehydrogenase deficiency. Conversely, in hypertension associated with salt-wasting congenital adrenal hyperplasia, e.g., 21-hydroxylase deficiency, PRA is markedly increased and PA is low. If PRA and PA are both decreased in this condition, the likely explanation is overtreatment with mineralocorticoid such as 9-α-fludrocortisone.

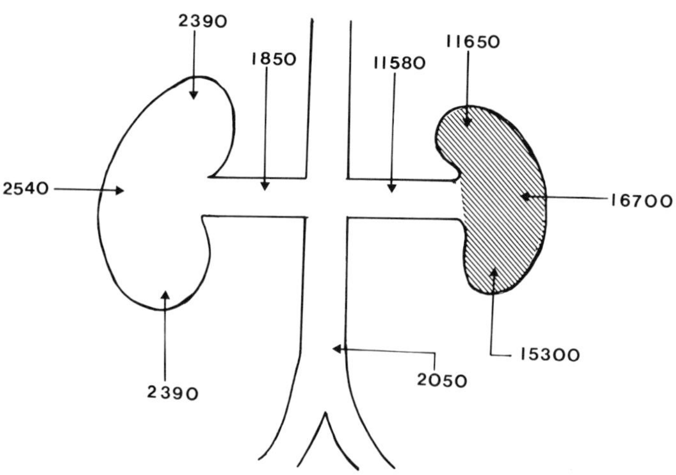

Figure 46.4. Main and segmental renal vein renin measurements in child with left-sided renal artery stenosis. PRA (in ng A1 l^{-1} h^{-1}) in main renal veins, segmental renal veins, and inferior vena cava demonstrates lateralization of renin release to left kidney (left to right main renal vein ratio: 6.25) and suppression of right kidney (right main renal vein to IVC ratio: 0.90).

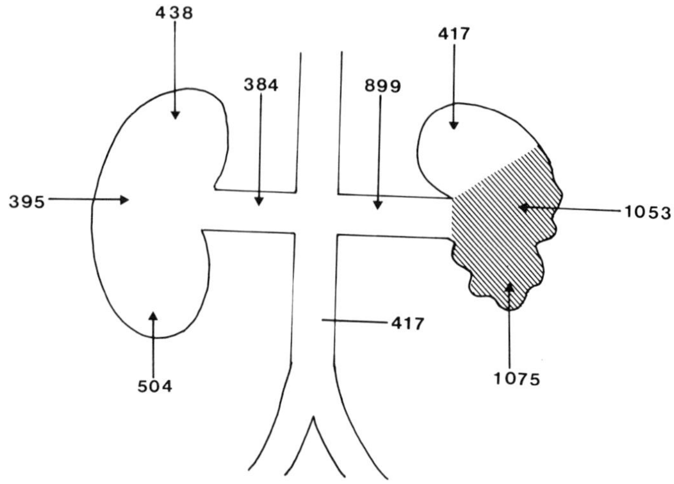

Figure 46.5. Main and segmental renal vein renin measurements in child with left-sided reflux nephropathy. PRA (in A1 l^{-1} h^{-1}) in main renal veins and segmental renal veins, and IVC demonstrates localization of renin release to left kidney but also defines local region of excess release in lower and mid zones of kidney with suppression of upper pole.

Pharmacological Blockade of the Renin Angiotensin System

Pharmacological blockade of angiotensin II may have diagnostic value (Fig. 46.6). Saralasin (1-sar-8-ala-angiotensin II), a competitive angiotensin II inhibitor, is used in certain types of hypertension to identify the RAAS as the cause (45, 46). If infusion of saralasin intravenously under controlled conditions decreases blood pressure and increases PRA, the test is positive. Although the test also may be helpful in children, it must be interpreted with caution. When using this test it is important to avoid salt-depletion of the patients because this can cause a false-positive result (47). We recommend using the test only in the hypertensive child in whom the peripheral PRA is equivocal and additional conformation of a renin component is required. Because it is time-consuming and prone to error, we do not recommend it for general use.

The oral converting enzyme inhibitor, captopril (SQ 14225) (48), initially looked promising as another diagnostic test for hyperreninemic hypertension; however, its ability to lower blood pressure in a variety of conditions independent of its effect on PRA has caused concern about its value in diagnosis. The hypotensive response to captopril has been used in renovascular disease to predict the outcome of surgical treatment (49). The response to an oral dose of captopril may help in identifying the children who have raised PRA values (50).

Urine and Plasma Catecholamines

The commonest screening test for pheochromocytoma is the measurement of urinary vanillylmandelic acid (VMA), although a normal level does not exclude the diagnosis. Most patients with a pheochromocytoma have markedly elevated levels of catecholamines and both deaminated and *o*-methylated metabolites in their urine (51). Of the two urine metabolites of catecholamines urinary metanephrine excretion is a more reliable test for pheochromocytoma (29). With sensitive and specific

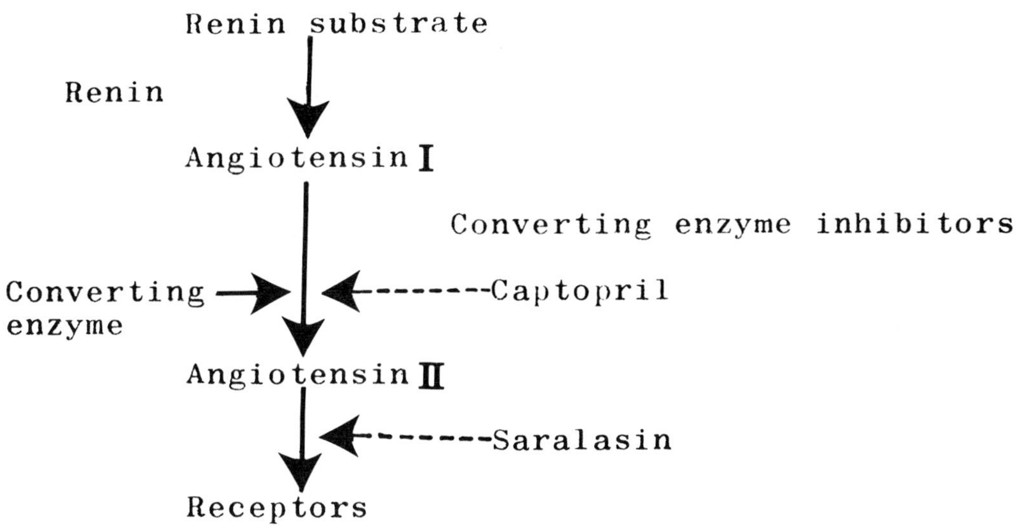

Figure 46.6. Diagrammatic representation of renin-angiotensin system showing sites of blockade by saralasin and captopril.

radioenzymatic techniques, it is possible to measure circulating catecholamines; this method is even more reliable than that for urinary metanephrine excretion and is extremely accurate (52). In view of this, it is now policy to diagnose pheochromocytoma by measuring plasma catecholamines. Plasma norepinephrine measurements are invariably raised in patients with pheochromocytoma irrespective of the level of blood pressure (29, 51).

Pharmacological Catecholamine Blockade

The hypotensive response to the intravenously administered short-acting α-blocker, phentolamine, has been used as a diagnostic test. A lack of specificity (false-negatives up to 50% and false-positives up to 10%) limits its usefulness. There also is a risk of a precipitous fall of pressure, which has caused death. An alternative therapeutic trial of oral phenoxybenzamine also gives misleading results. Neither is recommended.

Vena Caval Catecholamine Measurements

Localization of a catecholamine-producing tumor may prove difficult. Vena caval catheterization and multiple site sampling for plasma catecholamine estimations have proved to be a useful adjunct to other investigative procedures and may, in addition to confirming the presence of a single tumor, identify hitherto unknown multiple lesions (Fig. 46.7) (29).

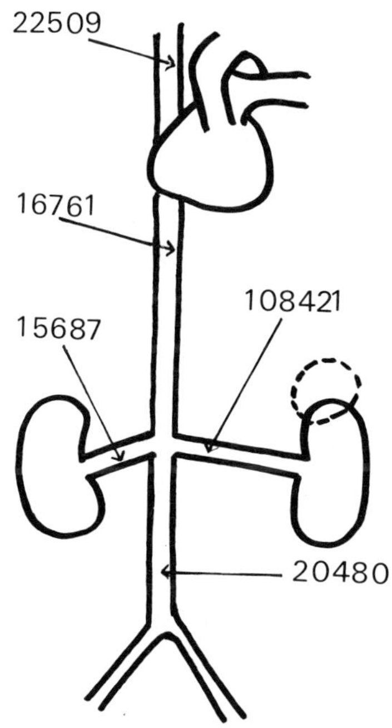

Figure 46.7. Vena caval and renal vein catecholamine measurements in a child with a left-sided adrenal pheochromocytoma. Norepinephrine (in pg/ml) in left renal vein confirms excess release from adrenal on that side draining into renal vein.

Urine Steroid Analysis

The analysis of 24-hour urine for steroids may prove valuable in investigations of endocrine hypertension. Excess mineralocorticoids are present in 11-β- and 17-α-hydroxylase deficiency with characteristic changes in glucocorticoids and sex steroids (53). Similarly, in Conn's syndrome, excess urine aldosterone is demonstrated, but without the findings seen in patients with steroid biosynthetic blockade. In the group of patients with low renin hypertension who do not come under the previous categories, the use of mass spectrometric–gas chromatographic analysis allows detection of minor but characteristic changes due to the decreased metabolism of cortisol; this allows the diagnosis of cortisol 11β-hydroxysteroid dehydrogenase deficiency to be made (34, 35).

Other Investigative Procedures for Endocrine Hypertension

Various stimulation and suppression tests are available for investigating Cushing's and Conn's syndromes, as well as low renin hypertension (for further details see References 53 and 54). Sampling from adrenal veins may be helpful in localizing the source of excess aldosterone secretion in Conn's syndrome; the process is similar to renal vein renin sampling for renin-dependent hypertension.

CAUSES

The causes of hypertension in children are divided into those that cause transient and those that cause sustained hypertension. The causes of severe and, in most cases, sustained hypertension in 326 children admitted to the Hospital for Sick Children are cited in Table 46.4.

Transient Hypertension

Many conditions that may be associated with acute and usually short-lived increases in blood pressure do not produce sustained hypertension at a later stage. Nevertheless, during the acute phase, the blood pressure may be of sufficient severity to require treatment in its own right.

Within this category, as in other childhood hypertensive states, renal disease predominates (Table 46.5). Hypertension is common in acute glomerulonephritis and in Henoch-Schönlein nephritis; it is present in one third of patients with the hemolytic uremic syndrome, and it is frequent in acute renal failure from any cause. The increased blood pressure in these circumstances usually is due to salt and water retention; however, in some situations, especially in the presence of renal ischemia or arteriolar damage, there is a contribution from the renin-angiotensin system.

Following urological surgery, transient hypertension often develops; it may be caused by disturbance of the renal pedicle or kidney with release of renin.

Hypertension during relapse of nephrotic syndrome is important and often misunderstood. It may be caused by the underlying disease state, for example, membranoproliferative glomerulonephritis with salt retention secondary to extensive renal parenchymal damage, or it may be iatrogenically caused by steroid therapy or overvigorous plasma replacement. A common and often overlooked cause, however, is hypovolemia with massive angiotensin release, which causes peripheral vasoconstriction to such an extent that, even though intravascular volume is diminished, blood pressure rises. The treatment, paradoxically, is ECF volume-repletion using plasma or saline; with repletion the blood pressure and plasma angiotensin II levels fall. A similar response may occur in any patient with chronic ECF volume depletion, e.g., patients with severe burns and those with renal and gastrointestinal salt-wasting states. It may be particularly confusing in salt-wasting congenital adrenal hyperplasia when mineralocorticoid is being administered.

Hypertension also is seen in the presence of raised intracranial pressure due to tumor, infection, injury, and in association with convulsions. In these circumstances, disturbance of the medullary vasomotor center, which modifies sympathetic nervous system activity, may play a role, but other factors, including changes in circulatory levels of the vasoactive hormones renin and vasopressin, also may be important. Sudden increases in blood pressure occur in the Guillain-Barré syndrome, poliomyelitis, and familial dysautonomia, probably for similar reasons.

Any of the following may cause significant but transient hypertension: lead poisoning; treatment with corticosteroid or sympathomimetic mediators; the contraceptive pill; or excess administration of blood, plasma, or saline.

Table 46.4.
Causes of Severe Hypertension in Children at the Hospital for Sick Children, London (1971–1983)

Diagnosis		Number of children	Percent
Coarse renal scarring	Chronic pyelonephritis	60	18.4
	Obstructive uropathy and neuropathic bladder	56	17.2
Glomerulonephritis		76	23.3
Renovascular disease		31	9.5
Coarctation of aorta		29	8.9
Renal polycystic disease		18	5.5
Hemolytic uremic syndrome		13	4.0
Idiopathic (essential)		11	3.4
Catecholamine excess states		9	2.8
Wilms tumor		8	2.4
Miscellaneous		15	4.6
		326	100

Table 46.5.
Causes of "Transient" Hypertension

Acute glomerulonephritis	
Henoch-Schönlein nephritis	
Hemolytic uremic syndrome	
Acute renal failure	
Following urological surgery	
Following renal transplantation	
Acute hypovolemia	Nephrotic relapse; Burns; Renal, adrenal and gastrointestinal saline depletion
Central nervous system disease	Tumor; Infection; Injury; Fits
Guillain-Barré syndrome	
Poliomyelitis	
Familial dysautonomia	
Hypercalcemia	
Lead poisoning	
Drug therapy or overdose	Corticosteroid; Sympathomimetic; Contraceptive pill
Excess administration of	Blood; Plasma; Saline

Sustained Hypertension

Sustained hypertension in childhood, especially if severe, is also likely to be secondary to renal disease (4). The main causes are given in Table 46.6. The most common underlying factor is activation of the RAAS. In the very young, coarctation of the aorta predominates. ECF volume overexpansion is the underlying factor in many cases of renal insufficiency.

Coarctation of the Aorta

Coarctation is observed in approximately 10% of children with sustained hypertension (1). The cause of hypertension is complex and not fully understood. Mechanical obstruction is the simplest explanation. The role of the renin-angiotensin system is controversial; there is evidence to implicate angiotension II in those patients in whom leg pressures are higher than normal for age (55). A hypotensive response to the angiotensin II competitive antagonist, saralasin, in this group tends to support this hypothesis (56). Diagnosis of coarctation is based on the findings of upper limb hypertension associated with delayed femoral pulses and a blood pressure gradient of 20 mm Hg or more between arms and legs.

Coarctation may be more extensive and involve the abdominal aorta

Table 46.6.
Causes of Sustained Hypertension in Childhood

Coarctation of aorta	
Chronic renal failure	
Renin-dependent hypertension	Renovascular disease Renal parenchymal disease Renal tumors
Catecholamine excess hypertension	Pheochromocytoma Neuroblastoma
Corticosteroid excess hypertension	Congenital adrenal hyperplasia Conn's and Cushing's syndromes Low-renin hypertensive states
Essential hypertension	

as well. When this occurs, there is a considerable risk of the renal arteries being involved by narrowing at their origins or in a more diffuse intrarenal fashion akin to that observed in fibromuscular dysplasia (Fig. 46.8). In this situation the hypertension is likely to be renin-dependent. Neurofibromatosis (57) and Takayasu disease (58, 59) are well-recognized causes of abdominal aortic narrowing associated with renovascular disease. Narrowing of the abdominal aorta has followed abdominal irradiation of children for malignancy (60).

The most appropriate treatment for coarctation of the thoracic aorta is surgical repair (61). There is, however, uncertainty about the optimum age for surgical correction. Currently, infants presenting in congestive cardiac failure with coarctation associated with a shunt urgently require surgical intervention. Those with simple coarctation are best operated on when older, probably between 4 and 8 yr of age (61). Preoperative hypotensive therapy is not recommended unless an accelerated hypertensive state is present. When this is the case, drug therapy to lower blood pressure is indicated, although caution must be exercised to avoid compromising renal and lower limb perfusion. Postoperative hypertension occurs frequently, but the cause remains unclear. A transient, reactive hypertension, rising to a peak within 36 hr of surgery, may occur after an initial drop of blood pressure. A second type of hypertensive manifestation is more delayed but lasts longer, up to one to three weeks on occasion. Hypertension in the early postoperative period is closely related to the postcoarctectomy syndrome. This is associated with abominal pain, ileus, and manifestations of mesenteric arteritis (62, 63). The role of autoregulatory mechanisms and the effect of a gradient across the renal arteries consequent to increased aortic blood flow and the changed nature of that flow remains uncertain. Treatment with hypotensive agents may be necessary.

Coarctation of the abdominal aorta requires very different surgical management. By-pass procedures using prosthetic grafts and, more recently, intraluminal angioplasty have been performed; their use depends on the area of narrowing. The anatomical relationship between the aortic pathology and the renal arteries is important when planning therapy. If the coarcted area is below the origin of the renal arteries, the aorta alone may be dealt with; however, if the renal arteries arise from the narrowed aorta or are affected by renovascular disease, they will have to be dealt with at the same time as the aorta.

Volume-Dependent Hypertension

Sustained volume-dependent hypertension occurs only when renal function is severely reduced. Chronic renal failure (CRF) from any cause may be associated with hypertension caused by salt and water overload.

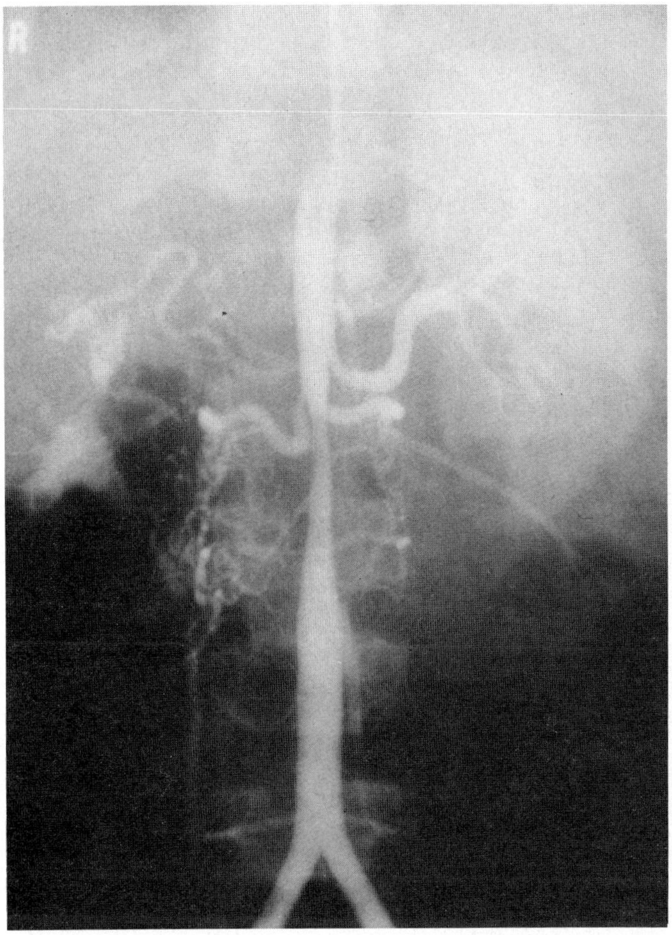

Figure 46.8. Flush aortogram in boy with neurofibromatosis demonstrating extensive narrowing of abdominal aorta, severe intrarenal artery disease on right, and proximal stenosis of left main renal artery. This boy's hypertension was cured by dilating his aorta and left renal artery and by right nephrectomy.

The treatment goal is to reduce ECF volume by dietary salt restriction, diuretics, and dialysis. Although in some cases there is evidence of an abnormal relationship between circulating renin and exchangeable sodium (64), in others hyperreninemia is an important contributor (10). The hypertension in chronic renal failure is most often ECF volume-dependent and responsive to its reduction. When renin is a contributing cause (65), drugs that specifically block angiotensin, converting enzyme, or bilateral nephrectomy may be used (62, 66). (See Chapter 53B.) The diagnosis usually is inferred from the presence of CRF, the absence of other factors, and response to therapy to lower ECF volume.

Renin-dependent Hypertension

Hypertension associated with activation of the RAAS (see also Chapter 16A) affects the largest group of severely hypertensive children. Within this category are various forms of renovascular disease, a range of renal parenchymal disorders, and renin-secreting tumors (67). Secondary hyperaldosteronism with hypokalemia occurs in most instances. Malignant hypertension from any cause is likely to stimulate renin release secondary to vascular damage; in this situation, hyperreninemia may not be the initiating cause but will increase blood pressure level. Three distinct entities are associated with renin-dependent hypertension in children.

Renovascular Disease. Renovascular hypertension results from a lesion or lesions that impair blood flow to a part or all of one or both kidneys (1). It constitutes between 4.5% and 11.5% of cases of secondary hypertension in children (1), tending to present more commonly in younger children. At the Hospital for Sick Children, between 1971 and 1983, 31 of 326 (9.5%) patients had renovascular disease. It is frequently curable and second only to coarctation as a cause of surgically remediable hypertension in children (68). The most common abnormality is some form of renal artery stenosis, which occurs in association with idiopathic hypercalcemia (69), Marfan's syndrome (70), the rubella syndrome (71), Takayasu's (pulseless) disease (68), and neurofibromatosis (72).

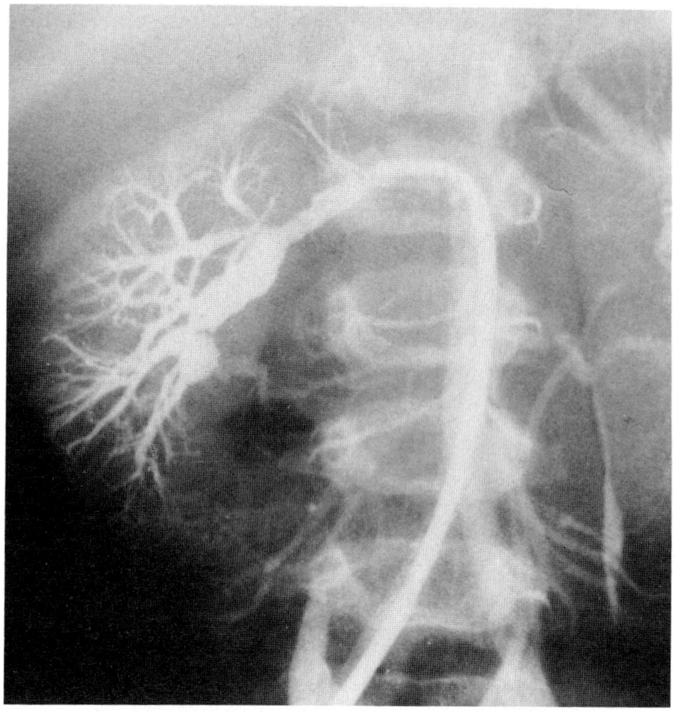

Figure 46.9. Selective renal angiogram showing fibromuscular dysplasia affecting right renal artery with poststenotic dilatation.

Approximately 70% of children with renovascular hypertension have fibromuscular dysplasia (60, 68, 73). The current classification is based on the arterial layer in which the lesions predominate. As a result lesions may be characterized as intimal hyperplasia or fibroplasia and, if the media is mainly affected, as fibromuscular dysplasia. The lesions result in areas of arterial narrowing alternating with aneurysmal sections giving rise to "string of beads" appearance (Fig. 46.9). The cause is unknown. Stenosis due to intimal proliferation is well recognized in neurofibromatosis (1); on the other hand there are familial cases reported without this association (74). Although a main renal artery may be affected in isolation, it is common to have bilateral disease (Fig. 46.10). Intrarenal arterial involvement also is common (Fig. 46.11) (68, 74). The latter occurs at times without main renal artery pathology and can masquerade as coarse renal scarring or chronic pyelonephritis (75).

Other causes of renovascular hypertension in children include renal artery aneurysm (74), arteriovenous fistulas, and renal artery disruption after trauma (68). In neonates the causes include renal artery thrombosis associated with the use of umbilical artery catheters (76) and renal artery embolization from thrombosis of the ductus arteriosus (76). We have seen hypertensive renovascular disease in children with the Feuerstein-Mims syndrome, the Klippel-Trenaunay-Weber syndrome, periarteritis nodosa, the hemolytic uremic syndrome, and post abdominal radiation. Children with renal artery anomalies also may have abnormalities elsewhere, including the mesenteric, splenic, and hepatic arteries in addition to the critically important arteries that supply the brain (Fig. 46.12).

External compression of a renal artery or arteries may cause hyperten-

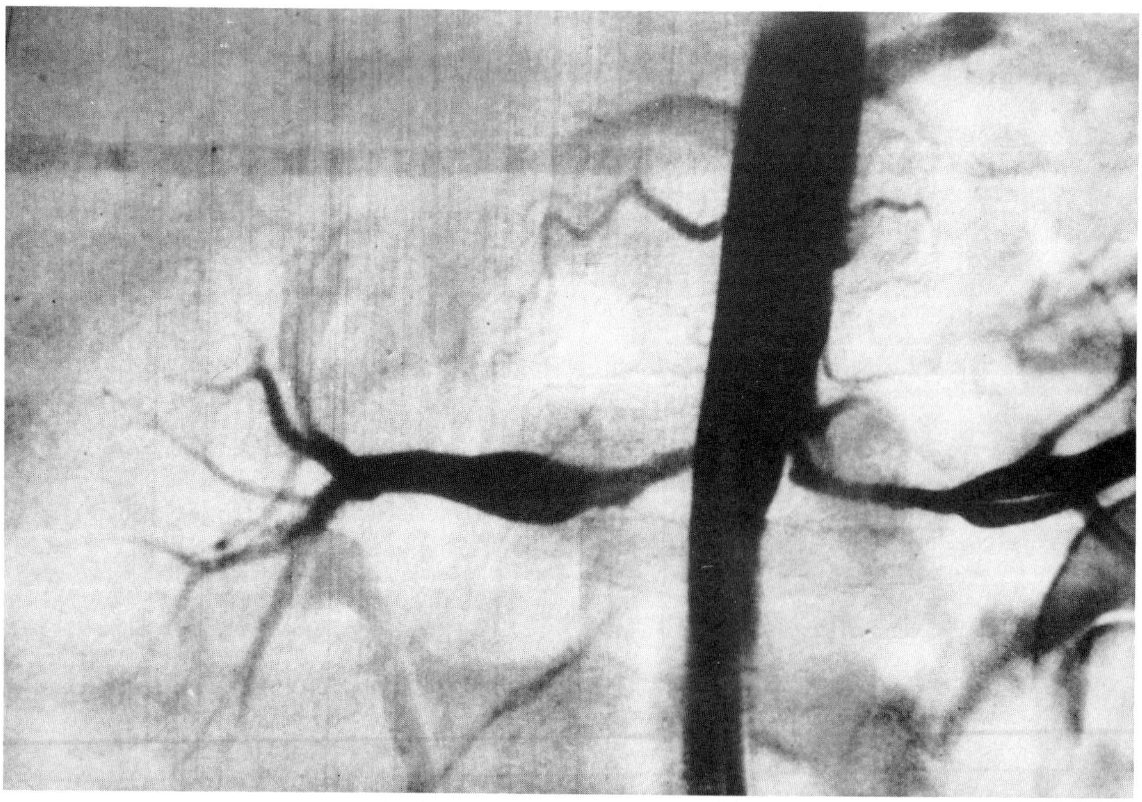

Figure 46.10. Flush aortogram showing bilateral main renal artery stenosis in girl with neurofibromatosis.

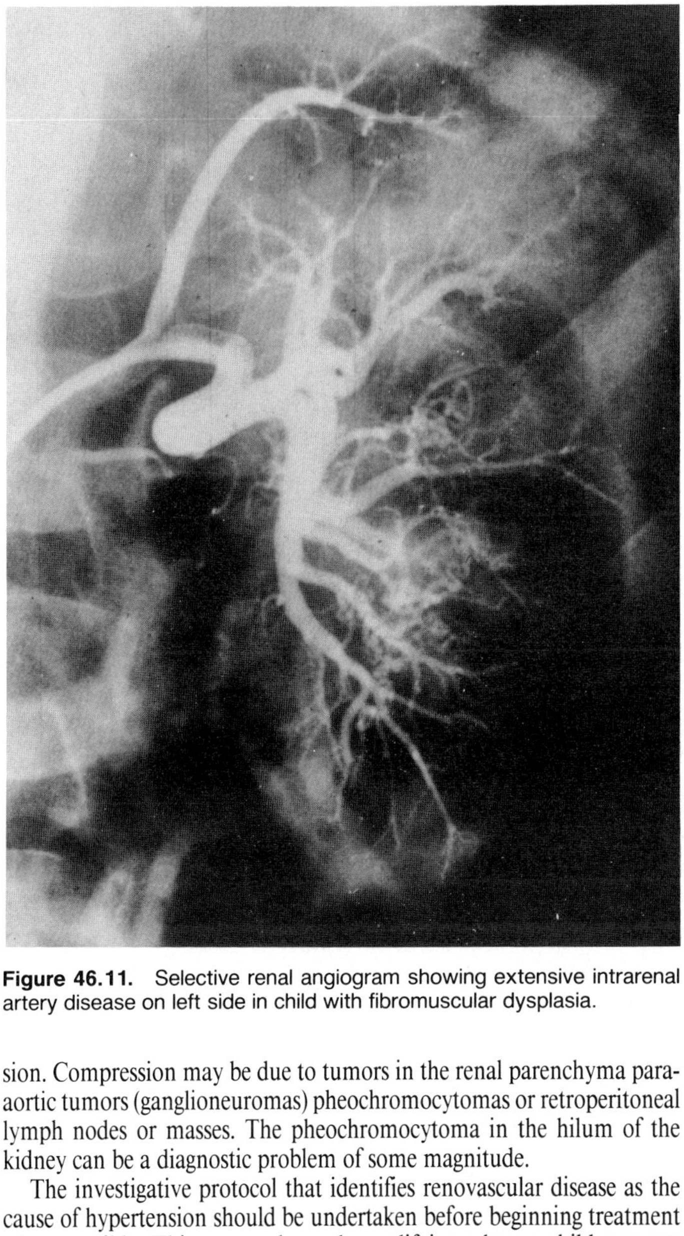

Figure 46.11. Selective renal angiogram showing extensive intrarenal artery disease on left side in child with fibromuscular dysplasia.

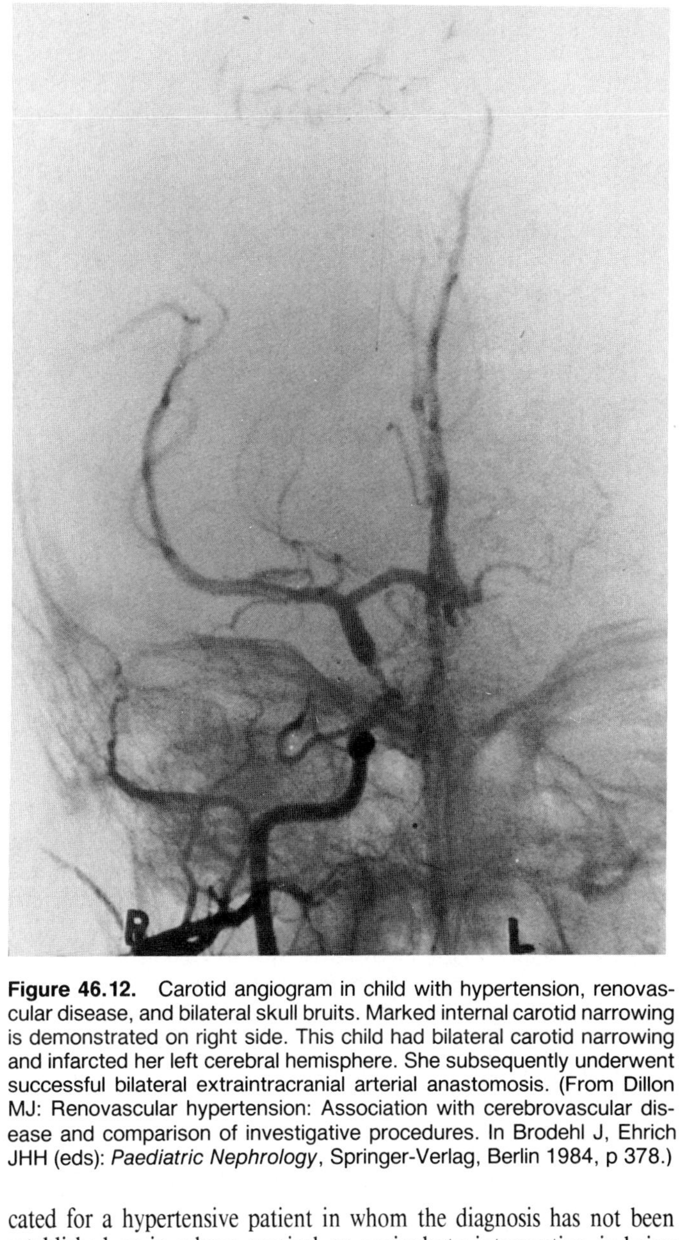

Figure 46.12. Carotid angiogram in child with hypertension, renovascular disease, and bilateral skull bruits. Marked internal carotid narrowing is demonstrated on right side. This child had bilateral carotid narrowing and infarcted her left cerebral hemisphere. She subsequently underwent successful bilateral extraintracranial arterial anastomosis. (From Dillon MJ: Renovascular hypertension: Association with cerebrovascular disease and comparison of investigative procedures. In Brodehl J, Ehrich JHH (eds): *Paediatric Nephrology*, Springer-Verlag, Berlin 1984, p 378.)

sion. Compression may be due to tumors in the renal parenchyma para-aortic tumors (ganglioneuromas) pheochromocytomas or retroperitoneal lymph nodes or masses. The pheochromocytoma in the hilum of the kidney can be a diagnostic problem of some magnitude.

The investigative protocol that identifies renovascular disease as the cause of hypertension should be undertaken before beginning treatment when possible. This approach needs modifying when a child presents with severe or malignant hypertension requiring urgent control. Clinical examination should be followed by evaluation of plasma chemistries, a urinalysis, a chest roentgenogram, and ECG. Recommended initial renal imaging consists of abdominal ultrasound and a ^{99m}Tc-DMSA scan, sometimes followed by a standard IVU if more renal anatomical detail is required, a VCU if there is a history of urinary infections or vesicoureteric reflux needs to be excluded (see also Chapter 37), or both. A supine PRA and PA and plasma catecholamine measurements complete the initial investigations. The abundant data produced by these procedures will help the clinician in the next stage of the evaluation.

US and IVU can fail to detect abnormalities even in the presence of extensive renovascular disease, although asymmetry of renal size and parenchymal loss may be demonstrated. The ^{99m}Tc-DMSA scan is more likely to identify pathological conditions in this situation and is particularly effective in localizing the sites of intrarenal ischemia as regions of diminished isotope uptake in the renal parenchyma. PRA will be increased in the majority of cases with or without an increased PA. Plasma catecholamines will be normal.

Renal vein renin sampling and selective renal angiography are indicated for a hypertensive patient in whom the diagnosis has not been established or in whom surgical or angioplasty intervention is being considered. A main renal vein renin ratio of 1.5 or more associated with contralateral renin suppression (demonstrated by a contralateral kidney to IVC renin ratio of <1.3) would indicate asymmetric renin release and suggest a surgical cure of hypertension if pathology is lateralized and surgical treatment feasible. Surgical or angioplasty correction may be indicated if segmental renal vein renin values identify local sources of renin release in the supposedly normal contralateral kidney due to intrarenal artery pathology. The flush aortogram coupled with selective renal arteriograms will demonstrate the anatomical site or sites of stenosis; these findings coupled with the renal vein renins and DMSA scan findings allow rational decisions to be made concerning surgical treatment. Good correlations have been demonstrated between renal arteriograms, segmental renal vein renin values, and DMSA scan findings in children with renovascular disease (19). (See also Chapter 20.)

In some patients with equivocal peripheral renin values, a saralasin (45) or similar test using captopril (50) may be indicated to help clarify whether there is a renin component to the hypertension. This may be especially valuable when hypotensive therapy with renin-suppressing agents such as β-blockers has been used.

The association between renal arterial lesions and vascular pathology elsewhere in the body may make it mandatory to undertake more extensive angiographic evaluations (77). The presence of cranial or carotid bruits or localizing neurological features on presentation might justify additional procedures. Several patients have had cerebral, vertebral or carotid artery narrowing in addition to renovascular disease (Fig. 46.12) (77).

The appropriate sequence of events in managing identified childhood renovascular hypertension is first to control blood pressure with drugs (Chapter 47) and then to consider surgery. Surgery may cure the condition or significantly lower drug requirements, which is especially important when required dosages cause serious side effects.

Renovascular disease may be managed surgically by nephrectomy, partial nephrectomy, revascularization by reconstructive vascular surgery (68, 78), intraluminal dilatation or angioplasty (79, 80), autotransplantation (74), and embolization (78). The ideal lesion is a unilateral, short-segment, renal artery stenosis with no evidence of intrarenal or contralateral renal disease by ^{99m}Tc-DMSA scan and angiography. Criteria for lateralization of renin release should be demonstrated before surgery. Bilateral main renal artery stenoses also are amenable to revascularization. These may be undertaken sequentially in some cases; a reversal of the main renal vein renin ratios may follow the initial intervention. Similarly, intrarenal segmental artery stenosis or stenoses may be dealt with by intraluminal angioplasty, heminephrectomy, or embolization.

The surgical techniques used in renal revascularization include saphenous vein by-pass grafts, autogenous arterial grafts, splenorenal anastomosis, hepatic-renal artery anastomosis, internal iliac renal anastomosis, and insertion of Dacron grafts. Renal autotransplantation to the pelvis and ex vivo surgery followed by repositioning of the kidney, have also been done (68, 74, 81, 82). Recently, transluminal angioplasty has been used (79, 80). In this procedure a balloon catheter is used to dilate the stenotic area and thus correct a stenosis.

When severe renal artery stenosis is associated with a small, poorly functioning kidney, nephrectomy may be preferable; however, the small kidney should be demonstrably responsible for the hypertension and it should be clear that the function of the contralateral kidney will not be compromised by removal of the small kidney. A renal scan to assess relative renal function is useful for this purpose.

It is also important to determine whether there are other arterial lesions outside the kidneys. Mesenteric or cranial artery stenosis may cause regional ischemia if blood pressure is lowered. Cerebrovascular stenoses occur in association with neuroectodermal syndromes, e.g., neurofibromatosis and the Feuerstein-Mims syndrome. Surgical treatment of these conditions may be feasible (77).

Renal Parenchymal Disease. Among the many parenchymal diseases that cause renin-induced hypertension, the most common (33% to 67%) in children is pyelonephritic scarring (2). It is associated with vesicoureteral reflux and urinary tract infection (UTI) in early life (83). At the Hospital for Sick Children over the past 12 years, 116 of 326 children (36%) admitted with severe hypertension had reflux nephropathy: of these, 56 also had some form of obstructive uropathy. Hypertension usually is a late sequel (7), rarely developing in the first five yr of life. In some cases the malignant phase is first detected in late childhood when there has been no prior history of UTI. Approximately 10% of children with renal scarring become hypertensive (36, 84).

Although increased PRA is a major factor causing hypertension in children with reflux nephropathy, other factors may contribute. Renin is commonly elevated once hypertension has developed (85) and may not return to normal, adjusted for age, in children with renal scarring, even though the children are normotensive (32). Renal scarring, by damaging the medulla, may also decrease vasodilator hormones, e.g., prostaglandins, and thereby contribute to the hypertension.

Other parenchymal renal diseases, e.g., chronic glomerulonephritis; the hemolytic uremic syndrome, dysplastic, hypoplastic, and polycystic kidneys (9), are associated with renin-induced hypertension. Hypertension also occurs after irradiation. Segmental hypoplasia (Ask-Upmark kidney) may be associated with renovascular disease (86, 87). Renal venous thrombosis may be followed by renin-induced hypertension later in life.

When hypertension is associated with CRF, the role of renin-induced hypertension must be distinguished from the role of volume-dependent hypertension. When parenchymal disease is associated with scarring or renal dysplasia, the evaluation does not differ greatly from that for renovascular disease. When reflux nephropathy is suspected an IVU and VCU are recommended. Arteriography is recommended only when there is doubt about the nature of the renal scarring. Diagnostic arteriography will probably not be necessary unless there is doubt about the nature of the renal scarring. Divided renal vein renin studies will be indicated only if surgery is being considered to control blood pressure; i.e., if there were lateralized pathology and the relative function of the kidneys was such that removal of the affected kidney was feasible. Segmental renal vein renin studies may be indicated when blood pressure is difficult to control with drugs and the presence of scarring points to a segmental lesion.

Surgical decompression of cysts in infantile polycystic disease incidentally reduced blood pressure in one infant with massive kidneys, although the procedure was done to alleviate abdominal distention.

Renal Tumors. Renin-induced hypertension may be associated with nephroblastoma (88), juxtamedullary cell tumor-hemangiopericytomas (89), and renal hamartomas (90).

The hypertension in Wilms' tumor may be renin induced from arterial compression and from excessive renin production by the tumor itself (88, 91). Hemangiopericytomas are small tumors that are difficult to locate. However, their removal cures the hypertension they have caused (1, 89).

Catecholamine Excess

Sustained hypertension due to excess catecholamine arises from a tumor of the neural crest, i.e., pheochromocytoma, neuroblastoma, or ganglioneuroma. The importance of these tumors is out of proportion to their incidence, but they are a cause of hypertension that can be defined clearly. Following their removal, blood pressure returns to normal.

Pheochromocytomas account for 2% of the cases of secondary hypertension in children (1). Boys are affected twice as often as girls; two thirds of the tumors are in the adrenal medulla (92). The most frequent extraadrenal sites are near the adrenal gland at the aortic bifurcation and in the renal hilum (92). At least 155 pediatric cases of pheochromocytoma have been reported (93). Hypertension is sustained in 88% (92). The clinical symptoms include headaches (75%), sweating (67%), nausea and vomiting (48%), visual disturbances (37%), abominal pain (32%), polydipsia and polyuria (31%), convulsions (22%), and acrocyanosis (22%) (92).

Although pheochromocytomas are usually sporadic, they are occasionally familial and have been associated with von Recklinghausen's disease, von Hippel-Lindau's disease (29), and type 1 and 2 multiple endocrine neoplasia syndromes (94, 95, 96). The multiple endocrine neoplasia syndrome type 2 (Sipple's syndrome) has been divided into type 2A (medullary thyroid carcinoma, pheochromocytoma, hyperparathyroidism) and type 2B, in which patients have a Marfanlike habitus with neuromas on skin, tongue, and lips (96). The inheritance of these conditions is autosomal dominant. The long-term outlook for cure of pheochromocytomas is good, and the incidence of malignancy is low (5% to 10%) (1).

The diagnosis of catecholamine-producing tumors can be established by demonstrating increased urinary excretion of catecholamines and their metabolites or, more precisely, by measuring plasma catecholamine levels. Localizing the tumor may be difficult, especially if multiple sites are involved. A combination of US, arteriography (after full α-adrenergic blockade), computerized tomography; ^{131}I MIBG scintigraphy, and vena caval catecholamine sampling usually is sufficient to localize the lesion or lesions. However, invasive procedures must be undertaken *only after adequate α-sympathetic blockade* and, sometimes, after β-sympathetic blockade as well. Blood pressure during the procedures should be carefully monitored and phentolamine, labetalol, or sodium nitroprusside should be available for immediate injection if there is a hypertensive crisis.

The treatment of catecholamine-producing tumors is surgical. A hypertensive child with neuroblastoma requiring surgical removal may require the same pharmacological blockade that is appropriate for pheochromocytoma.

Decisions concerning surgery for pheochromocytoma depend on preoperative localization and feasibility of intervention. Preoperatively α-blockade must be effected and β-blockade may be needed to counteract the effect of α-blockade-induced tachycardia or to counter the effects of dopamine and epinephrine that may be produced by the lesion. During the days required to attain α-blockade, a generous salt intake facilitates ECF volume expansion. Surgery should be undertaken with arterial and central venous lines in place, adequate supplies of appropriate hypotensive agents (phentolamine, labetalol, sodium nitroprusside), and supplies of blood, plasma and saline to fill the vascular space if necessary. Halothane or similar anesthesia that does not elicit sympathetic activity is favored.

Handling the tumor can produce catastrophic increases in blood pressure even in patients thought to be adequately blocked. Theoretically, if α-blockade is complete for some time preoperatively, blood pressure should not fall when the tumor is removed. However, blood pressure does usually fall because circulating vasoconstrictors dramatically decrease and vasodilatation caused by phenoxybenzamine and propranolol ensues. The initial danger comes when the veins of the tumor are ligated; a progressive drop over many hours may require ECF volume repletion. Sympathetic blockade should be discontinued as soon as the tumor is removed. Blood pressure is labile for several days even with these precautions.

Corticosteroid Excess

Corticosteroid excess is a relatively rare cause of hypertension in childhood. Apart from extraneously administered corticosteroids, it results from certain types of congenital adrenal hyperplasia; 11-β and 17-α-hydroxylase deficiencies (33); Conn's syndrome caused by an aldosterone-producing tumor or bilateral adrenal hyperplasia, Cushing's syndrome, and a syndrome of apparent mineralocorticoid excess. PRA suppression and hypokalemia are hallmarks of steroid hypertension.

In adrenal hyperplasia the hypertension is caused by accumulated mineralocorticoids: deoxycorticosterone (DOC) and compound S in 11-β-hydroxylase deficiency (33) and 17-desoxysteroids in 17-α-hydroxylase deficiency (33). The treatment goal is to replace cortisol and suppress ACTH and thus suppress mineralocorticoid secretion.

In Conn's syndrome, aldosterone is autonomously produced by the adrenal gland. Sodium retention, plasma volume expansion, hypertension, and renin suppression follow. The condition is extremely rare in childhood (97). Bilateral adrenal hyperplasia is the usual cause of corticosteroid induced hypertension in children.

The diagnosis is made by finding high PA, low PRA, and K wasting in a NaCl-replete state. Distinction between bilateral hyperplasia and a tumor is made by US, CT scanning, iodocholesterol scans, or by adrenal venous aldosterone and cortisol sampling. Surgery is the treatment of choice for the tumor; medical therapy is advisable for hyperplasia.

In childhood, hypertension is common in Cushing's syndrome—21 of 26 children in one report (98). The cause probably is multifactorial. The mineralocorticoid effect of excess cortisol, increased vascular reactivity to vasoconstrictors, and increased renin substrate may contribute (53). In childhood, Cushing's syndrome is most commonly caused by an adrenal tumor that overproduces glucocorticoids and androgens.

In some children ACTH is increased, causing adrenocortical hyperplasia and this condition is known as Cushing's disease. It is identified when plasma cortisol levels are suppressible. The primary abnormality in Cushing's disease is ACTH hypersecretion; in Cushing's syndrome, it is adrenal hypersecretion. Radiological studies of the adrenals including arteriography, venography, ultrasonography, and computerized tomography also assist in making the correct diagnosis. Androgen excess suggests adrenal carcinoma. Treatment depends on the underlying cause.

Surgery is indicated in Cushing's syndrome caused by an adrenal tumor. Since inhibition of the hypothalamic-hypophyseal system will cause the contralateral gland to be atrophic, it is essential to prepare patients for surgery as one would for a total adrenalectomy (54). Surgery is best performed after reducing the hypercortisolism by preoperative treatment with o,p′ DDD (1,1-dichloro-2 [*o*-chlorophenyl]-2-(*p*-chlorophenyl) ethane). For an adrenal adenoma unilateral adrenalectomy usually cures the patient. In Cushing's disease, total bilateral adrenalectomy (99) with subsequent life-long steroid supplement is recommended. Medical therapy with drugs such as cyproheptadine might obviate the need for surgery (54).

In the syndrome of apparent mineralocorticoid excess there is hypertension, hypokalemia, suppression of renin, and no oversecretion of any known hormones. The syndrome appears to be familial (100). Hypertension and hypokalemia have responded to triamterine therapy in some cases (101). Response to spironolactone has suggested the presence of an unidentified mineralocorticoid (102). Ulick and coworkers (103) demonstrated an abnormal pattern of urinary excretion of dihydrometabolites of cortisol and an increase in compounds with 5-α relative to 5-β stereochemistry; they then postulated a deficiency of cortisol 11-β-hydroxysteroid dehydrogenase as the primary defect. This has been confirmed in patients with similar clinical presentations (34, 35, 104). The condition has been fatal (104).

The cause of the hypertension of this condition remains unknown. Whether conversion of cortisol to cortisone normally protects the kidneys from the mineralocorticoid action of cortisol metabolites or whether there is increased sensitivity to the action of certain steroids that normally would not cause NaCl retention and K loss remains uncertain.

The condition is identified by the low PRA value and a normal or low PA; urine steroid analysis by mass spectrometry gas chromatographic analysis is needed for confirmation. Treatment with spironolactone, triamterine, dexamathasone, or all three is beneficial (see Chapter 47).

Essential Hypertension

A diagnosis of essential hypertension is made in preadolescent children only after other known causes are excluded. The prevalence is difficult to ascertain but is less than 3% of children and in most of these the hypertension is mild. Familial aggregation of blood pressure, tracking correlations, sib-sib correlations, and relationships to height, weight and ponderosity are described in Chapter 45.

In essential hypertension, urinary kallikrein levels are low (105), and plasma catecholamines are elevated (106). The role of the kinin-kallikrein system is unclear; autonomic hyperactivity may be important in the early stages of essential hypertension in some patients. The excess circulating catecholamine may be the cause or merely a consequence of essential hypertension.

The question of whether impairment of sodium-potassium membrane transport exists in essential hypertension is a controversial subject. Garay and coworkers (107) have shown a low red cell sodium-potassium net flux ratio in individuals with essential hypertension compared with normal individuals or patients with secondary hypertension. Cannessa and coworkers (108) found that sodium stimulated efflux from red cells, as lithium-sodium exchange in cells preloaded with lithium was abnormally fast in patients with essential hypertension compared with normotensive subjects. Others postulate that essential hypertension is caused by an inherited variability in the ability of the kidney to eliminate sodium (109). This produces a high level of sodium transport inhibition that helps the kidney to eliminate sodium but secondarily causes a rise in intracellular sodium and calcium, particularly of the smooth muscles of arterioles. The latter leads to increased arteriolar tone with the consequent increase in blood pressure (109, 110).

References

1. Leumann EP: Blood pressure and hypertension in childhood and adolescence. Ergebnisse der Inneren Medizin und Kinderheilkunde 43:109, 1979.
2. Still JL, Cottom D: Severe hypertension in childhood. Arch Dis Child 42:34, 1967.
3. Uhari M, Saukkonen AL, Koskimies O: Central nervous system involvement in servere arterial hypertension in childhood. Eur J Pediatr 132:141, 1979.
4. Londe S: Causes of hypertension in the young. Pediatr Clin North Am 25:55, 1978.
5. Rames LK, Clarke WR, Conner WE, et al: Normal blood pressures and the evaluation of sustained blood pressure elevation in childhood. The Muscatine Study. Pediatrics 61:245, 1978.
6. Calnan M, Peckham CS: Incidence of insulin dependent diabetes in the first sixteen years of life. Lancet 1:589, 1977.
7. Heale WF: Hypertension and reflux nephropathy. Aust Pediatr J 13:56, 1977.
8. Dillon MJ: Recent advances in evaluation and management of childhood hypertension. Eur J Pediatr 132:133, 1979.
9. Gill DG, Mendes da Costa B, Cameron JS, et al: Analysis of 100 children with severe and persistent hypertension. Arch Dis Child 51:951, 1976.
10. Dillon MJ: Hypertension in childhood. Update 17:1409, 1978.
11. Lloyd AVC, Jewett DE, Still JL: Facial paralysis in children with hypertension. Arch Dis Child 41:191, 1966.
12. Hulse JA, Taylor DSI, Dillon MJ: Blindness and paraplegia in accelerated hypertension of childhood. Lancet 2:553, 1979.
13. Jellinek EH, Painter M, Princas J, Ross-Russell R: Hypertensive encephalopathy with cortical disturbance of vision. Q J Med 33:239, 1964.
14. Ledingham JGG, Rajagopalan B: Cerebral complications in the treatment of accelerated hypertension. Q J Med 48:25, 1979.
15. Taylor D, Ramsay J, Day S, Dillon M: Infarction of the optic nerve head in children with accelerated hypertension. Br J Ophthalmol 65:153, 1981.
16. Bingham JB, Maisey MN: An evaluation of the use of 99mTc-dimercaptosuccinic acid (DMSA) as a static renal imaging agent. Br J Radiol 51:599, 1978.
17. Merrick MV, Uttley WS, Wild SR: The detection of pyelonephritic scarring in children by radioisotope imaging. Br J Radiol 53:544, 1980.
18. Dillon MJ, Gordon I, Shah V: 99Tc DMSA scanning and segmental renal vein renin estimations in children with renal scarring. In Hodson CJ, Heptinstall RH, Winberg J (eds): Contributions to Nephrology, Vol. 39, Reflux Nephropathy Update: 1983. Basel, Karger, 1984, p 20.
19. Stringer DA, de Bruyn R, Dillon MJ, Gordon I: Comparison of aortography, renal vein renin sampling, radionuclide scans, ultrasound and the IVU in the investigation of children renovascular hypertension. Br J Radiol 57:111, 1984.
20. Gordon I: Renal diagnostic imaging. In Williams DI, Johnston JM (eds): Paediatric Urology, ed 2, London, Butterworths, 1982, p 11.
21. Diffey BL, Hall FM, Corfield JR: The 99m Tc-DTPA dynamic renal scan with deconvolutional analysis. J Nucl Med 17:352, 1977.
22. Piepsz A, Denis R, Ham HR, et al: A simple method for measuring separate glomerular filtration rate using a single injection of 99m Tc DTPA and the scintillation camera. J Pediatr 93:769, 1978.
23. O'Reilly PH, Testa HJ, Lawson RS, et al: Diuresis renography in equivocal urinary tract obstruction. Br J Urol 50:76, 1978.
24. Bierwaltes WH, Lieberman LM, Ansari AN, Nishiyama H. Visualization of human adrenal glands in vivo by scintillation scanning. J Am Med Assoc 216:275, 1971.
25. Sisson JC, Frager MS, Valk TW, Gross MD, et al: Scintigraphic localization of pheochromocytoma. N Engl J Med 305:12, 1981.
26. Hillman BJ, Ovitt TW, Nudelman S, et al: Digital video subtraction angiography of renal vascular abnormalities. Radiology 139:277, 1981.
27. Ludwig JW, Verhoeven LHJ, Engles PHC: Digital video subtraction angiography (DVSA) equipment. Angiographic technique in comparison with conventional angiography in different vascular areas. Br J Radiol 55:545, 1982.
28. Khoury GA, Irving JD, Farrington K, et al: Digital vascular imaging and selective renin sampling in evaluation of vascular anatomy in renal transplant recipients. Br Med J 286:1003, 1983.
29. Sever PS, Roberts JC, Snell ME: Phaeochromocytoma. Clin Endocrinol Metab 9:543, 1980.
30. Robson AM: Special diagnostic studies for the detection of renal and renovascular forms of hypertension. Pediatr Clin North Am 25:83, 1978.
31. Dillon MJ, Ryness JM: Plasma renin activity and aldosterone concentration in children. Br Med J 4:316, 1975.
32. Savage JM, Dillon MJ, Shah V, et al: Renin and blood pressure in children with renal scarring and vesicoureteric reflux. Lancet 2:441, 1978.
33. New MI, Levine IS: Adrenocortical hypertension. Pediatr Clin North Am 25:67, 1978.
34. Shackleton CHL, Honour JW, Dillon MJ, et al: Hypertension in a four-year-old child: gas chromatographic and mass spectrometric evidence for deficient hepatic metabolism of steroids. J Clin Endocrinol Metab 50:786, 1980.
35. Honour JW, Dillon MJ, Levin M, Shah V: Fatal low renin hypertension associated with disturbance of cortisol metabolism in a 5 month-old infant. Arch Dis Child 58:1018, 1983.
36. Wallace DMA, Rothwell DL, Williams DI: The long-term follow-up of surgically treated vesicoureteric reflux. Br J Urol 50:479, 1978.
37. Stockigt JR, Noakes CA, Collins RD, et al: Renal vein renin in various forms of renal hypertension. Lancet 1:1194, 1972.
38. Godard C: Predictive value of renal-vein renin measurements in children with various forms of renal hypertension: an international study. Helv Paediatr Acta 32:49, 1977.
39. Dillon MJ, Shah V, Barratt TM: Renal vein measurements in children with hypertension. Br Med J 2:168, 1978.
40. Gerdts KG, Shah V, Savage JM, Dillon MJ: Renal vein renin measurements in normotensive children. J Pediatr 95:953, 1979.
41. Schambelan M, Glickman M, Stockigt JR, Biglieri EG: Selective renal-vein renin sampling in hypertensive patients with segmental renal lesions. N Engl J Med 290:1153, 1974.
42. Dillon MJ: Renal vein renin determinations in evaluating hypertensive children. In Gruskin AB, Norman ME (eds): Developments in Nephrology, 3, Pediatric Nephrology. The Hague, Martinus Nijhoff, 1981, p 127.
43. Vivian G, Stringer D, de Bruyn R, et al: 99 Tc DMSA scans in renovascular hypertension in childhood. In Raynaud C (ed): Nuclear Medicine and Biology, Paris, Pergamon Press, 1982, p 2663.
44. Dillon MJ: Application of study of the renin angiotensin system to paediatric pathology. In Giovennelli G, New MI, Gorini S (eds): Hypertension in Children and Adolescents, New York, Raven Press, 1981, p 137.
45. Streeten DHP, Anderson GH, Freiberg JM, Dalakos TG: Use of an angiotensin II antagonist (Saralasin) in the recognition of "angiotensinogenic" hypertension. N Engl J Med 292:657, 1975.
46. Baer L, Parr-Carrillo J, Radichevich I, Williams GS: Detection of renovascular hypertension with angiotensin II blockade. Ann Intern Med 86:257, 1977.
47. Favre L, Boerth RC, Braren V, Dean RH, Hollifield JW: Angiotensin II blockade by Saralasin in the evaluation of hypertension in children. Kidney Int 15:Suppl 9, 75, 1979.
48. Vidt DG, Bravo EL, Fouad FM: Captopril. N Engl J Med 306:214, 1982.
49. Atkinson AB, Brown JJ, Cumming AMM, et al: Captopril in renovascular hypertension: long-term use in predicting surgical outcome. Br Med J 284:689, 1982.
50. Daman Willems C, Uchiyama M, Shah V, et al: Therapeutic and diagnostic usage of captopril in childhood. Int J Pediatr Nephrol 5:125, 1984.
51. Bravo EL, Tarazi RC, Gifford RW, Stewart BH: Circulating and urinary catecholamines in pheochromocytoma. N Engl J Med 301:682, 1979.
52. Henry DP, Starman BJ, Johnson DG, Williams RH: A sensitive radioenzymatic assay for norepinephrine in tissues and plasma. Life Sci 16:375, 1975.
53. Levine LS, New MI: Endocrine aspects of hypertension. In Brook CGD (ed): Clinical Paediatric Endocrinology, Oxford, Blackwell Scientific, 1981, p 479.
54. Forest MG: Adrenal steroid excess. In Brook CGD (ed): Clinical Paediatric Endocrinology, Oxford, Blackwell Scientific, 1981, p 429.
55. Cugini P, Mancini A, Meucci T, et al: Evidence of an angiotensinogenic mechanism for generalised hypertension associated with coarctation of the aorta. In Giovannelli G, New MI, Gorini S (eds): Hypertension in Children and Adolescents, New York, Raven Press, 1981, p 319.
56. Parker FB, Farrell B, Streeton DHP, et al: Hypertensive mechanisms in coarctation of the thoracic aorta. Proceedings of the World Congress of Paediatric Cardiology, London, Abstract 130, 1980.
57. Mueller-Wiefel DE: Renovasculare hypertension bei neurofibromatose von Recklinghausen. Monatsschr Kinderheilkd 126:113, 1978.

58. Lee KS, Sohn KY, Hong CY, et al: Primary arteritis (pulseless disease) in Korean children. Acta Paediatr Scand 56:526, 1967.
59. Wiggelinkhuizen J, Cremin BJ: Takayasu arteritis and renovascular hypertension in childhood. Pediatrics 62:209, 1978.
60. Stanley P, Gyepes MT, Olson DL, Gates GF: Renovascular hypertension in children and adolescents. Radiology 129:123, 1978.
61. Goldring D: Cardiovascular form of hypertension: coarctation of aorta in the infant and child. In Giovannelli G, New MI, Gorini S (eds): Hypertension in Children and Adolescents, New York, Raven Press, 1981, p 209.
62. Ingelfinger JR: Pediatric Hypertension. Philadelphia, W B Saunders, 1982.
63. Ho ECK, Moss AJ: The syndrome of "mesenteric arteritis" following surgical repair of aortic coarctation. Pediatrics 49:40, 1972.
64. Davies DL, Beevers DG, Briggs JD, et al: Abnormal relation between exchangeable sodium and the renin-angiotensin system in malignant hypertension and in hypertension with chronic renal failure. Lancet 1:683, 1973.
65. Weidmann P, Maxwell MH: The renin-angiotensin aldosterone system in terminal renal failure. Kidney Int 8:suppl 5, 219, 1975.
66. Brunner HR, Gavras H, Turini GA, et al: Long term treatment of hypertension in man by orally active angiotensin-converting enzyme inhibitor. Clin Sci Molecular Med 55, Suppl 4, 293, 1978.
67. Dillon MJ: Renin and hypertension in childhood. Arch Dis Child 49:831, 1974.
68. Fry WJ, Ernst CB, Stanley JC, Brink B: Renovascular hypertension in the pediatric patient. Arch Surgery 107:692, 1973.
69. Wiltse HE, Goldbloom RB, Antia AU, et al: Infantile hypercalcemia syndrome in twins. N Engl J Med 275:1157, 1966.
70. Loughridge LW: Renal abnormalities in the Marfan syndrome. Q J Med 28:531, 1959.
71. Menser MA, Dorman DC, Reye RDK, Reid RR: Renal artery stenosis in the rubella syndrome. Lancet 1:790, 1966.
72. Bourke E, Gatenby PBB: Renal artery dysplasia with hypertension in neurofibromatosis. Br Med J 3:681, 1971.
73. Lawson JD, Boerth R, Foster JH, Dean RH: Diagnosis and management of renovascular hypertension in children. Arch Surg 112:1307, 1977.
74. Kaufman JJ, Goodwin WE, Waisman J, Gyepes MT: Renovascular hypertension in children. Report of seven cases treated surgically including two cases of renal auto-transplantation. Am J Surg 124:149, 1972.
75. Dillon MJ, Gordon I, Ransley PG, Risdon RA: Pyelonephritic scars not due to chronic pyelonephritis. Int J Pediatr Nephrol 3:113, 1982.
76. Adelman RD: Neonatal hypertension. Pediatr Clin North Am 25:99, 1978.
77. Dillon MJ: Renovascular hypertension: Association with cerebrovascular disease and comparison of investigative procedures. In Brodehl J, Ehrich JHH (eds): Paediatric Nephrology, Springer-Verlag, Berlin 1984, p 378.
78. Johnston JH: Renal arterial disease. In Williams DI, Johnston JH (eds): Paediatric Urology, ed 2 London, Butterworths, 1983, p 73.
79. McCook TA, Mills SR, Kirks DR, et al: Percutaneous transluminal renal artery angioplasty in a 3½ year old girl. J Pediatr 97:958, 1980.
80. Goertz KK, Linshaw MA, Lee KR, et al: Transluminal arterial dilation of a post-surgical stenosis of renal artery implant in a child with recurrent hypertension. Pediatrics 69:489, 1982.
81. Stoney RJ, Cooke PA, String ST: Surgical treatment of renovascular hypertension in children. J Pediat Surg 10:631, 1976.
82. Sinaiko A, Najarian J, Michael AF, Mirkin BL: Renal autotransplantation in treatment of bilateral renal artery stenosis: relief of hypertension in an 8 year old boy. J Pediatr 83:409, 1973.
83. Smellie JM, Normand ICS: Bacteriuria, reflux and renal scarring. Arch Dis Child 50:581, 1975.
84. Holland NH, Kotchen T, Bhathena D: Hypertension in children with chronic pyelonephritis. Kidney Int 8 (suppl 5):243, 1975.
85. Dillon MJ, Smellie JM: Peripheral plasma renin activity, hypertension and renal scarring in children. In Hodson CJ, Heptinstall RH, Winberg J (eds): Contributions to Nephrology. Reflux Nephropathy Update: 1983, Basel, Karger, 1984, p 68.
86. Royer P, Broyer M, Habib R, Nouaillie Y: L'hypoplasie segmentaire du rein chez d'enfant. In Actualities Nephrologiques de l'Hopital Necker. Paris, Flammarion, 1971, p 151.
87. Bernstein J: Renal hypoplasia and dysplasia. In Edelmann CE (ed): Pediatric Kidney Disease, Boston, Little, Brown, 1978, p 541.
88. Ganguly A, Gribble J, Tyne B, et al: Renin secreting Wilms' tumour with severe hypertension: report of a case and brief review of renin-secreting tumors. Ann Intern Med 79:835, 1973.
89. Robertson PW, Klidjian A, Harding LK, et al: Hypertension due to a renin-secreting tumour. Am J Med 43:963, 1967.
90. Hirose M, Arakawa K, Kikuchi M, et al: Primary reninism with renal hamartomatous alteration. J Am Med Assoc 230:1288, 1974.
91. Mitchell JD, Baxter TJ, Blair-West JR, McCredie DA: Renin levels in nephroblastoma (Wilms' tumour). Report of a renin secreting tumour. Arch Dis Child 45:376, 1970.
92. Stackpole RH, Melicow MM, Uson AC: Pheochromocytoma in children: report of 9 cases and review of the first 100 published cases with follow-up studies. J Pediatr 63:315, 1963.
93. Louis C, Dickmann L, Brisse B, Meuller KM: Beitrag zum Phaochromocytom im kindersalter. Zeitschrift fur Kinderheilkunde 119:197, 1975.
94. Sipple JH: The association of pheochromocytoma with carcinoma of the thyroid gland. Am J Med 31:163, 1961.
95. Keiser HR, Beaven MA, Doppman J: Sipple's syndrome. Medullary thyroid carcinoma, pheochromocytoma and parathyroid disease. Ann Intern Med 78:561, 1973.
96. Lips KJM, Veer J van der S, Struyvenberg A, et al: Bilateral occurrence of pheochromocytoma in patients with multiple endocrine neoplasia syndrome Type 2A (Sipple's syndrome). Am J Med 70:1051, 1981.
97. New MI, Peterson RE: Aldosterone in childhood. In Levine SZ (ed): Advances in Pediatrics, Chicago, Yearbook Medical Publishers, 1968, p 111.
98. Loridan L, Senior E: Cushing's syndrome in infancy. J Pediatr 75:349, 1969.
99. McArthur RG, Hayles AB, Salassa RM: Childhood Cushing's disease: results of bilateral adrenalectomy. J Pediatr 95:214, 1979.
100. Liddle AW, Bledsoe T, Coppage WS: A familial renal disorder simulating primary aldosteronism but with negligible aldosterone secretion. Trans Assoc Am Physicians 76:199, 1967.
101. Aarskog D, Stea KF, Thorson T, Wefring KW: Hypertension and hypokalemic alkalosis associated with under production of aldosterone. Pediatrics 76:199, 1963.
102. New MI, Levine LS, Biglieri EG, et al: Evidence for an unidentified steroid in a child with apparent mineralocorticoid hypertension. J Clin Endocrinol Metab 44:924, 1977.
103. Ulick S, Ramirez LC, New MI: An abnormality in steroid reductive metabolism in a hypertensive syndrome. J Clin Endocrinol Metab 44:799, 1977.
104. Fischer TJW, Otter BJ, Monnens LAH, et al: Low renin, low aldosterone hypertension and abnormal cortisol metabolism in a 19 month old child. Horm Res 16:107, 1982.
105. Lawton WJ, Fitz AE: Urinary kallikrein in normal renin essential hypertension. Circulation 56:856, 1977.
106. Mongeau JG, Davignon A, Lamarre A, de Champlain J: Plasma catecholamines in normotensive children and in children with essential hypertension. In Gruskin AG, Norman ME (eds): Developments in Nephrology, 3 Pediatric Nephrology, The Hague, Martinus Nijhoff, 1981, p 116.
107. Garay RP, Elghozi JL, Dagher G, Meyer P: Laboratory distinction between essential and secondary hypertension by measurement of erythrocyte cation fluxes. N Engl J Med 302:769, 1980.
108. Canessa M, Adragna N, Solomon HS: Increased sodium-lithium counter transport in red cells of patients with essential hypertension. N Engl J Med 302:772, 1980.
109. de Wardener HE, MacGregor GA: The natriuretic hormone and essential hypertension. Lancet I:1450, 1982.
110. Reuter H, Blaustein MP, Hausler G: Na-Ca exchange and tension development in arterial smooth muscle. Philos Trans R Soc Lond B 265:87, 1973.

CHAPTER 47

Drug Treatment of Hypertension

M. J. DILLON

The medical management of hypertension is controversial owing to the steady introduction of new drugs. Choice of therapy depends on severity of the hypertension, its underlying cause, and the experience of the physician with the drugs. The therapeutic choices include dietary manipulations, a variety of pharmacological agents, and specific treatment of the underlying disease causing hypertension.

GENERAL MANAGEMENT

Patients with moderate-to-severe hypertension require antihypertensive therapy. Patients also may need general advice regarding diet, exercise, and life-style; those with mild hypertension may need only these nonpharmacological strategies.

The benefit from dietary NaCl restriction is controversial; current evidence suggests that reducing sodium chloride intake may lower blood pressure (1) in some but not all cases (2). Severe salt restriction, as in the Kempner rice diet (3), is effective, but the diet is unpalatable and modern diuretic and dialysis treatment have superseded it. Antihypertensive drugs may be effective without salt restriction, but avoiding table salt and salty processed foods is recommended. Many popular "junk foods" are salty, e.g., a meal of a popular hamburger and chips contains 95 mmol of NaCl before any table salt is added (1); these foods should be avoided or limited. Potassium supplementation has a hypotensive role (4), and a high-K diet or K supplementation may be valuable in managing essential hypertension except in states of chronic renal failure (CRF) or other forms of hyperkalemia. In obese hypertensive patients, weight loss alone can lower blood pressure and make the control of hypertension easier, even without sodium restriction (5). Obese adolescents tend to have a greater salt and calorie intake than those of normal weight (6). Both NaCl restriction and weight control are sensible recommendations.

Exercise probably should be discouraged when blood pressure is poorly controlled but encouraged when control is established. Sporting activities are appropriate except for highly competitive games for some patients. Jogging and other forms of modest regular exercise reduce blood pressure in adults with essential hypertension (7). Behavioral therapy using relaxation techniques or biofeedback may reduce blood pressure but probably is impractical in children.

M. J. Dillon MB FRCP DCH, Consultant Physician and Pediatric Nephrologist, Hospital for Sick Children, Great Ormond Street, London WC1

In many instances, it is valuable to give the child's parents instructions for measuring blood pressure at home and assure the availability of the necessary equipment. Both patient and physician thus acquire useful information for effective medical management.

INDICATIONS FOR ANTIHYPERTENSIVE THERAPY

Severe hypertension in childhood should be treated because the incidence of morbidity and mortality is high without treatment (8, 9). A dilemma arises when considering milder forms of hypertension. In addition to the degree and constancy of hypertension, the presence of risk factors, e.g., obesity and a family history of hypertension, are important (10). When a child is symptomatic or when there is evidence of proteinuria, cardiomegaly, or left ventricular hypertrophy or if the cause is known to lead to progressive hypertension, treatment is indicated. The balance is between the advantages of controlling blood pressure relative to the disadvantages of the side effects of therapy, i.e., the complications of antihypertensive drugs or surgical procedures. This is sometimes difficult to predict; a period of observation with and without therapy may be useful.

ANTIHYPERTENSIVE DRUGS

There are many antihypertensive drugs. The treatment regimens have been used mainly in adults, but dosage recommendations for children are now available for most of these agents. These drugs may be classified as follows: (a) centrally acting agents, (b) ganglionic blocking agents, (c) postganglionic adrenergic blocking agents, (d) β-adrenergic blocking agents, (e) α-adrenergic blocking agents, (f) vasodilators, including calcium antagonists, (g) renin angiotensin inhibitors, and (h) diuretics (Fig. 47.1). Dosages are given in Tables 47.1 and 47.2.

Centrally Acting Agents

Clonidine

Clonidine is an adrenoceptor agonist, which lowers blood pressure by stimulating brain stem vasodepressor α-receptors. Sympathetic outflow is inhibited, and blood pressure falls (11). Plasma renin activity (PRA) decreases. Some peripheral α-receptor stimulation can cause a transient pressor response when clonidine is given intravenously. Side effects

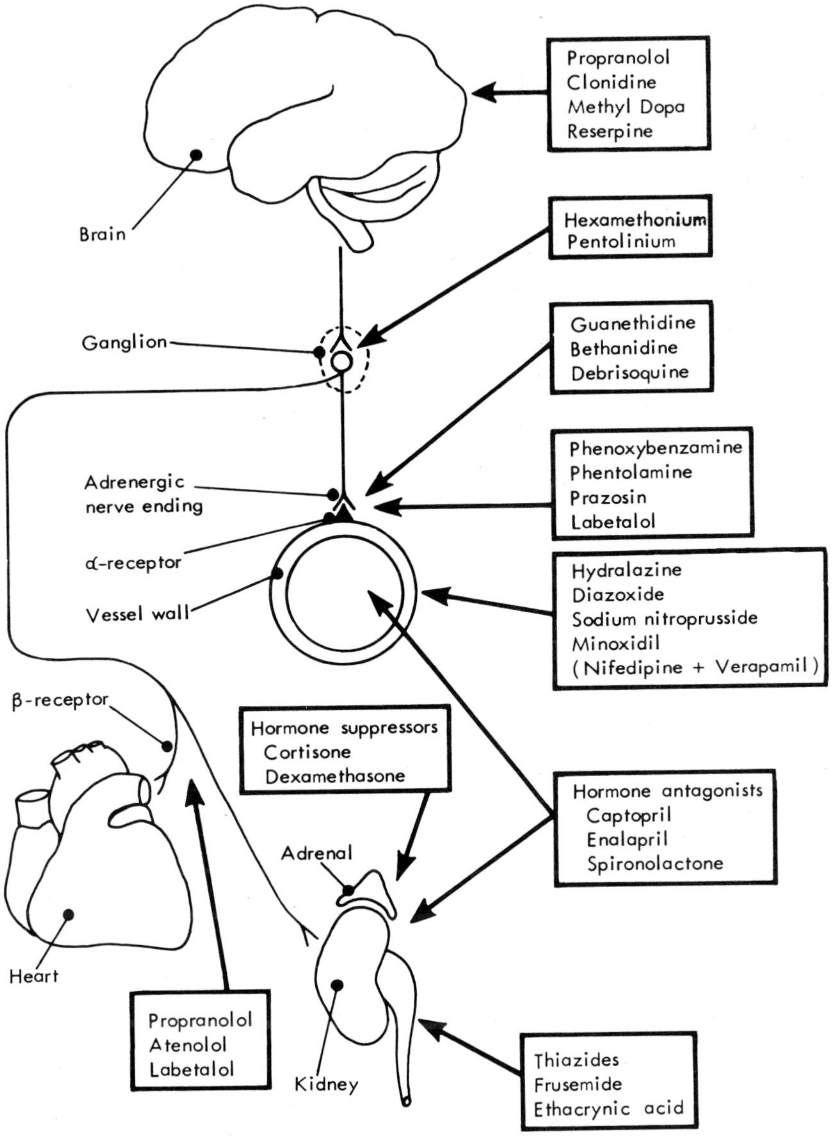

Figure 47.1. The sites of action of antihypertensive agents. (From Dillon MJ: Modern management of hypertension. In Meadow R (ed): Advances in Paediatrics, No. 7, 1984, Churchill Livingstone, Edinburgh, p. 35.

Table 47.1.
Drug Treatment of Acute Hypertensive Emergency[1]

Drug	Dose	Action	Comment
Labetalol	1–3 mg/kg per h IV	α- and β-blocker	Drug of choice
Sodium nitroprusside	0.5–8.0 μg/kg/min IV	Direct vasodilator	Drug of choice
Diazoxide	2–10 mg/kg IV (bolus)	Direct vasodilator	Second-line drug
Hydralazine	0.1–0.2 mg/kg IV or IM	Direct vasodilator	Second-line drug
Clonidine	2–6 μg/kg IV	Central α-adrenergic stimulator	Second-line drug
Verapamil	1–10 mg/kg/h IV	Calcium channel inhibitor	Limited experience in children
Furosemide	1–2 mg/kg IV	Loop diuretic	Diuretic of choice
Phentolamine	0.1–0.2 mg/kg IV	α-blocker	Valuable in pheochromocytoma
Captopril	0.1–0.3 mg/kg/dose (oral)	Converting enzyme inhibitor	Second-line drug
Minoxidil	0.1–0.2 mg/kg/dose (oral)	Direct vasodilator	Second-line drug

[1] See text for details. (From Dillon MJ: Modern management of hypertension. In Meadow R (ed): Recent Advances in Paediatrics, No. 7, 1984, Churchill-Livingstone, Edinburgh, p 35.)

Table 47.2.
Drug Treatment of Moderate-to-Severe Hypertension[1]

Drug	Oral Dose Initial (per kg/day)	Oral Dose Maximum (per kg/day)	Action	Comment
Propranolol	1–2 mg	10–12 mg	β-blocker	Drug of choice
Hydralazine	1–2 mg	8 mg	Direct vasodilator	Drug of choice
Prazosin	0.05–0.1 mg	0.4 mg	α-blocker	Drug of choice
Captopril	0.3 mg	5 mg	Converting enzyme inhibitor	Second-line drug
Minoxidil	0.1–0.2 mg	1–2 mg	Direct vasodilator	Second-line drug
Chlorothiazide	10 mg	40 mg	Diuretic	Drug of choice in mild hypertension
Hydrochlorothiazide	1 mg	4 mg	Diuretic	Drug of choice in mild hypertension
Furosemide	0.5–1.0 mg	15 mg	Loop diuretic	Drug of choice with vasodilator agents and in renal failure
Clonidine	5 μg	30 μg	Central α-adrenergic stimulator	Third-line drug
Methyldopa	5 mg	40 mg	Central α-adrenergic stimulator	Third-line drug
Phenoxybenzamine	1 mg	4 mg	α-adrenergic blocker	Drug of choice in pheochromocytoma
Spironolactone	1 mg	3 mg	Competitive aldosterone antagonist	Drug of choice in some mineralocorticoid excess states
Triamterine	2 mg	6 mg	Nonsteroidal potassium sparing agent	Of value in certain mineralocorticoid excess states
Atenolol	1 mg	2 mg	Cardioselective β blocker	β-blocker for use in the presence of asthma
Nifedipine	0.25 mg	1 mg	Calcium channel inhibitor	Limited experience in children, valuable in essential hypertension

[1] See text for details. (From Dillon MJ: Modern management of hypertension. In Meadow R (ed): Recent Advances in Paediatrics, No. 7, 1984, Churchill Livingstone, Edinburgh, p 35.)

include dryness of the mouth, drowsiness, nausea, constipation, and depression. The drug's most important complication is the withdrawal syndrome; there is a sharp rise in blood pressure if treatment is abruptly stopped. This may require phentolamine to control blood pressure. In children where adherence to therapy may be uncertain, the risks are greater.

Clonidine has a role when other agents are contraindicated. It can be given orally or intravenously (Tables 47.1 and 47.2).

Methyldopa

Methyldopa is converted to α-methyl noradrenaline and initially was thought to act by diminishing peripheral sympathetic neurohumoral transmission by acting as a false transmitter. The drug's main site of action, however, is the brain stem, where α-methyl noradrenaline stimulates central α-blood pressure lowering receptors (12). Methyldopa also lowers PRA.

Side effects include nasal stuffiness and dryness of the mouth, somnolence, or fatigue and depression. A positive direct Coombs' test develops in 20% of patients; in this event treatment should only be stopped if hemolytic anemia develops. Occasionally hepatocellular dysfunction, lupuslike reactions, and colitis have been reported.

Methyldopa, which was extremely popular, is not now recommended as a first-line drug for children because of these effects on mood. Although it is available for intravenous use, other more appropriate drugs are preferred (Table 47.2).

Ganglionic Blocking Agents

Hexamethonium, Pentolinium, and Trimethaphan

Hexamethonium, pentolinium, and trimethophan are not recommended. They act by blocking sympathetic and parasympathetic ganglia and produce such severe side effects that they have been completely superseded in pediatric practice by sodium nitroprusside and labetalol (see section on labetalol).

Postganglionic Adrenergic Blocking Agents

Guanethidine, Bethanidine, and Debrisoquine

Guanethidine, bethanidine, and debrisoquine are not recommended. They act at postganglionic nerve endings and interfere with release of the neurotransmitter noradrenaline (13). The major side effect is postural hypotension, which is sufficiently troublesome to discourage the use of these drugs in children.

Reserpine

Reserpine was once used extensively; now it is not recommended. It acts on neuronal storage vesicles in adrenergic nerve terminals, causing peripheral and central nervous system depletion of catecholamine stores (14). It also suppresses PRA. Side effects include depression, nightmares, sleepiness, nasal congestion, and gastrointestinal upsets.

β-adrenergic Blocking Agents

Propranolol

Propranolol is the best-known β-adrenergic blocking agent. It acts by competitive inhibition of catecholamines on β-receptor-mediated effects on heart and kidney, at presynaptic β-receptors of postganglionic nerve endings, and in the central nervous system. The result is diminished cardiac output, inhibited renin release, impaired neurotransmitter noradrenaline release, and reduced efferent sympathetic activity from the brain (15). The side effects include bradycardia, bronchospasm (especially in children with a history of asthma), mild decrease in renal blood flow, sodium and water retention, Raynaud's phenomenon, nightmares, hallucinations, nausea, diarrhea, and lethargy (14, 16). Occasionally it causes hypoglycemia which can be a major problem in children with juvenile diabetes.

The frequency of these adverse effects is low, however, and propranolol is therefore still a preferred drug because of its effectiveness. (Table 47.2)

Cardioselective β-Blockers

There is no evidence that any β-blocker is more effective than any other in lowering blood pressure when given in appropriate dosages; however, some such as atenolol are considered to be cardioselective. This or a similar preparation is preferred when β-blockade is required in a patient with a history of mild asthma, but even this preparation should be administered cautiously to these patients. Non-β-blocking hypotensive therapy should be used in patients with severe asthma. Atenolol has a long half-life and can be given once a day (17).

α-Adrenergic Blockers

Phenoxybenzamine

Phenoxybenzamine is a long-acting α-adrenergic blocking agent usually given orally, although an intravenous preparation is available. The drug has a long half-life, i.e., >24 hr, perhaps because it binds irreversibly to its receptors. Adverse reactions include postural hypotension, reflex tachycardia, miosis, nasal stuffiness, inhibition of ejaculation, feelings of weakness and tiredness, and, in some patients, nausea and vomiting (16, 18).

Phenoxybenzamine is a drug of choice in catecholamine excess states; often it is given in combination with the β-blocking agent propranolol (Table 47.2).

Phentolamine

Phentolamine is a rapidly acting α-blocking agent for intravenous use that is effective within 30 sec and whose action lasts 30 to 60 min. The hypotensive action usually is apparent only for 10 to 15 min, and its main use is in hypertensive emergencies associated with pheochromocytomas. It also has been used diagnostically to identify catecholamine excess states by the hypotensive response to intravenous injection (Table 47.1).

Prazosin

Prazosin has an α-adrenergic blocking action with selectivity for postsynaptic receptors (19). It was initially classified as a direct-acting vasodilator, but this mechanism has not been confirmed. The feedback control of neuronal adrenaline release by presynaptic receptors remains intact; thus the tachycardia, increased cardiac output, and hyperreninemia seen with conventional α-blocking agents are not seen with prazosin (16). The half-life of the drug in plasma is three to four hr, but the antihypertensive effects last longer, so twice daily doses are effective.

Side effects are mild, although a troublesome "first dose" phenomenon is seen at times, usually resulting from acute postural hypotension. Other adverse effects including headache, lethargy, weakness, palpitations, and nausea. Prazosin combined with a β-blocker is a drug of choice in children, especially when hydralazine is unsuitable. Prazosin is interchangable with phenoxybenzamine for treating catecholamine excess hypertension (Table 47.2).

Labetalol

α- and β-adrenoreceptor blockade characterize the pharmacological actions of labetalol (20), although it is less active at α- than at β-adrenoreceptors. It may be administered intravenously or orally. It is particularly valuable in children as an intravenous preparation for treating acute hypertensive emergencies (21) and in the management of catecholamine excess states.

Side effects of intravenous therapy include hypotension, heart failure and, in asthmatics, bronchospasm. Long-term use may be associated with headaches, tiredness, depression, dizziness, micturition difficulties, epigastric pain, nausea, vomiting, and skin rash.

This is a drug of choice for treating hypertensive emergencies, but as yet it appears to have no clear advantage over alternative therapy for chronic long-term oral use (Table 47.1).

Vasodilators

Hydralazine

Hydralazine is a direct, vasodilating agent acting on arteriolar smooth muscle (22). It reduces peripheral vascular resistance and hence systemic blood pressure. Afferent and efferent sympathetic pathways remain intact, and as a result, there is reflex tachycardia and increased cardiac output. Renin release is stimulated. The absence of effect on the venous circulation ensures a satisfactory venous return on standing with little postural hypotension.

Hydralazine is eliminated primarily by liver acetylation; the varied rate of this process is genetically determined. Fast acetylators require higher doses for blood pressure control than slow acetylators (23). Although the plasma half-life is two to four hr in most persons, the antihypertensive action is longer because the drug or its metabolites are retained in vessel walls. Twice daily doses are therefore possible, although usually the drug is administered every six to eight hr. In practice, knowledge of acetylation status is not essential before commencing therapy.

Side effects include flushing, headache, tachycardia, palpitations, increased cardiac output, and salt and water retention. A lupus erythematosus-like reaction consisting of arthralgia, fever, rash, and malaise is dose-related and disappears when the drug is discontinued. This reaction is associated with DNA antibodies in serum but not with renal or central nervous system complications (24).

Hydralazine can be administered orally or parenterally. As an oral agent, it is a preferred drug for children (Tables 47.1 and 47.2).

Minoxidil

Minoxidil is a powerful direct vasodilator acting on systemic arterioles (25). It has been used successfully in the management of severe childhood hypertension (14, 26).

The serum half-life is approximately 4 hr, but its hypotensive effect lasts for 12 to 24 hr. It stimulates renin release predominantly by activating β-adrenergic receptors (25).

Side effects include headache, flushing, tachycardia, palpitations, increased cardiac output, and salt and water retention. Hypertrichosis is induced, most prominently across the forehead but also on the trunk and limbs; this disappears within two to three months of discontinuing therapy (14).

Minoxidil is not recommended as a first-line hypotensive agent in children but is a valuable second-line drug in resistant hypertensive states (Tables 47.1 and 47.2).

Diazoxide

Diazoxide is a nondiuretic thiazide with a direct vasodilator action (27). It is usually administered by intravenous bolus injection to overcome the binding by plasma proteins, but it can also be used orally. The effect of an intravenous bolus may last for 12 hr or more; however, the serious risks of hypotension occurring shortly after injection require that it be used with caution.

Side effects, apart from hypotension, include salt and water retention, hyperglycemia, hyperuricemia, hypertrichosis, nausea, vomiting, and an unusual metallic taste in the mouth.

This is a second-line drug for treatment of hypertensive emergencies in children. It has a role if administered as small repeated bolus injections (Table 47.1).

Sodium Nitroprusside

Sodium nitroprusside acts as a direct vasodilator on capacitance vessels, thus causing arteriolar vasodilation (28). It also causes venous dilatation and hence has the ability to produce marked hypotension. Given intravenously it acts within seconds, and its effect lasts for a matter of minutes. Sodium nitroprusside rarely causes tachycardia, unlike the other vasodilators described in this section. The drug has been used widely and successfully in children (29, 30) to treat acute hypertensive emergencies.

Nitroprusside is metabolized to cyanide and thiocyanate, and the latter can accumulate in renal failure. Cyanide intoxication is rare; it may occur when the patient receives an excessive dose or has liver impairment. A practical disadvantage of the drug is its inactivation by light and the need to protect against this when it is being used.

This is a drug of choice for treating the acute hypertensive emergency in children (Table 47.1).

Calcium Antagonists

The calcium channel-inhibiting drugs have been developed to treat essential hypertension. The basis for their use is that in hypertension elevated intracellular sodium in arteriolar walls is believed to lead to increased arteriolar tone by raising intracellular free calcium (31); blocking calcium entry reverses this effect. Two drugs serve this purpose: verapamil (32) and nifedipine (33). These agents have not been used extensively in pediatrics, but they may provide an alternative to standard antihypertensive drugs in the future (Table 47.1 and 47.2).

Renin-Angiotensin System (RAS) Blocking Agents

Intravenous Drugs

Hypotensive agents that specifically block the renin angiotensin system (RAS) have special advantages in the treatment of hypertension caused by excess angiotensin II production. Saralasin, a competitive angiotensin II antagonist and SQ 20881, an angiotensin-converting enzyme inhibitor, have hypotensive effects; but because they can only be administered parenterally, they are not suitable for routine clinical use.

Captopril

The development of captopril (34), an orally effective agent that inhibits the conversion of angiotensin I to angiotensin II, has had major clinical implications.

Captopril is rapidly absorbed and metabolized; its peak blood levels are reached in 30 to 90 min (35), and it has a half-life of less than two hr. The main route for clearance is renal; consequently the dose is less in renal failure. The mechanism of action is complex and probably involves an increase in the vasodilator bradykinin as well as a decrease in the vasopressor angiotensin II. An increase in PRA and a decrease in aldosterone production occur while it is administered.

Adverse effects are few but include neutropenia in 0.3% of patients, proteinuria (35), reversible renal failure in patients with preexisting renal impairment (36) or renovascular disease (37); skin rashes, angioedema of the face, and disturbance of taste also occur.

Captopril has been used successfully in children (38), and although currently not the drug of choice in childhood hypertension, it has the potential to become so, particularly in renin-dependent hypertensive states (Table 47.2).

Enalpril (MK 421)

Enalpril (MK 421) is another orally active converting enzyme inhibitor (39) that is effective in lowering blood pressure in hypertensive adults (40). It has not yet been used to treat children.

Diuretics

Thiazides

The major action of the thiazide group of diuretics is to inhibit Na transport in the early distal tubule causing increased urinary sodium and water excretion and extracellular fluid volume depletion. Associated hemodynamic changes suggest in addition a possible modification of vascular reactivity to catecholamines and angiotensin and a decrease in cardiac output (41). These drugs are well absorbed from the gastrointestinal tract; peak serum levels are two to four hr after a dose, and clearance is primarily renal. Chlorothiazide and hydrochlorothiazide can maintain maximal diuretic effect by being administered every 12 hr.

The major adverse effect seen with thiazide therapy is hypokalemia, which may require potassium supplementation. Other side effects reported in adults, e.g., hyperglycemia, hyperuricemia, and hypercalcemia have not been reported as major problems in children (41). Occasionally skin rashes and other more serious allergic reactions have been seen (16) (Table 47.2).

Loop Diuretics

Furosemide is the most important of the loop diuretics, but ethacrynic acid, bumetanide, and indanone act in a similar way. The major site of action of these agents is the ascending limb of the loop of Henle, where inhibition of active Cl reabsorption occurs. They are potent diuretics, and their use is usually restricted to patients with significant fluid retention as a part of their disease or as a result of the other hypotensive therapy being used.

The main side effects of furosemide and ethacrynic acid are hypokalemia, volume depletion, and ototoxicity. Ototoxicity is related to high blood levels, and the risk is greatest in patients with renal insufficiency (14). Permanent hearing loss has been reported with both furosemide and ethacrynic acid; possibly the risk is greater with the latter. Reported interstitial nephritis with furosemide was reversed on drug withdrawal (42).

Furosemide is the recommended diuretic in this category for use in children (Tables 47.1 and 47.2).

Distal Tubule Diuretics

Spironolactone and triamterine are the two diuretics within this category that have therapeutic value in children.

Spironolactone is a competitive antagonist of aldosterone and is valuable in patients with aldosterone excess (adrenal adenoma or hyperplasia) and in some patients with low renin hypertension in which mineralocorticoidlike substances may play a part (14). Side effects include hyperkalemia, gynecomastia, and menstrual irregularities.

Triamterine, a nonsteroidal K-sparing agent, is used in clinical states similar to those in which spironolactone is appropriate; its action is independent of aldosterone antagonism. It is particularly helpful in low renin hypertension caused by cortisol 11 β-hydroxysteroid dehydrogenase deficiency (43). Its major side effect is hyperkalemia in the presence of renal insufficiency (Table 47.2).

PRINCIPLES OF THERAPY

Hypertensive Crisis

Indications and Risks

Emergency management is indicated when the level of blood pressure is a threat to life or to the function of vital organs. Drugs with rapid action are necessary but require careful administration to prevent sudden hypotension and resulting failure of autoregulatory mechanisms (44–46).

Until recently, intravenous diazoxide was the choice for the emergency treatment of hypertension; however, the incidence of hypotension after bolus injections of diazoxide has changed the approach; drugs that can be infused to finely control blood pressure during the critical early phase of management are preferred. Sodium nitroprusside (30) and labetalol (21) are both effective; labetalol may be more appropriate for initial use because its method of administration is simpler. Alternative parenteral agents such as intravenous verapamil (47) and clonidine (48) have been advocated but are seldom required if sodium nitroprusside or labetalol is available. Orally administered hypotensives, e.g., minoxidil (26), diazoxide (49), captopril (38), and nifedipine (33), have proved effective in treating malignant hypertension but lack the prompt response and fine control available with intravenous preparations.

Clinical Management

The hypertensive child requiring emergency treatment has a blood pressure raised to such an extent that neurological, cardiac, or renal complications may develop or may have already developed. Of these stroke is the most forbidding.

When treatment has to be initiated, the cause of hypertension frequently is unknown. It is usually necessary, therefore, to undertake investigative procedures at the same time as therapy, depending on the patient's clinical status. From the clinical examination clues to hypertension causation (see Chapter 46) may be detected and baseline observations made, especially those relating to the central nervous system. A check of visual acuity and pupillary reaction is important before beginning treatment. A pretreatment blood sample for peripheral PRA, PA, and catecholamine concentrations may be valuable.

If the child is having a convulsion, a suitable anticonvulsant should be administered intravenously and steps taken to reduce blood pressure by intravenous labetalol or sodium nitroprusside (50). Labetalol should be infused initially at the rate of 1 mg/kg/hr. If an adequate response is obtained, the infusion should be stopped until blood pressure rises again. If no response occurs within 30 min, the rate of infusion should be incrementally increased by 1 mg/kg/hr up to a maximum of 3 mg/kg/hr (Table 47.1). The duration of the hypotensive response varies but can be up to six hr.

Sodium nitroprusside, by contrast, is only effective while it is being administered. The starting dose is 0.5 μg/kg/min; this is incrementally increased as needed up to 8.0 μg/kg/min (Table 47.1). The infusion bottle and drip tubing need to be protected from light by aluminum foil during treatment.

Throughout this early phase of management blood pressure should be monitored frequently. The sphygmomanometer cuff must be the appropriate size and the defined limits of blood pressure values that justify change in treatment must be clear. The object is to reduce blood pressure sufficiently to avoid hypertensive complications yet to maintain it at a level that permits autoregulatory mechanisms to function and that ensures an adequate blood supply to the brain or other viscera (44). To achieve this, blood pressure should be decreased in the first 6 hr by not more than one third of the total reduction planned by a further third over the next 12 to 36 hr and the final third over the following 2 to 4 days. An intravenous line should be available during the first few days of this period so that saline or plasma can be administered rapidly if blood pressure drops unexpectedly. A central venous line also is valuable to monitor central venous pressure for detecting volume overload or depletion.

Many children with severe hypertension on presentation have ECF depletion; the administration of diuretics at that point is contraindicated because severe hypotension may ensue. Unless saline overload is obvious, as confirmed by cardiopulmonary congestion, it is probably safer to reserve diuretics until the hypertensive state is stabilized (50).

Repeated checks on visual acuity and pupillary reactions to light are essential because the risk of infarcting the optic nerve heads of children with accelerated hypertension is considerable (44, 51). The loss of vision or pupillary reaction to light as blood pressure is reduced is an emergency that justifies raising the blood pressure by intravenous saline or plasma. Dexamethasone may be required, and even a stellate ganglion block should be considered to improve blood flow through the branches of the ciliary arteries supplying the optic nerve.

Before stabilizing blood pressure it is probably wise to use just one hypotensive agent. Introducing several drugs simultaneously leads to unpredictable responses to incremental dose increases with the risks that these entail. There are times, however, when more than one agent has to be administered to control blood pressure adequately; the prolonged use of an ineffectual medication is ill advised. Once safe control is achieved, an oral maintenance antihypertensive regimen can gradually begin (Fig. 47.2). Appropriate further investigations can then be undertaken and decisions concerning therapy considered.

Medical Management of Moderate-to-Severe Chronic Hypertension

Management of moderate-to-severe hypertension in childhood depends somewhat on the underlying cause. Unlike hypertensive emergencies, there is time to identify the cause and to prescribe accordingly. Since the majority of children in this category have renin-dependent hypertension, few patients need alternative special therapy. Those that do include patients with coarctation of the aorta, renal failure, and catecholamine and corticosteroid excess hypertension. Notable among these are patients on dialysis therapy or those who have undergone renal transplantation.

Except for special category patients, most children can be managed effectively on a combination of vasodilator and β-blocking drugs with or without a diuretic. Hydralazine and propranolol or prazosin and propranolol are effective therapeutic combinations and have been used extensively. A cardioselective β-blocker may need to be prescribed instead of propranolol when bronchospasm is likely. A loop diuretic is often necessary to offset the salt and water retention that occurs with the

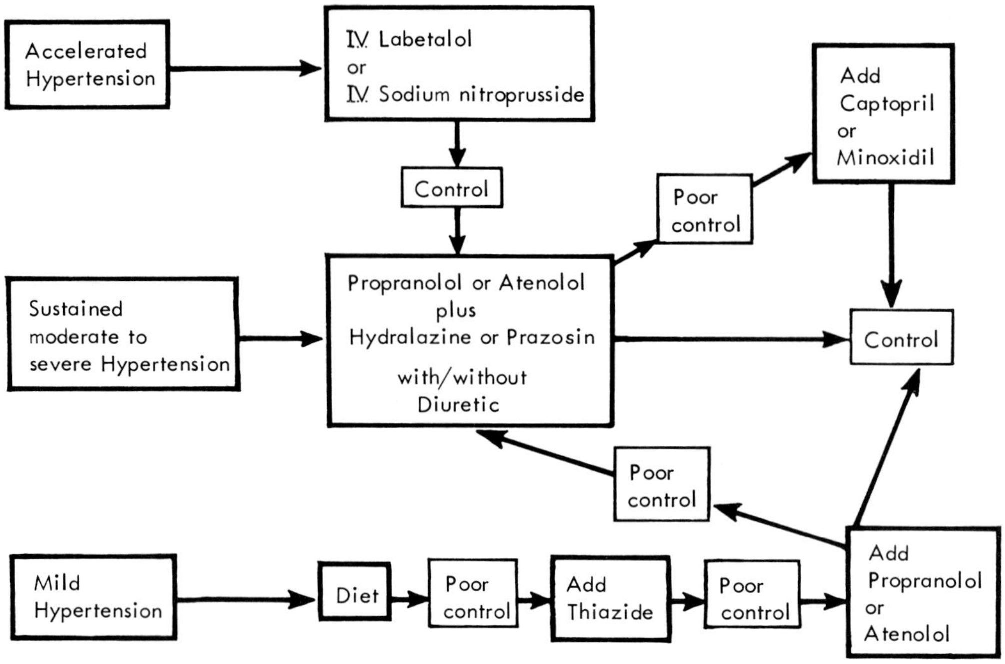

Figure 47.2. Flow chart of treatment in childhood hypertension. (From Dillon MJ: Modern management of hypertension. In Meadow R (ed): Advances in Paediatrics, No. 7, 1984, Churchill Livingstone, Edinburgh, p. 35.

use of peripheral vasodilators. Additional agents that may be added, if blood pressure is poorly controlled, include captopril or minoxidil. In view of its side effects, minoxidil probably should be reserved for refractory hypertensive problems and should be combined with a β-blocking agent and a diuretic. Captopril has considerable potential as a first-line treatment in combination with a diuretic. It may become the drug of choice in childhood hypertension when hyperreninemia is suspected. (See Figure 47.2 and Table 47.2 and previous text for dosages and side effects.)

Hypertension of Chronic Renal Failure

The hypertension associated with chronic renal failure is discussed in detail in Chapter 53B. Medical management depends on the underlying cause, the degree of renal impairment, the relative contributions of ECF volume overload and of the RAS to the hypertensive state. Other factors such as steroid therapy and the use of blood transfusions also are important. Before end-stage renal disease (ESRD), treatment usually consists of a combination of dietary NaCl limitation, diuretics, and antihypertensive agents such as propranolol and hydralazine. Hypertensive crises should be treated on their merits as outlined on p 763. With time, however, as renal failure advances to end-stage renal disease the major objective of management becomes controlling ECF volume by restricting salt and water intake and removing extra ECF by dialysis and ultrafiltration. In some patients blood pressure will not be adequately controlled by this means; there will be evidence of increased activity of the RAS. Some form of additional antihypertensive therapy may be required; captopril is a potentially valuable drug for this purpose. Alternatively, nephrectomy to remove renin-secreting kidneys that have little of no excretory function may be necessary. (See References 16 and 48 for more detail.)

Catecholamine Excess Hypertension

In catecholamine excess states associated with hypertension, phenoxybenzamine and propranolol is the most useful therapeutic combination. β-blockade in addition to α-blockade may be necessary to offset the tachycardia following the use of α-blocking agents; it also may have a role in blocking the effects of circulating epinephrinelike substances. Full α-blockade is critical before any invasive investigation. Prazosin may be interchangeable with phenoxybenzamine as the α-blocking agent (18). An adequate dietary intake of salt is recommended to restore ECF volume.

Corticosteroid Excess Hypertension

In congenital adrenal hyperplasia caused by 11-hydroxylase or 17-hydroxylase deficiency, the hypertension can be treated with hydrocortisone, which suppresses the production of abnormal mineralocorticoids. In Conn's syndrome due to adrenal hyperplasia, spironolactone is the drug of choice. It has a role preoperatively if the underlying cause is an adenoma. In Cushing's syndrome, some mineralocorticoid excess may be present, which would justify the use of spironolactone; however, it is usually necessary to treat these patients with standard hypotensives as well. In low renin hypertension due to cortisol 11-β-hydroxysteroid dehydrogenase deficiency presenting with severe hypokalemic alkalosis, treatment should include spironolactone and triamterine. (See Table 47.2 and previous text for dosages and side effects.)

Treatment of Mild Hypertension

Mild hypertension poses the greatest dilemma in determining treatment. It is important to balance the risks of prolonged drug therapy against those of leaving mild hypertension untreated. Decisions about treatment depend on the height of the blood pressure, its constancy, its cause, the presence or absence of various risk factors, and whether the child or adolescent is symptomatic or has evidence of target organ involvement. As has been mentioned in the section on general management, simple nonpharmacological measures may be tried first, e.g., weight reduction and dietary sodium restriction by avoiding table salt and salty processed foods.

Pharmacological agents, however, may be necessary. The first choice probably is a thiazide diuretic used alone. A β-blocking agent, e.g., propranolol or a calcium channel-inhibiting drug (e.g., nifedipine) if blood pressure is not controlled may be added if the diuretic drug is ineffective. It is important to stress to the patient that alternative drugs are available if unpleasant side effects occur. A commitment to drug treatment probably should be made only when the patient understands that treating an asymptomatic disease is important and that side effects, if they appear, usually can be reversed by changing therapy.

References

1. McGregor GA, Markandu ND, Best FE, et al: Double-blind randomized crossover trial of moderate sodium restriction in essential hypertension. Lancet 1:351, 1982.
2. Watt GCM, Edwards C, Hart JT, Hart M, et al: Dietary sodium restriction for mild hypertension in general practice. Br Med J 286:432, 1983.
3. Kempner W: The treatment of hypertensive vascular disease with rice diet. Am J Med 4:545, 1948.
4. Parfrey PS, Vandenburg MJ, Wright P, et al: Blood pressure and hormonal changes following alteration in dietary sodium and potassium in mild essential hypertension. Lancet 1:59, 1981.
5. Reisin E, Abel R, Modan M, et al: Effect of weight loss without salt restriction on the reduction of blood pressure in overweight hypertensive patients. N Engl J Med 298:1, 1978.
6. Ellison RC, Sosenko JM, Harper GP, et al: Obesity, sodium intake, and blood pressure in adolescents. Hypertension 2(42):78, 1980.
7. Boyer JL, Kasch FW: Exercise therapy in hypertensive men. J Am Med Assoc 211:1668, 1970.
8. Still JL, Cottom D: Severe hypertension in childhood. Arch Dis Child 42:34, 1967.
9. Uhari M, Saukkonen AL, Koskimies O: Central nervous system involvement in severe arterial hypertension in childhood. Arch Dis Child 42:34, 1967.
10. Julius S: Clinical and physiological significance of borderline hypertension in youth. Pediatr Clin North Am 25:35, 1978.
11. Pettinger WA: Clonidine, a new antihypertensive drug. N Engl J Med 293:1179, 1973.
12. Van Zwieten PA: The central action of antihypertensive drugs mediated via central alpha receptors. J Pharm Pharmacol 25:89, 1973.
13. Woosley RL, Nies AS: Guanethidine. N Engl J Med 295:1053, 1976.
14. Sinaiko AR, Mirkin BL: Clinical pharmacology of antihypertensive drugs in children. Pediatr Clin North Am 25:137, 1978.
15. Hollifield JW, Sherman K, Vander Zwagg R, Shand DG: Proposed mechanisms of propranolol's antihypertensive effect in essential hypertension. N Engl J Med 294:68, 1976.
16. Ingelfinger JR: Pediatric Hypertension. Philadelphia, W B Saunders Co Ltd, 1982.
17. Floras JS, Jones JV, Hassan MO, Sleight P: Ambulatory blood pressure during once daily randomised double-blind administration of atenolol, metoprolol, pindolol and slow-release propranolol. Br Med J 285:1387, 1982.
18. Sever PS, Roberts JC, Snell ME: Phaeochromocytoma. Clin Endocrinol Metab 9:543, 1980.
19. Graham RM, Pettinger WA: Prazosin. N Engl J Med 300:232, 1979.
20. Britain RT, Levy GP: A review of the pharmacology of labetalol, a combined alpha and beta adrenoceptor blocking drug. Br J Clin Pharmacol 3 (Suppl):681, 1976.
21. Cumming AMM, Davies DL: Intravenous labetalol in hypertensive emergency. Lancet 1:929, 1979.
22. Koch-Weser J: Hydralazine. N Engl J Med 295:320, 1976.
23. Zacest R, Koch-Weser J: The relation of hydralazine plasma concentration to dosage and hypotensive action. Clin Pharmacol Ther 13:420, 1972.
24. Perry HM: Late toxicity to hydralazine resembling systemic lupus erythematosis or rheumatoid arthritis. Am J Med 54:58, 1973.
25. Pettinger WA: Minoxidil and the treatment of severe hypertension. N Engl J Med 303:922, 1980.
26. Pennisi AJ, Takahashi M, Bernstein BH, et al: Minoxidil therapy in children with severe hypertension. J Pediatr 90:813, 1977.
27. Koch-Wesser J: Diazoxide. N Engl J Med 24:1271, 1976.
28. Palmer RF, Lasseter KC: Sodium nitroprusside. N Engl J Med 292:294, 1975.
29. Gordillo-Paniagua G, Velasquez-Jones L, Martini R, Valdes-Bolanos E: Sodium nitroprusside treatment of severe arterial hypertension in children. J Pediatr 87:799, 1975.
30. Luderer JR, Hayes AH Jr, Dubnsky O, Berlin CM: Long-term administration of sodium nitroprusside in childhood. J Pediatr 91:490, 1977.
31. Reuter H, Blaustein MP, Hausler G: Na-Ca exchange and tension development in arterial smooth muscle. Philos Trans R Soc Lond B265:87, 1973.
32. Buhler FR, Lennart Hulthen U, Kiowski W, Bolli P: Greater antihypertensive efficacy of the calcium channel inhibitor verapamil in older and low renin patients. Clin Sci 63 (Suppl 8):439S, 1982.
33. Bertel O, Conen D, Radu EW, et al: Nifedipine in hypertensive emergencies. Br Med J 286:19, 1983.
34. Ondetti MA, Rubin B, Cushman DW: Design of specific inhibitors of angiotensin-converting enzyme: new class of orally active antihypertensive agents. Science 194:441, 1977.
35. Vidt DG, Bravo EL, Fouad FM: Captopril. N Engl J Med 306:214, 1982.
36. Woodhouse K, Farrow PR, Wilkinson R: Reversible renal failure during treatment with captopril. Br Med J 2:1146, 1979.
37. Hricik DE, Browning PJ, Kopelman R, et al: Captopril-induced functional renal insufficiency in patients with bilateral renal-artery stenosis or renal artery stenosis in a solitary kidney. N Engl J Med 308:373, 1983.
38. Griswold W, McNeal R, O'Connor D, et al: Oral converting enzyme inhibitor in malignant hypertension. Arch Dis Child 57:235, 1982.
39. Patchett AA, Harris E, Tristram EW, et al: A new class of angiotensin-converting enzyme inhibitors. Nature 288:280, 1980.
40. Hodson GP, Brown JJ, Davies DL, et al: Converting-enzyme inhibitor enalapril (MK 421) in treatment of hypertension with renal artery stenosis. Br Med J 285:1697, 1982.
41. Mirkin BL: Antihypertensive drugs: mechanisms of action and therapeutic application in children. In Giovannelli G, New MI, Gorini S (eds): Hypertension in Children and Adolescents. New York, Raven Press, 1981, p 223.
42. Fuller TJ, Barcenas CG, White MG: Diuretic-induced interstitial nephritis. J Am Med Assoc 235:1998, 1976.
43. Shackleton CHL, Honour JW, Dillon MJ, et al: Hypertension in a four-year-old child: gas chromatographic and mass spectrometric evidence for deficient hepatic metabolism of steroids. J Clin Endocrinol Metab 50:786, 1980.
44. Hulse JA, Taylor DSI, Dillon MJ: Blindness and paraplegia in accelerated hypertension of childhood. Lancet 2:553, 1979.
45. Ledingham JGG, Rajagopalan B: Cerebral complications in the treatment of accelerated hypertension. Q J Med 48:25, 1976.
46. Dillon MJ: Recent advances in evaluation and management of childhood hypertension. Europ J Pediatr 132:133, 1979.
47. Scharer K, Alatas H, Bein G: Die behandlung der renalen hypertension mit verapamil. Kindesalter Monatsschrift fur Kinderheilkunde 125:706, 1977.
48. Scharer K, Rauh, W, Ulmer HE: The management of hypertension in children with chronic renal failure. In Giovannelli G, New MI, Gorini S (eds): Hypertension in Children and Adolescents. New York, Raven Press, 1981, p 239.
49. Kincaid-Smith P: Renal disease and hypertension. Med Clin North Am 61:611, 1977.
50. Dillon MJ: Modern management of hypertension. In Meadow R (ed): Recent Advances in Paediatrics, No. 7. Edinburgh, Churchill Livingstone, 1984, p 35.
51. Taylor D, Ramsay J, Day S, Dillon M: Infarction of the optic nerve head in children with accelerated hypertension. Br J Ophthalmol 65:153, 1981.

11

Reduced Renal Function

CHAPTER **48**

Acute Renal Failure

T. M. BARRATT

Acute renal failure (ARF) is a sudden reduction in renal function to a level insufficient to maintain homeostasis. Several reviews (1–3) and recent accounts of the condition in children are available (4–6). The cardinal feature is a reduction in glomerular filtration rate (GFR), usually but not invariably accompanied by oliguria (urine volume <500 ml/1.73 m^2SA/24 hr; in infants <0.5 ml/kg/hr). The secretion of urine depends on the adequacy of the blood supply to the kidney, the integrity of the renal parenchyma, and the patency of the urinary passages. Thus there is merit in the time-honored if simplistic classification of ARF as prerenal, renal, or postrenal (Table 48.1). In practice, however, the distinction between prerenal oliguria and acute tubular necrosis (ATN) may be blurred; in individual cases many factors may be operative, and episodes of ARF may be superimposed on preexisting renal disease (acute-on-chronic renal failure).

The epidemiology of ARF in children is influenced by many factors, the principal being standards of living and health care in the community. ARF is common in underdeveloped countries, usually ATN resulting from the salt and water depletion of gastroenteritis. In developed countries, ARF is rare in childhood, and the experience of any individual unit will be colored by patterns of referral rather than by the relative incidence of the various disorders in the community as a whole.

At the Hospital for Sick Children, London, there is a strong tradition of pediatric urology, and these cases, therefore, comprise a large proportion of the infants with ARF (Table 48.2) (7). In recent years, however, with improved standards of neonatal care, more of these babies are diagnosed early, before uremia or urinary tract infection (UTI) has supervened. Now the most common cause of ARF in infants at the Hospital for Sick Children is cardiopulmonary bypass surgery (Table 48.3) (8).

PATHOGENESIS

Prerenal Factors

If renal perfusion pressure falls, renal blood flow and GFR decline, but tubular reabsorption of salt and water continues. Thus there is oliguria with "good quality" urine: osmolality >300 mosm/kg and urine-plasma urea concentration ratio >5 but with a urine sodium concentration <20 mmol/L. These features are summarized in the fractional excretion of sodium (FENa), derived from the sodium/creatinine clearance ratio (9):

$$\text{FENa} = (\text{UNa}/\text{PNa})/(\text{Ucr}/\text{Pcr}) \times 100 \qquad (1)$$

In adults with prerenal ARF, FENa is 0.4 ± 0.1% (SD) and with ATN, 7.0 ± 1.4% (10); similar occurrences have been observed in children (11). Such kidneys exhibit a diuretic response to furosemide or mannitol and recover rapidly when renal perfusion is restored; it is worthy of note that the administration of a diuretic obscures the urinary evidence of hypoperfusion.

In most cases the circulatory failure underlying the renal hypoperfusion will be evident, with hypotension, poor peripheral circulation, and an increased core-skin temperature gap (12). The low cardiac output may arise from a low filling pressure (central venous pressure:CVP) resulting from hypovolemia: extracellular fluid (ECF) volume contraction caused by salt and water loss as with gastroenteritis; plasma volume contraction caused by the hypoalbuminemia of the nephrotic syndrome, liver failure, burns, or blood loss. Alternatively, the heart itself may be responsible, in which case the CVP may be raised. Accurate evaluation of the CVP is thus critical in the assessment of ARF in shocked children. Although bedside examination of the jugular venous pulse or review of the cardiac silhouette on chest roentgenogram may be helpful, it is frequently preferable to measure the CVP directly.

Renal Factors

Parenchymal causes of ARF may be classified under the following headings: arterial, venous, glomerular, tubular, and interstitial (Table 48.1). Of these, the renal tubule—being the major site of energy consumption within the kidney—is the most susceptible to ischemic or toxic insults and is the most common site of damage responsible for ARF; therefore, it will be considered first.

Tubular Lesions

Necrosis. The common necrotic condition is ATN, but the terminology is not entirely satisfactory, as necrosis is not always evident histologically, and the term has acquired clinical usage connoting established ARF without obstruction and with no arterial, venous, glomerular, or interstitial lesion sufficient to explain it (13).

The major pathophysiological event appears to lie in the renal circulation, and the term vasomotor nephropathy is gaining currency (14). The underlying feature is decreased renal cortical perfusion, possibly as a consequence of intranephron feedback inhibition resulting from in-

Table 48.1.
Acute Renal Failure (ARF): Pathogenesis

1. Prerenal factors: renal hypoperfusion
   - Hypovolemia
   - Cardiac insufficiency
2. Renal factors
   - Arterial
     - Thromboembolism
     - Arteritis
     - Hemolytic-uremic syndrome (HUS)
   - Venous: renal venous thrombosis (RVT)
   - Glomerular: acute glomerulonephritis (AGN)
     - Exudative
     - Cresentic
   - Tubular
     - Acute tubular necrosis (ATN): ischemic (vasomotor nephropathy) or nephrotoxic
     - Obstructive: crystal nephropathy
   - Interstital
     - Acute interstitial nephritis (AIN)
     - Pyelonephritis
3. Postrenal factors: obstructive nephropathy
   - Congenital
   - Acquired
4. Preexisting factors
   - Acute-on-chronic renal failure
   - End-stage renal failure with acute presentation

Table 48.2.
ARF in Infants <1 yr admitted to the Departments of Nephrology and Urology of the Hospital for Sick Children, London, 1971–1980 (7)

Etiology	Number	Dialyzed	Died
Prerenal and ATN (excluding cardiac cases)	36	13	15
RVT	16	6	2
HUS	15	9	1
UTI (± septicemia): normal urology	16	7	6
abnormal urology	25	6	3
Obstructive uropathy	84	7	8
Polycystic disease	4	2	3
Renal agenesis	3	0	3
Total	199	50	41

Table 48.3.
ARF Complicating Cardiopulmonary Bypass Surgery in Patients Needing Dialysis in the Cardiothoracic Department, Hospital for Sick Children, London, 1978–1979 (8)

Age	Number (N)	ARF	
		n (%N)	Died (%n)
<28 days	21	6 (29)	3 (50)
28 days–1 yr	134	10 (7.6)	5 (50)
>1 yr	304	8 (2.6)	3 (38)
Total	456	24 (5.3)	11 (46)

creased sodium concentration in the tubular fluid at the macula densa. There is evidence of involvement of the renin-angiotensin system in this regulatory mechanism (15). Infusion of dopamine at low rates dilates the renal vasculature and is beneficial, so long as perfusion pressure is maintained.

The parallels of ATN with the physiological characteristics of the infant kidney are worthy of note: the low GFR, decreased outer cortical perfusion, decreased proximal reabsorption of sodium, and increased plasma renin activity (16). The neonatal kidney has been said to be "half way to acute renal failure" (5).

There are two types of tubular lesion in ATN. With nephrotoxins such as mercuric chloride, there is confluent proximal tubular necrosis with an intact basement membrane, whereas with ischemia the tubular necrosis is more distal and patchy with focal ruptures of the basement membrane (17). In children, most cases of ischemic ATN arise from diarrheal dehydration, nephrotic hypovolemia, burns, gram-negative septicemia, perinatal asphyxia, and cardiopulmonary bypass surgery. Nephrotoxic ATN may result from the accidental ingestion of, for example, carbon tetrachloride, from hemoglobinemia, or the myoglobinuria of rhabdomyolysis, or may be iatrogenic as a result of an adverse drug reaction, especially to such antibiotics as gentamicin or some cephalosporins. Some cases of ATN are multifactorial, whereas no cause is apparent in others. The situation following cardiopulmonary bypass surgery is particularly complex, with many factors complicating the principal problem of renal hypoperfusion. Younger children and those with complex heart lesions requiring long bypass times are most at risk, with an overall mortality rate of 50% (Table 48.3) (8).

In the shocked patient, ATN is deemed to exist when renal function does not return in spite of adequate restoration of the circulation. In practice, such a diagnosis is not always easy to make, especially in infants. Hypovolemia is difficult to assess, CVP measurements are not easy to obtain accurately, and adequacy of cardiac output (particularly after cardiopulmonary bypass surgery) is hard to evaluate. Some authors distinguish between "incipient" ATN, in which renal function does not improve with restored perfusion but urine flow responds to diuretics, in contrast to "established" ATN, in which the oliguria is resistant to all measures (18).

Maintenance of adequate hydration and the prior administration of diuretics reduces the incidence of ATN in high-risk situations. For example, the addition of mannitol to the pump-priming fluid improves renal function in children after cardiopulmonary bypass surgery (19). Whether the administration of diuretics during the phase of incipient ATN is beneficial remains controversial, but it does have the advantage of easing the problems of salt and water overload and hyperkalemia (20).

The oliguric phase of ATN is shorter in children than in adults and may escape notice. Some patients are never oliguric but pass urine of insufficient quantity to prevent uremia; such polyuric cases have a better prognosis (21). During the recovery period there may be a diuretic phase with inappropriate losses of salt and water. Often, however, this represents excretion of fluid retained during the oliguric phase, perhaps compounded by the excessive administration of intravenous fluids on the mistaken assumption that the child is volume-depleted. Ultimate recovery is complete.

Obstruction. Tubular obstruction due to crystalluria is an important cause of ARF, for many cases are preventable. Uric acid nephropathy may complicate the treatment of leukemia and other malignancies; rarely, these disorders may present with ARF before any treatment has been proffered. Treatment with alkali and allopurinol reduces this problem, but management of ARF in these cases is complicated by the metabolic effects of cell destruction, particularly hyperkalemia and hyperphosphatemia. Sulfonamide crystalluria is now a rarity as a cause of ARF. An occasional case of primary hyperoxaluria presents with renal failure in infancy, and oxalate deposition with ARF is a feature of ethylene glycol poisoning.

Arterial Disorders

Obstruction. Renal arterial occlusion is a rare cause of ARF in childhood; it may occur as a complication of umbilical artery catheterization in the neonate and be associated with hypertension. Bilateral renal artery stenosis may present with ARF, as may thrombotic, embolic, or stenotic lesions in a solitary kidney. Small vessel disease is a feature of polyarteritis, though renal failure, if present, is usually the result of associated glomerulonephritis.

Hemolytic Uremic Syndrome. The hemolytic uremic syndrome (HUS) is characterized by platelet and fibrin deposition with endothelial proliferation that, in its severe form, results in afferent arteriolar obstruction (Chapter 27). There is sudden onset of a microangiopathic hemolytic anemia, thrombocytopenia, and renal failure (22). The disorder is heterogeneous, with an epidemic form occurring in younger children in summar months and associated with diarrhea, which has a good prognosis. This is in contrast to a sporadic form of insidious onset in older children, sometimes recurrent or familial, and carrying a worse prognosis for renal function (23). This heterogeneity is reflected in the histopathological findings. In mild cases there is glomerular capillary thrombosis, but in the severe forms endothelial proliferation with arteriolar obstruction is prominent, and occasionally there is complete cortical necrosis (24). The effect of the afferent arteriolar obstruction is to reduce nephron perfusion; ARF in this condition is associated with a low FENa. Current research suggests that there is a deficiency of prostacyclin, which predisposes to platelet aggregation (25); a circulating inhibitor of prostacyclin production seems to present in children with the sporadic but not the epidemic form of HUS (26).

Venous Obstruction

The neonatal kidney is particularly susceptible to renal venous thrombosis (RVT), perhaps in part due to high vascular resistance (Chapter 4).

The condition may complicate perinatal crises, particularly in infants of diabetic mothers, or it may be the consequence of severe dehydration (particularly if associated with hypernatremia), cyanotic congenital heart disease, or the nephrotic syndrome (27). The thrombosis starts in peripheral intrarenal veins, so thrombectomy is hardly ever appropriate. The clinical picture is of an unwell oliguric infant with gross macroscopic hematuria (an important distinguishing point from ATN), very firm enlargement of the kidneys and, almost invariably, thrombocytopenia. It is difficult to confirm the diagnosis rigorously, for renal venograms carry some risk and may exacerbate the condition. The affected kidney shrivels up, coming to resemble radiologically a kidney with chronic pyelonephritis though without vesicoureteric reflux, and may cause hypertension. However, even if there is complete anuria or both kidneys seem affected, recovery is still possible, for ATN may coexist and be responsible for the anuria, with the venous infarction being patchy.

Of 25 infants seen at the Hospital for Sick Children in London from 1971 to 1980 and diagnosed as having RVT on the clinical grounds stated, 15 apparently had a bilateral condition, yet all but 2 survived. Fourteen of the survivors had renal damage evident on follow-up urography, and three also had adrenal calcification, a legacy of neonatal adrenal hemorrhage, which is also a form of venous infarction (7).

Medullary necrosis in infants can be regarded as a related lesion in which the venous infarction is confined to the medulla, and the predisposing conditions are similar (28). An important consideration is that in sick infants radiological contrast media may cause the lesion, particularly in doses >3 ml/kg, as for example with angiocardiography (29). The medullary necrosis is typically accompanied by salt-wasting in the recovery phase. This may result in permanent caliceal clubbing similar to that of chronic pyelonephritis, except that there is no overlying cortical scar.

Acute Glomerulonephritis (AGN)

ARF necessitating dialysis occurs in a few patients with poststreptococcal AGN (Chapter 30). The diagnosis is suggested by the history: hematuria with granular casts, proteinuria, and a low plasma C3 concentration. The biopsy appearance is of an acute exudative glomerulonephritis with polymorph infiltration; however, persistent hypocomplementemia is also a feature of mesangiocapillary glomerulonephritis, which may present occasionally with ARF.

Crescentic nephritis is a serious prognostic finding in patients with ARF. It is not an entity in its own right but is a manifestation of severe glomerular injury in various forms of glomerulonephritis that are usually less aggressive: postinfectious, mesangiocapillary (dense deposit variety), Henoch-Schönlein syndrome, polyarteritis, the Goodpasture syndrome, and idiopathic cases. As the incidence of poststreptococcal AGN declines, the proportion of cases with more severe glomerular lesions increases. It is usually prudent to undertake a renal biopsy early in the course of ARF in a child with features of glomerular disease in order to identify the possible treatable disorders, e.g., anticoagulation and immunosuppression for crescentic nephritis and plasmapheresis for the Goodpasture syndrome (Chapter 33).

Interstitial Disease

Acute Interstitial Nephritis (AIN). Acute interstitial nephritis (AIN) arises as a side effect of drugs, a complication of a systemic illness such as juvenile rheumatoid arthritis, or may be idopathic. It is important to identify this condition by biopsy, as it is usually amenable to treatment, either by removing the offending agent or with corticosteroids (Chapter 33).

Pyelonephritis. Bacterial infection of the kidney is rarely sufficient to cause ARF but may be an important contributory factor in obstructive uropathy. This can occur both by direct parenchymal involvement and by introducing a prerenal element with salt and water losses from vomiting and fever. Septicemia is frequently complicated by ARF, partly on the basis of ATN and may be associated with disseminated intravascular coagulation (DIC). Overwhelming infection in the neonate, particularly in males, and principally with *Escherichia coli*, causes septicemia, hematogenous pyelonephritis, DIC, ARF, and sometimes meningitis.

Postrenal Factors

Congenital Factors. Urinary tract obstruction is usually congenital and therefore long-standing but may present as an emergency precipitated into ARF by infection or saline depletion (30). The obstruction is usually intravesical. A posterior urethral valve (Chapter 38) is the most common lesion in male infants, but it may be in the upper urinary tract if there is a solitary functioning kidney.

Acquired Obstructive Lesions. Stones, developing in a solitary kidney or bilaterally, may present as ARF and have an infective or a metabolic basis (Chapter 42). Nonopaque stones resulting from disorders of purine metabolism are a difficult diagnostic problem.

Preexisting Factors

Acute-on-chronic Renal Failure. If there is underlying chronic renal failure (CRF), minor factors may precipitate crises. Such factors include salt depletion, hypertension, UTI, urinary obstruction, and hypercalcemia. They are important to recognize, for they may confer an element of reversibility on what otherwise appears to be end-stage renal disease.

End-stage Renal Failure with Acute Presentation. Occasionally a child with CRF may present for the first time in advanced uremia. Clues of chronicity may be given by poor growth, anemia, and uremic osteodystrophy. Almost any type of chronic nephropathy may present in this manner; however, a silent insidious progression to end-stage renal failure in later childhood is rather typical of medullary cystic disease.

DIAGNOSIS

History

Clues to the underlying pathology of the renal failure may be found in the history. A history of UTI is suggestive of a urological disorder. In males, the character of the urinary stream is of particular importance, although in infants a significant urethral obstruction may be present even with apparently normal micturition. Diarrhea and vomiting suggest saline depletion but can also be a prelude to ATN, RVT, or HUS and can themselves be caused by pyelonephritis or uremia. Exposure to drugs and other nephrotoxins should be reviewed. An upper respiratory infection suggests AGN.

Examination

The physical examination is conducted with two principal problems in mind: the severity of the uremia and the underlying cause. The state of consciousness is impaired in advanced uremia, and many children with this condition have convulsions. Respiratory drive may be poor in infants with overwhelming multisystem disorders, of which ARF is only one facet, and assisted ventilation is often necessary. Hyperventilation (Kussmaul's respiration) is a consequence of metabolic acidosis. Assessment of blood pressure and circulation provides a good guide to the state of hydration. Hypertension and peripheral or pulmonary edema result from salt and water overload, whereas hypotension and diminished skin turgor indicate salt and water depletion.

Enlarged kidneys may represent hydronephrosis, cystic disease, or venous infarction, but pyelonephritis or ATN may also cause some increase in renal size. A full bladder suggests infravesical obstruction.

Monitoring

Careful recording of blood pressure, daily weight, and fluid balance are essential in all cases. A daily record of nutrient intake is important for all but the most transient cases. A venous line will usually be established, but oral administration of fluids and nutrients is preferable if tolerated. In sicker patients, an electrocardiographic monitor, CVP line, and skin and rectal temperature probes will be necessary. Bladder catheterization need not be routine unless there is an obstructive element but is often helpful initially to evaluate the situation. At this stage, complex intravenous schedules are usually necessary to maintain fluid balance and nutrition. For the very sick child in whom ARF is but one aspect of a catastrophic illness, the full panoply of intensive care is required, with arterial pressure monitoring, regular blood gas analysis, and facilities for intubation and intermittent positive pressure ventilation, and possibly for intracranial pressure monitoring as well.

Investigations (Table 48.4)

Blood and Urine

Plasma concentrations of electrolytes, urea, creatinine, calcium, magnesium, and phosphorus are estimated to indicate the severity of the biochemical disturbances. Blood gas analysis reveals the degree of metabolic acidosis and the adequacy of ventilation. Hemoglobin determination and white blood cell and platelet counts provide useful information because anemia with fragmented erythrocytes and thrombocytopenia is characteristic of HUS, although it also occurs with septicemia and RVT. A blood culture is almost always indicated.

Every drop of urine should be preserved for analysis. Routine tests for blood and protein should be supplemented by microscopy to look for red blood cells, casts, white blood cells, bacteria, and crystals. The urine should be cultured, and evidence of UTI is often a pointer to underlying urological disease. The osmolality and the urea, creatinine, and sodium concentrations should be measured to distinguish between prerenal and renal causes of oliguria.

Table 48.4.
Routine Investigations

Blood:	Hemoglobin and erythrocyte morphology
	White blood count and differential
	Platelet count
	Sodium, potassium, bicarbonate
	Urea, creatinine
	Calcium, magnesium, phosphorus
	Total protein, albumin
	Blood gases
	Blood culture
	C3
Urine:	Routine testing for blood and protein
	Microscopy for erythrocytes, leukocytes, casts, and crystals
	Culture
	Osmolality
	Sodium, urea, creatinine
Imaging:	Chest roentgenogram
	Plain abdominal roentgenogram
	Roentgenogram of wrists, hand, and knee
	Renal and bladder ultrasound

Imaging

The radiological investigation of ARF has been transformed by the advent of ultrasound, which in experienced hands can be used reliably to exclude hydronephrosis and provides important information about the state of the renal parenchyma. It facilitates, for example, the immediate recognition of underlying chronic renal disease or obstructive nephropathy. It is much easier to undertake the ultrasound study before a peritoneal catheter is inserted, if time permits.

If hydronephrosis is detected, the next investigation is a micturating cystourethrogram, leaving the child on catheter drainage if an infravesical obstruction, such as urethral valves, is demonstrated. A plain roentgenogram of the abdomen is needed to exclude opaque calculi and may give some information on the renal outlines. Roentgenograms of the chest and of the hand and wrist for osteodystrophy should also be performed. In due course, a ^{99m}Tc-DTPA gamma-camera renal scan will provide information about renal perfusion and the relative function of the two kidneys.

With these techniques, the intravenous urogram has a lesser role to play than formerly in diagnosing the underlying cause of ARF. It is sometimes difficult to fit into the hectic schedule of resuscitation and diagnosis but should be considered later. It is often helpful in the precise anatomical definition of obstructive lesions. Similarly, there is still a place occasionally for cystoscopy and retrograde examination, for example, in the diagnosis of nonopaque calculi.

MANAGEMENT

Resuscitation

The general principles of intensive care prevail, each system being reviewed in turn (Table 48.5).

Table 48.5.
Resuscitation in ARF

Condition	Treatment
Circulatory collapse	Plasma or normal saline 20 ml/kg IV Dopamine 1–10 μg/kg/min IV
Hyperkalemia	Ca gluconate (10%) 0.5 ml/kg IV Ca resonium 1 g/kg/day, oral or rectal Insulin 0.1 U/kg and glucose 0.3 g/kg IV
Convulsions	Diazepam 0.25 mg/kg IV
Hypocalcemia	Ca gluconate (10%) 0.5 ml/kg IV
Hypomagnesemia	Magnesium sulfate (50%) 0.1 ml/kg IM
Acidosis	$NaHCO_3$ 2 mmol/kg IV
Hypertension	Hydrallazine 0.2 mg/kg IV Labetalol 1–4 mg/kg/hr IV infusion
Overload	Furosemide 1–5 mg/kg IV
Hyperphosphatemia	Aludrox 1 ml/kg/24 hr oral
Sepsis	Gentamicin 2 mg/kg IV loading dose

Ventilation

Ventilatory assistance may be necessary immediately. There may be inadequate ventilatory drive caused by severe illness, convulsions, or the consequences of anticonvulsant therapy. Pulmonary edema accompanied by desaturation is best managed by elective ventilation with positive end-expiratory pressure.

Circulation

Volume depletion with hypotension and no evidence of raised CVP requires rapid volume expansion with plasma or normal saline, 20 ml/kg. A good intravenous line is essential. If hypotension persists in spite of an adequate CVP (<5 mm Hg), an initial dopamine infusion of 1 μg/kg/min, gradually increased to a maximum of 10 μg/kg/min, should be tried. The lower dose appears to have a specific dilating effect on the renal vasculature (31). If poor peripheral perfusion persists, with a wide temperature gap between peripheral and core temperature, and raised arterial pressure and CVP, then vasoconstriction can be inferred and a vasodilator, such as intravenous hydralazine, 0.2 mg/kg, may be appropriate (Table 48.6).

Usually a raised blood pressure with oliguria implies salt and water overload. If peripheral circulation is good, or there is peripheral or pulmonary edema or raised CVP as well, there is no doubt about the situation. Intake of salt and water should be minimized. Furosemide, 1 to 5 mg/kg, should be given intravenously; if the response is poor, dialysis is indicated. When hypertension persists in spite of attempts at volume depletion, the blood pressure should be controlled with oral propranolol and hydralazine, 2 mg/kg/day of each. However, β-blockers should be avoided if there is pulmonary edema or evidence of cardiac failure. If the control of hypertension seems an urgent matter, for example with encephalopathy, then parenteral hydralazine, 0.2 mg/kg intravenously, can be used. In the presence of severe hypertension without other evidence of salt and water overload, diazoxide is best avoided; a labetalol infusion, 1 to 4 mg/kg/hr until the desired control is achieved, is preferable.

Pulmonary edema resulting from hypertension and volume overload is a deceptively dangerous situation. Such patients require vigorous treatment and careful monitoring of blood gases. They may require assisted ventilation.

Circulatory collapse may be due to arrhythmia complicating hyperkalemia: children with ARF should be connected to an electrocardiographic monitor until stable. Hyperkalemia is suggested by tall peaked T waves. It may be counteracted in emergency by intravenous administration of 10% Ca-gluconate, 0.5 ml/kg. A cation exchange resin (preferably in the calcium phase), 1 g/kg administered by mouth or as an enema, and correction of acidosis tend to counteract hyperkalemia. The use of glucose and insulin, although effective in driving potassium into the cells, is sometimes accompanied by troublesome hypoglycemia.

Table 48.6.
Oliguria and Circulatory Status

BP	CVP	Skin temperature	Interpretation	Treatment
↓	↓	↓	Hypovolemia	Volume expansion
↓	↑	↓	Cardiac	Inotropic support
↑	N or ↑	↓	Vasoconstriction	Vasodilator
N or ↑	N or ↑	N	Renal	Diuretics/dialysis

(Modified from Trompeter RS, et al: Renal transplantation in very young children. Lancet 1:373, 1983.)

Neurological Status

Children with ARF frequently convulse. Many possible causes should be considered, e.g., uremia, hyponatremia, hypernatremia, hypocalcemia, hypomagnesemia, and hypertension. Convulsions also may be part of the syndrome responsible for ARF, e.g., meningitis complicating septicemia or cerebral edema. Convulsions during dialysis may be caused by a rapid fall in plasma urea concentration, leading to an osmotic gradient across the blood-brain barrier with fluid shifts into the brain—the dysequilibrium syndrome. Many anticonvulsants tend to accumulate in renal failure; the safest and most effective is intravenous diazepam, 0.25 mg/kg.

Phosphate retention in ARF leads to reciprocal hypocalcemia and tetany. In infants, convulsions are a more usual consequence of low plasma calcium. Acidosis protects from tetany associated with hypocalcemia; thus, rapid correction of acidosis by infusion of sodium bicarbonate may aggravate the problem. In infants, ARF also may be complicated by convulsions caused by hypomagnesemia; in older children and adults the plasma magnesium concentration tends to rise. The hyperphosphatemia can be temporarily controlled with aluminum hydroxide gel, 0.5 to 1 ml/kg/day.

Acidosis

A severe uncompensated metabolic acidosis should be treated with intravenous sodium bicarbonate 2 mmol/kg (an 8.4% solution contains 1 mmol/ml), provided volume overload and hypertension have been controlled. The sodium bicarbonate solution should be diluted. It is often useful to ensure that the bulk of the sodium is given as bicarbonate rather than as chloride during resuscitation.

Sepsis

In many cases of ARF there is demonstrable or suspected sepsis, often with a gram-negative organism in the urinary tract and bloodstream. Gentamicin is the most useful antibiotic; however, it should be remembered that it is excreted by the kidney and, in plasma concentrations >10 μg/ml, it is ototoxic and nephrotoxic. A loading dose of 2 mg/kg should be given intravenously. Subsequently, the blood level may be maintained by adding gentamicin to the dialysate in a concentration of 10 μg/ml.

Conservative Management

Energy Requirement

The objective is to minimize the rate of deterioration of the biochemical state of the child by providing an adequate intake of protein and energy to maintain a satisfactory balance between anabolism and catabolism; at the same time the input of surplus nutrients that contribute to the load presented for renal excretion should be limited. To some extent, the retention of metabolites in growing tissues relieves the kidney of its excretory burden. McCance (32) has described growth as "the third kidney," but, to this end, an adequate energy intake is essential.

Fluid and nutrient requirements are both related to metabolic rate and to energy requirements; the latter therefore become a primary reference standard for the child. Energy requirements can be derived from Tables of Recommended Dietary Allowance (33), or roughly calculated without resorting to surface area estimations as follows (34):

Body weight	1 to 10 kg :	100 kcal/kg/24 hr
Plus	11 to 20 kg :	50 kcal/kg/24 hr
Plus	>20 kg :	20 kcal/kg/24 hr

Thus, a 40 kg child requires $10 \times 100 + 10 \times 50 + 20 \times 20 = 1900$ kcal/24 hr.

A "renal feed" has been described that is composed of glucose polymer and lipid, which provides 3 kcal/ml water (6). Frequently, intravenous nutrition is necessary. Its institution should not be delayed if there is gastrointestinal intolerance. All intravenous fluids should contain 10% glucose, and intravenous fat emulsions should be given if an inadequate energy intake is protracted, the platelet count is normal, and there are no coagulation abnormalities.

Protein

In ARF, about 8% of the total calories required should come from protein. As the calorific value of protein is 4 kcal/g, this implies a protein intake of 2 g/100 kcal. In the past, undue attention was paid to dietary protein restriction in the conservative management of ARF. It is now apparent that the main priority should be the maintenance of adequate nutrition from the first day of the illness. The dialysis regime should be tailored to permit this. If protein intake is poor, L-amino acids (1 g/100 kcal) should be administered parenterally, provided there is no hepatic disturbance. Given such parenteral nutrition, improved survival rates of patients with ARF are well documented (35, 36). This important consideration sometimes gets lost in the other aspects of intensive care.

Fluids

In health, water requirements for maintenance are 100 ml/100 kcal, of which 25% is accounted for by insensible losses. In ARF, therefore, fluid intake should be reduced to 25 ml/100 kcal plus the previous day's urine volume. The oral route is preferable to the parenteral, if tolerated, as better nutrition can be provided. Intake of sodium and potassium should be reduced.

Drugs

With the advent of renal failure, many drug dosage schedules require modification. The prescription sheet should be reviewed with care, with particular regard to antibiotics, especially the penicillins and aminoglycosides, cardiac glycosides, and anticonvulsants, particularly phenobarbitone.

Dialysis

Indications

The decision to treat by dialysis is determined less by arbitrary criteria of blood chemistry than by an assessment of the probable course of the renal failure. Dialysis is indicated if the child is hypercatabolic or if a prolonged period of oliguria is expected. If a quick return of renal function seems likely, conservative management may suffice and dialysis can be deferred. In practice, diuretic-resistant saline overload is perhaps the most important indication because correction of acidosis or anemia is impossible under such circumstances without dialysis.

Techniques

Until recently, there has been little question that peritoneal dialysis is preferable to hemodialysis in the management of children with ARF, although there have always been a few patients in whom, for such technical reasons as a burst abdomen, peritoneal dialysis is impossible. The technical difficulties of hemodialysis in small children have included access to the circulation, the large blood volume of the artificial kidney relative to that of the child, and hyperefficient dialysis causing the disequilibrium syndrome. An even greater problem, however, has been that the relative infrequency with which hemodialysis is required in small children has hindered the acquisition of the expertise necessary for the safe use of the artificial kidney by pediatric renal units. The development of maintenance hemodialysis programs in children has opened the door to new technical solutions and some of the problems have now been overcome (37).

Suitable pediatric arterial and venous shunts are available, and pediatric dialyzers, which require less than 10% of the infant's blood volume for priming, have been developed. It is important to relate the efficiency of the dialyzer to the size of the child; urea clearances of 2 to 3 ml/kg/min are satisfactory. Nevertheless, even with these developments, it is likely that in the immediate future most renal centers will rely on peritoneal dialysis for the treatment of ARF in children.

Another choice has to be made regarding the type of peritoneal catheter used. For most children with ARF, when short periods of dialysis are anticipated, the standard "stiff" catheter inserted by paracentesis is appropriate; however, if protracted periods of dialysis seem likely or if the situation appears end-stage, the insertion of a soft silastic Tenckhoff catheter (38) under direct vision may be preferable.

Peritoneal Dialysis

Under light sedation and local anesthesia and with strict aseptic technique, the peritoneal cavity is first filled with dialysate fluid (about 30 mg/kg body weight) through a small needle. This maneuver reduces the risk of a perforated viscus. The peritoneal catheter itself should be moderately flexible, contain an internal stylet, and have perforations that do not extend more than 3 cm from the tip. In infants, it is often more convenient to insert the catheter in the left flank rather than the customary subumbilical position, because it may be difficult to bury the perforations below the peritoneum in the latter site. There is also an increased risk of perforation of the bladder, which in infants is an abdominal rather than pelvic organ. A small skin incision is made, and the catheter is inserted into the peritoneal cavity (it helps if the abdominal wall of the infant is made tense by crying) and advanced toward the pelvis.

Some modifications of the standard adult equipment are required for infants, e.g., a special catheter, a burette to measure the input volume, and a heating coil to minimize heat loss during dialysis. Ideally, the administration set should be manufactured as a single piece and not improvised from other intravenous equipment, since junctions and three-way taps are potent sources of infection (39).

Dialysis Regimen

Commercially available dialysate fluids may be used at all ages. A sodium concentration of 130 mEq/L is usually optimum. The glucose concentration should not exceed 2 g/100 ml, since higher concentrations cause such a rapid withdrawal along the osmotic gradient into the peritoneal cavity that hypovolemic shock can ensue.

Potassium should be added in a concentration of 4 mEq/L if its serum level is not elevated. Lactate is the usual metabolizable anion;

however, the sick anoxic neonate may fail to convert it to bicarbonate and develop lactic acidosis. It is then necessary to prepare a dialysate containing bicarbonate instead.

A cycle volume of about 25 to 50 ml/kg body weight is usually satisfactory, but the amount tolerated varies in different children. Overdistention of the peritoneum is dangerous because it may cause respiratory embarrassment or, in the infant, apneic attacks. Under most circumstances, it is convenient and adequate to use hourly cycles, i.e., allowing the fluid to run into the peritoneum for 10 min, to dwell for 20 min, and then to drain for 30 min. On this regimen, with a dialysate glucose concentration of 1.4 g/100 ml, the drainage usually exceeds the input by about 10%. Assuming insensible losses of 20 ml/kg/day, this permits a fluid intake of about 120 ml/kg/day plus the urine volume. Hypercatabolic states necessitate shorter cycles, which are best achieved by shortening the drainage phase since the efficiency of dialysis is related to the volume of fluid passing through the peritoneal cavity in unit time.

Accurate recording of the fluid balance, estimated from dialysis input and return, is important but susceptible to cumulative errors. The most useful observations are the child's weight and circulatory status, particularly blood pressure. Conversely, when repeated weighing is difficult, e.g., in children on mechanical ventilators or when other factors influence the cardiovascular signs of hydration (as after cardiac surgery), control of fluid balance may become difficult and CVP measurement is essential.

Opinions differ as to whether a child should be dialyzed continuously through the same catheter as long as it is functioning, until renal function returns, or whether it is preferable to dialyze the child intensively for 48 hr and remove the catheter, reinserting it later if necessary. At issue are the relative hazards of infection on the one hand and tampering with an effective system on the other, perhaps unnecessarily running the risk of repeated catheter insertion.

Complications

Bleeding after insertion of the catheter is usually not as troublesome as it may at first appear, unless the child has received anticoagulants. If bleeding does occur, it is helpful to add a small amount of heparin (200 IU/L) to the dialysate to prevent blockage of the catheter. Bowel perforation is unusual if the peritoneum is first filled with dialysate, but it may occur if the gut is grossly distended and is probably best managed by surgical exploration in young children. Difficulties in drainage of dialysate are infrequent in small children, probably because the omentum is not well developed and does not wrap around the catheter. Leakage around the catheter predisposes to infection and may be troublesome if subcutaneous edema develops, so the catheter should be resited. Although infection is reasonably easy to eradicate in older children, it is more serious in infants because septicemia can disseminate from a peritoneal focus. At the first suggestion of peritonitis, antibiotics should be added to the dialysate in a concentration that exceeds the minimum inhibitory concentration of the infecting organism and is yet less than the toxic blood level.

References

1. Brenner BM, Stein JH: Acute Renal Failure, Contemporary Issues in Nephrology, Vol. 6, New York, Churchill Livingstone, 1980.
2. Chapman A (ed.): Acute Renal Failure, Clinics in Critical Care Medicine, Vol. 1, Edinburgh, Churchill Livingstone, 1980.
3. Andreucci V (ed.): Acute Renal Failure, The Hague, Martinus Nijhoff, 1985.
4. Barratt TM, Rigden SPA: Acute renal failure. In Paediatric Urology, Williams DI, Johnston, JH (eds.): 2nd ed., London, Butterworths, 1982, p 27.
5. Chantler C: Renal failure in childhood. In Renal Disease, Black DAK, Jones NF (eds.): ed. 4. Oxford, Blackwell, p 825.
6. Haycock GB: Acute renal failure in infancy and childhood. In Acute Renal Failure, Andreucci V (ed.): The Hague, Martinus Nijhoff, 1985.
7. Barratt TM: Renal disease in the first year of life. Rec Adv Renal Med 2:197, 1982.
8. Rigden SPA, Barratt TM, Dillon MJ, et al: Acute renal failure complicating cardiopulmonary bypass surgery. Arch Dis Child, 57:425, 1982.
9. Espinel CH: The FENa test. JAMA 236:579, 1976.
10. Miller TR, Anderson JR, Linas SL, et al: Urinary diagnostic indices in acute renal failure: a prospective study. Ann Intern Med 89:47, 1978.
11. Mathew OP, Jones AS, James E, et al: Neonatal renal failure: usefulness of diagnostic indices. Pediatrics 65:57, 1980.
12. Aynsley-Green A, Pickering D: Use of central and peripheral temperature measurement in the care of the critically ill child. Arch Dis Child 49:471, 1974.
13. Kerr DNS: Acute renal failure. In Renal Disease, Black DAK, Jones NF (eds): ed. 4. Oxford, Blackwell, 1979, p 437.
14. Oken DE: Pathogenetic mechanisms of acute renal failure. In Pediatric Kidney Disease, Edelmann CM (ed): Boston, Little Brown, 1978, p 189.
15. Thurau K, Boylan JW, Mason J. Pathophysiology of acute renal failure. In Black DAK, Jones NF (eds): Renal Disease: ed 4, Oxford, Blackwell, 1979, p 64.
16. Spitzer A: Renal physiology and functional development. In Pediatric Kidney Disease, Edelmann CM (ed): Boston, Little Brown, 1978, p 25.
17. Oliver J, McDowell M, Tracey A: The pathogenesis of acute renal failure with traumatic and toxic injury. Renal ischemia, nephrotoxic damage and the ischemuric episode. J Clin Invest 30:1307, 1951.
18. Ledingham JGG: Acute renal failure. In Oxford Textbook of Medicine Weatherall DJ, Ledingham JGG, Warrell DA (eds.): Oxford University Press, p 111.
19. Rigden SPA, Dillon MJ, de Leval M, et al: A randomized controlled trial of the effect on postoperative renal function of prophylactic administration of mannitol during cardiopulmonary bypass surgery. Clin Nephrol 21:148, 1984.
20. Levinsky NC, Bernard DB, Johnston PA: Enhancement of recovery of acute renal failure: effects of mannitol and diuretics. In Contemp Issues Nephrol 6:163, 1980.
21. Anderson RJ, Linas SL, Berns AS, et al: Nonoliguric acute renal failure. N Engl J Med 296:1134, 1977.
22. Fong JSC, de Chadarevian JP, Kaplan BS: Haemolytic uraemic syndrome: current concepts and management. Ped Clin North Am 29:835, 1982.
23. Trompeter RS, Schwartz R, Chantler C, et al: Haemolytic uraemic syndrome in childhood: an analysis of prognostic features. Arch Dis Child 58:101, 1983.
24. Habib R, Levy M, Gagnadoux MF, Broyer M: Prognosis of the haemolytic uraemic syndrome in children. In Maxwell MH (ed): Adv Nephrol, 13:99, 1982.
25. Remuzzi G, Marchesi D, Mecca G, et al: Haemolytic-uraemic syndrome: deficiency of plasma factor(s) regulating prostacyclin activity? Lancet 2:871, 1978.
26. Levin M, Elkon KB, Nokes TJC, et al: Inhibitor of prostacyclin production in sporadic haemolytic uraemic syndrome. Arch Dis Childh 58:703, 1983.
27. Arneil GC: Renal venous obstruction. In Pediatric Kidney Disease Edelmann CM (ed): Boston, Little Brown p 1104, 1978.
28. Davies DJ, Kennedy A, Roberts C: Medullary necrosis in infancy and childhood. J Pathol 99:125, 1969.
29. Gruskin AB, Oetlicker OH, Wolfish NM, et al: Effects of angiography on renal function in infants and piglets. J Pediat 76:41, 1970.
30. Barratt TM, Williams DI: Obstructive uropathy in children. In Black DAK, Jones NF (eds): Renal Disease, ed 4. Oxford, Blackwell 1979, p 804.
31. Henderson IS, Beattie TJ, Kennedy AC: Dopamine hydrochloride in oliguric states. Lancet, 2:827, 1980.
32. McCance RA: The maintenance of stability in the newly born. 1. Chemical exchange. Arch Dis Child 34:361, 1959.
33. Department of Health and Social Security: Recommended Intakes of Nutrients for the United Kingdom. London, Stationery Office, 1969.
34. Holliday MA, Segar WE: The maintenance need for water in parenteral fluid therapy. Pediatrics 19:823, 1957.
35. Abel RM, Beck CH, Abbott WM, et al: Improved survival from acute renal failure after treatment with intravenous essential L-amino acids and glucose. Results of a prospective double-blind study. N Engl J Med 288:695, 1973.
36. Toback FG: Amino acid treatment of renal failure. In Acute Renal Failure, Brenner BM, Stein JH (eds): New York, Churchill-Livingstone, 1980, p 202.
37. Hodson EM, Kjellstrand CM, Mauer SM: Acute renal failure in infants and children: outcome of 53 patients requiring haemodialysis treatment. J Pediatr, 93:756, 1978.
38. Tenckhoff H, Schechter H: A bacteriologically safe access device. Trans Am Soc Artif Intern Org 14:181, 1968.
39. Donaldson MDC, Spurgeon P, Haycock GB, Chantler C: Peritoneal dialysis in infants. Brit Med J 286:759, 1983.
40. Trompeter RS, Bewick M, Haycock GB, Chantler C: Renal transplantation in very young children. Lancet 1:373, 1983.

CHAPTER 49

Progressive Loss of Renal Function

CYRIL CHANTLER
MALCOLM HOLLIDAY

INTRODUCTION

The loss of renal function is attended by adaptive renal and metabolic responses that initially compensate for the loss so that at first there are no clinical consequences. These adaptive responses provide insight into the mechanisms underlying the clinical signs that develop as loss of function progresses, and they are a guide to therapy as well.

In the early stage of the process, therapy is aimed principally at limiting the injury to the kidney; in the latter stages, its aim is to prevent or treat the metabolic consequences that follow from the loss of renal function. Since normal renal function is an essential factor in the tolerance to the generous ranges of intake of many nutrients, loss of function reduces that range (1). Therapy is, in part, adjustment of diet to nutrient intake within these narrower limits (Chapter 1).

Nutrition therapy, which originally focused on the control of the metabolic consequences of chronic renal failure (CRF) by regulating intake to fit tolerance, becomes a major consideration in therapy that is designed to slow the rate of loss of residual function (2, 3). For this purpose, nutrition therapy is considered early in the course of disease.

For children, therapy also is aimed at maximizing growth potential. This is particularly important in the first year of life because poor growth is common in this period; growth retardation at this time limits the growth potential, leading to permanent short stature (4).

This chapter describes the epidemiology of progressive renal disease, the renal and metabolic adaptations to loss of function, the nature of growth retardation, and strategies for assessing and treating chronic renal insufficiency (CRI), when function is <50% of normal, or CRF, when it is <25% normal. Later chapters in this section address dialysis and renal transplantation therapy, osteodystrophy, and other complications.

EPIDEMIOLOGY

Incidence and Prevalence

Neither incidence nor prevalence of renal disease with loss of function is well defined in children. Geography, economic status, and racial susceptibility to renal disease have a profound effect on incidence; children in those countries that have the greatest level of malnutrition have a higher prevalence of renal disease (Chapter 22).

The incidence of progressive renal disease that leads to CRF in childhood is not known. Some idea is gained from the incidence of end-stage renal disease in children, although obviously a large number of children with progressive renal disease develop end-stage renal disease beyond childhood. Earlier estimates of the incidence of end-stage renal disease in children in Western Europe and the United States varied from three to six children per million total population (MTP) (5–7). Those statistics, derived from death certificate surveys, overestimated the incidence of children suitable for treatment because they included children with multiorgan failure who could not be treated. Current studies have identified 1.5 to 3.0 children per million total population <16 yr of age who could benefit from treatment (8–11), which compared with 40 or more adults per million total population <60 yr of age who would benefit.

In some countries, the incidence of end-stage renal disease in adults is increasing as criteria for treatment broaden to include patients with diabetes, cancer, or other high-risk groups and those >60 yr of age (12). Similarly, the incidence in patients entering pediatric nephrology centers for dialysis and transplantation is increasing as low-birth-weight infants with renal disease and older children survive and are referred to pediatric nephrologists, when in the past they would not have been.

Of particular interest is a group of infants with dysplasia, polycystic disease, or obstructive uropathy who are detected by sonography of the mothers predelivery. These infants are detected early and have reduced function but often have been undetected in the past. They contribute less to the incidence of end-stage renal disease in childhood but are adding to the children with loss of function who benefit from conservative treatment and may need dialysis or transplantation later. The current incidence of end-stage renal disease in children relative to their own population is from three to six per million child population (mcp) among the five countries in Europe who provide 70% of childhood cases to the end-stage renal disease registry (13) (Table 49.1).

The prevalence in Switzerland of CRF in children from 6 months to 16 yr was ascertained in 1974. The survey identified 28 children nation-

Table 49.1.
Incidence and Prevalence of End-Stage Renal Disease and Distribution among Treatment Modalities of Children <15 Yr of age Reported by Five European Countries (includes 70% of children in the European Dialysis and Transplant Registry)[a]

	Incidence MCP[b]	Prevalence MCP[b]	Distribution of total cases			Total no. of cases
			HD[c]	PD[d]	p̄TX[e]	
				% of Total		
Federal Republic of Germany	3.5	30.2	44	4	52	376
France	5.7	48.2	55	3	43	591
Italy	2.8	21.0	59	10	31	280
Spain	3.4	24.5	63	5	32	236
United Kingdom	5.2	32.2	26	14	60	409

[a] Incidence derived from new cases added in 1983; prevalence is cumulative patients alive in 1983 who were <15 yr of age at time of entry and were alive on Dec. 31, 1983 (13).
[b] Per million children population.
[c] HD = Hemodialysis.
[d] PD = Peritoneal dialysis.
[e] p̄TX = Post transplant.

wide who had a plasma creatinine (P_{Cr}) >2 mg/dl (170 mmol/liter) for a prevalence of 18.5/mcp (8). This figure does not include children with lesser degrees of impairment.

The prevalence of end-stage renal disease also can be derived from the data of the European Dialysis and Transplant Registry, from the cumulative number of children on dialysis or post transplant who are being observed in each of the countries with the largest populations (13) (Table 49.1). The number of patients <15 yr who are being treated range from 21 to 48/mcp among the five countries. Approximately half of these children were on hemodialysis therapy, a small percent were on peritoneal dialysis therapy, and 45% had functioning renal grafts post transplant (Table 49.1). The percent on peritoneal dialysis therapy is increasing.

The distribution of affected children according to age also is important. The European Dialysis and Transplant Registry from five countries reported that <10% of children with end-stage renal disease were <3 yr of age, 10% were between 3 and 6.0, 20% between 6 and 9.0, and 60% were between 9 and 15.0 years (Table 49.2) (13).

In France, of 2502 children with renal disease admitted to the Hôpital des Enfants Malàdes over a 10-yr period, 270 developed CRF. Of these, 182 reached end-stage renal disease in that period and 124 were still <15 yr of age; 16% of these 124 were <5 yr of age (10). From these, it is estimated that 1 of 6/mcp who develop end-stage renal disease each year will be <5 yr of age. The trends in neonatal care may cause this estimate to increase.

The information made available from the European Dialysis and Transplant Registry is valuable in planning and evaluating therapy. Comparable information from other countries would benefit planning for the care of children in those countries.

Services

Because CRF and end-stage renal disease are rare in children, it has been suggested that a limited number of specialized children's centers should be responsible for their care rather than an occasional child being treated in a center for adults. Data from the European Dialysis and Treatment Registry have shown better patient survival on dialysis and better patient and graft survival following cadaver donor renal transplantation for children treated in specialized centers (13). The advent of continuous ambulatory peritoneal dialysis (CAPD) that facilitates home care makes this suggestion more practical to implement whenever care for children is planned.

Table 49.2.
Age Distribution of Children <15.0 yr with End-Stage Renal Disease in Five European Countries in 1983 (13)

	Age (yr)				
	0–3.0	3–6.0	6–9.0	9–12.0	12–15.0
			% of total		
Federal Republic of Germany	5	8	28	23	36
France	5	10	19	30	37
Italy	17	10	19	17	38
Spain	5	11	13	34	37
United Kingdom	4	9	15	26	47

These children's centers should have other specialized services associated with each unit, e.g., pediatric nurses, social workers, dietitians, educational and psychological staff, as well as the capacity and experience for urological procedures and renal transplantation for children. These provisions are expensive but less so when the better results are considered against long-term costs that ensue from less adequate services.

A reasonable population base for a pediatric center would be 8 to 10 million people, or 2.5 million children, providing an admission rate of about 15 children per year. This pattern creates difficulties and costs for families who have to travel long distances. Financial support for these nonmedical costs is required. Flexible arrangements for shared care with local pediatricians and general nephrology units can do much to offset expenses and increase effectiveness of care.

The resources required to treat end-stage renal disease are expensive; as a result there is a positive correlation between the per capita gross national product and the number of patients accepted for chronic dialysis (14). Very likely there is an inverse correlation with the incidence of CRF. Economic growth, which permits programs for the treatment of end-stage renal disease is associated with a fall in age-corrected prevalence and mortality from renal disease.

Many countries cannot afford or have decided not to accord priority to the treatment of all patients with end-stage renal disease; difficult selection decisions for treatment thus have to be made (15). Among adults, the marginal decisions tend to be made at the expense of the elderly or those with extrarenal complications (15). Among children, those with multiple handicaps or those <5 yr of age in whom potential

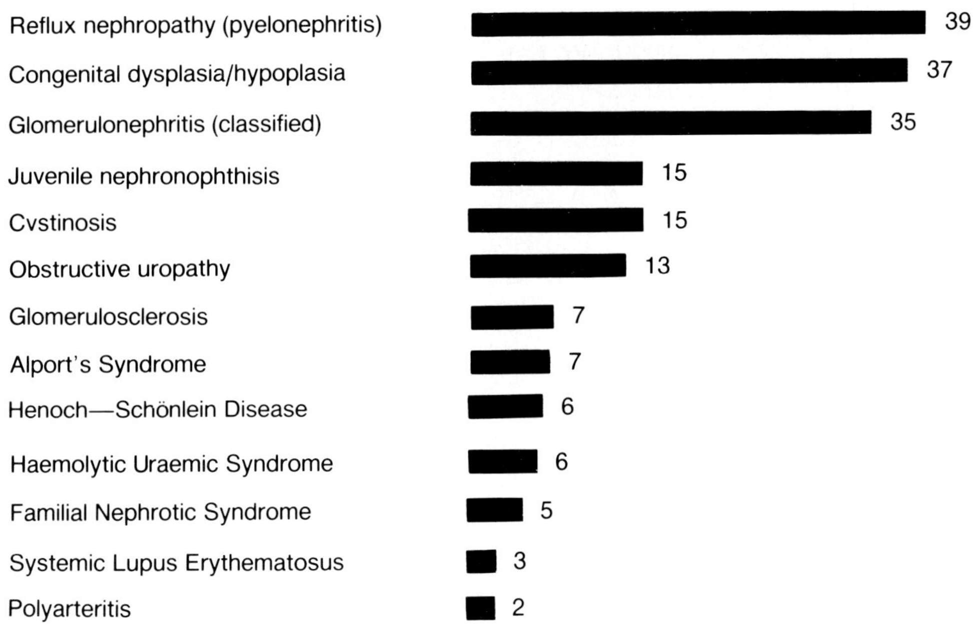

1 each; Shunt nephritis, Lawrence-Moon-Biedl Syndrome, Mitochondrial myopathy, Wilms' tumor, Cortical necrosis.

Figure 49.1. Primary renal disease leading to chronic renal failure in 195 children at Guy's Hospital.

difficulties in treatment are greatest are often denied treatment. Such unfortunate discrimination is perhaps inevitable when economic resources are limited. It is, however, difficult for the physician to accept these limitations, and it may be construed as part of the physician's responsibility to the individual with end-stage renal disease who consults him or her to do all that can be done to ensure that such limitations are minimal.

Causes

The causes of renal disease appear to vary according to country. For example, in the United Kingdom, reflux nephropathy is the most common single disease entity to cause end-stage renal disease in children (11) (Fig. 49.1). Not surprisingly, congenital and familial rather than acquired renal diseases are more common causes of CRF in children (7, 8, 10, 11, 16); however, progression to end-stage renal disease is more rapid with some forms of acquired disease. Leumann (8) noted that 86% of children with CRF had congenital disease, whereas only 44% of those with end-stage renal disease had congenital disease. Table 49.3 shows the distribution of diagnoses of children starting treatment for end-stage renal disease in seven European countries, each having >100 children receiving treatment for end-stage renal disease in 1980 (16). Differences among specific countries may represent different prevalence of disease or simply a different diagnostic terminology. Acquired glomerulonephritis in some form, for example, is a cause in <30% and some form of dysplasia or anatomical defect is responsible for >50% if pyelonephritis is included under this heading. For children <5 yr of age with end-stage renal disease, the distribution differs only slightly when the larger categories are considered.

Table 49.3.
Distribution of Primary Renal Diseases in Children with End-Stage Renal Disease Entered into the European Dialysis and Transplant Registry (16)

	Children <5 yr	All children (<15)
Renal hypoplasia	12	12
Pyelonephritis/interstitial nephritis (includes reflux and obstruction)	15	22
Heredofamilial diseases (includes cystic diseases)	14	16
Glomerulonephritis	21	31
Multisystems disease	14	7
Renal vascular disease	4	2
Other causes	15	6
Cause uncertain	6	4
Total	101	100
Total number of cases	263	3,342

STAGES OF DISEASE

The loss of renal function progresses through several stages defined by clinical characteristics but related to the percent of residual function remaining. Residual function is expressed in relation to estimates of residual glomerular filtration rate (GFR); residual potential is estimated as a percent of normal nephron number or residual filtration potential (Fig. 49.2) (17). The average change in single nephron GFR and the residual nephron number determine the residual function (18, 19). Residual filtration potential is the filtration surface area or filtration coefficient (K_F) and its capacity to increase.

Impaired Renal Function

In the early stage, residual renal function is between 80% and 50% and residual potential is between 50% and 25% of normal. Single nephrectomy to donate a kidney reduces nephron number to 50% and residual function to 70% to 80%, i.e., GFR in the remaining kidney increases to 1.4 to 1.6 times normal. The loss in function does not have a measurable clinical effect except for a slight increase in microprotein-

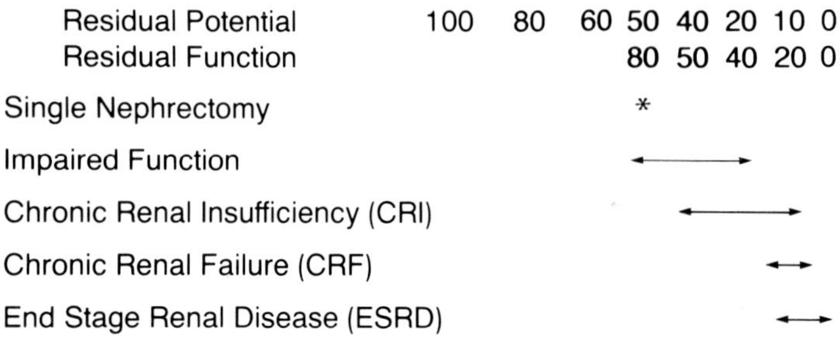

Figure 49.2. Stages of renal disease in terms of residual potential and residual function as progressive loss of function proceeds (see text).

uria and blood pressure in males observed 10 or more years post nephrectomy (20).

With further ablation the single nephron GFR in rats increases to approximately twice normal, which is the average maximum for this adaptive response (18). At this level of reduced function in humans, clinical signs are rarely detected. The important feature of this period is that up to 70% of the number of nephrons are lost or filtration potential is damaged without the development of clinical signs.

Chronic Renal Insufficiency

Chronic renal insufficiency (CRI) defines the stage in which residual function is between 50% and 25% of normal. Residual potential is <30% of normal. Changes in plasma concentration are present, and Ca absorption is impaired (21). Tolerances to variations in nutrient intake are demonstrably reduced. Clinical response to intercurrent illness or other major stresses, e.g., dehydration, hyperkalemia, or acidosis, may be more dramatic; acute renal failure secondary to dehydration is more likely to occur. In children, growth rate often is retarded (22). When residual function is <50%, progressive loss of function is likely and conservative management to protect residual function is indicated (23).

Chronic Renal Failure

Chronic renal failure (CRF) describes residual function <30%, and residual potential usually is <15% of normal. Metabolic abnormalities that reflect an adaptation to loss of function develop. Osteodystrophy, anemia, and hypertension are common and, on ordinary diets, azotemia approaches levels that are associated with uremic symptoms (see following section). Conservative management is indicated to control metabolic abnormalities. Patients who adhere to rigorous conservative therapeutic regimens may maintain customary activities with residual function <5% (23).

Uremia

Uremia is the symptom complex associated with renal failure characterized by anorexia, nausea, somnolence, and malaise (24). These progress to vomiting, convulsions, coma, and gastrointestinal bleeding if not treated. Cardiac failure and arrhythmias are common. Patients who are being treated do not progress to this stage unless an intercurrent illness induces a catabolic response to precipitate these symptoms. The symptoms are reversed by dialysis or stringent conservative management.

End-Stage Renal Disease

End-stage renal disease defines the stage at which dialysis therapy or renal transplantation begins. Because the criteria for undertaking either therapy are not agreed on, patients may have as much as 20% or as little as 2% residual function when classified as end-stage renal disease patients.

RENAL ADAPTATION

Loss of renal function initiates a hypertrophy response with a corresponding increase in functional capacity. The magnitude of the response varies in relation to the percent of nephrons lost, the nature of the underlying disease, and the metabolic effects imposed by diet or stress (25).

Hypertrophy Response

There is a prompt response to the removal of nephron mass by uninephrectomy. In rats and dogs, uninephrectomy is followed within minutes by increases in fractional excretion of NaCl, K, and water by the contralateral kidney (26). Increases in renal blood flow (RBF) and residual GFR occur as promptly (27) or later (26). Within hours, signs of renal growth, RNA, new membrane, and cell protein synthesis are detectable (28). The increase is greater as more kidney tissue is removed (18) but reaches a ceiling when size and function per nephron double (29). Glomerular size increases. The largest factor to cause the increase in renal weight is the increase in proximal tubular mass. Distal tubular mass is less affected. The process is nearly complete in rats after three weeks. Renal functional response to unilateral nephrectomy in humans nears completion in a few weeks (30); the increase after two to four years is not much greater (31).

Glomerular Response

Hemodynamic and Morphological Change. The glomerular response to reduced renal mass is an increase in glomerular capillary blood flow and single nephron GFR; an increase in capillary surface area and in glomerular ultrafiltration coefficient (K_f) are less well documented (32, 33). The change in single nephron GFR is a product of the net hydraulic pressure ($\Delta P = P_{GC} - P_T$) when P_T = tissue back pressure and a change in single nephron K_f ($SN \cdot K_f$).

$$\text{Single nephron GFR} = SN \cdot K_f \times \Delta \overline{P} \quad (1)$$

The response to removal of five sixths of renal mass in rats is associated with the appearance of blebs in the capillary surface (Fig. 49.3, *A*) followed by mesangial hypercellularity and thickening, progressing to segmental sclerosis (Fig. 49.3, *B*) (32).

When loss of function is secondary to glomerulonephritis, the general process is similar, but the effect of disease on the glomerular capillary surface modifies the response. Disease causes greater splay in single nephron GFR owing to greater splay in $SN \cdot K_f$ and in single nephron renal plasma flow (SN · RPF) (33, 34). With time, as noted, the hypertrophic response also lowers $SN \cdot K_f$ so that the destructive process seen with severe ablation is likely to be accelerated when glomerulonephritis causes loss of function. SN · GFR may be normal or decreased instead of two times normal. In patients with lupus glomerulonephritis whose GFR averaged 50% of normal, K_f was reduced more and ΔP was increased. The level of injury, i.e., change in K_f in all these conditions, is underestimated by measurement of GFR (34). When C_{Cr} is used to evaluate the loss of functional potential, the underestimation is greater because an increasing fraction of creatinine is cleared due to increased tubular secretion. In nearly one third of the instances where C_{IN} was below normal, C_{Cr} was in the normal range (Fig. 49.4) (35).

In rats, ablation of the kidney followed by glomerular capillary hyperfiltration and hypertension led to microproteinuria, then to heavy proteinuria as glomerular damage progressed. This process in rats is ameliorated by lowering dietary protein to levels unsuitable for growth but satisfactory for maintenance. With low dietary protein capillary hyperperfusion, hyperfiltration, and hypertension are less and the rate of progression of injury is slowed (32).

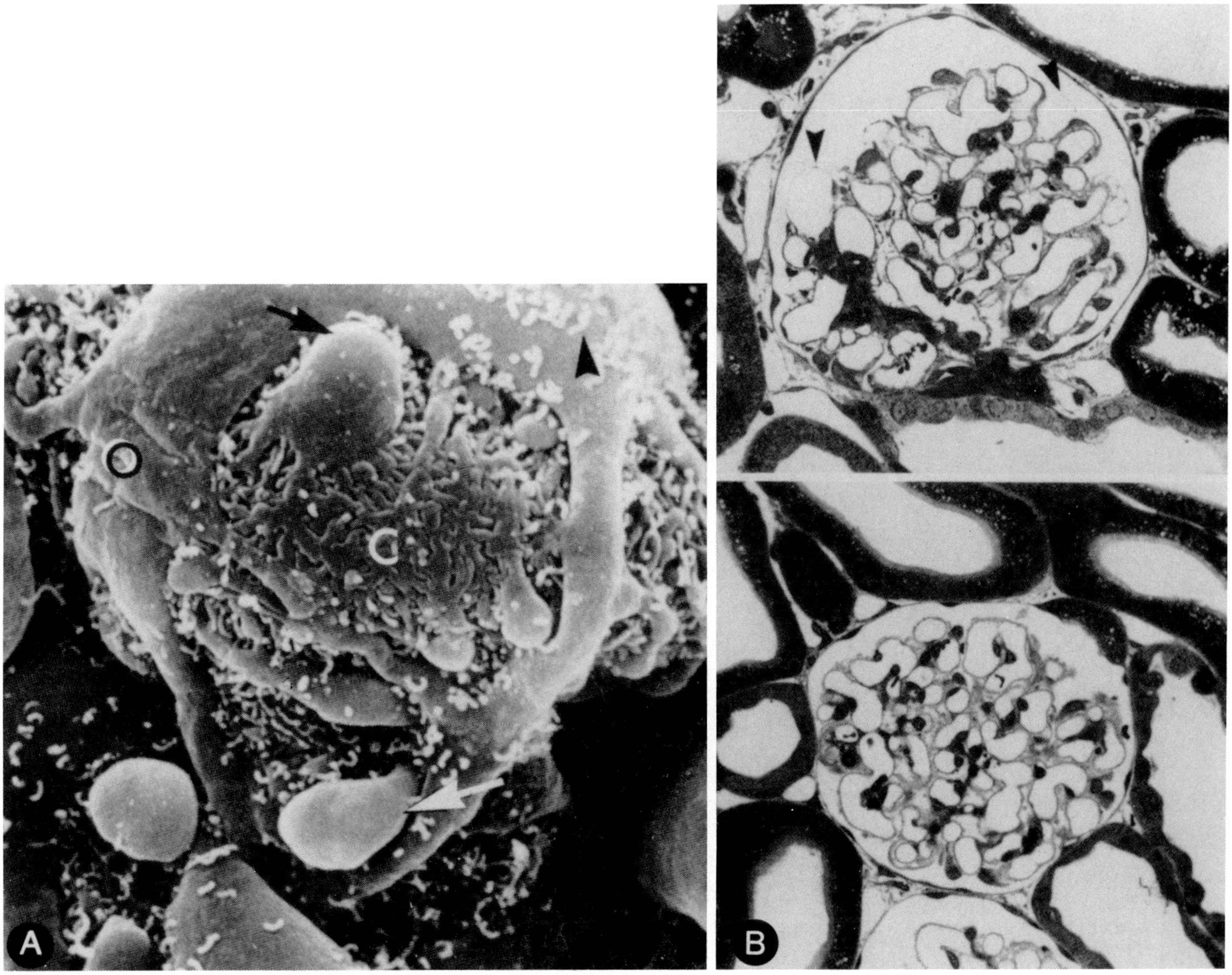

Figure 49.3. **A,** Scanning electron micrograph of a glomerulus from a "remnant kidney" rat fed a high-protein diet. Arrows point to blebs in the capillary. Sample taken seven days after renal ablation. **B,** Light micrograph of a glomerulus from remnant kidney. Rats on high-protein diet (top) and on low-protein diet (bottom) seven days after renal ablation. Arrow points to blebs. Mesangial matrix is increased. (With permission from the American Physiological Society.) (2)

What implication these findings have in clinical practice is not clear, but preliminary studies (see below) indicate that lowering dietary protein in patients with renal disease slows progression of the disease.

The fact that the C_{Cr} (35) or S_{Cr} underestimates the loss of GFR, and that glomerular damage, as estimated by a decrease in K_f, is more extensive than is measured even by accurate measurements of GFR makes it difficult to detect damage from conventional indices until the damage or loss in nephrons is extensive (see Fig. 49.2). Because the normal values for S_{Cr} in infants are low (Table 49.4) and accuracy of measurement is less at these levels, this problem is greater in infants (36).

Renal Reserve. When fed a meal high in protein (1 g/kg) individuals with normal kidneys increase GFR and C_{Cr} two to three hr after feeding by an average of 40% (Fig. 49.5). This response is viewed as reserve capacity responding to acute hyperfiltration. Normal individuals on a vegetarian diet have lower resting GFR and the same or greater reserve (37). Individuals with renal injury and hyperfiltration, i.e., diabetics with normal-to-elevated GFR and those with normal or reduced resting GFR secondary to disease, have lost this reserve (38) (Fig. 49.5). Even patients who have been kidney donors or who have recovered completely from acute glomerulonephritis have lost reserve (Fig. 49.6) (39). How useful this test will be in clinical practice is not clear, but the findings emphasize that adaptive response to loss of glomerular capillary surface obscure the extent of damage; when S_{Cr} is elevated as a consequence of glomerular injury, much damage has occurred and the process of injury is likely to progress.

Effect of Dietary Factors. Lowering dietary phosphorus (P) in rats with a five sixths nephrectomy also has protected residual renal function from further decline (40). The effect of the normal higher P diet is to increase renal tubular calcification and accelerate loss of function. The net effect of dietary P causing progression is similar to the effect of protein, but the pathological condition induced differs. As in the case of dietary protein, the effect is magnified as residual function declines (41); also as in the case of protein, the protective effect in rats has only been reported when the intake has been reduced to levels well below the requirement for growth (42). The relative role of protein and phosphorus in accelerating loss of function in experimental nephritis or remnant

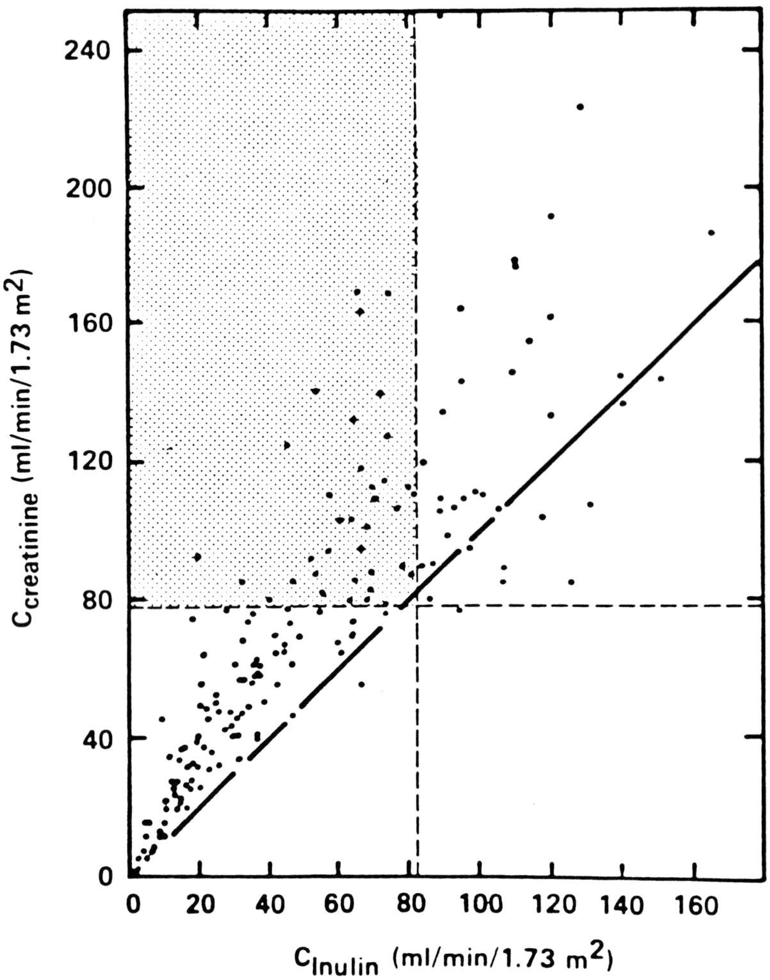

Figure 49.4. Comparing C_{Cr} with C_{IN} in 171 patients with various types of renal disease. Lower limit of normal values for C_{IN} (82 ml/min/1.73 m^2) in control population is defined by vertical broken line. Points to left are below normal. Points to left that are above horizontal broken line define C_{IN} values that are below normal range but within normal range for C_{Cr} (lower limit = 77 ml/min/1.73 m^2). In many instances C_{Cr} is in normal range when C_{IN} is low. (From Shemesh O, Golbetz H, Kriss JP, Myers BD: Kidney Int 28:830, 1985.)

Table 49.4.
Plasma creatinine levels[a] = mean for normal renal function (GFR), upper limit (+2 SD), and projected levels when renal function reduced to various levels of normal function (2)[b]

Age	Stature (cm)	P_{Cr} − normal values		P_{Cr} with reduced function-% normal		
		Mean	M + 2 SD	50	25	12.5
		mg/dl		*mg/dl*		
2–26 wks	60	0.39	0.55	0.78	1.6	3.2
.5–2 yr	70	0.32	0.46	0.64	1.3	2.6
6 year	114	0.43	0.59	0.86	1.7	3.3
12 year	147	0.59	0.78	1.12	2.2	4.4
Adult (F)	163	0.77	1.01	1.54	3.1	6.2
Adult (M)	174	0.97	1.22	1.94	3.9	7.8

[a] Approximates true creatinine.

[b] These projections do not take into account the increasing fraction of creatinine that is secreted as GFR declines. This may lower values by 20% to 60%.

kidneys in rats is disputed (32, 42). Patients placed on a low protein–low P diet followed for a year showed a decrease in serum parathyroid hormone (PTH) and an apparent slowing of the rate of loss of renal function (43).

Other clinical studies also report that lowering dietary protein and P slows progression of disease as measured by a change in the slope of $1/S_{Cr}$ versus time (44–45). A controlled study showed that patients with CRI who were prescribed a diet providing 0.6 g/kg/day of protein and a low P diet had less reduction in C_{Cr} than those maintained on the average higher intake; patients with CRF in this study also were protected and fewer progressed to end-stage renal disease (46, 47).

Effect of Pharmacological Factors. The effect of renal ablation on progressive loss of residual function in rats has been blunted by the use of agents that lower blood pressure (48). Enalapril, a drug that inhibits the enzymatic conversion of angiotensin I to angiotensin II, lowered P_{GC} in rats without significantly lowering single nephron GFR. The degree of glomerular injury was thereby reduced (49). A similar protective effect was observed in rats with renal ablation that were treated with a thromboxane inhibitor. In this study, it was proposed that glomerular injury caused by thromboxane-induced platelet deposition was inhibited by giving a thromboxane inhibitor (50). From this work, these authors have proposed a scheme for the pathogenesis of progressive glomerulosclerosis in the remnant kidney model in rats (Fig. 49.7).

Tubular Response

The response of proximal and distal tubules to ablation differ.

Proximal Tubule. The major increase in renal mass with hypertrophy is an increase in proximal tubules; following uninephrectomy or five

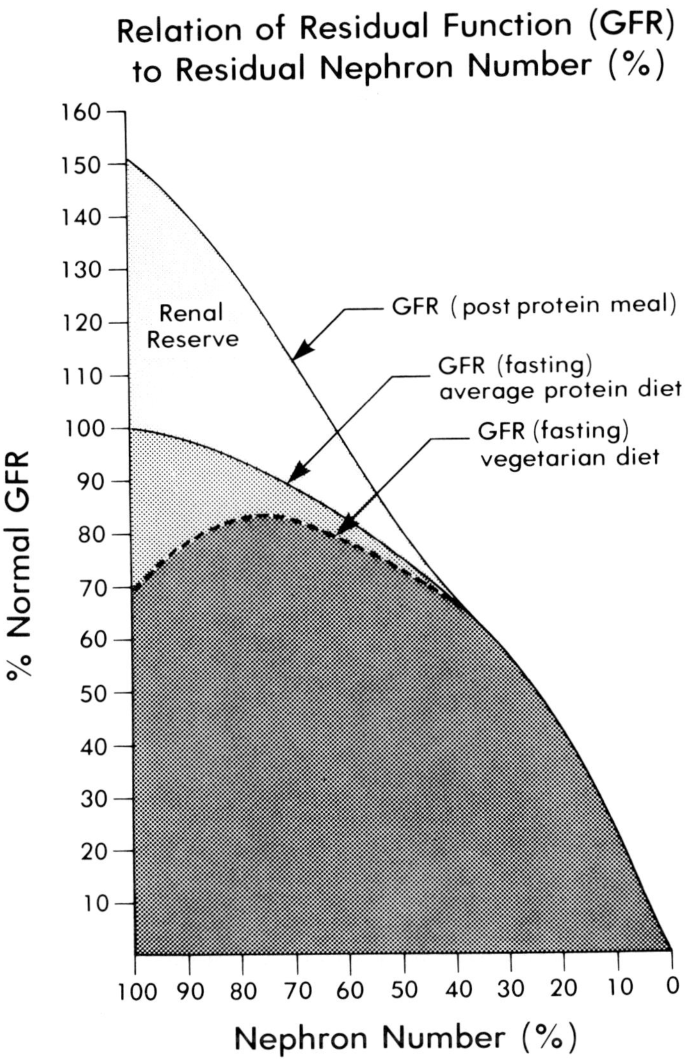

Figure 49.5. Idealized drawing defining curve for fasting GFR for normal individuals and those with progressive loss of function on average but abundant protein diet and the increase observed when a protein meal is fed—the renal reserve. Note renal reserve is lost when half the glomeruli are removed following uninephrectomy (37) Lowest curve is that defined by vegetarians who with normal nephron numbers have a low fasting GFR but a comparable reserve (38).

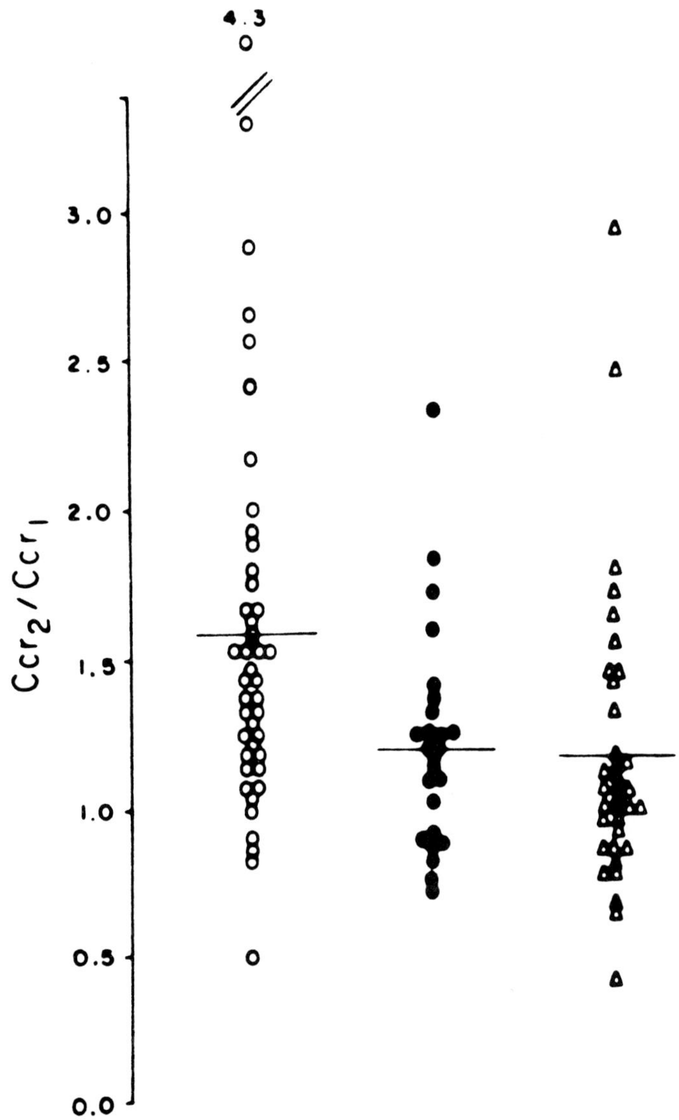

Figure 49.6. Relation of C_{Cr} post protein feeding (C_{Cr2}) to C_{Cr} postabsorptive (C_{Cr1}) in normal subjects (open circles), normal postnephrectomy kidney donors (closed circles), and patients recovered from acute poststreptococcal glomerulonephritis (open triangles). Average fasting C_{Cr} values for three groups were the same. Only first group had average increase in C_{Cr2}/C_{Cr1} that exceeded 1.1. (From Rodriguez-Iturbe B, Herrera J, Garvia R: Lancet 2:461, 1985.) (39)

sixths nephrectomy in rats, these elongate and increase in diameter. The increase in size is in proportion to the increase in single nephron GFR and glomerular size; the tubule handles a corresponding increase in glomerular filtrate. The distribution in the hypertrophy response among nephrons appears to be fairly uniform, as judged by the distribution in glomerular counts in different regions of the kidney (51). These findings contrast with the changes that occur in chronic glomerulonephritis in humans (52) and in experimentally induced renal injury (19). Fractional absorption of filtrate is proportional to single nephron GFR in the remnant kidney model (29). On the other hand, single nephron GFR varies in experimental renal disease: glomerulotubular balance is sustained, owing to reciprocal differences in postglomerular plasma flow rate, pressure that modulates single nephron proximal absorption to single nephron GFR, and P_{GC} (53).

Distal Nephron. Change in size in the distal nephron with renal ablation is less than that observed in the proximal (29); however, renal ablation causes changes in enzyme levels and in transport characteristics in this portion of the nephron, increasing the relative capacity for K and of hydrogen ion excretion (54, 55). Papillectomy, i.e., removal of the medulla, prevents these increases and consequently prevents these adaptive responses (56).

Adaptation of Tubular Function

The excretory function of the kidney responds to change in input from diet and metabolism by change in tubular function as well as by change in size. As residual function declines, the capacity to respond is limited or, as defined by Talbot and his associates, the homeostatic limits are narrowed (Fig. 49.8) (57). As single nephron GFR increases, solute load per nephron increases. The adaptations that respond to changes in input when kidney function is normal also operate when nephron numbers decline. In general, reabsorption from the proximal convolution balances single nephron GFR (29, 53) and renal controls sensitive to intake operate in the distal nephron (25). Total input and renal output stay the same, but the effect of a change in input on the adaptive responses is magnified (51). The overall adaptations adjust output to

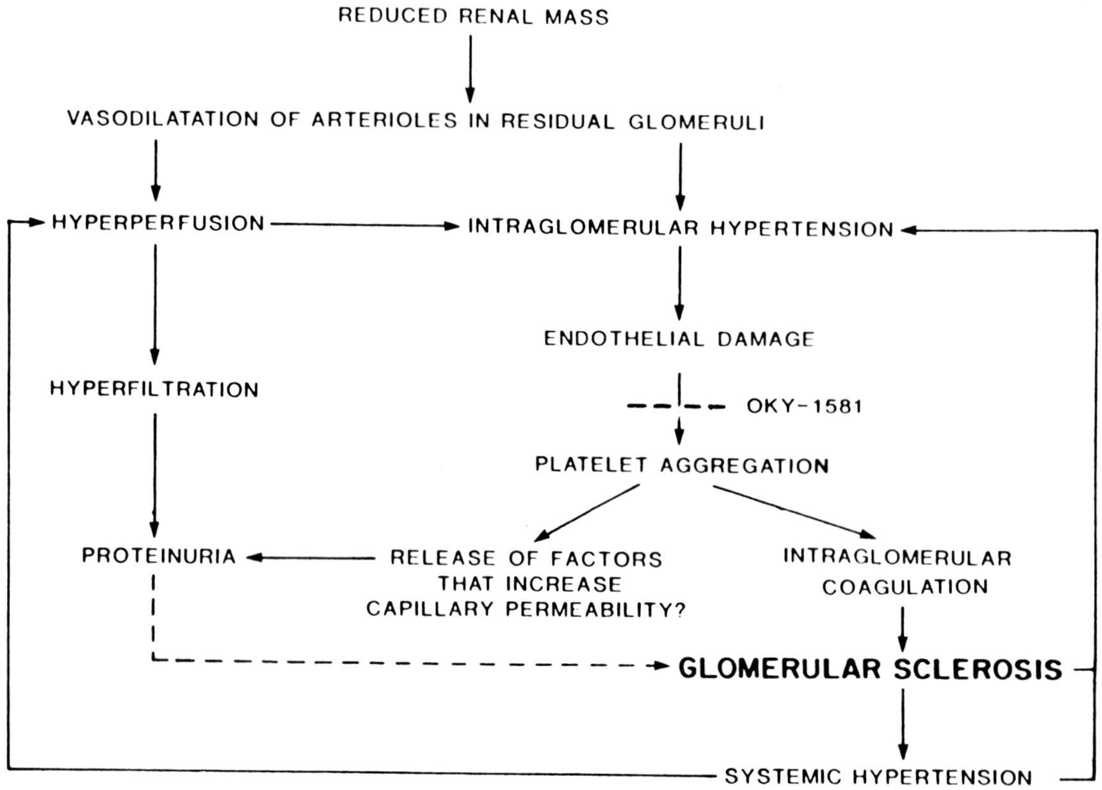

Figure 49.7. Schematic of proposed pathway for progressive glomerular injury in remnant kidney rats. The thromboxane inhibitor (OKY-1581) interferes with a major pathway of injury. (From Purkerson ML, Valdes A, Yates J, et al: Proc Nat Acad Sci 82:193, 1985.)

equal intake. These entail change in concentration of solutes in extracellular fluid (ECF), as occurs in the case of urea; adaptations in glomerular and proximal tubule function to sustain glomerulotubular balance; and change in distal tubular function to control electrolyte excretion. Regulation of P reabsorption is a proximal function.

NaCl

Tolerance. NaCl balance is maintained over a considerable range of salt intake with residual function of <30% and even <10%. To gain perspective, it is well to recall the remarkable range of tolerance for salt intake and output with normal kidney function (2 to 1000 mEq/day in adults) which extends well outside the range of intakes encountered in most diets 40 to 200 mEq/day (1000 to 5000 mg Na).

In one study of patients with an average of 10% residual function, salt intake changed from 7 to 3.5 g (120 to 60 mEq), and NaCl balance was sustained with little change in GFR, blood pressure, or ECF volume. Change beyond this range was reportedly poorly tolerated (58). However, sudden reductions in NaCl intake are poorly tolerated in patients with CRF (59), but in a small series of adults reductions made gradually over six months were well tolerated (60).

How NaCl balance is achieved in patients with CRF has been the focus of many studies. Overall balance is maintained by regulating Na reabsorption (Na_R) to Na filtered (Na_F), so that Na excreted (Na_E) equals Na intake (Na_I), i.e., ($Na_F - Na_R = Na_E = Na_I$. Within the range of intakes in most western diets (40 to 200 mEq/day), change in Na_I does not affect GFR or Na_F.

When salt intake is reduced from 200 to 40 mEq/day in a normal individual (Table 49.5), Na_R increases (from 19,800 to 19,960 or from 99% to 99.8% of Na_F) and effects a large relative change in Na_E (from 200 to 40 mEq/day or from 1% to 0.2% of Na_F). These changes are reflected in single nephron GFR as well. When residual function is 10% of normal and intake is reduced from 200 to 40 mEq/day, Na_R increases (from 1800 to 1960 mEq/day or from 90% to 98% Na_F) to effect a decrease in Na_E (from 200 to 40 mEq/day or from 10% to 2% of Na_F).

Viewed in terms of SN function in the state of renal ablation, where $SN \cdot Na_F$ is 140×10^{-7} mEq/min, the normal $SN \cdot NaR$ is 126 rather than the 69.4×10^{-7} mEq/min, and Na_E is 14 instead of $.76 \times 10^{-7}$ mEq/min noted for normal function. The relative increase in $SN \cdot Na_E$ is, of course, greater. When salt intake is reduced from 200 to 40 mEq/day, $SN \cdot Na_R$ is 137.2×10^{-7}/min instead of 126; $SN \cdot Na_E$ is 2.8 instead of $.14 \times 10^{-7}$ mEq/min. When compared with the normal, single nephron handling of Na is increased, i.e., SN_F, SN_R, and SN_E.

When translated into changes in tubular function, these examples cannot be so clearly stated. Drawing on micropuncture studies in rats with remnant kidney or with renal disease, where $SN \cdot Na_F$ is increased or decreased, proximal reabsorption changes proportionately (19, 29, 53) but not quite as much as $SN \cdot Na_F$ leaving, by inference, disproportionate Na to be delivered beyond. Even if change in proximal reabsorption is proportional to change in Na_F a larger, absolute volume of filtrate and more NaCl per nephron is delivered beyond this level (Table 49.6). The facultative or regulated excretion of Na is believed to occur beyond the proximal (25). Making the assumption that 40% or 4000 mEq of Na_F is delivered distally in normal individuals, 3800 mEq are reabsorbed and 200 mEq are excreted. When salt intake is reduced, making the assumption that neither Na_F nor distal delivery are affected, distal reabsorption increases to 3960 mEq, and 40 mEq are excreted reducing excretion to balance intake. Viewed in terms of single nephron function, changes in single nephron reabsorption of Na in the distal nephron increases from 24.3 to 24.86 meq $\times 10^{-7}$.

When intake is 200 mEq/day and residual function is 10% of normal, the amount delivered per nephron is two times normal. The amount reabsorbed is 1.5 times normal and the amount excreted is 20 times

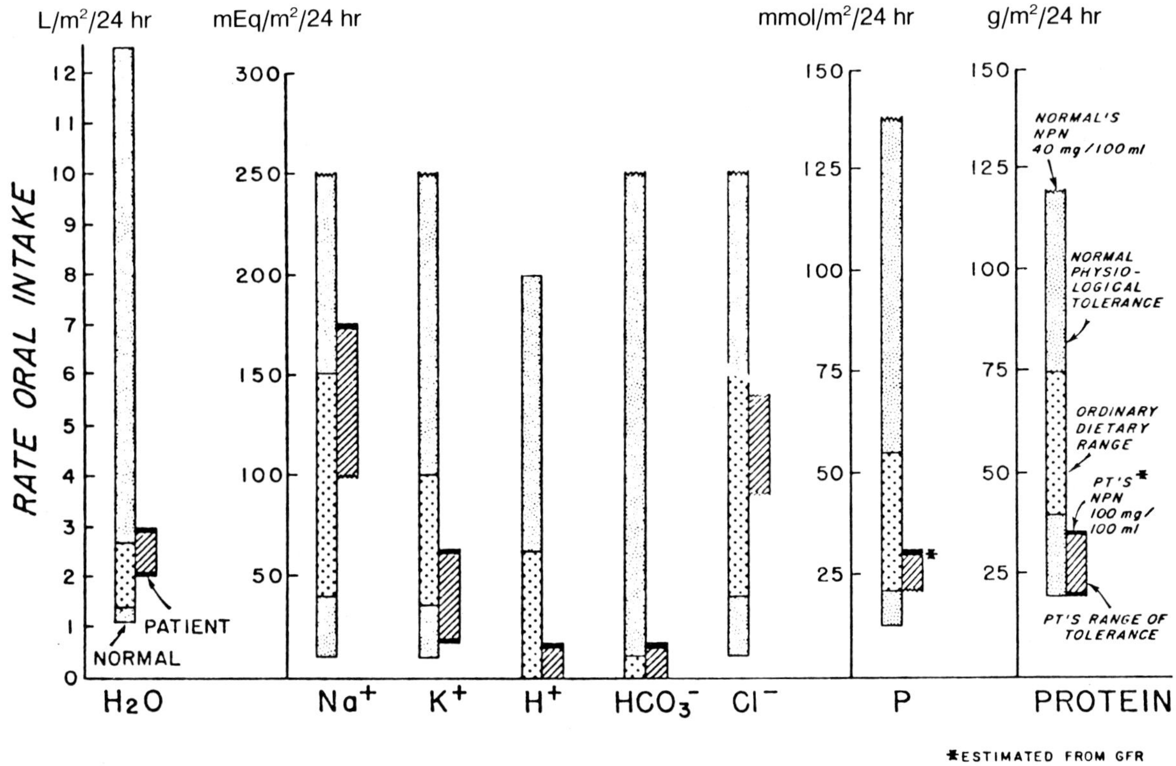

Figure 49.8. Comparison of maximal tolerances, ordinary dietary ranges, and tolerances of patient with chronic renal failure for water and certain other nutrients. From Talbot NB, Richie RH, Crawford JD: *Metabolic Homeostasis: a Syllabus for Those Concerned with the Care of Patients.* Cambridge, MA, Harvard University Press, 1959.)

Table 49.5.
Effect of change of NaCl intake from 200 to 40 mEq/day on Renal Handling of NaCl (see text for abbreviations)

Intake/output mEq/day	Normal function		Residual function[a,b]	
	Na_I mEq/day (%)[c]	SN·Na mEq × 10^{-7}/min	Na_I mEq/day (%)[c]	SN·Na mEq × 10^{-7}/min
200				
Na_F	20,000	70.0	2000	140
Na_R	19,800 (99)	69.4	1800 (90)	126
Na_E	200 (1)	0.6	200 (10)	14
40				
Na_F	20,000	70.00	2000	140
Na_R	19,960 (99.8)	69.86	1960 (98)	137.2
Na_E	40 (0.2)	0.14	40 (2)	2.8

[a] 10% of normal.
[b] Residual nephron number = 5%; single nephron GFR = 200% normal.
[c] % of filtered Na.

Table 49.6.
Theoretical Effect of Change in NaCl Intake from 200 to 40 mEq/day on Distal Nephron Handling of NaCl

Intake/output mEq/day	Normal function		Residual function[b,c]	
	Na_I mEq/day	SN·Na mEq × 10^{-7}/min	Na_I mEq/day	SN·Na mEq × 10^{-7}/min
200				
Distal Na delivery	4000	25.0	400	50
Distal Na reabsorption	3800	24.3	200	36
Na_E[a]	200	0.7	200	14
40				
Distal Na delivery	4000	25.0	400	50.0
Distal Na reabsorption	3960	24.86	380	47.2
Na_E	40	0.14	20	2.8

[a] 10% of normal.
[b] Residual nephron number = 5%; single nephron GFR = 200% normal.
[c] Na_E = excreted Na.

normal. When intake is reduced to 40 mEq/day, the amount reabsorbed is 1.65 times normal and the amount excreted per nephron is, again, 20 times normal.

It is not clear at this time whether the control of these changes in distal nephron NaCl reabsorption is effected through the operation of a special natriuretic factor of renal failure or whether natriuretic factors that operate in normal or through local or short loop factors regulate reabsorption in CRF (see Chapters 5 and 6). For example, in the case where residual function is 10% of normal and distal delivery is increased, flow past the macula densa is greater and this has an effect on renin release and on active Na and Cl reabsorption (61). Similarly, in that case, if K intake is maintained, Na, K-ATPase increases to effect greater Na-K exchange (62).

Atrial natriuretic peptides are peptide hormones that are stored in cells in the auricles; on release, they cause natriuresis. The actions of atrial natriuretic peptides have been considered in four categories: (a) renal hemodynamics (GFR) and electrolyte excretion, (b) smooth muscle relaxant, (c) hypotensive agent, and (d) inhibition of the action of renin (62). High levels have been reported in patients with congestive heart failure (63) and Na retention and in children on hemodialysis who were volume overloaded (64). In the latter case, fluid removal by dialysis lowered the levels. Its action on the kidney in patients with renal failure is not defined but may be explained by an acute increase in single nephron GFR. It appears to act in response to acute changes in ECF volume and atrial pressure more than to chronic changes in NaCl intake (63).

Tolerance to change in NaCl intake is reduced in patients with CRF in approximate proportion to the degree of loss of renal function (58), and the time required to adjust to a change in intake is prolonged (60). However, tolerance (the capacity to adjust output to intake) obviously exists within the range of a patient's intake or the patient develops symptoms of NaCl retention or depletion.

Retention. Patients with CRF who maintain an average Na intake beyond their tolerance develop an expanded ECF volume, hypertension, and/or progressive glomerular injury. For these patients, lowering dietary NaCl is valuable. The development of hypertension, an expanded ECF volume, or both may be subtle and only an awareness to look for both and relate the finding to NaCl intake gives the clinician the indication for therapy.

In severe CRF, concentration of Na in muscle cells also increases (65). The factors that underlie this change are removed by a low-protein diet or dialysis therapy within weeks; they reappear with inadequate (twice weekly) dialysis. This form of retention is a function of uremic toxicity, not NaCl overload.

Depletion. The prevalence of Na-wasting as NaCl in patients with CRF is disputed. The usual level of Na intake (>40 mEq/day) is sufficient to accommodate to some salt-wasting. As noted, abrupt reductions in NaCl intake to <40 mEq/day in patients with CRF leads to losses in body NaCl or ECF volume (59); graduated reduction in NaCl intake over several months does not (60). Therefore, most patients with CRF are kept on a NaCl intake >40 mEq/day (>1000 mg Na); abrupt changes in Na intake are avoided. Acute illnesses may dispose patients with CRF to NaCl loss and ECF volume contraction, with profound reduction in GFR and blood pressure. The decrease in GFR is sometimes irreversible.

A less frequent occurrence is overt NaCl-wasting, which requires salt supplementation. This is more common in children with renal dysplasia, medullary cystic disease, or obstructive uropathy. Tubular dysfunction impairs Na_R, particularly in the distal nephron, so that salt-wasting is the result (66). Several mechanisms may contribute; hyporeninemia, hypoaldosteronism, or resistance to aldosterone action are factors in some patients. When this is the case, hyponatremia, resistant hyperkalemia, and hyperchloremic acidosis are characteristic. This complication is more common in infants with congenital disease and in adults with diabetic nephropathy (67). Destruction of the distal nephron by disease is analogous to the effects of papillectomy described in experimental animals (56) and causes salt-wasting and hyperkalemia.

The clinical consequences of salt-wasting, leading to contracted ECF volume, range from subtle malaise and, in children, poor weight gain, to weight loss, hypotension, and obvious signs of dehydration. Abrupt withdrawal or omission of a salt supplement may precipitate the more extreme manifestations.

The tests for proximal and distal tubular function relating to NaCl and water, described in Chapter 19, have not been applied systematically to children with CRF, although a recent review provides some information (68).

Potassium

The range of tolerance for variations in K intake is nearly as great as that for Na. The principal control of K excretion is Na-K-ATPase activity in the renal medulla. In normal individuals, Na-K-ATPase regulates K excretion to balance dietary K (62). The regulation of Na-K-ATPase is significantly, but not totally, dependent on aldosterone, so it is less efficient when hypoaldosteronism is present (Chapter 7). With loss of function, changes in Na-K-ATPase continue to regulate K excretion (69), but the overall range of tolerance is reduced. Nonetheless, within the range of intakes commonly encountered in adults (50 to 100 mEq/day) balance is possible; change in K_s is uncommon until CRF is well advanced (function <20%), except for the special circumstances noted below.

Hyperkalemia. Hyperkalemia is prone to occur when the renin-angiotensin-aldosterone (RAA) system is impaired. This may occur in patients with hyporeninemia and hypoaldosteronism associated with interstitial nephritis (67) or congenital disease (68). Hyperkalemia occurs in patients with CRF when they become dehydrated and delivery of Na beyond the proximal is reduced. Obviously it is more likely to occur as CRF progresses or K intake or input from catabolic events increases. Patients on dialysis who are anephric have lower basal aldosterone levels and lower responses to ACTH and change in posture (70) because the RAA system is no longer active or because hepatic blood flow and, hence, metabolic clearance of aldosterone is increased (71), or because heparin inhibits aldosterone biosynthesis. These changes in aldosterone activity may affect the cellular distribution of Na and K and contribute to hyperkalemia. Anephric patients treated with peritoneal dialysis have normal responses (72) (Chapter 7).

Hypokalemia. Hypokalemia is uncommon in patients with reduced renal function. It may occur in CRF when clearance values are high and there is increased delivery of bicarbonate or other poorly reabsorbed anions to the distal nephron, as occurs in cystinosis. Patients treated with diuretics or those in whom K is restricted may become hypokalemic (Chapter 7). This is likely to occur in patients who have been malnourished and who become anabolic when they are treated with a parenteral or enteral formula low in K (73).

Hydrogen Ion

Acid base regulation by the kidney may be affected in several ways in patients with renal disease. Like K regulation, acid base regulation remains effective until CRF is advanced, unless renal tubular acidosis (RTA) develops with the underlying disease process, as often occurs in conjunction with hyperkalemia (Chapter 34).

Acidosis. As CRF progresses, acidosis may develop because proximal bicarbonate reabsorption is impaired (74); this leads to hyperchloremic acidosis and urine pH values of >6.0. Acidosis also develops when the compensatory ability to excrete ammonia is insufficient to buffer hydrogen ion that is excreted, in which case sulfate and organic acid are excreted as Na salts, and H+ and Cl− are retained, causing hyperchloremic acidosis; urine pH may be <5.0 (75). In both instances, alkali therapy is needed to correct the acidosis. In the latter, a low-protein, low-P diet may lower net acid intake and be effective (Chapter 8).

Renal tubular bicarbonate reabsorption is depressed by PTH, and this may contribute to bicarbonate-wasting (76). In chronic renal acidosis, bone alkali is titrated, leading to loss of bone mineral and the excretion of urinary calcium. This is prevented by giving alkali (77). When clearance is very low, sulfate, phosphate, and organic acids are retained and the undetermined anions in plasma are increased, usually when residual function is <10%. In this instance, lowering net acid intake is more effective than giving bicarbonate. In practical terms, this means lowering dietary protein, which lowers the intakes of sulfur amino acids and phosphorus.

Alkalosis. Metabolic alkalosis in CRF is uncommon. It usually develops in response to NaCl losses that are inadequately replaced; if alkali is given (and sometimes even in its absence), contraction alkalosis develops. The ECF volume contraction may be secondary to gastrointestinal or renal NaCl losses. In one case, extensive replacement of protein-rich ascitic fluid losses with blood bank plasma diluted with sodium citrate led to Cl deficiency and contraction alkalosis. A salt-free diet supplemented with alkali may have this effect; this also occurred when a commercial Cl-deficient formula was distributed inadvertently.

Water

Regulation of water excretion by the kidney is impaired relatively late in renal disease (78). The concentrating capacity is diminished as CRI progresses to CRF. Some of this loss is attributed to medullary injury, hyperemia, or both so the usual hyperosmolal state of the medulla is compromised. The osmotic diuresis induced by the relatively high load of urea delivered to each nephron as CRF progresses also is a factor. There is some evidence that cyclic AMP response to ADH is reduced (79). The usual result is that urine is dilute to isotonic. Under these conditions, the ability to excrete a standard water load (20 ml/kg) is retained, but the time required for its excretion is increased, i.e., the rate of excretion of free water is reduced in proportion to the reduction in GFR (68). On the other hand, patients with CRF generally reduce urine osmolality to the same low level as that of healthy individuals (68, 78).

Some children and fewer adults develop a vasopressin-resistant hyposthenuria analogous to the congenital form of nephrogenic diabetes insipidus (Chapter 35). Because GFR is low, the absolute degree of polyuria is less than that observed with familial nephrogenic diabetic insipidus but often is sufficient to be evident as polyuria. In infants, its expression may be subtle (80). We have seen at least one case associated with salt-wasting.

Phosphorus

The relation between PTH and phosphate excretion is complex and incompletely understood. PTH secretion is stimulated both by the hypocalcemia that results from depressed intestinal absorption of calcium (21) and directly from P intake (81–84). It has been postulated that transient hyperphosphatemia following P ingestion triggers PTH secretion (84). A recent study clearly shows the daily pattern of serum P in patients with CRI to parallel that of normal individuals and for the values to be less, not more, than normal (Fig. 49.9). Although changing dietary P causes a parallel change in the levels of PTH (82), the effect is not mediated by changes in plasma P (P_P) (83), as had been originally proposed (84).

Plasma levels of 1,25 vitamin D are reduced in children with CRI; in adults, levels are reduced only when they reach the stage of CRF (83). Giving vitamin D to children with CRF increases both Ca and Pi absorption. Lowering dietary Pi causes the plasma level of 1,25 vitamin D to increase; raising it results in the converse. There is an inverse relation between the levels of PTH and 1,25 vitamin D in response to changes in dietary Pi intake. These occur with insignificant changes in plasma Ca or P_P (83).

Urea Nitrogen

Net urea nitrogen (UN) production or UN appearance is a function of net dietary protein N intake; production of nonurea N products, e.g., creatinine and uric acid, change little if at all with changes in dietary protein. In practice, where body protein N is stable, UN production equals dietary N intake corrected for a relatively constant fraction of N lost in stool and skin secretion and the urinary nonurea N. Total nonurea N production is between 25 and 30 mg/kg/day in most stable states. Net UN production/kg/day is approximately equal to N intake per kilogram minus 30 mg (23).

UN excretion is a function of its concentration in plasma (and body water) and its renal clearance. Its clearance is equal to GFR less a variable fraction that is passively reabsorbed in the medulla. There is no renal adaptation to UN excretion as renal function declines; UN concentration in body water is a function of net urea synthesis and renal clearance. Output usually reflects input of dietary N (Fig. 49.10). As concentration of UN rises and, hence, load per nephron increases, the osmotic properties of urea begin to affect uptake of tubular fluid (85). As this occurs, UN clearance (C_{UN}) increases relative to GFR; with adequate hydration it is approximately 70% of GFR (86). When there is a brisk water diuresis, C_{UN} is also 70% of GFR in normal individuals (87).

Creatinine

Creatinine is excreted by glomerular filtration and tubular secretion (35). When GFR is normal, the tubular secretion is about 20% of the filtered creatinine, i.e., $U_{Cr}V$ = 120% filtered creatinine. As GFR declines, the percent of $U_{Cr}V$ that is secreted rises in a variable way to an average of 160% of filtered creatinine when GFR is 40 to 80 ml/min/1.73 m^2; it may reach values that are >200% of filtered creatinine when GFR is <40 ml/min/1.73 m^2. Consequently, the C_{Cr} as a measure of residual GFR tends to progressively overestimate GFR and underestimate rate of progression. As P_{Cr} increases, significant catabolism of creatinine develops so that $U_{Cr}V$ is less than total creatinine production (88), which also causes P_{Cr} or its reciprocal to overestimate GFR.

The use of the reciprocal of P_{Cr} to follow the course of renal disease derives from the assumptions that $U_{Cr}V$ is constant over time and that C_{Cr} bears a consistent relation to GFR. Since these assumptions are subject to significant and variable exceptions, this method of following the residual GFR is prone to considerable inaccuracy. The tendency for the reciprocal of P_{Cr} to define a linear relation with time (Chapter 19) in adults observed >1 yr is caused by several factors that tend to average out. Empirically, the relation of $1/P_{Cr}$ versus time was linear in 80% of adults (89) and 64% of children (90) observed for several years. Predicting GFR from height and P_{Cr} is reliable in children for clinical purposes (91) but following change in GFR in children from $1/P_{Cr}$ for short-term studies, this method probably is impractical because the accuracy of the prediction is not satisfactory for such a short period (92).

Hormones and the Kidney

The renal hormones—renin, prostaglandins, kallikreins, 1,25 dihydroxyvitamin D (1,25D), and erythropoietin—adjust differently as renal function declines. (Dunn [93] provides an excellent review of renal endocrinology.) With ablation or loss of nephrons, as occurs with glomerulonephropathy, renin production usually maintains the capacity for normal responses to physiological stimuli. In certain instances, however, hyporeninemia results (67). In renal failure, the action of locally acting hormones and autocoids, i.e., prostaglandins and kallikreins, are thought to play a role in regulating NaCl excretion to balance intake as function declines (Chapters 6 and 16). The capacity to synthesize vitamin D into 1,25D is impaired in proportion to the loss of function (94) (Chapter 52). The effect of CRF upon erythropoietin activity is described in Chapter 53B.

The role of the kidney in metabolizing peptides constitutes a principal mode of clearance for many peptide hormones, e.g., insulin, somatostatin, glucagon, calcitonin, growth hormone, prolactin, and parathormone. The clearance is effected by interaction of hormone in the peritubular circulation with receptors on the basolateral surface of renal tubular cells and to a lesser degree by filtration and removal by interaction with the brush border of these cells. Renal clearance accounts for between 30% to 60% total clearance of most of these hormones, and this relation continues despite reduction in function to <30% of normal. The frac-

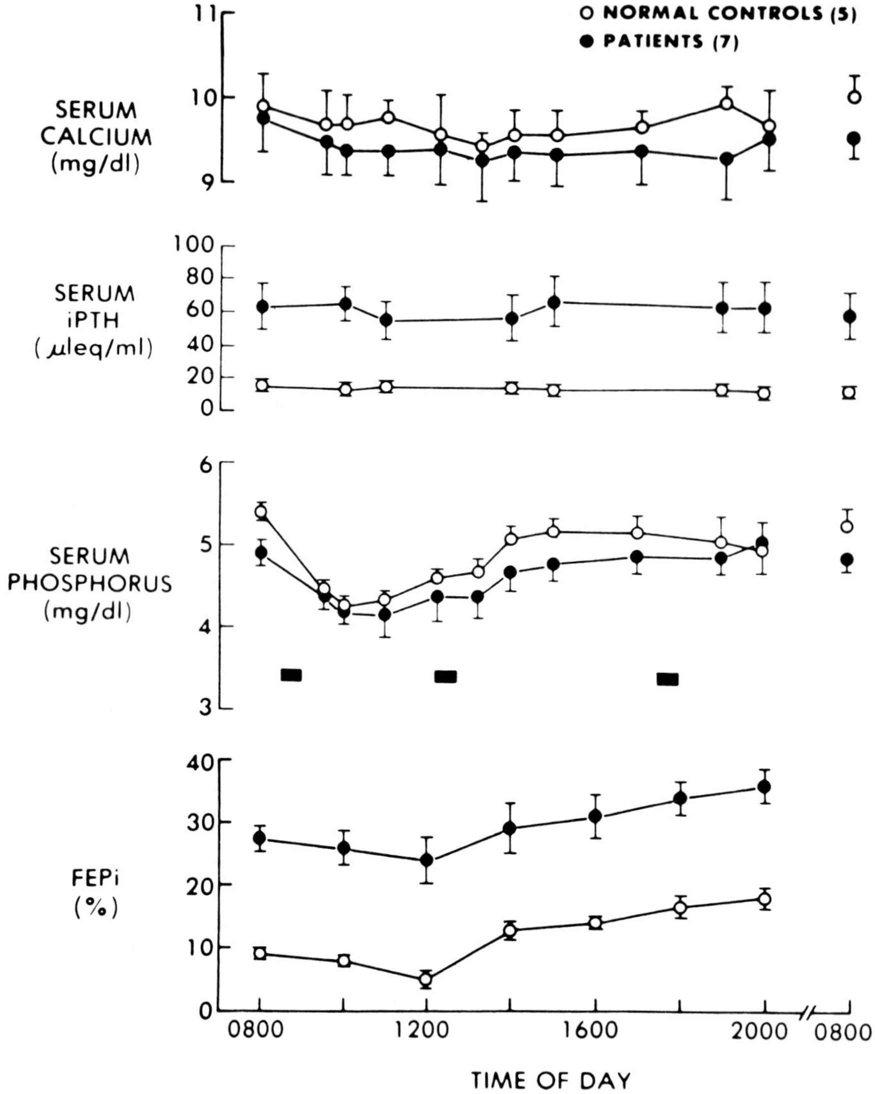

Figure 49.9. Diurnal pattern serum Ca, iPTH, Sp, and FePi of normal children (n = 5) age 5 to 15 yr of age (C_{Cr} = 116 ± 8 ml/min/1.73 m^2) and children with chronic renal failure (n = 7) age 6 to 17 yr of age (C_{Cr} = 45 ± 4 ml/min/1.73 m^2). Note serum P values in patients invariably are normal or low, although P intakes were 1200 mg/day for 2 days. With dietary P restriction and supplementation average fasting values changed less than (.5) 5 mg/dl. (From Portale AA, Booth BE, Halloran BP, et al: J Clin Invest 73:1580, 1984.)

tional clearance of hormones is relatively constant despite wide differences in plasma levels, attesting to the large capacity the kidney has for clearance in this manner, e.g., insulin half-life is not prolonged until GFR is <20% of normal (95, 96). In CRF, fragments of hormone may be immunoreactive, but they may be biologically less active or compete with active hormone and diminish or alter the response to normal hormone (94), e.g., parathormone and glucagon.

Renal Metabolism

The kidney is the predominant site of more than 25 enzymes, which with CRF are diminished in varying degrees (97) affecting metabolic pathways. Renal neutral peptidase is the principal enzyme used to degrade several peptide hormones. Loss of the peptidase reduces the clearance of the hormones. Myoinositol, a potential uremic toxin when its level is increased (see p 34), has a reduced clearance because the enzyme that degrades it, myoinositol oxygenase, is greatly reduced.

The principal site for serine synthesis is in the kidney. Low plasma serine levels are common in patients with CRF. Serine is integral to the biosynthesis of cysteine in hepatic gluconeogenesis. The effect of the low levels of serine in CRF is not known. Creatine synthesis is slowed by a deficiency of arginine:glycine amidinotransferase. Carnitine synthesis is impaired by deficiency of γ-butyrobetaine hydroxylase. Whether the low level of carnitine characteristic of patients on hemodialysis is a factor in the hypertriglyceridemia is being investigated. Although carnitine supplements may be beneficial, a suitable trial to test its efficacy and safety has not yet been reported.

METABOLIC ADAPTATION

Metabolic adaptation in CRI succeeds in averting clinical signs from loss of function unless stress exceeds adaptive capacity. The adaptation in CRF when GFR is <30% often is insufficient to avoid clinical signs related to metabolic abnormalities. The metabolic abnormalities in intermediary metabolism are complex and interrelated and are affected by the level of calories, carbohydrate, fat, and protein that are eaten.

Energy

A feature of CRF in adults is lassitude and reduced physical activity. Anorexia and reduced food intake also are common. It has been difficult to know whether malaise induces inactivity and loss of appetite, or loss of appetite induces calorie deficiency and malaise follows. In a given patient, either or both mechanisms may operate. Where there are signs of calorie malnutrition, i.e., reduced skinfold thickness or overt wasting, calorie deprivation may be an important factor in the clinical picture, and calorie supplementation may be beneficial (98). This occurs more often in younger children than it does in older children or adults.

Uremia often is described as a state of exaggerated catabolic response to stress. In terms of energy metabolism, this response would anticipate a higher resting metabolic rate and less efficient use of calories and protein for growth. Resting or basal oxygen consumption has not been elevated in rats with CRF (99); however, in careful pair-feeding studies, growth rate and storage of fat and protein relative to food intake was impaired (100).

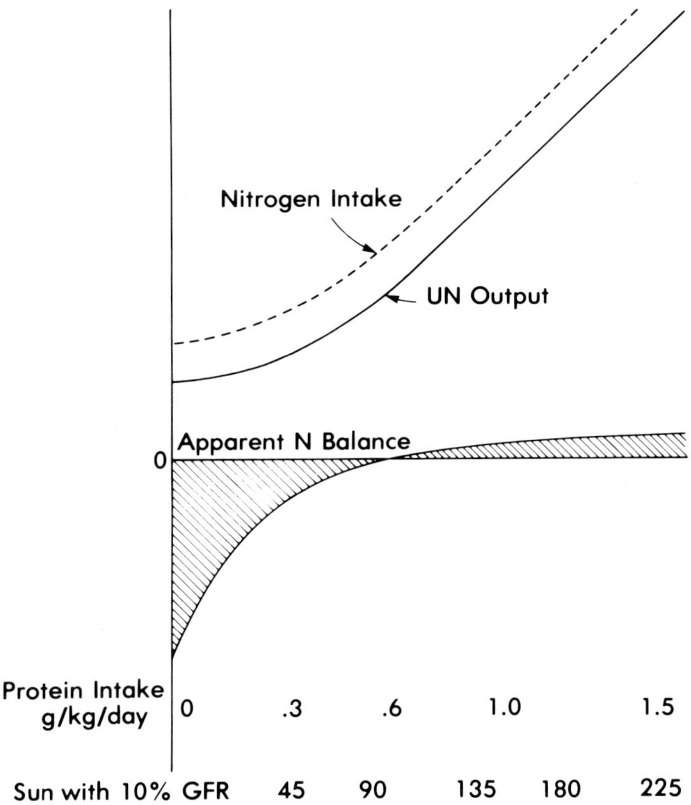

Figure 49.10. Diagram describing change in UN output (appearance) in relation to N intake and N balance when dietary N is changed.

Several studies have reported abnormalities in oxidative metabolism caused by CRF. These are included in a review of muscle bioenergetics and various factors that may cause myopathy (101). Experimental uremia has been associated with uncoupling of oxidative phosphorylation (102) and with changes in intestinal mitochondrial respiration (103).

Carbohydrate

Hyperinsulinemia and resistance to insulin-mediated glucose disposal are well-recognized aspects of CRF. Hyperinsulinemia is seen when residual renal function is about 30% normal; at that stage, it appears to be a compensatory response to resistance to insulin-mediated glucose disposal, inasmuch as glucose homeostasis is intact because there is extra insulin. As CRF failure progresses, glucose disposal is impaired despite hyperinsulinemia. This may be evident as fasting hyperglycemia (104) but more commonly is demonstrated when a glucose load is given, as is done in conventional glucose tolerance tests or when hyperglycemic or euglycemic clamps are done. Many of these studies are done in patients with residual function of 10% to 15% and just before dialysis. With dialysis, the defect in glucose disposal improves, even though with dialysis residual renal clearance values are still <15% of normal (105). The defect in glucose disposal is not due to impaired insulin binding but instead is an intracellular defect of insulin action. The site of the resistance is peripheral tissues—muscle and adipose tissue. Lactate release and Pi uptake also are affected, whereas K uptake is not (106). The effect of uremia on insulin-mediated amino acid uptake and protein synthesis is discussed below.

The effect of CRF on insulin-mediated glucose disposal, studied in children using a glucose clamp technique, was ameliorated by lowering dietary Pi (107) or by lowering dietary protein (108). Both measures improved insulin response, i.e., hyperinsulinemia increased, which accounted for much or all of the effect of these strategies on glucose disposal (Table 49.7). The problem of glucose intolerance has two parts: early, when there is a need for more insulin and hyperinsulinemia results, and later, when there is a failure to make enough insulin so that glucose intolerance results. The second effect responds to dialysis (105) or to reduced dietary Pi or dietary protein (107, 108).

The effect of CRF on glucose mobilization and metabolism in times of fasting or stress is less well defined. The general assumption (see previous section) is that CRF exaggerates the catabolic response to stress. In terms of carbohydrate metabolism this would anticipate a high rate

Table 49.7.
Effects of Uremia and of Dietary Treatment on Metabolism of Glucose (M), Plasma Insulin Levels (I), the Ratio M/I and PTH Levels in Patients Studied Using the Hyperglycemic Clamp (see Text)

	Adult controls	Pubertal uremic children	Pubertal uremic children on phosphate restriction	Pubertal uremic children on protein restriction	Pubertal uremic children on CAPD
M (mmol/kg/min)	0.067 ± 0.002	0.035 ± 0.003[b]	0.053 ± 0.005[a]	0.076 ± 0.006	0.065 ± 0.010
I (μU/ml)	44 ± 9	42 ± 2	56 ± 4	76 ± 14	52 ± 5
M/I (X1000)	1.54 ± 0.12	0.82 ± 0.05[b]	0.95 ± 0.04[b]	1.18 ± 0.22	1.33 ± 0.20
PTH (ng/l)	160 ± 20	2010 ± 690[a]	180 ± 50	310 ± 100	850 ± 250[a]
n	6	8	7	6	5

[a] $p < 0.05$.
[b] $p < 0.01$ of adult controls.

of hepatic glucose production, increased gluconeogenesis from lactate and amino acids, and a higher rate of release of these substrates from muscle. Glucose release from the perfused liver of rats with CRF, i.e., residual function about 30%, that had fasted 48 hr, was slightly increased but this was not associated with a greater extraction of gluconeogenic amino acids or of glucose production from alanine (109). In fed CRF rats, however, glutamine and alanine release from muscle increased (110), whereas we found no change in perfused hind limb (111).

Humans, having residual C_{Cr} of about 15%, have either normal (105) or increased (112) hepatic glucose output. Amino acid uptake by the liver may be normal or increased, but the fraction of glucose formed from gluconeogenic amino acids is increased (112).

Glycolysis may be impaired in CRF by reduced activity of the enzyme phosphofructokinase, which is a rate-limiting step in the conversion of glucose to pyruvate (113). This reduction in activity has been attributed to a specific inhibitor identified in uremic serum (114).

Fat

Hypertriglyceridemia and, less commonly, hypercholesterolemia occur in CRF. Hepatic production of triglycerides continues at a normal rate, but their plasma clearance is reduced secondary to decreased activity of plasma lipoprotein lipase. This may be related to glucose intolerance. Substituting fat for carbohydrate in the diet is associated with a fall in plasma triglyceride concentration (115). Hypercholesterolemia is reduced in children whose diet is low in cholesterol and high in polyunsaturated fat (El Bishti, Chantler, unpublished observations).

Mobilization of fatty acids may be limited in CRF by the antilipolytic action secondary to hyperinsulinemia (116). The plasma concentrations of free fatty acids (FFA) and glycerol tend to be low in adults and children on regular dialysis (116, 117), although plasma fatty acid concentrations rise with adequate dialysis (116). A few children with CRF become obese with high-carbohydrate diets in spite of decreased cell masses and diminished statural growth (118). The obesity may be associated with hyperglycemia and raised plasma insulin concentrations; it is more commonly seen in sedentary adults but observed in some infants with CRF who are tube-fed excess calories (119).

Protein

The consequences of reduced renal function are most evident in their effect on protein metabolism. Uremia describes toxicity from retention of end products of protein metabolism. Although the toxicity of urea itself is minimal, the level of UN is a sensitive index to the clinical toxicity of dietary protein in CRF. Adding to the importance of protein metabolism is the hypothesis that in CRI, dietary protein is a factor in accelerating the loss of residual function (see p 777). In this section, protein metabolism in CRF is discussed in relation to toxicity, muscle-wasting, abnormalities in amino acid metabolism, and the relation these may have to energy and carbohydrate metabolism.

Toxicity

The symptoms characteristic of uremia—mental confusion, nausea, vomiting, and bleeding—are the most obvious clinical expressions of uremic toxicity. They appear when UN level in plasma is between 100 and 200 mg/dl (35 to 60 mmol/liter), and function is <20% of normal—usually much less. The symptoms commonly develop as a consequence of an intercurrent illness in someone with CRF who has been stable. These symptoms may be reversed by lowering dietary protein (120) or assuring adequate carbohydrate intake or by dialysis.

Uremic toxins (121) are a large class of compounds designated as such because they are retained in uremia and their removal by dialysis reverses uremic symptoms. Most of them are nitrogen-containing compounds; their collective toxicity is apparent from the relief of symptoms that follow the introduction of a very-low-protein diet to uremic patients (120). The toxins have been studied by isolation and identification from uremic plasma or dialysate fluid and measuring the effect these isolated compounds or fractions have, using both in vivo and in vitro studies.

Compounds <500 Da. Compounds having a molecular weight <500 Da are readily dialyzable, and many potential ones have been chemically identified. The more important ones are urea, guanine compounds, aliphatic amines, polyamines, and myoinositol. When plasma UN levels are sustained at >300 mg/dl by adding urea to dialysate of patients on chronic dialysis therapy, some symptoms of uremia develop. Whether a lower level causes more subtle symptoms or simply is an index to the presence of other toxins is not clear. Guanidinosuccinic acid is the only guanidino compound of proven toxicity; it affects platelet adhesion and its removal corrects the bleeding disorder associated with defective platelet adhesion observed in some uremic patients (122). Aliphatic amines and polyamines, which may be derived from intestinal bacteria, are likely clinical toxins. Polyamines have many potential toxicities; their role as inhibitors of erythropoiesis is of particular interest (123).

An interesting class of compounds are those that displace other ligands bound to albumin; some of the displaced ligands in the unbound state are believed to be toxic (124).

Compounds >500 and <3000 Da. Compounds >500 and <3000 Da are less well characterized chemically; they often are termed "middle molecules" because their dialysance is decidedly less than those <500 Da and their clearance is more time-dependent. They have been classified according to fractions of uremic plasma or dialysate separated by gel filtration and chromatography. Most are chemically unidentified; many are peptides. They often are described in terms of the specific inhibitory effect they demonstrate, although some fractions have more than one effect. Among the inhibitory actions studied are the following (121): Fractions isolated by gel filtration inhibit the action of serum, somatomedin, or insulin to stimulate cartilage growth (125). Adipocytes from uremic rats have a depressed rate of hexose transport and glucose oxidation (126), although insulin-binding characteristics are normal. These defects were corrected when these cells were incubated in normal media. Conversely, adipocytes from normal rats incubated in uremic serum in time developed depressed transport rates. The inhibitors of these processes probably are peptides (127).

Inhibitors of cell proliferation, neurotoxins, and intermediary metabolism have been demonstrated in isolated tissue preparations or cell culture and are being investigated. What role these play in the clinical syndrome of CRF in humans is not clear; efforts to isolate and counter the action of these compounds are in progress (121).

Muscle-wasting

A reduced muscle mass is commonly described as a part of CRF. Muscle mass measured by total body K (128), by intracellular water minus bromide space (129), and by anthropometry (130) is reduced in patients with CRF. The reduction may be caused by physical inactivity, poor calorie intake, or by metabolic disturbances affecting protein synthesis and degradation. These, in turn, can have more direct causes: infection leads to catabolic stress and anorexia; toxins from catabolism may depress protein synthesis or increase degradation, either in a catabolic or an anabolic phase (131).

Exaggerated response to catabolic stress often is cited as characteristic of patients with CRF and those on dialysis therapy; documentation of the exaggerated catabolism is poor. The general clinical impression is that patients with CRF take longer to recover, either because the weight loss and loss of body protein associated with infection are greater, the anabolic response is less, or both. In uremic rats that fasted 48 hr, muscle protein synthesis, degradation, or both measured in vivo (132) and in perfused muscle preparations (133), are greater. Feeding or giving glucose abolishes the difference. Both protein synthesis and breakdown, studied in isolated incubated muscles, are affected by uremia (134). Although insulin-mediated uptake of α-amino isobutyric acid is inhibited both in vivo and in vitro by uremia in rats (135), the in vivo uptake of most amino acids, notably the branched chain amino acids, is not affected when insulin is given during a euglycemic clamp test (105).

In a preliminary report, muscle protein degradation rates were shown to vary inversely with total body fat in control and uremic rats; uremic rats, having less body fat, had higher degradation rates. Giving uremic rats higher calorie intakes that caused body fat to increase also restored muscle protein degradation rates to those seen in controls (131). This provocative finding should stimulate an inquiry into the relation between body fat and protein breakdown rates in patients with CRF.

Amino Acid Imbalance

Alterations in plasma amino acid concentrations are common in CRF. Reduction in fasting plasma branched chain amino acids—leucine, valine, isoleucine, and tyrosine—are commonly observed (136, 137). The low values may not be rate-limiting for growth because growth improves when a low-protein diet supplemented by an amino acid and keto-acid mixture is fed to uremic children, even though the low plasma concentrations of branched chain amino acids do not change (138). Reduction in threonine, lysine, and histidine varies. Serine, a nonessential amino acid, also is usually low. Elevation in methylhistidine and citrulline reflects their reduced clearances. Elevation of glycine, citrulline, alanine, glutamine, glutamate, proline, ornithine, and aspartate varies; glycine and citrulline levels tend to be increased because their conversion to serine and arginine, respectively, by renal metabolism is reduced (139). The reduction in fasting plasma branched chain amino acids is associated with reductions in the ketoanalog of the branched chain amino acids (140).

The interrelations of these changes with alanine and pyruvate (Fig. 49.11) point to a defect in metabolism that may contribute to muscle-wasting. The rate of pyruvate and lactate release is reduced; alanine release is accelerated (141). Leucine, which influences protein synthesis in vitro in the absence of insulin (142), may be deficient and affect protein synthesis, However, the fasting level of leucine in muscle intracellular (ICF) in patients with CRF is normal. Fasting muscle free valine and tyrosine levels are low (143). These findings have led to the proposal that valine and phenylalanine (the precursor for tyrosine) is two to three times recommended amounts. Supplementing the diet with extra valine and tyrosine improves the fasting amino acid levels in plasma and muscle (144) (Table 49.8) and appears to improve N balance and clinical status (145).

Values obtained in a fasting, i.e., postabsorptive, state reflect the ambient levels when the source of input into both plasma and muscle free amino acid pools is net tissue catabolism. A more sensitive assessment of the relation between diet and free amino acid pools in relation to muscle protein metabolism is obtained when these levels are measured after a low-protein meal feeding (146). Under these conditions, the stress of synthesis is measured with a low input of amino acids from the diet and a net output into muscle protein.

In a preliminary study, we showed that the difference in postfeeding plasma amino acids between normal infants and infants with CRI were greater than those seen in the fasting state (Table 49.9). On the other hand, valine- and tyrosine-supplemented low protein diets did not improve growth rates in young uremic rats (147).

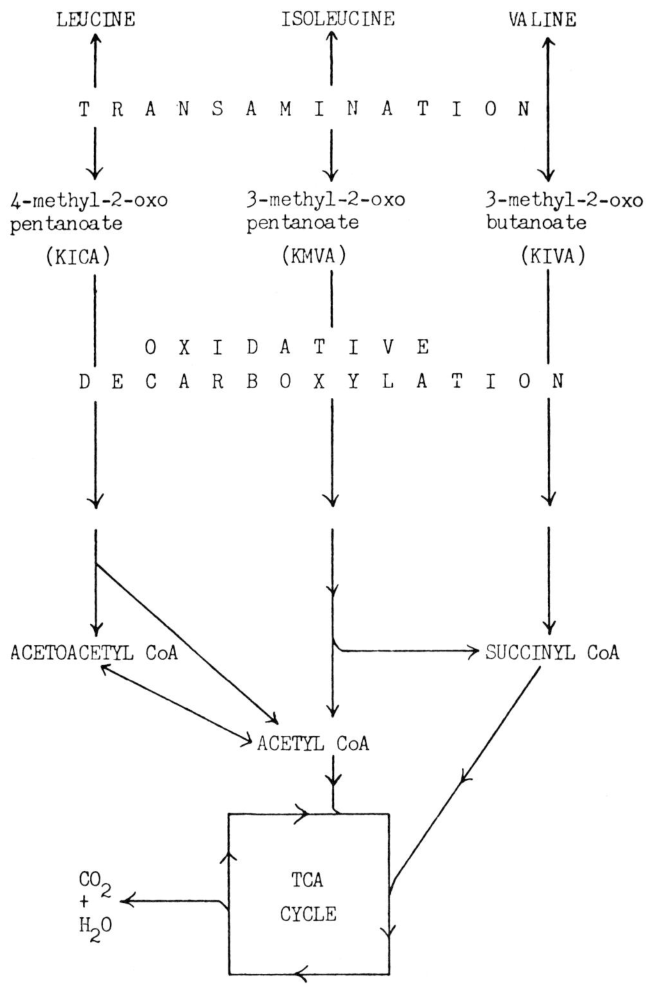

Figure 49.11. Metabolic pathways of leucine, isoleucine, and valine to their respective ketoanalogs and thence to oxidative decarboxylation and entry into tricarboxylic acid (TCA) cycle.

Table 49.8.
Comparison of Effects of Valine, Tyrosine-enriched Amino Acid Supplement (NA) Versus Standard Essential Amino Acid Formulation (EA) on Plasma and Muscle-free Amino Acids[a]

	Intake-% RDA[c]		Plasma (% of Control Values)		Muscle (% of Control Values)	
	EA	NA	EA	NA	EA	NA
LEU	165	140	55[b]	80	90	95
VAL	170	250	60[b]	100	55[b]	80
PHE	200	140	90	120	85	95
TYR	(60)[c]	(270)[c]	95	100	45[b]	65

[a] Adapted from Alvestrand et al (143). The intake provided by diet plus formulation of each amino acid relative to the RDA (211) is noted.
[b] Significantly below normal.
[c] RDA derived from suggested percent of phenylalamine intake as tyrosine.

Dietary Protein

The optimum dietary protein or protein amino acid mix for adult patients with CRF is not known (17). Very-low-protein diets (0.3 to 0.4 g/kg/day) relieve symptoms of uremia but do not sustain muscle mass

Table 49.9.
Effect of CRF upon Plasma AA Levels

	Ratio of CRF: Normal AA value	
	Fasting	3 hr post feeding
VAL	0.98	0.89
LEU	0.90	0.80
TYR	0.84	0.79
TRP	0.55	0.59
MET	0.91	0.71
LYS	0.60	0.56

[a] Children measured in fasting state and three hr after feeding 25% daily intake using a whey:casein formula providing 8% of calories as protein.

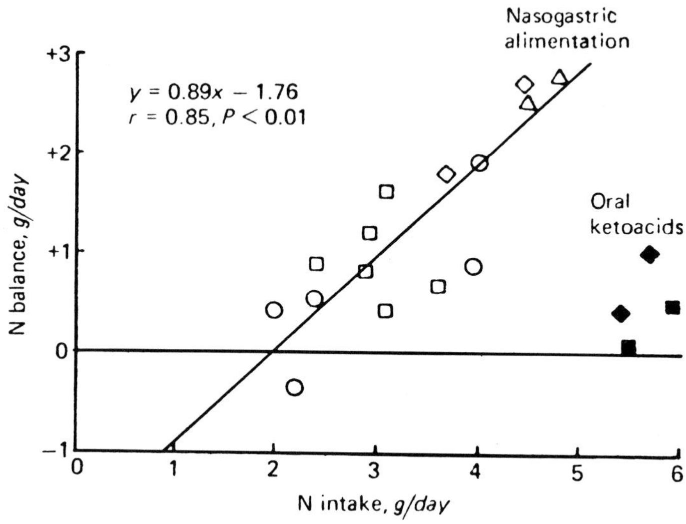

Figure 49.12. Relation of N balance to N intake of patients on amino acid–ketoacid supplements given orally (solid symbols) and by nasogastric feeding at night (open symbols). Note that neutral N balance with nasogastric feeding was achieved with intakes of ~2 g N/day, whereas 5 to 6 g N/day were required when intake was oral. (From Abras E, Walser M: Kidney Int 22:392, 1982.)

and body protein N at normal levels and are associated with negative N balance in some normal subjects (148, 149); more protein (0.6 g/kg/day) in moderately uremic patients does sustain N balance in moderately depleted patients (145, 148). Very-low-protein diets supplemented with a standard mix of essential amino acids also marginally sustains body protein N in depleted patients, and a modified amino acid mix in which extra tyrosine and valine are given appears to do so more effectively (145).

Very-low-protein diets (0.3 g/kg/day) and supplements of essential amino acids and ketoanalogs of amino acids also sustain N balance in patients with severe CRF, i.e., residual function <5% (150). The efficiency of N utilization improved even more when a synthetic amino acid–ketoanalog mixture was given overnight by tube and a very-low-protein diet allowed during the day (151) (Fig. 49.12). Children fed a reduced protein diet and given an amino acid–ketoanalog supplement showed improved growth even though calorie intake was unchanged (138). When very-low-protein diets and amino acid (152) or amino acid–ketoanalog supplements (153) have been used in place of no diet therapy, the rate of progression has been slowed. This is only true when S_{Cr} is <8 mg/dl. In one controlled study low-protein diets were effective in retarding the rate of loss of C_{Cr} (46, 47).

GROWTH AND DEVELOPMENT

Characteristics of Growth Retardation

Prevalence

Growth retardation is the outstanding complication of impaired renal function in childhood. In 1890, Dr. James Goodhart noted that growth retardation may be symptomatic of renal disease for "serious disease of the kidneys frequently fails in (other) symptoms" (154). More than half the children with CRF who reach end-stage renal disease are growth-retarded, i.e., are >2 SD below mean height for age (155–161). The average stature of young men and women treated for end-stage renal disease during childhood is >3 SD below the mean (161). Children with congenital renal disease tend to be more affected than those with acquired disease, because the rate of growth in this period is greater (4, 158) and the prevalence of renal tubular dysfunction is more common (68, 155, 161).

Pattern

Growth of fetuses with reduced renal mass in utero tends to be normal, so that length and weight at birth are near normal. Because both polyhydramnios and oligohydramnios are associated with impaired growth and both are associated with renal anomalies, the prevalence of low birth weight increases in fetuses with renal anomalies. There is, as well, an increased incidence of renal disease in low-birth-weight infants; hence, the distribution of body weight and length in infants with reduced renal function is skewed to the left (159, 160).

Growth in early infancy is retarded in half the patients referred with reduced renal function. Although growth velocity after 2 yr of age was often nearly normal in this study, there was a tendency for SD scores to shift down with time (162, 163). This was more marked in children with obstructive uropathy than it was in infants with simple reduced renal mass. Growth retardation occurred predominantly among children with a GFR of <25 ml/1.73 m^2 (158). Although relative height, as measured by the SDS for height, remains stable with growth in children whose SDS is negative, height deficit increases because the value of 1 SD tends to increase (Chapter 2). For example, a child who remains at −3.0 SD scores from 2 to 12 yr of age increases the difference between his or her height and average from 8 to 20 cm (Table 49.10). The tendency for a negative SDS to increase slowly, both in children with CRF and those on dialysis, describes an even greater increase in height deficit (164).

Stature after transplantation frequently maintains the same SDS (165); but catchup growth is uncommon and height deficit tends to increase (Table 49.10). Therapy to promote growth is needed early in childhood (158); although normal growth does occur, (Fig. 49.13) it is unfortunately not the rule.

The poor growth of the child with CRF usually is associated with delay in skeletal maturation (166, 167), especially in those with early onset of CRF. The delay averages about two yr but can be as great as six yr (167, 168). This delay may extend the potential for recovery of growth (164); however, apparent delay may be due in part to disordered bone growth that occurs in uremia, as well as to true delay, as occurs in malnutrition (Chapter 2), so the potential in any given case is hard to assess.

Between infancy and puberty there is a tendency for skeletal maturation and height to advance in parallel, thus the potential for catchup growth diminishes. Untreated renal osteodystrophy is associated with reduction in growth while skeletal maturation continues (166) (see Chapter 52).

In children who are on dialysis during puberty, skeletal maturation advances more rapidly than chronological age and height potential is further limited (169). Following transplantation, (165, 170–172) adolescents with a history of poor growth and bone maturation that exceeds 12 yr at the time of transplantation grow poorly (173). In younger children, growth following transplantation is better, but this may be because growth retardation is more severe or because younger, less affected bone has more growth potential. Normal growth following transplant has been observed in some older, severely growth-retarded children with bone ages >12 yr (174). Some children with end-stage renal disease and delay in skeletal maturation continue to grow at an age when growth in normal children has ceased; this prolonged growth period enables some catchup growth to be achieved (168, 175).

Table 49.10.
Relationship Between SDS and Height Deficit of Children at Different Ages who Maintain Score of −3.0 SDS using UK Data[a]

Age (yr)	Value of 1 SD	Height (cm)	Normal height (cm)	Height deficit[b] (cm)
United Kingdom				
1	2.69	68.2	76.3	8.1
2	3.30	76.0	85.9	9.9
4	4.30	88.7	101.6	12.9
6	5.14	99.2	114.6	15.4
8	5.73	109.0	126.2	17.2
10	6.20	118.3	136.9	18.6
12	6.48	127.5	146.9	19.4
14	6.59	140.8	160.6	19.8
United States				
10	6.20	118.9	137.5	18.6
12	7.51	127.2	149.7	22.5
14	8.48	127.7	163.1	25.4

[a] Data for 10–14 yr using US data also given. SDS for distance curves during puberty are greater in US.
[b] Ht deficit = Normal Ht − Obs Ht.

Sexual maturation is delayed in CRF (9, 176). Its onset correlates better with skeletal than with chronological age (168). The mean age of onset of menarche for girls on dialysis and those with a functioning renal transplant is 15.1 yr, whereas that of healthy girls is 13.4 yr (9).

Causes

Various factors have been implicated in the growth retardation of CRF (155–157, 175) (Table 49.11). Severe growth retardation is invariable in children with Fanconi's syndrome and cystinosis. The causes of the severe growth retardation (177) that accompany cystinosis are many and include bicarbonate-wasting (178), polyuria, and polydipsia (156, 179), K deficiency, hypophosphatemia (180), osteomalacia and osteodystrophy (181), and salt-wasting (66). Each of these in isolation may cause poor growth and, when corrected, lead to growth resumption. However, success in attacking all of these and improving growth in children with cystinosis has not been reported. Indomethacin, which reduces the increased fractional Na excretion in cystinosis, may improve growth along with other measures (182).

Table 49.11.
Causes of Growth Failure in Children with Renal Disease (177)

Tubular disease	Chronic renal insufficiency
Hypophosphatemia (180)	Anemia (183)
Osteomalacia and osteodystrophy (181)	Hypertension (184)
Bicarbonate-wasting (RTA) (178)	Energy deficiency (98)
NaCl-wasting (66)	Metabolic and hormonal changes (177)
Vasopressin resistant diabetes insipidus (156, 179)	

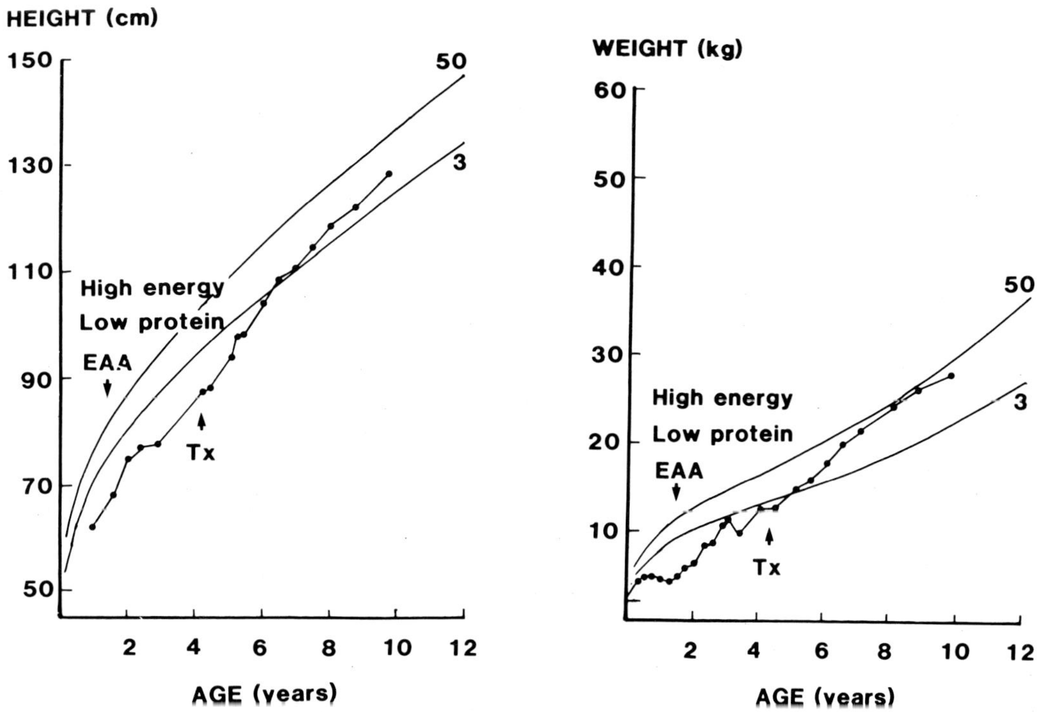

Figure 49.13. Growth curves for height and weight of a child with chronic renal failure who showed some improvement on a low-protein diet supplemented with essential amino acids; further improvement occurred following renal transplant. Similar curves are sometimes seen in children with CRF following calorie supplementation, vitamin D therapy, alkali and NaCl supplementation.

CRI causes changes in body composition that indirectly affect growth (Table 49.12). Anemia is often profound, especially in children on dialysis; however, few data relating anemia and growth retardation in CRI are available. Reduced oxygen delivery to cells may affect growth, which improves with other forms of chronic anemia when an active transfusion policy is instituted (183). Uncorrected hypertension (184) may be associated with poor growth in CRI. Chronic acidosis, like other factors associated with poor growth, may be causative. Early studies showed that most growth-retarded children with CRI were acidotic (155), but the association is not invariable and correction of acidosis does not always improve growth. However, children with growth retardation secondary to uncomplicated RTA experience catchup growth when acidosis is corrected (Chapter 34).

Because the capacity to conserve NaCl is reduced in CRI, NaCl-wasting can be a factor in retarding growth, particularly in children with obstructive uropathy or renal dysplasia. In some infants with CRI the provision of extra NaCl in the diet will improve growth (66).

Renal osteodystrophy slows growth. Correction of osteomalacia with vitamin D (185) or its active metabolites (181), suppression of secondary hyperparathyroidism by parathyroidectomy (186) with calcitriol (187), or by reducing P (82), appears to improve growth. The reduction in dietary phosphorus lowers PTH and raises 1,25 dihydroxyvitamin D levels in serum (83).

Anorexia is common in CRI. When the energy intake is <80% of RDA, the energy intake correlates with growth. Increasing energy intake above this level improves growth but usually does not restore stature to normal (98). Increasing energy intake in children whose intake is already adequate will not improve growth and will cause obesity (188).

The role that abnormalities in protein metabolism play in retarded growth are not known. Muscle mass, often reduced in children and adults with CRF, reflects impairment in the ability to sustain net gain in body protein N that is usually associated with growth. Factors associated with the reduced muscle mass (impaired protein synthesis, resistance to insulin action that may affect other insulinlike growth hormones, and increased muscle breakdown) may contribute to poor weight gain and retarded growth (131). Lower N intake in the form of a low-protein diet supplemented with essential amino acids and amino acid–ketoanalog and a low P intake are associated with improved growth (138).

Psychological and Social Development

CRF leads to psychological problems in some children; those on chronic hospital dialysis are most obviously affected (189–192). Most children and their families find dialysis a considerable stress (193). Young children have difficulty accepting such painful procedures as fistula needling, which may generate aggression toward parents and staff and lead to anxiety for all concerned. This aggression may be followed by withdrawal or refusal to cooperate, which also can make dialysis very difficult for all. This conflict can be a factor in reduced food intake. It affects growth, sexual maturation, schooling, and inhibits the child's social development. The problems for parents of children on dialysis are considerable, for their whole way of life is affected and other children in the family also suffer. Faced with these problems, it is reassuring that many children and families survive the experience so well. In one survey of adults who had been treated in childhood for an average of 11 yr, most were working full- or part-time in a variety of jobs that were not dissimilar to those of their peers. Many, particularly the women, were married and leading normal social lives. More families thought the experience had improved rather than adversely affected family life.

Renal transplantation is the preferred method of treatment in terms of improving developmental levels and promoting social maturation. Long-term survival rates of children following transplant are superior to those of children on hospital dialysis. Successful renal transplantation allows better rehabilitation (189–197) and is associated with fewer psychosocial problems. Although renal transplantation is a time of great stress, rehabilitation within 12 months of a successful transplant generally is good; some problems, e.g., steroid side effects, poor growth, and anxiety over rejection, remain (Chapter 51).

Intellectual performance may be reduced in adults with end-stage renal disease (195). The few studies in children suggest a similar effect (196, 197). Renal transplantation is associated with a "one time" improvement in developmental score. The long-term effects on later development of CRF that starts in infancy have not been studied longitudinally. The prevalence of significant developmental retardation appears to be increased. This may be caused by metabolic and hormonal abnormalities, the frequently associated disturbances in fluid and electrolyte balance, or the social factors noted. Reports that a progressive encephalopathy develops in infants with CRF (198) may be related to a variety of factors to which aluminum intoxication has been added (199).

ASSESSMENT

The assessment of children with loss of renal function entails following residual renal function, the clinical state of the child relative to the consequences of the loss of function, growth and development, and the underlying disease process. In general, residual renal function should be

Table 49.12.
Effects of Chronic Renal Insufficiency on Body Composition and Functions

Energy	Protein	Hormones	Skeletal mass	Other Nutrients
Poor intake Glucose intolerance with reduced peripheral glucose metabolism Plasma triglycerides increased Glycerol reduced	Reduced cell mass and cell protein Reduced protein synthesis and tendency to protein catabolism Reduced plasma, albumin, transferrin, etc. Reduced plasma branched chain amino acids and ketoacids Reduced tyrosine/phenylalanine ratio	Increased plasma insulin Increased growth hormone Increased somatomedin (radioreceptor assay) Decreased somatomedin (bioassay) Increased glucagon Cortisol levels normal or slightly raised Testosterone reduced with raised FSH and LH Plasma catecholamines normal or raised Parathyroid hormone increased	Osteomalacia Osteitis fibrosa cystica	Calcitriol reduced Pyridoxine reduced Plasma zinc variably reduced

followed whenever it has reached a level of <50% normal, i.e., CRI, regardless of the cause, because the course thereafter is likely to be continued loss of residual function. The clinical state also is important to observe during this period, as is growth and development. These should be followed more assiduously once residual function is <30%, i.e., CRF.

Renal Function

The conventional method for screening for loss of renal function is to evaluate S_{Cr} and BUN. Unfortunately, these do not increase to levels outside the normal range until residual function is <70% and residual nephron number or functional potential may be <35% of normal (see p 778). Therefore, the finding of an elevated S_{Cr} and evidence of irreversible renal injury is sufficient to conclude that <35% of functional potential may remain and the patient has CRI.

Once the latter is established, it is recommended that residual renal function—glomerular and tubular—be followed as described in Chapter 19. A decrease in S_{Cr} usually is evidence of improvement in function and of underlying disease; in the neonatal period, it is evidence of normal maturation and hypertrophy compensating for loss of renal function. A S_{Cr} that is stable but elevated may be evidence of stability; however, residual function may be declining and compensatory mechanisms overshadow the decline. Better measures of renal function and the effect of disease are needed to monitor the course of events in a patient with chronic renal disease and to evaluate the efficacy of interventions.

Observing the course of patients by plotting the reciprocal of S_{Cr} against time in adults is insensitive to change over the shorter periods when interventions are being tested, even though it is helpful in the long term as an index of rate of progression (92). The slope, if linear, is an underestimate of the rate of decline. Nonetheless, over periods of two or more years, the slope of $1/S_{Cr}$ versus time is linear in 80% of the cases in adults (89) and 64% of children (90). For normal children the estimate of clearance, using height/S_{Cr}, is an accurate predictor of GFR (91, 200), but the relatively poor precision makes it difficult to evaluate changes of 20% even under ideal conditions. Single-injection methods for measuring GRF may be an improvement, but the coefficient of variation (± 20%) limits the usefulness of this method for serial quantitative assessment (201, 202). Conventional clearance methods may be used when more precise measurements of change are needed, but these also require experienced personnel and excellent technique to obtain a coefficient of variation that is <10% (35). For infants and for patients with dilated ureters, a five-hr infusion of inulin and calculation of C_{IN} from input and S_{IN} provides accuracy and precision equal to that obtained with the conventional clearance methods (203).

Metabolic

Clinical Function Assessment

Metabolic assessment entails the monitoring of clinical, anthropometric, radiological, biochemical, and dietary data, usually done infrequently in children with CRI and more regularly in children with CRF.

A brief clinical history and examination, measurement of blood pressure, and urine culture when relevant should occur at one- to three-month intervals, depending on the clinical condition. Care must be taken in prescribing certain antibiotics, e.g., aminoglycosides and certain other drugs, such as digoxin or phenobarbital, whose renal excretion is reduced in renal failure and where accumulation causes toxicity. The Na and K content of antibiotics is noted (see Chapter 17).

Attention is paid to the presence of edema or evidence for ECF volume depletion. Pubertal status, when appropriate, should be assessed annually. The impact of the disease and its treatment (including dietary management) on the child and family should be discussed regularly with psychological, social, and nutritional assistance provided where necessary. School attendance and achievements, both intellectual and physical, should be observed; it is useful to ask to see school reports. Nutritional management cannot be separated from general clinical management. Integrating these aspects of care is time-consuming and each clinic visit occupies one half to one hour of physician time as well as the time of others. This is emphasized because providing less inevitably leads to less than optimal care. Conferences following assessment are important to coordinate care.

Anthropometric Assessment

Height, weight, skinfold thickness (205, 206) at the biceps and subcapsular sites and upper arm circumference are measured regularly (Chapter 2). Weight-for-height index is a measure of muscle and adipose tissue relative to height; when it is low, it provides a useful indication of malnutrition. A low value may be obscured, however, by an increase in ECF volume. Cell mass and weight for height ratios in children with CRF correlate ($r = 0.71$) (129). Skinfold thickness and arm circumference measurements provide estimates of body fat; these are good indicators for dietary energy sufficiency (98, 130). Deriving muscle mass from arm circumference is a relatively insensitive measure, but there are no good alternatives at present.

Radiological Assessment

Radiographs of the hand-wrist or knee are obtained at three- to six-month intervals for evaluating renal osteodystrophy; bone maturation score is evaluated annually (204). Bone absorptiometry, for measuring bone density, potentially is a better method that awaits evaluation (207) (see also Chapter 52).

Laboratory Assessment

A blood count, serum ferritin for Fe status, and red cell folate should be assessed initially and intermittently thereafter. Plasma electrolytes, S_{UN}, S_{Cr} Ca, P, alkaline phosphatase, and serum proteins should be assessed at each visit; fasting triglycerides and cholesterol should be measured occasionally.

A 24-hr urine collection, analyzed for creatinine, urea, Na, K, Ca and P concentration, is useful in monitoring children with CRF. A spot urine can provide useful estimates in infants with reduced function because intake of nutrients in the form of formula is relatively consistent. Because creatinine excretion in infants is approximately 10 to 15 mg/kg/day, it is possible to estimate the daily excretion of Na, K, P, and UN from a spot urine, although the confidence limits for the accuracy of the estimate have not been established. UN appearance plus urinary NH_3 N plus 20 mg N to allow for nonurea N losses per kilogram per day should predict N intake per kilogram per day when a steady state exists (see Fig. 49.10). On the other hand, the use of UN appearance and estimates of N intake from diet records, to derive a term for N balance, is grossly unreliable. Errors of measurement of both items preclude an estimate of N balance that has any validity, since balance represents a small difference between two large numbers, each of which can have a large error. For example, the difference between an N intake of 300 mg/kg/day (1.8 g protein) having a random error of estimate of ±60 mg and a UN appearance rate of 290 mg/kg/day, with an error of estimate of ±58 mg (20%), could range from +128 to −108 in more than half the instances and as great as +256 to −216 if the range of error is within 2 SD of the estimates. Even careful N balance studies performed at different levels of protein intake have a systematic error because N intake is usually overestimated, N losses are underestimated and, therefore, the higher the intake, the greater the apparent N retention (208). UN + NH_3N appearance rate is only useful as a check on the estimate of N intake determined by diet analysis.

The Na content of the urine provides a check on Na intake; it also can be valuable in identifying and managing infants and children with renal Na-wasting. This is also true for K.

The S_{UN} depends on urea clearance and on intake. Only rarely does acute gain or loss of body protein N affect S_{UN}. When the effect of catabolic stress on S_{UN} is significant, it can be estimated from UN appearance (209). Following major surgery, adults maintained on glucose excrete 6 g UN per day (210). Walser (209) has suggested than S_{UN} concentration should not exceed 90 mg/dl (30 mmol/liter); where protein intake is above requirement or there is excessive catabolism with a negative N balance, steps should be taken to lower S_{UN}. A high S_{UN} or S_{UN}:S_{Cr} ratio in a patient with CRF may mean that the protein intake is more than is necessary and protein restriction may be beneficial. Determinations of serum transferrin and albumin or the measurement of other nutrition-sensitive plasma proteins in patients with CRF provide an additional and useful assessment of the adequacy of protein nutrition (130).

A 24-hr urine collection and a fasting (postabsorption) blood sample (150) analyzed for P and creatinine enables the calculation of the fractional excretion of P (FE_{Pi}) and the theoretical threshold Tm_{PO_4}/GFR (Chapter 19). Tm_{PO_4}/GFR is more accurately estimated from a two- to three-hour urine collection taken in the morning, with a fasting blood sample obtained at approximate midpoint. This also is more convenient and less subject to urine collection errors and the effects of diurnal variations in U_PV than obtaining a 24-hr collection. The child voids on rising, notes the time, drinks a water load (20 ml/kg), and comes to the hospital; a blood sample is obtained, the child voids and the timed sample measured. Both fractional excretion of P (FE_P and Tm_P/GFR provide useful indices in clinical practice for assessing the adequacy of control of secondary hyperparathyroidism. The former is a more sensitive test of urinary P excretion relative to P intake in patients with CRF; the latter defines the tubular reabsorption capacity relative to GFR and is particularly useful in observing patients with primary parathyroid disease (see Chapter 9).

Dietary

Dietary intake of the following nutrients should be monitored at one- to three-month intervals: energy, Na, K, Ca, P, and protein—the last for quality and quantity. This is done by prospective recording of the weight or volume of all items consumed over a three-day period; usually, cooperation can be obtained if the recordings are not undertaken too frequently. Intake of specific nutrients can be calculated from standard tables of food composition, using any of several food composition tables and a computer programmed for that purpose. Intakes can then be compared with the RDA (211, 212) (Table 49.13). The three-day prospective dietary assessment method has been validated by comparing the dietary record with a double bag analysis of all food consumed (correlation coefficient for energy $r = 0.92$, for protein $r = 0.92$, mean discrepancy 11% (213).

Growth and Development

The assessment of growth in children is done by an assessing stature and weight:height ratios. Noting the progress of sexual maturation is also important (Chapter 2). Developmental assessment is useful in children with CRF, particularly those <5 yr of age.

Statural growth over time traditionally is measured against standard growth curves (Fig. 49.13). When growth retardation places a child under the fifth centile, there is advantage in expressing the child's stature in height (or length) SD score for age (164, 215). Growth over time should

Table 49.13.
Recommended Daily Allowances for Children with Chronic Renal Insufficiency[a,b]

Age (yr)	Height (cm)	Energy (kcal/kg)	Minimal Protein (g/kg)	Calcium (mg)	Phosphorus (mg)
0–0.1	55	120	2.2	400	200
0.1–0.5	63	110	2.0	500	400
0.5–1	72	100	1.8	600	500
1–2	81	1100	18	700	700
2–4	96	1300	22	800	800
4–6	110	1600	29	900	900
6–8	121	2000	29	900	900
8–10	131	2200	31	1000	1000
10–12	141	2450	36	1200	1200
12–14 M	151	2700	40	1400	1400
12–14 F	154	2300	34	1300	1300
14–18 M	170	3000	45	1400	1400
14–18 F	159	2350	35	1300	1300
18–22 M	175	2800	42	800	800
18–22 F	163	2200	33	800	800

[a] Sources of Data: Dept of Health and Social Services (UK), 1969 (211); National Academy of Science, Recommended Dietary Allowances (US) (212).

[b] At least 25% of energy should be provided by carbohydrate and at least 3% should be as enriched polyunsaturated fatty acids. An adequate vitamin and trace element intake is required. Phosphorus intake or absorption can be reduced according to plasma phosphorus concentration and or renal phosphorus handling. Sodium and potassium intake depend on renal function but for normal children, an intake of 1.5–2.5 mmol/kg body weight per day is recommended.

be expressed in terms of change in height SD score (164) and as SD score for growth velocity (214). This method is much superior to the use of height expressed as percent of normal growth (Chapter 2).

THERAPY

Therapy in patients with reduced renal function has, as a guiding principle, the adjustment of intake to be between the limits of need and tolerance that has been set by the injury to the kidney. Intolerance includes intakes that accelerate renal injury or cause metabolic abnormalities, including retarded growth. Medical management includes treatment of the complications of CRF:bone disease (see Chapter 52), anemia, and hypertension (Chapter 53A), which have both nutritional and pharmacological components.

Electrolytes and Water

Regulating intake of electrolytes (Na, Cl, K, and alkali) has been an important aspect of CRF therapy. Although loss of excretory function often requires reducing intake of the electrolytes Na, Cl, and K, tubular dysfunctions may require selective supplementation, particularly in infants.

NaCl

The indications for giving supplemental salt (NaCl) are subtle and, it is our impression, are commonly overlooked. Poor weight gain may be the only sign; a high S_{UN}:S_{Cr} adjusted for age and diet, or clinical signs of salt depletion are present only some of the time. A tendency to hyponatremia or hyperkalemia may indicate a hyporeninemic or hypoaldosterone state (66–68). Measuring fractional excretion of Na may provide a clue that FE_{Na} is high relative to intake and level of residual function.

Giving supplemental salt (2 to 15 mEq/kg/day) and noting improvement is the only sure method of establishing the need for a NaCl supplement. We have found as much as 15 meq/kg to be needed in a few children. Fludrocortisone has proved useful in some adults and children with CRI and hypoaldosteronism (67).

Alkali

Renal acidosis caused by bicarbonate-wasting or inability to make ammonia is evident as RTA or hyperchloremic metabolic acidosis. The clinical manifestation may be simply poor weight gain. Treatment of hyperchloremic acidosis associated with CRF usually is successful when 2 to 4 mEq/kg/day of alkali are given, generally as $NaHCO_3$. Occasionally, when acidosis occurs in CRF, larger doses are needed (Chapter 34). Very occasionally, $KHCO_3$ is needed when K-wasting occurs with CRI in Fanconi's syndrome.

Renal acidosis, with an increased anion gap caused by sulfate and phosphate retention, occurs only late in CRF when dietary protein is excessive; lowering dietary protein and P are recommended.

Potassium

K supplementation in CRI is rarely needed. In cystinosis or conditions in which secondary hyperaldosteronism is present, e.g., following intensive diuretic therapy, K supplementation may be needed. Usually 2 to 4 mEq/kg/day as KCl or as K bicarbonate, if renal acidosis is also present, is sufficient. S_K should be monitored closely.

Hyperkalemia is more commonly the problem in children with severe CRF or those with hyporeninemia or hypoaldosteronism. Dietary K can be estimated from K excretion either from 24-hr or spot urine checks. If K excretion exceeds 2 mEq/100 kcal of intake, a diet can be offered that is lower in K. Kayexalate will lower S_K, but its use indicates a marginal level of K control. If K intake and excretion are low and dialysis is not otherwise indicated, renin and aldosterone concentrations should be measured to try to determine whether treating Na-wasting and K retention with mineral corticoid is rational. Propranolol or other β-blockers used for hypertension may predispose to hyperkalemia.

Water

Vasopressin-resistant hyposthenuria occurs with dysplasia and obstructive uropathy. Children with CRF and vasopressin-resistant hyposthenuria who cannot take extra water in response to thirst may develop hypernatremia, but free water loss usually is not that great. We have seen vasopressin-resistant hyposthenuria and salt-wasting occur together. Usually the only therapy needed for the hyposthenuria is sensitivity to the child's vulnerability to water deprivation and appropriate advice to avoid the occurrence of free water deprivation, excess salt intake, or administration of x-ray contrast media. When salt or protein intake or both are inappropriately high, lowering them will lessen the requirement for water.

Nutrition

Signs similar to those of protein energy malnutrition are still reported as common in patients with CRF and patients on dialysis (130), but defining requirements for individual nutrients is difficult. Although CRF and dialysis modify nutrient requirements, the reference base from which to start is the RDA (211, 212). The nutritional aspects of managing patients with renal failure have been reviewed (130, 216).

Energy

RDA values represent the recommended intake for healthy children; the requirement for individuals of the same age and height may vary by ±50%. Prescribing energy requirements, therefore, is difficult in principle. In practice, calorie supplements are recommended when intakes are <80% of RDA and are associated with poor growth or decreased skinfold thickness. Supplements usually equal 15% to 20% of RDA (98). Energy supplements improve total energy intake and, by blunting appetite, reduce the intake of other nutrients (167). They should not be urged when their use is associated with tension and anxiety. Supplements containing fat are useful because of their high caloric density. Hypertriglyceridemia, which is common in CRI, may respond to substitution of dietary fat for carbohydrate (115) or may require a more formal investigation. When there are signs of inadequate energy intake, nighttime tube feedings are recommended (119). These assure delivery of a balanced and adequate diet with low psychological cost; some children pass their own tube. Nagging about meals is greatly reduced or, as one mother noted, "the battle of the mouth is over." Overnight feedings also may improve the efficiency of dietary N utilization (151) (Fig. 49.9). However, when tube feedings are used, oral stimulation is important to avoid developing eating disorders later.

Protein, Amino Acid, and Amino Acid–Ketoanalog Supplements

Protein intake in children with CRI usually is in excess of RDA (138), though low intake occasionally is noted. The RDA for protein is increased if low-quality protein is used in the diet (211), e.g., when the amino acid score of the average dietary protein is 70, the RDA is increased to 1.43 (1/0.7). RDA in the United Kingdom and the United States make generous allowance for this, so that adjustments in individual cases are not necessary. When low-protein diets are used without supplements, deficiency of an essential amino acid may develop.

The standard practice in treating adults who are given very-low-protein diets (1 g/100 kcal) or 4% calories as protein (.4 g/kg/day) and amino acid supplements is to give two to three times the RDA for each essential amino acid in the same formula as that proposed by Rose (217). There are no controlled studies testing variations from this, and the results are ambiguous. Our recommendation for children with CRI is to meet the RDA of the United Kingdom or United States diet for protein for children and adults. For infants, it is recommended that formulas conform to standard recommendations of the American Academy of Pediatrics (218).

It is difficult to get young children to eat very-low-protein diets and an adequate energy intake (118). One of us has used a diet calculated to provide a minimum protein intake according to height, with a protein energy ratio of 1.25 g/100 kcal (5% of calories from protein); nonselected protein was supplemented with an equal amount of essential amino acids. The regimen was administered to seven children over a period of six months and was associated with a marked reduction in S_{UN} and a positive N balance; however, the strict protein limitation could not be maintained, S_{UN} rose, and by the end of the study the average protein consumption was 1.9 g/100 kcal. Protein nutrition assessed by plasma transferrin concentration, weight for height ratios, and measurement of intracellular water was maintained, but growth did not improve. The one child who showed improvement in height maintained a protein calorie ratio of 1.4 g/100 kcal and an S_{UN} of <60 mg compared with an average S_{UN} of 135 mg/dl for the whole group (118).

In another study using a low-protein diet supplemented with an amino acid–ketoanalog mixture, growth velocity increased in all seven children studied. The diet was designed to provide minimum N intake equivalent to protein intake of 1.3 g/100 kcal of a nonselected protein supplemented with an amino acid–ketoanalog mixture, raising the total protein amino acid–ketoanalog intake. The more liberal allowance of nonselected protein permitted reasonable adherence to the diet, with an average protein amino acid–ketoanalog intake of 1.7 g/100 kcal having the N equivalent of 1.5 g/100 kcal. S_{UN} stabilized at 60 mg/dl and plasma transferrin, upper arm circumference, and body cell mass improved. Examination of the data relating N balance to S_{UN} from a study of low-protein amino acid–supplemented diet shows a correlation coefficient of −.73 but with considerable scatter; no individual with a S_{UN} >85 mg/dl was in positive balance (138).

A high S_{UN} does not preclude normal growth; however, the experience cited suggests that attempts should be made to reduce the S_{UN} to <60 mg/dl by reducing the dietary protein intake. Infants may be given 1.3 to 1.6 g/100 kcal (5% of calories as protein), using high-quality protein or nonselected protein with amino acid supplements while maintaining an adequate or high-energy intake and monitoring plasma transferrin and albumin for evidence of protein malnutrition (17).

There are two practical and one theoretical advantages in using ketoacid supplements (139). They permit a higher consumption of nonselected protein while keeping N intake low. They provide enough essential amino acids as the amino acid-ketoanalog supplement to meet minimum requirements, and the diet is a high-calcium and low-phosphorus one that aids in suppressing secondary hyperparathyroidism. The theoretical advantage is the assumption that the ketoacids of the branched chain amino acids, especially ketoleucine, reduces protein degradation and stimulates protein synthesis (210).

Current formulations have not demonstrated any advantage of ketoacid diets over amino acid diets in promoting N balance (145, 150).

Calcium, Phosphorus, Vitamin D

Because the anorexia of CRI may reduce Ca intake below RDA and diets low in P also are low in Ca, Ca supplements are recommended. Some Ca preparations, such as effervescent tablets, contain Na; if Na restriction is required, then Na-free Ca preparations are recommended.

Excess dietary P can be reversed in severe CRF in children (82) and adults (43) by feeding a low P diet supplemented with phosphate binders to prevent intestinal absorption of P. The selection of Al compounds as a binder for P has been questioned because of the risk of Al toxicity to bone (207) and to brain (199).

There is uncertainty about when to start vitamin D therapy. Because Ca absorption is impaired when residual function is <50%, there is a theoretical basis for giving supplements at that point; however, risks of hypervitaminosis D and hypercalcemia are restraining factors. There is general agreement that vitamin D therapy may be given to sustain S_{Ca} in the normal range; some recommend that S_{Ca} be maintained between 10.5 and 11.5 mg/dl. There is also uncertainty about which preparation of vitamin D is preferable. Vitamin D_2 and D_3 are used infrequently because each has a very long half-life; the dose has varied between 20,000 and 200,000 U/day. Dihydrotachysterol after transformation increases intestinal absorption of Ca and is effective in treating renal osteodystrophy in children; the dose is 0.125 to 1.5 mg/day. The analog 25(OH) vitamin D has reversed hypocalcemia: the dose is 100 μg/day; it lowered PTH levels in two studies in children. The analog 1-α-(OH)D is converted to $1,25(OH)_2$ vitamin D in the liver and is effective as the natural hormone: the dose is 1 to 2 μg/day. The renal hormone $1,25(OH)_2$, deficient in CRF, is highly effective in improving Ca reabsorption, raising S_{Ca}, and lowering PTH. It has a very short half-life, so skipped doses leave the patient with no carryover effect. Hypercalcemia from overdose is, however, rapidly reversed; the initial dose is 0.25 μg/da for children > 12 kg (219) (see also Table 52.2, p 872).

Other Vitamins

Vitamin intake derived from conventional diets for healthy children usually is adequate. For infants, supplementation with vitamin D and iron are recommended (218). For children with CRI, dietary intake may be modified by anorexia or by prescription, so vitamin intake is likely to be inadequate (220). Further signs of deficiency point to an increased requirement for pyridoxine (220). For children on dialysis, dietary modification and loss of folate during dialysis may lead to signs of folate depletion (221); a standard multivitamin supplement is therefore recommended (216). The value of vitamin supplements specially designed for patients with CRF relative to less expensive daily supplements has not been tested.

Trace Minerals

The trace mineral content of food is variable; the food preparation techniques (e.g., soaking or boiling vegetables) that are often recommended for patients with CRF may lower the trace mineral levels even more. Fe deficiency may occur because of low Fe intake or losses from covert bleeding or blood loss related to hemodialysis or laboratory studies. On the other hand, anemia from other causes is common, and Fe overload is a potential complication of long-standing CRF and dialysis therapy. Serum ferritin is the best means for detecting Fe deficiency and for determining the need for therapeutic doses of Fe (222).

Zn deficiency is difficult to assay in patients with CRF; however, as with iron, dietary restrictions and losses of Zn from blood loss may lead to deficiency. Assaying plasma, red cells, or hair for Zn is not a certain measure of Zn status (223). Results from controlled studies suggest a prevalence of Zn deficiency, but clinical guidelines for its use are not well developed.

Cu deficiency may develop in patients with CRF, and supplementation is sometimes recommended. Special trace mineral supplements have been given, but the benefits have not been documented.

PROGNOSIS AND PROSPECTS

The irreversible loss of renal mass, as demonstrated by imaging or biopsy associated with an elevation of S_{Cr} to levels outside normal, indicates substantial loss of functional capacity. This loss may foretell further loss secondary to dietary and other adaptive responses. Currently there is great interest in determining how diet modification or drug therapy can slow or arrest the rate of loss of residual function (224). Diet modification and drug therapy are thought to be most compelling early in CRI. Factors affecting growth of children also are important early in CRI (163). By contrast, the metabolic disturbances attributed to CRF occur late, when residual function is <30% and functional reserve is less. In this period, therapeutic measures are directed to restoring the patient to a better functional state and forestalling the development of complications associated with CRF i.e. uremia. Although these measures may also arrest disease progression, it is less likely.

For children, arresting progression and improving growth through early intervention are sometimes possible and will become more so. Whenever practical new interventions develop which might realize these goals, they should be subjected to appropriate controlled trials to avoid the risk of negative outcomes (225).

The prognosis of children with end-stage renal disease is slowly improving. Dialysis therapy (Chapter 50) and renal transplantation (Chapter 51) are slowly improving prospects for children treated by these methods. Nonetheless, long-term projections are not encouraging; in children with growth retardation the prognosis remains especially poor. Early detection and treatment of CRI, if proven effective, should assure better growth and development and forestall or avert the development of end-stage renal disease.

References

1. Holliday MA: Management of the child with renal insufficiency. In Lieberman E. (ed): Clinical Pediatric Nephrology Philadelphia, Lippincott, 1976.
2. Brenner BM, Meyer TW, Hostetter TH: Dietary protein intake and the progressive nature of kidney disease: the role of hemodynamically mediated glomerular injury in the pathogenesis of progresive glomerular sclerosis in aging, renal ablation, and intrinsic renal disease. N Engl J Med 307:652, 1982.
3. Haut LL, Alfrey AC, Suggenheim S, et al: Renal toxicity of phosphate in rats. Kidney Int 17:722, 1980.
4. Rizzoni G, Basso T, Setari M: Growth in children with chronic renal failure on conservative treatment. Kidney Int 26, 52, 1984.
5. Meadow SR, Cameron JS, Ogg CS: Regional service for acute and chronic dialysis of children. Lancet 2:707, 1970.
6. Potter D, Belzer FO, Rames L, et al: Treatment of chronic uremia in childhood: transplantation. Pediatrics 45:432, 1970.
7. Scharer K: Incidence and causes of chronic renal failure in childhood. Proc Eur Dial Transpl Assoc 8:211, 1971.
8. Leumann EP: Die chronische niereninsuffizienz im Kindesalter. Schweiz Med Wschr 106:244, 1976.
9. Broyer M, Donckerwolcke RA, Brunner FP, et al: Combined report on regular dialysis and transplantation of children in Europe 1980. Proc Eur Dial Transpl Assoc 18:60, 1981.
10. Habib R, Broyer M, Benmaiz H: Chronic renal failure in children. Nephron 11:209, 1973.
11. Chantler C, Carter JR, Bewick M, et al: Ten years experience with chronic hemodialysis and renal transplantation in children. Arch Dis Child 55:435, 1980.
12. Taube DH, Winder EA, Ogg CS, et al: Successful treatment of middle aged and elderly patients with end stage renal disease. Br Med J 286:2018, 1983.
13. Rizzoni G, Broyer M, Brunner FP, et al: Combined report on dialysis and transplantation of children in Europe, XIII, 1983. Proc EDTA 21:91, 1985.
14. Relman AS: Treatment of end stage renal disease—free but not equal. N Engl J Med 303:996, 1980.
15. Wing AJ: Why don't the British treat more patients with kidney failure. Br Med J 287:1157, 1983.
16. Donckerwalcke RA, Broyer M, Brunner FP, et al: Combined report on regular dialysis and transplantation in children in Europe, XI, 1981. Proc Eur Dial Transpl Assoc 19:61, 1982.
17. Holliday MA: Protein intake, renal function and growth in renal failure. In Mitch WE, Brenner BM, Stein J (eds): The Progressive Nature of Renal Disease: Contemporary Issues in Nephrology New York: Churchill, Livingston, 1985, p 245.
18. Kaufman JM, DiMeola HJ, Siegel NJ, et al: Compensatory adaptation of structure and function following progressive renal ablation. Kidney Int 6:10, 1974.
19. Kramp RA, MacDowell M, Gottschalk CW, et al: A study by microdissection and micropuncture of the structure and function of the kidneys and the nephrons of rats with chronic renal damage. Kidney Int 5:147, 1974.
20. Hakim RM, Goldszer RC, Brenner BM: Hypertension and proteinuria: Long-term sequelae of uninephrectomy in humans. Kidney Int 25:930, 1984.
21. Coburn JW, Slatapolsky E: Vitamin D, parathyroid hormone and renal osteodystrophy. In Brenner BM, Rector FC, (eds): The Kidney. Philadelphia, WB Saunders, 1981.
22. Betts PR, Magrath G: Growth pattern and dietary intake of children with chronic renal insufficiency. Br Med J 2:189, 1974.
23. Walser M: Conservative management of the uremic patient. In Brenner BM, Rector RC, (eds): The Kidney. Philadelphia, WB Saunders, 1981.
24. Schreiner GE, Maher JF: p. 15, In Uremia: Biochemistry Pathogenesis and Treatment. Springfield, IL, Charles C Thomas, 1963.
25. Hayslett JP: Functional adaptation to reduction in renal mass. Physiol Rev 59:137, 1979.
26. Peters G: Compensatory adaptation of renal function in the unanesthetized rat. Am J Physiol 205:1042, 1963.
27. Potter DE, Leumann EP, Sakai T, et al: Early responses of glomerular filtration rate to unilateral nephrectomy. Kidney Int 5:131, 1974.
28. Toback FG, Smith PD, Lowensteen LM: Phospholipid metabolism in the initiation of renal compensatory growth after acute reduction in mass. J Clin Invest 54:91, 1974.
29. Hayslett JP, Kashgarian M, Epstein FH: Functional correlates of compensatory renal hypertrophy. J Clin Invest 47:774, 1968.
30. Pabico, RC, McKenna BA, Freeman RB: Renal function before and after unilateral nephrectomy in renal donors. Kidney Int 8:166, 1975.
31. Ogden DA: Donor and recipient function 2–4 years after renal homotransplantation. A paired study of 28 cases. Ann Intern Med 67:998, 1976.
32. Hostetter TH, Olson JL, Rennke HG, et al: Hyperfiltration in remnant nephrons: a potentially adverse response to renal ablation. Am J Physiol 241:F85, 1981.
33. Maddox DA, Bennet CM, Deen WM, et al: Determination of glomerular filtration rate in experimental glomerulonephritis in the rat. J Clin Invest 55:305, 1975.
34. Friedman S, Strober S, Field EH, et al: Glomerular capillary wall function in human lupus nephritis. Am J Physiol 246:F-580, 1984.
35. Shemesh O, Golbetz H, Kriss JP, Myers BD: Limitations of creatinine as a filtration marker in glomerulopathic patients. Kidney Int 28:830, 1985.
36. Clayton BE, Jenkins P, Round JM: Paediatric Chemical Pathology. Oxford, Blackwell Scientific Publications, 1980, p 60.
37. Bosch JP, Saccagge A, Lauer A, et al: Renal functional reserve in humans: effect of protein intake of glomerular filtration rate. Am J Med 75:943, 1983.
38. Bosch JP, Lauer A, Glabman S: Short-term protein loading in assessment of patients with renal disease. Am J Med 77:873, 1984.
39. Rodriguez-Iturbe B, Herrera J, Garvia R: Response to acute protein load in kidney donors and in apparently normal postacute glomerulonephritis patients: evidence for glomerular hyperfiltration. Lancet 2:461, 1985.
40. Ibels LS, Alfrey AC, Haut L, et al: Preservation of function in experimental renal disease by dietary restriction of phosphate. N Engl J Med 298:122, 1978.
41. Kaslinsky ML, Haut L, Buddington B, et al: Preservation of renal function in experimental glomerulonephritis. Kidney Int 17:293, 1980.
42. Alfrey AC: Prevention of renal failure in experimental renal disease. Am J Kidney Dis 1:315, 1981.
43. Barsotti G, Morelli E, Gianoni A, et al: Restricted phosphorus and nitrogen intake to slow the progression of renal failure: a controlled trial. Kidney Int 24 (suppl 16): S-278, 1983.
44. Mitch WE, Walser M, Stein TI, et al: The effect of a keto acid-amino acid supplement to a restricted diet on the progression of chronic renal failure. N Engl J Med 311:623, 1984.
45. Maschio G, Oldrizzi L, Tessitore N, et al: Effects of dietary protein and phosphorus restruction on the progression of early renal failure. Kidney Int 22:371, 1981.
46. Rosman JB, Meijer S, Sluiter WJ, terWee PM, et al: Prospective randomised trial of early dietary protein restriction in chronic renal failure. The Lancet 2:1291, 1984.
47. Rosman JB, Stinter WJ, Donker Ab JM: Dietary protein restriction in chronic renal failure (letter). Lancet 1:465, 1985.
48. Purkerson ML, Hofsten PE, Klahr S: Pathogenesis of the glomerulopathy associated with renal infarction in rats. Kidney Int 9:407, 1976.
49. Anderson S, Meyer TW, Rennke HG, et al: Control of glomerular hypertension limits glomerular injury in rats with reduced renal mass. J Clin Invest 76:612, 1985.
50. Purkerson ML, Valdes A, Yates J, et al: Inhibition of thromboxane synthesis ameliorates the progressive kidney disease of rats with subtotal renal ablation. Proc Nat Acad Sci 82:193, 1985.
51. Kaufman JM, Siegel NJ, Hayslett JP: Functional and hemodynamic adaptation to progressive renal ablation. Circ Res 36:286, 1975.
52. Oliver J: Architecture of the Kidney in Chronic Bright's Disease. New York, Hoeber, 1939.
53. Ichikawa I, Hoyer JR, Seiler MW, et al: Mechanism of glomerulotubular balance in the setting of heterogeneous glomerular injury. Preservation of a close functional linkage between individual nephrons and surrounding vasculature. J Clin Invest 69:185, 1982.
54. Katz AI, Epstein FH: The role of sodium-potassium activated adenosine triphosphatase in the reabsorption of sodium by the kidney. J Clin Invest 46:1999, 1967.
55. MacLean A, Hayslett JP: Adaptive changes to ammonia excretion after reduction of nephron population. Am Soc Nephrol 10:77A, 1977.
56. Finkelstein FO, Hayslett JP: Role of medullary structures in the functional adaptation of renal insufficiency. Kidney Int 6:419, 1974.
57. Talbot NB, Richie RH, Crawford JD: Metabolic Homeostasis: a Syllabus for Those Concerned with the Care of Patients. Cambridge, MA, Harvard University Press, 1959.
58. Slatapolsky E, Elkan IO, Weerts C, et al: Studies on the characterization of the control system governing sodium excretion in uremic man. J Clin Invest 47:521, 1968.
59. Nickel JF, Lowrance PB, Leiffer, et al: Renal function, electrolyte excretion and body fluids in patients with chronic renal insufficiency before and after sodium deprivation. J Clin Invest 32:68, 1953.
60. Danovitch GM, Bourgoiguie J, Bricker NS: Reversibility of the "salt-losing" tendency of chronic renal failure. N Engl J Med 296:14, 1977.
61. Davis JO, Freeman RH: Mechanisms regulating renin release. Physiol Rev 56:1, 1976.
62. Silva P, Hayslett JP, Epstein FH: The role of Na-K activated adenosine triphosphatase in potassium adaptation. J Clin Invest 52:2665, 1973.
63. Laragh JH: Atrial natriuretic hormone, the renin-aldosterone axis and blood pressure-electrolyte homeostasis. N Engl J Med 313:1330, 1985.
64. Rascher W, Tulassay T, Lang RE: Atrial natriuretic peptide in plasma of volume overloaded children in chronic renal failure. Lancet 2:303, 1985.

65. Knockel JP, Selden DW: The pathophysiology of uremia. In Brenner BM, Rector FC (eds): The Kidney. Philadelphia, WB Saunders, 1981, p 2150.
66. Raine DN, Roy J: A salt-losing syndrome in infancy. Arch Dis Child 37:548, 1962.
67. Schambelin M, Sebastian A, Biglieri EG: Prevalence, pathogenesis, and functional significance of aldosterone deficiency in hyperkalemic patients with chronic renal insufficiency. Kidney Int 17:89, 1980.
68. Rodriguez-Soriana J, Arant BS, et al: Fluid and electrolyte imbalances in children with chronic renal failure. Am J Kidney Dis 7:268, 1986.
69. Schon DA, Silva AP, Hayslett JP: Mechanism of potassium excretion in renal insufficiency. Am J Physiol 227:1323, 1974.
70. Williams GH, Bailey G, Hampers CL, et al: Studies on the metabolism of aldosterone in chronic renal failure and anephric man. Kidney Int 4:280, 1973.
71. Mitra S, Genuth SM, Berman LB: Aldosterone secretion in anephric patients. N Engl J Med 286:61, 1972.
72. Corval P, Bertagna X, Bedrossian J: Increased steroid metabolic clearance rate in anephric patients. Acta Endocrinol 75:756, 1974.
73. Abitbol CL, Holliday MA: Total parenteral nutrition in anuric children. Clin Nephrol 5:153, 1976.
74. Schwartz WB, Hall PW III, Hayes RM, et al: On the mechanism of acidosis in chronic renal disease. J Clin Invest 38:39, 1959.
75. Simpson DP: Control of hydrogen ion homeostasis and renal acidosis. Medicine 50:503, 1971.
76. Muldowney FF, Carroll D, Donohoe JF, et al: Correction of renal bicarbonate wasting by parathyroidectomy. Q J Med 40:487, 1971.
77. Litzow JR, Lemann J Jr, Lennon EJ: The effect of treatment of acidosis on calcium balance in patients with chronic azotemia renal disease. J Clin Invest 46:280, 1967.
78. Kleeman CR, Hewitt WL, Guze LB: Pyelonephritis. Medicine 39:3, 1960.
79. Fine LG, Schlondorff D, Trizna W, et al: Functional profile of the isolated uremic nephron. J Clin Invest 52:1519, 1978.
80. Holliday MA, Egan TJ, Morris RC, et al: Pitressin-resistant hyposthenuria in chronic renal disease. Am J Med 42:378, 1967.
81. Slatopolsky E, Bricker NS: The role of phosphorus restriction in the prevention of secondary hyperparathyroidism in chronic renal disease. Kidney Int 4:141, 1973.
82. Mak RHK, Turner C, Thompson T, et al: Suppression of secondary hyperparathyroidism in children with chronic renal failure by high dose phosphate binders $CaCO_3$ vs $Al(OH)_3$. Br Med J 291:623, 1985.
83. Portale AA, Booth BE, Halloran BP, et al: Effect of dietary phosphorus on circulating concentrations of 1,25 dihydroxyvitamin D and immunoreactive parathyroid hormone in children with moderate renal insufficiency. J Clin Invest 73:1580, 1984.
84. Slatapolsky E, Cagler S, Pennell JP, et al: On the Pathogenesis of hyperparathyroidism in chronic experimental renal insufficiency in the dog. J Clin Invest 50:492, 1971.
85. Platt R: Structural and functional adaptation in renal failure. Br Med J 1:1313, 1952.
86. Lavender S, Hilton PJ, Jones NF: The measurement of glomerular filtration rate in renal disease. Lancet 2:1216, 1969.
87. Smith HW: Excretion of urea. In The Kidney. New York, Oxford University Press, 1951, p 78.
88. Jones JD, Burnett PD: Creatinine metabolism in humans with decreased renal function. Clin Chem 30:1204, 1974.
89. Rutherford WE, Blondin J, Miller JP, et al: Chronic progressive renal disease: Rate of change of serum creatinine concentration. Kidney Int 11:62, 1977.
90. Leumann EP: Progression of renal insufficiency in pediatric patients: estimation from serum creatinine. Helvet Paediatr Acta 33:35, 1978.
91. Counahan R, Chantler C, Ghazali S, et al: Estimation of glomerular filtration rate from plasma creatinine concentration in children. Arch Dis Child 51:875, 1976.
92. Barratt TM, Chantler C, Lederman S, et al: Assessment of renal function. Am J Kidney Dis 7:347, 1986.
93. Dunn MJ: Renal Endocrinology. Baltimore, Williams & Wilkins, 1983.
94. Portale AA, Booth BE, Tsai HC, et al: Reduced plasma concentration of $1,25(OH)_2D$ in children with moderate renal insufficiency. Kidney Int 21:627, 1982.
95. Emmanouel D, Lindeimer MD, Katz AI: Pathogenesis of endocrine abnormalities in uremia. Endoc Rev 1:28, 1980.
96. Emmanoeuel DS, Katz AI, Lindheimer MD: Renal catabolism of hormones. In Dunn MJ (ed): Renal Endocrinology. Baltimore, Williams and Wilkins, 1983, Chapter 14.
97. Affarah HB, Chawla RK, Bleier JC, et al: The loss of renal enzymes: a risk factor for nutritional and metabolic disorders. In Cummings NB, Klahr S (eds): Chronic Renal Disease New York and London, Plenum Medical Book, 1985, Chapter 56.
98. Arnold WC, Danford D, Holliday MA: Effects of calorie supplementation on growth in children with uremia. Kidney Int 24:205, 1983.
99. Adelman RD, Holliday MA: Oxygen consumption in the azotemic rat. Am J Clin Nutr 30:565, 1977.
100. Mehls O, Ritz E, Gilli G, et al: Nitrogen metabolism and growth in experimental uremia. Intl J Pediatr Nephrol 1:34, 1980.
101. Brautbar N: Skeletal myopathy in uraemia: abnormal energy metabolism. Kidney Int 24:S81, 1983.
102. Glaze RP, Morgan JM, Morgan RE: Uncoupling of oxidative phosphorylation by ultrafiltrates or uremic serum. Proc Soc Exper Biol Med 12:172, 1967.
103. Russell JE, Avioli LV: The effect of chronic uremia on intestinal mitochondrial activity. J Lab Clin Med 84:317, 1974.
104. DeFronzo RA, Andres R, Edgar P, et al: Carbohydrate metabolism in uremia: a review. Medicine 52:469, 1973.
105. DeFronzo RA, Smith D, Alvestrand A: Insulin action in uremia. Kidney Int 124:S102, 1983.
106. Westervelt FB: Insulin effect in uremia. J Lab Clin Med 74:79, 1969.
107. Mak RHK, Haycock G, Thompson T, et al: The role of secondary hyperparathyroidism in the glucose intolerance of chronic renal failure. J Clin Endocrinol Metab 60:229, 1985.
108. Turner C, Mak R, Thompson T, et al: Hormonal changes after short term low protein diet with ketoacid supplements in adolescents with chronic renal failure. Williamsburg, VA, Proceedings 4th International Congress in Nutrition and Metabolism in Renal Disease, 1985, p. 75.
109. Delmey JA, Rutherford WE, Klahr S, et al: Studies on the role of the liver and splanchnic tissues in the production of carbohydrate intolerance in uremia. Metabolism 30:658, 1981.
110. Garber AJ: Skeletal muscle protein and amino acid metabolism in experimental chronic uremia in the rat. J Clin Invest 62:623, 1978.
111. Powell D, Holliday MA: Effects of insulin on hemicorpus preparations from normal and uremic rats (abstract). Kidney Int 23:218, 1983.
112. Deferrari G, Garibotto G, Robando C, et al: Glucose interorgan exchange in chronic renal failure. Kidney Int 24:S115, 1983.
113. Guarnieri G, Togo G, deMarchi S, et al: Muscle hexokinase and phosphofructokinase activity in chronically uremic patients. In Giordano C, Friedman EA (eds): Uremia Milano, Wichtig, 1981, p 278.
114. Dzurik R, Hupkova V, Cernacek P, et al: The isolation of an inhibitor of glucose utilization from the serum of uremic subjects. Clin Chim Acta 46:77, 1973.
115. Sanfelippo ML, Swenson AS, Reaven GM: Response of plasma triglycerides to dietary changes in patients on hemodialysis. Kidney Int 14:180, 1978.
116. Roth DA, Meade RC, Barboriah JJ: Glucose insulin and free fatty acids in uremia. Diabetes 22:111, 1973.
117. El Bishti M, Counahan R, Bloom SR, et al: Hormonal and metabolic responses to intravenous glucose in children on regular haemodialysis. Am J Clin Nutr 31:1865, 1978.
118. Chantler C, El Bishti M, Counahan R: Nutritional therapy in children with chronic renal failure. Am J Clin Nutr 33:1682, 1980.
119. Conley SB, Brewer ED, Gandy S, et al: Chronic continuous peritoneal dialysis in very small children with end stage renal disease: achievement of normal growth rates. Clin Res 29:903A, 1981.
120. Giovannetti S, Maggiore O: A low nitrogen diet with proteins of high biological value for severe chronic uraemia. Lancet 1:1000, 1964.
121. Powell D, Bergstrom J, Dzurik R, et al: Toxins and inhibitors in chronic renal failure. Am J Kidney Dis 7:292, 1986.
122. Horowitz HI, Stein DM, Cohen BD: Further studies on the platelet-inhibitory effect of guanidinosuccinic acid and its role in uremic bleeding. Am J Med 49:336, 1970.
123. Radke HW, Rege AB, leMarche MB, et al: Identification of spermine as an inhibitor of erythropoiesis in patients with chronic renal failure. J Clin Invest 67:1623, 1981.
124. Gulyassy PF, Depner TA: Imparied binding of drugs and exogenous ligands in renal diseases. Am J Kidney Dis 11:578, 1983.
125. Phillips LS, Fusco AC, Unterman TG, et al: Somatomedin inhibitor in uremia. J Clin Endocrinol Metab 59:764, 1984.
126. Maloff BL, McCaleb ML, Lockwood DH: Cellular basis of insulin resistance in chronic uremia. Am J Physiol 245:E178, 1983.
127. McCaleb ML, Izzo MS, Lockwood DH: Characterization and partial purification of a factor from uremic serum that induces insulin resistance. J Clin Invest 75:391, 1985.
128. Ericsson F, Carlmark B: Potassium in whole body, skeletal muscle and erythrocytes in chronic renal failure. Nephron 33:173, 1983.
129. Jones RWA, Rigden SP, Barratt TM, et al: The effects of uremic renal failure in infancy on growth, nutritional status and body composition. Pediatr Res 16:784, 1982.
130. Harvey KB, Blumenkrantz MJ, Levine SE, et al: Nutritional assessment and treatment of chronic renal failure. Am J Clin Nutr 33:1586, 1980.
131. Wassner SJ, Bergstrom J, Bruselow SW, et al: Protein metabolism in renal failure: abnormalities and possible mechanism. Am J Kidney Dis 7:285, 1986.
132. Holliday MA, Chantler C, MacDonnell R, et al: Effect of uremia on nutritionally-induced variations in protein metabolism. Kidney Int 11:236, 1977.
133. Li JB, Wassner SJ: Protein synthesis and degradation in skeletal muscle of chronic uremic rats. Kidney Int 29:1136, 1986.
134. Harter HR, Karl IE, Klahr S, et al: Effects of reduced renal mass and dietary protein

intake on amino acid release and glucose uptake by rat muscle in vitro. J Clin Invest 64:513, 1979.
135. Arnold WC, Holliday MA: Tissue resistance to insulin stimulation of amino acid uptake in acutely uremic rats. Kidney Int 16:124, 1979.
136. Counahan R, El-Bishti M, Chantler C: Oral essential amino acids in children on regular hemodialysis. Clin Nephrol 9:11, 1978.
137. Delaporte C, Jean G, Broyer M: Free plasma and muscle amino acids in uremic children. Am J Clin Nutr 31:1647, 1978.
138. Jones RWA, Dalton N, Turner C, et al: Oral essential amino and ketoacid supplements in children with advanced chronic renal failure. Kidney Int 24:95, 1983.
139. Walser M: Therapeutic aspects of branched-chain amino and keto acids. Clin Sci 66:1, 1984.
140. Dalton RN, Chantler C: Relationship between branched-chain amino and alpha-keto acids in blood in uraemia. Kidney Int 16:S61, 1983.
141. Chantler C, Jones RWA, Dalton N: Amino acid and protein metabolism in chronic renal failure. In Gruskin AB, Norman WE (eds): Developments in Nephrology—3. Paediatric Nephrology. Proc. 5th International Paediatric Nephrology Symposium 1980. Boston: Martinas Nijhoff, 1981, p 310.
142. Buse MG, Reid SS: Leucine a possible regulator of protein turnover in muscle. J Clin Invest 58:1251, 1975.
143. Alvestrand A, Bergstrom S, Furst P, et al: The effect of oral essential amino acid supplementation on muscle and plasma amino acids in chronic uremia. Kidney Int 14:323, 1978.
144. Alvestrand A, Furst P, Bergstrom J: Plasma and muscle free amino acids in uremia: influence of nutrition with amino acids. Clin Nephrol 18:297, 1982.
145. Alvestrand A, Ahlberg M, Furst P, et al: Clinical results of long-term treatment with a low protein diet and a new amino acid preparation in patients with chronic uremia. Clin Nephrol 19:67, 1983.
146. MacLean WC, Placko RP, Graham GG: Postprandial plasma free amino acid changes in preschool children consuming exclusively rice protein. J Nutr 109:1285, 1979.
147. Powell DR, Speigel N, Harrah J, Holliday MA: Effect of valine and tyrosine supplements on growth of rats with renal failure. Kidney Int 27:249, 1985.
148. Kopple JD, Coburn JW: Metabolic studies of low protein diets in uremia. I. Nitrogen and potassium. Medicine 52:583, 1973.
149. Hyne BEB, Powell E, Lee HA: The effect of calorie intake on nitrogen balance in chronic renal failure. Clin Sci 43:679, 1974.
150. Mitch WE, Abras E, Walser M: Long-term effects of a new ketoacid-amino acid supplement in patients with chronic renal failure. Kidney Int 22:48, 1982.
151. Abras E, Walser M: Nitrogen utilization in uremia patients fed by continuous nasogastric infusion. Kidney Int 22:392, 1982.
152. Alvestrand A, Ahlberg M, Bergstrom J: Retardation of the progression of renal insufficiency in patients treated with low protein diets. Kidney Int 24:S268, 1983.
153. Mitch WE, Walser M, Stein TI, et al: The effect of a keto acid-amino acid supplement to a restricted diet on the progression of chronic renal failure. N Engl J Med 311:623, 1984.
154. Goodhart JF: Two clinical lectures on albuminuria. Br Med J 1:1183, 1890.
155. West CD, Smith WC: An attempt to elucidate the cause of growth retardation in renal disease. Am J Dis Child 91:460, 1956.
156. Bergstrom WH, DeLeon AS, Van Gemund JJ: Growth observations in renal disease. Pediatr Clin North Am 11:563, 1964.
157. Stickler GB, Bergen BJ: A review: short stature in renal disease. Pediatr Res 7:978, 1973.
158. Betts PR, Magrath G: Growth pattern and dietary intake of children with chronic renal insufficiency. Br Med J 2:189, 1974.
159. Scharer K, Chantler C, Brunner FO, et al: Combined report on regular dialysis and transplantation of children in Europe 1975. Proc Euro Dial Transpl Assoc 13:59, 1976.
160. Potter DE, Griefer I: Statural growth of children with renal disease. Kidney Int 14:334, 1978.
161. Chantler C, Broyer M, Donckerwolcke RA, et al: Growth and rehabilitation of long survivors of treatment for end stage renal failure in childhood. Proc Euro Dial Transpl Assoc 18:329, 1981, vol 18.
162. Kleinknecht C, Broyer M, Huit D, et al: Growth and development of non-dialyzed children with chronic renal failure. Kidney Int 24(suppl 15):40, 1983.
163. Rizzoni G, Broyer M, Guest C, et al: Growth retardation in children with chronic renal disease: scope of the problem. Am J Kidney Dis 8:256, 1986.
164. Barrett TM, Broyer M, Chantler C, et al: Assessment of growth. Am J Kidney Dis 8:340, 1986.
165. Bosque M, Munian A, Bewick M, et al: Growth after renal transplants. Arch Dis Child 58:110, 1983.
166. Broyer M, Kleinknecht C, Loirat C, et al: Maturation osseuse et developpement pubertaire chez l'enfant et l'adolescent en dialyse chronique. Proc Euro Dial Transpl Assoc 9:181, 1972.
167. Betts PR, White RHR: Growth potential and skeletal maturity in children with chronic renal insufficiency. Nephron 16:325, 1976.
168. Donckerwolcke RA, Chantler C, Brunner FP, et al: Combined report on regular dialysis and transplantation of children in Europe 1977. Proc Euro Dial Transpl Assoc 15:77, 1978.
169. Broyer M, Kleinknecht C, Loirat C, et al: Growth in children treated with long term hemodialysis. J Pediatr 84:642, 1974.
170. Pennisi AJ, Costin G, Phillips LS, et al: Linear growth in long term renal allograft recipients. Clin Nephrol 8:415, 1977.
171. Lewy JE, New MI: Growth in children with renal failure. Am J Med 58:65, 1975.
172. Ingelfinger JR, Grupe WE, Harmon WE, et al: Growth in acceleration following renal transplantation in children less than 7 years of age. Pediatrics 68:255, 1981.
173. Fine RN, Malekzadeh MH, Pennisi AJ, et al: Long term results of renal transplantation in children. Pediatrics 61:641, 1978.
174. Lilly JR, Giles G, Hurwitz R, et al: Renal homotransplantation in pediatric patients. Pediatrics 47:548, 1971.
175. Chantler C: Renal failure in childhood. In Black D, Jones NF (eds): Renal Disease ed 4. Oxford, Blackwell, 1979, p 825.
176. Broyer M, Donckerwolcke RA, Brunner FP, et al: Combined report on regular dialysis and transplantation of children in Europe 1980. Proc Euro Dial Transpl Assoc 18:60, 1981.
177. Chantler C, Holliday MA: Growth in children with renal disease with particular reference to the effects of calorie malnutrition, a review. Clin Nephrol 1:230, 1973.
178. Nash MA, Torrado AD, Greifer I, et al: Renal tubular acidosis in infants and children. J Pediatr 80:738, 1972.
179. Hillman DA, Neyzi O, Porter P, et al: Renal (vasopressin resistant) diabetes insipidus. Pediatrics 21:430, 1958.
180. Glorieux FH, Scriver CR, Reade TM, et al: Prevention of dwarfism and rickets in X-linked hypophosphatemia. N Engl J Med 287:481, 1972.
181. Chesney RW, Moorthy AV, Eisman JA, et al: Increased growth after long term oral 1-alpha-25 vitamin D in childhood renal osteodystrophy. N Engl J Med 298:238, 1978.
182. Haycock GB, Al-Dahhan J, Mak RHF, et al: Effect of indomethacin on clinical progress and renal function in cystinosis. Arch Dis Child 57:934, 1982.
183. Brook CGD, Thompson EN, Marshall WC, et al: Growth in children with thalassemia major and effect of two different transfusion regimes. Arch Dis Child 44:612, 1969.
184. Caliguiri LA, Shapiro AP, Holliday MA: Clinical improvement in chronic renal hypertension in children. Pediatrics 31:758, 1963.
185. Dent CE, Harper C, Philpot CR: Treatment of renal glomerular osteodystrophy. Q J Med 30:1, 1961.
186. Mak RHK, Turner C, Powell H, et al: Reversal and prevention of secondary hyperparathyroidism in children with chronic renal failure. Int J Pediatr Nephrol 3:131, 1982.
187. Balsan S, Gueris J, Levy D, et al: Suppressive effect of 1-alpha-hydroxyvitamin D^3 on the hyperparathyroidism of children on maintenance hemodialysis. Metab Bone Dis Pediatr Res 1:15, 1978.
188. Betts PR, MacGrath G, White RHR: Role of dietary energy supplementation on growth of children with chronic renal failure. Br Med J 1:773, 1977.
189. Khan A, Herndon M, Ahmadian S: Social and emotional adaptations of children with transplanted kidneys and chronic hemodialysis. Am J Psychiatr 127:114, 1971.
190. Korsch BM, Fine RN, Gruskin CM et al: Experiences with children and their families during extended hemodialysis and kidney transplantation. Med Clin North Am 18:625, 1971.
191. Rambault G: Psychological aspects of chronic renal failure and hemodialysis. Nephron 11:252, 1973.
192. Wolters WHG, Bonekamp ALM, Donckerwolcke R: Experiences in the development of a hemodialysis course for children. J Psychosom Res 17:271, 1973.
193. Wass VJ, Barralt TM, Baillod RM, et al: Home dialysis in children. Lancet 1:242, 1977.
194. Korsch BM, Negrete VF, Gardner JE, et al: Kidney transplantation in children: psychosocial followup study on child and family. J Pediatr 83:399, 1973.
195. Osberg JW, Meares GJ, McKee DC, et al: Intellectual functioning in renal failure and chronic dialysis. J Chronic Dis 35:445, 1982.
196. Rasbury WC, Fennell RS, Morris MK: Cognitive functioning of children with end stage renal disease before and after successful transplantation. J Pediatr 102:589, 1983.
197. Crittenden MR, Holliday MA, Piel CF, Potter DE: Intellectual development of children with renal insufficiency and end stage renal disease. Int J Pediatr Nephrol 6:275, 1985.
198. Rotundo A, Nevins TE, Lipton M, et al: Progressive encephalopathy in children with renal failure. Kidney Int 21:586, 1982.
199. Trompeter RS, Polinsky MS, Andreoli SA, Fennell RS: Neurological complications of renal failure. Am J Kidney Dis 8:318, 1986.
200. Schwartz GH, Haycock GM, Edelman CM: A simple estimate of glomerular

filtration rate derived from body length and plasma creatinine. J Pediatr 58:259, 1976.
201. Davies JG, Taylor CM, White RHR, Marshall T: Clinical limitations of the estimation of glomerular filtration rate from height: plasma creatinine ratio: a comparison with simultaneous ^{51}Cr edetic acid slope clearance. Arch Dis Child 57:607, 1982.
202. Morris MC, Allanby CW, Toseland P, et al: Evaluation of a height/plasma creatinine formula in the measurement of glomerular filtration rate. Arch Dis Child 57:611, 1982.
203. Cole BR, Giangiacomo J, Inglefinger J, Robson AM: Measurement of renal function without urine collection. N Engl J Med 287:1109, 1972.
204. Potter DE, Broyer M, Chantler C, et al: Measurement of growth in children with renal insufficiency. Kidney Int 14:378, 1978.
205. Gurney JM, Jelliffe DB: Arm anthropometry in nutritional assessment, nomogram for rapid calculation of muscle circumference and cross sectional muscle and fat areas. Am J Clin Nutr 27:1052, 1974.
206. Frisancho AR: Triceps skinfold and upper arm muscle size norms for assessment of nutritional status. Am J Clin Nutr 27:1052, 1974.
207. Chesney RW, Mazess RB, Rose RG, et al: Bone mineral status measured by direct photon absorptiometry in childhood renal disease. Pediatrics 60:864, 1977.
208. Wallace WM: Nitrogen content of the body and its relation to retention and loss of nitrogen. Fed Proc 18:1125, 1959.
209. Walser M: Determinants of ureagenesis, with particular reference to renal failure. Kidney Int 17:709, 1980.
210. Sapir DG, Stewart PM, Walser M, et al: Effects of alpha ketoisocaproate and of leucine in nitrogen metabolism in postoperative patients. Lancet 1:1010, 1983.
211. National Research Council, Food and Nutrition Board: Recommended Dietary Allowances ed 9. 1980. Washington, DC: National Academy of Sciences.
212. Department of Health and Social Security: Recommended Intakes of Nutrients for the United Kingdom. Reports of the Public Health and Medical Subjects No. 120. London, H.M. Stationary Office, 1969.
213. Brown HE: The evaluation of a new diet for children on hemodialysis. MSC thesis. London, Queen Elizabeth College 1976.
214. Roche AF, Hines JH: Incremental growth charts. Am J Clin Nutr 33:2041, 1980.
215. Tanner JM, Daves PSW: Clinical longitudinal standards for height and height velocity for North American Children. J Pediatr 107:317, 1985.
216. Holliday MA, McHenry-Richardson K, Potale A: Nutritional management of chronic renal disease. Med Clin North Am 63:945, 1979.
217. Rose WC: The amino acid requirements of adult man. Nutr Abstr Rev 27:631, 1957.
218. American Academy of Pediatrics, Committee on Nutrition: Commentary on breast feeding and infant formulas including proposed standards for infant formulas. Pediatrics 57:278, 1976.
219. Dabbagh S, Chesney RW: Treatment of Renal Osteodystrophy During Childhood in End Stage Renal Disease in Children. In Fine R, Gruskin A (eds.). Philadelphia, WB Saunders Co, 1984, p 225.
220. Dobblestein H, Korner WF, Merupel W, et al: Vitamin B6 deficiency in uremia and its implications for the depression of the immune response. Kidney Int 5:233, 1974.
221. Siddiqui J, Freeburger R, Freeman RM: Folic acid hypersegmented polymorphonuclear leukocytes and the uremic syndrome. Am J Clin Nutr 23:11, 1970.
222. Bell JD, Kincaid WR, Morgan RG, et al: Serum ferritin assay and bone marrow iron stores in patients on maintenance hemodialysis. Kidney Int 17:242, 1980.
223. Atkin-Thor E, Goddard BW, O'Nion J, et al: Hypoguesia and zinc depletion in chronic dialysis patients. Am J Clin Nutr 31:1948, 1978.
224. Mitch WE: The progressive nature of renal disease. In Brenner BM, Stein JH (eds): Contemporary Issues in Nephrology. New York, Churchill Livingston 1986, vol 14.
225. Silverman W; Human Experimentation: A Guided Step into the Unknown. Oxford UK, Oxford University Press, 1985.

CHAPTER 50 Dialysis Therapy

50A Hemodialysis

R. A. DONCKERWOLCKE
C. CHANTLER

PHYSIOLOGY

Dialysis therapy is used to control body fluid solute concentration and to regulate body fluid volume. During the process, dissolved particles from one fluid compartment are diffused to another across a semipermeable membrane that permits the passage of water and small molecules; plasma proteins and cells are too large to pass through the pores of the membrane. During dialysis treatment, dissolved particles and water move from the patient to the dialysate or vice versa, depending on the concentration, size, and electric charge of the dissolved particles. The transfer of water is regulated by osmotic pressure and of solute and water and by hydraulic pressure. The technical characteristis of the dialyzer greatly affect solute and water transfer. The technical assessment of dialyzer performance should include data on the rate of solute removal, ultrafiltration characteristics, and the compliance of the blood compartment.

Solute Removal Rate

"Dialysance" describes the function of the artificial kidney and defines the rate of exchange of a substance between blood and dialysate per minute and per unit blood-dialysate concentration gradient (1). The equation for calculating dialysance (1) is:

$$D = \frac{Q_B\ (C_{BI} - C_{BO})}{C_{BI} - C_{DI}} \qquad (1)$$

C = concentration of solute
BI = blood inflow
BO = blood outflow
DI = dialysate inflow
Q_B = blood flow rate (ml/min)

To calculate the solute removal rate of artificial kidneys, using single-pass dialysate systems, the equation can be simplified:

$$D = Q_B\ \frac{(C_{BI} - C_{BO})}{C_{BI}} \qquad (2)$$

The term "clearance" is commonly used to indicate dialyzer solute removal rates because of the similarity of artificial kidney dialysance in the single-pass system (continuous inflow of fresh dialysate) and the clearance concept used for evaluation of the function of the natural kidney.

Alterations in blood and dialysate flow rates affect the clearance of the dialyzer. Dialysate flow is usually fixed at a high rate, at least two times blood flow rates, to obtain a maximum solute concentration gradient. At low blood flow rates, clearance equals the blood flow rate; at higher (>100 ml/min) blood flow rates, clearance depends on dialyzer characteristics. Clearance increases when transmembrane pressure (hydraulic pressure) is raised to increase ultrafiltration of salt and water from the blood compartment. The removal of solute and water by ultrafiltration rather than by diffusion is termed "convection."

The characteristics of the dialyzer affecting solute removal are membrane surface area, membrane permeability, and flow geometry. The rate of movement of the solute from one compartment to another across the dialysis membrane is termed the "mass transfer rate" (1).

$$N = K \sum A\ (\Delta C) \qquad (3)$$

N = mass transfer rate (mol/min)
K = overall mass transfer coefficient (cm/min)
A = membrane area (cm^2)
ΔC = logarithmic mean concentration gradient, blood to fluid (mol/cm^3)

The overall mass transfer coefficient is determined by the sum of the resistances to solute passage through blood, across the membrane, and into the dialysis fluid. The membrane resistance depends on membrane thickness and chemical composition. For cellulose membranes (cellophane, Cuprophan), membrane resistance only slightly affects low-molecular-weight solute transfer rate but is an important barrier to the transfer of middle molecules. Noncellulose membranes, such as polymethylmethacrylate and polyacrylonitrile, have low resistance to solute transfer, particularly for middle molecular solutes, and facilitate ultrafiltration. Therefore, dialyzers with high permeability may be used only with devices to regulate the rate of ultrafiltration. Large surface area dialyzers have higher solute removal rates, in particular for middle molecules.

The geometry of blood and dialysate flow affect the solute concentration gradient and thereby determine mass transfer rate. Large concentration gradients are established using single-pass dialysate flow and countercurrent flow of blood and dialysate.

Ultrafiltration

The rate at which water is removed from the patient during dialysis is related to osmotic pressure and especially to the hydraulic pressure gradient between blood and dialysate. The oncotic pressure difference between blood and dialysate is small (19 to 28 mm Hg) and, therefore, the influence of plasma protein concentration on ultrafiltration may be disregarded. Solutes such as glucose added to the dialysate increase the osmotic pressure gradient and increase ultrafiltration. The difference in hydraulic pressure between blood and dialysate is designated as transmembrane pressure (TMP).

$$TMP = P_B - P_D \quad (4)$$

P_B = average blood compartment pressure
P_D = average dialysate pressure

The blood compartment pressure depends on the blood flow resistance and can be increased by constricting the venous blood line. Using parallel flow dialyzers, the required TMP is obtained by modifications of the dialysate (negative) pressure.

The ultrafiltration rate (UFR) can be calculated from the following equation:

$$UFR\ (ml/hr) = k_{UF} \cdot TMP\ (mm\ Hg) \quad (5)$$

k_{UF} = ultrafiltration constant (ml/mm Hg TMP); it is a characteristic of each dialyzer and is related to membrane hydraulic permeability and membrane surface area.

Blood Circuit

The blood compartment volume of the dialyzer is an important factor in selecting a dialyzer for a patient. The volume of the blood compartment changes with the transmembrane pressure according to the compliance. An increase in volume is associated with a larger cross-sectional area of the blood flow and a decreased diffusion of small molecules. For pediatric dialysis the blood compartment volume should be as small as possible, and compliance should be minimal. During dialysis the extracorporeal blood volume of the dialyzer and blood lines should not exceed 10% of patient's blood volume.

The resistance to blood flow is governed by the viscosity of blood and the geometry of the blood pathway. Dialyzers with a small number of long pathways have high resistance to blood flow. A dialyzer with high internal resistance has a high obligatory ultrafiltration rate.

Blood loss in the dialyzer contributes significantly to anemia and is caused by membrane rupture, clotting in the dialyzer, and retention of blood at the termination of dialysis. The requirements for low extracorporeal blood volume are not always compatible with low internal resistance and minimal residual blood loss in the dialyzer.

Dialyzers

Three types of dialyzers are used: flat plate (disposable and nondisposable), coil, and hollow-fiber dialyzers. The requirements for an ideal hemodialyzer are high clearances for small and middle molecules, negligible loss of vital solutes, adequate ultrafiltration, low residual blood volume, high reliability, nontoxicity, low cost, and potential for reuse (2).

Flat plate dialyzers are assembled in layers and use plates or mesh structures to support the membranes. Blood and dialysate flow in opposite directions. Pediatric versions have low blood volume and compliance. Ultrafiltration is obtained by negative dialysate pressure. These dialyzers have low blood flow resistance.

Coil dialyzers consist of cellulose tubing concentrically wound with a mesh supporting screen around a central core. Several pediatric versions have been made with reduced membrane surface area. They have large blood volume and compliance. Because of high internal blood flow resistance with high ultrafiltration rates, coils are not suitable for dialysis of children.

Hollow-fiber dialyzers consist of hollow fibers with various wall thicknesses. Increasing the number of fibers increases membrane surface area. Several disposable hollow-fiber dialyzers may be used for dialysis in children. They have low internal resistance and predictable ultrafiltration rates. Blood compartment volumes are small and without compliance. Table 50A-1 shows characteristics of disposable hollow fiber and flat plate dialyzers suitable for pediatric dialysis.

Dialysate

The optimum concentration for electrolytes in the dialysate is not known. Matching of the dialysis fluid to the patient's individual needs is desirable. The ideal approach may be to vary the composition of the dialysate throughout each dialysis, allowing progressive and smooth normalization of extracellular fluid (ECF) during dialysis (3). Urea and Na diffusion are the major determinants of changes in osmolality of the ECF during dialysis. The concentration of Na in the dialysate should be chosen to minimize the extent and rate of changes in osmolality.

Low Na^+ concentration in the dialysate increases dialysis side effects, probably because the rapid fall in ECF osmolality is associated with an increase in intracellular fluid volume at the expense of the plasma and ECF volume. High concentrations induce thirst and increase interdialytic weight gain.

Table 50A-1.
Characteristics of disposable pediatric dialyzers

Dialyser	Blood compartment volume (ml)	Compliance (ml/100 mm Hg)	Ultrafiltration coefficient (ml/hr/mm Hg)	Surface area (m^2)	Urea clearance at Q_B of * 50 (ml/min)	75	100	150	200
Gambro mini-minor	20	6	0.50	0.23	30	37	51	—	—
Gambro minor	30	10	1.70	0.41	43	59	67	77	100
RP-6 (all layers)	150	—	—	1.00	—	—	88	109	—
CDAK 0.6	53	0	0.84	0.60	—	50	83	105	118
Asahi 0.3	30	0	1.25	0.30	43	59	73	93	—
Asahi 0.6	55	0	3.00	0.60	49	69	88	100	—

* Data collected with in vivo studies at Q_D = 500 ml/min.

Determination of the K^+ concentration in the dialysate depends on dietary K^+ intake, frequency, and duration of dialysis, and residual renal function. Hyperkalemia is still an important cause of death in children on regular dialysis treatment. Patients with dietary K^+ restriction and appropriate dialysis treatment will have acceptable predialysis K^+ levels (<5.5 mmol/L) when the dialysis fluid contains 1.5 mmol potassium/L.

To avoid variations in the Ca^{++} concentration of the dialysis fluid, pretreatment of the water supply with water softeners, deionizers, or reverse osmosis is required. Patients with end-stage renal disease (ESRD) often are in negative Ca balance, and dialysis will cause additional Ca loss. Raising the calcium concentration of the dialysate to 1.75 mmol/L or more will result in the transfer of calcium from the dialysate to the patient; however, the administration of vitamin D_3 metabolites and oral calcium supplementation is preferred because of the beneficial effect of vitamin D on bone.

A dialysis fluid Ca^{++} concentration of 1.4 to 1.5 mmol/L is recommended. Acetate is frequently used to replace bicarbonate in the dialysate because of the relative insolubility of calcium in bicarbonate solutions. If acetate is reabsorbed from the dialysate at a higher rate than the maximal amount that can be metabolized, toxic effects may occur; acetate retention decreases peripheral vascular resistance and depresses cardiac output, causing blood pressure to fall.

CLINICAL MANAGEMENT OF REGULAR HEMODIALYSIS IN CHILDREN

Hemodialysis is a safe and efficient mode of renal replacement (4) for children with end-stage renal disease. Its successful use requires adapting techniques and equipment to meet the special requirements of children.

The Pediatric Dialysis Center

Special facilities are required to treat children with hemodialysis. Although the basic principles and procedures are the same in adults and children, equipment and methods have to be scaled to the patient's size. Hemodialysis in children requires flexibility in equipment use and treatment strategy. Pediatric patients not only require individualized dialysis treatment but also emotional support appropriate to their age group. Therefore, pediatric units must have a relatively high staff to patient ratio, and the staff should include pediatric nephrologists, nurses experienced in dialysis of children, a dietitian, a hospital school, and a social worker. Pediatric surgery and urology are required along with psychiatry services and the support of a general pediatric unit (5).

Equipment should include a large variation of dialyzers, allowing safe dialysis of children as small as 6 kg and as large as 50 kg. Small children need continuous monitoring with sensitive weight scales, cardiac monitoring, and Doppler blood pressure equipment (6).

Vascular Access. Adequate vascular access for maintenance hemodialysis is essential. The conditions to be fulfilled by an ideal vascular access are (7):

1. Preservation of normal vasculature
2. Least interference with normal physical activities
3. Easy access to puncture that allows adequate blood flow through the dialyzer.
4. Low complication rate
5. Long survival rates

Although external arteriovenous cannulae have been used extensively for chronic dialysis in children, the short life and frequent complications (thrombosis, infections) have limited the use of shunts to acute hemodialysis and to small children, for whom other forms of access are often unavailable. Adult shunt tips placed in proximal vessels (brachial and femoral artery) are preferred for long-term access in children <15 kg body weight. When the femoral artery is used, a segment of the saphenous vein can be anastomosed to the artery and then cannulated, so that arterial integrity is preserved (8). Shunts in proximal vessels lead to high blood flow and increases hemodynamic stress, but shunt survival is considerably better than if pediatric shunt tips are used to construct distal AV shunts.

Temporary vascular access while awaiting maturation of arteriovenous fistulae can be created with a percutaneous indwelling catheter into the subclavian or femoral veins (9). Between dialyses, heparin infusion, using a portable pump, will maintain catheter patency (9). The catheter should be removed after being in place for three to four weeks. Single-needle technique or double-lumen subclavian cannula is used for dialysis (10).

AV fistulae have a low complication rate and are the first choice for vascular access in pediatric patients. The Brescia-Cimino radiocephalic fistulae at the wrist provides ideal vascular access. The side-(artery) to-end (vein) anastomosis should be preferred to the end-to-end anastomosis because of the better flow through the hand when the distal portion of the artery remains patent. In small children, microsurgical techniques allow construction of arteriovenous fistulae (11). A brachial fistula may be performed, but in children whose forearm vessels are unsuitable for arteriovenous anastomosis, complications often occur.

Single-needle technique is often necessary in children because the vein to be punctured is short, but this technique increases the extracorporeal blood volume and reduces the efficiency of dialysis. Saphenous vein autografts, umbilical vein, and polytetrafluoroethylene (PTFE) grafts are efficient alternatives if the forearm vessels are not suitable for fistula creation (12–14). Insertion in the thigh between the superficial femoral artery and proximal saphenous vein will improve graft survival, but the graft should be placed superficially to avoid cannulation problems. Excellent results are obtained in children by using autogenous saphenous vein grafts inserted in a loop configuration in the forearm (12). Saphenous vein grafts placed between brachial artery and cephalic veins are frequently complicated by aneurysmal dilatation, and the patency in small children is poor (11).

Choice of Dialyzer and Blood Lines

The choice of dialyzer in treating children is governed by the blood volume and the clearance characteristics of the dialyzer. The extracorporeal blood volume of the dialyzer and blood lines should at no time exceed 10% of the child's blood volume calculated as 70 ml/kg. For anephric patients the priming volume should be <7% of the patient's blood volume. Calculation of extracorporeal blood volume should take account of compliance during ultrafiltration.

Blood lines with volumes varying between 35 and 75 ml are commonly used. Pediatric blood lines with 3 mm diameter tubing will restrict blood flow to <75 ml/min. If higher blood flows are required, special short blood lines with larger inner diameters reduce extracorporeal blood volume.

Hollow-fiber dialyzers have low blood compartment volumes and no compliance. Multilayer flat plate dialyzers allow a number of blood compartments to be clamped off; thus, size of these dialyzers may be adapted to the size of the patient. To obtain efficient clearances of small molecules like urea and creatinine, a ratio dialyzer surface area to patient surface area of 0.75 has been proposed (5).

Overefficient dialysis can be avoided by restricting the urea clearance to <3 to 4 ml/min/kg. Excessively high solute removal leads to the disequilibrium syndrome, with a rapid decrease in the serum osmolality without an equally fast decrease in intracellular osmolality of the brain, which causes cerebral edema. Symptoms include headache, abdominal pain, nausea, vomiting, muscle cramps, and convulsions (15).

Although blood flow rates must be indivdually determined for each patient, general guidelines may be used, based on patient's weight—uremic young children (<5 yr old) are often malnourished and underweight for height (16). Percentile charts should be used to determine the ideal weight according to body height and build of the child using the formula: Blood flow = 2.5 × Body wt (kg) + 100 for children 10–40 kg. In children who weigh <10 kg, blood flow rates should not exceed 100 ml/min, whereas in children >40 kg blood flow rates up to 250 ml/min can be used.

Excessive interdialytic weight gain from excessive NaCl and water intake is relatively frequent and potentially dangerous in children on regular dialysis. Assessment of dry weight is sometimes difficult.

Ultrafiltration

Ultrafiltration should be planned carefully and continuously monitored. Special devices for regulating ultrafiltration are useful in children. Continuous weight recording is less reliable because weight changes may be caused by food and fluid intake, fluid loss by vomiting, and by shifting of blood into or out of the dialyzer when dialyzer compliance causes changes in extracorporeal blood volume. Ultrafiltration during each dialysis should be <5% of body weight to avoid severe hypotension during dialysis. Hypovolemia, the major cause of hypotension during the dialysis session, and the decrease in plasma osmolality, which induces a water shift from the vascular toward the interstitial and intracellular space, aggravate hypovolemia. Dissociation of dialysis and ultrafiltration allows a much larger degree of weight loss without hypotension in fluid-overloaded children (17). During sequential ultrafiltration and dialysis, a period of ultrafiltration precedes or follows standard dialysis using the same dialyzer. Ultrafiltration is effected by increasing transmembrane pressure generated by a negative pressure across the nonblood side of the dialyzer's membrane or a positive pressure on the blood side of the membrane while the dialysate bypasses the dialyzer. Transmembrane pressure differences up to 500 mm Hg must be used. Although excellent ultrafiltration without serious side effects is obtained by this method, this procedure should be restricted to fluid-overloaded patients and care should be taken not to reduce the required dialysis time for solute removal (18).

Management of Regular Dialysis

Before dialysis begins the procedure should be explained to the child through drawings and by having the child attend a dialysis session of other children. The dialysis should be adjusted to the individual need of the child. These requirements are not only determined by the size of the patient but also by individual variations in dialysis tolerance. Careful observation of the patient and close monitoring of vital signs during the dialysis procedure is necessary. Allocation of a specific nurse to each patient allows accurate observation of the patient's physical and emotional response to treatment. Agitation, color changes, yawning, nausea, and abdominal pain often precede vomiting and hypotension. In small children, blood pressure and weight are measured frequently.

General heparinization can be effected by administration of a bolus of 50 U heparin/kg body weight at the beginning of dialysis, followed by continuous infusion of 50 U heparin/kg/hr. Because of wide variations in heparin requirements, the optimal heparin dosage for each patient should be established by determinations of whole blood activated clotting time during the first three hemodialyses the patient receives.

In small children, weighing <10 kg, the priming fluid of the dialyzer is transfused into the patient at the beginning of the dialysis procedure. In larger children the priming fluid is discharged unless the patient did not gain weight during the interdialytic period. At the end of dialysis the extracorporeal blood is transfused back into the patient. Only small amounts of saline (<50 ml) are used for the dialyzer washback procedure.

The requirement for dialysis is proportional to the metabolic rate because the intake of all nutrients is proportional to metabolic rate. Metabolic rate is proportional to body surface area (BSA), and the BSA of a child is greater in relation to body weight than for an adult. Because of the relatively high need for calories, protein, and fluids related to body weight, the child will accumulate metabolic waste products at a greater rate than adults. Therefore, pediatric patients need more dialysis in relation to their body weight than adults. Children without significant residual kidney function are often dialyzed three times weekly or more.

The duration of dialysis is determined by the time required for adequate fluid and solute removal. Pedatric dialyzers have small ultrafiltration coefficients and, therefore, dialysis times are often determined by fluid removal requirements. In patients with a moderately restricted protein intake (<1.3 g/kg/day), adequate solute removal is achieved with three to five hours' dialysis three times weekly. In Table 50A-2 the proposed combinations of dialysis time, dialyzer size, and blood flow rates according to patient's size are summarized. The importance of correct selection of the dialysis, lines, and time on dialysis cannot be overemphasized. Dialyzers that are too large lead to hypotension on dialysis or hypertension after washback, whereas too small dialyzers cause unnecessarily extended time on dialysis or inadequate dialysis (18a).

To counteract the decrease in serum osmolality during dialysis, the intravenous infusion of mannitol at 1 g/kg/dialysis has been advocated. Although mannitol infusion reduces the osmolality decrease during dialysis, it does not affect the fall of blood pressure during ultrafiltration, but the severity of dialysis-related side effects is reduced (19). Mannitol administration leads to mannitol retention, and the residual mannitol accumulates, reaching a steady-state level within a few dialyses. At this level, an amount equal to that infused will be removed during dialysis, and it will be inefficient to prevent the decrease in osmolality. To avoid accumulation, mannitol should be administered less than once weekly. The effects of mannitol accumulation on the patient are not known (20).

Vascular instability, hypotension, and other side effects of dialysis

Table 50A-2.
Proposed Combinations of Dialysis Time, Dialyzer Size, and Bloodflow Rates According to Patient's Size

Patient				Dialyzer				
Age yr	Weight (kg)	BSA (m^2)	Blood volume ml	S.A. (m^2)	Max extracorporeal blood volume (ml)	Blood flow (ml/min)	Max Cl_{BUN} (ml/min)	Time (hr) dialysis (predialysis urea) 20–10 mmol/l
2	11	0.50	770	0.37	75	125	44	3–5
4	17	0.75	1190	0.56	115	145	68	3–5
9	28	1.00	1960	0.75	190	170	112	3–5
14	43	1.30	3010	0.98	300	190	172	3–5

may be minimized by using bicarbonate rather than acetate dialysate (21, 22). Because bicarbonate dialysate results in more optimal corrections of acid base balance, it may also have long-term patient benefits, with the possibility of better bone mineralization and growth in children.

Modification in composition and flow rate of the dialysate will affect symptoms associated with dialysis. Improved tolerance to hemodialysis can be obtained using 400 mg/dl glucose-enriched dialysate, which reduces the fall in serum osmolality during dialysis (15). These symptoms are also reduced by high sodium dialysis (145 mmol sodium/L); this improvement is due to maintenance of normal plasma sodium and osmolality levels following dialysis (23). Recirculation of the dialysate and low flow single pass (dialysate flow <200 ml/min) will increase tolerance to ultrafiltration and decrease dialysis side effects; however, this will result in a reduced clearance for small molecular weight solutes.

Hypovolemia on dialysis is exacerbated by the failure of vasoconstriction to maintain blood pressure. Fluid removal by ultrafiltration alone is associated with an increase in peripheral vascular resistance (23a). The cause of this difference is not known, but various factors such as acetate toxicity or failure of catecholamine levels to rise and the higher temperature of blood returning to the body after dialysis have been implicated. Hypovolemia with hypotension should be treated with the infusion of 0.9% saline, 20% mannitol, or albumin solutions. It can, however, be avoided if sequential ultrafiltration and dialysis are used, if fluid removal during dialysis is neither too large nor too fast, if solute removal is not excessive, and if the child is monitored carefully so that the earliest symptoms are detected and controlled.

Hypertension in a child with ESRD may be caused by volume overload or excessive vasoconstriction. When the latter is due to excessive renin production, nephrectomy or preferably the administration of the angiotensin-converting enzyme inhibitor captopril may be necessary. Measurement of ECF volume, peripheral perfusion judged from toe temperature, plasma renin concentration, and the response to fluid removal on dialysis help to determine whether the hypertension should be treated with more vigorous dialysis or with captopril (5). Other hypotensive drugs should rarely, if ever, be necessary. β-blockade with propranolol should be avoided because of the interference with the ability of the vascular system to respond to fluid removal during dialysis to maintain cardiac output and blood pressure. If a child on dialysis has congestive cardiac failure, it usually means that the management is inadequate and digoxin should not be prescribed.

Hypertension occurring during dialysis may be associated with volume overload that requires more ultrafiltration or to excessive vasoconstriction that requires a vasodilator such as hydralazine. Clinical examination with attention to the filling pressure in the neck veins and monitoring toe temperature to judge peripheral perfusion enable the correct action to be determined.

The prevention of symptoms and complications during dialysis requires good interdialytic management, avoiding excessive changes in body composition (see p 804) proper equipment and time on dialysis, and careful supervision during the procedure. A child with end-stage renal disease on regular hemodialysis should wish and be able to eat freely during dialysis and to concentrate on school work or other activities. Between dialyses he or she should feel well, have a reasonable appetite, and be active. Good management is essential if these aims are to be achieved.

Assessment of Dialysis Adequacy

A high blood urea nitrogen (BUN) may mean excessive protein intake, inefficient clearance by the dialyzer, or acute illness and catabolism. Usually the first of these can be detected by diet history and confirmed by an estimate of net urea nitrogen production or appearance that, in a stable clinical state, is approximately equal to nitrogen intake (equation 6). The second of these also can be detected by an estimate from pre- and postdialysis BUN and change in weight using the equation for UN removal:

$$(BUN_I - BUN_F \times 0.55 \text{ Body wt} + (BUN_I \times (wt_I - wt_F)) \qquad (6)$$

or the more elaborate equation for urea generation (24).

The presence of an acute catabolic state is usually evident from clinical findings.

Using the kinetic model to estimate protein intake provides a slightly more accurate estimate of dietary protein intake and, hence, "protein catabolic rate." The inaccuracies in any system that attempts to derive nitrogen (N) balance from the difference between estimated N (protein) intake and urea N appearance rate (25) precludes the use of this method in determining the need for changing dietary protein. This decision should be made on clinical signs and laboratory values of albumin and transferrin (see Chapter 11). Poor removal of urea, as determined from the simple equation or from the urea kinetic model, is an indication for a change in dialysis mode. Detecting true catabolic states is only possible from clinical evaluation. It is an unusual occurrence and is associated with infection or injury.

Growth failure may be a symptom of inadequate dialysis; the effect of changing dialysis therapy on growth is a way to assess the effect of the change (26). Symptoms of inadequate dialysis may appear in some patients despite satisfactory urea and urate levels, although the latter have been used to assess adequacy. Urate levels in one study was inversely correlated with growth (27). Middle molecules, a group of substances of molecular weights between 500 to 2000 daltons, accumulate in uremia. The role of these middle molecules in toxicity is poorly documented. Although a relationship with some symptoms of uremia, such as infection, neuropathy, and malnutrition, has been proposed, correlations between the level of middle molecules in plasma and these clinical symptoms have not been established (28).

The middle molecule hypothesis has greatly affected dialysis procedure and stimulated the use of dialyzers that are highly efficient in removing molecules with a molecular weight of 500 to 2000 daltons, but its value remains unmeasured. Babb and coworkers (29) devised a dialysis index to express middle molecule removal during dialysis and by residual renal function. From this, for any patient-dialyzer combination, the required weekly dialysis time, allowing adequate middle molecule removal, can be assessed. For this index, removal rate for middle molecules is estimated by in vitro clearances of vitamin B_{12}; clearances for a solute of molecular weight 1000 and for creatinine are included. Reference is standard Kiil dialysis providing 29.0 l per week of vitamin B_{12} clearance, 31.0 l per week of solutes of molecular weight, 1000, and 77.4 1/week of creatinine clearance (30).

$$D_I = \frac{\text{Prescribed Kd Td} + \text{KrCr} \cdot \text{Twk}}{\text{Kiil reference (SA/1.73 m}^2)} \qquad (7)$$

Kd = dialyzcr clcarancc (ml/min)
Kr = renal clearance (ml/min)
Td = time dialysis/week
Twk = time/week
Cr = creatinine

Despite modification of dialyzers, according to the middle molecule hypothesis, its validity is not established; assessment of dialysis efficiency by the dialysis index alone is inappropriate and it may be of no use.

Nutrition

Dietary management of the child on dialysis is required. Food intake is often reduced by anorexia, which may be caused by altered taste sensation, tension and anxiety, hypertension, or the metabolic abnormalities of chronic renal failure. Whenever possible, these factors should be corrected.

Adequate nutrition should provide sufficient and balanced nutrients without exceeding their restricted tolerance. Despite adequate dialysis, reduced tolerance will require dietary restrictions. The caloric requirements for children on dialysis are unknown. If the energy intake is <80% of the RDA for height, additional energy intake should be provided. Extra energy supplements consisting of fat and carbohydrate are used to increase total energy intake.

Recommended protein intake for adults on hemodialysis is 1 g/kg/day, which is 20% more than the RDA for normal individuals (0.8 g/kg/day). For adults also receiving 35 kcal/kg, the RDA for calories for sedentary individuals, this is 10% to 12% of total calories as protein. Lacking more definitive information on children, the dietary protein calories should be between 10% and 12% of total calories; calorie intake should equal at least 80% of the RDA for calories for that age (see Chapters 10A and 11).

Salt (NaCl) intake of patients on dialysis should be limited so that weight gain between dialyses is not excessive. This usually means limiting Na intake to <1.5 mEq/kg/day, which entails a weight gain of 10 g/kg/day or 20 to 30 g/kg between dialyses if no salt is excreted by residual kidney function. When there are signs of salt-wasting (see Chapter 50), salt supplements are recommended.

For Ca, a net positive balance from dialysis is achieved by having dialysis concentration set at 1.5 to 1.75 mmol/L (6–7 mg/dl). Oral calcium supplements of 20 to 40 mg/kg of elemental Ca also are helpful. These are preferably given as calcium lactate or gluconate. Dietary phosphorus should be limited; this requires skillful menu development, phosphate binders, or both. Restriction should be implemented with a view to maintaining or returning serum parathormone (PTH) levels to normal.

Potassium intake of adult patients on dialysis is recommended to be <100 mmol/day or 1.5 mmol/kg/day. In anephric states this poses a load of 3 to 4.5 mmol/kg between dialyses, much of which is retained in cells.

Treatment of osteodystrophy requires administration of vitamin D products, such as dihydrotachysterol, 1-α- or 1,25 dihydroxycholecalciferol. Inadequate dietary intake and losses during dialysis treatment may result in deficiency of water-soluble vitamins. Daily administration of supplemental B complex, vitamin C, and folic acid is recommended.

Regular assessment of the adequacy of nutrition of the child on dialysis is required. An analysis of dietary intake should be performed monthly through the use of three-day diet histories and checked by calculating net urea nitrogen production or appearance rate.

References

1. Henderson LW: Hemodialysis: rationale and physical principles. In Brenner BM, Rector FC (eds): The Kidney, ed 1. Philadelphia, WB Saunders, 1976.
2. Hoenich NA, Kerr DNS: Dialysers. In Drukker W, Parsons FM, Maher JF (eds): Replacement of Renal Function by Dialysis, ed 2. Boston, Martinus Nijhoff Publishers, 1983.
3. Parsons FM, Stewart WK. The composition of dialysis fluid. In Drukker W, Parsons FM, Maker JF (eds): Replacement of Renal Function by Dialysis, ed 2. Martinus Nijhoff Publishers, Boston, 1983.
4. Broyer M, Gagnadoux MF, Bacri JL, Laborde K: Problems of long-term dialysis in children. In Gruskin AB, Norman HE (eds): Pediatric Nephrology. Boston, Martinus Nijhoff Publishers, 1981.
5. Donckerwolcke RA, Chantler C, Broyer MJC: Paediatric Dialysis. In Drukker W, Parsons FM, Maher JF (eds): Replacement of Renal Function by Dialysis, ed 2. Boston, Martinus Nijhoff Publishers, 1983.
6. Langfield BM, Meyer RM, Shideman JR, Kjellstrand CM: Hemodialysis of children less than 10 kilograms. Dial Transplant 10:789, 1981.
7. Kinnaert P: Access in children. In Kootstra G, Jörnin PJG (eds): Access Surgery. Lancaster, MTP Press Ltd., 1983.
8. Butt KMH: Blood Access. Clin Nephrol 9:138, 1978.
9. Harmon WE, Meyer A, Grupe WE: Substitution of a percutaneous vascular access for repeated hemodialysis in children. In Bulla M (ed): Renal Insufficiency in Children. Berlin, Springer-Verlag, 1982.
10. Bregman H, Hoover M: The double lumen subclavian cannula. A unique concept in vascular access. Dial Transplant 11:1065, 1982.
11. Gagnadoux ME, Pascal B, Bronstein M, et al: Arteriovenous fistulae in small children. Dial Transplant 9:318, 1980.
12. D'Apuzzo VC, Gruskin CM, Brennan CP, et al: Saphenous vein autograft arteriovenous fistula for extended hemodialysis in children. Acta Paediatr Scand 62:28, 1973.
13. Hussey JL: Experience with 30 human umbilical cord grafts as conduits for hemodialysis. Dial Transplantation 9:341, 1980.
14. Applebaum H, Shashikumar VL, Somers LA, et al: Improved hemodialysis access in children. J Pediatr Surg 15:764, 1980.
15. Mauer SM, Lynch RE: Hemodialysis techniques for infants and children. Pediatr Clin North Am 23:843, 1976.
16. Broyer M, Donckerwolcke RA, Brunner FP, et al: Combined report on regular dialysis and transplantation of children in Europe, Proc EDTA 20:76, 1983.
17. McMann BJ, de Leon LB, Weiss LS, Moore ES: Negative-pressure hydrostatic ultrafiltration in children. Dial Transplant 7:1170, 1978.
18. Ing TS, Vilbar RM, Shin KD, et al: Predialytic isolated ultrafiltration. Dial Transplant 7:557, 1978.
18a. Donckerwolcke RA, Chantler C, Broyer M, et al: Combined report on regular dialyses and transplanation of children in Europe. Proc EDTA 17:87, 1979.
19. Rosa AA, Shideman G, McHugh R, et al: The importance of osmolality fall and ultrafiltration rate on hemodialysis side effects. Nephron. 27:134, 1981.
20. Swamy AP, Cestero RVM: Mannitol and maintenance hemodialysis. Artificial Organs 3:116, 1979.
21. Van Stone GC, Cook J: The effect of bicarbonate dialysate in stable chronic hemodialysis patients. Dial Transplant 8:703, 1979.
22. Hampl H, Wolfgruber M, Pustelnik A, et al: Comparison of the circulatory stability in children during acetate and bicarbonate dialysis. Ed M Bulla, Berlin, Springer-Verlag, 1982.
23. Stewart WK, Fleming LW, Manuel MA: Benefits obtained by the use of high sodium dialysate during maintenance haemodialysis. Proc EDTA 9:111, 1972.
23a. Chantler C, Trompetar R, Rigden S, et al: Vascular stability during hemodialysis, Proc of the 6th International Symposium of Pediatric Nephrology. Paediatric Nephrology. Springer Verlag, 1984.
24. Sargent JA: Kinetic modeling in the guidance of dialysis therapy. Dial Transplant 8:1101, 1979.
25. Harmon WE, Spinozzi N, Meyer A, Grupe WE: The use of protein catabolic rate to monitor pediatric hemodialysis. Dial Transplant 10:324, 1981.
26. Gardiner AOP, Sawyer AN, Donckerwolcke RA, Haycock GB, et al: Assessment of dialysis requirement for children on regular haemodialysis. Dial Transplant 11:754, 1982.
27. Broyer M, Kleinknecht C, Loirat C, et al: Growth in children treated with long-term hemodialysis. J Pediatr 84:642, 1974.
28. Navarro G, Contreras P, Touraine JL, et al: Are "middle molecules" responsible for toxic phenomena in chronic renal failure. Nephron 32:301, 1982.
29. Babb AL, Strand MJ, Uvelli DA, et al: Quantitative description of dialysis treatment: a dialysis index. Kidney Inter. 7 (suppl 23), 1975.
30. Gotch FA: A quantitative evaluation of small and middle molecule toxicity in therapy of uremia. Dial Transplant 9:183, 1980.

50B Hemofiltration and Other Methods of Blood Purification

D. E. MÜLLER-WIEFEL

Although hemodialysis and peritoneal dialysis have been for many years the only methods for blood purification, new techniques have developed during the early 1970s, but the experience in the pediatric age group has been limited.

HEMOFILTRATION

Principles

Convective transport comparable to glomerular function, rather than diffusion as in conventional dialysis, is the mechanism of blood purification in hemofiltration (Fig. 50B.1). Glomerular filtration is imitated by using an artificial filter with a membrane cutoff >20,000 daltons and a filtration pressure of 200 to 500 torr (1). Clearance of high-molecular-weight substances, such as middle molecules, is better than in hemodialysis but that of low molecular weight substances is worse (Fig. 50B.2). The clearance (C_{HF}) can be calculated by the product of filtration flow rate (Q_F) and the sieving coefficient (S), which is the ratio of filtrate (C_F) and blood (C_B) concentration (2).

$$C_{HF} = Q_F \cdot S = \frac{Q_F \cdot C_F}{C_B} \qquad (1)$$

In contrast to the kidney, the loss of fluid and solvents in hemofiltration cannot be compensated for by tubular reabsorption. The loss of water and electrolytes therefore must be balanced by the infusion of a modified Ringer lactate solution, although the recycling of the hemofiltrate after different procedures of absorption is under study (3–6). To avoid fluid imbalance the substitution has to be carefully monitored and adjusted according to the amount of filtrate. This is achieved by a gravimetric or a volumetric method in which the filtered volume directly regulates the volume of replacement solution. The replacement fluid is infused before the blood has passed the filter (predilution method) or afterwards (postdilution method). Although the clearance of small-molecular-weight substances is better in the predilution method, the amounts of substitution fluid are three times higher than in the postdilution method (7). A bacterial filter is interposed to avoid bacterial contamination and pyrogenic reactions (8). The filtered volume not registered (and therefore not substituted) is reflected by the weight loss of the patient.

This body weight loss in hemofiltration now can be monitored exactly with a microprocessor system in which the desired weight loss is set in advance and achieved in a linear manner through the procedure (Fig. 50B.3). The safe monitoring of hemofiltration enables it to be used for home treatment (9, 10).

Indications

Hemofiltration is indicated for the short-term treatment of acute renal failure as well as for the long-term treatment of chronic renal failure (CRF) especially in children with (a) extreme overhydration (including diuretic-resistant cardiac failure); (b) intractable hypertension; (c) uremic neuropathy; (d) hemosiderosis; and (e) dialysis discomfort. Hemofiltration should be considered for intoxication, especially by substances with a molecular weight ranging between 1000 and 20,000 daltons, such as occur in hepatic coma.

Technique

In principle, hemofiltration is possible in all age groups. The smallest child we have treated had a body weight of 9 kg (11). The vascular access used for pediatric hemodialysis is suitable for hemofiltration (12). A single-needle system can be used with an integrated double-pump system (Hemoprocessor, Sartorius) (13). The vascular access must guarantee a sufficient rate of blood flow, which is the main determinant of the filtration flow rate. Blood flow rates <150 ml/m^2/min are unsatisfactory and result in extremely long treatment. Different filters characterized by the asymmetric construction of their membranes are available for hemofiltration (Table 50B.1). A low ratio of filling volume and filtration flow combined with low-molecular-weight cutoff seems to be most suitable for children (SN 40041/2, Sartorius). Residual blood volume in filters is comparable to that in dialyzers (12). The filtration flow rate that can be achieved ranges between 50 and 100 ml/min/m^2 and depends on hematocrit and protein concentration. Accordingly, the substitution volume is about 15 L/m^2 within a period of four hr. This means a substitution volume of 50% of body weight that, with the postdilution method, is sufficient to prevent uremic symptoms in children treated three times per week (12). The substitution solutions have sodium concentrations ranging between 135 and 160 mmol/L, potassium concentrations of between 0 and 4 mmol/L, and calcium concentrations between 1 and 2 mmol/L. The preferred substitution solution consists of 140 mmol/L Na, 2 mmol/L K, 2.1 mmol/L Ca, 1.5 mmol/L Mg,

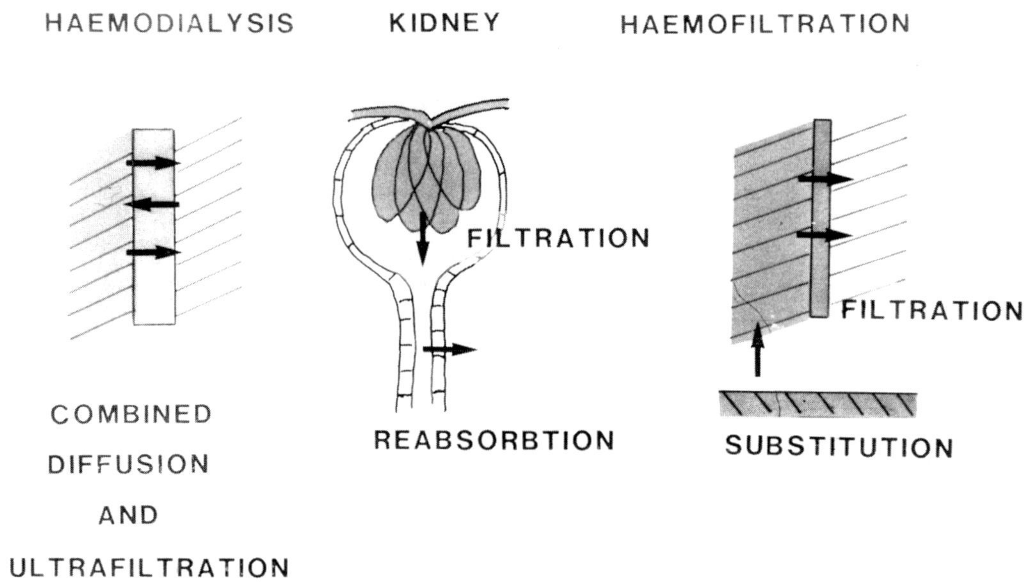

Figure 50B.1. Comparison of the principle of hemofiltration with those of natural kidney and hemodialysis.

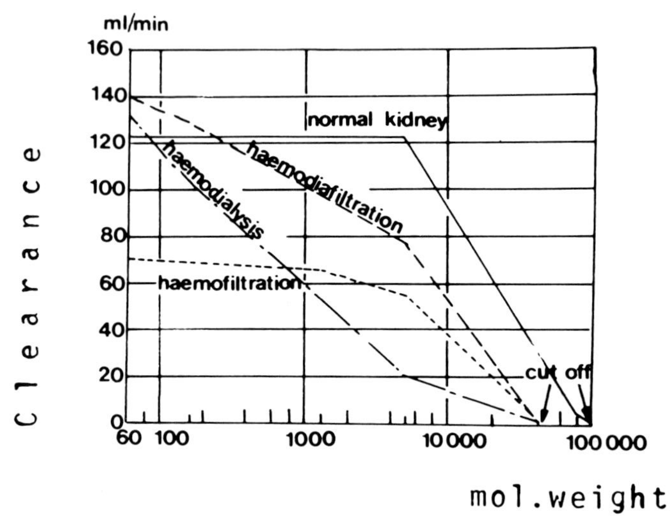

Figure 50B.2. Clearance characterization of different methods of blood purification.

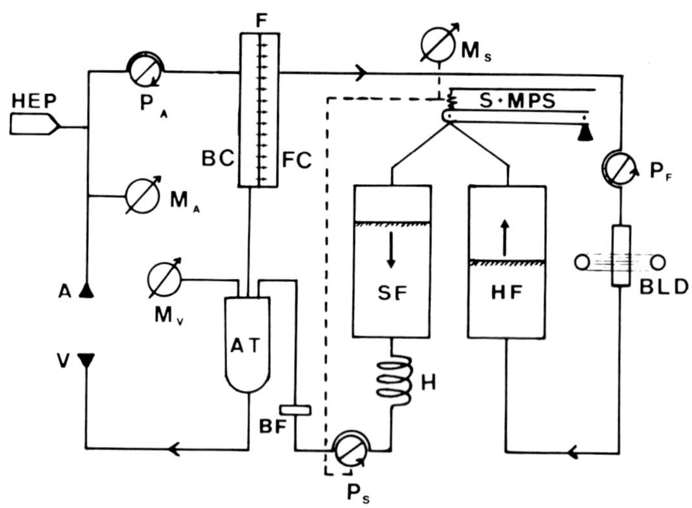

Figure 50B.3. Flow diagram of hemofiltration. A = arterial, V = venous blood access; F = filter; BC = blood, FC = filtrate compartment; HF = hemofiltrate; SF = substitution fluid; S = scales; MPS = microprocessor system; H = heater; HEP = heparinization; AT = air trap; BF = bacterial filter; BLD = blood leak detector; P = pump, M = monitor: A = arterial, V = venous, F = filtration, S = substitution.

112 mmol/L Cl and 35 mmol/L lactate (HF 23, Fa. Fresenius). The heparin dose needed is comparable to that required in hemodialysis.

Results

By the end of 1982 hemofiltration was documented as the mode of treatment in more than 1500 patients with end-stage renal failure (14).

Hemofiltration is well tolerated by children (11, 12, 15, 16). The frequency of side effects is lower than in conventional hemodialysis. Blood pressure is well maintained, without tachycardia during treatment, with a constant rate of fluid removal controlled by computer-controlled monitoring. In children in acute renal failure with an excessive fluid overload, fluid equal to 10% of body weight can be removed within one hr without discomfort. Hemofiltration is therefore a valuable technique for treating patients with dialysis-induced hypotension and those with fluid overload (17). We could not account for the good cardiovascular tolerance of hemofiltration by changes in the concentration of vasoactive hormones in plasma (renin, aldosterone, cortisone, noradrenaline, adrenaline), which were only minimally different from those found during hemodialysis, although in adults an increase in peripheral resistance has been noted (18, 19, 20). Moreover, oxygen supply to the tissues does not seem to be improved by hemofiltration compared with hemodialysis. A shift to the left in the oxygen dissociation curve of hemoglobin because of decreased erythrocyte organic phosphates may result from hemoconcentration during hemofiltration (21). No decrease in arterial oxygen pressure was found during hemofiltration (22, 23), suggesting absence of complement activation and leukocyte sequestration within the lungs (24). The minor decrease in plasma osmotic pressure during hemofiltration, compared with the major increase in plasma oncotic pressure during hemodialysis, is thought to contribute to the better cardiovascular tolerance of hemofiltration in adults (25).

Severe overload hypertension resistant to dialysis and drugs can be

Table 50B.1.
Membrane Characteristics of Different Hemofiltration Filters

Membrane	Type	Name	Filling volume (ml)	Surface area (m^2)	Cutoff (daltons)	Filtrate flow[1] (ml/min)
Triacetate	Flat membrane	Hemofilter Sartorius SM 40041	17	0.3	20,000	60
Triacetate	Flat membrane	Hemofilter Sartorius SM 40042	28	0.6	20,000	80
Polyacrylnitril	Flat membrane	RP 6 Rhône Poulenc	150	1.0	40,000	50
Polyacrylnitril	Hollow fiber	Asahi PAN 1.50	95	1.4	40,000	
Polysulfone	Hollow fiber	Amicon Diafilter	70	0.6	50,000	65
Polysulfone	Hollow fiber	Hemoflow F40 Fresenius AG	45	0.65	50,000	150
Polyamide	Hollow fiber	Gambro fiber Hemofilter FH 202	82	1.2	60,000	85
Polyamide	Hollow fiber	Gambro fiber Hemofilter FH 303	112	1.6	60,000	100

[1] Q_B = 200 ml/min; TMP = 500 mm Hg.

controlled by hemofiltration (26). The negative sodium balance without decrease of plasma sodium concentration with little change in plasma renin activity probably plays an essential role (25). Whereas the balance of the substituted solutes is dependent on body weight loss, the balance of nonsubstituted substances depends on the total filtered volume (12). Using the substitution solution mentioned previously, calcium balance remains positive even in the presence of a high loss of body weight (3 Kg) whereas there is a progressive negative sodium balance when body weight loss exceeds 1 kg. With ultrafiltration of 15 L, 16 g glucose and 3.6 g amino acids are removed (12). These losses are easily compensated by food intake.

Long-term investigations in children indicate that hormone depletion does not occur despite hormone removal. Peripheral insulin activity is improved by hemofiltration (27). Children on hemofiltration continue to grow. Calcium balance is positive, phosphate and parathyroid hormone are removed (28). Phosphate binders usually can be reduced.

The number of children on hemofiltration is too small to allow rigorous comparison with hemodialysis, although the overall results appear to be comparable. Despite the high clearance of middle molecules, no obvious improvement in anemia is observed in children (12) or adults (29). Iron elimination after chelation with deferoxamine is better in hemofiltration than in hemodialysis (30).

Complications

Use of hemofiltration has been inhibited by the costs of commercially available solutions required for high-volume substitution and the risks of bacterial and pyrogenic contamination. In adults, deaths have been attributed to septicemia, which has not been reported in children (8). Bacterial filters should be used between the substition bags and the patient. The risk of aluminum intoxication increases with duration of storage (E. Quellhorst, personal communication). Fluid imbalances are prevented by accurate monitoring systems (Hemoprocessor, Sartorius) which exactly regulate the substitution volume. Allergic reactions seldom occur (11, 31).

SPONTANEOUS ARTERIOVENOUS HEMOFILTRATION (SAVH)

Spontaneous arteriovenous hemofiltration (SAVH) is a modification of hemofiltration accomplished by a capillary filter placed between an arterial and venous line, commonly the femoral artery and femoral vein, or a Scribner shunt at any other location. As the procedure does not work with a single-needle system, which is the method of choice for vascular access in acute renal failure in childhood, the use of SAVH is limited. The total extracorporeal blood volume is low (about 50 ml). A blood pump is unnecessary in a patient with normal blood pressure; a blood flow of 20 ml/min will allow filtration of up to 300 ml/hr (Fig. 50B.4). SAVH is performed without any monitoring devices (32). Close supervision is mandatory to avoid fluid imbalance. The filters (e.g. FH 22 Gambro) must be changed at least every second day (33).

HEMODIAFILTRATION

Principles

Hemodiafiltration is the simultaneous combination of hemodialysis and hemofiltration (34–36). Mass transport across the membrane consists of a diffusive component to remove low-molecular-weight substances and a convective component to remove middle molecules; the rates of removal achieved are higher than by hemodialysis or hemofiltration alone (37). Clearances to be obtained can be calculated as follows:

$$C_{HDF} = C_{HD} + C_{HF} - \frac{C_{HD} \times C_{HF}}{C_{MAX}} \qquad (2)$$

where C represents the clearances by hemodiafiltration HDF, hemodialysis HD, hemofiltration HF, and the maximal clearance (MAX) (38).

The clearance characteristics closely resemble those of the normal human kidney (Fig. 50B.2). This method of blood purification enables treatment time to be reduced by one third (using equipment presently

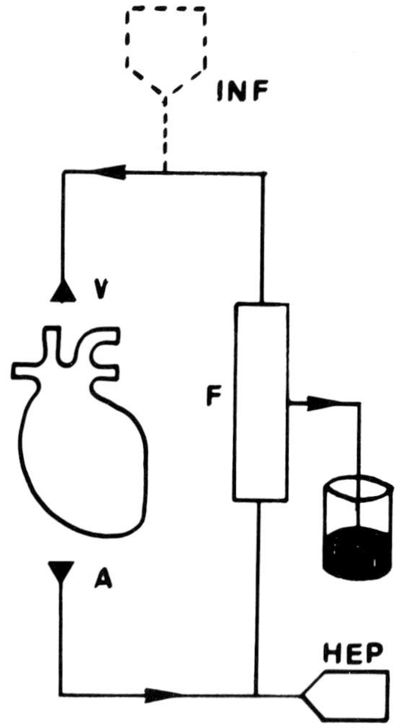

Figure 50B.4. Flow diagram of arteriovenous hemofiltration. A = arterial, V = venous blood access; F = filter; INF = facultative infusion; HEP = heparinization.

available) without deterioration in the patient's general condition (39–41). Experience with HDF in childhood is limited but encouraging (42).

Indications

Indications for hemodiafiltration in children are comparable to those for hemofiltration, but the advantage of a shorter treatment time, usually three hours, three times/week, has to be considered.

Technique

Hemodiafiltration uses high-flux membranes, such as polyacrylnitril, cellulose acetate, cuprophane, or polysulfone. The first hemodiafiltration filter developed for use in children consists of polysulfone. It has a filling volume of 45 ml and a surface area of 0.65 m^2 (F-40 polysulfone, Fa. Fresenius) (TCB 50B-A). The ultrafiltration rate is controlled by an ultrafiltration system, which is integrated into the dialysis monitor (A-2008 c, Fa. Fresenius) or is separate (Rhodial system, Fa. Hospal). In children the ultrafiltration rate should not exceed one third of the rate of blood flow, otherwise a high transmembrane pressure is needed that can develop "secondary" membranes that diminish the clearance capacity. In addition, high pressures lead to increased hemolysis and blood CO_2 loss. The substitution fluid is the same as that used for hemofiltration. The volume needed with the postdilution method depends on the desired body weight loss and ranges between 2 and 2.5 $L/m^2/hr$ in children. Nowadays, exact fluid substitution without using bed scales can be achieved by an automatic balance system (ABG, Fa, Fresenius) programmed to regulate the desired weight loss and duration of treatment (Fig. 50B.5). Dialysate flows of 500 ml/min of acetate or bicarbonate solutions must be sustained.

Results

Hemodiafiltration in children is efficient and well tolerated. Fluid removal is achieved without hypotensive episodes. In spite of shorter treatment times, BUN and S_{Cr} levels decreased and Hb values increased. Moreover, in adult patients on regular hemodiafiltration the dialysis index and motor nerve conduction velocity increased by >10% (34, 35). Changes in acid base and electrolyte balance seem to depend more on the composition of the substitution and dialysis fluid than on the method itself. Hormonal depletion syndromes were not detected during hemodiafiltration. Hemodiafiltration membranes, like those used for hemofiltration alone, are biocompatible (24). Polysulfone membranes are not associated with a drop in leukocyte or thrombocyte counts or in serum complement fractions C3 or C4 (43). Costs, however, are higher because of more expensive equipment and supplies. Home hemodiafiltration has not yet been reported in children.

HEMOPERFUSION

Principles

During hemoperfusion the blood is passed through an adsorbent material, such as activated charcoal, to remove toxic components. The charcoal is usually microencapsulated by various polymer membranes to decrease the risk of embolism and depletion of formed blood elements (Table 50B.2). Activated carbon has a large surface area and high porosity with pores varying from 20 nm (micropores) to 500 nm (macropores). Low-molecular-weight compounds are adsorbed most rapidly through the polymer coating and reach adsorption equilibration most rapidly. The adsorption of high-molecular-weight compounds is decreased by the rate of diffusion through the polymer coating. After diffusion, solute adsorption occurs by a process of internal diffusion through the macropores into the micropores. Other adsorbent agents used are uncoated and uncharged polystyrene resins (Hemoresin, Braun), which have a specific adsorptive attraction for lipid-soluble solutes. Due to saturation of adsorptive sites, there is a progressive decrease of the adsorptive capacity so that the system becomes ineffective after six hr (44).

Indications

Hemoperfusion is particularly effective in removing poisons that are lipid-soluble, highly protein-bound, or poorly distributed in plasma water (45–47) (Table 50B.3). Repeated treatments may be necessary. Hemoperfusion has been used in hepatic coma, but plasma exchange appears to be more effective.

Technique

The adsorber columns are connected by regular pediatric dialyzer lines to either side of an AV shunt or to two venous catheters. Single-needle devises should not be used in hemoperfusion. Because of the relatively high extracorporeal blood volume it is recommended that the system be primed with heparinized blood after rinsing. Because high blood flow rates are required, blood access should be selected to meet this requirement. Both arterial and venous pressure should be monitored; a pressure difference of more than 100 mm Hg indicates that clotting has occurred within the column and the adsorber should be changed or the procedure stopped at once because of the risk of embolism. A dialyzer with the adsorber may be used in series (48). Hemoperfusion usually is terminated after three to four hr and fresh-frozen plasma and platelet concentrate are infused (Fig. 50B.6).

Complications

The risk of severe thrombocytopenia, charcoal embolism, leukopenia, fibrinogenopenia, and hypocalcemia have been reduced by the use of polymer-coated charcoal; however, mild thrombocytopenia secondary to platelet retention on the charcoal column occurs in the majority of children. Hypotension can be treated by fluid substitution. Hypothermia may be a problem in infants.

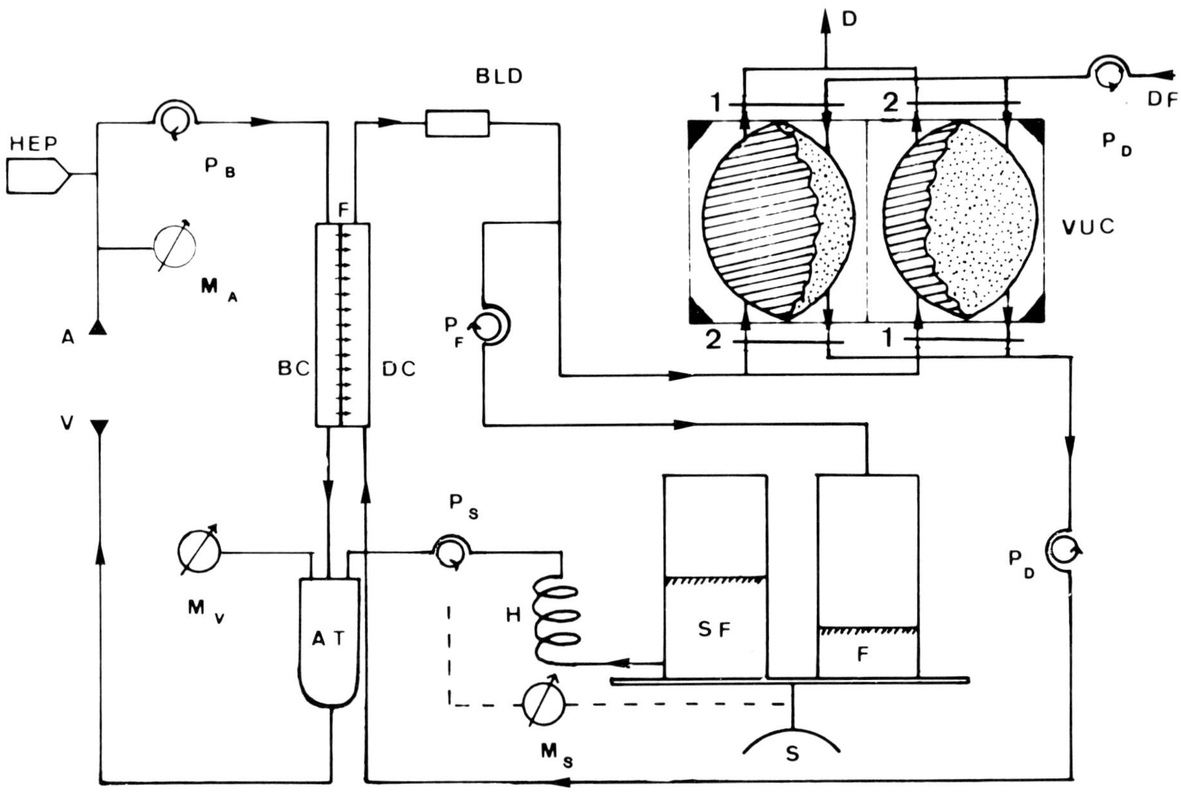

Figure 50B.5. Flow diagram of hemodiafiltration. A = arterial, V = venous blood access; F = filter, BC = blood, DC = dialysis compartment; VUC = volumetric ultrafiltration control; DF = dialysis fluid = □; D = dialysate = ▨; 1 – = membrane; position 1 – = closed (2 – = open) and 2 – = closed (1 – = open) are changing one after the other, so that the amount of dialysate is exactly equal to the amount of dialysis fluid; F = filtrate; SF = substitution fluid; S = scales; H = heater; HEP = heparinization; AT = air trap; BLD = blood leak detector; P = pump: B = blood, F = filtration, D = dialyzer, S = substitution; M = monitor: A = arterial, S = substitution, V = venous.

Table 50B.2.
Types of Charcoal Hemoperfusion Systems

Hemoperfusion device	Producer	Charcoal content (g)	Coating material	Priming volume (ml)
Haemacol 300	Smith/Nephew/Fresenius	300	Acrylic hydrogel	305
Haemacol 100 Pediatric	Smith/Nephew/Fresenius	120	Acrylic hydrogel	100
Adsorba 300 C	Gambro	300	Cellulose acetate	260
Hemosorba	Asahi	200	Collodion	140

PLASMAPHERESIS

Principles

Plasmapheresis is a procedure for separating the total plasma from the cell compartment of whole blood and eliminating not only low-, but also very high-molecular-weight compounds involved in the pathogenesis of a variety of predominantly immunological diseases and intoxications. The plasma is replaced by a protein-electrolyte solution or fresh-frozen plasma (therapeutic plasma exchange) or reinfused after specific detoxification procedures (plasma perfusion) (49, 50).

In centrifugal plasma exchange, a unit of whole blood is withdrawn from the patient and centrifuged off-line. The supernatant plasma is discarded while packed cells are resuspended and returned to the patient. This discontinuous mode of treatment is less suitable for children because blood volume changes are high. Continuously separating centrifugal separators have now been developed, nevertheless, the high extracorporeal volumes used and the development of thrombocytopenia favor, in children, the use of membrane plasma separation using synthetic membrane filters (Table 50B.4) with high molecular cutoffs to separate plasma from the whole blood. Membrane plasma separation is not only used for therapeutic plasma exchange but also for plasma perfusion which may be performed in three different ways. The first of these, the removal of proteins well identified in size (antibasement membrane antibodies), is achieved by cascade or double-step filtration using two types of filters with different cutoff points, the first one with a high and the second one with a low cutoff (Table 50B.4). The low-molecular-weight fraction is returned to the patient, reducing the requirement for replacement fluid. The second modification eliminates immunologically well-defined antibodies (acetylcholinesterase inhibitor antibody in myasthenia gravis) by immunoadsorption in which the second filter consists of adsorbed substances directed against the single protein. When cryoglobulin is involved in the pathogenesis of a disease, the third modification, cryopheresis, may be performed. Following a routine plasma separation, the plasma is cooled to +4 °C and refiltered through a second membrane, through which the precipitated cryoglobulins cannot pass (51).

Table 50B.3.
Drugs Removed by Hemoperfusion Better than by Dialysis

Analgesics	Dibenzepine
Paracetamol	Diethylpentenamide*
Phenacetin	Diphenhydramine
Phenylbutazone	Ethchlorvynol*
Antibiotics/anticancer agents	Glutethimide*
Adriamycin	Heroin
Chloramphenicol	Methaqualone
Chloroquine	Methyprylon
Methotrexate	Nitrazepam
Cardiovascular agents	Oxazepam
Digitoxin*	Thioridazine
Digoxin	Trifluoperazine
Procainamide*	Poisons
Quinine	Carbon Tetrachloride
Theophylline	Diquat
Hypnotics/psychotropic drugs	Mercury
Amitriptyline*	Organophosphates
Amphetamine	Paraquat
Barbiturates*	Strychnine
Bromisovalum*	Trichloroethylene
Carbamazepine	*Advantage of resins over charcoal proven
Carbromal*	
(Chlor)promazine	
(Des)ipramine	
Diazepam	

Indications

In principle, plasmapheresis may be indicated in the following circumstances:

1. Removal of specific (auto) antibodies (Goodpasture's syndrome,

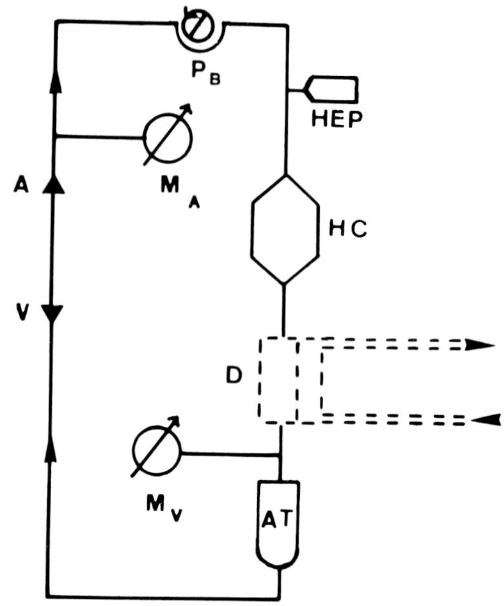

Figure 50B.6. Flow diagram of hemoperfusion. A = arterial, V = venous blood access; HC = hemoperfusion column; D = facultative dialysis system; AT = air trap; P_B = blood pump; M = monitor: A = arterial, V = venous, HEP = heparinization.

Table 50B.4.
Filters used in Plasmapheresis

Trade name	Source	Membrane material	Surface area (m²)	Priming volume (ml)
Plasma filters				
Plasmaflux P1	Fresenius AG	Polypropylene	0.25	30
Plasmaflux P2	Fresenius AG	Polypropylene	0.50	48
Fiber Plasmafilter PP	AB Gambro	Polypropylene	0.38	36
Hemaplex BT 900	Dideco s.p.a.	Polypropylene	0.20	18
CPS-10	Travenol Lab., Inc.	Polypropylene	0.17	17
Curesis	Organon Teknika	Polypropylene	0.12	12
Plasmaflo AP-05-H	Asahi Inc.	Cellulose diacetate	0.50	68
Plasmafilter	Cordis Dow Inc.	Polyethylene	0.70	66
MPS 0250	Mitsubishi Rayon Co. Ltd.	Polyethylene	0.50	45
Plasmax PS-05	Toray Ind., Inc.	Polymethylmetacrylate	0.50	59
Plasmax PS-02	Toray Ind., Inc.	Polymethylmetacrylate	0.15	19
PVA Filter type SA	Kuraray Co., Ltd.	Polyvinyl alcohol	0.60	68
Fiber Plasmafilter PC-1000	AB Gambro	Polycarbonate	0.27	24
TPE Plasma Separator	Cobe Lab., Inc.	Polyvinyl chloride	0.13	18
Teijin Plasma Separator TP	Teijin Ltd.	Polymer alloy	0.40	32
Cascade filters				
PF Prototype	Enka AG	Cellulose acetate	1.00	121
Eval Filter Type 4A	Kuraray Co., Ltd.	Ethylene vinyl alcohol	1.00	80
Plasmax AS-08	Toray Ind., Inc.	Polymethylmetacrylate	0.80	98
Plasmaflo AP-07-K	Asahi Inc.	Cellulose diacetate	0.75	103
Cryofilters				
Plasma ASC-08	Toray Ind., Inc.	Polymethylmetacrylate	0.80	87
PVA Filter, type SN	Kuraray Co., Ltd.	Polyvinyl alcohol	0.60	88
PVA Filter, type MN	Kuraray Co., Ltd.	Polyvinyl alcohol	0.40	71

systemic lupus erythematosus (SLE), myasthenia gravis, TTP, immune hemolytic anemia)

2. Removal of circulating immune complexes (SLE, rheumatic arthritis, Schönlein-Henoch purpura (HSP), Guillain-Barré Syndrome, rapidly progressive glomerulonephritis (RPGN))

3. Removal of mediators of inflammatory processes (globulins, fibrinogen, complement, CRP)

4. Removal of specific pathologic proteins (Waldenström, multiple myeloma, hyperlipidemia)

5. Removal of toxins bound to protein (drugs, hepatic coma, mushroom poisoning)

6. Substitution of plasma components by fresh-frozen plasma (TTP, hemolytic-uremic syndrome).

A list of conditions in which plasma exchange has been attempted is given in Table 50B.5. Those diseases in which the positive effect of plasma pheresis is no longer disputed are underlined. Because of the high molecular weight (1 to 4 × 10^6 daltons) of the proteins that must be removed, we favor those filters with the highest sieving coefficient (Plasmaflux, Fresenius) (52) and do not recommend reusing a filter.

Only a few reports exist concerning plasma exchange in childhood. Diseases in which therapeutic plasma exchange has been reported to be useful include lupus erythematosus (53, 54), Goodpasture's syndrome (55), RPGN (56), PSH (57), FSS, HUS (57, 58), hyperlipidemia (59), vascular graft rejection (60), polyarteritis, rheumatoid arthritis (61), autoimmune hemolytic anemia (62, 63), and dermatomyositis (64, 65). These studies however, were not standardized or prospective, lack controls, and do not include follow-up: further experience is necessary before the indications for therapeutic plasma exchange in pediatric practice are clear (66) (see also Chapter 29).

Technique

Plasmapheresis can be performed in children with a subclavian vein catheter. Maximal blood flow should not exceed 120 ml/min using the filters mentioned in Table 50B.4. To avoid a transmembrane pressure of >100 mm Hg, the filtration flow should not exceed one third of the blood flow. High transmembrane pressures cause hemolysis and create secondary membranes that diminish the sieving coefficient. Total filtration volume per session is usually equal to the total blood volume, and larger volumes do not significantly increase protein removal (67). The concentration (x_t) of a substance (x) after a certain time of treatment (t) is given by the equation:

$$x_t = x_0 e^{-rt} \tag{3}$$

Table 50B.5.
Pediatric Indications for Plasmapheresis

Diagnosis	Substances to be removed	Time of indication
Renal		
Goodpasture (like) syndrome	Antibasement membrane antibodies (AB)	At diagnosis (in combination with immunosuppression)
Rapidly progressive glomerulonephritis	Circulating immuncomplexes (CIC)	At diagnosis (in combination with immunosuppression)
Systemic lupus erythematosus	Antinuclear AB, CIC	Renal failure resistant to steroids
Purpura Schönlein-Henoch	CIC, IgA, IgG	Renal failure and/or nephrotic syndrome with crescents (>75%)
Vascular transplant rejection	AB involved in cytotoxicity	Corticoresistance
Hematological		
Idiopathic thrombocytopenia	Platelet AB	Uneventful high-dose Ig treatment
Posttransfusion purpura	Platelet AB	At diagnosis
Immune hemolytic anemia	Red-cell auto-AB	Unresponsiveness to other management
F VIII AB Hemophilia	F VIII AB	Severe bleeding
Neurological		
Myasthenia gravis	Antiacetylcholine-receptor AB	Acute crisis, uneventful immunosuppression
Guillain Barré syndrome	CIC	Rapid progression
Metabolic		
Familial Hypercholesterinemia[1]	Cholesterol, LDL	Progressive skin xanthomas
Refsum's disease	Phytanic acid	Clinical signs under dietary treatment
Fabry's disease	Ceramide trihexoside	N.S.A.
Poisons		
Intoxication by herbicides, drugs, mushrooms	Herbicides, drugs, mushrooms	At diagnosis
Hepatic coma	Endogenous toxins	At diagnosis
Endocrinological		
Thyroid storm	T3, T4	Unresponsive to conventional treatment
Skin + connective tissue		
Rheumatoid arthritis	IgM AB	Insufficient drug effects in extra-articular manifestations
Pemphigus	Auto AB to epidermal cell-membrane glycoproteins	Failure of conservative treatment

[1] Preferably immunoadsorption.

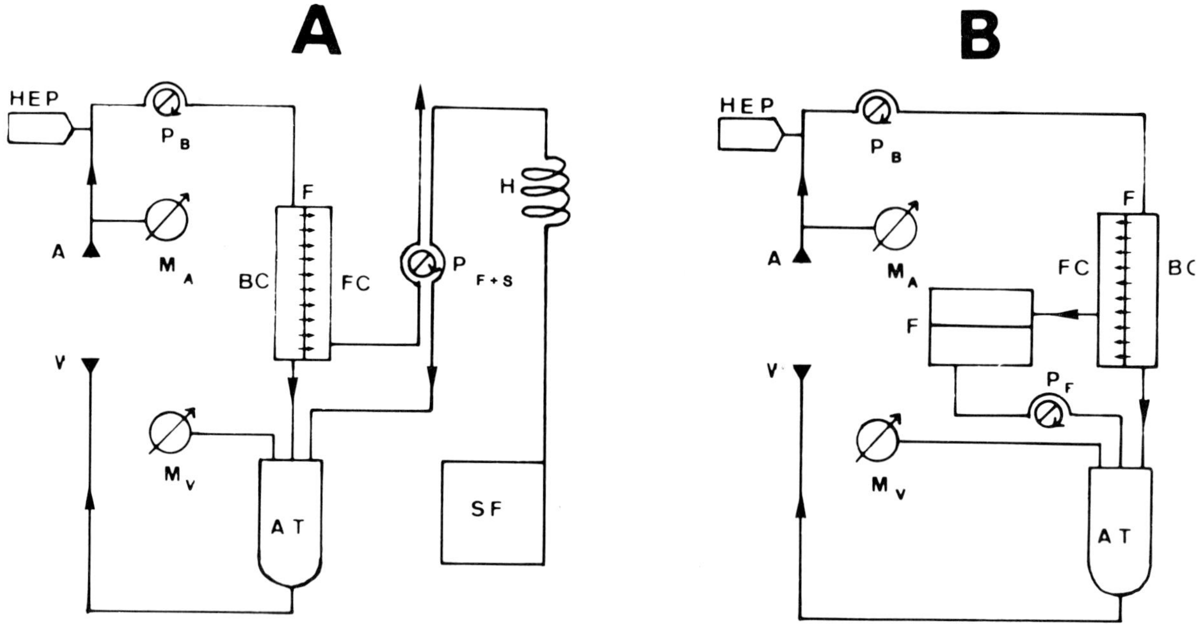

Figure 50B.7. Flow diagram of membrane plasma separation. A, Therapeutic plasma exchange. B, Plasmaperfusion: A = arterial, V = venous blood access; F_1 = first filter; F_2 = second filter (cascade filter, cryofilter, immune adsorption filter); BC = blood, FC = filtrate compartment; SF = substitution fluid; H = heater; HEP = heparinization; AT = air trap; P = pump, M = monitor: B = blood, F = filtration, S = substitution, A = arterial, V = venous.

where x_0 denotes the initial concentration of x and r the fractional rate of exchange, as defined by the equation [68]:

$$r = \frac{\text{exchange volume/hr}}{\text{plasma volume}} \tag{4}$$

This relationship is valid only if the amount of the substance catabolized during the exchange procedure is equal to the sum of the amount synthesized and the amount shifted from the extravascular into the intravascular compartment.

The exact simultaneous substitution of equal amounts of the replacement fluid is easily achieved with a double pump system (Fig. 50B.7) (A-2008 PF, Fresenius; Separa BT-796, Dideco/Bellco) (69). Albumin solutions are preferred to fresh-frozen plasma unless the substitution of a plasma component is desired, e.g., in hemolytic uremic syndrome and hepatic coma. The concentration of the albumin infused should be equivalent to the patient's serum concentration so that the oncotic pressure remains constant. Larger quantities of heparin are used in membrane plasma separation than in hemodialysis, but with normal liver function and alternate-day treatment clotting factors and immunoglobulins are resynthesized adequately.

Complications

Immunoglobulins are decreased by 40% and fibrinogen by 50% during each treatment, so that daily treatment increases the risk of infection and bleeding. Treatment should not be started when fibrinogen concentrations are <100 mg/dl. Intermittent thrombocytopenia is more common with the centrifugal than with the membrane method, in which the decrease is about 14% (51). The risk of hepatitis (5%) can be diminished using albumin replacement solution. The high incidence of septic complications reported in PPH is probably partly caused by the immunosuppressive drugs used to decrease resynthesis of pathological proteins. Allergic reactions in between 0.7% and 12% of patients have been reported (67). Fever, shivers, hypertension, cardiac arrhythmia and hypocalcemia when citrate is used for anticoagulation are occasional problems. The incidence of all side effects is between 5% and 25% (51).

References

1. Quellhorst EA: Ultrafiltration and hemofiltration, practical applications. In Drukker W, Parsons FM, Maher JF (eds): Replacement of Renal Function. Martinus Nijhoff Publishers Boston The Hague Dordrecht Lancaster, p 265.
2. Henderson LW: Biophysics of ultrafiltration and hemofiltration. In Drukker W, Parsons FM, Maher JF (eds): Replacement of Renal Function. Martinus Nijhoff Publishers Boston The Hague Dordrecht Lancaster, 1983, p 242.
3. Armstrong VW, Fuchs C, Klüver H, et al: A synthetic resorcinol-formaldehyde resin for the absorption of urea from hemofiltrate. Contrib Nephrol 32:181, 1981.
4. Rawer P, Krausch D, Schütterle G: Urea degradation with hollow-fiber bound urease and ammonium-ion removal with macrocyclic polyethers. Contrib Nephrol 32:186, 1981.
5. Shaldon S, Beau MC, Deschodt G, et al: Three years of experience with on-line preparation of sterile pyrogen-free infusate for hemofiltration. Contrib Nephrol 32:161, 1981.
6. Schünemann B, Nebendahl K, Schunk O, et al: Regeneration of hemofiltrate using an absorption and electrochemical oxidation system. Contrib Nephrol 32:192, 1981.
7. Henderson LW: Pre vs. post dilution hemofiltration. Clin Nephrol 2:120, 1979.
8. Frei U, Koch KM: Fever and shock during hemofiltration. Contrib Nephrol 36:107, 1982.
9. De Fremont JF, Morniére P, Pruna A, et al: Long-term evaluation of hemofiltration at home. Contrib Nephrol 32:119, 1981.
10. Shaldon S: Progress from Haemodialysis. Nephron 27:2, 1981.
11. Müller-Wiefel DE, Klare B, Querfeld U, et al: Hemofiltration in childhood. In Bulla M (ed): Renal Insufficiency in Children. Berlin, Heidelberg, New York, Springer 1982, p. 217.
12. Müller-Wiefel DE, Rauh W, Wingen AM, et al: Hemofiltration in children. Contrib Nephrol 32:128, 1982.
13. Verpooten GA, van Waeleghem JP, Pollet D, et al: Single needle hemofiltration. Contrib Nephrol 32:170, 1981.
14. Wing AJ, Broyer M, Brunner FP, et al: Combined report on regular dialysis and transplantation in Europe, XIII, 1982. Proc EDTA 20:5, 1983.
15. Edefonti A, Galato R, Saccaggi A, et al: Clinical impact of hemofiltration (HF) on dialysis discomfort in children. Int J Pediatr Nephrol 3, 1982.
16. Giani M, Picca M, Saccaggi A, et al: Use of urea kinetic model and haemofiltration to improve nitrogen balance in haemodialyzed children. Proc EDTA 20:201, 1983.
17. Davison AM, Roberts TG, Mascie-Taylor BH, Lewins AM: Hemofiltration for profound dialysis-induced hypotension: removal of sodium and water without blood-pressure change. Br Med J 285:87, 1982.
18. Baldamus CA, Ernst W, Fassbinder W, Koch KM: Differing haemodynamic stability

due to differing sympathetic response: Comparison of ultrafiltration, haemodialysis and haemofiltration. Proc EDTA 17:205, 1980.
19. Hampl H, Paeprer H, Unger V, Kessel MW: Haemodynamics during haemodialysis, sequential ultrafiltration and hemofiltration. J Dialysis 3:51, 1979.
20. Quellhorst E, Schuenemann B, Borghardt J, et al: Influence of hemofiltration on blood pressure regulation. Clin Nephrol 3:150, 1979.
21. Müller-Wiefel DE, Klare B, Schärer K: Effect of haemofiltration (HF) and haemodialysis (HD) on erythrocyte organic phosphates in uremic patients. Proc EDTA 16, 723, 1979.
22. Schaefer K, Ryzlewicz T, Sandri M, et al: Effect of hemofiltration on acid-base status and ventilation. Contrib Nephrol 32:69, 1982.
23. Schaefer K, von Herrath D, Hüfler M: Stable PO_2 during hemofiltration in spite of a drop in leucocytes. Letter to the Editor. Nephron 32:377, 1982.
24. Böhler J, Kramer P, Götze O, et al: Leucocyte counts and complement activation during pump-driven and arteriovenous hemofiltration. Contrib Nephrol 36:15, 1982.
25. Quellhorst E: Hämofiltration—Differentialindikation zur Hämodialyse unter Berücksichtigung hämodynamischer und metabolischer Aspekte. Klin Wochenschr 57, 1061, 1979.
26. Fischbach M, Schohn D, Jahn H, Geisert J: Deux observations d'hypertension artérielle maligne, chez des enfants hémodialysés, traitée par hémofiltration. Ann Pediatr 29, 9, 666, 1982.
27. Kishimoto T, Ezaki K, Yamagami S, Maekawa M: Glucose tolerance and erythrocyte insulin receptors in undialyzed patients and patients on maintenance hemodialysis and hemofiltration. Contrib Nephrol 32:97, 1981.
28. Pierides AM, Giacherio D, Schniepp B, Burritt M: Calcium, phosphorus and parathyroid hormone metabolism in chronic hemofiltration. Contrib Nephrol 32:77, 1981.
29. Quellhorst E, Schuenemann B, Borghardt J: Hemofiltration: current clinical applications and evolution of techniques. Renal Physicians Association. Northeastern Meeting Proceedings, 2:1, 1978.
30. McCarthy JT, Libertin CR, Mitchell JC, Fairbanks VF: Hemosiderosis in a dialysis patient. Treatment with hemofiltration and deferoxamine chelation therapy. Mayo Clin Proc 57:439, 1982.
31. Nicholls AJ, Platts MM: Anaphylactoid reactions due to hemodialysis, hemofiltration, or membrane plasma separation. Br Med J 285, 1607, 1982.
32. Kramer P, Kaufhold G, Gröne HJ, et al: Management of anuric intensive care patients with arteriovenous hemofiltration. Int J Artif Organs 3:225, 1980.
33. Dodd NJ, O'Donovan RM, Bennett-Jones DN, et al: Arteriovenous haemofiltration: a recent advance in the management of renal failure. Br Med J 287:1008, 1983.
34. Leber HW, Wizemann V, Goubeaud G, et al: Simultaneous hemofiltration/hemodialysis: an effective alternative to hemofiltration and conventional hemodialysis in the treatment of uremic patients. Clin Nephrol 9:115, 1978.
35. Sprenger KBG: Review Article: Haemodiafiltration. Life Support Systems 1:127, 1983.
36. Streicher E, Schneider H: Stofftransport bei Hämodiafiltration. Nieren- und Hochdruckkrankheiten 12:339, 1983.
37. Sprenger KGB: Measurement of mass transport during hemodiafiltration. In Schütterle G, Wizemann V, Seyffart G (eds): Hemodiafiltration, Proceedings 1. Symposion Giessen. Oberursel, Verlag Hygieneplan, 1981, p 49.
38. Granger A, Vantard G, Vantelon J, Perrone B: A mathematical approach of simultaneous dialysis and filtration (SDF). Proc Eur Soc Artif Intern Organs 5:174, 1978.
39. Kunitomo T, Kirkwood RG, et al: Clinical evaluation of postdilution dialysis with a combined ultrafiltration (UF)-hemodialysis (HD) systems. Trans Am Soc Artif Intern Organs 24:169, 1978.
40. Leber HW, Wizemann V, et al: Simultaneous hemofiltration/hemodialysis: an effective alternative to hemofiltration and conventional hemodialysis in the treatment of uremic patients. Clin Nephrol 9:115, 1978.
41. Ota K, Suzuki T, et al: Short time hemodiafiltration using polymethylmethacrylate hemodiafilter. Trans Am Soc Artif Intern Organs 24:454, 1978.
42. Fischbach M, Attal Y, Geisert J: Hemodiafiltration versus hemodialysis in children. A twelve months experience. Int J Pediatr Nephrol 3:151, 1984.
43. Streicher E, Schneider H: Polysulphone membrane mimicking human glomerular basement membrane. Lancet II, 1136, 1983.
44. Papadopoulou ZL, Novello AC: The use of hemoperfusion in children. Past, present, and future. Pediatr Clin North Am 29:1039, 1982.
45. Seyffart G: Poison index. Dialysis and hemoperfusion in poisonings. Ed. Fresenius Foundation, Bad Homburg, Bindernagel Friedberg/Hessen 1977. 2nd. revised supplement 1983.
46. Haddad LM, Winchester JF: Clinical management of poisoning and drug overdose. Philadelphia, Saunders, 1983.
47. Freundlich M, Cynamon H, Tamer A, et al: Clinical and laboratory observations. Management of chloramphenicol intoxication in infancy by charcoal hemoperfusion. J Pediatr 103:485, 1983.
48. Graben N, Sohn J, Pistor K: Treatment of life-threatening exogenous intoxications in infants and children by combination of hemoperfusion through charcoal or resin and hemodialysis. In Bulla M (ed): Dialysis and Kidney Transplantation in Children. Melsungen, Bibliomed, 1979, p 197.
49. Siebert HG: Plasma exchange. Plasmapheresis-plasmaseparation. Stuttgart, New York, Schattauer, 1980.
50. Gurland HJ, Heinze V, Lee HA: Therapeutic plasma exchange. Berlin Heidelberg New York, Springer, 1981.
51. Gurland HJ, Samtleben W, Blumenstein M: Review Article: Therapeutic plasmapheresis; present state and future aspects. Life Support Systems 1:61, 1983.
52. Gurland HJ, Lysaght MJ, Samtleben W, Schmidt B: Comparative Evaluation of Filters Used in Membrane Plasmapheresis. Nephron 36:173, 1984.
53. Johannessen A, Gutteberg T, Husby G: Plasma exchange in the treatment of severe, childhood onset systemic lumpus erythematosus. Acta Paediatr Scand 71:347, 1982.
54. Michalk D, Scharf J, Waldherr R: Plasmaseparation als effektive Behandlung der Glomerulonephritis bei Lupus erythematodes. Klin Pädiatr 195:418, 1983.
55. Brandis M, Offner G, Krohn HP, Schnaidt U, Sterzel RB, Stangel W: Plasmapheresis in a 13 year old girl with Goodpasture-like syndrome. In: Bulla M: Dialysis and kidney transplantation in children. Bibliomed, Melsungen, 1979, p 171.
56. Michalk DV, Scharf J, Stehr K: The role of plasmapheresis in the treatment of autoimmune diseases (AID) and rapidly progressive glomerulonephritis (RPGN). Eur J Pediatr 141:179, 1983.
57. Holland PC, Dillon MJ, Welsh A, Barratt TM: Plasma exchange in renal disease in children. Eur J Pediatr 141:180, 1983.
58. Gillor A, Bulla M, Roth B, et al: Plasmapheresis as a therapeutic measure in hemolytic-uremic syndrome in children. Klin Wochenschr 61:363–367, 1983.
59. Witztum JL, Williams JC, Ostlund R, et al: Successful plasmapheresis in a 4-year-old child with homozygous familial hypercholesterolemia. J Paediatr 97:615, 1980.
60. Müller-Wiefel DE, Bonzel KE, Wartha R, et al: Therapeutic plasma exchange in children with vascular kidney graft rejection. (in preparation)
61. Brewer EJ, Nickeson RW Jr, Rossen RD, et al: Plasma exchange in selected patients with juvenile rheumatoid arthritis. J Paediatr 98:194, 1981.
62. Bernstein ML, Schneider BK, Naiman JL: Plasma exchange in refractory acute autoimmune hemolytic anemia. J Pediatr 98:774, 1981.
63. Andersen O, Taaning E, Rosenkvist J, et al: Autoimmune haemolytic anaemia treated with multiple transfusions, immunosuppressive therapy, plasma exchange, and desferrioxamine. Acta Paediatr Scand 73:145, 1984.
64. Anderson LR, Ziter FA: Plasmapheresis via central catheter in dermatomyositis: a new method for selected pediatric patients. J Pediatr 98:240, 1981.
65. Dau PC, Bennington JL: Plasmapheresis in childhood dermatomyositis. J Pediatr 98:237, 1981.
66. Singsen BH: Plasmapheresis: a pediatric perspective. J Pediatr 98:232, 1981.
67. Sprenger KBG: Continuous membrane plasma separation: three years of experience. Life Support Systems 1:235, 1983.
68. Calabrese LH, Clough JD, Krakauer RS, Hoeltge GA: Plasmapheresis therapy of immunologic disease: report of nine cases and review of the literature. Cleve Clin Q 47:53, 1980.
69. Bambauer R, Jutzler GA, Mauch H, et al: Ein vereinfachtes Plasmapherese-Behandlungsverfahren. Nieren- und Hochdruckkrankheiten 10:126, 1981.

50-C Peritoneal Dialysis

J. W. BALFE

Peritoneal dialysis was first performed in 1923 (1) and by the late 1940s was used extensively in the treatment of acute and chronic renal failure (CRF) (2, 3). It fell into disfavor as a treatment for CRF during the 1960s, however, because it required an abdominal puncture for each dialysis (4). The repeated punctures were uncomfortable for the patient and time-consuming for the physician, and bowel perforation and peritonitis were significant risks (4). The success of arteriovenous shunts and improvements in the hemodialysis technique relegated peritoneal dialysis to a second-line mode of treatment for end-stage renal disease (ESRD) (5).

The necessity for repeated abdominal punctures was circumvented by the development of a permanent peritoneal catheter designed in 1964 (6) and modified in 1968 (7). The production of an automatic peritoneal cycler (8) in 1966 made it more acceptable because dialysis could be done at home. The reverse osmosis peritoneal dialysis system introduced in 1972 (9) greatly reduced the cost of the procedure, making it competitive with hemodialysis.

Peritoneal dialysis was used in a number of centers for patients with specific indications, e.g., no vascular access sites, unstable cardiovascular status, and inability to use heparin (10). It became an alternative to hemodialysis for most patients with the development of continuous ambulatory peritoneal dialysis (CAPD) in 1976 (11). By June 1983, 7800 CAPD patients in the US were being managed in 582 centers (K. D. Nolph and B. Prowant, personal communication), accounting for 12% of the chronic dialysis population in the United States. The percent of total dialysis that is done as CAPD varies widely among different countries. Data in children are scarce; in the United States patients <20 years old on CAPD represent 5.3% of the CAPD population (12). More recently, modifications of the CAPD technique have been introduced that combine nighttime automated with daytime long-dwell CAPD in a system called continuous cyclic peritoneal dialysis (CCPD) (13, 14).

PHYSIOLOGY OF PERITONEAL DIALYSIS

The physiological principle of peritoneal dialysis is based on an exchange of solute and water between blood and dialysis fluid by diffusion and ultrafiltration. The rate of exchange is a product of the character and surface area of the membrane and the dialysance and filtration properties of the solutes. The variables are the surface area of the peritoneal membrane, its dialysance characteristics, and the nature of the solute gradients between dialysate and plasma flow that transport them.

Peritoneal Surface Area

The results from three studies vary considerably (15–17) but two report values for infants (~450 cm^2) per kilogram of body weight that are approximately twice those of adults and correspond to the ratio of energy expenditure per kilogram of body weight of infants to adults (2.5:1).

Peritoneal Membrane

The movement of solutes between peritoneal capillaries and dialysate fluid is across a number of resistance sites (18). The capillary wall (R2, Fig. 50C.1) provides the major resistance to dialysis exchange. The filtration characteristics of the capillary membranes differ from those of hemodialysis membranes, allowing plasma proteins to be filtered into dialysis fluid (19). The peritoneal interstitium (R4, Fig. 50C.1) is a network of aqueous channels that traverse the mucopolysaccharide and collagenous gels of the interstitial space—also a major resistance site in the peritoneal membrane. Dehydration of the peritoneal gel by hypertonic fluids increases resistance (20); hypotonic fluids have the reverse effect (21). The mesothelium of the peritoneum presents little resistance (22). The stagnant films (R6, Fig. 50C.1) within the peritoneal cavity create resistance that would be lessened by agitation or stirring of the dialysate.

Transport of Solute

There are two types of passive transport across the semipermeable peritoneal membrane: diffusion and convection (23). Diffusion is the transport of solute down a concentration gradient independent of osmotic gradient. Convective transport involves two components: solvent movement across the peritoneal membrane and solute movement or solvent drag, which entrains solute within a solvent stream, i.e., ultrafiltration. The driving force of ultrafiltration is the osmotic rather than the concentration gradient. The osmotic gradient is created in the dialysate by

Table 50C.1
CAPD as a Percentage of the Total Chronic Dialysis Census*

Geographical Area	%
Australia and New Zealand	30
Canada	28
Great Britain	26
Scandinavia	20
United States	12
Spain	10
Belgium	8
France	8
Netherlands	8
Others	<8

*Personal communication, K. D. Nolph and N. Prowant

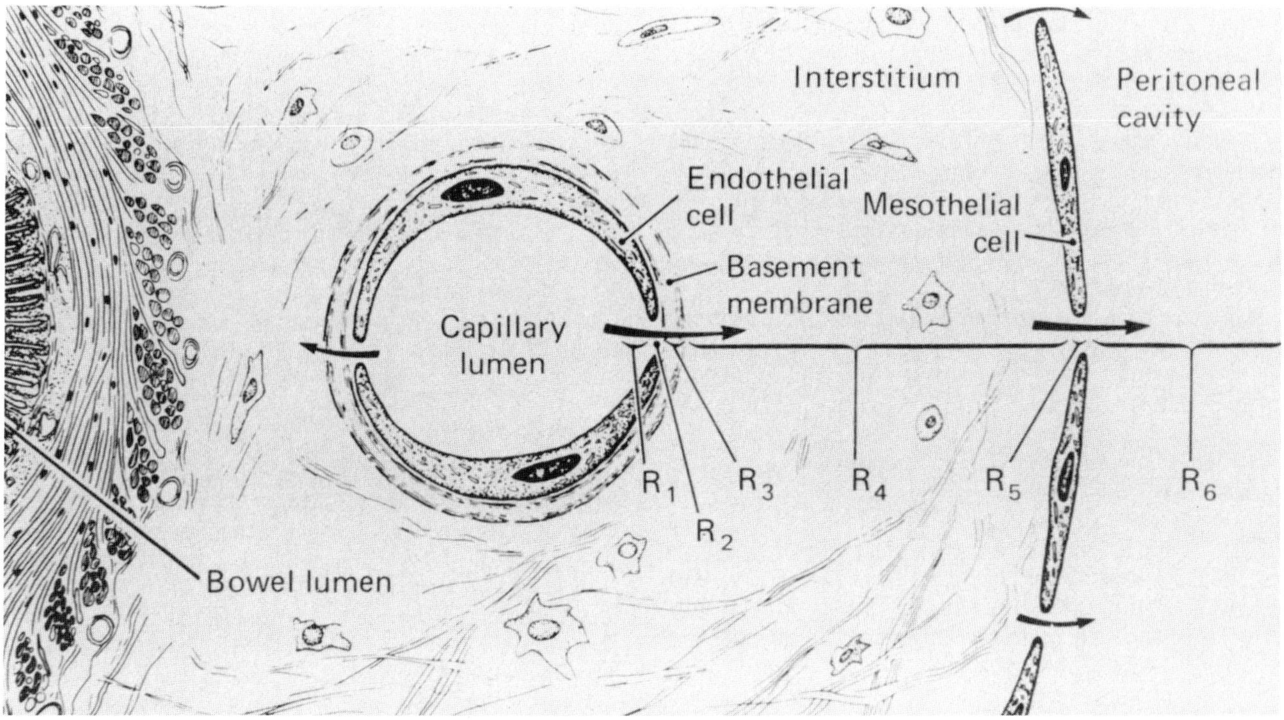

Figure 50C.1. Resistance sites to solute movements from peritoneal capillaries to dialysate. R1 = stagnant fluid films in capillary blood, R2 = capillary endothelium, R3 = capillary basal membranes, R4 = peritoneal interstitium, R5 = mesothelium and R6 = stagnant fluid films within the peritoneal cavity. (From Nolph et al: New directions in peritoneal dialysis concepts and applications. Kidney Int [Suppl 10]:S-111, 1980.)

adding glucose. The overall transfer of solute is the sum of diffusion and convection transport and is termed mass transfer of solute.

The rate of removal of solute is expressed as clearance. Clearance is estimated by the general clearance formula:

$$\text{Clearance} = \frac{C_D Q_D}{C_p} \quad (1)$$

where C_D = concentration of solute in the dialysate at the time of drainage;
Q_D (flow rate) = volume of dialysate per exchange time (ml/min); and
C_p = concentration of solute in plasma at the midpoint of the exchange time.

A more accurate measure of solute transport by diffusion is derived from the equation (24, 25)

$$\Delta B = \frac{-V_b V_D}{V_b + V_b} \times \left[\frac{\ln 1 - C_D \dfrac{(V_D + V_b)}{C_B V_b}}{t} \right] \quad (2)$$

where ΔB = dialysance of whole blood (ml/min);
V_b = volume of distribution of solute outside the peritoneal space (ml);
V_D = volume of dialysate removed at the end of an exchange (ml);
C_D = concentration of solute in dialysate at midpoint of exchange;
C_B = concentration of solute in plasma at midpoint of exchange;
and t = time in minutes.

This formula assumes that: (a) no ultrafiltration occurs; (b) the volume of distribution of solute does not change during the dialysis; and (c) solute diffusion is uniform during the study period.

We can measure the dialysance of solutes of differing molecular weights in a single exchange. A relative permeability index can be derived for each of the solutes as a function of a reference solute.

$$\text{Index} = \frac{\text{Dialysance solute } (x)}{\text{Dialysance solute } (y)} = \frac{\text{Permeability } (x)}{\text{Permeability } (y)} \times \frac{\text{Membrane area}}{\text{Membrane } (y)} \quad (3)$$

Using large-molecular-weight solutes and a short dwell-time, clearance without ultrafiltration approximates the overall permeability-surface area product or dialysance. The results for clearance and dialysance, however, are different when using small-molecule solutes and a long dwell-time (26).

The amount of water ultrafiltered is related to the time for inflow, dwell, and outflow, and the size of the osmotic gradient. The volume effectively ultrafiltered is measured by the difference between input and output dialysate volume. This may not be accurate because it depends on complete removal of dialysis fluid. By adding a nonabsorbable marker to the dialysate and measuring its change in concentration with time, one can measure the ultrafiltration rate. Substances currently used are radioiodinated serum albumin ($R^{131}ISA$), isotopically tagged dextran 70, and inulin (27).

Ultrafiltration is less effective in an infant than it is in an older child or adult, and net uptake of fluid is common due to a rapid fall in dialysis osmolality (28). Glucose concentration is lower in dialysate removed from patients <6 years of age than it is in older children, so that ultrafiltration is compromised (29).

Hypernatremia and hyperchloremia develop when a large quantity of fluid is rapidly ultrafiltered because the sieving coefficients of sodium and chloride cause their removal from extracellular fluid (ECF) relative to that of water to be slow (30). The sieving coefficient is the ratio of the concentration of solute in ultrafiltrate to the concentration in plasma water (31). To prevent hypernatremia, dialysate containing a Na concentration less than plasma water is used (32) and dwell-time is extended to at least one hr.

Hyponatremia occurs in a number of infants on CAPD who ingest a dilute solution; fluid is removed as isotonic NaCl; to offset this, the dialysate NaCl concentration may be increased to a value above that of plasma (33, 34) and salt added to the formula so that the water intake to provide nutrients, less insensible and urinary free water loss, is associated with a proportional intake of NaCl.

Techniques of mathematical modeling have been used (35) to simulate the patient–peritoneal dialysis system. The peritoneal membrane is characterized by two parameters: the mass transfer-area coefficient (MTAC) for transport by diffusion and the reflection coefficient (RC) for ultrafiltration. Results from studies on adults (31) are being compared with preliminary results from studies on children (36, 37).

Peritoneal dialysis is successful when performed with a long dwell-time because molecules are given time to equilibrate between plasma and dialysate. Naturally, small molecules equilibrate faster than large ones (Fig. 50C.2). Middle molecules (mol wt 500 to 5000) are removed better by long-dwell than short-dwell peritoneal dialysis (38). If middle molecules play a causal role in the uremic syndrome, this property of long-dwell dialysis is clinically important.

CHRONIC PERITONEAL DIALYSIS

Chronic peritoneal dialysis (CPD) is simple, effective, and less expensive than chronic hemodialysis. It is particularly attractive for children because the size of the patient is not a contraindication; other advantages are freedom from thrice-weekly in-center hemodialysis sessions (permitting regular school attendance), freedom to return home while awaiting a renal transplant—even if the home is some distance from the center, and freedom to go away on a prolonged vacation with parents.

Because of its ease of initiation, CPD naturally attracts more patients with new problems. A wider range of patients will be treated with peritoneal dialysis, and some children will electively remain on dialysis for longer periods of time. In pediatrics, dialysis and transplantation are considered together.

Some children in whom transplantation is not possible will remain on dialysis indefinitely. We do not know how long a person can remain on CPD. A number of adults have been treated >5 years; we have children who have been managed this way for >4 years. There are reports of membrane failure, which usually manifests as inability to ultrafilter water and sodium and chloride but solute removal is adequate.

Catheters Types

For all types of CPD a catheter made of Silastic rubber is used. Various models have been developed in an effort to avoid the catheter drifting upward in the abdominal cavity and becoming less efficient (Fig. 50C.3).

We prefer the straight, single-cuffed, Tenckhoff catheter (39). The adult size is used for children >30 kg body weight; the pediatric size for those between 10 to 30 kg; the neonatal size for infants <10 kg. In all three sizes, the Dacron felt cuff is fixed 5 cm from the first drainage holes.

We do not use the double-cuffed catheter. Although the second cuff is intended to prevent bacteria from migrating into the tunnel, leading to tunnel infection, we have had no problems with tunnel infections when using a single cuff. The distal cuff is also meant to prevent the catheter from sliding and thus irritating the skin at the exit site and producing infections. We see exit site infections, but they are managed easily. We have had to replace only one catheter for this reason.

We have used the Toronto Western catheter and the column-disc

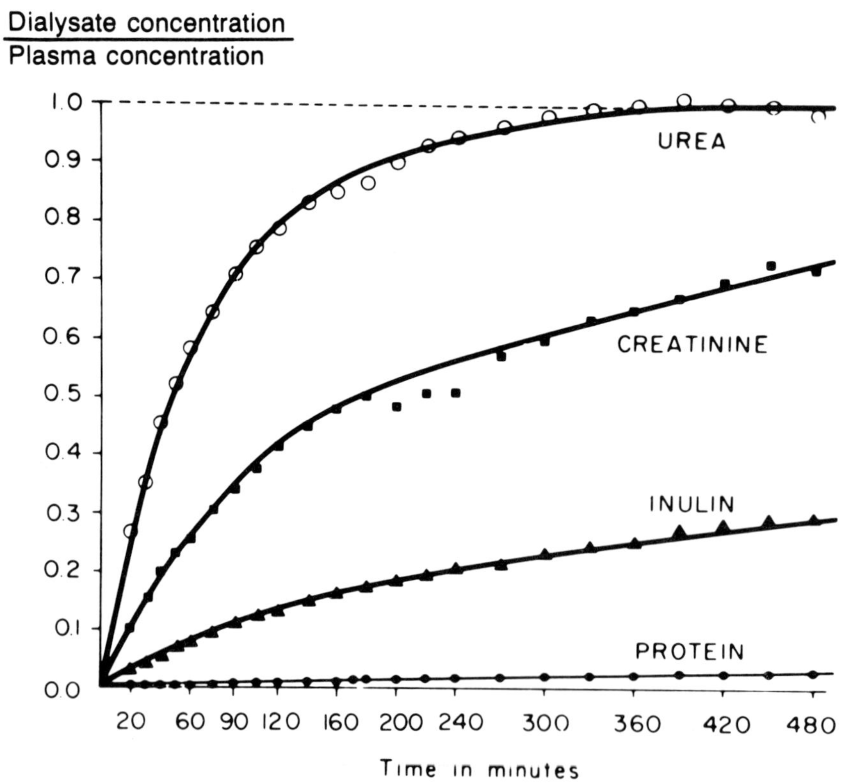

Figure 50C.2. Dialysate/plasma concentration ratios for urea, creatinine, inulin and protein from frequent samples throughout an entire 8-hour dwell. (From Popovich et al: Continuous ambulatory peritoneal dialysis. Ann Intern Med 88:449, 1978.)

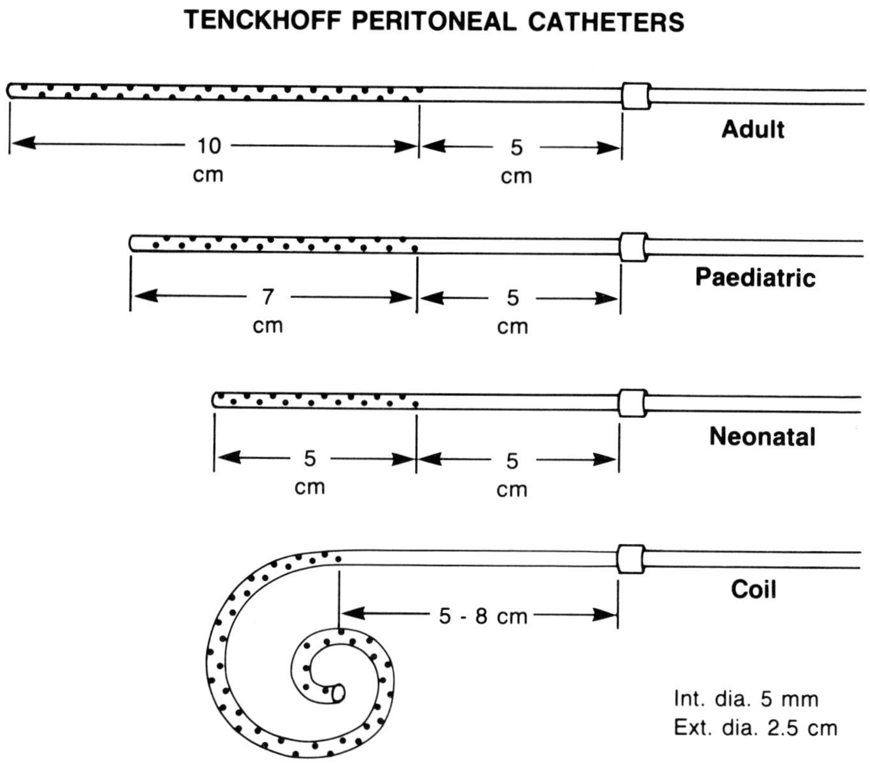

Figure 50C.3. Tenckhoff catheters of various sizes. All these catheters are used at our center, except the curled catheter.

catheter occasionally in cases of early catheter failure. There have been few controlled trials to establish which is the best catheter (40).

Catheter Insertion

There are numerous techniques for catheter insertion (41). In most centers catheters are inserted by a surgeon; in some, by the pediatric nephrologist. General anesthesia is commonly used in younger children, but local anesthesia is preferred when practical.

A small midline abdominal incision is made below the umbilicus (Fig. 50C.4), and the catheter tip is directed toward the pelvis. Care must be taken not to advance the catheter too far, thus pushing the tip cephalad and increasing the possibility of omental obstruction; special attention is required for the child <20 kg body weight.

In all cases, we secure the peritoneum around the catheter with a purse-string suture and bury the Dacron cuff between the peritoneum and the rectus abdominis muscle. A 7 cm tunnel, created lateral to the umbilicus, leads the catheter from the peritoneum to the skin exit site. The position of the catheter is checked radiographically and its water tightness and function are checked by irrigation and gravity drainage before the patient leaves the operating room.

It has been suggested (42) that the catheter be inserted more laterally, i.e., splitting the rectus muscle, being careful to avoid the inferior epigastric artery in order to have more tissue in which to bury the cuff. This reduces the likelihood of leakage.

Although omentectomy has been recommended to improve catheter drainage, the omentum has not caused problems in children in our experience and we have found omentectomy generally unnecessary. The risk of the procedure appears small, however, it may be useful in older patients or when a previous catheter has been obstructed by a large omentum.

We initiate dialysis immediately, using a small volume with no dwell-time. The availability of the automated small-volume dialyzer makes

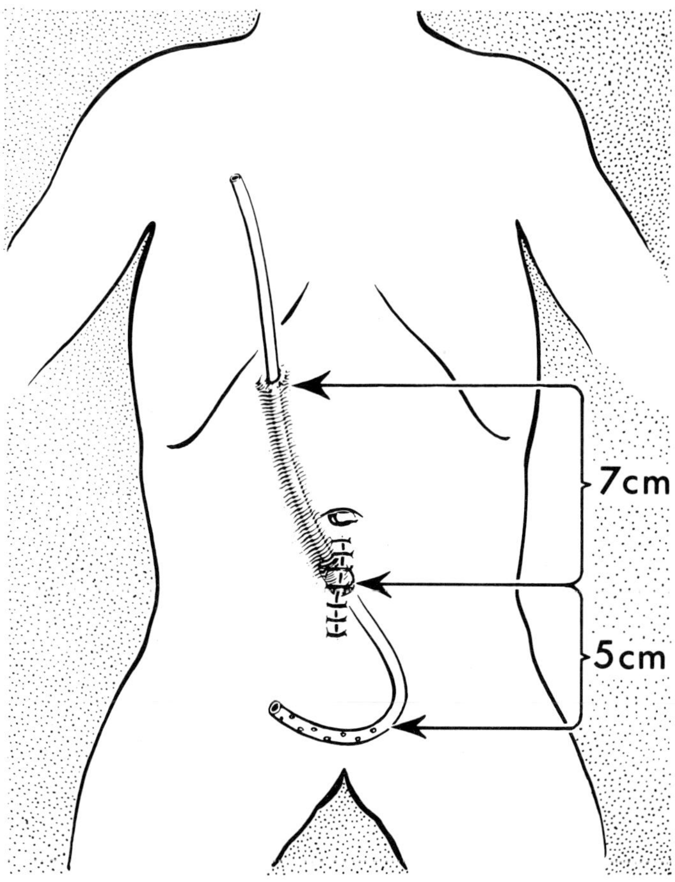

Figure 50C.4. A chronic Tenckhoff catheter in an infant. The single cuff is positioned at the middle arrow.

Table 50C.2
Protocol for Insertion of a New Tenckhoff Catheter

1. Infuse 10 ml/kg body weight 1.5% dialysate (containing heparin 500 IU/L and cephalothin 250 ml/l) with no dwell time for 4 hours.
2. If the dialysate is clear and draining well, start infusion, using a 10-minute dwell time for 6 hours.
3. After the "break in" (steps 1 & 2):
   a) For patients who do not need immediate dialysis or entrance into CAPD training:
      —inject 3 ml (1000 IU/ml) heparin into the catheter and cap it off;
      —irrigate the catheter twice weekly.
   b) For patients in need of immediate dialysis and/or entrance into CAPD training, infuse dialysate:
      —using 1 hour dwell-time for 24 hours;
      —using 2 hour dwell-time for 24 hours;
      —using 4 hour dwell-time for 24 hours.
4. Gradually increase the exchange volume over 3 days:

Patient Weight (kg)	Volume (ml)	
	Initial	Final
10	100	300
20	250	500
30	300	750
40	400	1000

5. After 24 hours of 4–6 hour dwell time, CAPD may be started and prophylactic cephalothin discontinued.

this approach practical. After the first few hours, the fluid is permitted to dwell in the abdomen and gradually the dwell-time and the volume of dialysate are increased.

Table 50C.2 describes the protocol used immediately before and after catheter insertion. Prophylactic antibiotics (we use tobramycin 1.5 mg/kg body weight intravenously and cephalothin 20 mg/kg body weight intravenously) are recommended before surgery. Heparin (500 IU/L) and cephalothin (250 mg/L) are added to the dialysate used immediately after surgery (see Protocol).

TYPES OF PERITONEAL DIALYSIS

Chronic Intermittent Peritoneal Dialysis (CIPD)

There are three types of peritoneal dialysis. There are surprisingly few reports of pediatric chronic intermittent and peritoneal dialysis (CIPD) programs. One of the earliest was described in 1968 (43); seven children, 6 to 14 yr old, were managed from three to eight months. The children were dialyzed only when their clinical condition deteriorated. The first pediatric program of home CIPD, using permanent catheters and automatic cyclers, was started in Seattle in the same year (44), and several other centers have subsequently described their experience (45–50).

Apparatus

In North America, the Lasker Cycler (51) (American Medical Products Corporation—AMP, Fairfield, N.J.) is used most frequently. This is a simple, gravity-type machine with a central pole and eight hooks, each one holding a 2 L bag of dialysate. It has a heater box, a cycler, and an outflow or drainage container. There are two timers, one for the "fill cycle," which includes time to drain into and dwell in the peritoneal cavity, and one for the cycle to drain the fluid out of the cavity. A counterbalance scale monitors the volume of fluid draining out. The machine is inexpensive, but running costs are high because commercially purchased bags of dialysate are used. Another disadvantage is that it is an open system, and thus there is an increased risk of peritonitis.

The reverse osmosis type of machine (52) (Physio-Control Company, Seattle, Wash.) produces its own sterilized, deionized water from tap water. A proportioning pump mixes 19 parts of this warmed, sterile water with 1 part of a concentrated solution of electrolyte and dextrose. The machine must be sterilized once every week with a formaldehyde solution. Such machines are expensive, but the operating costs and incidence of peritonitis are relatively low.

The gravity-type cycler (AMP) can be modified for small children who may be able to accommodate only 200 to 300 ml of dialysate in the peritoneal cavity. The volume permitted to flow is determined by placing a flexible plastic bag between two rigid metal heater plates, which are separated by placing four rigid spacers of equal length between them. The volume of fluid entering the bag varies with the length of the spacers. One manufacturer (JM Sounds, Automatic Peritoneal Cycler, Toronto, Ont.) also uses a timing device to adjust the flow rate, so that a flow rate of 300 ml/min can be achieved by setting the time. To achieve accuracy, air must be removed from the tubing during the initial cycle. Even though the volume control bag can be filled in 1 min, the initial drainage cycle should be set for at least 10 min to permit the fluid to warm.

The amount of peritoneal dialysis clearance required is affected by the amount of residual renal function. Most in-center patients (adults and children) require two 20-hr dialysis periods per week. Each cycle has a 20-min dwell-time. There can be many variations in the dialysis scheduling. Patients with some renal function maintain acceptable biochemistries with less dialysis.

Home CIPD. In a home CIPD program for adults, both the Lasker Cycler and a reverse osmosis-type machine have been used (53). The patients were dialyzed for four 8- to 12-hr sessions per week, using 24 L dialysate per session, overnight if possible. Another group (54) reported their home CIPD experience with adults, using a similar technique.

There is limited experience in home CIPD programs for children. From 1968 to 1970 we did in-center CIPD using the repeated puncture technique. Every 10 days the child received intermittent peritoneal dialysis (IPD) for 48 hr. Potter and coworkers (50) started home CIPD training several days after catheter insertion in an outpatient unit and required 7 to 11 training sessions, using Drake-W-6001 machines for 12 hr overnight, three times per week.

With the AMP automatic cycler (46), home training was completed in one to two weeks and, during training, dialysis was done each day; gradually, medical supervision was withdrawn until the parents and patient were self-sufficient. Children were dialyzed for 12 exchanges, three times per week, using 1200 ml/m^2 (maximum 2 L) volume and a 30-min dwell-time. Automatic cyclers that can deliver small volumes and long dwell-times are needed for children because of catheter "break-in" and also for the expected popularity of continuous cyclic peritoneal dialysis. An automated long-dwell pediatric cycler recently has become available (AMP, Fairfield, N.J.).

Continuous Ambulatory Peritoneal Dialysis (CAPD)

In continuous ambulatory peritoneal dialysis (CAPD), the principle of dialysis is simple, but the management of patients requires experienced personnel who are dedicated to its use. CAPD is now very popular in North America. Approximately 25% to 30% of adults on chronic dialysis in Canada are managed by CAPD. Physicians tend to believe the CAPD technique is simple and often start a program without adequate preparation. A hastily introduced CAPD program can end in failure for the program and unfortunate complications for the patients. Success

Table 50C.3
Indications for CAPD in Children

1. Small child or infant in whom HD is difficult;
2. Living a distance from a nephrology center;
3. Expected to remain on dialysis for a long time (e.g., elevated titer of preformed cytotoxic antibodies, treated Wilms' tumor);
4. No vascular access site available for HD;
5. Unstable cardiovascular system (e.g., arrhythmia, cardiomyopathy, reduced cardiac output);
6. End-stage diabetic renal failure (rare in children); or
7. Preference of patient/parent/physician.

demands an experienced team, including a knowledgeable physician, experienced nurses, a dietitian, and a social worker; members of the team should be sent to an experienced center for training.

CAPD is not a substitute for a renal transplant; however, it allows the nephrologist to properly prepare the patient for surgery. At present, it seems reasonable to persist with CAPD in infants and children as long as the child thrives physically and mentally. In some cases, for social or medical reasons, transplant surgery will be performed sooner.

Selection Criteria for CAPD

Selection criteria for CAPD vary from center to center. It is important to explain the various types of dialysis to the patient and family, then come to a collective decision on which mode is appropriate. Currently, most of the children at our center are managed by CAPD (Table 50C.3). There are few contraindications for CAPD in children. A patient with diverticulitis is considered unsuitable, but this is a rare complicating illness. We have used CAPD in patients with ureterostomies and even one with a colostomy without any major complications related to the stomas. If a patient or a family is disinclined to go on CAPD, there is no pressure placed on them. The technique requires considerable effort on the part of the patient or parent and will not succeed in the unenthusiastic family.

The prerequisites that have been outlined for a CAPD program for adults (55) are also essential for a pediatric unit, but pediatric programs have unique needs as well. A CAPD program should be coordinated with other modes of dialysis. The program should have its own nurses, who have had previous training in hemodialysis and in-center peritoneal dialysis. The patient-to-nurse ratio appears to be approximately 8 to 10 children to one nurse.

Facilities

We recommend (a) a training room with proper plumbing, (b) nurse's office, (c) a storage room for dialysate, supplies, and cyclers, (d) a room for parents to stay in during training, and (e) a backup room to treat patients with peritonitis during training.

Appropriately trained nurses provide in-hospital training and care of patients and follow-up of outpatients. This includes periodic hospital visits, home visits, and frequent telephone checks. A renal dietitian, who is experienced with CRF patients and aware of the extra nutritional requirements of CAPD patients, is important. The services of a social worker experienced in renal problems can help the patient and family cope with CAPD. This help is especially important to the family of an infant.

Patient or Parent Training

The break-in period following catheter placement is around four days, and the CAPD training period about two weeks. The exchange technique is taught to the patient or parent under close supervision during the first week of training and done under less supervision during the second week. The procedure in the second week is now done by the patient or parent under supervision of the nurse, who teaches the patient bag, tube, and dressing change techniques, and the practical physiological aspects of dialysis and general care. Signs of peritonitis and its early treatment also must be learned.

Home Follow-up

Once the patient is sent home we maintain close contact by telephone. Initially, we see the child every two weeks, then every four weeks when practical. The physician reviews the daily record sheet kept by the patient (or parent), noting blood pressure, weight change, and problems. Physical examination includes special attention to hydration and the catheter exit site. The patient is advised about correct "dry weight" and the types of dialysis fluid required to maintain that weight. The nurse changes the connecting tube or supervises the bag changing technique. The dietitian advises on food intake, especially protein and energy intake.

We recommend keeping four-day home records every four or eight weeks. When appropriate, the family physician participates in the patient's care. Samples for appropriate blood and bacteriological tests can be done under his or her supervision. In some instances, the family physician assumes total care of patients, especially for those living a great distance from the center; the nephrology center is available for consultation, often by telephone.

Catheter Care

The care of the catheter has changed. Initially, the wound was covered and twice weekly the catheter and exit site were cleaned meticulously with povidone-iodine solution and covered with an Airstrip bandaid. Over the past year, many centers, including ours, changed because the application of solution to an exit site plus a dressing prevented the natural formation of a cleanly epithelialized site. We recommend that patients scrub the exit site with a soft povidone-iodine sponge and, after rinsing, apply 3% hydrogen peroxide and rinse again. Finally, the exit site is dried and a circle of povidone-iodine solution is painted around it. We recommend daily catheter care and showering before care at least every two days.

Continuous cyclic peritoneal dialysis (CCPD)

Despite financial deterrents, continuous cycle peritoneal dialysis (CCPD) continues to grow in popularity and is expected to attract a percentage of the chronic dialysis population. Improved automated cyclers suitable for children will soon be available; however, the major cost of CCPD is for the disposable plastic bags and tubings. The cost of CAPD in 1980 to 1981 was set (62) at $19,600 (US)/yr compared with $54,300 (US) for in-center hemodialysis at their institution. CCPD tubings and bags would add another $15,000 to $20,000/yr. These costs will fall with time.

Experience with CCPD in adults and children is limited. This technique uses an automated cycler with a prolonged dwell-time during the evening and night (three exchanges of three hr each in adults) and an extended 15-hr ambulatory dwell during the day. A significant amount of dialysate is absorbed during the day when 1.5% dextrose dialysate is used, so that 4.25% dextrose dialysate is commonly used. CCPD is as efficient as CAPD in removing small molecules, but this may not be the case for middle molecules.

In North Carolina (14) and Texas (13), encouraging possibilities are reported for CCPD. Lum in Colorado and Fine in California use the technique for children and have each managed over 20 patients, aged three months to 18 years (personal communications). Usually, five exchanges have been required during the evening.

A relatively inexpensive long-dwell cycler is produced by AMP. It has three volume settings (250, 500, 750 ml), and the timing can be set from one min to 9.9 hr. Older AMP cyclers can be modified for a prolonged dwell-time, with volumes of 1, 1.5, and 2 L.

It is premature to compare CCPD with CAPD physiologically. It has been recommended (56) that all patients be managed initially by CAPD for three months, then select those who can be transferred to CCPD.

Some aspects of CCPD should be noted. Because there are only two disconnections per day, a reduction in peritonitis should be anticipated, but similar peritonitis rates have been observed in CCPD and CAPD patients: one episode per 9.4 patient-months versus one episode per 7 patient-months, respectively. Parent fatigue and the inconvenience of performing a bag change during the day, i.e., at day care or school, may be less.

In summary, a comparison of CAPD with CCPD is premature. Indeed the two may be used interchangeably in the same patient. Some recommend the patients be managed initially by CAPD and in time select those suitable for CCPD (56). Although CCPD involves fewer disconnections, the incidence of peritonitis in CCPD is 1 per 9.4 patient-months compared with 1 per 7 patient-months in one series (57). Parent fatigue may be less with CCPD because exchanges are fewer. A combination of the two methods that reduces interference with school activities may be useful in selected cases.

CLINICAL MANAGEMENT OF CHILDREN ON CHRONIC PERITONEAL DIALYSIS

Dialysis Frequency and Clearance

CAPD is able to maintain body biochemistry in a relative steady state comparable to that provided by hemodialysis (58–62). There is, however, no consensus on what constitutes adequate dialysis treatment. Uremia is thought to be secondary to accumulated waste products and the search for the "uremic toxin(s)" continues. Clearance of small molecules, such as urea and creatinine, is lower with CAPD, but since it is performed every day, weekly clearance values are the same as for hemodialysis and creatinine values are comparable. Some CAPD patients claim to feel better than they did on hemodialysis. Although this may be related to superior removal of middle molecules, which are believed to contain the putative uremic toxins, evidence for this is lacking.

If the measurement of middle molecules is an index of adequacy of dialysis, it is unfortunate that this assay is unavailable in most centers. Most physicians rely on the concentration of plasma urea and creatinine and the clinical condition of the patient (nausea, vomiting, blood pressure) to assess adequacy.

Three factors limit how much clearance can be provided by CAPD: (a) the volume of dialysate that the patient can accommodate; (b) the frequency of exchange; and (c) the nature of the peritoneal membrane. It seems that except in infants, using more than five exchanges per day defeats the usefulness, and fewer than three exchanges is not sufficient.

Three-liter exchanges, three per day in adults, are being tested (63). Usually four exchanges are performed unless a patient has sufficient residual kidney function, so that appropriate chemistries can be maintained with three exchanges. For an adult with renal failure, defining the adequacy of dialysis by the BUN level appears to be satisfactory (64). For children, however, rather than prescribing clearance based on abdominal size, available bag size and energy reserve of the patient or parent to do the exchanges, it is preferable to set a minimum clearance value, such as creatinine clearance >6 ml/min/1.73 m^2 (9 L/day/1.73 m^2).

Table 50C.4
Biochemical Control in 13 Children Managed by CAPD >12 Months

Test	Mean Level ± SD		p Value
	Before CAPD	On CAPD	
Urea (mmol/l)	36.1 ± 6.8	24.3 ± 7.1	<0.005
Creatinine (μmol/l)			
<6 years old	698 ± 194	424 ± 115	<0.001
>6 years old	1043 ± 203	902 ± 248	NS*
Urate (mmol/l)	428 ± 24	327 ± 48	<0.001
Magnesium (mml/l)	1.05 ± 0.15	1.35 ± 0.15	<0.001
Calcium (mmol/l)	2.15 ± 0.18	2.38 ± 0.25	<0.02
Phosphate (mmol/l)	1.61 ± 0.68	1.52 ± 0.52	NS
Triglycerides (mmol/l)	2.43 ± 0.50	3.37 ± 0.59	<0.001

*NS = not significant

Serum Chemistries

Plasma chemistries of our patients before dialysis and after 12 months of CAPD are shown in Table 50C.4. Plasma urea nitrogen (P_{UN}) is maintained in the 50 to 100 mg/dl (urea 18–35 mM) range for all ages, and plasma creatinine (P_{Cr}) for adolescents at <10 mg/dl (<1200 mM), and, for younger children, between 5 and 8 mg/dl (440–700 mM) (65).

Plasma Na (P_{Na}) in children in CAPD generally is normal (61, 62). Na concentration in the dialysate is less than that in plasma after four hr (66). In rapid cycle peritoneal dialysis (>1 cycle/hr) hypernatremia may develop (67), but in CAPD and CCPD this does not occur. We have observed hyponatremia in some infants whose net loss of Na exceeded that of water because formula intake was low in Na and ultrafiltrate removal of Na was high (68).

Patients who tend to develop hyperkalemia between hemodialysis treatments may do better on CAPD (34). In fact, many adults on CAPD tend toward hypokalemia and require K supplementation. Severe hypokalemia has been reported (69), but children on CAPD usually have normal P_K. P_K levels are elevated in some children, who then require dietary K restriction and sometimes K exchange resins.

Blood total CO_2 values in 73 children from four pediatric CAPD centers (70) were normal (23.5 mmol/L), whereas the plasma magnesium was high (1.4 mmol/L). Magnesium concentration in our patients increased after one yr of CAPD (1.05 to 1.35 mmol/L, normal = 0.65 to 1.00 mmol/L). The dialysate solution contained 0.75 mmol/L magnesium and 35 mEq/L lactate. Kohaut (70) has suggested that magnesium concentration be reduced and lactate concentration be increased in the dialysate. The consequences of mild hypermagnesemia are not known (71).

Plasma albumin concentration is used to assess nutritional status (72, 73). Plasma albumin concentration did not decrease in our patients. Protein loss in the dialysate was greater in children <6 years of age than in older patients (0.30 ± 0.06 versus 0.14 ± 0.02 g/kg body weight) (29); similar results in children have been reported by others (60, 62). Adults on CAPD lose 8.8 ± 1.7 g protein per day in the dialysate (74). Albumin accounted for 50% to 79% of this loss and IgG for 5% to 28%. They concluded that this was not a major protein loss and could be made up by dietary protein intake.

Plasma albumin levels are determined by many factors, e.g., synthetic and catabolic rates, losses in urine and stool, plasma volume, and distribution of albumin between plasma and interstitial fluid (75). Uremia per se affects albumin metabolism (76). Some of our younger patients on CAPD have hypoalbuminemia (33). For one child we added amino acid to the dialysate and discontinued intravenous albumin supplementation that was being used to treat hypoalbuminemia and edema (77).

Our patients have experienced a significant rise in serum triglyceride concentration with CAPD (Table 50C.4). The increase does not correlate with obesity. Elevation of serum cholesterol and triglyceride levels has been observed by others (60, 62). Serum triglycerides in the first three months of CAPD have been reported (78) as 257 ± 59 mg/dl, reaching a plateau during the second and third three-month periods (422 ± 32 and 427 ± 69 mg/dl, respectively). The hypertriglyceridemia has been attributed to increased absorption of dextrose from the dialysate (79). When use of dialysate with 4.25% dextrose was decreased, the triglyceride level decreased also (80, 81). Regular exercise and dietary carbohydrate restriction have also been suggested (19).

Calcium and phosphorus plasma levels are discussed under renal osteodystrophy.

Growth

Poor growth is commonly associated with chronic renal insufficiency (82). At birth the height is normal or subnormal. During infancy, generally a period with a high growth velocity, linear growth is poor and falls away from the mean normal height for age. After six months to three yr, the growth curve deviates less from the norm but the negative standard deviation score (SDS) tends to worsen. Between ages 2 and 11 yr, height velocity maintains a nearly stable negative SDS but catchup growth does not occur (see also Chapter 2). For this reason, efforts to improve growth in the first 6 or 12 months of life are critical (84).

Growth is usually poor in children managed by hemodialysis (85–87); after a successful renal transplant it may improve, yet catchup growth is rare (88). Previously, early dialysis was technically difficult for small children and infants, but CAPD has now made dialysis available to all children, even newborns.

We studied the linear growth of 17 children (range 0.4 to 18.5 yr; mean ± SD 9.3 ± 6.2 yr) compared with 18 children on hemodialysis and 20 children who had received transplants (89). Assessing growth, using the growth velocity index (GVI) based on bone age:

$$\left(\text{GVI}[\%] = \frac{\text{Observed height gain}}{\text{Expected height gain}} \times 100\right), \qquad (4)$$

Ten CAPD patients had a GVI >80%, six had a GVI of 50% to 80%, and one had GVI <50%. GVI in patients on CAPD was significantly better than it was in children on hemodialysis ($p < 0.01$) and did not differ significantly from children who had received a renal transplant.

Encouraging results on growth in children managed by CAPD are also being reported by others (78, 90, 91). Adequate and even catchup growth has been achieved when hyperparathyroidism was controlled and adequate energy and protein intake provided (90).

In a preliminary report (92), improved growth rate has been reported in very small children using CAPD or a modified CAPD technique. Seven to nine exchanges a day are done; formula is given by a nasogastric tube to ensure 90 to 150 kcal and 3.5 to 4.5 g protein/kg body weight/day (92). Lesser amounts may be more appropriate.

Although growth is a desirable goal in the management of children with CRI, poor growth per se is not an absolute indication for dialysis or transplantation. The report of 23 children with CRF in the first year of life (93), 20 of whom developed profound neurological abnormalities, led to a proposal for early transplantation to prevent these abnormalities. Although this may be effective, other results differ. Improved nutrition, which may necessitate tube feeding, early dialysis, or both, is another option (see also Chapter 49).

Nutrition

Nutrition is intimately related to growth. Conservative management of CRF frequently necessitates the restriction of some nutrients, which can lead to poor food intake, malnutrition, and disturbance in growth. Adequate intake of calories is important for growth in children on hemodialysis (94).

Defining an adequate protein intake is difficult. Excessive dietary protein may speed the progression of renal failure (95), so protein restriction may be indicated, but not to less than the minimum requirement (see Chapter 10). The protein requirements for the child on CAPD must take into account the losses in the dialysate.

Anorexia is observed in CRF (83) and is a frequent problem for CAPD patients, especially infants (58, 60, 96). The mechanism or mechanisms for the anorexia are speculative, such as intermittent elevations of blood sugar and their metabolic consequences, the removal of essential nutrients in the dialysate, and the sensation of satiety from a full abdomen.

The recommended dietary protein intake for the adult on CAPD is 1.2 to 1.3 g/kg body weight (97, 98); for children on CAPD 1.5 g/kg body weight is the minimum requirement (58, 60), whereas in infants 2.5 to 3.5 g/kg body weight is proposed (93a).

The energy and protein intake of 11 children in our program was assessed from four-day home food records (89). The energy intake for three children was <80% of the recommended daily nutritional intake (RDNI) (99); in addition, two of the three had an inadequate protein intake (<1.5 g/kg body weight/day), and all three grew poorly.

Twelve children managed by CAPD had a total caloric intake of 68 kcal/kg/body weight/day, which included dialysate glucose absorption (60). Their energy intake was 82% of the recommended dietary allowance (RDA) (98) for children of the same height and sex, and protein intake was 2.4 ± 0.9 g/kg body weight/day. In our patients, the glucose absorption through the dialysate was 2.74 ± 1.05 g/kg body weight/day for children <6 years old and 1.49 ± 0.72 for children >6 years old (29). A glucose absorption of 128 ± 61 g/day is reported in adults on CAPD (79). Extra energy intake causes obesity in some adults and children, but in some the extra energy intake may be useful in improving growth. Energy supplements probably are indicated when skin fold thickness is below normal and average intake <80 RDA, (see Chapter 49).

Glucose in the dialysate disturbs lipid metabolism; thus, preliminary trials of amino acid dialysate as an alternative osmotic agent have been done (101). More recently, there has been interest in the use of amino acid dialysate for protein nutrition. In acute studies (five hr), we measured changes in plasma amino acid concentrations, comparing 1% to 2% amino acid dialysate (Travasol, Baxter-Travanol) (102). Long-term studies in children and adults are necessary to test the efficacy of intraperitoneal amino acid. Oral supplements of essential amino acids in children on hemodialysis produced no measurable changes (103); however, the two clinical situations are not comparable.

Renal Osteodystrophy (ROD)

Renal osteodystrophy (ROD) connotes a constellation of skeletal abnormalities seen in patients with CRF. Children appear more susceptible than adults. Radiological evidence of ROD was detected (104) in 15 of 19 children who had developed ESRD. Dialysis prolongs life in children with renal failure, so the possibility exists of worsening bone disease (see Chapter 52).

Because of the steady state environment CAPD provides, many clinicians anticipated that it would reduce the severity of bone disease. Early reports in adults showed deterioration (105); however, improvement of histological ROD has been reported (106) in patients who received supplemental calcium and vitamin D when necessary and underwent parathyroidectomy as required. None received aluminum-containing phosphate binders. The serum concentration of 25-hydroxyvitamin D fell appreciably after nine months of dialysis. It has been shown (107) that 25-hydroxyvitamin D was lost in the dialysate of children on CAPD.

We assessed 15 children on CAPD from 0.3 to 2.4 yr of age (108). All had received 1,25 dihydroxyvitamin D_3 and aluminum hydroxide. In nine who received supplemental calcium, plasma calcium increased to high-normal levels; however, parathyroid overactivity was suppressed in only one patient. At the start of CAPD, nine patients had hyperparathyroid bone disease as revealed on roentgenogram, and three also had rickets. At the end of CAPD therapy, the hyperparathyroid lesions were healed in three, improved in four, and worse in two. The rachitic lesions healed in two patients and improved in one; however, two of the six children who started with no bone disease developed hyperparathyroid bone lesions and two others developed rickets.

Apparently, CAPD plus management of ROD can improve skeletal development. The proper Ca level in the dialysate and the types of vitamin D that should be given remain to be established. Currently dialysates contain 6.5–7.0 mg/dl (3.25 to 3.5 mEq/L) calcium. There is serious concern that Al can cause bone disease and dementia (109). Thus, dietary restriction of P and giving $CaCO_3$ as supplements are alternative treatments for hyperphosphatemia (see also Chapters 49 and 52).

In our patients, growth velocity was higher in those without roentgenographic evidence of bone disease. Vitamin D supplementation appears to improve growth in children with CRF (110, 111, 112), but more work is necessary to define the contribution of vitamin D deficiency relative to that of other abnormalities that affect growth.

COMPLICATIONS OF CONTINUOUS AMBULATORY PERITONEAL DIALYSIS

Peritonitis

One major disadvantage of CAPD is the relatively high rate of peritonitis. In experienced centers, the incidence is one episode per 11.1 treatment months (113).

Without underestimating the seriousness of peritonitis, one must appreciate that in most CAPD patients it is relatively easy to treat. Its start is insidious, with symptoms such as nausea or vague abdominal pain, but in a few hours the patient can be in a fair amount of abdominal discomfort. Suddenly, the dialysate becomes cloudy. After antibiotic therapy, the symptoms generally subside quickly. The classic triad for the diagnosis of peritonitis (abdominal pain, fever, cloudy peritoneal fluid) is not present invariably. Criteria for diagnosing peritonitis are described by Nolph and Sorkin (114) (Table 50C.4).

Our patients or their parents are trained to diagnose and r early treatment of peritonitis at home and are instructed

Table 50C.5
Complications of CAPD

Peritonitis
Hernia
Obesity (adults)
Hyperlipidemia
Hyponatremia
Orthostatic hypotension
Catheter dislocation and obstruction
Exit site infection
Tunnel infection
Dialysate leak around the catheter
Low back pain
Burn out
Anorexia

Table 50C.6
Diagnosis[109] and Treatment of Peritonitis

Required — cloudy dialysate with abdominal symptoms
— dialysate white cell count >100/mm^3
— dialysate neutrophils >50%

May be present but not required — Gram stain positive
— positive culture
— fever

1. Obtain a 10-ml specimen of dialysate for Gram stain, culture and sensitivity on centrifuged sample and cell count and differential on uncentrifuged sample.
2. Do 3 exchanges of dialysate without antibiotic using no dwell time (flushes).
3. Resume CAPD every six hours:
   a) If a gram-positive organism is present, add cephalothin 500 mg/l of dialysate to first exhange; for the following exchanges add cephalothin 250 mg/l of dialysate. Continue for 14 days.
   b) If a gram-negative organism is present, add tobramycin 1.7 mg/kg body weight to the first dialysate exchange; for the following exchanges add 8 mg/l of dialysate. Continue for 7 days.
   c) If no organism is detected on gram stain, add cephalothin 500 mg/l of dialysate plus tobramycin 1.7 mg/kg body weight for the first exchange; for the following exchanges, add cephalothin 250 mg/l and tobramycin 8 mg/l of dialysate. Continue the cephalothin for 14 days and the tobramycin for 7 days.
4. Add heparin (500–1000 IU/l) to the dialysate containing the antibiotic until the fluid is clear and/or no fibrin clots are present.
5. Repeat the cell count and differential as appropriate (at 7 or 14 days) after onset of treatment for peritonitis (earlier if indicated).

immediately if they suspect peritonitis. If the signs are suggestive, we instruct them to lavage the peritoneal cavity three times, using three quick bag exchanges, and to inject antibiotics into the next bag of dialysate (Table 50C.6). The cloudy bag is brought to the hospital for a cell count, Gram stain, and culture. The patient is examined by a physician and usually remains in the hospital for a few days. Generally, it is not necessary to give antibiotics intravenously, as blood cultures are usually negative and good serum levels of antibiotics are achieved through intraperitoneal administration (115). Rarely, we have managed patients entirely as outpatients.

Tobramycin and cephalothin have been used successfully by many centers for a number of years; other antibiotics may be used when necessary (Table 50C.7) (116). One should be cautious in adding a new or untried medication to the dialysate as it may damage the peritoneal membrane.

Many cases of peritonitis are believed to be secondary to contamination of the connecting tube spike. Skin organisms such as *Staphylococcus epidermidis* and *S. aureus* are frequently reported as causal agents; however, *S. viridans*, which is usually found in the oropharynx but not on the skin, also has been observed often (117). In children, gram-negative organisms are infrequent; in adults, these organisms are a serious concern as they may be a sign of a bowel rupture due to diverticulitis.

Eosinophilic peritonitis has been reported by a number of centers (118). The eosinophils are noted soon after CAPD begins; no cause has been found, though allergy to some constituent of the peritoneal dialysis system is believed to be responsible (119). It may resolve spontaneously or intraperitoneal hydrocortisone has been used successfully (120).

Fungal peritonitis is usually refractory to treatment, e.g., by intraperitoneal amphotericin B (121). Usually the catheter must be removed for a period of timc. Wc had one case of *Candida albicans* peritonitis that occurred one week after renal transplantation in a patient who had been managed on CAPD. The catheter was removed after intraperitoneal amphotericin B failed to resolve the infection; however, the transplant

Table 50C.7
Antibiotic Dosage for Patients on CAPD (Per Liter of Dialysate, Unless Otherwise Indicated)

Antibiotic	Loading Dose	Maintenance Dose
tobramycin	1.7 mg/kg/bag	8 mg
cephazolin	500 mg	250 mg
ampicillin	500 mg	50 mg
cloxacillin	1,000 mg	100 mg
penicillin	1,000,000 U	50,000 U
ticarcillin	1,000 mg	100 mg
co-trimoxazole		
sulfamethoxazole	400 mg	25 mg
trimethoprim	80 mg	5 mg
clindamycin	300 mg	50 mg
amikacin	125 mg	25 mg
vancomycin	10 mg/kg IV (max 1,000 mg) IV or 500 mg/L I.P.	30 mg
amphotericin B*		5 mg
5-fluorocytosin		100 mg
rifampin PO	10–20 mg/kg; given BID	

* Of questionable value.

failed and six weeks later a new catheter was inserted with no complications.

Sterile or culture-negative episodes of peritonitis have been reported (122). All centers are concerned when they are unable to culture the causal bacteria from the cloudy dialysate; some centers encounter this problem more frequently than others. Whether this reflects laboratory variability or different causal agents from center to center is not clear.

The best treatment of peritonitis is prevention, thus, careful teaching of sterile technique to the patient or parent cannot be overemphasized. When the spike has been contaminated, it must be sterilized by soaking in povidone-iodine for five min or the tube must be replaced.

Obviously, a fail-safe mechanism would be desirable. A millipore filter has reduced the rate of peritonitis (123, 124). Such a filter is commercially available (Peridex CAPD Filter, Millipore Corporation, Bedford, Mass.), but results of clinical trials are limited (125). Clinical trials are being performed on an ultraviolet sterilization apparatus (Travenol CAPD Ultraviolet Germicidal System, Deerfield, Ill.).

The incidence of peritonitis must be reduced for CAPD to be of lasting benefit. In 29 children managed by CAPD (126), the incidence was one episode per 12.5 patient-months, which is similar to our own experience (29). How centers analyze their incidence of peritonitis should be standardized. The usual method of pooling the number of CAPD treatment months from a particular center and factoring it by the number of episodes of peritonitis needs reevaluation. An approach has been presented that statistically analyzes CAPD peritonitis data that enables centers to compare their results and assess the efficiency of their techniques in preventing infection (127) by using life-table analysis and considering the first episode of peritonitis as an end event.

Hernia

Various types of hernias have been reported in children and adults on CAPD. We observed the development of most hernias as a consequence of CAPD in the first two yr of our program, usually in younger patients. Hernias in young children were inguinal, umbilical, or incisional (near the catheter exit site or in the areas of previous abdominal surgery). We have been able to defer repair of umbilical and incisional hernias until the time of renal transplantation; however, because inguinal hernias worsen with time we repair them when they develop. Surgery does not seriously upset the CAPD routine.

Some centers perform a peritoneogram at the time of the Tenckhoff catheter insertion and proceed to herniorrhaphy at that time if a patent tunica vaginalis is observed.

Blood Pressure Control

Orthostatic hypotension is observed more often in adult CAPD patients than it is in children, possibly because ultrafiltration is more efficient in adults. Although it seems that a large quantity of sodium might be removed by CAPD, the loss is not as great as suspected because of autoregulation of sodium balance (34). However, five adult CAPD patients have been reported (128) who were troubled by hypotension and had experienced symptomatic improvement through NaCl supplements. They attributed the beneficial effect of salt to expanded blood volume and increased sympathetic tone, as assessed by plasma norepinephrine levels. Symptomatic hypotension has been found (62) in 3 of 20 children on CAPD, in whom the mean blood pressure was 110/74 mm Hg compared with 129/79 for hemodialysis patients ($p < 0.005$ for systolic pressure).

CAPD was used successfully by Oreopoulos for blood pressure control in an adult with malignant hypertension, a high-renin state (personal communication). However, of the three children (aged 1, 5, 7 yr) in our series with ESRD resulting from the hemolytic uremic syndrome (which also produces a high-renin state), two were given captopril and one had bilateral nephrectomy to control hypertension (129). Nine of our 17 children received antihypertensives before CAPD; during CAPD, the medications were discontinued in six and reduced in two, and one patient had orthostatic hypotension. Antihypertensive drugs were used in 39% of children on CAPD in one study (62).

In spite of such difficulties, CAPD usually provides good blood pressure control for most adults and children. Components of the renin-angiotensin system in dialysate return have been demonstrated (130). Others report (60) excellent blood pressure control in children: of 13 patients receiving antihypertensive treatment before CAPD, only one child required treatment for hypertension while on CAPD.

The dialysis prescription and diet therapy for blood pressure control are variable. Salt and water intake, the amount removed by ultrafiltration, as well as urinary volume, are important factors. In addition, the activity of a renin-angiotensin system (native kidneys) also affects blood pressure. Therefore, one must assess the burden of bag changes (better fluid removal) and the risk of drug therapy in gaining control of blood pressure in children.

Burnout

Burnout is a term frequently heard in pediatric CAPD centers. CAPD for a child becomes a family affair and sometimes makes too many demands on the family.

Children >12 years are physically and mentally able to perform their own bag changes and to accept the responsibility for performing most of the CAPD routine. In fact, many become fastidious about their technique. We encourage parents to learn the CAPD technique as well, so they can do one daily bag change, preferably at one extreme of the day, permitting the patient to get more sleep at night. This is particularly important to the patient receiving four exchanges per day.

Nonetheless, in time many patients become weary of the repetitious routine and become slack about technique. It is important to watch for signs of burnout to prevent sloppy technique and resultant peritonitis. We sometimes admit a patient to the hospital for a short period while the nurses assume CAPD responsibilities; however, this is not a cost-effective remedy since the patient is not sick. Home helpers to perform the routine would be more appropriate; CCPD may be another remedy.

The parents of the younger patient, especially an infant, are at the highest risk for burnout. This occurs not only because anorexia, a problem in renal failure, is made worse with CAPD—the parent (usually the mother) must do four daily bag changes—but because the parent must spend considerable time feeding the child. Again, CCPD may be a solution. Also, some health workers or housekeepers, are necessary to help these families. It is essential to decrease the family's CAPD work burden, since prolonged use of CAPD may permit the infant to develop physically and mentally for a renal transplant at a more opportune time.

Anorexia and Tube Feeding

Anorexia

CRF is associated with nausea, vomiting, and anorexia, and CAPD permits the physician to prescribe a relatively free diet. Thus, we have bcome sensitive to anorexia in infants and children managed by CAPD. Insistence on adequate intake of energy and protein has produced even more feeding problems.

The specific cause or causes of anorexia related to renal failure and CAPD are not known. The periodic elevations of blood glucose from the glucose in the dialysate, the feeling of abdominal fullness from the dialysate, the hormonal changes produced by renal failure or CAPD, and the loss of essential nutrients in the dialysate all have been suspected. Further investigative work is necessary in this area.

Tube Feeding

The time consumed and the psychic trauma to the parent and child in attempting to feed the child has popularized tube feeding to infants and children with CRF. Guillot and coworkers (131) reported their experience with chronic renal enteral nutrition. Currently, we are comparing nasogastric and gastrostomy tube feedings. Three young children who required a gastrostomy tube also had esophageal reflux; consequently, plication of the fundus of the stomach is being performed during the same surgery. Frequently, nasogastric tube feeding precedes the gastrostomy and the possibility of the tube itself producing the reflux should be considered.

Many parents are pleased with tube feeding. It is easier, and improved nutrition and growth are frequently observed. The psychological consequences of tube feeding are unknown, so the physician must weigh the risks of malnutrition against the loss of oral gratification from eating.

RENAL TRANSPLANTATION FOR PATIENTS ON CONTINUOUS AMBULATORY PERITONEAL DIALYSIS

The preferred treatment for ESRD in childhood is a successful renal transplant. The difficulty is in establishing the correct time to perform the transplant. Success rates for transplantation in older children and adults are comparable (132). Some children prefer to proceed directly to a renal transplant with only a short period on dialysis. For such patients, hemodialysis appears preferable to CAPD until a cadaveric graft or a kidney from a live donor is available. Some children, however, may elect to finish the school year, and CAPD should provide them with enough free time to succeed at school.

A few years ago, some centers were reluctant to transplant CAPD patients for fear of infection. Enough experience has now accumulated in adults (132, 133) and children (134, 135) to say with confidence that these patients will encounter no more serious posttransplant complications than other recipients. In 23 of our children managed by CAPD before transplantation the actuarial graft survival was similar to that of children on hemodialysis, and patients who received no pretransplantation dialysis (Fig. 50C.5) (134). Although preoperative blood transfusions

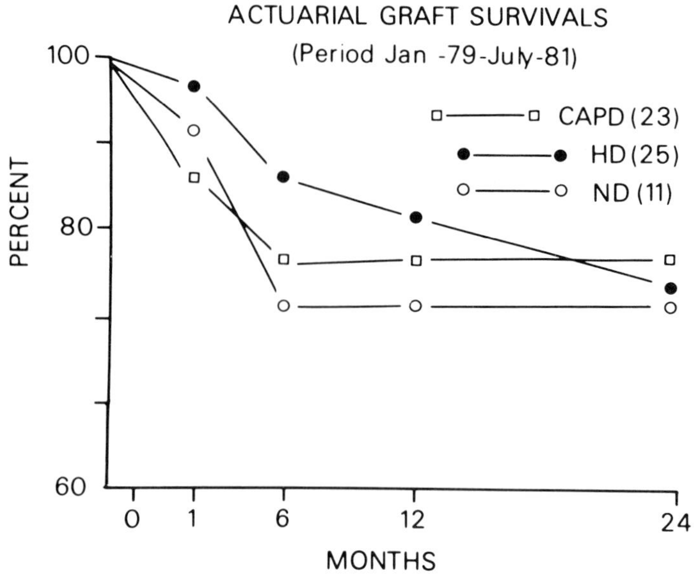

Figure 50C.5. Actuarial survival of graft in patients on either CAPD, HD, or no dialysis (ND). (From Stefanidis et al: Renal transplantation in children treated with continuous ambulatory peritoneal dialysis. Perit Dial Bull 3:5, 1983.)

may have a major beneficial effect on allograft survival (136), our CAPD children had received fewer transfusions than those treated with hemodialysis (1/2.6 CAPD treatment-months versus 1/1.5 treatment-months, $p < 0.005$).

Results for renal transplantation for the very young or very small patient, i.e., <2 years old, <10 kg body weight, have not been encouraging (137, 138). Recent results indicate that in highly specialized centers reasonably good results can be achieved in the very young (135, 136); yet for the present in many centers CPD in the very young seems preferable to enhance the likelihood of successful transplant surgery.

Graft Survival

A major concern in pediatric renal transplantation centers is the selection of an appropriate-sized graft for a child. If the graft is too large, the risk of underperfusion exists, which could result in infarction or thrombosis of the allograft. In addition, the GFR may be too large for the recipient, causing rejection that is undiagnosed, since increased plasma creatinine concentration (still our best index of rejection) may not be apparent. On the other hand, hyperfiltration or hyperperfusion of a graft too small for the recipient may also be injurious to the kidney. Apparently, grafts from donors <2 years and from anencephalic infants should not be used (139).

Does CAPD improve graft survival? Eleven of 12 children managed by CAPD before transplantation had a functioning allograft compared with only 7 of 21 children who had received hemodialysis (135). Subsequent studies report no differences; it appears that CAPD certainly is not a risk factor for renal transplantation.

Catheter Removal Following Transplant

The Tenckhoff catheter causes no problems after transplantation. If allograft acute tubular necrosis occurs, peritoneal dialysis can be used, provided the graft is extraperitoneal and the membrane is intact. We frequently observe postoperative ascites in ex-CAPD patients; the catheter facilitates drainage if necessary. Fever is also common, caused by infection or rejection. If the catheter is suspected as a site of infection, it should be removed. The removal time is variable. We remove it at transplantation if a vascular access is available or good graft function is certain or, otherwise, at a later, elective time, usually about one to two weeks after transplant surgery. Others remove the catheter two to three months after the surgery.

SUMMARY

CAPD can ensure growth comparable to that observed in the renal transplant patient. With improved nutrition, both orally and peritoneally, growth on peritoneal dialysis will be further enhanced; however, it places a tremendous burden on the family and child. "Although dialytic therapy for children with ESRD may be considered biologically successful, with a survival rate of 94% at 5 yr, serious deficits in short-term and long-term psychosocial development persist" (146).

CAPD and CCPD will have much to offer the child with serious CRF in the future; however, several aspects still require investigation or solution:

1. Prevention of parent or child fatigue. Should we be organizing teams of home peritoneal dialysis helpers to prevent burnout?
2. Improvement in the patient's nutrition. Will measures such as tube feeding and intraperitoneal amino acids, enhance growth and total well-being?
3. The role of trace metals in chronic CPD. Are they required as supplements to the diet or dialysate?
4. The different functions of the peritoneal membrane related to age.
5. Cost of peritoneal dialysis. Can it be reduced?
6. In-line filters and mechanisms to prevent peritonitis. A fail-safe device is needed.
7. Selection of patients or families best suited for peritoneal dialysis.
8. Prevention of ROD by establishing the correct calcium concentration in the dialysate, the correct type and amount of vitamin D, and the need for calcium supplementation and by identifying improved phosphate binders so aluminum can be excluded from therapy.

References

1. Ganter G: Über die Beseitigung giftiger Stoffe aus dem Blute durch Dialyse. Münch Med Wschr 70:1478, 1923.
2. Odel HM, Ferris DO, Power MH: Peritoneal lavage as an effective means of extrarenal excretion: a clinical appraisal. Am J Med 9:63, 1950.
3. Boen ST: Overview and history of peritoneal dialysis. Dial Transplant 6(2):12, 1977.
4. Oreopoulos DG: Renewed interest in chronic peritoneal dialysis. Kidney Int 13:S117, 1978.
5. Tenckhoff H: Peritoneal dialysis today: a new look. Nephron 12:420, 1974.
6. Palmer RA, Quinton WE, Gray JE: Prolonged peritoneal dialysis for chronic renal failure. Lancet 1:700, 1964.
7. Tenckhoff H, Schechter H: A bacteriologically safe peritoneal access device. Trans Am Soc Artif Intern Organs 14:181, 1968.
8. Lasker N, McCauley EP, Passarotti CT: Chronic peritoneal dialysis. Trans Am Soc Artif Intern Organs 12:94, 1966.
9. Tenckhoff H, Meston B, Shilipetar G: A simplified automatic dialysis system. Trans Am Soc Artif Intern Organs 18:436, 1972.
10. Oreopoulos DG: Chronic peritoneal dialysis. Clin Nephrol 9:165, 1978.
11. Popovich RP, Moncrief JW, Decherd JB, et al: The definition of a novel portable, wearable equilibrium peritoneal dialysis technique. Abstr Am Soc Artif Intern Organs 5:64, 1976.
12. National Registry, United States of America. Patient Population Demographic and Selected Outcome Measures for the Period January 1, 1981 through December 31, 1982. (Representing follow-up of 4,858 patients).
13. Price CG, Suki WN: Automated prolonged dwell peritoneal dialysis. Southeastern Dialysis & Transplantation Association 15:32, 1980 (abstract).
14. Diaz-Buxo JA, Walker CD, Farmer CD, et al: Continuous cyclic peritoneal dialysis (CCPD). Abstracts, Am Soc Nephrol 13:38A, 1980.
15. Esperanca MJ, Collins DL: Peritoneal dialysis efficiency in relation to body weight. J Pediatr Surg 1:162, 1966.
16. Putiloff PV: Materials for the study of the laws of growth of the human body in relation to the surface areas of the different systems; the trial on Russian subjects of planigraphic anatomy as a means for exact anthropometry—one of the problems of anthropology. Siberian Branch of the Russian Geographic Society, October 29, 1884, Omsk, 1886.
17. Henderson LW: The problem of peritoneal membrane area and permeability. Kidney Int 3:409, 1973.
18. Nolph KD, Miller F, Rubin J, Popovich R: New directions in peritoneal dialysis concepts and applications. Kidney Int [Suppl 10]:S-111, 1980.
19. Nolph KD, Sorkin M, Rubin J, et al: Continuous ambulatory peritoneal dialysis: three-year experience at one center. Ann Intern Med 92:609, 1980.
20. Wayland H, Silberberg A: Blood to lymph transport. Microvasc Res 15:367, 1978.
21. Rubin J, Nolph KD, Arfani D, et al: Clinical studies with a nonvasoactive peritoneal dialysis solution. J Lab Clin Med 93:910, 1979.
22. Tsilibary EC, Wissig SL: Absorption from the peritoneal cavity: SEM study of the mesothelium covering the peritoneal surface of the muscular portion of the diaphragm. Am J Anat 149:127, 1977.
23. Bresler EH, Groome LJ: On equations for combined convective and diffusive transport of neutral solute across porous membranes. Am J Physiol 241:F469, 1981.
24. Henderson LW, Nolph KD: Altered permeability of the peritoneal membrane after using hypertonic peritoneal dialysis fluid. J Clin Invest 48:992, 1969.
25. Boen ST: Peritoneal Dialysis in Clinical Medicine. Springfield, IL, Charles C Thomas, 1964.
26. Henderson LW: Peritoneal dialysis. In Massry SG, Sellers AL (eds): Clinical Aspects of Uremia and Dialysis. Springfield, IL, Charles C Thomas, 1976, p 555.
27. Daugirdas JT, Ing TS, Gandhi VC, et al: Kinetics of peritoneal fluid absorption in patients with chronic renal failure. J Lab Clin Med 95:351, 1980.
28. Kohaut EC, Alexander SR: Ultrafiltration in the young patient on CAPD. In Moncrief JW, Popovich JW (eds): CAPD Update: Continuous Ambulatory Peritoneal Dialysis. New York, Masson, 1981, p 221.
29. Balfe JW, Irwin MA, Oreopoulos DG: An assessment of continuous ambulatory peritoneal dialysis (CAPD) in children. In Moncrief JW, Popovich RP (eds): CAPD Update: Continuous Ambulatory Peritoneal Dialysis. New York, Masson, 1981, p 211.
30. Raja RM, Cantor RE, Boreyko C, et al: Sodium transport during ultrafiltration peritoneal dialysis. Trans Am Soc Artif Intern Organs 18:429, 1972.
31. Henderson L: Ultrafiltration with peritoneal dialysis. In Nolph KD (ed): Peritoneal Dialysis, (Developments in Nephrology 2). The Hague, Martinus Nijhoff, 1981, p 124.
32. Raja R, Kramer MS, Rosenbaum JL, et al: Evaluation of hypertonic peritoneal dialysis solutions with low sodium. Nephron 11:342, 1973.
33. Watson AR, Vigneux A, Willumsen J, Balfe JW: Continuous ambulatory peritoneal dialysis in children less than five years old. Eur J Pediatr 140:149, 1983 (abstract # 111).
34. Nolph KD, Sorkin MI, Moore H: Autoregulation of sodium and potassium removal during continuous ambulatory peritoneal dialysis. Trans Am Soc Artif Intern Organs 26:334, 1980.
35. Pyle WK, Moncrief JW, Popovich RP: Peritoneal transport evaluation in CAPD. In Moncrief JW, Popovich RP (eds): CAPD Update: Continuous Ambulatory Peritoneal Dialysis. New York, Masson, 1981, p 35.
36. Popovich RP, Pyle WK, Rosenthal DA, et al: Kinetics of peritoneal dialysis in children. In Moncrief JW, Popovich RP (eds): CAPD Update: Continuous Ambulatory Peritoneal Dialysis. New York, Masson, 1981, p 227.
37. Popovich RP, Moncrief JW, Nolph KD, et al: Continuous ambulatory peritoneal dialysis. Ann Intern Med 88:449, 1978.
38. Bergström J, Asaba H, Fürst P, Lindholm B: Middle molecules in chronic uremic patients treated with peritoneal dialysis. In Gahl GM, Kessel M, Nolph KD (eds): Advances in Peritoneal Dialysis, Proceedings of the Second International Symposium on Peritoneal Dialysis, Berlin, June 16–19, 1981. (International Congress Series No. 567). Amsterdam, Excerpta Medica, 1981, p 47.
39. Vigneux A, Hardy BE, Balfe JW: Chronic peritoneal catheter in children—one or two dacron cuffs? Peritoneal Dial Bull 1:151, 1981.
40. Rottembourg J, Jacq D, Vonlanthen M, et al: Straight or curled Tenckhoff peritoneal catheter for continuous ambulatory peritoneal dialysis? Peritoneal Dial Bull 1:123, 1981.
41. Alexander SR, Tank ES: Surgical aspects of continuous ambulatory peritoneal dialysis in infants, children and adolescents. J Urol 127:501, 1982.
42. Helfrich GB, Winchester JF: What is the best technique for implantation of a peritoneal catheter? Peritoneal Dial Bull 2:132, 1982.
43. Feldman W, Baliah T, Drummond KN: Intermittent peritoneal dialysis in the management of chronic renal failure in children. Am J Dis Child 116:30, 1968.
44. Counts S, Hickman R, Garbaccio A, Tenckhoff H: Chronic home peritoneal dialysis in children. Trans Am Soc Artif Intern Organs 19:157, 1973.
45. Potter DE: Comparison of peritoneal dialysis and hemodialysis in children. Dial Transplant 7:800, 1978.

46. Brouhard BH, Berger M, Cunningham RJ, et al: Home peritoneal dialysis in children. Trans Am Soc Artif Intern Organs 25:90, 1979.
47. Gagnadoux MF, Hernandez MA, Broyer M, et al: La dialyse péritonéale chronique: alternative de l'hémodialyse itérative chez l'enfant. Arch Fr Pediatr 34:860, 1977.
48. Baluarte HJ, Grossman MB, Polinsky MS, et al: Experience with intermittent home peritoneal dialysis (IHPD) in children. Pediatr Res 14:994, 1980 (abstract).
49. Lacke C, Senekjian HO, Knight TF, et al: Twelve months' experience with continuous ambulatory and intermittent peritoneal dialysis. Arch Intern Med 141:187, 1981.
50. Potter DE, McDaid TK, Ramirez JA: Peritoneal dialysis in children. In Atkins RC, Thomson NM, Farrell (eds): Peritoneal Dialysis. Edinburgh, Churchill Livingstone, 1981, p 356.
51. Lasker N: Chronic peritoneal dialysis. Pa Med 74:67, 1971.
52. Tenckhoff H, Merton B, Shilipetar G: A simplified automatic peritoneal dialysis system. Trans Am Soc Artif Intern Organs 18:436, 1972.
53. Fenton SSA, Cattran DC, Barnes NM, Waugh KJ: Home peritoneal dialysis: a major advance in promoting home dialysis. Trans Am Soc Artif Intern Organs 23:194, 1977.
54. Karanicolas S, Oreopoulos DG, Pylypchuk G, et al: Home peritoneal dialysis: 3 years' experience in Toronto. Can Med Assoc J 116:266, 1977.
55. Oreopoulos DG: Requirements for the organization of a continuous ambulatory peritoneal dialysis program. Nephron 24:261, 1979.
56. Fine RN: CCPD in pediatrics. In Current Status of CCPD. A Synopsis of the Symposium presented by St. Elizabeth's Hospital, Cambridge, MA, November 19, 1982. American Medical Products Corporation, 1983, p 6.
57. Lum GM: Peritoneal dialysis in children: a 6-year comparative analysis. Eur J Pediatr 140:150, 1983 (abstract # 115).
58. Alexander SR, Tseng CH, Maksym KA, et al: Clinical parameters in continuous ambulatory peritoneal dialysis for infants and children. In Moncrief JW, Popovich RP (eds): CAPD Update: Continuous Ambulatory Peritoneal Dialysis. New York, Masson, 1981, p 195.
59. Guillot M, Clermont MJ, Gagnadoux MF, Broyer M: Nineteen months' experience with continuous ambulatory peritoneal dialysis (CAPD) in children: main clinical and biological results. In Gahl GM, Kessel M, Nolph KD (eds): Advances in Peritoneal Dialysis, Proceedings of the Second International Symposium on Peritoneal Dialysis, Berlin, June 16–19, 1981 (International Congress Series No. 567). Amsterdam, Excerpta Medica, 1981, p 203.
60. Salusky IB, Lucullo L, Nelson P, Fine RN: Continuous ambulatory peritoneal dialysis in children. Pediatr Clin North Am 29:1005, 1982.
61. Eastham EJ, Kirpalani H, Francis D, et al: Paediatric continuous ambulatory peritoneal dialysis. Arch Dis Child 57:677, 1982.
62. Baum M, Powell D, Calvin S, et al: Continuous ambulatory peritoneal dialysis in children: comparison with hemodialysis. N Engl J Med 307:1537, 1982.
63. Twardowski ZJ, Prowant BF, Nolph KD, et al: High volume, low frequency continuous ambulatory peritoneal dialysis. Kidney Int 23:64, 1983.
64. Lowrie EG, Laird NM, Parker TF, Sargent JA: Effect of the hemodialysis prescription on patient morbidity. Report from the National Cooperative Dialysis Study. N Engl J Med 305:1176, 1981.
65. Gotch FA: A quantitative evaluation of small and middle molecule toxicity in therapy of uremia. Dial Transplant 9:183, 1980.
66. Nolph KD, Twardowski ZJ, Popovich RP, Rubin J: Equilibration of peritoneal dialysis solutions during long-dwell exchanges. J Lab Clin Med 93:246, 1979.
67. Shen FH, Sherrard DJ, Scollard D, et al: Thirst, relative hypernatremia, and excessive weight gain in maintenance peritoneal dialysis. Trans Am Artif Intern Organs 24:142, 1978.
68. Canoud B, Liendo-Liendo C, Mion C: Etude cinetique in vivo de l'ultrafiltration en dialyse peritoneale avec exchange prolonges. Methode et premiers resultats cliniques. J Urol Nephrol 85:897, 1979.
69. Rostand SG: Profound hypokalemia in continuous ambulatory peritoneal dialysis. Arch Intern Med 143:377, 1983.
70. Kohaut EC, Balfe JW, Potter D, et al: Hypermagnesemia and mild hypocarbia in pediatric patients on continuous ambulatory peritoneal dialysis. Peritoneal Dial Bull 3:41, 1983.
71. Cooke RE, Boyden DG, Haller E: The relationship of acidosis and growth retardation. J Pediatr 57:326, 1960.
72. James WPT, Hay AM: Albumin metabolism: effect of the nutritional state and dietary protein intake. J Clin Invest 47:1958, 1968.
73. Rothschild MA, Oratz M, Schreiber SS: Albumin metabolism. Gastroenterology 64:324, 1973.
74. Blumenkrantz MJ, Gahl GM, Kopple JD, et al: Protein losses during peritoneal dialysis. Kidney Int 19:593, 1981.
75. Blumenkrantz MJ, Kopple JD, Gutman RA, et al: Methods for assessing nutritional status of patients with renal failure. Am J Clin Nutr 33:1567, 1980.
76. Bianchi R, Mariani G, Giuseppina M, Carmassi F: The metabolism of human serum albumin in renal failure on conservative and dialysis therapy. Am J Clin Nutr 31:1615, 1978.
77. Oreopoulos DJ, Balfe JW, Khanna R, et al: Further experience with the use of amino acid containing dialysate (Amino-Dianeal) in peritoneal dialysis. In Moncrief JW, Popovich RP (eds): CAPD Update: Continuous Ambulatory Peritoneal Dialysis. New York, Masson, 1981, p 109.
78. Fennell RS, Orak JK, Garin EH, et al: Continuous ambulatory peritoneal dialysis in a pediatric population. Am J Dis Child 137:388, 1983.
79. Grodstein GP, Blumenkrantz MJ, Kopple JD, et al: Glucose absorption during continuous ambulatory peritoneal dialysis. Kidney Int 19:564, 1981.
80. Chan MK, Baillod RA, Chuah P, et al: Three years' experience of continuous ambulatory peritoneal dialysis. Lancet 1:1409, 1981.
81. Flynn CT, Shadur CA: A comparison of continuous ambulatory peritoneal dialysis in diabetic and nondiabetic patients. Am J Kidney Dis 1:15, 1981.
82. Stickler GB, Bergen BJ: A review: short stature in renal disease. Pediatr Res 7:978, 1973.
83. Betts PR, Magrath G: Growth pattern and dietary intake of children with chronic renal insufficiency. Br Med J 2:189, 1974.
84. Broyer M: Growth in children with renal insufficiency. Pediatr Clin North Am 29:991, 1982.
85. Cameron JS: The treatment of chronic renal failure in children by regular dialysis and by transplantation. Nephron 11:221, 1973.
86. Broyer M, Kleinknecht C, Loirat C, et al: Growth in children treated with long-term hemodialysis. J Pediatr 84:642, 1974.
87. Chantler C, Broyer M, Donckerwolcke RA, et al: Growth and rehabilitation of long-term survivors of treatment for end-stage renal failure in childhood. Proc Eur Dial Transplant Assoc 18:329, 1981.
88. Bosque M, Munian A, Bewick M, et al: Growth after renal transplants. Arch Dis Child 58:110, 1983.
89. Stefanidis CJ, Hewitt IK, Balfe JW: Growth in children receiving continuous ambulatory peritoneal dialysis. J Pediatr 102:681, 1983.
90. Kohaut EC: Growth in children with end-stage renal disease treated with continuous ambulatory peritoneal dialysis for at least one year. Perit Dial Bull 2:159, 1982.
91. Conley SB, Brewer ED, Gandy S, et al: Normal growth in very small children on peritoneal dialysis: 18 months experience. 12th Annual Clinical Dialysis and Transplant Forum, Chicago, December 8–13, 1982. Am J Kidney Dis (Suppl 1):8, 1982.
92. Wassner, SJ, Abitbol C, Alexander S, et al: Nutritional requirements for infants with renal failure. Am JKidDis 7(4):300, 1986.
93. Rotundo A, Nevins TE, Lipton M, et al: Progressive encephalopathy in children with chronic renal insufficiency in infancy. Kidney Int 21:486, 1982.
94. Simmons JM, Wilson CJ, Potter DE, Holliday MA: Relation of calorie deficiency to growth failure in children on hemodialysis and the growth response to calorie supplementation. N Engl J Med 285:653, 1971.
95. Hostetter TH, Rennke HG, Brenner BM: Compensatory renal hemodynamic injury: a final common pathway of residual nephron destruction. Am J Kidney Dis 1:310, 1982.
96. Balfe JW, Irwin MA: Continuous ambulatory peritoneal dialysis in pediatrics. In Legrain M (ed): Continuous Ambulatory Peritoneal Dialysis, Proceedings of an International Symposium, Paris, November 2nd and 3rd, 1979. Amsterdam, Excerpta Medica, 1980, p 131.
97. Blumenkrantz MJ: Protein and nitrogen metabolism during CAPD: comparison with haemodialysis. In Atkins RC, Thomson NM, Farrell PC (eds): Peritoneal Dialysis. Edinburgh, Churchill Livingstone, 1981, p 192.
98. Gahl GM, Baeyer HV, Averdunk R, et al: Outpatient evaluation of dietary intake and nitrogen removal in continuous ambulatory peritoneal dialysis. Ann Intern Med 94:643, 1981.
99. Canada Department of National Health and Welfare: Dietary Standards for Canada (rev. ed). Ottawa, Department of National Health and Welfare, 1975.
100. National Research Council, Committee on Dietary Allowances. Recommended Dietary Allowances (8th rev. ed). Washington, DC: National Academy of Sciences, 1974.
101. Oreopoulos DG, Crassweller P, Katirtzoglou R, et al: Amino acids as an osmotic agent (instead of glucose) in continuous ambulatory peritoneal dialysis. In Legrain M (ed): Continuous Ambulatory Peritoneal Dialysis, Proceedings of an International Symposium, Paris, November 2nd and 3rd, 1979. Amsterdam, Excerpta Medica, 1980, p 335.
102. Hanning RM, Balfe JW, Zlotkin SH: The efficacy of amino acid vs glucose dialysis in children on continuous ambulatory peritoneal dialysis. Pediatr Res 17 (4, pt. 2):350A, 1983 (abstract # 1580).
103. Counahan R, El-Bishti M, Chantler C: Oral essential amino acids in children on regular hemodialysis. Clin Nephrol 9:11, 1978.
104. Hsu AC, Kooh SW, Fraser D, et al: Renal osteodystrophy in children with chronic renal failure: an unexpectedly common and incapacitating complication. Pediatrics 70:742, 1982.

105. Calderaro V, Oreopoulos DG, Meema HE, et al: The evolution of renal osteodystrophy in patients undergoing continuous ambulatory peritoneal dialysis (CAPD). Proc Eur Dial Transplant Assoc 17:533, 1980.
106. Gokal R, Ramos JM, Ellis HA, et al: Histological renal osteodystrophy, and 25 hydroxycholecalciferol and aluminum levels in patients on continuous ambulatory peritoneal dialysis. Kidney Int 23:15, 1983.
107. Guillot M, Garabedian M, Lavocat C, et al: Evaluation of 25-hydroxyvitamin D and vitamin D binding protein losses in thirteen children on continuous ambulatory peritoneal dialysis. Int J Pediatr Nephrol, (in press).
108. Hewitt IK, Reilly BJ, Kooh SW, Balfe JW: Renal osteodystrophy in children undergoing continuous ambulatory peritoneal dialysis. J Pediatr, in press.
109. Parkinson IS, Ward MK, Feest TG, et al: Fracturing dialysis osteodystrophy and dialysis encephalopathy. An epidemiological survey. Lancet 1:406, 1979.
110. Chan JCM, Kodroff MB, Landwehr DM: Effects of 1,25-dihydroxyvitamin-D_3 on renal function, mineral balance, and growth in children with severe chronic renal failure. Pediatrics 68:559, 1981.
111. Chesney RW, Moorthy AV, Eisman JA, et al: Increased growth after long-term 1α,25-vitamin D_3 in childhood renal osteodystrophy. N Engl J Med 298:238, 1978.
112. Chesney, RW, Mehls O, Anast CS, et al: Renal osteodystrophy in children: the role of vitamin D, phosphorus and parathyroid hormone. AmJKidDis 7(4):275, 1986.
113. Williams C, Cattran D, Clayton S, et al: CAPD in Toronto—The first 5 years. Ann Roy Coll Phys Surg Can 16:384, 1983 (abstract).
114. Nolph KD, Sorkin MI: Continuous ambulatory peritoneal dialysis. In Brennen BM, Stein JH (eds): Chronic Renal Failure. New York, Churchill Livingstone, 1981, p 193.
115. Williams P, Khanna R, Vas S, et al: The treatment of peritonitis in patients on CAPD: to lavage or not? Perit Dial Bull 1:14, 1980.
116. Vas SI: Microbiologic aspects of chronic ambulatory peritoneal dialysis. Kidney Int 23:83, 1983.
117. Vas SI: Peritonitis during CAPD: a mixed bag. Perit Dial Bull 1:47, 1981.
118. Gokal R, Ramos JM, Ward MK, Kerr DNS: "Eosinophilic" peritonitis in continuous ambulatory peritoneal dialysis (CAPD). Clin Nephrol 15:328, 1981.
119. Humayun HM, Ing TS, Daugirdas JT, et al: Peritoneal fluid eosinophilia in patients undergoing maintenance peritoneal dialysis. Arch Intern Med 141:1172, 1981.
120. Leung ACT, Orange G, Henderson IS: Intraperitoneal hydrocortisone in eosinophilic peritonitis associated with continuous ambulatory peritoneal dialysis. Br Med J 286:766, 1983.
121. Bayer AS, Blumenkrantz MJ, Montgomerie JZ, et al: *Candida* peritonitis: report of 22 cases and review of the English literature. Am J Med 61:832, 1976.
122. Atkins RC, Humphery T, Thomson N, et al: Bacterial and 'sterile' peritonitis. Atkins RC, Thomson NM, Farrell PC (eds): In Peritoneal Dialysis. Edinburgh, Churchill Livingstone, 1981, p 272.
123. Mion C, Slingeneyer A, Liendo-Liendo C, et al: Reduction in incidence of peritonitis (P) associated with continuous ambulatory peritoneal dialysis (CAPD). Proc Clin Dial Transplant Forum 9:9, 1979.
124. Leahy TJ, Sullivan MJ, Slingeneyer A, Mion C: The efficiency of microbial retention by peritoneal dialysis filters. Trans Am Soc Artif Intern Organs 26:225, 1980.
125. Ash SR, Horswell R Jr, Heeter EM, Bloch R: Effect of the Peridex® filter on peritonitis rates in a CAPD population. Perit Dial Bull 3:89, 1983.
126. Fine RN, Salusky IB, Hall T, et al: Peritonitis in children undergoing continuous ambulatory peritoneal dialysis. Pediatrics 71:806, 1983.
127. Corey P: An approach to the statistical analysis of peritonitis data from patients on CAPD. Perit Dial Bull 1 (6) (suppl):S29, 1981.
128. Leenen FHH, Shah P, Boer WH, et al: Hypotension on CAPD: an approach to treatment. Peritoneal Dial Bull 3 (3) (suppl.):S33, 1983.
129. Powell HR, Rotenberg E, Williams AL, McCredie DA: Plasma renin activity in acute poststreptococcal glomerulonephritis and the haemolytic-uremic syndrome. Arch Dis Child 49:802, 1974.
130. Osmond DH, Loh AY, Dombros N, et al: Effects of continuous ambulatory peritoneal dialysis (CAPD) on the renin angiotensin system. Clin Res 26:870A, 1978.
131. Guillot M, Broyer M, Cathelineau L, et al: Nutrition entérale à débit constant en néphrologie pédiatrique. Résultats à long terme de son utilisation dans les néphroses congénitales, les cystinoses graves et les insuffisances rénales. Arch Fr Pediatr 37:497, 1980.
132. Fine RN: Transplantation in children. In Morris PJ (ed): Kidney Transplantation: Principles and Practice. London, Academic Press, 1979, p 353.
133. Moel DI, Butt KMH: Renal transplantation in children less than 2 years of age. J Pediatr 99:535, 1981.
134. DeShazo CV, Simmons RL, Bernstein DM, et al: Results of renal transplantation in 100 children. Surgery 76:461, 1974.
135. Arbus GS, Hardy BE, Balfe JW, et al: Cadaveric allografts in children aged 5 years or younger. Hospital for Sick Children, University of Toronto. Abstract. International Workshop in Recent Advances in Diagnosis and Treatment of Children with Chronic Renal Failure. Wichtig, Wichtig Editore, 1982.
136. Trompeter RS, Bewick M, Haycock GB, Chantler C: Renal transplantation in very young children. Lancet 1:373, 1983.
137. Iitake K, Martin LW, Cox JA, et al: Transplantation of cadaveric kidneys from anencephalic donors. J Pediatr 93:216, 1978.
138. Cardella CJ: The role of peritoneal dialysis in renal transplantation. In Fenton S, Kaye M, Price J (eds): The Treatment of End-Stage Renal Disease by Peritoneal Dialysis, A Monograph for the Canadian Clinician. Princeton Junction, 1982, p 119.
139. Gokal R, Ramos JM, Veitch P, et al: Renal transplantation in patients on continuous ambulatory peritoneal dialysis. Proc Eur Dial Transplant Assoc 18:222, 1981.
140. Stephanidis CJ, Balfe JW, Arbus GS, et al: Renal transplantation in children treated with continuous ambulatory peritoneal dialysis. Perit Dial Bull 3:5, 1983.
141. Alliapoulos JC, Ettenger RB, Salusky IB, et al: Improved allograft survival rates in patients undergoing continuous ambulatory peritoneal dialysis (CAPD). Pediatr Res 17:344A, 1983 (abstract # 1545).
142. Opelz G, Terasaki PI: Improvement of kidney-graft survival with increased numbers of blood transfusions. N Engl J Med 299:799, 1978.
143. Williams C, University of Toronto Collaborative Dialysis Group: CAPD in Toronto—an overview. Perit Dial Bull 3 (3) (suppl):S6, 1983.
144. Slingeneyer A, Canaud B, Mion C: Permanent loss of ultrafiltration capacity of the peritoneum in long-term peritoneal dialysis: an epidemiological study. Nephron 33:133, 1983.
145. Canadian Renal Failure Register 1981 Report. Kidney Foundation of Canada, 1982.
146. Weiss RA, Edelmann CM Jr: Children on dialysis. N Engl J Med 307:1574, 1982.

CHAPTER 51

Renal Transplantation

ROBERT B. ETTENGER
RICHARD N. FINE

INTRODUCTION

Renal transplantation usually is the goal of therapy for children with end-stage renal disease (ESRD) despite significant advances in dialysis therapy. A well-functioning kidney transplant improves psychological, social, and physical rehabilitation better than dialysis, but success is difficult to achieve. This chapter discusses the status of renal transplantation in children, emphasizing newer immunological strategies for improving the transplant outcomes.

INCIDENCE AND SURVIVAL

Incidence

The annual incidence of ESRD in children is approximately 1.5/million total population (1). If adolescents 16 to 21 yr of age and infants <1 yr old are included, this figure approaches 3/million children total population (2). Expressed another way, if the population is restricted to patients <15 yr of age, 25/million child population are being treated in European countries with well-developed ESRD facilities (3). From 1972 to the present, transplantation has been used in an increasing proportion of these children. According to the European Dialysis and Transplant Association (EDTA), in 1981 approximately 43% of children treated for ESRD had functioning transplants compared with 28% in 1972 (4).

Survival

The outcome of renal transplantation in children is comparable to that in adults for both patient and graft survival. Krakauer and associates have analyzed the efficacy of dialysis and transplantation in ESRD patients who began therapy between 1977 and 1980 (5). Table 51.1 shows comparable patient and allograft survival when comparing young (<10 yr old) or older children (11 to 20 yr) with the composite figure for patients >21 yr of age. Within the pediatric age group, patient survival appears to improve with increasing age while allograft outcome remains roughly comparable in all age groups (5, 6), except those <1 yr of age. As in adults (7), patient survival appears to be superior following living-related donor transplantation compared with first cadaver transplantation or dialysis (6). Currently, survival following first cadaveric transplant and dialysis is comparable in children aged 5 to 10 yr at all time intervals after transplant. At present, survival data for pediatric patients on chronic ambulatory peritoneal dialysis (CAPD) is too limited to allow comparison with children receiving renal transplants.

Over the past few years, the results of renal transplantation have started to improve with newer immunological manipulations; however, the survival of patients has been improving at an even greater rate, in large part because of a changing philosophy of medical care, which emphasizes less the saving of the kidney at all costs and stresses more the curtailment of aggressive immunosuppression in the failing renal transplant, the critically ill patient, or both (8).

CRITERIA FOR ACCEPTABILITY

Recipient Age

Cerelli and coworkers (9) reported the successful transplantation with a cadaver donor graft in a 9-month old girl who developed ESRD as a result of the hemolytic uremic syndrome. In contrast, experience with four infants, 6 weeks to 12 months of age, who received cadaver donor transplants was bad: all four died, leading the authors to conclude that the risk of transplantation in infants <1 yr of age required reevaluation (10).

The results of renal transplantation in children <1 yr and <5 yr of age have been reviewed. Of 13 infants 6 days to 12 months of age at the time of transplantation, 11 (85%) died and 2 had functioning grafts 13 and 44 months post transplant. Of the 4 infants whose grafts functioned initially, 1 died at three and one-half yr following transplant and 1 rejected the graft at 6 months following transplant; only 2 of 13 infants <1 yr of age at the time of transplantation survived with a functioning graft. Twelve of 13 infants received cadaver donor grafts, three of which were from anencephalic donors. Seventy-two children <5 yr of age received 92 grafts from 32 live-related and 60 cadaver donors; 19 had died (26%), and 43 had functioning grafts (60%) (12).

There was a striking difference in outcome depending on donor source. Of 32 live-related donor grafts in children <5 yr of age, 24 (75%) were functioning, whereas only 19 (32%) of 60 cadaver donor grafts were functioning (12). The advantage of live-related donor transplantation in children <5 yr of age was emphasized by Hodson and associates (13), who reported, cumulative four-yr patient survival rate of 77% and graft survival rates of 62% in 18 recipients. Conversely, the results of cadaver donor transplantation are poor (14). Only 1 of 12 infants, 1 to

Table 51.1. Patient and Allograft Survival Rates according to age of recipient

Age (yr)	Unrelated donor				Related donor			
	Patient survival (%)		Allograft survival (%)		Patient survival (%)		Allograft survival (%)	
	1 yr	3 yr	1 yr	3 yr	1 yr	3 yr	1 yr	3 yr
<10	89	80	58	46	93	89	80	71
11–20	92	87	59	46	97	95	77	68
21–>50	85	77	56	44	94	90	75	67

(Adapted from Krakauer H, et al; The recent U.S. experience in the treatment of end-stage renal disease by dialysis and transplantation. *N Engl J Med* 308: 1558, 1983.)

21 months of age, who received a cadaver donor graft had a functioning graft at the time of the report; 5 (42%) of the infants had died.

Recent reports (15, 16) are more encouraging. Trompeter and coworkers (15) described the results of 16 grafts (13 cadaver and 3 live-related donors) in 15 children <5 yr of age at transplantation; in a mean follow-up interval of 1.2 yr, 11 (75%) survived with functioning grafts and 4 (25%) had died. Growth postoperatively was encouraging, especially following initiation of alternate-day steroid therapy (ADT); however, only 4 of 10 children with a functioning graft for >3 months were above the 3rd centile growth curve, and only 4 of the 10 children exhibited catch-up growth. Of 39 cadaver donor grafts in 28 children <6 yr of age (16), 19 had functioning grafts and 6 (21%) had died after a mean follow-up period of 40 months. The causes of graft failure were primary nonfunction (25%), vascular thrombosis (25%), recurrent hemolytic uremic syndrome (20%), rejection (15%), and death (15%). Posttransplant growth appeared to parallel pretransplant growth in most of the children (around 80% of normal growth); however, only 4 (22%) were above the 10th percentile curve in stature.

From analysis of the preceding data, it is difficult to advocate cadaveric renal transplantation as the optimal treatment modality in young children with ESRD. The short-term outcome of cadaver donor transplantation in infants <1 yr of age has been rather dismal and, except for the recent reports (15, 16), the results of cadaver donor transplantation in young children between 1 and 5 yr of age have been disappointing. The long-term results of the latter two reports are difficult to assess, since the mean follow-up period was only 14 and 40 months, respectively.

The outcome of live-related, parental donor transplantation in children 1 to 5 yr of age has been more encouraging. Reports from Minnesota (13, 17) indicate that 18 of 28 (64%) initial live-related donor grafts were functioning; only 5 (18%) of the young children had died. The follow-up periods ranged from 13 to 75 months (13) and 20 to 112 months (17), respectively.

The last four reports stressed growth response following renal transplantation; however, few children sustained catch-up growth. In most of the recipients, status following transplant remained at the same standard deviation score or worsened.

The impact of renal transplantation on psychomotor development is difficult to assess. No serial measurements are included in any of the reports; however, of the 10 children with functioning grafts reported by Rizzoni and associates (12), 7 were attending regular school, 2, a school for handicapped children, and 1, a nursery school. Intellectual assessment of 15 children with functioning grafts (16) revealed 6 with high average, 5 average, 3 low average, and 1 mildly retarded. Miller and coworkers (17) indicated that all recipients had delayed psychomotor development at the time of transplantation. Following transplantation 8 of 10 recipients with a functioning graft were said to be functioning "at close to or at normal levels." Specific developmental test results were available in four recipients; two were functioning at a normal level for chronological age, and two were retarded.

The optimal treatment modality for the young child with ESRD is, therefore, difficult to determine. If a live-related donor is available, transplantation is an acceptable option. From available information, however, it is not possible to predict the long-term outcome of such an undertaking. Cadaver donor transplantation for children <1 yr of age should probably not be attempted according to available data. With the availability of some form of continuous peritoneal dialysis, these children can be managed until an adequate assessment of their psychomotor development can be made. If an infant is thriving with continuous peritoneal dialysis (CPD), it is probably reasonable to defer transplantation until a later date. Cadaver donor transplantation is a reasonable alternative to unsatisfactory dialysis therapy in children 1 to 5 yr of age.

Donor Age

Anencephalic Donors

To date, one or both kidneys from anencephalic donors have been used for transplantation in 19 recipients, aged 6 days to 18 years (Table 51.2). Of the 19 allografts, 12 (63%) never functioned, primarily due to poor perfusion secondary to vascular thrombosis; however, 4 of the remaining 7 allografts provided adequate long-term function. The longest survivor is a boy with prune belly syndrome who received a graft at 4 years of age; at 9½ yr of age his serum creatinine was 0.5 mg/dl and his height was between the 10th and 25th centile for chronological age (18).

The other three instances of long-term functioning of grafts from anencephalic infants include an infant who underwent surgery at 3 months, survived 3½ yr, and died of hypertensive encephalopathy (11, 14) and two children who were surviving one and one-half and three yr post transplant. Three additional grafts from anencephalic children functioned from one to three months.

In addition to the significant incidence of primary nonfunction, other problems surround the use of kidneys from anencephalic donors (18). There is a high incidence (15%) of urinary tract malformation (18). In addition, the anencephalic newborn may clinically deteriorate before a suitable histocompatible donor can be found (18). Although long-term successes have occurred using grafts from anencephalic donors, the high rate of primary nonfunction and other problems argue against their continued use.

Pediatric Donors

In an analysis of the results of 6883 kidney transplants from the American College of Surgeons/National Institute of Health (ACS/NIH) Registry according to donor age (19), graft survival was significantly better in those from the 11 to 20 and 21 to 30 yr of age donor group, when compared with those from older donors. A stepwise decline in graft survival rates was shown when the data were analyzed according to donor age by decades of life. This relationship between donor age and graft survival was confirmed by Morling and associates (20). Unfortunately, in neither of these studies were pediatric donors <10 yr of age included.

The use of cadaver kidneys from children <10 yr of age is controversial (21). A comparison of transplant outcome with cadaver kidneys from donors 0 to 5 yr of age with donors 6 to 10 and 11 to 20 yr of age showed that the survival rate for those from the 0 to 5 yr of age donor graft was less than it was for those from the other two age groups (22). Children who received grafts from pediatric donors 0 to 5 yr of age had poorer outcomes than those receiving grafts from donors 6 to 10 yr of age.

A recent report detailed the results of 440 consecutive cadaver donor grafts according to the decade of donor age (23). At 24 months post

Table 51.2. Transplantation in Infants Less Than 1 Yr of Age

Author	Age (Mo.)	Primary renal disease	Donor	Function (Mo.)	Outcome
Goodwin, et al (17a)	6 d	Prune belly syndrome	C, AN	NF	Died
Cerilli, et al (9)	5	HUS	C	13	Alive
De Shazo, et al (10)	12	—	C	—	Died
	5	—	C	—	Died
	4	—	C	—	Died
	1½	—	C	—	Died
Lawson, et al (449)	¼	—	C	NF	Died
	9	—	LD	—	Died
	12	—	C	—	Died
Kwun, et al (11)	1	PKD	C, AN	NF	Died
Moel and Butt (14)	3	CN	C, AN	6 R	Died
	8	OU	C	42 R	Died
Miller, et al (17)	11	OU	C	44	Alive

C = cadaver.
AN = anencephalic.
NF = nonfunction.
R = rejection.
d = days.
HUS = hemolytic-uremia syndrome.
PKD = polycystic kidney disease.
CN = cortical necrosis.
OU = obstructive uropathy.

transplant, the 0 to 10 and >51 yr of age donor groups had a 30% graft survival rate, whereas the other age groups had a 50% to 60% graft survival rate. Primary nonfunction contributed to the poor graft survival rate in the 0 to 10 age group, particularly with infant kidneys. In contrast, an analysis of the results of cadaver donor transplants from the EDTA between 1967 and 1981 showed that the 5-yr graft survival rate of 5993 grafts from donors 11 to 50 yr of age was almost identical (43.3%) to that of 626 grafts from donors <11 yr of age (43.6%) (24). The reasons for these discrepancies are not obvious; however, the proportion of donors <5 yr of age—especially those <1 yr of age—may account for the discrepancies.

Although the use of a single kidney from infants undergoing uretero-subarachnoid shunting for hydrocephalus provided adequate function in adult recipients (25), others have suggested (26) that en bloc transplantation of both cadaver kidneys from a child into adult recipients was advantageous. However, two studies, examining a total of 55 single kidneys from donors 1½ to 10 yr of age, demonstrated that such kidneys provided adequate renal function when transplanted into adult recipients (27, 28). In addition, serial measurements have been made of four kidneys from donors 4 to 5 yr of age, transplanted into adult recipients. The longitudinal axis of the kidneys measured 10.1 to 10.8 cm at the time of transplantation, and at five to nine months post transplant the grafts increased to 13.2 to 13.6 cm (28a).

One can conclude that a single cadaver kidney from an infant donor >1½ yr of age can provide adequate function for an adult recipient. The high incidence of complications with kidneys from infants <1 yr of age argues against their use, except perhaps under the special circumstances of an infant recipient (29).

Adult Donors

A report by Miller and associates (17) on renal transplantation in 12 children, weighing between 5400 and 8800 g, with grafts from adult donors indicates the technical feasibility of using adult kidneys for transplantation into very small recipients. Despite the technical feasibility of using an adult kidney in a very small child, we prefer to use pediatric cadaver kidneys for children weighing <10 kg; however, when immunological considerations dictate the use of adult kidneys in small children, this is practical.

Mental and Neurological Status

The infant with significant developmental delay and the child with severe mental retardation who has ESRD or progressive renal insufficiency pose a difficult problem. The major issues raised include the questions: Will preemptive introduction of ESRD care prevent or reverse the degree of intellectual impairment associated with uremia? Should the life of a child with severe mental retardation be prolonged by ESRD care? To what extent will the rigors of the treatment adversely affect the consciousness of the retarded child?

Although neurological disturbances in uremia have been appreciated for sometime, the magnitude of the problem has recently been noted in children. A distinct syndrome has been described (30) in six children, aged 26 months to 10 yr, with congenital renal disorders; this was characterized by myoclonus, dysarthria, seizures, dementia, and coma. The syndrome was evident when there was severe and persistent renal functional impairment (5 to 10 ml/min/1.73 m^2), despite dialysis and successful transplantation. Bale and coworkers (51) noted similar abnormalities in three children; however, the findings were initially observed when the GFR was 15 to 25 ml/min/1.73 m^2. Aluminum intoxication has been implicated (30); however, the cerebrospinal fluid Al concentration measured in one child was normal (31).

In a retrospective analysis of 23 children with chronic renal insufficiency (CRI) diagnosed before 1 yr of age (32), 20 of the 23 children had a progressive encephalopathy with developmental delay; four developed symptoms before receiving Al therapy, and all had symptoms before dialysis.

These reports suggest a deleterious effect of uremia on the developing brain, since all patients had evidence of renal functional impairment during the first year of life. It was suggested (31, 32) that earlier dialysis

in four patients following transplantation (66, 69). In our experience the degree of photophobia has remained unchanged.

In one study, hypothyroidism did not develop in any of nine children following transplantation (69). However, it occurred in one child followed by us six years post transplant. Those who are hypothyroid before transplantation require continued thyroid supplementation post transplant.

The growth of most children with cystinosis is severely retarded before transplantation. Although growth occurs post transplant, they remain severely growth retarded (70); however, pubertal development has been reported in children with cystinosis following successful transplantation (68, 70).

Although oxalosis may cause ESRD in infancy (71), few children with oxalosis have received renal allografts. The EDTA Pediatric Registry reporting on 25 children with oxalosis noted that five of nine post transplant patients had functioning grafts (3).

Because of the poor outcome of renal transplantation due to disease recurrence in the graft, patients with oxalosis were previously excluded as acceptable transplant candidates. Unfortunately the outlook with dialysis is also poor; tissue deposition of oxalate progresses, causing cardiac dysfunction and severe osteodystrophy. However, Leumann and associates (72) reported 3 yr survival of a cadaveric renal allograft in a 14-yr-old girl; successful cadaveric graft function for 10 yr was reported by Whelchel and coworkers (73) in a 43-yr-old woman who initially presented with oxalosis at age 19 yr. Both of these reports stress the importance of reducing the oxalate load with prophylactic pyridoxine, as well as daily dialysis preceding and following transplant if acute tubular necrosis or rejection occurs.

IMMUNOLOGICAL PARAMETERS AFFECTING ALLOGRAFT SURVIVAL

Histocompatibility

The success of kidney transplantation depends on many factors. One of the most important is the immune response of the recipient to histocompatibility antigens present in the donor but absent in the recipient. Histocompatibility antigens are genetically determined cell surface molecules distinctive for each individual. The histocompatibility antigens of all species include a system called the major histocompatibility complex (MHC), as well as a number of minor systems. Major and minor systems were originally designated in the mouse on the basis of the strength of rejection responses induced by skin and tumor grafts. The human MHC is called the HLA system (human leukocyte antigen), the antigens of which are present on virtually all nucleated cells, including all lymphocytes. The minor histocompatibility systems in humans are poorly defined but include several red cell antigen systems, e.g., Lewis, as well as antigens on vascular endothelial cells.

HLA Genetic Region

The HLA system, which is one of the most polymorphic genetic systems yet defined in humans, is on the short arm of chromosome 6 (Fig. 51.1). The phenotypic expression of HLA antigens follows a simple mendelian codominant pattern, i.e., if an allele is present on the chromosome, it is always expressed on the cell surface. The antigens inherited from a given parent on a single chromosome are referred to as a haplotype. (Fig. 51.2).

The HLA genetic region includes three categories of genes: those coding for serologically defined (SD) antigens (class I antigens: HLA-A, HLA-B, HLA-C); those inducing lymphocyte-defined (LD) antigens (Class II: HLA-D/-DR); and a group of genes coding for C2, C4, and factor B (C3 proactivator) of the complement system (class III antigens), as well as some enzymes. In addition, there are undoubtedly other genes coding for antigens important in transplant rejection that have not yet been defined in humans

Class I SD Antigens: HLA-A, -B, -C. These HLA antigens are cell membrane molecules, each consisting of two noncovalently linked glycoproteins. One glycoprotein is a 44,000 dl heavy chain that carries the antigen specificity and is variable. The other glycoprotein molecule is an 11,500 dl light chain β-2 microglobulin that is encoded by chromosome 15 (74). These SD antigens are detected by a standard microlymphocytotoxicity assay in which a known HLA antibody (usually a human serum) is incubated in the presence of rabbit complement with lymphocytes from the individual being typed (75).

Each HLA gene locus is polymorphic; over 50 well-defined class I HLA antigen specificities have been established (76). The HLA antigens are termed by numbers, e.g., HLA-A2, -A11, -B5, -B15. Every individual has two HLA haplotypes, one inherited from each parent, and each haplotype codes for three class I antigenic structures: A, B, and C. Therefore, the typing of one individual will reveal two HLA-A antigens,

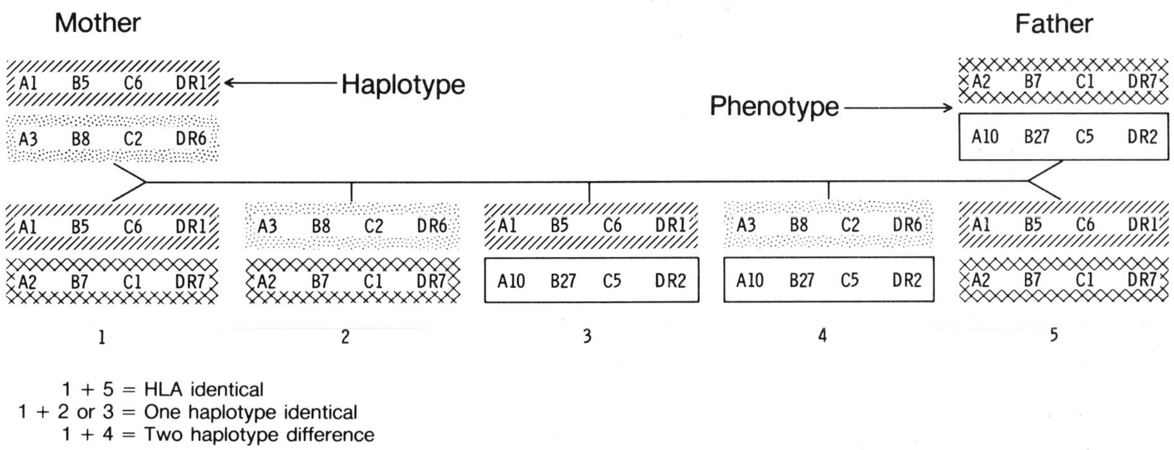

Figure 51.1. The major histocompatibility complex in humans is located on short arm of chromosome 6. This figure depicts locations of genes coding for class I and well-defined class II (D/DR) antigens, as well as those genes that govern production of some complement components. In addition, closely linked genes are responsible for development of several disease processes, including idiopathic hemochromatosis and congenital adrenal hyperplasia due to 21-hydroxylase deficiency. (cM = centimorgan map unit). (From Strom T B: The improving utility of renal transplantation in the management of end-stage renal disease. *Am J Med* 73:105, 1982.)

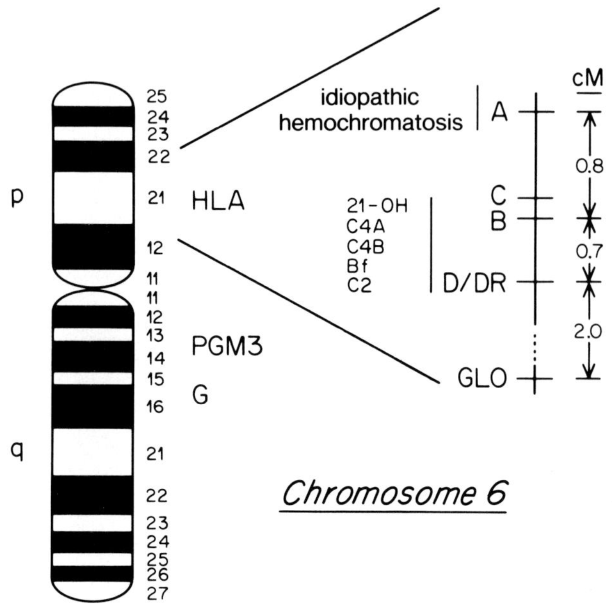

Figure 51.2. Genetics of HLA.

two HLA-B antigens, and two HLA-C antigens, although the last are less routinely typed. By simple mendelian inheritance, any given sibling pair has a 25% chance of having identical haplotypes; 50% will share one haplotype and the remaining 25% will be completely incompatible (Fig. 51.2).

Class II, LD Antigens: HLA-D/-DR. The class II HLA antigens consist of two noncovalently linked membrane glycoproteins, a 34,000 DA (Dalton) α-chain and a 29,000 DA β-chain. These antigens are also highly polymorphic. Class II antigens, termed HLA-D antigens, have a more restricted tissue distribution than class I antigens. They are present on B lymphocytes, monocytes, endothelial cells, activated T lymphocytes and sperm, but not on platelets or quiescent T lymphocytes. Mismatching for the HLA-D antigens between two populations of lymphocytes from different individuals stimulates a proliferative blastogenic response when these lymphocyte populations are cultured together; this is termed the mixed lymphocyte culture (MLC) reaction (77).

A series of antigens that are closely related, if not identical to HLA-D antigens, have been described recently. These antigens have been termed HLA-DR, for "D-related." These antigens are the targets of specific antibodies and, therefore, can be serologically identified in a manner similar to the HLA-A, -B, and -C antigens (78). The restricted cellular distribution of D-DR antigens makes it possible to use T-depleted, B cell–enriched lymphocytes for the typing. At least 10 HLA-DR specificities have been described and termed DR1 through DR10. Individual DR antigens are usually associated with corresponding HLA-D antigens; however, the precise relationship between HLA-D and HLA-DR is not yet clear. This association between D and DR determinants could represent identity or a high degree of linkage between two closely located gene loci. There are reports of dissociation between a specific D and a corresponding DR antigen, which supports the second theory.

Role of HLA Matching

Effect of HLA-A and HLA-B (class I) Matching

HI A-A and HLA-B matching is important in intrafamilial, living-related transplantation. The survival of allografts from HLA-identical siblings is far superior to the outcome of grafts from HLA haploidentical-related donors. The three-year graft survival rate ranges between 80% and 90% (79, 80) for intrafamilial HLA identical transplants, whereas our data (39) and that of others (79, 80) show a cumulative three-yr graft survival rate of 50% to 75% in intrafamilial haploidentical transplants. The importance of HLA matching in living-related transplantation is probably due to the fact that matching for the known HLA determinants within a family virtually assures compatibility for all gene products encoded within the haplotype. This is not the case when considering matching for HLA antigens in cadaver renal transplantation.

The value of HLA-A and -B matching in cadaver renal transplantation is less clear. Some single-center studies have demonstrated a correlation between HLA-A and -B matching and improved cadaver renal allograft outcome (81). In studies by Broyer and coworkers (81) in 130 children, the graft survival rate for three and four HLA-A and -B antigen-matched kidneys was 85% at five yr compared wtih 59% for grafts matched for 0, 1, or 2 HLA antigens. The multicenter Eurotransplant group found that improved HLA-A and -B matching significantly improved patient and graft survival in 2522 transplants (82). At five years, patient and graft survival rates with four antigen-matched grafts were 72% and 51%, respectively, whereas in grafts with no antigens matched, patient and graft survival rates were 54% and 32%, respectively ($p = 0.0005$) (82). In contrast, the multicenter study of Opelz and associates (83) found no effect on HLA-A and -B matching in 1697 transplants. Other studies have also found little or no effect of HLA-A and -B matching and graft outcome. In our experience with 178 first cadaver transplants in children, HLA-A and -B matching had no effect on the allograft survival rate (84), although a trend toward better outcome with improved matching was noted in the highly presensitized recipients, i.e., those with anti-HLA antibodies against more than 50% of a random panel of lymphocytes.

The overall effect of HLA-A and -B matching on cadaver renal allograft survival probably is highly variable; in comparison to the effect of HLA-DR matching on graft survival, it appears to be minimal.

Effect of HLA-DR (class II) Matching

Matching for HLA-DR antigens in cadaver renal transplantation appears to correlate well with allograft outcome (83, 85–89). Optimal DR matching is associated with significant improvement of graft outcome. This is true with DR matches (87, 88, 89) or mismatches (86, 89). Taken together, these reports show one-yr graft survival rates of 75% to 92% with optimal (2-DR) matched kidneys, compared with 41% to 56% with the poorest degree of DR matching (no DR antigen shared). Grafts mismatched for 1-DR antigen appear to do as poorly as those mismatched for 2-DR antigens (86–88). Thus, it appears the success of DR matching is an all-or-none phenomenon. The efficacy of DR matching makes sense on theoretical grounds. Class II antigens activate recipient helper T-lymphocytes, which leads to the production of interleukin-2, the release of a macrophage stimulant, and the formation of interleukin-1 and -2 receptors, which in turn propagate the rejection process through the generation of cytotoxic T-lymphocytes (90).

Optimal matching for DR antigens is feasible without significantly prolonging the waiting time on dialysis. Goeken and associates found that the mean waiting time for a DR-compatible kidney was approximately four months (91).

Effect of HLA Antigen Matching on Multiple Transplants

When multiple transplants are considered, most investigators have found no effect of HLA-A and -B matching on graft survival (83, 92); however, in our experience, there was a trend toward improved graft survival with better HLA-A and -B matching, particularly in highly

Table 51.4. Variables to be Considered in Selecting a Kidney Transplant Donor

Variable	Requirement
ABO blood groups	Compatibility mandatory
Rh blood group	Compatibility of doubtful importance
Class I (HLA A, B, C) matching	Cadaver grafts: minor importance Living-related grafts: major importance Broadly presensitized recipients: major importance
Class II (HLA DR) matching	Probably of major importance
Lewis antigen system	Lewis-negative recipient should receive Lewis-negative graft

presensitized patients (84, 92). HLA-DR matching had a beneficial effect on the outcome of second cadaver kidney transplants (83).

Immunological Selection of Donor

Since graft loss is most frequently due to rejection, immunological dissimilarities that provoke a rejection response should be avoided; however, even the best matches by our present histocompatibility criteria still have an appreciable failure rate because all variables have not been identified. Table 51.4 lists some of the more important recognized variables.

ABO Blood Group Antigens

Compatibility between the ABO blood groups of donor and recipient as applied in clinical transfusion is an absolute requirement for transplantation (93). Almost all transplants done across this barrier have led to the destruction of the graft with early vascular rejection (94), suggesting that these antigens are important histocompatibility antigens. A and B blood group antigens present on the endothelial cell surface of the kidney (95) probably serve as targets for the naturally occurring anti-A and -B antibodies of the recipients.

Successful crossing of the ABO barrier in living-related transplants has been reported in five of six cases following exhaustive plasmapheresis to lower the isohemagglutinin titers, administration of the relevant ABO antigen to bind residual antibody, and transfusion of donor platelets (96). This approach is still highly experimental.

Rhesus (Rh) Antigens

The role of Rh antigens in kidney transplantation is still debated. Their presence in kidney homogenates has been well documented (97); however, no difference has been found in graft survival between Rh-negative and Rh-positive recipients (98, 99). In fact, Huestis and Zukoski documented very good graft survival associated with the production of Rh antibodies following transplantation of Rh-positive kidneys to Rh-negative recipients (99). Nevertheless, some reports have shown approximately a 13% poorer graft survival rate in Rh-negative compared to Rh-positive recipients (100). We conclude that Rh antigens play, at most, a minor role in transplant immunology.

Lewis Antigens

Lewis-a and -b antigens have been identified on renal tubular epithelium (101). A large retrospective study showed a significant effect of Lewis antigen-matching on cadaver kidney graft survival (102). Lewis-negative recipients had an 8% lower graft survival rate than that of Lewis-positive recipients. Currently, matching for Lewis antigens is not practiced in clinical transplantation. Black recipients, who have a high incidence of being Lewis-negative, may benefit from prospective typing and matching for these antigens.

Endothelial-Monocyte System

The importance of an endothelial monocyte (E-M) antigen system has recently been recognized. These antigens are present on the plasma membrane of the endothelial cells (103) of peritubular capillaries and venules. The endothelial antigens crossreact with peripheral monocytes but not with lymphocytes (104, 105).

E-M antigens appear to be important in graft rejection since (a) pretransplant donor-specific antibodies against these antigens are associated with accelerated acute rejection in the absence of lymphocytotoxic antibodies (105), even in HLA-identical living-related transplants (106); (b) circulating anti-E-M antibodies appear in close temporal association with irreversible vascular rejection in about 50% of the patients (107); and (c) E-M antibodies can be eluted from rejected grafts (105, 107).

Matching for E-M antigens is not yet routinely practiced because of methodological difficulties and because all antimonocyte antibodies are not necessarily directed against endothelial cells of the peritubular capillaries (108).

Presensitization

Presensitization refers to preformed anti-HLA antibodies in the serum of the potential recipient, which may arise after a number of stimuli, e.g., pregnancy, infection, blood transfusion, or graft rejection. Two aspects of presensitization should be considered before transplantation: (a) the presence of specific presensitization against the donor in question and (b) the spectrum of presensitization against multiple HLA antigens, as represented by a lymphocyte panel.

Humoral Donor-specific, Presensitization: Lymphocyte Crossmatching (Table 51.5). It is extremely important to establish whether a recipient is specifically sensitized against a donor's histocompatibility antigens. Such presensitization, manifested by preformed lymphocytotoxic antibodies against the donor's HLA-A and -B antigens, results in hyperacute rejection (109–110). Presensitization is tested by a lymphocyte crossmatch between the recipient serum and the donor lymphocytes (110). The technique used in crossmatching is the standard complement-dependent microlymphocytotoxicity test (CDC) (75).

A negative lymphocyte crossmatch was previously considered an absolute prerequisite for transplantation; however, this requirement has

Table 51.5. Significance of Various Crossmatch Techniques in Renal Transplantation

Target cell	Significance
Donor T lymphocyte	1. Must be negative at time of transplant (109, 109a, 110) 2. May be acceptable if noncurrent serum is + but current serum is −. (121, 122, 123)
Donor B lymphocyte	
Room temperature incubation	Not associated with inferior allograft outcome (110a, 111, 111a)
"Cold" incubation	Not harmful (116, 117)
"Warm" incubation	May be harmful (118a, 119) but not invariably (83, 120, 120a)
Recipient autologous T and/or B lymphocytes	Not harmful (114, 114a, 117, 121)
Monocyte	Probably harmful (105, 106, 106a)

undergone modification. Most studies have shown that preformed antibodies against donor B but not donor T-lymphocytes are not associated with hyperacute rejection or inferior graft outcome (111). Occasional studies have reported different results, such as acute rejection or poorer graft survival rates, in B-cell crossmatch positive transplants (112). Some of these discrepant results occur because the B-lymphocyte crossmatch detects many different types of antibodies, such as (a) anti-DR antibodies; (b) anti-HLA-A, -B, or -C antibodies that are too weak to react against T-lymphocytes but will react with these antigens on the B-lymphocytes (113); (c) autoreactive antibodies (114); or (d) others, including anti-Lewis antibodies (115).

B-lymphocyte antibodies have been divided by the incubation temperature at which they react into "cold," i.e., 5 °C, or "warm" (37 °C) antibodies. Antibodies against B-lymphocytes reactive in the cold frequently are autoantibodies (114) that are not harmful (116) and may even be enhancing (117) to graft survival. The significance of warm anti-B cell antibodies is not clear (118). Although some have reported graft failure following positive "warm" B-cell crossmatches (119), others have found no difference in graft outcome (83, 120). Given the heterogeneity of the antibodies involved, positive B-lymphocyte crossmatches due to antibodies that are not deleterious, such as autoreactive antibodies, should be identified wherever possible (117, 121).

Despite adherence to the requirement for a negative pretransplant T-lymphocyte crossmatch, antibody-mediated rejection episodes and graft failure do occur. Possible explanations include (a) the presence of deleterious antibodies against antigenic systems not detected by lymphocyte crossmatching, e.g., the E-M system; (b) the presence of low levels of deleterious anti-HLA-A and -B antibody below the sensitivity threshold of the microlymphocytotoxicity test (122); (c) the existence of immunological memory allowing the secondary generation of donor-specific anti-HLA-A and -B antibodies that were previously present and then receded. Anti-HLA antibodies are known to appear and disappear over time and so may not be present and detectable at the time of transplant. A solution to this problem may lie in performing pretransplant crossmatching with noncurrent sera samples collected at frequent intervals, including the serum specimen with the broadest reactivity against a lymphocyte panel. However, it is still unclear whether a positive crossmatch using noncurrent sera is invariably predictive of graft rejection (123).

Donor-specific Cellular Presensitization. Renal allograft rejection can be cellularly mediated as well as antibody-mediated. A technique that can detect the presence of cellular immunity of the recipient against the donor is known as lymphocyte-mediated cytotoxicity (LMC). Almost all studies report a significant correlation between a positive LMC crossmatch and kidney graft loss from rejection (124). Although LMC is not used routinely in most renal transplant centers, it may ultimately become a standard pretransplant assay.

Presensitization against a Lymphocyte Panel. Testing for presensitization against a lymphocyte panel serves as a pretransplant screen of the individual's anti-HLA antibody status. All histocompatibility laboratories examine, at frequent intervals, sera of patients awaiting transplantation for the presence of CDC antibodies against HLA antigens represented by a lymphocyte panel.

The type of information obtained from the reactivity against a panel depends on the method by which the panel is selected. If the panel is randomly selected, the HLA antigens present have approximately the same frequency as that found in the general population, so the percentage of positive reactions yields information about the probability that a given recipient will have a positive crossmatch with a given donor. For example, if a patient's serum is reactive against 90% of a random panel, only 10% of potential cadaver donors can be expected to be crossmatch-negative. If, on the other hand, the panel is selected to contain all HLA antigens, the specificities of the anti-HLA antibodies may be more precisely determined, but the percentage of reactivity is less relevant than with the random panel. Some centers use this all-HLA panel to identify all of the antibody specificities an individual has generated (125). These data are then used to avoid transplanting kidneys that have antigens against which the recipient had made antibodies previously.

The significance in transplantation of broadly reactive lymphocytotoxic antibodies remains controversial. Does reactivity against a high percentage of a lymphocyte panel correlate with poor graft outcome despite a negative donor-specific crossmatch? Initial studies reported that sensitized patients, i.e., those reacting to more than 10% of a randomly selected panel, had a lower early graft survival rate than nonsensitized individuals (126) as detected by the tests available at the time. Other centers found a deleterious effect only among HLA-incompatible recipients (127). Still others found no correlation between pretransplant panel cytotoxicity and graft survival (128, 129). The reason for the discrepancies among units may relate to (a) the more recent use of multiple high-titer sera for lymphocyte crossmatches, as opposed to using only one current serum, and (b) more sensitive techniques to detect anti-HLA antibodies (128, 129).

Broad reactivity of multiple serum samples against a random lymphocyte panel does not necessarily predict graft survival; however, obtaining the results of such reactivity may serve to choose the most highly reactive serum for the crossmatch with the potential donor. It may also be of value in those centers where the cumulative list of specific antibodies produced by the recipient is considered at the time of transplant, i.e., a patient who in the past had antibodies against HLA-A2 would not receive a kidney with HLA-A2, even when the crossmatch was negative.

Living-Related Donors

HLA-Identical Donors

The best graft survival rate is obtained with live-related HLA-identical transplants. Graft survival is reported to be from 85% to 93% at 1 yr and 67% to 82% at 5 yr (131). Nevertheless, rejections do occur in HLA-identical transplants. Some are associated with a reactive MLC (131, 132), whereas others are accompanied by a negative MLC (130). Although the cause or causes are not clear for rejection in these "ideal" transplantations, some explanations have been offered. Patients with a negative MLC could have rejection secondary to donor-specific anti E-M antibody (106) or, occasionally, patients can be HLA-ABCD-identical and still be MLC-positive. HLA-identical siblings are considered the first choice for transplantation, if they are ABO-compatible, have a low MLC reactivity, and are crossmatch-negative. If the MLC is positive, it is not clear whether one should avoid such a transplant or attempt donor-specific transfusions.

HLA-Haploidentical Donors

Since the MHC is inherited in classic fashion, parents are obligatory HLA-haploidentical matches with their children, and each sibling has a 50% chance that another sibling is haploidentical (Fig. 51.2). Overall, renal allograft survival rates in haploidentical donor-recipient pairs are approximately 75% at one year (39, 79, 80), intermediate between that found in cadaver and HLA-identical living-related donor-recipient pairs. The MLC may be useful to evaluate the prognosis of transplantation in living-related HLA-haploidentical pairs. A good correlation is reported between pretransplant MLC reactivity and transplant outcome. Two-year cumulative graft survival rates of 80% to 90% were found when the MLC exhibited weak reactivity (133, 134). Graft survival rates similar to cadaver donor transplants are found with high reactivity in the MLC (133), although one pediatric series reports outstanding results in such a situation (135). Recently, the results of living-related HLA haploidentical transplants with high MLC reactivity have been greatly improved, using cyclosporine as immunosuppression (136) or pretransplant blood transfusions.

At most centers, siblings who are totally HLA mismatched are discouraged from being kidney donors, since theoretically their graft outcome should be no better than that achieved with cadaveric transplantation. However, at least one center has considered such donors preferable to parental donors (137) and the use of donor-specific transfusions in totally HLA-mismatched siblings has been promising (138).

Pretransplant Blood Transfusions

Many dialysis units once attempted to reduce the risk of presensitization by minimizing the number of blood transfusions given to patients with ESRD. However, it has been suggested (139) that contrary to what had been expected, pretransplant blood transfusions were associated with improved cadaver allograft survival rates. This finding has now been extensively confirmed (83, 140). The magnitude of the effect is remarkable. In one prospective study, untransfused cadaveric donor transplant recipients had a one-year survival rate of 20% while recipients receiving 10 or more transfusions had a rate of 89% (140). Transfusions appear to have their greatest effect by reducing accelerated rejection in the first months following transplantation (141).

Cadaveric Transplantation

There is no consensus as to the optimal number of third-party transfusions in cadaveric renal transplantation. The studies of Terasaki, Opelz, and their coworkers indicate that the effect can be correlated with the number of pretransplant transfusions, i.e., graft survival is poorest in untransfused recipients and improves as more transfusions are given (83, 140, 141). Their recent data suggest that approximately half of the total effect is conferred by one transfusion (140). The value of a single transfusion had been stressed previously by the Eurotransplant group, who showed maximal graft survival with only one leukocyte-poor transfusion (142). A recent multicenter study showed that most of the beneficial effect was present after five transfusions (141). Other recommendations regarding the optimal transfusion number have varied from one to five (142, 143), or ten (8).

The mechanism by which transfusions improve renal allograft survival is unknown. Possible explanations include (a) selection of "low responders" by their inability to produce anti-HLA antibodies in response to transfusions (144); (b) transfusion-induced production of antibodies (116, 117), e.g., antiidiotypic antibodies (145, 146), or other humoral substances, e.g., immune complexes, that mediate improved allograft survival; (c) induction of immunological unresponsiveness by cellular mechanisms, e.g., by inducing suppressor T-cells (147) or monocytes (148).

None of these mechanisms can account totally for the transfusion effect. In humans, leukocytes appear to be important, as leukocyte-poor blood, i.e., containing some leukocytes, is far superior to leukocyte-free blood (149). In fact, leukocytes have been successfully used as the only transfusion preparation (150). However, transfused erythrocytes may also result in immunological unresponsiveness (151) and improved transplant outcome (152). Even platelets have been reported to improve graft survival in rhesus monkeys (153). Whole blood or packed red blood cells appear to produce the most significant effect in humans (83, 154); however, some studies have found that frozen blood (155), and particularly frozen blood prepared by deglycerilization (156), has the same influence on graft survival as other preparations. It seems reasonable to conclude that transfusions must work through various mechanisms. Some are probably mediated by erythrocytes, whereas others may be mediated by leukocytes, platelets, or both.

There are few studies on the ideal amounts of blood and the timing of transfusion that will optimize transplant outcome. It has been proposed that transfusion given in the perioperative period may benefit cadaver graft outcome (157). In one study, previously untransfused recipients who received 2 units of blood at the time of transplantation surgery had a two-year cumulative graft survival rate of 76% compared with 36% in the untransfused control group (158). However, others have found that perioperative transfusions are associated with cadaver graft outcome that is intermediate between that seen with preoperative transfusions and no transfusion (159, 160). Similarly, in the large University of California, Los Angeles, multicenter study, perioperative blood transfusion significantly reduced the frequency of accelerated rejection only in recipients who had not received prior blood transfusions (83, 141). According to these studies, the advantages of perioperative transfusions are not as great as those attained with preoperative transfusions.

Sensitization Following Transfusions

The incidence and significance of anti-HLA antibodies generated by the transfusions is most important because, as noted previously, preformed antibodies in the recipient directed against the HLA-A or -B antigens of the kidney transplant donor can produce hyperacute rejection (110).

Opelz & associate found that the formation of broadly reactive lymphocytotoxins as a result of transfusions was relatively rare, particularly in patients without previous pregnancies (161). They showed that with up to 20 pretransplant transfusions, usually given as packed red blood cells, broadly reactive antilymphocyte antibodies, i.e., >90% reactivity against a random T-cell panel, were not found in any prospectively studied males or in females without previous pregnancies. Antibodies against a B-lymphocyte panel were found with greater frequency (161). Lymphocytotoxic antibodies occur after approximately one third of transfusions in uremic children, but only about 14% of all transfusions appear to result in anti-HLA antibodies directed against T-lymphocytes (162); the remainder of the sensitization is directed at B-lymphocytes (162). Significant sensitization is far more frequent following a rejected renal transplant (163). It therefore appears unlikely that a recipient will be rendered "untransplantable" because of prospective pretransplant transfusions only.

Are patients who develop cytotoxic antibodies against a lymphocyte panel in response to transfusion at increased risk to reject their renal transplant, even if the pretransplant crossmatch is negative? Patients who developed cytotoxic antibodies in response to transfusions had cadaver graft outcomes that were the same (164, 165) or better (140, 143) than those of untransfused graft recipients. Whether transfused patients develop preformed antibodies to B-lymphocytes, T-lymphocytes, or both, their one-year graft survival rate is still higher than the nontransfused recipients (166). In fact, many studies suggest that individuals who are highly presensitized by multiple transfusions have graft survival rates that are superior to (167) or, at the very least, almost equivalent to transfused patients who have remained unsensitized (140, 168). Some studies show some diminished graft survival with high levels of presensitization (83), although the percentage of well-functioning grafts is always superior to that of a comparable nontransfused group. Transfused patients who appear to be at increased risk for poor graft outcome are those who develop broadly reactive antibodies in response to only two to five transfusions (169). These patients have a one-year cadaver graft survival of approximately 20%. On the other hand, those with broadly reactive antibodies in response to a higher number of transfusions have one-year graft outcomes in the range of 50% to 75%.

Transfusion Effect in Living-Related Transplantation

The efficacy of preoperative transfusions in living-related transplantation has been less apparent. Since graft outcome is generally much better than with cadaveric transplantation, a transfusion effect may be more difficult to demonstrate statistically. It would be difficult to show a graft-enhancing effect of almost any adjunctive manipulation in renal transplantation between HLA-identical siblings (170) with a two-year graft survival that exceeds 90%.

Some reports have not shown a beneficial effect of "third-party" transfusions in one haplotype-matched living related transplantation (171), but the majority show a clear-cut benefit (169, 170, 172, 174). In one large series, third-party blood transfusions improved the two-year cumulative graft outcome from 50% to 75%. The effect was the same whether the recipient had received less or more than five transfusions (170). Third-party pretransplant transfusions have been reported to be of value when the MLC between donor and recipient is strongly reactive. Salvatierra and his colleagues found a one-year graft survival of 74% in 23 recipients who had third-party transfusions and only 18% in 11 recipients who had never received transfusions (174).

Another approach to improve graft outcome in these highly reactive donor-recipient pairs has been to use donor blood for pretreatment transfusion. Data in animals (175–178) and humans (150) show prolonged graft outcome. Transfused recipients who do not respond to the donor-specific transfusions (DST) by developing deleterious anti-HLA antibodies can receive transplants with a graft outcome approaching that obtained when using HLA-identical siblings as donors (179–181). One- and two-year graft survival rates of more than 90% have been reported in patients receiving DST and first living-related one-haploidentical renal transplants. In addition, rejection episodes are said to be milder in DST recipients, although first rejection episodes tend to occur earlier than in patients who have not received DST (182). Some centers perform DST for all one-haplotype living-related transplants regardless of the MLC reactivity (183), citing a smoother posttransplant course with DST. Other centers have continued to use MLC reactivity to determine whether a recipient should receive DST.

The major disadvantage of DST is the risk of developing deleterious antibodies against the histocompatibility antigens of the potential donors. Serial sera should be assiduously obtained from the DST recipient and frozen for subsequent lymphocytotoxic crossmatching with lymphocytes of the potential donor. Criteria for transplantation are negative T- and B-cell crossmatches on all sera by standard CDC testing (184). We have found that adverse presensitization develops in 29% of children receiving DST; this is comparable to most studies (32), but higher than that reported in some (180, 181).

In spite of rigorous screening protocols, immediate rejections have occurred, although rarely. These have been associated with negative crossmatches (184) or positive B-cell crossmatches at a 37°C incubation temperature (179). Such hyperacute rejection could be caused by an antibody against an antigen system that is not easily detectable, such as the E-M antigen system; alternatively, it could be caused by the presence of anti-HLA antibody below the level detectable by standard tests.

The mechanism or mechanisms by which DST improves graft outcome are not understood. The DST may segregate out a group of "high immunological responders," who are likely to reject the transplant; however, the uniform success rate of DST in the presence of varying sensitization rates (184–186) makes it unlikely that selection is the only operative mechanism. Preliminary evidence suggests that active immunological processes play an important part in the DST effect (187, 188).

Important modifications of DSTs have been introduced to diminish the chance of sensitization while preserving the beneficial effect. These include administering azathioprine (Imuran) during the DSTs (185) or using banked rather than fresh blood as the transfused substrate (186). Both of these modifications reduce the sensitization rate to only 10%.

The efficacy of DST has not yet been tested against third-party transfusions in a controlled randomized fashion. In addition, it is prudent to question the wisdom of performing a procedure that disqualifies almost one third of donors because of sensitization. This is particularly important in young children with ESRD, since they are so well rehabilitated with one-haplotype living-related donors (189). Some have questioned the need for DSTs in children (135). The real future of DST, particularly for children, will be in modifications such as those previously noted that can lower the sensitization rate to 10% or less while preserving its beneficial effects.

IMMUNOSUPPRESSION

Ideally, the optimal form of immunosuppression would be "specific," i.e., directed only against the graft. Such immunosuppression would reduce reactivity to the specific antigenic differences of the graft and would avoid general immunosuppression of the recipient's immune system. Although it is possible that blood transfusions may be a form of specific immunosuppression, it is generally conceded that a method for the reliable induction of specific immunosuppression in clinical transplantation is not yet available. Therefore, only nonspecific methods have been used.

The nonspecific methods of immunosuppression can be divided into three general categories: (a) pharmacological; (b) lymphoid depletion; and (c) heterologous antiserum.

Pharmacological Methods

Corticosteroids (Table 51.6)

Corticosteroids have been effective in reversing and in preventing rejection.

How corticosteroids work is not entirely clear. They cause a prompt

Table 51.6. Posttransplant Immunosuppression Utilizing Prednisone and Azathioprine (mg/kg/d)

Donor source	Immunosuppressive drug (mg/kg/d)	3 days Pre-TX	Day of TX (IV)	Week After transplant					
				1	4	8	12	26	52
Cadaver									ADT[a]
	Prednisone	—	10	0.5	0.4	0.3	0.25	0.18–0.25	0.5
	Azathioprine	—	2–3	1–2	1.5–3	2–3	2–3	2–3	2–3
Living-related								ADT[a]	ADT[a]
	Prednisone	0.5 (min. 20 mg)	10	0.5	0.4	0.25	0.18–0.25	0.5	0.3–0.5
	Azathioprine	2–3	2–3	1–2	1.5–3	2–3	2–3	2–3	2–3

[a] ADT = Alternate-day therapy.

but transient sequestration of circulating T-lymphocytes into lymphoid tissue (190). Helper T-lymphocytes are markedly sequestered, but there is no change in the distribution of suppressor T-lymphocytes (191). Steroids diminish production of cytotoxic T-lymphocytes from precursor cells and may also diminish the cytotoxic action of such killer T-cells (192). Humoral immunity is much less affected (193). Many of the effects of corticosteroids on cell-mediated immunity may be due to depression of interleukin-2 (194, 195), a lymphokine that helps to activate cytotoxic T-lymphocytes. Corticosteroids also may improve graft outcome by their antiinflammatory actions, such as inhibiting lysozomal enzyme release by neutrophils (196) and decreasing the response of neutrophils and monocytes to chemotactic stimuli (197).

Prednisone is the most common corticosteroid used in transplantation. There is little evidence that one corticosteroid compound is superior to another, although one study suggests that prednisone may be somewhat more effective than other compounds in suppressing alloantigenic recognition. The maintenance doses employed vary widely from center to center. In 1973, McGeown surveyed the transplant centers in the United Kingdom and found the initial maintenance daily dose of prednisone or prednisolone varied between 20 and 1000 mg (198).

Because of the wide dosage range, it seems appropriate to question the efficacy of prophylactic corticosteroids in the prevention of rejection. Kreis & coworkers (199) reported in 1978 the results of a nonrandomized study in which 53 recipients were given prophylactic corticosteroid and 54 were given corticosteroids only at the time of the first rejection episode. The incidence of irreversible rejection episodes was similar in the two groups and at six months post transplant, 79% and 76%, respectively, of the grafts were functioning. On the other hand, the occurrence of late acute rejection after abrupt discontinuation of corticosteroids because of noncompliance suggests that corticosteroids do forestall at least some rejection (200). Most transplant centers continue to use maintenance corticosteroid therapy following transplantation, but in light of the above data and steroid side effects, which are particularly troublesome in children, it is reasonable to examine the amount of steroids administered. McGeown & coworkers (201) reported a 76% actuarial graft survival rate for 151 transplants in 141 recipients between 1968 and 1978 using a maintenance dose of 20 mg prednisone for the initial six months post transplant. The value of this low-dosage maintenance corticosteroid was indicated by the minimal mortality related to infection post transplant. A controlled trial subsequently has confirmed that graft and patient survival are not adversely affected by low-dose maintenance corticosteroid therapy. Moreover, the side effects of corticosteroids, especially avascular necrosis of bone, are reduced (202).

Corticosteroids are also used to treat rejection episodes. Initially, high-dose oral prednisone was used, but the report of Bell & associates (203) in 1971 stimulated interest in the use of high-dose intravenous methylprednisolone. The authors used 1 g intravenous prednisolone to treat 18 episodes of acute rejection; 15 of these episodes were reversed (86%); 6 reversed after 1 g, 8 after 2 g, and 1 after 3 g. These authors suggested that this mode of therapy was associated with fewer side effects than the standard treatment with oral corticosteroids (203). Many centers adopted this form of therapy and used methylprednisolone dosages as high as 30 mg/kg daily for three days. Kauffman & coworkers (204) reevaluated the need for high-dose intravenous corticosteroid therapy in 48 recipients with acute rejection episodes who were randomized into a high-dose (30 mg/kg) or a low-dose (3 mg/kg) treatment protocol. The number of irreversible rejection episodes, recipient deaths, and serum creatinine level at three months post transplant was similar in the two groups; however, the total dose of corticosteroid administered was significantly lower in the low-dose (12.3 mg/kg) compared with the high-dose group (117 mg/kg) (204).

High-dose intravenous methylprednisolone and high-dose oral prednisone appear to be equally effective in reversing acute rejection (205). Although some investigators have shown that high-dose intravenous methylprednisolone therapy is accompanied by fewer side effects (205), others claim less toxicity with oral antirejection therapy.

Growth suppression occurs with a daily dose of prednisone >8.5 mg/m^2. Because of the growth-suppressive effects of daily corticosteroids, alternate day (ADT) therapy has been effectively used (206–208). In general, growth velocity improved, and side effects were reduced without a concomitant increase in the incidence of rejection.

The precise method and timing of conversion to ADT vary from report to report. Hoda & associates initiated ADT at three months post transplant (207), whereas McEnery and coworkers suggested initiating ADT during the initial six months post transplant (208). Our procedure is to switch to ADT at six months post transplant if the recipient has not manifested any rejection episodes or to wait until one year if the clinical course during the first six months is marked by rejection episodes (Table 51.6).

We administer 2¼ to 2½ times the daily dose on alternate days. If graft function remains stable, we gradually reduce the dose at three-month intervals to an amount equivalent to 1½ to two times the previous daily dosage (Table 51.6).

A recent report from the EDTA Pediatric Registry analyzed the effects of ADT in 28 children and compared the data with those obtained in 66 children receiving daily corticosteroid therapy. The incidence of hypertension was significantly higher (75% versus 43%) in the group receiving daily corticosteroid therapy, and the incidence of rejection was similar in both groups: 19% and 18%, respectively (209). Growth in 11 prepubertal children receiving ADT was significantly better than in 23 children receiving daily therapy. ADT reduced the incidence of hypertension as well as the incidence of hypercholesterolemia. The mean percentage of normal growth in 28 children on ADT improved (206).

There is thus ample evidence that ADT is associated with reduced side effects and somewhat improved growth. Nevertheless, some investigators have suggested that the transition to ADT predisposes to allograft rejection (209). However, two controlled studies in adults have concluded that maintenance ADT was not associated with an increased incidence of rejection episodes or with a greater loss of renal function when compared with patients on daily steroids (210, 211).

Is it possible to safely discontinue corticosteroids at any time following transplantation? Lorkkegaard & coworkers (212) in 1976 discontinued prednisone in 47 recipients with unimpaired graft function who were >2 yr post transplant and receiving about 10 mg prednisone daily. Eighteen had no complications; 9 sustained irreversible loss of function. In another study, prednisone was tapered at a rate of 1 mg/month in 10 patients receiving 10 mg daily who had stopped azathioprine electively. Four of the 10 sustained a loss of function at a dosage of <7 mg/day; only 1 of them regained function following resumed treatment (213). More recently, success in tapering and discontinuing prednisone in patients who were continued on azathioprine was reported (214). Slowly tapering the dose by 1 mg/month in patients who had had stable renal function for at least two years, these workers were able to discontinue prednisone in more than half of 80 patients (214).

It is still not clear whether tapering steroid therapy should be attempted or whether it is advisable to continue steroid therapy at a low ADT dosage. This question may become less important with the introduction of cyclosporin A.

Azathioprine (Imuran) (Table 51.6)

This drug is an S-imidazolyl derivative of 6-mercaptopurine and was first used in 1963 to inhibit graft rejection in humans (215). It appears to prevent rejection episodes, but does not abort continuing rejection. Cessation of azathioprine early in the posttransplant course is accompanied by a high rate of graft failure (216); however, withdrawal at a later date because of side effects did not affect graft survival in two studies (216, 217), but results in a third were adverse (218).

Azathioprine competes with inosinic acid for enzyme binding in the synthesis of nucleic acids. Because cell division and proliferation occur in response to antigenic stimulation, immune suppression may be mediated by interference with DNA synthesis in antigen-stimulated and -activated lymphocytes, by blockade of RNA synthesis, or both (219). Numerous T-cell functions are inhibited by azathioprine, including reactivity in the MLC (220), cytotoxic T-cell activity (219), and suppressor T-cell activity (221). Azathioprine also inhibits the cytotoxic activity of the so-called natural killer lymphocytes and lymphocytes that are active in antibody-dependent cellular cytotoxicity (222) and appears to inhibit primary antibody synthesis (223).

Azathioprine is used in a dosage range of 1 to 3 mg/kg/day. The higher dosage is used when there is no sign of toxicity; the lower dosage is used when side effects are noted. Because azathioprine is metabolized rapidly by the liver, the dosage need not be changed rapidly with changes in renal function; however, we lower the dosage to 1.0 to 1.5 mg/kg/dose immediately after transplantation or during chronic rejection, when patients may be more sensitive to its myelosuppressive effects.

Bone marrow suppression is the most common side effect associated with azathioprine therapy—usually manifested as leukopenia (216), less commonly as thrombocytopenia and megaloblastic anemia (224, 225). Bone marrow suppression is particularly common when azathioprine is used with other myelosuppressive drugs, such as trimethoprim-sulfamethoxazole (226). The concurrent use of azathioprine and allopurinol, a xanthine oxidase inhibitor, may increase immunosuppression and cause severe myelosuppression (227). Bone marrow depression almost always diminishes when the drugs are discontinued; azathioprine can then be used safely at a lower dosage (225). Leukopenia with azathioprine therapy also is common in patients with hypersplenism. In this situation, pretransplant splenectomy has been recommended (225).

Other complications of azathioprine include infection, particularly viral infection. With varicella or other herpes infections, the dose should be lowered or discontinued. Liver toxicity may be a complication of azathioprine (228). We discontinue its use when liver enzyme levels are elevated. Other reported side effects include alopecia. It may be a factor in the higher incidence of malignant disease post transplant (229, 230).

Cyclosporine (Cyclosporin-A, Sandimmune)

Cyclosporine is a highly stable, 11-amino-acid, cyclic polypeptide initially developed as an antifungal agent from soil fungi; Borel and associates noted its significant immunosuppressive characteristics (231). Initial clinical studies in human transplantation have been encouraging, although side effects appear to be significant.

Cyclosporine is a potent suppressor of allograft rejection in several species (232). Although it is a potent antilymphocyte agent (233); it is only weakly toxic to other hematopoetic cells (234). It acts predominantly on T-lymphocytes, inhibiting many of their responses and preventing generation of cytotoxic T-lymphocytes in vitro (233, 235), although it does not inhibit their activity once they have been generated (236). Although inhibiting the activity of helper T-lymphocytes, cyclosporine allows the expression of antigen-specific suppressor cells (233, 237). It has been suggested that cyclosporine interferes with an internal signal, triggered by antigen, which causes the T-lymphocyte to produce lymphokines, especially interleukin-2 (238). Since the presence of donor antigen is necessary to maintain an active state of immunosuppression toward the allograft, at least a portion of cyclosporine's activity may represent a donor-specific suppression, with resultant specificity for only those lymphocytes mediating allograft rejection (233, 239).

Cyclosporine was first used by Calne & coworkers (240); although there were successful outcomes, there were also high morbidity and mortality rates. More recent studies have demonstrated that its administration is associated with improved graft survival without high complication rates. The multicenter controlled European Trial (241) showed, after a minimum of one-year follow-up, that the graft survival rate was 20% higher with cyclosporine than with conventional therapy (72% versus 52%). The Canadian controlled trial found a one-year actuarial graft survival of 80% in the cyclosporine-treated group compared with 64% in the group receiving standard therapy (242). Single-center trials also have shown cyclosporine to be effective (243–245). Najarian and coworkers reported an 83.5% graft survival at 22 months (244). Although this figure was not significantly different from their results using standard therapy (including a 14-day course of high-dose antilymphocyte globulin), they found a much lower incidence of infectious complications, particularly cytomegalovirus, with cyclosporine use (244).

In children, the experience with cyclosporine has been limited. Three renal allograft recipients who were given cyclosporine, had rejected one or more previous grafts, and had broadly reactive lymphocytotoxic antibodies have maintained functioning grafts four to six & one-half months post transplant; serum creatinine levels ranged from 1.1 to 1.7 mg/dl (246). Other experiences with cyclosporine in children also have validated its efficacy, with excellent graft survival and good renal function (247).

The major problem with cyclosporine has been the high incidence of nephrotoxicity associated with its use (233, 241, 242, 244). The nephrotoxicity does not appear to be progressive, is dose-dependent, and seems to be reversible in response to decrements in dose (244). The use of cyclosporine blood levels is helpful in determining the dosage and in avoiding nephrotoxicity (233); however, blood levels alone do not differentiate cyclosporine nephrotoxicity from rejection (248). Flechner & associates combined clinical indices, e.g., a slow, sustained rise in creatinine that reversed with dosage reduction, with drug levels to distinguish rejection from nephrotoxicity (248a). Histological changes in biopsies by conventional or fine-needle aspiration have helped identify cyclosporine bound to the tubular cell (249).

Nephrotoxicity may prove to be a limiting factor in the use of cyclosporine for cadaveric renal transplantation. In a randomized clinical trial reported by the Canadian Multicenter Transplantation Study Group (239), cadaveric graft outcome with cyclosporine was no better than standard therapy in those kidneys that had a prolonged (>24 hr) pulsatile machine perfusion time or a surgical anastomosis time of >45 min. There was a trend in the cyclosporine-treated patients toward a greater incidence and duration of acute posttransplant tubular necrosis and primary nonfunction (247). Flechner & associates noted, however, that although more impaired graft function in the early posttransplant period may occur with cyclosporine, graft survival rates at one year were not affected adversely (250).

Other important side effects of cyclosporine administration include hypertension, hyperkalemia, reversible hepatotoxicity, tremor, hirsutism, gum hypertrophy, hyperasthesia, and gastrointestinal intolerance with nausea. The susceptibility to infections appears to be less than that observed with conventional immunosuppression (244). One of the greatest concerns with cyclosporine has been the increased incidence of lymphoma with its use. In a summary of European experience, 13 lymphomas were found among 1400 patients treated with the drug (251); the Canadian trial group found an incidence of <1% (242). Some of the lymphomas have been attributed to vigorous immunosuppression, which allows unchecked proliferation of Epstein-Barr virus-transformed B-lymphocytes (252). The incidence of lymphoma appears to be linked to the combined use of cyclosporine with other immunosuppressive agents (251).

Whereas some have used cyclosporine without giving steroids (253), a number of centers now use cyclosporine with low-dosage prednisone (233, 242, 244). This appears desirable since allograft function, particularly early allograft function, may be superior (242); however, it is not clear from controlled studies whether low-dosage prednisone improves ultimate graft outcome or whether the increased immunosuppression increases the risk of adverse side effects without significantly increasing graft survival. In treating children, the question of using steroids with cyclosporine may be particularly vexing since both steroids and a low GFR may be associated with poor growth.

Antilymphocyte Preparations

Antilymphocyte globulin (ALG) and antithymocyte globulin (ATG) have been evaluated extensively in human renal transplantation. Most experience has been gained with preparations obtained by immunizing horses or rabbits with human lymphocytes of different origins (254, 255). In experimental animals, ALG and ATG prolong renal allograft survival; however, its efficacy when used in human renal transplantation is less clear. Most studies suggest that ALG or ATG will forestall most first rejections while either is being given. However, conflicting evidence exists concerning efficacy of early ALG or ATG use when efficacy is assessed by transplant survival, number of rejection crises, or decrease in steroid dosage (254, 255).

The conflicting evidence can be attributed in part to differing dosages and to different potencies of preparations or batches (rabbit ATG appears to be particularly potent and well tolerated) (219, 254). The results of controlled studies on the efficacy of ATG or ALG in improving long-term graft function also are conflicting. A multicenter study from the United Kingdom found a 10-day course of a moderately potent ALG preparation had no effect on allograft survival (257); however, the Canadian multicenter trial (258) and single-center studies (259) suggest that a 10- to 14-day course of a potent ALG preparation may improve one-year allograft survival.

Although routine prophylactic use of ALG and ATG is controversial, their use with rejection episodes (260) may be effective, even some that resist high-dosage steroids alone (261). Treating rejection with ATG for 15 consecutive days at a dosage of 10 mg/kg improved outcome (260). High-potency rabbit ATG also was reported to be effective in reversing acute rejection (262). Their use with a lower dosage of steroids to treat rejection episodes (263) may reduce the risk of growth failure in children post transplant.

Side effects of ALG and ATG include fever and pain at the site of injection; these symptoms diminish in severity as treatment progresses. Other side effects include thrombocytopenia and sensitization to horse protein with attendant urticaria, hypotension or, occasionally, serum sickness or anaphylaxis (219). ATG or ALG has been associated with a higher incidence of viral infections, particularly cytomegalovirus infections (264).

With monoclonal antibody technology, mouse antibodies with activity against specific subsets of human T-lymphocytes have been developed. Monoclonal antibodies directed against certain antigens present on all T-lymphocytes, i.e., OKT_3 or T_{12}, have been successfully used to reverse acute rejection episodes (265). Preliminary work in simians examines whether monoclonal antibodies to particular T-lymphocyte subsets, e.g., helper T-lymphocytes, cytotoxic-suppressor T-lymphocytes, prevent or treat renal allograft rejection (266). One major problem with these agents is that they induce antimouse antibodies that inactivate the original monoclonal antibodies (266).

Agents That Interrupt Coagulation

Because vascular thrombosis and glomerular fibrin deposits occur in rejecting grafts, interruption of the coagulation process has been attempted, but with little success. In a controlled trial using dipyridamole & warfarin, there was no beneficial effect on graft function or survival rate (267), although the histological appearance of the glomeruli and vasculature of the treatment group was improved. A similar controlled study (268) with only dipyridamole failed to demonstrate any beneficial effect on the graft survival rate or on the histological appearance of the graft.

Nonpharmacological Immunosuppression

Plasmapheresis

Plasmapheresis is a potential treatment for acute vascular rejection unresponsive to steroids. Acute vascular rejection may be mediated by antibodies (269); therefore, it seemed possible that the removal of these antibodies would help prevent allograft failure. Early uncontrolled studies suggested a favorable response to plasmapheresis, but no significant improvement was observed in long-term overall graft survival (270). A controlled study of 24 patients with histologically proven severe vascular rejection failed to show improved outcome in patients treated with plasma exchange and bolus methylprednisolone versus those treated with methylprednisolone alone (271, 272).

Judged by these results, plasma exchange therapy does not appear to be effective in treating acute rejection; it may be useful under special circumstances, such as the inadvertently mismatched ABO blood group transplant, when there is a need to remove isohemagglutinins. This has been tried in ABO mismatched living-related transplants with some apparent benefit (96).

Irradiation

Total body irradiation was initially the method of immunosuppression used for renal transplantation. It was abandoned because the incidence of infectious complications, was high. Interestingly, one of the recipients has had a functioning graft >22 yr; the only immunosuppression used in his case was 350 rads of total body irradiation. Local graft irradiation has been used both prophylactically and to treat rejection with equivocal results. A controlled study of local graft irradiation used in 83 rejection episodes in 64 grafts demonstrated no benefit when used in conjunction with high-dose steroid therapy to reverse rejection episodes (273).

The long-term immunosuppressive effects of total lymphoid irradiation (TLI) in patients with Hodgkin's disease stimulated interest in TLI as adjunctive immunosuppression in renal graft recipients. Although no controlled studies have been performed to validate the efficacy of TLI, recent results are promising; a one-year 72% graft and 78% patient survival rate was obtained in 20 recipients including some children who had rejected an initial graft in < one year. The major difficulty in using TLI is the requirement that it be given close to the time the cadaver graft is placed. There also is a potential for lymphoid malignancies; however, this method of immunosuppression may be helpful as adjunctive therapy in children who have rejected one or more grafts.

Splenectomy

The immunosuppressive effect obtained by pretransplant splenectomy is controversial. A controlled study by Fryd & coworkers (275) demonstrated a 12% improvement in cadaver donor and 14% improvement in live-related donor grafts with pretransplant splenectomy in patients who were >16 yr of age.

The incidence of overwhelming infection in children post splenectomy

Table 51.7. Immunological Tests that Can Be Used to Monitor Host Reactivity to Transplanted Kidney

I. Specific Antidonor Activity
  A. Humoral
    1. Complement-dependent cytotoxicity (CDC)
      a. Against unfractionated lymphocytes
      b. Against B-lymphocytes
    2. Antibody-dependent cellular cytotoxicity (ADCC) against donor lymphocytes
  B. Cellular
    1. Lymphocyte-mediated cytotoxicity against donor lymphocytes
    2. Mixed lymphocyte culture reactivity vs donor lymphocytes
    3. Fine-needle aspiration biopsy
II. Nonspecific immune activity
  A. Antibodies generated against a B-Lymphocyte panel
  B. Spontaneous blastogenesis
  C. Enumeration of T lymphocytes
    1. Total
    2. "Active"
  D. Enumeration of T lymphocyte subsets

makes splenectomy a risky procedure in potential recipients. Although prophylactic antibiotic therapy may prevent overwhelming infection, it is important to recognize that prophylaxis is often omitted by the patient.

POSTTRANSPLANT IMMUNOLOGICAL MONITORING

A number of assays have been used to monitor the immunological reaction of the host to the transplanted kidney. The rationale for immunological monitoring post transplant includes (a) early detection of a rejection episode; (b) separating renal failure episodes into those due to rejection versus those due to other causes; and (c) differentiating rejection episodes that are amenable to high-dose immunosuppressive therapy from those that are resistant (Table 51.7).

Immunological monitoring involves two basic types of assays, detecting either specific host antidonor immune activity or nonspecific host immunological activation.

Specific Antidonor Immunological Activity

Humoral Activity

Complement-dependent Cytotoxic Antibody. Complement-dependent cytotoxic (CDC) antibody in the recipient serum against donor peripheral blood lymphocytes is strongly associated with rejection. False-positive results are infrequent (276–278); however, the sensitivity is not always great enough to provide accurate diagnosis (276). A CDC-positive test persists for a long time after the rejection episode, which also limits the usefulness of this test (278).

Antibody-dependent Cell-mediated Cytotoxicity. Antibody-dependent cell-mediated cytotoxicity (ADCC) is a sensitive test for IgG antibodies directed against donor HLA and non-HLA lymphocyte antigens. A strong correlation between acute rejection episodes and positive ADCC noted by some (277, 279) has not been confirmed by others (278, 280); however, persistence of a positive ADCC test, despite high-dose steroid treatment for rejection, is associated with vascular rejection and graft loss (277). A negative CDC and ADCC assay may be useful in excluding rejection.

Anti-B Cell Antibody. The presence of donor-specific anti-B-cell antibodies, detected by CDC (281) or by other (282) assays correlates with acute rejection, but the value of these results has not been confirmed (277, 283).

Cellular Activity

Lymphocyte-mediated Cytotoxicity. The lymphocyte-mediated cytotoxicity (LMC) test uses recipient lymphocytes as effector cells and donor lymphocytes labeled with ^{51}Cr as targets. A good correlation between LMC activity and clinical rejection has been reported by some (278, 279) but not by others (277). These discrepancies may be due to variations in techniques, e.g., different incubation time and type of donor cells used as targets.

Mixed Lymphocyte Culture. The mixed lymphocyte culture (MLC) is decreased at the time of rejection by some; however, others have not found it very specific or sensitive (283a). Some of the decrease in MLC reactivity after transplantation may be due to immunosuppression therapy.

Fine-Needle Aspiration Biopsy. A method of fine-needle aspiration (FNA) biopsy of the renal allograft was first described in the early 1960s and has been used subsequently in Europe (283). A 23-gauge spinal needle is inserted directly into the graft and 50 to 100 μl of renal cortical transudate is aspirated. The procedure is nearly risk-free and can be performed at the bedside. Processing of the sample requires centrifugation to obtain a cellular button, staining the button with May-Grünwald–Giemsa stain, and examination by light microscopy.

Renal parenchymal cells normally constitute 10% to 20% of the sample and include tubular, endothelial, and glomerular cells. With rejection, all of these cells undergo characteristic changes. Evidence for rejection is an increase in immunologically mediated cells: polymorphonuclear cells, lymphocytes, plasma cells, monocytes, and macrophages. Lymphocytes increase with mild and reversible rejection, and lymphoblasts and plasmablasts increase with rejection of increasing severity and duration. In severe rejections, monocytes constitute nearly 50% of the immunological cells. The results are quantified by determining the cellular increment (CI), which is a numerical value for the immunological cells in the graft and the gradation of the rejection episode. This technique has detected rejection from CI three to five days before any increase in the serum creatinine. This method has been used to effect an earlier and, in some cases, a longer antirejection regimen. Improved graft survival has been reported using this approach (284). With minor modifications this technique can be used successfully in small children and adolescents (285). In this series, the FNA biopsy CI reliably predicted rejection, as manifested by a rise in the serum creatinine level, with no false-negative results.

Nonspecific Immune Activity

Panel-reactive Anti-B Cell Antibody. The generation of anti-B cell antibodies against a lymphocyte panel has been associated with rejection episodes (283). Approximately 20% of tests show false-positive or -negative results.

Spontaneous Blastogenesis (SB). SB measures the spontaneous rate of DNA synthesis in recipient lymphocytes. A significant increase occurs prior to or concomitant with rejection (286). Although other factors may make SB rise somewhat, it is possible to correlate the intensity of SB reactivity with rejection (287).

Enumeration of T-lymphocyte Subsets. Observations in posttransplant patients treated with ATG suggest that a low level of circulating T-lymphocytes correlates with the absence of rejection (288), but this is not the case when other immunosuppressive agents are used. High "active" T-cell levels (a subpopulation of T-cells that possess high-affinity receptors for sheep red blood cells) may be useful in indicating rejection activity (289).

Functional T-lymphocyte subsets may be identified by using monoclonal antibodies. Monoclonal antibodies have been developed for total

T-lymphocytes (OKT_3, Leu_1); T helper/inducer cells (Th) (OKT_4, Leu_3); T suppressor/cytotoxic cells (Tscy) (OKT_8, Leu_2); and other cells with functions less well defined. A good correlation is found between Th/Tscy ratio and rejection, if the recipient does not have very low total T-cell levels (<150/mm^3) or an HLA identical donor (191, 290, 291). A strong overall correlation was reported between the irreversibility of graft injury and a low (<1.0) Th/Tscy ratio (291); 78% of rejection episodes with a low ratio were irreversible compared with only 6% of episodes accompanied by a normal or high Th/Tscy ratio (>1.0). However, other reports have not found predictability between the Th/Tscy ratio and rejection to be that reliable (292). Various factors could account for this discrepancy, e.g., CMV infection (293), the presence of immature cells containing both Th and Tscy markers (290), or an inadequate sample of T-lymphocytes (292). Despite these limitations, enumerating T-lymphocyte subsets may be helpful in monitoring for rejection episodes and for predicting reversibility.

RETRANSPLANTATION

The survival rate at five years after transplant for second and third allografts in 75 retransplants was similar to that obtained for first allografts, i.e., ± 45%. All third and fourth allografts failed within the first posttransplant month. The primary factor influencing allograft survival was recipient presensitization. The survival rate for recipients who were not presensitized, i.e., cytotoxic antibodies against <5% of a lymphocyte panel, or moderately presensitized (5% to 50% of the panel) was significantly better than that observed in highly presensitized recipients, i.e., those with antibodies to >50% of the panel. HLA-A and -B antigen compatibility led to improved graft survival rates in these highly presensitized recipients (92). Other factors affecting allograft rejection in multiple renal transplants include HLA-DR compatibility and possibly blood transfusions given before the first transplant (294).

TECHNICAL CONSIDERATIONS

The Small Child

Except for the small child, <20 kg, the technical aspects of renal transplantation in children are similar to those in adults. In the small child, depending on size, the graft can be placed extraperitoneally with the vascular anastomosis to the iliac or hypogastric vessels or transabdominally using the aorta and vena cava for anastomosis. Although some authors (295) have advocated the transabdominal approach when placing adult kidneys into children who weigh <20 kg, it has been our experience that this is required only in children weighing <10 kg. Appropriate-aged pediatric cadaver kidneys can always be placed extraperitoneally.

Intraoperative fluid management is critical when placing an adult kidney into a small child. Careful monitoring of the central venous and arterial pressure is necessary to maintain an adequate vascular volume. Whole blood, 100 to 250 ml, should be administered as a bolus before opening the vascular anastomoses to avoid hypotension resulting from opening the anastomosis. Hypotension predisposes to primary graft malfunction and vascular thrombosis.

Central-to-peripheral temperature measurements, as an indication of perfusion of peripheral tissues, is advocated (15). A decrease in the peripheral tissue temperature is indicative of vasoconstriction. If the vascular volume is normal under these circumstances, a vasodilator can be administered to assure adequate perfusion of the graft (15).

The ureter is reimplanted into the bladder if the bladder is adequate; if not, an ileal conduit is an acceptable alternative.

Bilateral Nephrectomy

Bilateral nephrectomy is not a prerequisite to renal transplantation and should be done for specific indications. The advantage of the production of erythropoetin (296), 1, 25 dihydroxy vitamin D (297), and added urine output are indications against routine nephrectomies; uncontrollable renin-dependent hypertension, persistent massive proteinuria in nephrotic children, and persistent pyelonephritis are indications for nephrectomy despite its disadvantages. Neither persistent vesicoureteral reflux nor hydronephrosis secondary to ureterovesical or ureteropelvic junction obstruction are indications for nephrectomy; corrective surgery is preferred.

When bilateral nephrectomy is indicated, it is best performed before renal transplant. Doing it at the time of transplantation lengthens the procedure and makes postoperative fluid and electrolyte management more difficult.

POSTOPERATIVE MEDICAL COMPLICATIONS

Infection

Infections are more frequent and severe in the immunosuppressed patient and are the most frequent cause of death after transplantation (298). Children may be less prone than adults to infection following steroid therapy (299). Although common bacterial infections occur in transplant recipients, infections with unusual organisms, such as *Serratia marcescens* and *Lysteria monocytogenes* also occur (300).

The herpes group of viruses: cytomegalovirus (CMV), herpes virus hominis (HVH), varicella zoster (VZV), and Epstein-Barr virus (EBV), are the most frequent pathogens causing infection post transplant. CMV infection is common, occurring in more than 60% of patients during the first year post transplant (264, 301). Infection with CMV is characterized by prolonged fever, leukopenia, thrombocytopenia, pulmonary symptoms, and hepatic dysfunction (302). Reduced graft function is due to a characteristic glomerulopathy (303). Since it takes two to three weeks to culture the virus from the throat, urine, blood, or bone marrow aspirate or to demonstrate a rise in the CMV antibody titer, it is frequently difficult to diagnose CMV infection. It is important to differentiate CMV infection from rejection because with CMV the dose of steroids should be reduced; increasing the dosage to treat rejection will enhance virus dissemination, prolong the illness, and increase its severity (303). Strategies have been suggested to reduce the risk or minimize the effects of CMV infection post transplant. Because a primary CMV infection is usually more severe than a secondary one, dialysis patients who are serially tested for antibodies and are seronegative should receive a transplant only from a seronegative donor (303a). Some interferon preparations, used prophylactically, may prevent CMV infection (304, 305).

Feldhoff and associates (306) described 19 episodes of varicella infection among 160 children post transplant over 11 yr; 8 had severe infection and 1 died. They observed an association between continuing azathioprine therapy with severity of disease. Therefore, it is recommended that azathioprine be withheld from the onset of symptoms until 24 to 48 hr after new vesicle formation has ceased.

Pneumonia—bacterial, viral, fungal, or protozoan—is a serious complication following transplantation. A transtracheal aspiration or open lung biopsy may be necessary to identify the pathogen. At times, several agents, e.g., CMV and *Pneumocystis*, are involved (307). Prophylactic trimethoprim-sulfamethoxazole therapy has significantly reduced the incidence of *Pneumocystis* in the immunocompromised patient (308).

Hepatic dysfunction following transplantation may be due to azathioprine toxicity (309) or to viral hepatitis, e.g., CMV, hepatitis A, B, or non-A, non-B (310). Children who develop persistent hepatitis B antigenemia during dialysis are candidates for transplantation (311), but precautions should be taken to prevent cross infection. More than 90% of the children are positive for hepatitis B "e" antigen, a marker of infectivity (312). The progressive liver disease that occurs in adults has not been reported in children with persistent antigenemia (311).

Hypertension

Hypertension in children posttransplant is related to many factors (313). In the immediate post transplant period, hypertension usually is related to hypervolemia, especially in patients with acute tubular necrosis and minimal urinary output. Hypertension is frequent with acute rejection and usually resolves with reversal of the rejection episode. It occurs with chronic rejection as well. Control of blood pressure is important to prevent deterioration of allograft function.

Hypertension in association with declining renal function any time after the first three months may be due to the renal artery stenosis. Angiography is diagnostic, and correction of the stenotic lesion will relieve the hypertension and usually improve allograft function (313). However, the surgical intervention may lead to graft loss (314). Transluminal angioplasty has been used to correct renal artery stenosis (315).

Hypertension in the patient with intact native kidneys may present a difficult diagnostic problem. Differential plasma renin determinations generally are not helpful. Native kidney removal should be considered only if the hypertension fails to respond to antihypertensive agents, e.g., captopril or minoxidil (316). (see Chapter 47). Although captopril is effective in lowering blood pressure, it may also reduce renal function in patients with renal artery stenosis of the donor kidney (316).

Steroid Toxicity

Cataracts

The incidence of posterior subcapsular lenticular opacities is related to the dosage of steroids and may be as high as 55% in children who have had a functioning allograft for more than one year (317). Visual impairment is uncommon, but 10% to 15% of patients with steroid-induced cataracts may require operative correction. These cataracts appear to progress little when the patient is on a low-maintenance dose of steroids.

Hyperlipidemia

Hyperlipidemia is present in the majority of children post transplant; type II and IV patterns are commonly noted (318, 319). The degree of hypercholesterolemia and steroid dosage is correlated (318). Because hyperlipidemia is a risk factor for cardiovascular disease, it would seem prudent to lower serum lipids to normal levels by reducing the steroid dosage and by other means (320).

Aseptic Necrosis

Aseptic necrosis of bone occurs in 5% to 20% of children post transplant (321–323). Any bone may be affected; however, the femoral head or femoral condyles are most commonly affected; multiple bone involvement is common. Of the 28 patients affected in the three reports, 18 had involvement of at least one femoral head. Pain usually is the initial complaint and may antedate x-ray findings by as long as nine months. Occasionally, asymptomatic aseptic necrosis is detected by roentgenogram.

The cause of aseptic necrosis is not known; a relationship with steroid therapy has been postulated, but in the three reports mentioned, no correlation between steroid dosage and aseptic necrosis was noted. Secondary hyperparathyroidism also is associated. It is our impression that the incidence of aseptic necrosis has decreased, as steroid dosage has been reduced and as management of pretransplant osteodystrophy has improved. Treatment is directed to relieving symptoms. Reducing steroid dosage once aseptic necrosis has developed has little benefit. Total hip replacement is indicated for unremitting aseptic necrosis of the femoral head. Surgery should be advised before the patient becomes depressed by persistent pain and decreased mobility.

Malignancy. Malignant disease is six times more frequent in post transplant patients than in the general population: some neoplasms, e.g., reticulum cell sarcoma of the central nervous system, occur almost exclusively in the immunosuppressed patient. It has been suggested that EBV infection may contribute to the occurrence of lymphoproliferative disease in the post transplant patient (252). The incidence and type of cancer noted in long-term follow-up of children is shown in Table 51.8. Although prevalence data are not available it appears to be lower in children than in adults.

GROWTH AND PUBERTAL DEVELOPMENT

Growth

The hope that a renal transplantation might lead to improvement in growth velocity has not been uniformly fulfilled. Growth in 41 children observed for three to eight years post transplant and receiving daily steroid therapy increased to normal in only 12%. Factors implicated in the poor response included the residual growth potential at the time of transplantation, the level of allograft function, and steroid dosage (324).

Children with a bone age >12 yr at the time of renal transplantation grow minimally, if at all post transplant whether they receive daily (324) or alternate-day (207) steroid therapy. More recent EDTA reports, however, have noted that substantial growth may occur post transplant in children with a bone age >12 yr. The reason for the difference is not apparent.

Growth post transplant is better in those children who received an allograft before 7 yr of age (331); 6 of 10 children who received a transplant between 11 and 45 months of age had normal or catch-up growth following transplantation. Because growth failure in the child with CRF often occurs in infancy (325), it may be appropriate to consider young children with CRF for early renal transplantation in order to improve growth potential following transplantation.

Table 51.8. Malignancy in Pediatric Allograft Recipients

Author	# Patients	Follow-up (yr)	Malignancy
De Shazo, et al (10)	100	10	None
Weil, et al (333)	57	13	Reticulum cell sarcoma of brain (1)
Martin, et al (336)	77	12½	None
Arbus, et al (16)	78	10	Hepatocarcinoma (1)
Chantler, et al (329)	75	10	Rhabdomyosarcoma (1)
Potter, et al (1)	145	15	None
Novello and Fine (335)	257	14½	Lymphoangiomatosis (1) Rhabdomyosarcoma (1) of prostate Adenocarcinoma of (1) thyroid Carcinoma in situ of cervix (2) Basal cell carcinoma of skin (2)

Impaired allograft function inhibits growth (327). Patients with a GFR <60 ml/min/1.73 m^2 grow poorly following transplantation. Somatomedin levels in children post transplant correlated with GFR. Relatively minimal reduction in allograft function may mediate growth impairment by decreased somatomedin activity.

The mechanism by which steroid therapy suppresses growth is not known. With alternate-day therapy growth velocity improves (208). Growth post transplant is improved by maintaining optimal allograft function and using alternate-day steroid therapy. The possible benefit of renal transplantation at an earlier age on subsequent growth has not been evaluated.

Pubertal Development

As a general rule, sexual maturation proceeds following renal transplantation. Pubertal development in 24 children who had a bone age <12 yr at the time of transplantation was reported during the three and one-half to eight-year follow-up period (326). Ten remained prepubertal, nine were progressing through puberty, and five had progressed normally to puberty.

In female patients who were pubertal before transplantation and became amenorrheic during the course of CRI, menses usually returned within 6 to 12 months post transplant. Adolescent patients should be given appropriate contraceptive information in the early posttransplant period (327).

Pubertal development in 12 boys post transplant was delayed (327 A). Stage of puberty as defined by Tanner correlated more closely with bone age. Serum testosterone and luteinizing hormone concentration were normal; serum follicle-stimulating hormone concentration in those recipients with a serum creatinine level <2.0 mg/dl was normal, but it was elevated when renal function was reduced. Interestingly, androgens produced by the adrenal gland were decreased, presumably because of depressed function secondary to steroid therapy. Exogenous androgen therapy may be helpful in those male recipients with delayed puberty, but guidelines have not been developed.

LONG-TERM OUTCOME

The 5- and 10-yr allograft survival rates reported in six studies are summarized in Table 51.9. Survival for five years in children does not guarantee continued survival. Allograft loss from chronic rejection continues despite adequate function five years post transplant. Indolent immunological injury probably occurs in every recipient; the child over a normal life span needs second or third allografts.

REHABILITATION (Table 51.10)

Rehabilitation of children following successful renal transplant is excellent. Of 296 children who received a renal transplant, 91% were attending school full-time (3). Of 86 patients at least one year post transplant, only 8% were not involved in vocational or educational programs or employed (39). Children and families following a successful renal transplant usually return to their previous psychological and social status within 1 yr (39).

Fertility and the effects of pregnancy are important questions for adolescents and adults who were treated for ESRD in childhood. Although successful pregnancy is common, there are risks to both mother and offspring. (Table 51.11). Reduction in allograft function occurs in 12% of patients, being more frequent in those who had impaired function before pregnancy. The renal impairment may improve after parturition, but more often function stabilizes or deteriorates further. Preeclampsia occurs in 25% of patients and is more frequent in those with preexistent hypertension, renal functional impairment, or both (327).

Approximately one half of newborns born to renal allograft recipients are premature by weight. The incidence of infections, congenital malformations (330), and physical and developmental delay in the children of these pregnancies is not increased (329). There also do not appear to be any increased complications in children fathered by renal transplant recipients (330). Infants born to transplant recipients receiving azathioprine should not be breast-fed, as this drug is secreted in breast milk and may be harmful to the infant.

Table 51.9. Long-term Outcome

Author	# Patients	% Actuarial graft survival			
		Live-related		Cadaver	
		5 yr	10 yr	5 yr	10 yr
De Shazo, et al (10)	100		74		44
Fine, et al (328)	69	73[a]		39[a]	
Chantler, et al (329)	75	55		43[b]	
Arbus, et al (16)	78				59
Potter, et al (1)	145		55		31

[a] Actual.
[b] 3 yr.

Table 51.10. Rehabilitation in 103 Pediatric Renal Transplant Recipients with Functioning Allografts for at Least 1 Year

Status	Number of patients	
School		
Preschool	1	
Elementary or secondary	49	
Performance		
Above average		13
Average		34
Below average		2
Handicapped programs	5	
Orthopedically		4
Mentally retarded		1
College	20	
Vocational rehabilitation	4	
Employment	14	
Full-time		8
Part-time		6
Child-rearing (mothers)	6	
No meaningful activity	4	
Total	103	

Table 51.11. Pregnancy in Renal Allograft Recipients: Effects on Mother and Offspring

Mother	Offspring
(allograft recipient)	
Spontaneous abortion (6%)	Gestation (by dates)
Reduction in allograft function (12%)	Term (47%)
Premature rupture of membranes (5%)	Preterm (52%)
Preeclampsia and/or eclampsia (26%)	Postterm (1%)
Urinary tract infection (12%)	Weight <2500 g (50%)
Delivery	Respiratory distress syndrome (47%)
Spontaneous vaginal (68%)	
Cesarean section (32%)	

References

1. Potter DE, Holliday MA, Piel CF, et al: Treatment of end-stage renal disease in children: a 15 year experience. Kidney Int 18:103, 1980.
2. Fine RN: Transplantation in children In Morris P (ed): Kidney Transplantation—Principles and Practice. London, Grune & Stratton Ltd, 1984, p. 589.
3. Donckerwolcke RA, Chantler C, Broyer M, et al: Combined report on regular dialysis and transplantation of children in Europe 1979, Proc Eur Dial Transpl Assoc 17:87, 1980.
4. Broyer M, Donckerwoldke RA, Bunner FP, et al: Combined report on regular dialysis and transplantation of children in Europe, 1980. Proc Eur Dial Transpl Assoc 18:60, 1981.
5. Krakauer H, Grauman JS, McMullan C: The recent U.S. experience in the treatment of end-stage renal disease by dialysis and transplantation. N Engl J Med 308:1558, 1983.
6. Donckerwolcke R, Broyer M, Brunner F, et al: Combined report on regular dialysis and transplantation of children in Europe XI, 1981. Proc Eur Dial Transpl Assoc 19:61, 1982.
7. Vollmer VM, Wahl PW, Blagg CR: Survival with dialysis and transplantation in patients with end-stage renal disease. N Engl J Med 308:1553, 1983.
8. Strom TB: The improving utility of renal transplantation in the management of end-stage renal disease. Am J Med 73:105, 1982.
9. Cerilli GJ, Nelsen C, Dorfmann L: Renal homotransplantation in infants and children with the hemolytic-uremic syndrome. Surgery 71:66, 1972.
10. DeShazo CV, Simmons RL, Bernstein DM, Results of renal transplantation in 100 children. Surgery 76:461, 1974.
11. Kwun YA, Butt KMH, Kim KH, et al: Successful renal transplantation in a 3 month old infant. Pediatrics 92:426, 1978.
12. Rizzoni G, Malekzadeh MH, Pennisi AJ, et al: Renal transplantation in children less than five years of age. Arch Dis Child 55:532, 1980.
13. Hodson EM, Najarian JS, Kjellstrand CM, et al: Renal transplantation in children ages 1 to 5 years. Pediatrics 61:458, 1978.
14. Moel DI, Butt KMH: Renal transplantation in children less than 2 years of age. J Pediatr 99:535, 1981.
15. Trompeter RS, Haycock GB, Bewick M, Chantler C: Renal transplantation in very young children. Lancet 1:373, 1983.
16. Arbus GS, Galiwango J, DeMaria JE, Churchill BM: The first 10 years of dialysis—transplantation at the Hospital for Sick Children. Can Med Assoc 120:659, 1980.
17. Miller LC, Bock GH, Lum CT, Mauer SM: Transplantation of the adult kidney into the very small child. Long term outcome. J Pediatr 1010:675, 1982.
17a. Goodwin WE, Kaufman JJ, Mims MM, et al: Human renal transplantation. I. Clinical experiences with six cases of renal homotransplantation. J Urol 89:13, 1963.
18. Iitaka K, Martin LW, Cox JA, et al: Transplantation of cadaver kidneys from anencephalic donors. J Pediatr 93:216, 1978.
19. Darmady EM: Transplantation and the ageing kidney. Lancet 2:1046, 1974.
20. Morling N, Ladefoged J, Lnage P, et al: Kidney transplantation and donor age. Tissue Ant 6:163, 1975.
21. Fine RN, Brennan LP, Edelbrock HH, et al: Use of pediatric cadaver kidneys for homotransplantation in children. JAMA 210:477, 1969.
22. Merkel FK, Ing TS, Ahmadian Y, et al: Transplantation in and of the young. J Urol 111:679, 1974.
22a. Glass NR, Stillman RM, Butt KMH, Kountz SL: Results of renal transplantation using pediatric cadaver donors. Surgery 85:504, 1979.
23. Hong JH, Shirani K, Arshad A, et al: Influence of cadaver donor age on the success of kidney transplants. Transplantation 32:532, 1981.
24. Van der Vliet JA, Cohen B, Kootstra G: Transplantation of pediatric cadaver kidneys. Transpl Proc 14:74, 1982.
25. Murray JE, Wilson RE, O'Conner NE: Evaluation of long-functioning human kidney transplants. Surgery 124:509, 1967.
26. Andersen OS, Jonasson O, Merkel FK: En bloc transplantation of pediatric kidneys in adult patients. Arch Surg 108:35, 1974.
27. Kootstra G, West JC, Dryburgh P, et al: Pediatric cadaver kidneys for transplantation. Surgery 83:333, 1978.
28. Boczko S, Tellis V, Veith FJ: Transplantation of children's kidneys into adult recipients. Surg Gynecol Obstet 146:387, 1978.
28a. Silber SJ: Renal transplantation between adults and children. Differences in renal growth. JAMA 228: 1143, 1974.
29. Bart KJ, Macon EJ, Whittier FC, et al: Cadaveric kidneys for transplantation. A paradox of shortage in the face of plenty. Transplantation 31:379, 1981.
30. Baluarte HR, Gruskin AB, Hiner LB, et al: Encephalopathy in children with chronic renal failure. Proc Clin Dial Transpl Forum 7: 95, 1977.
31. Bale JF Jr, Siegler RL, Bray P: Encephalopathy in young children with moderate chronic renal failure. Am J Dis Child 234:581, 1980.
32. Rotundo A, Nevins TE, Liptonk M, et al: Progressive encephalopathy in children with chronic renal insufficiency in infancy. Kidney Int 21:486, 1982.
33. Francis VR, Fine RN, Korsch BM: Physiologic and social adjustment to extended haemodialysis and renal homotransplantation in 42 children. Proc Eur Dial Transpl Assoc 7:366, 1970.
34. Korsch BM, Fine RN, Negrete VF: Non-compliance in children with renal transplants. Pediatrics 61:872, 1978.
35. Beck DE, Fennell RS, Yost RL, et al: Evaluation of an educational program on compliance with medication regimens in pediatric patients with renal transplants. J Pediatr 96:1094, 1980.
36. Negrete VF, Fine RN, Korsch BM: Non-compliance with immunosuppressive medication in renal transplants. Arzt Und Patient Jan, pp 20–23, 1980.
37. Penn I: Renal transplantation for Wilm's tumor: report of 20 cases. J Urol 12:793, 1979.
38. DeMaria JE, Hardy BE, Brezinski A, Churchill BM: Renal transplantation in patients with bilateral Wilm's Tumor. J Pediatr Surg 14:577, 1979.
39. Fine RN, Edelbrock HH, Riddell H, et al: Renal transplantation in children. Urology 9:61, 1977.
40. Makker SP, Kirson IJ: Renal transplantation in a child with Burkitt's lymphoma. Arch Intern Med 140:278, 1980.
41. Warshaw BL, Edelbrock HH, Ettenger RB, et al: Renal transplantation in children with obstructive uropathy. J Urol 123:737, 1980.
42. Firlet CF: Use of defunctionalized bladders in pediatric renal transplantation. J Urol 116:634, 1976.
43. Butt KM, Myer A, Kountz SL, Waterhouse K: Renal transplantation in patients with posterior urethral valves. J Urol 116:708, 1976.
44. Firlet CF, Merkel FK: The application of ileal conduits in pediatric renal transplantation. J Urol 118:647, 1977.
45. Levitt SB, Coberwal D, Kogan SJ, et al: Use of pre-existing ureterocutaneous anastomoses as conduits in renal allotransplantation. Urology 13:377, 1979.
46. Kreiger JN, Brem AS, Kaplan MR: Urinary tract infection in renal transplantation. Urology 15:362, 1980.
47. Porter KA, Dossetor JE, Marchioro TL, et al: Human renal transplants. I. Glomerular changes. Lab Invest 16:153, 1967.
48. Hsui HC, Suzuki Y, Churg J, Grishman E: Ultra-structure of the glomerular basement membrane in long term renal allografts with transplant glomerular disease. Histopathology 4:351, 1980.
49. Ettenger RB, Heuser ET, Malekzadeh MH, et al: Focal glomerulosclerosis in renal allografts. Am J Dis Child 131:1347, 1977.
50. Cameron JS: Glomerulonephritis in renal transplants. Transplantation 34:237, 1982.
51. Cosyns JP, Pirson Y, Squifflet JP, et al: De novo membranous nephropathy in human renal allografts: report of nine patients. Kidney Int 22:177, 1982.
52. Levy M, Charpentier B: De Novo membranous glomerulonephritis in renal allografts: report of 19 cases in 1550 transplant recipients. Transplant Proc 15:1099, 1983.
53. Leumann EP, Briner J, Donckerwolcke RAM, et al: Recurrence of focal segmental glomerulosclerosis in the transplanted kidney. Nephron 25:65, 1980.
54. Malekzadeh MH, Heuser EP, Ettenger RB, et al: Focal glomerulosclerosis and renal transplantation. J Pediatr 95:249, 1979.
55. Habib R, Hebert D, Gagnadoux MF, Broyer M: Transplantation in idiopathic nephrosis. Trans Proc 14:489, 1982.
56. Maizel SE, Sibley RK, Horstman JP, et al: Incidence and significance of recurrent focal segmental glomerulosclerosis in renal allograft recipients. Transplantation 32:512, 1981.
57. Zimmerman CE: Renal transplantation for focal segmental glomerulosclerosis. Transplantation 29:172, 1980.
58. Pinto J, Lacerda G, Cameron JS, et al: Recurrence of focal segmental glomerulosclerosis in renal allografts. Transplantation 32:83, 1981.
59. Hoyer JR, Kjellstrand CM, Simmons RL, et al: Successful renal transplantation in 3 children with congenital nephrolytic syndrome. Lancet 1:1410, 1973.
60. Pennisi AJ, Heiser ET, Malekzadeh MH, et al: Renal transplantation in children with membranoproliferative glomerulonephritis. VII International Congress of Nephrology, Montreal, 1978.
61. Amend WJC Jr, Vincenti F, Feduska NJ, et al: Recurrent systemic lupus erythematosus involving renal allografts. Annu Intern Med 94:444, 1981.
62. Levy M, Ami Moussa R, Habib R, et al: Anaphylactoid purpura and transplantation. (in press).
63. Baliah T, Kim KH, Anthone S, et al: Recurrence of Henoch-Schönlein purpura glomerulonephritis in transplanted kidneys. Transplantation 18:343, 1974.
64. Herdman RC, Uriza RE: Hemolytic-uremic syndrome. In (Rubin MI, Barrat TM eds): Pediatric Nephrology. Baltimore, Williams and Wilkins, 1975, p. 189.
65. Folman R, Arbus GS, Churchill B, et al: Recurrence of the hemolytic uremic syndrome in a 3½ year old child, 4 months after second renal transplantation. J Clin Nephrol 10:121, 1978.
66. Mahoney CP, Striker GE, Hickman RO, et al: Renal transplantation for childhood cystinosis. N Engl J Med 283:397, 1970.

67. Malekzadeh MH, Neustein HB, Schneider JA, et al: Cadaver renal transplantation in children with cystinosis. Am J Med 63:525, 1977.
68. Broyer M, Guillot M, Gubler MC, Habib R: Infantile cystinosis: a reappraisal of early and late symptoms. In Crosnier J, Grunfeld JP, Maxwell MD (eds): Advances in Nephrology Year Book 10:137, 1981.
69. Langlois RP, O'Regan S, Pelletier M, Robitaille P: Kidney transplantation in uremic children with cystinosis. Nephron 28:273, 1981.
70. Malekzadeh MH, Pennisi AJ, Phillis L, et al: Growth and endocrine function in children with cystinosis following renal transplantation. Trans A.S.A.I.O. 24:278, 1978.
71. Morris MC, Chambers TL, Evans PWG, et al: Oxalosis in infancy. Arch Dis Child 57:224, 1982.
72. Leumann EP, Wemann W, Largiader F: Prolonged survival after renal transplantation in primary hyperoxaluria of childhood. Clin Nephrol 9:29, 1978.
73. Whelchel JD, Alison DV, Luke RG, et al: Successful renal transplantation in hyperoxaluria: a report of two cases. Transplantation 35:161, 1983.
74. Carpenter CB, Strom TB: Transplantation: immunogenetic and clinical aspects. Part I. Hosp Pract 17:125, 1982.
75. Terasaki PI, Bernoco D, Park MS, et al: Microdroplet testing for HLA-A,B,C and D antigens. Am J Clin Pathol 69:103, 1978.
76. Garavoy MR: Immunogenetic association in nephrolytic states. In Brenner BM, Stein JH (eds): Contemporary Issues in Nephrology: Nephrotic Syndrome. New York, Edinburgh, London, and Melborne, Churchill Livingstone, 1982, p 259.
77. Yunis EJ, Amos DB: Three closely linked genetic systems relevant to transplantation. Proc Nat Acad Sci USA 68:3031, 1971.
78. Van Rood JJ, van Leeuwen A, Keuning JJ, et al: The serological recognition of the human MLC determinants using a modified cytotoxicity technique. Tissue Antig 5:73, 1975.
79. Opelz G, Mickey MR, Terasaki PI: Calculations on long term graft and patient survival in human kidney transplantation. Transplant Proc 9:27, 1977.
80. Solheim BG, Flatmark A, Halvorsen S, et al: Influence of HLA, A,B,C and D matching and pretransplant blood transfusions on kidney graft survival. Transplant Proc 11:748, 1979.
81. Broyer M, Gagnadoux MF, Buerton D, et al: Importance of HLA-A, B matching in kidney transplantation in children. Transplantation 30:310, 1980.
82. Persijn GG, Cohen B, Lansbergen Q, et al: Effect of HLA-A and HLA-B matching on survival of grafts and recipient after renal transplantation. N Engl J Med 307:905, 1982.
83. Opelz G, Terasaki PI: International study of histocompatibility in renal transplantation. Transplantation 33:87, 1982.
84. Ettenger RB, Jordan SC, Malekzadeh MH, et al: Immunologic considerations in renal transplantation. In Gruskin AB, Norman ME (eds): Developments in Nephrology: Pediatric Nephrology, Proc. Vth International Pediatric Nephrology Symposium. The Hague, Martinus Nijhoff, 3:364, 1981.
85. Svejgaard A: DR matching and cadaver kidney transplantation. Transplantation 33:1, 1982.
86. Moen T, Albrechtsen D, Flatmark A, et al: Importance of HLA-DR matching in cadaveric renal transplantation: a prospective one center study of 170 transplants. N Engl J Med 303:850, 1980.
87. Goeken NE, Thompson JS, Corry RJ: A 2-year trial of prospective HLA-DR matching. Effects on renal allograft survival and rate of transplantation. Transplantation 32:522, 1981.
88. Ayoub G, Terasaki PI: HLA-DR matching in multicenter, single-typing laboratory data. Transplantation 33:515, 1982.
89. Ting A, Morris PJ: Powerful effect of HLA-DR matching on survival of cadaveric renal allografts. Lancet 2:282, 1980.
90. Strom TB, Carpenter CB: Transplantation. Immunogenetic and clinical aspects. Part II. Hosp Pract 18:135, 1983.
91. Goeken NE, Shulak JA, Nghiem DD, et al: Feasibility of optimal HLA-DR matching: a retrospective view. Transplantation 34:297, 1982.
92. Fine RN, Malekzadeh MH, Pennisi AJ, et al: Renal retransplantation in children. J Pediatr 95:244, 1979.
93. Dausset J, Rapaport FT: The role of blood group antigens in human histocompatibility. Ann Acad Sci 129:498, 1966.
94. Wilbrandt R, Tung KSK, Deodhar SD, et al: ABO blood group incompatibility in human renal homotransplantation. Am J Clin Pathol 51:15, 1969.
95. Bariety J, Oriol R, Hinglais N, et al: Distribution of blood group antigen A in normal and pathologic human kidneys. Kidney Int 17:820, 1980.
96. Alexandre G: Successful renal transplantation across the ABO blood-group barrier. Am Soc Transpl Surgeons, 9th Annual Scientific Meeting. Chicago, 1983.
97. Boorman KE, Dodd BE: The group-specific substances A,B, M,N, and Rh: their occurrence in tissues and body fluids. J Pathol 55:329, 1943.
98. Annual Report, National Organ Matching Service. United Kingdom, 1974–1975.
99. Huestis DW, Zukoski CF: Secondary stimulation of Rh antibodies by kidney allografts from Rh-positive donors. Vox Sang 24:524, 1973.
100. Opelz G, Terasaki PI: Cadaver kidney transplants in North America: analysis 1978. Dial Trans 8:167, 1979.
101. Oriol R, Cartron JP, Cartron J, et al: Biosynthesis of ABH and Lewis antigens in normal and transplanted kidneys. Transplantation 29:184, 1980.
102. Oriol R, Opelz G, Chun C, et al: The Lewis system and kidney transplantation. Transplantation 29:397, 1980.
103. Paul LC, van Es LA, Fleuren G: Demonstration of transplantation antigens on the endothelium of peritubular capillaries in renal allografts by the immunoperoxidase method. Transplantation 28:72, 1979.
104. Moraes JR, Stastny P: A new antigen system expressed in human endothelial cells. J Clin Invest 60:449, 1977.
105. Paul LC, Class FHJ, van Es LA, et al: Accelerated rejection of a renal allograft associated with pretransplantation antibodies directed against donor antigens on endothelium and monocytes. N Engl J Med 100:1258, 1979.
106. Cerilli GJ, Galouzis LB, de Francis ME: Clinical significance of antimonocyte antibody in kidney transplant recipients. Transplantation 32:495, 1981.
106a. Etheredge EE, Bettonville P, Sicard GA, et al: Immunologic studies of rejection of HLA-identical renal allografts in sib pairs. Transplant Proc 15:1057, 1983.
107. Paul LC, van Es LA, van Rood JJ, et al: Antibodies directed against antigens on the endothelium of peritubular capillaries in patients with rejecting renal allografts. Transplantation 27:175, 1979.
108. Baldwin WM, Claas FHJ, Paul LC, et al: All monocyte antigens are not expressed on renal endothelium. Tissue Antig 21:254, 1983.
109. Kissmeyer-Nielsen F, Olsen S, Peterson VP, et al: Hyperacute rejection of kidney allografts, associated with pre-existing humoral antibody. Lancet 2:662, 1966.
109a. Williams GM, Hume DM, Hudson RP Jr, et al: Hyperacute renal-homograft rejection in man. N Engl J Med 279:611, 1968.
110. Patel R, Terasaki PI: Significance of the positive crossmatch test in kidney transplantation. N Engl J Med 280:735, 1969.
110a. Ettenger RB, Terasaki PI, Opelz G, et al: Successful renal allografts across a positive crossmatch for donor B lymphocyte alloantigens. Lancet 2:56, 1976.
111. Ettenger RB, Uittenbogaart ChH, Pennisi AJ, et al: Long term cadaver allograft survival in the recipient with a positive B lymphocyte crossmatch. Transplantation 27:315, 1979.
111a. Lobo PI, Westervelt FB, Rudolf LE. Kidney transplantability across a positive cross-match. Cross match assays and distribution of B lymphocyte in donor tissues. Lancet 1:925, 1977.
112. Dejelo CL, Williams TC: B cell cross-match in renal transplantation. Lancet 2:241, 1977.
113. Richiardi P, Diotallevi T, Matejc T, et al: HLA antibodies cytotoxic only for B lymphocytes. Tissue Antig 10:323, 1977.
114. Ettenger RB, Jordan SC, Fine RN: Autolymphocytotoxic antibodies in patients on dialysis awaiting renal transplantation. Transplantation 32:248, 1981.
114a. Jeannet M, Vassali P, Hufschmid MF: Enhancement of human kidney allografts by cold B lymphocyte cytotoxins. Transplantation 29:174, 1980.
115. Hudelson B, Liu J, Ocariz J, et al: Lymphocytotoxic anti-Lewis bh antibody. Transplantation 31:449, 1981.
116. Iwaki Y, Terasaki PI, Park MS, et al: Enhancement of human kidney allografts and B-cold lymphocyte cytotoxins. Lancet 1:1228, 1978.
117. Ettenger RB, Jordan SC, Fine RN: Cadaver renal transplant outcome in recipients with autolymphocytotoxic antibodies. Transplantation 35:429, 1983.
118. Ettenger RB, Malekzadeh MH, Pennisi AJ, et al: B lymphocyte crossmatching: lack of effect on transplant outcome based on incubation temperature. Proc Dial Transplant Forum 9:197, 1979.
118a. Salvatierra O, Vincenti F, Amend W, et al: Pretreatment with donor-specific blood transfusions in related recipients with high MLC. Transplant Proc 13:142, 1981.
119. Blank JL, Leo CM, Sollinger HW, et al: B-warm-positive crossmatch: a contraindication for transplantation in living related transplants undergoing donor specific transfusion. Transplantation 33:212, 1982.
119a. Ahern AT, Artruc SB, DellaPelle P, et al: Hyperacute rejection of HLA-AB-identical renal allografts associated with B lymphocyte and endothelial reactive antibodies. Transplantation 33:103, 1982.
120. Deierhoi MN, Ting A, Morris PJ: Successful renal transplantation despite warm B cell antibodies. Transplantation 36:207, 1983.
120a. Vaidya S, Orosz CG, Cerrilli J, et al: The clinical significance of donor specific B cell antibody following donor-specific blood transfusion in renal transplantation. Transpl Proc 16:1447, 1984.
121. Ting A: The lymphocytotoxic crossmatch test in clinical renal transplantation. Transplantation 35:403, 1983.
122. Thorsby E, Ettenger RB, Garavoy M: Pretransplant immunologic considerations. Transpl Proc 16:1649, 1984.
123. Cardella CJ, Falk JA, Peters P, et al: Do repeated blood transfusions prevent

successful transplantation in highly sensitized potential transplant recipients? Transplant Proc 14:359, 1982.
124. Garovoy MR, Frnaco V, Zschaeck D, et al: Direct lymphocyte mediated cytotoxicity as an assay of presensitization. Lancet 1:573, 1973.
125. Garovoy MR, Myrburgh SJ, Cooper CM, et al: Computer analysis of presensitization and cross-reacting antibodies. Transplant Proc 9:1811, 1977.
126. Opelz G, Mickey MR, Terasaki PI: HLA and kidney transplant: re-examination. Transplantation 17:371, 1974.
127. Van Hoof JP, Schippers HMA, van der Steen GJ, et al: Efficacy of HL-A matching in Eurotransplant. Lancet 2:1385, 1972.
128. Cross DE, Whittier FC, Weaver P, et al: A comparison of the antiglobulin versus extended incubation time crossmatch: results in 223 renal transplants. Transplant Proc 9:1803, 1977.
129. Fuller TC, Cosimi AB, Russel PS: Use of an antiglobulin-ATG reagent for detection of low levels of alloantibody improvement of allograft survival in presensitized recipients. Transplant Proc 10:463, 1978.
130. Braun WE, Straffon RA: Long-term results in 35 HLA-identical siblings and 3 HLA-identical parent-child renal allograft recipients. Nephron 22:232, 1978.
131. Seigleer HF, Ward FE, McCoy RE, et al: Long-term results with forty-five living related renal allograft recipients genotypically identical for HLA. Surgery 81:274, 1977.
132. Etheredge EE, Shons AR, Schmidtke JR, et al: Mixed leukocyte culture reactivity and rejection in renal transplantation in HLA-identical siblings. Transplantation 17:538, 1974.
133. Cochrum K, Salvatierra O, Blezer FO: Correlation between MLC stimulation and graft survival in living related and cadaver transplants. Ann Surg 180:617, 1974.
134. Garovoy MR, Person A, Carpenter CB: Correlation of mixed lymphocyte culture (MLC) reactivity and graft survival in 1 haploitype matched recipients. Proc Clin Dial Transplant Forum 8:209, 1978.
135. Papdopoulou ZL, Turner MA, Helfrich BG: Successful pediatric renal transplantation without donor specific transfusion (DST). 15th Annual Meeting of the American Society of Nephrology. Chicago, 1982, p 201A.
136. Flechner SM, Kerman RH, Van Buren CT, et al: The high risk haploidentical living related recipient: transplantation without blood transfusions and steroid withdrawal using cyclosporine. Transplant Proc 15:442, 1983.
137. Najarian JS: Immunologic aspects of organ-transplantation. Hosp Pract 17:61, 1982.
138. Salvatierra O Jr, Iwaki F, Vincenti F, et al: Update of the University of California at San Francisco experience with donor-specific blood transfusions. Transplant Proc 14:363, 1982.
139. Dossetor JB, MacKinnon KJ, Gault MH, et al: Cadaver kidney transplants. Transplantation 5:844, 1967.
140. Opelz G, Graver B, Terasaki PI: Induction of high kidney graft survival rate by multiple transfusions. Lancet 1:1223, 1981.
141. Terasaki PI, Perdue S, Ayoub G, et al: Reduction of accelerated failures by transfusion. Transpl Proc 14:251, 1982.
142. Persign GG, Van Hoof JP, Kalff MW, et al: Effect of blood transfusion and HLA matching on renal transplantation in the Netherlands. Transpl Proc 5:503, 1977.
143. Feduska NJ, Vincenti F, Amend WJ, et al: Do blood transfusions enhance the possibility of a compatible transplant? Transplantation 27:35, 1979.
144. Solheim BG: The role of pre-transplant blood transfusions. Transpl Proc 11:138, 1979.
145. Singal DP, Joseph S, Szewezuk MR: Possible mechanisms of the beneficial effect of pretransplant blood transfusion on renal allograft survival in man. Transpl Proc 14:316, 1982.
146. Fangelli L, Singal DP: Blood transfusion may induce anti-T cell receptor antibodies in renal patients. Transpl Proc 14:319, 1982.
147. Kerman RH, Van Buren CT, Payne W, et al: Influence of blood transfusions on immune responsiveness. Transpl Proc 14:335, 1982.
148. Lenhard V, Massen G, Serfert P, et al: Characterization of transfusion induced suppressor cells in prospective kidney allograft recipients. Transpl Proc 14:329, 1982.
149. Persijn GG, van Leeuwen A, Parlevliet J, et al: Two major factors influencing kidney graft survival in Eurotransplant: HLA DR matching and blood transfusion. Transpl Proc 13:150, 1981.
150. Newton WT, Anderson CB: Attempted enhancement in patients undergoing renal allotransplantation. Arch Surg 114:1007, 1979.
151. Keown PA, Descamps B: Improved renal allograft survival after blood transfusion: a non-specific erythrocyte-mediated immunoregulatory process? Lancet 1:20, 1979.
152. Van Es AA, Marquet RL, Van Rood JJ, et al: Influence of a single blood transfusion on kidney allograft survival in unrelated rhesus monkeys. Transplantation 26:325, 1978.
153. Borleffs JCC, Neuhaus P, van Rood JJ, et al: Platelet transfusions have a positive effect on kidney allograft survival in rhesus monkeys inducing cytotoxic antibodies. Transpl Proc 15:985, 1983.
154. Spees EK, Vaughn WK, Williams GM, et al: Effects of blood transfusion on cadaver renal transplantation. Transplantation 30:455, 1980.
155. Green WF, Niblack GD, Johnson HK, et al: Multifactorial analysis of factors influencing graft survival in recipients of living-related renal allografts. Transpl Proc 14:282, 1982.
156. Fuller TC, Dlmonico FL, Cosimi AB, et al: Impact of blood transfusion on renal transplantation. Ann Surg 187:211, 1978.
157. Siller CR, Lockwood BL, Sinclair NR, et al: Beneficial effect of operation day blood transfusion on human renal allograft survival. Lancet 1:169, 1978.
158. Williams KA, Ting A, French ME, et al: Preoperative blood transfusion improves cadaveric renal allograft survival in non-transfused recipients. Lancet 1:104, 1980.
159. Corry RJ, West JC, Hunsicker LG, et al: Effect of timing of administration and quantity of blood transfusion on cadaver renal transplant survival. Transplantation 30:425, 1980.
160. Feduska NJ, Amend WJ, Vincenti F, et al: Blood transfusions before and on the day of transplantation: effects on cadaver graft survival. Transpl Proc 14:302, 1982.
161. Opelz G, Graver B, Mickey MR, et al: Lymphocytotoxic antibody responses to transfusion in potential kidney transplant recipients. Transplantation 32:177, 1981.
162. Ettenger RB: Pretransplant blood transfusion and renal transplantation outcome. In Fine RN (moderator): Renal Transplantation update Ann Int Med 100:246, 1984.
163. Morris PJ, Mickeyu MR, Singal DP, et al: Serotyping for homotransplantation. XXII. Specificity of cytotoxic antibodies developing after renal transplantation. Br Med J 1:758, 1969.
164. Opelz G, Terasaki PI: Dominant effect of transfusions on kidney graft survival. Transplantation 39:153, 1980.
165. Sanfilippo F, Vaughn WK, Bollinger RR, et al: The relationship of transfusion and presensitization with graft and patient survival. Transpl Proc 14:287, 1982.
166. Iwaki Y, Terasaki PI, Heintz R, et al: Report of the pre-sensitization workshop. Transpl Proc 14:417, 1982.
167. Kreis H: Selection of a donor. In Hamburger J, Crosnier J, Bach JF, Kreis H (eds): Renal Transplantation Theory and Practice. Baltimore, London, Williams and Wilkins, 1981, p 36.
168. Suchia G, Mercurial F, Scalamogna M, et al: Comparative effects of pregnancy, transfusion and prior graft rejection on sensitization and renal transplant results. Transplantation 34:360, 1982.
169. Opelz G, Terasaki PI: Improvement of kidney graft survival with increased numbers of blood transfusion. N Engl J Med 299:799, 1978.
170. Solheim BG, Flatmark A, Halvorsen S, et al: Effect of blood transfusions on renal transplantation: study of 191 consecutive first transplants from living related donors. Transplantation 30:281, 1980.
171. Fehrman I: Pretransplant blood transfusions and related kidney allograft survival. Transplantation 34:46, 1982.
172. Brynger H, Frisk B, Ahlmen J, et al: Blood transfusion and primary graft survival in male recipients. Scand J Urol Nephrol (suppl) 42:76, 1977.
173. Opelz G, Terasaki PI, Graver B, et al: Correlation between number of pretransplant blood transfusions and kidney graft survival. Transpl Proc 11:145, 1979.
174. Salvatierra O, Vincenti F, Amend W, et al: What about blood transfusions in living related transplantation? Proc Am Soc Nephrol p 178A, 1979.
175. Halasz NA, Orloff MJ, Hirone F: Increased survival of renal homografts in dogs after injection of graft donor blood. Transplantation 2:453, 1964.
176. Marquet RL, Heystek GA, Tinbergen WJ: Specific inhibition of organ allograft rejection by donor blood. Transpl Proc 3:708, 1971.
177. Fabre JW, Morris PJ: The effect of donor strain blood pretreatment on renal allograft rejection in rats. Transplantation 14:608, 1972.
178. Okazaki H, Maki T, Wood ML, et al: Prolongation of skin allograft survival in H_2K and I region-incompatible mice by pretransplant blood transfusion. Transplantation 32:111, 1981.
179. Salvatierra O, Vincenti F, Amend W, et al: Deliberate donor specific blood transfusions prior to living-related renal transplantation: a new approach. Ann Surg 192:543, 1980.
180. Mendez R, Iwaki Y, Mendez R, et al: Seventeen consecutive successful one haplotype matched living related first renal transplants using donor specific blood transfusion. Transplantation 33:621, 1982.
181. Schweitzer R, Bow L, Generas D, et al: Serologic considerations in donor-specific transfusion therapy for kidney transplantation. Transpl Proc 14:374, 1982.
182. Amend W, Vincenti F, Feduska N, et al: Unusual renal transplant rejections in recipients of pre-transplant, donor-specific transfusion. Am Soc Nephrol p 157A, 1980.
183. Salvatierra O Jr: Donor-specific blood transfusions. Medical Staff Conference, University of California, San Francisco. West J Med 138:398, 1983.
184. Ettenger RB, Kerman R, Arnett J, et al: Sensitization after donor-specific transfusions for live-related renal transplantation. Transpl Proc 15:943, 1983.

185. Anderson CB, Sicard GA, Etheredge EE: Pretreatment of renal allograft recipients with azathioprine and donor-specific blood products. Surgery 92:315, 1982.
186. Light JA, Metz S, Oddenino K, et al: Donor specific transfusion with diminished sensitization. Transplantation 34:352, 1982.
187. Cochrum K, Hanes D, Potter D, et al: Improved graft survival with donor-specific transfusion pretreatment. Transpl Proc 13:190, 1981.
188. Leivestad T, Flatmark A, Hirschberg H, et al: Effect of pre-transplant donor-specific transfusions in renal transplantation. Transpl Proc 14:370, 1982.
189. Miller LC, Bock GH, Lum CT, et al: Transplantation of the adult kidney into the very small child: long-term outcome. J Pediatr 100:675, 1982.
190. Fauci AS, Dale DC: The effect of in vivo hydrocortisone on subpopulation of human lymphocytes. J Clin Invest 53:240, 1974.
191. Cosimi AB, Calvin RB, Burton RC, et al: Monoclonal antibodies for immunologic monitoring and treatment in recipients of renal allografts. N Engl J Med 305:308, 1981.
192. Balow JE, Hunninghake GW, Fauci AS: Corticosteroids in human lymphocyte mediated cytotoxic reactions. Transplantation 23:322, 1977.
193. Keown PA, Essery GL, Stiller CR, et al: Mechanisms of immunosuppressions by cyclosporin. Transpl Proc 13:386, 1981.
194. Gillis S, Crabtree GR, Smith KM: Glucocorticoid-induced inhibition of T cell growth factor production. I. The effect on mitogen induced lymphocyte proliferation. J Immunol 123:1624, 1979.
195. Suthanthiran M, Kaye WA, Rubin AL, Stenzel KH: Interleukin-z profiles in renal graft recipients. Transpl Proc 16:1473, 1984.
196. Goldstein IM: Effects of steroids on lyposomes. Transpl Proc 7:21, 1975.
197. Dale DC, Fauci AS, Wolff SM: Alternate-day prednisone: leukocyte kinetics and susceptibility to infections. N Engl J Med 291:1154, 1974.
198. McGeown M: Immunosuppression for kidney transplantation. Lancet 2:310, 1973.
199. Kreis H, Lacombe M, Noel LH, et al: Kidney graft rejection: Has the need for steroids to be reevaluated. Lancet 2:1353, 1978.
200. Fine RN: Renal transplantation in children. Proc Eur Dial Transpl Assoc 18:321, 1981.
201. McGeown M, Kennedy JA, Loughridge WGG: One hundred kidney transplants in the Belfast City Hospital. Lancet 1:876, 1971.
202. Chan L, French MF, Oliver DO, Morris PJ: High and low-dose prednisolone. Transpl Proc 13:336, 1981.
203. Bell PRF, Calman KC, Wood RFM, et al: Reversal of acute clinical and experimental organ rejection using large doses of intravenous prednisolone. Lancet 1:876, 1971.
204. Kauffman HD, Stormstad AS, Sampson D, et al: Randomized steroid therapy of human kidney transplant rejection. Transpl Proc 11:36, 1979.
205. Gary D, Shepherd H, Deer A, et al: Oral versus intravenous high-dose steroid treatment of renal allograft rejection. Lancet 1:117, 1978.
206. Pennisi AJ, Malekzadeh MH, Uittenbogaart CH, et al: Alternate day corticosteroid therapy in pediatric renal transplant recipients. VIIth International Congress of Nephrology, Montreal, 1978.
206a. Reimold EW: Intermittent prednisone therapy in children and adolescents after renal transplantation. Pediatrics 52:235, 1983.
207. Hoda Q, Hasinoff DJ, Arbus GS: Growth following renal transplantation in children and adolescents. Clin Nephrol 3:6, 1975.
208. McEnery PT, Gonzalez LL, Martin LW, West CD: Growth and development of children with renal transplants: use of alternate day steroid therapy. J Pediatr 83:806, 1973.
209. Leb DE: Alternate day prednisone treatment may increase kidney transplant rejection. Proc Dial Transpl Forum 9:136, 1978.
210. Dumler F, Levin NW, Szego G, et al: Long-term alternate day steroid therapy in renal transplantation. Transplantation 34:78, 1982.
211. McDonald FD, Horenstexn ML, Mayor GB, et al: Effect of alternate day steroids on renal transplant function: a controlled study. Proc Eur Dial Transpl Assoc 13:216, 1976.
212. Lorkkegaard H, Hessthaysen J: Permanent withdrawal of prednisone in necro-kidney transplantation. Proc Eur Dial Transpl Assoc 13:216, 1976.
213. Naik RB, Abdeen H, English J, et al: Prednisolone withdrawal after 2 years in renal transplant patients receiving only this form of immunosuppression. Transpl Proc 11:39, 1979.
214. Steinman TI, Brown RS, Yager HM, et al: Effect of tapering and discontinuing prednisone in kidney transplant recipients. Chicago, American Society of Transplant Physicians, 1983, p 40.
215. Murray JE, Merrill JP, Harrison JH, et al: Prolonged survival of human kidney homografts by immunosuppressive drug therapy. N Engl J Med 268:1315, 1963.
216. Haesslein HC, Peirce JC, Lee HM, et al: Leukopenia and azathioprine management in renal homotransplantation. Surgery 71:598, 1972.
217. Dandavino R, Trunet P, Descamps B, et al: Prolonged withdrawal of azathioprine in kidney transplantation. Transpl Proc 10:655, 1978.
218. Toussaint C, Kinnaert P, Vereerstraeten P, et al: Azathioprine is necessary in kidney transplantation. Transplantation 34:78, 1982.
219. Bach JF: Immunosuppression. In Hamburger J, Crosnier J, Bach JF, Kreiss H (eds): Renal Transplantation, Theory and Practice. Baltimore, Williams and Wilkins, 1981, p 89.
220. Bach MA, Bach JF: Activities of immunosuppressive agents in vitro. II. Different timing of azathioprine and methotrexate in inhibition and stimulation of mixed lymphocyte reactions. Clin Exp Immunol 11:89, 1972.
221. Dimitriv A, Fauci AS: Differential sensitivity of human lymphocyte subpopulations to azathioprine. Transpl Proc 10:878, 1979.
222. Prince HE, Ettenger RB, Dorey F, et al: Azathioprine suppression of natural killer cell activity and antibody dependent cellular cytotoxicity in renal transplant recipients. Transpl Proc 16:1475, 1984.
223. Galanaud P, Crevon MC, Duclos H, et al: New data on the effect of azathioprine at the cellular level. Adv Nephrol 6:371, 1980.
224. De Clerk YA, Ettenger RB, Ortega JA, et al: Macrocytosis and pure RBC anemia caused by azathioprine. Am J Dis Child 134:377, 1980.
225. Fisher KA, Makajan SK, Hill JL, et al: Prediction of azathioprine intolerance in transplant patients. Lancet 1:828, 1973.
226. Bradley PP, Warden GD, Maxwell JG, et al: Neutropenia and thrombocytopenia in renal allograft recipients treated with trimethoprim-sulfa-methoxazate. Ann Intern Med 93:560, 1980.
227. Elion GB, Callahan S, Nathan H, et al: Potentiation by inhibition of drug degradation: 6 substituted purines and xanthine oxidase. Biochem Pharmacol 12:85, 1963.
228. Ireland P, Rashid A, Von Lichtenberg F: Liver disease in kidney transplant patients receiving azathioprine. Arch Intern Med 132:29, 1973.
229. Penn I: Tumor incidence in human allograft recipients. Transpl Proc 11:1047, 1979.
230. Hoy WE, Packman CH, Freeman RB: Evolution of acute leukemia in renal transplant patient—relationship to azathioprine. Transplantation 33:333, 1982.
231. Borel JF: Comparative study of in vitro and in vivo drug effects on cell mediated cytotoxicity. Immunology 31:631, 1976.
232. Calne RY: Immunosuppression for organ grafting; observations on cyclosporin. Immunol Rev 46:113, 1979.
233. Morris PJ: Cyclosporin A: overview. Transplantation 32:349, 1981.
234. Calne RY, White DJG, Thriu S, et al: Cyclosporin A in patients receiving renal allografts. Surg Gynecol Obstet 145:729, 1978.
235. Leapman SB, Filo RS, Smith EJ, et al: Differential effects of cyclosporin A on lymphocyte subpopulations. Transpl Proc 13:405, 1981.
236. Hess AD, Tutschka PJ: Effect of cyclosporin A on human lymphocyte responses in vitro. I. CS-A allows for the expression of alloantigen-activated suppressor cells while preferentially inhibiting the induction of cytolytic effective lymphocytes in MLR. J Immunol 124:2601, 1980.
237. Hess AD, Tutschka PJ, Santos GW: Effect of cyclosporin A on human lymphocyte responses in vitro. II. Induction of specific alloantigen unresponsiveness mediated by a nylon wool adherent suppressor cell. J Immunol 126:961, 1981.
238. Lafferty KJ, Borel JF, Hodgkin P: Cyclosporin A: models for the mechanism of action. Transpl Proc 15:2242, 1983.
239. Homan WP, Williams KA, Millard PR, et al: Studies on the immunosuppressive properties of cyclosporin A in rats receiving renal allografts. Transplantation 31:423, 1981.
240. Calne RY, Rolles K, White DJG, et al: Cyclosporin A initially as the only immunosuppressant in 34 recipients of cadaveric organs: 32 kidneys, 2 pancreases and 2 livers. Lancet 2:1033, 1979.
241. European Multicenter Trial Group: Cyclosporin in cadaveric renal transplantation: one year follow-up of a multicenter trial. Lancet 2:986, 1983.
242. The Canadian Multicentre Transplant Study Group: A randomized clinical trial of cyclosporine in cadaveric renal transplantation. N Engl J Med 309:809, 1983.
243. Ferguson RM, Rynasiewicz J, Sutherland D, et al: Cyclosporin A in renal transplantation: a prospective randomized trial. Surgery 92:175, 1982.
244. Najarian J, Ferguson RM, Sutherland DER, et al: A prospective trial of the efficacy of cyclosporine in renal transplantation at the University of Minnesota. Transpl Proc 15:438, 1983.
245. Starzl TE, Weil R III, Iwatsuki S, et al: The use of cyclosporin A and prednisone in cadaver kidney transplantation. Surg Gynecol Obstet 151:17, 1980.
246. Starzl TE, Iwatsuki S, Malatack JJ, et al: Liver and kidney transplantation in children receiving cyclosporin A. J Pediatr 100:681, 1982.
247. Conley SB, Brewer ED, Van Buren CT, Kahan BD: Renal transplantation using cyclosporine in pediatric recipients 3 to 17 years old. Transpl Proc 15:2528, 1983.
248. Orocz CG, Ferguson RM, Olson S, Ascher N: A novel assay for C_sA Activity in patient's serum. Transpl Proc 16:1624, 1984.
248a. Flechner S, Van Buren C, Kerman RH, Kahan BD: The nephrotoxicity of cyclosporine in renal transplant recipients. Transpl Proc 15:2689, 1983.
249. Von Willibrand E, Hyary P: Cyclosporin A deposits in renal allografts. Lancet 2:189, 1983.

250. Flechner SM, Payne WD, Van Buren C et al: The effect of cyclosporine on early graft function in human renal transplantation. Transplantation 36:268, 1984.
251. Beveridge T: Cyclosporin A: an evaluation of clinical results. Transpl Proc 15:433, 1983.
252. Hanto DW, Frizzera G, Gail-Peczalska KJ: Epstein-Barr virus–induced B cell lymphoma after renal transplantation. N Engl J Med 306:913, 1982.
253. Calne RY, Rolles K, White DJG, et al: Cyclosporin A in clinical organ grafting. Transpl Proc 13:349, 1981.
254. Mannick JA, Davis RC, Cooperband SR, et al: Clinical use of rabbit antihuman lymphocyte globulin in cadaver-kidney transplantation. N Engl J Med 284:1109, 1971.
255. Uittenbogaart CH, Robinson BJ, Malekzadeh MH, et al: The use of antithymocyte globulin (dose by rosette protocol) in pediatric renal allograft recipients. Transplantation 28:291, 1979.
256. Kerman RH, Floyd M, Van Buren CT, et al: Improved allograft survival of strong immune responder—high-risk recipients with adjunctive antithymocyte globulin therapy. Transplantation 30:450, 1980.
257. Bell RF, Blamey RW, Briggs JD, et al: Medical Research Council trial of antilymphocyte globulin in renal transplantation: a multicenter randomized double-blind placebo controlled clinical investigation. Transplantation 35:539, 1983.
258. Taylor HE, Ackman CFD, Horowitz I: Canadian clinical trial of antilymphocyte globulin in human cadaver renal transplantation. Can Med Assoc J 115:1205, 1976.
259. Novick AC, Braun WE, Stinmuller D, et al: A controlled randomized double-blind study of antilymphoblast globulin in cadaver renal transplantation. Transplantation 35:175, 1983.
260. Filo RS, Smith EJ, Leapman SB: Therapy of acute cadaveric renal allograft rejection with adjunctive antithymocyte globulin. Transplantation 30:445, 1980.
261. Hardy MA, Nowygrod R, Elberg A, et al: Use of ATG in treatment of steroid-resistant rejection. Transplantation 29:162, 1980.
262. Hoitsma AJ, Reekers P, Kreeftenberg JG, et al: Treatment of acute rejection of cadaveric renal allografts with rabbit antithymocyte globulin. Transplantation 33:12, 1982.
263. Streem SB, Novick AC, Braun WE, et al: Low-dose maintenance prednisone and antilymphoblast globulin for the treatment of acute rejection: a steroid sparing approach to immunosuppressive therapy. Transplantation 35:420, 1983.
264. Rubin RH, Cosimi AB, Hirsch MS, et al: Effects of antithymocyte globulin on cytomegalovirus infection in renal transplant recipients. Transplantation 31:143, 1981.
265. Carpenter CB: Third international immunologic monitoring symposium: workshop summary. Transpl Proc 15:1995, 1983.
266. Jonker M, Goldstein G, Balner H: Effects of in vivo administration of monoclonal antibodies specific for human T cell subpopulations on the immune system in a rhesus monkey model. Transplantation 35:521, 1983.
267. Mathew TH, Kincaid-Smith P, Clyne DM, et al: A controlled trial of oral anticoagulants and dipyridamale in cadaveric organ allografts. Lancet 1:1307, 1974.
268. Anderson M, Dewar P, Fleming LB, et al: A controlled trial of dipyridamole in human renal transplantation and an assessment of platelet function studies in rejection. Clin Nephrol 2:93, 1974.
269. Carpenter CB, d'Apice AJF, Abbas AK: The role of antibodies in the rejection and enhancement of organ allografts. Adv Immunol 22:1, 1976.
270. Naik RB, Ashlin R, Wilson C, et al: The role of plasmapheresis in renal transplantation. Clin Nephrol 11:245, 1979.
271. Kirubakaram MG, Disney APS, Norman J, et al: A controlled trial of plasmapheresis in the treatment of renal allograft rejection. Transplantation 32:164, 1981.
272. Allen NH, Dyer P, Geoghegan T, et al: Plasma exchange in acute renal allograft rejection: a controlled trial. Transplantation 35:425, 1983.
273. Pilepich MV, Dicard GA, Breaux SR, et al: Renal graft irradiation in acute rejection. Transplantation 35:208, 1983.
274. Rynasiewicz JS, Sutherland DER, Ferguson RM, et al: Total lymphoid irradiation and kidney transplantation: a clinical experience. Transplant Proc 13:417, 1981
275. Fryd DS, Sutherland DER, Simmons RL, et al: Results of a prospective randomized study on the effect of splenectomy versus no splenectomy in renal transplant patients. Transpl Proc 13:48, 1981.
276. Descamps B, Gagnon R, Debray-Sachs M, et al: Lymphocyte dependent and complement dependent antibodies in human renal allograft recipients. Transplant Proc 7:635, 1975.
277. Gailliunas P, Suthanthiran M, Person A, et al: Post-transplant immunologic monitoring of the renal allograft recipient. Transplant Proc 10:609, 1978.
278. Stiller CR, Sinclair NR, Stc, Abrahams S, et al: Anti-donor immune responses in prediction of transplant rejection. N Engl J Med 294:978, 1976.
279. Garovoy MR, Gailliunas P, Carpenter CB, et al: Immunologic monitoring of transplant rejection: correlation of in vitro assays with morphologic changes on transplant biopsy. Nephron 22:208, 1978.
280. Grunnet N, Kristensen T: Antibody and lymphocyte mediated immunological recipient versus donor reactions before and after human renal transplantation: a prospective study. Transplant Proc 10:531, 1978.
281. Soulillou JP, Peyrat MA, Guenel J: Association between treatment resistant kidney allograft rejection and post-transplant antibodies to donor B-lymphocyte alloantigens. Lancet 1:354, 1978.
282. Bakkaloglu A, Sandilands GP, Briggs JD, et al: Inhibition of Fc rosette formation by serum of patients with renal allograft rejection. Lancet 2:430, 1977.
283. Ettenger RB, Terasaki PI, Ting A, et al: Anti-B lymphocytotoxins in renal-allograft rejection. N Engl J Med 295:305, 1976.
283a. Bach ML, Engstrom MA, Bach FH, et al: Specific tolerance in human kidney allograft recipients. Cell Immunol 3:161, 1972.
284. Hayry P, von Willebrand E: Cytological evaluation of in-situ inflammatory response of rejection in human renal transplantation. Transplant Proc 13:81, 1981.
285. Tabak MA, DuPuis MA, Ettenger RB, Fine RN: Fine needle aspiration biopsy: experience in a pediatric population. In Kreis H, Droz D (eds.): Renal Transplant Cytology. Wichtig-Editore, Milan. P. 105, 1984.
286. Anderson CB, Codd JE, Graff RJ, et al: Lymphocyte activation after renal transplantation. Transplantation 16:68, 1973.
287. Vessela RL, Pierce GE, Barth RF, et al: Correlation of spontaneous leukocyte blastogenesis with human renal allograft rejection. Transplantation 23:277, 1977.
288. Cosimi AB, Delmonico FL, Burdick JF, et al: Individualized management of immunosuppression according to serial monitoring of immunocompetence. Transplant Proc 10:647, 1978.
289. Kerman RH, Floyd M, Van Buren CT, et al: Correlation of non-specific immune monitoring with rejection or impaired function of renal allografts. Transplantation 32:16, 1981.
290. Binkley WF, Valenzuela R, Braun WE, et al: Flow cytometry quantitation of peripheral blood (PB) T-cell subsets in human renal allograft recipients. Transplant Proc 15:1163, 1983.
291. Colvin RB, Cosimi AB, Burton RC, et al: Circulating T-cell subsets in 72 human renal allograft recipients: the $OKT^{4+}/OKT_8{}^{+}$ cell ratio correlates well with reversibility of graft injury and glomerulopathy. Transplant Proc 15:1166, 1983.
292. Walzer WC, Anaise RJ, Bachovaroff RJ, Rapaport FT: Lymphocyte subpopulations in renal transplantation. Transplant Proc 16:1544, 1984.
293. Carney WB, Rubin RH, Hoffman RA, et al: Analysis of T lymphocyte subsets in cytomegalovirus mononucleosis. J Immunol 126:2114, 1981.
294. Persign GG, Lansbergen O, D'Amaro J, et al: Blood transfusion and second kidney allograft survival. Transplantation 32:392, 1981.
295. Lum CT, Fryd DS, Potter TA, Najarian JS: Results of kidney transplantation in the young child. Transplantation 34:167, 1982.
296. Van Ypersele de Strihou C, Stragier A: Effect of bilateral nephrectomy on transfusion requirements of patients undergoing chronic dialysis. Lancet 2:705, 1969.
297. Ettinger CW: Calcium absorption after nephrectomy in a uremic patient. N Engl J Med 291:458, 1974.
298. Fine RN: Treatment of end stage renal disease. Pediatr Ann 10:65, 1981.
299. Roth D, Freundlich M, Kyriakides GK et al: Immunological considerations in renal transplantation in young patients. Transplantation 37:612, 1984.
300. Avner ED, Harmon WE, Grupe WE, et al: Mortality of chronic hemodialysis and renal transplantation in pediatric end-stage renal disease. Pediatrics 67:412, 1981.
301. Marker SC, Howard RJ, Simmons TL, et al: Cytomegalovirus infection: a quantitative prospective study of three hundred twenty consecutive renal transplants. Surgery 89:660, 1981.
302. Fine RN, Grushkin CM, Malekzadeh M, Wright HT, Jr: Cytomegalovirus post-transplantation in children. Arch Surg 105:564, 1972.
303. Richardson WP, Colvin RB, Cheeseman SH, et al: Glomerulopathy associated with cytomegalovirus viremia in renal allografts. N Engl J Med 305:58, 1981.
303a. Betts RF, Freeman RB, Douglas RG Jr, Falley TE: Clinical manifestations of renal allograft derived primary cytomegalovirus infection. Am J Dis Child 131:759, 1977.
304. Cheeseman SH, Rubin RH, Stewart JA, et al: Controlled clinical trial of prophylactic human leukocyte interferon in renal transplantation: effects on cytomegalovirus and herpes simplex infections. N Engl J Med 300:1345, 1979.
305. Hirsch MS, Schooley RT, Cosimi AB, et al: Effects of interferon-alpha on cytomegalovirus reactivation syndromes in renal transplant recipients. N Engl J Med 308:1489, 1983.
306. Feldhoff CM, Balfour HH, Simmons RL, et al: Varicella in children with renal transplants. J Pediatr 98:25, 1981.
307. Rosen PP, Martini N, Armstrong D: Pneumocystis carinii pneumonia: diagnosis by lung biopsy. Am J Med 58:794, 1975.
308. Hughes WT, Feldman S, Sanyal SK: Treatment of pneumocystis carinii pneumonitis with trimethoprin-sulfamethoxazole. Can Med Assoc J 112:475, 1975.
309. Malekzadeh MH, Grushkin CM, Wright HT Jr, Fine RN: Hepatic dysfunction post-transplantation in children. J Pediatr 81:279, 1972.
310. Ware AJ, Luby JP, Eigenbrodt EH, et al: Spectrum of liver disease in renal transplant recipients. Gastroenterology 68:755, 1975.

311. Fine RN, Malekzadeh MH, Pennisi AJ, et al: HBs antigenemia in renal allograft recipients. Ann Surg 185:411, 1977.
312. Ettenger RB, Tong MJ, Landing BH, et al: Hepatitis B infection in pediatric dialysis and transplant patients. Significance of E antigen. J Pediatr 97:550, 1980.
313. Malekzadeh MH, Brennan LP, Payne VC Jr, Fine RN: Hypertension after renal transplantation in children. J Pediatr 86:370, 1975.
314. Ehrlich RM: Surgical complications of renal transplantation. In Fine RN, (moderator): Renal Transplantation Update. Ann Int Med 100:246, 1984.
315. Barth KH, Brusilow SW, Kaufman SL, Ferry FT: Percutaneous transluminal angioplasty of homograft renal artery stenosis in a 10-year-old girl. Pediatrics 67:675, 1981.
316. Curtis JJ, Luke RG, Whelchel JD, et al: Inhibition of angiotensin-converting enzyme in renal transplant recipients with hypertension. N Engl J Med 308:377, 1983.
317. Wilson WA, Fine RN: Long-term follow-up of cataracts in children after renal transplantation. Am Ophthalmol Soc 1:8, 1979.
318. Pennisi AJ, Heuser ET, Mickey MR, et al: Hyperlipidemia in pediatric hemodialysis and renal transplant patients (and coronary artery disease). Am J Dis Child 130:957, 1976.
319. Saldanha LF, Hurst KS, Amend JC Jr, et al: Hyperlipidemia after renal transplantation in children. Am J Dis Child 130:951, 1976.
320. Goldberg AP, Haigers JM, Delmez JA, et al: Exercise training improves abnormal lipid and carbohydrate metabolism in hemodialysis patients. Trans Am Soc Artif Intern Organs 25:431, 1979.
321. Uittenbogaart CH, Isaacson AS, Stanley P, et al: Aseptic necrosis after renal transplantation in children. Am J Dis Child 132:765, 1978.
322. Potter DE, Genant HK, Salvatierra O Jr: Avascular necrosis of bone after renal transplantation. Am J Dis Child 132:1125, 1978.
323. Hely D, Fennell RS III, Petty W, et al: Osteonecrosis of the femoral head and condyle in the post-transplantation courses of children and adolescents. Int J Pediatr Nephrol 3:297, 1982.
324. Pennisi AJ, Phillips LS, Costin G, et al: Linear growth in long-term renal allograft recipients. Clin Nephrol 8:415, 1977.
325. Betts PR, Magrath G: Growth pattern and dietary intake of children with chronic renal insufficiency. Br Med J 2:189, 1974.
326. Pennisi AJ, Costin G, Phillips LS, et al: Somatomedin and growth hormone studies: in pediatric renal allograft recipients who receive daily prednisone. Am J Dis Child 133:950, 1979.
327. Fine RN: Pregnancy in renal allograft recipients. Am J Nephrol 2:117, 1982.
327a. Ferraris J, Saenger P, Levine L, New M, Pang S, Saxena BB, Lewy JE: Delayed puberty in males with chronic renal failure. Kidney Int 18:344, 1980.
328. Fine RN, Malekzadeh MH, Pennisi AJ, et al: Long-term results of renal transplantation in children. Pediatrics 61:641, 1978.
329. Chantler C, Carter JE, Bewick M, et al: 10 years' experience with regular hemodialysis and renal transplantation. Arch Dis Child 55:435, 1980.
330. Penn I, Makowski EL, Harris P: Parenthood following renal and hepatic transplantation. Transplantation 30:397, 1980.
331. Inglefinger JR, Grupe WE, Harmon WE, et al: Growth acceleration following renal transplantation in children less than 7 years of age. Pediatrics 68:255, 1981.
332. Chantler C, Donckerwolke RA, Brunner FP, et al: Combined report on regular dialysis and transplantation of children in Europe, 1978. Proc Eur Dial Transpl Assoc 16:76, 1980.
333. Wiel T, Putnam CW, Porter KA, Starzl TE: Transplantation in children. Surg Clin North Am 56:467, 1976.
334. Arbus GS, Hardy BE, Balfe JW, et al: Cadaveric renal transplants in children under 6 years of age. Kidney Int 24:5, 1983.
335. Novello AC, Fine RN: Renal transplantation in children—a review. Int J Pediatr Nephrol 3:87, 1982.
336. Martin LW, McEnery PT, Rosenkrantz JG, et al: Renal homotransplantation in children. J Pediatr Surg 14:571, 1979.
337. Lawson RK, Talwalker YB, Musgrave JE, et al: Renal transplantation in pediatric patients. J Urol 113:225, 1975.
338. Kinnaert P, Persijn G, Cohen B, Van Geertruden J: Transplantation of kidneys from anencephalic donors. Transplant Proc 16:71, 1984.

CHAPTER 52

Renal Osteodystrophy

OTTO MEHLS
EBERHARD RITZ

INTRODUCTION

Pediatricians have known for decades that renal failure is associated with retarded growth and a peculiar form of metabolic bone disease (1–3), the clinical manifestations of which tend to be more severe in the growing skeleton of children than in adults. Lesions may appear earlier in the metaphyses, where rapid modeling occurs, than in other areas of the growing skeleton. This may also explain why orthopedic problems; e.g., epiphyseal slipping and metaphyseal fractures, are not uncommon in uremic children.

Since chronic hemodialysis and renal transplantation have become routine modalities of treatment for end-stage renal disease (ESRD), considerable interest has focused on the problems of growth disturbance and bone disease of uremic children, particularly because chronic hemodialysis fails to correct these abnormalities (4, 5).

DISTURBED Ca-P METABOLISM

Abnormalities in Chronic Renal Insufficiency (Residual Function 80% to 50% Normal)

Elevated immunoreactive parathormone (iPTH) levels occur even in early chronic renal insufficiency (CRI), i.e., in patients with 80% to 70% function or a glomerular filtration rate (GFR) of <80 ml/min/1.73 m^2 (Fig. 52.1) (6, 7). Elevation of iPTH levels may reflect accumulation of biologically inert material secondary to delayed catabolism of PTH fragments; however, we have found woven osteoid (Fig. 52.2) and other evidence of excessive PTH action on bone tissue in adult patients with early CRI (8). Furthermore, nephrogenous cAMP, evidence of excessive PTH action on target tissue, is increased in patients with a 60% to 50% function and mean GFR of 60 ml/min/1.73 m^2 (9).

The presence of hyperparathyroidism so early in CRI raises the question of what signal triggers PTH oversecretion (10). Levels of both serum Ca and P are low in the early phases of reduced renal function. Hypocalcemia in children with moderately elevated levels of serum creatinine may represent a stimulus, not necessarily the only one, for PTH hypersecretion at an early stage of CRI (10) (Fig. 52.3). As a result of the phosphaturic action of PTH, this hypersecretion is associated with hypophosphatemia (9). Although fasting hypophosphatemia has been found by most investigators, it may not be an adequate reflection of serum P levels throughout the day. In our own study, circadian serum P levels and their response to an oral phosphate load were normal. Fasting serum P was low in six patients with a mean GFR of 70 ml/min/1.73 m^2, and the changes of serum Pi in responses to oral phosphate were identical with those of healthy controls (Fig. 52.4) (11).

This finding is relevant to the hypothesis advanced by Bricker (12), who proposed that during progressive loss of nephrons, the kidney adapts to increased filtered loads of P, via PTH oversecretion. The latter was thought to be a "trade off" for the necessity to increase fractional P excretion when GFR falls progressively. Although hyperphosphatemia is present in advanced CRF (13), it has not been demonstrated to initiate the hyperparathyroidism early in CRI. The kidneys can adapt to changes in P load even in the absence of PTH; parathyroidectomized rats with subtotal nephrectomy display variations in renal Pi threshold in response to different dietary loads of phosphorus (14). Experiments employing proportional reductions of dietary P intake are, therefore, difficult to interpret since P intake itself alters renal P handling independently of PTH and influences the phosphaturic response to PTH.

The cause of hypocalcemia early in CRI has not been completely clarified. Massry and associates (15) hypothesized that circulating $1,25(OH)_2D_3$ levels were low in CRI and that these were ultimately responsible for the development of hypocalcemia and hyperparathyroidism. The response of serum $1,25(OH)_2D_3$ levels in CRI is somewhat controversial. Renal production of $1,25(OH)_2D_2$ falls in proportion to the fall in GFR (16). Slatopolsky coworker (17) reported $1,25(OH)_2D_3$ levels in the upper range of normal in adults with CRI, whereas others (18, 19) found these levels to be decreased. Studies in children show significantly decreased mean circulating $1,25(OH)_2D_3$ levels when GFR has fallen below approximately 50 ml/min/1.73 m^2, although individual levels may be within the range of normal (20–23).

However, levels of $1,25(OH)_2D_3$ that are in the normal range in early CRI may not be appropriate to the prevailing biochemical milieu. Early in CRI, impaired intestinal absorption of Ca, hypocalcemia, hyperparathyroidism, and fasting hypophosphatemia are all present and should stimulate renal 1-α-hydroxylase activity. Therefore, an abnormality in vitamin D metabolism may be an early event in CRI. In the healing phase of nutritional vitamin D deficiency with a comparable constellation of serum chemistries (24), $1,25(OH)_2D_3$ levels are very high. The inability

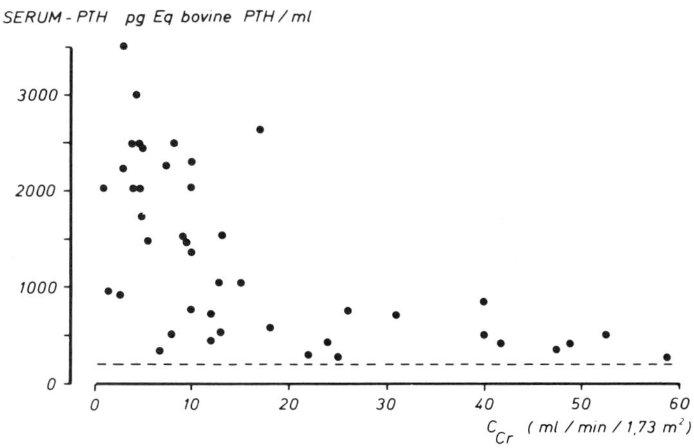

Figure 52.1. Relationship between serum PTH and C_{Cr} in untreated children with congenital renal diseases with varying levels of renal function. (From Mehls O, Ritz E: Early treatment of renal osteodystrophy. In Buccianti G (ed): Early Treatment of Renal Insufficiency. Contr Nephrol 37:17, 1983, with permission.)

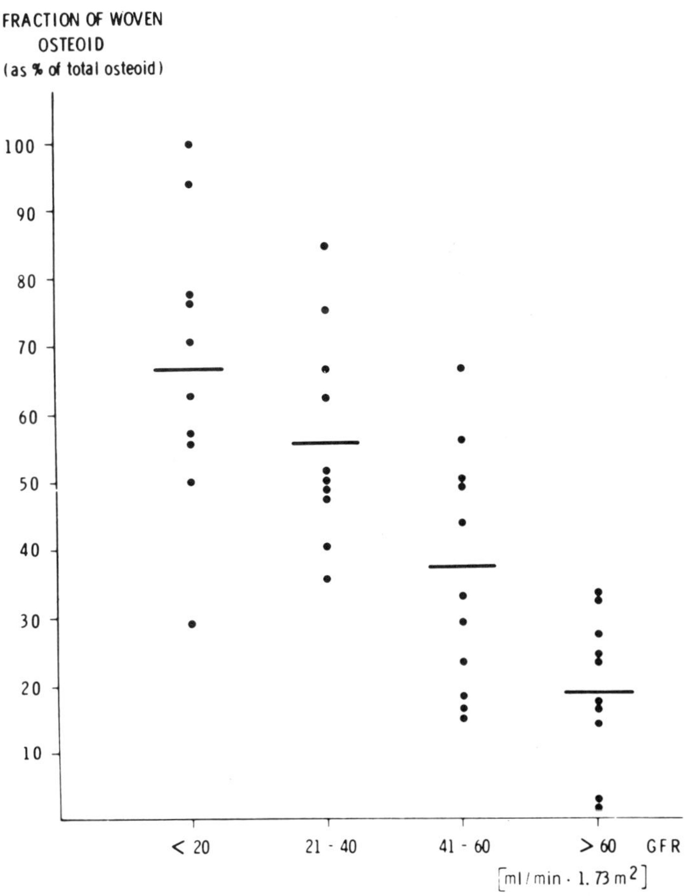

Figure 52.2. Fraction of woven osteoid as percent of total osteoid at various levels of GFR. There is some woven osteoid even in mild renal failure and a progressive increase with decreasing GFR. (From Malluche HH, et al: Bone histology in incipient and advanced renal failure. Kidney Int 9:355, 1976, with permission.)

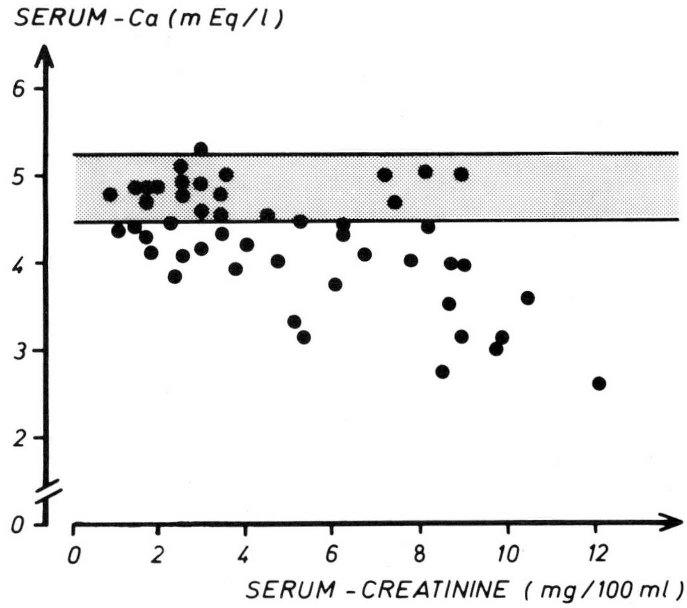

Figure 52.3. Relationship between serum levels of Ca and Cr in untreated children with congenital renal diseases and varying levels of renal function. (From Mehls O, Ritz E: Early treatment of renal osteodystrophy. In Buccianti G (ed): Early Treatment of Renal Insufficiency. Contr Nephrol 37:17, 1983, with permission.)

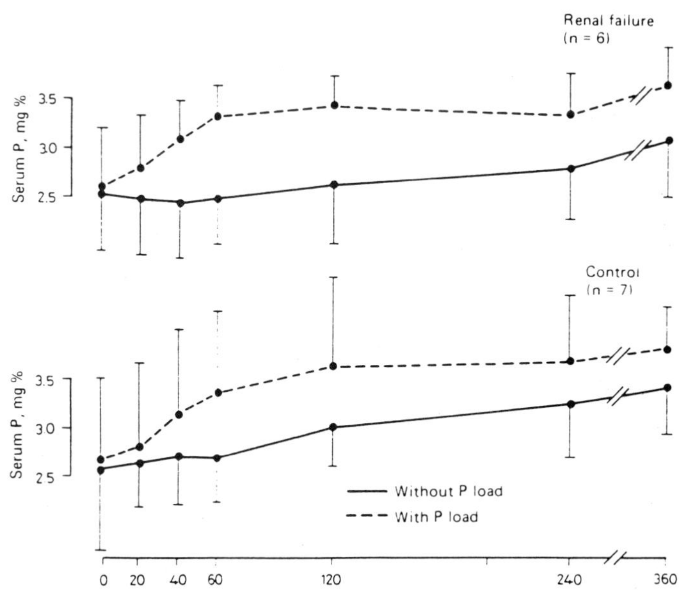

Figure 52.4. Serum Pi without and with oral phosphate load in patients with incipient renal failure (from Ritz E et al: Pathogenesis of renal osteodystrophy: role of phosphate and skeletal resistance to PTH. Adv Exp Med Biol 103:423, 1978).

of the organism even in early CRI to increase $1,25(OH)_2D$ production or to correct the abnormalities in Ca and P metabolism points to ineffective stimulation of renal 1 α-hydroxylase activity and possibly to resistance to the effects of $1,25(OH)_2D_3$, i.e., an altered dose-response relationship.

Administration of $1,25(OH)_2D_3$ to individuals with CRI increases intestinal absorption of Ca, urinary Ca excretion, and decreases iPTH levels (25). It is uncertain whether this represents the response to substitution of the hormone in a deficiency state or a pharmacological effect of $1,25(OH)_2D_3$.

The rise of ionized serum Ca in response to PTH is attenuated in early CRI (26), although there is an appropriate rise in fractional renal cAMP excretion. This resistance to the calcemic action of PTH may be the cause or the consequence of hyperparathyroidism. In many hormonal systems, down-regulation of hormone receptors occurs in response to sustained elevation in levels of that hormone. Bone cells lose responsiveness to PTH on continuous exposure (27, 28). This observation could provide an explanation for earlier findings (29) that the calcemic response to PTH is maintained in vitamin D–deficient rats when severe hyperparathyroidism is prevented by interfering with parathyroid blood supply. In experimental acute uremia, responsiveness of cartilage receptor-adenylate-cyclase complex to PTH in an in vitro system is diminished. This disturbance is present whether or not the parathyroid glands are intact or whether pharmacological doses of $1,25(OH)_2D_3$ were administered (30).

The cause of the diminished calcemic response to PTH in humans with CRI requires additional study. Rats with CRI show an early resistance to PTH action due only to hyperphosphatemia, whereas a more slowly appearing component of PTH resistance apparently is due to deranged vitamin D metabolism (31). Because of the interdependence of vitamin D and PTH actions, deranged vitamin D metabolism could play a role in PTH resistance. In some systems, vitamin D status influences PTH receptors (32).

In summary, early CRI is characterized by diminished intestinal absorption of Ca (33); hypocalcemia (6); hyperparathyroidism (6, 7) with incipient renal osteitis fibrosa (8); fasting hypophosphatemia (11, 23) secondary to PTH-induced lowering of renal Pi threshold (9); hypocalciuria (34), primarily because of PTH action on renal tubular reabsorption of Ca, diminished filtered load of Ca, or both, and inappropriately low $1,25(OH)_2D_3$ levels (15, 22, 23). These findings are integrated into a hypothetical pathogenetic sequence (Table 52.1).

Abnormalities in chronic renal failure (CRF)

In patients with chronic renal failure, (residual function <25% normal; GFR <30 ml/min/1.73 m^2), hyperphosphatemia is a consistent finding (Fig. 52.5). Either hypocalcemia or hypercalcemia may be present. The latter is occasionally observed in patients with extreme osteitis fibrosa, particularly after serum P levels have been lowered. In the past, the paradoxical occurrence of hyperparathyroidism in the presence of hypercalcemia was thought to indicate escape of parathyroid glands from suppression by high levels of ionized (so-called autonomous tertiary hyperparathyroidism). However, parathyroid hyperplasia may increase

Table 52.1
Hypothetical Pathogenetic Sequence of Changes in Ca and P Metabolism in CRD

Reduced renal mass
↓
Diminished basal renal 1-alpha-hydroxylase
↓
Inappropriate 1.25 $(OH)_2D_3$ levels
↓
Intestinal Ca absorption reduced
↓
Bone/extracellular fluid Ca equilibrium reset (hypocalcemia)
↓
PTH resistance
↓
Compensatory increase of PTH secretion
↓
Steady state:
Hypocalcemia
Hypophosphatemia
Hyperparathyroidism
(Normal) 1.25$(OH)_2D_3$ levels

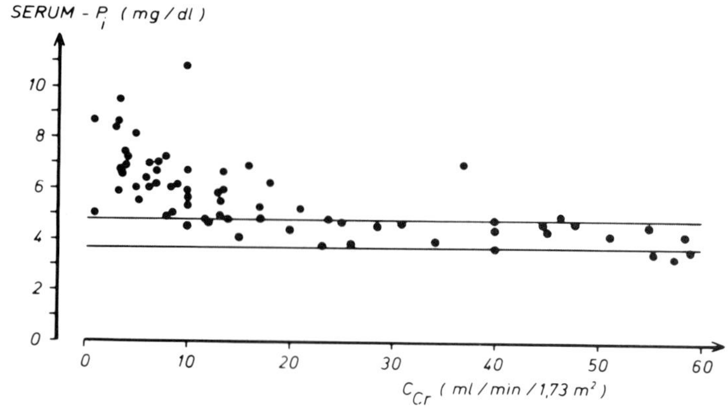

Figure 52.5. Relationship between serum phosphorus levels and creatinine clearance in untreated children with congenital renal diseases and varying levels of renal function (tubular disorders excluded). Serum levels are low at a clearance of 70 ml/min/1.73 m^2. They are above normal starting at a clearance below 25 ml/min/1.73 m^2. (From Mehls O, Ritz E: Early treatment of renal osteodystrophy. In Buccianti G (ed): Early Treatment of Renal Insufficiency. Contr Nephrol 37:17, 1983, with permission.)

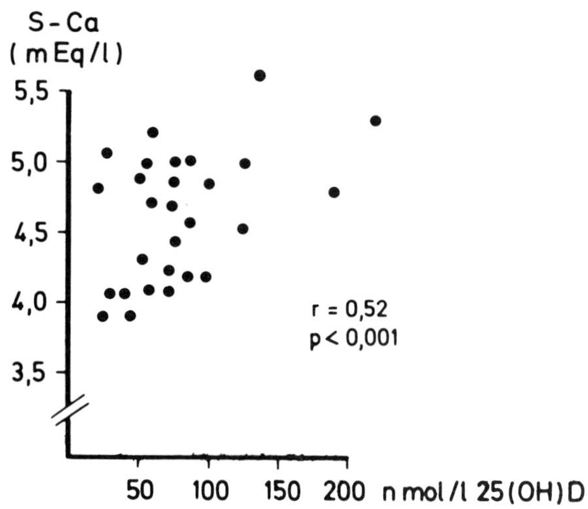

Figure 52.6. Relationship between serum Ca and serum 25(OH)D levels in children on maintenance dialysis. (Modified from Schmidt-Gayk H, et al: 25-OH-vitamin D in experimental and clinical uremia. Calcif Tissue Res 22 (Suppl): 430, 1977.)

non-Ca-suppressible basal PTH secretion to the extent that circulating PTH levels are sufficient to maintain increased bone resorption and hypercalcemia (35). Although high serum Ca levels correlate with histological evidence of osteitis fibrosa (31), low serum Ca levels are indicative of large amounts of osteoid in the skeleton of uremic patients (36). Furthermore, serum Ca and $25(OH)D_3$ levels are correlated (Fig. 52.6) (37).

In patients at this stage of renal failure, intestinal absorption of Ca usually is depressed (38), although with advanced hyperparathyroidism it may be elevated occasionally. When Ca intakes are high, net intestinal absorption rises because of transfer of Ca across the intestinal mucosa by diffusion. Because self-selected diets of children with CRF usually are low in Ca, they are at risk to negative Ca balance, which can be overcome by increasing Ca intake, by administering vitamin D metabolites, or both (Fig. 52.7). In addition, despite increased renal fractional excretion of Ca (39), urinary Ca excretion is severely depressed (40) except in states of renal salt-wasting (41).

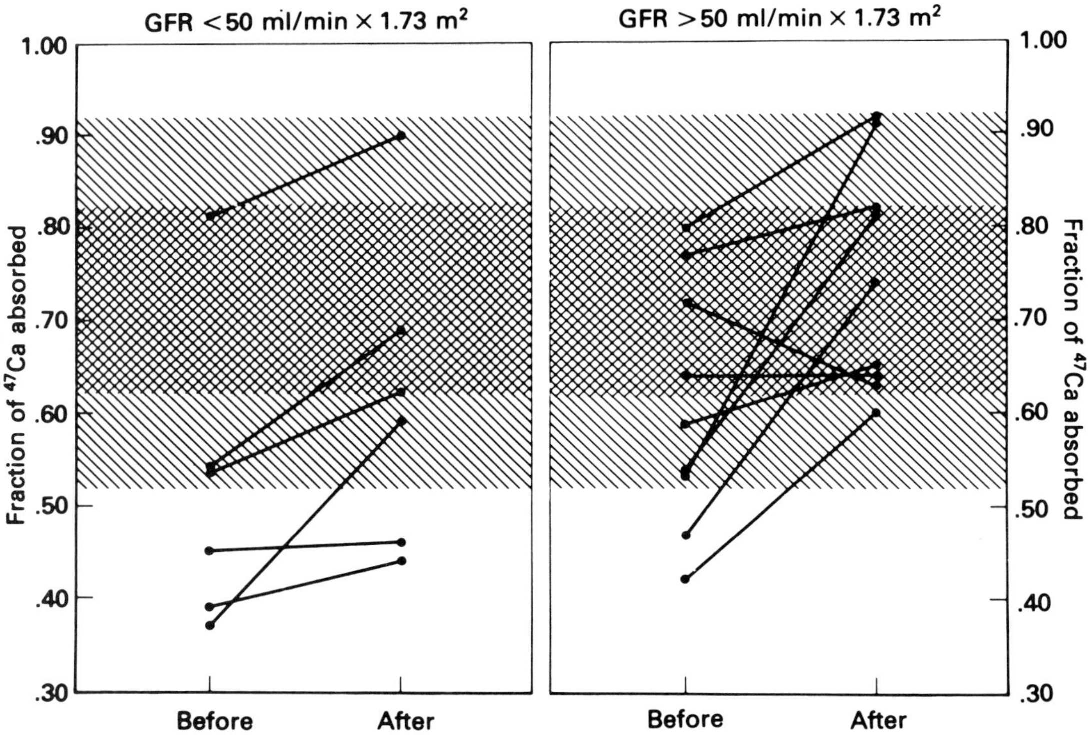

Figure 52.7. Fractional absorption of Ca measured by whole-body counting, double-dose technique in patients with incipient renal failure before and after vitamin D_3 therapy. Normal range indicated by shaded area (cross-hatched area, 1 SD; cross-hatched and lined area, 2 SD). (From Malluche HH, et al: Long-term administration of vitamin D steroles in incipient and advanced renal failure—effect on bone histology. Clin Nephrol 10:218, 1978, with permission.)

Elevated serum P_i levels in advanced CRF are influenced by alterations in dietary intake, increased skeletal resorption, or muscle catabolism. P_s levels fall when net intestinal absorption is reduced with administration of oral phosphate binders, after parathyroidectomy (42), or during an anabolic state. Net intestinal absorption of P is diminished (43) but may increase in response to administration of $1,25(OH)_2D_3$.

GENESIS OF DISTURBED Ca-P METABOLISM

Vitamin D

The kidney is the main site of conversion of 25(OH)D to $1,25(OH)_2D_3$ (44), although some extrarenal synthesis occurs. The alternative metabolite $24,25(OH)_2D$ is synthesized not only in the kidney but also in chondrocytes (45). Ablation of most nephrons, as occurs with CRF, impairs production of $1,25(OH)_2D$ (46) and possibly $24,25(OH)_2D$. Reduction in $1,25(OH)_2D$ may be caused in part by down-regulation of renal 1-α-hydroxylase activity by hyperphosphatemia (47) and possibly metabolic acidosis. Renal levels of 1-α-hydroxylase activity in rats with subtotal nephrectomy are reduced by NH_4Cl-induced acidosis (48). Circulating $1,25(OH)_2D$ levels decrease in proportion with reduction in renal mass in rats with subtotal nephrectomy (16). Patients with ESRD have low (18–23) levels of $1,25(OH)_2D$. The detectable levels in anephric subjects (49, 50) may be due to extrarenal synthesis of the hormone. Extrarenal synthesis of $1,25(OH)_2D_3$ is presumably not regulated by parathyroid status and demand for Ca and P, but is substrate-dependent. This may explain the finding that $1,25(OH)_2D_3$ levels rise in patients with terminal renal failure in response to the administration of $25(OH)D_3$ (50). However, identification by mass spectrum analysis of the compound in uremic serum which cochromatographs with 1,25 and binds to 1,25 receptors has not been carried out; therefore, identification of 1,25 in serum of anephric subjects remains tentative.

Low circulating $1,25(OH)_2D_3$ levels may contribute to several features of uremia, e.g., intestinal malabsorption of Ca and P (43), decreased calcemic response to PTH (26), development of renal osteodystrophy (51), abnormal metabolism of bone collagen (52), myopathy involving proximal muscles (53), and inefficient suppression of PTH secretion in response to increasing serum Ca (54). However, anephric patients do not necessarily exhibit osteomalacia as do patients with vitamin D deficiency (55), despite the near absence of $1,25(OH)_2D_3$. This paradox may be explained by the observation that $1,25(OH)_2D_3$ is formed by bone cells (56).

The extent to which circulating 24-R,$25(OH)_2D_3$ levels are low in patients with renal failure has been controversial (42, 57) and is important because 24-R,$25(OH)_2D_3$ may have biological actions not shared with $1,25(OH)_2D_3$ (58). Studies indicate that 24-R,$25(OH)_2D_3$ levels in adults (59) and children (48) with ESRD are subnormal and proportional to circulating $25(OH)D_3$ levels.

Levels of $25(OH)D_3$ usually are normal in uremic patients (18, 60, 61). Vitamin D-binding protein (DBP) is normal in patients with CRI except in those with the nephrotic syndrome (62).

Vitamin D metabolites exert important effects not only on the skeleton, intestine, and muscle but also on the hypophysis, pancreatic islet cells, salivary glands, mammary tissue, and testicular tissue (63). Changes in the effect of vitamin D (63) and $1,25(OH)_2D_3$ (64) on muscle may be related to some features of the myopathy of uremia (65). The presence of $1,25(OH)_2D_3$ receptors on tendon fibroblasts may explain disturbances in collagen cross-link maturation (66) and the occurrence of tendon rupture in uremic individuals (67). The gonadal actions of vitamin D metabolites may be relevant for the gonadal dysfunction in uremia (68).

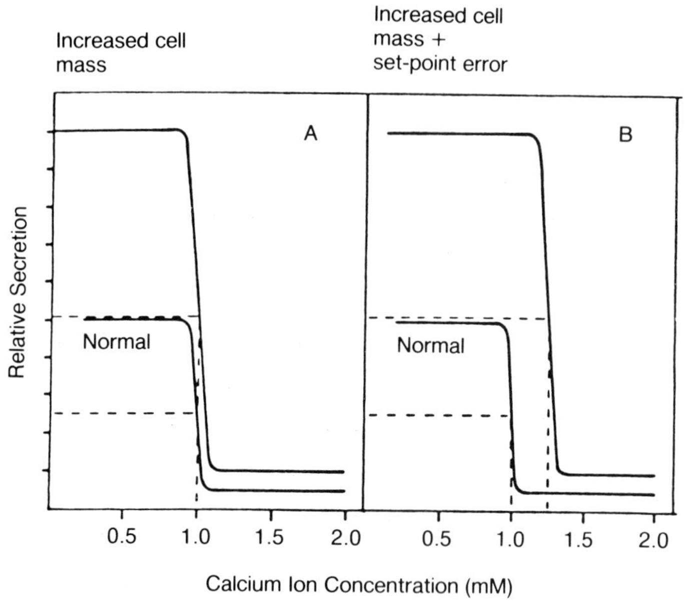

Figure 52.8. Diagrammatic representation of the relative rates of PTH secretion in relation to ionized calcium concentrations in the normal state and with secondary hyperparathyroidism (A = increased cell mass of parathyroid gland; B = increased cell mass and setpoint error). The "setpoint," or calcium concentration with 50% reduction in PTH release is indicated by the interrupted line. (After Morissey J et al. In Massry S, Maschio G (eds): Phosphate and other minerals. New York, Plenum Press, 1983.)

Abnormal levels of vitamin D metabolites probably play a role for several extraskeletal abnormalities observed in uremia.

Although circulating levels of 25(OH)D generally are normal, vitamin D deficiency from a number of causes is possible. These include reduced intake (60), reduced exposure to sunlight from indoor living (70, 71), reduced dermal conversion secondary to melanosis cutis (72), and loss of vitamin D-binding proteins (DBP) when proteinuria is severe (62, 73, 74). Administration of phenobarbital and other drugs that stimulate hepatic microsomal enzyme may lower 25(OH)D levels (75, 76).

Hyperparathyroidism

In renal failure, disturbances of PTH metabolism occur on several levels. PTH secretion increases (6, 7), secretory control of the parathyroids is abnormal (77), PTH catabolism is delayed (78), and PTH response in end-organs is abnormal (79, 80).

Serum Ca plays a central role in the control of PTH secretion in individuals with and without renal insufficiency. Because of the curvilinear relationship between serum ionized Ca and PTH (Fig. 52.8), PTH secretion is maximal even at modest degrees of hypocalcemia. Hypercalcemia suppresses secretion and diverts a greater proportion of PTH toward intraglandular proteolytic degradation. Hypomagnesemia stimulates and hypermagnesemia suppresses secretion of PTH. Although serum Ca is the major secretory signal, possible noncalcium secretory control by alternative signals, e.g., β-adrenergic or dopaminergic agonists, prostaglandins, calcitonin, histamine, and specifically vitamin D metabolites, is likely (81). β-2 agonists bind to parathyroid cell membranes and increase cAMP generation (82, 83). Although isoproterenol increases iPTH in animals (84) and humans (85), the effects of catecholamines on PTH secretion concern the secretory granule pool and apparently are not sustained. The consequences of β-adrenergic blockade on PTH secretion are highly controversial (84–86); no convincing evidence of long-term effect has been reported to date. Similarly, although blocking of histamine-dependent adenylate cyclase activity (87, 88) by H^2 antagonist (89) on parathyroid cell membranes has been shown, no consistent long-term effect of H_2 histaminergic blockade on PTH secretion has been noted (90, 91).

In contrast, recent evidence clearly points to an important role for $1,25(OH)_2D_3$ in the modulation of PTH secretion. Parathyroid cells contain a Ca-binding protein that is responsive to $25(OH)D_3$ (92). Various authors (93, 94) report cytosolic and nuclear receptors for vitamin D metabolites, and $1,25(OH)_2D_3$ and $24,25(OH)_2D_3$ modulate adenylate cyclase activity of plasma membranes of parathyroid cells (32).

Some confusion exists with respect to control of PTH secretion by vitamin D metabolites. In vitro PTH secretion is suppressed by $1,25(OH)_2D_3$ independent of ionized Ca (95). In vivo, no ionized Ca-independent change of iPTH was demonstrated in humans (96) or in rats (97, 98). Others (54) have administered $1,25(OH)_2D_3$ to uremic patients in whom Ca^{++} concentration was kept constant by peritoneal dialysis and reported a fall of iPTH, despite no change in plasma Ca^{++}. iPTH falls with administration of $1,25(OH)_2D_3$ to dialyzed patients (99), although it is difficult to dissociate the fall from a concomitant rise of ionized Ca. Recent work, however, suggests that PTH secretion is suppressed by $1,25(OH)_2D_3$ in humans before a rise in serum ionized Ca (54). Furthermore, with $1,25(OH)_2D_3$, sustained suppression of iPTH was noted. This would agree with previous reports of Bouillon (99), who noted only transient depression of iPTH with elevated ionized in dialyzed patients, but sustained suppression of iPTH with administration of vitamin D_3.

The mechanism of action of $1,25(OH)_2D_3$ on parathyroids may be complex. Vitamin D metabolites may increase the sensitivity of parathyroid glands to the ionized Ca signal (92). In addition, delayed effects of vitamin D metabolites on synthesis of cell organelles and on mitotic control of glandular cell mass may exist.

PTH levels are high in some uremic patients despite normocalcemia or even hypercalcemia. This may be caused by one or several of the following. Basal, i.e., non-calcium-suppressible PTH secretion may be high when parathyroid cell mass is increased (95) and may be sufficient to maintain a hyperparathyroid state (35). For example, in rats, following transplantation of a large number of autologous parathyroid glands, hypercalcemia develops (100). Parathyroid mass is strikingly increased in uremic patients (101). This continues even years after successful renal transplantation (102). In the course of long-standing renal failure, simple hyperplasia is followed by nodular hyperplasia and finally gross pseudoadenoma formation (103). The mechanisms that control parathyroid cell proliferation and parathyroid mass are not well defined. After surgical reduction of parathyroid mass, autotransplants of parathyroid glands continue to proliferate despite normocalcemia.

This may point to potential abnormalities of mitotic control of parathyroid glands in patients with renal hyperparathyroidism (104). Since primary hyperparathyroidism is present in an appreciable proportion of the normal population (105), e.g., 0.5% of the Scandinavian population, it is possible that a latent disturbance of parathyroid control is frequent and may be provoked under the "stimulus" of uremia. Increased parathyroid mass and non-calcium-suppressible basal PTH secretion may also account for the observation that after successful renal transplantation hypercalcemic hyperparathyroidism may continue despite reversal of uremia (102).

Another abnormality that may explain hypercalcemic hyperparathyroidism is a change in set-point, i.e., an elevation of the ambient Ca concentration necessary to half-maximally suppress PTH secretion (77, 106, 107). This change has been demonstrated in parathyroid adenoma cells (77, 106) and in parathyroid cells from uremic patients (108). Furthermore, Ca^{++} control of adenylate cyclase of parathyroid gland

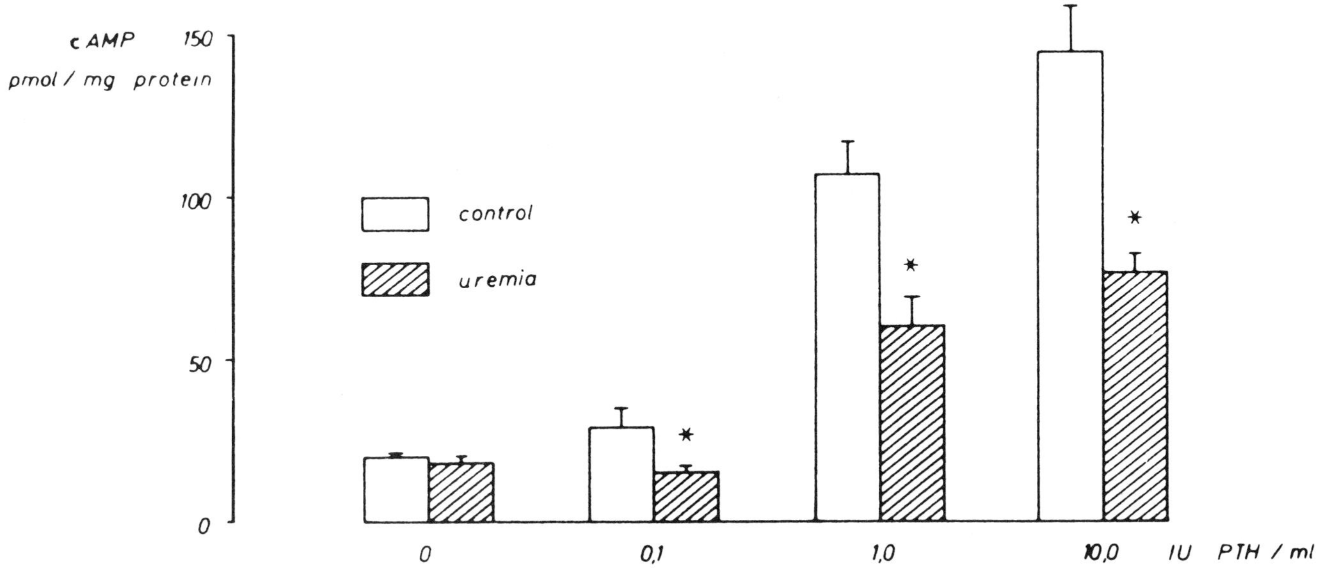

Figure 52.9. Effect of PTH on cAMP response of growth cartilage in vitro. The cAMP response is significantly blunted in uremia ($p < 0{,}01$; $n = 9$ in each group). (From Kreusser W, et al. Effect of parathyroid hormone, calcitonin and growth hormone on cAMP content of growth cartilage in experimental uremia. Eur J Child Invest 12:337, 1982.)

plasma membranes in uremia may be abnormal (109). Figure 52.8 shows the consequence of increased parathyroid gland mass with normal set-point, or a combination of the two abnormalities (86).

The intact 1.82 PTH is cleaved into peptide fragments, predominantly in liver and kidney (78, 110) and to a lesser extent in bone (111, 112). Renal elimination of carboxyterminal bioinactive fragments is delayed in patients with CRF (113), although liver degradation is not affected. This has important consequences for the interpretation of PTH radioimmunoassays because the epitope recognized by a given PTH antibody may comprise bioinactive material.

End-organ response to PTH is abnormal in uremia. Calcemic response to PTH, despite adequate increase of urinary cAMP, is impaired in patients with early or late CRF (26, 79). Treatment with $1{,}25(OH)_2D_3$ partly corrects this abnormality in dogs with ARF (80) and rats with CRF (26, 80). Correcting the resistance to PTH is an important goal in vitamin D therapy. Cartilage from rats with CRF has a disturbed response to PTH in vivo and in vitro (Fig. 52.9) but bone cells from the calvarium of rats with ARF do not (30, 114). The cartilage abnormality was present in rats treated with $1{,}25(OH)_2D_3$ and those that underwent parathyroidectomy (25). Therefore, it cannot be explained by disturbed interaction with $1{,}25(OH)_2D_3$ or down-regulation of PTH receptors alone. PTH has been implicated in the genesis of numerous facets of the uremic syndrome, e.g., anemia (115), disturbed thrombocyte function (116), and myocardiopathy (117), and has therefore been considered a "uremic toxin" (118).

Calcitonin (CT)

Increased levels of plasma CT may attenuate the effects of PTH on bone (119) by inhibiting PTH-induced osteoclastic bone resorption (120). Alkaline phosphatase and iPTH values are higher in uremic patients with low iCT (121). The iCT levels increase after bilateral nephrectomy, associated with a decrease in some indicators of bone turnover. However, therapeutic doses (100 MRC units) of CT failed to improve renal osteodystrophy (122) in one clinical study, and we did not observe any relation between iCT levels and quantitative bone histology in dialysis patients (123). The role of CT in uremic bone disease remains uncertain.

Other Factors

Osteomalacia

A relation has been noted between metabolic acidosis and bone disease, predominantly osteomalacia (124). The role of metabolic acidosis in the genesis of renal osteodystrophy is not clear (125, 126). In normal individuals made acidotic, Ca delivery from the skeleton and urinary Ca excretion increase (127). In children with RTA, tubular reabsorption of Ca is depressed, with little or no increase in intestinal absorption; there is, therefore, a net loss of skeletal Ca (128). In contrast, bone density (129, 130) and total body Ca (131) are normal or increased in patients with ESRD (see p 861).

Vitamin D Deficiency

The role of vitamin D deficiency in the genesis of osteomalacia in patients with CRF is uncertain. On the one hand, osteomalacia was only observed in nondialyzed uremic patients if and when circulating 25-OHD levels were low (132). On the other hand, we (133) and others (134) found no correlation between $25(OH)D_3$ levels and histological indices of osteomalacia. In a more recent report, no correlation was found between histological indices of bone disease and any of the circulating vitamin D metabolites (135). Deficiency of vitamin D or one of its metabolites cannot account for the genesis of osteomalacia in dialyzed patients, although this does not exclude vitamin D deficiency superimposed on uremia as a factor in the development of osteomalacia in some patients with ESRD (5). This problem may be resolved when the role of the local production of $1{,}25(OH)_2D$ by human bone cells and its role in the mineralization process is resolved (56).

Protein-calorie Malnutrition

Calorie deficiency occurs in some children with CRF. Malnutrition may be important for two reasons: (a) negative protein balance in malnourished hypercatabolic children may contribute to osteopenia as a result of reduced synthesis of bone matrix (136); (b) self-selected low-Ca diets may contribute to Ca deficiency. Another factor may be the effect of steroids, which are commonly used in children with the nephrotic syndrome who develop CRF or in children following renal transplantation. Steroid therapy is a major cause of pathological fractures, particularly of vertebrae and of bones of children with CRF who have osteonecrosis.

The various effects of steroids on vitamin D metabolism, bone matrix synthesis, and bone tissue turnover have been the subject of recent reviews (137, 138). In brief, steroid therapy diminishes intestinal absorption of Ca, stimulates release of PTH, increases bone resorption, and causes hypercalciuria. The defect in intestinal absorption of Ca occurs despite unchanged $1,25(OH)_2D_3$ levels. Intestinal absorption of Ca in those receiving steroid therapy is responsive to pharmacological doses of vitamin D (139). Steroids also depress synthesis of osteoid.

RENAL OSTEODYSTROPHY:HISTOLOGY

The histology of osteodystrophy in cancellous bone of children (4, 140) is the same as it is in adults (129), but osteodystrophy also affects the histology of the growth zone in the growing skeleton.

Cancellous Bone

CRI is a condition in which the structural integrity of the skeleton is sacrificed to maintain plasma Ca levels. Bone histology is characterized by two major patterns of bone tissue responses: osteomalacia and osteitis fibrosa. The preponderance of these varies, and in many patients the features of both are present. Transiliac bone biopsies show bone disease even in children with moderate reduction of GFR. Usually a progression of bone lesions is observed with decreasing GFR (Figs. 52.2, 52.10 to 52.12).

Abnormalities in bone surface morphology and remodeling dynamics may be accompanied by local or generalized alterations of bone mass, i.e., osteosclerosis or osteopenia.

Osteomalacia

In children, this feature is observed in the growth apparatus, as well as metaphysis and diaphysis, including iliac crest spongiosa as the usual sampling site. Histological findings correspond to those in the skeleton of adult osteomalacic patients. The features in the growth zone show similarities and differences with vitamin D–deficiency rickets. Osteomalacia is characterized by the abundance of broad resting lamellar seams of osteoid, which are covered by flat endosteal cells or osteoblasts without signs of cellular activity (129). Usually endosteal fibrosis is absent, and osteoclasts are scarce. The characteristic features of osteomalacia are evident from Fig. 52.13.

Osteitis Fibrosa

Osteitis fibrosa reflects the effects of excessive PTH action on bone cells and on skeletal remodeling. The histological features are characterized by increased osteoclastic resorption of the trabeculae from deeply

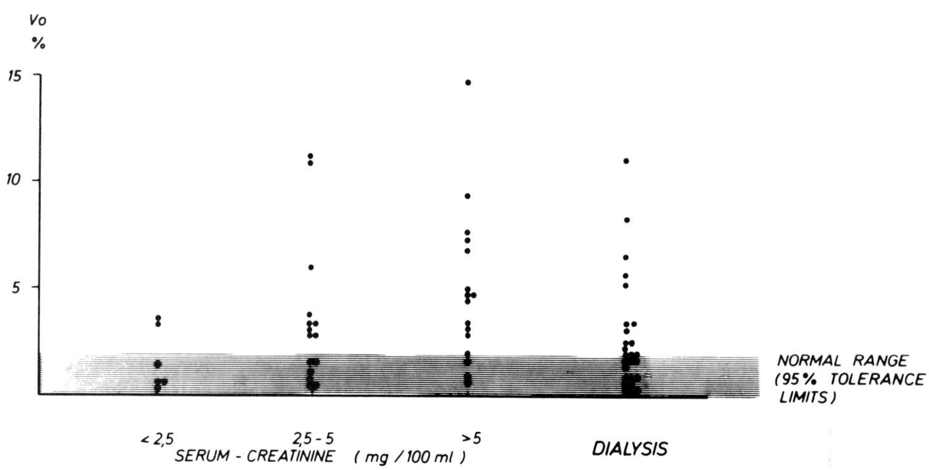

Figure 52.10. Osteoid volume (V_o) as percent of spongiosal volume (iliac crest biopsies) in children with renal insufficiency at various stages. There is an increase of osteoid with decreasing renal function. Normal range is indicated by shaded area.

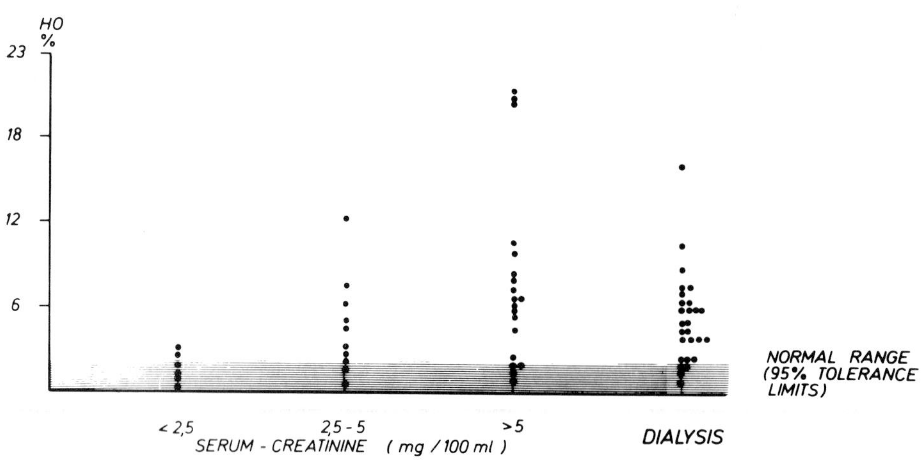

Figure 52.11. Active Howship's lacunae (HO) as fraction of trabecular surface (iliac crest biopsies) in children with CRI at various stages. Surface increases with active osteoclasts with decreasing renal function. Normal range is indicated by shaded area.

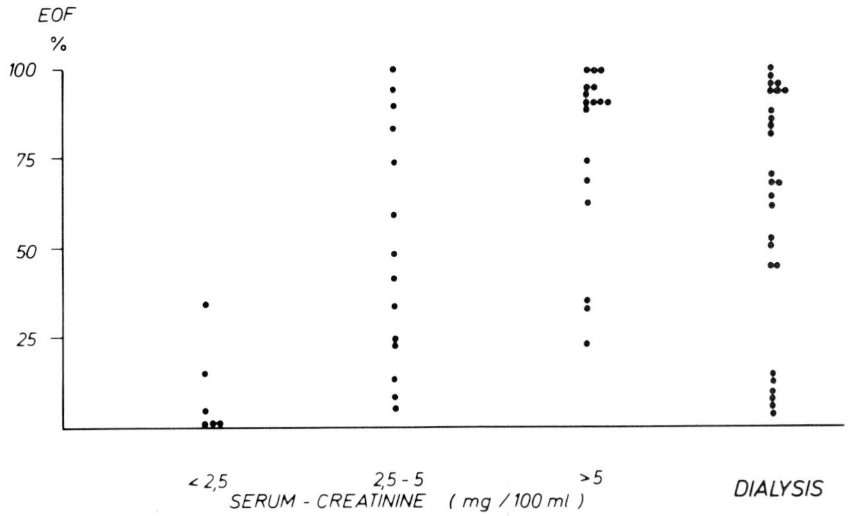

Figure 52.12. Endosteal fibrosis (EOF) as percent of trabecular surface covered by endosteal fibrosis (iliac crest biopsies) in children with CRI at various stages. The degree of endosteal fibrosis increases with decreasing renal function. In normal bone no endosteal fibrosis is seen.

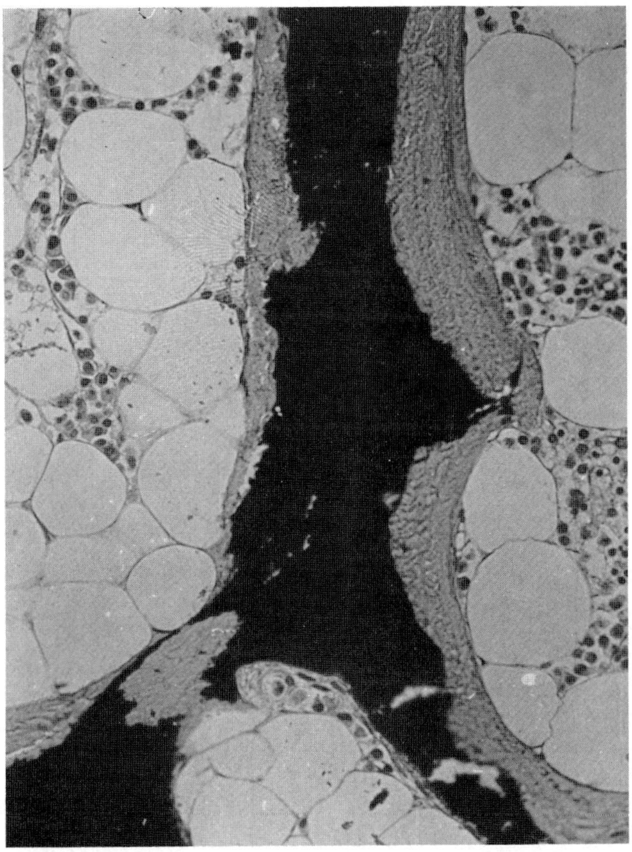

Figure 52.13. Renal osteomalacia. Undecalcified section. Krutsay stain, microphotograph (×130). Bizarre contours of the remnants of the well-mineralized premorbid trabecules (black) after osteoclastic surface resorption. Broad, resting osteoid seams (gray) with recognizable lamellar structure surrounded by normal fat marrow. No osteoblastic activity, no endosteal fibrosis. (From Ritz E, et al: Bone histology in renal insufficiency. In David DS (ed): Calcium Metabolism in Renal Failure and Nephrolithiasis. New York, John Wiley, 1977, p 197, with permission.)

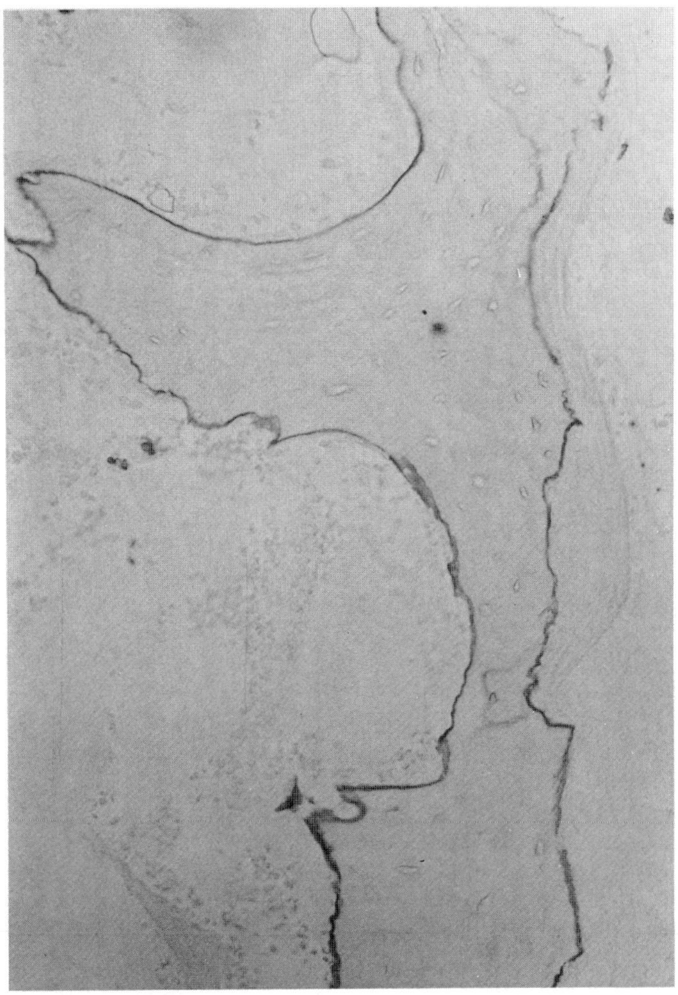

Figure 52.14. Photomicrograph of trabecular bone stained for aluminum. Aluminum is seen on red line (here black) at calcification front between mineralized bone and osteoid (Aluminum stain; ×270; Courtesy I.B. Salusky, M.D.).

penetrating resorption cavities or from intratrabecular dissecting tunnels. On the endosteal surface, patchy endosteal fibrosis, i.e., layers of coarse collagen fibers parallel to the trabecular surface, are common. Foci of more marked fibrosis are usually found over remodeling sites, e.g., resorption cavities or apposition fronts. Widespread replacement of hematopoetic or fat marrow by fibrous tissue (marrow fibrosis), the hallmark of osteitis fibrosa, is encountered only in a few patients with advanced osteitis fibrosa. In these patients there are foci of metaplastic fibrous bone formation in the fibrotic marrow space.

Increased bone apposition is reflected by an increased surface extension of active osteoid seams. As a rule, the osteoid deposited by osteoblasts under the influence of excess PTH does not exhibit mature lamellar osteoid but immature haphazard collagen structure, i.e., woven osteoid similar to that seen in embryonal bone or bone during growth or repair. Woven bone arises from woven osteoid and is characaterized by the appearance of numerous densely packed osteocytes with broad cytoplasmic seams. Bone turnover, measured with tetracycline double labeling (141) is high with numerous bone apposition fronts, whereas in osteomalacia turnover is low.

Aluminum (Al) Toxicity

Because Al toxicity of bone is now a recognized complication presenting as low turnover osteomalacia (142), it is advisable to routinely examine bone biopsies for the presence of Al by electron probe microanalysis (143) or an A1 stain (144) (Fig. 52.14). A1-induced osteomalacia is characterized by the absence of cellular endosteal activity with few osteoblasts or osteoclasts. In states of acute Al intoxication, little osteoid may be present in the face of no tetracycline uptake and no endosteal cell activity. Parathyroid status apparently plays a major role in determining Al distribution in bone tissue. Whereas in osteitis fibrosa, Al is diffusely distributed throughout the trabecula. Al is preferentially trapped at the osteoid bone interface in cases of low turnover osteomalacia (143, 144).

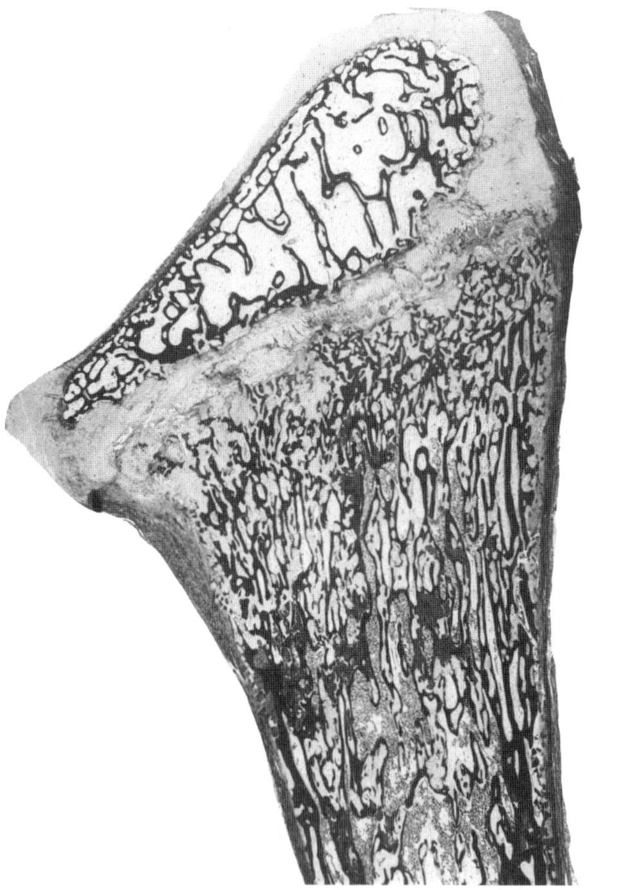

Figure 52.15. Growth zone of the distal radius in a 10-yr-old girl with renal hypoplasia and terminal renal failure. Microphotograph of undecalcified section, Masson-Goldner-stain (×3). Narrow irregular cartilage plate. Severe fibroosteoclasia with destruction of primary and secondary spongiosa. Incipient displacement of epiphysis toward ulnar side with erosion of its lower radial border. (From Krempien B et al: Morphological studies on pathogenesis of epiphyseal slipping in uremic children. Virchows Arch (Pathol Anat) 362:129, 1974, with permission.)

Growth Zone

Rickets

The hallmark of Vitamin D deficiency rickets is an increased width of the cartilaginous growth zone caused by the accumulation of cartilage cells in the area of degeneration. The longitudinal columnar arrangement of cartilage cells is lost. Mineralization in the zone of provisional calcification is reduced or absent, and the process of vascular invasion is deranged by lack of a scaffold for invading capillaries. Cartilage gradually merges with metaphyseal spongiosa, which is covered by thick osteoid seams; chondroid and osteoid mingle, giving rise to a broad zone of chondroosteoid (145).

Osteitis Fibrosa

In advanced renal osteitis fibrosa (146) the growth cartilage is narrow (Figs. 52.15 and 52.16); however, provisional calcification of cartilage ground substance is not consistently abnormal. The transition between epiphysis and metaphyseal bone is affected. Vascular invasion is virtually absent, and the growth cartilage zone is occluded by a bar of dense bone, which physically separates it from metaphyseal bone. In the metaphysis, trabeculae arise de novo by metaplastic formation from primitive fibrous tissue. These trabeculae differ from normal in several ways. They are not in physical contact with cartilage, are devoid of a chondroid core, and consist entirely of poorly mineralized woven bone that lacks the usual longitudinal orientation. Additional abnormalities are present at the periosteal surface of the metaphysis, where intensive osteoclastic resorption occurs. A continuous layer of cortical bone may no longer be recognizable, since compact bone is transformed into cancellous bone "cancellization").

Rickets versus Osteitis Fibrosa

The transitions from the pattern of rickets to that of osteitis were described by Pommer (147) in children with vitamin D-deficiency rickets. The pattern of osteitis fibrosa may supervene as hyperparathy-

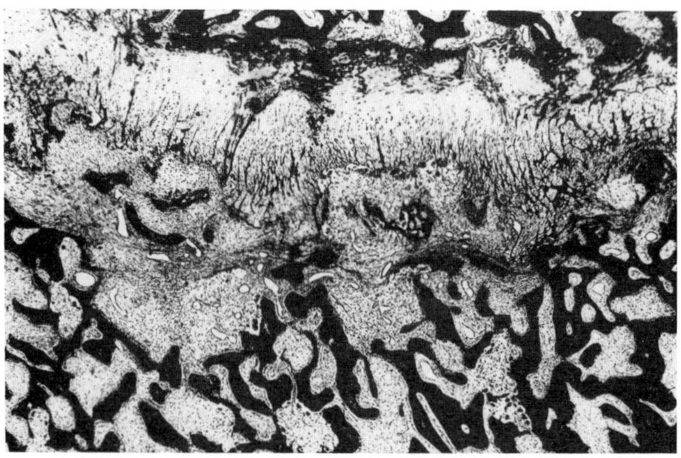

Figure 52.16. Detail from Figure 52.13. Microphotograph, Masson-Goldner-stain (×20). Note small cartilage plate with irregular border toward metaphysis. Destruction of primary and secondary spongiosa by dense fibrous tissue. Fibrous tissue provides plane of cleavage for slipping epiphysis. Defects within spongiosa are morphological substrates for widened radiolucent growth zone on roentgenograms.

roidism develops in patients with vitamin D deficiency, so that chondroosteoid disappears when chondroclastic and osteoclastic resorption become more intense. From the reports in the literature (148–151), primary hyperparathyroidism causes abnormalities in the epiphyses that are indistinguishable radiographically and, presumably, histologically, from the findings in CRF. Consequently, the lesions found in the growth zone are not simply a direct result of impaired vitamin D metabolism as is tacitly assumed by many authors.

Epiphyseal Slipping

The mechanisms of epiphyseal slipping can be understood from the underlying histology (Fig. 52.17). In bones with epiphyseal slipping, we found no histological evidence of traumatic separation (146). i.e., neither hemorrhage, callus formation, or rupture of the periosteal ring.

Epiphyseal slipping appears to be the result of a lateral movement of the epiphyseal structure in the wake of intensive destructive and reparative processes at the epiphyseal-metaphyseal junction (the histology of this zone resembles a Looser zone). The ultimate lateral movement of the epiphysis appears to be caused by failure of the trabeculae of the metaphyseal spongiosa to tightly interlock with the growth cartilage. This is caused by removal of the calcified chondroid by chondroclasts, by intensive resorption of spongiosal trabeculae by osteoclasts, or by a combination of both processes. In uremia, the plane of slippage is located in the metaphysis, whereas in idiopathic epiphysiolysis, the plane of cleavage is fibrous tissue within the damaged growth cartilage (151, 152).

MINERAL CONTENT OF THE SKELETON

Adults on dialysis have normal bone mineral content measured by bone mass (129, 130) or as total body Ca by neutron activation analysis (131). Adults with CRF or chronic acidosis, however, are in negative Ca balance (153).

Children with CRF are at risk of negative Ca balance because dietary Ca usually is reduced, vitamin D may be deficient and acidosis, if present, causes loss of bone mineral (128). Dialysis in children in which dialysate Ca is low may contribute to Ca loss.

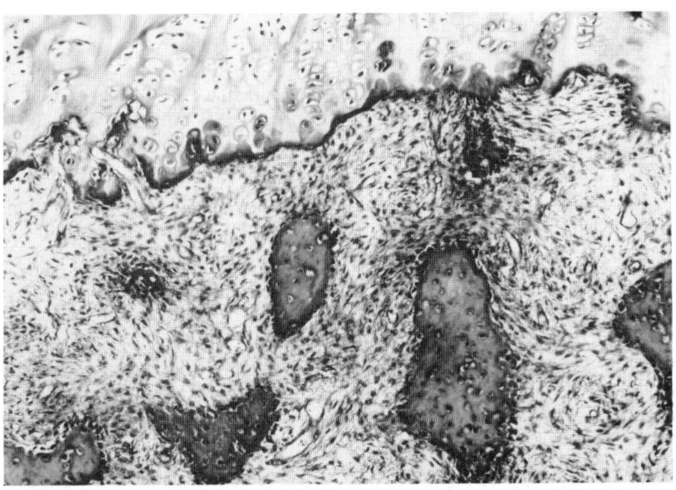

Figure 52.17. Growth zone of distal femur of a 12-yr-old boy with obstructive uropathy. Microphotograph, Masson-Goldner-stain (×125). Cluster formation of growth cartilage cells, separation of growth cartilage from primary spongiosa by fibrous tissue and woven bone. (With permission) [146]. (From Krempien B, et al: Morphological studies on pathogenesis of epiphyseal slipping in uremic children. Virchows Arch (Pathol Anat) 362:129, 1974, with permission.)

Mineral Content

Skeletal mineral content reflects cumulative Ca balance. Results vary, depending on whether children with CRF are compared with controls of the same age, height, weight, or bone age. Another problem is posed by skeletal heterogeneity, i.e., the divergent behavior of the diaphysis from that of the metaphysis, and of appendicular versus axial skeleton. Finally, the evaluation of mineral content poses technical problems. None of the existing procedures is ideal in this respect.

Photon Densitometry

For demineralization to be apparent on routine x-ray films, up to 40% of skeletal bone mineral must be lost (154). In children, the methods of whole-body neutron activation analysis and x-ray spectrophotometry have not been used. Only a few studies have been reported in which photon densitometry was used, the results of which are conflicting. Chesney and coworkers (155) found diminished mineral density of the radius and ulna in uremic children relative to age, sex, height, and weight-corrected normal values. Somewhat different findings were obtained by us in children with congenital renal diseases without a history of steroid treatment who were evaluated by ^{241}Am photon densitometry (Fig. 52.18). Forearm mineral density was low for age and appropriate for height when measured in the metaphysis, but low for age and height when measured in the diaphysis of the radius and ulna—an example of skeletal heterogeneity. The differences are explained by the development of dense osteosclerosis of spongy bone in the metaphysis, reflecting increased bone matrix and net mineral resorption that is not matched by mineral apposition in the cortical bone of the diaphysis.

The data on metaphyseal mineral content agree with previous findings of normal or high whole-body Ca content in adults with CRF (131). Although intestinal absorption of Ca is diminished in absolute terms, it is appropriate to the mineral demand of the slowly growing uremic skeleton, so that bone mass remains normal.

Barnett Nordin Index

In adult patients with secondary hyperparathyroidism, cortical thickness often decreases as a result of accelerated endosteal resorption. This can be quantified by using the Barnett Nordin Index (156) of the second metacarpal, which gives the thickness of cortical bone as a fraction of total metacarpal width. In uremic children, diminished cortical width or area (157) is not correlated with radiological evidence of renal osteodystrophy (Fig. 52.19), in contrast to findings in adults (158). On the other hand, both cortical area and radiographic bone lesions of osteitis fibrosa correlate positively with growth velocity (unpublished observations). Evidently secondary hyperparathyroidism does not invariably cause bone loss or demineralization. We noted no correlation between cortical thickness and bone biopsy findings or serum iPTH levels.

CLINICAL PRESENTATIONS

Myopathy

Uremic children often suffer from a specific type of metabolic myopathy characterized by asthenia (65), which affects proximal muscles of the pelvic and shoulder girdles primarily (159, 160). The weakness becomes apparent when they try to raise the arms or climb a flight of stairs. A positive Trendelenburg sign and waddling gait are common. Slipped femoral epiphyses or myopathy may cause a waddling gait. These findings now are uncommon because detection and treatment begin at earlier stages of disease. Children rarely complain of weakness, but on physical examination, it is commonly noted, e.g., the hand grip is affected. The myopathy improves with vitamin D therapy and its progress

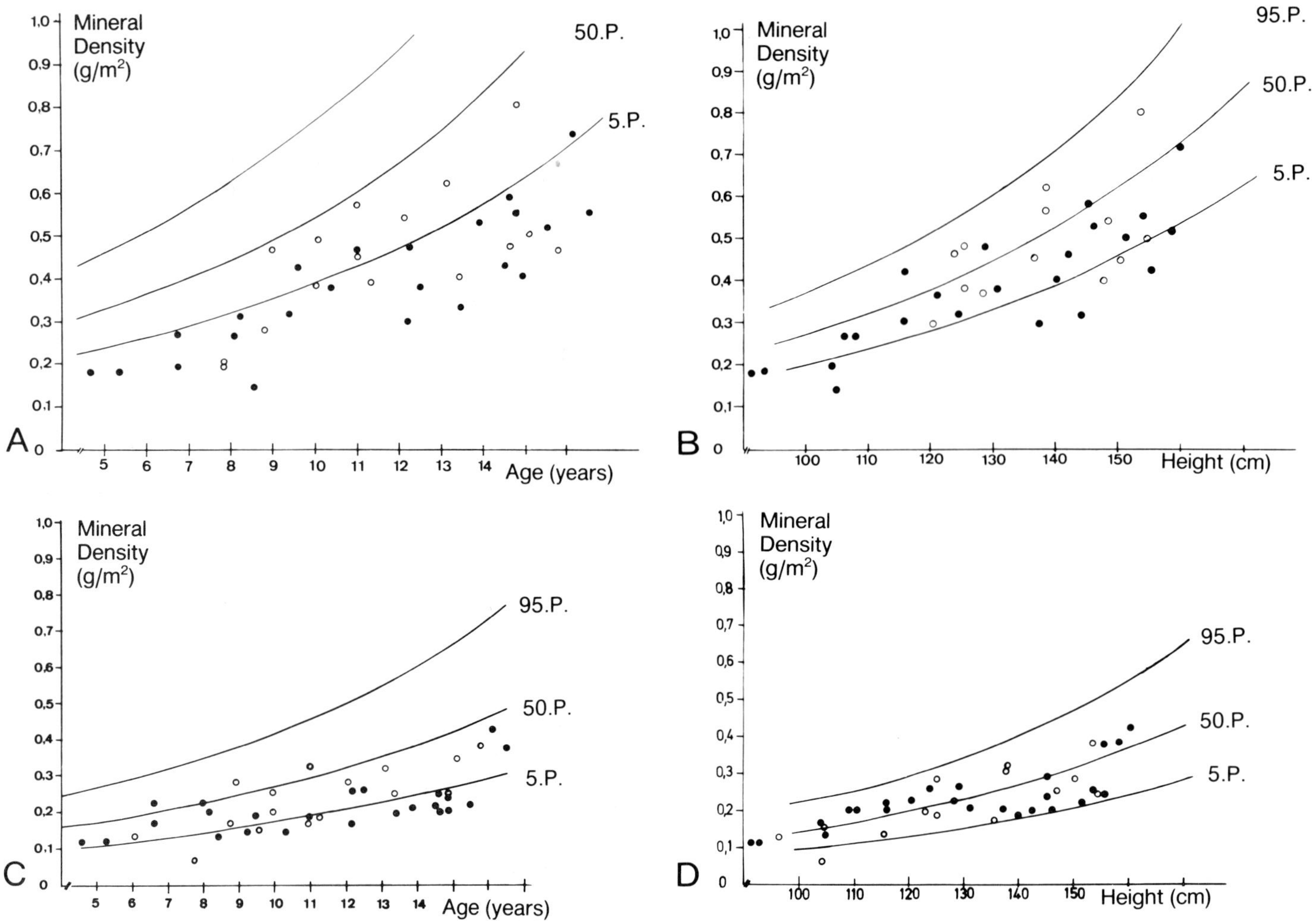

Figure 52.18. Forearm bone mineral density measured by photon-densitometry in children with CRF. Closed circles, in patients on dialysis; open circles, before dialysis. Bone mineral content is low for age when measured both in the metaphysis (B) and diaphysis (A). When corrected for height, bone mineral content is reduced only in diaphysis (C) but not in metaphysis (D). Dialysis patients tend to have lower bone mineral content in the diaphysis than uremic children under conservative treatment.

can be followed casually by changes in the hand grip. In adults with CRF, nonspecific atrophy of type II fiber with ultrastructural damage to the myofibrillar pattern and electromyographic changes in muscles are characteristic (161), but these changes were not present in the children with CRF (162).

Growth Retardation, Skeletal Deformities, and Other Physical Findings

Uremic children frequently are growth-retarded, i.e., they are below the third percentile of height for age (163). Hemodialysis therapy does not normalize growth (164) (see also Chapter 50).

In small children with CRF in whom CRI is not detected early, the findings resemble those of late rickets—rosary, Harrison's groove, and enlargement of wrists and ankles. Deformed extremities are due to bending of the metaphyses; bowing of the diaphyses of long bones usually is not seen. Craniotabes is rare because renal osteodystrophy usually develops after the first year of age.

In school-age children who are untreated, skeletal deformities include knock-knees, ulnar deviation of the hand, (Fig. 52.20), enlargement of wrists, ankles, medial end of clavicles and chondrocostal junctions.

Fractures of bones, vertebral collapse (165), and femoral neck fractures (166) are uncommon but are occasionally observed after seizures. Fractures must be distinguished from Looser zones, which are less commonly observed in children (5) (Fig. 52.21) than in adults.

The physical findings are greater than one would anticipate from patient complaints. Children with CRF probably restrict activity and avoid exercise so that complaints about bone pain are rare.

Young children almost never have soft tissue calcification, i.e., arterial, periarticular, or bursal calcifications (4, 167), although Ca_s and P_s levels in children with CRF are similar to those in adults (167). In children, the Ca-P product does not predict the risk of calcification. Infants and toddlers have a physiological Ca-P product of 70 mg/dl × mg/dl, which is considered the risk threshold for soft tissue calcification in adults. As in adults, hyperparathyroidism and a high Ca-P product may lead to pruritus, red eye syndrome, and corneal calcification (4).

Epiphyseal Slipping

Epiphyseal slipping, the most severe manifestation of renal osteodystrophy in the growing skeleton, has been common in children with ESRD whose abnormalities of Ca metabolism have not been treated appropriately (151, 159, 168–171). We observed slipped epiphyses in 10 of 33 new cases of CRF in children, but it developed in only 1 of 82 children on dialysis (159). With more effective treatment, the incidence has decreased dramatically in recent years.

Epiphyseal slipping tends to occur late in CRF and may become apparent within a very short time. Slipping has developed within three months, more commonly in children with congenital renal disease and CRF of long duration. Children with epiphyseal slipping have more profound hypocalcemia, more elevation of iPTH levels, and more severe osteitis fibrosa in the iliac crest bone (159).

The site is related to the patient's age and whether the child is crawling or walking. During the first year of life, the distal tibial epiphyses and both upper and lower femoral epiphyses are involved, but the distal radial and ulnar epiphyses are not. In older children, the upper femoral (Fig. 52.22) or radial and ulnar epiphyses or both usually are involved. During puberty, the forearm epiphyses is more commonly affected. Extreme hyperparathyroidism interferes with this age-dependent pattern, and epiphyseal slipping can occur in all growth zones.

Slipping is suspected when ulnar deviation or metaphyseal bowing of the long bones are present. Waddling gait, inability to walk, or painful limitation of movement of the hip joint are characteristic. The diagnosis is made by roentgenogram (see Figs. 52.20 to 52.22).

Epiphyseal slipping must be distinguished from traumatic metaphyseal fracture (166) (Fig. 52.23) and necrosis of the femoral head (172) (Fig. 52.24).

The late consequences of epiphyseal slipping are not well known. Late arthrosis of the hip joint is a possibility; malpositioned femoral heads appear to be prone to osteonecrosis following renal transplantation.

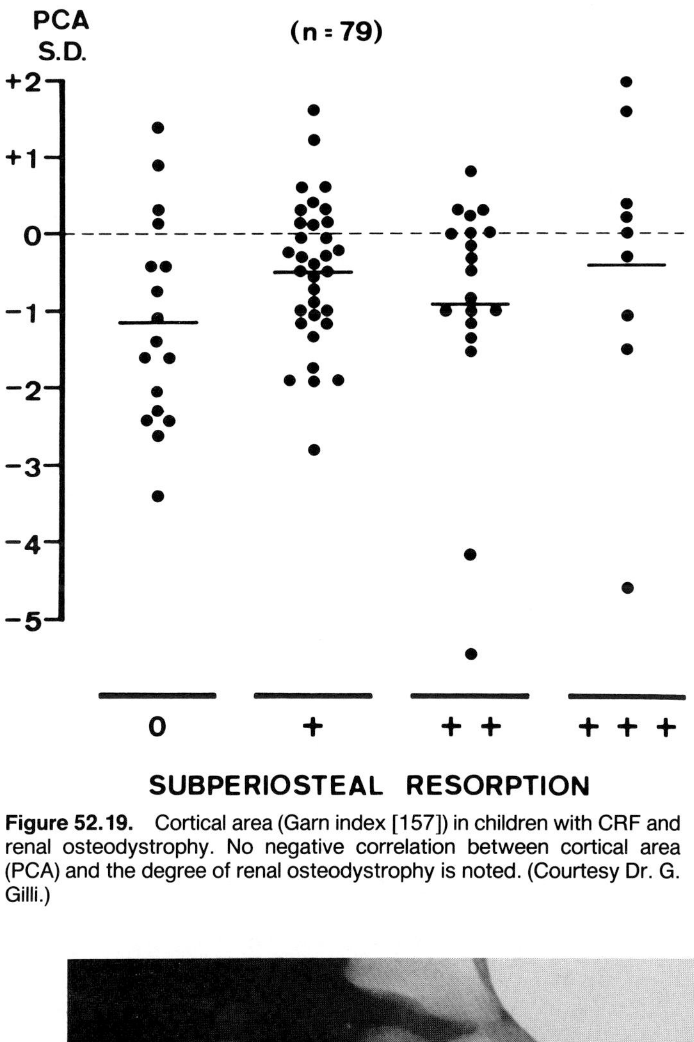

Figure 52.19. Cortical area (Garn index [157]) in children with CRF and renal osteodystrophy. No negative correlation between cortical area (PCA) and the degree of renal osteodystrophy is noted. (Courtesy Dr. G. Gilli.)

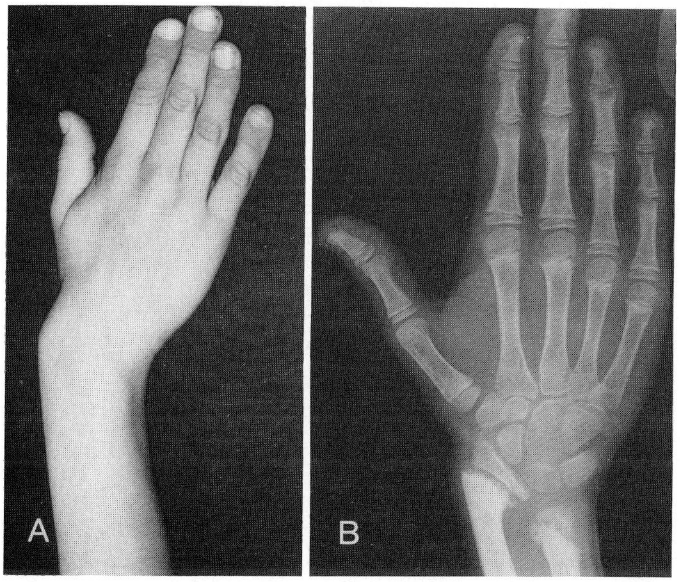

Figure 52.20. **A,** Ulnar deviation of right hand as clinical evidence of slipped epiphysis in severe renal osteodystrophy. Note pseudoclubbing of fingers. **B,** Roentgenogram of right hand skeleton after initiation of vitamin D therapy. Slipping of radial epiphysis toward ulnar side. Severe metaphyseal changes. Note severe subperiosteal resorption zones at cortex of metacarpals and acro-osteolysis of terminal phalanges. (From Mehls O, et al: Slipped epiphyses in renal osteodystrophy. Arch Dis Child 50: 545, 1975, with permission.)

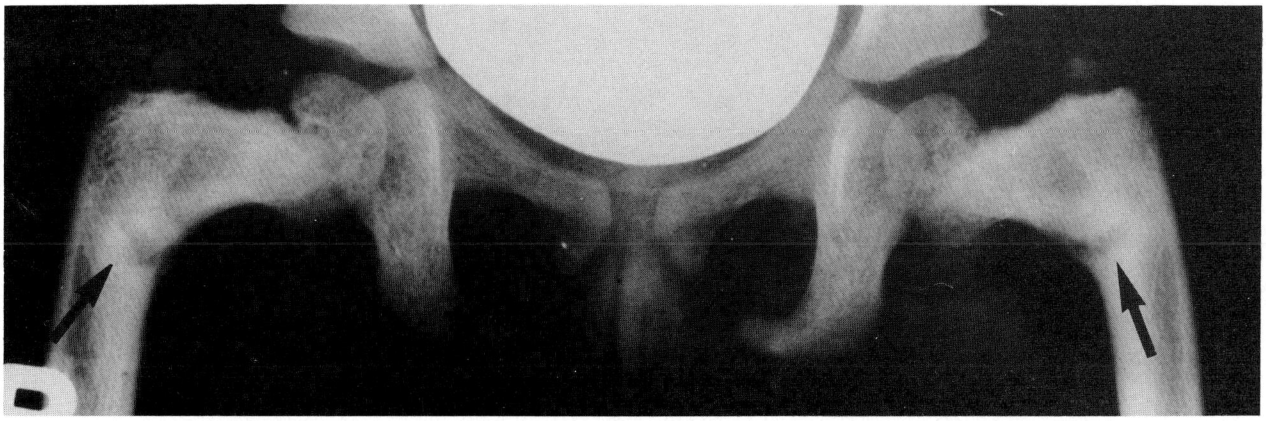

Figure 52.21. Bilateral Looser zones of medial proximal femora. Marked reduction of the collodiaphyseal angle and varus position of both femoral necks. Femoral necks are irregularly textured and outlined as consequence of severe osteodystrophy. Five-year-old girl with oligomeganephronic hypoplasia, C_{Cr} 25 ml/min/1.73 m^2. (From Mehls O, et al: Renal osteodystrophy in uremic children. Clin Endocrinol Metab 9:151, 1980, with permission.)

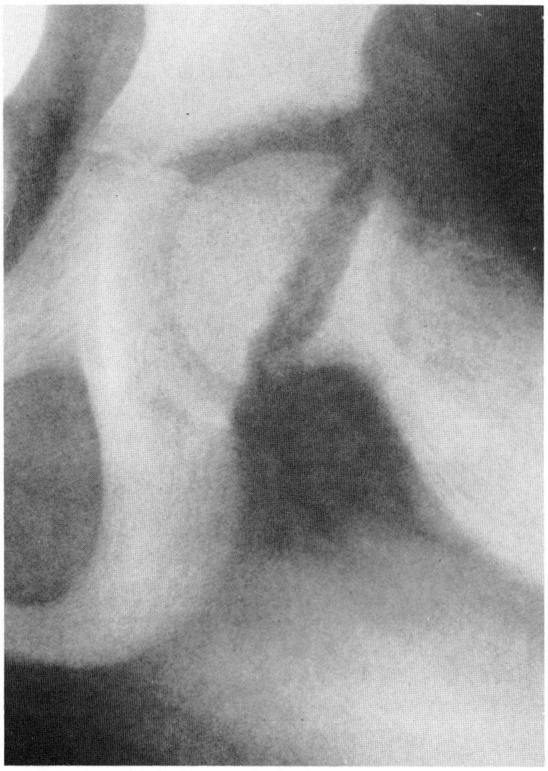

Figure 52.22. Severe epiphyseal changes and incipient slipping of the femoral head. Roentgenogram in frogleg position in a 9-year-old boy with nephronophthisis (serum creatinine 8.4 mg/dl). Radiolucent woolly metaphyseal texture underneath growth plate. Note also subperiostal resorption zones around femoral neck.

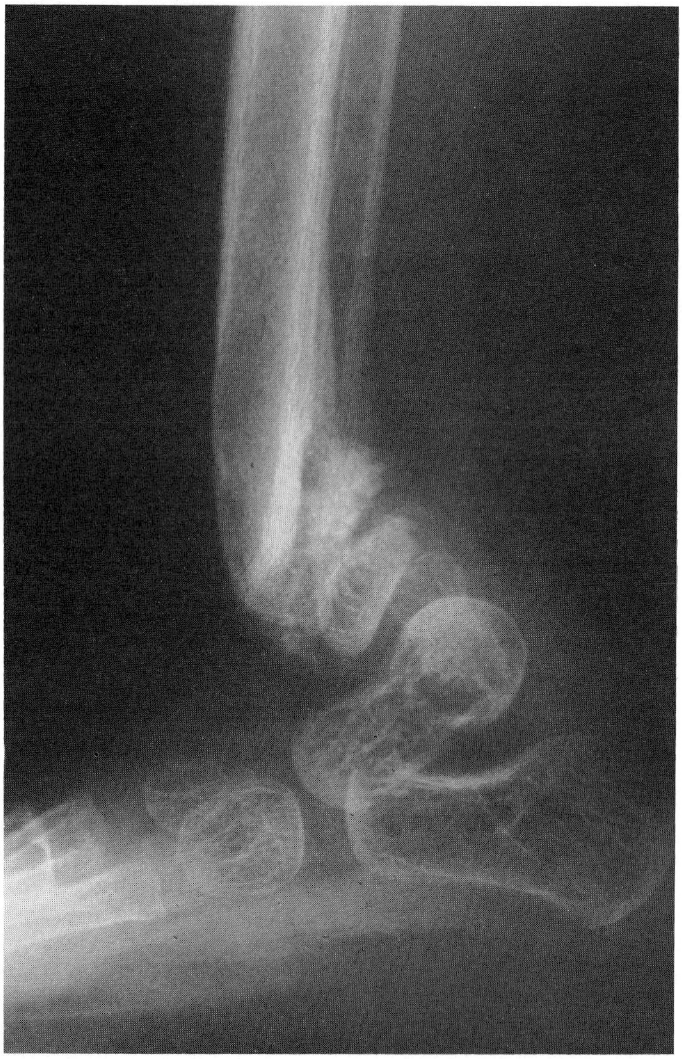

Figure 52.23. Metaphyseal fracture of distal tibia. Roentgenogram of left foot joint in 2½-yr-old boy. Tibial fracture following repeated microtraumata within metaphysis. Dorsal dislocation of epiphysis and adjacent metaphysis. Note by comparison with Figure 52.22 that there is no epiphyseal slipping at this site.

Osteonecrosis may develop in children with CRF with no history of steroid therapy and no antecedent epiphyseal slipping (Fig. 52.24) (172).

Dental Development

Peculiar abnormalities of dental development in children with CRF, particularly those conditions secondary to congenital disease, have been described (173, 174). Defects of enamel formation and dental deformities are characteristic. Resorption of alveolar bone may occur with hyperparathyroidism. It has been thought that resorption of lamina dura is a sensitive and early indicator of renal secondary hyperparathyroidism, but our controlled studies demonstrate that only severe resorptive lesions are indicative of hyperparathyroidism. Some resorption is also seen in normal controls or children with nephrotic syndrome and normal renal function.

Soft Tissue Calcifications

Extraosseous calcifications develop in older children and adults at sites subjected to trauma (elbow, shoulder, knuckles). These may present as tumorlike masses around articulations or bursae and cause acute arthritis, particularly of the intraphalangeal joints.

Occasionally, dermal or subcutaneous calcifications are observed. Arterial calcifications occur more commonly in arteries of the pelvis and extremities. Calcifications of viscera (myocardium, lungs) rarely cause clinical or x-ray signs (175) but are occasionally noted at autopsy (167, 176). Soft tissue calcification, common in adults with CRF, is rare in children (4, 147, 167, 177).

Bony Problems Unrelated to Uremia

Not all bone disease in a uremic child is uremic osteodystrophy. Uremic osteodystrophy may coexist with other processes like malnutrition, protein loss by nephrotic syndrome, steroid therapy, and acquired vitamin D deficiency. Furthermore, the presence of associated lesions should be considered.

The nail-patella syndrome is characterized by abnormal patellae and other skeletal abnormalities unrelated to CRF (178, 179). Glomerulosclerosis may be associated with multicentric osteolysis (Fig. 52.25) (180). Nephronophthisis is associated with metaphyseal chondrodysplasia (181). Primary oxalosis may cause focal osteolytic lesions secondary to oxalate-induced giant cell granulomas in the marrow, causing fractures (Fig. 52.26) (182). In contrast, cystinosis does not cause skeletal pathology; although cystine crystals are present in bone marrow macrophages (183).

Specific problems may arise when tubular dysfunctions, e.g., Fanconi's syndrome and RTA, are present. Impaired mineralization of bone matrix

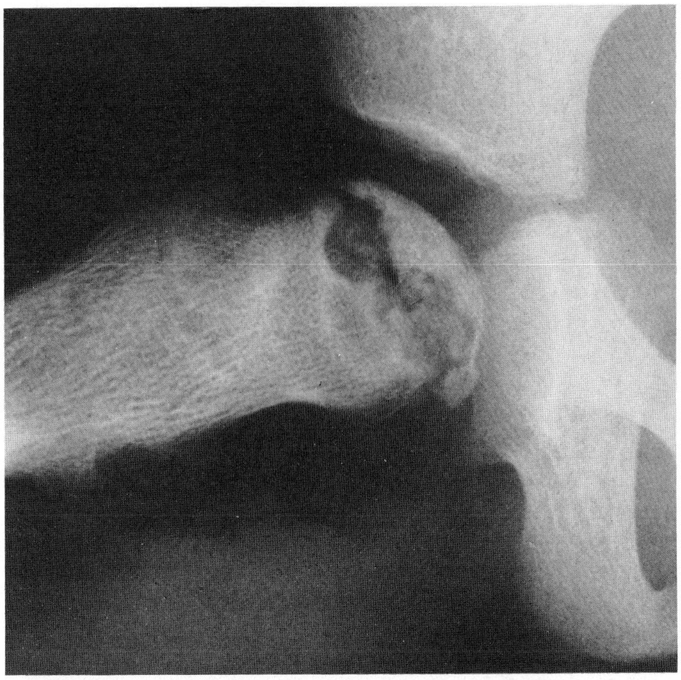

Figure 52.24. Femoral head necrosis in an 8-yr-old girl with oligomeganephronic hypoplasia and a serum creatinine of 3,3 mg/dl. Roentgenogram of right hip joint. Right femoral head is collapsed to small dense shell of bone; wide, irregularly fuzzy defects in metaphysis. Child had never received corticosteroids but in past had severe renal osteodystrophy that caused extreme coxavara at both sides. (From Mehls O, et al: Femoral head necrosis in uremic children without steroid treatment or transplantation. J Pediatr 6:926, 1981, with permission.)

is predominantly, if not exclusively, the result of hypophosphatemia (184). Renal generation of $1,25(OH)_2D_3$ is impaired in experimentally induced Fanconi's syndrome; low levels of 1,25(OH)D have been found in children with Fanconi's syndrome or RTA (185, 186), even when impairment of renal function was slight (186). These factors may contribute to osteomalacia and rickets in these children who later develop CRF (184, 187).

SERUM CHEMISTRIES AND ROENTGENOGRAMS

Serum Chemistry

Serum chemistry is of limited value to assess the severity and type of bone disease.

Calcium

Hypocalcemia is associated with abundant osteoid (81) and low levels of 25(OH)D; hypercalcemia usually points to advanced osteitis fibrosa but may also occur with Al toxicity, occasionally with vitamin A toxicity, or after immobilization (188).

Phosphorus

Hyperphosphatemia is common in ESRD and is associated with osteitis fibrosa, a high intake of milk products, or hypercatabolic states. Hyperphosphatemia occurs commonly with vitamin D therapy in children with CRF and is thought to result from vitamin D–stimulated intestinal P uptake. Hypophosphatemia is observed occasionally because of overzealous use of phosphate binders or from poor dietary intake. Hypophosphatemia may be perpetuated by obligatory P loss while on dialysis (189); its possible relation to osteomalacia is contested (81).

Immunoreactive PTH

iPTH levels must be interpreted with caution in uremic patients, because most available assays recognize breakdown products of the PTH as well. Presently, the reliability of radioimmunoassays leaves much to be desired. iPTH measurement is useful in differentiating between hypercalcemia from osteitis fibrosa and that due to other causes and may be useful in observing patients during therapy. When iPTH levels are normal or undetectable, the presence of Al intoxication should be suspected (190).

Serum Alkaline Phosphatase

Serum alkaline phosphatase, specifically the isoenzyme of bone, is an index of osteoblastic activity; it is elevated in states of high bone turnover and usually is found in osteitis fibrosa. Low alkaline phosphatase may point to Al intoxication (191, 192). Serial measurements of alkaline phosphatase are useful to monitor therapy, especially vitamin D therapy. Serum hydroxyproline (193) and bone Gla-protein (194) may become useful noninvasive indicators of bone metabolism, but their clinical value is not established.

Skeletal Roentgenograms

Because information obtained with serum biochemistry and physical examination is limited and bone histology is not readily available, skeletal roentgenograms are the most important source of information to diagnose and to monitor renal osteodystrophy (166, 195–198). Roentgenograms are useful to distinguish between the lesions of cortical bone (subperiosteal, intracortical, and endosteal bone resorption; periosteal neo-ostosis; acroosteolysis); and those of cancellous bone (focal accumulation of coarse trabeculae with blurred outlines sometimes associated with osteosclerosis or osteopenia). These lesions are similar in adults and children, but their intensity and rate of progression is greater in children because the rate of bone turnover in the growing skeleton is higher.

Cortical Bone Lesions

Radiolucent resorptive defects at the subperiosteal site are characteristic of osteitis fibrosa in the older child and adult. In our experience, they are rarely present in small children. Punched-out lesions at the outer contour of cortical bone, bridged by a mineralized outer lamella, may represent subperiosteal resorption or periosteal neoostosis (199)—both indicators of osteitis fibrosa. The sites of roentgenologically demonstrable subperiostal resorption differ with age, because they may become evident only at sites of high bone modeling, the rates of which in different bones vary with age and growth rate.

In uremia, bone is resorbed at the subperiosteal surface, along Haversian channels within cortical bone and from the endosteal surface. The circumferential outer lamella of tubular bones may be eroded and replaced by fibrous tissue or woven bone (200), particularly at sites of insertion of tendons or ligaments, e.g., at the phalangeal base, where some woven bone is found even in the normal skeleton. Osteoclastic "drill holes" on the bone surface are directed perpendicularly to the circumferential lamella. Roentgenograms give a characteristic "spicular" appearance in zones of acro-osteolysis (Fig. 52.25) and subperiosteal resorption (Fig. 52.27). The radial side of the middle phalanx of the second and third digit are most likely to develop signs of osteitis fibrosa in adults and older children but are uncommon in preschool children. They develop a fluffy indistinct delineation of the cortex, which may be the only x-ray finding. In this age group, subperiosteal resorption zones

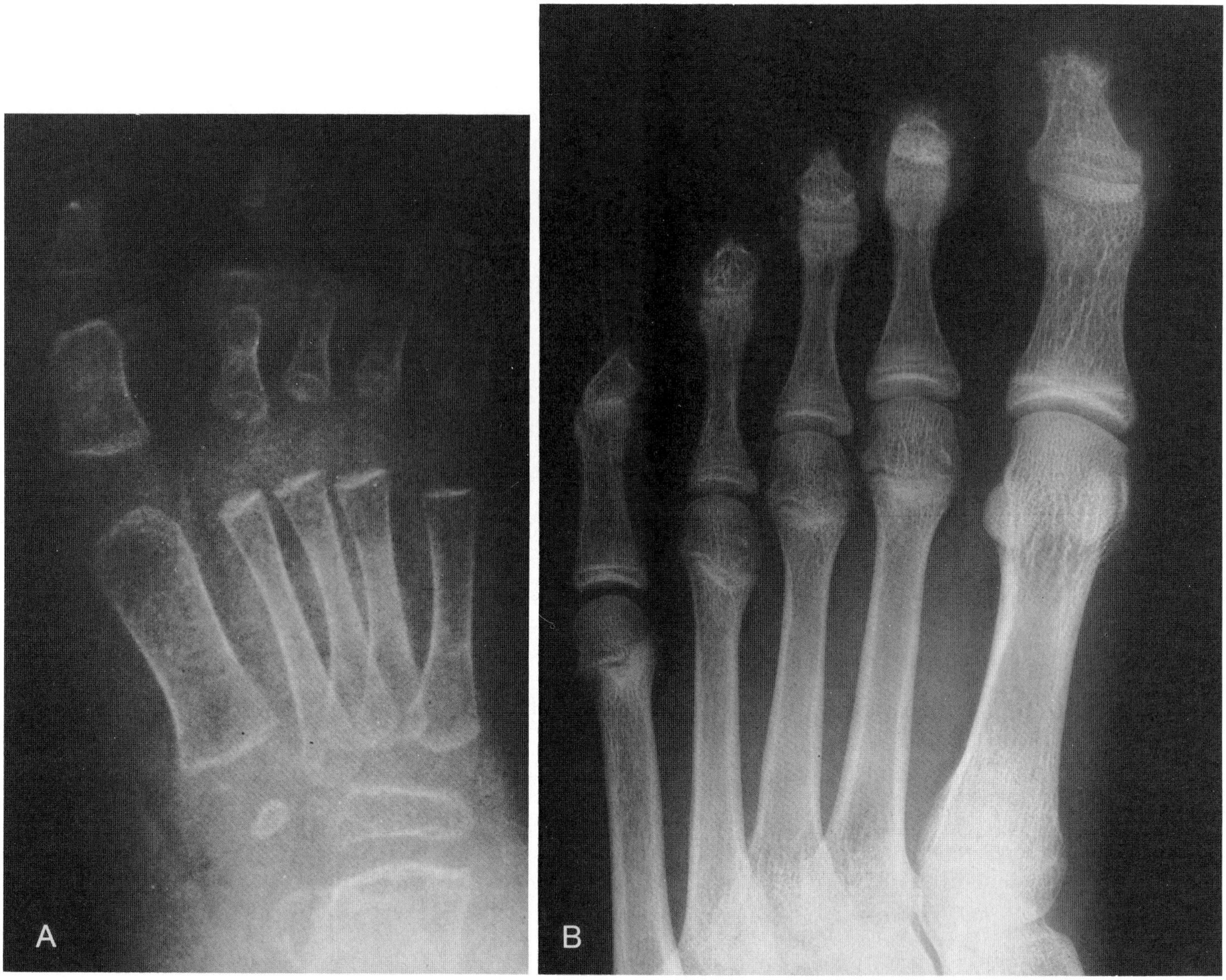

Figure 52.25. **A,** Multicentric osteolysis in a 2-yr-old girl with glomerulosclerosis. Terminal phalanges are partly or completely missing. This is caused by bone-forming defect and not by renal osteodystrophy. **B,** Acroosteolysis of terminal phalanges of left foot in a 9-yr-old girl with oligomeganephronic hypoplasia and severe renal osteodystrophy, serum creatinine 9.2 mg/100 ml. In contrast to **A** note that only the terminal part of end-phalanges is resorbed by severe osteitis fibrosa.

are seen at the lateral aspect of the distal radius and ulna and at the medial side of the upper tibia.

In long bones, the site of transition between metaphysis and shaft is a common site of bony erosion caused by a collar of active osteoclasts. These osteoclasts are present even in the normal skeleton. Such osteoclasts reduce the diameter of the epiphyseal growth plate to that of the diaphyseal shaft of bone. Exaggeration of this process in the metaphysis of the femoral neck in renal osteodystrophy causes the "rotten fence post" sign (201).

Resorptive lesions of the tuft of the terminal phalanges give rise to acro-osteolysis (Fig. 52.25). When erosion of the tuft is advanced, the terminal phalanx may collapse. The redundency of soft tissue then gives rise to the clinical sign of pseudoclubbing (Fig. 52.26).

Several characteristics of subperiosteal resorption zones can be understood from knowing the underlying histology. For example, mature lamellar bone at this site is replaced by poorly mineralized fibrous bone; with vitamin D therapy or parathyroidectomy, the original shape of bone is rapidly restored. When erosions are healing, bone mineral is first visible at the inner side of the periosteal tube; then a shell of bone separated from the cortex by a small radiolucent zone is noted. This zone corresponds to a layer of undermineralized fibrous tissue in histological sections. This phenomenon, occurring spontaneously or during therapy, is called periosteal neo-osteosis (see Fig. 52.28). With further healing, the radiolucent zone becomes dense, so that the thickness of the cortex apparently increases.

Within the core of cortical bone, osteoclastic activity is increased, and longitudinal resorption cavities arise along Haversian systems. Normal remodeling is not visible on roentgenogram because resorption cavities are rapidly filled with mature mineralized lamellar bone. Longitudinal cortical striation is visible on x-ray film (202) only when resorption cavities are filled with poorly mineralized lamellar bone, woven bone, or even fibrous tissue. Enlargement of Haversian channels of the metacarpals is not specific for secondary hyperparathyroidism; it is also noted during states of high bone turnover, even during the normal adolescent growth spurt.

Increased osteoclastic activity at the endosteal surface leads to endos-

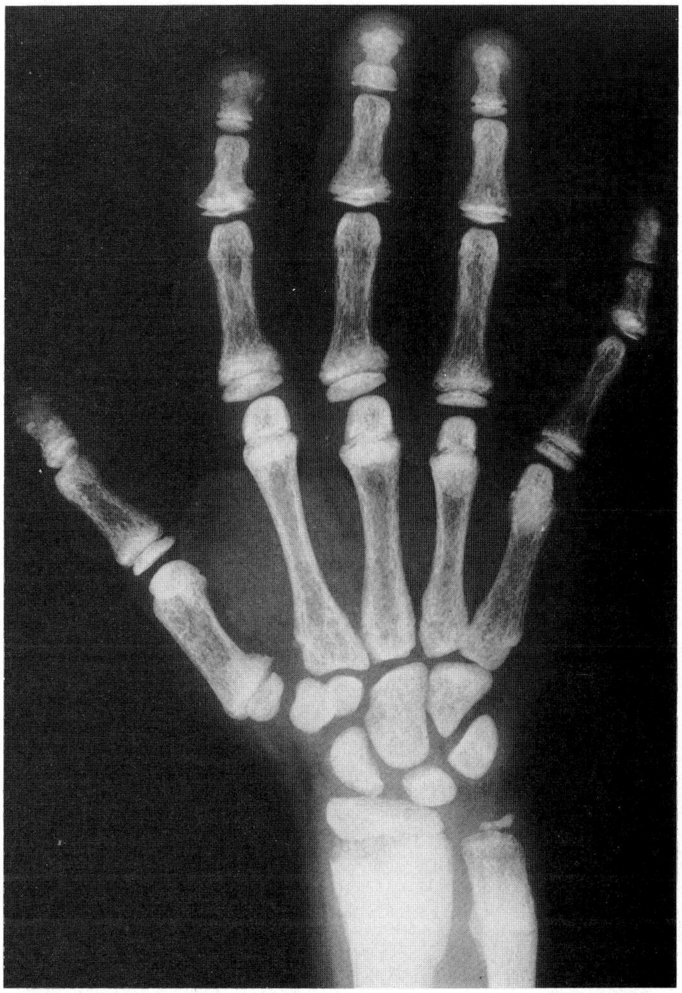

Figure 52.26. Skeletal changes caused by oxalosis. Right-hand skeleton of 12-yr-old girl with oxalosis and on hemodialysis since age 8 yr. Multifocal crippling fractures and patchy sclerosis are late consequences of long-standing oxalosis.

teal bone loss and cortical thinning. Cortical thinning is not a useful index of hyperparathyroidism in children. We did not find a correlation between cortical thickness (Garn index) and bone biopsy evidence of osteitis fibrosa.

Cortical bone erosions also are noted in several tight joints (syndesmosis), e.g., the acromioclavicular and sternoclavicular joints, the sacroiliac joint, the symphysis, the vertebral body adjacent to the disk, or the mandibular condyle adjacent to the temporomandibular joint.

Cancellous Bone Lesion

The number and diameter of trabeculae commonly are increased in uremic children. The contours of the trabeculae appear fuzzy, and the shape appears bizarre, which may be evidence of covering of the trabecular surface by osteoid and disorderly surface remodeling. Increased trabecular bone mass, i.e., osteosclerosis, is most readily demonstrable at skeletal sites where cancellous rather than cortical bone predominates: skull, vertebra, pelvis, and metaphyses of tubular bones. The typical signs of local osteosclerosis are the rugger-jersey spine, increased density of ossa iliaca or metaphyses of long bones, and sclerosis of the skull. The characteristic small resorptive defects in an osteosclerotic skull give rise to the sign of the "pepperpot" skull. Osteosclerosis usually becomes more readily apparent after vitamin D therapy.

Cyst formation (brown tumors) occur more commonly in children (203, 204) than in adults with CRF (166). They tend to occur within metacarpals, the distal femur, proximal tibia, and distal radius (see Fig. 52.29).

Looser Zones

The radiographic features of osteomalacia are far less characteristic than those of osteitis fibrosa. Looser zones (pseudofractures) are uncommon in children. They are characteristic of osteomalacia but not specific for it. They present as wide, straight bands of radiolucency abutting onto the cortex, perpendicular to the long axis of the bone; they usually are symmetrical and may have a narrow region of adjacent sclerosis (166). Preferential sites in children include the proximal femur (see Fig. 52.20) and upper and lower ends of the fibula and ribs. Looser zones are easily missed if the plane of projection is not perpendicular to the Looser zone. Skeletal scintigraphy will detect more Looser zones than are visible on roentgenograms.

Growth Zone (Epiphyses and Metaphyses)

The interpretation of the x-ray appearance of the epiphyseal growth plate of uremic children has been confused in the past because histological documentation was lacking. The relative contribution of osteitis fibrosa and rickets has not been defined clearly.

Ricketslike lesions were reported in primary hyperparathyroidism of children (148–151) and secondary hyperparathyroidism associated with target cell resistance to PTH (205). These cases may represent an independent manifestation of hyperparathyroidism, which induces a disturbance of endochondral ossification that may resemble rickets radiographically despite a different histopathogenesis.

It is not only the fast-growing lower femoral and upper tibial metaphyses that are affected in renal osteodystrophy, but also the slow-growing upper femoral and lower tibial metaphyses. An accurately aligned roentgenogram usually shows that the radiolucent zone is not caused by widening of the growth plate but by rarefication of the metaphyseal spongiosa. The metaphysis is the site of subendochondral and subperiosteal resorption and osteoclastic resorption of metaphyseal trabeculae, giving rise to an irregular radiolucent zone underneath the epiphysis.

Some authors have confused (197, 198) changes caused by hyperparathyroidism with those caused by rickets. In CRF, the lesions at the end of long bones commonly result from hyperparathyroidism and not rickets (146, 159). Although true rickets is documented in children with mild CRF (206), we have not confirmed its presence in histopathological studies of our children with advanced CRF (146). The subepiphyseal radiolucent area does not represent cartilage or chondro-osteoid tissue in the growth plate, as it does in vitamin D–deficiency rickets. Instead, it represents undermineralized woven bone or fibrous tissue in metaphyseal spongiosa, i.e., changes that reflect the action of PTH on the skeleton. If visible in properly aligned roentgenograms, the poorly delineated zone of provisional calcification interposed between growth cartilage and primary spongiosa permits assessment of the width of the growth cartilage, which is usually narrow (Fig. 52.29).

EFFECT OF TREATMENT—DIALYSIS AND RENAL TRANSPLANTATION

Hemodialysis

Maintenance hemodialysis permits some control of plasma Ca, Ca-P balance, and parathyroid secretion; however, metabolic bone disease continues in children on dialysis.

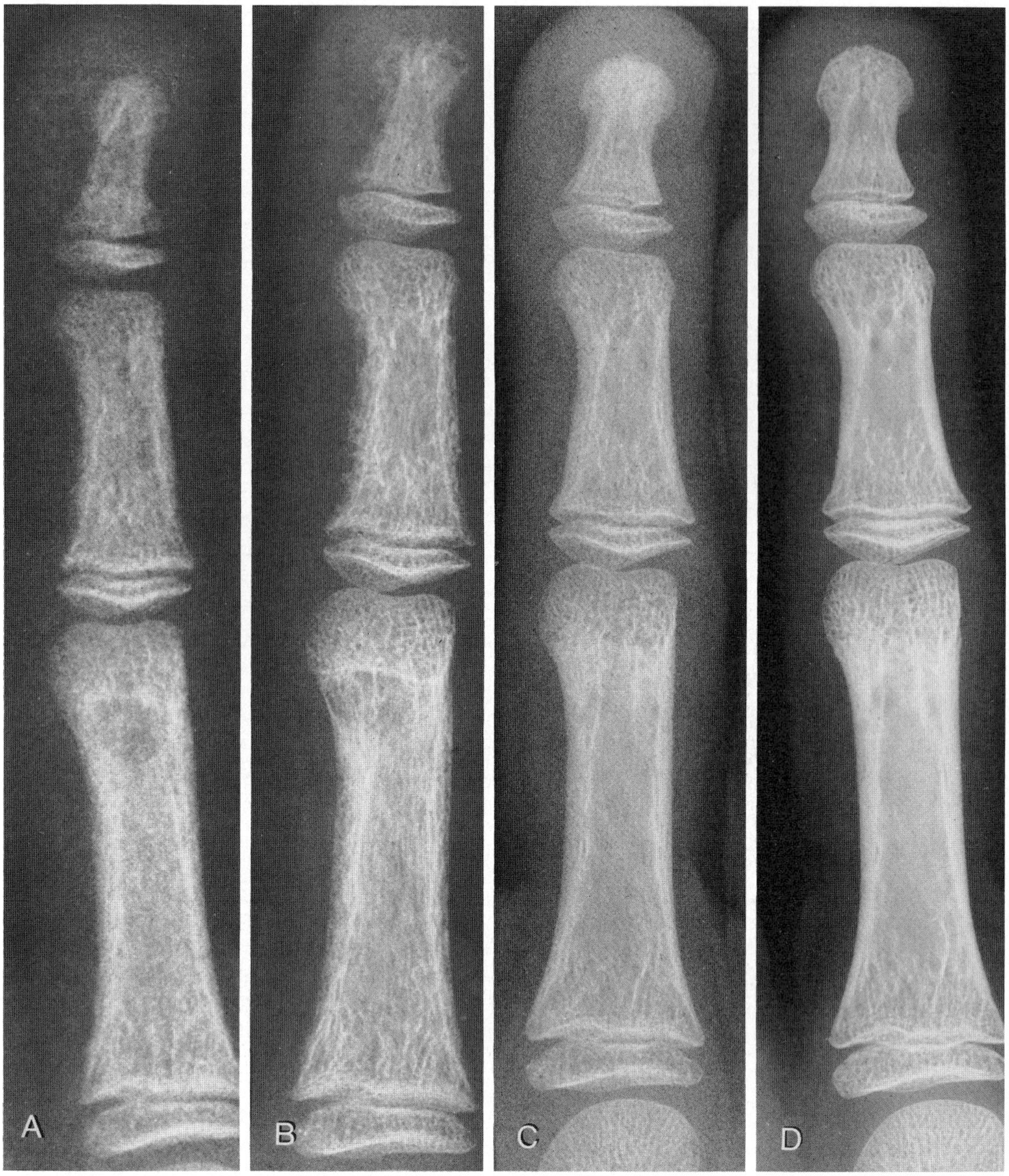

Figure 52.27. Subperiosteal resorption and periosteal neo-ostosis. Roentgenogram of right distal ulna of 16-yr-old boy with renal hypoplasia and serum creatinine of 12 mg/dl. Severe renal secondary hyperparathyroidism despite vitamin D treatment. Lateral side of ulna is eroded, but new bone formation is seen at inner side of periosteum, giving rise to periosteal neo-ostosis.

Ca Balance

During dialysis Ca balance depends on diffusive and convective Ca transfer across dialysis membranes. Diffusive transfer of Ca depends on its concentration gradient between plasma and dialysate and flow rates. Convective transfer of Ca depends on the rate of ultrafiltration. The magnitude of convective loss often is not appreciated, e.g., 3 kg per dialysis session 3 times weekly can cause the loss of 0.5 g Ca/week or 25 g/yr. There is little or no Ca gain by diffusion in normocalcemic patients when Ca concentrations of dialysate is 2.8 to 3.0 mEq/liter (5.6 to 6.0 mg/dl). In the interdialytic interval, net intestinal losses of 200 mg/week are estimated for patients on normal or low dietary intake of Ca (207). Therefore, it is advisable to use higher dialysate Ca concentrations to increase dialysis balance and offset convective and gastrointestinal losses. Adult patients on dialysis maintain a constant whole-body Ca, measured by neutron activation analysis, when dialysate Ca is 7.0 to 8.0 mg/dl. No data are available for children on dialysis; however, there is consensus that dialysate Ca for children should be the same.

Bone Mineral Content

Factors causing loss of body Ca in adults and children with CRF have been cited (p 854). We found reduced forearm mineral density in dialyzed children (208). In adult patients on dialysis, mineral loss from the appendicular skeleton progresses; this was partially reversed by high dialysate Ca or vitamin D therapy. Interpretation of measurements in the appendicular skeleton, however, are difficult because skeletal Ca may redistribute from cortical to cancellous bone and from appendicular to axial skeleton. Despite changes in the appendicular skeleton, whole body Ca content of patients on long-term hemodialysis, observed in our center for close to a decade, is normal (209).

Removal of P by dialysis usually is not sufficient to offset P uptake in

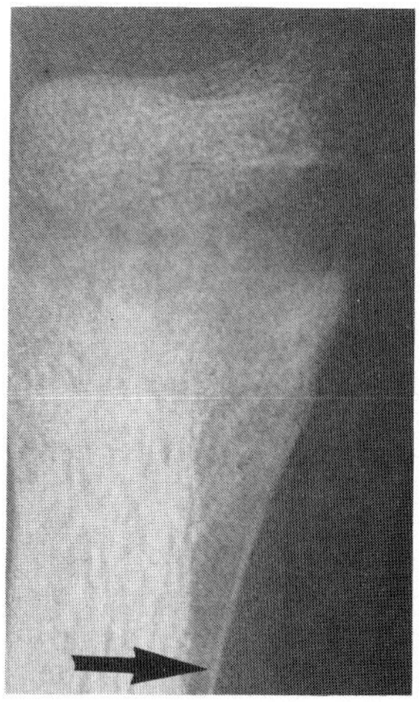

Figure 52.28. Brown tumor in renal osteodystrophy. Roentgenogram of right hand of 15-yr-old boy with nephronophthisis; serum creatinine 13 mg/dl. Brown tumor involves the fifth metacarpal. Cortical erosions threaten biomechanical stability bone. There are excessive lucent areas beneath the growth plates of the radius and ulna. (From Mehls O, Oppermann HC: Renale Osteopathien. In Diethelm L, Heuck F, Olsson O, et al (eds): Handbuch d. Medizinischen Radiologie Band V. Röntgendiagnostik der Skeletterkrankungen. Berlin-Heidelberg, Springer Verlag, 1983.)

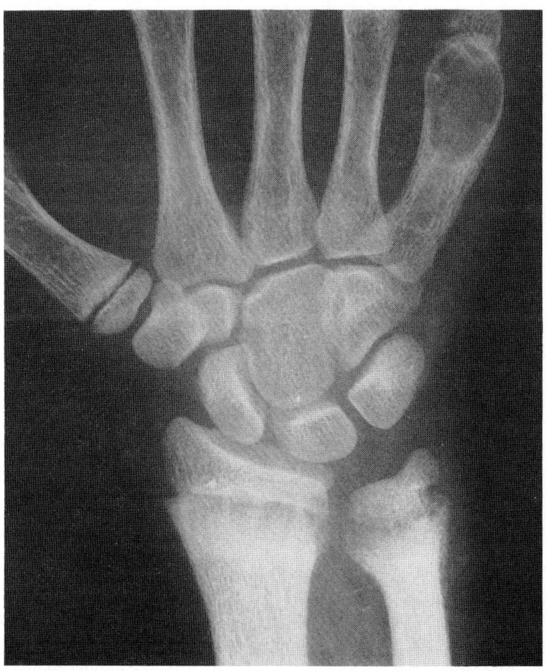

Figure 52.29. Index finger of a 12-yr-old girl with oligomeganephronic hypoplasia, serum creatinine 11,2 mg/100 ml. Roentgenograms before **(A)** one month **(B)**, three months **(C)**, and 15 months **(D)** after initiation of vitamin D therapy (20,000 IU vitamin D_3/day). Before therapy, one can see severe subperiosteal resorption zones, acroosteolysis and spongiosation of the cortical bone. At this time, border between cortical and spongy bone is no longer distinguishable. Coarse plump trabeculae of spongiosa. Rapid healing of bone lesions under vitamin D treatment. (From Mehls O., Oppermann H.-C. (204) with permission.)

the interdialytic interval when customary diets are used (210) without using phosphate binders. Because of the risk of Al toxicity, Al-containing phosphate binders should be administered with caution. We recommend using diets low in P and giving $CaCO_3$ as a phosphate binder.

Levels of iPTH are commonly elevated in children on dialysis, despite normal levels of total serum Ca and (according to histological evidence) increased osteoclastic bone resorption. However, parathyroidectomy is seldom done (<2% of our children on dialysis).

The prevalence of symptomatic bone disease and other manifestations of disturbed Ca metabolism in children on maintenance dialysis has markedly decreased in the past decade. However, osteodystrophy manifested as hyperparathyroidism and abnormal bone histology is still a major problem (4, 140, 211–213), although no systematic longitudinal studies are available. There is consensus that the histological lesions encountered in children with CRF are not changed by dialysis treatment. Restoring bone histology to normal with vitamin D therapy has not been reported.

At least 14% of children who are 2 to 5 yr old when dialysis begins develop disabling bone disease; x-ray evidence of bone disease was observed in 50% of children (214). We found x-ray abnormalities in 40% of our children, a prevalence that is higher than that in our adult patients on dialysis. Children on dialysis therapy for more than two years may develop osteopenia, cortical thinning of tubular bones, and spontaneous bone (rib, metacarpal) fractures. The role of Al intoxication is being worked out.

Hemofiltration

Despite past reports that control of hyperphosphatemia was easier with hemofiltration than with dialysis (215), little difference between the two has been shown with respect to phosphatemia (216, 217). During hemofiltration, Ca balance is determined by the partition of plasma Ca into ultrafiltrable and nonultrafiltrable Ca, Ca concentration in the substitution fluid, and overall fluid balance (volume of ultrafiltrable minus substituent). These points are of special importance for children in whom the volume exchanged in one hemofiltration session may correspond to 50% to 90% of body weight (218). To offset negative Ca balance in the interdialytic interval and convective Ca loss during hemofiltration, Ca concentration in the replacement fluid must be higher than in the ultrafiltrate. In clinical practice, Ca concentrations of 3.5 to 4.0 mEq/liter are used.

Removal of fragments of PTH by hemofiltration may be beneficial for controlling renal osteodystrophy; however, in a feedback-controlled system, it is doubtful whether removing a hormone will have more than a transient effect on circulating levels of bioactive hormone. Clinical studies (219, 220) have failed to document long-term changes of iPTH or bone disease that could not be explained by Ca-P balance. Vitamin D-binding protein (DBP) and $25(OH)D_3$ are not lost during hemofiltration because the cut-off point is 15,000 to 40,000 Dalton.

Continuous Ambulatory Peritoneal Dialysis (CAPD)

During recent years CAPD has become common practice for children needing dialysis. In preliminary and uncontrolled studies, growth and metabolic bone disease are better for children on CAPD compared with those on hemodialysis (221, 222). Other reports are less encouraging (223, 224).

Ca balance during CAPD is the net result of diffusive and convective Ca transport, depending on the concentration of diffusible Ca in plasma, Ca concentration in the dialysate, and fluid balance. Ca balance is negative when dialysate Ca is <6 mg/dl (<3.0 mEq/liter) although total S_{Ca} does not change (225). It increases only slightly, and ionized Ca levels remain low even though dialysate Ca concentration is raised to 3.5 mEq/liter (226). Higher dialysate Ca concentrations, vitamin D treatment, or both are recommended if the patient's weight gain requires excessive fluid removal by ultrafiltration and attendant Ca losses. Although decreases in iPTH are reported in patients on CAPD (227), there is a consensus that significant decreases in iPTH occur only when S_{Ca} increases (226, 228).

Protein loss into the dialysate fluid ranges between 0.1 and 0.3 g/kg/day and concurrently DBP and $25(OH)D_3$ are lost; however, the rate of loss usually does not exceed the rate of production. DBP and $25(OH)D_3$ levels did not change in adult patients on CAPD. Levels of $25(OH)D_3$ increase with time in these patients when they are given 50,000 U vitamin D_3/week (229, 229a).

Transplantation

Evolution of Hyperparathyroidism

After transplantation, evidence of renal hyperparathyroidism usually disappears in several weeks. In a few patients, however, particularly those with severe osteitis fibrosa, hypercalcemia may continue for months; this occasionally necessitates partial parathyroidectomy. Hypophosphatemia is common after transplantation; causes include persistent hyperparathyroidism and the hypophosphatemic effect of steroid therapy. The tubular phosphate threshold (TMP/GFR) is low and $1,25(OH)_2D$ levels may be inappropriately low in relation to serum Pi (230).

These comments apply to children with conventional immunosuppression, including steroids, following renal transplantation. Use of cyclosporin-A may diminish the requirement for steroids and improve results. Catch-up growth, which is rarely observed following renal transplant in children given steroids, is reported with cyclosporin-A (231). In these patients, bone alkaline phosphatase isoenzyme and osteoblasts in bone increase, which contrasts with experience in patients receiving steroids.

X-ray findings of renal osteodystrophy usually disappear within two months following renal transplantation (232); occasionally they persist for periods up to two years (227, 232a, 233). In our experience, these lesions disappear more slowly in children who have been on long-term (three years) dialysis therapy compared with those on therapy for shorter periods.

Osteopenia

High doses of steroids cause osteopenia. Severe osteopenia occurs in patients with the nephrotic syndrome who receive large doses of steroids before developing ESRD. Complications from steroid-induced osteopenia are infrequent, but we have observed vertebral collapse and static vertebral pain. Vitamin D metabolites marginally affects the prevalence of osteopenia in nonrenal patients receiving steroids (233a); the effect of $1,25(OH)_2D$ therapy given to adult patients post transplant, in a prospective controlled study, was marginal (234). In children, bone mineral content increases post transplant, possibly resulting from skeletal growth. We have not observed "catch-up mineralization," i.e., an increase in bone mineral density out of proportion to increase in height age.

The effect of renal transplantation on preexistent dialysis osteopenia is marginal. In our experience, dialysis osteopenia is usually not favorably affected. However, when cortical thinning results from secondary hyperparathyroidism, increased bone mass may be noted post transplant. Since this is correlated with improved growth velocity, we cannot exclude the possibility that the observed amelioration was secondary to improved growth.

Aseptic Bone Necrosis

The most serious complication following renal transplantation is aseptic bone necrosis. Its incidence varies from 3% to 45% (235, 236), with an overall frequency about 8%. Osteonecrosis usually appears within the first postoperative year, but may occur as late as five years after transplant (235). The mechanism by which this occurs is unknown. X-ray evidence of osteonecrosis occurs before transplantation in children (172) and adults (237), despite the fact that they had not been treated with steroids. Secondary hyperparathyroidism may play a role in the genesis of osteonecrosis. We believe that coxa vara in patients with uremia predisposes to osteonecrosis of the femoral head (172). Most investigators have not found a correlation between the incidence of osteonecrosis and the average, cumulative, or maximal steroid dosage (235). This observation does not exclude the possibility that corticosteroid therapy is the critical factor in the genesis of osteonecrosis. Recent observations that low-dosage steroid therapy (238) following transplantation is associated with virtually no osteonecrosis suggest that steroids are a necessary factor causing aseptic necrosis and that the threshold dose may be quite low (239).

The femoral head is the most common site affected in children. The femoral condyles are also commonly affected, followed by the os naviculare carpi, naviculare tarsi, talus, and calcaneus (235). Pain is the usual presenting symptom and sometimes may be noted months before x-ray signs appear. In other cases, lesions on roentgenogram may be present for months before symptoms develop. The diagnosis is made by roentgenogram. An early x-ray sign is a radiolucent line that parallels the articular surface of the femoral head; this line represents a fracture, and a resorption zone close to the articular cartilage. As the lesion progresses, the femoral head collapses, the articular cartilage is deformed, and "steps" are noted on x-ray film. Bone collapse and remodeling cause sclerosis and increased density that is evident on roentgenogram. Lesions also can be detected in an early phase using bone scintigraphy and ^{18}F or ^{99}Tc scans.

Al Toxicity

Al toxicity, recently recognized as an important cause of bone disease in patients on dialysis (240), results from Al contamination of dialysis water (241) or from ingestion of Al-containing oral phosphate binders (242). The syndrome is characterized by skeletal pain, proximal muscle weakness, and bone fractures unresponsive to vitamin D therapy. When vitamin D or $1,25(OH)_2$ is given, hypercalcemia often develops, but the osteomalacia does not heal. Al bone disease may be associated with Al encephalopathy and microcytic hypochromic anemia (243, 244).

It is tempting to speculate that high local concentrations of Al are toxic to osteoblasts and their microtubular system. A toxic effect on osteoblasts may explain the low alkaline phosphatase values (191, 192), loss of bone mass (192), and the presence of low turnover bone disease. Low turnover bone disease also results from low basal iPTH levels. PTH dose not increase in response to hypocalcemia. Al is stored in the parathyroid glands, and this may affect the control of PTH release (245). The interrelation between Al and parathyroid function is complex. Hyperparathyroidism favors intestinal absorption of Al, whereas accumulation of Al suppresses parathyroid function.

The diagnosis of Al bone disease may be made from elevated basal Al levels (243), from the response of Al levels to intravenous desferrioxamine (246), from the high Al content in bone (142), or from demonstration of Al in bone taken by biopsy (143, 144). Until 1983 most published information concerned adults on dialysis. Current reports describe severe rachetic lesions, especially in young children, including those with CRF who are not on dialysis therapy but who have been treated with Al-containing phosphate binders (242). There are no reports describing the effect of Al intoxication on growth; however, Al-intoxicated rats grow at a slower rate (Mehls and Ritz, unpublished observations).

Desferrioxamine is used to treat Al intoxication (246). For dialysis patients, treatment is intermittent during dialysis (247).

RENAL OSTEODYSTROPHY AND GROWTH

Although growth failure occurs in uremic children in the absence of evidence of bone disease, renal osteodystrophy is assumed as one cause of growth failure. Its effect on growth may be evaluated from growth response to therapy of osteodystrophy or from studying the effect that Ca-regulating hormones have on growth.

Vitamin D

Children on dialysis have had no consistent pattern of improvement in growth rate following treatment with vitamin D_3 (164, 248), 1-α-hydroxycholecalciferol (249), or $1,25(OH)_2D_3$ (250, 251). This contrasts to the response observed in isolated $1,25(OH)_2D_3$ deficiency, associated with vitamin D–dependent rickets (251a), in which catch-up growth, with subsequent attainment of normal stature, is observed in response to treatment with $1,25(OH)_2D_3$. The disappointing effect of $1,25(OH)_2D_3$ therapy on growth in children with CRF demonstrates that deficiency of $1,25(OH)_2D$ alone is not the major cause of growth failure despite anecdotal observations to the contrary in children with CRF (164). In these patients, unfortunately, the vitamin D status before therapy was not established. Because plasma $25(OH)D_3$ levels are frequently low in patients with renal failure, one cannot exclude the possibility that such children were vitamin D–deficient. This would explain the dramatic therapeutic response to vitamin D administration.

Growth has improved in children with CRF who were treated with $1,25(OH)_2D_3$ and who had previously failed to respond to high doses of vitamin D_3 (251b, 251c). However, in no instance has catch-up growth been reported. In some studies, the alleged growth-promoting effect of $1,25(OH)_2D_3$ could not be distinguished from the possible effect of a pubertal growth spurt. The growth-promoting effect of vitamin D therapy was transient. The growth curves on follow-up paralleled the third centile of age-corrected growth curves (252). In some of these communications, vitamin D status was not described. When one compares results of treatments with $1,25(OH)_2D_3$ with those of previous treatments with vitamin D_3, one has to use equipotent doses. Unfortunately, the potency ratio of $1,25(OH)_2D_3$ to cholecalciferol in humans is not known. At this point, a specific effect of $1,25(OH)_2D$ therapy on growth has not been established.

Although there is little clinical evidence for a growth-promoting action of vitamin D in children with CRF, growth rate in uremic rats is improved by vitamin D therapy (253). However, since energy intake also increased in rats treated with vitamin D_3, the effect may have been due to improved calorie intake, anabolism, and muscle growth (254). There is considerable uncertainty as to whether the growth-promoting action of vitamin D is mediated exclusively through $1,25(OH)_2D_3$ or whether action of other vitamin D metabolites, e.g., $24,25(OH)_2D_3$, is also required. We have found vitamin D_3 to have growth-promoting effect equal to that of $1,25(OH)_2D_3$ in dosages that had equal effects on serum Ca (254, 255).

Control of PTH

In general, children with the most severe degree of osteitis fibrosa are reported to be most growth-retarded (256); however, growth rate and severity of osteitis fibrosa as seen on roentgenogram do not correlate. Paradoxically, children with the highest growth rates soon develop severe resorptive lesions on skeletal roentgenograms, presumably because rapid skeletal growth unmasks osteitis fibrosa. Unfortunately, information on the relation between changing bone histology and the course of growth in this circumstance is not available.

Although it is generally claimed that children with primary hyperparathyroidism grow poorly, no published data evaluate this. Two clinical observations argue for a growth-promoting effect of PTH. When patients with primary hypoparathyroidism are treated with vitamin D therapy to maintain normal Ca_s, they do not grow normally, although Ca_s is normal. On the other hand, children with pseudohypoparathyroidism and osteitis fibrosa usually are tall (166) and have high circulating PTH concentrations. It is assumed that skeletal response to PTH to regulate growth is intact, whereas the renal response is not. PTH stimulation of growth cartilage is consistent with the finding that PTH induces mitosis in osteoprogenitor (257) or extraskeletal cells, e.g. thymocytes (258). In experimental uremia, responsiveness of growth cartilage cAMP to PTH in vivo or in vitro is diminished (30). Children with advanced renal osteitis fibrosa who grow little probably have destroyed the normal architecture of the growth zone (146). In some, parathyroidectomy was followed by improved growth rates (256, 259), but the improvement in growth rate lasted for no more than several months.

PATIENT MANAGEMENT BEFORE DIALYSIS AND TRANSPLANTATION

Children with CRI (GFR <50% or <60 ml/1.73 m^2)

"An ounce of prevention is better than a pound of cure." Prevention of renal osteodystrophy is intellectually appealing. Such prevention can be tried by maintaining normal serum chemistries to compensate for the failing renal function and by prophylactically administering $1,25(OH)_2D_3$ to compensate for the failing kidneys' endocrine role. Unfortunately, no controlled study on the efficacy of such prophylaxis has been reported.

Serum Pi is age-dependent declining from infancy to adolescence. This may be related to the need for retaining P during growth. Deficiency of dietary P interferes with skeletal growth; however, hyperphosphatemia is undoubtedly harmful in patients with CRF. In view of this dilemma, more information is necessary before more detailed recommendations can be made about P restrictions. It appears wise to maintain serum P levels of uremic children in the age-corrected normal range.

Hyperparathyroidism has been partially reversed by dietary restriction of P in adult patients with CRI (260); however, in children, the safety of interventions to limit dietary P is not proven and ideal intake of P has not been defined. The dietary sources of P are meat, dairy products, and prepared foods in which P is used in food processing. Average P intake in most western diets exceeds the recommended intake. Intake can be reduced by about 50% to 60% by adherence to lower protein and P diets that meet recommended intakes. Although low-protein diets may prevent progression of renal failure in experimental models of renal damage, the safety and efficacy of these diets in adults and children with CRI has not been established. In very young children, it is difficult to eliminate cow's milk from the diet, except by substituting low P infant milk-base formulas. With CRF, it is difficult to provide a diet that is adequate and maintains P_s in the normal range. Therefore, it becomes necessary to use oral phosphate binders in the form of Al-containing compounds. Because Al compounds have the potential to induce Al toxicity, alternative products have been developed. Ca-carbonate may simultaneously correct hypocalcemia and hyperphosphatemia; however, because of the risk of hypercalcemia, the dose required to correct hyperphosphatemia may not be tolerated. Ca-carbonate may be a useful adjunct to Al-containing phosphate binders. Mg-containing phosphate binders are not recommended because they may induce hypermagnesemia in patients with CRF (261). Al-free polyuronate compounds have been developed to prevent hyperphosphatemia, but their safety and efficacy have not been established.

Because of the risks of Al toxicity, serum Al levels should be monitored every few months in patients taking Al-containing phosphate binders. Basal and postdesferrioxamine Al levels should be monitored when unexplained neurological, skeletal, or hematological signs develop.

Although the efficacy of giving vitamin D or its metabolites to children with CRF to prevent bone disease and growth failure has not been demonstrated in prospective trials, prophylaxis with vitamin D seems reasonable on theoretical grounds (6). Since prolonged administration of vitamin D_3 in dosages sufficient to reverse intestinal malabsorption of Ca fails to normalize bone histology in adults (33) and children (O Mehls, unpublished observations), prophylaxis with vitamin D_3 presumably should be started when children have CRI (GFR <50%). This treatment is under investigation.

In our experience, 3000 to 5000 U/day of vitamin D_3 administered to children with CRI prevents severe osteodystrophy. We have not observed hypercalcemia or deterioration of renal function with this dose. Recent reports on potential nephrotoxicity of vitamin D unrelated to hypercalcemia (262) or hypercalciuria are not supported by more detailed follow-up studies (252, 263).

Children with Advanced CRF

In children with advanced CRF (GFR <25% normal or <30 ml/ 1.73 m^2), the signs of bone disease improve with treatment of any of the following: vitamin D_2 (264, 265) 25-hydroxy-vitamin D_3 (61, 211), 1-α-hydroxycholecalciferol (266–269), dihydrotachysterol (249, 270), or 1,25$(OH)_2D_3$ (271–274). All these compounds raise S_{Ca} decrease iPTH, and improve but do not completely correct histological evidence of osteitis fibrosa. They are less consistent in reversing the mineralization defect. The effect on S_{Ca} is accompanied by increased intestinal absorption and increased renal excretion of Ca. In addition, intestinal absorption of P is increased, which may lead to hyperphosphatemia. Muscular strength may improve.

All the metabolites are effective even in anephric patients. Each of these metabolites is bound by the 1,25$(OH)_2D_3$ receptor (275), and this may explain why each of them is effective. However, although extrarenal 1-α-hydroxylase has been demonstrated, the respective roles of extrarenal production of 1,25$(OH)_2D_3$ or contamination with other bioactive vitamin D metabolites have not been completely clarified. The effect of vitamin D therapy can be monitored by measuring serum and urinary Ca, serum alkaline phosphatase, iPTH and skeletal roentgenograms. Skeletal x-ray findings usually improve within two to four weeks, but the lesions usually do not heal completely for six months or more (Fig. 52.27). Bone lesions can best be monitored in sites where subperiosteal or epiphyseal lesions are evident. Bone biopsy is also useful.

Controversy exists as to whether 1,25$(OH)_2D_3$ is equipotent with vitamin D or metabolites in its action on the bone mineralization front (276–278), but this issue has not been investigated in children. It has been proposed that the effects on the skeleton obtained by vitamin D are not fully reproduced by 1,25$(OH)_2D$, implying that metabolites other than 1,25$(OH)_2D_3$, i.e., both 1,25 and 24,25$(OH)_2D$, are required for the full effect (277–279). This claim is not well substantiated; comparisons with full-dosage response curves are needed. We have not found differences in longitudinal growth (255), weight gain (254), and bone histology in experimental studies between vitamin D_3 and 1,25$(OH)_2D_3$; however, there are practical reasons to prefer one metabolite to the other.

Because of its short half-life, 1,25$(OH)_2D_3$ may be advantageous when fluctuations of S_{Ca} are anticipated, because hypercalcemia from overdose can be rapidly reversed. Reversal of hypercalcemia from overdose with 25$(OH)D_3$, and even more so with vitamin D_3, usually takes longer. The longer half-life of each of these compounds may be advantageous because efficacy is not compromised when the patient does not adhere to a prescribed schedule. The cost of 25$(OH)D_3$ and vitamin D_3 is less.

In clinical practice, the dose of any vitamin D metabolite must be adjusted to the patient's serum and urinary Ca responses. The increase in urinary Ca usually is marked before changes in S_{Ca} become apparent, even in patients with CRF (280). The danger of hypercalcemia is particularly great when bone alkaline phosphatase levels decrease one to three months after beginning treatment. Presumably, at this point the numbers of osteoblasts and the volume of osteoid in the skeleton decrease. Reduction of active osteoid will remove the "sink" for Ca so that hypercalcemia is more likely. This possibility is much greater if children are immobilized by bed rest at this point.

It is imperative to normalize S_p before beginning vitamin D therapy because all compounds increase intestinal absorption of P and may cause hyperphosphatemia and soft tissue calcification.

Representative daily doses for oral use in treating patients with osteodystrophy are in Table 52.2. The biological effect of the doses, i.e., calcemic and calciuric effect, outlast the presence of the metabolites in plasma. Although differences in drug action between oral and intravenous administration of drug have been demonstrated, their clinical relevance is not yet established.

In our experience, spectacular results can be obtained in children who have had x-ray signs of severe renal osteodystrophy and high serum levels of alkaline phosphatase. In contrast, patients without subperiosteal resorption and without radiolucency of metaphyses and normal serum alkaline phosphatase may develop osteopenia and fractures despite vitamin D treatment. These observations, made before appreciating the effects of Al toxicity, may reflect vitamin D unresponsiveness of Al osteopathy.

Control of PTH

In a few children (about 3%) with advanced renal hyperparathyroidism, subtotal parathyroidectomy may be required to control PTH oversecretion. Indications for this measure are uncontrolled hypercalcemia or severe osteitis fibrosa not controlled with the administration of vitamin D metabolites. One specific indication is calciphylaxis, i.e., the rapid appearance of cutaneous necrosis and signs of ischemia (281). These have been reversed by prompt parathyroidectomy (282).

There is little reported experience with parathyroidectomy in children with uremic osteodystrophy (283, 284). In the past, subtotal parathyroidectomy was preferred; currently, the preferred procedure is total parathyroidectomy and autotransplantation of residual parathyroid tissue into the forearm musculature underneath the fascia (284, 287). Autotransplantation can be done under local anesthesia, without any sequelae. Furthermore, additional parathyroid tissue should be cryopreserved in case the transplant fails to function properly. Uncontrolled growth of the parathyroid graft may require surgical intervention. In some reports, the uncontrolled growth of autografts was considered to be malignant (287).

After parathyroidectomy, hypocalcemia must be anticipated if severe bone disease is associated with an elevated alkaline phosphatase before

Table 52.2
Vitamin D treatment of renal osteodystrophy in advanced CRF. The doses are representative for all age groups.

	Prophylactic use	Therapeutic use
Vit D_3 (μg/day)	100–250	500–2000
25$(OH)D_3$ (μg/day)	12.5–25	50–150
1,25$(OH)_2D_3$ (μg/day)	0.12–0.25	1–2
1$\alpha$$(OH)D_3$ (μg/day)	0.25–0.50	2–4

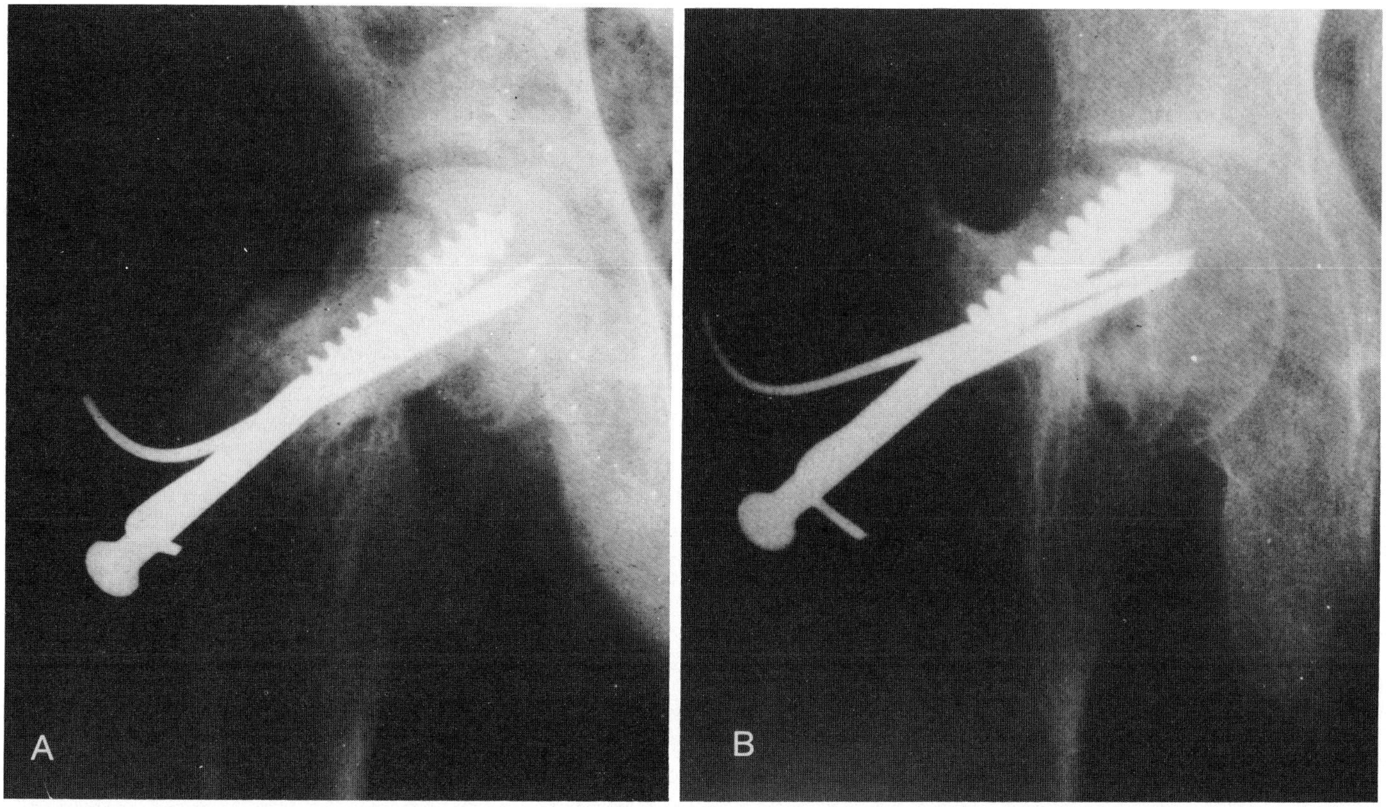

Figure 52.30. Surgical treatment of slipped epiphysis in a 12-yr-old girl with nephronophthisis, serum creatinine 8.3 mg/dl. **A,** Surgical attempt to fixate femoral head was mistakenly done before adequate treatment of metabolic bone disease by vitamin D. Note rotten fencepost sign at femoral neck. **B,** Fixation was not successful because of the fibrous transformation of bone tissue and a disastrous result was seen 3 months after.

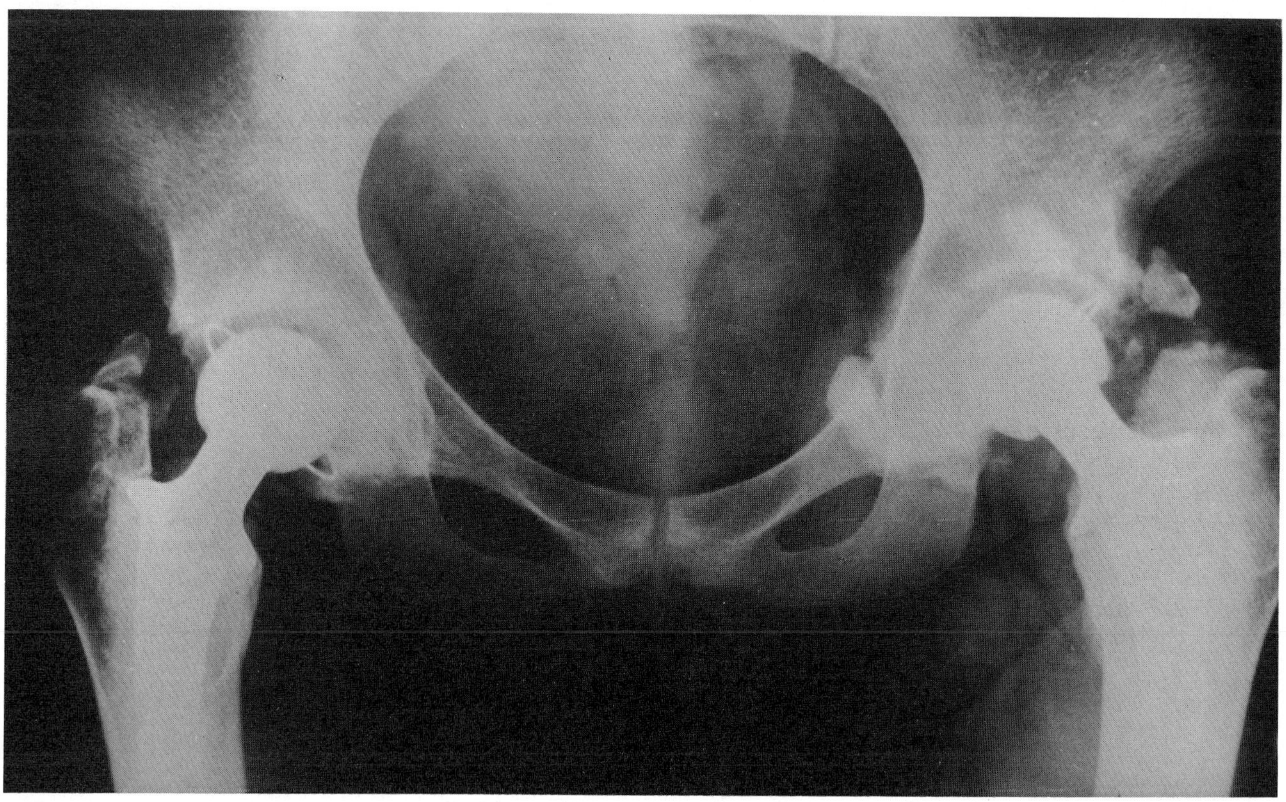

Figure 52.31. Total hip endoprosthesis because of bilateral femoral head necrosis in 19 yr old female patient who had kidney transplant three years earlier.

surgery, i.e., the "hungry bone syndrome." Hypocalcemia usually can be prevented by prior treatment with $1,25(OH)_2D_3$ and oral or ntravenous Ca supplements. When bone disease heals, as is evident from a fall in alkaline serum phosphatase, the dose of Ca supplements usually can be reduced. Several authors noted that after parathyroidectomy, severe osteitis fibrosa was replaced by osteomalacia (288). This occurs especially in patients with Al intoxication; therefore, the Al status of bone should be evaluated from a bone biopsy. If bone Al is increased, desferrioxamine treatment should be given to reduce bone Al (289).

Epiphyseal Slipping

Slipped femoral epiphyses present a therapeutic dilemma for which early surgical intervention has been recommended (169, 170, 290). Mechanical devices, e.g., wires, nails, and screws, have proved disastrous (see Fig. 52.30). These devices will not stabilize dislocated epiphyses when the femoral neck consists of fibrous bone or tissue (280). We recommend first consolidating metabolic bone disease by vitamin D therapy with or without parathyroidectomy. During treatment, children with incipient rather than overt slipped epiphysis need not be placed on bed rest unless they complain of pain, which rarely happens. With this treatment, even a slipped femoral head will be stabilized within a couple of weeks (280).

Surgical correction of any resulting deformity should be postponed until the osteodystrophy has healed. Corrective osteotomy prevents late arthrosis or femoral head necrosis (172). In cases in which hope for spontaneous correction of an abnormal collodiaphyseal angle can no longer be sustained, reconstruction by wedge osteotomy is recommended.

Bone Problems Following Renal Transplant

Most reports on osteopathy after transplantation are anecdotal. This is not surprising since the number of children post-renal transplant is small, e.g. 1255 in Europe in 1979 (291). Osteonecrosis of the femoral head is the most devastating skeletal complication after transplantation (235). With conventional immunosuppressive therapy, the overall incidence for osteonecrosis was 8% (292). We anticipate a fall in this percentage because the presently recommended dosage for steroids is less. This will be more likely if cyclosporine becomes the preferred therapy for immunosuppression. There are occasional reports of osteonecrosis of femoral heads with preexisting coxa vara or femoral slipping resulting from uremic osteodystrophy (172). Faulty alignment may predispose to development of osteonecrosis. It appears logical to correct these deformities before transplantation to prevent late epiphyseal necrosis.

In symptomatic patients, conservative measures (reduction in weightbearing) are indicated, but benefit from this procedure is not convincing. It is reasonable, and often sufficient, to treat the patient with analgesic drugs (but a negative effect of antiinflammatory agents on GFR of the transplant should be kept in mind). If patients are incapacitated by pain, total hip endoprosthesis may be necessary (Fig. 52.31). Experience reported by the EDTA (291), and our own observations attest to its efficacy. Despite preexisting metabolic bone disease and steroid osteoporosis, loosening of the prosthesis seems to be rare. In children, growth should be complete before endoprosthesis surgery is done.

References

1. Förster R: Über Schrumpfnieren im Kindesalter. Z Kinderheilk 26:38, 1887.
2. Lucas RC: On a form of late rickets associated with albuminuria, rickets in adolescents. Lancet 1:993, 1883.
3. Cameron HC: Case of osteomalacia and infantilism with renal deficiency. Proc R Soc Med 2:22, 1918.
4. Mehls O, Krempien B, Ritz E, et al: Renal osteodystrophy in children on maintenance hemodialysis. Proc Eur Dial Transpl Assoc 10:197, 1973.
5. Mehls O, Ritz E, Kreusser W, Krempien B: Renal osteodystrophy in uremic children. Clin Endocrinol Metab 9:151, 1980.
6. Mehls O, Ritz E: Early treatment of renal osteodystrophy. In Buccianti G (ed): Early treatment of renal insufficiency. Contr Nephrol 37:17, 1983.
7. Reiss E, Canterbury JM, Egdahl RH: Experience with a radioimmunoassay of parathyroid hormone in human sera. Trans Assoc Am Physicians 81:104, 1968.
8. Malluche HH, Ritz E, Lange HP, et al: Bone histology in incipient and advanced renal failure. Kidney Int 9:355, 1976.
9. Kleerekoper M, Cruz C, Bernstein RS, et al: The phosphaturic action of PTH in the steady state in patients? Adv Exper Med Biol 128:145, 1980.
10. Friis T, Hahnemann S, Weeke E: Serum calcium and serum phosphorus in uremia during administration of sodium phytate and aluminum hydroxide. Acta Med Scand 183:497, 1968.
11. Ritz E, Malluche HH, Krempien B, et al: Pathogenesis of renal osteodystrophy: role of phosphate and skeletal resistance to PTH. Adv Exper Med Biol 103:423, 1978.
12. Bricker NS: An exposition of the "trade off" hypothesis. N Engl J Med 286:1093, 1972.
13. Slatopolsky E, Caglar S, Pennell JP, et al: On the pathogenesis of hyperparathyroidism in chronic experimental renal insufficiency in the dog. J Clin Invest 50:492, 1971.
14. Caversazio G, Gloor HJ, Fleisch H, Bonjour JP: Parathyroid hormone independent adaptation of renal tubular phosphate transport to renal mass reduction. Kidney Int 17:856, 1980.
15. Massry SG, Ritz E, Verberckmoes R: Role of phosphate in the genesis of secondary hyperparathyroidism. Nephron 18:77, 1977.
16. Van Stone J, Frank DT, Brandsford WR: The effect of decreased renal function with and without renal mass on $1,25(OH)_2$ cholecalciferol production in rats. J Lab Clin Med 89:1168, 1977.
17. Slatopolsky E, Gray R, Adams ND, et al: Low serum levels of $1,25(OH)_2D_3$ are not responsible for the development of secondary hyperparathyroidism in early renal failure. Kidney Int 14:177, 1978.
18. Ogura Y, Kawaguchi Y, Sakai S, et al: Plasma levels of vitamin D metabolites in renal diseases. Contr Nephrol 22:18, 1980.
19. Haussler MR, Baylink DJ, Hughes MR, et al: The assay of 1-alpha-25-OH_2D_3: Physiologic and pathologic modulation of circulating hormone levels. Clin Endocrinol 5:151, 1976.
20. Chesney RW, Mazess RR, DeLuca HF: Long-term influence of calcitriol on growth patterns in childhood renal osteodystrophy. Rotterdam Excerptd Med 1980, p 28.
21. Chesney RW, Hamstra AJ, Mazess RB, et al: Circulating vitamin D metabolite concentrations in childhood renal diseases. Kidney Int 21:65, 1982.
22. Portale AA, Booth BE, Tsai HC, Morris RC Jr: Reduced plasma concentration of 1,25-dihydroxyvitamin D in children with moderate renal insufficiency. Kidney Int 21:627, 1982.
23. Portale AA, Booth BE, Halloran BP, Morris RC Jr: Effect of dietary phosphorus on circulating concentrations of 1,25-dihydroxyvitamin D and immunoreactive parathyroid hormone in children with moderate renal insufficiency. Clin Invest 73:1580, 1984.
24. Stanbury WS, Taylor CM, Lumb GA, et al: Formation of vitamin D metabolites following correction of human vitamin D deficiency. Observations in patients with nutritional osteomalacia. Min Electrol Metab 5:212, 1980.
25. Healy MD, Malluche HH, Goldstein DA, et al: Effects of long-term therapy with calciferol in patients with moderate renal failure. Arch Intern Med 140:1030, 1980.
26. Llach F, Massry SG, Singer FR, et al: Skeletal resistance to endogenous parathyroid hormone in patients with early renal failure. A possible cause for secondary hyperparathyroidism. J Clin Endocrinol Metab 41:339, 1975.
27. Heersche JNM, Martin R, Aurbach GD: Calcitonin and the formation of 3′5′ AMP in bone and kidney. Endocrinology 92:241, 1974.
28. Wong GL: Induction of metabolic changes and down regulation of bovine parathyroid hormone-responsive adenylate cyclase are dissociable in isolated osteoclastic and osteoblastic bone cells. J Biol Chem 254:779A, 1979.
29. Pavlovitch H, Fontaine O, Balsan S: Maintenance of a calcemic response to parathyroid hormone in vitamin D deficient rats by prevention of severe hyperparathyroidism. Calcif Tissue Res 23:277, 1977.
30. Kreusser W, Weinkauf R, Mehls O, Ritz E: Effect of parathyroid hormone, calcitonin and growth hormone on cAMP content of growth cartilage in experimental uremia. Eur J Child Invest 12:337, 1982.
31. Sommerville PJ, Kaye M: Resistance to parathyroid hormone in renal failure: role of vitamin D metabolites. Kidney Int 14:245, 1978.
32. Cloix JF, Ulmann A, Bachelet M, Funck-Brentano JL: Cholecalciferol metabolite binding in porcine parathyroid glands. Steroids 28:743, 1977.
33. Malluche HH, Ritz E, Werner E, Meyer-Sabellek W: Long-term administration of vitamin D steroles in incipient and advanced renal failure—effect on bone histology. Clin Nephrol 10:218, 1978.
34. Agus ZS, Gardner LB, Beck LH, Goldberg M: Effects of parathyroid hormone on

renal tubular reabsorption of calcium, sodium, and phosphate. Am J Physiol 224:1143, 1973.
35. Parfitt AM: Relation between parathyroid cell mass and plasma calcium concentration in normal and uremic subjects. Arch Intern Med 124:269, 1969.
36. Stanbury SW, Lumb GA: Parathyroid function in chronic renal failure. Q J Med 35:1, 1966.
37. Schmidt-Gayk H, Ritz E, Mehls O, et al: 25-OH-vitamin D in experimental and clinical uremia. Calcif Tissue Res 22 (suppl):430, 1977.
38. Coburn JW, Marcelo H, Kopple MH, et al: Study of intestinal absorption of calcium in patients with renal failure. Kidney Int 3:264–272, 1973.
39. Coburn JW, Popovtzer MM, Massry SG, Kleeman CR: The physiochemical state and renal handling of divalent ions in chronic renal failure. Arch Intern Med 124:302–311, 1969.
40. Lichtwitz A, Parlier R: Physiopathologie des troubles phosphocalciques dans l'insuffisance rénale. In Calcium et Maladies Métaboliques de l'Os, pp. 224–246. L'Expansion Scientifique Française, Paris, 1965.
41. Popovtzer MM, Massry SG, Coburn JW, Kleeman CR: The interrelationship between sodium, calcium and magnesium excretion in advanced renal failure. J Lab Clin Med 73:763–771, 1969.
42. Stanbury SW, Lumb GA: Metabolic studies of renal osteodystrophy. I. Calcium, phosphorus and nitrogen metabolism in rickets, osteomalacia and hyperparathyroidism complicating chronic uremia and the osteomalacia of the adult Fanconi syndrome. Medicine (Baltimore) 41:1, 1962.
43. Coburn JW, Brickman AS, Hartenbower DL, Norman AW: Intestinal phosphate absorption in normal and uremic man: effects of $1,25(OH)_2$vitamin D_3 and 1(OH)vitamin D_3. In Massry SG, Ritz E (eds): Phosphate Metabolism New York, Plenum, 1977, p 549.
44. Fraser DR, Kodicek E: Unique biosynthesis by kidney of a biologically active vitamin D metabolite. Nature (London) 228:764, 1970.
45. Garabedian M, Liebherr M, N'Gueyen TM, et al: In vitro production and activity of $24,25\text{-}OH_2D_3$ in cartilage and calvarium. Clin Orthop Rel Res 135:241, 1978.
46. Mawer EB, Taylor CM: Vitamin D metabolism in man, the role of the kidney. In Proceedings 5th International Congress of Nephrology, Montreal. S. Karger Publisher, 1978, p 469.
47. Tanaka Y, DeLuca HF: The control of 25-hydroxy-vitamin D metabolism by inorganic phosphorus. Arch Biochem Biophys 159:566, 1973.
48. Lee SW, Russell J, Avioli LV: 25-hydroxycholecalciferol to 1,25-dihydroxycholecalciferol: conversion impaired by systemic metabolic acidosis. Science 195:994, 1977.
49. Jongen MJM, van der Vijgh WJF, Lips P, Netelenbos JC: 1,25-hydroxy-vitamin D measurements in anephric subjects (abstract). 5th Workshop on Vitamin D, Williamsburg, VA, 1982, p 285.
50. Lund B, Clausen E, Friedberg M, et al: Serum 1,25-dihydroxy-vitamin D_3 in anephric, hemodialysed and kidney-transplanted patients. Effect of vitamin D_3 supplement. Nephron 25:30, 1980.
51. Stanbury SW: The role of vitamin D in renal bone disease. Clin Endocrinol 7 (suppl):258, 1977.
52. Avioli LV, Teitelbaum SL: The renal osteodystrophies. In Brenner BM, Rector FC (eds): The Kidney Philadelphia, Saunders, 1976, vol 2, p 1542.
53. Ritz E, Boland R, Kreusser W: Effects of vitamin D and parathyroid hormone on muscle: potential role in uremic myopathy. Am J Clin Nutr 33:1522, 1980.
54. Madsen S, Olgaard F, Ladefoged J: Direct feed-back regulation of PTH secretion by 1,25-dihydroxy-vitamin D_3 in renal failure: a controlled trial. Proc EDTA 17:557, 1980.
55. Bordier PJ, TunChot S, Eastwood JB, et al: Lack of histological evidence of vitamin D abnormality in the bones of anephric patients. Clin Sci 44:33, 1973.
56. Howard GA, Turner RT, Sherrard DJ, Baylink DJ: Human bone cells in culture metabolize 25-hydroxy-vitamin D to 1,25-dihydroxy-vitamin D_3 and 24,25-dihydroxy-vitamin D_3. J Biol Chem 256:7738, 1981.
57. Llach F, Brickman AS, Singer FR, Coburn JW: 24,25-Dihydroxycholecalciferol, a vitamin D sterol with qualitatively unique effects in uremic man. Metab Bone Dis Rel Res 2:11, 1979.
58. Kanis JA, Cundy T, Bartlett M, et al: Is 24,25-dihydroxycholecalciferol a calcium-regulating hormone in man? Br Med J 1.1382, 1978.
59. Haddad JG, Min C, Walgate J: Radioimmunoassay of human serum DBP and competitive binding protein radioassay of $24,25(OH)_2$ vitamin D_3. In De Gruyter Publisher, Vitamin D, Biochemical, Chemical and Clinical Aspects Related to Calcium Metabolism. Berlin, Norman AW (ed): 1977, p 463.
60. Offermann G, v Herrath D, Schaefer K: Serum 25-hydroxycholecalciferol in uremia. Nephron 13:269, 1974.
61. Langman CG, Mazur AT, Baron R, Norman ME: 25-Hydroxyvitamin D_3 (calcifediol) therapy of juvenile renal osteodystrophy. beneficial effect on linear growth velocity. J Pediatr 100:815, 1982.
62. Schmidt-Gayk H, Schmitt W, Grawunder C, et al: 25-hydroxy-vitamin D. Lancet 2:105, 1977.
63. Pointon JJ, Francis JJO, Smith R: Effect of vitamin D deficiency on sarcoplasmic reticulum function and troponin C concentration of rabbit skeletal muscle. Clin Sci 57:257, 1979.
64. Matthews C, Heimberg KW, Ritz E, et al: Effect of 1,25-dihydroxycholecalciferol on impaired calcium transport by the sarcoplasmic reticulum in experimental uremia. Kidney Int 11:227, 1977.
65. Ritz E, Kreusser W, Rambausek M, Mehls O: Myopathy in uremia. Proceedings of 6th International Workshop on phosphate and other minerals, Verona 1983. Adv Biol Med 78:435, 1984.
66. Lee SL, Liberman UA, Wientroub S: Is tendon another target organ for vitamin D? (abstract). 5th Workshop on Vitamin D. Williamsburg, VA, 1982, p 58.
67. Lotem M, Bernheim J, Confort B: Spontaneous rupture of tendons: a complication of hemodialyzed patients treated for renal failure. Nephron 21:201, 1978.
68. Kreusser W, Spiegelberg U, Ritz E, Kelly P: Decreased Leydig cell cAMP response to LH in acute and chronic uremia, a defect corrected by $1,25(OH)_2$ vitamin D_3 (submitted for publication).
69. Stanbury SW: Azotemic renal osteodystrophy. Clin Endocrinol Metab I:267, 1972.
70. Cook DB, Pierides AM, Shannan G: Seasonal variation of serum 25-hydroxy-vitamin D in patients with chronic renal failure treated by regular hemodialysis. Clin Chim A 76:251, 1977.
71. Sallman AL, Jacob AI, Hollis B, et al: Impaired photoproduction of vitamin D in uremia. In 14th Annual Meeting of the American Society of Nephrology, Washington DC, 1981, p 13A.
72. Stanbury SW, Mawer EB, Taylor CM, de Silva P: The skin, vitamin D and the control of its 25-hydroxylation. An attempted integration. Min Electrol Metabol 3:51, 1980.
73. Alon U, Chan JCM: Calcium and vitamin-D metabolism in nephrotic syndrome. Int J Pediatr Nephrol 4:115, 1983.
74. Alon U, Chan JCM: Calcium and vitamin D homeostasis in the nephrotic syndrome: current status. Nephron 36:1, 1984.
75. Pierides AM, Kerr DNS, Ellis HA, et al: 1-alpha-hydroxycholecalciferol in hemodialysis and renal osteodystrophy. Adverse effect of anticonvulsant therapy. Clin Nephrol 5:189, 1976.
76. Silver J, Davies TJ, Kupersmitt E, et al: Prevalence and treatment of vitamin D deficiency in children on anticonvulsant drugs. Arch Dis Child 49:344, 1974.
77. Brown EM, Wilson RE, Thatcher JG, Marynick SP: Abnormal calcium regulated PTH release in normal parathyroid tissue from patients with adenoma. Am J Med 71:565, 1981.
78. Martin KJ, Hruska KA, Lewis J, et al: The renal handling of parathyroid hormone. Role of peritubular uptake and glomerular filtration. J Clin Invest 60:808, 1977.
79. Massry SG, Coburn JW, Lee DBN, et al: Skeletal resistance to parathyroid hormone in renal failure; studies on 105 human subjects. Ann Intern Med 78:337, 1973.
80. Massry SG, Stein R, Garty J, et al: Skeletal resistance to calcemic action of parathyroid hormone: role of $1,25(OH)_2D_3$. Kidney Int 9:467, 1976.
81. Ritz E, Mehls O, Krempien B: Calcium and phosphorus metabolism in maintenance hemodialysis. In Hamburger J, Crosnier J, Grünfeld JP, Maxwell MH (eds): Advances in Nephrology 9. 1980, p 71.
82. Williams GA, Hargis GK, Bowser EN, et al: Evidence for a role of adenosine 3,5′-monophosphate in parathyroid hormone release. Endocrinology 92:687, 1973.
83. Hanley DA, Takatsuki K, Birnbaumer ME, et al: In vitro perfusion for the study of parathyroid hormone secretion. Effects of extracellular calcium concentration and beta-adrenergic regulation on bovine parathyroid hormone secretion in vitro. Calcif Tiss Res 32:19, 1980.
84. Blum JW, Fischer JA, Hunziker WH, et al: Parathyroid hormone response to catecholamines and to changes of extracellular calcium in cows. J Clin Invest 61:1113, 1978.
85. Kukreja SC, Hargis GK, Bowser EN: Role of adrenergic stimuli in parathyroid hormone secretion. J Clin Endocrinol Metab 40:478, 1975.
86. Morissey JJ, Cohn DV: Regulation of secretion of parathormone and secretory proteins from separate intracellular pools by calcium, dibutyryl cAMP and (1) isoproterenol. J Cell Biol 82:93, 1979.
87. Williams R, Longley RS, Hargis GK, et al: Effect of histamine on secretion of parathyroid hormone. Clin Res 27:704, 1979.
88. Brown EM: Histamine receptors in parathyroid adenomas. Clin Res 28:388A, 1980.
89. Abbond HE, Zimmerman D, Edis AJ, Dousa TP: Histamine and parathyroid cAMP accumulation. Clin Res 38:515, 1980.
90. Fiore CE, Lunetta M, Costa M, et al: Cimetidine and calciotropic hormones in normal subjects and in chronic renal failure. Min Metab Res 1:10, 1980.
91. Ljunghall S, Adami HO, Bjorklung O, et al: Serum concentration of parathyroid hormone in hyperparathyroid subjects during cimetidine treatment. N Engl J Med 303:1178, 1980.

92. Oldham SB, Fischer JA, Shen CH, Arnaud CD: Isolation and properties of a calcium binding protein from porcine parathyroid gland. Biochemistry 13:4790, 1974.
93. Henry HL, Norman AW: Studies of the mechanism of action of calciferol VII. Localisation of 1,25-dihydroxy-vitamin D_3 in chick parathyroid glands. Biochem Biophys Res Comm 62:781, 1975.
94. Brumbaugh PF, Hugues MR, Haussler MR: Cytoplasmic and nuclear binding components for 1,25-dihydroxy-vitamin D_3 in chick parathyroid glands. Proc Nat Acad Sci 72:4871, 1975.
95. Mayer GP, Habener JF, Potts JT Jr: Parathyroid hormone secretion in vitro. Demonstration of a calcium independent non-suppressible component of secretion. J Clin Invest 57:678, 1976.
96. Llach F, Coburn JW, Brickman AS, et al: Acute actions of 1,25-dihydroxy-vitamin D_3 in normal man. Effect on calcium and parathyroid status. J Clin Endocrinol Metab 44:1054, 1977.
97. Chertow BS, Baylink DJ, Wergedal JE, et al: Decrease in serum immunoreactive parathyroid hormone in rats and in parathyroid hormone secretion in vivo by 1,25-dihydroxycholecalciferol. J Clin Invest 56:668, 1975.
98. Tanaka Y, DeLuca HF, Ghazarian JG, et al: Effect of vitamin D and its metabolites on serum parathyroid hormone levels in the rat. Min Electrol Metab 2:20, 1979.
99. Bouillon R, Verberckmoes R, De Moor P: Influence of dialysate calcium concentration and vitamin D on serum parathyroid hormone during repetitive hemodialysis. Kidney Int 7:422, 1975.
100. Gittes RF, Radde IC: Experimental model for hyperparathyroidism: effect of excessive numbers of transplanted isologous parathyroid glands. J Urol 95:595, 1966.
101. Katz AJ, Hampers CJ, Merrill JP: Secondary hyperparathyroidism and renal osteodystrophy in chronic renal failure. Medicine 48:333, 1969.
102. David DS, Sakai S, Brennan BL, et al: Hypercalcemia after renal transplantation. Long-term follow-up data. N Engl J Med 289:398, 1973.
103. Mendes V, Jorgetti V, Nemeth J, et al: Secondary hyperparathyroidism in chronic hemodialysis patients. Proc EDTA 20:731, 1983.
104. Ritz E, Rambausek M, Kreusser W, Mehls O: Bone metabolism in renal disease. In Jones F, Peters DK (eds): Recent Advances in Renal Medicine New York, Churchill Livingstone, 1982, p 151.
105. Christenson T, Hellstroem K, Wengle B: Hypercalcemia and primary hyperparathyroidism. Arch Intern Med 137:1138, 1977.
106. Brown EM, Brennan MF, Hurwitz S, et al: Dispersed cells prepared from human parathyroid glands: distinct calcium sensibility of adenomas vs. primary hyperplasia. J Clin Endocrinol 46:267, 1978.
107. Habener JF: Responsiveness of neoplastic and hyperplastic parathyroid tissues to calcium in vitro. J Clin Invest 62:436, 1978.
108. Sherwood LM, Lundberg WB Jr, Targovnik JH, et al: Synthesis and secretion of parathyroid hormone in vitro. Am J Med 50:658, 1971.
109. Bellorin-Font E, Martin KJ, Freitag JJ, et al: Altered adenylate cyclase kinetics in hyperfunctioning human parathyroid glands. J Clin Endocrinol Metab 52:499, 1981.
110. Martin K, Hruska K, Greenwalt A, et al: Selective uptake of intact parathyroid hormone by the liver. Differences between hepatic and renal uptake. J Clin Invest 58:781, 1976.
111. Martin KJ, Freitag JJ, Conrades M, et al: Selective uptake of the synthetic aminoterminal fragment of bovine parathyroid hormone by isolated perfused bone. J Clin Invest 62:256, 1978.
112. Parsons JA, Robinson CJ: A rapid indirect hypercalcemic action of parathyroid hormone demonstrated in isolated perfused bone. In Talmage RV, Belanger LF (eds): Parathyroid Hormone and Thyrocalcitonin (Calcitonin). Amsterdam, Excerpta Medica, 1968, p 329.
113. Freitag J, Martin KJ, Hruska KA, et al: Impaired parathyroid hormone metabolism in patients with chronic renal failure. N Engl J Med 298:29, 1978.
114. Oda Y, Kurokawa K, Aznar E, et al: Effect of parathyroid hormone on cyclic AMP and cyclic AMP-dependent protein kinase activity in calvaria of acutely uremic rats. Min Electr Metab 6:210, 1981.
115. Müller-Wiefel DE, Mehls O, Schärer K: The role of hyperparathyroidism in the pathogenesis of renal anemia. Eur J Pediatr 141:63, 1983.
116. Remuzzi G, Benigni A, Dodesini P, et al: Parathyroid hormone inhibits platelet function. Lancet 2:1321, 1981.
117. Bogin E, Massry SG, Harary I: Effect of parathyroid hormone on rat heart cells. J Clin Invest 67:1215, 1981.
118. Massry SG: Does parathyroid hormone play the role of a uremic toxin in patients with chronic renal failure? In Hamburger J, Crosnier J, Grünfeldt JP, Maxwell MH (eds): Advances in Nephrology. Chicago, London, Year Book Medical, 1982, vol II, p 223.
119. Isaac R, Nivez MP, Piamba G, et al: Influence of calcium infusion on calcitonin and parathyroid hormone concentrations in normal and hemodialysed subjects. Clin Nephrol 3:14, 1975.
120. Heynen G, Kanis JA, Oliver D, et al: Evidence that endogenous calcitonin protects against renal bone disease. Lancet 2:1322, 1976.
121. Kanis JA, Earnshaw M, Heynen G, et al: Changes in histological and biochemical indexes of bone turnover after bilateral nephrectomy in patients on hemodialysis: evidence for a possible role of endogenous calcitonin. N Engl J Med 296:1073, 1977.
122. Delano BG, Baker R, Gardner B, Wallach S: A trial of calcitonin therapy in renal osteodystrophy. Nephron 11:287, 1973.
123. Malluche H, Faugere M, Ritz E: Does endogenous calcitonin protect against osteitis fibrosa in dialysis patients? Mineral Electrolyte Metal 12:113, 1986.
124. Cochran M, Bulusu L, Horsman A, et al: Hypocalcaemia and bone disease in renal failure. Nephron 10:113, 1973.
125. Kraut JA, Gordon E, Horst RL, et al: Effect of chronic metabolic acidosis on vitamin D metabolism in man. Kidney Int 1983, p. 644.
126. Weber HP, Gray RW, Dominguez JH, Lemann J Jr: The lack of effect of chronic metabolic acidosis on 25-OH-vitamin D metabolism and serum parathyroid hormone in humans. J Clin Endocrinol Metab 43:1047, 1976.
127. Lemann J Jr, Litzow JR, Lennon EJ: The effect of chronic acid loads in normal man: further evidence for the participating of bone mineral in the defense against chronic metabolic acidosis. J Clin Invest 45:1608, 1966.
128. Greenberg AJ, McNamara H, McCrory WW: Metabolic balance studies in primary renal tubular acidosis: effects of acidosis on external calcium and phosphorus balances. J Pediatr 69:610, 1966.
129. Ritz E, Malluche A, Krempien B, Mehls O: Bone histology in renal insufficiency. In David DS (ed): Calcium Metabolism in Renal Failure and Nephrolithiasis. New York, John Wiley, 1977, p 197.
130. Malluche HH, Ritz E, Lange HP, et al: Bone mass in maintenance haemodialysis. Prospective study with sequential biopsies. Eur J Clin Invest 6:265, 1976.
131. Letteri JM, Cohn SH: Total body neutron activation analysis in the study of mineral homeostasis in chronic renal disease. In David DD (ed): Calcium Metabolism in Renal Failure and Nephrolithiasis. New York, Wiley, 1977, p 249.
132. Eastwood JB, Harris E, Stamp TCB, de Wardener HW: Vitamin D deficiency in the osteomalacia of chronic renal failure. Lancet 2:1209, 1976.
133. Ritz E, Mehls O, Malluche HH, et al: Unanswered problems in uremic bone disease. In Norman AW, Schaeffer K, Grigoleit HG, et al (eds): Vitamin D and Problems Related to Uremic Bone Disease. Berlin, De Gruyter Publisher, 1975, p 497.
134. Offermann G, Schaefer K, Schulz A, Delling G: Immunoreaktives Parathormon, 25-Hydroxycholecalciferol und Knochenhistologie bei renaler Osteopathie. Klin Wschr 54:625, 1976.
135. Coburn JW, Brickman AS, Sherrard DJ, Wong EGC, Singer FR, Norman AW: Defective skeletal mineralization in uremia without relation to vitamin D, serum Ca or P. Kidney Int 12:455, 1977.
136. Falkner F: Nutrition and bone development. In Modern Problems in Pediatrics. Basel, Karger, 1975, vol 14, p 185.
137. Avioli LV, Hahn TJ: Steroid-induced osteopenia. In Copp DH, Talmage RV (eds): Endocrinology of Calcium Metabolism. Amsterdam, Excerpta Medica, 1978, p 23.
138. Ritz E, Kreusser W, Rambausek M: Effects of glucocorticoids on calciuria. In Avioli LV (ed): Glucocorticoids and Bone. New York, Plenum Press (in press).
139. Favus MJ, Walling MW, Kimbere DV: Effects of 1,25dihydroxycholecalciferol on intestinal calcium transport on cortisone treated rats. J Clin Invest 52:1680, 1973.
140. Mehls O, Ritz E, Krempien B, et al: Slipped epiphyses in renal osteodystrophy. In Norman AW (ed): Vitamin D and Problems Related to Uremic Bone Disease. Berlin, De Gruyter, 1975, p 553.
141. Frost HM: Histomorphometry of trabecular bone. I. Theoretical correction of appositional rate measurements. II. An empirical test of the theoretical correction for appositional rate measurements and definition of symbols for bone histomorphometry: Frostian system. In Meunier P (ed): Bone Histomorphometry. Toulouse, Imprimerie Fournié, 1977, p 361.
142. Alfrey AC, Hegg A, Miller N, et al: Interrelationship between calcium and aluminium metabolism in dialyzed uremic patients. Min Electrol Metab 2:81, 1979.
143. Cournot-Witmer G, Zingraff J, Plachot JJ, et al: Aluminium localisation in bone from hemodialysed patients: relationship to matrix mineralisation. Kidney Int 20:375, 1979.
144. Chesney RW, Mehls O, Ahast CS, et al: Renal osteodystrophy in children-vitamin D phosphorus PTH. Am J Kidney Dis 7:275, 1986.
145. Park EA: Observations on the pathology of rickets with particular reference to the changes at the cartilage shaft junctions of the growing bones. Bull NY Acad Med 15:495, 1939.
146. Krempien B, Mehls O, Ritz E: Morphological studies on pathogenesis of epiphyseal slipping in uremic children. Virchows Arch (Pathol Anat) 362:129, 1974.
147. Pommer G: Untersuchungen über Osteomalazie und Rachitis nebst Beiträgen über Kenntnis der Knochenresorption und—Apposition in verschiedenen Altersgruppen. Leipzig, Vogel, 1885.
148. Wood BSB, Gerorge WH, Robinson AW: Parathyroid adenoma in a child presenting as rickets. Arch Dis Child 33:46, 1958.

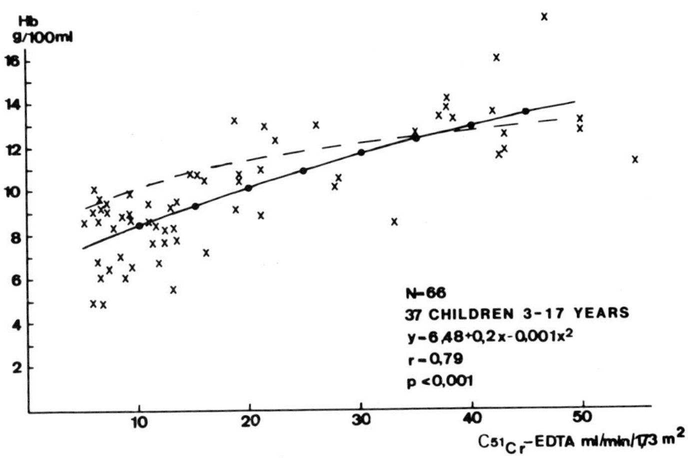

Figure 53A.1. Correlation between Hb concentration and GFR measured by ^{51}Cr-EDTA-clearace with the regression lines for children (——) and adults (- - -). (From Müller-Wiefel DE; Renale Anämie im Kindesalter. Untersuchungen zur, Pathogenese und Kompensation. Stuttgart, New York, G Thieme, 1982.)

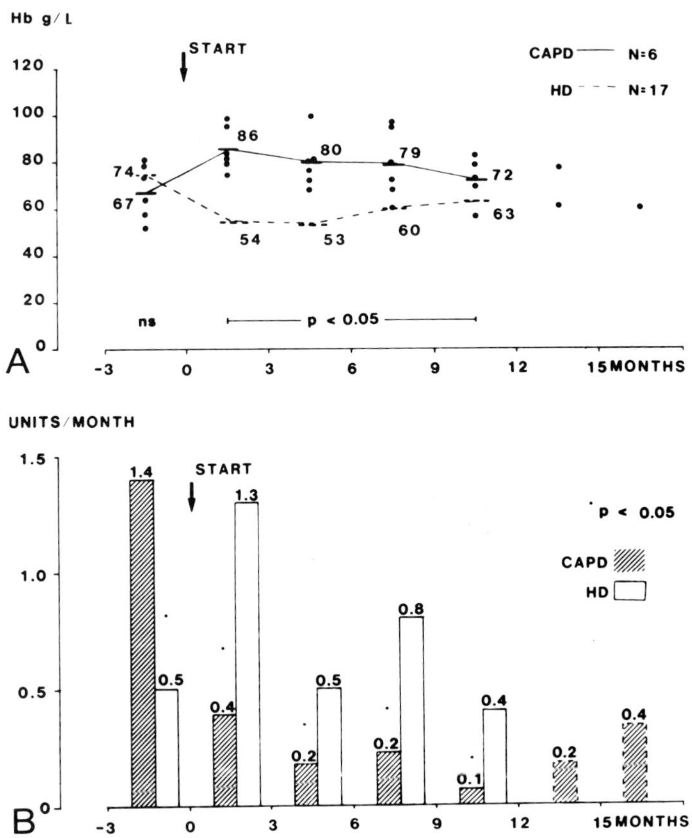

Figure 53A.2. **A**, Changes of Hb concentration in children during treatment by CAPD (——) and by home hemodialysis (- - -). **B**, Number of blood transfusions per month during the same periods of treatment by CAPD and by home hemodialysis. Values indicated are means of three-month periods.

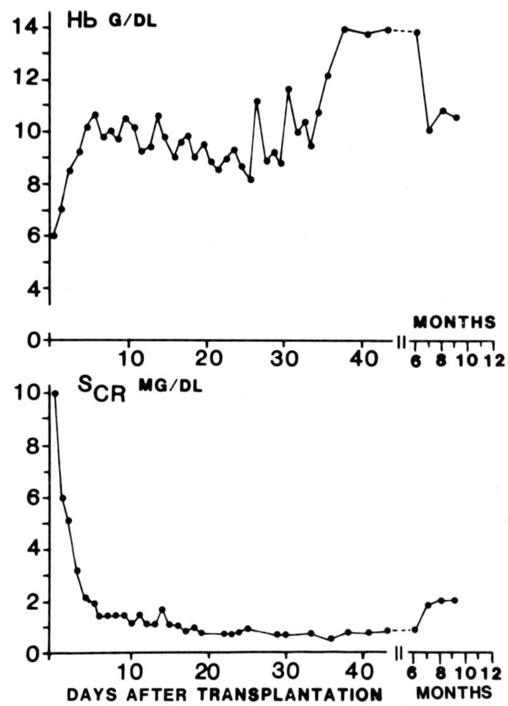

Figure 53A.3. Inverse relation between blood Hb and S_{Cr} concentrations following cadaver kidney transplantation in a bilaterally nephrectomized 14-year-old girl.

(CFU_e) (22). Various low- and high-molecular-weight toxins, which inhibit red blood cell proliferation, have been reported in uremia (23–26), and the influence of middle molecules (17, 27, 28) and of parathyroid hormone (PTH) (29, 30) is uncertain. Bone marrow depression caused by increased arsenic concentrations has been suggested (31). Aluminum (A1) intoxication causes a non-iron-deficient, microcytic, and hypochromic anemia, probably caused by disturbed heme synthesis, specifically involving δ-amino-levulinic acid dehydrogenase (32). The anemia is followed by toxic effects on the brain and bones.

Hemolysis. Erythrocyte life span, as measured by isotope techniques, is reduced to 55% of normal values in children with advanced CRF before start of dialysis (BUN >60 mg/dl) (15). Following institution of RDT, the life span increases, which suggests that the hemolysis is caused by the direct action of uremic toxins (33, 34). Hemolysis may also be related to other toxic agents, e.g., copper, zinc, nitrate, chloramine, and formaldehyde.

Blood Loss. Blood loss is an important factor (35). The Hb levels observed before and after start of RDT are related to the amount of blood loss. The labeling of erythrocytes by isotopes, e.g., ^{111}indium, has allowed losses to be measured precisely.

With conservative treatment, blood loss is mainly intestinal; in children with an S_{Cr} of 6 mg/dl it amounts to an average value of 7 ml/m^2 BSA/day (15). On RDT the mean intestinal loss is even higher (11 ml/m^2/day), corresponding to five times normal values; this is caused by heparin and other drugs, which influence the coagulation system, e.g., synthetic penicillins. In addition, children on RDT lose blood during the dialysis procedure either by cannulation or by trapping in the dialyzer or lines (15).

Compensatory Mechanisms

The compensatory mechanisms available to overcome the detrimental effects of anemia in uremic children are shown in Figure 53A.5. Cardiac output and pulmonary ventilation may increase. Reduced tissue oxygenation usually leads to a shift from oxy-Hb to its deoxygenated form, accompanied by increased production of erythrocyte 2,3-diphosphoglycerate (2.3-DPG), which increases free oxygen (O_2) delivery to tissues by

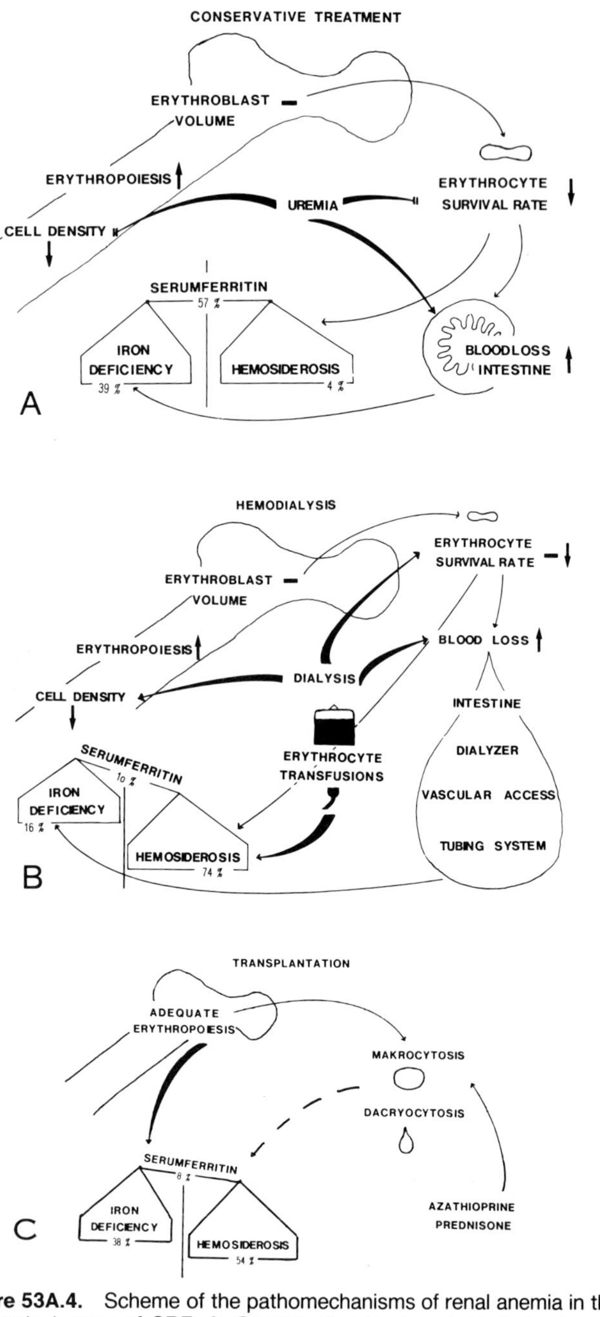

Figure 53A.4. Scheme of the pathomechanisms of renal anemia in the preterminal stage of CRF. **A**, Conservative treatment. **B**, during hemodialysis. **C**, After transplantation. Changes in serum ferritin levels are represented in left lower part of the figures. The percent distribution of low, normal, and increased ferritin levels is indicated for the respective pathological states (43). ↑ = increase, ↓ = decrease, — = unchanged.

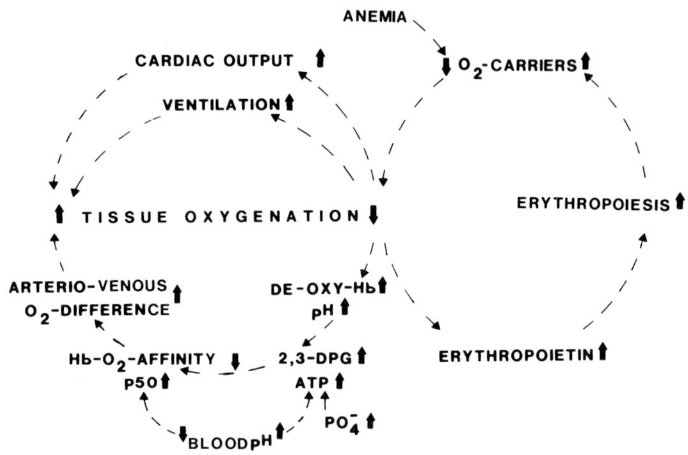

Figure 53A.5. Compensatory mechanisms in renal anemia. Indirect mechanisms are indicated on left, direct mechanisms on right. (From Müller-Wiefel DE: Renale Anämie im Kindesalter. Untersuchungen zur Pathogenese und Kompensation. Stuttgart, New York, G. Thieme, 1982.)

replacing O_2 in the Hb molecule at a specific binding site. The decreased oxygen affinity of Hb can be measured by a rise of half saturation pressure of Hb (p50) and by a shift of the Hb-O_2 dissociation curve to the right.

In contrast to children with other forms of chronic anemia, those with CRF or on RDT have no increased concentration of 2.3-DPG in erythrocytes and, even if corrected for pH, fails to show a compensatory rise of p50 (3). Although a negative correlation is found between Hb and 2.3-DPG concentration, this plays at a lower level compared to children without or with other forms of chronic anemia (36).

It is unclear if the insufficient rise of 2.3-DPG in children with CRF is caused by a relatively lower pH of uremic red blood cells or by a toxic inhibition of 2.3-DPG mutase. Erythrocyte 2.3-DPG in uremic children depends on blood pH and rises when acidosis is corrected during hemodialysis (36). Rapid correction of acidosis by short dialysis schedules or by bicarbonate decreases tissue oxygenation because the shift of the Hb-O_2 dissociation curve to the left cannot be counterbalanced by a rapid rise of organic phosphates in erythrocytes. Low concentrations of erythrocyte 2.3-DPG may also be caused by reduced levels of serum inorganic phosphate (12) and should be avoided in uremic patients.

Anemia should cause a rise in erythropoetin (EPO) production (37). Previously, it was thought that this rise did not occur in CRF. Through a sensitive fetal mouse liver cell assay, we found normal levels of plasma EPO before start of RDT, with an inverse correlation to Hb and p50 (38). With advancing CRF, however, the compensatory rise of EPO diminishes when it is compared to the response of children with nonrenal anemia (Fig. 53A.6). After start of RDT, this hormonal compensation fails completely, and it appears that then Hb levels are determined by the degree of EPO production. Soon after transplantation, EPO levels and their physiological regulation normalize; some transplanted patients even develop erythrocytosis, which might be caused by exaggerated EPO formation (39) or an increased EPO stem cell sensitivity (40).

Iron Metabolism

The introduction of radioimmunological assays to determine serum ferritin has increased the reliability of the assessment of body iron stores (41). Serum ferritin concentration now is regarded as a sensitive indicator of total iron stores in the reticuloendothelial system, predominantly in liver and spleen, and to a minor extent also in bone marrow of patients with CRF (41, 42) (Fig. 53A.7). It should be measured frequently in every child with CRF and provides a better indicator of body iron status than the estimation of serum iron iron-binding capacity or bone marrow iron deposition.

Iron Deficiency. Iron deficiency appears to be rare in children with CRF. Only a third of pediatric patients on conservative treatment and 7% on RDT have serum ferritin levels below the normal limit (40 μg/liter) when measured by a radioimmunometric assay in a heterologous antibody system (41, 43).

Iron Overload. Iron overload is a more critical problem than iron deficiency. About three quarters of children on dialyses and half of those

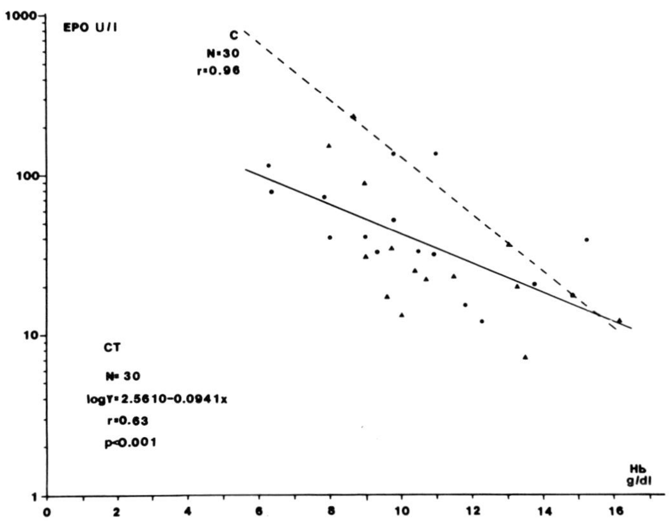

Figure 53A.6. Correlation between serum EPO and Hb concentrations in children with CRF on conservative treatment. The regression line (——) is compared with that of control children without renal failure (C – – –). (From Müller-Wiefel DE, Schärer K: Serum erythropoietin in children with chronic failure. Kidney Int 24 Suppl 15:70, 1983.)

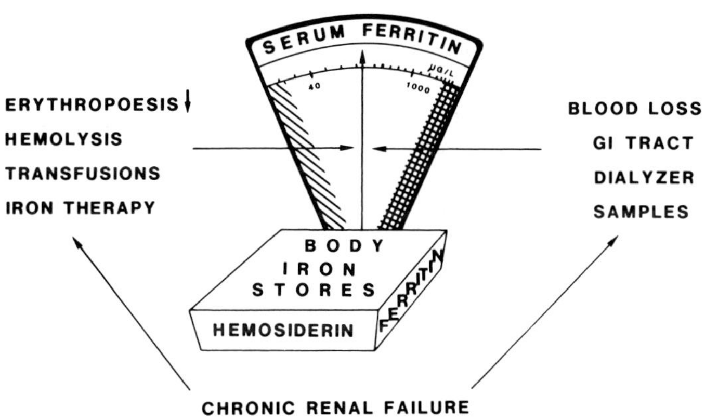

Figure 53A.7. Positive (left side) and negative (right side) influences of various intrinsic and extrinsic changes in body iron stores as reflected by serum ferritin concentrations in CRF.

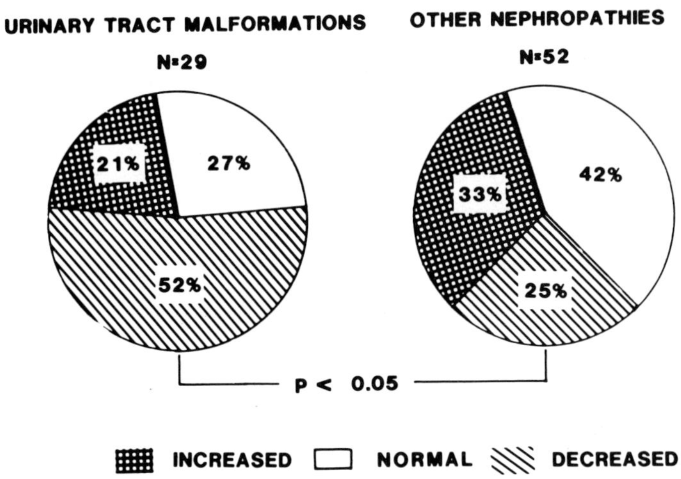

Figure 53A.8. Distributions of serum ferritin levels in children on conservative treatment with CRF caused by urinary tract malformations and by other (acquired) nephropathies.

with transplants showed clearly increased levels of serum ferritin (>1000 µg/liter) (43) with the associated risks of hemosiderosis and its effects on liver, heart, muscles, and endocrine function (43–46).

Serum ferritin concentrations are regulated by a number of factors that influence iron metabolism and transport (Fig. 53A.7). Increased concentrations result from reduced erythropoiesis, hemolysis, blood transfusions, iron therapy, and dysfunction of the reticuloendothelial system caused by hepatitis or other chronic infections; blood loss reduces ferritin levels. Iron stores also seem to depend on the type of primary kidney disease present; congenital uropathies are associated with lower ferritin levels than acquired nephropathies, at least before start of RDT (3) (Fig. 53A.8). Iron storage also is genetically determined, with a strong association between high ferritin levels and the hemochromatosis alleles of the HLA system (A3 and B7) in uremic children (47).

Therapy

Bone Marrow Hypoplasia

Bone marrow hypoplasia is most resistant to treatment. In adult patients with CRF, androgens and anabolic steroids have been used successfully to stimulate bone marrow activity (10, 11, 34), but they are not usually recommended in children in view of the virilizing and bone maturating actions of these agents. If tried, only agents such as oxandrolone, which has minimal virilizing effects, should be used, with careful monitoring for side effects, including hepatic toxicity. If EPO preparations become available in larger quantities, their potent stimulating effects on erythropoiesis should be subjected to clinical trial therapeutically.

Reducing Blood Loss

In children with CRF, blood losses can be reduced by limiting blood sampling for biochemical investigations, by careful cannulation during hemodialysis, and by complete washback of blood at the end of each dialysis session. The choice of appropriate dialyzers and tubing systems with low filling voulmes is important (15). Reduced frequency or duration of hemodialysis sessions can lower Hb levels (17). Splenectomy to diminish the degree of hemolysis should be avoided because of the risk of septicemia unless frank hypersplenism is present.

Continuous Ambulatory Peritoneal Dialysis

Higher Hb concentrations are associated with continuous ambulatory peritoneal dialysis (CAPD) (8, 48). The frequency of transfusions needed in children in CAPD was found to be one-fifth that required for children on hemodialysis (49). The reasons for this difference are not yet clear; blood losses on CAPD are lower and serum EPO levels higher (48, 49), whereas the degree of hemolysis is similar to that of patients on hemodialysis (50).

Oral Iron Therapy

Oral iron is always indicated if the serum ferritin concentration is low. The intestinal absorption of iron adapts well to the quantity of iron needed in CRF (51). Intravenous iron therapy is rarely indicated and may be dangerous (44). The usual daily oral dose of 5 mg/kg Fe-II is best given as sulfate and should be monitored by regular (monthly) serum ferritin determinations. As soon as the ferritin level exceeds 300 µg/liter (usually after three to six months), the supplements should be discontinued.

Iron-Binding Therapy

The indication for iron-binding therapy is still controversial. In our opinion, iron-binding therapy should be started in patients on RDT if iron overload is demonstrated by constant increase of serum ferritin levels >2000 μg/liter and in the absence of signs of liver dysfunction or chronic infection. Computer tomography of the liver may be helpful to confirm iron overload associated with increased density, i.e., above 65 Hounsfield units (43). Liver biopsy is indicated to confirm siderosis if hepatic dysfunction with raised serum transaminases is present. A dose of 1 g/m^2 BSA desferrioxamine intravenously is recommended at the end of each hemodialysis session as long as levels of serum ferritin are higher than 1000 μg/liter (43). During CAPD, adding desferrioxamine to the dialysis fluid will remove the iron (52). Similar therapy is indicated for aluminum-induced anemia. Desferrioxamine may produce anaphylactic reactions, nephrotoxicity and ocular abnormalities (53) and is associated with increased tendency for infections; therefore, it should be introduced only if iron overload is well documented.

Blood Transfusions

Blood transfusions aid kidney graft survival and can be given according to the clnical state of the child, though the risks of hepatitis, infection, hemosiderosis, and erythropoiesis suppression should be remembered. Transfusion is usually not necessary when Hb levels exceed 7 g/dl. If possible, young, unfrozen buffy-coat-free erythrocytes should be transfused. Bilateral nephrectomy, with loss of residual EPO production, should be avoided whenever possible (16, 34, 54).

Subtotal Parathyroidectomy (PTX)

Subtotal parathyroidectomy and intensive vitamin D therapy are known to improve renal anemia (55), although only about 50% of uremic patients show a clear-cut increase of Hb after PTX. The possible mechanisms for this improvement are summarized in Figure 53A.9. They include reducing bone marrow fibrosis, disappearance of toxic effects of PTH on erythroid precursor cells and erythrocytes, and decreased gastrointestinal blood loss from reduced platelet aggregation (30, 56).

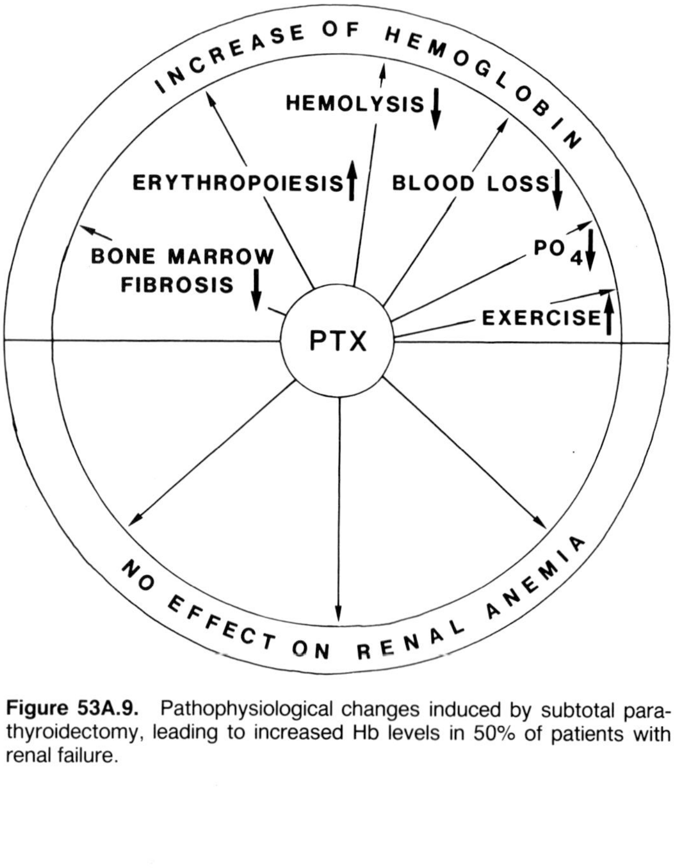

Figure 53A.9. Pathophysiological changes induced by subtotal parathyroidectomy, leading to increased Hb levels in 50% of patients with renal failure.

Other Therapy

Low plasma concentrations of folic acid or vitamin B_{12} or an increased proportion of peripheral macrocytes should be healed with supplements. Excessive hemolysis due to some toxic agents, such as formaldehyde, may be treated by altering dialysis technique.

Bleeding Abnormalities

Bleeding is a frequent complication of advanced CRF and is related mainly to platelet dysfunction (9a, 57).

Bleeding Time

In untreated uremic subjects, bleeding time is prolonged to 20 to 30 min. The exact cause for this is unknown, but a number of hemostatic abnormalities have been demonstrated: (a) thrombocytopenia occurs in about 50% of adult uremic patients; (b) a defect in platelet adhesion (58); (c) deficient platelet aggregation by ADP, epinephrine, and collagen caused by uremic plasma (59), as well as by substances known to accumulate in uremia, e.g., guanidinosuccinic acid; (d) decreased levels of platelet factor III, which is also inhibited by phenolic compounds in vitro; (e) various abnormalities of coagulation factors, e.g., decreased concentrations of factor VIII van Willebrand activity (60). In addition, a nondialyzable heat-labile factor was found in uremic plasma that inhibits the production of platelet prostaglandin (thromboxane A) and at the same time stimulates endothelial prostacyclin (PGI_2) (61, 62).

Elevated plasma concentrations of fibrinogen and coagulation factors II, VII, and X have been observed. Fibrinolysis is usually reduced due to low levels of plasminogen activators and high levels of urokinase inhibitors (63).

Bleeding time seems also to be influenced by other factors not directly involved in hemostasis, and uremic hemorrhages can be successfully treated by raising the packed red cell volume (64). A number of drugs frequently used in patients with CRF, such as heparin (62) and synthetic penicillins (65), may also influence the coagulation mechanisms (66) (Table 53A.1).

Hemodialysis

Regular hemodialysis improves platelet function in spite of the trauma of the extracorporeal circuit (67). Platelet aggregation and prostacyclin function is enhanced by hemodialysis in the presence of low molecular concentrations of arachidonic acid but reduced at high concentrations (68). Cyclic AMP concentration, which is high initially, falls rapidly during dialysis, leading to increased clotting tendency and resulting in a transient decrease of platelet counts due to increased consumption (57). In addition, hemodialysis results in a marked rise in antithrombin-III levels, attributed to the release of this factor from the vascular endothelium following heparin administration and platelet damage (69). This rise can be completely prevented by the use of prostacyclin (70). Finally, the interaction between blood, foreign surfaces, and anticoagulants used during dialysis will greatly influence the primary hemostatic defects in uremic patients. Detailed descriptions of these interactions and the practical conclusions derived for therapy have been reviewed (71).

Alterations of Leukocytes

Uremic individuals are believed to have an increased susceptibility to infections (72), although this may not be caused by uremia itself (73). Infection was the cause of death in 11% of pediatric patients treated by hospital hemodialysis in Europe and in 29% of all deaths after transplantation (74). Most infections encountered in uremic patients with severe renal failure are caused by commonly occurring bacteria rather than unusual opportunistic organisms. They appear to be the conse-

Table 53A.1.
Hematological Effects of Drugs Used in Children with Renal Failure

	Aplastic anemia	Hemolysis	Neutropenia	Thrombocytopenia	Coagulation disorder
Antibiotics					
Ampicillin			+	+	
Carbenicillin			+	D[a]	+
Cephalexin		+			
Cephalozin		+	+	+	
Chloramphenicol	+				
Gentamycin			+		
Penicillin		+	+	+	+
Tetracyclines				+	
Trimethoprim/Sulfamethoxazole			+	+	
Antihypertensives					
Hydrochlorthiazide			+	+	
Propranolol			+	+	
Methyldopa		+	+	+	

[a] D = platelet dysfunction.

quence of an impaired inflammatory response and reduced host defense with alterations in humoral immunity and in white blood cell function (72, 75).

Although the number of leukocytes in the peripheral blood is not reduced, the migration of polymorphonuclear cells into damaged tissues appears to be delayed, probably by acidosis. In addition, the chemotactic activity of polymorphonuclear cells was found to be decreased even after the introduction of hemodialysis (76). The phagocytic and bactericidal capacities of polymorphonuclear leukocytes are normal in renal failure when tested in vivo (77). Similarly, intracellular killing of bacteria phagocytosed by neutrophils appears to be normal or even enhanced by the nitroblue tetrazolium test.

The number of peripheral lymphocytes (B and T cells) is moderately reduced in uremic patients, but the mechanism for this is unclear (78). The blastogenic response of lymphocytes to mitogens has been near normal when studied with homologous serum but decreased in the presence of uremic serum, suggesting the absence of an intrinsic defect (72).

The function of the mononuclear phagocytic system appears also to be impaired in uremia (79). Mononuclear cells of uremic patients show a delayed appearance when studied by the Rebuck skin window technique (80). In addition, locomotion and phagocytic function are depressed in vitro when mononuclear cells are tested with uremic plasma. Humoral immunity also is disturbed in uremia, e.g., there is reduced production of serum antibodies after vaccination against hepatitis and other viruses.

Hemodialysis with cuprophan membranes is associated with a transient fall of thee neutrophil and monocyte cell count (20–30% of initial levels) which occurs within the first hour of dialysis with a nadir between 10 and 30 min (81, 82). A rapid rebound is observed in the neutrophil count but not in the monocyte count, which is less able to be restored from bone marrow reserves. The dramatic leukopenia induced by hemodialysis may be caused by activation of the complement system by contact of white cells with membranes and subsequent sequestration of leukocytes in the lung with pulmonary hypoxia (83). More recent studies, however, have demonstrated that there is no relation between the degree of leukopenia and the intensity of complement activation or with hypoxia (84). It has also been suggested that dialysis-induced leukopenia is caused by a transient increase in granulocyte adherence, depending on the type of membrane used (82), for it is much less with polyacrylnitrile and other membranes than with cuprophan. Neither the leukocyte count nor complement activation is altered significantly by hemofiltration (85).

Leukocytes obtained from CAPD dialysate failed to demonstrate any change in neutrophil or lymphocyte functions that might be responsible for peritoneal infections (86). After transplantation, the function of neutrophils and of the cells of the reticuloendothelial system is depressed, presumably by the action of immunosuppressive drugs (corticosteroids, azathioprin, ALG) (87). No fall in the leukocyte count has so far been reported in patients with cyclosporin A.

References

1. Schärer K, Müller-Wiefel DE: Renal anemia, a review. Int J Pediatr Nephrol 4:193, 1982.
2. Ulmer HE, Greiner H, Schüler HW, Schärer K: Cardiovascular impairment and physical working capacity in children with chronic renal failure. Acta Paediatr Scand 67:43, 1978.
3. Müller-Wiefel DE: Renale Anämie im Kindesalter. Untersuchungen zur Pathogenese und Kompensation. Stuttgart, New York, G Thieme 1982.
4. Schärer K, Brunner FP, von Dehn H, et al: Combined report on regular dialysis and transplantation of children in Europe, 1972. Proc EDTA 10:58, 1973.
5. Donckerwolcke RA, Chantler C, Broyer M, et al: Combined report on regular dialysis and transplantation of children in Europe, 1979. Proc EDTA 17:87, 1980.
6. Müller-Wiefel DE, Schärer K, Ulmer HE, et al: Verlauf der Anämie bei Kindern mit chronischer Niereninsuffizienz. Mschr Kinderheilk 124:323, 1976.
7. Santiago GC, Rao TKS, Laird NM: Effect of dialysis therapy on the hematopoietic system: the National Cooperative Dialysis Study Kidney Int 23 (suppl 13): 595, 1983.
8. Müller-Wiefel DE, Schärer K: Effects of chronic ambulatory peritoneal dialysis on renal anemia in children. 17th Int Congr Pediatr, Manila, 1983 vol 1, p 84 (abstract).
9. Kikuchi Y, Koyama T, Koyama Y, et al: Red blood cell deformability in renal failure. Nephron 30:8, 1982.

9a. Eschbach JW: Hematologic problems of dialysis patients. In Drukker W, Parsons FM, Maher JF (eds): Replacement of Renal Function by Dialysis, ed 2. Amsterdam, M Nijhoff, 1983, p 630.

10. Anagnostou A, Fried W: Anemia of renal disease. In Jepson JH (ed): Hematologic Problems in Renal Disease. Menlo Park, CA, Addison-Wesley, 1979, p 2.
11. Fisher JW: Mechanism of the anemia of chronic renal failure. Nephron 25:106, 1980.
12. Bursaux E, Broyer M, Poyart C, et al: Oxygen transport in children on maintenance hemodialysis. Clin Sci Mol Med 54:85, 1978.
13. Gusmano R, Perfumo F, Basile G, Ciardi MR: I problemi dell' ancmia nel bambino uremico. Minerva Nefrol 24:23, 1977.
14. Hellwege HH, Bläker F, Neth R: In vitro studies of bone marrow stem-cell function in uremic children. Eur J Pediatr 129:279, 1977.
15. Müller-Wiefel DE, Sinn H, Gilli G, Schärer K: Hemolysis and blood loss in children with chronic renal failure. Clin Nephrol 8:581, 1977.

16. Ortega JA, Malekzadeh MH, Dukes PP, et al: A beneficial effect of the in situ kidney on in vitro marrow erythropoiesis in chronic renal failure. Nephron 23:169, 1979.
17. Scigalla P, Gudim VI, Noack CH, et al: Zur Bedeutung der Mittelmolekülelimination aus dem Serum niereninsuffizienter Kinder für die Pathogenese der renalen Anämie. Dt Ges Wesen 35:170, 1980.
18. Müller-Wiefel DE, Swoboda R, Mehls O, Schärer K: Knochenmarkszellularität bei Kindern mit chronischer Niereninsuffizienz. In Van Dittrich P (ed): Aktuelle Probleme der Dialyseverfahren und der Niereninsuffizienz. Friedberg/Hessen, C Bindernagel, 1981, p 208.
19. Keyssner J, Hauswaldt C, Uhl N, Hunstein W: Testosteronbehandlung bei renaler Anämie. Schweiz Med Wschr 104:1938, 1974.
20. Fisher JW, Ohno Y, Barona J, et al: The role of serum inhibitors of erythroid colony forming cells in the mechanism of the anemia of renal insufficiency. In Murphy J (ed): In Vitro Aspects of Erythropoiesis. Berlin, New York, Heidelberg Springer, 1978, p 64.
21. Heilmann E, Graefe W, Steinhausen R: Effekt der Hämodialyse auf das Wachstumsverhalten hämatopoetischer Stammzellen in Methylcellulose-Kulturen bei terminaler Niereninsuffizienz. Nieren- und Hochruckkrankh 12:72, 1983.
22. McGonigle RJS, Boineau FG, Ohene-Frempong K, et al: The role of erythropoietin and inhibitors of erythropoiesis in the anemia of renal disease in children. Eur J Pediatr 140:163, 1983 (abstract).
23. Wallner SF, Kurnick JE, Ward HP, et al: The anemia of chronic renal failure and chronic disease. In vitro studies of erythropoiesis. Blood 47:561, 1976.
24. Gutman RA, Huang AT, Bouknight NS: Inhibitor of marrow thymidine incorporation from sera of patients with uremia. Kidney Int 18:715, 1980.
25. Radtke HW, Rege AB, La Marche MB, et al: Identification of spermine as an inhibitor of erythropoiesis in patients with chronic renal failure. J Clin Invest 67:1623, 1981.
26. Freedman MH, Cattran DC, Saunders EF: Anemia of chronic renal failure: inhibition of erythropoiesis by uremic serum. Nephron 35:13, 1983.
27. Asaba H, Alvestrand A, Bergström J, et al: Uremic middle molecules in non-dialysed azotemic patients: relation to symptoms and clinical biochemistries. Clin Nephrol 17:90, 1982.
28. Navarro J, Contreras P, Touraine JL, et al: Are "middle molecules" responsible for toxic phenomena in chronic renal failure? Nephron 32:301, 1982.
29. Massry SG: Role of parathyroid hormone in the pathogenesis of the uremic manifestations. Klin Wschr 57:1085, 1979.
30. Müller-Wiefel DE, Mehls O, Schärer K: The role of hyperparathyroidism in the pathogenesis of renal anemia. Eur J Pediatr 141:63, 1983.
31. Pershagen G, Hast R, Lins LE, Pehrsson U: Increased arsenic concentration in the bone marrow in chronic renal failure—a contributor to anemia? Nephron 30:250, 1982.
32. Wills MR, Savory J: Aluminum poisoning: dialysis encephalopathy, osteomalacia, and anemia. Lancet 2:29, 1983.
33. Giovanetti S, Barsotti G: Uremic intoxication. Nephron 14:123, 1975.
34. Koch KM, Patyna WD, Shaldon S, Werner E: Anemia of the regular hemodialysis patient and its treatment. Nephron 12:405, 1974.
35. Koch KM, Bechstein P, Fassbinder W, et al: Occult blood loss and iron balance in chronic renal failure. Proc EDTA 12:362, 1976.
36. Müller-Wiefel DE, Schärer K, Fischer W, Michalk D: Erythrocyte organic phosphates in anemia of renal failure in childhood. Eur J Pediatr 128:103, 1978.
37. Nathan DG, Sytkowski A: Erythropoietin and the regulation of erythropoiesis. N Engl J Med 308:520, 1983.
38. Müller-Wiefel DE, Schärer K: Serum erythropoietin in children with chronic renal failure. Kidney Int 24 (suppl) 15:S-70, 1983.
39. Wickre CG, Norman DJ, Bennison A, et al: Postrenal transplant erythrocytosis, a review of 53 patients. Kidney Int 23:731, 1983.
40. Heilmann E, Gottschalk D, Gottschalk I, Lison AE: Studies in polycythemia after kidney transplantation. Clin Nephrol 20:94, 1983.
41. Müller-Wiefel DE, Brendlein F, Ehrlich J, et al: Serumferritinbestimmung bei Kindern mit Eisenbilanzstörungen. Helv Paediatr Acta 37:254, 1982.
42. Ali M, Fayemi AO, Frascino J, et al: Failure of serum ferritin levels to predict bone marrow iron content after intravenous iron-dextran therapy. Lancet 1:652, 1982.
43. Müller-Wiefel DE, Waldherr R, Feist D, van Kaick G: The assessment of iron stores in children on regular dialysis treatment. Contr Nephrol 38:141, 1984.
44. Ali M, Fayemi AO, Rigolosi R, et al: Hemosiderosis in hemodialysis patients. An autopsy study of 50 cases. JAMA 244:342, 1980.
45. Bregman H, Gelfand MC, Winchester JF, et al: Iron-overload-associated myopathy in patients on maintenance haemodialysis: a histocompatibility-linked disorder. Lancet 2:882, 1980.
46. Koch KM, Hilfenhaus M, Bechstein PB: Therapy and monitoring of hypersiderosis in chronic renal insufficiency. Contr Nephrol (in press).
47. Müller-Wiefel DE, Lenhard V, Schärer K: Body iron stores in children with chronic renal failure in relation to HLA phenotypes. Proc EDTA 18:524, 1981.
48. Zappacosta AR, Caro J, Erslev A: Normalization of hematocrit in patients with end-stage renal disease on continuous ambulatory peritoneal dialysis: the role of erythropoietin. Am J Med 72:53, 1982.
49. Müller-Wiefel DE, Bonzel K, Wartha R et al: Renal anemia in children on CAPD. In Fine RN, Schäner K, Mehls O (eds): CAPD in children. Berlin, Springer 1985, p. 150.
50. Hefti JE, Blumberg A, Marti HR: Red cell survival and red cell enzymes in patients on continuous peritoneal dialysis (CAPD). Clin Nephrol 19:232, 1983.
51. Bezwoda WR, Derman DP, Bothwell TH, et al: Iron absorption in patients on regular dialysis therapy. Nephron 28:289, 1981.
52. Falk RJ, Mattern WB, Lamanna RW, et al: Iron removal during continuous ambulatory peritoneal dialysis using deferoxamine. Kidney Int 24:110, 1983.
53. Davies SC, Marcus RE, Hungerford JL, et al: Ocular toxicity of high-dose intravenous desferrioxamine. Lancet 2:181, 1983.
54. Caro J, Brown S, Miller O, et al: Erythropoietin levels in uremic nephric and anephric patients. J Lab Clin Med 93:449, 1979.
55. Better OS, Shasha SM, Winaver J, Chaimovitz C: Improvement in the anemia of hemodialysed patients following subtotal parathyroidectomy. Proc Am Soc Nephrol 9:1, 1976.
56. Potasman I, Better OS: The role of secondary hyperparathyroidism in the anemia of chronic renal failure. Nephron 33:229, 1983.
57. Frumin AM: Platelet function, coagulation and fibrinolysis. In Jepson JH (ed): Hematologic Problems in Renal Disease. Menlo Park, CA, Addison-Wesley 1979, p 2.
58. Remuzzi G, Livio M, Marchiaro G, et al: Bleeding in renal failure. Altered platelet function in chronic uremia only partially corrected by hemodialysis. Nephron 22:347, 1978.
59. Lindsay RM, Bolton CF, Clark WF, Linton AL: The effect of alterations of uremic retention products upon platelet and peripheral nerve function. Clin Nephrol 19:110, 1983.
60. Kazatchkine M, Sultan Y, Caen JP, Bariéty J: Bleeding in renal failure: a possible cause. Br Med J 2:612, 1976.
61. Remuzzi G, Marchesi D, Livio M, et al: Altered platelet and vascular prostaglandin generation in patients with renal failure and prolonged bleeding time. Thromb Res 13:1007, 1978.
62. Lindsay RM: Practical use of anticoagulants. In Drukker W, Parsons FM, Maher JF (eds): Replacement of Renal Function by Dialysis, ed 2. Amsterdam, M Nijhoff, 1983, p 201.
63. Panicucci F, Sagripanti A, Pinori E, et al: Comprehensive study of haemostasis in chronic uremia. Nephron 33:5, 1983.
64. Livio M, Gotti E, Marchesi D, et al: Uremic bleeding, role of anemia and beneficial effect of red cell transfusions. Lancet 2:1013, 1982.
65. Andrassy K, Scherz M, Ritz E, et al: Penicillin-induced coagulation disorder. Lancet 2:1039, 1976.
66. Hall CA: Hematologic effects of drugs used in the treatment of patients with renal disease. In Jepson JH (ed) Hematologic problems in renal disease, Menlo Park, CA, Addison-Wesley, 1979, p 270.
67. Lindsay RM, Moorthy AV, Koens F, Linton A: Platelet function in dialyzed and non-dialyzed patients with chronic renal failure. Clin Nephrol 4:52, 1975.
68. Remuzzi G, Benigni A, Dodesini P, et al: Platelet function in patients on maintenance hemodialysis: depressed or enhanced? Clin Nephrol 17:60, 1982.
69. Turney JH, Fewell M, Williams LC, et al: Paradoxical behaviour of antithrombin III during hemodialysis and its prevention with prostacyclin. Clin Nephrol 17:1, 1982.
70. Weston MJ: Prostacyclin in hemodialysis and charcoal haemoperfusion. Contr Nephrol 36: 68, 1983.
71. Mason RG, Chuang HYK, Mohammad SF: Extracorporeal thrombogenesis: mechanisms and prevention. In W Drukker, FM Parsons, JF Maher (eds) Replacement of renal function by dialysis, ed 2, Amsterdam, M Nijhoff, 1983, p 186.
72. Keane WF, Rau LR: Host defense and infectious complications in maintenance hemodialysis patients. In W Drukker, FM Parsons, JF Maher (eds) Replacement of renal function by dialysis, ed 2, Amsterdam, 1983, M Nijhoff, p 646.
73. Clarke IA, Ormrod DJ, Miller TE: Host immune status in uremia. Effect of uremia on resistance to bacterial infection. Kidney Int 24:66, 1983.
74. Broyer M, Donckerwolcke RA, Brunner FP, et al: Combined report on regular dialysis and transplantation of children in Europe 1982. Proc EDTA 20:79, 1983.
75. Galbraith PR: Leucokinetics and leucocyte function in renal disease. In Jepson J (ed): Hematologic Problems in Renal Disease. Menlo Park, CA, Addison Wesley, 1979, p 221.
76. Salant DJ, Glover AM, Anderson R, et al: Depressed neutrophil chemotaxis in patients with chronic renal failure and after renal transplantation. J Lab Clin Med 88:536, 1976.
77. Nelson J, Omrod DJ, Miller TE: Host immune status in uremia. IV. Phagocytosis and inflammatory response in vivo. Kidney Int 23:312, 1983.
78. Hoy WE, Cestero RVM, Treeman RB: Deficiency of T and B lymphocytes in uremic

subjects and parallel improvement with maintenance hemodialysis. Nephron 20:182, 1978.
79. Drutz DJ: Altered cell mediated immunity and its relationship to infection susceptibility in patients with uremia. Dial Transpl 8:320, 1979.
80. Ringoir S, van Looy L, van de Heyning P, Leroux-Roels G: Impairment of phagocytic activity of macrophages as studied by the skin window test in patients on regular hemodialysis treatment. Clin Nephrol 4:234, 1975.
81. Aljama P, Bird PAE, Ward MK, et al: Hemodialysis induced leucopenia and activation of complement: effect of different membranes. Proc EDTA 15:144, 1978.
82. Bauer H, Brunner H, Franz HE, Bultmann B: Leucocyte function tests during hemodialysis with different dialysis membranes. Contr Nephrol 36:9, 1983.
83. Jacob AI, Gavellas G, Zarco R, et al: Leucopenia, hypoxemia and complement function with different hemodialysis membranes. Kidney Int 18:505, 1980.
84. Vinuesa de SG, Resano M, Luno J, et al: Leucopenia, hypoxia and complement activation in hemodialysis, three unrelated phenomena. Proc EDTA 19:159, 1982.
85. Böhler J, Kramer P, Götze O, et al: Leucocyte counts and complement activation during pump-driven and arteriovenous hemofiltration. Contr Nephrol 36:15, 1983.
86. Rubin I, Lin LM, Lewis R, et al: Host defense mechanisms in continuous ambulatory peritoneal dialysis. Clin Nephrol 20:140, 1983.
87. Drivas G, Uldall PR, Wardle N: Reticuloendothelial function in renal allograft patients. Br Med J 3:743, 1975.

53B Cardiovascular Complications

KARL SCHÄRER AND HERBERT ULMER

Cardiovascular disease in children with CRF is an important cause of morbidity and mortality; EDTA statistics show that 63% of deaths in children treated by regular hemodialysis and 27% of those in transplanted children part were due to cardiovascular causes (1). Few studies of cardiovascular status in children with CRF are available (2), but atherosclerosis, ischemic heart disease, and bacterial endocarditis, which are important in adults (3), rarely occur.

Uremic Heart Disease

Uremic heart disease comprises all forms of cardiac involvement occurring in CRF. The term is preferable to cardiomyopathy (4, 5), which in our view should be reserved for histologically well-defined and clinically irreversible primary myocardial disease (6, 7). Uremic heart disease may be caused by complications of CRF, such as anemia or infection, or follow the construction of an arteriovenous fistula.

Cardiological review, including clinical examination, chest roentgenogram, and electrocardiogram, should be undertaken regularly in children with CRF, especially after dialysis or transplantation has become necessary. Echocardiography, phonocardiography, ergometry, and mechanocardiography are useful in the diagnostic evaluation. Table 53B.1 summarizes the data from a study using noninvasive diagnostic methods in 137 children with CRF observed consecutively during a three-year period (1976 to 1978) (6) and supplemented by a long-term followup (7).

Clinical Manifestations

The clinical manifestations of cardiac involvement in children with CRF are mainly those of heart failure and pericarditis.

Congestive heart failure was rarely found in our patients before the Scr reached 5 mg/dl but was present in 24% of all children on dialysis (Table 53B.1). Heart failure seems to be less common in children (6) than adults with ESRD (8). Increased heart size on chest roentgenogram was present in about half the children on conservative treatment and two thirds of those on hemodialysis. The range in cardiothoracic ratios in dialyzed patients may reflect the instability of fluid balance. Cardiomegaly is mainly a physiological adaptation to increase in stroke volume rather than the result of intrinsic cardiac dilatation. No significant correlation was observed between the cardiothoracic ratio and left ventricular performance assessed by mechanocardiography, though a close relation between echocardiographically determined dilatation and poor left ventricular performance has been found (9).

Ergometric testing reveals early derangement of cardiovascular function. Submaximal working capacity (PW 170) of children with CRF is reduced when Scr is between 2 to 5 mg/dl; it is not improved by dialysis (10, 11) (Fig. 53B.1). Anemia also affects working capacity, but the decrease in children on regular dialysis is caused by decreased aerobic capacity, whereas anaerobic metabolism is more or less unchanged (12), suggesting that factors other than cardiac dysfunction and anemia might be involved.

Electrocardiographic changes appear to be less frequent in children than in adults (6, 13, 14). Unequivocal signs of left ventricular hypertrophy were present in one third of children and were common when hypertension was present (Table 53B.2). Severe forms of resistance hypertrophy characterized by discordant T waves over the left precordium were found almost exclusively in association with excessive arterial hypertension and severe uremia (6).

Table 53B.1.
Prevalence (%) of Cardiovascular Manifestation in 137 Children with CRI According to Stage of Disease[a]

	Conservative treatment		Hemodialysis	Transplantation
	S_{Cr} <5 mg/dl	S_{Cr} >5 mg/dl		
Number of patients	40	41	42	14
Hypertension (%)	55	63	40	50
Cardiomegaly (%)	46	48	67	36
Left ventricular hypertrophy in ECG (%)	23	34	36	14
Heart failure (%)	10	39	24	7
Pericarditis (%)	—	7	14	—
Anemia (Hbg 7 g %, %)	5	27	52	—

[a] Each patient is ascribed only to the stage in which he was examined at first cardiological observation. Heart failure was defined by the presence of clinical signs and the requirement of digitalis medication. S_{Cr} = serum creatinine. (Data from Reference 79.)

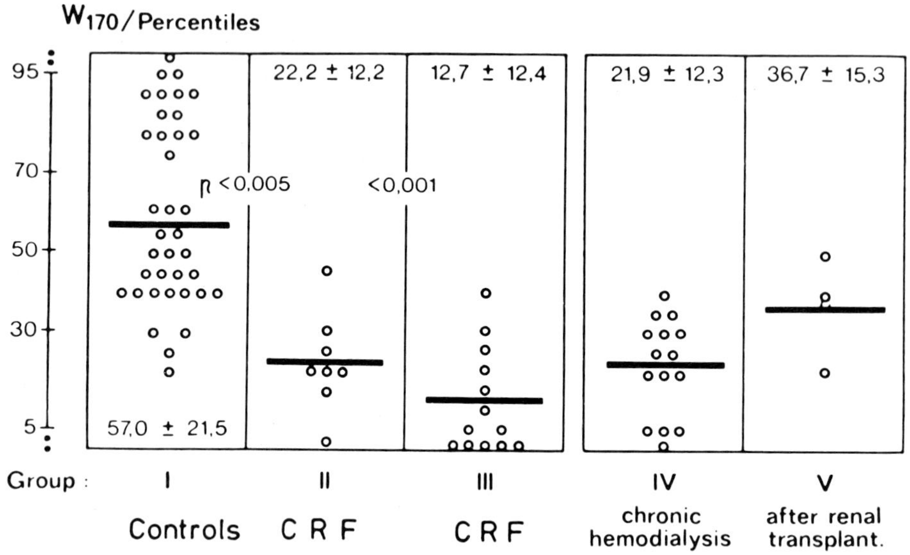

Figure 53B.1. Physical working capacity (W_{170}) in 40 children with CRF (groups II-V) and 22 control children (group I). The results are presented in percentiles related to the body surface area employing the nomograms of Adams et al (see ref. 10). Group II: S_{Cr} 2–5 mg/dl, group III: S_{Cr} above 5 mg/dl.

Table 53B.2.
Prevalence of Electrocardiographic Changes in 64 Children with Advanced CRF (Serum Creatinine >5 mg/dl) Before Start of Dialysis[a]

	Normotensive	Hypertensive
Number of patients	25	39
Mean serum creatinine (mg/dl)	8.0	10.1
Mean hemoglobin (g/dl)	7.3	7.8
ECG		
Left ventricular hypertrophy	20%	41%
ST depression	—	
Signs of hyperkalemia	24%	23%
Signs of hyperkalemia + hypocalcemia	4%	13%
Alterations of cardiac conduction and dysrhythmias	—	27%

[a] Data from Reference (6).

The characteristic changes of hyperkalemia were present transiently in 8, and those of hypocalcemia in 18 of 41 patients with Scr > 5 mg/dl before start of dialysis. These electrolyte disturbances are a predominant cause of cardiac arrhythmias (3). Atrioventricular blocks are always caused by drug therapy. Supraventricular and ventricular ectopic beats were present in only 3, and other forms of arrhythmias in 6 of 137 pediatric cases examined by routine electrocardiograms. The low frequency of dysrhythmias was related to restricted use of digitalis glycosides and β-blockers; however, detection of electrocardiographic changes is related to the frequency with which tracings are taken. Determining the incidence of cardiac arrhythmias requires long-term monitoring (15).

Alterations of the electrocardiogram during hemodialysis were less common in our pediatric patients than in adults. They consisted mainly of changes in the QT interval and depressed T-waves, whereas alterations of the ST segment and of R waves, described in adults as signs of ischemia or of sodium loss (13, 14), were absent.

One of the most striking cardiological findings in children, in contrast to adults with CRF, is the presence of heart murmurs, which are best analyzed by phonocardiography (Fig. 53B.2). Sometimes these murmurs mimic congenital heart disease (7). Holosystolic diamond-shaped murmurs are frequent and best heard along the left sternal border or over the aorta. They may be caused by functional aortic stenosis and usually are preceded by an early systolic ejection click originating from the dilated aortic root. Mesodiastolic or presystolic murmurs due to functional stenosis of a normal mitral valve may be detected. A few patients have transitory early diastolic murmurs characteristic of valvular aortic

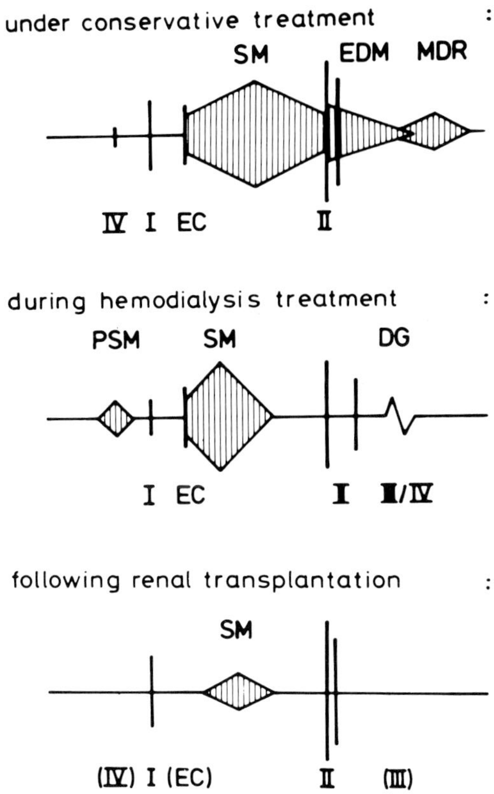

Figure 53B.2. Common phonocardiographic findings in children with CRF at various stages of the disease. I, II, III, IV: heart sounds; EC: ejection click; PSM: presystolic murmur; SM: systolic murmur; EDM: early diastolic murmur; MDR: mesodiastolic rumble; DG: diastolic gallop.

incompetence (7). Autopsy studies have shown no aortic valve abnormality in such cases (6, 16), and the murmur appears to be related to the combination of arterial hypertension, severe anemia, and overhydration.

Cardiac Function and Morphology

Some investigations in adult patients with CRF have assessed cardiac function by catheterization. In the predialytic stage and in the absence of fluid overload, cardiac output was normal (17). In contrast, after the start of hemodialysis, a significantly elevated cardiac index (cardiac output expressed in liters per minute per square meter) was observed (18–21). Stroke index is normal or increased (19), and the increased cardiac index is caused by an increase in stroke index and heart rate (21). Left ventricular end-diastolic pressures are elevated, suggesting cardiac failure from high output (19).

Gross abnormalities of myocardial function have not been detected in some studies of adult patients on hemodialysis (17, 22). Left ventricular dimensions and ejection fraction as parameters of systolic function as well as diastolic function were found to be normal when measured angiographically (21). Minor functional changes of cardiac dynamics were attributed to alterations of left ventricular preload, afterload, or both, depending on volume changes during the dialysis procedure or between dialysis sessions (6). In other studies, however, moderate-to-severe impairment of myocardial function ("cardiomyopathy") was found in up to 50% of adult patients on hemodialysis (4, 5, 8).

Cardiac function in children with CRF has usually been investigated by noninvasive techniques, i.e., by mechanocardiography (23) and echocardiography (9, 24, 25), whereas only rarely has angiography been undertaken (26).

The study of left ventricular cycle time sequences, i.e., of the systolic time intervals (STI) by mechanocardiography, provides a sensitive noninvasive way to assess left ventricular function (27).

In the study mentioned previously, 66 children were subjected repeatedly to mechanocardiography (6). A uniform pattern of decreased left ventricular performance was found, which was most marked in children on hemodialysis: preejection period (PEP) was prolonged, left ventricular ejection time (LVET) was shortened, and there was a marked increase in the ratio PEP/LVET, which reflects the ejection fraction as determined by angiography. Total electromechanical systole (QS2), which is the interval from onset of the QRS complex to closure of the aortic valve, reflected by the second heart sound, was unchanged. Similar results were found in adult patients (28) and in a longitudinal study of 11 children observed during three consecutive stages of CRF (7). On conservative treatment the mean ratio PEP/LVET was increased only slightly but increased up to 12 months on hemodialysis and returned to normal one year after transplantation (Fig. 53B.3). More than half of all PEP/LVET values on dialysis were above the 95th percentile (27). The majority of children treated by hemodialysis, although usually asymptomatic, suffer from uremic heart disease.

Echocardiography enables cardiac chamber size, cardiac output, and ventricular performance to be measured (2). In adult patients with CRF, right and left ventricular dilatation; concentric or asymmetric left ventricular hypertrophy and depressed ventricular function, with reduced ejection fraction; and depressed mean velocity of circumferential fiber shortening has been found (22, 28–31). Similar results have been found in children (2, 9, 24, 25, 32–34), though in the absence of cardiac failure, myocardial function usually is normal (34). Parameters of contractility improved after hemodialysis (25). Dilatation of the left heart with thickening of myocardial walls was prevalent in more advanced stages of CRF and in the presence of hypertension (32).

Asymmetrical septal hypertrophy with or without left ventricular outflow obstruction has been observed repeatedly in adults (31, 35) and children (6, 36) with CRF, usually associated with severe hypertension. In one of our cases this lesion disappeared about six months after transplantation when hypertension and anemia disappeared (7).

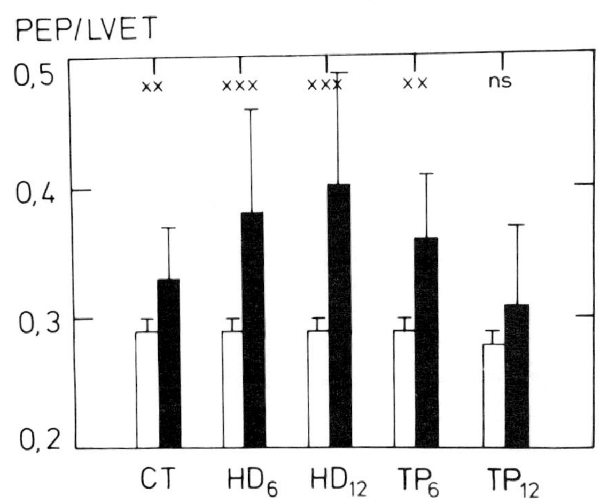

Figure 53B.3. Ratio of pre-ejection period–left ventricular ejection time in 11 children with CRF examined serially. Open columns: predicted normal values (27). Closed columns: values of patients. Data are given in means ± SD at following points: CT: conservative treatment; HD6, HD12: 6 and 12 months after start of hemodialysis, respectively; TP6, TP12: 6 and 12 months after transplantation, respectively; xx: $p < 0.01$; xxx: $p < 0.001$.

Pathogenesis

Numerous factors may affect cardiac function in CRF (3, 4). These include (a) volume overload caused by fluid retention anemia and/or construction of an arteriovenous fistula for hemodialysis; (b) increased pressure load from persistent hypertension; or (c) metabolic, endocrine, or nutritional factors.

Decreases in blood viscosity and increases in peripheral vasodilatation lead to diminished peripheral resistance and to increased cardiac output. Volume overload is worse in children with CRF because of their relatively severe anemia. If the hematocrit is increased to 30% by transfusions without raising blood volume, cardiac output is lowered to normal and peripheral resistance and blood pressure rise (37).

Arteriovenous communications for vascular access for hemodialysis lead to a decrease in peripheral vascular resistance with a compensatory rise in cardiac output to maintain blood pressure (3). Absolute flow rates in children with arteriovenous external shunts or fistulas are similar to those in adult patients (26, 38); therefore, a relatively higher proportion of total cardiac output is shunted. Fistula flow may increase with time, e.g., by formation of an aneurysm (39) or with exercise.

Measurements of fistula flow obtained by indirect methods, e.g., by calculation from the difference in cardiac output before and after external fistula occlusion (38), are difficult to interpret. Data on the rise of cardiac output after fistula formation are conflicting (40, 41). In children with external shunts, 2% to 10% of total cardiac output has been attributed to shunt flow (26). No significant increase in cardiac output was detected in nine children studied before and 8 to 12 weeks after constitution of a forearm fistula, though myocardial contractility fell (42). Apparently the proposed criterion for the development of cardiac failure (about 20% of cardiac output attributed to fistula flow) is rarely attained. Only a few children have been observed with overt cardiac insufficiency following fistula construction (26, 43, 44), and in a large series dealing with arteriovenous fistulae in children no case requiring closure of the communication (45) occurred. Cardiac deterioration should be anticipated, especially with large arteriovenous communication at proximal sites (3), and may be suspected if bradycardia follows temporary occlusion of the fistula referred to as the Nicaladini-Branham sign (3). Treatment is possible by banding of the fistula or operative revision.

The dialysis procedure may alter cardiac performance. The acute effects of hemodialysis on cardiac function have been investigated repeatedly in adult patients; findings have varied (18, 20, 22, 30, 46–49). In most studies, decreased cardiac output and pulmonary arterial pressure were noted. This fall apparently is due to ultrafiltration and corresponds to a decrease in end-systolic, end-diastolic, and stroke volumes following reduction in central blood volume (46, 47). Both ventricular preload and afterload usually decline during hemodialysis, indicating diminished pumping function without significant changes in myocardial contractility (22); however, in some cases with severe hypervolemia and cardiac failure, the dialysis may result in an increase in cardiac output (18, 48). At the end of the procedure, following reinfusion of the dialysis fluid, cardiac output usually rises so that its overall change is insignificant. Any factor that compromises cardiac function during dialysis, such as severe anemia, hypertension, or ischemic heart disease, is a further stress and may lead to anginal pain and ST depression in the electrocardiogram.

In children, decreased cardiac output and increased mean velocity of circumferential fiber shortening, interpreted as improvement of myocardial function, were found following dialysis (25).

Fourteen children were investigated by six serial measurements of systolic time intervals before, during, and after hemodialysis of six to eight hours' duration (6). The hemodynamic changes were separated into three phases (Fig. 53B.4). In the first period, corresponding to the removal of blood to the dialyzer, QS2, PEP, and LVET all decreased, indicating an increased inotropic reaction of the myocardium, probably by stimulated sympathetic activity. During the following period of dialysis, PEP rose steadily while QS2 remained unchanged and LVET diminished, which might be interpreted as a decreased inotropic state of the heart resulting from myocardial hypoxia or from a toxic action of acetate contained in the dialysis fluid (49). The ultrafiltration applied during dialysis removes plasma and thereby reduces ventricular preload which, according to Starling's law, is followed by a decreased contractile response. It is assumed that the opposite change of PEP and LVET during

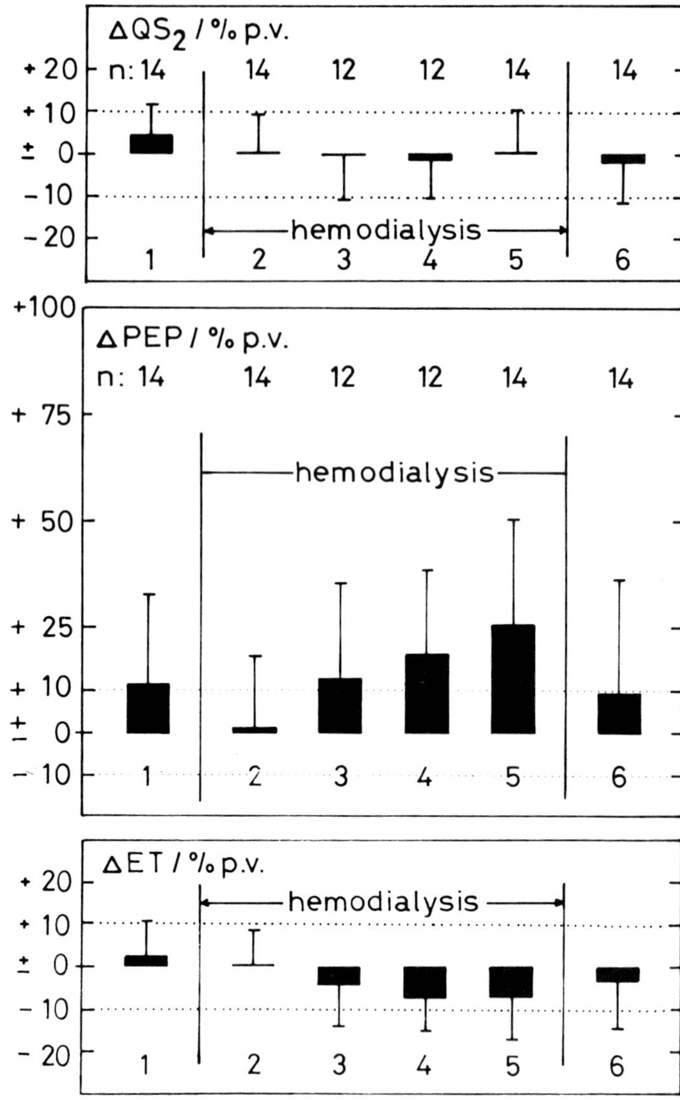

Figure 53B.4. Changes of total electromechanical systoles (ΔQS2), pre-ejection period (ΔPEP), and ejection time (ΔET) during the course of a hemodialysis session in 14 pediatric patients (age 5.5 to 20 yrs) without congestive heart failure. Mean Hb 6.7 g/dl. The patients were dialyzed for six to eight hours through an arteriovenous fistula. On the day of examination antihypertensive medication, applied to two patients, was omitted. The tracings were taken at the following times: 1: immediately before start of dialysis; 2: 30 to 45 min afterward; 3 and 4: at regular intervals on dialysis; 5: at end of dialysis before reinfusion of extracorporeal fluid; 6: after reinfusion, one hour after removing puncture needles. Mean values ± SD are indicated in percent deviation from mean normal values of systolic time intervals (27). (From Ulmer HE: Das Herz bei chronischer Niereninsuffizienz im Kindesalter, Heidelberg, Germany, University of Heidelberg, 1978, professorial thesis.)

hemodialysis is due purely to diminished ventricular filling without change in contractility. This is in agreement with recent work in adult patients (46, 50). In the third period after dialysis ceases, while the extracorporeal fluid is reinfused to the body, the preload increases again, thus improving ventricular performance. This explains the final drop of PEP shown in Figure 53B.4.

Myocardial contractility improves during dialysis but not during ultrafiltration (51). Sympathetic and hemodynamic responses to a constant volume removal by pure ultrafiltration, hemofiltration, acetate hemodialysis, and bicarbonate hemodialysis have been studied (52). Sympathetic response, resulting in an increase of total peripheral resistance, was qualitatively adequate with ultrafiltration and hemofiltration but not with either acetate or bicarbonate hemodialysis, which would explain the observed instability of the arterial system during hemodialysis. Echocardiographic studies in patients treated by CAPD have shown improved left ventricular function and hypertrophy with normalization of blood pressure and volume overload (53).

Hypertension frequently persists or even deteriorates after transplantation. Cardiac performance improves rapidly after a successful graft; fluid and electrolyte balance is restored and anemia and uremia are eliminated (54). Irreversible myocardial damage acquired during preceding renal disease or from hypertension may explain why some clinical, radiological, electrocardiographic, and hemodynamic changes persist. In our longitudinal study on children observed up to one year after transplantation, the ratio PEP/LVET gradually decreased after grafting, indicating a continuous improvement of left ventricular performance in 9 of 11 children (Fig. 53B.3). Echocardiographic studies in pediatric patients demonstrated a significant reduction of cardiac index and of end-diastolic diameter following transplantation, which was attributed to the general rise in Hb levels (55), which was associated with a rise in working capacity (Fig. 53B.1). However, maximal working capacity may remain diminished for a longer period of time, possibly because of insufficient training and secondary weight gain.

Metabolic and endocrine changes associated with CRF alter cardiac function (56). Whereas in acutely uremic animals the contractile force of the heart is increased, the experimental evidence for depressed cardiac function in chronic uremia is uncertain. Chronic excess of PTH has an inhibitory effect on the myocardium with decreased ATP synthesis, presumably because of calcium overload. Myocardial contractility improved following parathyroidectomy in dialyzed patients (4), although in more recent studies this effect was less convincing (57).

Abnormalities of the sympathetic nervous system may be another pathogenetic factor in uremic heart disease. Increased plasma catecholamines have been reported repeatedly in uremic adults, but in children with end-stage CRF, basal plasma adrenaline and noradrenaline levels usually are normal (58). There is some evidence that catecholamines increase resistance of the myocardium and other organs to catecholamines and that β-agonists alter the response of heart rate and myocardial contractility (56).

Further metabolic factors possibly related to the myocardial dysfunction in CRF include vitamin B_1 deficiency, elevated calcium/phosphate product, magnesium deficiency, iron deficiency or overload, excess of certain trace elements, such as cobalt (59), and depletion of taurine in heart muscle (60). Finally, some systemic disease, such as amyloidosis or oxalosis, may involve both heart and kidneys (3).

Treatment of Heart Failure

In dialyzed children, restriction of sodium and fluid intake between dialyses is of paramount importance (61). Hemodialysis should be performed at least three times per week to allow a reasonable tolerance for intermittent fluid intake. In cases of frank congestive heart failure or severe arterial hypertension, daily hemodialysis with high ultrafiltration or hemofiltration is indicated. In some cases, especially in those associated with hypertension, peritoneal dialysis is preferred because ultrafiltration is more gradual. Anemia should be corrected by transfusions of packed red cells.

In ESRD presenting with congestive heart failure, digitalis or related drugs are indicated only when there is an insufficient response to fluid removal by hemodialysis. The effect should be evaluated primarily by clinical guidelines, i.e., the disappearance of dyspnea, tachycardia, edema, hepatomegaly, hypertension, or cardiomegaly. Few believe that digoxin should be used prophylactically in the absence of congestive heart failure if signs of diminished myocardial performance occur (28). In our experience, there are three relative indications for digitalis treatment in children with CRF: (a) before construction of a large arteriovenous communication in children with impending heart failure before the start of intermittent hemodialysis: (b) with severe hypertension (>180/140 mm Hg) that does not immediately respond to the usual emergency treatment; (c) with specific cardiac dysrhythmias, e.g., atrial flutter or paroxysmal supraventricular tachycardia.

The two cardiac glycosides currently applied in CRF are digitoxin and digoxin. Digitoxin is almost completely bound to proteins and metabolized mainly in the liver, so only 10% of the dose applied is excreted in the urine. Since in CRF decreased renal clearance of digitoxin is well compensated for by an increase in hepatobiliary clearance (62, 63), a normal loading dose can be given, whereas the maintenance dose should be slightly reduced (64). The main disadvantage of this drug is its slow elimination (half-life eight days in uremic as in normal subjects).

For this reason, we and many others prefer digoxin. The normal half-life of 34 hr for this drug is increased up to 83 hr in anuric patients (65), because about 70% is excreted by the kidneys and extrarenal clearance does not fully compensate (62). In our experience, the following schedule of digoxin administration is useful and tolerated by most children with CRF: (a) loading dose 0.04 mg/kg intravenously, divided into four equal doses given over 24 to 48 hr; (b) maintenance dose 0.01 mg/kg/day intravenously x 1/serum creatinine (mg/100 ml) given in two daily doses. When given orally, the digoxin dose must be 25% higher and should be administered twice a day. The individual tolerance varies greatly and, therefore, serum levels should be measured twice a week; frequent electrocardiogram tracings (at least daily at the commencement of therapy) are mandatory.

The upper therapeutic digoxin level in adult patients with advanced CRF ranges between 1.5 and 2.8 μg/ml (66). Any increase of serum calcium or decrease of serum potassium or magnesium concentrations may sensitize the myocardium for cardiac glycosides. Acetyl-digoxin and methyl-digoxin are similar to digoxin but are better absorbed. Elimination of digoxin by hemodialysis is low because of high tissue binding; therefore, the maintenance dose has to be reduced to 20% of normal in dialyzed patients. If any signs of digitalis overdose develop, administration must be stopped completely and, if necessary, specific antiarrhythmic treatment should be started. In any case, these drugs should be used rarely, and the period of treatment should be kept as short as possible.

Pericarditis

Uremic pericarditis is an inflammatory process; fibrin forms and an effusion ensues. It may be observed in acute renal failure or in CRF (3, 4, 67). The presence of pericarditis may be diagnosed if there is an unequivocal pericardial friction rub noted by at least two physicians or, in the absence of the rub, chest pain consistent with pericarditis and echocardiographic evidence of an effusion (68).

The incidence of uremic pericarditis in two studies of children with CRF was 12% and 9% (69, 70). Over the last decade the incidence appears to have declined. Earlier recognition and earlier more intensive therapy have contributed to the improved prognosis (3).

Three forms of uremic pericarditis can be differentiated clinically (67, 70). The first form mainly occurs in nondialyzed patients with terminal CRF, presenting with a serous effusion rapidly increasing in size to produce cardiac tamponade if dialysis is not instituted immediately. In the second form, mainly observed during the first weeks or months on dialysis, the effusion is frequently hemorrhagic but sterile, and the response to inflammatory drugs usually is good. The third form appears following a systemic bacterial infection; usually more than 6 months after start of dialysis, the fluid effusion is purulent, and the prognosis is poor.

Clinical Manifestations

In uremic pericarditis clinical manifestations vary greatly and depend largely on the size of the effusion. The classic triad of precordial pain, friction rub, and cardiac failure was observed in only 5 of 12 children with uremic pericarditis (70). Fever is almost constant and often appears before other signs. Further frequent manifestations are cardiomegaly, sudden drop of hemoglobin and increased leukocyte count (Fig. 53B.5). Hypotensive episodes in the presence of large interdialytic weight gain have been described mainly in adult patients (3). In general, clinical features of pericarditis are more severe in patients on dialysis than in those on conservative therapy (71).

A friction rub heard by auscultation and documented by phonocardiography is typical but by no means constant. It occurred in only 58% of our cases (70). In adult patients it appears to be more common, and some authors regard it as an obligatory sign (72). Characteristically, the rub becomes louder when increased pressure is applied on the stethoscope or when body position is changed. In some cases, it is transient. The heart sounds are depressed only with larger effusions.

Electrocardiographic tracings regarded as typical (ST elevation, low voltage) are rare in children with pericarditis; on the other hand, cardiac dysrhythmias are frequent. Imaging diagnostic procedures are mandatory to evaluate the presence and size of the effusion. By fluoroscopy decreased motility of the left ventricle and altered cardiac contours after change in body position are observed. The lung fields appear clear, in sharp contrast to the pulmonary congestion observed with myocardial failure. Frequently, pleural effusions coexist.

Echocardiography is the most reliable diagnostic tool, although small effusions accompanied by a typical friction rub are frequently missed (72). Circumferential effusions of more than 10 mm in diameter are regarded as relevant in older children. Thickening of the pericardium without significant echo-free space may indicate subacute constrictive pericarditis, which remains a rare complication (71). Since a significant effusion can be found in about 50% of all (adult) cases with advanced CRF by echocardiography (72), this seems to be indicated in every patient entering this stage. When used immediately before start of dialysis, echocardiography detects an effusion with a size of 100 ml or more in 14% of adult patients (73).

Pathogenesis

Uremic toxins probably play a role in the pathogenesis of pericarditis in CRF, for it is less common if dialysis is adequate and responds to increasing the frequency of dialysis (3). Bacterial infections, e.g., from the site of vascular access, are responsible especially for the late forms of pericarditis. A viral etiology has also been postulated. Heparin used during hemodialysis may perpetuate the inflammatory process, causing repeated bleedings from the inflamed pericardial surface. Fluid overload as a result of intolerance to ultrafiltration may contribute. Uremic pericarditis has so far not been reported in children on CAPD. The pathogenetic role of an increased calcium-phosphorus product and of hyperparathyroidism is still in doubt (4, 72).

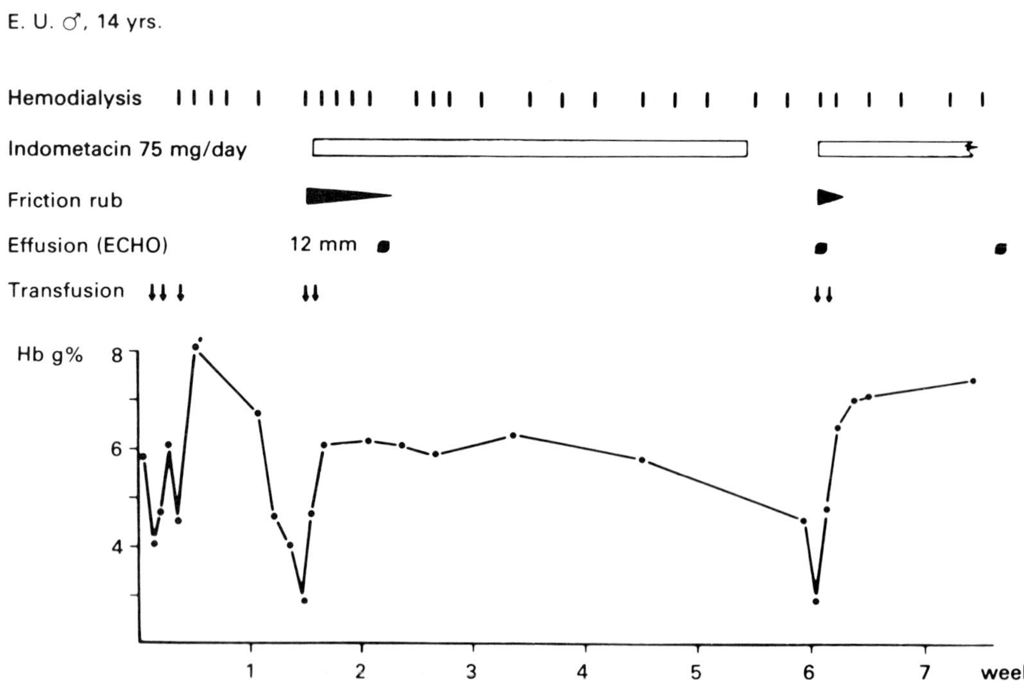

Figure 53B.5. Course of uremic pericarditis in a 14-yr-old boy who started hemodialysis treatment four weeks before onset of clinical signs. Course consists of fever, precordial pain, cardiomegaly, and sudden fall of Hb level; blood transfusions required before a friction rub and diagnosis of an effusion by echocardiography. Treatment by daily hemodialysis and indomethacin. After indomethacin was discontinued, pericarditis recurred following a fall in Hb.

Treatment and Prognosis

The treatment of uremic pericarditis is controversial. Bed rest and fluid restriction seem to be appropriate. Regular dialysis resolves pericarditis in 70% of cases. If pericarditis is discovered under dialysis treatment, daily sessions are indicated for one to two weeks, preferably with small-volume saline-primed dialyzers to avoid large changes in the intravascular volume (71). Regional or minimal heparinization should replace the systemic use of heparin, or the patient may be switched to peritoneal dialysis. Some authors, however, do not believe that increased dialysis is useful in patients who are already adequately dialyzed (68).

The additional use of antiinflammatory drugs is advocated for those patients who have no evidence of sepsis, high fever, or low blood pressure and still have significant effusion after three days of daily dialysis. Oral treatment by corticosteroids rapidly affects clinical signs but possibly promotes chronic constrictive pericarditis. Prednisone (1 mg/kg/day) appears to have a favorable effect, especially in severely ill patients on dialysis (70, 71). The administration of indomethacin (3 mg/kg/day) was reported to be successful in 50% to 87% of cases, but gastrointestinal side effects may limit its use (74). In a recent double-blind study using indomethacin, no favorable effect on uremic pericarditis was reported except for better temperature control (68). Both antiinflammatory drugs should be continued for at least three weeks because of the high tendency for recurrence (Fig. 53B.5). Digitalis is indicated for myocardial failure. If an infection cannot be excluded, antibiotics should be administered.

Operative intervention is indicated in patients with impending tamponade or with persistent large pericardial effusions unresponsive to dialytic and medical therapy. In these patients, a more aggressive approach should not be delayed; three of five children with cardiac tamponade died in our unit before 1975 when facilities were not yet satisfactory for intervention. Anterior pericardiectomy is the procedure preferred by most authors (3). Pericardiocentesis may be life-saving in acute cases with impending tamponade. It has a high rate of traumatic complications. A catheter is inserted 2 to 3 cm below the xiphoid process on the left of the median line and advanced immediately below the sternum in the direction of the right atrium. Concomitant electrocardiographic monitoring and cardiac resuscitation facilities are mandatory (71).

The prognosis of uremic pericarditis depends on the size and content of the effusion. Patients presenting with small amounts of pericardial fluid rarely develop major complications, whereas moderate or large effusions in dialyzed patients require invasive interventions (72). On conservative treatment the chest pain usually disappears within a few days, but the rub takes longer to subside (68). Recurrent episodes of pericarditis were noted in about a third of all patients (70).

Cardiac tamponade has become rare in recent years but may be life-threatening (69, 70, 75, 76). The signs of tamponade are more likely to develop in the presence of prolonged pain and rub, but the latter may also disappear while the amount of effusion is increasing (71). Clinically, impending tamponade is characterized by dyspnea relieved in the lateral supine position, severe precordial pain, lethargy, hypotension, tachycardia, paradoxical pulse, disappearance or drop of systolic blood pressure by 15 mm Hg during inspiration, congested neck veins, hepatomegaly, and diminished heart sounds with or without a rub. Tamponade is the most frequent cause of death, followed by cardiac arrhythmias and cardiac failure due to concomitant myocardial damage. Constrictive forms of uremic pericarditis have not been described in children.

The death rate due to pericarditis has declined remarkably in recent years, from 50% to 6–10% in adult patients (4, 71). From our experience it appears that the severity of uremic pericarditis and number of deaths caused by it have also decreased recently in children (77).

Hypertension

Prevalence and Causes

Most children with CRF develop some degree of hypertension during the course of illness (78, 79). In our experience, 79% of 119 children with moderate or severe degrees of CRF had high blood pressure or required antihypertensive drugs before dialysis was started (80) (Table 53B.3). Frequency and severity of hypertension vary considerably, depending on the primary renal disorder, the stage of renal dysfunction, and the mode of treatment. In children with glomerular disease or with reflux nephropathy, blood pressure tends usually to be higher than in those with most congenital kidney disorders (see Chapter 46). In the terminal stage, only a few patients retain a normal blood pressure. On regular hemodialysis 40% of our patients remained hypertensive or needed antihypertensive drugs, but the need for antihypertensive therapy rapidly declined with longer duration of treatment (79). After kidney transplantation, the proportion of children with above normal pressure readings ranges between 60% and 93% (81, 82).

Pathogenesis

The pathomechanisms leading to hypertension with progressive CRF have been reviewed recently (82, 83, 84) and are summarized in Fig. 53B.6. The main hemodynamic alteration responsible for hypertension in CRF is an increase in peripheral vascular resistance relative to the normal or high cardiac output. The development of hypertension is largely responsible for the myocardial dysfunction (Fig. 53B.7).

Table 53B.3.
Frequency and Course of Hypertension in 119 Children with CRF (GFR < 40 ml/min/1.73 m² before Dialysis) in Relation to Primary Renal Disease (University Children's Hospital, Heidelberg, 1970–1978)

	Number of patients		Number of patients with hypertensive crises	Mean Scr (mg/dl)[a] (number of patients analyzed in brackets)
	Total	Persistent hypertension		
Glomerulopathies	23	21	10	1.1 (17)
Chronic pyelonephritis with or without urinary tract malformations	29	23	6	2.4 (22)
Segmental renal hypoplasia	11	10	8	1.6 (10)
Renal hypoplasia with oligomeganephronia	14	9	0	4.4 (9)
Nephronophthisis	18	12	0	4.0 (11)
Polycystic kidneys	5	4	2	1.0 (4)
Other and unknown nephropathies	19	15	4	2.8 (14)

The mean values for serum creatinine (Scr) relate to the commencement of persistent hypertension.

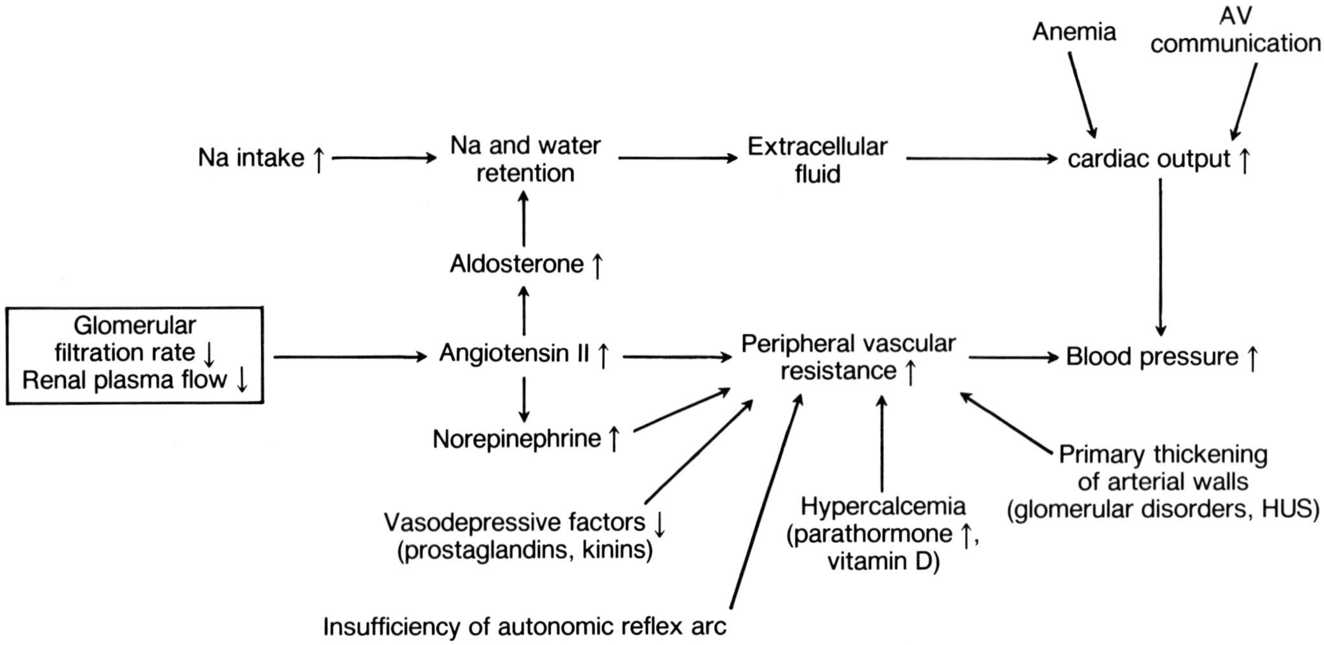

Figure 53B.6. Main pathogenetic factors leading to hypertension in chronic renal failure.

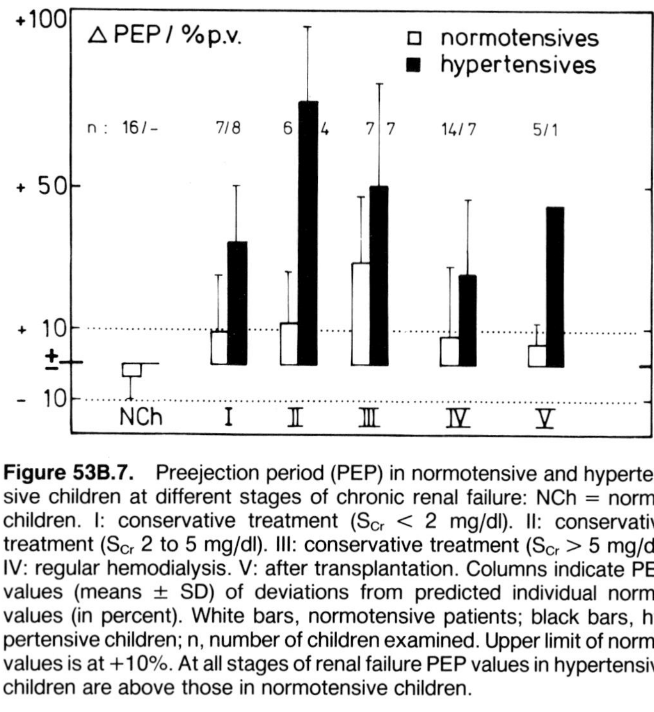

Figure 53B.7. Preejection period (PEP) in normotensive and hypertensive children at different stages of chronic renal failure: NCh = normal children. I: conservative treatment (S_{Cr} < 2 mg/dl). II: conservative treatment (S_{Cr} 2 to 5 mg/dl). III: conservative treatment (S_{Cr} > 5 mg/dl). IV: regular hemodialysis. V: after transplantation. Columns indicate PEP values (means ± SD) of deviations from predicted individual normal values (in percent). White bars, normotensive patients; black bars, hypertensive children; n, number of children examined. Upper limit of normal values is at +10%. At all stages of renal failure PEP values in hypertensive children are above those in normotensive children.

The predominant factor in the pathogenesis of hypertension in CRF is salt and water overload (84, 85). In children with CRF, before and after the start of dialysis, we found a close correlation between circulating blood volume and mean arterial pressure (86).

A secondary pathogenetic factor is excessive renin release from the kidneys. In most cases of hypertension in CRF it seems to be less important than volume overload, although plasma renin activity (PRA) and blood pressure are correlated when PRA is profiled against blood-volume and exchangeable sodium (87). For any given exchangeable sodium PRA, is on the average, more than twice as high in dialyzed adults with CRF and hypertension than it is in normal subjects (88). On the other hand, the response of renin secretion to upright stature or volume depletion during dialysis appears to be diminished in terminal uremia, probably because of autonomic insufficiency of the juxtaglomerular apparatus (83). In the preterminal stage of children with CRF, PRA ranged from low to extremely high values (89). Increased PRA is found in a high proportion of children with segmental renal hypoplasia (86), chronic glomerulonephritis, hemolytic uremic syndrome (90), and pyelonephritic shrunken kidneys (91). Children with CRF caused by nephronopthisis also tend to have high PRA levels, even in the presence of normal blood pressure, probably in response to excessive sodium loss; this hyperreninemia may persist in the ESRD when sodium wasting is no longer present (58). Stimulation of the renin-angiotensin system is an important cause of hypertension in the small group of hypertensive CRF patients with very high PRA levels who are refractory to salt depletion but normalize their blood pressure after bilateral nephrectomy (83).

PRA rises during hemodialysis and may sustain hypertension, since angiotensin levels are slow to fall while the patient is reaccumulating volume (92).

Basal levels of PRA and aldosterone did not differ significantly from control values in 15 children on hemodialysis, although a range from very low to high values was noted (58). Predialysis values for vasopressin concentration were significantly increased, whereas noradrenalin and adrenalin concentration, contrary to reports in adult patients, were normal. During dialysis sessions, PRA and catecholamine levels significantly increased while plasma aldosterone showed variable responses (93). There was a significant correlation between PRA and plasma aldosterone in children with terminal CRF, indicating that the renin-angiotensin system is a major determinant of aldosterone secretion even in ESRD. In this study blood pressure correlated only with PRA (post dialysis) but not with the other vasoactive hormones, which again stresses the prominent role of the renin-angiotensin system for blood pressure control in ESRD (58). (See also Chapter 16).

Disturbances of the sympathetic nervous system may contribute to hypertension as well as to orthostatic and dialysis-associated hypotension in CRF (87, 94). In pediatric patients the function of the autonomic nervous system has not been examined in detail; however, plasma levels of adrenalin and noradrenalin in children on regular dialysis treatment are not significantly different from controls, and the response to the volume depletion by hemodialysis and hemofiltration is adequate (58). Therefore, other factors must be sought to explain the hypotensive episodes frequently encountered during dialysis (84).

The mechanisms of posttransplant hypertension are multiple (81, 82). In the immediate postoperative period volume overload is frequently caused by administration of salt, water, and colloid, as well as glucocorticoids. Renin-mediated hypertension may occur.

Treatment

In the predialytic stage of CRF, control of hypertension is critical in delaying the progression of renal insufficiency. The principles of dietary and medical treatments are outlined in Chapter 49 and reviewed elsewhere (79, 82). Drug dosage should be adjusted according to the degree of renal dysfunction and the concomitant changes in half-life for each individual drug. In practice, a combination therapy using furosemide, propranolol, and hydralazine has proved to be appropriate for most children in the predialytic stage of CRF who are not responding to a single drug. In severe forms of hypertension resistant to conventional drug therapy captopril (95, 96) and minoxidil (97) have been used successfully. Unfortunately, side effects of these drugs are often severe, even with reduced dosages. Captopril may precipitate the further loss of renal function (98) (Chapter 17).

In the few hypertensive children with ESRD who resist any drug therapy, especially in the presence of very high PRA levels, dialysis treatment is mandatory. The main indication for dialysis (or hemofiltration) in such cases is intractable heart failure. Drug therapy should continue on regular dialysis as long as pressure readings are above normal values. Frequently, it is necessary to omit one dose of antihypertensives scheduled immediately before or during dialysis time in order to avoid hypotensive episodes.

In the majority of patients undergoing intermittent hemodialysis, ultrafiltration to dry weight is able to normalize blood pressure. Adequacy of dialysis should be checked regularly and the appropriate value of dry weight carefully evaluated. If necessary, additional fluid removal must be obtained by reducing interdialytic fluid intake, increasing ultrafiltration pressures, using dialyzers with larger surface areas or more effective dialytic membranes, lowering sodium concentration in the dialysate, or removing any additional factors that might increase pressure activity, e.g., ephedrine nose drops or large arteriovenous fistulae (61).

Only a few children with terminal CRF have such severe forms of hypertension that they cannot be controlled by appropriate dialysis with ultrafiltration and antihypertensive drugs. The proportion of such cases in adults is <5% (83). Frequently, these patients suffer from congestive heart failure, severe retinopathy, encephalopathy, wasting, and excessive thirst due to stimulation of the renin-angiotensin system.

References

1. Broyer M, Donckerwolcke RA, Brunner FP, et al: Combined report on regular dialysis and transplantation of children in Europe XII 1982. Proc EDTA 20:79, 1983.
2. O'Regan S: Cardiovascular abnormalities in pediatric patients with ESRD. In Fine RN, Gruskin AB (eds): End-stage Renal Disease in Children. Philadelphia, WB Saunders, 1984, p 359.
3. Comty CM, Shapiro FL: Cardiac complications of regular dialysis therapy. In Drukker W, Parsons FM, Maher JF (eds): Replacement of Renal Function by Dialysis. Boston, M. Nijhoff, 1983, p 595.
4. Drüeke T, Le Pailleur C, Zingraff J, Jungers P: Uremic cardiomyopathy and pericarditis. Adv Nephrol 9:33, 1980.
5. del Greco F: Cardiomyopathy and congestive heart failure. In Massry SG, Glassock RJ (eds): Textbook of Nephrology. Baltimore, Williams and Wilkins, 1983, p 732.
6. Ulmer HE: Das Herz bei chronischer Niereninsuffizienz im Kindesalter. Heidelberg, Germany, University of Heidelberg, 1978, professorial thesis.
7. Ulmer HE, Heupel EW, Schärer K: Long-term evaluation of cardiac function utilizing systolic time intervals in children with chronic renal failure. Int J Pediatr Nephrol 3:79, 1982.
8. Dongradi G, Dubois D, Becourt G, et al: Function myocardique de l'hémodialyse chronique: evaluation par mesure des intervalles de temps systoliques. Nouv Presse Méd 6:2039, 1977.
9. Blanchard WB, Fennell RS, Buciarelli RL, Victoria BE: Echocardiographic patterns in children and adolescents with chronic renal failure. Int J Pediatr Nephrol 1:222, 1980.
10. Ulmer HE, Greiner H, Schüler HW, Schärer K: Cardiovascular impairment and physical working capacity in children with chronic renal failure. Acta Paediatr Scand 67: 43, 1978.
11. Ono M: Exercise capacity of children with chronic renal failure. Japan J Nephrol 21:1089, 1979.
12. Bonzel KE, Weiss M, Mehls O, Schärer K: Aerobic capacity and maximal physical performance in children and adolescents on regular dialysis. Eur J Pediatr 141:262, 1984 (abstract).
13. Diskin CJ, Salzsieder KH, Solomon RJ, et al: Electrocardiographic changes following dialysis. Nephron 27:94, 1981.
14. Ono K, Hisana Y, Kikawa K: Effect of dialysate sodium concentration on the appearance of ischemic EKG patterns. Nephron 33:182, 1983.
15. Weber H, Schwarzer C, Stummvoll HK, et al: Chronic hemodialysis: high risk patients for arrhythmias? Nephron 37:180, 1984.
16. Storstein O, Örjavik O: Aortic insufficiency in chronic renal failure. Acta Med Scand 203:175, 1978.
17. Lewis BS, Milne F, Goldberg B: Left ventricular function in chronic renal failure. Br Heart I 38:1229, 1976.
18. Del Greco F, Simon NM, Goguska J, Walker C: Hemodynamic studies in chronic uremia. Circulation 40:87, 1969.
19. Capelli JP, Kasparian H: Cardiac work demands and left ventricular function in end-stage renal disease. Ann Int Med 86:261, 1977.
20. Pedersen T, Rasmussen K, Cleemann-Rasmussen K: Effect of hemodialysis on cardiac performance and transmural myocardial perfusion. Clin Nephrol 19:31, 1983.
21. Ikram H, Lynn KL, Bailey RR, Little PJ: Cardiovascular changes in chronic hemodialysis patients. Kidney Int 24:371, 1983.
22. Cohen MV, Diaz P, Scheuer J: Echocardiographic assessment of left ventricular function in patients with chronic anemia. Clin Nephrol 12:156, 1979.
23. Ulmer HE, Gilli G, Schärer K: Assessment of uremic cardiomyopathy in childhood by systolic time intervals. Pediatr Res 10:897, 1976 (abstract).
24. Ulmer HE, Knapp WH, Schärer K: Exercise tests and echocardiography in children with chronic renal failure. Pediatr Res 9:855, 1975 (abstract).
25. O'Regan S, Villemand D, Revillon L, et al: Effects of hemodialysis on myocardial function in pediatric patients. Nephron 25:214, 1980.
26. Potter P, Larsen D, Leumann E, et al: Treatment of chronic uremia in childhood. II. Hemodialysis. Pediatrics 46:678, 1970.
27. Ulmer HE, Heupel EW, Weckesser G: Mechanocardiographic assessment of systolic time intervals in normal children. Basic Res Cardiol 77:197, 1982.
28. Trznadel K, Luciak M, Wyszogrodzka M: The left ventricular systolic function after digoxin administration in patients with chronic renal failure. Clin Nephrol 13:231, 1980.
29. Schott CR, Le Sor JF, Kotler MN, et al: The spectrum of echocardiographic findings in chronic renal failure. Cardiovasc Med 3:215, 1978.
30. Miach PJ, Dawborn JK, Louis WJ, McDonald IG: Left ventricular function in uremia: echocardiographic assessment in patients on maintenance dialysis. Clin Nephrol 15:259, 1981.
31. Mehta BR, Ireland MA, Shin MF: Echocardiographic evaluation of cardiac size and function in dialysis patients. Clin Nephrol 20:61, 1983.
32. Palcoux JB, Palcoux MC, Jonan JP, et al: Echocardiographic patterns in infants and children with chronic renal failure. Int J Pediatr Nephrol 3:311, 1982.
33. Fischbach M, de Geeter B, Kieny R, Geisert J: Echocardiographic evaluation of children with chronic renal failure. Int J Pediatr Nephrol 2:148, 1981 (abstract).
34. O'Regan S, Matina D, Ducharme G, Davignon A: Echocardiographic assessment of cardiac function in children with chronic renal failure. Kidney Int 24 (suppl)16:S77, 1983.
35. Abbasi AS, Slaughter JC, Allen MW: Asymmetric septal hypertrophy in chronic hemodialysis patients. Circulation 54 (suppl II):190, 1976
36. Drukker A, Urbach J, Glaser J: Hypertrophic cardiomyopathy with end-stage renal disease and hypertension. Proc EDTA 18:542, 1981.
37. Neff MS, Kim KE, Persoff M, et al: Hemodynamics of uremic anemia. Circulation 43:876, 1971.
38. Révillon L, O'Regan S, Robitaille P, et al: The effects of Brescia-Cimino fistulas on cardiac function in transplanted pediatric patients. Clin Nephrol 12:26, 1979.

39. Kult J, Holtz G, Grosswendt J, Klütsch K: Der Anteil des Shunt-Volumens am Herzminutenvolumen bei regelmäßig hämodialysierten Patienten. Verh Dtsch Gesellsch Inn Med 77:1143, 1973.
40. Von Bibra H, Castro L, Autenrieth G, et al: The effects of arteriovenous shunts on cardiac function in renal dialysis patients—an echocardiographic evaluation. Clin Nephrol 9:205, 1978.
41. Andersen CB, Codd JR, Craff GM, et al: Cardiac failure and upper extremity arteriovenous dialysis fistulas. Arch Intern Med 136:292, 1976.
42. O'Regan S, Villemant D, Ducharme G, et al: Effects of Brescia-Cimino fistulae on myocardial function in pediatric patients. Dial Transpl 10:202, 1981.
43. Scigalla P, Devaux S, Zoellner K, Grossmann P: Erfahrungen mit verschiedenen Gefäßzugängen für die chronische Hämodialyse im Kindesalter. Dtsch Ges Wesen 30:133, 1975.
44. Erasmi H, Horsch S, Bodon P, et al: Shunt surgery in childhood. In Bulla M (ed): Renal Insufficiency in Children. Berlin, Heidelberg, New York, Springer 1982, p 169.
45. Gagnadoux MF, Pased B, Bronstein M, et al: Arteriovenous fistulae in small children. Dial Transpl 9:318, 1980.
46. Bornstein A, Gaasch WH, Harrington J: Assessment of the cardiac effects of hemodialysis with systolic time intervals and echocardiography. Am J Cardiol 51:332, 1983.
47. Gilmartin JJ, Duffy BS, Finnegan P, McCready N: Non-invasive study of left ventricular function in chronic renal failure before and after hemodialysis. Clin Nephrol 20:55, 1983.
48. Hung J, Harris PJ, Uren RF, et al: Uremic cardiomyopathy—effect of hemodialysis on left ventricular function in end-stage renal failure. N Engl J Med 302:547, 1980.
49. Chen TS, Freidman MS, Smith AJ, Del Monte ML: Hemodynamic changes during hemodialysis: role of dialysate. Clin Nephrol 20:190, 1983.
50. Kramer W, Wizemann V, Kindler M, et al: Influence of fluid removal rate during hemodialysis on left ventricular performance and exercise tolerance in patients with coronary artery disease. Clin Nephrol 21:280, 1984.
51. Cini G, Camici M, Pentimone F, Palla R: Echocardiographic hemodynamic study during ultrafiltration sequential dialysis. Nephron 30:124, 1982.
52. Baldamus CA, Ernst W, Frei U, Koch FM: Sympathetic and hemodynamic response to volume removal during different forms of renal replacement therapy. Nephron 31:324, 1982.
53. Leenen FHH, Smith DL, Khanna R, Oreopoulos DG: Changes in left ventricular anatomy and function on CAPD. Perit Dial Bull 3 (suppl):S26, 1983.
54. Lai KN, Barnden L, Mathew TH: Effect of renal transplantation on left ventricular function in hemodialysis patients. Clin Nephrol 18:74, 1982.
55. O'Regan S, Douste-Blazy MY, Ducharme G, et al: Renal transplantation and cardiac function in pediatric patients. Clin Nephrol 17:237, 1982.
56. Kreusser W, Klocker P, Rambausek M, Ritz E: Digitalis treatment in uremic patients. Contr Nephrol 41:255, 1984.
57. McGonigle RJS, Fowler MB, Timmis AB, et al: Uremic cardiomyopathy: potential role of vitamin D and parathyroid hormone. Nephron 36:94, 1984.
58. Rauh W, Hund E, Sohl G, et al: Vasoactive hormones in children with chronic renal failure. Kidney Int 24 (suppl 15):S-27, 1983.
59. Pehrsson SK, Lins LE: The role of trace elements in uremic heart failure. Nephron 34:93, 1983.
60. Michalk DE, Essich HJ, Böhles HJ, Schärer K: Taurine metabolism in experimental renal failure. Kidney Int 24 (suppl 15):S-16, 1983.
61. Donckerwolcke RA, Chantler C, Broyer M: Paediatric dialysis. In Drukker W, Parsons FM, Maher JF (eds): Replacement of Renal Function by Dialysis, ed 2. Boston, M Nijhoff, p 514.
62. Kramer P, Stroh E, Matthei D, et al: Increased digitalis tolerance in uremic patients. In Bodem G, Dengler HJ (eds): Cardiac Glycosides. Berlin, Heidelberg, New York, Springer 1978, p 304.
63. Grabensee B, Peters U, Risler T, Grosse-Brockhoff F: Digitoxin and digoxin in patients with chronic renal failure and on hemodialysis. In Bodem G, Dengler HJ (eds): Cardiac Glycosides. Berlin, Heidelberg, New York, Springer 1978, p 317.
64. Kreusser W, Mann J, Rambausek M, et al: Cardiac function in experimental uremia. Kidney Int 24 (suppl 15):S-83, 1983.
65. Ohnhaus EE, Vozeh S, Nüesch E: Absolute bioavailability of digoxin in chronic renal failure. Clin Nephrol 11:302, 1979.
66. Kramer W, Wizemann V, Kindler M, et al: Influence of fluid removal rate during hemodialysis on left ventricular performance and exercise tolerance in patients with coronary artery disease. Clin Nephrol 21:280, 1984.
67. Comty CM, Wathen RL, Shapiro FL: Uremic pericarditis. In Spodick DH (ed): Pericardial Diseases, Cardiovascular Clinics vol 7.3. Philadelphia, WB Saunders, 1976, p 219.
68. Spector D, Alfred H, Siedlecki M, Briefel G: A controlled study of the effect of indomethacin in uremic pericarditis. Kidney Int 24:670, 1983.
69. Gusmano R, Perfumo F, Formicucci L, Bertolini A: La pericarditide uremica in età pediatrica. Minerva Nefrol 24:239, 1977.
70. Ulmer HE, Gilli G, Schärer K: Urämische Perikarditis im Kindesalter. Nieren—und Hochdruckkrankh 9:193, 1980.
71. Shapiro FL, Comty CM: Pericarditis. In Massry SG, Glassock RJ (eds): Textbook of Nephrology. Baltimore, Williams and Wilkins, 1983, p 727.
72. Luft FC, Gilman IK, Weyman AE: Pericarditis in the patient with uremia: clinical and echocardiographic evaluation. Nephron 25:160, 1980.
73. Wray TM, Stone WJ: Uremic pericarditis: a prospective echocardiographic and clinical study. Clin Nephrol 6:295, 1976.
74. Minuth ANW, Nottebohm GA, Eknoyan G, Suki WN: Indomethacin treatment of pericarditis in chronic hemodialysis patients. Arch Intern Med 135:807, 1975.
75. Cohen EN, Brewer HW, Kaye M: Peritoneal dialysis for the treatment of pericorditis. Can Med Assoc J 102:1365, 1970.
76. Chaimovitz C, Abinader E, Bendely A, Better OS: Uremic cardiac tamponade in children. Am J Dis Child 122:172, 1971.
77. Ulmer HE, Brass H, Rupp M: Urämische Perikarditis. In Franz HE (ed): Blutreinigungsverfahren. Technik und Klinik ed 2. Stuttgart, Thieme, 1981, p 200.
78. Loirat C, Pillion G, Blum C: Hypertension in children: present data and problems. Adv Nephrol 11:65, 1982.
79. Schärer K, Rauh W, Ulmer HE: The management of hypertension in children with chronic renal failure. In Giovannelli G, New MI, Gorini S (eds): Hypertension in Children and Adolescents. New York, Raven Press, 1981, p 239.
80. Schärer K: Renal hypertension in childhood. Ann Nestlé 42:1, 1984.
81. Fennell RS III, Zalenski R, Geary DF, et al: Hypertension in a pediatric and adolescent population following kidney transplantation. Int J Pediatr Nephrol 2:89, 1981.
82. Ingelfinger JR: Hypertension in children. In Fine RN, Gruskin AB: End-stage Renal Disease in Children. Philadelphia, WB Saunders, 1984, p 340.
83. Weidmann P: Hypertension. In Massry SG, Glassock RJ (eds): Textbook of Nephrology. Baltimore, Williams and Wilkins, 1983, p 738.
84. White RP, Rubin AL: Blood pressure-control in chronic dialysis patients. In Drukker W, Parsons FM, Maher JF (eds): Replacement of Renal Function by Dialysis, ed 2. Amsterdam, M Nijhoff, 1983, p 575.
85. Schalekamp MADH, Schalekamp-Kuyken MPA, De Moor-Fruytier M, et al: Interrelationship between blood pressure, renin, renin substrate and blood volume in terminal renal failure. Clin Sci Mol Med 45:417, 1973.
86. Rauh W, Müller-Wiefel DE, Heide B, Schärer K: Hypertension bei chronischer Niereninsuffizienz im Kindesalter. Monatsschr Kinderheilk 125:1375, 1977.
87. Lilley JJ, Golden J, Slone RA: Adrenergic regulation of blood pressure in chronic renal failure. J Clin Invest 57:1190, 1976.
88. Weidmann P, Beretta-Piccoli C, Steffen F, et al: Hypertension in terminal renal failure. Kidney Int 9:294, 1976.
89. Rauh W, Oertel PJ: Endocrine function in children with ESRD. In Fine RN, Gruskin AB (eds): End-stage Renal Disease in Children. Philadelphia, WB Saunders, 1984, p 296.
90. Grunfeld B, Gimenez M, Liapchuc S, et al: Systemic hypertension and plasma renin activity in children with the hemolytic-uremic syndrome. Int J Pediatr Nephrol 3:211, 1982.
91. Dillon MJ, Smellie J, Shah V: Peripheral plasma renin activity, hypertension and renal scarring in children. In Hudson CJ, Heptinstall RH, Winberg T (eds): Reflux Nephropathy: update 1983. Contr. Nephrol 39:68, 1984.
92. Textor SC, Gavras H, Tifft CP, et al: Norepinephrine and renin activity in chronic renal failure: evidence for interacting roles in hemodialysis hypertension. Hypertension 3:294, 1981.
93. Ghione S, Fommei E, Clerico A, et al: Major determinants of plasma aldosterone levels in chronic uremia on dialytic treatment. Nephron 30:110, 1982.
94. Campese VM, Romoff MS, Levitan D, et al: Mechanisms of autonomic nervous system dysfunction in uremia. Kidney Int 20:246, 1981.
95. Bacri JL, Dechaux M, André JL et al: Captopril et hypertension artérielle sévère de l'enfant. Arch Fr Pédiatr 38:887, 1981.
96. Sinaiko AR, Mirkin BL, Hendrick DA, et al: Antihypertensive effect and elimination kinetics of captotril in hypertensive children with renal disease. J Pediatr 103:799, 1983.
97. Andreucci VE, Usberti M, Federico S, et al: Long-term follow-up of minoxidil therapy in refractory hypertension. A prospective trial in patients with various degrees of renal insufficiency. Clin Nephrol 19:55, 1983.
98. Colavita RD, Gaudio KM, Siegel NJ: Reversible reduction in renal function during treatment with captopril. Pediatrics 71:839, 1983.

53C Neurological Problems

RICHARD S. TROMPETER

The association between abnormal renal function and central nervous system (CNS) disease was recognized over 30 yr ago (1). Seizures and coma were frequent complications of acute uremia, whereas peripheral neuropathy and uremic encephalopathy were observed in progressive uremia, which was frequently terminal. In spite of the improvement in the quality and duration of life brought about by dialysis and transplantation, patients with renal failure continue to manifest a variety of neurological disorders. Patients with chronic renal failure (CRF), in whom dialysis is not yet a requirement, may exhibit neurological symptoms, including weakness, memory loss, an inability to concentrate, apathy, and lethargy. Such patients may also have peripheral neuropathy.

UREMIC NEUROPATHY

The polyneuropathy associated with CRF has long been recognized but before chronic dialysis became available, most patients with end-stage renal disease (ESRD) did not live long enough to develop a clinically apparent neuropathy. The overt clinical polyneuropathy is rarely recognized in early childhood. Uremic neuropathy is a distal, symmetrical, mixed polyneuropathy. Motor and sensory modalities are affected, and the lower limbs are most severely involved. The classic early manifestations include the "restless leg syndrome" characterized by a pricking sensation and pruritus. Muscle weakness and irritability are frequently encountered in undialyzed patients, often heralded by a loss of the deep tendon reflexes, particularly knee and ankle jerks. Sensory loss takes the form of "stocking and glove" anesthesia and includes the loss of pain, light touch, vibration, and pressure. Uremic neuropathy is not limited to impaired motor and sensory function; autonomic dysfunction is not uncommon, usually associated with postural hypotension and impaired sweating (2). Dialysis-related hypotension also has been associated with autonomic insufficiency (3).

The pathological changes associated with peripheral nerve pathology in uremia consist of axonal degeneration and segmental demyelination. There is a decrease in the number of nerve fibers and the thickness of individual fibers, in addition to a loss of myelin. Whether axonal degeneration or demyelination is the primary pathological event remains unresolved. Marked slowing of nerve conduction velocity and frequent improvement of symptoms following hemodialysis or transplantation tends to favor segmental demyelination as the primary lesion. Information on this problem in children on long-term hemodialysis is scarce, but recent opinion suggests nerve conduction defects are rare (4). The usefulness of motor nerve conduction velocity as an index of peripheral neuropathy is restricted by the day-to-day variation in conduction velocity from normal to abnormally low in the same individual.

UREMIC ENCEPHALOPATHY

The earliest sign of uremic encephalopathy is a nonspecific general depression of cerebral function. Vague headaches are common, and typically, periods of alertness and a feeling of well-being alternate with periods of depression and altered behavior. As renal function deteriorates, the signs of encephalopathy become more pronounced, with generalized weakness, anorexia, muscle cramps, asterixis, and speech disorders. A toxic psychosis mimicking any form of psychiatric illness also may develop. Further progression of renal failure may be associated with a seizure disorder and focal neurological signs may present, including disorders of cranial nerve function, cerebellar ataxia, and transient motor deficits, such as monoplegia, diplegia, or hemiplegia.

The cerebral changes associated with uremia are nonspecific and not infrequently relate to the underlying disease. Subdural hemorrhages occur in 1% to 3% of patients on dialysis, and intracerebral hemorrhages are present in approximately 6% of dialyzed patients who die, usually from causes associated with hypertension (5). No specific histological changes are found in the brain of uremic patients, but a generalized neuronal degeneration is frequently present, although variable in its location. Areas of necrosis and small intracerebral hemorrhages are seen in about 10% of uremic patients and focal glial proliferation in 2%.

Electroencephalograms (EEG) have been studied in many patients with CRF and demonstrate a generalized slowing of background frequencies, loss of normal α-rhythm, a shift in the percentage of frequencies from higher (>9 Hz) to lower (<7 Hz), and an increase in the index of spike and wave activity. After approximately six months of dialysis therapy or following successful renal transplantation, the EEG reverts to a normal pattern (6a).

Psychometric studies have shown that there is intellectual impairment in most dialysis patients with chronic renal insufficiency (CRI) (6). The resultant loss of intellectual function is influenced mainly by a deterioration in the performance IQ. Recently, the development of progressive CNS dysfunction in 20 of 23 children who developed CRI during the first year of life has been described (7). Whether this was caused by a neurotoxin, associated malnutrition, or severe electrolyte imbalance remains unclear; so far, similar experience has not been reported from other centers.

Pathophysiology

The cause of uremic encephalopathy and uremic polyneuropathy is uncertain, but most theories involve the role of one or more "uremic toxins" (8). The physiological and biochemical changes that occur as a consequence of renal failure are complicated, and there is a lack of correlation between the development and severity of neurological dysfunction and the levels of any single biochemical constituent in plasma or dialysate. The success of dialysis in reversing certain neurological manifestations of uremia was the basis for the theory of the toxic effects of low-molecular-weight dialyzable compounds, the so-called "middle molecules" (9). This hypothesis is controversial; experimental evidence from work in animals and human disputes it (10). One large group of toxic substances accumulating in the plasma and tissues of the uremic patient represent the end-product of protein metabolism (Table 53C.1). Increased catabolism and decreased excretion are responsible for their accumulation; however, attempts to reproduce the symptoms of uremia by injecting any one of these agents have been unsuccessful.

The severity of uremic encephalopathy correlates poorly with the degree of biochemical abnormalities in plasma. Acidosis is a constant feature of the uremic state, and cerebral acidosis has been suggested as a possible mechanism of encephalopathy; however, the pH of cerebrospinal fluid obtained from uremic patients is usually normal. The inhibition of cerebral enzyme activity, in particular ATPase, may have a direct bearing in the decrease in sodium flux and increase in potassium flux found in the brains of uremic individuals. The inhibition of ATPase by substance, such as methylguanidine and the phenolic acids, may predispose to the accumulation of inorganic phosphate, an anion that may act as neurotoxin in the uremic patient.

The elevated plasma concentrations of potential uremic toxins, e.g., urea, creatinine, PTH, myoinositol, transketolase, guanidine, and "middle molecules", have been correlated with motor nerve conduction velocity. To be considered a uremic toxin, the level of biochemical compound should correlate better with the measured peripheral nerve function than with the reduction of GFR. This criterion has not been satisfied to date (11).

Recent attention has focused on PTH as a potential neurotoxin (12); however, nerve conduction velocities in patients with acute or chronic renal failure are normal even in the face of high PTH levels. No beneficial effect has been noted following the recovery of renal function, chronic hemodialysis, or parathyroidectomy. Excess PTH may increase nerve and brain calcium concentration, but it is not clear whether it plays an important role in the mechanism of cerebral and nerve dysfunction.

The frequent occurrence of polyneuropathies in chronic debilitating illnesses may indicate that inadequate nutrition, vitamin deficiencies, or both may be important in the evolution of neurological symptoms in uremia. There is evidence to suggest that there is a critical period of brain growth in early infancy extending into the second year of life, during which malnutrition may produce irreversible damage (13). Clinically, the administration of high doses of water-soluble vitamins to dialysis patients has not been associated with clear evidence of improvement.

Table 53C.1
Potential "Toxins" Accumulating in Uraemia

Products of Protein Metabolism	Urea, Creatinine, Uric Acid, Free and Conjugated Amino Acids, Organic Acids, Aliphatic and Aromatic Amines, Phenols, Indoles, Myoinositol, Sorbitol, Sulfates, Polyamines, Middle Molecules.
Guanidine Compounds	Guanidine, Methylguanidine, Guanidinosuccinic Acid, Guanidinoacetic Acid, Guanidinoproprionic Acid, Guanidinobutyric Acid, Glycocyamine.
Hormones	Parathormone, Calcitonin, Glucagon, Natriuretic Hormone, Growth Hormone, Renin, Gastrin.
Metallic Ions	Aluminum, Tin, Lead, Cadmium, Zinc, Mercury, Manganese, Arsenic, Copper, Iron.
Enzyme and Vitamin Deficiencies	Transketolase, Thiamine

Dialysis Dementia and Aluminum Toxicity

In 1972, Alfrey and coworkers (14) described a progressive and fatal encephalopathy in the chronic hemodialysis patient, characterized by speech disturbances, dementia, myoclonus, asterixis, and convulsions. Postmortem studies of the CNS revealed no specific abnormalities; however, elevated Al levels have been demonstrated in the gray matter and blood of affected adults, suggesting Al intoxication as a possible cause for the encephalopathy (14, 15). Since 1977 there have been increasing reports of a similar clinical picture occurring in uremic children, none of whom were on dialysis (16–20).

The neurological signs develop gradually and within 6 to 11 months of the onset of symptoms; most patients are unable to communicate verbally. High levels of Al in the dialysate water are a consequence of the use of Al salts (alum) in water purification. Following epidemics, a decrease in the number of cases of dialysis dementia has been reported after removing Al with deionizers and reverse osmosis.

Gastrointestinal absorption following oral administration of aluminum hydroxide as a phosphate binding agent may also cause Al toxicity. To date, three cases of Al toxicity have been reported, of which two were fatal (18, 21, 22). One child died at the age of 11 months following an intractable seizure disorder, and the second died at the age of 8 yr with dementia. Serum Al levels in brain and CSF were elevated in these children, as well as serum levels in the third child, who developed a seizure disorder and dementia at the age of 31 months.

DIALYSIS DISEQUILIBRIUM SYNDROME

Dialysis disequilibrium characteristically occurs during hemodialysis, although it also may follow peritoneal dialysis and be a feature of the immediate postrenal transplantation period. The syndrome is particularly common in children (23). Using standard methods of dialysis, it is possible to correct most of the biochemical abnormalities in the uremic patient within a relatively short period of time. The efficiency of dialysis can be further increased by increasing blood or dialysate flow rates through the system, resulting in a rapid fall in the plasma urea concentration. A complex of neurological symptoms may ensue, including headache, nausea and vomiting, visual disturbances, disorientation and seizures, sometimes associated with wide swings in blood pressure.

Pathophysiology

The pathophysiology of this condition has been explained by the development of cerebral edema, which is transient. Experimental evidence has demonstrated that any osmotic gradients across the blood-brain barrier are short-lived. Arieff and associates (24), however, have postulated a rise in the intracellular osmolality of the brain caused by an unidentified solute classified as "idiogenic osmoles" (24). Early institution of dialysis, avoiding the need to lower the blood urea concentration dramatically, minimizes the risk of this complication. The prophylactic use of intravenous diazapam and infusions of mannitol (5 ml of a 20% solution of 1 g mannitol/kg body weight/hr throughout dialysis (double this concentration is given during the first hour of dialysis) are helpful in preventing disequilibrium in the previously undialyzed patient. A regimen employing short, frequent periods of dialysis combined with sequential ultrafiltration is beneficial in the management of such patients.

HYPERTENSIVE ENCEPHALOPATHY

Changes in systemic blood pressure do not materially influence cerebral blood flow. When blood pressure rises, cerebral vessels constrict; when the pressure falls they dilate and thus preserve blood flow. Severe hypertension results in a breakdown of this autoregulatory process, with resultant cerebral hyperemia that causes focal damage to the cerebral arterioles, increased permeability, and edema (25). There are no specific neurological symptoms of hypertension, and any neurological sign should be regarded as significant. Severe generalized headache is the most common complaint. Visual disturbances range from blurring of vision to transient cortical blindness, although permanent blindness due to infarction of the optic nerves has been reported in a vary small number of children (26).

Severe hypertension in childhood is most frequently secondary to renal parenchymal disease. An epileptic seizure was the initial presenting sign in over 40% of children with previously undetected arterial hypertension (27). It is encouraging that the long-term prognosis following a single episode of hypertensive encephalopathy is good, and no evidence of permanent neurologial damage is present (27).

Management

Management of the acute clinical state requires arresting the seizure activity, usually with diazapam. Intractable seizures may be treated with phenytoin, thus avoiding depression of brain stem functions (loading dose: 15 to 20 mg/kg given intravenously over 45 min in a dextrose-free vehicle to avoid the formation of microcrystals; therapeutic blood levels will be achieved for 12 hr; maintenance dose: 5 to 7 mg/kg/day in two divided doses). Regular monitoring of blood pressure is mandatory during the early stages of antihypertensive therapy to ensure gradual reduction and to avoid precipitous falls that may predispose to visual disturbances (26). Malignant hypertension is often associated with salt depletion, and saline infusion may be necessary in conjunction with vasodilatation if precipitous falls in blood pressure are to be avoided. Provided optimal control of blood pressure is achieved, the prescription of prophylactic anticonvulsants is not indicated following a single hypertensive seizure (see also Chapter 47).

COMPLICATIONS FOLLOWING RENAL TRANSPLANTATION

Neurological Disturbances

Neurological disturbances may follow the diuresis associated with a well-functioning kidney in the immediate postoperative period if the child has been inadequately dialyzed. A clinical picture analogous to that of the dialysis disequilibrium syndrome develops.

Immunosuppression with large doses of corticosteroids may cause hypertension or a toxic psychosis mimicking any form of psychiatric illness. The long-term administration of steroids may produce evidence of apparent cerebral atrophy on a brain scan, the clinical significance of which is uncertain (27).

Lymphoma

The risk of lymphoma in a patient who has received a renal transplant is about 35 times greater than normal; most such tumors are reticulum cell sarcomas (28). Of 138 cases of malignant disease reported in nearly 9000 renal transplant recipients, 10 (7.2%) had developed primary tumors of the brain after transplantation (29). Cerebral lymphoma has been reported in two patients, aged 14 and 20 yr, presenting at 5½ and 7 months, respectively, following transplantation (30) as has metastatic carcinoma to the brain from de novo malignant epithelial tumors. Lymphomas do not occur with greater frequency in patients who have received long-term immunosuppression for reasons other than transplantation, a finding that suggests factors other than chronic drug-induced immune deficiency are important. Four main hypotheses have been proposed to explain the increased incidence of cerebral tumors in transplant receipients: (a) sustained antigenic stimulation by the homograft; (b) direct damage from immunosuppressive drugs; (c) depression of normal immunological defense mechanisms; and (d) proliferation of oncogenic viruses (31).

Cytomegalovirus

Cytomegalovirus (CMV) is the most frequently diagnosed infectious complication following renal transplantation (32). Recovery of the virus can be obtained from 40% to 80% of transplant patients within the first four months after surgery. Typical neuropathological features of CMV have been found in the brains of some patients who died after renal transplantation (33). Although infection of infants and children with CMV is probably common, clinical disease is rare; to date, no clinical picture has been associated with the neuropathological findings.

Other Infections

Chronic immunosuppression favors the occurrence of other opportunistic infections as well as the reactivation of latent infections. Systemic infections with almost all types of fungi have been reported, presenting as meningitis and brain abscess. CNS involvement with toxoplasmosis has been observed, predominantly in adults presenting with the clinical features of encephalitis, meningoencephalitis, and intracerebral focal lesions.

Syndromes characterized by slowly progressive neurological disease, i.e., progressive multifocal leukoencephalopathy and central pontine myelolysis, have been recognized on postmortem studies of the brains in posttransplant patients. These histological changes may result from viral infection or from activation of a dormant virus in the CNS secondary to altered immunity in the host.

References

1. Roosen-Runge FC: Retardation of postnatal development of kidney in persons with early cerebral lesions. Am J Dis Child 77:185, 1949.
2. Tyler HR: Neurological aspects of uraemia: an overview. Kidney Int 55 (suppl 2): 188, 1975.
3. Kersh ES, Kronfield SJ, Unger A, et al: Autonomic insufficiency in uraemia as a cause of haemodialysis induced hypotension. N Engl J Med 290:650, 1974.
4. Chan CMJ, Eng G: Long-term haemodialysis and nerve conduction in children. Paediatr Res 13: 591, 1979.
5. Rotter W, Roettger P: Comparative pathologic-anatomic study of cases of chronic global renal insufficiency with and without haemodialysis. Clin Nephrol 1:257, 1974.
6. English A, Savager D, Britton PG, et al: Intellectual impairment in chronic renal failure. Br Med J 1:888, 1978.

6a. Teschan PE: On the pathogenesis of uraemia. Am J Med 48: 671, 1970.

7. Rotundo A, Nevins TE, Lipton M, et al: Progressive encephalopathy in children with renal failure. Kidney Int 21: 586, 1982.
8. Bergstrom J, Furst P: Uraemic toxins. Kidney Int 13 (suppl 8): 59, 1978.
9. Scribner BH, Farrell PC, Milutinovic J, Babb AL: Evolution of the middle molecule hypothesis. Proc 5th Int Cong Nephrol 5: 190, 1972.
10. Kjellstrand CM: Do middle molecules cause uraemic intoxication? Am J Kidney 1:51, 1981.
11. Nielson VK: The peripheral nerve function in chronic renal failure: a survey. Acta Med Scand 7 (suppl 573): 1974.
12. Massry SG: Is parathyroid hormone a uraemic toxin? Nephron 19:125, 1974.
13. Winick M: Malnutrition and brain development. J Paediatr 74:667, 1976.

14. Alfrey AC, Mishell JM, Burks J, et al: Syndrome of dyspraxia and multifocal seizures associated with chronic dialysis. Trans Am Soc Artif Organs 18: 257, 1972.
15. Alfrey AC, LeGendre GR, Kaehny WD: The dialysis encephalopathy syndrome. Possible aluminum intoxication. N Engl J Med 294:184, 1976.
16. Baluarte HR, Gruskin AB, Hiner LB, et al: Encephalopathy in children with chronic renal failure. Proc Clin Dial Transpl Forum 7:95, 1977.
17. Bale JF, Siegler RL, Bray PF: Encephalopathy in young children with moderate chronic renal failure. Am J Dis Child 134:581, 1980.
18. Nathan E, Pedersen SE: Dialysis encephalopathy in a nondialysed uraemic boy treated with aluminum hydroxide orally. Acta Paediatr Scan 69:793, 1980.
19. Geary DF, Fennell ES, Andriola M, et al: Encephalopathy in children with chronic renal failure. J Paediatr 96:41, 1980.
20. Foley C, Polinsky MS, Gruskin AB, et al: Encephalopathy in infants and children with chronic renal disease. Arch Neurol 38:656, 1981.
21. Griswood WR, Reznik V, Mendoza SA, et al: Accumulation of aluminium in a nondialyzed uraemic child receiving aluminium hydroxide. Paediatrics 71:56, 1983.
22. Randall ME: Aluminium toxicity in an infant not on dialysis. Lancet 1:1327, 1983.
23. Grushkin CM, Korsch B, Fine RN: Haemodialysis in small children. JAMA 221:869, 1972.
24. Arieff AI, Masry SG, Barrientos A, Kleeman CR: Brain water and electrolyte balance in uraemia: effects of slow and rapid haemodialysis. Kidney Int 4:177, 1973.
25. Byrom FB: The hypertensive vascular crisis. London, Heinemann, 1969, p 19.
26. Hulse JA, Taylor DSI, Dillon MJ: Blindness and paraplegia in severe childhood hypertension. Lancet 2:553, 1979.
27. Trompeter RS, Smith RL, Hoare RD, et al: Neurological complications of arterial hypertension. Arch Dis Child 57:913, 1982.
28. Hoover R, Fraumeni JF: Risk of cancer in renal transplant recipients. Lancet 1:983, 1971.
29. Jacobs C, Brunner FP, Bryngner H, et al: Malignant diseases in patients treated by dialysis and transplantation in Europe. Transpl Proc 13:729, 1981.
30. Schneck SA, Penn I: Cerebral neoplasms associated with renal transplantation. Arch Neurol 22:226, 1970.
31. Anonymous: Immunosuppression and intracerebral lymphomas. Lancet 2:143, 1971.
32. Rosenthal LJ, Clanton DJ: The involvement of human cytomegalovirus in renal transplantation. Dial Trans 10:915, 1981.
33. Shneck SA: Neuropathological features of human organ transplantation. 1. Probable cystomegalovirus infection. J Neuropathol Exp Neurol 24:415, 1965.

12

The Perinatal Period

CHAPTER 54

Development of Function in Fetal Kidney

JEAN E. ROBILLARD

INTRODUCTION

Development of human renal funtion proceeds through a series of successive and interdependent morphogenic and physiological changes.

The first evidence of a renal excretory system in the human embryo consists of individual paired tubules that arise from nephrotomes to form the pronephros. The human pronephros, which develops from the cephalic end of the nephrotome, is a rudimentary nonfunctional kidney that appears around the third week of gestation and undergoes complete involution within two weeks. The pronephros is of no significance as a functioning excretory organ since it has only a transitory existence. Its only role is to give rise to the mesonephric duct. The mesonephros arises more caudally along the nephrotome and consists of approximately 20 pairs of thick-walled tubules and glomeruli. By the fifth week of gestation the mesonephric kidneys are functional and are forming urine (1, 2). There are great variations among species in the functional contribution of the mesonephros during fetal life; however, in humans it degenerates completely by the eleventh to twelfth week of gestation as the metanephros begins functioning. The most important function of the mesonephros is to induce the formation of the ureteric bud that is required to form the metanephros. The mesonephros remains vestigial in humans and supplies tubules that become the ducts of the epididymis, the ductus deferens, and the ejaculatory duct in males. In females, the entire system regresses early in the third month to become nonfunctional vestigial ducts. A failure of mesonephric differentiation may lead to renal agenesis, renal hypoplasia, or congenital cyst and also to anomalous development of gonads and adrenal glands (see also Chapter 3).

Definite nephrons arise from the metanephros; their development depends on the interaction of the ureteric bud with the undifferentiated mesenchymal cell mass containing the contiguous nephrogenic ridges (nephrogenic blastema). Renal tubular function appears in the human metanephric kidney by about the ninth week of gestation; renal blood supply is also established by that time. By the 14th week of gestation the loop of Henle is functioning and tubular reabsorption is present. Nephron induction ceases by the thirty-sixth week of gestation and, at term, each of the human kidneys contains one million nephrons.

Knowledge of the mechanisms regulating renal function during fetal life is essential for the development of new concepts regarding fetal management during high-risk pregnancies and prevention of renal failure during the perinatal period. It is becoming evident that survival of premature infants weighing less than 1000 g is related in part to an understanding of the limitation imposed by the immature kidney. Until the last decade, knowledge of renal function in prenatal life was sparse because of the technical difficulties of obtaining reliable information from the fetus. Before development of the chronic fetal lamb preparation (3, 4), the study of fetal renal function was limited to the analysis of fetal and newborn urine (5, 6) and to the determination of renal clearances in experimental animals studied at the time of surgery (7–12). The development of the chronic fetal lamb model has permitted investigators to study the ontogeny of the fetal kidney in its normal environment without the effects of operative and anesthetic stresses.

RENAL BLOOD FLOW

The kidneys receive between 2.2% and 3.7% of the combined ventricular output in fetal lambs (13–16) and approximately 2.7% in fetal rhesus monkeys and baboons (17, 18). It also has been shown that the renal blood flow (RBF) is low during the last trimester of gestation in fetal lambs (19–21) and is associated with a high renal vascular resistance (RVR) and small filtration fraction when compared to newborn animals (19, 21) (Fig. 54.1). However, immediately after birth when the umbilical cord has been clamped, RBF values are similar in fetal and newborn lambs (19), suggesting that RBF does not change much at birth. On the other hand, RBF does increase significantly during the first week of postnatal life and thereafter (19, 21). This rise in RBF is associated with a significant drop in RVR and a significant rise in filtration fraction and in mean arterial blood pressure (21) (Fig. 54.1). However, the relative increase in blood pressure (88%) is less than the rise in RBF (292%); i.e., in the postnatal period factors other than blood pressure are responsible for the changes in RBF.

A portion of the work presented in this chapter has been supported by Public Health Service grants HD-11466 and HL-14388, and Iowa Heart Association Grant No. 85-G-21.

The intrarenal distribution of fetal glomerular blood flow is quantitatively different from that in the newborn (19, 21) (Table 54.1). First, the fetal glomerular perfusion rate (GPR) in fetal lambs remains the same across the cortex during the last third of gestation (21). Second, although cord clamping does not change RBF, it has a pronounced effect on intrarenal blood flow distribution. The quotient between inner and outer cortical glomerular blood flow decreases significantly at the time of birth (19). After birth, GPR values increase significantly in the outer zone of the cortex (zone I) although there are no changes in the inner cortex (zone IV) (Table 54.1) (21). Many factors may contribute to this increase in GPR after birth. The rise in GPR during postnatal maturation has been thought to be partially related to an increase in cardiac output (22). A close correlation between the redistribution of blood flow toward the outer cortex and the increase in arterial blood pressure during postnatal development (23) suggested that maturation of GPR might be related to the maturation of arterial blood pressure. However, Olbing and associates (24) were unable to confirm Kleinman and Reuter's results (23); more recently, Aperia and Herin (25) suggested that changes in arterial pressure do not necessarily relate to changes in GPR. Finally, other factors such as a decrease in glomerular vascular resistance, a decrease in hematocrit (26), a rise in total plasma protein concentration (27) and an increase in glomerular size also contribute to the increase in GPR that occurs in the postnatal period.

Factors Affecting Changes in the Fetal Renal Circulation

Renin-Angiotensin System

The renin-angiotensin system (RAS) has an important role in modulating the fetal circulation and renal hemodynamics (28–32). The vasopressor response (31) and the renal vascular reactivity (30) to exogenous angiotensin II (A-II) infusion are less in fetal lambs than in adult sheep. It has been suggested that decreased renal vascular reactivity to A-II during fetal life is secondary to a high receptor occupancy by endogenous A-II (30). Administration of A-II, which decreases renal blood flow, is associated with an increase in filtration fraction without changes in glomerular filtration rate (GFR), suggesting that A-II acts primarily by increasing the efferent arterial tone, as shown previously in adults (33).

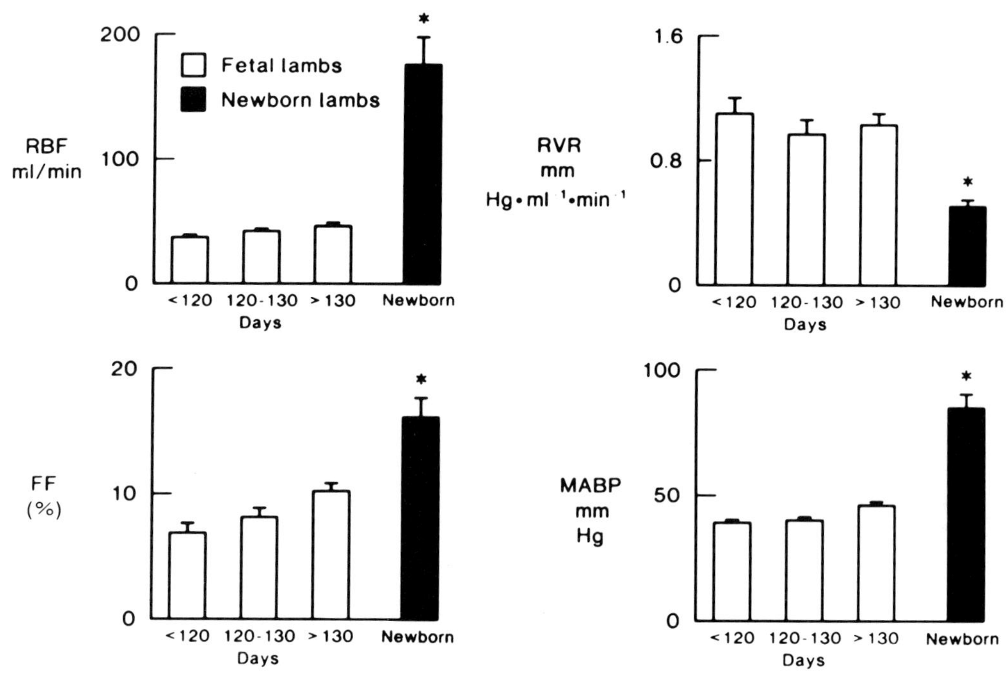

Figure 54.1. Renal hemodynamics values in fetal and newborn lambs. Newborn lambs were studied between 3 and 19 days postnatally. Values are expressed as means ± S.E.M. *, Newborn values are significantly different than fetal values ($p < 0.05$). (Adapted from Robillard et al: Pediatr Res 15:1248, 1981.) RBF, renal blood flow; RVR, renal vascular resistance; FF, filtration fraction; MABP, mean arterial blood pressure

Table 54.1
Mean Values of Glomerular Perfusion Rate (ml/min) in Fetuses and Newborns

	n^a	Zone I	Zone II	Zone III	Zone IV	*F*	*P*
Fetuses							
<120 days	10	61.4 ± 8.2[c]	72.5 ± 7.2	71.1 ± 7.6	70.5 ± 9.3	0.38	NS
120–130 days	10	81.7 ± 15.5	58.8 ± 8.2	61.6 ± 6.3	69.6 ± 7.5	1.03	NS
>130 days	9	69.2 ± 8.9	53.6 ± 4.2	55.6 ± 10.0	59.7 ± 4.7	2.02	NS
Newborns	8	206.9 ± 16.8	161.3 ± 20.7	119.5 ± 8.9	79.2 ± 13.8	12.18	<0.001
F^b		26.30	21.10	11.20	0.69		
P		<0.001	<0.001	<0.001	NS		

[a] n, number of kidneys studied.

[b] F, values for F distribution when the means of the four groups of animals or the means of each cortical zone are compared.

[c] Mean ± S.E.

The physiological significance of circulating endogenous A-II in modulating renal hemodynamics has been investigated recently in chronically catheterized fetal sheep (28, 32). Iwamoto and Rudolph (28), using saralasin, a competitive antagonist of angiotensin II, have shown that A-II exerts a tonic action on the fetal cardiovascular system at rest and plays an important role in controlling blood flow to the unbilical-placental circulation by maintaining blood pressure. More recently, Robillard and coworkers (32) confirmed these results and demonstrated that systemic administration of the angiotensin-converting enzyme inhibitor captopril does not affect renal hemodynamics in young fetal lambs (<120 days' gestation, term 145 days) but decreases renal vascular resistance in near-term fetuses (>130 days' gestation) and newborn lambs. Taken together, these results suggest that the renin-angiotensin system might have physiological significance during maturation, but that this role seems to be more important in near-term fetuses and postnatally than in early gestation.

It has been suggested that the RAS may have an important role in modulating fetal renal hemodynamics during stressful conditions (34–39). However captopril, which inhibits angiotensin II synthesis, does not protect against a decrease in RBF and a rise in RVR during fetal hypoxemia (37, 38). On the other hand, the RAS plays an important role in the response to hemorrhage in fetal sheep (33, 34, 36). The decrease in RBF associated with fetal hemorrhage (≅20% of fetoplacental blood volume) is abolished following administration of captopril. In contrast, RBF declines further during fetal hemorrhage following infusion of saralasin (36). The differences between these two studies (35, 36) may be explained by a rise in circulating bradykinin following captopril administration.

Arginine Vasopressin

Intravenous infusion of arginine vasopressin (AVP) increases blood pressure and decreases heart rate during the last trimester of gestation in fetal lambs (14, 40–42). Moreover, during exogenous AVP infusion, fetal plasma AVP concentration rises from 1.73 to 22.9 μU/ml and redistributes combined ventricular output. Blood flow to the gastrointestinal and peripheral circulation is reduced and that to the umbilical-placental, myocardial, and cerebral circulations is increased. However, infusion of AVP in two studies was not associated with significant changes in RBF nor RVR (14, 41). Because fetal lambs tend to be more sensitive to the pressor activity of AVP than adult sheep, vasopressin may have an important role in regulating hemodynamics (14) and renal function during hypoxemic episodes. AVP does play a significant role in modulating fetal cardiac output and blood pressure during hypoxemia but does not affect fetal renal hemodynamics as judged from studies using a specific vascular AVP-inhibitor ($d(CH_2)_5Tyr(Me)AVP$) (43).

Taken together, these studies do not support a role for AVP in modulating fetal renal hemodynamics at rest or during stressful conditions.

Prostaglandins

The presence of high concentrations of PGE_2, $PGF_{2\alpha}$ and metabolites of prostacyclin and thromboxane in urine of fetal lambs (39, 44–46) confirms biochemical estimates that the fetal kidney has the ability to synthesize and excrete prostaglandins (47). Terragno and associates (48) have suggested that prostaglandins produced by the fetal kidney may be involved in the regulation of renal blood flow and renal function since blood vessels dissected from fetal pig kidneys have higher capacity to produce and to release PGE_2 and PGI_2 than do those from mature pig kidney.

Prostaglandins produced by the fetal kidney may be important in modulating renal blood flow (44, 49, 50). Fetal RBF decreases transiently in the chronically catheterized fetal lamb preparation following administration of meclofenamate or indomethacin. The reduction in RBF is greater in the inner than in the outer portion of the fetal renal cortex (44). Moreover, because the reduction in RBF is associated with an increase in filtration fraction without appreciable change in GFR, it has been suggested that the prostaglandins act on the efferent arteriolar tone (44).

The role of prostaglandins as mediators of renal hemodynamic response to stress in fetuses is being investigated. For example, with increased urinary PGE and $PGF_{2\alpha}$, excretion rate increases during fetal hypoxemic stress (39); inhibitors of prostaglandin synthesis completely block the renal vasodilation seen during the acute phase of fetal hypoxemia (50). We have recently reported that renal prostaglandins are of primary importance in opposing the renal vasoconstriction associated with fetal hypoxemia (51).

Kallikrein-Kinin

The physiological role of the renal kallikrein-kinin system in controlling RBF during fetal and postnatal life is just being investigated. Urinary kallikrein excretion rate expressed in milliesterase units per hour, absolute corrected for kidney weight, or GFR increases during fetal maturation and following birth. The rise in RBF observed during fetal maturation correlates with the increase in urinary kallikrein excretion rate (52). Inhibition of kininase II is associated with a decrease in renal vascular resistance in near-term fetal lambs, whereas administration of a competitive antagonist of A-II, [sar^1],[gly^8]-angiotensin II, does not (32). However, inference of a physiological role for the kallikrein-kinin system in modulating renal blood flow during development is still premature, since renal kinin production has not been determined yet.

Reflex Regulation and Sympathoadrenal Control of Renal Circulation

The functional status of the renal sympathetic pathway depends on the development of its several components, including renal adrenergic receptors, synaptic terminals capable of storing and releasing norepinephrine, and sympathetic ganglia able to transmit nerve impulses to intrarenal nerve terminals. However, little is known presently about the ontogeny of the renal sympathetic neurotransmission.

The adrenergic innervation of the dog kidney changes with growth from birth to two months of age (53). At birth, adrenergic fibers enter the kidney with the renal artery and follow the arterial supply into the inner cortex. The outer portion of the cortex, which continues active nephrogenesis until two weeks of age, contains only single adrenergic fibers. The outer medulla, unlike the cortex, does not contain nerve fibers at birth, although the vasa recta are present. Nerve fibers begin to join vasa recta by about three weeks of age (53). Development of the rat kidney during postnatal development is similar (54).

Comparable studies have not been done during fetal life. But there is indirect evidence suggesting that the fetal sympathetic nervous system does not become fully functional until late in gestation (55). Moreover, Zink and Van Petten (56) have suggested that the fetal kidney becomes innervated late in gestation, since tyramine, which stimulates the release of norepinephrine from sympathetic nerve terminals, has no effect on fetal renal blood flow, whereas direct infusion of norepinephrine produces renal vasoconstriction (56, 57). On the other hand, Zimmerman (58) has observed innervation of the distal convoluted tubules in 13- to 16-week-old human fetuses.

Despite its relative immaturity, the sympathetic nervous system participates in the control of renal circulation during fetal life. A recent study by Robillard and coworkers (51) has demonstrated that renal denervation attenuated the renal vasoconstriction associated with fetal

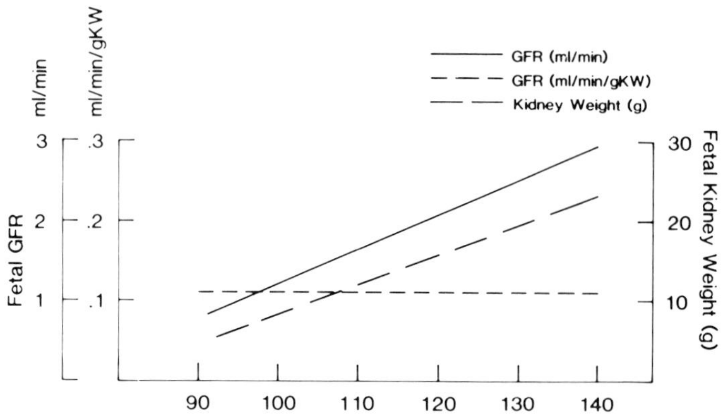

Figure 54.2. Maturation of glomerular filtration rate (GFR) in fetal lamb. GFR is expressed in units of ml/min (——) and units of $ml \cdot min^{-1} \cdot g$ kidney wt^{-1} (– – –). Rate of kidney growth is also known (— —). (From data of Robillard et al: Am J Obstet Gynecol 122:601, 1975.)

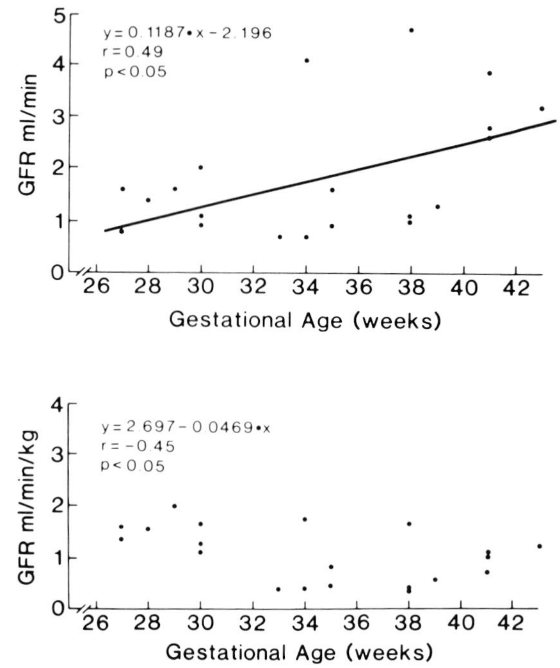

Figure 54.3. Glomerular filtration rate (GFR) in premature infants studied during the first 24 hr after birth and expressed in absolute values (ml/min) or corrected for body weight (ml/min/kg). (Adapted from Leake RD, Trygstad CW: Pediatr Res 11: 959, 1977.)

hypoxemia in chronically catheterized fetal lambs during the last trimester of gestation.

GLOMERULAR FILTRATION RATE

Pattern of GFR Maturation

During fetal life, GFR is low and increases in relation to fetal age (3, 59–62); in chronically catheterized fetal lambs, the fetal GFR, increases 2.5 times during the last trimester of gestation (60, 61). During fetal life GFR increases at the same rate as body weight (3, 60); that is, GFR in milliliters per minute per kilogram of body weight does not change (Fig. 54.2). After birth GFR increases disproportionately to body weight or kidney weight (63, 64).

The developmental pattern of GFR in preterm infants follows closely the observations made in sheep in utero. GFR (ml/min) in newborn infants delivered between 27 and 43 weeks of gestation and measured in the first 24 hr after birth correlates with gestational age (65, 66). However, when GFR is expressed as a function of body weight (ml/min/kg), there is a slight decrease (Fig. 54.3), comparable to the change in GFR measured in utero in sheep. The mean GFR in premature infants studied during the first 24 hr after birth (65) expressed as a function of body weight (1.07 ± 0.12 ml/min/kg) is very close to values found in chronically catheterized fetal lambs (1.14 ± 0.08 ml/min/kg) (61) studied during the last third of gestation.

The increase in GFR in premature infants studied after the first 24 hr of life, is disproportionately higher than the concomitant increase in body weight (65, 67). This pattern of GFR maturation is similar to that described in full-term newborn infants.

Although factors modulating GFR during fetal life are not well known, the increase in GFR at any stage must depend on the surface area for filtration (S), effective filtration pressure (P_{UF}) and capillary filtration coefficient (K_f). K_f is a function of the effective hydraulic permeability of the glomerular capillary wall (k) and the surface area (S) available for filtration. These interrelationships are expressed by the equations $GFR = K_f \cdot P_{UF} = k \cdot S \cdot P_{UF}$, (68) (see also, Chapter 4).

These factors have not been quantified yet in fetuses; however, it appears that low GFR (25), low K_f (69), and capillary hydraulic pressure (P_{GC}) (70, 71) all contribute to the low GFR characteristic of gestation. The importance of each of these variables has been quantified in relation to GFR in newborn animals (72). The increase in GFR (25 times) that occurs after birth depends predominantly on an increase in the glomerular surface area (8 times), and, to a lesser extent, on a rise in P_{UF} (2.5 times). Changes in hydraulic permeability of the glomerular capillary (1.3 times) contribute only minimally to the postnatal rise in GFR.

During fetal life, the increase in GFR does not correlate with glomerular perfusion rate (glomerular plasma flow) at any cortical level (21); however, fetal GFR increases as kidney weight increases; i.e., increasing fetal GFR depends on the development of new nephrons. Humoral factors, e.g., angiotensin II, vasopressin, and prostaglandins, influence fetal GFR by affecting the efferent arteriolar glomerular flow (31, 41, 44). In summary, the increase in GFR that occurs during maturation is the combination of the effects of factors promoting and opposing filtration. During fetal life, active nephrogenesis, changes in renal vascular resistance, progressive increase in the function of the superficial nephrons, and modification of forces involved in the ultrafiltration process are factors that influence the development of glomerular function.

SODIUM CHLORIDE METABOLISM

The percent of filtered Na excreted (FE_{Na}) is high early in gestation and decreases as gestation advances. The fractional excretion of Na decreases from 11% at 130 days' gestation to 5% near term (145 days) in chronically catheterized fetal lambs (61). The clearance of NaCl and of other solutes is always high in the fetus (73) and the urinary Na^+/K^+ ratio decreases as a function of gestational age (74, 75) (see also Chapters 5 and 56) (Fig. 54.4). These findings are similar to those in infants (76–79). In infants at less than 30 weeks' gestation, the fractional excretion of Na is over 5% in the first three days of life but in term newborns this decreases to 0.2% (79) (Fig. 54.5).

Renal tubular immaturity (80, 81), large extracellular fluid (ECF) volume (82), presence of circulating natriuretic factor (83), and relative tubular insensitivity to circulating aldosterone (84) have been proposed as factors to explain the high rate of urinary NaCl excretion during fetal

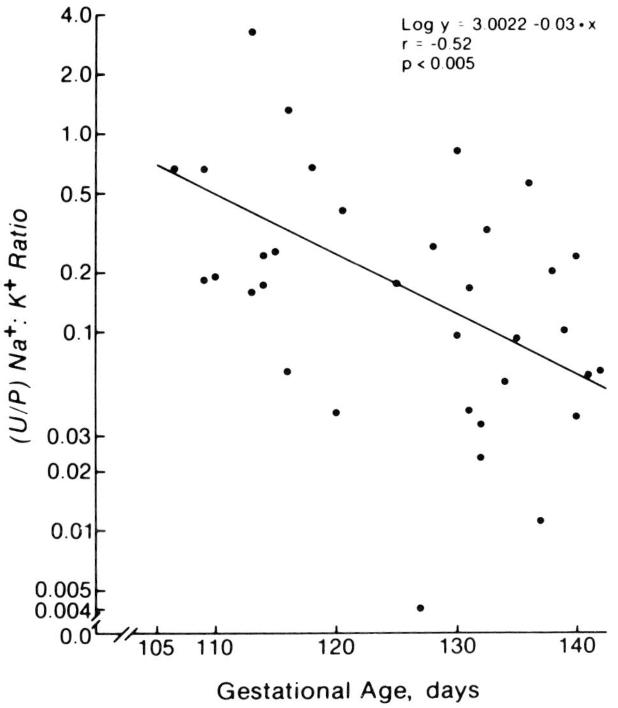

Figure 54.4. Relationship between gestation age and (U/P)Na^+:K^+ ratio. (U/P)Na^+:K^+ = ratio of (U/P)Na^+ over (U/P)K^+. (From Robillard et al: Develop Pharmacol Ther 1:201, 1980.)

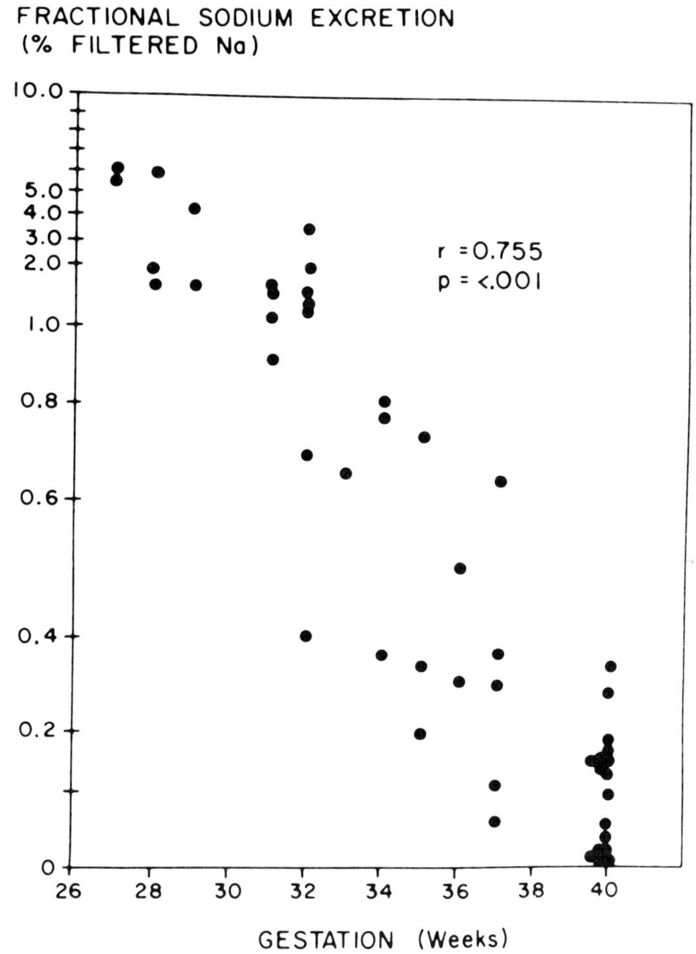

Figure 54.5. Correlation between fractional excretion of sodium (FE_{Na^+}) and conceptional age. (U/P), urine over plasma. (From Siegel S, Oh W: Acta Paediatr Scand 65:481, 1976.)

life and in premature infants. Based on morphological evidence, a relatively inadequate tubular surface area for reabsorption has been proposed (80). Since there is glomerular preponderance relative to tubules during fetal development (80), it has been postulated that a functional glomerulotubular imbalance may be partly responsible for the decreased tubular function in fetal lambs (61). More recently, Merlet-Benichou and associates (73) demonstrated in fetal guinea pigs that there is a phase of functional glomerular preponderance in the early stages of superficial nephron maturation followed by a phase of tubular catchup. On the other hand, evidence derived from studies in newborn dogs (63) and guinea pigs (86) does not support this hypothesis.

The large ECF volume during fetal life has been suggested as a potential factor controlling NaCl reabsorption by the fetal kidney. The contraction of fetal ECF volume following peritoneal dialysis decreases FE_{Na} from 10% to 6%; however, physical factors other than the contraction of ECF volume alone may have influenced these results. On the other hand, the fetal kidney does respond appropriately to volume expansion; isotonic saline produces an increase in GFR and a decrease in fractional sodium reabsorption.

Sodium-potassium–activated adenosine triphosphatase (Na-K-ATPase) plays a role in the reabsorption of NaCl (87–89). The activity in most segments of the immature nephrons is lower than it is in corresponding segments of the mature nephron (90, 91), which may influence Na reabsorption.

Aldosterone contributes to Na reabsorption by the fetal kidney (59, 74, 75, 92). The fetal adrenal gland synthesizes and secretes aldosterone in vitro following stimulation by angiotensin II (93), or adrenocorticotrophin (ACTH) (93) or by increasing K concentration (94). Elevating plasma angiotensin II during the last trimester of gestation in fetal lambs, stimulates aldosterone secretion (31, 95, 96), but elevating ACTH (97, 98) or K infusion (99) does not. On the other hand, ACTH is an important modulator of aldosterone secretion during fetal hypoxemia (100).

Our knowledge regarding the maturation of the renal response to aldosterone during fetal life is limited. Urinary Na:K ratio decreases as the fetus matures (Fig. 54.4) at the time that fetal plasma aldosterone levels increase (Fig. 54.6). Merlet-Benichou and de Rouffignac (59) have suggested that the increased Na reabsorption observed during maturation and postnatally may be secondary to an increase in plasma aldosterone level. Administration of exogenous aldosterone stimulates distal Na reabsorption and increases K excretion in fetal lambs (74, 92, 101). The increase in renal tubule sensitivity to aldosterone during development may be related to aldosterone induction of Na-K-ATPase and the inductive process may be mediated by glucocorticoid receptors (90).

Prostaglandins may have an important role in modulating sodium homeostasis during development. Prostaglandins (PGE_2 and PGI_2) have potent natriuretic properties (102), and urinary excretion of prostaglandin in the chronically catheterized fetal lamb is elevated during fetal life (32, 44, 52). Inhibition of prostaglandin synthesis by indomethacin produces an increase in fetal urinary NaCl excretion (44) that is contrary to its effect in adults (102). Despite a decrease in fetal renal blood flow, endogenous prostaglandins appear to have an effect on fetal tubular sodium chloride opposite to that seen in adults. Most prostaglandins synthesized in the kidney are natriuretic, and indomethacin reduces NaCl excretion (102).

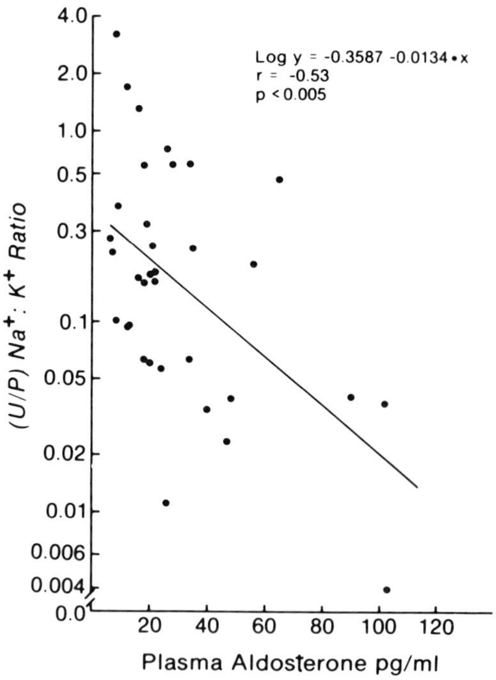

Figure 54.6. Relationship between plasma aldosterone concentration and (U/P)Na^+:K^+ ratio during fetal life. (U/P)Na^+:K^+ = ratio of (U/P)Na^+ over (U/P)K^+. (From Robillard et al: Develop Pharmacol Ther 1:201, 1980.)

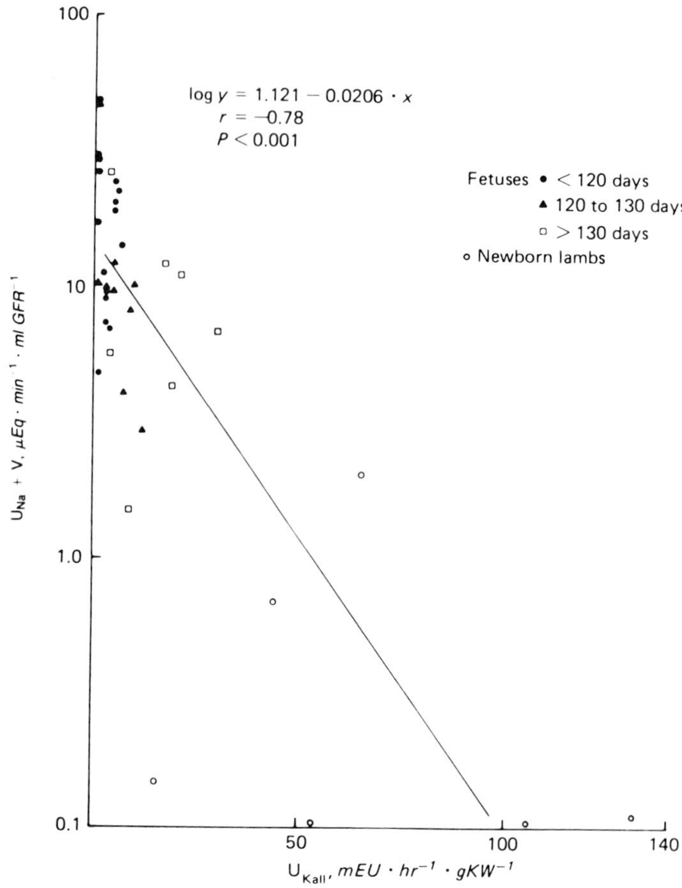

Figure 54.7. Log linear relationship of urinary sodium excretion (U_{Na} + V) corrected for GFR and urinary kallikrein (U_{Kall}) excretion rate corrected for kidney weight (KW). (From Robillard et al: Kidney Int 22:594, 1982.)

Although indomethacin-induced natriuresis is contrary to its effect in adults, natriuresis without kaliuresis in response to indomethacin does occur in adult animals (103, 104). Development stage or experimental conditions may alter the effects of endogenous renal prostaglandins on NaCl transport.

The renal kallikrein-kinin system appears to participate directly in the control of electrolyte and water excretion (105). During fetal life urinary kallikrein excretion rate corrected for kidney weight increases as gestation progresses and continues to increase after birth (52). The rise in fetal urinary kallikrein excretion rate follows closely an increase in plasma aldosterone concentration. The urinary kallikrein excretion rate varies inversely with urinary NaCl excretion (Fig. 54.7).

Renal oxygen consumption is also an important factor regulating Na reabsorption in the immature kidney. In newborn rats, Na reabsorption depends on oxygen consumption (106). The observation that NaCl excretion increases during fetal hypoxemia (39) but not during fetal hemorrhage (34) led us to speculate that O_2 content is an important determinant in the ability of the fetal nephron to reabsorb Na. Recent studies by Iwamoto and coworkers (85) tend to support this observation.

WATER METABOLISM

In mammals, urine produced by the fetal kidney is hypotonic to plasma (8, 10, 11, 59, 107–111) until very late in gestation (11, 111). In fetal lambs urine osmolality increases after 130 days' gestation (term 145 days); this parallels an increase in urinary urea and nonurea solute (111) (Fig. 54.8). The changes that occur in urine composition during the last part of gestation are not accompanied by major changes in the electrolyte composition of fetal plasma. On the other hand, the percentage of both filtered water excreted (V/GFR) and free water clearance corrected for GFR (CH_2O/GFR) decrease significantly after 130 days' gestation (Fig. 54.9); i.e., free water reabsorption by the fetal kidney increases in late gestation.

Factors that control renal tubular reabsorption of water during fetal life have been reviewed (112, 113). The antidiuretic hormone, vasopressin, is present in the posterior pituitary during fetal life (114, 115), e.g., as early as the 11th week of gestation in humans (116). During human and ovine parturition there is a release of vasopressin by the fetus (117–120). Both volume and osmoreceptor controls of vasopressin secretion are functional in the last trimester of gestation in the lamb fetus (121, 122). On the other hand, the fetal nephron is less sensitive to vasopressin than is the adult nephron. The capacity of the fetal kidney to concentrate urine increases with gestation (41, 85, 123, 124) (Fig. 54.10). Urine osmolality during vasopressin infusion was one third that seen in adult sheep for the same plasma concentration of circulating AVP (Fig. 54.11); i.e., renal tubule response to vasopressin during fetal life is impaired. The smaller vasopressin stimulation of cyclic-AMP early during development (125–128) may be an important factor contributing to the limited renal concentrating ability in immature animals. Prostaglandin E_2, found in high concentration in fetal lamb urine (44, 45), may inhibit vasopressin action on water flow.

The structural immaturity of the medulla, characterized by a short loop of Henle (129) and the relatively increased blood flow to the medulla (24, 130, 131), probably limits the development of an osmotic gradient in the medulla of the fetal kidney. The capacity to reabsorb NaCl by the ascending limb of the loop of Henle and generate a hypotonic urine

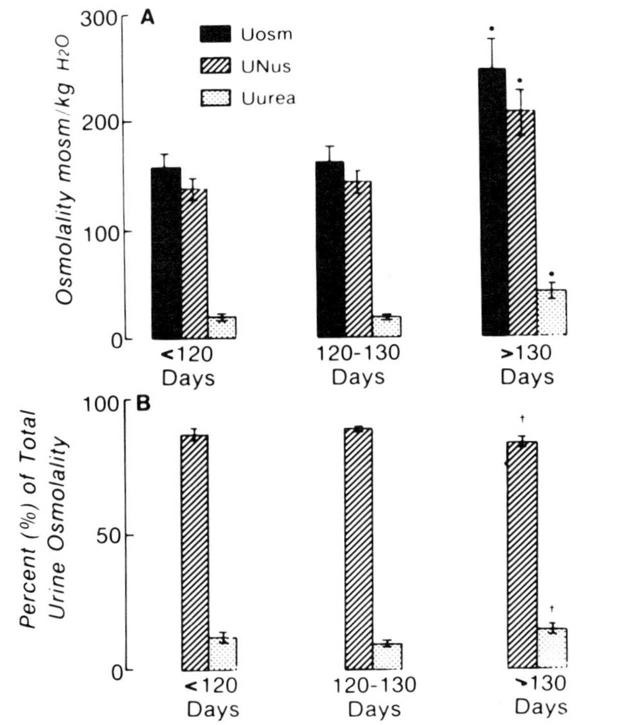

Figure 54.8. A, Fetal urine composition at different gestational ages. U_{osm}, urine. *, $p < 0.05$ when fetuses of 130 days are compared either with fetuses <120 days or between 120 and 130 days. **B**, Percent of urea (U_{urea}) and nonurea solute (U_{NUS}) to total urine osmolality. †, $p < 0.02$ when fetuses >130 days are compared with fetuses between 120 to 130 days. (From Robillard et al: In Spitzer A (ed): The Kidney during Development. New York, Masson 1982, p 205.)

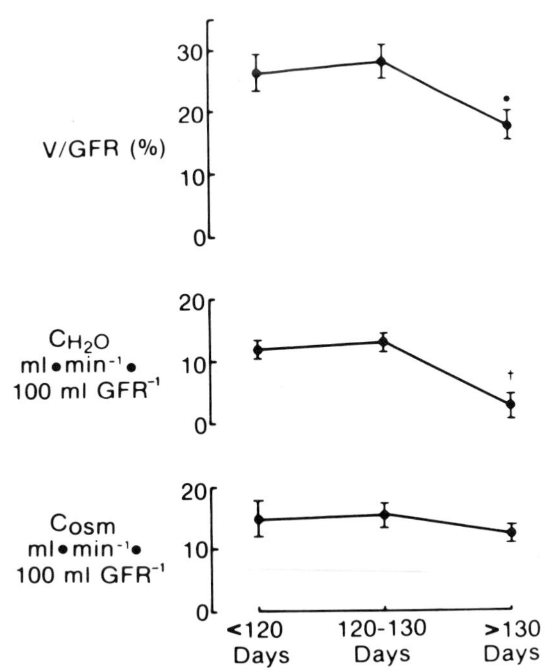

Figure 54.9. Summary of fetal osmolar and water clearances at different gestational ages. V/GFR, fractional water excretion (%); C_{H_2O}/GFR, free water clearance corrected for 100 ml GFR; C_{osm}, GFR, osmolar clearance corrected for 100 ml GFR. *, $p < 0.05$; †, $p < 0.01$ when fetuses >130 days are compared either with fetuses <120 days or between 120 to 130 days. (From Robillard et al: In Spitzer A (ed.): The Kidney during Development. New York, Masson 1982, p 205.)

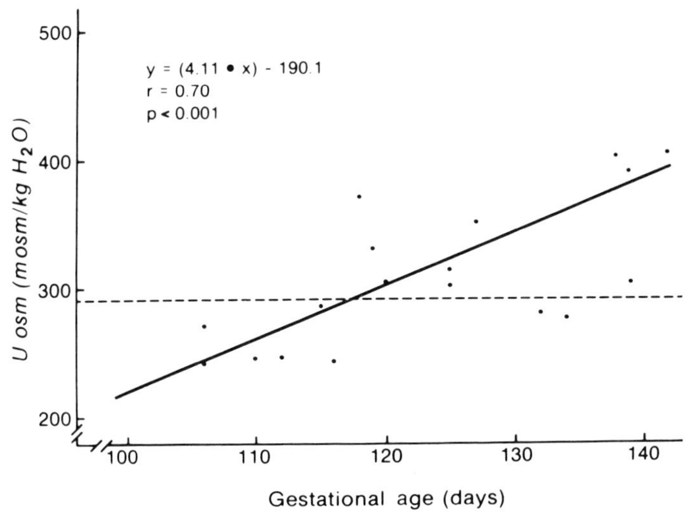

Figure 54.10. Relationship between fetal gestational age and fetal urine osmolality during AVP infusion. Dotted line represents mean plasma osmolality (291 ± 1.45) during AVP infusion. (From Robillard et al: Am J Physiol 238:F407, 1980.)

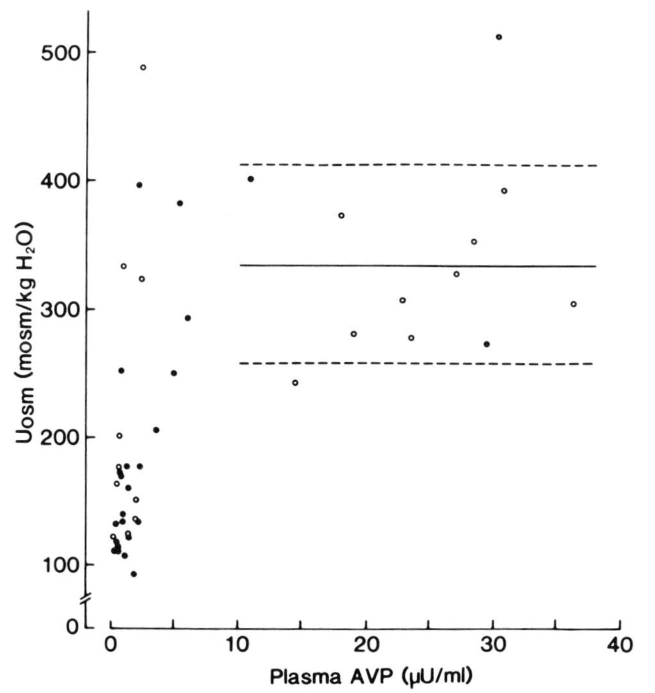

Figure 54.11. Relationship of plasma AVP to urine osmolality. Regression line for P_{AVP} values below 6 μU/ml was expressed by the formula $U_{osmol} = 135 + (35 \cdot P_{AVP})$. Coefficient of correlation for this relationship ($r = 0.50$) was statistically significant ($p < 0.005$). Broken lines represent ± 1 standard deviation from mean U_{osmol} value (solid line) for P_{AVP} levels above 6 μU/ml. (From Robillard et al: Am J Physiol 238:F407, 1980.)

(132–134) is not fully developed in rats 12 to 25 days of age. An intrarenal solute and osmolar gradient is present in fetal lamb kidneys by early midgestation (135–137), i.e. the countercurrent multiplier system is functional by midgestation. Moreover, since the blood flow in the immature kidney is distributed to a greater extent to the juxtamedullary glomeruli, whose efferent arterioles supply the vasa recta of the medulla, the high flow of blood through the vasa recta may disperse the intrarenal

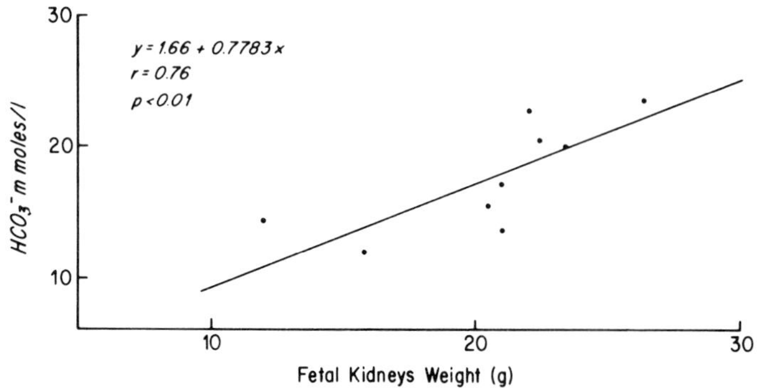

Figure 54.12. Relationship between fetal kidney weight and plasma bicarbonate at threshold. (From Robillard et al: Pediatr Res 11:649, 1977.)

solute gradient normally found in the medulla of more mature animals. As a consequence the medullary interstitium of the fetus does not become as hypertonic as that of the newborn or adult. The fetal kidney participates in maintaining fetal osmolar and volume homeostasis in its unique environment. Outside that environment, problems arise.

Hypoxemia affects fetal and neonatal renal concentrating ability. Urine osmolality (U_{osm}) increases and free water clearance decreases are associated with fetal hypoxemia (39, 138, 139) and fetal asphyxia (140, 141) in lambs. Moreover, U_{osm} during fetal hypoxemia correlates closely with gestational age. The higher U_{osm} in near-term fetal lambs (>130 days; term 145 days) and the higher proportion of near-term than young fetuses (<120 days) showing increased free-water reabsorption during hypoxemia does not seem to be related to the presence of lower plasma arginine vasopressin (AVP) concentrations in young than in near-term fetuses (39), but more on the increased ability of the fetal nephron to respond to AVP as gestation advances (41). Furthermore, factors other than increased AVP secretion alone may influence the ability of the fetal kidney to reabsorb free water during hypoxemia. A decrease in GFR in adult dogs produces an increase in U_{osm} in the absence of ADH (142); however, fetal GFR did not change significantly in hypoxemia (39). Decreased RBF (143), increased concentration of circulating catecholamines, and stimulation of the renal nerves (144) are factors known to affect renal water reabsorption in older animals. However, the influences these factors have on the antidiuretic response to hypoxemia during fetal life are not known.

ROLE OF KIDNEY IN ACID BASE METABOLISM DURING FETAL LIFE

The regulation of acid base homeostasis by the mature kidney involves the reabsorption of filtered bicarbonate and the excretion of hydrogen ion as titrable acid and ammonium. During fetal life the maternal kidneys and lungs (through the placenta) play the major role in modulating fetal response to acidosis; however, knowledge of the fetal kidney's ability to regulate acid-base metabolism is necessary to understand the characteristics of acid-base balance in premature infants.

Bicarbonate Reabsorption

The values of plasma bicarbonate at threshold for renal bicarbonate excretion are lower in fetal lambs than in nonpregnant adult ewes; the mean values for plasma bicarbonate at threshold are 17.7 ± 1.4 mmol/liter in fetuses and 28.7 ± 1.7 in adult ewes. The level of plasma bicarbonate at threshold increases significantly with fetal kidney weight (Fig. 54.12) (82).

The large fetal ECF volume may be a major determinant in the decreased reabsorption of bicarbonate. Depletion of fetal ECF volume produces a rise in bicarbonate and electrolyte reabsorption; this suggests that the low threshold for bicarbonate by the fetal kidney is related to the expanded ECF volume and is not due solely to a limited capacity to increase bicarbonate or sodium reabsorption.

The low threshold for renal bicarbonate reabsorption in fetuses probably is not due to lack of fetal renal carbonic anhydrase activity. Acetazolamide, a carbonic anhydrase inhibitor, infused in fetal lambs during the last trimester of gestation, causes significant increase in urinary excretion of bicarbonate and K and in urinary pH. From these results we propose that renal carbonic anhydrase enzyme is present and active during the last third of gestation and does not limit the capacity of the fetal kidney to reabsorb bicarbonate (145).

Urinary Acidification and Hydrogen Ion Excretion

The excretion of titrable acid and ammonium per unit of body weight is considerably less in the fetal lamb and primates than it is in adults (146–148). The fetal renal response to infusion of HCl led to an increase in hydrogen ion excretion in a manner qualitatively similar to that in adults (146).

The response of the fetal lamb kidney to an infusion of sodium sulfate (Na_2SO_4), a poorly reabsorbable anion, produced a clear-cut pH gradient between blood and urine without the production of a metabolic acidosis (149). These findings suggest that the low level of renal reabsorption of Na^+ in exchange for H^+ in the fetus explains the observed low level of net acid excretion.

References

1. Gersh I: The correlation of structure and function in the developing mesonephros and metanephros. Contrib Embryol 26:35, 1937.
2. Stanier MW: The function of the mammalian mesonephros. J Physiol (Lond) 151:472, 1960.
3. Gresham EL, Rankin JHG, Makowski EL, et al: An evaluation of fetal renal function in a chronic sheep preparation. J Clin Invest 51:149, 1972.
4. Rankin JHG, Gresham EL, Battaglia FC, et al: Measurement of fetal renal inulin clearance in a chronic sheep preparation. J Appl Physiol 32:129, 1972.
5. Jacque L: De la genese des liquides amniotique et allantoidien; cryoscopie et analyses chimiques. Arch Intern Physiol 3:463, 1905.
6. Makepeace AW, Smith F, Dailey ME, Carrol MP: The nature of the amniotic fluid. A comparative study of human amniotic fluid and maternal serum. Surg Gynecol Obstet 53:635, 1931.
7. Alexander DP, Nixon DA: Plasma clearance of *p*-aminohippuric acid by the kidneys of foetal, neonatal and adult sheep. Nature 194:483, 1962.
8. Alexander DP, Nixon DA: Reabsorption of glucose, fructose, and mesoinositol by the foetal and postnatal sheep kidney. J Physiol (Lond) 167:480, 1963.
9. Alexander DP, Nixon DA, Widdas WF, Wohlzogen FX: Gestational variations in the composition of foetal fluids and foetal urine in the sheep. J Physiol (Lond) 140:1, 1958.
10. Alexander DP, Nixon DA, Widdas WF, Wohlzogen FX: Renal function in the sheep foetus. J Physiol (Lond) 140:14, 1958.
11. Chez RA, Smith FG, Hutchinson DL: Renal function in the intrauterine primate fetus. Am J Obstet Gynecol 90:128, 1964.
12. Smith FG, Adams FH, Bordon M, Hilburn J: Studies of renal function in the intact fetal lamb. Am J Obstet Gynecol 96:240, 1966.
13. Gilbert RD: Control of fetal cardiac output during changes in blood volume. Am J Physiol 238:H80, 1980.
14. Iwamoto HS, Rudolph AM, Keil LC, Heymann MA: Hemodynamic responses of the sheep fetus to vasopressin infusion. Circ Res 44:430, 1979.
15. Rudolph AM, Heymann MA: Circulatory changes during growth in the fetal lamb. Circ Res 26:289, 1970.
16. Siimes ASI, Creasy RK, Heymann MA, Rudolph AM: Cardiac output and its

distribution and organ blood flow in the fetal lamb during ritodrine administration. Am J Obstet Gynecol 132:42, 1978.
17. Behrman RE, Lees MH, Peterson EN, et al: Distribution of the circulation in the normal and asphyxiated fetal primate. Am J Obstet Gynecol 108:956, 1970.
18. Paton JB, Fisher DE, Peterson EN, et al: Cardiac output and organ blood flows in the baboon fetus. Biol Neonate 22:50, 1973.
19. Aperia A, Broberger O, Herin P, Joelsson I: Renal hemodynamics in the perinatal period. Acta Physiol Scand 99:261, 1977.
20. Beguin F, Dunnihoo DR, Quilligan EJ: Effect of carbon dioxide elevation on renal blood flow in the fetal lamb in utero. Am J Obstet Gynecol 119:630, 1974.
21. Robillard JE, Weismann DN, Herin P: Ontogeny of single glomerular perfusion rate in fetal and newborn lambs. Pediatr Res 15:1248, 1981.
22. Aperia A, Broberger O, Herin P: Maturational changes in glomerular perfusion rate and glomerular filtration rate in lambs. Pediatr Res 8:758, 1974.
23. Kleinman LI, Reuter JH: Maturation of glomerular blood flow distribution in the newborn dog. J Physiol (Lond) 228:91, 1973.
24. Olbing H, Blaufox MD, Aschinberg LC, et al: Postnatal changes in renal glomerular blood flow distribution in puppies. J Clin Invest 52:2885, 1973.
25. Aperia A, Herin P: Development of glomerular perfusion rate and nephron filtration rate in rats 17–60 days old. Am J Physiol 228:1319, 1975.
26. Schrier RW, Earley LE: Effects of acute changes in hemotocrit on renal hemodynamics and sodium excretion in hydropenic and volume-expanded dogs. J Clin Invest 49:1656, 1970.
27. Vereerstraeten P, Taussaint C: Effects of plasmapheresis on renal hemodynamics and sodium excretion in dogs. Pflugers Arch Eur J Physiol 306:92, 1969.
28. Iwamoto HS, Rudolph AM: Effects of endogenous angiotensin II on the fetal circulation. J Develop Physiol 1:283, 1979.
29. Iwamoto HS, Rudolph AM: Effects of angiotensin II on the blood flow and its distribution in fetal lambs. Circ Res 48:183, 1981.
30. Robillard JE: Changes in renal vascular reactivity to angiotensin-II during development in fetal newborn and adult sheep: role of A-II vascular receptors occupancy. Pediatr Res 17:355A, 1983.
31. Robillard JE, Gomez RA, Van Orden DE, Smith FG Jr: Comparison of the adrenal and renal responses to angiotensin II in fetal lambs and adult sheep. Circ Res 50:140, 1982.
32. Robillard JE, Weismann DN, Gomez RA, et al: Renal and adrenal responses to converting-enzyme inhibition in fetal and newborn life. Am J Physiol 244:R249, 1983.
33. Levens NR, Peach MJ, Carey RM: Role of the intrarenal renin-angiotensin system in the control of renal function. Circ Res 48:157, 1981.
34. Gomez RA, Meernik JG, Kuehl WD, Robillard JE: Developmental aspects of the renal response to hemorrhage during fetal life. Pediatr Res 18:40, 1984.
35. Gomez RA, Robillard JE: Developmental aspects of the renal responses to hemorrhage during converting-enzyme inhibition in fetal lambs. Circ Res 54:301–312, 1984.
36. Iwamoto HS, Rudolph AM: Role of renin-angiotensin system in response to hemorrhage in fetal sheep. Am J Physiol 240:H848, 1981.
37. Robillard JE, Ayres NA, Nakamura K: Effects of reninangiotensin system inhibition on renal hemodynamics and renal function during hypoxemia in fetal lambs (in preparation).
38. Robillard JE, Gomez RA: Effect of angiotensin-II blockade on glomerular and renal hemodynamics during hypoxemia. Pediatr Res 15:699, 1981 (abstract).
39. Robillard JE, Weitzman RE, Burmeister L, Smith FG Jr: Developmental aspects of the renal response to hypoxemia in the lamb fetus. Circ Res 48:128, 1981.
40. Alexander DP, Bashore RA, Britton HG, Forsling ML: Antidiuretic hormone and oxytocin release and antidiuretic hormone turnover in the fetus, lamb, and ewe. Biol Neonate 30:80, 1976.
41. Robillard JE, Weitzman RE: Developmental aspects of the fetal renal response to exogenous arginine vasopressin. Am J Physiol 238:F407, 1980.
42. Rurak DW: Plasma vasopressin in fetal lambs. J Physiol (Lond) 256:36P, 1975.
43. Ayres NA, McWeeny O, Robillard JE: The role of arginine vasopressin in modulating the cardiovascular response in hypoxemic fetal lambs. Pediatr Res 18:134A, 1984.
44. Matson JR, Stokes JB, Robillard JE: Effects of inhibition of prostaglandin synthesis on fetal renal function. Kidney Int 20:621, 1981.
45. Walker D, Mitchell MD: Prostaglandins in the urine of foetal lambs. Nature (London) 271:161, 1978.
46. Walker D, Mitchell MD: Presence of thromboxane 2 and 6-ketoprostaglandin F_1 in the urine of fetal sheep. Prostaglandins Med. 3:249, 1979.
47. Pace-Asciak CR: Prostaglandin biosynthesis and catabolism in the developing fetal sheep kidney. Prostaglandins 13:661, 1977.
48. Terragno NA, McGiff JC, Terragno A: Prostaglandin (PGI_2) production by renal blood vessels: relationship to an endogenous prostaglandin synthesis inhibitor (EPSI). Clin Res 26:545, 1978 (abstract).
49. Heymann MA, Rudolph AM: Effects of acetylsalicylic acid on the ductus arteriosus and circulation in fetal lambs in utero. Circ Res 38:418, 1976.
50. Millard RW, Baig H, Vatner SF: Prostaglandin control of the renal circulation in response to hypoxemia in the fetal lamb in utero. Circ Res 45:172, 1979.
51. Robillard JE, Nakamura, KT, DiBona GF: Role of renal nerves as a major renal ischemic factor during fetal hypoxemia. Am J Physiol 250:F294–F301, 1986.
52. Robillard JE, Lawton WJ, Weismann DN, Sessions C: Developmental aspects of the renal kallikrein-like activity in fetal and newborn lambs. Kidney Int 22:594, 1982.
53. McKenna OC, Angelakos ET: Development of adrenergic innervation in the puppy kidney. Anat Rec 167:115, 1970.
54. Grignolo A, Seidler FJ, Bartolome M, et al: Norepinephrine content of the rat kidney during development: alterations induced by perinatal methadone. Life Sciences 31:3009, 1982.
55. Lebowitz EA, Novick JS, Rudolph AM: Development of myocardial sympathetic innervation in the fetal lamb. Pediatr Res 6:887, 1972.
56. Zink J, Van Petten GR: Noradrenergic control of blood vessels in the premature lamb fetus. Biol Neonate 39:61, 1981.
57. Assali NS, Holm LW, Sehgal N: Regional blood flow and vascular resistance of the fetus in utero. Am J Obstet Gynecol 83:809, 1962.
58. Zimmerman HD: Elektronenmikroskopische befunde zur innervation des nephron nach untersuchungen an der fetalen nachniere des menschen. Z Zellforsch 129:65, 1972.
59. Merlet-Benichou C, de Rouffignac C: Renal clearance studies in fetal and young guinea pigs: effect of salt loading. Am J Physiol 232:F178, 1977.
60. Robillard JE, Kulvinskas C, Sessions C, et al: Maturational changes in the fetal glomerular filtration rate. Am J Obstet Gynecol 122:601, 1975.
61. Robillard JE, Sessions C, Kennedey RL, et al: Interrelationship between glomerular filtration rate and renal transport of sodium and chloride during fetal life. Am J Obstet Gynecol 128:727, 1977.
62. Robillard JE, Sessions C, Kennedey RL, Smith FG Jr: Maturation of the glucose transport process by the fetal kidney. Pediatr Res 12:680, 1978.
63. Horster M, Valtin H: Postnatal development of renal function: Micropuncture and clearance studies in the dog. J Clin Invest 50:779, 1971.
64. Kleinman LI, Lubbe RJ: Factors affecting the maturation of glomerular filtration rate and renal plasma flow in the newborn dog. J Physiol (Lond) 223:395, 1972.
65. Leake RD, Trygstad CW: Glomerular filtration rate during the period of adaptation to extrauterine life. Pediatr Res 11:959, 1977.
66. Guignard JP, Torrado A, DaCunha O, Gautier E: Glomerular filtration rate in the first three weeks of life. J Pediatr 87:268, 1975.
67. Leake RD, Trygstad CW, Oh W: Insulin clearance in the newborn infant: relationship to gestational and postnatal age. Pediatr Res 10:759, 1976.
68. Brenner BM, Ichikawa I, Dean WM: Glomerular filtration. In Brenner BM, Rector FC (eds): The Kidney Philadelphia, W.B. Saunders Co., 1981, p 289.
69. Tucker BJ, Blantz RC: Factors determining superficial nephron filtration in the mature, growing rat. Am J Physiol 232:F97, 1977.
70. Allison MEM, Lipham EM, Gottschalk CW: Hydostatic pressure in the rat kidney. Am J Physiol 223:975, 1972.
71. Spitzer A, Edelmann CM Jr: Maturational changes in pressure gradients for glomerular filtration. Am J Physiol 221:1431, 1971.
72. Spitzer A: Factors underlying the increase in glomerular filtration rate during postnatal development. In Spitzer A (ed): The Kidney During Development: Morphology and Function, New York, Masson 1982, p 127.
73. Merlet-Benichou C, Pegorier M, Muffat-Joly M, Augeron C: Functional and morphologic patterns of renal maturation in the developing guinea pig. Am J Physiol 241:F618, 1981.
74. Lingwood B, Hardy KJ, Coghlan JP, Wintour EM: Effect of aldosterone on urine composition in the chronically cannulated ovine foetus. J Endocrinol 76:553, 1978.
75. Robillard JE, Ramberg E, Sessions C, et al: Role of aldosterone on renal sodium and potassium excretion during fetal life and newborn period. Dev Pharmacol Ther 1:201, 1980.
76. Aperia A, Broberger O, Thodenius K, Zetterstrom R: Developmental study of the renal response to an oral salt load in preterm infants. Acta Paediatr Scand 63:517, 1974.
77. Arant B: Developmental patterns of renal functional maturation compared in the human neonates. J Pediatr 92:707, 1978.
78. Engelke S, Shah B, Vasan V, Page J: Sodium balance in very low birth-weight infants. J Pediatr 93:837, 1978.
79. Siegel S, Oh W: Renal function as a marker of human fetal maturation. Acta Paediatr Scand 65:481, 1976.
80. Fetterman GH, Shuplock NA, Philipp FJ, Gregg HS: The growth and maturation

of human glomeruli and proximal convolutions from term to adulthood. Pediatrics 35:601, 1965.
81. McCance RA, Widdowson EM: Renal function before birth. Proc Roy Soc B 141:488, 1953.
82. Robillard JE, Sessions C, Burmeister L, Smith FG: Influence of fetal extracellular volume contraction on renal reabsorption of bicarbonate in fetal lambs. Pediatr Res 11:649, 1977.
83. Hurley JK, Kirkpatrick SE, Pitlick PT, et al: Renal responses of the fetal lamb to fetal or maternal volume expansion. Circ Res 40:557, 1977.
84. Sulyok E, Nemeth M, Tenyi I, et al: Relationship between the postnatal development of the renin-angiotensin-aldosterone system and electrolyte and acid-base status of the NaCl-supplemented premature infants. In Spitzer A (ed): The Kidney During Development: Morphology and Function. New York, Masson, 1982, p 273.
85. Iwamoto HS, Rudolph AM: Metabolic responses of the kidney in fetal sheep: effect of acute and spontaneous hypoxemia. Am J Physiol 249:F836–F841, 1985.
86. Spitzer A, Brandis M: Functional morphologic maturation of the superficial nephrons. J Clin Invest 53:279, 1974.
87. Katz AI, Epstein FH: Physiologic role of Na-K-ATPase in the transport of cations across biologic membranes. N Engl J Med 278:253, 1968.
88. Kiil F: Na-K-ATPases as regulators of Na and water excretion. Scand J Clin Lab Invest 28:375, 1971.
89. Sachs G: Ion pumps in the renal tubule. Am J Physiol 233:F359, 1977.
90. Aperia A, Larsson L, Zetterstrom R: Hormonal induction of Na-K-ATPase in developing proximal tubular cells. Am J Physiol 241:F356, 1981.
91. Schmidt V, Horster M: Na-K-activated ATPase: activity maturation in rabbit nephron segments dissected in vitro. Am J Physiol 233:F55, 1977.
92. Siegel SR, Oakes G, Palmer S: Transplacental transfer of aldosterone and its effects on renal function in the fetal lamb. Pediatr Res 15:163, 1981.
93. Wintour EM, Brown EH, Denton DA, et al: In vitro and in vivo adrenal cortical steroid production by fetal sheep: effect of angiotensin II, sodium deficiency and ACTH. In Conti C (ed): Research on Steroids. Amsterdam, Elsevier/North Holland, 1977, vol VII, p 475.
94. Wintour, EM, Brown EH, Denton DA, et al: The ontogeny and regulation of corticosteroid secretion by the ovine foetal adrenal. Acta Endocrinol 79:301, 1975.
95. Robillard JE, Gomez RA, Meernik JG, et al: Role of angiotensin II on the adrenal and vascular responses to hemorrhage during development in fetal lambs. Circ Res 50:645, 1982.
96. Siegel SR, Oakes G, Palmer S: Effects of angiotensin II on blood pressure, plasma renin activity and aldosterone in fetal lambs. Dev Pharmacol Ther 3:144, 1981.
97. Alexander DP, Britton HG, James VHT, et al: Steroid secretion by the adrenal gland of foetal and neonatal sheep. J Endocrinol 40:1, 1968.
98. Brown EH, Coghlan JP, Hardy KJ, Wintour EM: Aldosterone, corticosterone, cortisol, 11-deoxycortisol and 11-deoxycorticosterone concentrations in the blood of chronically cannulated ovine foetuses: effect of ACTH. Acta Endocrinol 88:364, 1978.
99. Wintour EM, Barnes A, Cahiff F, et al: Potassium: aldosterone relationship in pregnant ewes and chronically cannulated ovine fetuses. Pediatr Res 13:265, 1979.
100. Robillard JE, Ayers NA, Gomez RA, et al: Factors controlling aldosterone secretion during hypoxemia in fetal lambs. Pediatr Res 18:607–611, 1984.
101. Robillard JE, Nakamura KT, McWeeny O, et al: Effects of aldosterone on urinary kallikrein and sodium excretion during fetal life. Pediatr Res 19:1048–1052, 1985.
102. Dunn MJ: Renal prostaglandins: influences on excretion of sodium and water, the renin angiotensin system, renal blood flow, and hypertension. In Brenner BM, Stern JH (eds): Hormonal Function and the Kidney, New York, Churchill Livingstone, 1979, p 89.
103. Kirschenbaum MA, Stein JH: The effect of inhibition of prostaglandin synthesis on urinary sodium excretion in the conscious dog. J Clin Invest 47:517, 1976.
104. Oliw E, Kover G, Larsson C, Auggard E: Indomethacin and diclotenac sodium increase sodium and water excretion after extracellular volume expansion in the rabbit. Eur J Pharmacol 49:381, 1978.
105. Carretero OA, Scicli AG: The renal kallikrein-kinin system. Am J Physiol 238:F247, 1980.
106. Elinder G, Aperia A: Renal oxygen consumption and sodium reabsorption during isotonic volume expansion in the developing rat. Pediatr Res 16:351, 1982.
107. Alexander DP, Nixon DA: The foetal kidney. Br Med Bull 17:112, 1961.
108. Boylan JW, Colbourn EP, McCance RA: Renal function in the foetal and newborn guinea-pig. J Physiol (Lond) 141:323, 1958.
109. Buddingh F, Parker HR, Ishizaki G, Tyler WS: Long-term studies of the functional development of the fetal kidney in sheep. Am J Vet Res 32:1993, 1971.
110. McCance RA, Stanier MW: The function of the metanephros of foetal rabbits and pigs. J Physiol (Lond) 151:479, 1960.
111. Robillard JE, Matson JR, Sessions C, Smith FG Jr: Developmental aspects of renal tubular reabsorption of water in the lamb fetus. Pediatr Res 13:1172, 1979.
112. Robillard JE, Matson JR: The premature nephron: physiologic characteristics and clinical implications. In Moss AJ (ed): Pediatric Update. New York, Elsevier/North Holland 1980, p 167.
113. Robillard JE, Weitzman RE, Fisher DA, Smith FG Jr: Developmental aspects of renal tubular reabsorption of water and fetal renal response to arginine vasopressin. In Spitzer A (ed): The Kidney During Development. New York, Masson 1982, p 205.
114. Froger JL, Aminot A, Blouquit-Debray MF, Roffi J: Antidiuretic activity in the fetal and newborn rabbit hypophysis. Biol Neonate 30:224, 1976.
115. Vizsolyi E, Perks AM: New neurohypophyseal principle in foetal mammals. Nature 223:1169, 1969.
116. Levina SE: Endocrine features in development of human hypothalamus hypophysis and placenta. General Compar Endocrinol 11:151, 1968.
117. Alexander DP, Bashore RA, Britton HG, Forsling ML: Maternal and fetal arginine vasopressin in the chronically catheterized sheep. Biol Neonate 25:242, 1974.
118. Alexander DP, Britton HD, Forsling ML, et al: The concentrations of adrenocorticotrophin, vasopressin and oxytocin in the foetal and maternal plasma of the sheep in the latter half of gestation. J Endocrinol 49:179, 1971.
119. Chard T, Hudson CN, Edward CRW, Boyd NRH: Release of oxytocin and vasopressin by the human fetus during labor. Nature 234:352, 1971.
120. Stark RI, Daniel SS, Husain KM, et al: Arginine vasopressin during gestation and parturition in sheep fetus. Biol Neonate 35:235, 1979.
121. Robillard JE, Weitzman RE, Fisher DA, Smith FG: The dynamics of vasopressin release and blood volume regulation during fetal hemorrhage in the lamb fetus. Pediatr Res 13:606, 1979.
122. Weitzman RE, Fisher DE, Robillard JE, et al: Arginine vasopressin response to an osmotic stimulus in the fetal sheep. Pediatr Res 12:35, 1978.
123. Lingwood B, Hardy KJ, Horacek I, et al: The effects of antidiuretic hormone on urine flow and composition in the chronically-cannulated ovine fetus. Q J Exp Physiol 63:315, 1978.
124. Wintour EM, Congiu M, Hardy KJ, Hennessy DP: Regulation of urine osmolality in fetal sheep. Q J Exp Physiol 67:427, 1982.
125. Joppich R, Schrader J, Haberle DA: Effect of antidiuretic hormone and dibutyryl cAMP upon the urinary concentrating capacity in neonatal piglets. Pediatr Res 14:1234, 1980.
126. Rajerison RM, Butlen D, Jard S: Ontogenic development of antidiuretic hormone receptors in rat kidneys: comparison of hormonal binding and adenylate cyclase activation. Mol Cell Endocrinol 4:271, 1976.
127. Schlondorff D, Weber H: Cyclic nucleotide metabolism in compensatory renal hypertrophy and neonatal kidney growth. Proc Natl Acad Sci USA 73:524, 1976.
128. Schlondorff D, Weber H, Trizna W, Fine LG: Vasopressin responsiveness of renal adenylate cyclase in newborn rats and rabbits. Am J Physiol 234:F16, 1978.
129. Speller AM, Moffat DB: Tubulo-vascular relationships in the developing kidney. J Anat 123:487, 1977.
130. Aschinberg LC, Goldsmith DI, Olbing H, et al: Neonatal changes in renal blood flow distribution in puppies. Am J Physiol 228:1453, 1975.
131. Jose PA, Logan AG, Slotkoff LM, et al: Intrarenal blood flow distribution in canine puppies. Pediatr Res 5:335, 1971.
132. Zink H, Horster M: Maturation of diluting capacity in loop of Henle of rat superficial nephrons. Am J Physiol 233:F519, 1977.
133. Jamison RL, Maffly RH: The urinary concentrating mechanism. N Engl J Med 295:1059, 1976.
134. Kokko JP: The role of the renal concentrating mechanisms in the regulation of serum sodium concentration. Am J Med 62:165, 1977.
135. Moore ES, Kaiser BA, Simpson EH, McMann BJ: Ontogeny of intrarenal solute gradients in fetal life. In Spitzer A (ed): The Kidney During Development: Morphology and Function. New York, Masson, 1982, p 223.
136. Forrest JN Jr, Stanier NW: Kidney composition and renal concentration ability in young rabbits. J Physiol (Lond) 187:1, 1966.
137. Stanier MW: Development of intrarenal solute gradients in foetal and postnatal life. Pflugers Arch 336:263, 1972.
138. Walker DW: Effect of hypoxia on glomerular filtration rate, urine flow and urine composition in chronically catheterized foetal lambs. J Physiol (Lond) 272:15P, 1977.
139. Walker DW: Renal function and micturition in fetal lambs and the effects of hypoxemia. Ann Rech Vet 8:497, 1977.
140. Daniel SS, Husain MK, Milliez J, et al: Renal response of fetal lamb to complete occlusion of umbilical cord. J Pediatr 131:514, 1978.
141. Daniel SS, Yeh MN, Bowe ET, et al: Renal response of the lamb fetus to partial occlusion of the umbilical cord. J Pediatr 87:788, 1975.
142. Levinsky NG, Davidson DG, Berliner RW: Effect of reduced glomerular filtration on urine concentration in the presence of antidiuretic hormone. J Clin Invest 38:730, 1959.

143. Berline RW, Davidson DG: Production of hypertonic urine in the absence of pituitary antidiuretic hormone. J Clin Invest 36:1416, 1957.
144. Korner PI: Effects of low oxygen and carbon monoxide on the renal circulation in unanesthetized rabbits. Circ Res 12:361, 1963.
145. Robillard JE, Sessions C, Smith FG Jr: In vivo demonstration of renal carbonic anhydrase activity in fetal lambs. Biol Neonate 35:253, 1978.
146. Smith FG Jr, Schwartz A: Response of the intact lamb fetus to acidosis. Am J Obstet Gynecol 106:52, 1970.
147. Vaughn D, Kirschbaum TH, Bersentes T, et al: Fetal and neonatal response to acid loading in the sheep. J Appl Physiol 24:135, 1968.
148. Moore ES, Kaiser BA: Renal function in fetal life. In Gruskin AB, Norman ME (eds): Pediatric Nephrology, Proceedings of the Fifth International Pediatric Nephrology Symposium. Boston, Martinus Nijhoff Pub., 1980, p 245.
149. Moore ES, de Lannoy C, Paton JB, Ocampo M: Effect of Na_2SO_4 on urinary acidification in the fetal lamb. Am J Physiol 223:167, 1972.

CHAPTER 55 The Adaptive Capacity of the Newborn

55A Water and Electrolyte

ANITA APERIA

Infants must adjust to extrauterine life with kidneys that are still somewhat immature. Low glomerular filtration rate (GFR), low capacity to vary Na and water transport, and low capacity to correct for metabolic acidosis are some of the limiting immaturities. Those limitations generally have few consequences for the healthy full-term infant fed a proper diet. During stress, however, inappropriate extrarenal losses of water and electrolytes and with renal disease the limitations of the neonatal kidneys often become apparent and produce unpredictable disturbances in water and electrolyte balance. During the last trimester of pregnancy, there is a rapid structural and functional development of the kidney. Disturbances of water and electrolyte balance are therefore more common in preterm than in full-term infants.

SALT AND WATER TRANSPORT IN THE DEVELOPING NEPHRON

GFR is low at birth and increases during the entire period of ontogeny (1, 2). In the proximal tubule there is an isotonic reabsorption of NaCl and water that is governed by active and passive forces. The NaCl reabsorptive capacity of the proximal tubule increases postnatally (3). The activity of NaKATPase, the enzyme that yields energy for active Na transport (4), also increases postnatally (5, 6, 7).

It has not yet been conclusively demonstrated that the fraction of filtrate reabsorbed in the proximal tubule is the same as in the adult nephron at all stages of maturation. Micropuncture of "late proximal" tubules has suggested that this is the case, but late proximal tubules are difficult to localize, especially in the young hydropenic animal (8, 9). In the first segment of the proximal tubule, Na reabsorption is coupled to bicarbonate reabsorption.

Micropuncture of early distal tubules has shown that the factional delivery of NaCl and water to this point is higher in the immature than in the mature nephron (10). The fractional reabsorption of sodium along the relatively water-impermeable distal nephron is as high in the immature as in the mature nephron during hydropenia, and it may be higher in the immature than in the mature nephron during extracellular volume expansion.

The differences between immature and mature tubular segments with regard to Na-transporting properties are schematically illustrated in Figure 55A.1. The heterogenous development of the Na-transporting capacity in proximal and distal tubular segments has implications for the renal control of salt balance. Because of the relatively high distal tubular Na reabsorptive capacity in the immature nephron, the natriuretic response to a salt load generally observed in the adult is blunted in the infant (Fig. 55A.2.).

The urinary concentrating capacity is low at birth in all mammalian species studied. The countercurrent system is less efficient due to immature transport properties of the thick ascending loop of Henle (11) and to short loops of Henle (12). Immature collecting duct cells have been shown to respond less well to antidiuretic hormone (13). In the adult kidney the pelvic spaces surrounding the papilla—the fornices—are narrower than in the developing kidney. This anatomical difference might contribute to the low concentrating capacity during ontogeny, since there now is evidence suggesting that the urine bathing the papilla enhances papillary (and urine) osmolality (14). The factors that can potentially contribute to the low concentrating capacity of the infant kidney are summarized in Figure 55A.3.

The concentrations of receptors for parathyroid hormone (15) and for aldosterone are high (16) in the distal tubule and the cortical collecting duct. Those segments have the capacity to finely adjust P, Ca, Na, and K balance. Not much is known about the development of those segments. Secretion of hydrogen ions also occurs from those distal segments.

There is a centrifugal structural development of the nephrons (17).

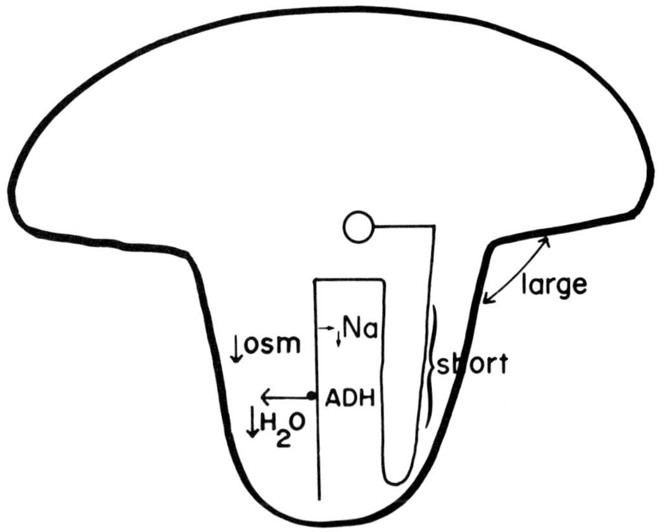

Figure 55A.1. Sodium transport during basal hydropenic conditions in immature (i) and mature (m) nephrons. The low sodium reabsorptive capacity of the proximal tubule and the loop of Henle might contribute to the natriuresis from the very immature kidney that is often observed during basal hydropenic conditions. (From Aperia A, Broberger O, Herin P, Zetterström R: Salt content in human breast milk during the three first weeks after delivery. Acta Paediatr Scand 68:441, 1979.)

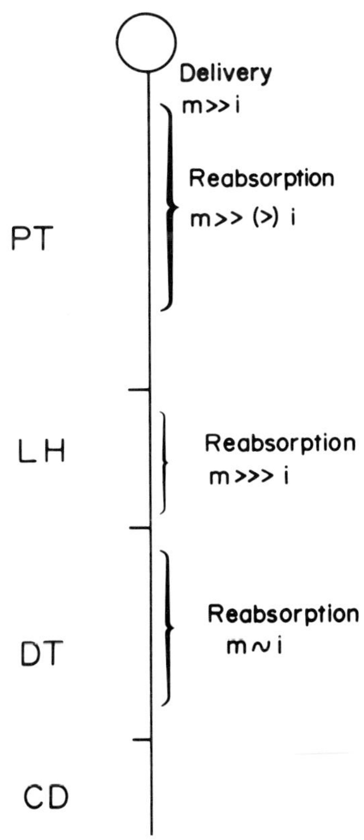

Figure 55A.2. Changes in Na transport following a salt load in immature (i) and mature (m) nephrons. In the immature salt-challenged kidney, the distal tubular Na reabsorption is still relatively high. The increased filtered load of sodium (32) and the decreased reabsorption of sodium in the proximal tubule and loop of Henle might therefore not be sufficient to produce natriuresis.

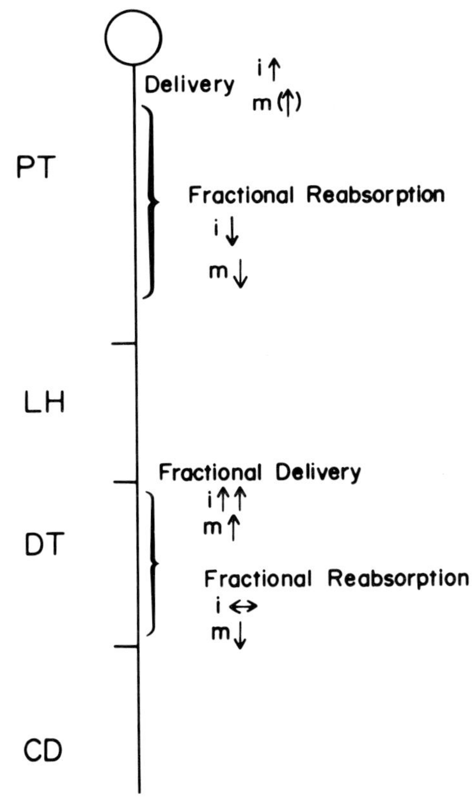

Figure 55A.3. The urinary concentrating capacity in the immature kidney is low for several reasons: The sodium reabsorption in the water-impermeable thick ascending limb of Henle is low. This contributes to a low interstitial osmolality. The loop of Henle is short, which reduces the efficiency of the countercurrent system. The end organ response to antidiuretic hormone is not fully developed, and the anatomical configuration of the kidney with relatively large pelvic spaces might prevent the final concentration of the pelvic urine.

The juxtamedullary nephrons are formed and start to function early in pregnancy, whereas the superficial nephrons are formed around birth. It is therefore possible for the juxtamedullary nephrons to reach their maximal functional capacity earlier than the superficial segments (18, 19). Since the water and electrolyte transporting properties of the juxtamedullary and the superficial nephrons differ (20), a grossly heterogeneous functional development of the kidney would have consequences for the control of body fluid and electrolyte homeostasis in infants.

RENAL WATER EXCRETION

Before discussing the possible limitations of the neonatal kidney to excrete water, we shall review some postnatal changes of the extrarenal factors that determine water balance. Because of the immaturity of the gastrointestinal system, the infant has to consume nutrients in a well-diluted suspension. This necessitates a high water turnover during at least the first six months of life. Experimental studies suggest that the mechanisms regulating intestinal water transport change in the neonatal period (21). Intestinal water transport, which is bidirectional, appears to be more readily influenced by passive pressure forces in infancy than later in life. Total body water is proportionally higher in the fetus than in the adult. The most rapid fall in body water occurs in late fetal life (22). It has therefore been suggested that some weight loss during the first week of life is physiological. The transepidermial water losses are relatively high in the neonatal period: they are highest in premature infants and decrease after birth as gestational age increases (23, 24, 25).

Newborn term infants can produce a urine that is only a little more concentrated than plasma even if they are given antidiuretic hormone (26). Since newborn infants do not respond to antidiuretic hormone, the syndrome of inappropriate ADH secretion does not generally exist during the first week of life. There is a rapid postnatal development of the urinary concentrating capacity, at least in infants with a gestational age above 30 weeks. At four to six weeks of age, infants with a gestational age above 30 weeks can produce an average urine osmolality of around 550 mosm/l when they are given antidiuretic hormone (26). The capacity to concentrate urine appears to increase exponentially during the first year of life. It reaches an adult level around the second year of life (27).

The control of water excretion is limited in the human infant, as in other newborn mammals (Fig. 55A.1). Newborn human infants are capable of producing antidiuretic hormone (28). The response to exogenously administered antidiuretic hormone is low. An immaturity of the end organ (collecting duct cells) response to antidiuretic hormone can therefore be assumed. The length of the loop of Henle changes in postnatal life in the human infant as well as in the rat pup. Physiological factors such as low protein intake and low urea availability might also reduce the capacity to concentrate the urine in the human infant. High protein intake has been shown to increase the urinary concentrating capacity in infants older than two months (29).

The production of an almost isotonic urine satisfies the infant's need for a high water turnover; thus one might question whether the low concentrating capacity during infancy is just a sign of immaturity. Studies in experimental animals suggest that development of the urinary concentrating capacity is accelerated at the time of weaning (30).

The low urinary concentrating capacity makes the infant more sensitive to extrarenal water losses. Dehydration occurs rapidly during intestinal water losses in infants; therefore diarrhea is a more serious condition with a higher mortality rate among infants than among older children. Since in general infants with a postconceptional age of more than 40 weeks have a high capacity to reabsorb Na but a low capacity to concentrate the urine, they are predisposed to larger net losses of water than of salt. It is therefore not surprising that the frequency of hypertonic dehydration is higher in infants than in older children and adults (31, 32) (see also Chapter 6).

It is well established that severe dehydration reduces the GFR in the adult kidney. The capacity to control electrolyte (and water) balance is thereby reduced, and a vicious cycle with regard to water and electrolyte homeostasis will be created in severe dehydration. There is evidence suggesting that the GFR of the infant kidney is even more sensitive to changes in the state of hydration than is the GFR of the adult kidney (33). Dehydration is therefore a common cause of prerenal failure in the neonate. It has been suggested that when renal failure occurs in respiratory distress syndrome, it may be attributed to dehydration (34).

In preterm infants the large transepidermal water losses during the first days of life might cause dehydration. A relatively high water intake has therefore been recommended. This argument must be balanced, however, against the presumed dangers of overhydration. The GFR is low at birth in both preterm and full-term infants (35, 36). It increases rather rapidly immediately after birth in infants with a gestational age above 34 weeks. In infants with a lower gestational age, the GFR remains low, generally less than 40 ml/1.73 m^2 BSA/min during the entire first month of life (36). The capacity of the preterm infant to excrete a very large water load is therefore limited. It has been suggested that overhydration of newborn infants increases frequency of patent ductus arteriosus (37), pulmonary edema (38) and bronchopulmonary dysplasia and alters regional blood flow predisposing to necrotizing enterocolitis as well (37). The tolerance of the neonatal kidney to low and high water intake is incompletely delineated. It is, however, a general experience that most infants can tolerate an intake as low as 100 ml/kg/da without developing dehydration and prerenal failure if no excessive extrarenal water loss occurs. It is also a general experience that most infants can take as much as 165 ml water/kg/day without developing harmful fluid retention. In some instances a higher fluid intake is necessary to satisfy the nutritional needs of the infant. The infants must then be carefully observed for inappropriate weight gains and for circulatory complications.

In countries with a hot climate, high transepidermial water losses might have to be considered throughout infancy. Traditionally most infants in developing countries with a hot climate are given extra water in addition to breast milk (39). The necessity of this regimen remains to be confirmed.

RENAL SODIUM AND POTASSIUM EXCRETION

The kidney is mainly responsible for the control of Na balance. NaCl tolerance is limited in newborn infants (40, 41). Newborn preterm infants and distressed full-term infants have a limited capacity to retain Na and to excrete excess Na. Healthy full-term infants tolerate retention of Na but cannot rapidly excrete excess Na.

Breast milk contains 10 to 20 mmol of sodium during the first two weeks after parturition and 5 to 6 mmol thereafter (42). If newborn preterm infants are fed pooled breast milk or a formula with a sodium concentration less than 10 mmol/L, their urinary Na excretion often exceeds their Na intake and they sustain a net loss of NaCl (43). They respond with an increased release of aldosterone and renin (44); however, because the endorgan response is reduced, the salt-retaining effect of those hormones is limited (43). A moderate hyponatremia is commonly associated with the loss of NaCl in infancy (45) because water intake remains high. It has been reported that hyponatremia results in growth retardation (46, 47); however, hyponatremia is generally overlooked as a clinical problem. It should be remembered, however, that in adults, longstanding hyponatremia has been shown to cause pontine lesions (48).

It is recommended that the diet of preterm infants be supplemented with NaCl, so that the total salt intake ranges between 2 and 3 mmol/kg/da. This is generally sufficient to keep them from developing a negative Na balance.

Healthy term infants are able to conserve salt when salt intake is as low as in human milk $<$10 mM/l. However, when the full-term infant develops a condition such as hypoxia or septicemia or has renal disease, urinary salt losses often become a prominent feature. Hyponatremia is a common manifestation of renal insufficiency in the neonate (49, 50, 51). This is not surprising. Sodium transport is the most energy-demanding process in the kidney. The activity of NaKATPase, the enzyme that yields energy for active sodium transport, is lower in the neonatal than in the adult kidney. Although the low enzyme activity appears to be sufficient for the maintenance of sodium balance during basal conditions, there is probably no reserve capacity to cope with hypoxia or cellular damage.

The capacity to retain Na, i.e., to increase Na reabsorption during a negative Na balance, is governed by mechanisms other than the reverse of the mechanism by which Na reabsorption is depressed during Na retention. Preterm infants, like term infants, are unable to excrete an Na load rapidly. This inability of the neonate to rapidly excrete a salt load was first observed by McCance and Widdowson in the 1950s in an experimental study (52) and since has been confirmed in clinical studies (53).

The capacity to excrete a salt load increases during infancy to reach adult levels between the first and the second year of life (54). The inability to rapidly excrete a salt load has been attributed to a heterogenous development of the nephrons with a poor coordination between different nephron segments (10, 55) and to the high levels of mineralcorticoid hormones found in infants (Fig. 55A.3) (56, 57).

Human breast milk gives the infant a constant supply of NaCl in low concentration. This is adequate for the healthy term newborn. If the term infant is given more Na, for instance cow's milk, for a longer period of time there is a risk of developing NaCl and water retention resulting in expanded plasma volume and edema; sometimes there is a more selective retention of NaCl resulting in hypernatremia (58). Hypernatremia is a complication to be avoided since it can cause cerebral hemorrhage as well as permanent damage to brain cells (59, 60). The mortality rate from hypernatremia is high. The incidence of hypernatremia is greater in more premature newborns, i.e., those having a lower gestational age (59).

Salt-sensitive hypertensive rats fed a high salt diet during prepubertal growth permanently alter blood pressure control and develop hypertension in later life, even though salt intake is controlled following puberty (61, 62). The long-term effect of a moderately positive salt and water balance in human infants remains to be elucidated. It is presently recommended though that full-term infants be given a NaCl intake that does not much exceed that provided by breast milk during the first months of life and that the Na intake should be increased slowly during the next 10 to 12 months.

Transient hyperkalemia is frequently observed in the neonatal period. In preterm infants with an otherwise uncomplicated course, serum potassium (K_s) levels above 6 are not uncommon (47).

Since K is primarily an intracellular ion, total K balance cannot be evaluated from K_s values. There is little information available on whether transcellular potassium transport changes during ontogeny (Chapter 7).

K intake is not excessive in the neonatal period. The Na/K ratio in breast milk decreases from 1 to ~0.6 (in mm) during the first weeks after parturition and then remains constant throughout lactation (42).

Urinary K excretion and the urinary Na/K ratio is higher in newborn *preterm* infants than in newborn *full-term* infants (43, 63). The higher urinary Na/K ratio might be an expression of low responsiveness to aldosterone, low NaKATPase activity in the Na reabsorbing tubular segments, or both. The result is a net loss of NaCl and a reduction in ECF volume during the early neonatal period; these are greater in preterm infants.

Changes in potassium balance also will influence the ionic transport in the intestine. In response to high potassium intake, the adult colon increases its NaKATPase activity and its rate of potassium secretion (64). Animal experiments have shown that the NaKATPase activity of the colon increases postnatally at least until weaning is completed (65). Although these responses are qualitatively appropriate, the effect upon balance is minimal. The kidney is the main regulator of total body K and serum K.

Since term infants generally have a pH and buffer base level lower than children or adults, a low intracellular pH also is likely. This may be a factor affecting distribution of potassium ions between cells and extracellular fluid and affecting the capacity for tubular secretion of potassium. These factors may contribute to the high extracellular potassium concentration in the neonatal period.

Transient hyperkalemia in infants usually is not considered to be a clinical problem; however, the daily potassium allowance should not much exceed that provided by breast milk.

RENAL PHOSPHATE AND CALCIUM EXCRETION

Radiological changes compatible with skeletal demineralization or rickets are frequently observed in preterm infants during their first year of life (66, 67). It is generally agreed that the bone changes are mainly due to an inadequate supply of Ca and P and that immature renal function is of relatively little importance for disturbances in Ca and P balance in the neonate.

Beginning with birth the serum Ca level gradually falls in normal infants fed human milk so that by the second or third day of life the level is lower than that found in older infants and children (68, 69). In most normal full-term infants the serum calcium level returns to normal by 10 days of life. The fall in Ca_s level is more pronounced in preterm and in distressed infants. The transient hypocalcemia has not yet been related to the function of parathyroid hormone, calciotonin, or 25 hydroxyvitamin D (68, 70). The parathyroid hormone level is low immediately after birth but increases rapidly thereafter and is generally above the adult range in infants older than 34 hr of age. It has been suggested that the renal response to parathyroid hormone is incompletely developed in preterm infants (71).

The capacity to excrete P is determined both by glomerular filtration rate and tubular transport mechanisms. Parathyroid hormone increases glomerular filtration rate and decreases tubular phosphate reabsorption. During the first week of life the fractional excretion of phosphate is higher in preterm than in full-term infants (72). The mechanism for this has not been determined. Immaturity of the proximal tubules and extracellular volume expansion have been suggested as contributory factors. After the first week of life, fractional excretion of phosphate is generally low in both preterm and in full-term infants (73). The fractional excretion of phosphate is lower in infants than in children (73) and lower in children than in adults (74). A low fractional excretion of phosphate has also been observed in growing rats, and it is generally regarded as appropriate to preserve phosphate for bone mineralization. Animal studies suggest that parathyroid hormone is not responsible for this adaptive response (75).

Available information suggests that under basal conditions fractional excretion of calcium is similar in infants and older children (76). The capacity of the infant kidney to cope with negative and positive calcium balance has, however, not yet been fully evaluated.

Since many preterm infants develop rickets, supplementation with phosphate, calcium, and vitamin D is generally used. Some neonatologists recommend a supplement with 1.25 dihydroxyvitamin D for preterm infants; however, a regimen of this kind or one with a very high calcium supplement requires careful monitoring of serum calcium levels since the upper limit of the renal capacity to excrete an excess of calcium has not yet been established in infants.

RENAL REGULATION OF ACID BASE BALANCE

Total blood CO_2 is lower in infants than in older children and adults, and it is lower in preterm than in term infants (77, 78). Renal immaturity contributes to the low blood CO_2 because the infant has a low capacity to reabsorb bicarbonate and a low capacity to excrete titratable acids (79, 80). Administration of ammonium chloride increases ammonia production in preterm and term infants (80), but the ammonia production might not be sufficient to compensate fully for a metabolic acidosis until the end of the second year of life (81).

It has been suggested that a relatively high extracellular volume and a tubular immaturity contribute to the relatively low bicarbonate reabsorption in neonates. Most of the bicarbonate is reabsorbed in the first 20%

of the proximal tubule. There is evidence suggesting that the low capacity of the proximal tubule to reabsorb bicarbonate during ontogeny is linked to its low capacity to reabsorb sodium. It has been observed in clinical studies that the decrease in sodium excretion that occurs with increasing postconceptional age parallels the decrease in urinary pH (82). It has also been demonstrated that sodium supplementation in preterm infants increases total CO_2 content and base excess (83).

In newborns with such conditions as hypoxia and septicemia or renal disease, bicarbonate reabsorption is further reduced. In RDS, an alkaline urine is generally excreted even in case of metabolic acidosis and hypocapnia (84). Metabolic acidosis is an earlier and more serious complication of renal insufficiency in the infant than in the adult. Metabolic bone disease and growth retardation are invariable complications during long-standing acidosis (85). It is therefore of utmost importance to detect chronic metabolic acidosis early and treat it with bicarbonate supplements. Primary renal tubular acidosis is generally symptomatic in infancy. Its clinical manifestations include vomiting, polyuria, dehydration, constipation, and failure to thrive (86).

It has not yet been settled whether metabolic acidosis should be corrected in infants who have total CO_2 values in the lower range of normal for postnatal and gestational age, but it is the general consensus today that if total CO_2 is above 14.5 mmol/L and tends to increase continuously, the metabolic acidosis will have no immediate effect on growth (78). The possibility that metabolic acidosis in preterm infants results in metabolic bone disease later has, however, not yet been properly evaluated. Since infants have a limited capacity to regulate acid base metabolism, they have a low tolerance for a daily load of nonvolatile acid. It is well established that ingestion of cow's milk, which has a higher protein and phosphorous content than human milk, often precipitates symptomatic acidosis in infants (77).

References

1. Aperia A, Herin P: Development of glomerular perfusion rate and nephron filtration rate in rats 17–60 days old. Am J Physiol 228:1319, 1975.
2. John E, Goldsmith DI, Spitzer A: Quantitative change in the canine glomerular vasculature during development: physiological implications. Kidney Int 20:223, 1981.
3. Aperia A, Larsson L: Correlation between fluid reabsorption and proximal tubule ultrastructure during development of the rat kidney. Acta Physiol Scand 105:11, 1979.
4. Jørgensen PL: Sodium and potassium ion pump in kidney tubules. Physiol Rev 60:864, 1980.
5. Schmidt U, Horster M: Na-K-activated ATPase activity maturation in rabbit nephron segments dissected in vitro. Am J Physiol 233:F55, 1977.
6. Aperia A, Larsson L, Zetterström R: Hormonal induction of Na-K-ATPase in developing proximal tubular cells. Am J Physiol 10:F356, 1981.
7. Igarashi Y, Aperia A, Larsson L, Zetterström R: A time course study of changes in NaKATPase activity in developing proximal tubules induced by betamethasone. Am J Physiol 245:F232–F237, 1983.
8. Spitzer A, Brandis M: Functional and morphologic maturation of superficial nephrons: relationship to total kidney function. J Clin Invest 53:279, 1974.
9. Elinder G: Effect of isotonic volume expansion on proximal tubular Na and fluid reabsorption in the developing rat kidney. Acta Physiol Scand 112:83, 1981.
10. Aperia A, Elinder G: Distal tubular sodium reabsorption in the developing rat kidney. Am J Physiol 9:F487, 1981.
11. Horster M: Loop of Henle functional differentiation in in vitro perfusion of the isolated thick ascending segment. Pflügers Arch 378:15, 1978.
12. Edwards BR, Mendel DB, La Rochelle FT, et al: Postnatal development of urinary concentrating ability in rats: changes in renal anatomy and neurohypophysical hormones in the kidney during development. In Spitzer A (ed): The Kidney during Development. Masson 1982, p 233.
13. Schlondorf D, Wever H, Trizna W, Fine LG: Vasopressin in responsiveness of renal adenylate cyclase in newborn rats and rabbits. Am J Physiol 234:F16, 1978.
14. Bonventre JV, Roman RJ, Lechene C: Effect of urea concentration of pelvic fluid on renal concentrating ability. Am J Physiol 239:F609, 1980.
15. Morel F: Sites of hormone action in the mammalian nephron. Am J Physiol 240:F159, 1981.
16. Vandewalle A, Farman N, Bencsath P, Bonvalet JP: Aldosterone binding along the rabbit nephron: an autoradiographic study on isolated tubules. Am J Physiol 240:F172, 1981.
17. Potter EL: Normal and abnormal development of the kidney. Chicago, Year Book Medical Publishers, 1972.
18. De Rouffignac C, Monnens L: Functional and morphological maturation of superficial and juxtamedullary nephrons in the rat. J Physiol. 262:119, 1976.
19. Dlouha H, Bibr B, Jezek J, Zicha J: Single nephron glomerular filtration rate ratios of superficial, intercortical and juxtamedullary nephrons in rats during development. Pflügers Arch 366:277, 1976.
20. Jacobsson HR: Characteristics of volume reabsorption in rabbit superficial and juxtamedullary proximal convoluted tubules. J Clin Invest 64:410, 1979.
21. Younoszai MK: Development of water and electrolyte transport in the small intestine. In Lebenthal E (ed): Textbook of Gastroenterology and Nutrition in Infancy. New York, Raven Press, 1981, p 615.
22. Friis-Hansen B: Body composition during growth: biochemical data and in vivo measurements. Pediatrics 47:264, 1971.
23. Bell EF, Gray JC, Weinstein MR, Oh W: The effects of thermal environment on heat balance and insensible water loss in low-birth-weight infants. J Pediatr 96:452, 1980.
24. Hammarlund K, Sedin G: Transepidermal water loss in newborn infants. III. Relation to gestational age. Acta Paediatr Scand 68:795, 1978.
25. Hammarlund K, Sedin G, Strömberg B: Transepidermal water loss in newborn infants. VII. Relation to postnatal age in very preterm and full-term appropriate for gestational age infants. Acta Paediatr Scand 71:369, 1982.
26. Svenningsen NW, Aronson AS: Postnatal development of renal concentration capacity as estimated by DDAVP-test in normal and asphyxiated neonates. Biol Neonate 25:230, 1974.
27. Polacek E, Vocel J, Neugebauerova L, et al: The osmotic concentrating ability in healthy infants and children. Arch Dis Child 40:291, 1965.
28. Pohjavuori M, Fyhrquist F: Hemodynamic significance of vasopressin in the newborn infant. J Pediatr 97:462, 1980.
29. Edelmann CM Jr, Barnett HL, Troupkou V: Renal concentrating mechanisms in newborn infants, effect of dietary protein and water content, role of urea, and responsiveness to antidiuretic hormone. J Clin Invest 39:1062, 1960.
30. Falk G: Maturation of renal function in infant rats. Am J Physiol 181:157, 1955.
31. Paneth N: Hypernatremic dehydration of infancy. Am J Dis Child 134:785, 1980.
32. Hill ID, Mann MD, Bowie MD: Hypernatraemic dehydration: a prospective study in children with diarrhoeal disease. S Afr Med J 59:479, 1981.
33. Elinder G, Aperia A, Herin P, Källskog Ö: Effect of isotonic volume expansion on glomerular filtration rate and renal hemodynamics in the developing rat kidney. Acta Physiol Scand 108:411, 1980.
34. Guignard JP, Torrado A, Mazouni SM, Gautier E: Renal function in respiratory distress syndrome. J Pediatr 88:845, 1976.
35. Guignard JP, Torrado A, Gautier E: Glomerular filtration rate in the first three weeks of life. J Pediatr 87:268, 1975.
36. Aperia A, Broberger O, Elinder G, et al: Postnatal development of renal function in preterm and full-term infants. Acta Paediatr Scand 70:183, 1981.
37. Bell EF, et al: Effect of fluid administration on the development of symptomatic patent ductus arteriosus and congestive heart failure in premature infants. N Engl J Med 302:598, 1980.
38. Brown ER, et al: Bronchopulmonary dysplasia: possible relationship to pulmonary edema. J Pediatr 92:982, 1978.
39. Almroth SG: Water requirements of breast-fed infants in a hot climate. Am J Clin Nutr 31:1154, 1978.
40. Spitzer A: The role of the kidney in sodium homeostasis during maturation. Kidney Int 21:539, 1982.
41. Aperia A: Salt and water metabolism in the perinatal period. In Battaglia FC, Boyd RDH (eds): Pediatrics, Vol 2, Perinatal Medicine. London, Butterworth and Co (Publishers) Limited, 1983, p 113.
42. Aperia A, Broberger O, Herin P, Zetterström R: Salt content in human breast milk during the three first weeks after delivery. Acta Paediatr Scand 68:441, 1979.
43. Aperia A, Broberger O, Herin P, Zetterström R: Sodium excretion in relation to sodium intake and aldosterone excretion in newborn preterm and full-term infants. Acta Paediatr Scand 68:813, 1979.
44. Sulyok E, Nemeth M, Tenyi I, et al: Postnatal development of renin-angiotensin-aldosterone system, RAAS, in relation to electrolyte balance in premature infants. Pediatr Res 13:817, 1979.
45. Roy RN, Chance GW, Radde IC, et al: Late hyponatremia in very low birth-weight infants (<1.3 kg). Pediatr Res 10:526, 1976.
46. Chance GW, Radde IC, Willis DM, et al: Postnatal growth of infants of <1.3 kg birth weight: effects of metabolic acidosis, of caloric intake, and of calcium, sodium, and phosphate supplementation. J Pediatr 91:787, 1977.
47. Day GM, Radde IC, Balfe JW, Chance GW: Electrolyte abnormalities in very low birth weight infants. Pediatr Res 10:522, 1976.

48. Burcar PJ, Norenberg MD, Yarnell PR: Hyponatremia and central pontine myelinolysis. Neurology 27:223, 1977.
49. Mathew OP, Jones AS, James E, et al: Neonatal renal failure: usefulness of diagnostic indices. Pediatrics 65:1, 1980.
50. Norman ME, Asadi FK: A prospective study of acute renal failure in the newborn infant. Pediatrics 63:3, 1979.
51. Reimold EW, Don TD, Worthen HG: Renal failure during the first year of life. Pediatrics 59:987, 1977.
52. McCance RA, Widdowson EM: The response of the newborn puppy to water, salt and food. J Physiol 141:81, 1958.
53. Aperia A, Broberger O, Thodenius K, Zetterström R: Renal response to an oral sodium load in newborn full-term infants. Acta Paediatr Scand 61:670, 1972.
54. Aperia A, Broberger O, Thodenius K, Zetterström R: Development of renal control of salt and fluid homeostasis during the first year of life. Acta Paediatr Scand 64:393, 1975.
55. Rodriguez-Soriano J, Vallo A, Castillo G, Oliveros R: Renal handling of water and sodium in infancy and childhood: a study using clearance methods during hypotonic water diuresis. Kidney Int 20:700, 1981.
56. Dillon MJ, Gillin MEA, Ryness JM, De Swiet M: Plasma renin activity and aldosterone concentration in the human newborn. Arch Dis Child 51:537, 1976.
57. Van Acker KJ, Scharpe SL, Deprettere AJR, Neels HM: Renin-angiotensin-aldosterone system in the healthy infant and child. Kidney Int 16:196, 1979.
58. Taitz LS, Byers HD: High calorie/osmolar feeding and hypertonic dehydration. Arch Dis Child 47:257, 1972.
59. Simmons MA, Adcock EW, Bard H, Battaglia FC: Hypernatremia and intracerebral hemorrhage in neonates. N Engl Med 291:6, 1974.
60. Macaulay D, Watson M: Hypernatraemia in infants as a cause of brain damage. Arch Dis Child 42:485, 1967.
61. Dahl LK, Heine M, Tassinari L: Effects of chronic excess salt ingestion. J Exper Med 115:1173, 1962.
62. Bianchi G, Baer PG, Fox U, Guidi E: The role of the kidney in the rat with genetic hypertension. Postgrad Med J 53:123, 1977.
63. Sulyok E, Varga E, Györy E, et al: On the mechanism of renal sodium handling in newborn infants. Biol Neonate 37:75, 1980.
64. Hayslett JP, Binder HJ: Mechanism of potassium adaptation. Am J Physiol 243:F103, 1982.
65. Marin L, Aperia A: Water and electrolyte transport in the developing colon. J Pediatr Gastroenterol Nutr 3:471–474, 1984.
66. Eek S, Gabreielsen LH, Halvorsen S: Prematurity and rickets. Pediatrics 20:63, 1957.
67. Chesney RW, Hamstra AJ, DeLuca HF: Rickets of prematurity, supranormal levels of serum 1.25-dihydroxy-vitamin D. Am J Dis Child 135:34, 1981.
68. Hillman LS, Rojanasathit S, Slatopolsky E, Haddad JG: Serial measurements of serum calcium, magnesium, parathyroid hormone, calcitonin and 25-Hydroxy-Vitamin D in premature and term infants during the first week of life. Pediatr Res 11:739, 1977.
69. David L, Anast CS: Calcium metabolism in newborn infants. J Clin Invest 54:287, 1974.
70. Steichen JJ, Tsang RC, Gratton TL, et al: Vitamin D homeostasis in the perinatal period, 1.25-dihydroxyvitamin D in maternal, cord, and neonatal blood. N Engl J Med 302:315, 1980.
71. Mallet E, Basuyay J-P. Brunelle P, et al: Neonatal parathyroid secretion and renal receptor maturation in premature infants. Biol Neonate 33:304, 1978.
72. Arant B: Developmental patterns of renal functional maturation compared in the human neonate. J Pediatr 92:705, 1978.
73. Brodehl J, Gellissen K, Weber H-P: Postnatal development of tubular phosphate reabsorption. Clin Nephrol 17:163, 1982.
74. Kruse K, Kracht U, Göpfert G: Renal threshold phosphate concentration ($TmPO_4$/GFR). Arch Dis Child 57:217, 1982.
75. Caverzasio J, Bonjour J-P, Fleisch H: Tubular handling of P_i in young growing and adult rats. Am J Physiol 242:F705, 1982.
76. Day GM, Chance FW, Radde IC, et al: Growth and mineral metabolism in very low birth weight infants. II. Effects of calcium supplementation on growth and divalent cations. Pediatr Res 9:568, 1975.
77. Kildeberg P: Disturbances of hydrogen ion balance occurring in premature infants. I. Early types of acidosis. Acta Paediatr Scand 53:505, 1964.
78. Schwartz GJ, Haycock GB, Chir B, et al: Late metabolic acidosis: a reassessment of the definition. J Pediatr 95:102, 1979.
79. Edelmann CM Jr, Rodriguez-Soriano J, Biochis H, et al: Renal bicarbonate reabsorption and hydrogen ion excretion in normal infants. J Clin Invest 46:1309, 1967.
80. Svenningsen NW: Renal acid-base titration studies in infants with and without metabolic acidosis in the psotneonatal period. Pediatr Res 8:659, 1974.
81. Monnens L, Schretlen E, vanMunster P: The renal excretion of hydrogen ions in infants and children. Nephron 12:29, 1974.
82. Sulyok E, Heim T, Soltesz G, Jaszai V: The influence of maturity on renal control of acidosis in newborn infants. Biol Neonate 21:418, 1972.
83. Sulyok E, Nemeth M, Tenyi I, et al: Relationship between the postnatal development of the renin-angiotensin-aldosterone system and the electrolyte and acid-base status in the sodium chloride supplemented premature infant. Acta Paeditrica Academiae Scientiarum Hungaricae 22:109, 1981.
84. Torrado A, Guignard JP, Prod'hom LS, Gautier E: Hypoxemia and renal function in newborns with respiratory distress syndrome (RDS). Helv Paediatr Acta 29:399, 1974.
85. McSherry E, Morris RC: Attainment and maintenance of normal stature with alkali therapy in infants and children with classic renal tubul acidosis. J Clin Invest 61:509, 1978.
86. Rodriguez-Soriano J, Vallo A, Castillo G, Oliveros R: Natural history of primary distal renal tubular acidosis treated since infancy. Pediatrics 101:669, 1982.

55B Nutrition

WILLIAM C. HEIRD

NUTRITIONAL ADAPTATION

The fetus, in utero, receives necessary nutritional substrates from the mother through the placenta. The major substrates are glucose and amino acids (1). Only a small fraction, if any, of the fetus' energy requirement is met directly by fat, although it is likely that a variety of ketoacids and other organic acids derived from fat are used as energy substrates. At birth, the situation changes abruptly. Since the continuous supply of nutrients from the placenta is no longer available, the infant's ongoing needs must be met by the metabolism of endogenous nutrient stores or exogenously administered nutrients. In either case, lipid becomes a much more important energy substrate than it was in utero.

The switch to using lipid does not occur abruptly. Immediately after birth, the infant's limited glycogen stores are used as a continuing source of glucose, as in acute starvation. In addition, even the prematurely born infant is capable of mounting a gluconeogenic response, i.e., converting endogenous protein into amino acids and subsequently to glucose. Nonetheless, the infant's blood glucose concentration inevitably drops considerably during the first few hours after birth. It is not clear whether this is caused primarily by residual insulin released before birth, persistent insulin release characteristic of the in utero situation, slow adaptation of extrauterine glucose homeostatic mechanisms, or a combination of these factors.

The hormonal milieu of the fetus in large part is determined by the hormonal milieu of the mother; however, it is clear that the fetus, particularly during the latter part of gestation, also is able to mount independent endocrinological responses. Although not absolutely necessary, perhaps, the hormonal changes associated with the stress of birth, i.e., increased secretion of catecholamines and adrenal corticosteroids by the infant, the mother, or both, theoretically could contribute to the successful adaptation to extrauterine life. Catecholamines as well as glucagon enhance glycogenolysis, whereas catecholamines and the corticosteroids promote breakdown of endogenous protein to provide amino acids as gluconeogenic substrates. These hormones also counter the effects of insulin, which tends to inhibit fat utilization. Subsequently, when insulin levels are lower, endogenous lipid stores can be used to help meet ongoing energy needs. Use of the endogenously released lipid in turn sets the stage for subsequent use of the lipid content of breast milk or formula.

Generally, it is thought that the newborn infant requires greater amounts of all nutrient than the fetus; however, the magnitude of these differences is not known. Resting energy expenditure roughly doubles over the first few days of life (2). In part, this increase represents greater requirements for response to cold stress and for activity. There is no convincing evidence that the basal energy expenditure of the newborn infant is greater than that of the fetus, but theoretically the hormonal changes at birth should result in greater needs. Since the magnitude and quality of intrauterine growth and growth during the first few weeks following birth are similar, the newborn infant's energy needs for growth should not be very different from those of the fetus. The greater protein requirement of the infant compared to that of the fetus probably reflects the relative inefficiency of the infant compared with the fetus.

The first few days of life are associated with a number of other dramatic changes as well. The changes in circulation as well as the pulmonary changes that occur at birth have been studied extensively and are reasonably well understood. Changes that occur in other organ systems, however, are less well understood. At birth, for example, the gastrointestinal tract and the kidneys, neither of which is used extensively in utero, must assume responsibility, respectively, for digestion and absorption of exogenous nutrients and for excreting waste products produced by metabolism of these nutrients. Knowledge concerning the changes in these organs at birth are derived primarily from studies in animals (3). One of the most revealing studies is that of Widdowson and coworkers (4); it describes a marked increase in intestinal mucosal mass and kidney weight of piglets during the first 24 hr of life. Such studies, along with descriptions of histological and enzymatic changes in the gastrointestinal tract and the kidney during gestation, permit the development of theories concerning the functional changes in these organs in the human infant. Logically speaking, these changes should facilitate intestinal absorption of nutrients needed by the infant as well as the renal excretion of the waste products produced from metabolism of these nutrients.

In general, the infant born at term has few difficulties adapting to the changes in nutrient substrate necessitated by birth. Such infants have well-developed sucking and swallowing mechanisms and, in the absence of severe birth trauma or congenital anomalies, can be fed shortly after birth. Prematurely born infants, on the other hand, frequently experience difficulties. These infants, particularly the more immature infants, have neurological and other developmental deficits (e.g., uncoordinated sucking and swallowing, ineffective gastric emptying, and ineffective intestinal peristalsis) that limit the volume of exogenous nutrients that can be administered through the gastrointestinal tract; many also have immature metabolic processes that limit use of absorbed nutrients. Nonetheless, with appropriate management, i.e., careful attention to the route of nutrient delivery and the composition of the nutrient intake, prematurely born infants have surprisingly few difficulties with nutritional adaptation to extrauterine life.

Because the endogenous nutrient stores of prematurely born infants are limited, appropriate early nutritional management is of major importance. Based on body composition data (5), the 1000 g infant has endogenous energy reserves of approximately 250 kcal. Assuming an energy expenditure of 50 to 60 kcal/kg/day, this is sufficient to permit survival for only four or five days without exogenous nutrients (Fig. 55B.1). Endogenous reserves of the 2000 g infant are somewhat greater (i.e., approximately 600 kcal/kg), due largely to a greater fat content. These are sufficient to enable survival for 10 to 12 days without exogenous nutrients. The term infant weighing 3500 g is much less vulnerable; endogenous energy reserves (approximately 1650 kcal/kg) are sufficient to enable survival for close to a month.

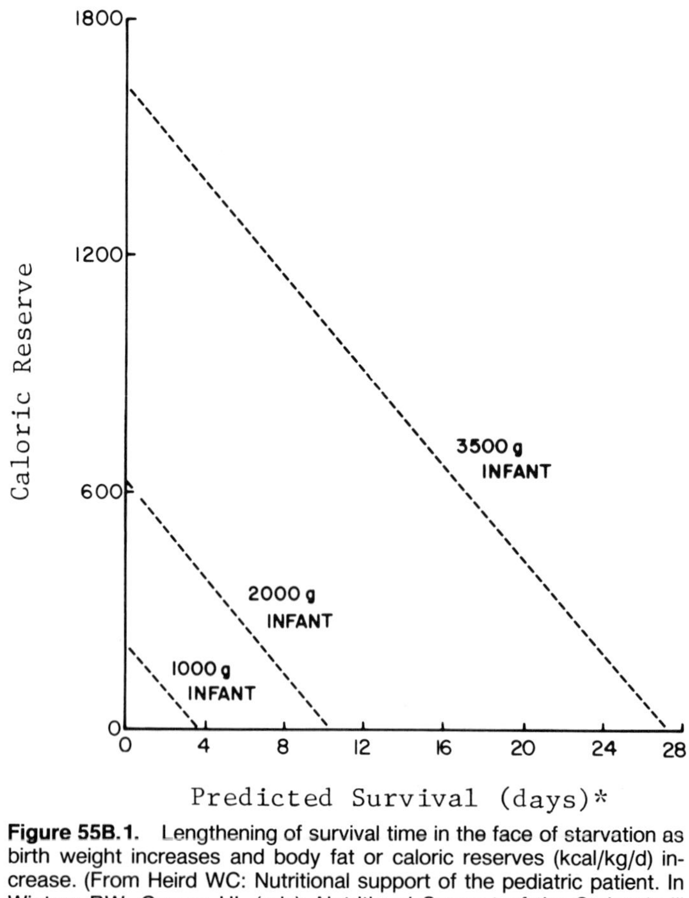

Figure 55B.1. Lengthening of survival time in the face of starvation as birth weight increases and body fat or caloric reserves (kcal/kg/d) increase. (From Heird WC: Nutritional support of the pediatric patient. In Winters RW, Greene HL (eds): Nutritional Support of the Seriously Ill Patient. New York, Academic Press, 1983, p. 157.)

Such calculations, of course, are based on a number of assumptions. The major one, perhaps, is the assumption that energy needs remain constant in the face of inadequate intake, i.e., that the infant does not "adapt" to starvation or semistarvation as does the older child (see Chapter 10). Nonetheless, the predictions derived from such calculations are borne out by clinical experience. Within the context of this chapter, the greatest value of these calculations, perhaps, is to illustrate the newborn infant's limited adaptive mechanisms for inadequate exogenous nutrient intake and to highlight the need for early intervention to assure that ongoing nutrient needs, particularly maintenance needs, are met.

NUTRIENT REQUIREMENTS

Most agree that human milk is the optimal intake for the normal term infant. In fact, the growth rate of infants fed human milk usually is the standard against which alternative nutritional regimens are judged. The age at which human milk should be supplemented is less unanimously agreed upon; although more enthusiastic proponents of human milk advocate its adequacy for the first year of life, most feel that supplementation after about four months of age is desirable. The infant who is breast-fed exclusively for the first four months of life, on average, receives protein and energy intakes, respectively, of ~2 g/kg/d, and 100 to 120 Kcal/kg/d. These intakes probably are the minimal intakes of protein and energy compatible with adequate nutrition, particularly if human milk is replaced by an artificial formula; however, these intakes may not be adequate for all infants, e.g., malnourished infants or those with chronic illness.

There is much less agreement concerning the nutrutional needs of the low-birth-weight infant. Some feel that the growth rate achieved with human milk fed at 180 to 200 ml/kg/d is sufficient. Others, however, feel that the goal should be to continue the intrauterine growth rate. The fact that human milk contains insufficient amounts of protein, calcium, sodium, and perhaps zinc to allow accumulation of these nutrients at the intrauterine rate, even if absorption of each is complete, prevents consolidation of these two views (7, 8).

Data to support the obviously logical concept that continuation of the intrauterine growth rate during extrauterine life is necessary or efficacious are lacking. Until such data are available, however, the possibility that failure to maintain the intrauterine growth rate may result in delayed growth and development of maturing organ systems cannot be discounted. On the other hand, some data suggest that the amount of protein required to assure continuation of the intrauterine growth rate may exceed the low-birth-weight infant's metabolic tolerance (9). If so, the resulting metabolic derangements (e.g., acidosis, hyperaminoacidemia) may exert equally deleterious effects on growth and development of various organ systems.

The adequacy of the protein content of human milk for low-birth-weight infants has been questioned since the demonstration, some 40 years ago, that such infants fed artificial formulas of high protein content gain weight more rapidly than those fed human milk (10). This study, however, did not address the possibility that all or part of the greater weight gain might be due to water retention secondary to the greater electrolyte and mineral intake of infants fed the high protein formula. Subsequent studies demonstrated that at least part of the weight gain attributed solely to the greater protein intake probably was due to water retention (11). Nonetheless, most clinical studies designed to differentiate between the effects of protein and mineral intake indicate a direct relationship between protein intake and growth.

In addition to lower growth rates, infants fed banked human milk (protein intake, approximately 2 g/kg/d) have lower plasma albumin concentrations than those fed protein intakes of 2.25 or 4.5 g/kg/d (9). However, they do not exhibit clinical signs of hypoalbuminemia. The protein content of milk produced by mothers who deliver prematurely is some 20% higher than that of mothers who deliver at term (12), and low-birth-weight infants who are fed their own mother's milk (13) as well as those fed banked milk of mothers who deliver prematurely (14) appear to gain weight at the intrauterine rate. Thus, the protein intake of these infants, i.e., approximately 2.7 g/kg/d, probably is the best estimate of the minimal intake compatable with adequate nutrition.

The foregoing discussion illustrates the general lack of concrete information concerning the goals of nutritional management, and therefore the nutrient requirements of the low-birth-weight infant. The Committee on Nutrition of the American Academy of Pediatrics, however, has made tentative recommendations based on the existing information (Table 55B.1). Until further information is available, these recommendations provide useful guidelines for judging the adequacy of any nutritional regimen. Human milk fed in reasonable volumes (up to 200 ml/kg/24 hr) does not provide the recommended intakes of a number of nutrients, namely, protein, sodium, calcium, and possibly zinc. Some who prefer to provide the potential nonnutritional advantages of human milk routinely provide supplemental sodium and calcium or a formula supplement. Another approach is to be aware of the potential inadequacies of human milk and institute adequate monitoring to detect hyponatremia, hypocalcemia, inadequate skeletal mineralization, or all these conditions; should any occur, supplementation obviously is indicated.

Table 55B.1.
Recommended Nutrient Intakes of Low-Birth-Weight-Infants (16)

Nutrient	Recommended intake
Energy[a]	120 kcal/kg/d
Protein	2.25–5.0 g/kg/d
Minerals	
Sodium[b]	2.25–3.5 mEq/kg/d
Potassium	2–3 mEq/kg/d
Calcium	200–250 mg/kg/d
Phosphorus	110–125 mg/kg/d
Zinc	0.6 mg/kg/d (0.5 mg/100 kcal)
Manganese	6.0 mg/kg/d (5.0 mg/100 kcal)
Copper	108 mg/kg/d (90 mg/100 kcal)
Iron[c]	2–3 mg/kg/d
Iodine	6.0 mg/kg/d (5.0 mg/100 kcal)
Vitamins	
Vitamin A	300–900 IU/kg/d (250/750 IU/100 kcal)
Vitamin K	4.8 mg/kg/d (4 mg/100 kcal)
Thiamine	48 mg/kg/d (40 mg/100 kcal)
Riboflavin	72 mg/kg/d (60 mg/100 kcal)
Niacin	300 mg/kg/d (250 mg/100 kcal)
Pyridoxine	42 mg/kg/d (35 mg/100 kcal)
Pantothenic acid	360 mg/kg/d (300 mg/100 kcal)
Vitamin B_{12}	0.18 mg/kg/d (0.15 mg/100 kcal)
Biotin	1.8 mg/kg/d (1.5 mg/100 kcal)
Folic acid	50 mg/d
Vitamin C	35 mg/d
Vitamin D	500 IU/d
Vitamin E[d]	0.84 IU/kg/d (0.7 IU/100 kcal)

[a] Linoleic acid should constitute 3% of total energy intake.
[b] Infants weighing <1500 g at birth may require 4–8 mEq/kg/d.
[c] Iron supplement probably is not required before two months of age; if given before this age, vitamin E intake should be increased.
[d] Some recommend 5–25 $IU \cdot d^{-1}$; total intake should be 1.0 IU per gram of linoleic acid.

DELIVERY NUTRIENT REQUIREMENTS TO LOW-BIRTH-WEIGHT

For most low-birth-weight infants, the foregoing discussion is largely academic. The infants' underlying illness as well as a number of neurophysiological deficiencies (i.e., poor or unsustained suck, uncoordinated swallowing mechanism, delayed gastric emptying, and poor intestinal motility) make delivery of any enteral nutritional regimen within the first several days of life virtually impossible. For these infants, many feel that a nutritional regimen that prevents catabolism and allows some increment in lean body mass is satisfactory. This more realistic goal for the first several days of life can be achieved in sick low-birth-weight infants with a parenteral regimen that provides 60 kcal/kg/d, an amino acid intake of 2.5 g/kg/d, and necessary electrolytes, minerals, and vitamins (15). A similar regimen delivered enterally, of course, should produce the same results.

Various methods of delivering nutrients by the intravenous route (total parenteral nutrition) as well as methods of delivering feedings by the gastrointestinal tract (e.g.) continuous nasogastric or transpyloric infusions) have been proposed as alternatives to more conventional feeding techniques. Although no one method is likely to be ideal for all situations, a combination of these methods of nutrient delivery, allowing the particular clinical problems of an individual infant to be the basis for selecting the method of delivery, should improve nutritional management. In many infants, a combination of conventional as well as these less conventional methods of feeding permits delivery of sufficient nutrients to supprt "normal" growth.

Within reason, every infant should be given a trial at conventional feeding—i.e., tolerated nipple or gavage feedings of human milk and/or a special formula plus intravenous supplementation with 5% to 10% glucose solutions. If adequate nutrients cannot be delivered in this way, a trial of continuous nasogastric or transpyloric infusion seems warranted. Tolerated enteral feedings delivered conventionally or by continuous infusion also can be supplemented by intravenous infusions of appropriate mixtures of glucose, amino acids, and lipid. In the event that enteral feedings are not tolerated, parenteral administration of a balanced nutritional mixture deserves serious consideration. A regimen that provides 75 kcal/kg/d plus amino acids, electrolytes, minerals, and vitamins can be delivered by peripheral vein infusion without imposing an unreasonable fluid load. Since such a regimen almost certainly maintains existing body composition, it is particularly applicable for infants who are likely to tolerate enteral intake within a brief period of time. Use of a central vein catheter allows delivery of a more concentrated nutrient mixture and is particularly useful in situations associated with prolonged intolerance of enteral feedings.

References

1. Hahn P: Nutrition of the newborn. In Slavell (ed): Perinatal Physiology. Plenum Medical, 1978, p 357.
2. Hill JR, Rahimtulla KA: Heat balance and the metabolic rate of newborn babies in relation to environmental temperature and the effect of age and of weight on basal metabolic rate. J. Physiol. (Lond):180, 1965.
3. Grand RJ, Watkins JB, Torri FM: Development of the human gastrointestinal tract. (a review). Gastroenterology 70:790, 1976.
4. Widdowson EM, Columbo VE, Astavanis CA: Changes in the organs of pigs in response to feeding for the first 24 hours after birth. II. The digestive tract. Biol Neonate 28:272, 1976.
5. Widdowson EM: Growth and composition of the fetus and newborn. In Asali NS (ed): Biology of Gestation. II. The fetus and neonate. New York, Academic Press, 1968, p. 1–49.
6. Heird WC, Anderson TL: Nutritional requirements and methods of feeding low birth weight infants. Curr Probl Pediatr 7:3, 1977.
7. Tyson JE, Lasky RE, Mize CE, et al: Growth, metabolic response and development in very low birth weight infants fed banked human milk or enriched formula. 1. Neonatal findings. J Pediatr 103:95, 1983.
8. Schanler RJ, Ohio W: Nitrogen and mineral balance in preterm infants fed human milk or formula. J Pediatr Gast Nutr 4:214, 1985.
9. Raiha NCR, Heinonen K, Rassin DK, Gaull GE: Milk protein quantity and quality in low birth weight infants. 1. Metabolic response and effects on growth. Pediatrics 57:659, 1976.
10. Gordon HH, Levine SZ, McNamara H: Feeding of premature infants. A comparison of human and cow's milk. Am J Dis Child 73:442, 1947.
11. Kagan BM, Hess, JH, Lundeen E, et al: Feeding premature infants—a comparison of various milks. Pediatrics 15:373, 1955.
12. Atkinson SA, Beryan MH, Anderson GH: Human milk: difference in nitrogen concentration in milk from mothers of term and premature infants. J Pediatr 93:67, 1978.
13. Atkinson SA, Bryan MH, Anderson GH: Human milk feeding in premature infants: protein, fat and carbohydrate balances in the first two weeks of life. J Pediatr 99:617, 1981.
14. Gross SJ: Growth and biochemical response of preterm infants fed human milk or modified infant formula. N Engl J Med 308:237, 1983.
15. Anderson TL, Muttart CR, Bieber MA, et al: A controlled trial of glucose vs. glucose and amino acids in premature infants. J Pediatr 94:947, 1979.
16. Heird WC: Nutritional support of the pediatric patient. In Winters RW, Greene HL, (eds): Nutritional support of the seriously ill patient. New York, Academic Press, 1983, p 157.
17. Committee on Nutrition, American Academy of Pediatrics: Nutrition needs of low-birth-weight infants. Pediatrics 75:976, 1985.

CHAPTER 56

Neonatal Nephrology

JEAN-PIERRE GUIGNARD

Renal disease in the neonate results from specific problems of inherited, congenital, and acquired disorders that interact in the physiology of the developing kidney and the metabolic characteristics of the newborn infant, thus endowing the clinical practice of neonatal nephrology with features quite distinct from the rest of renal medicine in childhood.

PRESENTATION OF RENAL PROBLEMS

The presence of renal pathology in a newborn infant may be suggested by the patient's familial, gestational, and neonatal history, clinical observations, laboratory findings, or all of these.

Familial History

A few familial renal diseases may manifest themselves during the neonatal period or may be present but asymptomatic, for example, infantile or adult polycystic kidney disease, nephrogenic diabetes insipidus, and congenital nephrotic syndrome. In several families, the parents or siblings of infants with bilateral renal agenesis or dysgenesis have been found to have less severe kidney malformations such as unilateral renal agenesis or the same fetal renal agenesis-dysgenesis as that of the index patients (1). A high incidence of severe vesicoureteric reflux has been observed among siblings of a child with reflux (2–5). Ultrasonographic screening is mandatory in these families.

Gestational History

Oligohydramnios

The presence of oligohydramnios suggests renal agenesis, hypoplasia or dysplasia, or severe obstruction of the urinary tract as with prostatic urethral valves. The lack of amniotic fluid around the fetus is responsible for the nonrenal features of a syndrome that includes altered facies, aberrant hand and foot positioning, pulmonary hypoplasia, and late fetal growth deficiency. The complete expression of this "fetal compression syndrome," or Potter's syndrome, is seen with renal agenesis (6).

Polyhydramnios

Excess amniotic fluid (more than 2 liters) indicates severe swallowing difficulties caused by neurological disturbances or upper alimentary tract obstructive disorders. As many as 50% of patients with esophageal atresia or tracheoesophageal fistula also have renal malformations. Polyhydramnios may also result from nephrogenic diabetes insipidus or from severe congenital Bartter's syndrome.

Hypertrophied Placenta

A placenta weighing more than 25% of the infant at birth is observed in the Finnish type of congenital nephrotic syndrome. This condition, transmitted by an autosomal recessive gene, is often associated with prematurity and fetal distress. Prenatal diagnosis is suggested by an elevation of α-fetoprotein in amniotic fluid and, less confidently, in maternal blood (7).

Umbilical Cord Anomalies

The presence of a single umbilical artery and, to a lesser extent, a velamentous insertion of the umbilical cord, is associated with a high incidence of various congenital malformations (8), which reaches approximately 30% in cases of a single umbilical artery. No organ system seems to be involved more frequently than others. Associated anomalies of the urinary system include renal hypoplasia and aplasia, hydronephrosis, double renal pelvis, stricture of the ureter, and extrophy of the bladder (8).

Perinatal Problems

Fetal distress in utero, a difficult delivery, perinatal asphyxia, or severe stress may result in acute tubular necrosis, renal venous thrombosis, and renal failure.

Antenatal Ultrasound

An increasing number of fetuses with urological abnormalities are being detected by antenatal ultrasound examination (9) (see Chapter 57).

Micturition

Micturition occurs during delivery or soon after birth in a third of all neonates. Ninety-two percent of newborn infants pass urine during the first 24 hr of life, and 99% within the first 48 hr (10). A urological or renal disturbance is likely if no diuresis has occurred by the 72nd hr of life. Severe dehydration is the most common cause of oligoanuria. In the absence of dehydration, a delay in micturition may indicate a failure of urine formation or an obstruction of the urinary tract. The conditions associated with each are given in the following list (11):

1. Failure of urine formation:
   Bilateral renal agenesis
   Postnatal intravascular hypovolemia
   Restriction of oral fluid

Cortical necrosis
Tubular necrosis
Bilateral renal vein thrombosis
Congenital nephrotic syndrome
Congenital nephritis
Congenital pyelonephritis

2. Obstruction to urine flow:
   Imperforate prepuce
   Urethral strictures
   Urethral diverticulum
   Hypertrophy of the verumontanum
   Neurogenic bladder
   "Megacystis syndrome"
   Ureterocele
   Extrinsic tumor compressing bladder outlet

A urinary stream that is weak or jerky is suggestive of bladder outflow obstruction or dysfunction. An acceptable stream does not, however, eliminate the possibility of lesser degrees of obstruction. The presence of residual urine in the bladder must be looked for by bladder palpation and percussion and confirmed by ultrasonography.

Urine Flow Rate

A healthy infant excretes 15 to 30 ml/kg/24 hr of urine during the first two days of life and 25 to 120 ml/kg/24 hr during the next four weeks (12, 13) (Table 56.1). Urine volume depends on the infant's solute excretion. The relation between urine volume, urine osmolality, and urine solute excretion is shown in Figure 56.1 (14). Oliguria is defined as a urine output of less than 1.0 ml/kg/hr (15).

A postnatal loss of birth weight greater than 10% in a normally fed infant whose urine osmolality is below 200 mosm/kg H_2O (specific gravity 1.005) may be the first sign of nephrogenic diabetes insipidus. A urine osmolality above 350 mosm/kg H_2O (specific gravity 1.010) does not exclude the diagnosis of diabetes insipidus, as some urine concentration may be achieved by the dehydrated infant in the absence of vasopressin.

Gross Hematuria

Gross hematuria in the neonate is rare, and the cause often remains unknown. It may be the consequence of a wound in the area of the meatus, of a urological malformation, of cystic and dysplastic disorders, or of acquired renal vascular disorders such as renal venous thrombosis and corticomedullary necrosis. The following list indicates renal disorders associated with hematuria (16):

1. Vascular disorders:
   Acute tubular necrosis (vasomotor nephropathy)
   Corticomedullary necrosis
   Renal venous thrombosis
   Microemboli
   Adrenal hemorrhage
2. Cystic diseases:
   Infantile polycystic disease
   Adult polycystic disease
   Cystic dysplasia/multicystic kidney
3. Hydronephrosis:
   Obstruction
   Severe ureteral reflux

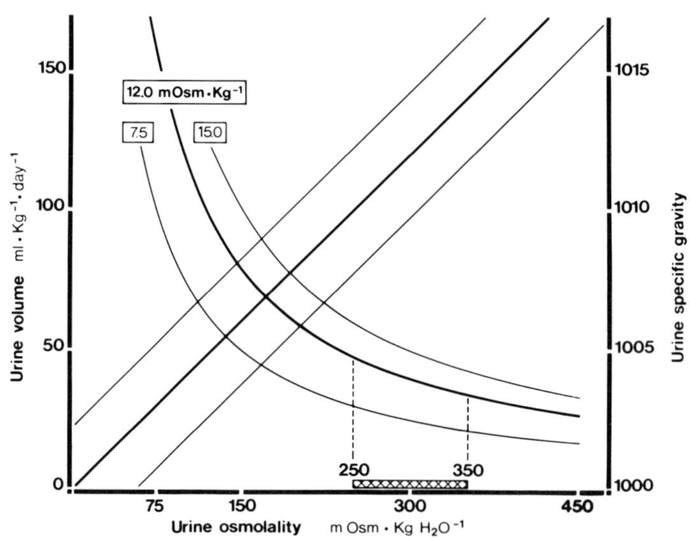

Figure 56.1. Relation between urine volume, urine osmolality, and urine solute excretion. Isopleths describe daily urine solute excretion of 12 mosm/kg BW per day, 15 mosm/kg BW per day (high solute excretion rate), and 7.5 mosm/kg per day (low solute excretion rate). The relation between urine osmolality and urine-specific gravity is shown with its confidence limits. (Modified from Roy RN, Sinclair JC: Hydration of the low birth-weight infant. Clin Perinatol 2:393, 1975.)

Table 56.1.
Normal Values of Renal Function

	Age of infant				
	Premature infant	Term infant			
	First 3 days	First 3 days	2 weeks	8 weeks	1 yr
Daily excretion of urine					
ml/kg/24 hr	15–75	20–75	25–120	80–130	40–100
% of fluid intake	40–80	40–80	50–70	45–65	40–60
Voiding size					
ml/kg per voiding	4–6	4–6	4–7	4–6	3–6
Maximal urine osmolality					
mosm/kg H_2O	400–500	600–800	800–900	1000–1200	1200–1400
Glomerular filtration rate					
ml/min per 1.73 m^2	10–15	15–20	35–45	75–80	90–110

Adapted from references 12, 13, 32, 33, 53, and 151.

4. Interstitial nephritis:
   - Infection
     - Sepsis
     - Urinary tract infection
   - Drugs (?)
     - Penicillins
     - Aminoglycosides
     - Anticonvulsants
     - Diuretics
5. Tumors:
   - Wilms' tumor
   - Mesoblastic nephroma and fetal hamartomas
   - Angiomas
6. Glomerulonephritis:
   - Infection-mediated
   - Immunologically mediated (?)

The presence of high uric acid concentrations and uric acid crystals in the urine of neonates may make it reddish or pink. This condition must be distinguished from the "red diaper syndrome," in which an intestinal bacteria, *Serratia marcescens*, is responsible for the coloration of the diaper.

Physical Examination

General Configuration

The face may show the classic Potter facies with wide-set eyes, beaked nose, low-set ears, and a prominent fold arising from the inner canthus (Fig. 56.2). Potter facies is associated with renal agenesis. Isolated anomalies of the external ear may accompany obstructive uropathy. Abnormalities of chest such as pectus excavatum, widely spaced nipples, pneumomediastinum, and pneumothorax with respiratory distress may also be associated with obstructive uropathy.

Extrophy of the bladder is a severe abnormality of the abdominal wall and lower urinary tract. Extrophy of the cloaca can be associated with an abnormality of the upper urinary tract.

Examination of the genitalia is important. Abnormal drainage of the urinary tract may be associated with ambiguous genitalia. The presence of hypospadias or epispadias is associated with an increased incidence of urinary tract abnormalities, including urethral meatal stenosis.

Examination of the anus may reveal an imperforate anus, which is often associated with urological abnormalities.

Examination of the lumbosacral area and thoracic spine may demonstrate kyphosis, scoliosis, spina bifida, or myelomeningocele, all malformations associated with an increased number of genitourinary anomalies.

Abdominal Palpation

Renal masses may be demonstrated in 0.5% to 0.8% of infants (17). Most are related to the kidneys or urinary tract (Table 56.2) (18, 19). Several techniques have been recommended for identifying an abdominal mass, but bimanual palpation is the method of choice. The left kidney of the newborn infant is often palpable, but this does not necessarily

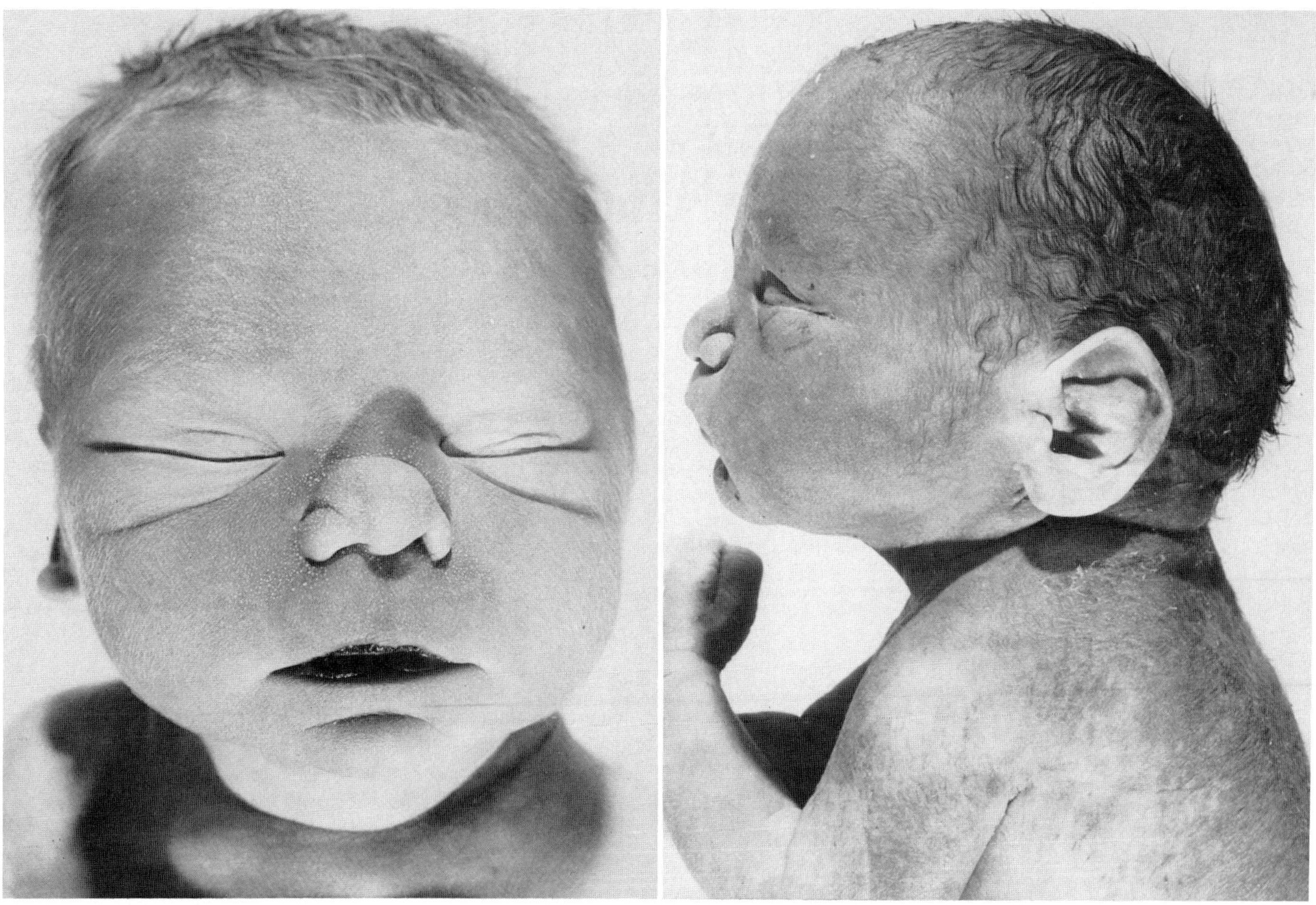

Figure 56.2. The facies in Potter syndrome.

Table 56.2.
Neonatal Abdominal Masses

Type of mass	Percent of total
Renal masses	55
Hydronephrosis	
Multicystic dysplastic kidney	
Polycystic kidney disease	
Mesoblastic nephroma	
Renal ectopia	
Renal vein thrombosis	
Nephroblastomatosis	
Wilms' tumor	
Genital masses	15
Hydrometrocolpos	
Ovarian cyst	
Gastrointestinal masses	15
Duplication	
Volvulus	
Complicated meconium ileus	
Mesenteric-omental cyst	
"Pseudocyst" proximal to atresia	
Nonrenal retroperitoneal masses	10
Adrenal hemorrhage	
Neuroblastoma	
Teratoma	
Hepatosplenobiliary masses	5
Hemangioendothelioma	
Hepatoblastoma	
Hepatic cyst	
Splenic hematoma	
Choledochal cyst	
Hydrops of gallbladder	

(From Kirks DR, Merten DF, Grossman H, Bowie JD: Diagnostic imaging of pediatric abdominal masses: an overview. Radiol Clin North Am 19:527, 1981, reprinted with permission.)

have a pathological significance. When present, a renal mass must be confirmed by ultrasonography, which may reveal polycystic kidneys, multicystic dysplasia, renal venous thrombosis, renal tumors, horseshoe kidneys, hydronephrosis, or a large bladder secondary to urethral valves (20). Addition of renal scintigraphy with delayed images (24 hr) allows a more accurate diagnosis (21). Enlarged kidneys do not necessarily carry a grave prognosis, as the condition may be transient and reflect reversible intratubular obstruction (22). Weakness or absence of the abdominal muscles is seen in the prune belly syndrome, characterized by a large hypotonic bladder, dilated prostatic urethra, massive reflux, and renal dysplasia (23). Pulmonary hypoplasia secondary to oligohydramnios and intestinal malrotation are anomalies frequently associated with the prune belly syndrome.

Edema

The main causes of edema in the newborn are as follows:

1. Physiological
2. Cardiac
3. Renal
4. Miscellaneous
   - Hypoxia in utero
   - Hyaline membrane disease
   - Erythroblastosis fetalis
   - Umbilical vein thrombosis
   - Lymphedema
   - Congenital ascites (chylous ascites, cirrhosis, peritonitis)
   - Vitamin E deficiency
   - Hypomagnesemia and hypocalcemia
   - Cystic fibrosis
   - Hypoparathyroidism
   - Turner's syndrome

The edema may be physiological, have a cardiac or a renal origin or be caused by a disturbance of capillary permeability.

Physiological edema appears on the second day of life of premature neonates and diminishes steadily during the first week. The pathogenesis is unknown; it may be an exaggerated example of the normally high volume of extracellular fluid characteristic of the newborn, but it has been suggested that immaturity of the renal sodium-handling mechanisms contributes to a transitory sodium retention, with consequent changes in extracellular fluid balance. The phenomenon is more marked in premature infants.

Sodium retention with edema may occur whenever cardiac output is reduced. A variety of congenital cardiac abnormalities may cause cardiac failure and edema.

Two mechanisms are implicated in the pathogenesis of renal edema. First, fluid and salt retention may be a result of renal failure: severe hypoxemia, obstructive uropathy, and renal venous thrombosis are common causes of such edema in the neonate. Second, edema may be caused by decreased plasma oncotic pressure, in turn secondary to hypoalbuminemia resulting from gastrointestinal or renal loss. Heavy proteinuria is observed in congenital nephrotic syndromes secondary to microcystic disease, congenital syphilis, toxoplasmosis, cytomegalovirus, nephroblastoma, renal venous thrombosis, and mercury intoxication.

Retention of water leading to edema with hyponatremia occurs when excessive free water is given to infants with inappropriate secretion of antidiuretic hormone (ADH) accompanying pulmonary or cerebral disorders.

Hydrops Fetalis

Hydrops fetalis denotes generalized edema of the neonate at birth. It may be accompanied by ascites or pleural effusions. It results from alterations in the physical forces that govern the movement of fluid across the capillary wall (24). Hydrops fetalis is a nonspecific finding in a variety of maternal and fetal disorders (25). It is often associated with polyhydramnios. Nonimmune causes of hydrops fetalis are now responsible for at least 75% of the cases. Renal causes include congenital malformations of the urinary tract or parenchyma. Urinary obstruction may be internal, caused by ureteral or urethral valves and stenosis, or external, as with compression of the ureter by congenital retroperitoneal fibrosis. Polycystic and dysplastic kidneys are sometimes associated with polyhydramnios, ascites, and occasionally hydrops fetalis. The congenital nephrotic syndrome of the Finnish type produces generalized edema in the early newborn period, rather than in the fetus. Congenital infections such as syphilis, toxoplasmosis, and cytomegalic inclusion disease may result in hydrops fetalis and congenital nephrotic syndrome.

Ascites in Newborn

The accumulation of fluid in the peritoneal cavity during extrauterine life must be distinguished from other fetal abdominal fluid collections, such as distended urinary bladder, cysts, cystic kidneys, or hydrops. The main causes leading to or associated with the ascites include abnormalities of the gastrointestinal, portohepatic, or genitourinary tracts (26). Erythroblastosis fetalis is sometimes a cause of marked ascites without significant generalized edema. Chylous ascites is occasionally congenital in origin. Ascites may occur in cases of hepatic cirrhosis, fetal peritonitis (syphilitic or meconial), agenesis of intraabdominal organs, imperfora-

Table 56.3.
Renal Anomalies in Trisomy Syndromes

Trisomy	Renal anomaly
11	Dysplastic multicystic kidneys
13–15	Bilateral hydronephrosis
	Renal cysts
16–18	Horseshoe kidneys
	Hydronephrosis
	Dysplastic multicystic kidneys
	Renal cortical cysts
	Abnormal nodule of renal blastema
21	Agenesis/hypoplasia

tion of the anus, and rupture of renal and intraabdominal cysts. About 25% of neonatal ascites is caused by urinary tract disease. Most cases of urinary ascites are due to the presence of posterior urethral valves and obstruction. Complex caudal anomalies, usually anorectal and urethral atresia, and miscellaneous lesions that include bladder outlet flaps, ureterocele, ureteral atresia, myelomeningocele with neurogenic bladder, extrinsic lesions such as presacral neuroblastoma, and spontaneous rupture of the bladder (27) may occasionally cause urinary ascites. Transient fetal ascites may be an important feature of the prune belly syndrome. The cause-and-effect relationship between obstruction of the urinary tract and the formation of ascitic fluid is obscure. Direct communication between the dilated urinary tract and the peritoneal cavity or transudation from the distended urinary tract have been postulated. The rapid equilibration between the plasma and ascitic fluid makes it difficult to demonstrate the presence of urine in the ascitic fluid. Erect and supine roentgenograms of the abdomen and ultrasonography help in defining the presence of ascitic fluid. Its opacification by leakage of contrast material during cystography or intravenous urography may lead to striking relative radiolucency of the liver. This phenomenon may be an important clue to the differential diagnosis of the cause of neonatal ascites (28).

Nonspecific Signs

Renal disease often presents with nonspecific signs, which may be referred to the gastrointestinal, respiratory, or central nervous systems. Refusal to eat, weight loss, diarrhea, respiratory distress secondary to pulmonary hypoplasia with pneumothorax, fever, irritability, and convulsions may all be the first sign of renal disease. Jaundice may point to urinary tract infection.

Renal malformation or dysfunction may be part of a complex malformation syndrome in which various structures and organs are involved. The renal malformations include various uropathies, horseshoe kidneys, cystic kidneys, hypoplasia, dysplasia, and agenesis. They may be found in association with chromosomal abnormalities (Table 56.3), single-gene mutation syndromes, and sporadic malformation syndromes or may result from teratogenic causes. They are described in more detail in Chapter 24.

Intestinal abnormalities are also often associated with anomalies of the urinary system. They include anal, colonic, duodenal, and esophageal atresia, Meckel's diverticulum, abnormalities of the internal genitalia, pulmonary hypoplasia, congenital heart disease.

INVESTIGATION

Laboratory tests, imaging studies, or both may be necessary to confirm or exclude renal involvement in a sick neonate. The results must be interpreted in relation to the conceptional and the postnatal age of the child.

Urinalysis

Hematuria

The normal newborn infant excretes less than three red cells per cubic millimeter of urine, corresponding to less than three red cells per high-power field. Significant hematuria is defined as more than 10 red cells per cubic millimeter. Conditions associated with microscopic or macroscopic hematuria are listed on p 922.

Leukocyturia

The urine of the newborn infant contains less than 25 (male) or 50 (female) white cells per cubic millimeter. Increased leukocyturia is found in febrile patients, in renal parenchymal diseases, in renal vascular disorders, and during severe infectious episodes. Pyuria is often associated with urinary tract infection but is not pathognomonic.

Proteinuria

Proteinuria varies with gestational age (29) (Table 56.4) and postnatal age (30) (Table 56.5). It is slightly higher in premature than in term neonates. Transient proteinuria is often present during the first three to five days of life. From then on, proteinuria is usually below 0.15 mg/kg/hr. The following renal disorders are associated with proteinuria in the neonate (16):

- Physiological proteinuria
- Vascular disorders
  - Renal venous thrombosis
  - Corticomedullary necrosis
- Neonatal nephrotic syndrome
  - Hereditary diseases
    - Finnish-type
    - Onycho-osteodysplasia (nail-patella syndrome)
    - Severe infantile sialidosis
  - Infectious diseases
    - Syphilis
    - Toxoplasmosis
    - Cytomegalovirus
  - Drugs
    - Mercury compounds
    - Other drugs?

Glucosuria

The urine of the healthy term normoglycemic neonate contains only trace amounts of glucose. A congenital tubular disorder should be suspected if glucosuria is present and the plasma glucose concentration is not raised. Because of the low glucose renal threshold in low-birth-

Table 56.4.
Proteinuria in Relation to Gestational Age

Gestational age (weeks)	Proteinuria (mg/m^2 per h)[a]
<28	0.86 (0.2–1.33)
30	2.08 (0–9.40)
32	2.32 (0–5.22)
34	2.48 (0–13.07)
36	1.27 (0–4.60)
40	1.29 (0–6.14)

[a] Proteinuria: mean (range) values observed in the first 48 hr of life. (From Arant BS: Developmental patterns of renal functional maturation compared in the human neonate. J Pediatr 92:705, 1978, with permission).

Table 56.5.
Urinary Concentration of Proteins in Single Urine Specimens in Relation to Postnatal Age[a]

Age (days)	Total protein (mg/liter)	Albumin (mg/liter)	β_2-microglobulin (mg/liter)	α-amino N (mg α-amino N/liter)	Creatinine (mmol/liter)
1	494 (103–2360)	143 (14–1510)	0.28 (0.02–3.69)	172 (75–399)	4.1 (0.8–22)
5	176 (39–798)	21 (4–97)	1.04 (0.07–16.30)	110 (36–335)	2.5 (0.5–14)
15	55 (10–324)	6 (1–33)	0.34 (0.02–6.16)	51 (20–133)	0.5 (0.1–3)
43	46 (12–185)	4 (1–18)	0.13 (0.01–1.61)	46 (17–125)	0.5 (0.09–3)

[a] Mean (range). (From Karlsson FA, Hardell L-I, Hellsing K: Prospective study of urinary proteins in early infancy. Acta Paediatr Scand 68:663, 1979.)

weight infants, significant glucosuria may be observed at a plasma concentration of 150 mg/dl (8.3 mmol/liter) (31). A few premature neonates may even present with glucosuria at plasma concentrations below 100 mg/dl (5.5 mmol/liter) (29), a finding that probably reflects heterogeneity of immature nephrons.

pH

Even in the first days of life, urine pH changes in response to plasma bicarbonate concentration (Fig. 56.3). Most neonates have a urinary pH of about 6 during the first days of life. Excretion of an inappropriate alkaline urine in the presence of metabolic acidosis is observed in neonates with severe respiratory distress syndrome (32) and in the various syndromes of renal tubular acidosis.

Bacteriuria

Urine culture is essential in any neonate presenting with symptoms suggesting urinary tract infection (UTI). The diagnosis of UTI depends on the demonstration of a significant number of organisms in a properly collected urine specimen. The urinary concentration of bacteria considered as presenting true infection varies according to the method used for urine collection (see p 935).

Specific Gravity and Osmolality

There is a linear correlation between urinary osmolality and specific gravity (Fig. 56.1). This relationship is altered by the presence of proteins, glucose, or radiological contrast agents in the urine. The newborn infant is able to decrease urine osmolality to values as low as 50 mosm/kg H_2O in response to hypotonic loading. Premature infants infused with 5% to 10% glucose usually excrete urine with osmolalities below 100 mosm/kg H_2O. The concentrating mechanism of the term newborn infant is not fully developed, and urinary osmolality cannot be increased above 700 to 800 mosm/kg H_2O in response to dehydration (33). Following DDAVP administration, 10 μg, newborn infants increased urine osmolality to 385 $\pm$ 25 mosm/kg H_2O by the age of 1 to 3 weeks and to 566 $\pm$ 50 mosm/kg H_2O by the age of 4 to 6 weeks. Maximal urine osmolality was slightly less in premature infants, with value of 359 at 1 to 3 weeks and 524 at 4 to 6 weeks (34). Pyelonephritis, renal failure, hypokalemia, and hypercalcemia can all disturb the urinary concentration ability. Disturbances in dilutional capacity are observed in the syndrome of inappropriate secretion of ADH, in hypoaldosteronism, in hypothyroidism, in renal failure, and during distal diuretic blockade.

Blood Tests

Creatinine

The plasma creatinine concentration is elevated at birth, its level reflecting the mother's plasma concentration (35). A rapid decrease in creatinine concentration is observed during the first days of life (36), its value stabilizing around 0.40 mg/dl (35 μmol/liter) (range: 0.14–0.70 mg/dl) at the end of the first week of life (Fig. 56.4) (37). The plasma creatinine concentration at birth is definitely higher in very low birthweight infants, and appears to be inversely related to gestational age.

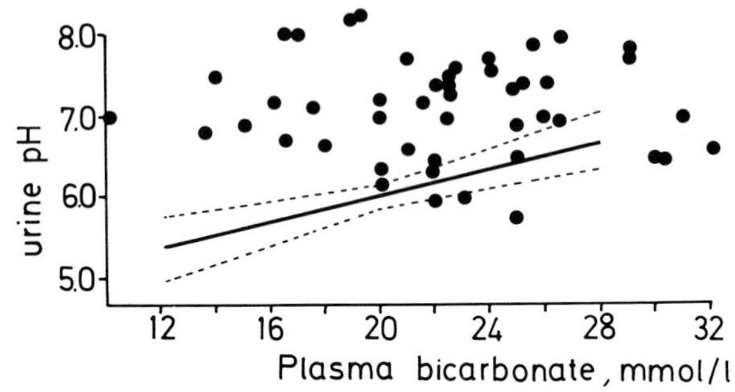

Figure 56.3. Relation between urinary pH and plasma bicarbonate during first 72 hr of life of control premature neonates (regression line and 95% confidence limits) and hypoxemic newborn infants presenting with severe RDS (dots). (From Torrado A, Guignard J-P, Prod'hom LS, Gautier E: Helv. Paediatr. Acta 29:399, 1974, with permission.)

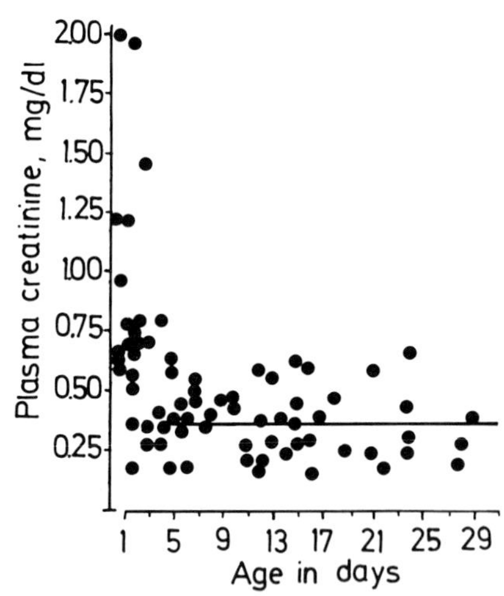

Figure 56.4. Plasma creatinine concentrations during first month of life. (From Feldman H, Guignard J-P: Plasma creatinine in the first month of life. Arch Dis Child 57:123, 1982, with permission.)

Urea

The plasma urea concentration of the newborn is below 40 mg/dl (7.0 mmol/liter). A progressive rise in this parameter may indicate a functional or an organic renal disturbance. Urea concentration is, however, markedly affected by extrarenal factors, particularly protein intake and metabolism.

Sodium

Hyponatremia is not an uncommon finding in the newborn, particularly in high-risk neonates. It may be secondary to impaired excretion of free water or to sodium-wasting.

Impaired water excretion has been observed in the following conditions:

1. Inappropriate secretion of ADH secondary to cerebral distress (asphyxia, meningitis, subdural or subarachnoid hematoma or hemorrhage, encephalitis) or drug toxicity (barbiturates, isoproterenol, indomethacin, carbamazepine)
2. Prerenal failure secondary to cardiac insufficiency
3. Adrenal failure

Salt-wasting is observed in the following conditions:

1. Preterm infants with a high fractional sodium excretion rate may develop negative sodium balance when sodium excretion rate exceeds sodium intake (38–41). The immaturity of the proximal tubule reabsorptive function, along with resistance of the distal tubule to aldosterone (38), probably accounts for the tendency of very-low-birth-weight infants to develop severe salt depletion. By contrast, term infants whose proximal reabsorption is also immature reabsorb a greater fraction of filtered sodium in the distal tubule (42), probably under the effect of high plasma aldosterone concentrations. Late hyponatremia occurs in very-low-birth-weight infants (<1300 g) given only 1.3 mmol/kg/24 hr of sodium, and can be prevented by giving additional sodium (3 to 4 mmol/kg/24 hr) (43). Late hyponatremia is transient and disappears in a few weeks.
2. Aldosterone deficiency, as seen in the adrenogenital syndrome or selective defects of aldosterone biosynthesis, and resistance to aldosterone effect can lead to hyponatremia. Transient pseudohypoaldosteronism has been described in infants presenting with obstructive uropathy and urinary tract infection (44, 45).
3. Diuretics, when given to the mother before birth or to the newborn, can induce hyponatremia by inducing sodium depletion or by interfering with the diluting mechanism.
4. Extrarenal losses, as seen in vomiting, diarrhea, and cystic fibrosis, can also be responsible for hyponatremia.

Hypocalcemia

Early neonatal hypocalcemia defined as total calcium <8.0 mg/dl (2.0 mmol/liter) in a full-term infant or <7.0 mg/dl (1.75 mmol/liter) in the premature infant during the first three days of life is seen in one third of preterm low-birth-weight infants and of infants with birth asphyxia. Early neonatal hypocalcemia appears to be a physiological phenomenon due neither to an impairment of parathormone secretion nor of vitamin D activation (46). Recent studies suggest that because of a close relationship between sodium and calcium excretion in the premature neonate, the aggressive administration of sodium to sick hypocalcemic premature neonates may aggravate the risk of hypercalciuria with early-onset neonatal hypocalcemia (47).

Bicarbonate

In normal conditions, the plasma bicarbonate concentration is determined by the renal bicarbonate threshold. This threshold is low in the newborn, especially in premature infants. The plasma bicarbonate concentration is therefore about 21 to 23 mmol/liter in the term neonate and 19 to 22 mmol/liter in the preterm infant.

In the very-low-birth-weight infant an even lower bicarbonate threshold can lead to normal bicarbonate plasma concentrations as low as 14.5 mmol/liter (48). The ability of these infants to excrete a load of acid is, however, appropriate, and these so-called "acidemic" low-birth-weight babies, whose growth rate is appropriate, must be considered normal. The state of volume expansion present at this age or renal immaturity may account for the depression of bicarbonate threshold. This condition, sometime defined as *late metabolic acidosis*, is transient and does not need treatment.

A state of acute or chronic renal failure may lead to metabolic acidosis by decreasing hydrogen ion excretion and inducing a state of positive hydrogen ion balance.

Metabolic acidosis may also be caused by a renal tubular defect affecting the proximal tubule, the distal tubule, or both. The excretion of an alkaline urine in the presence of metabolic acidosis points to a tubular defect (see Chapter 19).

Uric Acid

Serum uric acid levels are often elevated at birth and decrease during the first days of life (49). Concentrations are more elevated in premature infants and decrease with conceptional age. Values of 7.71, 6.04, and 5.19 mg/dl (459, 359, and 309 μmol/liter) have been recorded on the first day of life of newborn infants with gestational age of 29 to 33, 34 to 37, and 38 to 40 weeks, respectively. Fractional excretion of uric acid is inversely related to conceptional age, decreasing from 30% at 30 weeks of conceptional age to 18% at 40 weeks (50). Serum uric acid concentrations increase with stress such as hypoxia and perinatal asphyxia. Acute renal failure and renal uric acid infarctions have been described in hyperuricemic stressed neonates (51, 52). The excretion of dilute and often alkaline urine by the newborn infant decreases, however, the likelihood of uric acid precipitation and allows the excretion of large amounts of uric acid without harmful effect.

Glomerular Filtration Rate

Glomerular filtration rate (GFR) may be estimated by measuring the standard clearance of inulin or creatinine. Both techniques require accurate urine collection. The former method is the most accurate but requires a constant infusion of an exogenous marker and cannot be used in clinical practice (53, 54).

Creatinine is the most commonly used marker of GFR. Its clearance approximates inulin clearance (55). The values of GFR generated by creatinine clearance must, however, be interpreted with caution. The variability of plasma creatinine concentration during the first weeks of life decreases the accuracy of creatinine clearance. Furthermore, because of the low level of creatinine in the blood of infants, small variations in laboratory measurements may spuriously alter the estimated creatinine clearance.

The indirect methods for estimating GFR without urine collection, as for instance the constant infusion or the single injection of glomerular markers, do not offer definitive advantage. The results they give during the first weeks of life differ from those obtained by measuring the standard clearance of inulin (56, 57). The results of the constant infusion method can be improved by constantly infusing inulin for at least 24 hr (57). Although obviating the need for urine collection, this technique is difficult to perform in clinical routine. Clearance techniques are discussed in more detail in Chapter 19. The development of GFR in relation to gestational age and postnatal age is illustrated in Figures 56.5 and 56.6. Normal values of GFR in the infant are given in Table 56.1.

Imaging Studies

See Chapter 20 for additional discussion.

Ultrasonography

Ultrasonography, a noninvasive technique, is the method of choice for determining the size and position of the kidneys and bladder. It can define a palpable abdominal mass as fluid-filled, cystic, or solid, thus orienting the diagnosis toward obstructive uropathy, cystic disease, or tumor. Ultrasonography is particularly useful in patients with nonfunctioning or poorly functioning kidneys. The diagnosis of bilateral hydronephrosis, distended obstructed bladder, or cystic disease can be made antenatally by ultrasonographic examination (9). This may help reduce morbidity and mortality by allowing prompt surgical correction of an obstructed kidney that otherwise might have undergone irreparable damage or become infected, producing lethal sepsis. The prenatal diagnosis of a distended bladder in the fetus may, however, lead to the dilemma of whether to provoke a premature delivery in order to salvage an obstructed kidney. Although sonar may not be completely hazard-free, it is certainly safer than ionizing radiations.

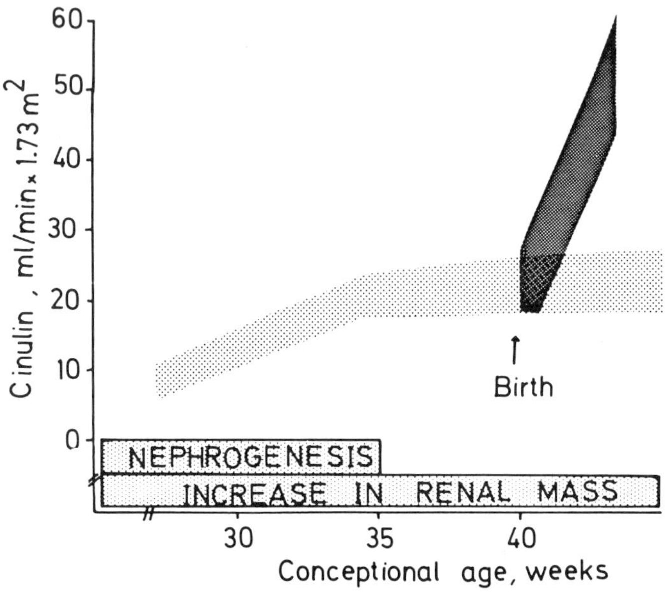

Figure 56.5. Maturation of GFR in relation to conceptional age. (From Guignard J-P: The neonatal stressed kidney. In Gruskin AB, Norman ME (eds): Pediatric Nephrology. Martinus Nijhoff, 1981, with permission.)

Voiding Cystourethrography

Voiding cystourethrography with a contrast agent or a radioisotopic marker such as technetium 99m pertechnetate is indicated in all neonates with urinary tract infection or lower urinary tract symptoms. It will demonstrate the presence of vesicoureteric reflux and will outline the bladder, prostatic urethral valves, or other urethral diseases.

Renal Scintigraphy

Scintigraphy provides information on kidney structure and function. The most widely used labeled complexes are ^{99m}Tc DTPA, ^{99m}Tc DMSA, and ^{131}I orthoiodohippurate. They are useful in diagnosing vascular disorders, obstructive uropathies, and renal parenchymal injury. Information on GFR, renal perfusion, and drainage are best obtained with DTPA and ^{123}I orthoiodohippurate. Excellent imaging studies are obtained with DMSA.

Computed Tomography

Computed tomography uses ionizing radiations; it adds little to the information provided by ultrasonography, except in the case of solid tumors.

Intravenous Urography

Intravenous urography is of limited value during the first two weeks of life (58) but may be informative after this period. It permits the delineation of the renal parenchyma and urinary tract. Because of the limited concentrating capacity of the kidney in the neonatal period, the dose of the contrast agent must be increased up to 4 ml of a 50% solution per kilogram of body weight. The newborn must be well hydrated before the examination because of the high osmotic load of the contrast medium. Complications include ischemia of the renal cortex, papillary or medullary necrosis, and pulmonary edema.

RENAL FUNCTION DURING NEONATAL RESPIRATORY DISORDERS

Perinatal asphyxia or hypoxemia, as seen in severe idiopathic respiratory distress syndrome or in secondary respiratory distress syndrome after complicated or traumatic deliveries, can profoundly affect renal

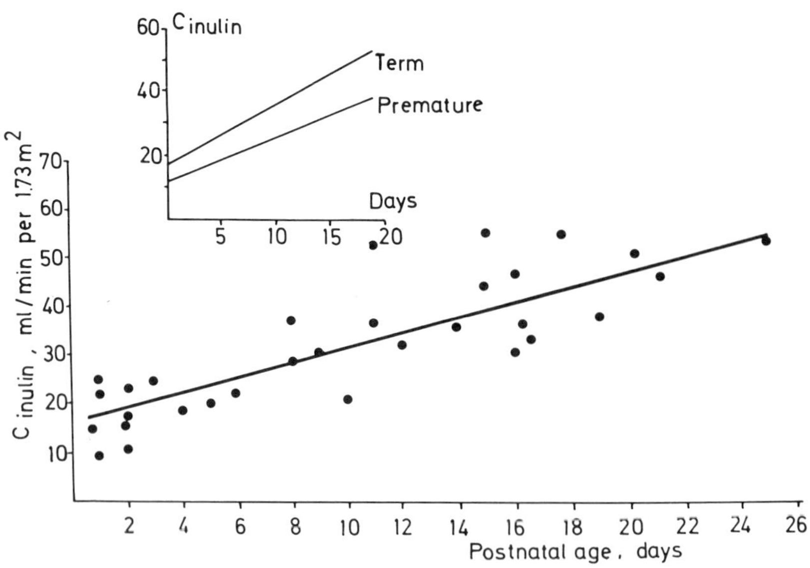

Figure 56.6. Postnatal maturation of GFR in term and preterm neonates (From Guignard J-P: The neonatal stressed kidney. In Gruskin AB, Norman ME (eds): Pediatric Nephrology. Martinus Nijhoff, 1981, with permission.)

function, with impairment of renal perfusion, GFR, and tubular function (32, 59–62). Hypotension, hypovolemia, metabolic acidosis, and respiratory acidosis are often present in hypoxic patients and may all contribute to the renal functional changes observed (Fig. 56.7).

The asphyxiated infant also often presents with signs of cardiovascular failure. This may be secondary to peripheral vasoconstriction and myocardial failure resulting from hypoxia and acidosis. Blood volume can be decreased, but most infants suffering from perinatal asphyxia have a normal or even increased blood volume (63). Several postnatal asphyxia is complicated by metabolic acidemia due to the accumulation of organic acids.

Oliguria and Renal Insufficiency

Severe or prolonged hypoxemia causes oliguria (32, 64). The urine-plasma osmolality ratio is greater than unity, indicating impaired dilution in hypoxemic neonates as compared to control infants (32). Decreased urine flow may be due to decrease in effective intravascular volume secondary to pooling of large amounts of fluid in the lung, increased circulating vasopressin levels, decreased GFR, or all three (61). A correlation has been observed between the decrease in urine output and the lowest plasma oxygen tension recorded before or during the urine collection period (32); however, an increase in urine output appears to occur before an improvement in alveolar-arterial oxygen gradient. This suggests that the improvement in the respiratory condition is secondary to renal excretion of fluid previously pooled in the lungs.

Renal hypoperfusion with decreased GFR has been observed in patients presenting with severe respiratory distress syndrome (RDS) (61). The decrease in renal perfusion appears to be related to the severity of RDS. Creatinine clearance measurements or single inulin injection studies have shown normal values in well-hydrated neonates with moderate RDS (65, 66). The low GFR present in severely hypoxemic neonates may be responsible for the impairment of free-water excretion. Alternatively, an increased release of ADH could be responsible. Increased levels of ADH have been reported in infants with RDS and in those suffering from perinatal asphyxia.

Impaired Tubular Function

Several features suggest impaired tubular function in hypoxemic neonates, e.g., significant tubular proteinuria (67), the increased fractional excretion rate of sodium and β_2-microglobulin (68), decreased maximal urinary concentrating ability (34), and impaired renal acidification (32, 69). A state of renal tubular acidosis has indeed been observed in these patients who acidify their urine poorly even in the presence of metabolic acidosis.

The pathogenesis of the asphyxia–hypoxemia-induced renal impairment is not yet clear. Pathological studies in deceased patients have not shown any significant lesion except in severely asphyxic neonates who can present with cortical-medullary necrosis. Prerenal factors are probably partly responsible for the development of renal insufficiency in some of the patients. Volume expansion can improve the state of renal perfusion. Stimulation of the renin-angiotensin system has been demonstrated in human neonates with RDS and in hypoxemic adults, as well as in fetal animals. Studies in fetal lambs also indicate that hypoxia increases the release of catecholamines and arginine vasopressin (70, 71). The renal vasoconstriction with consequent hypoperfusion of the kidney may also be induced, at least in part, by the treatment of the primary disease. Both positive-pressure ventilation (72) and constant positive-airway pressure (CPAP) (73,74) have been reported to interfere with renal function (Fig. 56.7).

Mechanical Ventilation. Experimental studies have clearly shown

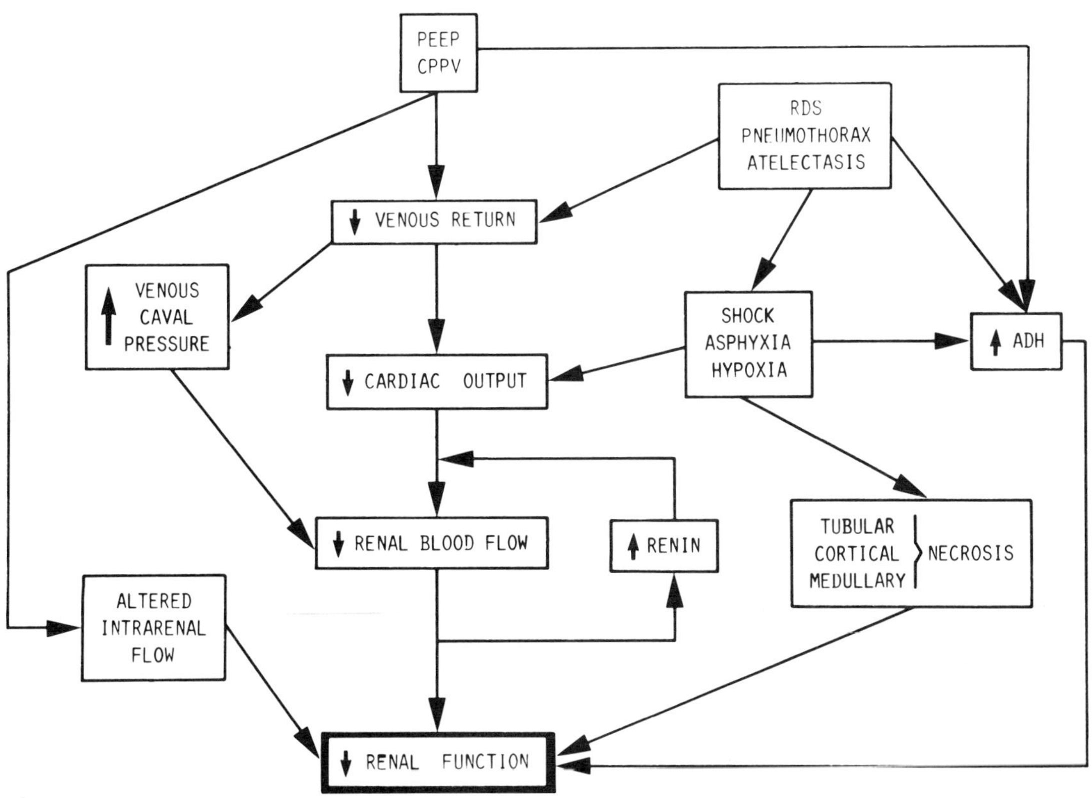

Figure 56.7. Pathophysiology of neonatal renal changes secondary to respiratory disorders. Abbreviations: PEEP = positive end-expiratory pressure; CPPV = continuous positive-pressure ventilation; RDS = respiratory distress syndrome; ADH = antidiuretic hormone.

that conventional ventilators with positive end-expiratory pressure can impair renal function in dogs, swine, newborn goats, monkeys, or lambs. Continuous positive-pressure ventilation decreases urine output, sodium excretion, glomerular filtration rate, and effective renal plasma flow. In the dog, these changes do not occur in a denervated kidney, suggesting that they are mediated through increased renal sympathetic nervous activity (75). The changes are associated with an increase in intrapleural pressure, a decrease in cardiac filling pressure, and a depression of cardiac output. Positive-pressure ventilation also alters intrarenal distribution of blood flow, leading to decreased perfusion of cortical nephrons and increased perfusion of juxtamedullary nephrons. These alterations may be secondary to increases in circulating levels of vasopressin, angiotensin, and catecholamines.

Constant Positive Airway Pressure (CPAP). CPAP decreases urine flow rate, sodium excretion, and glomerular filtration rate in experimental animals without necessarily affecting cardiac output, mean arterial pressure, or heart rate (73, 74). The same applies to human neonates breathing at end-expiratory pressures of 6 cm H_2O or more (76).

The renal complications associated with hypoxemic disorders are self-limiting when the respiratory condition improves. Recent advances in the management of neonatal respiratory disorders have considerably improved the associated renal disturbances.

Management of Asphyxiated or Hypoxic Neonate

The asphyxiated newborn infant often presents with cardiac failure, hypoxia, and metabolic acidosis. Blood volume may be decreased. When hypovolemia is suspected to be the cause of decreased urine output, volume expansion is required. It should be performed with great caution because of the possibility of myocardial damage. In the preterm infant, rapid expansion may also increase the risk of intracranial hemorrhage (77). When volume expansion is required, it can be achieved by infusing 5 to 10 ml/kg BW of plasma or blood.

The metabolic acidosis present in hypoxic infants may result in myocardial depression, pulmonary hypertension, and renal vasoconstriction. Acidosis can be corrected by the slow infusion of isotonic or 0.5 M sodium bicarbonate. To avoid CO_2 retention, it is important to establish adequate ventilation before bicarbonate administration.

With severe perinatal asphyxia, fluid retention may result from renal failure, excessive ADH secretion, or both. The resultant increase in total body fluids may further aggravate the heart failure, increase the risk of brain edema, and also diminish pulmonary function by increasing lung fluid. It is therefore essential to avoid overhydration of infants who suffered perinatal asphyxia. Daily fluid administration must initially be restricted to 40 to 60 ml/kg BW until adequate diuresis is established. In heart failure, inotropic agents such as dopamine or dobutamine may be indicated. Fluid intake should be increased to 120 to 150 ml/kg/24 hr only after adequate diuresis is established (2 to 3 ml/kg/hr) and body weight starts to decrease.

Management of Infants with RDS

Adequate hydration with maintenance of optimal respiratory and cardiovascular condition are mandatory in infants with RDS. Since lung function appears to improve after the onset of diuresis (78), attempts should be made to improve the renal condition. Restoration of cardiac output, blood volume, and blood pressure is critical. Attempts to accelerate the diuresis by administering furosemide or generous amounts of fluid (more than 160 ml/kg/day) can have a potent diuretic effect without acutely improving cardiorespiratory function (79) or increase the risk of patent ductus arteriosus with congestive heart failure, as well as that of necrotizing enterocolitis (80). The improved lung function sometimes noted after furosemide administration could reflect improved pulmonary compliance (81). Fluid intakes providing 80 to 100 ml/kg/24 hr are probably acceptable to achieve a physiological negative water balance with an anticipated weight loss of approximately 10% during the first week of life while maintaining adequate renal perfusion. Fluid balance should be closely monitored and urine flow rate measured at 6-hr intervals. Urine osmolality should be determined regularly. An increase in osmolality above isotonicity indicates impaired renal perfusion and points to the need for actively restoring cardiac output.

Recent advances in RDS management have considerably improved the renal function in RDS and its prognosis. The prerenal failure may, however, lead to parenchymal injury, resulting in acute tubular necrosis or, in severe forms, acute cortical necrosis.

ACUTE RENAL FAILURE

Acute renal failure (ARF) is characterized by a sudden decrease in glomerular filtration rate, which leads to disturbances in water, electrolytes, and acid-base homeostasis and to accumulation of nitrogen end-products. ARF may be secondary to acute circulatory insufficiency, without structural renal damage, to severe renal parenchymal injury or to acute urinary tract obstruction. The following list indicates conditions that may cause acute renal failure in the neonate:

Prerenal Conditions: Hypovolemia, hypotension, and hypoxemia are responsible for a decrease in renal perfusion.

a. Dehydration: inadequate fluid intake, vomiting, diarrhea, phototherapy, high environmental temperature.
b. Blood loss, clamping of the aorta during cardiac surgery, hypovolemia secondary to fluid shifts.
c. Perinatal asphyxia, severe respiratory distress.
d. Congestive cardiac failure, polycythemia.

Intrarenal Conditions: Glomerular, tubular, and vascular structures are injured.

a. Vascular disorders: renal venous or renal artery thrombosis.
b. Acute renal necrosis: cortical, medullary, or papillary necrosis secondary to renal ischemia, nephrotoxic agents, hemoglobinuria.
c. Congenital nephropathies: bilateral renal agenesis, dysgenesis or hypoplasia, infantile polycystic disease, congenital nephrotic syndrome.
d. Acute pyelonephritis.

Postrenal Conditions: The condition is secondary to ureteral or urethral obstruction.

Most cases of ARF in neonates are preventable if the predisposing factors are treated early and adequately.

Clinical Presentation

The clinical signs of ARF vary in the newborn infant (82–87). Oliguria, defined as urine output of less than 1.0 ml/kg/hr, is usually the first sign of ARF. A normal urine output does not, however, exclude the diagnosis of ARF, as diuresis may be well maintained despite a decreased GFR (88). Symptoms associated with ARF relate to the factors producing ARF or to the pathophysiological consequences of renal failure:

1. Symptoms determined by the disorder responsible for ARF: dehydration, hypotension, cardiac failure, asphyxia, shock, primary and secondary respiratory distress syndrome, large renal masses, Potter's facies, palpable bladder, urinary ascites.
2. Symptoms secondary to renal failure: poor feeding, vomiting, edema, anemia, hyperventilation, cardiac arrhythmia, seizures, hypertension, hypertensive encephalopathy.

The cardinal features of the uremic syndrome are not always present or discernible in the high-risk neonate with ARF. The diagnosis must therefore be considered in any baby with shock, dehydration, sepsis, or malformation syndrome.

Causes

Prerenal ARF

The neonatal kidney may be more sensitive to changes in perfusion and less able to withstand substantial changes in renal arterial pressure. Prerenal failure develops when autoregulation fails to compensate for decreases in renal perfusion pressure. Correction of the cause rapidly returns renal function to normal. Prompt recognition of this form of ARF is important, as prolonged uncorrected renal hypoperfusion may lead to ischemic reactions at the cellular level, with consequent edema of the vascular and tubular cells.

Intrinsic Causes

In intrinsic ARF, vascular, glomerular, and tubular structures are injured. Acute renal necrosis is often seen after prolonged renal ischemia secondary to major perinatal disorders. Neonatal asphyxia, meconium aspiration, hemorrhage, sepsis, and shock are the most frequent causes (86, 87). Acute renal failure is an important complication of cardiac surgery in young infants (89). Other causes of intrinsic ARF include vascular disorders, which can occur spontaneously or be precipitated by iatrogenic maneuvers. Renal artery thrombosis has been observed after catheterization of the umbilical artery. It may result in ARF or cause severe arterial hypertension. Renal venous thrombosis is frequently associated with a prenatal or postnatal insult. The risk is increased with hypovolemia, hypotension, and hypoxemia. It occurs more frequently in infants from diabetic mothers. It can be a complication of angiography and may be precipitated by potent loop diuretics. Congenital nephropathies such as the nephrotic syndrome or cystic dysplasia can result in impaired renal function. Acute functional changes are often superimposed on chronic structural damage. Interstitial nephritis, congenital or acquired, allergic or infectious, can profoundly affect renal function. It is often secondary to generalized septicemia. ARF may develop as a consequence of pigment-associated renal insult, as seen during hemoglobinuria or myoglobinuria (90), or may be associated with polycythemia (91). Hyperbilirubinemia has been reported to decrease GFR (92), but the claim has not been confirmed (93). In animal studies, conjugated bilirubin appears to sensitize the kidney to the effects of anoxic damage (94).

Postrenal Failure

Obstruction to urine flow may cause ARF. Except in patients with a single kidney or with bilateral parenchymal disease affecting kidney function, obstruction must be bilateral to produce significant renal failure. Renal dysplasia or cysts are observed in a high proportion of neonates with obstructive malformations of the urinary tract. Obstructive renal failure is a treatable form of ARF, but the concomitant presence of structural parenchymal abnormalities may darken the prognosis after relief of the obstruction.

Differential Diagnosis

Oliguria is usually the hallmark of ARF, but urine volume may be well maintained in some circumstances (88). The absence of oliguria generally excludes prerenal events as sole causes of the renal failure. Osmotic diuresis, mineralocorticoid deficiency, diabetes insipidus, partial urinary tract obstruction, and postobstructive diuresis may all be associated with a sustained urine output, even though creatinine rises. Normal urine volumes in newly recognized azotemia characterize chronic renal failure. Complete anuria rarely occurs in prerenal or intrinsic renal failure. When caused by intrinsic renal disease, anuria is an ominous indicator of such causes as acute bilateral renal arterial or venous occlusion or bilateral cortical necrosis.

The accumulation of nitrogen end-products confirms the presence of ARF, which is characterized by the following changes:

1. Plasma urea: concentration above 50 mg/dl (8.3 mmol/liter) with a daily increase above 10 mg/dl (1.7 mmol/liter).
2. Plasma creatinine: concentration above 1.0 mg/dl (88 μmol/liter) with a daily increase above 0.2 mg/dl (18 μmol/liter).

Values of creatinine plasma concentration should be interpreted with caution during the first weeks of life. Elevated levels are found at birth, the newborn plasma creatinine reflecting the mother's values. Concentration in the neonate has been shown to reach steady levels by the fifth day of life (37). The rate of increase in plasma creatinine may also be very variable among neonates with renal failure, creatinine production being less, for example, in malnourished infants whose muscle mass is reduced.

Assessment of urinary sediment may help in diagnosing ARF. An active sediment with renal tubular epithelial cells, cellular debris, casts, red blood cells, and proteinuria indicates intrinsic renal disease. The absence of cellular elements and proteins in the urine is most compatible with prerenal or postrenal azotemia.

Considerable information may be obtainable from the urine composition assessment. Tests of tubular function have proven helpful in separating prerenal from acute intrinsic renal oliguria (95, 96) (Table 56.6). These tests are based on the assumption that tubules of the hypoperfused ischemic kidney respond appropriately to intense stimuli for salt and water retention. Oliguria is an appropriate physiological response in such instances. Urine osmolality is a more reliable index of concentrating ability than specific gravity, as it is only influenced by the number of particles dissolved in the urine and not by the size of the molecules. Urine osmolalities above 400 mosm/kg H_2O suggest prerenal failure, whereas osmolalities below 400 suggest intrinsic renal damage. The urine-to-plasma osmolar ratio is more specific than urine osmolality alone. Values above 2 indicate prerenal failure; values below 1.0 suggest intrinsic renal failure.

The renal handling of sodium may also help in differentiating prerenal from intrinsic renal failure. The normal hypoperfused kidney avidly reabsorbs sodium, thus decreasing its urinary concentration. In patients with renal damage, the renal tubular capacity to reabsorb sodium is impaired, and its concentration is elevated above 40 mmol/liter. The scatter of values is, however, very large. The assessment of the fractional excretion of sodium (FE_{Na}) gives more precise information on the oliguria. A FE_{Na} below 2% occurs in prerenal failure. Its value is increased above 2.5% in patients with intrinsic renal failure. The overlap is minimal (95, 96). Falsely high fractional excretion rate values can be

Table 56.6.
Diagnostic Indices in Neonates with Oliguria

Index suggestive of	Prerenal insufficiency	Intrinsic failure	References
U_{Na} (mmol/liter)[a]	31 ± 20	63 ± 35	85, 95
U/P Na[b]	0.2 ± 0.1	0.5 ± 0.2	85, 95
U/P urea[c]	30 ± 18	6 ± 3	85, 95
U/P osm[d]	>2.0	<1.0	86, 87
FE_{Na} (%)[e]	0.8 ± 0.6	4.8 ± 1.4	96
RFI[f]	1.0 ± 0.2	7.2 ± 1.3	96

[a] U_{Na}: urine sodium concentration.
[b] U/P Na: urine to plasma sodium ratio.
[c] U/P urea: urine to plasma urea ratio.
[d] U/P osm: urine to plasma osmolality ratio.
[e] FE_{Na}: fractional excretion of Na.
[f] RFI: renal failure index = U_{Na} × P/U creatinine.

observed if a large sodium load is given or if diuretics are administered. Caution should be exercised when applying these indices to very premature neonates, for elevated FE_{Na} is normally present in the first days of life of preterm infants, occasionally reaching values as high as 5%. The renal failure index gives information similar to that obtained by FE_{Na} (Table 56.6).

Although urinary indices may help in differentiating prerenal from intrinsic renal failure, they are usually obtained only after treatment of the patients has already started. A therapeutic trial of volume expansion often provides the best method for defining the nature of the ARF (see section on treatment). Prerenal oliguria rapidly responds to volume expansion with saline or plasma. Failure of fluid administration to restore urine output suggests intrinsic renal failure or obstruction (85).

Imaging Studies

Ultrasonography is useful in evaluating poorly functioning or nonfunctioning kidneys. Renal agenesis, renal hypoplasia, renal masses, hydronephrosis, cystic kidneys, and bladder distention can be precisely identified. Voiding cystourethrography is useful in defining the obstructive causes of ARF such as posterior urethral valves and stricture, obstruction of the ureters, ureterocele, and severe vesicoureteric reflux.

Excretory urography is of limited value in the diagnosis of ARF. The osmotic load of the contrast agent may aggravate the cellular dehydration and have a nephrotoxic effect. When indicated, intravenous urography should be performed with the new nonionic contrast agents, the osmolality of which is close to 450 mosm/kg H_2O and thus much lower than that of standard agents.

Radioisotopic scanning and renograms may be useful in evaluating the size, position, and function of poorly functioning kidneys. The renal parenchymal phase of the renogram is prolonged in renal tubular necrosis. Renal angiography may be indicated when renal arterial or venous thrombosis is suspected, but the procedure carries a substantial risk, related in part to the use of hypertonic contrast agents (97, 98). Digital subtraction angiography may prove to be useful.

Treatment of ARF

Confirmation of ARF Type (Fig. 56.8)

Whenever possible, the cause of ARF should be precisely defined and prerenal factors such as hypovolemia, hypotension, and hypoxemia should be rapidly corrected. Adequate ventilation and hydration are mandatory. When dehydration is present, the fluid deficit should be corrected initially by the administration of 20 to 40 ml/kg of a solution over 2 hr; solution composition is determined by the nature of the dehydration. The use of an isotonic saline solution or an isotonic sodium solution containing 20 to 25 mmol/liter of bicarbonate is a safe method of rehydration. If the state of renal failure is prerenal, diuresis should begin in the next few hours.

If diuresis does not ensue rapidly after correcting the fluid deficit and if some doubt persists concerning the state of hydration, administering plasma at a rate of 20 ml/kg over 2 hr can be tried. If the oligoanuria persists despite a normal state of hydration, administration of powerful loop diuretics, furosemide or ethacrynic acid, 2 to 5 mg/kg, may occasionally produce diuresis in prerenal as well as in postrenal or intrinsic ARF. Diuretic administration, however, does not provide much diagnostic insight, and the natriuretic effect may worsen previously dehydrated infants. The administration of mannitol has also been recommended in older children and adults, either to differentiate prerenal from intrinsic ARF or to improve the renal circulation. Its usefulness in prerenal ARF is questionable, and the cerebral risk of an acute rise in plasma osmolality in very premature infants may be substantial.

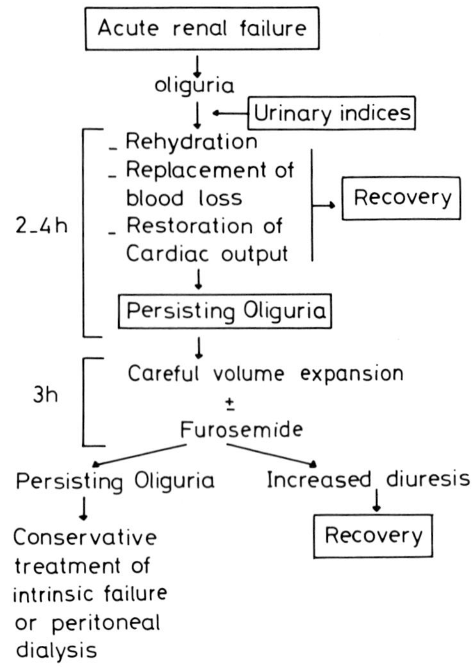

Figure 56.8. Management of acute renal failure.

Table 56.7.
Normal Water Losses in Neonates

	Water (ml/kg/24 hr)		
	<1500 G	1500–2500 G	>2500 G
Losses			
Basal insensible water loss	30–60	15–35	15–25
Stool	5–10	5–10	5–10
Urine[a]	50–100	50–100	50–100
Increment for phototherapy	20	20	20

[a] Urinary water loss is calculated as that needed at a urine osmolality of 150 to 300 mosm/kg H_2O when renal solute excretion equals 15 mosm/kg BW/day. This is also the urine volume required at a urine osmolality of 75 to 150 mosm/kg H_2O when urine solute excretion equals 7.5 mosm/kg/day. (Modified from Roy NR, Sinclair JC: Hydration of the low birth-weight infant. Clin Perinatol 2:393, 1975.)

Persistence of oligoanuria despite therapeutic maneuvers indicates the presence of renal parenchymal lesions. Conservative treatment of the ARF is indicated.

Conservative Management

The aim of conservative management is to maintain fluid balance (Tables 56.7 and 56.8). Body weight is the best guide, and the infant should be weighed every 8 to 12 hr. Fluid balance should be maintained by infusing an hourly volume equal to the urine output plus insensible water loss, which approximates 0.7 to 1.0 ml/kg/hr in the full-term infant but is greater (on a body weight basis) in low-birth-weight neonates (Table 56.7) (82).

Water losses increase with phototherapy, and 0.6 to 0.8 ml/kg/hr must be added to the normal insensible losses. Insensible water loss decreases if the neonate is on the ventilator.

Caloric needs can rarely be met in oligoanuric infants, so a daily loss of 0.2% to 1.0% of body weight is expected. An increase in body weight or a steady body weight reflects overhydration. Insensible water losses should be replaced with 10% glucose (555 mmol/liter) intravenously.

Table 56.8.
Fluid and Electrolyte Requirements in the Neonatal Period

Infant age	Water (ml/kg/24 hr)	
	Premature	Term
Day		
1	60–70	70
2	80–90	75
3	100–110	80
4	120–150	85
5	125–150	90
Weeks 2–4	150	120
Electrolytes (mmol/kg/24 hr)		
Sodium	2–4	2–4
Potassium	2–3	2–3
Chloride	3–5	3–5
Calcium	3–4	1–1.5
Phosphorus	2–3	0.8–1.2
Magnesium	0.25–0.50	0.2–0.3

Treatment of Complications

Hyponatremia. The hyponatremia observed in ARF is most often due to excessive water intake coupled with the inability of the kidney to excrete free water. Thus the dilutional hyponatremia must not be corrected by sodium administration, but rather by decreasing the administration of free water. If the hyponatremia is so severe ($P_{Na} < 120$ mmol/liter) or has occurred so rapidly that central nervous system symptoms such as lethargy and seizures develop, a rapid form of treatment is required. Administration of furosemide (2 mg/kg IV) and hypertonic sodium (20 ml/kg of 1.5% NaCl) should raise serum sodium concentration and cause excretion of excess water. This treatment should be reserved for emergency situations and should be followed by fluid restriction.

Hyperkalemia. Hyperkalemia is a life-threatening disturbance that must be rapidly corrected. The serum potassium level should be determined immediately and a base line electrocardiogram obtained. The ECG must be monitored continuously if there is any sign of cardiac toxicity. Ventricular arrhythmia or cardiac arrest may occur whenever the classic sine wave of hyperkalemia is present. Once ARF is suspected, potassium intake from all sources should be avoided.

Patients with mild hyperkalemia can be treated with exchange resins (kayexalate) administered orally or rectally in a dose of 1 g/kg every 6 hr. The resin is diluted in 10 ml of 70% sorbitol. One gram of kayexalate removes approximately 1 mmol of potassium from the body.

The fastest method of reversing the effects of hyperkalemia is to antagonize the peripheral neuromuscular effects of potassium. This can be achieved by raising the extracellular calcium concentration. Ten percent calcium gluconate is given intravenously at a rate of 0.5 to 1.0 ml/kg over 2 to 4 min under ECG surveillance. Calcium therapy has an onset of action within minutes, but the effect does not last.

Redistribution of potassium from the extracellular space into the intracellular space is also an effective acute treatment of hyperkalemia. This can be achieved by administering 2 ml/kg of 8.4% sodium bicarbonate. Infusion of 25% glucose in a central vein can also be used to drive potassium into the cells. Alkalinization and glucose therapy have an onset of action within 30 min and last for several hours.

Acidosis. Metabolic acidosis occurs when acids produced by the catabolism of dietary and tissue proteins are retained. Only severe systemic acidosis with base deficits greater than 8 mmol/liter or serum pH values below 7.20 should be corrected. The number of millimoles of sodium bicarbonate needed to correct the acidosis can be approximated by the classic formula: 0.3 × body weight (kg) × base deficit (mmol/liter). The calculated deficit should be corrected over the ensuing 12 hr. As a rule, administration of 1.0 ml/kg of 0.5 M $NaHCO_3$ raises the serum bicarbonate concentration by approximately 1 mmol/liter. Overzealous correction of acidosis may result in fluid overload, intracranial hemorrhage in the premature newborn infant, and a decrease in ionized calcium leading to tetany, which may necessitate the intravenous administration of calcium gluconate.

Hypocalcemia. Hypocalcemia often develops early in the course of ARF. Symptomatic or severe hypocalcemia (total serum calcium <7 to 8 mg/dl or 1.75 to 2.00 mmol/liter) is treated by intravenous administration of 10% calcium gluconate, 1.0 ml/kg, over 5 to 10 min, with ECG monitoring, or, if not available, cardiac rate monitoring for evidence of bradycardia. Large doses of calcium are often necessary to raise serum calcium. Oral administration of calcium carbonate, 50 mg/kg/24 hr, may be necessary.

Hyperphosphatemia. Plasma phosphorus levels are elevated in most neonates with ARF. They should be decreased by oral administration of aluminum hydroxyde, 60 to 100 mg/kg/day, or calcium carbonate, 50 mg/kg/day. The doses are adjusted to maintain a normal serum phosphorus concentration below 6 mg/dl (2.0 mmol/liter).

Anemia. Severe symptomatic anemia may be cautiously corrected by administering 10 ml/kg BW of freshly packed red cells over 2 days. The risk of congestive heart failure should be kept in mind.

Hypertension. The most frequent cause of arterial hypertension is fluid overload. The condition usually responds to fluid restriction. Hypotensive drugs should be used with caution in persistent hypertension. Furosemide may be useful to increase sodium excretion. It must be given in large doses of 5 to 10 mg/kg if neonates with depressed GFR are to respond. The dose must not be repeated in nonresponders, as the drug can produce ototoxic effects. In hypertensive emergencies, blood pressure may be decreased by means of potent vasodilators such as hydralazine (0.2 to 1.0 mg/kg), diazoxide (5 mg/kg), or sodium nitroprusside (0.1 to 8.0 μg/kg/min), or by captopril (1 mg/kg) (99).

Convulsions. Seizures are usually secondary to an electrolyte imbalance, to rapid changes in serum osmolality, plasma pH, and bicarbonate, and to intracranial hypertension. Hyponatremia, hypoglycemia, hypomagnesemia,and hyperphosphatemia have all been associated with seizures. Hypocalcemia often presents as seizures rather than tetany. Preventive measures should include control of hypertension, reduction of fluid overload, correction of electrolyte abnormalities, and administration of calcium gluconate before correction of metabolic acidosis. If the infant presents with convulsions, an adequate airway should be maintained. Anticonvulsive therapy consists of the administration of intravenous diazepam, 0.3 mg/kg, or intravenous phenobarbital, 6 mg/kg. If no vein is available for puncture, seizures can be stopped by giving diazepam in a rectal solution (5 mg/dose). Phenytoin, 10 to 25 mg/kg, in a slow intravenous injection, can be used when phenobarbital or diazepam does not stop the seizures.

Infections. Infections are frequent in infants presenting with ARF, and sepsis is a frequent cause of death. Diagnosis of infection requires a high degree of suspicion. Fever can be absent, and blood cells counts may be misleading. Hypotension, tachycardia, and evidence of continued hypercatabolism may all be early signs of sepsis. Cultures should be obtained, and catheter sites examined for evidence of phlebitis. If the infant's clinical condition is deteriorating, antibiotics should be administered without waiting for the culture results. Antibiotics should be directed toward gram-negative organisms and *Staphylococcus aureus*. In general, gentamicin and cephalothin are indicated. Ticarcillin and clindamycin are indicated for anaerobic organisms. Full doses are given initially. Subsequent maintenance doses are adjusted to the level of glomerular filtration rate; when possible serum drug levels should be obtained.

Nutrition. Conservative regimes are extremely restrictive in oligoanuric infants. All efforts should be made to provide 100 kcal and 1 to 2 g of proteins per kilogram by infusing 20% to 40% dextrose in water, along with essential amino acids and lipids. When oral feeding is possible, breast milk or a low-protein formula should be given, along with high calorie substances with low osmolalities and polyunsaturated fats (100, 101).

Dialysis

Most patients presenting with ARF can be treated conservatively. Dialysis is indicated if ARF lasts for more than a week or if intractable complications such as fluid overload, congestive heart failure, hypertension, incipient pulmonary edema, and progressive uremia develop. The following chemical abnormalities may also be an indication for dialysis: plasma sodium below 120 mmol/liter, plasma potassium above 8.0 mmol/liter, severe acidosis with plasma bicarbonate below 12 mmol/liter, plasma urea above 0.3 g/dl (50 mmol/liter), and plasma creatinine above 10 mg/dl (900 μmol/liter).

Hemodialysis. Hemodialysis can be performed in newborn infants (102, 103). Blood access may be achieved through the umbilical vessels, the brachial artery, the jugular vein, the femoral artery, and the saphenous vein. Small volume blood lines and dialyzers have been developed; these require as little as 24 ml to prime, i.e., 10% of the blood volume of a 3 kg infant. Although hemodialysis is technically feasible in newborn infants, the outcome is generally very poor in the severe cases for which it is required.

Peritoneal dialysis. Peritoneal dialysis is the method of choice in neonates. It can be rapidly and safely carried out with minimal equipment, does not overstress the cardiovascular system, and does not require heparin therapy. Because it has a high peritoneal surface area/body weight ratio (383 cm^2/kg in the infant versus 177 cm^2/kg in adults), peritoneal dialysis is very efficient in the young infant (104).

For peritoneal dialysis, a special soft catheter (Tenckhoff pediatric catheter) or a Holter ventricular catheter is used to give access to the abdominal cavity. To avoid the risk of bladder puncture, the bladder should be emptied by catheterization. Following local anesthesia, the catheter is introduced 2 cm below the umbilicus in the midline or in the left flank, either percutaneously or through a small laparotomy incision. The catheter is fixed by a purse string suture to ensure its stability and to avoid fluid leakage and tacking between abdominal wall layers. After warming to 37 °C, the dialysate solution is infused by gravitational flow or by an infusion pump. Exchange volumes of 30 to 50 ml/kg BW are used. Dialysis cycles are usually of one to three hours duration. Early diagnosis of peritonitis is achieved by regular dialysate cultures, white cell counts, and determination of the dialysate protein concentration. These tests must also be performed whenever the dialysate is cloudy. Practical approaches to peritoneal dialysis are given in Chapter 48.

Clinical Course of ARF

Recovery or partial recovery from ARF is indicated by a progressive increase in urine output, which may supervene after up to three weeks of oliguria. Even though a polyuric phase can occur at this stage, the glomerular filtration rate in these catabolic infants may not be sufficient to prevent a further increase in plasma urea and creatinine concentrations. The urine resembles the glomerular filtrate and, as large amounts of electrolytes such as sodium and potassium may be lost during this phase, the risk of dehydration and hypoelectrolytemia is ever present.

Prognosis

The prognosis of ARF depends largely on the nature and severity of the underlying disease, the skill in correcting the chemical disturbances associated with ARF, and the expertise in managing these high-risk neonates. Infection is still a common cause of death in ARF. Prerenal failure has a good prognosis if the predisposing factors can be rapidly corrected. Patients with acute renal tubular necrosis usually have complete recovery. The recovery is less likely when there is cortical, medullary, or corticomedullary necrosis. Intrinsic renal failure may have a poor outcome, the degree of recovery of renal function depending on the nature of the parenchymal lesion. Patients with congenital structural defects are often left with a state of chronic renal failure. Hypertension may persist after the acute phase of ARF and be associated with a state of chronic renal insufficiency. Postrenal failure has a favorable prognosis provided the obstruction can be corrected early, before the occurrence of parenchymal lesions.

The management of neonates with ARF is a therapeutic challenge. Many patients have severe problems of cardiac and respiratory function in addition to the primary ARF. These infants are best managed in specialized units where a multidisciplinary approach can be offered.

URINARY TRACT INFECTION

Incidence and Manifestations

Urinary tract infection (UTI) is found in approximately 0.7% of term neonates (105) and in 2.2% to 3.4% of premature, postmature, and high-risk neonates (106). Infected boys outnumber girls fivefold. The sex ratio is due to the frequency of congenital anomalies in boys and a greater susceptibility of male infants to infection. It has been suggested that the predominance of males in neonatal infections (mostly caused by gram-negative bacilli) is related to a sex-linked factor in host susceptibility, possibly located on the X chromosome and involving synthesis of immunoglobulins.

The clinical manifestations of UTI in the neonate are highly variable, ranging from asymptomatic bacteriuria to septicemia (Table 56.9) (106, 107). Gastrointestinal symptoms are frequent and include poor feeding, failure to thrive, vomiting, and diarrhea. Other symptoms are fever, lethargy, irritability, and dehydration. Cyanosis, convulsions, and jaun-

Table 56.9.
Symptoms of Neonatal Urinary Tract Infection

	Total number	%
Total number of neonates	1762	100
Infected neonates	43	2.4
Symptomatic infections	34	1.9
Asymptomatic infections	9	0.5
Incidence of symptoms in infected neonates		
Vomiting	16	37
Weight loss, dehydration	13	30
Fever	9	21
Diarrhea	6	14
Palpable kidneys	6	14
Poor feeding	5	12
Jaundice	16	37
Metabolic acidosis	9	21
Miscellaneous	15	35

(Adapted from Maherzi M, Guignard J-P, Torrado A: Urinary tract infection in high-risk newborn infants. Pediatrics 62:521, 1978.)

dice are sometimes observed. The kidneys are palpable in at least 20% of cases.

Diagnosis

The diagnosis of UTI depends on the demonstration of a significant number of organisms in a properly collected urine specimen. Urine can be collected by spontaneous micturition in a bag, by spontaneous stream-voiding, or by suprapubic bladder puncture.

An adhesive bag should be applied after careful desinfection of the external genitalia with 0.02% chlorhexidine or, more simply, soapy water. Irrigation of the preputial folds is recommended, as they can act as a reservoir for bacteria. Rinsing with sterile water is necessary to remove the desinfectant solution or soap. A sterile plastic bag is then fixed to the perineal region. Any sample containing more than 10^4 organisms per milliliter is suspect, and a further sample should be obtained. A finding of less than 10^4 colonies per milliliter is considered to represent urine contamination. When the urine contains 10^5 or more colonies per milliliter, the diagnosis of UTI is highly probable, but the urine should be reexamined by bladder aspiration (108). In the male infant, a satisfactory midstream urine specimen can occasionally be collected without a bag.

Suprapubic aspiration is easy to perform in infants if the bladder is full. The bladder must thus be percussed before the procedure; loss of urine is prevented by compressing the penis in the male or the urethra in the female with a finger in the rectum. The skin of the lower abdomen is cleaned with 0.02% chlorhexidine or 70% alcohol. The puncture is performed 1 cm above the symphysis, in the midline. A 2-cm, 21-gauge needle is used. It is directed toward the fundus at an inclination of 60°. The urine is gently aspirated in a 5-ml syringe and immediately placed on the culture plate. The growth of even a single colony on the culture plate is proof of UTI (107).

The reliability of a urine specimen obtained by bladder catheterization is not better than that of a bag specimen. The method should not be used because of the danger of iatrogenic infection (109).

Bacteriology

Escherichia coli is the organism most frequently responsible for UTI in the neonatal period (Table 56.10) followed by *Klebsiella pneumoniae* and *Proteus mirabilis* (106). Other organisms such as the coliforms (*Aerobacter aerogenes*, *A. paracolon*), the *Pseudomonas* species, and the enterococci are also encountered. The presence of two bacterial species in the urine, usually a sign of contamination in older children, is observed in a few neonates, even when the urine is obtained by suprapubic aspiration (106). This intriguing finding could be related to the neonatal pattern of local antibody synthesis, for secretory IgA is detectable only after several weeks of postnatal life.

Table 56.10.
Bacteriology in High-risk Neonates with Urinary Tract Infection Diagnosed by Bladder Puncture

Organisms	% of cases
Escherichia coli	67
Klebsiella pneumoniae	21
Proteus	2
E. coli + *Proteus*	5
E. coli + *Klebsiella*	2
E. coli + enterococcus	2

(Adapted from Maherzi M, Guignard J-P, Torrado A: Urinary tract infection in high-risk newborn infants. Pediatrics 62:521, 1978.)

Pyuria is frequently associated with bacteriuria. It is not, however, pathognomonic of UTI (108) and simply reflects the inflammation of the urinary tract. Microscopic hematuria is sometimes also found in neonates with UTI, especially in high-risk neonates, where it may be related to hypoxic perinatal distress rather than to UTI.

Predisposing Abnormality Factors

Malformations of the urinary tract represent the most important predisposing factor in the pathogenesis of UTI. Vesicoureteric reflux (VUR), hydronephrosis, ureterocele, ureteropelvic obstruction, or urethral valves are present in about 50% of neonates with UTI (106, 110, 111). They produce stasis of urine and thus favor UTI.

Vesicoureteric Reflux

Vesicoureteric reflux (VUR) (see also Chapter 37) is a common anomaly and may be present in as many as 0.5% of normal neonates (3). It usually disappears spontaneously in the first year of life, for with maturation, the path of the ureter through the wall elongates, producing an effective antireflux valve. The severity of reflux varies. It may be limited to the lower ureter or be associated with gross dilatation of the ureter, the renal pelvis, and calyces. The prevalence of gross reflux is greater among siblings of a child with VUR (2, 4, 5). Vesicoureteric reflux, like obstructive uropathies, is a threat to the integrity of the renal parenchyma. Infected vesicoureteric reflux is frequently associated with renal parenchymal scarring (112, 113). A sterile reflux also appears to produce scarring when associated with high back pressure (114).

In some neonates, VUR is limited to the lower ureter or to the pelvis. In others, reflux extends into the renal parenchymal (113). Intrarenal reflux (IRR) is demonstrated by parenchymal opacification during excretory cystography. The importance of IRR is that its presence is a prerequisite to the development of pyelonephritic scarring. IRR occurs in renal segments drained by predisposed "refluxing papillae" which are present in two thirds of healthy infants (112). These papillae permit reflux of infected urine into the parenchyma, thus initiating progressive scarring. Neonates with reflux should be given prophylactic antibiotherapy to prevent the scarring that appears to develop very early in life. Atrophic kidneys are sometimes present at birth and are frequently associated with malformations of the urinary tract. The scarring in them probably reflects dysplasia. It may be difficult at a later age to determine to what extent "reflux nephropathy" is due to dysplasia or to postnatally acquired pyelonephritic scarring.

Obstructive Uropathy

A poor urinary stream or distended bladder in a neonate with UTI suggests urinary tract obstruction. In the male infant, posterior urethral valves or prune belly syndrome may be present, but in females the commonest obstructive lesion in the lower urinary tract is an ectopic ureterocele. If infected, these babies require bladder catheterization and antibiotics; urological consultation is urgently needed as well (see Chapter 38). If the urine is sterile, the hesitation to undertake diagnostic cystography should be resisted until the follow-up urological plan has been formulated.

Investigation

All newborn infants with proven UTI must undergo imaging studies. Ultrasonography should come first. It can detect obstructive uropathy, severe VUR, scarred kidneys, and a distended bladder—all conditions frequently associated with UTI. It is particularly useful if renal function is poor and can be performed in the presence of UTI.

Voiding cystourethrography with a contrast agent is also indicated in all neonates with UTI. It will demonstrate the presence of VUR and will outline the bladder and urethra. Intravenous urography will permit delineation of the renal parenchyma and urinary tract. It is of limited value in the first two weeks of life. (See Chapter 20 for additional discussion.)

Therapy

When limited to the lower urinary tract, the infection may be treated by oral amoxycillin, 20 to 50 mg/kg/day in three or four doses, for a total of seven days. This will rapidly eradicate the infection if the bacteria are sensitive. If the urine is not sterile within three days, the antibiotics should be changed according to the sensitivity of the organism. Neonates with UTI and VUR should be treated by amoxycillin, 20 to 50 mg/kg/day in three or four doses for seven days, followed by oral amoxycillin, 10 to 20 mg/kg/day in two doses, or sulfonamides, 50 mg/kg/day in two doses. The latter should, however, be avoided if jaundice is present. Prophylaxis should be continued as long as the reflux and the associated risk of renal scarring persist.

UTI associated with an obstructive malformation of the urinary tract must be treated by intravenous amoxycillin, 20 to 50 mg/kg/day in three or four doses. Because of the risk of scarring, the obstruction must be relieved after the shortest possible delay. Prophylaxis is usually recommended for some weeks after the surgical procedure.

When the infection reaches the renal parenchyma, the risks are increased, and the infection should be treated vigorously. Intravenous amoxycillin, 50 to 100 mg/kg/day, possibly associated with gentamicin, 3.5 to 7.5 mg/kg/day in two doses, should be administered for 10 days. If there is generalized septicemia as well, the therapy should consist of gentamicin, 3.5 to 7.5 mg/kg/day, and amoxycillin, 50 to 100 mg/kg/day, for 10 days. To avoid toxic drug dosage in these neonates, whose GFR is usually depressed below its normal low level, plasma concentrations of gentamicin should be monitored. The plasma creatinine should also be determined regularly to detect a nephrotoxic effect of gentamicin and to adapt the dose.

RENAL NECROSIS

Renal necrosis may involve the cortex (115), the medulla (116, 117), or the papilla (118–120). Cortical and medullary necrosis are often associated.

Etiology

Most of the precipitating factors that produce vasomotor nephropathy (prerenal insufficiency) may cause renal necrosis. Impaired renal perfusion results in ischemic tissue damage and necrosis. Prolonged hypoxia, asphyxia, and shock are the major factors in development of cortical, medullary, and papillary necrosis in the neonate (Fig. 56.9). Renal necrosis has been described after septic and hemorrhagic shock, severe anemia, perinatal asphyxia, erythroblastosis fetalis, and placental hemorrhage. It is often associated with disseminated intravascular coagulation.

Renal medullary necrosis has been described following angiographic hypertonic contrast agents. Severe hyperbilirubinemia has been associated with medullary necrosis, and a direct effect of unconjugated bilirubin on medullary tissue has been implicated. Papillary necrosis in the newborn infant has occurred after asphyxia. hyperbilirubinemia, and hemorrhagic, septic, and asphyxic shock. The diagnosis is usually made post mortem, but a few infants have survived.

Clinical Presentation

Cortical and medullary necrosis present as anuria or oligoanuria arising in the clinical settings previously mentioned. The kidneys are

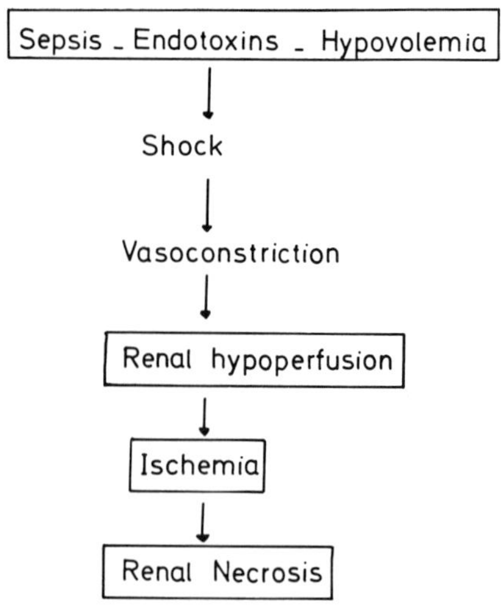

Figure 56.9. Pathophysiology of renal necrosis.

usually mildly enlarged. Microscopic hematuria is always present, often accompanied by proteinuria, and the urine is sometimes grossly bloody. Thrombosis of the renal vein is a frequent accompanying event. Clinically, cortical necrosis cannot be differentiated from medullary necrosis in the acute phase. In surviving cases, a concentrating defect with salt-wasting is observed after medullary or papillary necrosis (121).

Diagnosis

Cortical and medullary necrosis must be differentiated from acute tubular necrosis, renal venous and arterial thrombosis, and renal infarction due to arterial embolism. The diagnosis is not easy and is often only made retrospectively. Imaging studies are helpful in demonstrating the presence of the kidneys and absence of obstruction by ultrasonography and assessing kidney function by the isotope renogram. If residual function is sufficient, an IVU can confirm the suspicion of medullary necrosis. A prolonged nephrogram with heavy opacification of the pyramids is seen early in the course of the disease, whereas pyelocalyceal deformity is a late sequel. Calcification of necrotic cortical tissue occurs rapidly and may permit a retrospective diagnosis of cortical necrosis (115). Angiographic studies may help to differentiate renal necrosis from venous thrombosis, but radiological studies using hypertonic contrast material should be avoided, as they may exacerbate the renal damage.

Prognosis

Bilateral cortical necrosis is often fatal (115). Recovery of renal function is unusual; when it does occur the lesion is usually patchy. Survival of kidney function may be due to a relative sparing of deep nephrons. Hypertension and chronic renal failure may ensue. The concentrating defect seen in medullary and papillary necrosis is sometimes permanent and may represent a risk of dehydration in surviving infants. The defect is attributed to a permanent loss of juxtamedullary nephrons and disruption of the medullary and papillary tissue.

RENAL VENOUS THROMBOSIS

Renal venous thrombosis (RVT) is a severe condition primarily affecting the neonate and frequently secondary to perinatal stress. Thrombosis of the renal venous tree is more common than primary renal vein thrombosis.

Incidence

RVT predominantly affects neonates, 75% of cases occurring during the first month of life (122). It is not always recognized during life, and it has been found in 2% to 3% of routine neonatal postmortem examinations. Newborn male infants are more often affected than girls (1.9:1), but the reason is unknown.

Etiology

RVT is often associated with an hyperosmolar state secondary to dehydration (diarrhea and shock), with the use of hypertonic contrast material, with perinatal asphyxia, with polycythemia due to congenital heart disease, with pyelonephritis, and septicemia. It occurs more frequently in infants of prediabetic or diabetic mothers, in infants presenting with congenital renal anomalies, a stressful delivery, and prenatal or postnatal distress.

Pathogenesis

The renal vessels appear vulnerable to thrombosis under circumstances of hemoconcentration, hyperviscosity, and hyperosmolality. Formation of local microthrombi generally begins in the peripheral renal veins, such as the interlobular veins and vasa recta, and then extends to the renal veins, suprarenal veins, and occasionally to the inferior vena cava. The thrombosis may be unilateral or bilateral.

Clinical Signs

Gross or microscopic hematuria, oligoanuria, and renal insufficiency are cardinal signs of severe renal venous thrombosis. Anemia is sometimes present. Signs and symptoms of the primary underlying disorders may be observed. Anorexia, diarrhea, vomiting, tachypnea, pallor, and shock may be present. Large palpable kidneys are found in most affected infants. Blood pressure is usually normal or low in the acute phase of RVT but may increase later. Laboratory findings reveal a pronounced anemia in a third of infants, with thrombocytopenia in 90%. Red cell fragmentation is seen on blood films. Low plasma levels of fibrinogen, factor V, and plasminogen are often found, along with elevated fibrin degradation products, reflecting active intravascular coagulation.

Differential Diagnosis

The differential diagnosis is that of large hematuric kidneys, i.e. cortical, medullary, and papillary necrosis, hydronephrosis, acute obstruction, and nephroblastoma. The presence of hematological features of disseminated coagulation and the history may help the diagnosis.

Ultrasonography is the method of choice for visualizing a nonfunctioning kidney. It detects a diffuse increase in echogenicity of the renal parenchyma with loss of the normal central pelvicalyceal echo pattern. IVU, when performed, is abnormal in most cases and is valuable in reinforcing the diagnosis of RVT, but it should not be performed in the acute phase of RVT, as it can irreversibly worsen the condition of the infant. Later, an IVU will show the extent of shrinkage of the damaged kidney. Selective venography precisely delineates vascular thrombosis but carries a high risk in these very sick patients. Isotope renography and standard renal clearances may be useful to document the function of the unaffected kidney or the recovery in the affected kidney.

Therapy

Conservative management of RVT is that of renal insufficiency and may require dialysis. The use of heparin has been recommended, but data from controlled studies are not available. Anticoagulant therapy should be considered when there is evidence of continuing intravascular coagulation, such as persisting thrombocytopenia, increased fibrin degradation products, a fall in fibrinogen and factor V plasma levels. Heparin may be given as an initial bolus injection of 100 IU/kg followed by 25 IU/kg/hr. Infusion rate is adjusted to bring the capillary bleeding time to between 240 and 300 sec, or the activated partial thromboplastin time to values 1.5 to 2 times normal. Heparin therapy is continued until the thrombocyte counts and coagulation factors become normal.

There is no indication for surgery during the acute phase of RVT, as the fibrosed thrombi may eventually partly recanalize. Hypertension, when present in a late stage, may respond to captopril. If the damaged kidney is not functional a few months after onset of RVT, nephrectomy should be considered to avoid refractory hypertension requiring the use of potent but toxic hypotensive agents.

Prognosis

The mortality rate for RVT is substantial but is considerably decreased by appropriate medical and surgical management (123, 124). Apart from hypertension, which may develop months after the onset of RVT, other complications include chronic renal failure, tubular dysfunction, and medullary or papillary necrosis.

Prevention

The use of hyperosmolar solutions must be avoided and states of dehydration rapidly corrected. Infants undergoing imaging studies must be adequately hydrated. The risk of developing RVT must be borne in mind when treating infants from diabetic mothers and those presenting with cyanotic congenital heart disease.

ARTERIAL HYPERTENSION

Arterial hypertension is a rare condition in the neonate, in whom it causes a high risk of cardiorespiratory failure, cerebral distress, and growth failure (99). Improvement in blood pressure monitoring in newborns helps in the early detection of hypertension. Adequate aggressive management of elevated blood pressure may improve the prognosis.

Measurement of Blood Pressure

The difficulty of measuring blood pressure accurately and noninvasively has been overcome recently with the Doppler technique (see Chapter 45). This method has now largely replaced older techniques such as the flush method, the auscultatory, or the palpatory sphygmomanometer method, all of which give blood pressure values slightly lower than those measured by the Doppler method (125, 126).

The Doppler ultrasound method detects blood flow and arteriolar wall oscillation by a transducer. The ultrasonic device is incorporated underneath a 4 to 5 cm cuff assembly. The Doppler technique accurately estimates systolic blood pressure but is less precise for diastolic blood pressure determination. Comparison with direct intra-arterial measurement (umbilical artery) in low-birth-weight infants shows an overestimation of blood pressure values of approximately 5 mm Hg by the Doppler technique (humoral artery) (127). A recently developed low-frequency sensing device needs further trials (128).

Factors Affecting Blood Pressure

Blood pressure is low at birth (129). It increases with age by about 1 to 2 mm Hg per day within the period of three to eight days and by about 1 mm Hg per week between ages 5 to 7 weeks (Table 56.11). There is a significant relationship between blood pressure at 5 days and blood pressure at 6 weeks. At 6 weeks, systolic blood pressure is close to 95 $\pm$ 10 mm Hg in awake infants. The level of blood pressure is influenced by the state of wakefulness. It is approximately 6 mm Hg lower in babies asleep than awake. There is significant correlation between birth weight or gestational age and systemic blood pressure during the first 12 hr of life (130, 131) (see Chapter 45).

Table 56.11.
Blood Pressure[a] in Relation to Postnatal Age and Level of Consciousness

State of animation	Days 3	Days 6	Days 8–10	Weeks 6
Awake	72 ± 6	77 ± 10	88 ± 17	96 ± 11
Asleep	68 ± 7	72 ± 9	75 ± 9	89 ± 11
P95[b] awake	95			113

[a] Arterial systolic blood pressure (X ± SD) measured by the Doppler technique.

[b] P95: percentile 95.

(Modified from de Swiet M, Fayers P, Shinebourne EA: Systolic blood pressure in a population of infants in the first year of life: the Brompton study. Pediatrics 65:1028, 1980.)

Causes of Arterial Hypertension

Neonatal hypertension is secondary to congenital malformations or to acquired diseases: (56).

1. Congenital Malformations
   - Renovascular:
     - Renal artery stenosis
     - Renal artery hypoplasia
     - Abdominal aortic atresia
   - Cystic renal diseases:
     - Infantile polycystic disease
     - Adult polycystic disease (?)
     - Multicystic dysplastic disease (?)
   - Reflux/obstructive nephropathies
   - Neuroblastoma
   - Coarctation of the aorta
2. Acquired Diseases
   - Renovascular:
     - Thrombo-embolic renal artery complications secondary to umbilical artery catheterization, thrombosis of ductus arteriosus
   - Closure of abdominal wall defects
   - Adrenal hemorrhage with renal artery compression
   - Adrenal carcinoma
   - Seizures in preterm infant
   - Central nervous system disorders
   - Drug-induced hypertension:
     - Phenylephrine eyedrops
     - Infants of drug-dependent mothers

Renal Artery Thrombosis

Thrombosis of the renal artery is most commonly observed after umbilical artery catheterization and has been reported to occur in 3% to 10% of cases (132, 133). This complication appears related to the duration of the indwelling catheter, is observed more frequently when the catheter tip is placed in high position at or above the L1 level, and is favored by the injection of hyperosmolar solutions. The catheter tip should be positioned at the aortic bifurcation and whenever possible removed within 72 hr. Idiopathic renal artery thrombosis has been associated with thrombosis of the ductus arteriosus. Complete obstruction of the renal artery by thrombi results in total infarction of the kidney without hypertension. Frequently, however, the kidney has viable areas supplied by collateral capsular vessel leading to renin release by these underperfused areas and consequent hypertension. Unilateral or bilateral renal enlargement may be observed. Urinalysis reveals hematuria and proteinuria. Plasma renin activity is usually elevated. The diagnosis is confirmed by angiographic and radionuclide evaluation. Medical treatment with captopril or β-blockers is indicated, and only those cases with unilateral renal involvement refractory to hypotensive agents benefit from nephrectomy (134).

Renal Artery Embolism

A thrombosed ductus arteriosus may cause renal artery embolism (135). Diagnosis is confirmed by angiographic studies and renal arteriography. Treatment is similar to that of renal artery thrombosis.

Renal Artery Stenosis

An intrinsic stenosis or an extrinsic compression of a renal artery can induce renin-dependent hypertension (136). Stenosis of the renal artery is sometimes associated with hypoplasia or total atresia of the abdominal aorta. High plasma renin levels are frequently observed. Renal scintigraphy and early urographic pictures will confirm the diagnosis. Medical management by captopril or nephrectomy in resistant cases can control the hypertension. Arterioplasty is not possible at this age.

Urological Malformation

Severe hydronephrosis secondary to bilateral reflux, posterior urethral valves, ureteropelvic obstruction, and ureterovesical stenosis is rarely associated with hypertension (137, 138). Activation of the renal pressor system may be responsible. Ureteropelvic junction obstruction causes hypertension in young dogs but not in adult dogs. Chronic pyelonephritic damage may already be present in early life and be the cause of the elevated blood pressure.

Closure of Abdominal Wall

Hypertension has been observed in newborns following closure of abdominal wall defects (139). The elevated blood pressure appears related to the size of the defect, the extent of hypoplasia of the abdominal wall, and the degree of traction required for closure of the defect. Possible mechanisms responsible for this hypertension include compression of the renal parenchyma or vasculature producing ischemia and renin release, compression or traction on the nerve supply, and increased catecholamine release. The condition is transient, and antihypertensive therapy is usually only required for three to six months.

Drug-induced Hypertension

Hypertension has been described after the intranasal use of 10% phenylephrine, a potent vasoconstrictor. It is absorbed across thin mucous membranes such as the eye or nose, thus entering the circulation directly and avoiding first-pass inactivation by the liver. Severe hypertension (180/100 mm Hg) has been observed after administering phenylephrine, 0.6 mg/kg in 20 min (140).

Elevated systolic blood pressure has been observed in neonates born from heroin- or methadone-addicted mothers (141). The increase in blood pressure was transient and lasted up to 21 days. An increase in plasma renin activity secondary to increased β-adrenergic activity has been described. Propanolol is the treatment of choice.

Coarctation of the Aorta

Tight coarctation of the aorta, proximal to the ductus arteriosus, may be responsible for severe hypertension in the newborn (142). When the stenosis is distal to the ductus, it is manifested by intractable congestive heart failure rather than by hypertension. Plasma renin is sometimes elevated. Surgical treatment can correct this hypertension, but the major concern of undertaking repair during infancy is the risk of recoarctation. The principal potential benefit of early intervention is reducing the incidence of persistent postoperative hypertension.

Adrenal Causes

Neonatal hypertension has been described after rupture of an adrenal hematoma in the perirenal space compressing the renal artery. The hematoma sometimes presents as a huge abdominal mass. Echotomography is useful in establishing the diagnosis.

An endogenous or exogenous excess of mineralocorticoids or glucocorticoids may be responsible for high blood pressure (143). A neuroblastoma with catecholamine excess may cause hypertension in the neonatal period.

Central Nervous System Disorders

Intracranial hypertension and other neurological disorders can elevate blood pressure. A moderate increase in blood pressure is also present during seizures (144).

Prematurity

Idiopathic hypertension has been detected in 5% of high-risk premature neonates during a three-month follow-up after discharge from an intensive care unit, suggesting that these infants may be at risk for the development of hypertension (145).

Clinical Manifestations

Hypertension may be asymptomatic, produce nonspecific symptoms such as failure to thrive, or cause significant cardiorespiratory and neurological disturbances. The following are symptoms associated with systemic hypertension:

1. Asymptomatic manifestations
2. Failure to thrive
3. Cardiorespiratory manifestations
   Tachypnea, cyanosis
   Congestive heart failure, cardiomegaly, hepatosplenomegaly
4. Neurological manifestations
   Lethargy, coma, tremors, floppiness, hypertonicity
   Apnea, opithotonos, seizures
   Intracranial hemorrhage, asymmetric reflexes, hemiparesis
5. Renal manifestations
   Volume depletion, dehydration, sodium-wasting
6. Peripheral manifestations
   Impaired vascular perfusion, decreased pulse, peripheral cyanosis, vasomotor instability
7. Fetal manifestations
   Pulmonary arterial hypertension (?)

These symptoms are usually secondary to well-known complications of systemic hypertension. Hypertensive retinopathy was observed in 11 of 21 hypertensive infants studied by indirect ophthalmoscopy. Inverse ratio of venous to arterial caliber, vascular tortuosity, superficial and deep hemorrhages, and exudates were found. These findings appeared to resolve after control of the hypertension (146). Other possible complications are less well established but have been documented in recent experimental studies. Fetal systemic hypertension could, for instance, lead to increased pulmonary vascular smooth muscle with consequent postnatal persistent pulmonary hypertension (147). In the premature newborn beagle, intraventricular hemorrhage may result from a moderate but rapidly induced elevation of systemic blood pressure (148). Sodium-wasting secondary to high-pressure diuresis has been described in a neonate with severe renovascular hypertension (149).

Renal enlargement suggests polycystic kidneys, multicystic dysplasia, obstructive uropathy, renal tumor, or adrenal hematoma compressing the renal artery. A faint systolic bruit is occasionally heard in the flank in cases of renal artery stenosis. Vasomotor instability manifested by peripheral cyanosis, cool extremities, and decreased pulses has been described.

Treatment

Treatment of hypertension in the neonate requires experience and should be instituted in a specialized neonatal unit. Whenever possible, treatment should be directed at the underlying cause. The aim of symptomatic treatment is to lower blood pressure to acceptable levels and not necessarily to normalize blood pressure. Mild hypertension may respond to diuretics, especially when salt retention is an aggravating factor. Intravenous furosemide or oral thiazides are used at dosages indicated in Table 56.12. More severe hypertension may require the use of β-blockers. High dosages are often required and appear to be well tolerated. The long-term effect of β-blockers on the development of endocrine and other systems is unknown. Other agents such as hydralazine and α-methyldopa can be used to control mild-to-severe hypertension. The use of calcium antagonists such as verapamil and nifedipine in infants is still under investigation, but may prove valuable for the treatment of chronic hypertension as well as acute hypertensive crises. The same applies to captopril, an oral inhibitor of the angiotensin I converting enzyme, which may be valuable in controlling severe renovascular hypertension (150). It should, however, be administered with caution to patients in whom the risk of a critically low level of renal perfusion can be increased by the drug.

Hypertensive crises must be treated vigorously, as they carry a significant risk of intracranial hemorrhage and heart failure. Captopril and nifedipine may be used orally. The effect of captopril is potentiated by volume depletion and may thus be optimalized by simultaneous intravenous injections of furosemide. Potent vasodilators such as diazoxide or sodium nitroprusside can be life-saving. Sodium nitroprusside needs to be constantly infused to titrate blood pressure but has the advantage of having a rapid onset and a short half-life.

Surgical Treatment. Unilateral nephrectomy should be reserved for those infants with unilateral involvement whose hypertension remains severe after an adequate trial of medical treatment.

Follow-up. Blood pressure must be measured at regular intervals after the onset of hypertension, and drug dosage must be adapted to the weight of the infant. Renal growth must be assessed by sonography, and functional development by renal clearance tests. Side effects of hypertensive agents must be carefully searched for.

Prognosis

The morbidity and mortality rates of neonatal hypertension are high. Death may be caused by severe uncontrollable hypertension or by

Table 56.12.
Antihypertensive Agents

	Route of administration	Dosage (mg/kg/day)
Hydrochlorothiazide	Oral	1–3
Furosemide	Oral, IV	1–10
Hydralazine	Oral, IV	0.2–4
α-methyldopa	Oral, IV	5–40
Diazoxide	IV	2–5
Propranolol	Oral, IV	0.5–2.0
Na-nitroprusside	IV	1–10
Captopril	Oral	0.1 0.5 (?)

(Modified from Adelman RD: Neonatal hypertension. Pediatr Clin North Am 25:99, 1978.)

concomitant problems related to the primary disease. In a significant number of infants, medication can be completely discontinued in the months or years following onset of treatment. Such was the case for 13 of 17 patients reported recently (99), the majority of them presumably suffering from renal artery thrombosis. Morbidity may also be related to drug-resistant hypertension or to drug side effects. Surgery in these severely ill infants also carries a high risk.

DRUGS AND THE NEONATAL KIDNEY

Pharmacokinetics

At birth, GFR approximates 17 ml/min × 1.73 m^2 SA in term neonates. It is lower in premature infants below 35 weeks' gestation, GFR bearing a linear relationship to gestational age during weeks 28 to 35 and then leveling off up to the time of birth (Fig. 56.5). GFR matures rapidly during the first month of life, its value doubling within the first two weeks of life (53). The velocity of maturation appears similar in term and preterm neonates (52, 151, 152). The slope of maturation of GFR during the first month of life is shown in Figure 56.6.

Because of the rapid changes in GFR and tubular functional maturation, dosages of drugs that are eliminated by glomerular filtration or secreted by the tubules must be adapted according to the level of renal function (153, 154). For drugs eliminated only by glomerular filtration, the theoretical approach is similar to that present when considering older children with renal failure.

Management of the very sick neonate often requires use of potent drugs that can impair renal function. Alternatively toxic drug levels may result if drug dosage is not adapted to the low level of GFR present in the neonate. Drugs commonly used in neonatal units and that may act on or interfere with renal function are described in the following section.

Drugs Given to Neonates

Furosemide

Furosemide is excreted by glomerular filtration and secreted by a weak organic acid tubular transport mechanism, both of which are immature in the neonate. Furosemide acts from within the tubular lumen. The overall effect of furosemide in the neonate is similar to that observed in mature kidneys; however, the onset of action is seen about one hour instead of 10 min in adults, and the duration is six hr instead of two hr (155). The relatively prolonged action of furosemide in neonates is due to their low GFR and limited renal tubular secretion. This also explains the less intense diuretic action of furosemide in the newborn infant and the need for relatively larger doses. A dose of 1 mg/kg administered to six low-birth-weight infants (1500 g) aged 10 to 57 days produced a net loss averaging 28 ml/kg of H_2O, 3.5 mmol/kg of sodium, and 0.3 mmol/kg of potassium with an increase in excretion of free water (156). The remarkable variability in the magnitude of response to furosemide in sick neonates, as well as its decreased efficacy in hypoxemic neonates, probably relates to the depression of GFR in these conditions.

Displacement of bilirubin from albumin has been described with chlorothiazide, ethacrynic acid, and furosemide administration (157). The increase is, however, probably not clinically significant when ethacrynic acid and furosemide are used at the recommended dosage.

Besides promoting natriuresis and diuresis, furosemide also promotes calcium excretion. Prolonged furosemide administration has been associated with renal calcifications in neonates given furosemide in a dose of at least 2 mg/kg/day for at least 12 days. Urinary tract infection increased the risk of calcification. Dissolution of the renal calcifications and a sharp decrease in urinary calcium excretion occurred when chlorothiazide was administered subsequently (158). Secondary hyperparathyroidism and bone disease have been described after long-term administration of furosemide to preterm infants (159).

Furosemide increases the incidence of patent ductus arteriosus in premature infants with the respiratory distress syndrome, probably through a prostaglandin-mediated process (160). Some claim, however, that furosemide prevents the renal side effects of indomethacin given to premature infants with patent ductus arteriosus without affecting the efficacy of indomethacin in the closure of the ductus (161).

Dopamine

The renal effect of dopamine in newborn infants is not well established. Dopamine, 0.5 to 2.0, μg/kg/min, significantly increases urine flow, creatinine clearance, and sodium excretion by the preterm infant. Once given to hypotensive preterm neonates with severe hyaline membrane disease, dopamine (2 to 8 μg/kg/min) increased systolic and diastolic blood pressure and improved diuresis. Heart rate increased only at doses of 8 μg/kg/min (162). The effect of low doses of dopamine could be mediated by a fall in prolactin levels. It has been claimed that dopamine blunts the renal tubular side effects of indomethacin, returning sodium excretion and urine flow to normal without affecting the renal vasoconstriction induced by indomethacin (163). The use of dopamine is not always associated with improved renal function, and the renal benefits of dopamine in high-risk neonates still await confirmation.

Tolazoline

Tolazoline is an α-adrenergic blocking agent sometimes used as a pulmonary vasodilator in persistent pulmonary hypertension in the neonate (164). This condition is characterized by right-to-left shunting through the foramen ovale and ductus arteriosus, leading to severe hypoxemia. A striking improvement in the plasma oxygen tension and in the clinical condition of sick neonates may follow the administration of tolazoline. Tolazoline also has histamine-like properties and a direct nonadrenergic relaxant effect on smooth muscles. In the anesthetized rabbit, it increases the systemic blood pressure and decreases urine flow, electrolyte excretion, GFR, and renal blood flow (165). The increase in blood pressure is best explained by an increase in cardiac output due to direct sympathicomimetic stimulation of the heart, by peripheral vasoconstriction, or by both. The increase in renal vascular resistance and the consequent decrease in renal perfusion seem to represent a partial α-agonist action of tolazoline. A recent report describes the occurrence of acute renal failure in two neonates treated with tolazoline (166). This effect is usually transient, but because of the associated oliguria, it adversely affects the management of the sick infants.

Indomethacin

Inhibition of prostaglandin synthesis has been recommended for the pharmacological closure of the ductus arteriosus in premature infants. This treatment has been associated with undesirable side effects, most notably transient renal dysfunction such as oliguria, increased serum creatinine and urea concentrations, and decreased sodium excretion. Studies in rabbits and newborn lambs have shown that the acute administration of prostaglandin synthetase inhibitors alters renal blood flow and intrarenal blood flow distribution (167). It also decreases water excretion by reducing the inhibitory action of prostaglandins on vasopressin. In babies with patent ductus arteriosus, administration of indomethacin (0.1 to 0.2 mg/kg repeated twice at 8 or 24 hr intervals) has been shown to induce a variable decrease in urine flow rate, GFR, free-water clearance, and electrolyte excretion rate, the arterial blood pressure remaining constant (168, 169). These effects are transient, and the altered functions return to pretreatment values within one or two weeks after stopping the drug (170–172).

Anticonvulsants

The intravenous administration of diazepam may provoke a transient decrease in renal blood flow, GFR, and urine flow in the infant (173). Acute urine retention has been described after phenobarbital administration to the newborn (174).

Aminoglycosides

Aminoglycosides are excreted mainly by glomerular filtration. Dosages must therefore be adapted to the low level of GFR present at birth and modified subsequently according to the increasing rate of filtration. Gentamicin half-life bears an inverse correlation to gestational age, so conceptional age rather than postnatal age must be considered when adjusting the dose (175). Because of the striking increase in GFR in the first month of life, dosage that may be toxic at birth can become inadequate a few weeks later.

The aminoglycosides are concentrated in the renal cortex. Their nephrotoxicity is well established in adults, in whom it is associated with depression of GFR and direct tubular damage. Gentamicin-associated nephrotoxicity is generally considered to be infrequent in neonates. This concept was inferred from the failure of plasma creatinine to increase after 7 to 10 days of therapy (176) More recent studies, using specific creatinine determination, have shown, however, that several infants receiving gentamicin substantially increase their plasma creatinine concentration during treatment (37, 177) or show elevated urinary tubular enzyme concentration (178). The premature kidney, the cortex of which is underperfused, could be relatively protected against gentamicin accumulation.

Contrast Agents

Major renal side effects such as renal artery thrombosis, medullary necrosis, ischemia, and renal insufficiency have been associated with the use of hypertonic radiographic contrast material in infants (97, 98). The usual dose of these contrast agents, the osmolality of which ranges from 1300 to 1950 mosm/kg H_2O, can abruptly raise the infant's plasma osmolality by 20 to 110 mosm/kg H_2O and produce intraventricular hemorrhage in premature infants. Radiographic studies should thus be performed with prudence during the neonatal period and only after adequate hydration of the infant. The use of nonionic contrast agents with osmolalities around 450 mosm/kg H_2O markedly reduces the risk of toxicity in neonates.

Maternal Drugs

Captopril

Persistent fetal anuria has been observed in a neonate whose mother had been given captopril at the 26th week of gestation (179). Drug administration had been rapidly followed by the disappearance of amniotic fluid. Systemic hypotension and peripheral vasodilatation were present at birth. The deleterious effect of captopril, which rapidly crosses the placental barrier, is confirmed by animal studies that show a markedly elevated perinatal mortality in newborn rabbits and lambs whose mothers had been treated with captopril (180, 181). The pathogenesis of the anuria could include interference with the renin-angiotensin system, the prostaglandins, or bradykinin.

Ritodrine

Ritodrine hydrochloride, a β-adrenergic agonist, is used commonly to inhibit premature onset of labor. Ritodrine crosses the placenta readily, leading to umbilical cord blood concentrations from 30% to 100% of maternal venous values. Administration of 60 to 260 (mean 230) mg of ritodrine in the 12 to 23 hr before delivery has been reported to decrease inulin clearance and increase plasma renin activity and urine-arginine vasopressin excretion on the first day of life of 15 low-birth-weight infants (182). The effect was not present on the sixth day of life. No other signs of renal dysfunction, such as oliguria or disturbances in water and electrolyte homeostasis, were observed, however. The clinical significance of these findings thus remains to be defined.

References

1. Roodhooft AM, Birnholz JC, Holmes LB: Familial nature of congenital absence and severe dysgenesis of both kidneys. N Engl J Med 310:1341, 1984.
2. Addor N-C, Pescia G, Guignard JP, Genton N: Etude familiale du reflux vésico-urétéral. J Génét Hum 32:91, 1984.
3. International Reflux Study Committee: Medical versus surgical treatment of vesicoureteral reflux. Pediatrics 67:392, 1981.
4. De Vargas A, Evans K, Ransley P, et al: A family study of vesicoureteric reflux. J Med Genet 15:85, 1978.
5. Lewy PR, Belman AB: Familial occurrence of nonobstructive, noninfectious vesicoureteral reflux with renal scarring. J Pediatr 86:851, 1975.
6. Thomas IT, Smith DW: Oligohydramnios, cause of the nonrenal features of Potter's syndrome, including pulmonary hypoplasia. J Pediatr 84:811, 1974.
7. Aula P, Rapola J, Karjalainen O, et al: Prenatal diagnosis of congenital nephrosis in 23 high-risk families. Am J Dis Child 132:984, 1978.
8. Bjoro K, Jr: Vascular anomalies of the umbilical cord. II. Perinatal and pediatric implications. Early Hum Dev 8:279, 1983.
9. Gruenewald SM, Crocker EF, Walker AG, Trudinger BJ: Antenatal diagnosis of urinary tract abnormalities: correlation of ultrasound appearance with postnatal diagnosis. Am J Obstet Gynecol 148:278, 1984.
10. Sherry SN, Kramer I: The time of passage of the first stool and first urine by the newborn infant. J Pediatr 46:158, 1955.
11. Moore ES, Galvez MB: Delayed micturition in the newborn period, J Pediatr 80:867, 1972.
12. Douglas Jones M, Gresham EL, Battaglia FC: Urinary flow rates and urea excretion rates in newborn infants. Biol Neonate 21:321, 1972.
13. Goellner MH, Ziegler EE, Fomon SJ: Urination during the first three years of life. Nephron 28:174, 1981.
14. Roy RN, Sinclair JC: Hydration of the low birth-weight infant. Clin Perinatol 2:393, 1975.
15. Jain R: Acute renal failure in the neonate. Pediatr Clin North Am 24:605, 1977.
16. Brem AS: Neonatal hematuria and proteinuria. Clin Perinatol 8:321, 1981.
17. Museles M, Gaudry CL, Bason WM: Renal anomalies in the newborn found by deep palpation. Pediatrics 47:97, 1971.
18. Henderson, KC, Torch EM: Differential diagnosis of abdominal masses in the neonate. Pediatr Clin North Am 24:557, 1977.
19. Kirks DR, Merten DF, Grossman H, Bowie JD: Diagnostic imaging of pediatric abdominal masses: an overview. Radiol Clin North Am 19:527, 1981.
20. Evans BB: Obstructive uropathy in the neonate. Clin Perinatol 8:273, 1981.
21. Chevalier RL, Campbell F, Brenbridge ANA: Nephrosonography and renal scintigraphy in evaluation of newborn with renomegaly. Urology 24:96, 1984.
22. Stapleton FB, Hilton S, Wilcox J, Leopold GR: Transient nephromegaly simulating infantile polycystic disease of the kidneys. Pediatrics 67:554, 1981.
23. Moerman P, Fryns J-P, Goddeeris P, Lauweryns JM: Pathogenesis of the prune-belly syndrome: a functional urethral obstruction caused by prostatic hypoplasia. Pediatrics 73:470, 1984.
24. Giacoia GP: Hydrops fetalis (fetal edema). Clin Pediatr 19:334, 1980.
25. Beckwitt Turkel S: Conditions associated with nonimmune hydrops fetalis. Clin Perinatol 9:613, 1982.
26. Lord JM: Foetal ascites. Arch Dis Child 28:398, 1953.
27. McDonald J, Murphy AV: Neonatal ascites from spontaneous rupture of the bladder. Arch Dis Child 50:956, 1975.
28. Colodny AH, Griscom NT: Clue to diagnosis of neonatal urinary ascites. Relative radiolucency of liver shadow. Urology 11:295, 1978.
29. Arant BS: Developmental patterns of renal functional maturation compared in the human neonate. J Pediatr 92:705, 1978.
30. Karlsson FA, Hardell L-I, Hellsing K: Prospective study of urinary proteins in early infancy. Acta Paediatr Scand 68:663, 1979.
31. Stonestreet BS, Rubin L, Pollak A, et al: Renal functions of low birth weight infants with hyperglycemia and glucosuria produced by glucose infusions. Pediatrics 66:561, 1980.
32. Torrado A, Guignard J-P, Prod'hom LS, Gautier E: Hypoxaemia and renal function in newborns with respiratory distress syndrome (RDS). Helv Paediat Acta 29:399, 1974.

33. Edelman CM, Barnett HL, Troupkou V: Renal concentrating mechanisms in newborn infants. Effect of dietary protein and water content, role of urea, and responsiveness to anti-diuretic hormone. J Clin Invest 39:1062, 1960.
34. Svenningsen NW, Aronson AS: Postnatal development of renal concentration capacity as estimated by DDAVP-test in normal and asphyxiated neonates. Biol Neonate 25:230, 1974.
35. Manzke H, Spreter von Kreudenstein P, Dörner K, Kruse K: Quantitative measurements of the urinary excretion of creatinine, uric acid, hypoxanthine and xanthine, uracil, cyclic AMP, and cyclic GMP in healthy newborn infants. Eur J Pediatr 133:157, 1980.
36. Sertel H, Scopes J. Rates of creatinine clearance in babies less than one week of age. Arch Dis Child 48:717, 1973.
37. Feldman H, Guignard J-P: Plasma creatinine in the first month of life. Arch Dis Child 57:123, 1982.
38. Aperia A, Broberger O, Herin P, Zetterström R: Sodium excretion in relation to sodium intake and aldosterone excretion in newborn pre-term and full-term infants. Acta Paediatr Scand 68:813, 1979.
39. Sulyok E, Németh M, Tényi I, et al: Postnatal development of renin-angiotensin aldosterone system, RAAS, in relation to electrolyte balance in premature infants. Pediatr Res 13:817, 1979.
40. Engelke SC, Shah, BL, Vasan U, Raye JR: Sodium balance in very low-birth-weight infants. J Pediatr 93:837, 1978.
41. Ross B, Cowett RM, Oh W: Renal functions of low birth weight infants during the first two months of life. Pediatr Res 11:1162, 1977.
42. Rodriguez-Soriano J, Vallo A, Castillo G, Oliveros R: Renal handling of water and sodium in infancy and childhood: a study using clearance methods during hypotonic saline diuresis. Kidney Int 20:700, 1981.
43. Roy RN, Chance GW, Radde IC, et al: Late hyponatremia in very low birthweight infants (<1.3 kilograms). Pediatr Res 10:526, 1976.
44. Rodriguez-Soriano J, Vallo A, Oliveros R, Castillo G: Transient pseudohypoaldosteronism secondary to obstructive uropathy in infancy. J Pediatr 103:375, 1983.
45. Heijden AJ, Versteegh FGA, Wolff ED, et al: Acute tubular dysfunction in infants with obstructive uropathy. Acta Paediatr Scand 74:589, 1985.
46. Salle BL, Glorieux FH, Delvin EE, et al: Vitamin D metabolism in preterm infants. Acta Paediatr Scand 72:203, 1983.
47. Brown DR, Steranka BH: Renal cation excretion in the hypocalcemic premature human neonate. Pediatr Res 15:1100, 1981.
48. Schwartz GJ, Haycock GB, Edelmann CM, Spitzer A: Late metabolic acidosis: a reassessment of the definition. J Pediatr 95:102, 1979.
49. Ravio KO: Neonatal hyperuricemia. J Pediatr 88:625, 1976.
50. Stapleton FB: Renal uric acid clearance in human neonates. J Pediatr 103:290, 1983.
51. Ahmadian Y, Lewy PR: Possible urate nephropathy of the newborn infant as a cause of transient renal insufficiency. J Pediatr 91:96, 1977.
52. Manzke H, Eigster G, Harms D, et al: Uric acid infarctions in the kidneys of newborn infants. Eur J Pediatr 126:29, 1977.
53. Guignard J-P, Torrado A, Da Cunha O, Gautier E: Glomerular filtration rate in the first three weeks of life. J Pediatr 87:268, 1975.
54. Coulthard MG, Ruddock V: Validation of inulin as a marker for glomerular filtration in preterm babies. Kidney Int 23:407, 1983.
55. Stonestreet BS, Bell EF, Oh W: Validity of endogenous creatinine clearance in low birthweight infants. Pediatr Res 13:1012, 1979.
56. Fawer CL, Torrado A, Guignard JP: Single injection clearance in the neonate. Biol Neonate 35:321, 1979.
57. Coulthard MG: Comparison of methods of measuring renal function in preterm babies using inulin. J Pediatr 102:923, 1983.
58. Martin DJ, Gilday DL, Reilly BJ: Evaluation of the urinary tract in the neonatal period. Radiol Clin North Am 13:359, 1975.
59. Svenningsen NW: Single injection polyfructosan clearance in normal and asphyxiated neonates. Acta Paediatr Scand 64:87, 1975.
60. Svenningsen NW: Renal acid-base titration studies in infants with and without metabolic acidosis in the postneonatal period. Pediatr Res 8:659, 1974.
61. Guignard J-P, Torrado A, Mazouni SM, Gautier E: Renal function in respiratory distress syndrome. J Pediatr 88:845, 1976.
62. Dauber IM, Krauss AN, Symchych PS, Auld PAM: Renal failure following perinatal anoxia. J Pediatr 88:851, 1976.
63. Yao AC, Lind J: Blood volume in the asphyxiated term neonate. Biol Neonate 21:199, 1972.
64. Cort RL: Renal function in respiratory distress syndrome. Acta Paediatr Scand 51:313, 1961.
65. Siegel SR, Fisher DA, Oh W: Renal function and serum aldosterone levels in infants with respiratory distress syndrome. J Pediatr 83:854, 1973.
66. Broberger U, Aperia A: Renal function in idiopathic respiratory distress syndrome. Acta Paediatr Scand 67:313, 1978.
67. Miltényi M, Pohlandt F, Bóka G, Kun E: Tubular proteinuria after perinatal hypoxia. Acta Paediatr Scand 70:399, 1981.
68. Aperia A, Broberger U: Beta-2-microglobulin, an indicator of renal tubular maturation and dysfunction in the newborn. Acta Paediatr Scand 68:669, 1979.
69. Allen AC, Usher R: Renal acid excretion in infants with the respiratory distress syndrome. Pediatr Res 5:345, 1971.
70. Robillard JE, Weitzman RE, Burmeister L, Smith FG, Jr: Developmental aspects of the renal response to hypoxemia in the lamb fetus. Circ Res 48:128, 1981.
71. Lewis AB, Evans WN, Sischo W: Plasma catecholamine responses to hypoxemia in fetal lambs. Biol Neonate 41:115, 1982.
72. Moore ES, Galvez MB, Paton JB, et al: Effects of positive pressure ventilation on intrarenal blood flow in infant primates. Pediatr Res 8:792, 1974.
73. Marquez JM, Douglas ME, Downs JB, et al: Renal function and cardiovascular responses during positive airway pressure. Anesthesiology 50:393, 1979.
74. Fewell JE, Norton JB Jr: Continuous positive airway pressure impairs renal function in newborn goats. Pediatr Res 14:1132, 1980.
75. Fewell JE, Bond GC: Renal denervation eliminates the renal response to continuous positive-pressure ventilation. Proc Soc Exp Biol Med 161:574, 1979.
76. Tulassay T, Machay T, Kiszel J, Varga J: Effects of continuous positive airway pressure on renal function in prematures. Biol Neonate 43:152, 1983.
77. Goldberg RN, Chung D, Goldman SL, Bancalari E: The association of rapid volume expansion and intraventricular hemorrhage in the preterm infant. J Pediatr 96:1060, 1980.
78. Langman CB, Engle WD, Baumgart S, et al: The diuretic phase of respiratory distress syndrome and its relationship to oxygenation. J Pediatr 98:462, 1981.
79. Marks KH, Berman W, Friedman Z, et al: Furosemide in hyaline membrane disease. Pediatrics 62:785, 1978.
80. Bell EF, Warburton D, Stonestreet BS, Oh W: Effect of fluid administration on the development of symptomatic patent ductus arteriosus and congestive heart failure in premature infants. N Engl J Med 302:598, 1980.
81. Najak ZD, Harris EM, Lazzara A, Pruitt AW: Pulmonary effects of furosemide in preterm infants with lung disease. J Pediatr 102:758, 1983.
82. Rahman N, Boineau FG, Lewy JE: Acute renal failure in the perinatal period. Clin Perinatol 8:241, 1981.
83. Reimold EW, Don TD, Worthen HG: Renal failure during the first year of life. Pediatrics 59:987, 1977.
84. Anand SK, Northway JD, Crussi FG: Acute renal failure in newborn infants. J Pediatr 92:985, 1978.
85. Anand SK: Acute renal failure in the neonate. Pediatr Clin North Am 29:791, 1982.
86. Aschinberg LC, Zeis PM, Hageman JR, Vidyasagar D: Acute renal failure in the newborn. Crit Care Med 5:36, 1977.
87. Norman ME, Asadi FK: A prospective study of acute renal failure in the newborn infant. Pediatrics 63:475, 1979.
88. Grylack L, Medani C, Hultzen C, et al: Nonoliguric acute renal failure in the newborn. Am J Dis Child 136:518, 1982.
89. Chesney RW, Kaplan BS, Freedom RM, et al: Acute renal failure: an important complication of cardiac surgery in infants. J Pediatr 87:381, 1975.
90. Haftel AJ, Eichner J, Haling J, Wilson ML: Myoglobinuric renal failure in a newborn infant. J Pediatr 93:1015, 1978.
91. Herson VC, Raye JR, Rowe JC, Philipps AF: Acute renal failure associated with polycythemia in a neonate. J Pediatr 100:137, 1982.
92. Broberger U, Aperia A: Renal function in infants with hyperbilirubinemia. Acta Pediatr Scand 68:75, 1979.
93. Engle WD, Arant BS, Jr: Neonatal hyperbilirubinemia and renal function. J Pediatr 100:113, 1982.
94. Baum M, Stirling GA, Dawson J: Further study into obstructive jaundice and ischaemic renal damage. Br Med J 2:229, 1969.
95. Mathew OP, Jones AS, James E, et al: Neonatal renal failure: usefulness of diagnostic indices. Pediatrics 65:57, 1980.
96. Torrado A: Acute renal failure in neonates. In Brodehl J, Ehrich E (eds): Paediatric Nephrology. Heidelberg, Springer Verlag, 1984, p 65.
97. Gilbert EF, Khoury GH, Hogan GR, Jones B: Hemorrhagic renal necrosis in infancy: relationship to radiopaque compounds. J Pediatr 76:49, 1970.
98. Gruskin AB, Oetliker OH, Wolfish NM, et al: Effects of angiography on renal function and histology in infants and piglets. J Pediatr 76:41, 1970.
99. Adelman RD: Neonatal hypertension. Pediatr Clin North Am 25:99, 1978.
100. Abitbol CL, Holliday MA: Total parenteral nutrition in anuric children. Clin Nephrol 5:153, 1976.
101. Takala J, Kekomäki M: Parenteral nutrition in anuria of infancy: evidence for sustained net protein synthesis. JPEN 7:45, 1983.
102. Kjellstrand CM, Mauer SM, Buselmeier TJ, et al: Haemodialysis of premature and newborn babies. Proc. EDTA 10:349, 1973.
103. Mauer SM, Lynch RE: Hemodialysis techniques for infants and children. Pediatr Clin North Am 23:843, 1976.

104. Zamora J, Martínez F, Mendizábal S, Simón J: Diálisis peritoneal en el recién nacido. An Esp Pediat 13:477, 1980.
105. Edelmann CM, Ogwo JE, Fine BP, Martinez AB: The prevalence of bacteriuria in full-term and premature newborn infants. J Pediatr 82:125, 1973.
106. Maherzi M, Guignard J-P, Torrado A: Urinary tract infection in high-risk newborn infants. Pediatrics 62:521, 1978.
107. Bergström T, Larson H, Lincoln K, Winberg J: Studies of urinary tract infections in infancy and childhood. J Pediatr 80:858, 1972.
108. Abbott GD: Neonatal bacteriuria—the value of bladder puncture in resolving problems of interpretation arising from voided urine specimens. Aust Paediatr J 14:83, 1978.
109. Guignard J-P: Urinary infection after micturating cystography. Lancet 1:103, 1979.
110. Bensman A, Baudon JJ, Jablonski JP, Lasfargues G: Uropathies diagnosed in the neonatal period: symptomatology and course. Acta Paediatr Scand 69:499, 1980.
111. Drew JH, Acton CM: Radiological findings in newborn infants with urinary infection. Arch Dis Child 51:628, 1976.
112. Ransley PG, Ridson RA: Reflux and renal scarring. Br J Radiol 14:1, 1978.
113. Rolleston GL, Maling TMJ, Hodson CJ: Intrarenal reflux and the scarred kidney. Arch Dis Child 49:531, 1974.
114. Hodson J: Reflux nephropathy. Med Clin North Am 62:1201, 1978.
115. Leonidas JC, Berdon WE, Gribetz D: Bilateral renal cortical necrosis in the newborn infant: roentgenographic diagnosis. J Pediatr 79:623, 1971.
116. Chrispin AR: Medullary necrosis in infancy. Br Med Bull 28:233, 1972.
117. Davies DJ, Kennedy A, Roberts C: Renal medullary necrosis in infancy and childhood. J Pathol 99:125, 1969.
118. Chrispin AR, Hull D, Lillie JG, Ridson RA: Renal tubular necrosis and papillary necrosis after gastroenteritis in infants. Br Med J 1:401, 1970.
119. Husband P, Howlett KA: Renal papillary necrosis in infancy. Arch Dis Child 48:116, 1973.
120. Banister A, Hatcher GW: Renal tubular and papillary necrosis after dehydration in infancy. Arch Dis Child 48:36, 1973.
121. Anand SK, Northway JD, Smith JA: Neonatal renal papillary and cortical necrosis. Am J Dis Child 131:773, 1977.
122. Belman AB: Renal vein thrombosis in infancy and childhood. Clin Pediatr 15:1033, 1976.
123. Rasoulpour M, McLean RH: Renal venous thrombosis in neonates. Initial and follow-up abnormalities. Am J Dis Child 134:276, 1980.
124. Jobin J, O'Regan S, Demay G, et al: Neonatal renal vein thrombosis—a long-term follow-up after conservative management. Clin Nephrol 17:36, 1982.
125. Elseed AM, Shinebourne EA, Joseph MC: Assessment of techniques for measurement of blood pressure in infants and children. Arch Dis Child 48:932, 1973.
126. Virnig NL, Reynolds JW: Reliability of flush blood pressure measurements in the sick newborn infant. J Pediatr 84:594, 1974.
127. Dweck HS, Reynolds DW, Cassady G: Indirect blood pressure measurement in newborns. Am J Dis Child 127:492, 1974.
128. Reder RF, Dimich I, Cohen ML, Steinfeld L: Evaluating indirect blood pressure measurement techniques: a comparison of three systems in infants and children. Pediatrics 62:326, 1978.
129. de Swiet M, Fayers P, Shinebourne EA: Systolic blood pressure in a population of infants in the first year of life: the Brompton study. Pediatrics 65:1028, 1980.
130. Versmold HT, Kitterman JA, Phibbs RH, et al: Aortic blood pressure during the first 12 hours of life in infants with birth weight 610 to 4,220 grams. Pediatrics 67:607, 1981.
131. Hervé F, Murat I, de Gamarra E, et al: Pression artérielle chez le nouveau-né pendant les 72 premières heures de vie. Arch Fr Ped 39:777, 1982.
132. Neal WA, Reynolds JW, Jarvis CW, Williams HJ: Umbilical artery catheterization: demonstration of arterial thrombosis by aortography. Pediatrics 50:6, 1972.
133. Plumer LB, Kaplan GW, Mendoza SA: Hypertension in infants—a complication of umbilical arterial catheterization. J Pediatr 89:802, 1976.
134. Adelman RD, Merten D, Vogel J, et al: Nonsurgical management of renovascular hypertension in the neonate. Pediatrics 62:71, 1978.
135. Durante D, Jones D, Spitzer R: Neonatal renal arterial embolism syndrome. Pediatrics 89:978, 1976.
136. Ljungqvist A, Wallgren G: Unilateral renal artery stenosis and fatal arterial hypertension in a newborn infant. Acta Paediatr 51:575, 1962.
137. Carella JA, Silber I: Hyperreninemic hypertension in an infant secondary to pelviureteric obstruction treated successfully by surgery. J Pediatr 88:987, 1976.
138. Munoz AI, Baralt JFP, Melendez MT: Arterial hypertension in infants with hydronephrosis. Am J Dis Child 131:38, 1977.
139. Adelman RD, Sherman MP: Hypertension in the neonate following closure of abdominal wall defects. J Pediatr 97:642, 1980.
140. Saken R, Kates GL, Miller K: Drug-induced hypertension in infancy. J Pediatr 95:1077, 1979.
141. Dube SK, Jhaveri RC, Rosenfeld W, et al: Urinary catecholamines, plasma renin activity and blood pressure in newborns: effects of narcotic withdrawal. Dev Pharmacol Ther 3:83, 1981.
142. Goldring D: Treatment of the infant and child with coarctation of the aorta. Pediatr Clin North Am 25:111, 1978.
143. Robson AM: Special diagnostic studies for the detection of renal and renovascular forms of hypertension. Pediatr Clin North Am 25:83, 1978.
144. Perlman JM, Volpe JJ: Seizures in the preterm infant: effects on cerebral blood flow velocity, intracranial pressure, and arterial blood pressure. J Pediatr 102:288, 1983.
145. Sheftel DN, Hustead V, Friedman A: Hypertension screening in the follow-up of premature infants. Pediatrics 71:763, 1983.
146. Skalina ME, Annable WL, Kliegman RM, Fanaroff AA: Hypertensive retinopathy in the newborn infant. J Pediatr 103:781, 1983.
147. Levin DL, Hyman AI, Heymann MA, Rudolph AM: Fetal hypertension and the development of increased pulmonary vascular smooth muscle: a possible mechanism for persistent pulmonary hypertension of the newborn infant. J Pediatr 92:265, 1978.
148. Goddard J, Lewis RM, Armstrong DL, Zeller RS: Moderate, rapidly induced hypertension as a cause of intraventricular hemorrhage in the newborn beagle model. J Pediatr 96:1057, 1980.
149. Rosendahl W, Ranke M, Mentzel H: Sodium loss as leading sympton of renovascular hypertension in the newborn. Klin Wochenschr 58:953, 1980.
150. Bifano E, Post EM, Springer J, et al: Treatment of neonatal hypertension with captopril. J Pediatr 100:143, 1982.
151. Fawer C-L, Torrado A, Guignard J-P: Maturation of renal function in full-term and premature neonates. Helv Paediat Acta 34:11, 1979.
152. Guignard J-P: Renal function in the newborn infant. Pediatr Clin North Am 29:777, 1982.
153. Guignard J-P: Clinical implications of a low GFR. In Brodehl J, Ehrich J (eds): Pediatric Nephrology. Heidelberg, Springer Verlag, 1984, p 60.
154. Bräunlich H: Excretion of drugs during postnatal development. Pharmacol Ther 12:299, 1981.
155. Woo WR, Dupont C, Collinge J, Aranda JV: Effects of furosemide in the newborn. Clin Pharmacol Ther 23:266, 1978.
156. Ross BS, Pollak A, Oh W: The pharmacologic effects of furosemide therapy in the low-birth-weight infant. J Pediatr 92:149, 1978.
157. Wennberg RP, Rasmussen LF, Ahlfors CE: Displacement of bilirubin from human albumin by three diuretics. J Pediatr 90:647, 1977.
158. Hufnagle KG, Khan SN, Penn D, et al: Renal calcifications: a complication of long-term furosemide therapy in preterm infants. Pediatrics 70:360, 1982.
159. Venkataraman PS, Han BK, Tsang RC, Daugherty CC: Secondary hyperparathyroidism and bone disease in infants receiving long-term furosemide therapy. Am J Dis Child 137:1157, 1983.
160. Green TP, Thompson TR, Johnson DE, Lock JE: Furosemide promotes patent ductus arteriosus in premature infants with the respiratory-distress syndrome. N Engl J Med 308:743, 1983.
161. Yeh TF, Wilks A, Singh J, et al: Furosemide prevents the renal sides effects of indomethacin therapy in premature infants with patent ductus arteriosus. J Pediatr 101:433, 1982.
162. Seri I, Tulassay T, Kiszel J, et al: Cardiovascular response to dopamine in hypotensive preterm neonates with severe hyaline membrane disease. Eur J Pediatr 142:3, 1984.
163. Seri I, Tulassay T, Kiszel J, Csömör S: The use of dopamine for the prevention of the renal side effects of indomethacin in premature infants with patent ductus arteriosus. Int J Ped Nephrol 5:209, 1984.
164. Goetzman BW, Sunshine P, Johnson JD, et al: Neonatal hypoxia and pulmonary vasospasm: response to tolazoline. J Pediatr 89:617, 1976.
165. Naujoks S, Guignard J-P: Renal effects of tolazoline in rabbits. Lancet 2:1075, 1979.
166. Trompeter RS, Chantler C, Haycock GB: Tolazoline and acute renal failure in the newborn. Lancet 1:1219, 1981.
167. Dunn MJ, Zambraski EJ: Renal effects of drugs that inhibit prostaglandin synthesis. Kidney Int 18:609, 1980.
168. Catterton Z, Sellers B, Gray B: Inulin clearance in the premature infant receiving indomethacin. J Pediatr 96:737, 1980.
169. Cifuentes RF, Olley PM, Balfe JW, et al: Indomethacin and renal function in premature infants with persistent patent ductus arteriosus. J Pediatr 95:583, 1979.
170. Betkerur MV, Yeh, TF, Miller K, et al: Indomethacin and its effect on renal function and urinary kallikrein excretion in premature infants with patent ductus arteriosus. Pediatrics 68:99, 1981.
171. Seyberth HW, Rascher W, Hackenthal R, Wille L: Effect of prolonged indomethacin therapy on renal function and selected vasoactive hormones in very-low-birth-weight infants with symptomatic patent ductus arteriosus. J Pediatr 103:979, 1983.
172. John EG, Vasan U, Hastreiter AR, et al: Intravenous indomethacin and changes of renal function in premature infants with patent ductus arteriosus. Pediatr Pharmacol 4:11, 1984.

173. Guignard JP, Filloux B, Lavoie J, et al: Effect of intravenous diazepam on renal function. Clin Pharmacol Ther 18:401, 1975.
174. Levene MI: Retention of urine in the neonate possibly due to anticonvulsant drugs. Arch Dis Child 52:975, 1977.
175. Assael BM: Pharmacokinetics and drug distribution during postnatal development. Pharmacol Ther 18:159, 1982.
176. McCracken GH, Jones LG: Gentamicin in the neonatal period. Am J Dis Child 120:524, 1970.
177. Elinder G, Aperia A: Development of glomerular filtration rate and excretion of β_2-microglobulin in neonates during gentamicin treatment. Acta Paediatr Scand 72:219, 1983.
178. Adelman RD, Zakauddin S: Urinary enzyme activities in children and neonates receiving gentamicin therapy. Dev Pharmacol Ther 1:325, 1980.
179. Guignard J-P: Drugs and the neonatal kidney. Dev Pharmacol Ther 4:19, 1982.
180. Ferris TF, Weir EK: Effect of captopril on uterine blood flow and prostaglandin E synthesis in the pregnant rabbit. J Clin Invest 71:809, 1983.
181. Broughton Pipkin F, Symonds EM, Turner SR: The effect of captopril (SQ 14,225) upon mother and fetus in the chronically cannulated ewe and in the pregnant rabbit. J Physiol 323:415, 1982.
182. Hansen NB, Oh W, LaRochelle F, Stonestreet BS: Effects of maternal ritodrine administration on neonatal renal function. J Pediatr 103:774, 1983.

CHAPTER 57

Neonatal Urology

JOHN R. WOODARD
THOMAS S. PARROTT

UROLOGICAL ABNORMALITIES DIAGNOSED IN UTERO

Obstetrical Ultrasound and Antenatal Diagnosis

Ultrasonography during pregnancy reveals many fetal abnormalities that previously were diagnosed only after delivery. Because fluid-filled masses are easy to detect on sonography, obstructive uropathy and renal cystic disease are often found serendipitously in the fetus. Ultrasound during pregnancy has become routine in some centers (1), and its use is increasing in others. For this reason, the presentation of neonates with obstructive uropathy has changed, and many lesions are now known to exist at birth in spite of the absence of such classic signs of obstruction as an abdominal mass, hematuria, voiding dysfunction, or urinary tract infection (2–4). Pregnancies complicated by a fetal abnormality can be monitored closely, and delivery carried out at a center where expert neonatal, nephrological and urological care is available.

It is estimated that one fourth to one half of all pregnant women in the United States are examined at least once by ultrasound (5, 6). Despite its relatively widespread use, little is known of its potential long-term harmful effects on the fetus. The procedure should be used only when clinically indicated: there are no obvious short-term effects of ultrasound on the fetus, but there is a possibility of delayed or subtle consequences. Biological effects have been observed in animal and in vitro studies which, for the most part, cannot yet be extrapolated to the human (6). So far, there are no anecdotal reports of harmful effects in children exposed to ultrasound in utero.

Indications

Initially the indications for fetal ultrasonography were confined to concerns about the stage of pregnancy, fetal age or demise, multiple gestation, placental location, maternal medical problems, or obstetrical history indicating risk. The following is a generally accepted scheme of the current indications for fetal ultrasound (7).

Routine indications:
- Placental localization
- Gestational age
- Fetal position
- Multiple gestation

Indications of potential pathological conditions:
- Rh sensitization
- Amniocentesis
- Fetal death
- Maternal diabetes
- Previous congenital anomalies
- Exposure to teratogens
- Discrepancy in uterine size and dates
  - Oligohydramnios
  - Polyhydramnios
  - Intrauterine growth retardation

Incidence of Fetal Abnormalities

Fetal ultrasound in a large group of such "at risk" pregnancies revealed 16 cases of unsuspected fetal abnormalities, of which 5 were urological, an incidence of 0.2% (8). In another large study, 1.7% of "at risk" pregnant women bore an offspring with a urinary tract anomaly (9). Similarly, at an institution where over half of the deliveries were examined prenatally by ultrasound, the incidence of antenatally detected urological abnormalities was 0.1% (10).

Urological Abnormalities Detected

In the English litertaure from 1970 to 1981, there were 54 reported cases of obstructive uropathy or renal cystic disease detected antenatally (11). The reported abnormalities were cystic disease (autosomal dominant, recessive, and multicystic), ureteropelvic junction obstruction (UPJO), ureterovesical junction obstruction (UVJO), renal agenesis, primary megaureter, and urethral obstruction. Subsequently, cases of vesicoureteral reflux (VUR), paranephric cyst secondary to calyceal rupture, hydrocolpos with hydronephrosis, infundibular stenosis, cystic neuroblastoma, and adrenal cyst were also reported (1–3, 12).

Timing of Fetal Ultrasound

The urological abnormalities previously described may be detected as early as 12 to 15 weeks' gestation (13). Normal fetal kidneys, on the other hand, are difficult to identify early in pregnancy. In a large study involving 100 consecutive women between 11 and 40 weeks' gestation, the kidney was never positively identified in the first trimester. Between 15 and 26 weeks it was seen but was difficult to distinguish from surrounding tissue. Fat deposition in the renal sinus and pararenal space was thought to aid in identifying the kidney in the third trimester (14). The diagnosis of bilateral renal agenesis can be made by the 20th week. When the kidneys are not visualized by this time, failure to demonstrate the bladder within one to two hours after intravenous administration of furosemide to the mother is considered confirmatory (15). Obviously the gestational age at the time of sonography is important in accurately diagnosing fetal urinary tract abnormalities. It has been shown that the earlier in pregnancy the ultrasound is performed, the less reliable it is in detecting obstructive uropathy (2).

Errors in Diagnosis

Although in most instances the prenatal and postnatal diagnoses of obstructive uropathy or renal cystic disease correlate appropriately, there are a significant number of diagnostic errors. Not all large sonolucent retroperitoneal masses in the fetal abdomen are the result of obstructive uropathy. Physiological hydronephrosis, said to occur in the third trimester in 20% of pregnancies, may be a source of confusion (13). Some have used this as an argument against aggressive fetal intervention (16). Multicystic kidney and ureteropelvic junction obstruction are often confused. Whereas obstruction at the ureteropelvic junction has typical sonographic characteristics and is usually readily discernible from the most common form of multicystic kidney associated with upper ureteral atresia, there is a hydronephrotic form of multicystic kidney that can be impossible to differentiate sonographically from ureteropelvic junction obstruction. The severity of the embryological obstruction determines whether cystic disease or hydronephrosis develops, and little is known about the exact timing of these events. VUR has been infrequently diagnosed before birth, and significant reflux may be present even though the antenatal ultrasound findings are normal or show only minimal dilatation. Initially VUR may be an intermittent phenomenon and only later become persistent. It may then be associated with severe urinary tract dilatation (3). There are many other instances where the fetal ultrasound is reportedly normal and yet the child is born with significant obstructive uropathy (2). Additionally, in a large prospective series of maternal-fetal ultrasounds performed at 17 and 32 weeks' gestation, three of four cases with proven obstructive uropathy were not seen on the initial ultrasound (17). Further, significant obstructive uropathy may not be associated with classic hydronephrosis. Glazer and coworkers (18) were impressed with the variable sonographic appearance of fetuses with urethral obstruction, since most of their subjects demonstrated a relative lack of pelvicalyceal dilatation despite megaureter and even total urethral obstruction. Prenatal percutaneous antegrade pyelography has been successfully used to differentiate the level of obstruction in equivocal cases (19).

Significance of Oligohydramnios

Fetal urinary anomalies that prevent urine production lead to oligohydramnios, whereas those such as duodenal or esophageal atresia that inhibit fetal swallowing produce polyhydramnios. Both conditions should be detected by the experienced sonographer. A lack of sufficient amniotic fluid should lead to a careful examination of the fetal urinary tract. Oligohydramnios has been shown to result from renal agenesis, infantile polycystic disease, as well as from obstructive uropathy (9). The prognosis is poor when the diagnosis is made early, since only 2 normal-term infants were delivered from 37 cases of oligohydramnios in Campbell's series in which oligohydramnios was diagnosed before 26 weeks (9). More ominous is the review of the literature up to 1981, which failed to show a surviving infant in 15 reported cases of oligohydramnios, 11 having died shortly after delivery and 4 as a result of elective termination (11). Harrison and coworkers, based on an extensive series, feel that the obstructed fetus who presents with severe oligohydramnios very early in gestation may already have severe renal changes that make return of function unlikely and are pessimistic about fetal survival when amniotic fluid deficiency develops before the 20th week of gestation (12).

Relationship of Urinary Tract Obstruction, Renal Dysplasia and Pulmonary Hypoplasia

The concept that *treatment* of fetal obstructive uropathy before delivery may lessen the renal damage that results from the obstructive process has not yet been substantiated. One problem with fetal intervention arises from the fact that babies born with obstructive uropathy often have renal dysplasia in addition to hydronephrosis. Fetal intervention to avoid the deleterious effects of hydronephrosis would not be worthwhile if renal dysplasia is present as well. Likewise, infants born with obstructive uropathy often die of associated pulmonary hypoplasia rather than from renal insufficiency. These findings have challenged investigators to define the relationship between urinary tract obstruction, renal dysplasia, and pulmonary hypoplasia. Normal lung development seems to require at least a minimal volume of amniotic fluid. Deficiency of amniotic fluid prevents normal fetal lung expansion, probably because of simple compression (20). In congenital urinary tract obstruction, the massively distended urinary system elevates the diaphragm and the oligohydramnios results in a small intrauterine cavity that compresses the fetal thorax. This rather simplistic theory of the development of pulmonary hypoplasia by thoracic compression is not supported by several reports of severe oligohydramnios without lung deformity (7, 21). In the experimental animal, however, artificially induced bilateral hydronephrosis in late pregnancy resulted in severe pulmonary hypoplasia that was relieved by subsequent urinary decompression into the amniotic space (22). The problem with animal models of this type is that the surgical alteration has been created relatively late in gestation compared to the human counterpart, where it is thought that the developmental insult causing pulmonary hypoplasia occurs much earlier and results in structurally and functionally immature lungs (20). Late urinary tract decompression in the human may relieve the compression effect on the fetal thorax but could not be expected to alleviate the faulty pulmonary embryogenesis. Furthermore, no experimental or clinical studies to date have shown that unilateral congenital hydronephrosis produces pulmonary hypoplasia (13).

Beck, in a pioneering study, created total ureteral obstruction in fetal lambs and compared the renal histological findings between those whose obstruction dated from the first half of gestation to those from the last half (23). Renal dysplasia was found only in the early group, whereas hydronephrosis alone occurred in those obstructed later in gestation. Glick and coworkers, using a similar animal model, created total ureteral obstruction in the first half of gestation, and all obstructed kidneys were not only grossly hydronephrotic but dysplastic as well (24). The changes were thought similar to those seen in the human neonate with obstructive uropathy and renal dysplasia (Fig. 57.1).

In contrast with a purely obstructive etiology for renal dysplasia is the hypothesis of Mackie and Stephens, which postulates that a ureteral bud originating from an abnormal position on the Wolffian duct penetrates the metanephric blastema at a peripheral location and stimulates the development of disordered parenchyma resulting in renal dysplasia (25). Support for such "hereditary" types of renal dysplasia comes from an animal model in which early manipulation of the urinary tract is possible. Using the chick embryo, Maizels and Simpson denuded the ureteric buds of metanephric mesenchyme and produced primitive ducts, suggesting that renal dysplasia in the chick may be caused by nonobstructive phenomena (26). The most common type of cystic dysplasia, however, appears to be a developmental consequence of obstruction during active

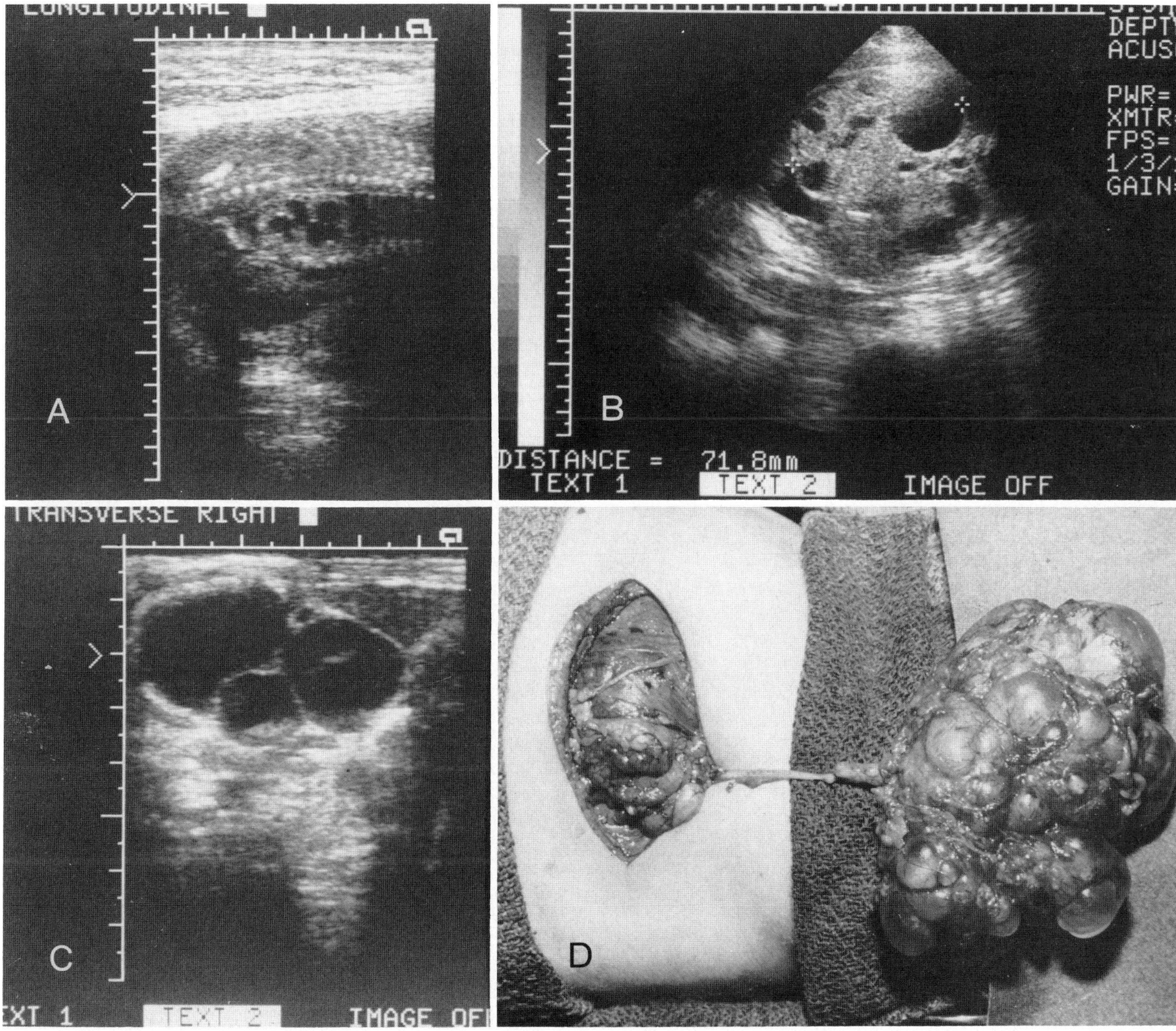

Figure 57.1. **A**, Maternal-fetal ultrasound at 22 weeks suggests hydronephrosis. **B**, At 34 weeks ultrasound looks more like multiple cysts. **C**, Neonatal ultrasound shows variable size of cystic structures. **D**, Multicystic dysplastic kidney: gross specimen.

nephrogenesis (27). The severity of renal dysplasia seems to depend on the timing in gestation and the degree of the obstruction. Certainly renal dysplasia secondary to early complete obstruction affects tubular and glomerular differentiation throughout the kidney and may not be reversible, although recent experimental data in the fetal lamb suggest that relief of obstruction created in the early second trimester may prevent the formation of renal dysplasia, which occurs invariably if such obstruction is not relieved (28). Caution must be used in extrapolating from these data in the experimental animal to the human, as the human fetal urinary tract in utero is rarely completely obstructed. Further, human fetal surgery for hydronephrosis in which dilated ureters due to posterior urethral valves were drained into the amniotic space by cutaneous ureterostomy at 21 weeks' gestation failed to reverse the presentation of renal dysplasia and pulmonary hypoplasia at delivery. The urinary tract was successfully decompressed, and the fetus continued to grow and develop in the three months before delivery; however, the renal and pulmonary damage was too advanced, and the infant died within a day of delivery (29). In fact, neither this modality nor shunts using percutaneously placed catheters from the fetal urinary tract to the amniotic space have been reported to prevent the associated renal dysplasia and pulmonary hypoplasia or to alter the course of abnormal urinary tract development.

Recommendations for Fetal Management

What should be the procedure once the diagnosis of a fluid-filled mass in the fetal abdomen is made on sonography? It is of paramount importance to decide whether it is genitourinary in origin. Most such masses involve the urinary tract, and other cystic lesions such as ovarian or choledochal cysts, dilated bowel loops associated with gastroschisis, omphalocele, or jejunal atresia can be distinguished by their location and the identification of normal kidneys (7). The next determinations to be made are (a) whether the condition is unilateral or bilateral, (b) the adequacy of amniotic fluid, and (c) whether the bladder can be visualized (9, 16, 31). Fetuses with congenital hydronephrosis may then be separated into four groups for management purposes: (a) unilateral hydronephrosis; (b) bilateral hydronephrosis with good function; (c) bilateral hydronephrosis with poor function; and (d) bilateral hydronephrosis with equivocal function (32).

Unilateral Hydronephrosis

Unilateral conditions with normal contralateral kidneys will have adequate amounts of amniotic fluid and the bladder will be observed to empty spontaneously at times. There is no evidence to suggest that unilateral hydronephrosis causes pulmonary hypoplasia. These patients can be observed carefully, and in utero intervention is not necessary except in unusual instances in which decompression at term of an exceptionally large mass may allow for vaginal delivery. Harrison and coworkers observed eight cases of unilateral hydronephrosis and normal amounts of amniotic fluid to near term (12). All eight did well, and six subsequently had successful pyeloplasties for ureteropelvic junction obstruction. In two, damage was severe enough to require nephrectomy. Likewise Mandell and coworkers observed seven patients with unilateral hydronephrosis to term, and all underwent successful operative correction in the newborn period (33). Similarly, eight successful pyeloplasties for unilateral ureteropelvic junction obstruction were performed in the newborn period by Parrott and coworkers (2). Three of these neonates were normal on physical examination. Pulmonary hypoplasia has not been associated with unilateral obstructive lesions, and renal dysplasia has not been averted by prenatal intervention with fetal ureterostomy or fetal shunt. Therefore, there appears to be no indication for percutaneous puncture of the fetal urinary system in them (34). The primary benefit from prenatal diagnosis of unilateral obstructive uropathy is to allow the families and physicians to choose the time, place, and conditions for optimal postnatal care. Hydronephrosis, which might cause progressive damage if undetected, can be managed operatively before urinary tract infection or other complications occur.

Bilateral Hydronephrosis with Good Function

When adequate amniotic fluid is present, the fetus with bilateral hydronephrosis can be presumed to have nearly normal renal, and pulmonary function and intervention need not be considered. Cases of apparently severe bilateral hydronephrosis and adequate amniotic fluid have been shown to resolve spontaneously as pregnancy progresses. Such cases as those reported by Harrison and coworkers demonstrated that fetal urinary tract dilatation is not necessarily progressive or harmful and that spontaneous resolution is possible (12). Serial ultrasound examinations are necessary to determine if the process is progressive, and the pregnancy should be observed carefully.

Bilateral Hydronephrosis with Poor Function

Bilateral hydronephrosis and oligohydramnios detected on initial sonography have in all instances caused fetal death from severe renal dysplasia and pulmonary hypoplasia. Furthermore, although technically feasible, shunts or open fetal decompression have failed to reverse the development of renal dysplasia or pulmonary hypoplasia in human (22, 29, 35). Harrison and coworkers used percutaneous external drainage of obstructed systems in an effort to predict potential recoverability of renal function when obstruction was diagnosed in the first half of pregnancy (22). Failure to produce significant urine after decompression allowed the prediction of a nonviable fetus, and the pregnancies were terminated.

Bilateral Hydronephrosis with Equivocal Function

The fetus with bilateral obstructive uropathy in whom amniotic fluid volume is initially normal but subsequently diminishes on ultrasonography constitutes the last group. In the rare case when these events are shown to occur before 32 weeks' gestation, fetal shunting may be of benefit. Once pulmonary maturity has been assured, however, the fetus is best managed ex utero with conventional urological maneuvers. In the fetus with obstructive uropathy, there is no evidence to suggest that relief of obstruction in utero will result in renal or pulmonary function beyond that achieved ex utero by pyeloplasty, vesicostomy, or ablation of posterior urethral valves (33). Furthermore, in utero intervention carries some risks to the fetus and mother, such as hemorrhage, sepsis, abortion, and premature labor. Until more is known of the natural history of congenital urinary tract dilatation in the fetus, as well as the measurement of fetal renal function and its recoverability following decompression, the experience accumulated to date suggests that only rarely is fetal intervention warranted. Most pregnancies complicated by fetal urinary tract dilatation should be managed with observation by serial ultrasound.

VISIBLE ANOMALIES OF THE ABDOMINAL WALL AND GENITALIA

Bladder Exstrophy

Although it occurs only once in 10,000 to 50,000 births, exstrophy (see also Chapter 43) is probably the most common bladder abnormality. In patients with its typical form, the remainder of the urinary tract is usually normal, although virtually all have an associated epispadias. Although the cause of exstrophy is unknown, it is certainly a fetal accident and not a developmental arrest (36). The result is a defect in the anterior abdominal wall filled with the open bladder (Fig. 57.2). The ureteral orifices can be seen as well as the entire urethra. In the male, the widely separated pubic symphysis results in an upward tilted, somewhat wide, and usually short, stubby penis. Typical exstrophy is part of a spectrum of anomalies involving the urogenital tract, musculoskeletal system and, occasionally, the intestinal tract. The variations include all degrees of epispadias, cloacal exstrophy, and superior vesical fissure (37, 38). Of infants born with this set of anomalies, approximately 60% have typical bladder exstrophy, 30% have some degree of epispadias, and only 10% have one of the less common variants such as cloacal exstrophy or superior vesicle fissure.

The results of reconstructive surgery for bladder exstrophy, when judged by continence and preservation of upper urinary tract integrity, have in the past been most discouraging (39). Before the 1970s a 10% to 20% success rate would have been considered the norm, with urinary diversion and compromised renal function being the more common result. In the past decade or so, however, an individualized staged approach has markedly improved functional closure of bladder exstrophy (40–42). Many surgeons now prefer to undertake the first stage during the first one to three days of life.

Cloacal Exstrophy

Unlike classic exstrophy, cloacal exstrophy (Fig. 57.3) remains a major and often frustrating challenge to the urological surgeon (see also Chapter 43). Until recently, most infants were expected to die. With improvements in intravenous alimentation, however, many of these infants now survive and present a problem to the reconstructive surgeon. Other major associated anomalies are common, particularly omphalocele and myelodysplasia. These infants are essentially missing a functioning large bowel, and the nutritional problem results from inadequate bowel length. In the male infant, the genitalia are usually hopeless insofar as future

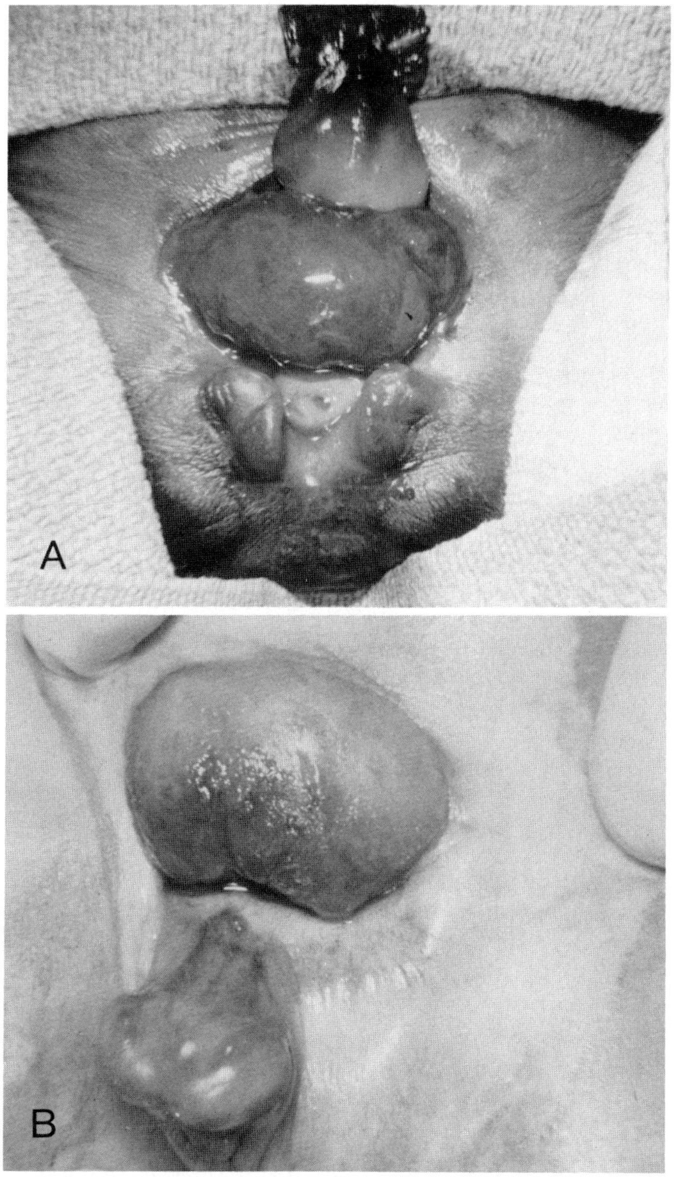

Figure 57.2. **A**, Female neonate with classic bladder exstrophy shown from above: umbilical cord; exstrophic bladder orifice between widely separated bifid clitoris. **B**, Male neonate with classic bladder exstrophy showing exstrophic bladder continuous with complete epispadias.

sexual function is concerned, and most of these should be reared as females.

Patent Urachus

The uncommon anomaly patent urachus results when, at the fourth to fifth gestational month, the urachus fails to close into a solid cord. The umbilical cord is usually distended at birth. After the cord sloughs off, urinary leakage may be noted from the umbilicus. The urachus may be obviously patent or may present as a wet umbilicus with umbilical granulation. Bladder outlet obstruction, particularly in boys with the prune belly syndrome, may contribute to failure of the urachus to close; however, only 14% of the reported cases of patent urachus have been found to have bladder outlet obstruction (43). The urine may drain continuously or intermittently. A voiding cystourethrogram (Fig. 57.4) is a useful study, not only to demonstrate the patent urachus but to also

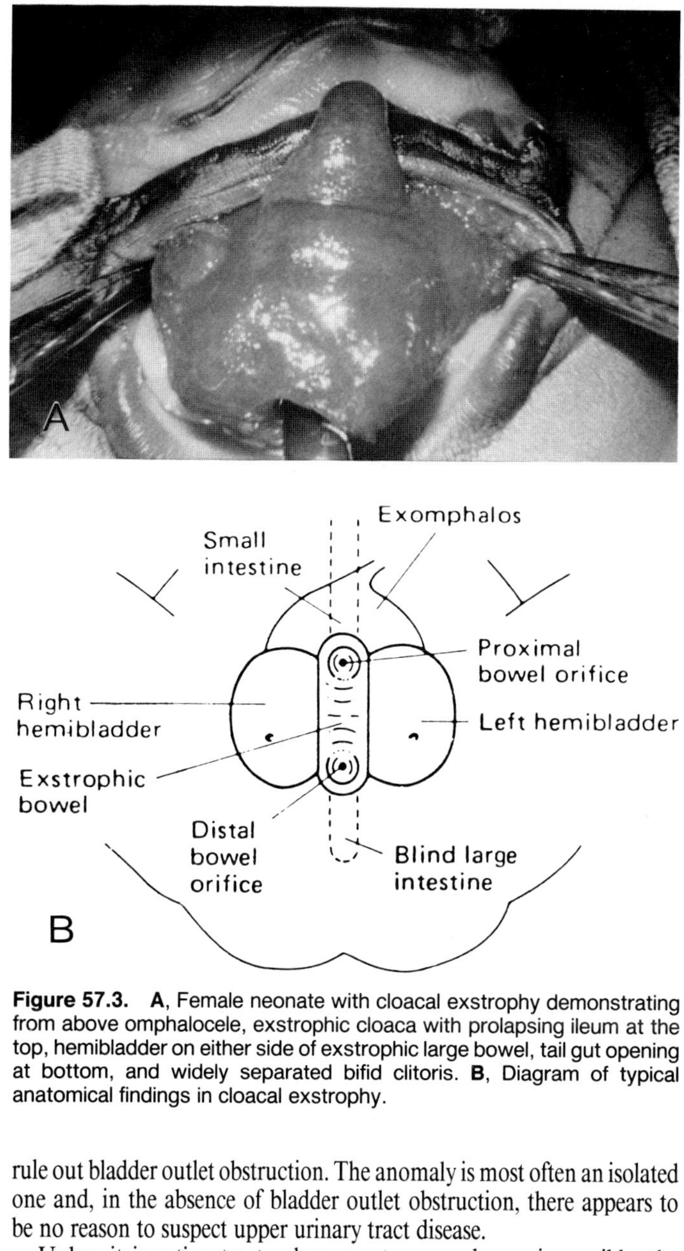

Figure 57.3. **A**, Female neonate with cloacal exstrophy demonstrating from above omphalocele, exstrophic cloaca with prolapsing ileum at the top, hemibladder on either side of exstrophic large bowel, tail gut opening at bottom, and widely separated bifid clitoris. **B**, Diagram of typical anatomical findings in cloacal exstrophy.

rule out bladder outlet obstruction. The anomaly is most often an isolated one and, in the absence of bladder outlet obstruction, there appears to be no reason to suspect upper urinary tract disease.

Unless it is a tiny tract, when spontaneous closure is possible, the urachus necessitates complete surgical excision of the tract as well as a small cuff of the bladder dome. This can usually be done extraperitoneally.

Urinary Ascites

An infant with ascites has a bulging abdomen in which radiological examination demonstrates gas-filled loops of bowel floating in a densely opaque background (Fig. 57.5). Although many conditions can produce ascites in infants, urine is the fluid most commonly found in the neonate (44), and obstructive uropathy is the usual underlying cause. Typically, the obstruction is in the lower urinry tract—most commonly in the posterior urethral valves of the male infant. It can, however, occur as a consequence of upper or lower tract obstruction in both males and females. The diagnosis is usually suspected from the bulging, tense abdomen, which frequently produces respiratory embarrassment and is confirmed by a plain abdominal roentgenogram.

Paracentesis is performed to aid in the diagnosis and, often, to

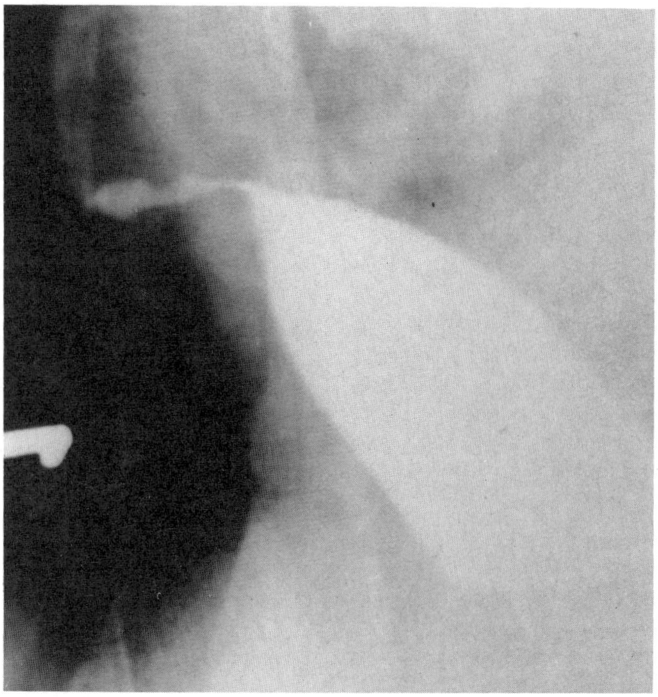

Figure 57.4. Voiding cystourethrogram showing patent urachus with contrast material extending from dome of bladder to umbilicus.

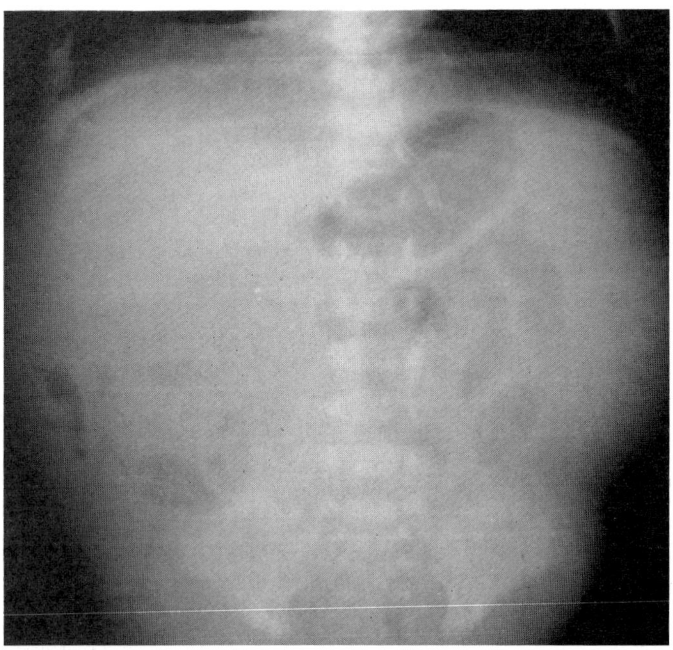

Figure 57.5. Plain abdominal x-ray film of neonate with urinary ascites. Shows typical ground glass appearance of abdomen with loops of intestinal gas floating in fluid.

temporarily relieve respiratory difficulty. If the ascites is urinary, the fluid should have a higher creatinine concentration than plasma. This difference may be slight, however, due to the dialyzing property of the peritoneal membrane. A voiding cystourethrogram and a renal abdominal ultrasound study should be done to localize the site of urinary obstruction.

It was previously thought that infants with posterior urethral valves having urinary ascites had a worse prognosis than those without ascites. This is probably not true. In fact, the upper tract decompression afforded by the intraperitoneal exstravasation may reduce renal damage (45). The urine may enter the peritoneal cavity by transudation or by direct communication between the retroperitoneum and the peritoneal cavity.

The treatment of urinary ascites is essentially the treatment of the obstructive lesion that formed it. A paracentesis may be necessary to control respiratory embarrassment initially while preparation is being made to decompress the urinary tract. Otherwise, the presence of ascites does not alter the management of the primary lesion (46, 47).

Congenital Absence of the Abdominal Musculature (Prune Belly Syndrome)

Congenital absence of the abdominal musculature, more commonly known as prune belly syndrome (Fig. 57.6), is usually readily apparent at birth. Although it occurs almost exclusively in boys and only once in 35,000 to 50,000 live births (48), few syndromes have presented greater interest or challenge for the urological surgeon. In addition to the flabby, lax abdominal wall, the syndrome is characterized by undescended testicles and dilated tortuous ureters, thus suggesting the eponym, "triad syndrome." Renal dysplasia, hydroureteronephrosis, and vesicoureteral reflux are common. The bladder is typically large and often empties poorly. Although the cause of the abdominal wall defect is unknown, recent speculation suggests it might be caused by fetal ascites. The more commonly held theory is that it results from a primary mesodermal error leading directly or indirectly to its various manifestations.

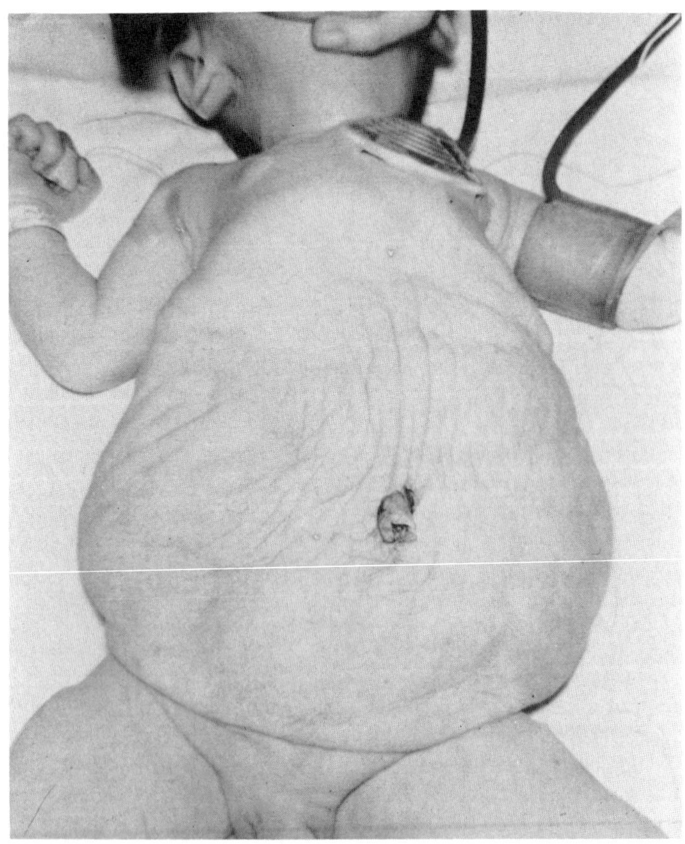

Figure 57.6. Typical appearance of infant with prune belly syndrome showing characteristic thin-wall, wrinkled abdomen and flared costal margins.

The management of patients with this syndrome is discussed in detail in Chapter 38. It might be emphasized, however, that the initial evaluation should avoid catheterization or other urological instrumentation because of the risk of bacterial contamination. Abdominal ultrasonography and perhaps excretory urography should be the initial urological studies. Pulmonary and renal function should be monitored closely, since pulmonary hypoplasia and renal dysplasia have played a major role in determining the ultimate fate of these infants.

Hypospadias

Occurring in approximately 8.2 per 1000 births, hypospadias is one of the more common urological abnormalities (see also Chapter 43). The milder forms are more common, and ventral curvature (chordee) is present in approximately one third of cases (49). Hypospadias results from failure of the urethral folds to fuse, an event that may place the meatus anywhere between the glans and the perineum (Fig. 57.7). A failure or deficiency of continuous hormonal production by the fetus at the appropriate gestational time or a cellular inability to fully use the testosterone produced by the fetus may play a role in its etiology (50, 51).

Infants with hypospadias should not be circumcised, since the preputial skin is necessary for surgical correction of the anomaly. Although the timing of surgical repair varies somewhat with the surgeon's preference, all agree that it should be completed before school age. Recently, there has been a tendency toward a much earlier repair, although most surgeons still wait until the patient is at least 1 yr of age (52, 53). Most cases are now repaired in a single-stage operation, and good cosmetic and functional results are likely.

Micropenis

Micropenis (Fig. 57.8) is a small, normally formed organ that is less than 2.5 cm in stretched length (54, 55). Since the embryological formation of the penis and its subsequent growth are both testosterone-dependent, micropenis apparently results from a defect in testosterone production, failure of testosterone to be converted to dyhydrotestosterone, or a failure of cell transport after the first trimester (56). Since micropenis may result from primary or secondary hypogonadism, affected infants need prompt endocrine evaluation so that proper management may be instituted. The evaluation should include a karyotype to document chromosomal sex. Serum luteinizing hormone, follicle-stimulating hormone, and testosterone levels should be obtained and human chorionic gonadotropin stimulation test done to distinguish primary from secondary hypogonadism.

Most patients with micropenis respond to testosterone. Once the diagnostic studies have been obtained, a course of systemic testosterone should be administered under the auspices of the endocrinologist (57). When the male infant with micropenis fails to respond to testicular stimulation or when corporal tissue is lacking and the penis can never be expected to develop into a sexually or cosmetically satisfactory organ, female sex assignment is appropriate. Therefore, an early and complete endocrine evaluation as well as a testosterone trial are important so that sex assignment can be decided at the earliest feasible time.

Ambigious Genitalia

It is not until about the seventh week that sexual differentiation in the human fetus begins. The critical factor appears to be a gene located on the short arm of the Y chromosome near the centromere. It is this gene that is responsible for the elaboration of the H-Y antigen, which can be identified on the surface of all male mammalian cells and may be essential for the development of a testis from the primitive indifferent gonad. The first evidence that a fetus is going to be male appears shortly after the seventh week, when the gonad begins to differentiate into a testis. The other aspects of male development apparently depend on this primary event. The fetal testis produces two hormonal substances, Müllerian inhibiting factor and testosterone. The former is responsible for disappearance of the Müllerian ductal system and the latter for male sexual differentiation. Some instances of intersexuality are caused, not by failure to make testosterone but by the inability of the tissues to respond. If the fetus is to develop as a female, the Müllerian ducts will differentiate into fallopian tubes and fuse distally to form the uterus and proximal vagina,

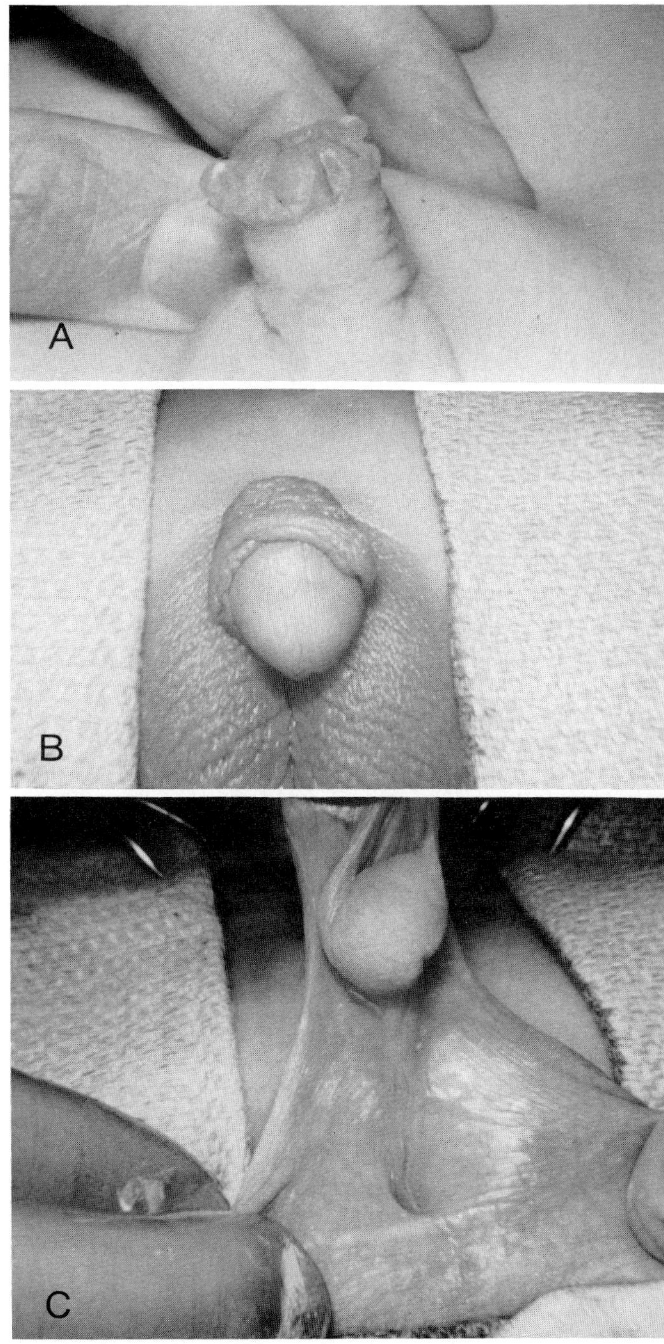

Figure 57.7. **A**, Neonate with mild, coronal hypospadias showing typical hooded prepuce. **B** and **C**, Infant with perineal hypospadias, severe chordee, and slight bifid scrotum.

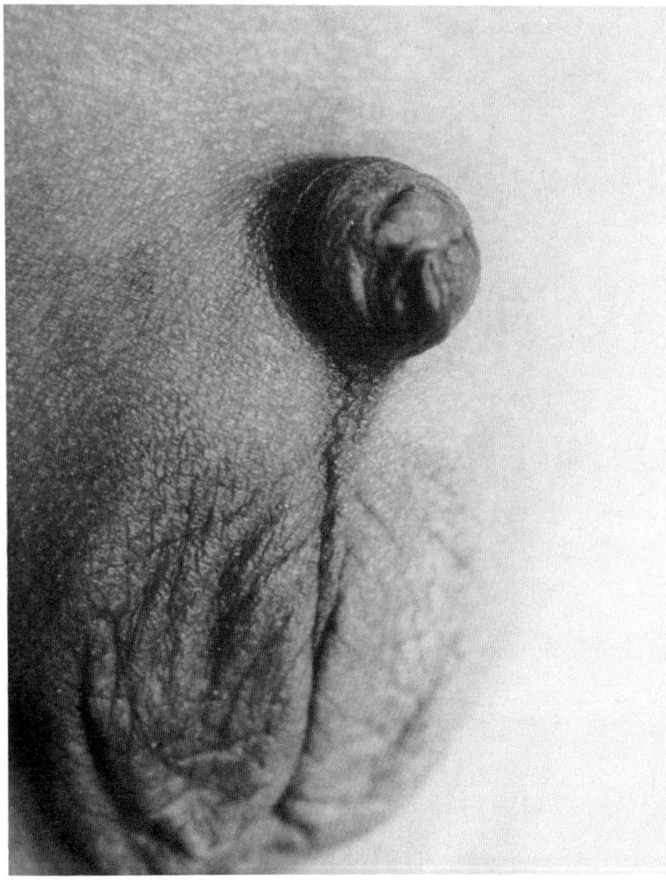

Figure 57.8. Typical micropenis. Phallus is 1.5 cm in stretched length and consists primarily of skin with virtually no corpora.

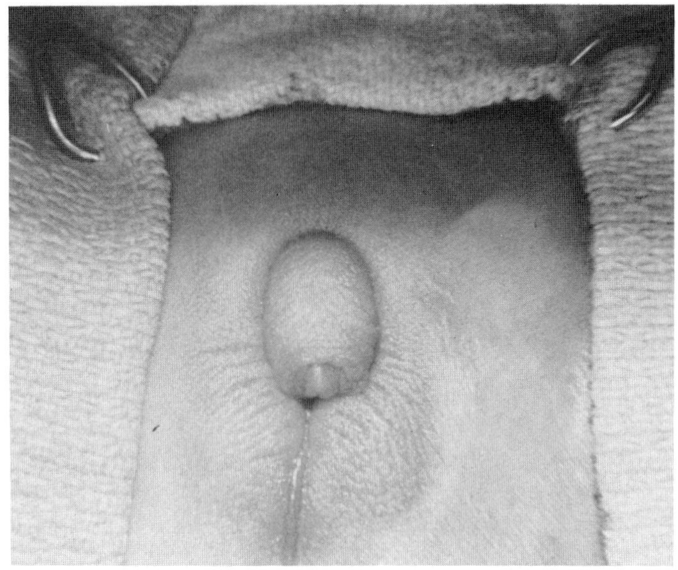

Figure 57.9. Typical appearance of ambiguous genitalia in genetic female neonate with congenital adrenal hyperplasia and adrenogenital syndrome. Note marked clitoral enlargement with prominent labioscrotal folds, which are rugose.

whereas the wolffian ducts will undergo atrophy and the external genitalia will feminize. By the end of the first trimester, the genitalia are fully formed.

Infants born with ambigious genitalia fall into one of five major categories: (a) female pseudohermaphrodite (ovary only), (b) true hermaphrodite (ovary plus testis), (c) male pseudohermaphrodite (testis only), (d) mixed gonadal dysgenesis (testis and streak gonad), (e) pure gonadal dysgenesis (streak gonad only). Another simple way of viewing ambigious genitalia is as overandrogenization of a female or underandrogenization of a male. The female pseudohermaphrodite then is a genetic female who has been exposed to excessive amounts of androgen at some point before the twelfth week of gestation. This might be exogenous exposure from a drug administered to the mother during the first trimester of pregnancy or endogenous from the fetal adrenal as in the adrenogenital syndrome (Fig. 57.9). The adrenogenital syndrome is particularly important in the consideration of infants with ambigious genitalia because of its relative frequency as the most common of the entities and also because of its potentially lethal nature in its salt-losing form. This is one of the reasons the evaluation of the intersex infant represents an urgent problem (58).

Epispadias

Epispadias (see also Chapter 43) alone is less common than complete bladder exstrophy with epispadias. In males, it varies in degree from balanitic to penile to subsymphyseal, depending on the location of the urethral meatus. Typically, the penis appears short and broad with dorsal tethering or chordee so that it lies in contact with the pubic skin (Fig. 57.10). The preputial skin is on the ventrum and less redundant than the typical dorsal hood in hypospadias. In the female (Fig. 57.11), the abnormality is less conspicuous on superficial examination; however, on spreading the labia it becomes apparent that the affected female has a wide separation of the clitoris so that it appears duplicated. The urethra is defective dorsally to a variable extent. The external defect is associated with some degree of separation of the symphysis pubis, which can be seen on an x-ray film of the pelvis. Of greater importance than the external defect in epispadias is the possibility of an incompetent bladder neck with total urinary incontinence commonly termed complete epispadias. Although it is important to obtain a voiding cystourethrogram in these patients, one may not be able to make a definite decision regarding the presence of incontinence during the neonatal period.

Urethral Duplication

Urethral duplication, or accessory urethra, may be complete or incomplete, depending on whether the accessory tract extends to the bladder. All types of urethral duplication are rare and typically present in one of three ways. The most common type has an accessory opening in the epispadic position (Fig. 57.12, *A*, *B*). Although it may not be evident during early infancy, the more dorsal tract may be incontinent. Those that present with hypospadias do not have a problem with continence and both urethras are ventral to the corpora. The most complicated presentation, commonly referred to as Y duplication, is characterized by a somewhat rudimentary urethra in the normal position with a glandular meatus and a second, somewhat larger, urethral channel opening into the rectum just inside the anus (Fig. 57.12, *C*). The latter variety is likely to escape diagnosis initially and also presents a more difficult therapeutic challenge to the surgeon (59).

Scrotal Mass

The differential diagnosis of a scrotal mass at birth includes testicular torsion, incarcerated inguinal hernia, and testicular neoplasm. Acute epididymitis does occur at this age but is rare and usually secondary to bacteremia. Occasionally, a testicular or scrotal hematoma will result from a traumatic delivery. Although testicular tumors can occur at any

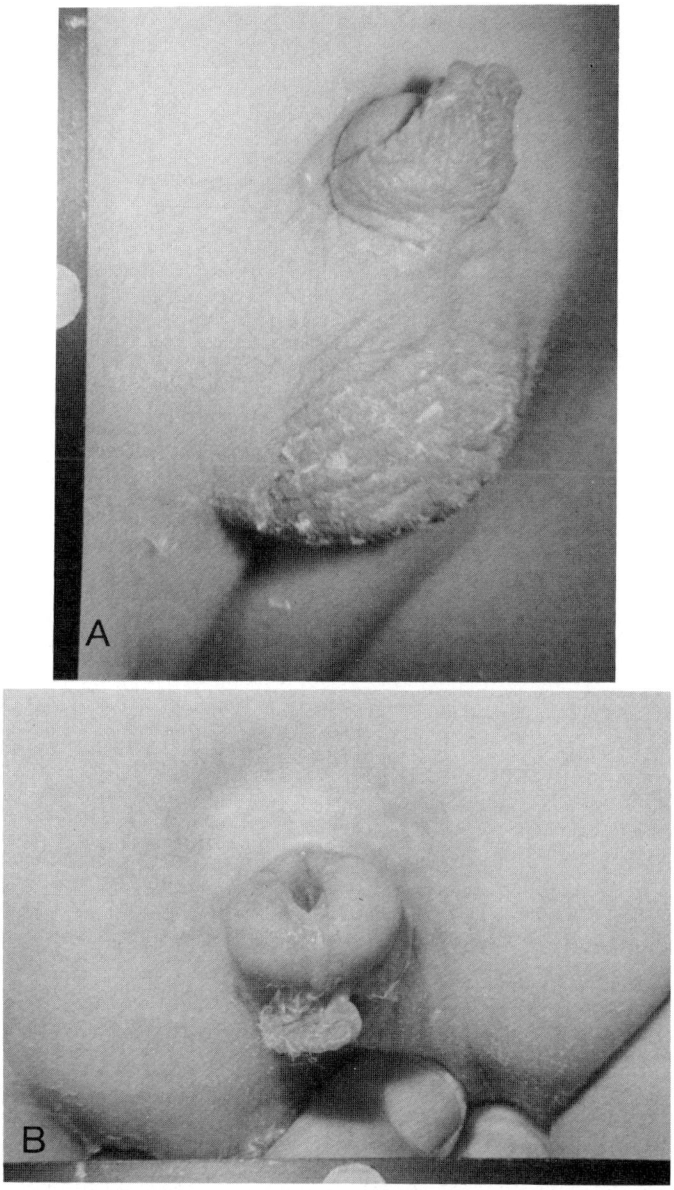

Figure 57.10. **A** and **B**, Typical appearance of penile epispadias with "dorsal chordee."

age, a significant percentage of childhood testis tumors are found in early infancy, the most common being benign teratomas (60). Neonatal testicular torsion is usually an in utero event and, consequently, the possibility of salvaging a viable testis is rare. The testis is vulnerable to torsion during the normal process of descent because of poor fixation of the tunica vaginalis as it moves through the inguinal canal (61, 62). The diagnosis can usually be made on the basis of physical examination by finding a hard, nontender, and usually discolored mass on the affected side.

Urogenital Sinus and Cloacal Disorders

Persistent urogenital sinus and cloaca are manifestations of developmental arrest during the formation of the primitive cloaca. In persistent cloaca, the urethra, vagina, and rectum drain into a common perineal outlet, whereas in persistent urogenital sinus (Fig. 57.13), the rectum has separated from the genitourinary tract and opens separately but often in

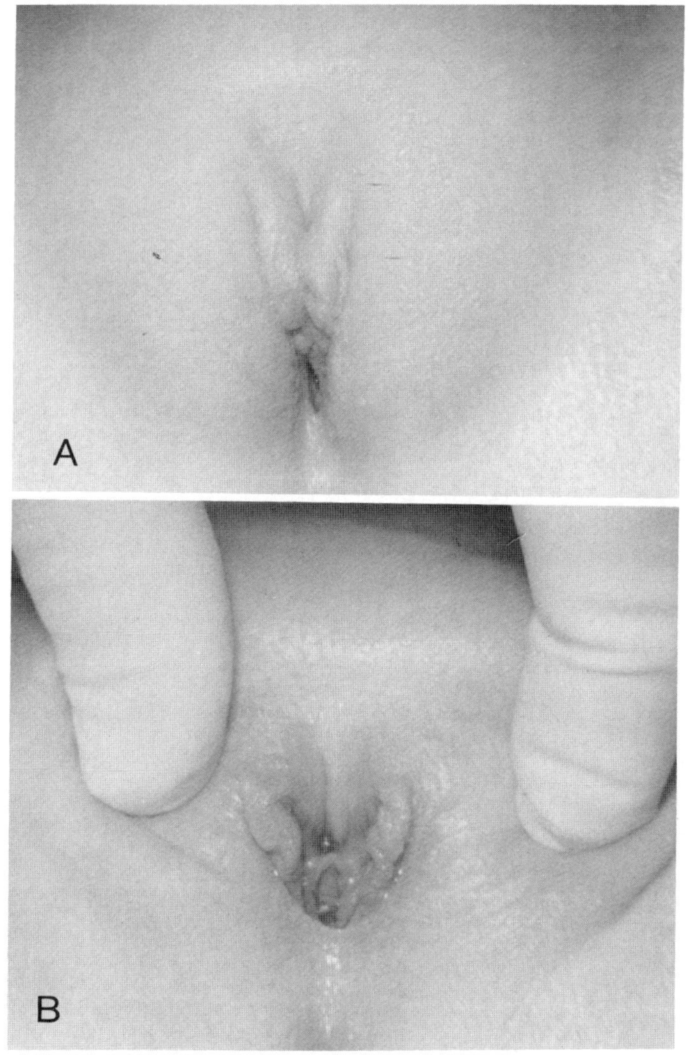

Figure 57.11. **A** and **B**, Female infant with subsymphyseal epispadias. Note bifid scrotum and patulous urethra.

a slightly anterior position. Both anomalies present major surgical problems (63).

Vaginal Agenesis

Vaginal agenesis is often unrecognized in the newborn infant. It results from lack of fusion of the caudal portions of the müllarian ducts. This anomaly may be associated with renal and ureteric malformations such as unilateral renal agenesis. Therefore, when vaginal agenesis is noted in the neonate, a renal ultrasound study is indicated (64).

"Vaginal" Cysts

Cystic bulges are occasionally seen at the vaginal or urethral orifice in neonates (Fig. 57.14). These may be simple periurethral inclusion cysts, which cause no immediate problems and may be excised at any opportune time; however, they may represent prolapse of an ectopic ureterocele. If the distinction is not evident on a simple external examination, a renal ultrasound or an excretory urogram should be obtained inasmuch as ectopic ureteroceles are generally associated with duplication anomalies with severe dilatation of the ureter and upper pole of the kidney on the involved side.

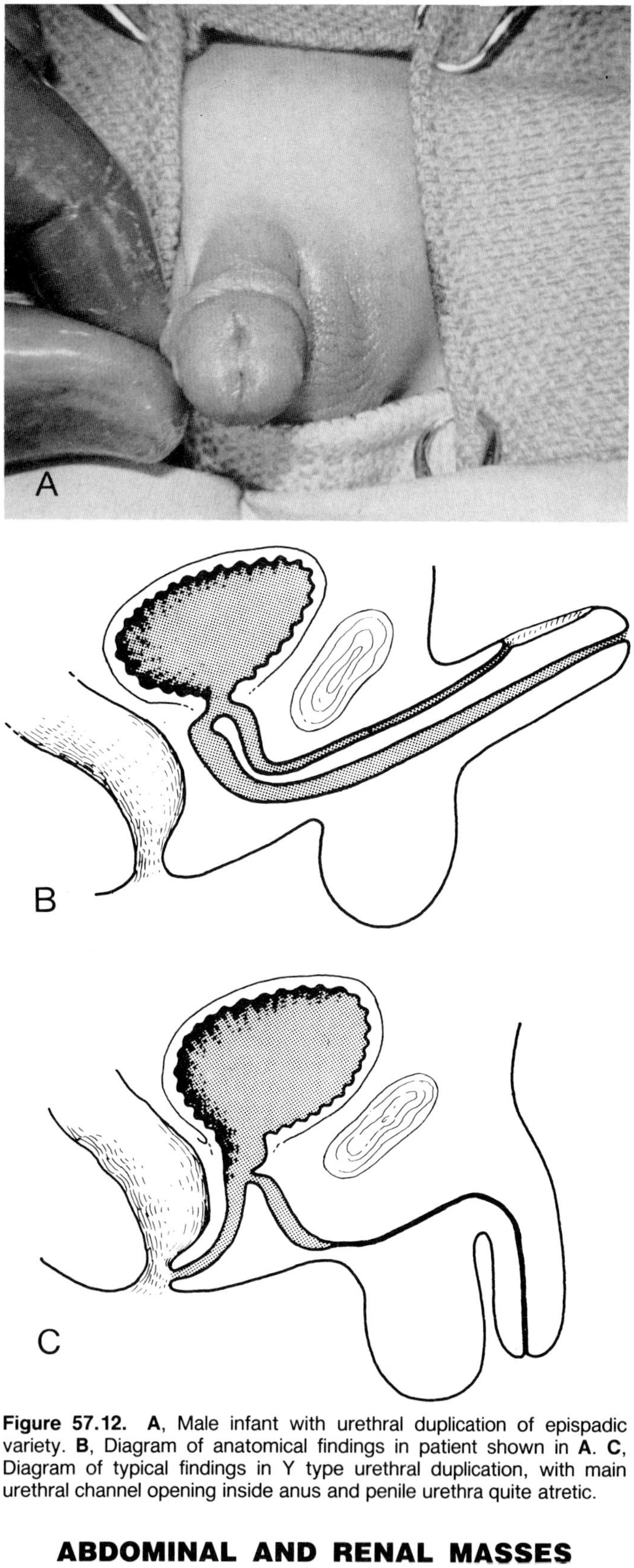

Figure 57.12. A, Male infant with urethral duplication of epispadic variety. B, Diagram of anatomical findings in patient shown in A. C, Diagram of typical findings in Y type urethral duplication, with main urethral channel opening inside anus and penile urethra quite atretic.

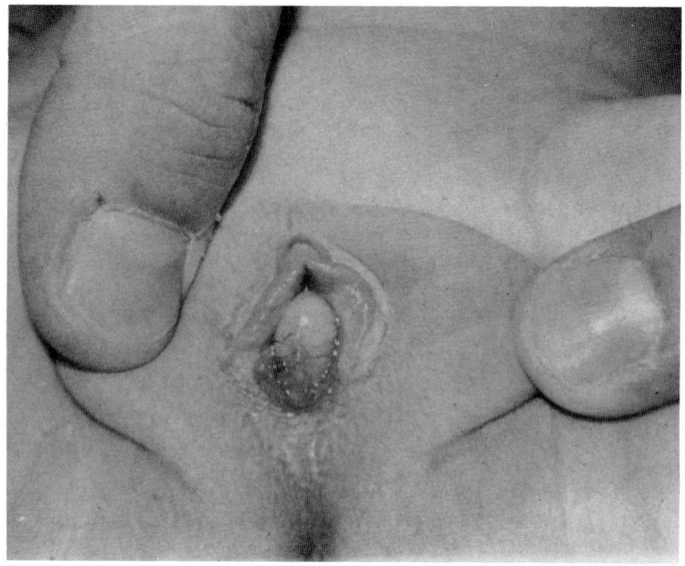

Figure 57.13. Typical appearance of female infant with persistent urogenital sinus with normal-appearing clitoris but otherwise hypoplastic-appearing introitus, often associated with anterior placement of anus.

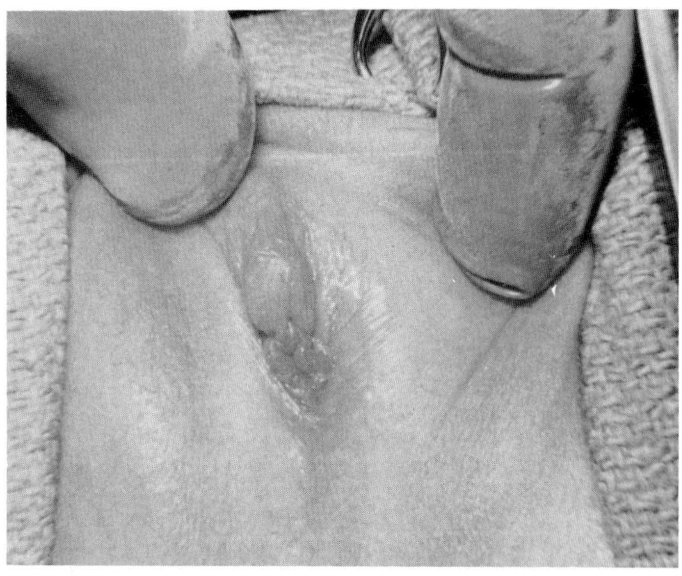

Figure 57.14. Cystic swelling presenting in vaginal orifice of female neonate. This cyst was a simple periurethral cyst, although it may be difficult to distinguish from prolapsing ectopic ureterocele.

ABDOMINAL AND RENAL MASSES

Neonatal Abdominal Mass

An abdominal mass is by far the most common sign ultimately leading to urological surgery in the neonate (65). Table 57.1 is a composite inventory derived from three published series reporting on neonatal abdominal masses and shows the relative frequency of the various entities that are likely to produce as an abdominal mass at this age (66–68). Well over 50% of these abdominal masses were of renal origin, and it should therefore be assumed that even a mass presenting anteriorally might arise from the retroperitoneal area. Hydronephrosis and multicystic kidney occurred with approximately equal frequency. Of all of the masses reported, 83% originated in the kidney, retroperitoneal area, or female genital tract. Only 17% were related to the liver or gastrointestinal tract. An accurate diagnosis is the first priority in managing the neonate with an abdominal mass. Careful abdominal palpation usually provides important information relative to the size, contour, location, and mobility of the mass and helps to determine its site of origin. For example, a mass in the epigastrium that moves with respiration is likely to be hepatic,

Table 57.1.
Frequency of Causes of Neonatal Abdominal Masses in 115 Patients[a]

Site and cause	No. of patients
Kidney	
Hydronephrosis	33
Multicystic kidney	35
Polycystic kidney	2
Renal vein thrombosis	3
Solid tumors	2
Retroperitoneum	
Neuroblastoma	7
Teratoma	2
Hemangioma	1
Bladder	
Urethral valves	1
Female genital tract	
Hydrocolpos	7
Ovarian cyst	5
Gastrointestinal tract	
Duplications	5
Giant cystic meconium peritonitis	2
Mesenteric cyst	1
Volvulus of ileum	1
Teratoma of stomach	1
Leiomyoma of colon	1
Hepatic or biliary tract	
Hemangioma of liver	2
Solitary cyst of liver	1
Hepatoma	1
Distended gallbladder	1
Choledochal cyst	1

[a] Data from Longino and Martin (65), Raffensperger and Abouseleiman (67), and Wedge, Grosfeld, and Smith (68).

omental, or gastric in origin. When masses are bilateral, which is not infrequent, they are more often of renal origin with hydronephrosis and polycystic kidneys being the more likely lesions. A smooth lower abdominal mass could represent a distended bladder, but in the female it might be of uterine or ovarian origin. In the past, the radiological examination began with a plain abdominal film followed by an excretory urogram; however, with the advent of ultrasonography and its refinements, the first step should be an ultrasound examination of the abdomen, since this involves neither ionizing radiation nor contrast material. The examination can be performed quickly and safely and is accurate in determining the presence or absence of a pathological mass (69). When a mass is detected, its size, location, internal consistency, and organ involvement can be determined. In the majority of cases, a specific diagnosis can be made. In other instances the information gained is valuable in directing further studies to arrive at the correct diagnosis in an expeditious manner. In many instances, when the mass is of renal origin, an excretory urogram or some other contrast study of the urinry tract may be necessary to complete the evaluation; however, the selection of radiological studies can be much more precise after sonography has been performed. Many neonatal abdominal masses require surgical intervention for therapeutic reasons or to finalize the diagnosis.

Hydronephrosis

Hydronephrosis (see also Chapter 38) is the most common cause of a neonatal abdominal mass and one of the most common abnormalities requiring surgical correction in the neonate. Most often it is due to obstruction at the ureteropelvic junction (Fig. 57.15, *A*). It is slightly more common in male infants and is bilateral approximately 25% of the time. When it is bilateral, one must ensure that bladder outlet obstruction does not exist. Primary obstruction at the ureterovesical junction is less likely to be recognized in the neonate. Congenital multicystic kidney (Fig. 57.16) is the lesion that most often must be distinguished from hydronephrosis, and this can usually be done by means of ultrasonography (Fig. 57.15, *B*). Ultrasonography is also helpful in localizing the site of the obstruction. The ureter is usually not readily identifiable with ureteropelvic junction obstruction, whereas it can be seen to be dilated in instances of ureterovesical obstruction. It may be necessary, however, to confirm sonographic findings with contrast urography—either intravenous (Fig. 57.15, *C*), antegrade, or retrograde studies—before corrective surgery is undertaken. Voiding cystourethrography is often also recommended since vesicoureteral reflux is an occasional finding. Once evaluation is complete and if obstruction appears to be functionally significant, treatment should be directed toward relieving obstruction and preserving renal function. Pyeloplasty and other reconstructive procedures in the newborn can be very successful, and the obstructed kidney should be preserved in the presence or even a thin rim of recognizable renal parenchyma.

It has been shown that even severe degrees of temporary hydronephrosis and hydroureter in the neonate can result from sepsis and that complete reversal may occur with proper antibiotic treatment (70, 71). This possibility must be borne in mine when evaluating the infant with hydronephrosis and urinary sepsis (72).

Multicystic Kidney

Multicystic kidney is the other of the two most common causes of neonatal abdominal masses. Its importance perhaps lies in its frequency and in the possibility of its being confused with hydronephrosis. It represents an extreme form of dysplasia associated with atresia of the ureter and has been classified as Potter Type II (73). On histological examination there is renal dysplasia, a reduced number of nephrons, and no normal renal parenchyma. It is usually unilateral, although some bilateral cases have been reported in association with Potter's facies (74). The cysts (Fig. 57.16, *A*) are relatively few, may be large and heterogenous in size, and are loosely bound together. The diagnosis is usually suspected from the nature of the palpable abdominal mass, and ultrasonography is required to confirm the diagnosis. Sonography usually demonstrates that the cysts do not communicate (Fig. 57.16, *B*) and thus distinguishes it from hydronephrosis. Excretory urography or renal radionuclide scan may be important to ensure normality of the contralateral kidney. There is some controversy among urological surgeons regarding the proper treatment of multicystic kidney once the diagnosis is made. The controversy concerns whether nephrectomy is indicated for final confirmation of the diagnosis or as definitive therapy. Although late complications from this lesion are poorly documented, many if not most of these multicystic kidneys are still removed when there is no contraindication to surgery or anesthesia.

Renal Vein Thrombosis

Although renal vein thrombosis (see also Chapter 56) may present as an abdominal mass, it also accounts for up to 20% of the cases of gross hematuria occurring in the first month of life (75). Approximately 40% of renal vein thrombosis cases in children occurred during the first two weeks of life. The diagnosis is usually suspected from the combination of abdominal mass, hematuria, thrombocytopenia, with typical findings on renal ultrasound examination. In the absence of sepsis or uncontrolled hemorrhage, the treatment is medical (76).

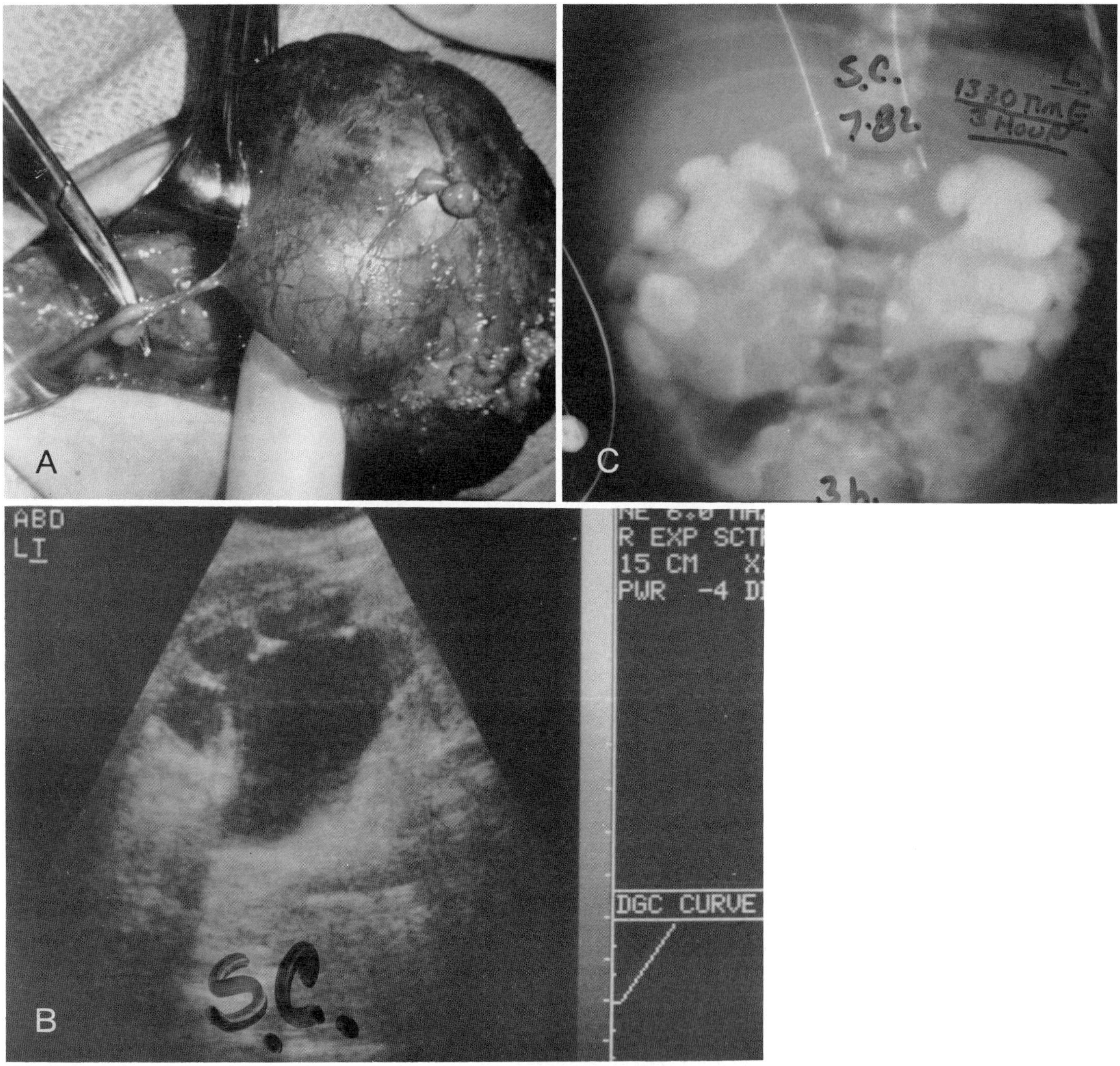

Figure 57.15. **A**, Typical hydronephrosis in neonate with distended and thinned renal parenchyma, marked distention of renal pelvis, and severe narrowing of ureteropelvic junction, which is site of obstruction. **B**, Renal ultrasound study in same patient showing distended calyces communicating with distended renal pelvis by a wide infundibular. No visualization of ureter. **C**, Intravenous pyelogram in same patient showing bilateral ureteropelvic junction obstruction with typical hydronephrosis and no visualization of ureters.

Massive Adrenal Hemorrhage

Small hemorrhages in the neonate's adrenal gland occur with surprising frequency and are found in 1% to 2% of those undergoing autopsy examination (77). Massive adrenal hemorrhage is a different entity and is much less common. In addition, it has a significant mortality rate (78, 79). The traumatic events of childbirth appear to be the principal causal factors; the right adrenal gland is more commonly involved than the left. The clinical features of massive adrenal hemorrhage are the presence of a mass in one or both flanks, signs of blood loss, and possibly urinary infection or sepsis. The abdominal ultrasound examination (Fig. 57.17) is particularly helpful in making the diagnosis and in subsequent surveillance. Although patients may do well on conservative treatment consisting of careful monitoring and fluid replacement, there is always the possibility of massive hemorrhage with vascular collapse and shock or of abscess within the hemorrhage. These complications require emergency surgical intervention (79, 80).

Renal Tumors

The most common solid renal tumor in childhood is nephroblastoma or Wilms' tumor. Although Wilms' tumors have been reported to occur

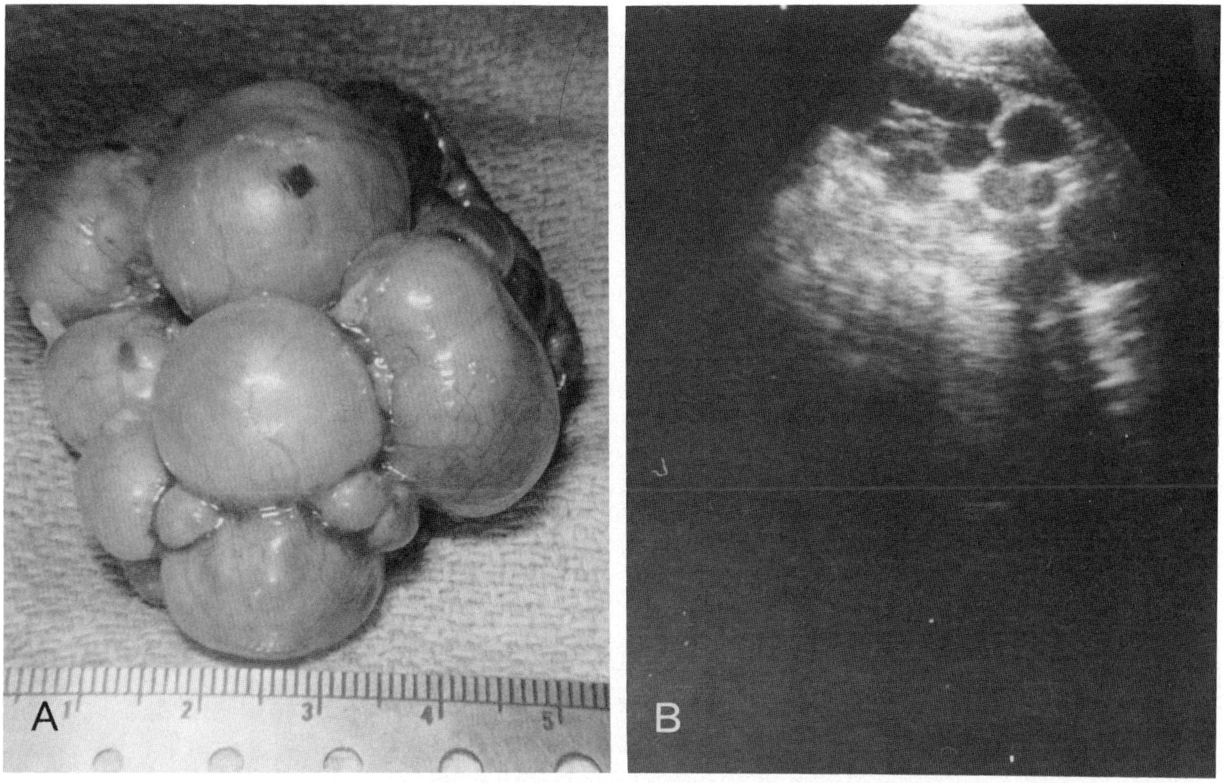

Figure 57.16. **A**, Typical appearance of congenital multicystic kidney associated with atretic ureter. Note varying sized of cyst and loose connections between cyst without indentifiable renal parenchyma. **B**, Abdominal ultrasound in same patient showing noncommunicating sonolucent cyst.

in neonates (81), most solid renal tumors in the neonate are mesoblastic nephromas. These predominantly mesenchymal tumors must be recognized as a different entity from Wilms' tumor to avoid the hazards of overtreatment (82). Mesoblastic nephroma is usually discovered because of an abdominal mass and has the pyelographic and sonographic features of other solid renal mass lesions. Surgical removal should cure the patient, since metastases do not occur. Further treatment with radiation, chemotherapy, or both is therefore contraindicated.

Hydrometrocolpos

Hydrometrocolpos is a rare but important abdominal mass occurring in the female neonate; it is produced by fluid distention of the vagina and uterus. The circumstances necessary for its development are vaginal obstruction with excessive secretion of the cervical glands in response to circulating maternal estrogen. In persistent urogenital sinus or cloacal abnormalities, urine contributes to the fluid accumulation. Hydrometrocolpos produces a mass that is large, firm, and midline in position. It arises from the pelvis and on rectal examination can be felt anterior to the rectum and posterior to the bladder. It commonly produces ureteral obstruction with hydronephrosis. A quick and accurate diagnosis depends on awareness of the condition by the examiner. Treatment should be aggressive (83). In general, the obstructive uropathy can be expected to resolve following satisfactory drainage of the uterus. Occasionally, however, surgical intervention is necessary for persistent urinary obstruction or for urinary sepsis.

Ovarian Cysts

An ovarian cyst must be considered a possible cause of an abdominal mass in the female infant (68). Most of these cysts are follicular and can be quite large. Malignant ovarian tumors during the neonatal period are rare. An ovarian cyst usually presents in the lower abdomen but may occasionally occupy the entire abdomen and resemble ascites. When smaller, they are usually mobile. Sudden complications such as torsion or rupture may produce an acute abdominal condition (66). Prompt surgical treatment is indicated, and an effort should be made to preserve a functional ovary by removing the cyst wall. This is particularly important in bilateral cases (84).

FAILURE TO PASS URINE

Failure to pass urine in the first 24 hr of life should arouse concern, since micturition occurs in two-thirds of all neonates within 12 hr of birth and in at least 90% of newborns during the first 24 hr (Table 57.2) (85). If voiding has not occurred by 24 to 48 hr, appropriate steps should be taken to define the cause of the anuria. The average infant excretes 15 to 60 ml of urine per 24 hr during the first two days of life and 50 to 100 ml/kg/day during the next four weeks. Oliguria, defined as passage of less than 0.5 ml/kg/hr after the first 24 hr, should also be promptly investigated for underlying causes (86).

Certain external malformations may indicate underlying urological causes for oliguria or anuria. Potter's facies, characterized by large, low-set and flabby ears and widely spaced eyes, is now well known as a sign of renal agenesis. These facies may also occur in some infants with prune belly syndrome, renal cystic disease, or severe urethral atresia and renal dysplasia. In fact, almost any severe renal malformation leading to profound oligohydramnios during pregnancy may be associated with varying degrees of Potter's facies, probably secondary to intrauterine compression. Furthermore, renal involvement should be considered in any neonate presenting with dysmorphic signs such as prune belly syndrome, abnormalities of the external ear, widely spaced nipples, imperforate anus, and spina bifida. In addition, palpable abdominal

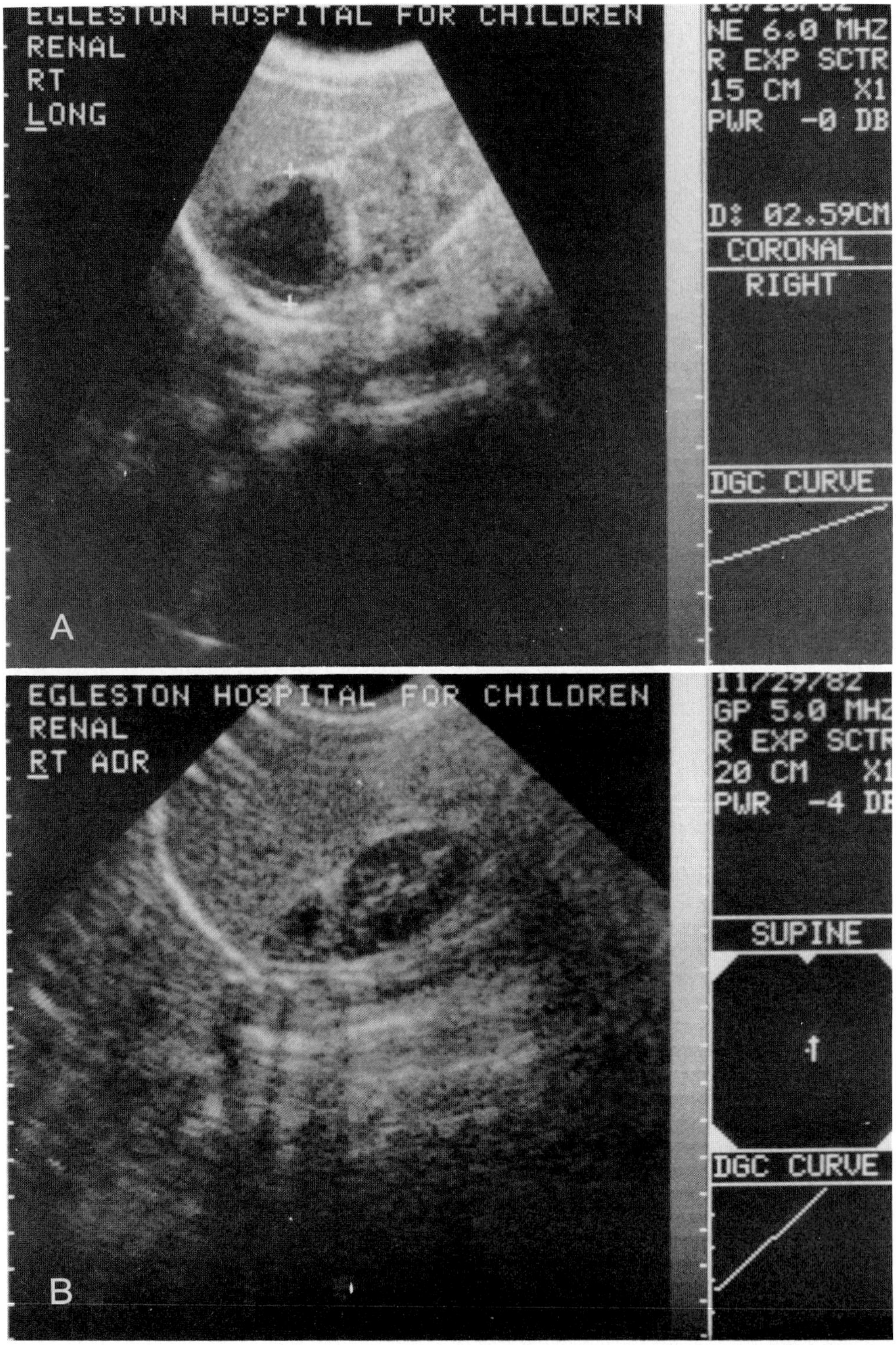

Figure 57.17. **A**, Abdominal ultrasound showing massive adrenal hemorrhage that is approximately equal in size to kidney to its right. Note sonolucency in center of hemorrhage with increased density around the periphery. **B**, Same patient two weeks later showing resolution in adrenal hemorrhage with decrease in size of mass.

masses associated with oliguria or anuria should suggest significant obstructive uropathy or renal cystic disease. Subtle clues such as a sacral-dermal sinus may indicate a spinal abnormality or a teratoma.

Prerenal Causes

Although renal abnormalities should be suspected when investigation for oligoanuria is undertaken, severe dehydration is the most common cause and may be associated with acute renal failure (86). Critically ill neonates, particularly those with respiratory distress syndrome, are subject to hypoperfusion of the kidneys caused by hemorrhage, shock, hypoxia, and congestive heart failure, all of which may lead to failure to pass urine. When the state of hydration is satisfactory or when hypoxia

Table 57.2.
Time of Urine Passage in 500 Neonates

Time (hr)	%
0–12	67.6
12–24	92.4
24–48	99.4
Over 48	0.6

Data from Sherry and Kramer (85).

is not a complication, a delay in micturition is most often caused by failure of urine production due to intrinsic renal disease or to an obstruction to urine flow.

Intrinsic Renal Disease

Infants with congenital renal anomalies with bilateral involvement such as agenesis, multicystic dysplasia, and autosomal recessive (infantile) polycystic disease often present with oliguria or anuria, but other characteristic clinical features usually suggest the underlying nature of the problem. The infant with oliguria and hematuria may signal a vascular catastrophe such as renal vein thrombosis, renal artery thrombosis, or renal cortical necrosis. Certain drugs, such as tolazoline and indomethacin, are often used in sick neonates; they may be nephrotoxic and lead to diminished urine output. Maternal administration of captopril during pregnancy has been reported to cause oligohydramnios, neonatal hypotension, and ultimately fetal anuria (86). Large doses of contrast agents used in cardiac catheterization are occasionally associated with acute renal failure and oliguria in neonates (87).

Obstruction to Urine Flow

Bilateral renal obstruction secondary to posterior urethral valves may delay micturition. A neonate with anuria and a palpably distended bladder should suggest the presence of just such an obstruction. A weak urinary stream, with or without a distended bladder, was the presenting sign or symptom in 15% of neonates requiring major urological surgery in the authors' experience (65). Neuropathic bladders in children with spina bifida may also be distended in the neonatal period, and if the defect is subtle, oliguria or anuria may be the initial sign of an abnormality. Severe bilateral upper tract obstruction from stenosis at the ureteropelvic junction may lead to diminished urine flow, and this obstruction may also exist in single kidneys or in those situations where the opposite kidney is nonfunctional due to multicystic dysplasia. Not all obstructions to urine flow are as potentially serious as those previously noted. Magnesium sulfate, administered to the mother for toxemia during delivery, may produce neuromuscular blockage in the infant, with generalized hypotonia and severe, although transient, bladder distention and delayed voiding (4).

HEMATURIA

It is an axiom in urological practice that microscopic or gross hematuria must be fully evaluated in all patients. In the newborn, hematuria is an emergency. Gross hematuria at this age is rare, as evidenced by only 35 neonatal admissions to the Children's Memorial Hospital in Chicago for that reason between 1950 and 1967 (75). The sign usually reflects underlying pathological conditions that are often treatable. Careful investigation is mandatory. Table 57.3 lists causes of hematuria in the neonate (88). The vascular disorders that present with gross or microscopic hematuria include renal cortical necrosis, renal vein thrombosis, and renal artery thrombosis. Acute cortical necrosis is a serious disorder manifested by hematuria, oliguria, hyposthenuria, and azotemia

Table 57.3.
Causes of Hematuria

1. Vascular
   Cortical necrosis
   Venous thrombosis
2. Cystic
   Polycystic kidney disease
   Multicystic kidney
3. Urinary tract obstruction
4. Urinary tract infection
5. Glomerulonephritis ?
6. Tumor
   Wilms' tumor
   Angioma
7. Drugs
   Penicillins
   Aminoglycosides
   Heparin
8. Trauma
   Birth
   Surgical
9. Coagulopathy
   Sepsis
   Hypoxia

(89). Recovery, of course, depends on the amount of renal tissue that has become necrotic.

Renal Vein Thrombosis

Renal vein thrombosis (see also Chapter 56) usually presents with an enlarged kidney in addition to hematuria. Besides the obvious hematuria, many infants display evidence of disseminated intravascular coagulation associated with decreased platelet counts.

Renal Artery Thrombosis

Thrombosis of the renal artery is rare and usually associated with hypertension and possibly congestive heart failure (90). There may be azotemia with each of these conditions.

Miscellaneous

A number of developmental anomalies may present with hematuria but rarely in the neonatal period; these include Wilms' tumor, renal angioma, obstructive uropathy, polycystic kidneys, and multicystic dysplastic kidneys. Renal ultrasound and excretory urography are diagnostic procedures useful in differentiating these disorders. The various obstructive uropathies, both upper and lower tract, may be associated with hematuria, although in the neonatal period other symptoms are usually more prominent. Medications administered to the neonate, particularly some antibiotics, may produce hematuria. Neonatal glomerulonephritis may also be a cause. There are many possible nonrenal causes of hematuria, such as generalized bleeding secondary to heparin administration or to disseminated intravascular coagulation. Various types of birth trauma, as well as urinary infection with cystitis, may produce blood cells in the urine.

References

1. Sarda P, Bard H, Teasdale F, et al: The importance of an antenatal ultrasonographic diagnosis of correctable fetal malformations. Am J Obstet Gynecol 147:443, 1983.
2. Parrott TS, Woodard JR, Hawkins B, et al: The influence of obstructive uropathy. (Submitted for publication.)

3. Dell'Agnola CA, Tomaselli V, Ferazzi E, et al: Perinatal ultrasound monitoring: early detection and treatment of congenital uropathy. Br J Urol 55:469, 1983.
4. Woodard JR: Signs and symptoms of urological disease in neonates. Dial Pediatr Urol 2:3, 1979.
5. Brent RL: Ultrasonography in fetal diagnosis. Pediatr Ann 10:49, 1981.
6. Bolsen B: Question of risk still hovers over routine use of ultrasound. JAMA 247:2195, 1982.
7. Canty TG, Leopold GR, Wolf DA: Maternal ultrasonography for the antenatal diagnosis of surgically significant neonatal anomalies. Ann Surg 194:353, 1981.
8. Parrott TS: Prenatal diagnosis of fetal urologic conditions. Dial Pediatr Urol 2:2, 1979.
9. Campbell S, Pearce JM: Ultrasound visualization of congenital malformations. Br Med Bull 39:322, 1983.
10. Cass A, Smith S, Gobec C, et al: Prenatal diagnosis of fetal urinary tract abnormalities by ultrasound. Urology 18:197, 1981.
11. Hadlock FP, Deter RL, Carpenter R, et al: Sonography of fetal urinary tract anomalies. Am J Roentgenol 137:261, 1981.
12. Harrison MR, Golbus MS, Filly RA, et al: Management of the fetus with congenital hydronephrosis. J Pediatr Surg 17:728, 1982.
13. Kramer SA: Current status of fetal intervention for congenital hydronephrosis. J Urol 130:641, 1983.
14. Bowie JD, Rosenberg ER, Androetti RF, et al: The changing sonographic appearance of fetal kidneys during pregnancy. J Ultrasound Med 2:505, 1983.
15. Wladimiroff JW: Effect of furosemide on fetal urine production. Br J Obstet Gynecol 82:221, 1975.
16. Gruenwald SM, Crocker EF, Walker AG, et al: Antenatal diagnosis of urinary tract anomalies: correlation of ultrasound appearance with postnatal diagnosis. Am J Obstet Gynecol 148:278, 1984.
17. Kullendorf CM, Larsson LT, Jorgensen C: The advantage of antenatal diagnosis of intestinal and urinary tract malformations. Br J Obstet Gynecol 91:144, 1984.
18. Glazer GM, Filly RA, Callen PW: The varied sonographic appearance of the urinary tract in the fetus and newborn with urethral obstruction. Radiology 144:563, 1982.
19. Gore RM, Callen PW, Filly RA, et al: Prenatal percutaneous antegrade pyelography in posterior urethral valves: sonographic guidance. Am J Roentgenol 139:994, 1982.
20. Wigglesworth JS, Desai R, Guerrini P: Fetal lung hypoplasia: biochemical and structural variations and their possible significance. Arch Dis Child 56:606, 1981.
21. Bellinger M: Fetal intervention for obstructive uropathy. Dial Pediatr Urol 5:6, 1982.
22. Harrison MR, Nakayama DK, Noall R, et al: Correction of congenital hydronephrosis in utero. II. Decompression reverses the effects of obstruction on the fetal lung and urinary tract. J Pediatr Surg 17:965, 1982.
23. Beck AD: The effect of intra-uterine urinary obstruction upon the development of the fetal kidney. J Urol 105:784, 1971.
24. Glick PL, Harrison MR, Noall RA, et al: Correction of congenital hydronephrosis in utero. III. Early mid-trimester ureteral obstruction produces renal dysplasia. J Pediatr Surg 18:681, 1983.
25. Mackie GG, Stephens FD: Duplex kidneys: a correlation of renal dysplasia with position of the ureteral orifice. J Urol 114:274, 1975.
26. Maizels M, Simpson SG: Primitive ducts of renal dysplasia induced by culturing ureteral buds denuded of condensed renal mesenchyme. Science 21:509, 1983.
27. Bernstein J: The morphogenesis of renal parenchymal development. Pediatr Clin North Am 18:394, 1971.
28. Glick PL, Harrison MR, Adzick NS, et al: Correction of congenital hydronephrosis in utero IV: In utero decompression prevents renal dysplasia. J Pediatr Surg 19:649, 1984.
29. Harrison MR, Golbus MS, Filly RA, et al: Fetal surgery for congenital hydronephrosis. N Engl J Med 306:591, 1982.
30. McFayden IR, Wigglesworth JS, Dillon MJ: Fetal urinary tract obstruction: is active intervention before delivery indicated? Br J Obstet Gynecol 90:342, 1983.
31. Harrison MR, Filly RA, Parer JT, et al: Management of the fetus with a urinary tract malformation. JAMA 246:635, 1981.
32. Kramer SA: Detection and management of hydronephrosis in utero. In Kelalis PP, King LR, Belman AB (eds): Clinical Pediatric Urology. Philadelphia, WB Saunders, 1985, p 434.
33. Mandell J, Kinard HW, Mittlestaedt CA, et al: Prenatal diagnosis of unilateral hydronephrosis with early postnatal reconstruction. J Urol 132:303, 1984.
34. Duckett JW: Fetal intervention for obstructive uropathy. Dial Pediatr Urol 5:8, 1982.
35. McFayden IR: Obstruction of the fetal urianry tract: a role for surgical intervention in utero. Br Med J 288:459, 1984.
36. Muecke EC: The role of the cloacal membrane in exstrophy: the first successful experimental study. J Urol 92:659, 1964.
37. Marshall VF, Muecke EC: Variations in exstrophy of the bladder. J Urol 88:766, 1962.
38. Turner WR, Ransley PG, Bloom DA et al: Variants of the exstrophic complex. Urol Clin North Am 7:493, 1980.
39. Williams DI, Keeton J: Vesicle exstrophy: twenty years experience. Br J Surg 60:203, 1973.
40. Duckett JW, Caldamone AA: Bladder and urachus. In Kelalis PP, King LR, Belman AB (eds): Clinical Pediatric Urology, ed 2. Philadelphia, WB Saunders, 1985, p 726.
41. Jeffs RD, Exstrophy. In Harrison HJ, Gittes RF, Perlmutter AD, et al (eds): Campbell's Urology, ed 4. Philadelphia, WB Saunders, p 1672, 1978.
42. Jeffs RD, Guice SL, Oesch I: The factors in successful exstrophy closure. J Urol 127:974, 1982.
43. Herbst WP: Patent urachus. South Med J 30:711, 1937.
44. Moncada R, Cooper RA, Reynes CJ, et al: Neonatal urine ascites associated with urinary outlet obstruction: another survivor. Br J Radiol 46:1005, 1973.
45. Trulock TS, Finnerty DP, Woodard JR: Neonatal bladder rupture: case report and review of literature. J Urol 133:271, 1985.
46. Greenfield SP, Hensle TW, Berdon WE, et al: Urinary extravasation in the newborn male with posterior urethral valves. J Pediatr Surg 17:751, 1982.
47. Woodard JR: Neonatal and perinatal emergencies. In Harrision HJ, Gittes RF, Perlmutter AD, et al (eds): Campbell's Urology. Philadelphia, WB Saunders, 1978, p 1855.
48. Garlinger P, Ott J: Prune belly syndrome—possible genetic implications. Birth Defects 10:173, 1974.
49. Sweet RA, Shrott HG, Kurland R, et al: Study of the incidence of hypospadias in Rochester, Minnesota, 1940–1970, and a case controlled comparison of possible etiologic factors. Mayo Clin Proc 49:52, 1974.
50. Knorr D, Beckman D, Bidlingnaier F, et al: Plasma testosterone in male puberty. II. HCG stimulation test in boys with hypospadias. Acta Endocrinol (Copenhagen) 90:365, 1979.
51. Aarskog D: Maternal progestins as a possible cause for hypospadias. N Engl J Med 300:75, 1979.
52. Manley CV, Epstein ES: Early hypospadias repair in children under one year of age. J Urol 128:1273, 1982.
53. Belman AB, Kass EJ: Hypospadias repair in children under one year of age. J Urol 128:1273, 1982.
54. Feldman KW, Smith DW: Fetal phallic growth and penile standards for newborn male infants. J Pediatr 86:395, 1975.
55. Schonfeld WA, Beebe GW: Normal growth and variation in the male genitalia from birth to maturity. J Urol 48:759, 1942.
56. Jirasek JE, Raboch J, Uher J: The relationship between the development of gonads and external genitals in human fetuses. Amer J Obstet Gynec 101:830, 1968
57. Burstein S, Grumbach MM, Kaplan SL: Early determination of androgen-responsiveness is important in the management of microphallus. Lancet 2:983, 1979.
58. Allen TD: Disorders of sexual differentiation. Urology 7: (suppl) 1–32, 1976.
59. Woodhouse CRJ, Williams DI: Duplication of the lower urinary tract in children. Br J Urol 51:481, 1979.
60. Giebink GS, Ruymann FB: The varied sonographic appearance of the urinary tract in the fetus and newborn with urethral obstruction. Radiology 144:563, 1974.
61. Cumming CD, Hyndman CW, Deacon JSR: Intra-uterine testicular torsion: not an emergency. Urology 14:603, 1979.
62. Gerkins GR, Noe HN, Hollabaugh RS, et al: Spermatic cord torsion in the neonate. J Urol 129:121, 1983.
63. Bartholomew TH, Gonzales ET: Urologic management in cloacal dysgenesis. Urology 11:549, 1978.
64. Griffin JE, Edwards C, Madden JD et al: Congenital absence of the vagina. The Mazer-Rokitansky-Kuster-Hauser syndrome. Ann Intern Med 85:224, 1976.
65. Parrott TS, Woodard JR: Urologic surgery in the neonate. J Urol 116:506, 1976.
66. Longino LA, Martin LW: Abdominal masses in the newborn infant. Pediatrics 21:596, 1958.
67. Raffensperger J, Abouseleiman A: Abdominal masses in children under one year of age. Surgery 63:514, 1968.
68. Wedge JJ, Grosfeld JL, Smith JP: Abdominal masses in the newborn: 63 cases. J Urology 106:770, 1971.
69. Wilson DA: Ultrasound screening for abdominal masses in the neonatal period. Am J Dis Child 136:151, 1982.
70. Alton DJ: Pelvoureteric obstruction in childhood. Radiol Clin North Am 29:4, 1977.
71. Lebowitz RL, Griscom NT: Neonatal hydronephrosis: 146 cases. Radiol Clin North Am 15:49, 1977.
72. Pais VM, Retik AB: Reversible hydronephrosis in the neonate with urinary sepsis. N Engl J Med 192:465, 1975.
73. Potter EL: Normal and abnormal developments of the kidney. Chicago, Year Book Medical Publishers, 1972.
74. Williams DI: Renal anomalies. In Williams DI (ed): Urology in Childhood. New York, Springer-Verlag, 1974, p 70.
75. Emanuel B, Aronson N: Neonatal hematuria. Am J Dis Child 120:204, 1974.

76. Belman AB, Susmano DF, Burden JJ, et al: Nonoperative treatment of unilateral renal vein thrombosis in the newborn. JAMA 211:1165, 1970.
77. Black J, Williams DI: Natural history of adrenal hemorrhage in the newborn. Arch Dis Child 48:183, 1973.
78. Sober I, Hirsch M: Unilateral massive adrenal hemorrhage in the newborn infant. J Urol 93:430, 1965.
79. Eckloff O, Grotte G, Garulf H, et al: Perinatal hemorrhagic necrosis of the adrenal gland. Pediatr Radiol 4:31, 1974.
80. Rajani K, Shapiro SR, Goetzman BW: Adrenal abscess: complication of supportive therapy of adrenal hemorrhage in the newborn. J Pediatr Surg 16:677, 1980.
81. Hartenstein H: Wilms' tumor in the newborn infant. J Pediatr 35:381, 1949.
82. Richmond H, Dougall AJ: Neonatal renal tumors. J Pediatr Surg 5:513, 1970.
83. Ramenofski ML, Raffensperger JG: An abdominal perineal vaginal pullthrough for definitive treatment of hydrometrocolpos. J Pediatr Surg 6:381, 1971.
84. Aamed S: Neonatal and childhood ovarian cysts. J Pediatr Surg 6:702, 1971.
85. Sherry SN, Kramer I: The time of passage of first stool and first urine by the newborn infant. J Pediatr 46:158, 1955.
86. Guignard JP: Renal function in the newborn infant. Pediatr Clin North Am 29:4, 1982.
87. Anand SK: Acute renal failure in the neonate. Pediatr Clin North Am 29:4, 1982.
88. Brem AS, Lewy JE: Neonatal hematuria. Perinatal Care 2:42, 1978.
89. Kurnetz R, Burstein J: Neonatal blood loss in hematuria. J Pediatr 84:452, 1974.
90. Woodard JR, Patterson JM, Brinsfield D: Renal artery thrombosis in newborn infants. Am J Dis Child 114:191, 1967.

Index

Pages numbers followed by "t" or "f" denote tables and figures, respectively.